Contents

JONES & BARTLETT LEARNING

2020

Nurse's Drug Handbook

Nineteenth Edition

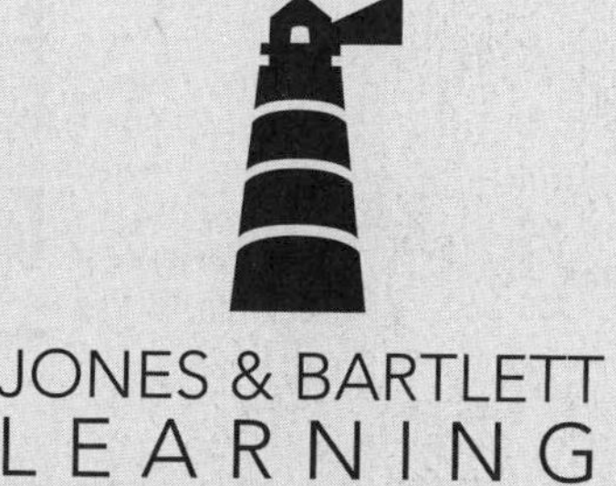

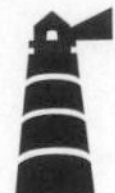

World Headquarters
Jones & Bartlett Learning
5 Wall Street
Burlington, MA 01803
978-443-5000
info@jblearning.com
www.jblearning.com

Jones & Bartlett Learning books and products are available through most bookstores and online booksellers. To contact Jones & Bartlett Learning directly, call 800-832-0034, fax 978-443-8000, or visit our website, www.jblearning.com.

Substantial discounts on bulk quantities of Jones & Bartlett Learning publications are available to corporations, professional associations, and other qualified organizations. For details and specific discount information, contact the special sales department at Jones & Bartlett Learning via the above contact information or send an email to specialsales@jblearning.com.

Production Credits
VP, Product Management: Amanda Martin
Director of Product Management: Matthew Kane
Product Manager: Teresa Malmberg
Product Assistant: Melina Leon
Senior Project Specialist: Vanessa Richards
Digital Project Specialist: Angela Dooley
Marketing Manager: Lindsay White
Product Fulfillment Manager: Wendy Kilborn
Composition and Project Management: S4Carlisle Publishing Services
Cover Design: Michael O'Donnell
Senior Media Development Editor: Troy Liston
Rights Specialist: John Rusk
Cover Image: © ajt/Shutterstock
Printing and Binding: LSC Communications
Cover Printing: LSC Communications

ISBN: 978-1-284-16790-0

6048

Printed in the United States of America
23 22 21 20 19 10 9 8 7 6 5 4 3 2 1

Mechanism-of-Action Illustrations *(continued)*

Drugs with illustrated mechanisms of action	Drugs with similar mechanisms of action
isosorbide dinitrate, isosorbide mononitrate	nitroglycerin
lanthanum carbonate	sevelamer hydrochloride
linezolid	none
memantine hydrochloride	none
milrinone lactate	none
nateglinide	repaglinide
olmesartan medoxomil	irbesartan, losartan potassium, valsartan
omeprazole	esomeprazole magnesium, lansoprazole, pantoprazole sodium, rabeprazole sodium
orlistat	none
palonosetron hydrochloride	alosetron, dolasetron, granisetron, ondansetron
phenelzine sulfate	isocarboxazid
spironolactone	none
tacrine hydrochloride	donepezil hydrochloride, galantamine hydrobromide, rivastigmine tartrate
teriparatide	none
vasopressin	desmopressin acetate
ziconotide	none

Reviewers and Clinical Consultants

Reviewers

Peter J. Ambrose, PharmD
Clinical Professor
Los Angeles–Orange County Area Clerkships
University of California
San Francisco, California

Michael C. Barros, PharmD, BCPS, CACP
Clinical Assistant Professor of Pharmacy Practice
Temple University School of Pharmacy
Clinical Pharmacist, Heart Failure/Transplant
Temple University Hospital
Philadelphia, Pennsylvania

Edward M. Bednarczyk, PharmD
Clinical Assistant Professor
Pharmacy Practice and Nuclear Medicine
State University of New York at Buffalo
Buffalo, New York

Cristina E. Bello, PharmD
Assistant Professor of Pharmacy Practice
College of Pharmacy
Nova Southeastern University
Fort Lauderdale, Florida

Scott M. Bonnema, PharmD
Consultant Pharmacist
Emissary Pharmacy and Infusion
Casper, Wyoming

Felesia R. Bowen, RN, MS, PNP-C
Clinical Nurse Specialist
Children's Hospital at Robert Wood Johnson University Hospital
New Brunswick, New Jersey

Cynthia Burman, PharmD
Clinical Assistant Professor
School of Pharmacy
Temple University
Philadelphia, Pennsylvania

Jason M. Cota, PharmD, MS, BCPS
Assistant Professor
Department of Pharmacy Practice
University of the Incarnate Word
Feik School of Pharmacy
Infectious Diseases
Clinical Pharmacist
Brooke Army Medical Center
San Antonio, Texas

Kimberly A. Couch, PharmD
Clinical Pharmacy Specialist, Infectious Diseases
Department of Pharmacy
Christiana Care Health System
Newark, Delaware

Brenda S. Frymoyer, RN, MSN
Clinical Nurse Specialist
Berks Cardiologists, Inc.
Reading, Pennsylvania

Jason Gallagher, PharmD, BCPS
Associate Professor
Clinical Specialist, Infectious Diseases
Director, Infectious Diseases Pharmacotherapy Residency
Temple University
Philadelphia, Pennsylvania

Kimberly A. Galt, PharmD, FASHP
Associate Professor of Pharmacy Practice
Director
Drug Information Services
Co-Director
Center for Practice Improvement and Outcomes Research
Creighton University
Omaha, Nebraska

John Gatto, RPh
Clinical Pharmacist
Eckerd Pharmacy
Owego, New York

Deborah L. Green, RN, MSN
Director
Medical Telemetry-CHF Program
Moses H. Cone Health System
Greensboro, North Carolina

Ronald L. Greenberg, PharmD, CPS
Clinical Pharmacy Coordinator
Fairview Ridges Hospital
Burnsville, Minnesota

Jan K. Hastings, PharmD
Assistant Professor
College of Pharmacy
University of Arkansas for Medical Science
Little Rock, Arkansas

Michael D. Hogue, PharmD
Assistant Professor of Pharmacy Practice
McWhorter School of Pharmacy
Samford University
Clinical Coordinator
Walgreens Drug Store
Birmingham, Alabama

Kimberly A. Hunter, PharmD
Assistant Professor of Pharmacy Practice
Albany College of Pharmacy
Albany, New York

William A. Kehoe, Jr., PharmD, CPS, FCCP
Professor of Clinical Pharmacy and Psychology
School of Pharmacy and Health Sciences
University of the Pacific
Stockton, California

Julienne K. Kirk, PharmD, CPS, CDE
Assistant Professor
Department of Family Medicine
School of Medicine
Wake Forest University
Winston-Salem, North Carolina

Peter G. Koval, PharmD, BCPS
Clinical Pharmacist
Moses H. Cone Family Practice
Greensboro, North Carolina

Lisa M. Krupa, RN-C, CEN, FNP
Nurse Practitioner
Medical Specialists
Munster, Indiana

Amista A. Lone, PharmD
Clinical Assistant Professor
College of Pharmacy
University of Arizona
Tucson, Arizona

Jennifer L. Lutz, PharmD
Pharmacy Resident
Samuel S. Stratton Veterans Affairs Medical Center
Albany, New York

T. Donald Marsh, PharmD, FASCP, ASHP
Director
Department of Pharmacotherapy
Mountain Area Health Education Center
Asheville, North Carolina

Patrick McDonnell, PharmD
Assistant Professor of Clinical Pharmacy
School of Pharmacy
Temple University
Philadelphia, Pennsylvania

Kenyetta N. Nesbitt, PharmD
Assistant Professor
Wayne State University
Detroit, Michigan

Catherine M. Oliphant, PharmD
Assistant Professor of Pharmacy Practice
School of Pharmacy
University of Wyoming
Laramie, Wyoming

Vinita B. Pai, PharmD
Assistant Professor of Clinical Pharmacy
College of Pharmacy
Ohio State University
Columbus, Ohio

David J. Quan, PharmD
Clinical Pharmacist
University of California, San Francisco
San Francisco, California

Brenda M. Reap-Thompson, RN, MSN
Assistant Clinical Professor
Drexel University
Philadelphia, Pennsylvania

Nancy Jex Sabin, RN, MSN, APRN
Clinical Assistant Professor
University of San Diego
San Diego, California

Elizabeth Sloand, PhD, RN, PNP-BC
Assistant Professor
School of Nursing
Johns Hopkins University
Baltimore, Maryland

Craig Williams, PharmD
Clinical Specialist
Wishard Memorial Hospital
Assistant Professor of Clinical Pharmacy
School of Pharmacy
Purdue University
Indianapolis, Indiana

Clinical Consultants

Madeline Albanese, RN, MSN
Nurse Educator
Hospital of the University of Pennsylvania
Philadelphia, Pennsylvania

Sheree M. Fitzgerald, RN-C, MSN, CNA
Program Coordinator
Ancora Psychiatric Hospital
Hammonton, New Jersey

Maryann Foley, RN, BSN
Independent Consultant
Flourtown, Pennsylvania

Grace Hukushi, RN, BSN, LNC
Critical Care Nurse
Nursing Enterprises, Inc.
Brick, New Jersey

Sammie Justesen, RN, BSN
Independent Nurse Consultant
Providence, Utah

Catherine T. Kelly, RN, PhD, CCRN, CEN, ANP
Faculty
School of Nursing
Mount Saint Mary College
Newburgh, New York

Sharon Kumm, RN, MN, CCRN
Assistant Professor
School of Nursing
University of Kansas
Kansas City, Kansas

Leanne McQuade, RN, BSN, CEN
Staff Nurse
Emergency Department
Doylestown Hospital
Case Manager
CAB Medical Consultant
Doylestown, Pennsylvania

Pamela S. Ronning, RN, MPA
Program Coordinator
Kirkhof College of Nursing
Grand Valley State University
Allendale, Michigan

Maureen Ryan, RN, CS, MSN, FNP
Assistant Professor
Grand Valley State University
Allendale, Michigan
Nurse Practitioner
Emergency Department
St. Mary's Hospital
Grand Rapids, Michigan

Julie M. Smith, RN, BA
Staff Nurse
Radiology-Heart Station
Rancocas Hospital
Willingboro, New Jersey

Aaron J. Strehlow, RN, PhD, FNP
Administrator and Director of Clinical Services
UCLA School of Nursing
Health Center at the Rescue Mission
Los Angeles, California

Maria Wilson, RN, MSN, CCRN
Staff Nurse
Emergency Department
Chestnut Hill Hospital
Philadelphia, Pennsylvania

How to Use This Book

Jones & Bartlett Learning *Nurse's Drug Handbook* gives you what today's nurses and nursing students need: accurate, concise, and reliable drug facts. This book emphasizes the vital information you need to know before, during, and after drug administration. The information is presented in easy-to-understand language and organized alphabetically, so you can find what you need quickly.

What's Special

In addition to the drug information you expect to find in each entry (see "Drug Entries" for details), the *Nurse's Drug Handbook* boasts these special features:

- **The design** makes it easy to find the most need-to-know drug information, such as indications, dosages, dosage adjustments, and warnings.
- **The size** makes the *Nurse's Drug Handbook* easy and convenient to carry and use.
- **Practical trim size** allows the book to open flat so you can find the information you need without wrestling with a book that wants to close. You can hold the book in one hand, see complete pages at a glance, and use your other hand to document or perform other activities.
- **Introductory material** reviews essential general information you need to know to administer drugs safely and effectively, including an overview of pharmacology and the principles of drug administration. In addition, the five steps of the nursing process are explained and related specifically to drug therapy.
- **Highly useful illustrations** throughout the text help you visualize selected mechanisms of action by showing how drugs work at the cellular, tissue, and organ levels. In addition, the inside front cover features a table listing all the drugs whose mechanisms of action are illustrated, as well as other drugs with the same mechanisms of action.
- **No-nonsense writing style** speaks in everyday language and uses the terms and abbreviations you typically encounter in your practice and your studies. To avoid sexist language, we alternate between male and female pronouns throughout the book.
- **Up-to-date drug information** includes the latest FDA-approved drugs, new and changed indications, new warnings, and newly reported adverse reactions.
- **Dosage adjustment,** headlined in color, alerts you to expected dosage changes for a patient with a specific condition or disorder, such as advanced age or renal impairment.
- **Warning,** displayed in color, calls attention to important facts that you need to know before, during, and after drug administration. For example, in the alatrofloxacin entry, this feature informs you that the drug is usually reserved for hospitalized patients and is given for no more than 2 weeks because of the high risk of severe liver damage.
- **Easy-to-use tables** showing route, onset, peak, and duration (see page *xv* for more details), and other tables in the appendices provide a time-saving way to track and check information. The appendices give you an overview of the most important facts and nursing considerations for important drug groups, including insulin preparations and oral allergen extracts, selected antihistamines, ophthalmics, topical drugs, antivirals, antineoplastic drugs, interferons, and antihypertensive combination drugs, as well as selected obstetrical drugs and vitamins. You'll also find handy instructions for calculating drug dosages and I.V. flow rates.

Drug Entries

The *Nurse's Drug Handbook* clearly and concisely presents all the vital facts on the drugs that you'll typically administer. To help you find the information you need quickly, drug entries are organized alphabetically by generic drug name—from abatacept to zonisamide. For ease of use, every drug entry follows a consistent format. However, if specific details are unknown or don't apply, the heading isn't included so you can go right to the next section.

GENERIC AND TRADE NAMES

First, each entry identifies the drug's main generic name, as well as alternate generic names. (For drugs prescribed by trade name, you can quickly check the comprehensive index, which refers you to the appropriate generic name and page.)

Next, the entry lists the most common U.S. trade names for each drug. It also includes common trade names available only in Canada, marked (CAN).

CLASS, CATEGORY, AND SCHEDULE

Each entry lists the drug's pharmacologic and therapeutic classes. With this information, you can compare drugs in the same pharmacologic class but in different therapeutic classes, and vice versa.

The entry also lists the FDA's pregnancy risk category, which categorizes drugs based on their potential to cause birth defects. (For details, see *FDA pregnancy risk categories*.)

However, effective after June 30, 2015, new prescription drugs submitted to the FDA for approval will no longer be allowed to use the lettering system to categorize drugs based on their potential to cause birth defects. Instead, a new, more comprehensive text will be required in the label to explain the risks. Prescription drugs currently using the lettering system to identify potential for a drug to cause birth defects will be gradually phased into the new labeling requirement. Labeling of over-the-counter drugs will remain unchanged and is not affected by the FDA-mandated change.

Where appropriate, the entry also includes the drug's controlled substance schedule. (For details, see *Controlled substance schedules*, page *xv*.)

FDA pregnancy risk categories

Each currently prescribed drug may be placed in a pregnancy risk category based on the FDA's estimate of risk to the fetus. If the FDA hasn't provided a category, the *Drug Handbook* notes that the drug is "Not classified." The categories range from A to X, signifying least to greatest fetal risk. Note that pregnancy risk categories will no longer be used in drug labeling for drugs approved after June 30, 2015, and existing drug labels that use the category will be gradually phased into the new labeling requirements.

A Controlled studies show no risk

Adequate, well-controlled studies with pregnant women have failed to demonstrate a risk to the fetus in any trimester of pregnancy.

B No evidence of risk in humans

Adequate, well-controlled studies with pregnant women haven't shown increased risk of fetal abnormalities, despite adverse findings in animals, or, in the absence of adequate human studies, animal studies show no fetal risk. The chance of fetal harm is remote, but remains possible.

C Risk can't be ruled out

Adequate, well-controlled human studies are lacking, and animal studies have shown a risk to the fetus or are lacking as well. A chance of fetal harm exists if the drug is given during pregnancy, but the potential benefits may outweigh the risk.

D Positive evidence of risk

Studies in humans, or investigational or postmarketing data, have shown fetal risk. Nevertheless, potential benefits from the drug's use may outweigh risks. For example, the drug may be acceptable if needed in a life-threatening situation or to treat a serious disease for which safer drugs can't be used or are ineffective.

X Contraindicated in pregnancy

Studies in animals or humans, or investigational or postmarketing reports, have shown positive evidence of fetal abnormalities or risks that clearly outweigh any possible benefit to the patient.

Controlled substance schedules

The Controlled Substances Act of 1970 mandated that certain prescription drugs be categorized in schedules based on their potential for abuse. The greater their potential for abuse, the greater the restrictions on their prescription. The controlled substance schedules range from I to V, signifying highest to lowest abuse potential.

I High potential for abuse

No accepted medical use exists for schedule I drugs, which include heroin and lysergic acid diethylamide (LSD).

II High potential for abuse

Use may lead to severe physical or psychological dependence. Prescriptions must be written in ink or typewritten and must be signed by the prescriber. Oral prescriptions must be confirmed in writing within 72 hours and may be given only in a genuine emergency. No renewals are permitted.

III Some potential for abuse

Use may lead to low-to-moderate physical dependence or high psychological dependence. Prescriptions may be oral or written. Up to five renewals are permitted within 6 months.

IV Low potential for abuse

Use may lead to limited physical or psychological dependence. Prescriptions may be oral or written. Up to five renewals are allowed within 6 months.

V Subject to state and local regulation

Abuse potential is low; a prescription may not be required.

INDICATIONS AND DOSAGES

This section lists FDA-approved therapeutic indications. For each indication, you'll find the applicable drug form or route, age group (adults, adolescents, or children), and dosage (which includes amount per dose, timing, and duration, when known and appropriate).

ROUTE, ONSET, PEAK, AND DURATION

Quick-reference tables show the drug's onset, peak, and duration (when known) for each administration route. The onset of action is the time a drug takes to be absorbed, reach a therapeutic blood level, and elicit an initial therapeutic response. The peak therapeutic effect occurs when a drug reaches its highest blood concentration and the greatest amount of drug reaches the site of action to produce the maximum therapeutic response. The duration of action is the amount of time the drug remains at a blood level that produces a therapeutic response.

MECHANISM OF ACTION

This section concisely describes how a drug achieves its therapeutic effects at cellular, tissue, and organ levels, as appropriate. Illustrations of selected mechanisms of action lend exceptional clarity to sometimes complex processes.

INCOMPATIBILITIES

In this section, you'll be alerted to drugs or solutions that are incompatible with the topic drug when mixed in a syringe or solution, or when infused through the same I.V. line.

CONTRAINDICATIONS

An alphabetical list details the conditions and disorders that preclude administration of the topic drug.

INTERACTIONS

This section includes drugs, foods, and activities (such as alcohol use and smoking) that can cause important, problematic, or life-threatening interactions with the topic drug. For each interacting drug, food, or activity, you'll learn the effects of the interaction.

ADVERSE REACTIONS

Organized by body system, this section highlights common, serious, and life-threatening adverse reactions.

NURSING CONSIDERATIONS

Warnings, general precautions, and key information that you must know before, during, and after drug administration are

Teaching your patient about drug therapy

Your teaching about drug therapy will vary with your patient's needs and your practice setting. To help guide your teaching, each drug entry provides key information that you must teach your patient about that drug. For all patients, however, you also should:

- ✓ Teach the generic and trade name for each prescribed drug that he'll take after discharge—even if he took the drug before admission.
- ✓ Clearly explain why each drug was prescribed, how it works, and what it's supposed to do. To help your patient understand the drug's therapeutic effects, relate its action to her disorder or condition.
- ✓ Review the drug form, dosage, and route with the patient. Tell him whether the drug is a tablet, suppository, spray, aerosol, or other form, and explain how to take it correctly. Also, tell him how often to take the drug and for what length of time. Emphasize that he should take the drug exactly as prescribed.
- ✓ Describe the drug's appearance, and explain that scored tablets can be broken in half for safe, accurate dosing. Warn the patient not to break unscored tablets, because doing so may alter the drug dosage. If your patient has trouble swallowing capsules, explain that she can open ones that contain sprinkles and take them with food or a drink but that she shouldn't do this with capsules that contain powder. Also, warn her not to crush or chew enteric-coated, extended-release, sustained-release, or similar drug forms.
- ✓ Teach the patient about common adverse reactions that may occur. Advise him to notify the prescriber at once if a dangerous adverse reaction, such as syncope, occurs.
- ✓ Warn her not to suddenly stop taking a drug if she's bothered by unpleasant adverse reactions, such as a rash and mild itching. Instead, encourage her to discuss the reactions with her prescriber, who may adjust the dosage or substitute a drug that causes fewer adverse reactions.
- ✓ Because drugs may cause adverse reactions (such as dizziness and drowsiness) that can impair the patient's ability to perform activities that require alertness, help him develop a dosing schedule that prevents these adverse reactions.
- ✓ Inform the patient which adverse reactions resolve with time.
- ✓ Teach the patient how to store the drug properly. Let him know if the drug is sensitive to light or temperature and how to protect it from these elements.
- ✓ Instruct the patient to store the drug in its original container, if possible, with the drug's name and dosage clearly printed on the label.
- ✓ Inform the patient which devices to use—and which to avoid—for drug storage or administration. For example, warn him not to take liquid cyclosporine with a plastic cup or utensils.
- ✓ Teach the patient what to do if she misses a dose. Generally, she should take a once-daily drug as soon as she remembers—provided that she remembers within the first 24 hours. If 24 hours have elapsed, she should take the next scheduled dose, but she should not double the dose. If she has questions or concerns about missed doses, tell her to contact the prescriber.
- ✓ Provide information specific to the prescribed drug. For example, if a patient takes a diuretic to manage heart failure, instruct him to weigh himself daily at the same time of day, using the same scale, and wearing the same amount of clothing. Or, if the patient takes digoxin or an antihypertensive drug, teach him how to measure his pulse and blood pressure and how to record the measurements. Then instruct him to bring the diary to his regular appointments so the prescriber can monitor his response to the drug.
- ✓ Advise the patient to refill prescriptions promptly, unless she no longer needs the drug. Also instruct her to discard expired drugs because they may become ineffective or even dangerous over time.
- ✓ Warn the patient to keep all drugs out of the reach of children at all times.

detailed in this section. Examples include whether a pill can be crushed and how to properly reconstitute, dilute, store, handle, or dispose of a drug.

Patient teaching information is also included here. You'll find important guidelines for patients, such as how and when to take each prescribed drug, how to spot and manage adverse reactions, which cautions to observe, when to call the prescriber, and more. To save your time, however, this section doesn't repeat basic patient-teaching points. (For a summary of those, see *Teaching your patient about drug therapy,* page *xvi,* and *Federal guidelines for drug disposal,* page *xvii.*)

New to this edition, life-threatening adverse reactions are now highlighted to draw attention to how serious the adverse reaction is.

In short, Jones & Bartlett Learning *Nurse's Drug Handbook* is designed expressly to give you more of what you need. It puts vital drug information at your fingertips and helps you always stay current in this critical part of your practice or studies.

Federal guidelines for drug disposal

Give patients these important instructions for properly disposing of their unwanted prescription drugs:

- ✓ Take unused, unneeded, or outdated prescription drugs out of their original containers and throw them in the trash.
- ✓ Consider mixing discarded prescription drugs with a substance like coffee grounds or used cat litter and putting them in impermeable, nondescript containers, such as empty cans or sealable bags.
- ✓ Flush prescription drugs down the toilet only if the label or accompanying patient information specifically tells you to do so.
- ✓ See if your community has a pharmaceutical take-back program that allows citizens to bring unused drugs to a central location for proper disposal.

Foreword

Safe, effective drug therapy is one of your most important responsibilities. Not infrequently, a patient's life will depend on your ability to give drugs accurately and safely. In addition, you must keep up with the latest drug information, including newly approved drugs and recently reported life-threatening adverse reactions, as well as those drugs withdrawn from the market after widespread use.

Despite all the drug information available, medication errors remain one of the greatest threats to patients' well-being and a leading cause of lawsuits against nurses, physicians, and hospitals.

Your Responsibilities in Drug Therapy

Your basic responsibilities in drug therapy include the following:

- Administer the right drug in the right dose by the right route at the right time to the right patient using the right preparation and administration.
- Know the therapeutic use, dosage, interactions, adverse reactions, and warnings of each administered drug.
- Be aware of newly approved drugs that may be prescribed.
- Know about changes to existing drugs, such as new indications and dosages and recently discovered adverse reactions and interactions.
- Concentrate fully when preparing and administering drugs.
- Respond promptly and appropriately to serious or life-threatening adverse reactions, interactions, and complications.
- Instruct each patient about the drug, how it's administered, which effects it causes or may cause, and which reactions to watch for and report.

Several factors may reduce your ability to meet these basic responsibilities—and contribute to medication errors. First, hospitals and other healthcare facilities have budget constraints that may result in elimination of professional nursing positions or the hiring of less qualified technicians to fill them. This forces the remaining nurses to care for more patients. Second, many hospital patients are older and more acutely ill, and they typically receive more complex drug therapy than ever. Together, these factors place greater demands on you—increasing your stress level, reducing the time you have to concentrate on drug administration, and increasing your risk of making medication errors or overlooking serious adverse reactions or interactions.

The same factors reduce your time and energy for learning the latest drug facts—which you need to have at your command. You must have this information at your fingertips because your next patient may need a recently approved drug or a complex and unfamiliar drug regimen.

How can you balance your limited time with your need to know the latest developments?

Meeting Your Needs

Nurses and students need a reliable, accurate, easy-to-use, quick-reference drug book. They need a book clearly written by and for nurses that has been reviewed by experts in nursing and pharmacology. You hold such a book in your hands: Jones & Bartlett Learning *Nurse's Drug Handbook*, with features that are always current.

The content of *Nurse's Drug Handbook* was developed, written, and edited by experienced practicing nurses. Expert consultants, reviewers, and advisors—both nurses and pharmacists—help ensure the accuracy and reliability of the information covered in each entry and help target that information to your needs. What's more, every drug fact is checked against the most prominent drug references today, including the drug's package insert approved by the FDA, *American Hospital Formulary Service Drug Information, Drug Facts and Comparisons, The Physicians' Desk Reference*, the FDA's website of new drug approvals, and the USP DI's *Drug Information for the Health*

Care Professional. In addition, to help you quickly access much-needed information, the book is organized alphabetically by generic drug name, follows a consistent format, and is concise.

To ensure that you're always current, Jones & Bartlett Learning *Nurse's Drug Handbook* is updated every year. This newest edition contains:

- Important new drug entries in the main part of the book and in the appendices.
- New drug facts on hundreds of existing entries, including updated information on new indications and dosages, new incompatibilities and interactions, new adverse reactions, and new nursing considerations.
- Hundreds of patient-teaching guidelines and suggestions.

And as always, you'll find the same color-coded, highly readable type that reduces eyestrain as you speed to the information you need.

Getting More from Your Drug Reference Handbook

Whether you currently work in or are preparing to work in acute care, home care, long-term care, or another healthcare setting, you'll want your own copy of the *Nurse's Drug Handbook.* That's because this book can help you:

- Reduce your risk of medication errors because you'll have easy access to accurate, reliable drug information that's relevant to your practice.
- Stay current on the most up-to-date drug developments of the year.
- Improve your drug administration skills and patient care before, during, and after drug therapy.
- Quickly detect and manage serious or life-threatening adverse reactions and complications or prevent them from occurring.
- Save time because you won't have to sift through volumes of information to find what you need, search for a book that's up-to-date, or look through several drug handbooks to get enough information.
- Increase your confidence about drug administration and enhance your professional interactions with other healthcare team members.
- Ensure the delivery of safe, effective care.
- Improve the depth and quality of your patient teaching.

Reaping the Rewards

Your patients deserve the best and safest care possible—and you deserve to have the tools to deliver that care. Whether you're a student or an experienced clinician, Jones & Bartlett Learning *Nurse's Drug Handbook* will help you provide safe, effective drug therapy because of its practical, easy-to-understand, accurate, and reliable information on virtually all the drugs you're likely to administer.

This handbook has aided thousands of nurses in their patient care. Take it with you to the clinical setting, share it with your peers, and use it to enhance your present and future position in the nursing profession.

Kathleen Dracup, RN, FNP, DNSc, FAAN
Dean and Professor
School of Nursing
University of California, San Francisco
San Francisco, California

Overview of Pharmacology

Understanding the basics of pharmacology is an essential nursing responsibility. Pharmacology is the science that deals with the physical and chemical properties, and biochemical and physiologic effects, of drugs. It includes the areas of pharmacokinetics, pharmacodynamics, pharmacotherapeutics, pharmacognosy, and toxicodynamics.

The *Nurse's Drug Handbook* deals primarily with pharmacokinetics, pharmacodynamics, and pharmacotherapeutics—the information you need to administer safe and effective drug therapy (discussed as follows). Pharmacognosy is the branch of pharmacology that deals with the biological, biochemical, and economic features of naturally occurring drugs. Toxicodynamics is the study of the harmful effects that excessive amounts of a drug produce in the body; in a drug overdose or drug poisoning, large drug doses may saturate or overwhelm normal mechanisms that control absorption, distribution, metabolism, and excretion.

Drug Nomenclature

Most drugs are known by several names—chemical, generic, trade, and official—each of which serves a specific function. (See *How drugs are named.*) However, multiple drug names can also contribute to medication errors. You may find a familiar drug packaged with an unfamiliar name if your institution changes suppliers or if a familiar drug is newly approved in a different dose or for a new indication.

Drug Classification

Drugs can be classified in various ways. Most pharmacology textbooks group drugs by their functional classification, such as psychotherapeutics, which is based on common characteristics. Drugs can also be classified according to their therapeutic use, such as antipanic or

How drugs are named

A drug's chemical, generic, trade, and official names are determined at different phases of the drug development process and serve different functions. For example, the various names of the commonly prescribed anticonvulsant divalproex sodium are:

- Chemical name: pentanoic acid, 2-propyl-, sodium salt (2:1), or ($C_{16}H_{31}O_4Na$)
- Generic name: divalproex sodium
- Trade name: Depakote
- Official name: divalproex sodium delayed-release tablets, USP

A drug's chemical name describes its atomic and molecular structure. The chemical name of divalproex sodium—pentanoic acid, 2-propyl-, sodium salt (2:1), or $C_{16}H_{31}O_4Na$ (pronounced valproate semisodium)—indicates that the drug is a combination of two valproic acid compounds with a sodium molecule attached to only one side.

Once a drug successfully completes several clinical trials, it receives a generic name, also known as the nonproprietary name. The generic name is usually derived from, but shorter than, the chemical name. The United States Adopted Names Council is responsible for selecting generic names, which are intended for unrestricted public use.

Before submitting the drug for FDA approval, the manufacturer creates and registers a trade name (or brand name) when the drug appears ready to be marketed. Trade names are copyrighted and followed by the symbol ® to indicate that they're registered and that their use is restricted to the drug manufacturer. Once the original patent on a drug has expired, any manufacturer may produce the drug under its own trade name.

A drug's official name is the name under which it's listed in the United States Pharmacopoeia (USP) and the National Formulary (NF).

antiobsessional drugs. Drugs within a certain therapeutic class may be further divided into subgroups based on their mechanisms of action. For example, the therapeutic class antineoplastics can be further classified as alkylating agents, antibiotic antineoplastics, antimetabolites, antimitotics, biological response modifiers, antineoplastic enzymes, and hormonal antineoplastics.

Pharmacokinetics

Pharmacokinetics is the study of a drug's actions—or fate—as it passes through the body during absorption, distribution, metabolism, and excretion.

ABSORPTION

Before a drug can begin working, it must be transformed from its pharmaceutical dosage form to a biologically available (bioavailable) substance that can pass through various biological cell membranes to reach its site of action. This process is known as absorption. A drug's absorption rate depends on its route of administration, its circulation through the tissue into which it's administered, and its solubility—that is, whether it's more water soluble (*hydrophilic*) or fat soluble (*lipophilic*).

Although drugs may penetrate cellular membranes either actively or passively, most drugs do so by *passive diffusion*, moving inertly from an area of higher concentration to an area of lower concentration. Passive diffusion may occur through water or fat. Passive diffusion through water—*aqueous diffusion*—occurs within large water-filled compartments, such as interstitial spaces, and across epithelial membrane tight junctions and pores in the epithelial lining of blood vessels. Aqueous diffusion is driven by concentration gradients. Drug molecules that are bound to large plasma proteins, such as albumin, are too large to pass through aqueous pores in this way. Passive diffusion through fat—*lipid diffusion*—plays an important role in drug metabolism because of the large number of lipid barriers that separate the aqueous compartments of the body. The tendency of a drug to move through lipid layers between aqueous compartments often depends on the pH of the medium—that is, the ability of the water-soluble or fat-soluble drug to form weak acid or weak base.

Drugs with molecules that are too large to readily diffuse may rely on active *diffusion*, in which special carriers on molecules, including peptides, amino acids, and glucose, transport the drug through the membranes. However, some molecules with selective membrane carriers can expel foreign drug molecules; this is why many drugs can't cross the blood–brain barrier.

Drug absorption begins at the administration route. The three main administration route categories are enteral, parenteral, and transcutaneous. Depending on its nature or chemical makeup, a drug may be better absorbed from one site than from another.

Enteral Administration

Enteral administration consists of the oral, nasogastric, and rectal routes.

Oral: Drugs administered orally are absorbed in the GI tract and then proceed by the hepatic portal vein to the liver and into the systemic circulation. Although generally considered the preferred route, oral drug administration has a number of disadvantages:

- The oral route doesn't always yield sufficiently high blood concentrations to be effective.
- Bioavailability may be less than optimal because of incomplete absorption and first-pass elimination (the part of metabolism that occurs during transit through the liver before the drug reaches the general circulation).
- Drug absorption may be incomplete if the drug is degraded by digestive enzymes or the acidic pH in the stomach or if it's excreted from the liver into the bile.
- Food in the GI tract, gastric emptying time, and intestinal motility may also impede drug absorption.

Nasogastric: Drugs administered through a nasogastric tube enter the stomach directly and are absorbed in the GI tract.

Rectal: Rectal drugs and suppositories also enter the GI tract directly after being inserted in the rectum and absorbed through the rectal mucosa. After being absorbed into the lower GI tract, rectal drugs enter the circulation through the inferior vena cava, bypassing the liver and thus avoiding first-pass metabolism. Suppositories, however, tend to travel upward into the rectum, where veins, such as the superior hemorrhoidal vein, lead to the liver. As a result, drug absorption by this route is often unreliable and difficult to predict.

Parenteral Administration

Parenteral routes may be used whenever enteral routes are contraindicated or inadequate. These routes include intramuscular (I.M.), intravenous (I.V.), subcutaneous, and intradermal administration. Drug absorption is much faster and more predictable after parenteral administration than after enteral administration.

I.M.: Drugs administered by the I.M. route are injected deep into the muscle, where they're absorbed relatively quickly. The rate of drug absorption depends on the vascularity of the injection site, the physiochemical properties of the drug, and the solution in which the drug is contained.

I.V.: I.V. drug administration involves injecting or infusing the drug directly into the blood circulation, allowing for rapid distribution throughout the body. This route usually provides the greatest bioavailability.

Subcutaneous: Drugs administered by the subcutaneous route are injected into the connective tissue just below the skin and are absorbed by simple diffusion from the injection site. The factors that affect I.M. absorption also affect subcutaneous absorption. Absorption by the subcutaneous route may be slower than by the I.M. route.

Intradermal: Drugs administered intradermally, such as purified protein derivative (PPD), are injected into the dermis, from which they diffuse slowly into the local microcapillary system.

Transcutaneous Administration

Transcutaneous drug administration allows drug absorption through the skin or soft-tissue surface. Drugs may be inhaled, inserted sublingually, applied topically, or administered by the eyes, ears, nose, or vagina.

Inhalation: Inhaled drugs may be given as a powder and aerosolized or mixed in solution and nebulized directly into the respiratory tract, where they're absorbed through the alveoli. Inhaled drugs are usually absorbed quickly because of the abundant blood flow in the lungs, though some inhaled drugs have low systemic absorption.

Sublingual: Sublingual drug administration involves placing a tablet, troche, or lozenge under the tongue. The drug is absorbed across the epithelial lining of the mouth, usually quickly. This route avoids first-pass metabolism.

Topical: Topical drugs—creams, ointments, lotions, and patches—are placed on the skin and then cross the epidermis into the capillary circulation. They may also be absorbed through sweat glands, hair follicles, and other skin structures. Absorption by the skin is enhanced if the drug is in a solution.

Ophthalmic: Ophthalmic drugs include solutions and ointments that are instilled or applied directly to the cornea or conjunctiva as well as small, elliptical disks that are placed directly on the eyeball behind the lower eyelid. The movements of the eyeball promote distribution of these drugs over the surface of the eye. Although ophthalmic drugs produce a local effect on the conjunctiva or anterior chamber, some preparations may be absorbed systemically and therefore produce systemic effects.

Otic: Drops administered into the external auditory canal, otic drugs are used to treat infection or inflammation and to soften and remove ear wax. Otic solutions exert a local effect and may result in minimal systemic absorption with no adverse effects.

Nasal: Nasal solutions and suspensions are applied directly to the nasal mucosa by instillation or inhalation to produce local effects, such as vasoconstriction to reduce nasal congestion. Some nasal solutions, such as vasopressin, are administered by this route specifically to produce systemic effects.

Vaginal: Vaginal drugs include creams, suppositories, and troches that are inserted into the vagina, sometimes using a special applicator. These drugs are administered locally to treat such conditions as bacterial and fungal infections.

DISTRIBUTION

Distribution is the process by which a drug is transported by the circulating fluids to various sites, including its sites of action. To ensure maximum therapeutic effectiveness, the drug must permeate all membranes that separate it from its intended site of action. Drug distribution is influenced by blood flow, tissue availability, and protein binding. Drugs that cannot distribute to the tissues in which they are needed are not effective.

METABOLISM

Drug metabolism is the enzymatic conversion of a drug's structure into substrate molecules or polar compounds that are either less active or inactive and are readily excreted. Drugs can also be synthesized to larger molecules. Metabolism may also convert a drug to a more toxic compound. Because the primary site of drug metabolism is the liver, children, the elderly, and patients with impaired hepatic function are at risk for altered therapeutic effects.

Biotransformation is the process of changing a drug into its active metabolite. Compounds that require metabolic biotransformation for activation are known as *prodrugs*. During phase I of biotransformation, the parent drug is converted into an inactive or partially active metabolite. Much of the original drug may be eliminated during this phase. During phase II, the inactive or partially active metabolite binds with available substrates, such as acetic acid, glucuronic acid, sulfuric acid, or water, to form its active metabolite. When biotransformation leads to synthesis, larger molecules are produced to create a pharmacologic effect.

EXCRETION

The body eliminates drugs by both metabolism and excretion. Drug metabolites—and, in some cases, the active drug itself—are eventually excreted from the body, usually through bile, feces, and urine. The primary organ for drug elimination is the kidney. Impaired renal function may alter drug elimination, thereby altering the drug's therapeutic effect. Other excretion routes include evaporation through the skin, exhalation from the lungs, and secretion into saliva and breast milk.

A drug's elimination half-life is the amount of time required for half of the drug to be eliminated from the body. The half-life roughly correlates with the drug's duration of action and is based on normal renal and hepatic function. Typically, the longer the half-life, the less often the drug has to be given and the longer it remains in the body.

Pharmacodynamics

Pharmacodynamics is the study of the biochemical and physiologic effects of drugs and their mechanisms of action. A drug's actions may be structurally specific or nonspecific. Structurally specific drugs combine with cell receptors, such as proteins or glycoproteins, to enhance or inhibit cellular enzyme actions. Drug receptors are the cellular components affected at the site of action. Many drugs form chemical bonds with drug receptors, but a drug can bond with a receptor only if it has a similar shape—much the same way that a key fits into a lock. When a drug combines with a receptor, channels are either opened or closed and cellular biochemical messengers, such as cyclic adenosine monophosphate or calcium ions, are activated. Once activated, cellular functions can be turned either on or off by these messengers.

Structurally nonspecific drugs, such as biological response modifiers, don't combine with cell receptors; rather, they produce changes within the cell membrane or interior.

The mechanisms by which drugs interact with the body are not always known. Drugs may work by physical action (such as the protective effects of a topical ointment) or chemical reaction (such as an antacid's effect on the gastric mucosa), or by modifying the metabolic activity of invading pathogens (such as an antibiotic) or replacing a missing biochemical substance (such as insulin).

AGONISTS

Agonists are drugs that interact with a receptor to stimulate a response. They alter cell physiology by binding to plasma membranes or intracellular structures. *Partial agonists* can't achieve maximal effects even though they may occupy all available receptor sites on a cell. *Strong agonists* can cause maximal effects while occupying only a small number of receptor sites on a cell. *Weak agonists* must occupy many more receptor sites than strong agonists to produce the same effect.

ANTAGONISTS

Antagonists are drugs that attach to a receptor but don't stimulate a response; instead, they inhibit or block responses that would normally be caused by agonists. *Competitive antagonists* bind to receptor sites that are also compatible with an agonist, thus preventing the agonist from binding to the site. *Noncompetitive antagonists* bind to receptor sites that aren't occupied by an agonist; this changes the receptor site so that it's no longer recognized by the agonist. *Irreversible antagonists* work in much the same way that noncompetitive ones do, except that they permanently bind with the receptor.

Antagonism plays an important role in drug interactions. When two agonists that cause opposite therapeutic effects, such as a vasodilator and a vasoconstrictor, are combined, the effects cancel each other out. When two antagonists, such as morphine and naloxone, are combined, both drugs may become inactive.

Pharmacotherapeutics

Pharmacotherapeutics is the study of how drugs are used to prevent or treat disease. Understanding why a drug is prescribed for a certain disease can assist you in prioritizing drug administration with other patient care activities. Knowing a drug's desired and unwanted effects may help you uncover problems not readily apparent from the admitting diagnosis. This information may also help you prevent such problems as adverse reactions and drug interactions.

A drug's *desired effect* is the intended or expected clinical response to the drug. This is the response you start to evaluate as soon as a drug is given. Dosage adjustments and the continuation of therapy often depend on your accurate evaluation and documentation of the patient's response.

An *adverse reaction* is any noxious and unintended response to a drug that occurs at therapeutic doses used for prophylaxis, diagnosis, or therapy. Adverse reactions associated with excessive amounts of a drug are considered drug overdoses. Be prepared to follow your institution's policy for reporting adverse drug reactions.

An *idiosyncratic response* is a genetically determined abnormal or excessive response to a drug that occurs in a particular patient. The unusual response may indicate that the drug has saturated or overwhelmed mechanisms that normally control absorption, distribution, metabolism, or excretion, thus altering the expected response. You may be unsure whether a reaction is adverse or idiosyncratic. Once you report the reaction, the pharmacist usually determines the appropriate course of action.

An *allergic reaction* is an adverse response that results from previous exposure to the same drug or to one that's chemically similar to it. The patient's immune system reacts to the drug as if it were a foreign invader and may produce a mild hypersensitivity reaction, characterized by localized dermatitis, urticaria, angioedema, or photosensitivity. Allergic reactions should be reported to the prescriber immediately and the drug should be discontinued. Follow-up care may include giving drugs, including antihistamines and corticosteroids, to counteract the allergic response.

An *anaphylactic reaction* involves an immediate hypersensitivity response characterized by urticaria, pruritus, and angioedema. Left untreated, an anaphylactic reaction can lead to systemic involvement, resulting in shock. It's often associated with life-threatening hypotension and respiratory distress. Be prepared to assist with emergency life-support measures, especially if the reaction occurs in response to I.V. drugs, which have the fastest rate of absorption.

A *drug interaction* occurs when one drug alters the pharmacokinetics of another drug—for example, when two or more drugs are given concurrently. Such concurrent administration can increase or decrease the therapeutic or adverse effects of either drug. Some drug interactions are beneficial. For example, when taken with penicillin, probenecid decreases the excretion rate of penicillin, resulting in higher blood levels of penicillin. Drug interactions also may occur when a drug's metabolism is altered, often owing to the induction of or competition for metabolizing enzymes. For example, H_2-receptor agonists, which reduce secretion of the enzyme gastrin, may alter the breakdown of enteric coatings on other drugs. Drug interactions due to carrier protein competition typically occur when a drug inhibits the kidneys' ability to reduce excretion of other drugs. For example, probenecid is completely reabsorbed by the renal tubules and is metabolized very slowly. It competes with the same carrier protein as sulfonamides for active tubular secretion and so decreases the renal excretion of sulfonamides. This particular competition can lead to an increased risk of sulfonamide toxicity.

Special Considerations

Although every drug has a usual dosage range, certain factors—such as a patient's age, weight, culture and ethnicity, gender, pregnancy status, and renal and hepatic function—may contribute to the need for dosage adjustments. When you encounter special considerations such as these, be prepared to reassess the prescribed dosage to make sure that it's safe and effective for your patient.

CULTURE AND ETHNICITY

Certain drugs are more effective or more likely to produce adverse effects in particular ethnic groups or races. For example, blacks with hypertension respond better to thiazide diuretics than do patients of other races; on the other hand, blacks also have an increased risk of developing angioedema with angiotensin-converting enzyme (ACE) inhibitors. A patient's religious or cultural background also may call for special consideration. For example, a drug made from porcine products may be unacceptable to a Jewish or Muslim patient.

ELDERLY PATIENTS

Because aging produces certain changes in body composition and organ function, elderly patients present unique therapeutic and dosing problems that require special attention. For example, the weight of the liver, the number of functioning hepatic cells, and hepatic blood flow all decrease as a person ages, resulting in slower drug metabolism. Renal function may also decrease with aging. These processes can lead to the accumulation of active drugs and metabolites as well as increased sensitivity to the effects of some drugs in elderly patients. Because they're also more likely to have multiple chronic illnesses, many elderly patients take multiple prescription drugs each day, thus increasing the risk of drug interactions.

CHILDREN

Because their bodily functions aren't fully developed, children—particularly those under age 12—may metabolize drugs differently than adults. In infants, immature renal and hepatic functions delay metabolism and excretion of drugs. As a result, pediatric drug dosages are very different from adult dosages.

The FDA has provided drug manufacturers with guidelines that define pediatric age categories. Unless the manufacturer provides a specific age range, use these categories as a guide when administering drugs:

- neonates—birth up to age 1 month
- infants—ages 1 month to 2 years
- children—ages 2 to 12
- adolescents—ages 12 to 16.

PREGNANCY

The many physiologic changes that take place in the body during pregnancy may affect a drug's pharmacokinetics and alter its effectiveness. Additionally, exposure to drugs may pose risks for the developing fetus. Before administering a drug to a pregnant patient, be sure to check its assigned FDA pregnancy risk category, or the new more comprehensive text for drugs approved after June 30, 2015, and intervene appropriately.

Principles of Drug Administration

Because there are thousands of drugs and hundreds of facts about each one, taking responsibility for drug administration can seem overwhelming. One way that you can enhance your understanding of the principles of drug administration is to *associate, ask*, and *predict* during the critical thinking process. For example, associate each drug with general information you may already know about the drug or drug class. *Ask* yourself why a drug is administered by a certain route and why it's given multiple times throughout the day rather than only once. Learn to *predict* a drug's actions, uses, adverse effects, and possible drug interactions based on your knowledge of the drug's mechanism of action. As you apply these principles to drug administration, you'll begin to intuitively know which facts you need to make rational clinical decisions.

Prescriptions for patients in hospitals and other institutions typically are written by a physician on a form called the *physician's order sheet* or they're directly input into a computerized system with an electronic signature. Drugs are prescribed based not only on their specific mechanisms of action but also on the patient's profile, which commonly includes age, ethnicity, gender, pregnancy status, smoking and drinking habits, and use of other drugs.

"Rights" of Drug Administration

Always keep in mind the following "rights" of drug administration: the right drug, right time, right dose, right patient, right route, and right preparation and administration.

RIGHT DRUG

Many drugs have similar spellings, different concentrations, and several generic forms. Before administering any drug, compare the exact spelling and concentration of the prescribed drug that appears on the label with the information contained in the medication administration record or drug profile.

Regardless of which drug distribution system your facility uses, you should read the drug label and compare it to the medication administration record at least three times:

- before removing the drug from the dispensing unit or unit dose cart
- before preparing or measuring the prescribed dose
- before opening a unit dose package (just before administering the drug to the patient).

RIGHT TIME

Various factors can affect the time that a drug is administered, such as the timing of meals and other drugs, scheduled diagnostic tests, standardized times used by the institution, and factors that may alter the consistency of blood levels and drug absorption. Before administering any p.r.n. drug, check the patient's chart to ensure that no one else has already administered it and that the specified time interval has passed. Also, document administration of a p.r.n. drug immediately.

RIGHT DOSE

Whenever you're dispensing an unfamiliar drug or are in doubt about a dosage, check the prescribed dose against the range specified in a reliable reference. Be sure to consider any reasons for a dosage adjustment that may apply to your particular patient. Also, make sure you're familiar with the standard abbreviations your institution uses for writing prescriptions.

RIGHT PATIENT

Always compare the name of the patient on the medication record with the name on the patient's identification bracelet. When using a unit dose system, compare the name on the drug profile with that on the identification bracelet.

RIGHT ROUTE

Each drug prescription should specify the administration route. If the administration route is missing from the prescription, consult the prescriber before giving the drug. Never substitute one route for another unless you obtain a prescription for the change.

RIGHT PREPARATION AND ADMINISTRATION

For drugs that need to be mixed, poured, or measured, be sure to maintain aseptic technique. Follow any specific directions included by the manufacturer regarding diluent type and amount and the use of filters, if needed. Clearly label any drug that you've reconstituted with the patient's name, the strength or dose, the date and time that you prepared the drug, the amount and type of diluent that you used, the expiration date, and your initials.

Administration Routes

Drugs may be administered by a variety of routes and dosage forms. A particular route may be chosen for convenience or to maximize drug concentration at the site of action, to minimize drug absorption elsewhere, to prolong drug absorption, or to avoid first-pass metabolism.

Different dosage forms of the same drug may have different drug absorption rates, times of onset, and durations of action. For example, nitroglycerin is a coronary vasodilator that may be administered by the I.V., sublingual, oral, or buccal route, or as a topical ointment or disk. The I.V., sublingual, and buccal forms of nitroglycerin provide a rapid onset of action, whereas the oral, ointment, and disk forms have a slower onset and a prolonged duration of action.

Drug administration routes include the enteral, parenteral, and transcutaneous routes.

ENTERAL

The enteral route consists of oral, nasogastric, and rectal administration. Drugs administered enterally enter the blood circulation by way of the GI tract. This route is considered the most natural and convenient route as well as the safest. As a result, most drugs are taken enterally, usually to provide systemic effects.

Oral

- *Tablets:* Tablets, the most commonly used dosage form, come in a variety of colors, sizes, and shapes. Some tablets are specially coated for various purposes. Enteric coatings permit safe passage of a tablet through the stomach, where some drugs may be degraded or may produce unwanted effects, to the environment of the intestine. Some coatings protect the drug from the destructive influences of moisture, light, or air during storage; some coatings actually contain the drug, such as procainamide; still others conceal a bad taste. Coatings are also used to ensure appropriate drug release and absorption. Some tablets shouldn't be crushed or broken because doing so may alter drug release.
- *Capsules:* Capsules are solid dosage forms in which the drug and other ingredients are enclosed in a hard or soft shell of varying size and shape. Drugs typically are released faster from capsules than from tablets.
- *Solutions:* Drugs administered in solution are absorbed more rapidly than many of those administered in solid form; however, they don't always produce predictable drug levels in the blood. Some drugs in solution should be administered with meals or snacks to minimize their irritating effect on the gastric mucosa.
- *Suspensions:* Suspensions are preparations consisting of finely divided drugs in a suitable vehicle, usually water. Suspensions should be shaken before administration to ensure the uniformity of the preparation and administration of the proper dosage.

Nasogastric

Drugs administered through a nasogastric or gastrostomy tube enter the stomach directly, bypassing the mouth and esophagus. They're usually administered in liquid form because an intact tablet or capsule could cause an obstruction in a gastric tube. Sometimes a tablet may be crushed or a capsule opened for nasogastric administration; however, doing so will affect the drug's release. You may need to consult a pharmacist to determine which tablets can be crushed or capsules opened.

Rectal

Some enteral drugs are administered rectally—as suppositories, solutions, or ointments—to provide either local or systemic effects. When inserted into the rectum, suppositories soften, melt, or dissolve, releasing the drug contained inside them. The rectal route may be preferred for drugs that are destroyed or inactivated by the gastric or intestinal environment or that irritate the stomach. It also may be indicated when the oral route is contraindicated because of vomiting or difficulty swallowing. The drawbacks of rectal administration include inconvenience, noncompliance, and incomplete or irregular drug absorption.

PARENTERAL

In parenteral drug administration, a drug enters the circulatory system through an injection rather than through GI absorption. This administration route is chosen when rapid drug action is desired; when the patient is uncooperative, unconscious, or unable to accept medication by the oral route; or when a drug is ineffective by other routes. Drugs may be injected into the joints, spinal column, arteries, veins, and muscles. However, the most common parenteral routes are the intramuscular (I.M.), intravenous (I.V.), subcutaneous (SubQ), and intradermal (I.D.) routes. Drugs administered parenterally may be mixed in either a solution or a suspension; those mixed in a solution typically act more rapidly than those mixed in a suspension. Parenteral administration has several disadvantages: The drug can't be removed or the dosage reduced once it has been injected, and injections typically are more expensive to administer than other dosage forms because they require strict sterility.

Intramuscular

I.M. injections are administered deep into the anterolateral aspect of the thigh (vastus lateralis), the dorsogluteal muscle (gluteus maximus), the upper arm (deltoid), or the ventrogluteal muscle (gluteus medius). I.M. injections typically provide sustained drug action. This route is commonly chosen for drugs that irritate the subcutaneous tissue. The drug should be injected as far as possible from major nerves and blood vessels.

Intravenous

In I.V. drug administration, an aqueous solution is injected directly into the vein—typically of the forearm. Drugs may be administered as a single, small-volume injection or as a slow, large-volume infusion. Because drugs injected I.V. don't encounter absorption barriers, this route produces the most rapid drug action, making it vital in emergency situations. Except for I.V. fat emulsions used as nutritional supplements, oleaginous preparations aren't usually administered by this route because of the risk of fat embolism.

Subcutaneous

The subcutaneous route may be used to inject small volumes of medication, usually 1 ml or less. Subcutaneous injections typically are given below the skin in the abdominal area, lateral area of the anterior thigh, posterior surface of the upper arm, or lateral lumbar area. Injection sites should be rotated to minimize tissue irritation if the patient receives frequent subcutaneous injections—as, for example, in a patient who takes insulin.

Intradermal

Common sites for intradermal injection are the arm and the back. Because only about 0.1 ml may be administered intradermally, this route is rarely used except in diagnostic and test procedures, such as screening for allergic reactions.

TRANSCUTANEOUS

In transcutaneous administration, a drug crosses the skin layers from either the outside (dermal) or the inside (mucocutaneous). This route includes sublingual, inhalation, ophthalmic, otic, nasal, topical, and vaginal administration.

Sublingual

In sublingual administration, tablets are placed under the tongue and allowed to dissolve. Nitroglycerin is commonly administered by this route, which allows rapid drug absorption and action. The sublingual route also avoids first-pass metabolism.

Inhalation

Some drugs may be inhaled orally or nasally to produce a local effect on the respiratory tract or a systemic effect. Although drugs given by inhalation avoid first-pass hepatic metabolism, the lungs can also serve as an area of first-pass metabolism by providing respiratory conversion to more water-soluble compounds.

Ophthalmic

Ophthalmic solutions and ointments are applied directly to the cornea or conjunctiva for enhanced local penetration and decreased systemic absorption. These drugs usually are used in eye examinations and to treat glaucoma. Ophthalmic solutions pose a greater risk of drug loss through the nasolacrimal duct into the nasopharynx than ophthalmic ointments do.

Otic

Otic solutions are instilled directly into the external auditory canal for local penetration and decreased systemic absorption. These drugs, which include anesthetics, antibiotics, and anti-inflammatory drugs, usually require occlusion of the ear canal with cotton after instillation.

Nasal

Nasal solutions and suspensions are applied directly to the nasal mucosa for enhanced local penetration and decreased systemic absorption. These drugs are usually used to reduce the inflammation typically associated with seasonal or perennial rhinitis.

Topical

Topical drugs—including creams, ointments, lotions, and pastes—are applied directly to the skin. Transdermal delivery systems, usually in the form of an adhesive patch or a disk, are among the latest developments in topical drug administration. Because they provide slow drug release, these systems are typically used to avoid first-pass metabolism and ensure prolonged duration of action.

Vaginal

Vaginal troches, suppositories, and creams are inserted into the vagina for slow, localized absorption. Body pH that differs from blood pH causes drug trapping or reabsorption, which delays drug excretion through the renal tubules. Vaginal secretions are alkaline, with a pH of 3.4 to 4.2, whereas blood has a pH of 7.35 to 7.45.

Drug Therapy and the Nursing Process

A systematic approach to nursing care, the nursing process helps guide you as you develop, implement, and evaluate your care and ensures that you'll deliver safe, consistent, and effective drug therapy to your patients. The nursing process consists of five steps, including assessment, nursing diagnosis, planning, implementation, and evaluation. Even though documentation is not a step in the nursing process, you're legally and professionally responsible for documenting all aspects of your care before, during, and after drug administration.

Assessment

The first step in the nursing process, assessment involves gathering information that's essential to guide your patient's drug therapy. This information includes the patient's drug history, present drug use, allergies, medical history, and physical examination findings. Assessment is an ongoing process that serves as a baseline against which to compare any changes in your patient's condition; it's also the basis for developing and individualizing your patient's plan of care.

DRUG HISTORY

The patient's drug history is critical in your planning of drug-related care. Ask about his previous use of over-the-counter and prescription drugs, as well as herbal remedies. For each drug, determine:

- the reason the patient took it
- the prescribed dosage
- the administration route
- the frequency of administration
- the duration of the drug therapy
- any adverse reactions the patient may have experienced and how he handled them.

Also determine if the patient has a history of drug abuse or addiction. Depending on his physical and emotional state, you may need to obtain the drug history from other sources, such as family members, friends, other caregivers, and the medical record.

PRESENT DRUG USE

Ask about the patient's current use of over-the-counter and prescription drugs, as well as herbal remedies. As you did in the drug history, find out the specific details for each drug (dosage, route, frequency, and reason for taking). Also ask the patient if he thinks the drug has been effective and when he took the last dose.

If the patient uses herbal remedies, similarly explore the use of these products, because herbs may interact with certain drugs. Also ask about the patient's use of recreational drugs, such as alcohol and tobacco, as well as illegal drugs, such as marijuana and heroin. If the patient acknowledges use of these drugs, be alert for possible drug interactions. This information also may provide you with insight about the patient's response—or lack of response—to his current drug treatment plan.

Try to find out if the patient has any other problems that might affect his compliance with the drug treatment plan, and intervene appropriately. For instance, a patient who is unemployed and has no health insurance may fail to fill a needed prescription. In such a case, contact an appropriate individual in your facility who may be able to help the patient obtain financial assistance.

Be sure to ask the patient if his drug treatment plan requires special monitoring or follow-up laboratory tests. For example, patients who take antihypertensives need to have their blood pressure checked routinely, and those who take warfarin must have their prothrombin time tested regularly. Other patients must undergo periodic blood tests to assess their hepatic and renal function. Determine whether the patient has complied with this part of his treatment plan, and ask him if he knows the results of the latest monitoring or laboratory tests.

ALLERGIES

Find out if the patient is allergic to any drugs or foods. If he has an allergy, explore it further by determining the type of drug or food that triggers a reaction, the first time he experienced a reaction, the characteristics of the reaction, and other related information. Keep in mind that some patients consider annoying symptoms, such as indigestion, an allergic reaction. However, be sure to document a true allergy according to your facility's policy to ensure that the patient doesn't receive that drug or any related drug that may cause a similar reaction. Also, document allergies to foods because they may lead to drug interactions or adverse drug reactions. For example, sulfite is a food additive as well as a drug additive, so a patient with a known allergy to sulfite-containing foods is likely to react to sulfite-containing drugs.

MEDICAL HISTORY

While reviewing your patient's medical history, determine if he has any acute or chronic conditions that may interfere with his drug therapy. Certain disorders involving major body systems, such as the cardiovascular, GI, hepatic, and renal systems, may affect a drug's absorption, transport, metabolism, or excretion and interfere with its action; they also may increase the incidence of adverse reactions and lead to toxicity. For each disorder identified, try to determine when the condition was diagnosed, what drugs were prescribed, and who prescribed them. This information can help you determine whether the patient is receiving incompatible drugs and whether more than one prescriber is managing his drug therapy.

Ask a female patient if she is or may be pregnant or if she is breastfeeding. Many drugs are safe to use during pregnancy, but others may harm the fetus. Also, some drugs are distributed into breast milk. If your patient is or might be pregnant, check the FDA's pregnancy risk category for the prescribed drug and notify the prescriber if the drug may pose a risk to the fetus. If the patient is breastfeeding, find out if the drug is distributed in breast milk and intervene appropriately.

PHYSICAL EXAMINATION FINDINGS

As part of the physical examination, note the patient's age and weight. Be aware that age determines the dosage of certain drugs, such as sedatives and hypnotics, whereas weight determines the dosage of others, including some I.V. antibiotics and anticoagulants. As you perform the physical examination, note any abnormal findings that may point to body organ or system dysfunction. For example, if you detect liver enlargement and ascites, the patient may have impaired hepatic function, which can affect the metabolism of a drug he's taking and lead to harmful adverse or toxic effects. Also note whether a body organ or system appears to be responding to drug treatment. For example, if a patient has been taking an antibiotic to treat chronic bronchitis, thoroughly evaluate his respiratory status to measure his progress. Be sure to assess the patient for possible adverse reactions to the drugs he's taking.

Assess the patient's neurologic function to make sure that he can understand his drug regimen and carry out required tasks, such as performing a fingerstick to obtain blood for glucose measurement. If the patient can't understand essential drug information, you'll need to identify a family member or another person who is willing to become involved in the teaching process.

Nursing Diagnosis

Based on information derived from the assessment and physical examination findings, the nursing diagnoses are statements of actual or potential problems that a nurse is licensed to treat or manage alone or in collaboration with other members of the healthcare team. They're worded according to guidelines established by NANDA International.

One of the most common nursing diagnoses related to drug therapy is *knowledge deficit*, which indicates that the patient doesn't have sufficient understanding of his drug regimen. However, adverse reactions are the basis for most nursing diagnoses related to drug administration. For example, a patient receiving an opioid analgesic might have a nursing diagnosis of *constipation* related to decreased intestinal motility or *ineffective breathing* pattern related to respiratory depression. A patient receiving long-term, high-dose corticosteroids may have a risk for *impaired skin integrity* related to cortisone acetate or *self-concept disturbance* related to physical changes from prednisone therapy. Many antiarrhythmics cause orthostatic hypotension and thus may place an elderly patient at *high risk for injury* related to possible syncope. Broad-spectrum antibiotics, especially penicillin, may lead to the overgrowth of *Clostridium difficile*, a bacterium that is normally present in the intestine. This overgrowth in turn may lead to pseudomembranous colitis, characterized by abdominal pain and severe diarrhea. The nursing diagnoses in such a case might include *potential for infection* related to bacterial overgrowth, *alteration in comfort* related to abdominal pain, and *fluid balance deficit* related to diarrhea.

Planning

During the planning phase, you'll establish expected outcomes—or goals—for the patient and then develop specific nursing interventions to achieve them. Expected outcomes are observable or measurable goals that should occur as a result of nursing interventions and sometimes in conjunction with medical interventions. Developed in collaboration with the patient, the outcomes should be realistic and objective and should clearly communicate the direction of the plan of care to other nurses. They should be written as behaviors or responses for the patient, not the nurse, to achieve and should include a time frame for measuring the patient's progress. An example of a typical expected outcome is, *The patient will accurately demonstrate self-administration of insulin before discharge*. Based on each outcome statement you establish, you'd then develop appropriate nursing interventions, which might include drug administration techniques, patient teaching, monitoring of vital signs, calculation of drug dosages based on weight, and recording of intake and output.

Implementation

As you implement the nursing interventions, be sure to stringently follow the classic rule of drug administration: administer the right dose of the right drug by the right route to the right patient at the right time. Also, keep in mind that you have a legal and professional responsibility to follow institutional policy regarding standing orders, prescription renewal, and the use of nursing judgment. During the implementation phase, you'll also begin to evaluate the patient's expected outcomes and nursing interventions and make necessary changes to the plan of care.

Evaluation

Evaluation is an ongoing process rather than a single step in the nursing process. During this phase, you evaluate each expected outcome to determine whether or not it has been achieved and whether the original plan of care is working or needs to be modified. In evaluating a patient's drug treatment plan, you should determine whether or not the drug is controlling the signs and symptoms for which it was prescribed. You also should evaluate the patient for psychological or physiologic responses to the drug, especially adverse reactions. This constant monitoring allows you to make appropriate and timely suggestions for changes to the plan of care, such as dosage adjustments or changes in delivery routes, until each expected outcome has been achieved.

Documentation

You're responsible for documenting all your actions related to the patient's drug therapy, from the assessment phase to evaluation. Each time you administer a drug, document the drug name, dose, time given, and your evaluation of its effect. When you administer drugs that require additional nursing judgment, such as those prescribed on an as-needed basis, document the rationale for administering the drug and follow-up assessment or interventions for each dose administered.

If you decide to withhold a prescribed drug based on your nursing judgment, document your action and the rationale for it, and notify the prescriber of your action in a timely manner. Whenever you notify a prescriber about a significant finding related to drug therapy, such as an adverse reaction, document the date and time, the person you contacted, what you discussed, and how you intervened.

A

abacavir sulfate

Ziagen

Class and Category

Pharmacologic class: Nucleoside reverse transcriptase inhibitor (NRTI)
Therapeutic class: Antiretroviral
Pregnancy category: Not classified

Indications and Dosages

➤ *As adjunct to treat human immunodeficiency virus (HIV) infection*

ORAL SOLUTION, TABLETS

Adults. 600 mg once daily or 300 mg twice daily in combination with other antiretroviral agents.
Children, infants 3 months of age and over. 16 mg/kg once daily or 8 mg/kg twice daily in combination with other antiretroviral agents. *Maximum*: 600 mg daily.

DOSAGE ADJUSTMENT For patients with mild hepatic impairment, dosage reduced to 200 mg twice daily and only oral solution used to ensure accurate dosage.

Mechanism of Action

Blocks an HIV enzyme called reverse transcriptase, which is responsible for starting or increasing the speed of a chemical reaction. By blocking this enzyme, HIV is prevented from multiplying.

Contraindications

Hypersensitivity to abacavir or its components, moderate or severe hepatic impairment, presence of HLA-B*5701 allele

Interactions

DRUGS

methadone: Possibly increased methadone clearance

Adverse Reactions

CNS: Anxiety, chills, depression, dizziness, fatigue, fever, headache, lethargy, malaise, migraines, paresthesia, sleep disorders
CV: Edema, elevated triglyceride levels, **hypotension**, **MI**
EENT: Conjunctivitis, ENT infections, mouth ulcerations, pharyngitis
ENDO: Cushingoid appearance, fat redistribution, hyperglycemia
GI: Abdominal pain, diarrhea, elevated liver enzymes, gastritis, hyperamylasemia, **liver failure**, nausea, **pancreatitis**, **severe hepatomegaly with steatosis**, vomiting
GU: Renal dysfunction, **renal failure**
HEME: Anemia, **neutropenia**, **leukopenia**, **thrombocytopenia**
MS: Achiness, arthralgia, elevated CPK levels, musculoskeletal pain, myalgia, myolysis
RESP: Adult respiratory distress syndrome, bronchitis, cough, dyspnea, pneumonia, **respiratory failure**, viral respiratory infections
SKIN: Erythema multiforme, rash, **Stevens–Johnson syndrome**, **toxic epidermal necrolysis**
Other: Anaphylaxis, **lactic acidosis**, lymphadenopathy, **multiorgan failure**, nonspecific pain

Nursing Considerations

- Check to be sure patient has been screened for the HLA-B*5701 allele prior to initiating abacavir therapy, because carriers of this allele are at greater risk of developing serious and sometimes fatal hypersensitivity reactions to abacavir.
- Know that a past medical history of an allergic reaction to abacavir, including any abacavir-containing product, is a contraindication for the use of abacavir therapy.
- Use caution when administering abacavir to patients with known risk factors for liver disease.
- Use cautiously in patients with coronary artery disease, because an increase in myocardial infarctions has occurred within 6 months of initiating abacavir therapy.
- Be aware that a scored tablet is available for pediatric patients weighing 14 kg or more, provided the child can swallow tablets.

WARNING Monitor patient closely for any hypersensitivity reaction. If present, notify prescriber immediately and expect drug to be discontinued, especially if a hypersensitivity reaction cannot be ruled out. Obesity, prolonged nucleoside exposure, and being a woman have been identified as risk factors. Know that a hypersensitivity reaction to abacavir usually presents with at least two of the following signs or symptoms: constitutional symptoms (achiness, fatigue, generalized malaise), fever, GI symptoms (abdominal pain, diarrhea, nausea, vomiting), rash, or respiratory symptoms (cough, dyspnea, pharyngitis). Other signs and symptoms that may be present include arthralgia, edema, headache, lethargy, myalgia, myolysis, and paresthesia. Know that adult respiratory distress syndrome, anaphylaxis, hypotension, renal failure, and respiratory failure have also occurred in association with an abacavir-induced hypersensitivity reaction and death has occurred.

- Monitor patient's liver enzymes periodically, as ordered, and monitor patient for any signs and symptoms of lactic acidosis or liver dysfunction such as severe hepatomegaly with steatosis, which may become life-threatening. Be aware that incidence is higher in women and in the presence of obesity. If present, notify prescriber, and expect abacavir therapy to be discontinued even in the absence of marked transaminase elevations.
- Be aware that immune reconstitution syndrome has occurred in patients treated with combination antiretroviral therapy, including abacavir. The inflammatory response predisposes susceptible patients to opportunistic infections such as cytomegalovirus infection, *Mycobacterium avium* infection, *Pneumocystis jiroveci* pneumonia, or tuberculosis. Autoimmune disorders such as Graves' disease, Guillain–Barré syndrome, or polymyositis have also occurred. Report sudden or unusual adverse reactions to prescriber.
- Observe patient for redistribution of body fat, including breast enlargement, central obesity, development of buffalo hump, facial wasting, and peripheral wasting, which may produce a cushingoid-type appearance.

PATIENT TEACHING

- Instruct patient/parents/caregiver to administer drug exactly as prescribed. If a dose is missed, have patient take it as soon as it is remembered. Stress importance of not doubling the next dose or taking more than the prescribed dose.

WARNING Review the warning card and medication guide with patient/parents/caregiver on how to recognize a hypersensitivity reaction. Stress importance of stopping abacavir at the first sign of a hypersensitivity reaction and notifying prescriber.

- Instruct patient/parents/caregiver on the signs and symptoms of lactic acidosis and liver dysfunction. Advise patient to stop taking abacavir if present and notify prescriber.
- Advise patient/parents/caregiver to inform prescriber of any signs or symptoms of an infection, as well as any unusual, persistent severe, or unusual adverse reactions.
- Instruct a mother not to breastfeed while she is receiving abacavir therapy, as drug is present in human milk.
- Warn patient that fat distribution may occur with abacavir therapy.
- Tell women of childbearing age to report a known or suspected pregnancy.

abaloparatide

Tymlos

Class and Category

Pharmacologic class: Parathyroid hormone analogue
Therapeutic class: Anti-osteoporotic
Pregnancy category: Not classified

Indications and Dosages

➤ *To treat postmenopausal women with osteoporosis who are at high risk for fracture, such as a history of multiple risk factors for fracture, have already sustained an osteoporotic fracture, or who have failed or are intolerant to other available osteoporosis therapy*

SUBCUTANEOUS INJECTION

Adult postmenopausal women. 80 mcg once daily.

Route	Onset	Peak	Duration
SubQ	Unknown	0.51 min	Unknown

Mechanism of Action

Acts as an agonist at the PTH1 receptor, which activates the cAMP signaling pathway in target cells to increase bone mineral density and content. This in turn increases bone strength at vertebral and/or nonvertebral sites.

Contraindications

Hypersensitivity to abaloparatide or its components

Interactions

DRUGS

None

Adverse Reactions

CNS: Dizziness, fatigue, headache, vertigo
CV: Orthostatic hypotension, palpitations, tachycardia
GI: Abdominal pain (upper), nausea
GU: Hypercalciuria, urolithiasis
Other: Anti-abaloparatide antibodies, elevated uric acid levels, **hypercalcemia**, injection site reactions (severe edema, pain, redness)

Nursing Considerations

- Know that abaloparatide and parathyroid hormone analogues such as teriparatide should not be given for more than 2 years cumulatively during patient's lifetime because of the potential risk of osteosarcoma.
- Be aware that abaloparatide should not be given to patients at increased risk for osteosarcoma. These risks include bone metastases or skeletal malignancies, hereditary disorders predisposing to osteosarcoma, open epiphyses, Paget's disease of bone or unexplained elevations of alkaline phosphatase, or prior external beam or implant radiation therapy involving the skeleton.
- Know that abaloparatide should not be given to women with preexisting hypercalcemia or who have an underlying hypercalcemic disorder, such as primary hyperparathyroidism, because of the risk of exacerbating hypercalcemia.
- Administer abaloparatide only as a subcutaneous injection into the periumbilical region of the abdomen at about the same time every day. Never give intramuscularly or intravenously. Rotate injection site daily. Give first several doses where patient can lie down or sit down, as orthostatic hypotension may occur.
- Monitor patient for orthostatic hypotension for at least 4 hours after each dose.
- Monitor patient's serum calcium levels, as ordered, because drug may increase calcium levels, causing hypercalcemia, hypercalciuria, and urolithiasis. If preexisting hypercalciuria or urolithiasis is suspected, expect to measure the patient's urinary calcium excretion, as ordered.
- Ensure that patient is receiving supplemental calcium and vitamin D if dietary intake is inadequate.

PATIENT TEACHING

- Inform patient that abaloparatide should not be given more than 2 years cumulatively in patient's lifetime because of a potential risk for osteosarcoma. Tell patient to immediately report persistent localized pain or occurrence of a new soft tissue mass that is tender to touch.
- Instruct patient or caregiver how to administer a subcutaneous injection using the abaloparatide pen and how to properly dispose of the needle and pen.
- Emphasize the importance of not sharing the drug or needles with others. Also tell patient not to transfer the contents of the pen to a syringe.
- Tell patient the pen must be discarded after 30 days of use, even if it still contains unused solution.
- Advise patient to change positions slowly for at least 4 hours after abaloparatide has been given and to watch for a drop in her blood pressure with position changes. Symptoms to be alert for include dizziness, nausea, or a rapid heart rate. If present, tell patient to lie down or sit until symptoms pass.
- Instruct patient to report signs and symptoms of high calcium levels such as constipation, lethargy, muscle weakness, nausea, or vomiting. Inform patient that she will need to have her calcium level checked routinely.
- Review dietary sources of calcium and vitamin D. Inform patient that calcium and vitamin D supplementation will be needed if dietary intake is insufficient.

abatacept

Orencia

Class and Category

Pharmacologic class: Selective costimulation modulator
Therapeutic class: Anti-arthritic (psoriatic, rheumatic)
Pregnancy category: Not classified

Indications and Dosages

➤ *To reduce signs and symptoms, induce major clinical response, inhibit progression of structural damage, and improve physical function in patients with moderate to severe active rheumatoid arthritis as monotherapy or concomitantly with disease-modifying antirheumatic drugs (DMARDs) other than tumor necrosis factor (TNF) antagonists; to treat active psoriatic arthritis*

I.V. INFUSION

Adults weighing more than 100 kg (220 lb). *Initial:* 1,000 mg infused over 30 min, repeated at 2 and 4 wk after the first infusion and every 4 wk thereafter.
Adults weighing 60 to 100 kg (132 to 220 lb). *Initial:* 750 mg infused over 30 min, repeated at 2 and 4 wk after the first infusion and every 4 wk thereafter.
Adults weighing less than 60 kg (132 lb). *Initial:* 500 mg infused over 30 min, repeated at 2 and 4 wk after the first infusion and every 4 wk thereafter.

SUBCUTANEOUS INJECTION

Adults. Following a single I.V. loading dose as per body weight categories listed above for treatment of rheumatoid arthritis, 125 mg given within a day, followed by 125 mg once wk. 125 mg once wk for treatment of rheumatoid arthritis when I.V. loading dose is not used or to treat psoriatic arthritis.

DOSAGE ADJUSTMENT For patient transitioning from I.V. therapy to SubQ injection, first SubQ dose should be administered instead of the next scheduled I.V. dose.

➤ *To reduce signs and symptoms of moderate to severe active polyarticular juvenile idiopathic arthritis as monotherapy or concomitantly with methotrexate*

I.V. INFUSION

Children ages 6 to 17 weighing more than 100 kg (220 lb). *Initial:* 1,000 mg infused over 30 min, repeated at 2 and 4 wk after the first infusion and every 4 wk thereafter.
Children ages 6 to 17 weighing 75 to 100 kg (165 to 220 lb). *Initial:* 750 mg infused over 30 min, repeated at 2 and 4 wk after the first infusion and every 4 wk thereafter.
Children ages 6 to 17 weighing less than 75 kg (165 lb). *Initial:* 10 mg/kg infused over 30 min, repeated at 2 and 4 wk after the first infusion and every 4 wk thereafter.

SUBCUTANEOUS INJECTION

Children age 2 and over weighing 50 kg (110 lb) or more. 125 mg once wk.
Children age 2 and over weighing 25 kg (55 lb) to less than 50 kg (110 lb). 87.5 mg once wk.
Children age 2 and over weighing 10 kg (22 lb) to less than 25 kg (55 lb). 50 mg once wk.

Mechanism of Action

Inhibits T-cell activation by binding to CD80 and CD86 to block interaction with CD28. CD28 is part of the costimulatory signal needed for full activation of T cells. Activated T cells have been implicated in the pathogenesis of rheumatoid arthritis. With decreased proliferation of T cells, inflammation and other evidence of rheumatoid arthritis decrease.

Incompatibilities

Don't infuse abatacept solution with other drugs in the same intravenous line concurrently because it is not known whether the drugs may interact.

Contraindications

Hypersensitivity to abatacept or its components

Interactions

DRUGS

live-virus vaccines: Possibly decreased response to vaccine, and risk of infection with live virus
tumor necrosis factor antagonists: Increased risk of serious infection

Adverse Reactions

CNS: Dizziness, fever, headache
CV: Hypertension, **hypotension**
EENT: Nasopharyngitis, rhinitis, sinusitis
GI: Abdominal pain, diarrhea, diverticulitis, dyspepsia, nausea
GU: Acute pyelonephritis, UTI
MS: Back or limb pain
RESP: Bronchitis, COPD worsening, cough, dyspnea, pneumonia, upper respiratory tract infection, wheezing
SKIN: Cellulitis, flushing, pruritus, rash, urticaria
Other: Anaphylaxis, antibody formation against abatacept, herpes simplex, herpes zoster infection, flu-like symptoms, **malignancies**, serious infections such as **sepsis**, varicella infection

Nursing Considerations

- Screen patient for latent tuberculosis with a tuberculin skin test before starting abatacept. If test is positive, expect to provide treatment, as ordered, before starting abatacept. Also screen patient for hepatitis B. If present, expect abatacept to be withdrawn because antirheumatic therapies such as abatacept may reactivate hepatitis B.
- Review patient's immunization record, and make sure all immunizations are current before therapy starts. Drug may blunt effectiveness of some vaccines and increase the risk of infection with live viruses.
- Use cautiously in patients with a history of recurrent infections, underlying conditions that may predispose them to infection, or existing chronic, latent, or localized infection. They have an increased risk of infection with abatacept therapy.
- Use cautiously in patients with COPD and monitor respiratory status closely because abatacept may worsen COPD and increase the risk of adverse respiratory reactions.
- Know that tumor necrosis factor antagonists shouldn't be given with abatacept because of an increased risk of serious infection.
- Prepare for I.V. injection, by reconstituting each vial with 10 ml of sterile water for injection, directing the stream of sterile water to the glass wall of the vial to minimize foaming. Use only the silicone-free disposable syringe provided with each vial because a siliconized syringe may cause translucent particles to form in solution. Also use an 18- to 21-gauge needle. After injecting sterile water into vial, gently swirl vial until contents are completely dissolved. To minimize foaming, don't shake. Vent the vial with a needle to dissipate any foam that may be present.
- Dilute further the reconstituted solution with 0.9% sodium chloride injection to achieve a final solution volume of 100 ml. Slowly add solution into infusion bag or bottle using the same silicone-free disposable syringe provided with each vial. Mix gently. Do not shake the bag or bottle.
- Give I.V. dose after dilution over 30 minutes using an infusion set and a sterile, nonpyrogenic, low protein-binding filter with a pore size of 0.2 μm.
- Be aware that once fully diluted, I.V. solution may be kept for 24 hours at room temperature or refrigerated. If reconstituted solution isn't used within 24 hours, discard.
- Watch patient closely for infusion-related reactions that may occur within 1 hour of the start of the infusion. Adverse reactions to be alert for include dizziness, headache, and hypertension. Less commonly a patient may experience cough, dyspnea, flushing, hypersensitivity, hypotension, nausea, pruritus, rash, and wheezing. Notify prescriber if present, but know that most patients need not discontinue abatacept because of these events unless severe.
- Administer subcutaneous injection using only the supplied 125 mg/ml single-dose prefilled glass syringe or the prefilled ClickJect autoinjector. Know that the 125 mg/syringe or autoinjector are never to be used for intravenous infusion.
- Rotate sites and never give in areas where the skin is tender, bruised, red, or hard.
- Monitor patient closely for evidence of hypersensitivity reaction such as dyspnea,

pruritus, rash, urticaria, or wheezing after administering abatacept. If present, notify prescriber, and provide emergency care, as ordered.
- Monitor patient closely for evidence of infection or malignancy because abatacept inhibits T-cell activation, increasing the risk of both.

PATIENT TEACHING

- Instruct patient receiving abatacept subcutaneously on how to administer the drug. Inform patient that injection sites should be rotated and should never be administered in an area where the skin is tender, bruised, red, or hard.
- Instruct patient self-administering abatacept subcutaneously to use a puncture-resistant container for disposal of needles and syringes. Have patient check with her community guidelines for correct way to dispose of a sharps container and stress the importance of not recycling the sharps container.
- Instruct patient not to receive immunizations with live vaccines during abatacept therapy and for 3 months afterward.
- Advise patient to tell prescriber of all medications being taken, including over-the-counter drugs and other biologic drugs.
- Emphasize need to report any evidence of infection or hypersensitivity to prescriber.
- Alert patient that abatacept may increase the risk of maligancy.
- Warn patient to avoid crowds and people with infections.
- Inform women to report known or suspected pregnancy. Encourage patient to register with the pregnancy exposure registry by calling 1-877-311-8972 if pregnancy occurs.

acamprosate calcium

Class and Category

Pharmacologic class: Amino acid neurotransmitter analogue
Therapeutic class: Alcohol deterrent
Pregnancy category: C

Indications and Dosages

➤ *To maintain abstinence from alcohol for alcohol-dependent patients who are abstinent at the start of treatment*

E.R. TABLETS

Adults. 666 mg three times daily.
DOSAGE ADJUSTMENT For patients with moderate renal impairment (creatinine clearance of 30 to 50 ml/min), initial dosage reduced to 333 mg three times daily.

Route	Onset	Peak	Duration
P.O.	Unknown	3–8 hr	Unknown

Contraindications

Hypersensitivity to acamprosate or its components, severe renal impairment (creatinine clearance 30 ml/min or less)

Interactions

DRUGS

None

Adverse Reactions

CNS: Abnormal thinking, amnesia, anxiety, asthenia, chills, depression, dizziness, headache, insomnia, paresthesia, somnolence, **suicidal ideation**, syncope, tremor
CV: Chest pain, hypertension, palpitations, peripheral edema, vasodilation
EENT: Abnormal vision, dry mouth, pharyngitis, rhinitis, taste perversion
GI: Abdominal pain, anorexia, constipation, diarrhea, flatulence, increased appetite, indigestion, nausea, vomiting
GU: **Acute renal failure**, decreased libido, impotence
HEME: **Leukopenia**, lymphocytosis, **thrombocytopenia**
MS: Arthralgia, back pain, myalgia
RESP: Bronchitis, cough, dyspnea
SKIN: Diaphoresis, pruritus, rash
Other: Flu-like symptoms, infection, weight gain

Mechanism of Action

Chronic alcoholism may alter the balance between excitation and inhibition in neurons in the brain; acamprosate restores it.

When the neurotransmitter gamma-aminobutyric acid (GABA) binds to its receptors in the CNS, it opens the

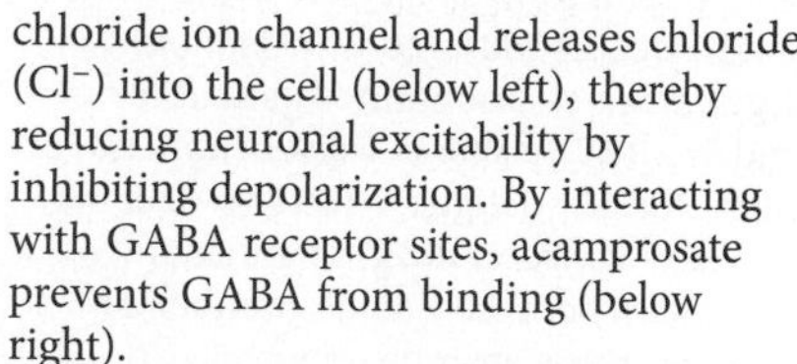

chloride ion channel and releases chloride (Cl^-) into the cell (below left), thereby reducing neuronal excitability by inhibiting depolarization. By interacting with GABA receptor sites, acamprosate prevents GABA from binding (below right).

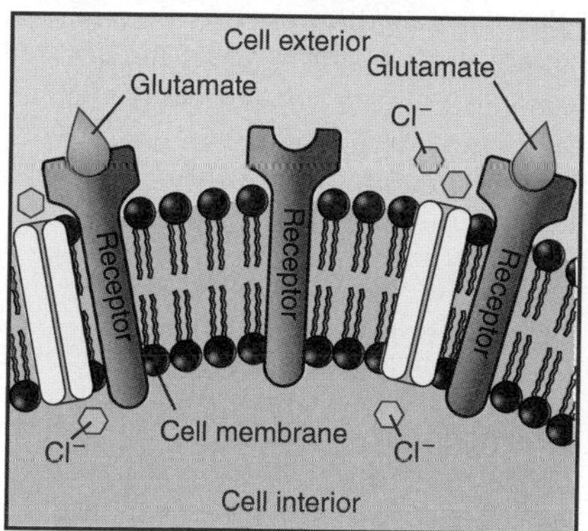

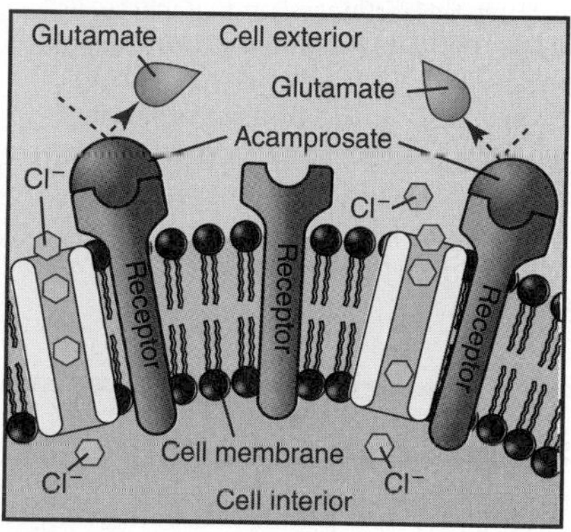

When glutamate binds to its receptors, it closes the chloride ion channel, increasing neuronal excitability by promoting depolarization (below left). This imbalance fosters a craving for alcohol. By interacting with glutamate receptor sites, acamprosate prevents glutamate from binding (below right).

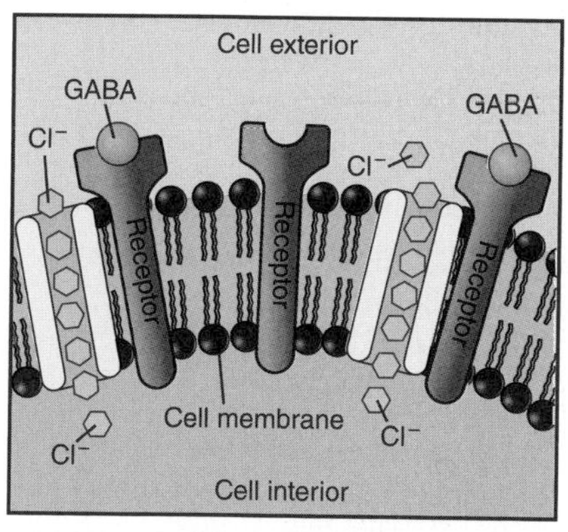

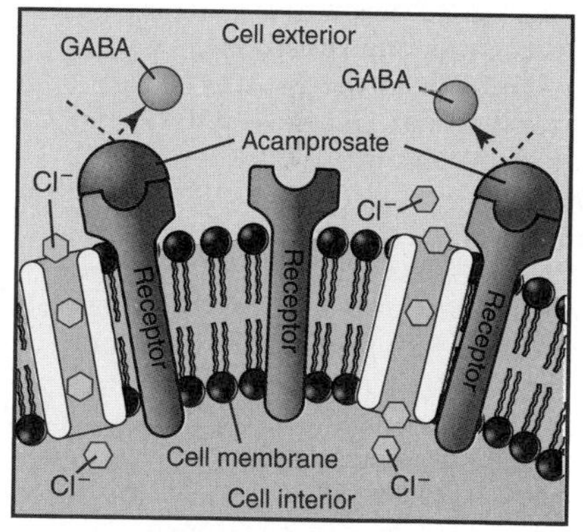

Nursing Considerations

- Know that acamprosate should start as soon as possible after patient has undergone alcohol withdrawal and achieved abstinence.
- Continue to give acamprosate even during periods of alcohol relapse, as ordered.

PATIENT TEACHING

- Instruct patient to take acamprosate exactly as prescribed, even if a relapse occurs, and to seek help for a relapse.
- Tell patient to take tablet whole and not to crush, split, or chew it.

- Warn patient that acamprosate won't reduce symptoms of alcohol withdrawal if relapse occurs followed by cessation.
- Urge caregivers to monitor patient for evidence of depression (lack of appetite or interest in life, fatigue, excessive sleeping, difficulty concentrating) or suicidal tendencies because a small number of patients taking acamprosate have attempted suicide.
- Advise patient to use caution when performing hazardous activities until adverse CNS effects of drug are known.
- Tell female patient to notify prescriber if she is or intends to become pregnant while taking acamprosate; the drug may need to be stopped because fetal risks are unknown.

acarbose

Glucobay (CAN), Precose

Class and Category

Pharmacologic class: Alpha-glucosidase inhibitor
Therapeutic class: Oral antidiabetic
Pregnancy category: B

Indications and Dosages

➤ *As adjunct to diet and exercise to control blood glucose level in type 2 diabetes mellitus*

TABLETS

Adults. *Initial:* 25 mg three times daily with first bite of each meal. *Maintenance:* Increased at 4- to 8-wk intervals, as needed. *Maximum:* 50 mg three times daily for patients weighing 60 kg (132 lb) or less; 100 mg three times daily for patients weighing more than 60 kg.

DOSAGE ADJUSTMENT For patients at increased risk for gastrointestinal adverse effects, initial dosage started at 25 mg once daily with frequency increased gradually until 25 mg three times daily is reached.

Mechanism of Action

Inhibits action of alpha-amylase and alpha-glucoside enzymes. Normally, alpha-amylase hydrolyzes complex starches to oligosaccharides in the small intestine and alpha-glucoside hydrolyzes oligosaccharides, trisaccharides, and disaccharides to glucose and other monosaccharides in the brush border of the small intestine. In diabetic patients, acarbose inhibits these actions and delays glucose absorption, reducing blood glucose level after meals.

Contraindications

Chronic intestinal disease, cirrhosis, colonic ulceration, conditions that may deteriorate because of increased gas formation in intestines, diabetic ketoacidosis, digestive or absorption disorders, history of bowel obstruction, hypersensitivity to acarbose or its components, inflammatory bowel disease, partial intestinal obstruction

Interactions

DRUGS

calcium channel blockers, corticosteroids, digestive enzymes (such as pancreatin), diuretics, estrogen, intestinal adsorbents (such as activated charcoal), isoniazid, nicotinic acid, oral contraceptives, phenothiazines, phenytoin, sympathomimetics, thyroid hormones: Possibly decreased therapeutic effects of acarbose
digoxin: Decreased serum level and therapeutic effects of digoxin
insulin, sulfonylureas: Decreased insulin action, possibly increased risk of hypoglycemia

Adverse Reactions

CV: Edema
GI: Abdominal distention and pain, diarrhea, elevated liver enzymes, flatulence, **fulminant hepatitis**, **hepatotoxicity**, ileus, intestinal wall gas-filled cysts, jaundice
HEME: Thrombocytopenia
SKIN: Erythema, exanthema, rash, urticaria

Nursing Considerations

WARNING Be aware that acarbose isn't recommended for patients with significant renal dysfunction and a serum creatinine level above 2 mg/dl.

- Check blood glucose level often, as ordered, if patient is receiving acarbose and a sulfonylurea or insulin to enhance glucose control.
- Store drug in sealed container in cool environment.
- Expect to decrease dosage to control GI upset.
- Monitor glycosylated hemoglobin level as ordered every 3 months for first year to evaluate glucose control and patient compliance and then periodically thereafter.
- Monitor serum liver enzyme levels every 3 months during first year of therapy and periodically thereafter, as ordered, because acarbose may increase serum liver enzymes.

PATIENT TEACHING

- Explain importance of self-monitoring glucose level during acarbose therapy.
- Teach patient to recognize hypoglycemia and hyperglycemia.
- Warn patient that noncompliance with treatment can increase risk of diabetic complications, including neuropathy, retinopathy, and renal insufficiency.
- Explain that temporary insulin therapy may be needed if fever, trauma, infection, illness, surgery, or other stress alters blood glucose control.
- Warn patient not to take other drugs within 2 hours of acarbose unless specifically instructed by prescriber.
- Tell him to consult prescriber before taking OTC drugs during acarbose therapy.
- Advise patient who also takes another antidiabetic to carry glucose with him at all times in case hypoglycemia occurs.

acetaminophen

Oral or rectal: Abenol (CAN), Acephen, Actamin Maximum Strength, Actimol Children's (CAN), Actimol infant (CAN), Altenol, Aminofen, Apra, Atasol (CAN), Cetafen, Children's Mapap, Children's Nortemp, Dolono, Febrol, Feverall, Genapap, Genebs, Mapap, Pediaphen (CAN), Pyrecot, Pyrigesic, Redutemp, Silapap, Tylenol, Tylenol 8-hr Arthritis Pain Caplets, Tylenol Extra Strength Caplets; Parenteral: Ofirmev

Class and Category

Pharmacologic class: Nonsalicylate, para-aminophenol derivative
Therapeutic class: Antipyretic, nonopioid analgesic
Pregnancy category: B

Indications and Dosages

➤ *To relieve mild to moderate pain*

REGULAR STRENGTH (325 MG): CAPLETS, CAPSULES, CHEWABLE TABLETS, ELIXIR, GELCAPS, LIQUID SOLUTION, SPRINKLES, SUSPENSION, TABLETS

Adults and children 12 yr and over. 640 or 650 mg every 4 to 6 hr, as needed. *Maximum:* 3,250 mg (5 doses) in 24 hr.

EXTRA STRENGTH (500 MG) CAPLETS OR TABLETS

Adults. 1,000 mg every 6 hr, as needed. *Maximum:* 3,000 mg in 24 hr.

8-HR (650 MG) CAPLETS

Adults. 1,300 mg every 8 hr. *Maximum:* 3,900 mg in 24 hr.

CHEWABLE TABLETS, ORAL SUSPENSION, SYRUP

Children age 12 and over weighing 43.5 kg (96 lb) or more. 640 mg every 4 hr, as needed. *Maximum:* 3,200 mg (5 doses) in 24 hr.

Children age 11 weighing 32.6 kg (72 lb) to 43 kg (95 lb). 480 mg every 4 hr, as needed. *Maximum:* 2,400 mg (5 doses) in 24 hr.

Children age 9 to 10 weighing 27 kg (60 lb) to 32 kg (71 lb). 400 mg every 4 hr, as needed. *Maximum:* 2,000 mg (5 doses) in 24 hr.

Children age 6 to 8 weighing 21.5 kg (48 lb) to 26.5 kg (59 lb). 320 mg every 4 hr, as needed. *Maximum:* 1,600 mg (5 doses) in 24 hr.

Children age 4 to 5 weighing 16 kg (35 lb) to 21 kg (47 lb). 240 mg every 4 hr, as needed. *Maximum:* 1,200 mg (5 doses) in 24 hr.

Children age 2 to 3 weighing 10.9 kg (24 lb) to 15.9 kg (35 lb). 160 mg every

4 hr, as needed. *Maximum:* 800 mg (5 doses in 24 hr.

SUPPOSITORIES

Adults and adolescents. 650 mg every 4 to 6 hr, as needed. *Maximum:* 3,900 mg in 24 hr.

Children ages 6 to 12. 325 mg every 4 to 6 hr, as needed. *Maximum:* 1,625 mg in 24 hr.

Children ages 3 to 6. 120 mg every 4 to 6 hr, as needed. *Maximum:* 600 mg in 24 hr.

Children ages 1 to 3. 80 mg every 4 to 6 hr, as needed. *Maximum:* 400 mg in 24 hr.

Children ages 6 to 11 months. 80 mg every 6 hr, as needed. *Maximum:* 320 mg in 24 hr.

➤ *To relieve mild to moderate pain; to manage moderate to severe pain with adjunctive opioid analgesics*

I.V. INFUSION (OFIRMEV)

Adults and adolescents age 13 and over weighing 50 kg (110 lb) or more. 650 mg administered over 15 min every 4 hr, as needed, or 1,000 mg administered over 15 min every 6 hr, as needed. *Maximum:* 4,000 mg in 24 hr.

Adults and children age 2 and over weighing less than 50 kg (110 lb). 12.5 mg/kg administered over 15 min every 4 hr, as needed, or 15 mg/kg (up to 750 mg) administered over 15 min every 6 hr, as needed. *Maximum:* 75 mg/kg (up to 3,750 mg) in 24 hr.

➤ *To reduce fever*

I.V. INFUSION (OFIRMEV)

Adults and adolescents age 13 and over weighing 50 kg (110 lb) or more. 650 mg administered over 15 min every 4 hr, as needed, or 1,000 mg administered over 15 min every 6 hr, as needed. *Maximum:* 4,000 mg in 24 hr.

Adults and children age 2 and over weighing less than 50 kg (110 lb). 12.5 mg/kg administered over 15 min every 4 hr, as needed, or 15 mg/kg (up to 750 mg) administered over 15 min every 6 hr, as needed. *Maximum:* 75 mg/kg (up to 3,750 mg) in 24 hr.

Infants 29 days to 2 years. 15 mg/kg every 6 hr, as needed. *Maximum:* 60 mg/kg/day with minimum dosing interval of 6 hr.

Premature neonates at least 32 weeks gestational age and up to 28 days. 12.5 mg/kg every 6 hr, as needed. *Maximum:* 50 mg/kg/day with minimum dosing interval of 6 hr.

DOSAGE ADJUSTMENT For patient with severe renal impairment (creatinine clearance 30 ml/min or less), dosing interval increased and total daily dosage reduced. For patient with mild to moderate hepatic impairment, total daily dosage reduced.

Route	Onset	Peak	Duration
P.O., P.R., I.V.	Varies	1–3 hr	3–4 hr

Mechanism of Action

Inhibits the enzyme cyclooxygenase, blocking prostaglandin production and interfering with pain impulse generation in the peripheral nervous system. Acetaminophen also acts directly on temperature-regulating center in the hypothalamus by inhibiting synthesis of prostaglandin E_2.

Incompatibilities

Don't mix parenteral acetaminophen with any other medication. Diazepam and chlorpromazine are physically incompatible with parenteral acetaminophen.

Contraindications

Hypersensitivity to acetaminophen or its components, severe hepatic impairment, severe active liver disease

Interactions

DRUGS

anticholinergics: Decreased onset of acetaminophen action

barbiturates, carbamazepine, hydantoins, isoniazid, rifampin, sulfinpyrazone: Decreased therapeutic effects and increased hepatotoxic effects of acetaminophen

dasatinib, imatinib: Possibly increased risk of hepatotoxicity

lamotrigine: Possibly decreased therapeutic effects of these drugs

oral contraceptives: Decreased effectiveness of acetaminophen

probenecid: Possibly increased therapeutic effects of acetaminophen
propranolol: Possibly increased action of acetaminophen
warfarin: Possibly increased international normalized ratio
zidovudine: Possibly decreased zidovudine effects

ACTIVITIES

alcohol use: Increased risk of hepatotoxicity

Adverse Reactions

CNS: Agitation, anxiety, fatigue, fever, headache, insomnia
CV: **Hypotension**, hypertension, peripheral edema
EENT: **Stridor (parenteral form)**
ENDO: **Hypoglycemic coma**
GI: Abdominal pain, constipation, diarrhea, **hepatotoxicity**, jaundice, nausea, vomiting
GU: Oliguria (parenteral form)
HEME: **Hemolytic anemia (with long-term use), leukopenia, neutropenia, pancytopenia, thrombocytopenia**
MS: Muscle spasm (parenteral form)
RESP: Parenteral form: **atelectasis**, dyspnea, plural effusion, **pulmonary edema**, wheezing
SKIN: **Acute generalized exanthematous pustulosis**, blisters, pruritus, rash, reddening, **Stevens–Johnson syndrome**, **toxic epidermal necrolysis**, urticaria
Other: **Anaphylaxis**, **angioedema**, hypersensitivity reactions; for parenteral form: hypoalbuminemia, **hypokalemia**, **hypomagnesemia**, hypophosphatemia, injection-site pain

Nursing Considerations

- Use acetaminophen cautiously in patients with hepatic impairment or active hepatic disease, alcoholism, chronic malnutrition, severe hypovolemia, or severe renal impairment.
- Know that before and during long-term therapy including parenteral therapy, liver function test results, including AST, ALT, bilirubin, and creatinine levels, as ordered must be monitored because acetaminophen may cause hepatotoxicity. Ensure that the daily dose of acetaminophen from all sources does not exceed maximum daily limits.
- Monitor renal function in patient on long-term therapy. Keep in mind that blood or albumin in urine may indicate nephritis; decreased urine output may indicate renal failure; and dark brown urine may indicate presence of the metabolite phenacetin.
- Store suppositories under 26.6°C (80°F).

WARNING Do not confuse a dose in milligrams with a dose in milliliters when preparing and administering the parenteral form of acetaminophen. Also, make sure the dose is based on the patient's weight and infusion pumps are properly programmed.

- Be aware that patients weighing 50 kg (110 lb) or more and requiring 1,000-mg doses of parenteral acetaminophen (Ofirmev) can have the dose administered by inserting a vented intravenous set through the septum of the 100-ml vial. Further dilution is not required. For doses less than 1,000 mg, the appropriate dose must be withdrawn from the vial and placed into a separate container prior to administration to prevent inadvertent overdose. Place small-volume pediatric doses up to 60 ml in a syringe and administer over 15 minutes using a syringe pump.
- Monitor the end of a parenteral infusion to prevent possibility of air embolism.
- Use parenteral drug within 6 hours once vacuum seal of glass vial has been penetrated or contents transferred to another container.

WARNING Be aware that Pediaphen is a concentrated form of acetaminophen containing 80 mg/0.8 ml (standard liquid forms contain 32 mg/ml). Make sure to use correct concentration and dosage of liquid acetaminophen because serious adverse reactions can result from confusing concentrated form with regular liquid form.

PATIENT TEACHING

- Tell patient that tablets may be crushed or swallowed whole.
- Know that concentrated infant drops are being phased out and are no longer manufactured, but may still be available.

- Instruct patient to read manufacturer's label and follow dosage guidelines precisely. Explain that infants' and children's acetaminophen liquid aren't equal in drug concentration and aren't interchangeable. Until concentrated infant drops are completely phased out, parents should use extra caution to ensure the correct dose is given with strength being used. Tell them to use only the measuring device that comes with the bottle to help ensure accurate dosage.
- Caution patient not to exceed recommended dosage or take other drugs containing acetaminophen at the same time because of risk of liver damage. Advise him to contact prescriber before taking other prescription or OTC products because they may contain acetaminophen.
- Teach patient to recognize signs of hepatotoxicity, such as bleeding, easy bruising, and malaise, which commonly occurs with chronic overdose.

WARNING **Caution patient that serious skin reactions, although rare, may occur even with first-time use and any time acetaminophen is used, even if no skin reactions occurred with a previous use of drug. Tell patient that if a skin rash, redness, or blisters occur, he should stop using drug and seek emergency treatment immediately.**

- Inform patient that acetaminophen may cause reduced fertility in both females and males.

acetazolamide

acetazolamide sodium

Class and Category

Pharmacologic class: Carbonic anhydrase inhibitor
Therapeutic class: Anticonvulsant, antiglaucoma, diuretic
Pregnancy category: C

Indications and Dosages

➤ *To treat chronic simple (open-angle) glaucoma*

E.R. CAPSULES
Adults. 500 mg twice daily.
I.V. INJECTION, TABLETS
Adults. 250 to 1,000 mg daily (divided for doses exceeding 250 mg).

➤ *As short-term therapy to treat secondary glaucoma; to treat acute angle-closure glaucoma preoperatively when delay of surgery is needed in order to lower intraocular pressure*

E.R. CAPSULES
Adults. 500 mg twice daily.
I.V. INJECTION, TABLETS
Adults. 250 mg twice daily or every 4 hr; or 500 mg initially, followed by 125 to 250 mg every 4 hr for severe acute glaucoma. Oral therapy usually started after initial I.V. dose.

➤ *To treat edema caused by congestive heart failure*

I.V. INJECTION, TABLETS
Adults. *Initial:* 250 to 375 mg or 5 mg/kg daily in morning. *Maintenance:* 250 to 375 mg or 5 mg/kg on alternate days or for 2 days followed by a drug-free day.

➤ *To treat drug-induced edema*

I.V. INJECTION, TABLETS
Adults. 250 to 375 mg once daily for 1 to 2 days alternating with a day of rest.

➤ *To treat seizures, including generalized tonic–clonic, absence, and mixed seizures, and myoclonic jerk patterns*

I.V. INJECTION, TABLETS
Adults. 8 to 30 mg/kg daily in divided doses. *Optimal:* 375 to 1,000 mg daily. When used with other anticonvulsants, intially, 250 mg daily, increased as needed to optimal dosage.

➤ *To prevent or relieve symptoms of acute mountain sickness*

E.R. CAPSULES, TABLETS
Adults. 500 to 1,000 mg daily in divided doses, given 24 to 48 hr before ascent and continued for 48 hr or longer while at high altitude, as needed, to control symptoms.

Route	Onset	Peak	Duration
P.O. (E.R.)	2 hr	8–12 hr	18–24 hr
I.V.	2 min	15 min	4–5 hr

Mechanism of Action

Inhibits the enzyme carbonic anhydrase, which normally appears in the eyes' ciliary processes, brain's choroid plexes, and kidneys' proximal tubule cells. In the eyes, enzyme inhibition decreases aqueous humor secretion, which lowers intraocular pressure. In the brain, inhibition may delay abnormal, intermittent, and excessive discharge from neurons that cause seizures. In the kidneys, it increases bicarbonate excretion, which carries out water, potassium, and sodium, thus inducing diuresis and metabolic acidosis. This acidosis counteracts respiratory alkalosis and reduces symptoms of mountain sickness, including headache, dizziness, nausea, and dyspnea.

Contraindications

Chronic noncongestive closed-angle glaucoma; cirrhosis; hyperchloremic acidosis; hypersensitivity to acetazolamide, sulfonamides, other sulfonamide derivatives, or their components; hypokalemia; hyponatremia; severe hepatic, renal, or adrenocortical impairment; suprarenal gland failure

Interactions

DRUGS

amphetamines, methenamine, phenobarbital, procainamide, quinidine: Decreased excretion and possibly toxicity of these drugs
corticosteroids: Increased risk of hypokalemia
cyclosporine: Increased cyclosporine level, possibly nephrotoxicity or neurotoxicity
diflunisal: Possibly significantly decreased intraocular pressure
lithium: Increased excretion and decreased effectiveness of lithium
primidone: Decreased serum and urine primidone levels
salicylates: Increased risk of salicylate toxicity

Adverse Reactions

CNS: Ataxia, confusion, depression, disorientation, dizziness, drowsiness, fatigue, fever, flaccid paralysis, headache, lassitude, malaise, nervousness, paresthesia, **seizures**, tremor, weakness
EENT: Altered taste, tinnitus, transient myopia
GI: Anorexia, constipation, diarrhea, **hepatic dysfunction**, **melena**, nausea, vomiting
GU: Crystalluria, decreased libido, glycosuria, hematuria, impotence, **nephrotoxicity**, phosphaturia, polyuria, renal calculi, renal colic, urinary frequency
HEME: Agranulocytosis, **hemolytic anemia**, **leukopenia**, **panyctopenia**, **thromboctyopenia**, **thrombocytopenic purpura**
SKIN: Photosensitivity, pruritus, rash, **Stevens–Johnson syndrome**, urticaria
Other: Acidosis, hyperuricemia, **hypokalemia**, weight loss

Nursing Considerations

- Use acetazolamide cautiously in patients with calcium-based renal calculi, diabetes mellitus, gout, or respiratory impairment.
- Know that acetazolamide may increase risk of hepatic encephalopathy in patients with hepatic cirrhosis.
- Reconstitute each 500-mg vial with at least 5 ml sterile water for injection. Use within 12 hours because drug has no preservative unless refrigerated (use within 3 days).
- Monitor blood tests during acetazolamide therapy to detect electrolyte imbalances.
- Monitor fluid intake and output every 8 hours and body weight daily to detect excessive fluid and weight loss.

PATIENT TEACHING

- Advise patient to avoid hazardous activities if dizziness or drowsiness occurs.
- Instruct patient who takes high doses of salicylates to notify prescriber immediately about evidence of salicylate toxicity, such as anorexia, tachypnea, and lethargy.
- Tell patient if she plans to mountain climb, urge her to descend mountain gradually and to seek immediate medical care if symptoms of mountain sickness occur.

acetohydroxamic acid

Lithostat

Class and Category

Pharmacologic class: Urease inhibitor
Therapeutic class: Antagonist to bacterial enzyme urease
Pregnancy category: X

Indications and Dosages

➤ *As an adjunct to antimicrobial therapy to treat chronic UTI caused by urea-splitting bacteria*

TABLETS

Adults. *Initial:* 12 mg/kg daily in divided doses every 6 to 8 hr on an empty stomach. *Usual:* 250 mg three or four times daily for a total of 10 to 15 mg/kg daily. *Maximum:* 1,500 mg daily. **Children.** *Initial:* 10 mg/kg daily in divided doses on an empty stomach, increased or decreased as tolerated and needed.

DOSAGE ADJUSTMENT For a patient with a creatinine clearance level above 1.8 mg/dl, dosage interval increased to every 12 hours and maximum daily dosage decreased to 1 g.

Mechanism of Action

Inhibits urease, the enzyme that catalyzes urea's hydrolysis to carbon dioxide and ammonia in urine infected with urea-splitting bacteria. This action reduces the urine ammonia level and pH, enhancing antimicrobial drug effectiveness.

Contraindications

Contributing disorder that's treatable by surgery or appropriate antimicrobial therapy, hypersensitivity to acetohydroxamic acid or its components, inadequate renal function (serum creatinine level above 2.5 mg/dl or creatinine clearance below 20 ml/min), risk of pregnancy, UTI caused by non–urease-producing organisms, UTI that could be controlled by appropriate antimicrobial therapy

Interactions

DRUGS

iron: Decreased intestinal absorption of iron, decreased effects of iron and acetohydroxamic acid

ACTIVITIES

alcohol use: Increased risk of severe rash 30 to 45 minutes after drinking alcohol

Adverse Reactions

CNS: Anxiety, depression, fever, headache, lack of coordination, malaise, nervousness, slurred speech, tiredness, tremor
CV: Deep venous thrombosis, palpitations, superficial phlebitis
EENT: Pharyngitis, sudden change in vision
GI: Anorexia, nausea, vomiting
HEME: Hemolytic anemia, reticulocytosis, **unusual bleeding**
RESP: Dyspnea, **pulmonary emboli**
SKIN: Ecchymosis, hair loss, nonpruritic macular rash

Nursing Considerations

- Use acetohydroxamic acid cautiously in patients with anemia or chronic renal disease and those who've had phlebitis or thrombophlebitis.
- Be aware that risk of adverse psychomotor effects increases if patient drinks alcohol or takes drugs that affect alertness and reflexes, such as analgesics, antihistamines, narcotics, sedatives, and tranquilizers.

WARNING **Be aware that acetohydroxamic acid chelates with dietary iron. If patient has iron deficiency anemia, expect to administer I.M. iron as needed during acetohydroxamic acid therapy.**

- Monitor follow-up laboratory tests to check hepatic and renal function and urine pH, as ordered.

PATIENT TEACHING

- Instruct patient to take drug at same time each day, as prescribed.
- Tell patient to take a missed dose up to 2 hours after scheduled time. If more than 2 hours have passed, he should wait for next scheduled dose and shouldn't double that dose.
- Warn patient not to take drug with alcohol or iron and to consult prescriber before taking it with any other drug.
- Instruct patient to avoid hazardous activities during therapy.

acetylcysteine

Acetadote, Acetylcysteine 10% or 20%, Cetylev, Parvolex (CAN)

Class and Category

Pharmacologic class: L-cysteine derivative
Therapeutic class: Antidote (for acetaminophen overdose), mucolytic
Pregnancy category: B

Indications and Dosages

➤ *To liquefy abnormal, thickened, or viscid mucus secretions in chronic pulmonary disorders (including bronchiectasis, bronchitis, cystic fibrosis, and emphysema) and in pneumonia, pulmonary complications of cardiovascular or thoracic surgery, and tracheostomy care*

SOLUTION BY DIRECT INSTILLATION INTO TRACHEOSTOMY (ACETYLCYSTEINE)

Adults and children. 1 to 2 ml of 10% or 20% solution instilled every 1 to 4 hr, as needed.

SOLUTION BY INHALATION (ACETYLCYSTEINE)

Adults and children. 1 to 10 ml of 20% solution or 2 to 20 ml of 10% solution nebulized through face mask, mouthpiece, or tracheostomy every 2 to 6 hr. *Usual:* 3 to 5 ml of 20% solution or 6 to 10 ml of 10% solution three or four times daily.

➤ *To treat acetaminophen overdose*

EFFERVESCENT TABLETS (CETYLEV), SOLUTION P.O. (ACETYLCYSTEINE)

Adults and children. *Loading dose:* 140 mg/kg. *Maintenance:* 70 mg/kg 4 hr after loading dose and then every 4 hr to a total of 17 doses.

I.V. INFUSION (ACETADOTE)

Adults and children weighing 41 kg (90.2 lb) or more. 150 mg/kg in 200 ml of diluent infused over 60 min, followed by 50 mg/kg in 500 ml of diluent infused over 4 hr, followed by 100 mg/kg in 1,000 ml of diluent infused over 16 hr.

Adults and children weighing 20 kg (44 lb) to 41 kg (90.2 lb) 150 mg/kg in 100 ml of diluent infused over 60 min, followed by 50 mg/kg in 250 ml of diluent infused over 4 hr, followed by 100 mg/kg in 500 ml of diluent infused over 16 hr.

Children weighing 5 kg (11 lb) to 20 kg (44 lb). 150 mg/kg in 3 ml/kg of diluent infused over 60 min, followed by 50 mg/kg in 7 ml/kg of diluent infused over 4 hr, followed by 100 mg/kg in 14 ml/kg of diluent infused over 16 hr.

Mechanism of Action

Decreases viscosity of pulmonary secretions by breaking disulfide links that bind glycoproteins in mucus. Reduces liver damage from acetaminophen overdose. Usually, acetaminophen's toxic metabolites bind with glutathione in the liver, which detoxifies them. When acetaminophen overdose depletes glutathione stores, toxic metabolites bind with protein in liver cells, killing them. Acetylcysteine maintains or restores levels of glutathione or acts as its substitute, which reduces liver damage from acetaminophen overdose.

Incompatibilities

Don't give acetylcysteine with nebulization equipment if drug can contact copper, iron, or rubber. Don't give drug with amphotericin B, ampicillin sodium, chlortetracycline, chymotrypsin, erythromycin, hydrogen peroxide, iodized oil, oxytetracycline, tetracycline, or trypsin.

Contraindications

Hypersensitivity to acetylcysteine or its components, no contraindications when used as antidote

Interactions

DRUGS

activated charcoal: Possibly adsorption and decreased effectiveness of oral acetylcysteine

nitroglycerin: Increased effects of nitroglycerin and possibly significant headache and hypotension

Adverse Reactions

CNS: Chills, dizziness, drowsiness, fever, headache

CV: Edema, hypertension, **hypotension**, tachycardia

EENT: Rhinorrhea, stomatitis, **stridor**, tooth damage

GI: Anorexia, constipation, **hepatotoxicity**, nausea, vomiting

RESP: Bronchospasm, chest tightness, cough, **hemoptysis**, **respiratory distress**, shortness of breath, wheezing

SKIN: Clammy skin, erythema, facial flushing, pruritus, rash, urticaria

Other: Anaphylaxis, **angioedema**

Nursing Considerations

- Know that acetylcysteine should be used cautiously in patients with asthma or a history of bronchospasm because drug may adversely affect respiratory function.

WARNING Treating acetaminophen overdose with intravenous therapy may require adjusting total administered volume, as ordered, for patients weighing less than 40 kg (88 lb) and for those who need fluid restriction, to avoid fluid overload and possibly fatal hyponatremia or seizures.

- Be aware that it may be necessary to dilute 20% inhalation or instillation solution with normal saline solution or sterile water when acetycysteine is used to liquefy secretions. The 10% solution may be used undiluted.
- Follow guidelines for product prescribed when treating acetaminophen overdose. For example, dissolve appropriate number of 2.5 g and/or 500 mg effervescent tablets (Cetylev) in water (for patients weighing 19 kg or less, dissolve in 100 ml of water; for patients weighing 20 to 60 kg, dissolve in 150 ml of water; and, for patients weighing 60 kg or more, dissolve in 300 ml of water). Once tablets are dissolved, administer oral solution immediately. For oral solution form (acetylcysteine), dilute 20% oral solution with cola or other soft drink to a concentration of 5%, and use within 1 hour.
- Dilute parenteral solution (Acetadote) with D_5W or half-normal saline (0.45% sodium chloride) solution for injection following manufacturer guidelines because dilution is based on dosage. Acetadote may turn from colorless to slight pink or purple once the stopper is punctured, but color change has no effect on product quality.
- Keep in mind that acetylcysteine is most effective if given within 24 hours of acetaminophen ingestion. For specific instructions, contact a regional poison center at 1-800-222-1222 or a special health professional assistance hotline at 1-800-525-6115.
- Repeat dose as prescribed, if patient vomits loading dose or any maintenance dose within 1 hour of administration.
- Keep in mind that suicidal patient may not provide reliable information about vomiting. Watch such a patient to ensure that he ingests all of prescribed dosage.
- Watch for signs of hepatotoxicity (altered coagulation, easy bruising, and prolonged bleeding time), during treatment for acetaminophen overdose.
- Be aware that acetylcysteine may have a disagreeable odor, which disappears as treatment progresses.
- When drug is given intravenously, acute flushing and erythema of the skin may occur within 30 to 60 minutes of administration and often resolves spontaneously even with continued infusion of drug. However, monitor patient closely for acute hypersensitivity reactions regardless of form of drug administered, such as hypotension, rash, shortness of breath, and wheezing. If present, immediately stop administration of drug, notify prescriber, and provide supportive care according to protocol.
- Have patient wash his face and rinse his mouth at the end of each nebulization treatment because nebulization causes sticky residue on face and in mouth.
- Be aware that an open vial of solution may turn light purple but that this doesn't alter its effectiveness.
- Refrigerate opened vials and discard after 96 hours.
- Assess type, frequency, and characteristics of patient's cough. Particularly note sputum. If cough doesn't clear secretions, prepare to perform mechanical suctioning.
- Monitor patient for tachycardia.

PATIENT TEACHING

- Tell patient receiving acetylcysteine intravenously that facial redness or flushing may occur but usually resolves on its own.
- Instruct patient to notify prescriber immediately about nausea, rash, or vomiting, as well as feeling dizzy or lightheaded, shortness of breath, or wheezing.
- Warn patient about acetylcysteine's unpleasant smell; reassure him that it subsides as treatment progresses.
- Urge patient prescribed drug to loosen mucus, to consume 2 to 3 L of fluid daily unless contraindicated by another condition, to decrease mucus viscosity.
- Instruct female patient who is breastfeeding to consider pumping and discarding her milk for 30 hours after acetylcysteine administration.

acitretin

Soriatane

Class and Category

Pharmacologic class: Second-generation retinoid
Therapeutic class: Antipsoriatic
Pregnancy category: X

Indications and Dosages

➤ *To treat severe psoriasis*

CAPSULES

Adults. 25 to 50 mg once daily with the main meal.

Route	Onset	Peak	Duration
P.O.	Unknown	2–5 hr	Unknown

Mechanism of Action

Binds to several retinoid receptors to regulate gene transcription. Exactly how the action of this second-generation retinoid allows normal growth and development of skin is unknown.

Contraindications

Alcohol consumption; blood donation; breastfeeding; chronic hyperlipidemia; concurrent use of etretinate, methotrexate, or tetracycline; hypersensitivity to acitretin, other retinoids, or their components; pregnancy; severe hepatic or renal impairment

Interactions

DRUGS

methotrexate: Increased risk of hepatitis
oral contraceptives containing only progestin: Possibly decreased effectiveness of oral contraceptive
phenytoin: Possibly decreased protein binding of phenytoin
sulfonylureas: Possibly increased risk of hypoglycemia
tetracyclines: Possibly increased intracranial pressure
vitamin A and other oral retinoids: Increased risk of hypervitaminosis A

ACTIVITIES

alcohol use: Increased risk of adverse reactions and acitretin toxicity

Adverse Reactions

CNS: Aggression, **CVA**, depression, fatigue, headache, hyperesthesia, hypotonia, insomnia, **intracranial hypertension**, paresthesia, peripheral neuropathy, rigors, somnolence, **suicidal ideation**, thirst
CV: Chest pain, decreased high-density lipoproteins, edema, elevated cholesterol or triglyceride levels, **MI**, **thromboembolism**
EENT: Abnormal or blurred vision, blepharitis, conjunctivitis, corneal epithelial abnormality, decreased night vision, deafness, dry eyes or mouth, earache, epistaxis, eye pain, gingival bleeding, gingivitis, increased saliva, photophobia, sinusitis, stomatitis, taste perversion, tinnitus, ulcerative stomatitis
ENDO: Hot flashes, hyperglycemia
GI: Anorexia, abdominal pain, diarrhea, elevated liver enzymes, **hepatitis**, **hepatotoxicity**, nausea, **pancreatitis**
GU: Vulvovaginitis
HEME: Capillary leak syndrome, **hemorrhage**, **increased bleeding time**
MS: Arthralgia, arthrosis, back pain, hyperostosis, myalgia, myopathy
SKIN: Abnormal skin or hair texture, alopecia, bullous eruption, cold or clammy skin, dermatitis, diaphoresis, dry or peeling skin, erythematous rash, **exfoliative dermatitis**, erythroderma, flushing, fragility or thinning of skin, loss of eyelashes or eyebrows, photosensitivity, pruritus, purpura, pyogenic granuloma, rash, scaling, seborrhea, skin fissure or ulceration
Other: Hypervitaminosis A, increased appetite

Nursing Considerations

WARNING Don't give acitretin to a pregnant woman, a woman contemplating pregnancy, or a woman who may not use reliable contraception during drug therapy and for at least 3 years afterward because acitretin causes major fetal abnormalities.

- Make sure patient has had two negative urine or serum pregnancy tests with a sensitivity of at least 25 mIU/ml before receiving acitretin. First test should be obtained when decision is made to use acitretin and second test during first 5 days of the menstrual period just before acitretin therapy starts. For patients with amenorrhea, second test should be done at least 11 days after the last act of unprotected sexual intercourse (which means without using two effective forms of contraception simultaneously).

- Check to make sure female patient of childbearing age has signed the patient agreement and informed consent form before starting acitretin therapy.
- Obtain a lipid profile, as ordered, before acitretin therapy starts and every 1 to 2 weeks for up to 8 weeks or until lipid effects are known. In high-risk patients, such as those with diabetes, obesity, or a history of alcohol abuse and those taking acitretin long-term, check lipid profile periodically throughout therapy.
- Monitor liver enzymes, as ordered. If hepatotoxicity is suspected, expect to stop drug and investigate cause.
- Monitor patient closely for capillary leak syndrome demonstrated by localized or generalized edema, weight gain, fever, hypotension, and myalgias. If present, notify prescriber and expect to obtain laboratory studies for evidence of neutrophilia, hypoalbuminemia, and an elevated hematocrit. If confirmed, discontinue acitretin therapy, as ordered.
- Prepare patient for periodic bone radiography if she takes acitretin long term or she develops a skeletal disorder because ossification abnormalities can occur, especially of the vertebral column, knees, and ankles.
- Monitor patient's eyes for abnormalities throughout therapy. Expect patient to stop drug and have an ophthalmologic examination if eye abnormalities occur.
- Monitor patient for evidence of increased intracranial pressure, such as papilledema, headache, nausea, vomiting, and visual disturbances. If papilledema occurs, stop drug therapy immediately and obtain a neurologic evaluation, as ordered. Patient should never receive a tetracycline while taking acitretin because combined use can increase intracranial pressure.
- Assess patient for suicidal ideation because depression and other psychiatric symptoms, including thoughts of self-harm, may occur with acitretin use. Expect drug to be discontinued if psychiatric symptoms develop.
- Be aware that significantly lower doses of phototherapy are needed during acitretin therapy because drug increases the risk of erythema. If patient develops serious skin reactions, notify prescriber and expect acitretin therapy to be discontinued.

PATIENT TEACHING

WARNING Warn women of childbearing age that acitretin causes major fetal abnormalities.

- Inform woman of childbearing age that she must have a pregnancy test before acitretin therapy starts, every month during acitretin therapy, and every 3 months for 3 years after therapy stops.
- Emphasize to woman of childbearing age that she must use two effective forms of contraception simultaneously unless she has chosen absolute abstinence or has had a hysterectomy. This must begin at least 1 month before acitretin therapy starts and continue throughout therapy and for at least 3 years after therapy ends.
- Caution women taking oral contraceptives that some prescribed and OTC drugs, including herbal supplements such as St. John's wort, may interfere with oral contraceptives. Urge her to tell prescriber about all drugs she takes.
- Alert female patient of childbearing age that any method of birth control can fail, including tubal ligation, and that microdose progestin "minipill" preparations are not recommended to be taken with acitretin. Tell her to seek immediate medical care on how to obtain emergency contraception if sexual intercourse occurs without using 2 effective forms of contraception simultaneously.
- Caution patient not to consume alcohol or products that contain alcohol during acitretin therapy and for 2 months after therapy ends.
- Inform patient that regular blood tests will be needed to monitor liver function. Tell him to notify prescriber if any of the following develops: nausea and vomiting, loss of appetite, dark urine, or whites of eyes or skin turns yellow.
- Warn patient, male or female of any age, not to donate blood during acitretin therapy and for at least 3 years after it ends.

- Review acitretin medication guide with patient, and answer the patient's questions.
- Inform patient that psoriasis may worsen during initial treatment and that full effects of drug may not be seen for up to 3 months.
- Caution patient to avoid hazardous activities until drug's CNS and ophthalmic effects are known.
- Inform patient that tolerance to contact lenses may decrease during acitretin therapy and for a period of time after treatment ends.
- Advise patient not to take more than the minimum recommended daily allowance of vitamin A during acitretin therapy because of the risk of vitamin A toxicity.
- Caution patient not to use sun lamps and to avoid excessive exposure to sunlight because the effects of UV light are enhanced by retinoids such as acitretin.
- Tell patient to notify prescriber of any new skin changes that become serious or prolonged, as acitretin therapy may need to be discontinued, if present.

aclidinium bromide

Tudorza Pressair

Class and Category

Pharmacologic class: Anticholinergic
Therapeutic class: Bronchodilator
Pregnancy category: C

Indications and Dosages

➤ *To provide long-term maintenance treatment of bronchospasm associated with chronic obstructive pulmonary disease (COPD), including chronic bronchitis and emphysema*

INHALATION AEROSOL

Adults. 1 inhalation (400 mcg) twice daily.

Mechanism of Action

Inhibits muscarinic receptor, M3, in smooth muscle in the airways to produce bronchodilation.

Contraindications

Hypersensitivity to aclidinium or its components, severe hypersensitivity to milk proteins

Interactions

DRUGS

other anticholinergics: Potential additive effect

Adverse Reactions

CNS: Dysphonia, headache
CV: Cardiac failure (rare), cardio-respiratory arrest (rare), first degree AV block, tachycardia
EENT: Blurred vision, dry mouth, nasopharyngitis, rhinitis, sinusitis, stomatitis, worsening of glaucoma
ENDO: Hyperglycemia
GI: Diarrhea, nausea, vomiting
GU: Worsening of urinary retention
RESP: Cough, **paradoxical bronchospasm**
SKIN: Pruritus, rash, urticaria
Other: Anaphylaxis, angioedema, immediate hypersensitivity reaction

Nursing Considerations

- Use aclidinium with extreme caution in patients with known hypersensitivity reactions to atropine or severe hypersensitivity to milk proteins as aclidinium may produce a similiar reaction.
- Use aclidinium cautiously in patients with narrow-angle glaucoma or urinary retention because drug can make these conditions worse.

WARNING Monitor patient closely, especially after first dose, for signs and symptoms of hypersensitivity such as anaphylaxis, angioedema, bronchospasms, pruritus, rash, shortness of breath and urticaria because aclidinium may cause an immediate hypersensitivity reaction. Be prepared to treat such a reaction, as ordered and expect drug to be discontinued.

PATIENT TEACHING

- Caution patient that aclidinium is not intended to be used as a rescue inhaler for the treatment of acute episodes of bronchospasms. Instruct patient that if bronchospasms occur while using aclidinium, he or she should stop using aclidinium and immediately notify the prescriber.
- Teach patient how to get the inhaler ready by pressing the green button all the way down and then releasing it. Next, patient should check the control window on the inhaler to make sure it has turned green. If it is still red, tell patient to press the green button again. Then instruct how to use the inhaler by first breathing

out completely, then putting lips tightly around the mouthpiece and breathing in quickly but deeply through the mouth. Patient should hear a click but should keep breathing in to be sure the full dose is received. After removing mouthpiece, patient should check the control window again to be sure it has now turned to red.
- Inform patient that some people may taste the medicine during their inhalation but that an extra dose should not be taken if the patient is not able to taste the medication
- Emphasize importance of not allowing the powder to get into eyes when using the inhaler because this may cause blurring of vision and pupil dilation.

WARNING Review signs and symptoms of an allergic reaction to drug. Emphasize need to stop taking drug and the importance of seeking immediate emergency care.
- Advise patient with narrow-angle glaucoma to notify prescriber if eye pain or discomfort, blurred vision, visual halos or colored images in association with red eyes from conjunctival congestion and corneal edema occur at any time with aclidinium therapy and to stop using the drug until seen by prescriber.

acyclovir

Sitavig, Zovirax

acyclovir sodium

Zovirax I.V.

Class and Category

Pharmacologic class: Nucleoside analogue
Therapeutic class: Antiretroviral
Pregnancy category: B

Indications and Dosages

➤ *To treat initial episodes of herpes genitalis*

CAPSULES, ORAL SUSPENSION, TABLETS

Adults. 200 mg every 4 hr, 5 times daily for 10 days.

OINTMENT 5%

Adults. Applied to completely cover all lesions (about ½-inch ribbon of ointment per 4 square inches of surface area) every 3 hr, 6 times daily for 7 days.

➤ *To treat severe initial episodes of herpes genitalis*

I.V. INFUSION

Adults and adolescents. 5 mg/kg infused at a constant rate over 1 hr, every 8 hr for 5 days.

➤ *To suppress unusually frequent recurrent episodes of herpes genitalis (6 or more episodes per year)*

CAPSULES, ORAL SUSPENSION, TABLETS

Adults. 200 mg three times daily, increased if breakthrough occurs up to 200 mg, 5 times daily. Alternatively, 400 mg twice daily.

➤ *To treat recurrent episodes of herpes genitalis intermittently*

CAPSULES, ORAL SUSPENSION, TABLETS

Adults. 200 mg every 4 hr, 5 times daily for 5 days.

➤ *To treat recurrent herpes labialis in immunocompetent patients*

BUCCAL TABLETS (SITAVIG)

Adults. 50 mg as a single dose to the upper gum region applied within 1 hr after onset of prodromal symptoms and before the appearance of any signs of herpes labialis.

CREAM 5%

Adults and adolescents. Applied 5 times daily for 4 days and initiated as soon as possible following onset of signs and symptoms.

➤ *To treat non-life-threatening mucocutaneous* Herpes simplex *virus infections in immunocompromised patients*

OINTMENT 5%

Adults. Applied to completely cover all lesions (about ½-inch ribbon of ointment per 4 square inches of surface area) every 3 hr, 6 times daily for 7 days.

➤ *To treat cutaneous and mucosal herpes simplex (HSV-1 and HSV-2) infections in immunocompromised patients*

I.V. INFUSION

Adults and adolescents. 5 mg/kg infused at a constant rate over 1 hr, every 8 hr for 7 days.
Children. 10 mg/kg infused at a constant rate over 1 hr, every 8 hr for 7 days.

➤ *To treat herpes simplex encephalitis*

I.V. INFUSION

Adults and adolescents. 10 mg/kg infused at a constant rate over 1 hr, every 8 hr for 10 days.
Children 3 months to 12 years. 20 mg/kg infused at a constant rate over 1 hr, every 8 hr for 10 days.

➤ *To treat neonatal herpes simplex virus infections*

I.V. INFUSION

Neonates birth to 3 months. 10 mg/kg infused at a constant rate over 1 hr, every 8 hr for 10 days.

➤ *To treat herpes zoster*

CAPSULES, ORAL SUSPENSION, TABLETS

Adults. 800 mg every 4 hr, 5 times daily for 7 to 10 days with treatment initiated within 72 hr of onset of lesions.

➤ *To treat* Varicella zoster *infections*

CAPSULES, ORAL SUSPENSION, TABLETS

Adults. 20 mg/kg (not to exceed 800 mg) 4 times daily for 5 days initiated within 24 hr of the appearance of rash.

➤ *To treat* Varicella zoster *infections in immunocompromised patients*

I.V. INFUSION

Adults and adolescents. 10 mg/kg infused at a constant rate over 1 hr, every 8 hr for 7 days.

Children. 20 mg/kg infused at a constant rate over 1 hr, every 8 hr for 7 days.

DOSAGE ADJUSTMENT

For patients with renal impairment who have genital herpes or *Herpes zoster* infections, oral dosage reduced or dosage interval increased as follows: if dosage is normally 200 mg every 4 hr 5 times daily and creatinine clearance is less than 10 ml/min, dosage interval increased to every 12 hr; if dosage is normally 400 mg every 12 hr and creatinine clearance is less than 10 ml/min, dosage reduced to 200 mg every 12 hr; if dosage is normally 800 mg every 4 hr and creatinine clearance is 10 to 25 ml/min, dosage interval increased to every 8 hr, and if creatinine clearance is less than 10 ml/min, dosage interval increased to every 12 hr. For patients receiving intravenous dosing, dosage reduced or dosage interval increased as follows: if creatinine clearance is 25 to 50 ml/min, dosage interval increased to every 12 hr; if creatinine clearance is 10 to 25 ml/min, dosage interval increased to every 24 hr; if creatinine clearance is 0 to 10 ml/min, dosage is reduced by 50% and dosage interval increased to every 24 hr. For patients receiving hemodialysis, an additional dose is given after each dialysis.

Mechanism of Action

Several actions (inhibition of DNA polymerase, premature termination of DNA synthesis and thymidine kinase specificity) combine to inhibit herpes virus replication.

Contraindications

Hypersensitivity to acyclovir or valacyclovir or any of their components

Interactions

DRUGS

cimetidine, probenecid: Possibly increased acyclovir plasma concentrations

mycophenolate mofetil: Increased plasma concentration of both drugs

Adverse Reactions

CNS: Agitation, asthenia, ataxia, **coma**, confusion, dizziness, **encephalopathy**, fever, hallucinations, headache, malaise, paresthesia, psychotic symptoms, **seizures**, somnolence, tremor

CV: Peripheral edema

EENT: Visual abnormalities

GI: Diarrhea, elevated liver enzymes, gastrointestinal distress, **hepatitis**, hyperbilirubinemia, jaundice, nausea, vomiting

GU: **Acute renal failure**, elevated blood creatinine and blood urea nitrogen, hematuria, **hemolytic uremic syndrome**, renal pain

HEME: Anemia, **leukopenia**, lymphadenopathy, **thrombocytopenia**, **thrombotic thrombocytopenic purpura**

MS: Myalgia

RESP: Dyspnea

SKIN: Alopecia, contact dermatitis (topical), eczema (topical), **erythema multiforme**, photosensitivity, pruritus, rash, **Stevens–Johnson syndrome**, **toxic epidermal necrolysis**, urticaria

Other: **Anaphylaxis**, **angioedema**, generalized pain

Nursing Considerations

- Know that acyclovir therapy should be initiated as soon as possible after signs and symptoms appear.
- Use caution when administering acyclovir to patients with dehydration or preexisting renal disease or who are receiving other nephrotoxic drugs, because of increased risk of renal impairment. Also use cautiously in patients with underlying neurologic disorders as well as electrolyte abnormalities, hepatic dysfunction, or significant hypoxia because, although

uncommon, encephalopathic changes have occurred with acyclovir administration.

- Ensure that patient receiving acyclovir is adequately hydrated before drug is given, to decrease risk of renal impairment.
- Prepare intravenous infusion by first dissolving the contents of a 10-ml vial containing 500 mg of acyclovir in 10 ml of sterile water for injection. The result is a concentration of 50 mg acyclovir per each milliliter. Shake the vial well to ensure that drug has been dissolved. Use reconstituted solution within 12 hr. Know that if refrigerated, a precipitate may form but will redissolve at room temperature.
- Remove reconstituted solution from vial and add to any appropriate intravenous solution at a volume to administer over 1 hr. Once diluted for administration, each dose should be used within 24 hr.
- Administer intravenous form of acyclovir only as an infusion over 1 hr to reduce risk of renal tubular damage. Never administer it intramuscularly, subcutaneously, or as an I.V. bolus or rapid injection.

WARNING Know that hemolytic uremic syndrome and thrombotic thrombocytopenic purpura have occurred in immunocompromised patients receiving acyclovir therapy and have resulted in death. Report any hematologic or renal dysfunction signs and symptoms to prescriber immediately.

PATIENT TEACHING

- Inform patient that acyclovir does not cure herpes infections but helps to manage the signs and symptoms.
- Tell patient prescribed buccal tablets that it is given as a single dose and should be placed onto the upper gum within 1 hr after the onset of prodromal symptoms and before the appearance of any signs of a cold sore. The tablet should not be chewed, crushed, sucked, or swallowed whole.
- Explain to patient receiving topical form of acyclovir how to apply the cream or ointment ordered, stressing need to completely cover entire lesion area and to apply only to affected areas. Tell patient to use a finger cot or rubber glove to apply to prevent transferring infection to other parts of his body or to other people. Tell patient to start therapy as early as possible following appearance of signs and symptoms. Instruct patient not to apply topical form to the inside of his mouth or nose or to put in his eyes.
- Instruct patient prescribed oral suspension form to use an accurate measuring device when measuring dosage.
- Stress importance of stopping drug therapy and seeking immediate medical attention if any signs and symptoms of an allergic reaction occur.
- Instruct patient to seek medical attention if his symptoms become severe or he experiences troublesome adverse reactions.
- Tell women of childbearing age to notify prescriber if pregnancy occurs or is suspected.
- Stress importance of maintaining adequate hydration throughout acyclovir therapy to reduce risk of kidney damage.
- Advise patient with genital herpes to avoid contact, including intercourse, when lesions and/or symptoms are present, to avoid infecting partner.
- Instruct patient who requires acyclovir therapy to manage recurrent genital herpes to initiate therapy at the first sign or symptom of an episode.

adalimumab

Humira

adalimumab-adbm

Cyltezo

adalimumab-adaz

Hyrimoz

adalimumab-atto

Amjevita

Class and Category

Pharmacologic class: Monoclonal antibody
Therapeutic class: Tumor necrosis factor (TNF) blocker
Pregnancy category: Not classified

Indications and Dosages

➤ *To reduce signs and symptoms, induce major clinical response, inhibit progression of structural damage, and improve physical function in patients with moderately to severely active rheumatoid arthritis; to reduce signs and symptoms, inhibit progression of structural damage, and improve physical function in patients with psoriatic arthritis; to reduce signs and symptoms in patients with active ankylosing spondylitis*

SUBCUTANEOUS INJECTION (AMJEVITA, CYLTEZO, HUMIRA, HYRIMOZ)
Adults. 40 mg every other wk.
DOSAGE ADJUSTMENT Dosage may be adjusted to 40 mg every wk, as needed and prescribed, for patients with rheumatoid arthritis not taking methotrexate.

➤ *To reduce signs and symptoms and induce and maintain clinical remission in patients with moderately to severely active Crohn's disease who have had an inadequate response to conventional therapy or who have stopped responding to or have become intolerant of infliximab*

SUBCUTANEOUS INJECTION (AMJEVITA, CYLTEZO, HUMIRA, HYRIMOZ)
Adults. *Initial:* 40 mg four times daily for 1 day or 40 mg twice daily for 2 consecutive days, followed by 80 mg on day 15. *Maintenance:* 40 mg every other wk starting on day 29.

➤ *To reduce signs and symptoms and induce and maintain clinical remission in children with moderately to severely active Crohn's disease who have had an inadequate response to conventional therapy or who have had an inadequate response to corticosteroids or immunomodulators such as azathioprine, 6-mercaptopurine, or methotrexate*

SUBCUTANEOUS INJECTION (HUMIRA)
Children age 6 and over who weigh 40 kg (88 lb) or more. *Initial:* 40 mg four times daily on day 1 or 40 mg twice daily for 2 days, followed by 80 mg on day 15 given in 2 divided doses of 40 mg each. *Maintenance:* 40 mg every other wk starting on day 29.
Children age 6 and over who weigh less than 40 kg (88 lb) but at least 17 kg (37 lb). *Initial:* 40 mg twice daily on day 1, followed by 40 mg on day 15. *Maintenance:* 20 mg every other wk starting on day 29.

➤ *To reduce signs and symptoms of moderately to severely active polyarticular juvenile idiopathic arthritis*

SUBCUTANEOUS INJECTION (HUMIRA)
Children age 2 and over who weigh 30 kg (66 lb) or more. 40 mg every other wk.
Children age 2 and over who weigh less than 30 kg (66 lb) but at least 15 kg (33 lb). 20 mg every other wk.
Children age 2 and over who weigh less than 15 kg (33 lb) but at least 10 kg (22 lb). 10 mg every other wk.

SUBCUTANEOUS INJECTION (AMJEVITA)
Children age 4 and over who weigh 30 kg (66 lb) or more. 40 mg every other wk.
Children age 4 and over who weigh less than 30 kg (66 lb) but at least 15 kg (33 lb). 20 mg every other wk.

SUBCUTANEOUS INJECTION (CYLTEZO, HYRIMOZ)
Children age 4 and over who weigh 30 kg (66 lb) or more. 40 mg every other wk.

➤ *To treat moderate to severe chronic plaque psoriasis in patients who are candidates for systemic therapy or phototherapy, and when other systemic therapies are less appropriate*

SUBCUTANEOUS INJECTION (AMJEVITA, HUMIRA, HYRIMOZ)
Adults. *Initial:* 80 mg followed 1 wk later with 40 mg. *Maintenance:* 40 mg every other wk.

➤ *To induce and sustain a remission in patients with moderate to severe active ulcerative colitis who have had an inadequate response to immunosuppressants such as azathioprine, corticosteroids, or 6-mercaptopurine*

SUBCUTANEOUS INJECTION (AMJEVITA, CYLTEZO, HUMIRA, HYRIMOZ)
Adults. *Initial:* 160 mg given as four 40-mg injections on day 1 or given as two 40-mg injections on day 1 and repeated on day 2, followed by 80 mg on day 15 and 40 mg on day 29. *Maintenance:* 40 mg every other wk.

➤ *To treat moderate to severe hidradenitis suppurativa*

SUBCUTANEOUS INJECTION (HUMIRA)
Adults and adolescents age 12 and over weighing 60 kg (132 lb) or more. *Initial:* 40 mg four times daily for 1 day or 40 mg twice daily for 2 consecutive days, followed by 80 mg on day 15. *Maintenance:* 40 mg weekly starting on day 29.
Adolescents age 12 and over weighing 30 kg (66 lb) to 60 kg (132 lb). *Initial:* 80 mg on day 1 followed by 40 mg on day 8.

Maintenance: 40 mg every other wk starting on day 22 from initial dose.

➤ *To treat noninfectious intermediate, posterior and panuveitis*

SUBCUTANEOUS INJECTION (HUMIRA)

Adults. *Initial:* 80 mg followed 1 wk later with 40 mg. *Maintenance:* 40 mg every other wk.

Children age 2 and over weighing 30 kg (66 lb) or more. 40 mg every other wk.

Children age 2 and over weighing less than 30 kg (66 lb) but at least 15 kg (33 lb). 20 mg every other wk.

Children age 2 and over weighing less than 15 kg (33 lb) but at least 10 kg (22 lb). 10 mg every other wk.

Mechanism of Action

Binds to tumor necrosis factor (TNF) to block interaction with p55 and p75 cell-surface TNF receptors, and lyses surface TNF-expressing cells in the presence of complement. TNF may be a major component of rheumatoid arthritis inflammation and joint destruction. Reduced TNF level in synovial fluid improves signs and symptoms and prevents further structural damage in rheumatoid arthritis. It also causes a decrease in levels of acute phase reactants of inflammation such as C-reactive protein, which may explain its useful in alleviating signs and symptoms in other inflammatory disease processes.

Contraindications

Active infection, hypersensitivity to adalimumab or its components

Interactions

DRUGS

abatacept, anakinra, rituximab: Possibly increased risk of serious infection and neutropenia in patients with rheumatoid arthritis

CYP450 substrates with narrow therapeutic index such as cyclosporine, theophylline, warfarin: Possibly altered effectiveness of these drugs

live vaccines: Increased risk of adverse vaccine effects

Adverse Reactions

CNS: Confusion, **CVA**, demyelinating disorders such as **Guillain–Barré syndrome**, or multiple sclerosis, fever, headache, **hypertensive encephalopathy**, paresthesia, **subdural hematoma**, syncope, tremor

CV: Arrhythmias, **atrial fibrillation**, **cardiac arrest**, chest pain, **congestive heart failure**, coronary artery disease, **deep vein thrombosis**, hypercholesterolemia, hyperlipidemia, hypertension, **MI**, palpitations, **pericardial effusion**, **pericarditis**, peripheral edema, **systemic vasculitis**, tachycardia

EENT: Cataract, optic neuritis, sinusitis

ENDO: Ketosis, parathyroid disorder

GI: Abdominal pain, cholecystitis, cholelithiasis, diverticulitis, elevated alkaline phosphatase level, elevated liver enzymes, esophagitis, gastroenteritis, **gastrointestinal hemorrhage**, **hepatic failure or necrosis**, **hepatitis**, **large bowel perforation**, nausea, **pancreatitis**, vomiting

GU: Hematuria, paraproteinemia, **pyelonephritis**, UTI

HEME: Agranulocytosis, **aplastic anemia**, **granulocytopenia**, **leukopenia**, lymphocytosis, **pancytopenia**, polycythemia, **thrombocytopenia**

MS: Arthritis (including pyogenic or septic arthritis); back, extremity, pelvic, or thorax pain; bone disorder, fracture, or necrosis; muscle spasms; myasthenia; prosthetic infections; synovitis

RESP: Asthma, bronchitis, **bronchospasm**, decreased pulmonary function, dyspnea, pleural effusion, pneumonia, **pulmonary embolism**, **pulmonary fibrosis** or tuberculosis, upper respiratory tract infection

SKIN: Alopecia, cellulitis, cutaneous vasculitis, erysipelas (red skin), **erythema multiforme**, herpes zoster, **lichenoid reaction**, **Merkel cell carcinoma**, new or worsening psoriasis, rash, **Stevens–Johnson syndrome**, urticaria

Other: Anaphylaxis; **angioedema**; antibody formation against adalimumab; bacterial, mycobacterial, fungal, parasitic, viral, and other opportunistic infections; benign or unspecified cysts or polyps; dehydration; flare-up of disease process; flu-like symptoms; healing abnormalities; injection-site erythema, hemorrhage, itching, pain, or swelling; lupus-like symptoms; **lymphomas and other malignancies such as breast, colon, lung,**

melanoma, and prostate; postsurgical infection; new onset or reactivation of tuberculosis; sarcoidosis; **sepsis**

Nursing Considerations

- Use adalimumab cautiously in patients with recurrent infection or increased risk of infection and in patients who live in regions where tuberculosis and certain mycoses, such as *Histoplasma*, are endemic. Be aware that *Legionella* and *Listeria,* two bacterial infections, also have occurred with tumor necrosis factor–alpha blockers such as adalimumab. Monitor patient closely because infections associated with tumor necrosis factor–alpha blocker therapy may involve multiple organ systems and become life-threatening.

WARNING Assess patient for signs and symptoms of an active infection before beginning adalimumab therapy. If patient has evidence of an active infection when drug is prescribed, therapy shouldn't start until the infection has been treated. Monitor all patients for infection during therapy, especially those receiving concomitant immunosuppressants. If a serious infection develops, the drug should be stopped.

- Ensure that children with juvenile idiopathic arthritis are up to date with current immunization guidelines prior to adalimumab therapy being started. However, know that they may receive vaccinations, except for live vaccines, while taking adalimumab, if needed. Be aware that the safety of administering live or live-attenuated vaccines in infants exposed to drug in utero is unknown.
- Use cautiously in a patient with a preexisting or recent onset of a central or peripheral nervous system demyelinating disorder such as multiple sclerosis, optic neuritis, or Guillain–Barré because, although rare, new onset or exacerbation of demyelinating disorders have occurred with adalimumab therapy. If this occurs, know that drug should be discontinued.
- Make sure patient has a tuberculin skin test before therapy starts. If skin test is positive, treatment of latent tuberculosis will start before adalimumab, as prescribed. Also, ensure that patient previously treated for tuberculosis, including prophylactic treatment, has a tuberculin skin test periodically throughout therapy, as adalimumab may induce new onset or reactivate tuberculosis.
- Review patient's medical and medication history and discuss with prescriber prior to starting adalimumab.
- Be aware that the needle cover of the syringe contains dry rubber. Don't handle if allergic to latex.
- Know that adalimumab must be refrigerated but may be left at room temperature with cap or cover on for about 15 to 30 minutes before injecting. Inject daily doses in separate sites in the abdomen or thigh. Rotate injection sites and do not give injections into an area where the skin is bruised, hard, red, or tender.
- Activate the protection device on needles of prefilled syringes delivered to institutions by holding the syringe in one hand and, with the other hand, sliding outer protective shield over exposed needle until it locks into place.
- Know that adalimumab may come in a single-use glass vial containing 40 mg (0.8 ml) of adalimumab referred to as an "institutional use vial" because the drug should only be given in a medical institution. Withdraw only one dose when using the "institutional use vial" and administer promptly. Since the vial does not contain preservatives, discard any unused portions.

WARNING Stop adalimumab immediately and tell prescriber if patient has an allergic reaction. Expect to provide supportive care.

- Watch closely for evidence of congestive heart failure (sudden, unexplained weight gain; dyspnea; crackles; anxiety), and notify prescriber if they occur.
- Monitor patient's CBC, as ordered, because adalimumab may have adverse hematologic effects. Notify prescriber about persistent fever, bruising, bleeding, or pallor.
- Be aware that, although rare, malignancies, especially lymphomas and leukemias, have occurred in patients receiving TNF blockers such as adalimumab. These malignancies have also occurred in children. Patients with rheumatoid arthritis, especially those with very active disease, and patients with Crohn's disease, ankylosing spondylitis,

psoriatic arthritis, or plaque psoriasis are at greatest risk. Monitor patients closely.

PATIENT TEACHING

- Inform patient that the first injection of adalimumab must take place with a healthcare professional present.
- Teach patient or caregiver how to give adalimumab as a subcutaneous injection at home, if applicable. Emphasize importance of injecting the full amount in the syringe to obtain the correct dose.
- Advise patient that the needle cover contains rubber and can cause a latex-induced allergic reaction if touched with bare hands.
- Provide patient or caregiver with a puncture-resistant container for disposal of needles and syringes at home.
- Instruct patient or caregiver to rotate injection sites in the abdomen and thigh and to avoid injecting in any area that's bruised, hard, red, or tender.
- Inform patient that prefilled syringes must be refrigerated (not frozen) but may be left at room temperature for 15 to 30 minutes before injecting to decrease injection discomfort. Keep the cap or cover on while allowing it to reach room temperature. Also keep syringe protected from light and stored in the original container.
- Urge patient to check expiration dates and not to use outdated drug. Also tell patient not to use a prefilled syringe if the liquid is cloudy, discolored, or has flakes or particles in it.
- Review signs and symptoms of an allergic reaction (difficulty breathing, rash, swollen face), and tell patient to seek emergency care immediately if these occur.
- Inform patient that injection-site reactions (such as bruising itching, rash, redness, and swelling) may occur but are usually mild and transient. Instruct him to apply a towel soaked with cold water on the injection site if it hurts or remains swollen. If reaction does not disappear or seems to worsen, tell patient to call prescriber immediately.
- Inform patient that tuberculosis may occur during adalimumab therapy. Instruct him to report persistent cough, wasting or weight loss, and low-grade fever to prescriber.
- Teach patient how to recognize evidence of infection and bleeding disorders and to tell prescriber if they occur; drug may need to be stopped. Advise patient to avoid people with infections and to have all prescribed laboratory tests.
- Inform patient that the risk of certain kinds of cancer, especially lymphomas, is higher in patients taking adalimumab but still rare. Emphasize the importance of follow-up visits and reporting an unusual or sudden onset of signs or symptoms.
- Caution patient against receiving live-virus vaccines while taking adalimumab because doing so may adversely affect the immune system.
- Inform patient that blood samples may be needed periodically, but especially around week 24 of therapy, to check for autoantibody development. Explain that adalimumab therapy will have to be stopped if it's detected.
- Instruct patient to report lupus-like signs and symptoms that, although rare, may occur during therapy, such as chest pain that doesn't go away, joint pain, a rash on arms or cheeks that's sensitive to the sun, or shortness of breath. Explain that drug may be stopped if these occur.
- Advise patient to inform all healthcare providers about adalimumab use and to inform prescriber about any OTC medications being taken, including herbal remedies and mineral and vitamin supplements.
- Instruct women of childbearing age to notify prescriber immediately if pregnancy is suspected or known, as adalimumab may affect the immune response of an uteroexposed newborn or infant. Also, emphasize the importance of telling pediatrician if adalimumab was taken any time during pregnancy, prior to having infant receive any vaccines.
- Encourage mother wishing to breastfeed infant to discuss with prescriber before doing so.

adefovir dipivoxil

Hepsera

Class and Category

Pharmacologic class: Nucleotide analogue
Therapeutic class: Antiviral
Pregnancy category: C

Indications and Dosages

➤ *To treat chronic hepatitis B in patients with evidence of active viral replication and either evidence of persistent elevations in serum aminotransferases (ALT or AST) or histologically active disease*

TABLETS

Adults and children age 12 and over. 10 mg once daily.

DOSAGE ADJUSTMENT For patients with a creatinine clearance between 30 and 49 ml/min, dosage interval changed to every 48 hr. For patients with a creatinine clearance between 10 and 29 ml/min, dosage interval changed to 72 hr. For patients receiving hemodialysis, dosage interval changed to every 7 days following dialysis.

Mechanism of Action

Inhibits hepatitis B virus (HBV) by competing with the natural substrate deoxyadenosine triphosphate and by causing DNA chain termination after its incorporation into viral DNA, which prevents replication.

Contraindications

Hypersensitivity to adefovir dipivoxil or its components

Interactions

DRUGS

drugs that are excreted renally or known to affect renal function, such as *aminoglycosides, cyclosporine, NSAIDs, tacrolimus, and vancomycin:* Possibly increased serum concentrations of adefovir or these drugs or both, increasing risk of adverse reactions

Adverse Reactions

CNS: Asthenia, headache
GI: Abdominal pain, diarrhea, dyspepsia, flatulence, nausea, **pancreatitis**, **severe acute exacerbations of hepatitis**, **severe hepatomegaly with steatosis**, vomiting
GU: Abnormal renal function, elevated creatinine level, **Fanconi syndrome**, **nephrotoxicity**, **proximal renal tubulopathy**, **renal failure**
MS: Bone pain, myopathy, osteomalacia
SKIN: Pruritus, rash
Other: **HIV resistance**, hypophosphatemia, **lactic acidosis**

Nursing Considerations

- Check to be sure HIV antibody testing has been done prior to starting adefovir therapy because treatment with anti-hepatitis B therapies, such as adefovir, may cause an emergence of HIV resistance.
- Use with extreme caution in patients with renal dysfunction. Check to ensure that patient's creatinine clearance is known before adefovir therapy begins and then rechecked periodically throughout therapy, because adefovir may cause a delayed nephrotoxicity that may require dosage interval to be lengthened or drug discontinued. Know that patients at higher risk include those having underlying renal dysfunction and patients taking concomitant nephrotoxic agents such as aminoglycosides, cyclosporine, NSAIDs, tacrolimus, and vancomycin.
- Use caution when administering adefovir to patient with liver dysfunction or known risk factors for liver disease.

WARNING Know that lactic acidosis and severe hepatomegaly with steatosis have occurred with adefovir therapy and death has occurred in some patients. Risk factors include presence of obesity, prolonged nucleoside exposure, and being a woman. However, know that lactic acidosis and severe hepatomegaly with steatosis have also occurred in patients with no known risk factors. Expect drug to be discontinued in any patient who develops clinical or laboratory findings suggestive of lactic acidosis or pronounced hepatotoxicity, even in the absence of marked transaminase elevations.

- Monitor patient throughout treatment for evidence of loss of therapeutic response. Indicators include increasing levels of HBV DNA over time after an initial decline below assay limit, progression of clinical signs or symptoms of hepatic disease and/or worsening of hepatic necroinflammatory findings, or return of persistently elevated ALT levels. These findings may require drug to be discontinued.
- Be aware that immune reconstitution syndrome has occurred in patients treated with combination antiretroviral therapy,

including adefovir. The inflammatory response predisposes susceptible patients to opportunistic infections such as cytomegalovirus infection, *Mycobacterium avium* infection, *Pneumocystis jiroveci* pneumonia, or tuberculosis. Autoimmune disorders such as Graves' disease, Guillain–Barré syndrome, or polymyositis have also occurred. Report sudden or unusual adverse reactions to prescriber.

- Expect patient to be closely monitored for at least several months after adefovir has been discontinued, because exacerbation of hepatitis may occur, some cases of which have been severe.

PATIENT TEACHING

- Instruct patient to take adefovir once daily. If he misses a dose, tell him to take it as soon as he remembers but not to double the next dose or take more than the prescribed dose.
- Advise patient that treatment with adefovir does not reduce the risk of transmission of HBV to others.
- Tell patient to report any new or worsening symptoms to prescriber immediately, because emergence of resistant hepatitis B virus may occur or disease may worsen during treatment.
- Instruct patient with hepatitis B on the importance of testing for HIV before therapy begins and then periodically throughout therapy to avoid development of resistance to HIV treatment.
- Warn patient with hepatitis B that acute severe exacerbations of hepatitis B may occur following discontinuation of adefovir. He should not discontinue drug without prescriber knowledge. Tell patient to report any reappearance of signs and symptoms of hepatitis B.
- Instruct mother not to breastfeed while she is receiving adefovir therapy, as drug is present in human milk.
- Tell women of childbearing age to report a known or suspected pregnancy.

WARNING Alert patient that severe conditions may develop while taking adefovir. Encourage him to stop taking drug and seek medical attention immediately if he experiences any persistent, severe, or unusual symptoms; especially abdominal pain, change in urine characteristics or urination pattern, loss of appetite, pale stools, muscle pain, or yellowing of the eyes.

adenosine

Adenocard, Adenoscan

Class and Category

Pharmacologic class: Nuceloside
Therapeutic class: Class V antiarrhythmic, diagnostic aid
Pregnancy category: C

Indications and Dosages

➤ *To convert paroxysmal supraventricular tachycardia (PSVT) to normal sinus rhythm*

I.V. INJECTION (ADENOCARD)

Adults and children weighing 50 kg (110 lb) or more. *Initial:* 6 mg by rapid peripheral I.V. bolus over 1 to 2 sec. If PSVT continues after 1 to 2 min, 12 mg given as rapid bolus and repeated in 1 to 2 min, if needed. *Maximum:* 12 mg as a single dose.

Children weighing less than 50 kg. *Initial:* 0.05 to 0.1 mg/kg by rapid central or peripheral I.V. bolus followed by a saline flush. If PSVT continues after 1 to 2 min, additional bolus injections are given, incrementally increasing dose by 0.05 to 0.1 mg/kg. Each bolus followed with a saline flush. Administration continued until PSVT converts to normal sinus rhythm or until patient reaches maximum single dose. *Maximum:* 0.3 mg/kg as a single dose.

➤ *Adjunct to thallium-201 myocardial perfusion scintigraphy in patients unable to exercise adequately during testing*

I.V. INJECTION (ADENOSCAN)

Adults.140 mcg/kg/min infused over 6 minutes continuously (total infused dose of 0.84 mg/kg).

Route	Onset	Peak	Duration
I.V.	Immediate	Immediate	Unknown

Mechanism of Action
Slows conduction time through the AV node and can interrupt AV node reentry pathways to restore normal sinus rhythm.

Incompatibilities
Don't mix adenosine with other drugs.

Contraindications
Hypersensitivity to adenosine or its components; second- or third-degree heart block or sick sinus syndrome, except in patients with a functioning artificial pacemaker

Interactions
DRUGS

carbamazepine: Increased degree of heart block
digoxin, verapamil: Possibly increased depressant effect on SA or AV node and increased risk of ventricular fibrillation
dipyridamole: Increased adenosine effects
methylxanthines, such as theophylline: Antagonized adenosine effects

FOODS

caffeine: Antagonized adenosine effects

Adverse Reactions
CNS: Apprehension, **CVA**, dizziness, headache, heaviness in arms, light-headedness, nervousness, paresthesia, **seizures**
CV: Atrial fibrillation, **bradycardia**, **cardiac arrest**, chest pain or pressure, **heart block**, hypertension, **hypotension**, **MI**, palpitations, **prolonged asystole**, tachycardia, **sinus exit block or pause**, **sustained ventricular tachycardia**, **torsades de pointes**, transient hypertension, **ventricular fibrillation**
EENT: Blurred vision, metallic taste, **throat tightness**
GI: Nausea, vomiting
MS: Jaw, neck, and back pain
RESP: Bronchoconstriction, **bronchospasm**, dyspnea, hyperventilation, **respiratory arrest**
SKIN: Diaphoresis, erythema, facial flushing, rash
Other: Injection-site reactions including pain, sensitivity reactions

Nursing Considerations
- Know that Adenoscan should not be given to patients with signs and symptoms of acute myocardial ischemia, as these patients may be at greater risk for serious cardiovascular reactions, including a myocardial infarction during a medical stress test.
- Inspect adenosine for crystals before use. If solution isn't clear, don't give it.
- Give Adenocard used to convert PSVT to normal sinus rhythm by rapid I.V. bolus over 1 to 2 seconds. Slower delivery can cause systemic vasodilation and reflex tachycardia. Give Adenoscan used as an adjunct to thallium-201 myocardial perfusion scintigraphy as a continuous peripheral intravenous infusion over 6 minutes. Know that the required dose of thallium-201 should be injected at the midpoint of the Adenoscan infusion. It is compatible with Adenoscan and may be injected directly into the Adenoscan infusion set.
- Expect prescriber to inject adenosine directly into a vein to make sure drug reaches systemic circulation. If given into an I.V. line, give drug as close to insertion site as possible and follow with rapid saline flush.

WARNING Don't give single doses of Adenocard more than 12 mg.

- Monitor heart rate and rhythm, blood pressure, and respiratory status often during adenosine therapy.
- Be aware that at the time of conversion to normal sinus rhythm, arrhythmias (such as premature atrial or ventricular contractions, sinus bradycardia, sinus tachycardia, or AV block) may occur for a few seconds, but they don't usually require intervention.

WARNING Stop drug use and notify prescriber immediately if severe respiratory difficulties develop or patient develops other signs of hypersensitivity such as chest discomfort, erythema, flushing, or rash.

- Store adenosine at room temperature. Discard unused portion.

PATIENT TEACHING

- Inform patient of increased risk for serious adverse effects. Instruct patient to report chest pain, palpitations, difficulty breathing, or severe headache during adenosine therapy.

- Warn patient that mild, temporary reactions may occur, such as flushing, nausea, and dizziness.

albuterol sulfate
(salbutamol sulphate)

AccuNeb, ProAir Digihaler, Proair HFA, ProAir Respiclick, Ventolin HFA, VoSpire ER

Class and Category

Pharmacologic class: Adrenergic
Therapeutic class: Bronchodilator
Pregnancy category: C

Indications and Dosages

➤ *To prevent exercise-induced bronchospasm*

INHALATION POWDER

Adults and children age 4 and over. Two inhalations 15 to 30 min before exercise.

➤ *To treat bronchospasm in patients with reversible obstructive airway disease*

E.R. TABLETS

Adults and children over age 12. *Initial:* 4 or 8 mg every 12 hr. *Maximum:* 32 mg daily in divided doses every 12 hr.
Children ages 6 to 12. *Initial:* 4 mg every 12 hr. *Maximum:* 24 mg daily in divided doses every 12 hr.

SYRUP

Adults and children over age 14. *Initial:* 2 to 4 mg (1 to 2 tsp) three or four times daily. *Maximum:* 32 mg daily in divided doses.
Children ages 6 to 14. *Initial:* 2 mg (1 tsp) three or four times daily. *Maximum:* 24 mg daily in divided doses.
Children ages 2 to 6. *Initial:* 0.1 mg/kg three times daily (not to exceed 2 mg three times daily), increased to 0.2 mg/kg three times daily (not to exceed 4 mg three times daily). *Maximum:* 12 mg daily in divided doses.

TABLETS

Adults and children over age 12. *Initial:* 2 or 4 mg three or four times daily. *Maximum:* 32 mg daily in divided doses.
Children ages 6 to 12. *Initial:* 2 mg three or four times daily. *Maximum:* 24 mg daily in divided doses.

DOSAGE ADJUSTMENT For elderly patients and patients sensitive to beta-adrenergic stimulation, initial dosage reduced to 2 mg (1 tsp) of syrup three or four times daily or 2 mg of tablets three or four times daily (up to 32 mg daily).

INHALATION SOLUTION

Adults and children age 12 and over. 2.5 mg three or four times daily, as needed, by nebulization over 5 to 15 min.
Children ages 2 to 12. *Initial:* 0.63 mg or 1.25 mg three or four times daily, as needed, by nebulization over 5 to 15 min.

➤ *To treat or prevent brochospasms in*

INHALATION POWDER

Adults and children age 4 and over. 1 inhalation every 4 hr to 2 inhalations every 4 to 6 hr.

INHALATION POWDER (PROAIR RESPICLICK)

Adults and children 4 yr and over. 1 inhalation every 4 hr or 2 inhalations every 4 to 6 hr.

Route	Onset	Peak	Duration
P.O. (E.R. tab)	30 min	2–3 hr	12 hr
P.O. (syrup)	Rapid	2 hr	Unknown
P.O. (tab)	30 min	2–3 hr	4–8 hr
Inhalation (powder)	5–15 min	50–55 min	3–6 hr
Inhalation (solution)	5–15 min	1–2 hr	3–6 hr

Contraindications

Hypersensitivity to albuterol or its components

Interactions

DRUGS

beta blockers: Inhibited effects of albuterol
bronchodilators (sympathomimetics), such as theophylline: Possibly adverse CV effects
digoxin: Decreased serum digoxin level
MAO inhibitors, tricyclic antidepressants: Increased vascular effects of albuterol
potassium-lowering drugs: Possibly hypokalemia
potassium-wasting diuretics: Possibly increased hypokalemia

Mechanism of Action

Albuterol attaches to $beta_2$ receptors on bronchial cell membranes, which stimulates the intracellular enzyme adenylate cyclase to convert adenosine triphosphate (ATP) to cyclic adenosine monophosphate (cAMP). This reaction decreases intracellular calcium levels. It also increases intracellular levels of cAMP, as shown. Together, these effects relax bronchial smooth-muscle cells and inhibit histamine release.

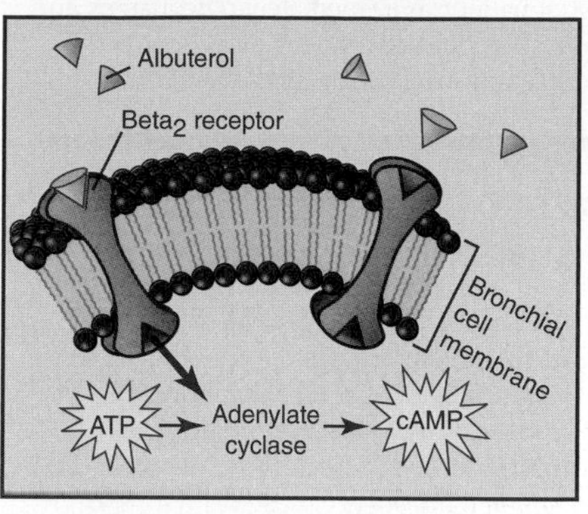

Adverse Reactions

CNS: Anxiety, dizziness, drowsiness, headache, hyperkinesia, insomnia, irritability, nervousness, tremor, vertigo, weakness
CV: **Angina**, **arrhythmias**, chest pain, hypertension, **hypotension**, palpitations
EENT: Altered taste, dry mouth and throat, ear pain, glossitis, hoarseness, **oropharyngeal edema**, pharyngitis, rhinitis, taste perversion
ENDO: Hyperglycemia
GI: Anorexia, diarrhea, dysphagia, heartburn, nausea, vomiting
GU: UTI
MS: Muscle cramps
RESP: **Bronchospasm**, cough, dyspnea, **paradoxical bronchospasm**, **pulmonary edema**
SKIN: Diaphoresis, flushing, pallor, pruritus, rash, urticaria
Other: **Angioedema**, **hypokalemia**, infection, **metabolic acidosis**

Nursing Considerations

- Administer pressurized inhalations of albuterol during second half of inspiration, when airways are open wider and aerosol distribution is more effective.

WARNING Use cautiously in patients with cardiac disorders, diabetes mellitus, digitalis intoxication, hypertension, hyperthyroidism, or history of seizures. Albuterol can worsen these conditions.

- Monitor serum potassium level because albuterol may cause transient hypokalemia.
- Be aware that drug tolerance can develop with prolonged use.

PATIENT TEACHING

- Teach patient how to use inhaler. Tell him if he is precribed Proair HFA to shake canister before use and to check that a new canister is working by spraying it the appropriate number of times (once to four times based on manufacturer instructions) into the air while looking for a fine mist. However, if patient is prescribed the ProAir Digihaler or ProAir Respiclick device, tell him that they do not require priming and these devices should not be used with a spacer or volume holding chamber.
- Instruct patient to wash mouthpiece with water once a week and let it air-dry if patient is using a Proair HFA device. However, if patient is using a ProAir Digihaler or ProAir RespiClick device, he should not wash or put these devices in water. Instead they should be cleaned by gently wiping the mouthpiece with a dry cloth or tissue, if needed. Tell patient to discard the ProAir Digihaler and ProAir RespiClick devices after 13 months from opening the foil pouch or after the expiration date, whichever comes first. The ProAir RespiClick device should also be discarded before 13 months from opening the foil pouch if the dose counter displays 0.
- Advise patient to wait at least 1 minute between inhalations if dosage requires more than one inhalation.
- Tell patient to check with his prescriber before using other inhaled drugs.
- Warn patient not to exceed prescribed dose or frequency. If doses become less effective, tell patient to contact his prescriber.

- Tell patient to immediately report signs and symptoms of allergic reaction, such as difficulty swallowing, itching, and rash.

alendronate sodium

Binosto, Fosamax

Class and Category

Pharmacologic class: Bisphosphonate
Therapeutic class: Bone resorption inhibitor
Pregnancy category: C

Indications and Dosages

➤ *To prevent postmenopausal osteoporosis*

TABLETS

Adults. 5 mg daily or 35 mg once/wk in the morning with a full glass of water at least 30 min before first food, drink, or other drugs.

➤ *To treat postmenopausal osteoporosis*

ORAL SOLUTION, TABLETS

Adults. 10 mg (tablet) daily or 70 mg (oral solution or tablet) once/wk in the morning with a full glass of water at least 30 min before first food, drink, or other drugs.

EFFERVESCENT TABLETS

Adults. 70 mg once/wk in the morning dissolved in 4 ounces of room-temperature water at least 30 min before first food, drink, or other drugs.

➤ *To treat Paget's disease of the bone in patients whose alkaline phosphatase level is twice the upper limit of symptomatic and at risk for further complications*

TABLETS

Adults. 40 mg daily with a full glass of water for 6 months. Treatment repeated following a 6 month post-treatment evaluation period, if needed, in patients who have failed to normalize their serum alkaline phosphatase levels or have relapsed based on increases in alkaline phosphatase.

➤ *To increase bone mass in men with osteoporosis*

ORAL SOLUTION, TABLETS

Adults. 10 mg (tablet) daily or 70 mg (oral solution or tablet) once/wk in the morning with a full glass of water at least 30 min before first food, drink, or other drugs.

EFFERVESCENT TABLETS

Adults. 70 mg once/wk in the morning dissolved in 4 ounces of room temperature water at least 30 min before first food, drink, or other drugs.

➤ *To treat glucocorticoid-induced osteoporosis in men and women who receive a daily glucocorticoid dosage of 7.5 mg or greater of prednisone and who have low bone-mineral density*

TABLETS

Adults. 5 mg daily in the morning with a full glass of water at least 30 min before first food, drink, or other drugs.

DOSAGE ADJUSTMENT Dosage for glucocorticoid-induced osteoporosis increased to 10 mg daily for postmenopausal women not receiving estrogen.

Route	Onset	Peak	Duration
P.O.	Unknown	Unknown	6 wk*

* After single 5-mg dose for osteoporosis; 6 months after single 5-mg dose for Paget's disease.

Mechanism of Action

Reduces activity of cells that cause bone loss, slows rate of bone loss after menopause, and increases amount of bone mass. May act by inhibiting osteoclast activity on newly formed bone resorption surfaces, which reduces the number of sites where bone is remodeled. Bone formation then exceeds bone resorption at these remodeling sites, which gradually increases bone mass. May also inhibit bone dissolution by binding to hydroxyapatite crystals, which are composed of calcium, phosphate, and hydroxide and give bone its rigid structure.

Contraindications

Esophageal abnormalities that delay esophageal emptying, such as achalasia or stricture; hypersensitivity to alendronate or its components; hypocalcemia; inability to stand or sit upright for at least 30 minutes

Interactions

DRUGS

antacids, calcium, iron, multivalent cations: Decreased absorption of alendronate
aspirin: Increased risk of GI distress
levothyroxine: Possibly slight decrease in bioavailability of alendronate

FOODS

any food: Delayed absorption and decreased serum level of alendronate

Adverse Reactions

CNS: Asthenia, dizziness, headache, vertigo
CV: Peripheral edema
EENT: Cholesteatoma of external auditory canal
GI: Abdominal distention and pain, constipation, diarrhea, dysphagia, **esophageal perforation** or ulceration, esophagitis, flatulence, gastritis, gastroesophageal reflux disease, heartburn, indigestion, **melena**, nausea, vomiting
MS: Arthralgia; femoral shaft or subtrochanteric fractures; focal osteomalacia; jaw osteonecrosis; joint swelling; muscle spasms; myalgia; severe bone, joint, and/or muscle pain
RESP: Asthma exacerbation
SKIN: Photosensitivity, pruritus, rash, **Stevens–Johnson syndrome**, **toxic epidermal necrolysis**
Other: Anaphylaxis, **hypocalcemia**

Nursing Considerations

- Prepare to administer effervescent form of alendronate by dissolving one tablet in 4 ounces of plain water (do not use mineral water or flavored water) that is at room temperature. Wait 5 minutes after effervescence stops and then stir the solution for about 10 seconds before handing to patient to ingest.
- Monitor patient's serum calcium level before, during, and after treatment. Expect hypocalcemia to be treated before alendronate therapy begins. If hypocalcemia occurs during therapy, expect prescriber to order a calcium supplement.
- Ensure adequate dietary intake of calcium and vitamin D before, during, and after treatment.
- Be aware that oral osteoporosis drugs such as alendronate may have the potential to increase the risk of esophageal cancer. While studies are underway to determine this potential, assess patient regularly for painful or difficulty swallowing, chest pain, or new or worsening heartburn; notify prescriber if present.

WARNING **Monitor patient closely, as alendronate may irritate upper GI mucosa, causing adverse reactions such as esophageal ulceration. To help minimize these reactions, have patient take drug with a full glass of water and remain upright for at least 30 minutes.**

- Monitor patient for jaw pain because alendronate may cause osteonecrosis of the jaw, with risk increasing as therapy duration becomes longer. Patients at increased risk include those who have poor oral hygiene, preexisting dental or periodontal disease, wear ill-fitting dentures, or require an invasive dental procedure. Patients are also at increased risk if they have a cancer diagnosis, concomitant therapy such as chemotherapy or corticosteroid therapy, or other illnesses, such as preexisting dental or periodontal disease, anemia, coagulopathy, or infection.

PATIENT TEACHING

- Advise patient to take alendronate in the morning with a full glass of water. Explain that beverages such as orange juice, coffee, and mineral water reduce alendronate's effects.
- Instruct patient who is prescribed the effervescent tablet form to dissolve the tablet in 4 ounces of room-temperature water (mineral water or flavored water should not be used). After the effervescence stops, tell the patient to wait 5 minutes and then stir the solution for about 10 seconds and ingest.
- Tell patient not to chew or suck on tablet to help reduce esophageal irritation.
- Instruct patient to wait at least 30 minutes after taking alendronate before eating, drinking, or taking other drugs. Teach patient to remain upright for 30 minutes after taking alendronate and until she has eaten the first food of the day.
- Encourage patient to consume adequate daily amounts of calcium and vitamin D.
- Instruct patient to report to prescriber any new or unusual pain in hip or thigh.
- Tell patient to inform dentist of alendronate therapy prior to dental work and to notify dentist of any signs of infection or delayed healing after an extraction.

• Instruct patient to report any difficulty swallowing or pain when swallowing, chest pain, or new or worsening heartburn to prescriber.
• Inform patient receiving the effervescent tablet form to be aware that each tablet contains 650 mg sodium, which is equivalent to approximately 1,650 mg of salt (sodium chloride) per tablet.

alfuzosin hydrochloride

Uroxatral, Xatral (CAN)

Class and Category

Pharmacologic class: Alpha$_1$ blocker
Therapeutic class: Benign prostatic hypertrophic
Pregnancy category: B

Indications and Dosages

➤ *To treat signs and symptoms of benign prostatic hyperplasia*

E.R. TABLETS

Adults. 10 mg daily taken with same meal each day.

Mechanism of Action

Selectively blocks alpha$_1$-adrenergic receptors in smooth muscle of the bladder neck and prostate. This causes relaxation, and blocks postsynaptic alpha$_1$ adrenoreceptors in the bladder base and neck, prostate, prostatic capsule, and urethra, preventing further action at these sites. These actions improve urine flow and bladder emptying and reduce urinary hesitancy, frequency, and nocturia.

Contraindications

Hypersensitivity to alfuzosin or its components, moderate or severe hepatic insufficiency, use with CYP3A4 inhibitors, such as itraconazole, ketoconazole, and ritonavir

Interactions

DRUGS

antihypertensives, nitrates: Possibly synergistic lowering of blood pressure and syncope
CYP3A4 inhibitors (such as itraconazole, ketoconazole, ritonavir): Increased alfuzosin effects
other alpha blockers: May potentiate alfuzosin action
PDE5 inhibitors: May cause symptomatic hypotension

Adverse Reactions

CNS: Dizziness, fatigue, headache
CV: Angina (preexisting coronary artery disease), **atrial fibrillation**, chest pain, edema, orthostatic hypotension, **QT-interval prolongation**, tachycardia
EENT: Intraoperative floppy iris syndrome, pharyngitis, rhinitis, sinusitis
GI: Abdominal pain, **cholestatic and hepatocellular liver injury**, constipation, diarrhea, indigestion, jaundice, **hepatotoxicity**, nausea, vomiting
GU: Impotence, priapism
HEME: Thrombocytopenia
RESP: Bronchitis, upper respiratory tract infection
SKIN: Flushing, pruritus, rash, **toxic epidermal necrolysis**, urticaria
Other: Angioedema, generalized pain

Nursing Considerations

• Use alfuzosin cautiously in patients who have symptomatic hypotension or who have had a hypotensive response to other drugs. Orthostatic hypotension (with or without symptoms such as dizziness) may occur within hours after alfuzosin administration.
• Use cautiously in patients with severe renal insufficiency; decreased drug clearance may increase risk of adverse reactions.
• Be aware that alfuzosin shouldn't be used to treat bladder symptoms in women.
• Know that alpha$_1$ blockers such as alfuzosin may predispose patients to intraoperative floppy iris syndrome during cataract surgery that may require surgical repair.
• Monitor patient for chest pain. If symptoms of angina pectoris occur or worsen, notify prescriber immediately and expect drug to be discontinued.

PATIENT TEACHING

• Emphasize need to take alfuzosin with a meal because absorption is decreased by 50% if taken on an empty stomach.
• Tell patient not to crush or chew tablets but to swallow them whole.
• Caution patient to avoid hazardous activities until drug's CNS effects are known and also

for several hours after taking dose; blood pressure may drop suddenly after use.
- Advise patient to change position slowly to minimize drop in blood pressure.

alirocumab

Praluent

Class and Category

Pharmacologic class: Human monoclonal antibody to PCSK9
Therapeutic class: Antihyperlipidemic
Pregnancy category: Not classified

Indications and Dosages

➤ ***Adjunct to diet and maximally tolerated statin therapy to treat heterozygous familial hypercholesterolemia or clinical atherosclerotic cardiovascular disease in patients who require additional lowering of LDL-C***

SUBCUTANEOUS INJECTION

Adults. *Initial:* 75 mg once every 2 wk, increased to 150 mg once every 2 wk, as needed. Alternatively, 300 mg once every 4 wk. *Maximum:* 150 mg once every 2 wk or 300 mg once every 4 wk.

Mechanism of Action

Proprotein convertase subtilisin kexin type 9 (PCSK9) binds to low-density lipoprotein receptors on the surface of hepatocytes for the purpose of degrading the receptors within the liver. Alirocumab inhibits the binding of PCSK9 therefore increasing the number of LDL receptors available to clear circulating low-density lipoproteins. This results in a lower LDL-C level.

Contraindications

Hypersensitivity to alirocumab or its components

Adverse Reactions

CNS: Confusion, memory impairment
EENT: Nasopharyngitis, sinusitis
GI: Diarrhea, elevated liver enzymes
GU: UTI
MS: Muscle spasms, musculoskeletal pain, myalgia
RESP: Bronchitis, cough
SKIN: Eczema, hypersensitivity vasculitis, pruritus, rash, urticaria
Other: Antialirocumab antibodies; flu-like symptoms; injection site reactions such as erythema, itching, pain, swelling, tenderness

Nursing Considerations

- Administer alirocumab by first allowing drug to warm to room temperature for 30 to 40 minutes before giving the injection. Injection should be administered as soon as possible after it has warmed up. Discard if the solution has been at room temperature for 24 hours or longer. Inject alirocumab into the patient's abdomen, thigh, or upper arm and rotate the injection sites.
- Monitor patient's LDL-C levels, as ordered, within 4 to 8 weeks after alirocumab therapy is begun or titrated to assess response
- Monitor patient for allergic reactions to alirocumab such as pruritus, rash, or urticaria. Be aware that some allergic reactions may become serious enough to require hospitalization. If signs or symptoms of a serious allergic reaction occurs, notify prescriber, expect to discontinue drug and provide supportive care, as ordered.

PATIENT TEACHING

- Inform patient that alirocumab therapy is not a substitution for dietary measures or statin therapy.
- Teach patient how to administer a subcutaneous injection. Tell patient to warm up the solution to room temperature 30 to 40 minutes before administering and to discard if left at room temperature for more than 24 hours.
- Instruct patient to administer the injection into his abdomen, thigh, or upper arm and to rotate the injection sites. Inform him that it may take up to 20 seconds to inject the drug. Caution him not to inject into areas of active skin disease, sunburned areas, or where an infection, inflammation, or rash is present. Warn patient not to coadminister drug with other injectable drugs at the same injection site. Advise him not to reuse the pen or syringe device and how to dispose it properly.
- Instruct patient who misses a dose to administer the injection within 7 days, and then resume his normal dosing schedule. However, if the missed dose is

not administered within 7 days of the normal dosing schedule, advise the patient to wait until the next dose is due.
- Advise patient to stop taking alirocumab, notify prescriber if an allergic reaction occurs, and seek medical care.

aliskiren

Rasilez (CAN), Tekturna

Class and Category

Pharmacologic class: Direct renin inhibitor
Therapeutic class: Antihypertensive
Pregnancy category: Not classified

Indications and Dosages

➤ *To treat hypertension*

ORAL PELLETS, TABLETS

Adults and children age 6 to 17 weighing 50 kg (110 lb) or more. 150 mg once daily, increased to 300 mg once daily, as needed.
Children age 6 to 17 weighing less than 50 kg (110 lb) but 20 kg (44 lb) or more. 37.5 or 75 mg daily. *Maximum:* 150 mg daily.

Route	Onset	Peak	Duration
P.O.	Unknown	1–3 hr	Unknown

Mechanism of Action

Inhibits renin secreted by the kidneys in response to decreased blood volume and renal perfusion. Renin cleaves angiotensinogen to form angiotensin I, which is converted to angiotensin II by ACE and non-ACE pathways. Angiotensin II is a powerful vasoconstrictor that induces release of catecholamines from the adrenal medulla and prejunctional nerve endings. It also promotes aldosterone secretion and sodium reabsorption. Together, these actions increase blood pressure. By inhibiting renin release, aliskiren impairs the renin–angiotensin–aldosterone system. Without the vasoconstrictive effect of angiotension II, blood pressure decreases.

Contraindications

Children under the age of 2; hypersensitivity to aliskiren or its components, presence of diabetes and concurrent angiotensin-converting enzyme inhibitor (ACEI) or angiotensin receptor blocker (ARB) therapy, pregnancy

Interactions

DRUGS

ACE inhibitors, ARBs: Increased risk of hyperkalemia, hypotension or renal dysfunction, especially in the elderly and patients who are volume-depleted or already have renal impairment
atorvastatin, cyclosporine, itraconazole, ketoconazole, verapamil: Increased aliskiren blood level
furosemide: Decreased blood furosemide levels
irbesartan: Decreased blood aliskiren level
NSAIDs: Increased risk of decreased renal function and hypotension
P-glycoprotein: Possible alteration in absorption and disposition of aliskiren at Pgp site
potassium-sparing diuretics, potassium supplements: Increased risk of hyperkalemia

FOODS

high-fat food: Decreased aliskiren absorption substantially

Adverse Reactions

CNS: Dizziness, fatigue, headache, **seizures**
CV: Hypotension, peripheral edema
EENT: Nasopharyngitis
GI: Abdominal pain, diarrhea, dyspepsia, elevated liver enzymes, gastroesophageal reflux, **hepatic dysfunction**, nausea, vomiting
GU: Elevated blood creatinine, renal calculi
HEME: Decreased hemoglobin and hematocrit
MS: Back pain
RESP: Increased cough, upper respiratory tract infection
SKIN: Erythema, pruritus, rash, **Stevens–Johnson syndrome**, **toxic epidermal necrolysis**, urticaria
Other: Anaphylaxis, **angioedema**, elevated creatine kinase or uric acid level, gout, hyperkalemia, hyponatremia

Nursing Considerations

- Be aware that aliskiren should not be used in patients with diabetes who are concurrently taking ARBs or ACEIs because of the increased risk of serious adverse effects such as renal dysfunction, hyperkalemia, and hypotension. Also know that aliskiren should not be given to patients with moderate renal impairment (glomerular filtration rate of less than 60 ml/min) who are also receiving ARB or ACEI therapy because renal impairment may worsen.

- Monitor patient's renal function closely, especially in patients receiving drugs such as ARBs, ACEIs, NSAIDs, potassium supplements or potassium-sparing diuretics that affect the renin–angiotensin system. Use aliskiren cautiously in patients whose renal function may depend in part on the activity of this system such as those with renal artery stenosis, severe heart failure, postmyocardial infarction, or who are elderly or experiencing volume depletion because aliskiren therapy increases the risk of renal dysfunction in these patients that could lead to acute renal failure.
- Take measures to correct volume or salt depletion from high-dose diuretic therapy before starting aliskiren, as ordered, to prevent hypotension. If hypotension occurs during aliskiren therapy, place patient in a supine position and give normal saline solution intravenously, as needed and prescribed.
- Expect to administer oral pellets for patients who are unable to swallow tablets. The pellets are dispensed in a capsule. Open the dispensing capsule, empty the contents onto a spoon, and then administer by mouth. Have patient swallow the pellets immediately. Follow with milk (dairy or soy-based) or water immediately without patient chewing or crushing the pellets. Make sure that no pellets remain in the dispensing capsule. Never give the capsule containing the oral pellets for patient to swallow and do not empty the contents of the capsule directly into patient's mouth. Alternatively, after opening the dispensing capsule, pellets can be immediately mixed with one or more teaspoons of milk that is dairy or soy-based, vanilla ice cream, vanilla pudding, or water as a dosing vehicle. Have patient take the contents of one dispensing capsule with one teaspoon of dosing liquid. Again, ensure that patient does not chew or crush the pellets in mouth but swallows the pellets immediately.

WARNING **Watch closely for angioedema of the head or neck. if angioedema occurs, discontinue aliskiren, notify prescriber, and provide supportive therapy until swelling has ceased. if swelling of the tongue, glottis, or larynx is involved, be prepared to give epinephrine solution 1:1,000 (0.3 to 0.5 ml), as prescribed, and provide measures to ensure a patent airway. Be aware that patient shouldn't receive aliskiren again.**

- Monitor serum electrolytes, especially potassium levels, as ordered in patients who already are experiencing renal insufficiency or who have diabetes because of increased risk for hyperkalemia in the presence of aliskiren therapy. Also monitor patients who are taking ARBs, ACEIs, or NSAIDs along with aliskiren because of increased risk of hyperkalemia.

PATIENT TEACHING

- Tell patient who is unable to swallow tablets that aliskiren can be taken by oral pellets. Tell him the pellets are dispensed in a capsule. After opening the dispensing capsule, tell him to empty the contents onto a spoon and then administer by mouth and swallow immediately. He should follow with milk (daily or soy-based) or water immediately without chewing or crushing the pellets. He should check to make sure that no pellets remain in the dispensing capsule. He should never take the capsule containing the oral pellets and he should never empty the contents of the capsule directly into his mouth. Alternatively, tell him the pellets, after opening the dispensing capsule, can be immediately mixed with one or more teaspoons of milk that is dairy or soy-based, vanilla ice cream, vanilla ice pudding, or water as a dosing vehicle. He should mix the contents of one dispensing capsule with one teaspoon of dosing liquid. Again, he should not chew or crush the pellets in mouth but swallow the mixture immediately.
- Advise patient to avoid high-fat meals while taking aliskiren because fat decreases drug absorption significantly.
- Instruct patient how to monitor blood pressure to determine effectiveness of aliskiren therapy.

- Explain that decreased blood pressure could lead to light-headedness, especially in the first few days of therapy. Advise patient to change positions slowly and, if light-headedness develops, to notify prescriber. Tell patient to stop taking aliskiren and to notify prescriber if she faints.
- Explain that light-headedness and fainting could also result from dehydration caused by inadequate fluid intake, excessive perspiration, diarrhea, or vomiting.
- Instruct patient to avoid using potassium supplements or potassium salt substitutes and to inform all prescribers about her aliskiren and ACE inhibitor or ARD therapy.

WARNING **Emphasize importance of stopping aliskiren and seeking immediate medical attention if patient has swelling of face, extremities, eyes, lips, or tongue, or if patient has trouble swallowing or breathing.**

- Instruct female patient to notify prescriber immediately if she is or could be pregnant because drug will need to be discontinued and another antihypertensive chosen. Also inform mothers that breastfeeding is not recommended while taking aliskiren, as drug can cause high potassium level, kidney impairment, and low blood pressure in a nursing infant.

allopurinol

Apo-Allopurinol (CAN), Lopurin, Purinol (CAN), Zyloprim

allopurinol sodium

Aloprim

Class and Category

Pharmacological class: Xanthine oxidase inhibitor
Therapeutic class: Antigout
Pregnancy category: C

Indications and Dosages

➤ *To treat primary gout and hyperuricemia*

TABLETS

Adults. *Initial:* 100 mg daily increased by 100 mg/wk until serum uric acid level is 6 mg/dl or less. Dosages above 300 mg daily given in divided doses. *Maximum:* 800 mg daily.

➤ *To treat secondary hyperuricemia caused by neoplastic disease*

TABLETS

Adults. 600 to 800 mg daily for 2 to 3 days, then adjusted to keep serum uric acid level within normal limits.
Children ages 6 to 10. 300 mg daily, adjusted after 48 hr, depending on response to treatment.
Children under age 6. 150 mg daily, adjusted after 48 hr, depending on response to treatment.

➤ *To treat recurrent calcium oxalate calculi*

TABLETS

Adults. 200 to 300 mg daily as a single dose or in divided doses, adjusted based on 24-hr urine urate level.

➤ *To treat increased serum and urine uric acid levels in patients with leukemia, lymphoma, and solid tumors whose cancer chemotherapy has increased those levels and who can't tolerate oral therapy*

I.V. INFUSION

Adults. 200 to 400 mg/m^2 daily as a single infusion or in equally divided infusions every 6, 8, or 12 hr. *Maximum:* 600 mg daily.
Children. 200 mg/m^2 daily as a single infusion or in equally divided infusions every 6, 8, or 12 hr.

DOSAGE ADJUSTMENT For patient with impaired renal function, dosage adjusted to 200 mg daily if creatinine clearance is 10 to 20 ml/min, 100 mg daily if creatinine clearance is 3 to 10 ml/min, or 100 mg every other day if creatinine clearance falls below 3 ml/min.

Route	Onset	Peak	Duration
P.O.	2–3 days	1–3 wk*	1–2 wk
I.V.	10–15 min	Unknown	5 hr

* For hyperuricemia; several months for gout attack prevention.

Mechanism of Action

Inhibits uric acid production by inhibiting xanthine oxidase, the enzyme that converts hypoxanthine and xanthine to uric acid. Allopurinol is metabolized to oxipurinol, which also inhibits xanthine oxidase.

Incompatibilities

Don't combine I.V. allopurinol in solution with amikacin, amphotericin B, carmustine, cefotaxime sodium, chlorpromazine hydrochloride, cimetidine hydrochloride, clindamycin phosphate, cytarabine, dacarbazine, daunorubicin hydrochloride, diphenhydramine hydrochloride, doxorubicin hydrochloride, doxycycline hyclate, droperidol, floxuridine, gentamicin sulfate, haloperidol lactate, hydroxyzine hydrochloride, idarubicin hydrochloride, imipenem-cilastatin sodium, mechlorethamine hydrochloride, meperidine hydrochloride, metoclopramide hydrochloride, methylprednisolone sodium succinate, minocycline hydrochloride, nalbuphine hydrochloride, netilmicin sulfate, ondansetron hydrochloride, prochlorperazine edisylate, promethazine hydrochloride, sodium bicarbonate, streptozocin, tobramycin sulfate, vinorelbine tartrate.

Contraindications

Hypersensitivity to allopurinol or its components

Interactions

DRUGS

ACE inhibitors: Increased risk of hypersensitivity reactions
amoxicillin, ampicillin: Increased risk of rash
azathioprine, mercaptopurine: Increased plasma levels of these drugs with increased risk of toxicity
chlorpropamide: Increased risk of hypoglycemia in patients with renal insufficiency
cyclophosphamide, other cytotoxic drugs: Enhanced bone marrow suppression
dicumarol: Increased half-life and anticoagulant action of dicumarol
thiazide diuretics: Possibly increased risk of allopurinol toxicity
uricosuric agents: Increased urinary excretion of uric acid

Adverse Reactions

CNS: Chills, drowsiness, fever, headache, neuritis, paresthesia, peripheral neuropathy, somnolence
CV: Vasculitis
EENT: Epistaxis, loss of taste
GI: Abdominal pain, diarrhea, dysphagia, elevated liver enzymes, gastritis, **granulomatous hepatitis**, **hepatic necrosis**, hepatomegaly, nausea, vomiting
GU: Exacerbated renal calculi, **renal failure**
HEME: **Agranulocytosis**, **aplastic anemia**, **bone marrow depression**, eosinophilia, leukocytosis, **leukopenia**, **thrombocytopenia**
MS: Arthralgia, exacerbation of gout, myopathy
SKIN: Alopecia; ecchymosis; jaundice; maculopapular, scaly, or exfoliative rash (sometimes fatal); pruritus; urticaria
OTHER: Drug hypersensitivity syndrome (DHS), drug reaction with eosinophilia and systemic symptoms (DRESS)

Nursing Considerations

- Obtain baseline CBC and uric acid level, as ordered, and review results of renal and liver function tests before and during allopurinol therapy.
- Reconstitute and dilute I.V. preparation to a concentration of 6 mg/ml or less.

WARNING Discontinue allopurinol and notify prescriber immediately at first sign of hypersensitivity reaction, such as rash, which may precede more severe reactions.

- Maintain a fluid intake to produce a daily urinary output of 2 L daily. Also, don't give vitamin C because the pH of urine should be kept neutral to slightly alkaline.
- Monitor patient for the development of a skin rash that may occur 1 week or more after allopurinal therapy is initiated. If present, notify prescriber immediately because this could be a sign of DRESS, which may become life-threatening. Expect drug to be discontinued.

PATIENT TEACHING

- Advise patient to take allopurinol after meals and to drink enough water (8 to 10 full glasses) to produce a daily urinary output of at least 2 L.

- Instruct patient to report unusual bleeding or bruising, chills, fever, gout attack, numbness, and tingling.
- Inform patient that acute gout attacks may occur more often early in allopurinol treatment and that results may not be noticeable for 2 weeks or longer.
- Instruct patient not to drive or perform hazardous tasks if drug causes drowsiness.
- Tell patient to notify prescriber immediately if a rash develops and to stop taking drug until the rash is evaluated.

almotriptan malate

Axert

Class and Category

Pharmacologic class: Selective serotonin receptor agonist (5-T_1)
Therapeutic class: Antimigraine drug
Pregnancy category: C

Indications and Dosages

➤ *To treat acute migraine*

TABLETS

Adults and adolescents ages 12 to 17. *Initial:* 6.25 or 12.5 mg as a single dose, repeated in 2 hr as needed. *Maximum:* 25 mg/24 hr or 4 migraine treatments/mo.

DOSAGE ADJUSTMENT For patient with impaired hepatic or renal function or patients receiving potent CYP3A4 inhibitors such as ketoconazole, initial dose reduced to 6.25 mg with maximum daily dose of 12.5 mg.

Mechanism of Action

May stimulate 5-HT_1 receptors on intracranial blood vessels and sensory nerves in trigeminal vascular system. By activating these receptors, almotriptan selectively constricts dilated and inflamed cranial blood vessels and inhibits production of proinflammatory neuropeptides. It also interrupts transmission of pain signals to the brain.

Contraindications

Basilar or hemiplegic migraine, cerebrovascular, or peripheral vascular disease, hypersensitivity to almotriptan or its components, hypertension (uncontrolled), ischemic or vasospastic coronary artery disease (CAD), use within 24 hours of other serotonin-receptor agonists or ergotamine-containing or ergot-type drugs

Interactions

DRUGS

ergotamine-containing drugs: Prolonged vasospastic reactions
erythromycin, itraconazole, ketoconazole, MAO inhibitors, ritonavir, verapamil: Possibly increased blood almotriptan level
selective serotonin reuptake inhibitors (such as citalopram, escitalopram, fluoxetine, fluvoxamine, paroxetine, sertraline), serotonin norepinephrine reuptake inhibitors (such as duloxetine, venlafaxine): Increased risk of serotonin syndrome

Adverse Reactions

CNS: Confusion, dizziness, headache, hemiplegia, hypoesthesia, malaise, paresthesia, restlessness, **seizures**, **serotonin syndrome**, somnolence, syncope, vertigo
CV: Angina pectoris, **coronary artery vasospasm**, hypertension, **ischemia**, **MI**, palpitations, tachycardia, vasodilation, **ventricular fibrillation or tachycardia**
EENT: Blepharospasm, dry mouth, oral hypoesthesia, swollen tongue, visual impairment
GI: Abdominal pain or discomfort, colitis, nausea
MS: Arthralgia, extremity coldness or pain, myalgia
SKIN: Cold sweat, diaphoresis, erythema
Other: Anaphylaxis, **angioedema**

Nursing Considerations

WARNING **Monitor patient with CAD for angina because almotriptan can cause coronary artery vasospasm. Because it may cause peripheral vasospastic reactions, such as ischemic bowel disease, watch for abdominal pain and bloody diarrhea.**

- Expect to give first dose of almotriptan in a medical facility for patient with risk factors for CAD but no known cardiovascular abnormalities.
- Obtain an ECG immediately after first dose of almotriptan, as ordered, in patient with risk factors for CAD because cardiac

ischemia can occur without causing clinical symptoms.
- Expect to give a lower dosage to patients with hepatic or renal dysfunction because of impaired drug metabolism or excretion.
- Monitor blood pressure regularly during therapy in patients with hypertension because almotriptan may produce a transient increase in blood pressure.

WARNING **Monitor patient for evidence of serotonin syndrome, such as agitation, chills, confusion, diaphoresis, diarrhea, fever, hyperactive reflexes, poor coordination, restlessness, shaking, talking or acting with uncontrolled excitement, tremor, and twitching. In its most severe form, serotonin syndrome can resemble neuroleptic malignant syndrome, which includes autonomic instability with possible fluctuations in vital signs, high fever, mental status changes, and muscle rigidity.**
- Monitor patients hypersensitive to sulfonamides for hypersensitivity to almotriptan because cross-sensitivity may occur.

PATIENT TEACHING
- Inform patient that almotriptan is used to treat acute migraine and that he shouldn't take it to treat nonmigraine headaches.
- Advise patient to consult prescriber before taking any OTC or prescription drugs.
- Advise patient not to take more than maximum prescribed dosage, as medication overuse can cause migraine-like daily headaches or a marked increase in frequency of migraine attacks requiring detoxification to treat, which could lead to withdrawal symptoms.
- Caution patient that drug may cause adverse CNS reactions, and advise him to avoid hazardous activities until he knows how drug affects him.
- Instruct patient to seek emergency care immediately for signs of hypersensitivity such as breathing difficulties, itching, or a rash; cardiac symptoms (such as heaviness, pain, pressure, or tightness in chest, jaw, neck, or throat); or if multiple new symptoms develop (such as diarrhea, high fever, incoordination, mental changes nausea, vomiting) after taking the drug.
- Advise women of childbearing age to notify prescriber if pregnancy is suspected or occurs. Also advise mothers who wish to breastfeed to discuss with prescriber first.

alogliptin

Nesina

Class and Category

Pharmacologic class: Dipeptidyl peptidase-4 (DPP-4) inhibitor
Therapeutic class: Oral antidiabetic
Pregnancy category: B

Indications and Dosages

➤ *To achieve control of glucose level in type 2 diabetes mellitus as monotherapy or in conjunction with combination therapy*

TABLETS

Adults. 25 mg once daily.

DOSAGE ADJUSTMENT For patients with moderate renal impairment (creatinine clearance less than 60 ml/min but equal to or greater than 30 ml/min), dosage decreased to 12.5 mg once daily. For patients with severe renal impairment (creatinine clearance less than 30 ml/min but equal to or greater than 15 ml/min) or patients with end-stage renal disease or who are on hemodialysis, dosage decreased to 6.25 mg once daily.

Mechanism of Action

Inhibits the dipeptidyl peptidase-4 enzyme to slow inactivation of incretin hormones. These hormones are released by the intestine in response to a meal. When blood glucose level is increased, incretin hormones increase insulin synthesis and release from pancreatic beta cells. One type of incretin hormone, glucagon-like peptide (GLP-1), also lowers glucagon secretion from pancreatic alpha cells, which reduces hepatic glucose production. These combined actions decrease blood glucose level in type 2 diabetes.

Contraindications

Diabetic ketoacidosis; hypersensitivity to alogliptin or its components including anaphylaxis, angioedema, or severe cutaneous adverse reactions; type 1 diabetes

Interactions

DRUGS

insulin, sulfonylureas: Possibly increased risk of hypoglycemia

Adverse Reactions

CNS: Headache
CV: Heart failure
EENT: Nasopharyngitis
ENDO: Hypoglycemia
GI: Acute pancreatitis, elevated liver enzymes, **fulminant hepatic failure**
MS: Arthralgia (disabling and severe), joint pain (severe)
RESP: Upper respiratory tract infection
SKIN: Rash, **Stevens–Johnson syndrome**, urticaria
Other: Anaphylaxis, **angioedema**, serum sickness

Nursing Considerations

- Use alogliptin cautiously in patients with a history of angioedema to another drug in the same class because it is not known if patient will be predisposed to angioedema with alogliptin therapy.
- Determine patient's history for prior history of heart failure and a history of renal impairment because drug may increase risk for heart failure.
- Assess patient's renal function before starting alogliptin therapy. Know that in moderate to severe renal dysfunction, dosage will need to be reduced.
- Assess patient's liver function before starting alogliptin therapy. If abnormalities are present, monitor patient closely for signs and symptoms of liver dysfunction. If patient develops anorexia, dark urine, fatigue, jaundice, or right upper abdominal discomfort during therapy, notify prescriber and expect liver enzymes to be assessed. If elevated, expect drug to be discontinued.
- Monitor patient for serious hypersensitivity reactions, including severe cutaneous adverse reactions. If present, notify prescriber, expect alogliptin to be discontinued, and provide supportive care, as ordered.
- Check patient's blood glucose level, as ordered, to determine effectiveness of alogliptin therapy.

WARNING Monitor patient for signs and symptoms of acute pancreatitis, such as acute upper abdominal pain, fever, nausea, and vomiting. If suspected, notify prescriber and expect alogliptin to be discontinued, if confirmed.

PATIENT TEACHING

- Emphasize the need to follow an exercise program and a diet control program during alogliptin therapy.
- Advise patient to notify prescriber immediately if he has trouble breathing, develops swelling or skin reactions such as hives, rash, or other cutaneous abnormalities.
- Inform patient that periodic blood tests will be done to determine effectiveness of drug.
- Teach patient how to monitor blood glucose level and when to report changes.
- Caution patient that taking other drugs used to decrease blood glucose level may lead to hypoglycemia. Review signs, symptoms, and appropriate treatment.
- Instruct patient to contact prescriber if he develops other illnesses, such as infection, or experiences trauma or surgery, because his diabetes medication may need adjustment.
- Advise patient to carry identification indicating that he has diabetes.
- Instruct patient to stop taking alogliptin and to report persistent severe abdominal pain, possibly radiating to the back, that may or may not be accompanied by vomiting.
- Alert patient that if severe joint pain occurs, he should notify prescriber as alogliptin may need to be discontinued.
- Review signs and symptoms of heart failure with patient and instruct her to notify prescriber immediately if present.

alosetron hydrochloride

Lotronex

Class and Category

Pharmacologic class: Selective serotonin 5-HT_3 receptor antagonist
Therapeutic class: Antidiarrheal
Pregnancy category: B

Indications and Dosages

➤ *To treat women with severe diarrhea-predominant irritable bowel syndrome (IBS) who have chronic IBS symptoms (usually lasting 6 months or longer) with no gastrointestinal tract anatomic or biochemical abnormalities present and who haven't responded to conventional therapy*

TABLETS

Adults. *Initial:* 0.5 mg twice a day for 4 wk, then increased up to 1 mg twice daily, if needed.

DOSAGE ADJUSTMENT For patient who develops constipation with initial dosage, drug discontinued until constipation is resolved and then re-started at 0.5 mg once a day.

Mechanism of Action

Inhibits activation of 5-HT_3 nonselective cation channels found in enteric neurons in the GI tract, thereby decreasing, colonic transit, secretions, and visceral sensations in the GI tract. These changes reduce GI pain and hyperactivity, symptoms that are prominent in diarrhea-predominant IBS.

Contraindications

Concomitant use with fluvoxamine, history of severe bowel disorders (chronic or severe constipation or sequelae from constipation, Crohn's disease, diverticulitis, GI perforation or adhesions, impaired intestinal circulation, intestinal obstruction or stricture, ischemic colitis, toxic megacolon, or ulcerative colitis), hypercoagulable state, hypersensitivity to alosetron or its components, severe hepatic impairment, thrombophlebitis

Interactions

DRUGS

cimetidine, clarithromycin, itraconazole, protease inhibitors, quinolones, telithromycin, voriconazole: Possibly increased alosetron level

fluvoxamine, ketoconazole: Increased blood alosetron level

Adverse Reactions

CNS: Anxiety, fatigue, headache, hypnagogic effects, malaise, temperature regulation disturbances

CV: Tachyarrhythmias

GI: Abdominal or GI discomfort and pain, abdominal distention, constipation (may be severe), diarrhea, dyspepsia, flatulence, **GI obstruction or perforation**, GI spasms or lesions, hemorrhoids, hemorrhoidal hemorrhage, hyposalivation, ileus, impaction, **ischemic colitis**, nausea, regurgitation and reflux, **small bowel mesenteric ischemia**, ulceration

GU: Urinary frequency

RESP: Breathing disorders

SKIN: Diaphoresis, rash, urticaria

Other: Nonspecific cramps or pain

Nursing Considerations

WARNING Be aware that alosetron is a restricted drug and is prescribed on a limited basis because of the potential for severe and life-threatening gastrointestinal complications. It should only be prescribed for women with severe IBS who have not responded to more conventional forms of treatment.

- Use alosetron cautiously in patients with mild to moderate liver dysfunction because alosetron is extensively metabolized in the liver.

WARNING **Monitor patient for constipation, especially if she's debilitated or elderly or takes drugs that decrease GI motility. Also watch for evidence of ischemic colitis, such as bloody diarrhea, new or worsening abdominal pain, or rectal bleeding. Serious adverse GI reactions may occur without warning. If they do, be prepared to stop alosetron therapy immediately. If discontinued for ischemic colitis, drug shouldn't be resumed later; however, a patient who no longer has constipation can resume it, if needed.**

- Expect drug to be discontinued if patient's IBS symptoms have not been adequately controlled after 4 weeks of treatment with 1 mg twice a day.

PATIENT TEACHING

- Explain that alosetron therapy can't begin until patient has read the medication guide that outlines drug's risks and benefits.
- Instruct patient not to start alosetron if constipated and to notify prescriber.
- Advise patient that serious adverse GI effects may occur without warning. Tell her to stop taking alosetron immediately and to notify prescriber if evidence of constipation or ischemic colitis arises. Tell

her to notify prescriber if constipation doesn't resolve after stopping drug.
- Inform patient that alosetron will be stopped after 4 weeks of 1 mg taken twice daily if it doesn't control IBS symptoms.

alprazolam

Alprazolam Intensol, Apo-Alpraz (CAN), Novo-Alprazol (CAN), Xanax, Xanax TS (CAN), Xanax XR

Class, Category, and Schedule

Pharmacologic class: Benzodiazepine
Therapeutic class: Anxiolytic, antipanic
Pregnancy category: D
Controlled substance schedule: IV

Indications and Dosages

➤ *To control anxiety disorders, relieve anxiety (short-term therapy), or treat anxiety associated with depression*

ORAL SOLUTION, ORALLY DISINTEGRATING TABLETS, TABLETS

Adults. *Initial:* 0.25 to 0.5 mg three times daily and increased, as needed, every 3 to 4 days. *Maximum:* 4 mg daily in divided doses.

DOSAGE ADJUSTMENT In elderly or debilitated patients or patients with advanced hepatic disease, initial dosage 0.25 mg twice daily or three times daily and increased gradually, as needed and tolerated.

➤ *To treat panic disorder*

ORAL SOLUTION, ORALLY DISINTEGRATING TABLETS, TABLETS

Adults. *Initial:* 0.5 mg three times daily, increased every 3 to 4 days by no more than 1 mg daily, based on patient response. *Maximum:* 10 mg in equally divided doses three or four times daily.

E.R. TABLETS

Adults. *Initial:* 0.5 to 1 mg daily in morning, increased every 3 to 4 days by no more than 1 mg daily, based on patient response. *Maximum:* 10 mg daily as single dose in morning.

Mechanism of Action

May increase effects of gamma-aminobutyric acid (GABA) and other inhibitory neurotransmitters by binding to specific benzodiazepine receptors in cortical and limbic areas of the CNS. GABA inhibits excitatory stimulation, which helps control emotional behavior. The limbic system contains many benzodiazepine receptors, which may help explain drug's antianxiety effects.

Contraindications

Acute angle-closure glaucoma; hypersensitivity to alprazolam, its components, or other benzodiazepines; itraconazole or ketoconazole therapy

Interactions

DRUGS

amiodarone, cyclosporine, diltiazem, ergotamine, isoniazid, macrolide antibiotics (clarithromycin, erythromycin), nicardipine, nifedipine, paroxetine, sertraline: Possible alteration in alprazolam plasma levels antacids: Altered alprazolam absorption rate
anticonvulsants; antidepressants; antihistamines; other benzodiazepines, CNS depressants, and psychotropics: Possibly increased CNS depressant effects
carbamazepine: Decreased plasma level of alprazolam and potential decreased effectiveness
cimetidine, fluoxetine, oral contraceptives, propoxyphene: Decreased alprazolam elimination and increased effects
digoxin: Possibly increased serum digoxin level, causing digitalis toxicity
itraconazole, ketoconazole: Possibly profoundly inhibited alprazolam metabolism
opioids: Increased risk of significant respiratory depression
phenytoin: Possibly increased serum phenytoin level, causing phenytoin toxicity

ACTIVITIES

alcohol use: Enhanced adverse CNS effects of alprazolam; increased risk of significant sedation and somnolence, especially if combined with an opioid

Adverse Reactions

CNS: Agitation, akathisia, confusion, depression, dizziness, drowsiness, fatigue, hallucinations, headache, insomnia, irritability, lack of coordination, light-headedness, memory loss, nervousness, paresthesia, rigidity, speech problems, syncope, tremor, weakness

CV: Chest pain, edema, **hypotension**, nonspecific ECG changes, palpitations, peripheral edema, tachycardia
EENT: Blurred vision, altered salivation, dry mouth, nasal congestion, tinnitus
ENDO: Galactorrhea, gynecomastia, hyperprolactinemia
GI: Abdominal discomfort, anorexia, constipation, diarrhea, elevated liver function test results, **hepatitis**, **hepatic failure**, nausea, vomiting
GU: Altered libido, urinary hesitancy
MS: Dysarthria, muscle rigidity and spasms
RESP: Hyperventilation, upper respiratory tract infection
SKIN: Dermatitis, diaphoresis, pruritus, rash, **Stevens-Johnson syndrome**
Other: Angioedema, weight gain or loss

Nursing Considerations

WARNING Be aware that opioid therapy should only be used concomitantly with alprazolam in patients for whom other treatment options are inadequate. If prescribed together, expect dosing and duration of the opioid to be limited. Monitor patient closely for signs and symptoms of decrease in consciousness, including coma, profound sedation, and significant respiratory depression. Notify prescriber immediately and provide emergency supportive care, as death may occur.

- Expect to give a higher dosage if patient's panic attacks occur unexpectedly or during such activities as driving.
- Plan to reduce dosage slowly when alprazolam is discontinued, as ordered, because use can lead to dependency.

PATIENT TEACHING

- Warn against stopping drug abruptly because withdrawal symptoms may occur.
- Instruct patient never to increase prescribed dose because of risk of dependency.
- Tell patient prescribed orally disintegrating tablets to use dry hands to remove tablet from bottle just prior to administration. Then she should immediately place the tablet on top of her tongue to dissolve. Inform patient that drinking a liquid beverage is not necessary after taking this form of alprazolam.

WARNING Warn patient not to consume alcohol or take an opioid during alprazolam treatment without prescriber knowledge, as severe respiratory depression can occur and may lead to death.

WARNING Inform patient about potentially fatal additive effects of combining alprazolam with an opioid. Instruct patient to inform all prescribers of alprazolam use, especially if pain medication may be prescribed.

- Advise patient to avoid driving and activities that require alertness until alprazolam's effects are known.
- Instruct female patient of childbearing age to notify prescriber immediately if she becomes or might be pregnant. Drug isn't recommended during pregnancy.

alteplase

(tissue plasminogen activator, recombinant)

Activase, Activase rt-PA (CAN), Cathflo Activase

Class and Category

Pharmacologic class: Tissue plasminogen activator (tPA)
Therapeutic class: Thrombolytic
Pregnancy category: Not classified

Indications and Dosages

➤ *To treat acute MI for reduction of mortality and incidence of heart failure*

I.V. INJECTION COMBINED WITH ACCELERATED I.V. INFUSION

Adults weighing more than 67 kg (148 lb). 15-mg bolus followed by 50 mg infused over 30 min and then 35 mg infused over next 60 min. *Maximum:* 100 mg.

Adults weighing 67 kg or less. 15-mg bolus followed by 0.75 mg/kg (up to 50 mg) infused over 30 min and then 0.5 mg/kg (up to 35 mg) infused over next 60 min. *Maximum:* 100 mg.

I.V. INJECTION COMBINED WITH 3-HOUR I.V. INFUSION

Adults weighing more than 65 kg (143 lb). 6 to 10 mg by bolus over first 1 to 2 min,

then as an infusion, 50 to 54 mg over remainder of first hour, 20 mg over second hour, and 20 mg over third hour. *Maximum.* 100 mg.
Adults weighing 65 kg or less. 0.075 mg/kg by bolus over first 1 to 2 min, then as an infusion, 0.675 mg/kg over remainder of first hour, 0.25 mg/kg over second hour, and 0.25 mg/kg over third hour. *Maximum:* 100 mg.

➤ *To treat acute ischemic stroke within 3 hr after onset of stroke symptoms and only after computed tomography or other diagnostic imaging method excludes intracranial hemorrhage.*

I.V. INJECTION COMBINED WITH I.V. INFUSION
Adults. 0.9 mg/kg infused over 60 min, with 10% of total dose given as bolus over first min. *Maximum:* 90 mg.

➤ *To treat acute massive pulmonary embolism*

I.V. INFUSION
Adults. 100 mg infused over 2 hr.

➤ To restore function of occluded central venous access devices

I.V. INJECTION (CATHFLO ACTIVASE)
Adults and children weighing 30 kg (66 lb) or more. 2 mg/2 ml instilled into occluded catheter; if unsuccessful, may repeat once after 2 hr.
Adults and children weighing less than 30 kg (66 lb). 110% of the lumen volume (not to exceed 2 mg/2ml) instilled into occluded catheter; if unsuccessful, may repeat once after 2 hr.

Route	Onset	Peak	Duration
I.V.	Immediate	20–120 min	4 hr

Mechanism of Action
Binds to fibrin in a thrombus and converts trapped plasminogen to plasmin. Plasmin breaks down fibrin, fibrinogen, and other clotting factors, which dissolves the thrombus.

Incompatibilities
Don't add other drugs to solution that contains alteplase.

Contraindications
For all indications: Active internal bleeding, arteriovenous malformation or aneurysm, bleeding diathesis, hypersensitivity to alteplase or its components, intracranial neoplasm, severe uncontrolled hypertension
For acute MI and pulmonary embolism only: History of stroke, intracranial or intraspinal surgery or trauma in past 3 months
For acute ischemic stroke only: Recent head trauma, recent intracranial or intraspinal surgery or trauma in past 3 months, recent stroke, seizure activity at onset of stroke, subarachnoid hemorrhage, suspicion or history of intracranial hemorrhage

Interactions
DRUGS
angiotensin-converting enzyme (ACE) inhibitors: Possible increased risk of angioedema
anticoagulants, antiplatets, vitamin K antagonists: Increased risk of bleeding

Adverse Reactions
CNS: **Cerebral edema or herniation**, **CVA**, fever, **seizures**
CV: **Arrhythmias (including bradycardia and electromechanical dissociation)**, **cardiac arrest**, **cardiac tamponade**, **cardiogenic shock**, **cholesterol embolism**, **coronary thrombolysis**, **heart failure**, **hypotension**, mitral insufficiency, **myocardial reinfarction or rupture**, **pericardial effusion**, **pericarditis**, **venous embolism or thrombosis**
EENT: Epistaxis, gingival bleeding, **laryngeal edema**
GI: **GI bleeding**, nausea, **retroperitoneal bleeding**, vomiting
GU: **GU bleeding**
HEME: **Bleeding that may be severe**
RESP: Pleural effusion, **pulmonary edema**, **pulmonary reembolization**
SKIN: Bleeding at puncture sites, ecchymosis, rash, urticaria
Other: **Anaphylaxis**, **angioedema**

Nursing Considerations
WARNING Know that treatment for acute ischemic stroke must begin within 3 hours after onset of stroke symptoms and only after computed tomography or other diagnostic imaging method excludes intracranial hemorrhage to avoid complications.
WARNING Monitor patient closely for hypersensitivity reactions which may be life-threatening (angioedema, laryngeal edema, rash, shock) during alteplase

administration and for several hours after infusion is completed. If hypersensitivity occurs, discontinue the alteplase infusion immediately and institute appropriate emergency interventions such as administering antihistamines, epinephrine, or intravenous corticosteroids as prescribed.

- Reconstitute alteplase with sterile water for injection only immediately before use. Swirl gently to dissolve powder; don't shake.

WARNING Know that alteplase can cause internal bleeding that could be severe and sometimes fatal, as well as external bleeding, especially at arterial and venous puncture sites. Avoid intramuscular injections and trauma to patient receiving drug. Discontinue alteplase immediately if serious bleeding occurs. Be aware that the following conditions increases risk: advanced age, especially if patient is currently receiving anticoagulant therapy; acute pericarditis; cerebrovascular disease; diabetic hemorrhagic retinopathy or other hemorrhagic ophthalmic conditions; hemostatic defects including those secondary to severe hepatic or renal disease; hypertension (diastolic above 110 mm/Hg or systolic above 175 mm Hg); pregnancy; recent gastrointestinal or genitourinary bleeding, intracranial hemorrhage, or trauma; septic thrombophlebitis or occluded AV cannula at seriously infected site; significant hepatic dysfunction; or subacute bacterial endocarditis.

- Minimize bleeding from noncompressible sites by avoiding internal jugular and subclavian venous puncture sites.
- Apply pressure at puncture site for at least 30 minutes, followed by a pressure dressing after administering alteplase.
- Assess blood pressure and heart rate and rhythm frequently during and after therapy.

WARNING Monitor continuous ECG for arrhythmias during drug therapy because alteplase therapy may cause arrhythmias from sudden reperfusion of the myocardium.

- Be aware that the use of thrombolytics such as alteplase can increase the risk of thromboembolic events in patients with high risk of left heart thrombus, such as patients with atrial fibrillation or mitral stenosis. Also know that the drug does not adequately treat underlyng deep vein thrombosis in patients with a pulmonary embolism. Watch this type of patient closely for re-embolization.
- Store reconstituted solution at room temperature (about 30°C [86°F]) or refrigerated (2.2° to 7.7°C [(36° to 46°F]).
- Know that the most common complication of thrombolytic therapy is bleeding and that pregnancy may increase this risk. Monitor pregnant patient closely for evidence of bleeding.

PATIENT TEACHING

- Tell patient to immediately report bleeding, including from the nose or gums.
- Advise patient to limit physical activity during alteplase administration to reduce risk of injury and bleeding.

aluminum carbonate

Basaljel

aluminum hydroxide

Alternagel, Alu-Cap, Alugel (CAN), Alu-Tab, Amphojel, Dialume

Class and Category

Pharmacologic class: Aluminum salt
Therapeutic: Antacid, phosphate binder
Pregnancy category: Not classified

Indications and Dosages

➤ *To treat hyperacidity associated with gastric hyperacidity, gastritis, hiatal hernia, peptic esophagitis, and peptic ulcers; to prevent phosphate renal calculus formation*

CAPSULES, SUSPENSION, TABLETS (ALUMINUM CARBONATE)

Adults. 2 capsules or tablets or 10 ml suspension every 2 hr up to 12 times daily, as needed.

CAPSULES, TABLETS (ALUMINUM HYDROXIDE)

Adults. 500 to 1,500 mg in divided doses 3 to 6 times daily, taken between meals and at bedtime.

SUSPENSION

Adults. 5 to 30 ml, as needed, taken between meals and at bedtime.

➤ *To reduce hyperphosphatemia in chronic renal failure*

ORAL SUSPENSION

Adults. 300 mg to 600 mg three times daily.

Children. 50 to 150 mg/kg/day in 4 to 6 divided doses.

Route	Onset	Peak	Duration
P.O.	Varies	Unknown	20–40 min*

* If fasting; at least 3 hr if given 1 hr after meals.

Mechanism of Action

Neutralizes or reduces gastric acidity, increasing stomach and duodenal alkalinity. Protects stomach and duodenum lining by inhibiting pepsin's proteolytic activity. Binds with phosphate ions in intestine to form insoluble aluminum–phosphate compounds, which lower blood phosphate level.

Contraindications

Hypersensitivity to aluminum or its components

Interactions

DRUGS

allopurinol, chloroquine, corticosteroids, diflunisal, digoxin, ethambutol, H_2*-receptor blockers, iron, isoniazid, penicillamine, phenothiazines, ranitidine, tetracyclines, thyroid hormones, ticlopidine:* Decreased effects of these drugs

benzodiazepines: Increased benzodiazepine effects

Adverse Reactions

CNS: Encephalopathy

GI: Constipation, **intestinal obstruction**, white-speckled stool

MS: Osteomalacia, osteoporosis

Other: Aluminum intoxication, electrolyte imbalances

Nursing Considerations

- Don't give aluminum hydroxide within 1 to 2 hours of other oral drugs.
- Know that two 0.6-g aluminum hydroxide tablets can neutralize 16 mEq of acid.
- Monitor patient's serum levels of sodium, phosphate, and other electrolytes, as appropriate.

PATIENT TEACHING

- Instruct patient to chew tablets thoroughly before swallowing and then to drink a full glass of water.
- Warn patient not to take maximum dosage for more than 2 weeks unless prescribed because doing so may cause stomach to secrete excess hydrochloric acid.
- Teach patient to prevent constipation with a high-fiber diet and increased fluid intake (2 to 3 L daily), if appropriate.
- Advise patient to notify prescriber about taking other medications and supplements before taking aluminum because of risk of interactions.
- Advise patient to notify prescriber if symptoms worsen or don't subside.

alvimopan

Entereg

Class and Category

Pharmacologic class: Peripherally acting mu-opiod antagonist

Therapeutic class: Bowel function restorative

Pregnancy category: B

Indications and Dosages

➤ *To accelerate GI recovery in hospitalized patients after partial large- or small-bowel resection with primary anastomosis*

CAPSULES

Adults. *Initial:* 12 mg 30 min to 5 hr before surgery, followed by 12 mg twice daily, starting the day after surgery for up to 7 days or until discharge. *Maximum:* 24 mg/day with a maximum of 15 doses total.

Route	Onset	Peak	Duration
P.O.	Unknown	2 hr	Unknown

Mechanism of Action

Competitively binds to selective mu-opioid receptors in GI tract, antagonizing peripheral effects of opioids on GI motility and secretion without reversing the central analgesic effects of opioid agonists. This action alleviates postoperative ileus by causing bowel function to return more quickly after part of bowel has been removed and an end-to-end anastomosis performed.

Contraindications

Complete gastrointestinal obstruction, hypersensitivity to alvimopan or its components, presence of gastric or pancreatic anastomosis, severe hepatic or renal impairment, use of opioids for more than 7 consecutive days immediately before alvimopan starts

Interactions

DRUGS

opioids given within previous 7 days at therapeutic doses: Increased risk of serious adverse reactions

Adverse Reactions

GI: Abdominal pain, constipation, diarrhea, dyspepsia, flatulence
GU: Urine retention
HEME: Anemia
MS: Back pain
Other: Hypokalemia

Nursing Considerations

- Don't give alvimopan to patients with severe hepatic or renal impairment or to patients having surgery to correct a complete bowel obstruction.
- Know that alvimopan is prescribed only for short-term use with maximum of 15 doses and is only dispensed in hospitals enrolled in Entereg Access Support and Education (EASE) program. Closely monitor number of doses given, and expect to stop drug when patient has received 15 doses or is discharged from hospital, because there is a potential risk for patient to experience a myocardial infarction if drug is used beyond 15 doses.
- Monitor patient's serum potassium level closely, as ordered, because drug may cause hypokalemia. Also check patient's hemoglobin level and hematocrit because drug has been associated with anemia.
- Monitor patient with mild to moderate hepatic or renal failure for evidence of high alvimopan levels, such as abdominal pain or cramping, diarrhea, nausea, and vomiting. Also monitor patients recently exposed to opioids, as they may be more sensitive to the effects of alvimopan and experience greater gastrointestinal effects. If present, alert prescriber.
- Monitor Japanese patients closely for possible adverse effects because alvimopan level may be higher in this population.

PATIENT TEACHING

- Explain the need to accurately describe long-term or intermittent use of opioid pain therapy, including any use of opioids in the week before receiving alvimopan. Taking alvimopan after such use may cause serious adverse GI reactions.
- Inform patient that the most common adverse effects of alvimopan are constipation, dyspepsia, and flatulence.
- Tell patient that drug is for in-hospital use only and will not be taken at home.

amantadine

Gocovri, Osmolex ER

amantadine hydrochloride

(adamantanamine hydrochloride)

Class and Category

Pharmacologic class: Dopamine agonist
Therapeutic class: Antidyskinetic, antiviral
Pregnancy category: C

Indications and Dosages

➤ *To manage symptoms of primary Parkinson's disease, postencephalitic Parkinsonism, arteriosclerotic Parkinsonism, and Parkinsonism caused by CNS injury from carbon monoxide intoxication*

CAPSULES, SYRUP, TABLETS (SYMMETREL)

Adults who do not have serious medical illnesses or who are not receiving high doses of other antiparkinson drugs. 100 mg twice daily and increased, as needed.

Adults with serious associated medical illnesses or who are receiving high doses of other antiparkinson drugs. 100 mg once daily, increased after 1 to several weeks to 100 mg twice daily, if needed. *Maximum:* 400 mg daily in divided doses.

➤ *To treat drug-induced extrapyramidal reactions*

CAPSULES, SYRUP, TABLETS (SYMMETREL)

Adults. *Initial:* 100 mg twice daily and then increased, as needed. *Maximum:* 300 mg daily in divided doses.

➤ *To prevent and treat respiratory tract infection caused by influenza A virus*

CAPSULES, SYRUP, TABLETS (SYMMETREL)

Adults up to age 65 and children age 12 and over. *Initial:* 200 mg daily or 100 mg twice daily and continued for at least 10 days following exposure or, if used in conjunction with inactivated influenza A virus vaccine, until protective antibody responses develop, continued for 2 to 4 wk after vaccine has been given. Treatment started as soon as possible, preferably within 24 to 48 hr after onset of signs and symptoms and continued for 24 to 48 hr after signs and symptoms disappear. *Maximum:* 200 mg daily.

Adults age 65 and over. 100 mg daily and continued for at least 10 days following exposure or, if used in conjunction with inactivated influenza A virus vaccine, until protective antibody responses develop, continued for 2 to 4 wk after vaccine has been given. Treatment should be started as soon as possible, preferably within 24 to 48 hr after onset of signs and symptoms, and should be continued for 24 to 48 hr after signs and symptoms disappear.

Children ages 9 to 12. 100 mg every 12 hr, started in anticipation of an influenza A outbreak and before or after contact with individuals with influenza A virus respiratory tract illness. Treatment started as soon as possible, preferably within 24 to 48 hr after onset of signs and symptoms and continued for 24 to 48 hr after signs and symptoms disappear. *Maximum:* 200 mg daily.

Children ages 1 to 9 2.2 to 4.4 mg/kg every 12 hr, started in anticipation of an influenza A outbreak and before or after contact with individuals with influenza A virus respiratory tract illness. Treatment started as soon as possible, preferably within 24 to 48 hr after onset of signs and symptoms and continued for 24 to 48 hr after signs and symptoms disappear. *Maximum:* 150 mg/day.

DOSAGE ADJUSTMENT (SYMMETREL) For all indications in adult patient with a creatinine clearance of 30 to 50 ml/min, 200 mg on day 1 and then 100 mg daily. For patient with a creatinine clearance of 15 to 29 ml/min, 200 mg on day 1 and then 100 mg every other day. For patient with creatinine clearance less than 15 ml/min or patient on hemodialysis, 200 mg weekly. For patients with congestive heart failure, orthostatic hypotension, or peripheral edema, dosage may have to be reduced. For patient who develops central nervous system adverse effects or other effects while taking 200 mg once daily dose, dosage split into 100 mg twice daily.

➤ *To treat dyskinesia in patients with Parkinson's disease receiving levodopa-based therapy*

E.R. CAPSULES (GOCOVRI)

Adults. *Initial:* 137 mg once daily at bedtime. After 1 wk, increased to 274 mg once daily at bedtime.

DOSAGE ADJUSTMENT (GOCOVRI) For patient with a creatinine clearance of 30 to 59 ml/min, initial dosage reduced to 68.5 mg once daily at bedtime, with maximum dosage not to exceed 137 mg once daily at bedtime. For patient with a creatinine clearance of 15 to 29 ml/min, dosage reduced to 68.5 mg once daily at bedtime with no increased dosage adjustment.

➤ *To treat Parkinson's disease; to treat drug-induced extrapyramidal reactions*

E.R. TABLETS (OSMOLEX ER)

Adults. *Initial:* 129 mg once daily in morning with dosage increased weekly to 322 mg. *Maximum:* 322 mg given as a 129 mg and 193 mg tablet in morning.

DOSAGE ADJUSTMENT (OSMOLEX ER) For patient with a creatinine clearance of 30 to 59 ml/min, dosage titration done every 3 weeks instead of weekly and dosing frequency increased to one dose every 48 hours. For patients with a creatinine clearance of 15 to 29 ml/min, dosage titration interval increased to every 4 weeks instead of weekly, and dosing frequency increased to one dose every 96 hours.

Route	Onset	Peak	Duration
P.O.	In 48 hr*	Unknown	Unknown

* Antidyskinetic action; antiviral action unknown.

Mechanism of Action

Affects dopamine, a neurotransmitter that is synthesized and released by neurons leading from substantia nigra to basal ganglia and is essential for normal motor function. In Parkinson's disease, progressive degeneration of these neurons reduces intrasynaptic dopamine. Amantadine may cause dopamine to accumulate in the basal ganglia by increasing dopamine release or by blocking dopamine reuptake into the presynaptic neurons of the CNS. Amantadine also may stimulate dopamine receptors or make postsynaptic receptors more sensitive to dopamine. These actions help control alterations in involuntary muscle movements, such as tremors and rigidity, that are associated with Parkinson's disease.

Amantadine may inhibit influenza A viral replication by blocking uncoating of virus and release of viral nucleic acid into respiratory epithelial cells. It also may interfere with early replication of viruses that have already penetrated cells.

Contraindications

Angle-closure glaucoma, hypersensitivity to amantadine or its components

Interactions

DRUGS

anticholinergics or other drugs with anticholinergic activity, other antidyskinetics, antihistamines, phenothiazines, tricyclic antidepressants: Possibly increased anticholinergic effects and risk of paralytic ileus

carbidopa-levodopa, levodopa: Increased effectiveness of these drugs

CNS stimulants: Excessive CNS stimulation, possibly causing arrhythmias, insomnia, irritability, nervousness, or seizures

hydrochlorothiazide, triamterene: Possibly decreased amantadine clearance and increased risk of toxicity

live-virus vaccines: Possibly interference with vaccine effectiveness

quinidine, quinine, trimethoprim-sulfamethoxazole: Increased blood amantadine level

ACTIVITIES

alcohol use: Possibly increased risk of CNS effects—including confusion, dizziness, and light-headedness—and orthostatic hypotension

Adverse Reactions

CNS: Agitation, anxiety, confusion, dizziness, drowsiness, fatigue, fever, hallucinations, insomnia, irritability, light-headedness, mental impairment, nervousness, **neuroleptic malignant syndrome**, nightmares, **suicidal ideation**, syncope

CV: Arrhythmias, cardiac arrest, orthostatic hypotension, peripheral edema, tachycardia

EENT: Blurred vision; dry mouth, nose, or throat; keratitis; mydriasis

GI: Constipation, diarrhea, dysphagia, nausea

GU: Dysuria, increased libido

HEME: Agranulocytosis, leukopenia, neutropenia

RESP: Acute respiratory failure, pulmonary edema, tachypnea

SKIN: Diaphoresis, livedo reticularis (purplish, netlike rash), pruritus

Other: Anaphylaxis; intense urges to perform certain activities, such as gambling or sexual acts

Nursing Considerations

- Be aware that amantadine should not be used as the first drug of choice to prevent or treat influenza A because of high levels of resistance to the drug that has developed over the past several years.
- Monitor patients who have a history of psychiatric illness or substance abuse because amantadine may worsen these conditions. Some patients taking amantadine have attempted suicide or had suicidal ideation.
- Monitor for weight gain and edema because drug may cause redistribution of body fluid.
- Be aware that amantadine may increase seizure activity in patients with a history of seizures.

WARNING Monitor patient for evidence of neuroleptic malignant syndrome during dosage reduction or discontinuation of therapy. These include fever, hypertension or hypotension, involuntary motor activity, mental changes, muscle rigidity, tachycardia, and tachypnea. Be prepared to provide supportive treatment and additional drug therapy, as prescribed.

- Be aware that patients receiving more than 200 mg daily are more likely to experience adverse or toxic reactions.
- Monitor patient for decreased drug effectiveness over time. If therapeutic response declines, expect to increase dosage or discontinue drug temporarily, as ordered.
- Assess patient regularly for skin changes because melanoma risk is higher in those with Parkinson's disease. It isn't clear whether the risk is increased by the disease or by its treatment.

PATIENT TEACHING

- Instruct patient to take amantadine exactly as prescribed and not to stop abruptly.
- Instruct patient taking Osmolex ER tablets to swallow tablets whole and not to chew, crush, or divide tablets. Advise patient to notify prescriber if drug becomes less effective.
- Tell patient to notify prescriber if influenza symptoms don't improve after 2 to 3 days.

WARNING Advise patient or family member to notify prescriber immediately if patient reveals thoughts of suicide.

- Encourage patient to avoid consuming alcohol during amantadine therapy because alcohol may increase the risk of confusion, dizziness, light-headedness, or orthostatic hypotension.
- Advise patient to avoid driving and other activities that require a high level of alertness until he knows how the drug affects him because it may cause blurred vision and mental impairment.
- Advise patient to change positions slowly to minimize effects of orthostatic hypotension.
- Tell patient to use ice chips or sugarless candy or gum to relieve dry mouth.
- Caution patient to resume physical activities gradually as signs and symptoms improve.
- Urge patient to have regular skin examinations by a dermatologist or other qualified health professional.
- Instruct patient to notify prescriber about intense urges, such as for gambling or sex, because dosage may need to be reduced or drug discontinued.

amikacin sulfate

Amikin, Arikayce

Class and Category

Pharmacologic class: Aminoglycoside
Therapeutic class: Antibiotic
Pregnancy category: D

Indications and Dosages

➤ *To treat serious gram-negative bacterial infections (including bone, burns, CNS, joint, intra-abdominal, postoperative infections, respiratory tract, skin and soft-tissue; neonatal sepsis; septicemia; and serious, complicated, and recurrent UTI) caused by* Acinetobacter, Enterobacter, Escherichia coli, Klebsiella, Proteus, Providencia, Pseudomonas, *and* Serratia; *and susceptible strains of* staphylococci *in patients allergic to other antibiotics, and in mixed staphylococcal/gram-negative infections*

I.V. INFUSION, I.M. INJECTION

Adults and children. 15 mg/kg daily in equal doses at equally spaced intervals (7.5 mg/kg every 12 hr or 5 mg/kg every 8 hr) for 7 to 10 days. I.V. infusion administered over 30 to 60 min.
Neonates. *Loading dose:* 10 mg/kg. I.V. infusion administered over 1 to 2 hr. *Maintenance:* 7.5 mg/kg every 12 hr for 7 to 10 days. I.V. infusion administered over 1 to 2 hr. *Maximum:* 15 mg/kg daily.

➤ *To treat uncomplicated UTI*

I.V. INFUSION, I.M. INJECTION

Adults. 250 mg twice daily for 7 to 10 days. I.V. infusion administered over 30 to 60 min.

DOSAGE ADJUSTMENT (AMIKIN) For patients with impaired renal function, loading dose of 7.5 mg/kg daily; then maintenance dosage based on creatinine clearance and serum creatinine level and given every 12 hr. For morbidly obese patients, dosage not to exceed 1.5 g daily.

➤ *To treat refractory* Mycobacterium avium *complex (MAC) lung disease for patients who did not achieve negative sputum cultures after a minimum of 6 consecutive months of a multi-drug background regimen therapy*

ORAL INHALATION (ARIKAYCE)

Adults. 590 mg once daily using the Lamira Nebulizer System.

Route	Onset	Peak	Duration
I.V.	Immediate	Unknown	Unknown
I.M.	Rapid	Unknown	Unknown

Mechanism of Action
Binds to negatively charged sites on bacteria's outer cell membrane, disrupting cell integrity. Also binds to bacterial ribosomal subunits and inhibits protein synthesis. Both actions lead to cell death.

Incompatibilities
Don't mix or infuse amikacin with other drugs.

Contraindications
Hypersensitivity to amikacin, other aminoglycosides, or their components

Interactions
DRUGS

general anesthetics: Increased risk of neuromuscular blockade
loop diuretics: Increased risk of ototoxicity
neuromuscular blockers: Possibly increased neuromuscular blockade and prolonged respiratory depression
penicillins: Possibly inactivation of or synergistic effects with amikacin
other nephrotoxic drugs: Increased risk of nephrotoxicity

Adverse Reactions
CNS: Drowsiness, headache, loss of balance, **neuromuscular blockade**, tremor, vertigo
EENT: Hearing loss, ototoxicity, tinnitus
GI: Nausea, vomiting
GU: Azotemia, dysuria, **nephrotoxicity**, oliguria or polyuria, proteinuria
MS: Acute muscle paralysis; arthralgia; muscle fatigue, spasms, and weakness
RESP: Apnea; *Inhalation form:* **bronchospasm**, exacerbation of underlying pulmonary disease, **hemoptysis**, **hypersensitivity penumonitis**
Other: Hyperkalemia

Nursing Considerations
- Expect to obtain results of culture and sensitivity testing before therapy begins.
- Obtain patient's weight prior to treatment for calculation of correct dosage.
- Prepare amikacin I.V. solution by adding contents of 500-mg vial to 100 or 200 ml of sterile diluent. Then infuse drug over 30 to 60 minutes for adults and children and 1 to 2 hours for neonates.
- Give I.M. injection in large muscle mass.
- Know that Arikayce is for oral inhalation use only. Administer by nebulization only using the Lamira Nebulizer System. Prior to opening glass vial, shake vial well for at least 10 to 15 seconds until the contents appear uniform and well mixed. Open the vial by flipping up the plastic top of the vial then pulling downward to loosen the metal ring. The metal ring and rubber stopper should be removed carefully. Then pour the contents of the vial into the medication reservoir of the nebulizer handset.
- Know that patients with asthma, brochospasm, chronic obstructive pulmonary disease, or known hyper-reactive airway disease, may need to be pretreated with a short-acting selective beta-2 agonist. This is because the drug has been associated with an increased risk of respiratory adverse reactions such as bronchospasm, exacerbation of underlying pulmonary disease, hemoptysis and hypersensitivity penumonitis.
- Watch for signs of ototoxicity, such as tinnitus and vertigo, especially during high-dosage or prolonged amikacin therapy.

WARNING **Assess renal function before and daily during therapy, as ordered because amikacin may produce nephrotoxic effects. To minimize renal tubule irritation, maintain hydration during therapy.**

- Be aware that amikacin may exacerbate muscle weakness in such conditions as myasthenia gravis and Parkinson's disease.

- Measure serum amikacin concentrations as ordered, usually 30 to 90 minutes after injection (for peak concentration) and just before administering next parenteral dose (for trough concentration).

PATIENT TEACHING

- Tell patient that daily laboratory tests are necessary during treatment.
- Instruct patient to report ringing in ears, hearing changes, headache, nausea, vomiting, and changes in urination.
- Instruct patient prescribed oral inhalation amikacin therapy how to administer drug. Tell patient that drug is to be administered by nebulization only using the Lamira Nebulizer System. Prior to opening glass vial, instruct patient to shake vial well for at least 10 to 15 seconds until the contents appear uniform and well mixed. Then patient should open the vial by flipping up the plastic top of the vial then pulling downward to loosen the metal ring. The metal ring and rubber stopper should be removed carefully. Then tell patient to pour the contents of the vial into the medication reservoir of the nebulizer handset and then follow manufacturer instructions on use of the nebulizer unit.
- Tell patient using oral inhalation form that if he misses a daily dose, he should administer the next dose the next day and not double the dose.

WARNING **Alert patient taking drug by oral inhalation to seek immediate medical attention if he experiences breathing difficulty.**

amiloride hydrochloride

Apo Amiloride (CAN), Midamor

Class and Category

Pharmacologic class: Potassium-sparing diuretic
Therapeutic class: Diuretic
Pregnancy category: B

Indications and Dosages

➤ *As adjunct to loop or thiazide diuretic therapy in patient with heart failure or hypertension to correct diuretic-induced hypokalemia or to prevent diuretic-induced hypokalemia that increases the risk of arrhythmias or other complications*

TABLETS

Adults. 5 to 10 mg daily as single dose; if hypokalemia persists, increased to 15 mg daily and then 20 mg daily.

Route	Onset	Peak	Duration
P.O.	2 hr	6–10 hr	24 hr

Mechanism of Action

Inhibits sodium reabsorption in distal convoluted tubules and cortical collecting ducts, causing sodium and water loss and enhancing potassium retention.

Contraindications

Hypersensitivity to amiloride or its components; impaired renal function; serum potassium level above 5.5 mEq/L; therapy with another potassium-sparing diuretic, such as spironolactone or triamterene, or a potassium supplement

Interactions

DRUGS

angiotensin-converting enzyme inhibitors, angiotensin II receptor antagonists, cyclosporine, enalapril, lisinopril, potassium products, spironolactone: Increased risk of hyperkalemia
digoxin: Decreased effectiveness of digoxin
lithium: Reduced renal clearance of lithium and increased risk of lithium toxicity
NSAIDs: Reduced diuretic effect of amiloride

FOODS

high-potassium food: Increased risk of hyperkalemia

Adverse Reactions

CNS: Confusion, depression, dizziness, drowsiness, **encephalopathy**, fatigue, headache, insomnia, nervousness, paresthesia, somnolence, tremor, vertigo
CV: Angina, **arrhythmias**, orthostatic hypotension, palpitations
EENT: Dry mouth, increased intraocular pressure, nasal congestion, tinnitus, vision disturbances
GI: Abdominal pain or fullness, anorexia, appetite changes, constipation, diarrhea, **GI bleeding**, heartburn, indigestion, jaundice, nausea, thirst, vomiting

GU: Bladder spasms, dysuria, impotence, loss of libido, polyuria
HEME: **Aplastic anemia, neutropenia**
MS: Arthralgia, muscle spasms or weakness
RESP: Cough, dyspnea
SKIN: Alopecia, pruritus, rash
Other: Dehydration, hyperchloremia, **hyperkalemia, hypernatremia, metabolic acidosis**

Nursing Considerations

- Administer amiloride with food to reduce GI upset and early in the day to minimize sleep interference from polyuria.
- Monitor renal function test results, fluid intake and output, and weight. Also monitor serum potassium level to detect hyperkalemia.

WARNING Don't administer amiloride with other potassium-sparing diuretics.

PATIENT TEACHING

- Warn patient to avoid high-potassium food and salt substitutes that contain potassium.
- Advise patient to consult prescriber before taking other drugs, including OTC remedies, especially sympathomimetics.
- Tell patient to report dizziness, trembling, numbness, and muscle weakness or spasms.
- Advise patient to increase fluid and fiber intake to prevent constipation.
- Warn patient to expect reversible hair loss and impotence.

aminocaproic acid

Amicar

Class and Category

Pharmacologic class: Aminohexanoic acid
Therapeutic class: Antifibrinolytic, antihemorrhagic
Pregnancy category: C

Indications and Dosages

➤ *To treat excessive bleeding caused by fibrinolysis*

ORAL SOLUTION, SYRUP, TABLETS

Adults. *Initial:* 5 g in first hour, followed by 1 to 1.25 g/hr to sustain drug plasma level of 0.13 mg/ml. *Maximum:* 30 g daily.

I.V. INFUSION

Adults. 4 to 5 g in 250 ml of diluent over 1 hr followed by continuous infusion of 1 g/hr (4 ml/hr) in 50 ml of diluent. Continued for 8 hr or until bleeding stops.

Route	Onset	Peak	Duration
P.O.	Rapid	Unknown	Unknown
I.V.	Immediate	Unknown	Under 3 hr

Mechanism of Action

Inhibits breakdown of blood clots by interfering with plasminogen activator substances and producing antiplasmin activity.

Contraindications

Active intravascular clotting such as in disseminated intravascular coagulation, hypersensitivity to aminocaproic acid or its components, upper urinary tract bleeding

Interactions

DRUGS

activated prothrombin, prothrombin complex concentrates: Increased risk of thrombosis
estrogens, oral contraceptives: Increased risk of hypercoagulation

Adverse Reactions

CNS: **CVA,** delirium, dizziness, hallucinations, headache, malaise, weakness
CV: **Bradycardia, cardiomyopathy,** elevated serum CK level, **hypotension,** ischemia, thrombophlebitis
EENT: Nasal congestion, tinnitus
GI: Abdominal cramps and pain, diarrhea, elevated AST level, nausea, vomiting
GU: Elevated BUN level, **intrarenal obstruction, renal failure**
HEME: **Agranulocytosis, leukopenia, thrombocytopenia**
MS: Myopathy
RESP: Dyspnea, **pulmonary embolism**
SKIN: Pruritus, rash
Other: Elevated serum aldolase levels, **hyperkalemia**

Nursing Considerations

- Be aware that patients on oral therapy prescribed tablet form may need up to 10 tablets during the first hour of treatment and tablets around the clock during continued treatment.
- Mix aminocaproic acid solution for intravenous infusion with sterile water for injection, normal saline solution, D_5W, or Ringer's solution.

WARNING **Avoid rapid I.V. delivery because it increases risk of hypotension and bradycardia.**

- Monitor neurologic status for drug-induced changes. Note that increased clotting may lead to stroke.

PATIENT TEACHING

- Tell patient that he'll be closely monitored during I.V. therapy and will have blood drawn for laboratory tests before, during, and after treatment.
- Advise patient who takes aminocaproic acid at home to report adverse reactions, take drug exactly as prescribed, and keep follow-up appointments with prescriber.

aminoglutethimide

Cytadren

Class and Category

Pharmacologic class: Adrenal steroid inhibitor
Therapeutic class: Adrenal steroid inhibitor
Pregnancy category: D

Indications and Dosages

➤ *To suppress adrenal function in patients with Cushing's syndrome who are waiting for surgery or for whom other treatment can't be used*

TABLETS

Adults. *Initial:* 250 mg every 6 hr. Increased as needed by 250 mg daily every 1 to 2 wk. *Maximum:* 2,000 mg daily.

Route	Onset	Peak	Duration
P.O.	3–5 days	Unknown	72 hr

Mechanism of Action

Inhibits the conversion of cholesterol to delta-5-pregnenolone, which is needed to produce certain hormones, including adrenal glucocorticoids, mineralocorticoids, estrogens, and androgens.

Contraindications

Hypersensitivity to aminoglutethimide, glutethimide or their components

Interactions

DRUGS

antidiabetics, dexamethasone, digoxin, medroxyprogesterone, synthetic glucocorticoids, theophylline, warfarin and other oral anticoagulants: Decreased effects of these drugs

Adverse Reactions

CNS: Dizziness, drowsiness, fever, headache
CV: **Hypotension**, orthostatic hypotension, tachycardia
ENDO: Adrenal insufficency, hypothyroidism, masculinization
GI: Anorexia, nausea
SKIN: Hair growth, morbilliform rash, pruritus, urticaria

Nursing Considerations

- Expect to reduce aminoglutethimide dosage or discontinue treatment if extreme drowsiness, severe rash, or excessively low cortisol level occurs.

WARNING **Monitor for signs of hypothyroidism, including lethargy, dry skin, and slow pulse. If prescribed, administer thyroid hormone supplement.**

- Monitor blood pressure for orthostatic or persistent hypotension.

PATIENT TEACHING

- Teach patient to recognize orthostatic hypotension (dizziness, weakness when moving from sitting to standing position) and to minimize it by rising slowly from a supine to an upright position.
- Tell patient to report dizziness, appetite loss, nausea, headache, or severe drowsiness. Warn him to avoid driving if drowsy.
- Instruct patient to take a missed dose as soon as remembered and to space out the day's remaining doses evenly.
- Advise patient that rash, sometimes accompanied by fever, may appear on day 10 of treatment and should subside by day 15 or 16. Tell him to report severe rash or one that doesn't disappear.

amiodarone hydrochloride

Cordarone, Nexterone, Pacerone

Class and Category

Pharmacologic class: Benzofuran derivative
Therapeutic class: Class III antiarrhythmic
Pregnancy category: D

Indications and Dosages

➤ *To treat life-threatening, recurrent ventricular fibrillation and hemodynamically unstable ventricular tachycardia when these arrhythmias don't respond to other drugs or when patient can't tolerate other drugs*

TABLETS (CORDARONE, PACERONE)

Adults. *Loading:* 800 to 1,600 mg daily in divided doses for 1 to 3 wk. *Maintenance:* 600 to 800 mg daily in divided doses for 1 mo; then if cardiac rhythm is stable, 400 mg daily given as a single dose or divided into 2 doses.

➤ *To treat or prevent life-threatening, recurrent ventricular fibrillation and hemodynamically unstable ventricular tachycardia when these arrhythmias don't respond to other drugs, when patient can't tolerate other drugs, or when oral amiodarone is indicated but patient is unable to take oral medication*

I.V. INFUSION (CORDARONE)

Adults. *Loading:* 150 mg over 10 min (15 mg/min) followed by 360 mg infused over 6 hr (1 mg/min). *Maintenance:* 540 mg infused over 18 hr (0.5 mg/min); then after the first 24 hr, 720 mg infused over 24 hr (0.5 mg/min), continued up to 2 to 3 wk, as needed. Rate may be increased in first 24 hr, if needed, but initial infusion rate shouldn't exceed 30 mg/min. Changed to oral form as soon as possible.

I.V. INFUSION (NEXTERONE)

Adults. *Loading:* 150 mg/100 ml premixed in dextrose over 10 min (15 mg/min) followed by 360 mg/200 ml premixed in dextrose infused over 6 hr (1 mg/min). *Maintenance:* 540 mg infused over 18 hr (0.5 mg/min) using 360 mg/200 ml premixed in dextrose; then after the first 24 hr, 720 mg infused over 24 hr (0.5 mg/min) using 360 mg/200 ml premixed in dextrose, continued up to 2 to 3 wk, as needed. Rate may be increased in first 24 hr, if needed, but initial infusion rate shouldn't exceed 30 mg/min. Changed to oral form as soon as possible.

➤ *To treat breakthrough episodes of ventricular fibrillation or hemodynamically unstable ventricular tachycardia*

I.V. INFUSION (NEXTERONE)

Adults. 150 mg/100 ml premixed in dextrose and infused over 10 min (15 mg/min).

Route	Onset	Peak	Duration
P.O.	2 days–3 wk	1–5 mo	Weeks–months
I.V.	Hours–3 days	1–3 wk	Weeks–months

Mechanism of Action

Acts on cardiac cell membranes, prolonging repolarization and the refractory period and raising ventricular fibrillation threshold. Drug relaxes vascular smooth muscles, mainly in coronary circulation, and improves myocardial blood flow. It relaxes peripheral vascular smooth muscles, decreasing peripheral vascular resistance and myocardial oxygen consumption.

Incompatibilities

To prevent precipitation, don't mix amiodarone 4 mg/ml admixed with aminophylline, amoxicillin sodium-clavulanic acid, ampicillin sodium-sulbactam sodium, argatroban, bivalirudin, cefamadole nafate, cefazolin sodium, ceftazidime, digoxin, furosemide, mezlocillin sodium, heparin sodium, imipenem-cilastatin sodium sodium, magnesium sulfate, micafungin, piperacillin sodium-tazobactam sodium, potassium phosphates, sodium bicarbonate, sodium nitroprusside, and sodium phosphates. Also, don't use plastic containers in series connections because this could result in an air embolism and don't use evacuated glass containers for admixing Cordarone because precipitation may occur.

Contraindications

Bradycardia that causes syncope (unless pacemaker present), cardiogenic shock, hypersensitivity to amiodarone or its components, SA node dysfunction, second- and third-degree AV block (unless pacemaker present)

Interactions

DRUGS

anticoagulants: Increased anticoagulant response and possibly serious bleeding

azole antifungals, antiarrhythmics, fluoroquinolones (selected ones), loratadine, macrolide antibiotics (selected ones), trazodone: Increased risk of prolonged QT interval and life-threatening arrhythmias such as torsades de points
beta blockers: Increased serum levels of beta blockers with increased risk of AV block, bradycardia, and hypotension
calcium channel blockers: Increased serum levels of these drugs and increased risk of AV block, bradycardia, and hypotension
cholestyramine, phenytoin, rifampin, St. John's wort: Decreased amiodarone level
cimetidine, protease inhibitors (selected ones): Increased amiodarone level
cyclosporine: Increased cyclosporine level
dabigatran, dextromethorphan, phenytoin: Possible increased serum levels of these drugs
dextromethorphan, methotrexate, phenytoin: Increased serum levels of these drugs and increased risk of toxicity if amiodarone is taken orally for more than 2 weeks
digoxin: Increased serum digoxin level and risk of digitalis toxicity
fentanyl: Increased serum fentanyl level with increased risk of bradycardia, decreased cardiac output, and hypotension
flecainide procainamide, quinidine: Increased serum levels of these drugs
HMG-CoA reductase inhibitors such as atorvastatin, lovastatin, and simvastatin: Increased risk of myopathy and rhabdomyolysis
ledipasvir/sofosbuvir, sofosbuvir/simeprevir: May cause serious symptomatic bradycardia
protease inhibitors: Possibly increased risk of elevated amiodarone levels and toxicity
rifampin, St. John's wort: Decreased serum amiodarone level and effectiveness
theophylline: Increased serum theophylline level; increased risk of theophylline toxicity

FOODS

grapefruit juice: Increased amiodarone level

Adverse Reactions

CNS: Abnormal gait, ataxia, confusion, delirium, demyelinating polyneuropathy, disorientation, dizziness, fatigue, fever, hallucinations, headache, insomnia, involuntary motor activity, lack of coordination, malaise, paresthesia, parkinsonian symptoms, peripheral neuropathy, **pseudotumor cerebri**, sleep disturbances, tremor
CV: Arrhythmias (including AV block, **bradycardia**, **electromechanical dissociation**, **torsades de pointes**, **and ventricular tachycardia or fibrillation)**, **cardiac arrest**, **cardiogenic shock**, edema, **heart failure**, **hypotension**, **QT prolongation**, vasculitis
EENT: Abnormal salivation, abnormal taste and smell, blurred vision, corneal microdeposits, dry eyes or mouth, halo vision, lens opacities, macular degeneration, optic neuritis, optic neuropathy, papilledema, permanent blindness, photophobia, scotoma
ENDO: Hyperthyroidism, hypothyroidism, syndrome of inappropriate ADH secretion, thyroid nodules, **thyroid cancer**
GI: Abdominal pain, anorexia, **cirrhosis**, constipation, diarrhea, elevated bilirubin or liver enzymes, hepatic failure, hepatitis, nausea, **pancreatitis**, vomiting
GU: Acute renal failure, decreased libido, epididymitis, impotence, **renal insufficiency**
HEME: Agranulocytosis, **aplastic or hemolytic anemia**, **coagulation abnormalities**, **neutropenia**, **pancytopenia**, spontaneous bruising, **thrombocytopenia**
MS: Muscle weakness, myopathy, **rhabdomyolysis**
RESP: Acute respiratory distress syndrome in postoperative setting; bronchiolitis obliterans organizing pneumonia; bronchospasm; **eosinophilic pneumonia; infiltrates that lead to** dyspnea, cough, **hemoptysis**, **hypoxia**, **pulmonary fibrosis**, **pulmonary alveolar hemorrhage**, **pulmonary interstitial pneumonitis**; crackles and wheezing; pleural effusion; pleuritis; pneumonia; pulmonary inflammation, **pulmonary fibrosis**; **respiratory arrest or failure**

SKIN: Alopecia, bluish gray pigmentation, bullous dermatitis, eczema, **erythema multiforme**, **exfoliative dermatitis**, flushing, photosensitivity, pruritus, **skin cancer**, solar dermatitis, **Stevens–Johnson syndrome**, **toxic epidermal necrolysis**, urticaria
Other: **Anaphylaxis including shock**, **angioedema**, **drug reaction with eosinophilia and systemic symptoms (DRESS)**, lupus-like syndrome

Nursing Considerations

- Check patient's implantable cardiac device (if present), as ordered, at the start of and during amiodarone therapy because drug may affect pacing or defibrillating thresholds.
- Dilute parenteral amiodarone in D_5W or normal saline solution and mix in polyvinyl chloride (PVC), polyolefin, or glass containers except for Nexterone, which is already premixed.
- Use an in-line filter during I.V. administration of amiodarone. Also use a central venous catheter whenever possible. A central venous catheter is required when infusion rate exceeds 2 mg/ml because drug may cause peripheral vein phlebitis at higher rates. Amiodarone I.V. must be given by volumetric infusion pump.
- Monitor amiodarone I.V. infusion closely because loading doses at higher concentrations and rates may cause acute renal failure, hepatocellular necrosis, and death.
- Know that infusion of up to 0.5 mg/min may be continued for 2 to 3 weeks, regardless of patient's age, left ventricular function, or renal function.
- Expect patient to be switched to oral therapy from intravenous therapy as soon as possible with dosage dependent on the dose of intravenous drug already administered. Monitor all patients but especially elderly patients closely when conversion to oral amiodarone is made for continued effectiveness.

WARNING **Be aware that amiodarone may cause or worsen pulmonary disorders that may develop days to weeks after therapy and progress to respiratory failure or even death. Expect to obtain chest x-ray and pulmonary function tests before therapy starts and then chest x-ray and follow-up exams every 3 to 6 months during therapy.**

- Monitor vital signs and oxygen level often during and after giving amiodarone. Keep emergency equipment and drugs nearby.

WARNING Monitor continuous ECG; check for increased PR and QRS intervals, arrhythmias, and heart rate below 60 beats/min because amiodarone may cause sinus arrest or symptomatic bradycardia and new ventricular arrhythmias or worsen existing arrhythmias as well as increasing resistance to cardioversion. Electrolyte imbalance or use of concomitant antiarrhythmics or other interacting drugs may increase the development of these arrhythmias. Expect to correct electrolyte imbalance, as ordered, prior to initiating treatment with amiodarone.

- Monitor serum amiodarone level, which normally ranges from 1.0 to 2.5 mcg/ml.
- Assess thyroid hormone levels; drug inhibits conversion of T_4 to T_3 and may cause drug-induced hyperthyroidism, thyrotoxicosis, and new or worsened arrhythmias. If new signs of arrhythmia occur, notify prescriber at once.
- Monitor liver enzymes, as ordered. If elevations become persistent and significant, notify prescriber and expect maintenance dosage to be reduced or drug discontinued.
- Be aware that patient should undergo regular ophthalmic examinations including funduscopy and slit-lamp examination during amiodarone therapy because drug can cause serious visual impairment including permanent blindness.

PATIENT TEACHING

- Explain that patient will need frequent monitoring and laboratory tests during treatment.
- Advise patient to report cough, dark urine, dyspnea, fainting, fatigue, light-headedness, nausea, swollen feet and hands, vomiting, wheezing, yellow sclerae or skin, or a sudden change in quality or rapidity of pulse.
- Instruct patient to report abnormal bleeding or bruising. Also tell patient to report any sign of visual impairment or decreased or increased levels of energy.
- Stress importance of informing all prescribers of amiodarone use, as serious drug interactions may occur.

- Advise patient to avoid corneal refractive laser surgery while taking drug.
- Warn female patient of childbearing age that amiodarone can cause fetal harm. Instruct her to use effective contraceptive measures and report suspected or known pregnancy immediately.
- Advise female patient who has been breastfeeding to discontinue nursing, because drug is excreted in human milk and may cause potential harm.
- Advise patient to avoid drinking grapefruit juice or taking St. John's Wort while receiving amiodarone.

amitriptyline hydrochloride

Elavil, Levate (CAN)

Class and Category

Pharmacologic class: Tricyclic antidepressant
Therapeutic class: Antidepressant
Pregnancy category: C

Indications and Dosages

➤ ***To relieve depression, especially when accompanied by anxiety and insomnia***

TABLETS

Adults. *Out-patient:* 75 mg daily in divided doses, increased to 150 mg daily, if needed. Increases made preferably with late afternoon and/or bedtime doses. Alternatively, 50 to 100 mg at bedtime, increased by 25 to 50 mg, as needed, in bedtime dose to 150 mg daily. *In-patient:* 100 mg daily, gradually increased to 300 mg daily, if needed. *Maintenance:* 40 to 100 mg daily at bedtime.

DOSAGE ADJUSTMENT Dosage reduced to 10 mg three times a day plus 20 mg at bedtime for adolescent and elderly patients.

Route	Onset	Peak	Duration
P.O.	14–21 days	Unknown	Unknown

Contraindications

Acute recovery phase after MI, concurrent therapy with cisapride, hypersensitivity to amitriptyline or its components, MAO inhibitor therapy within 14 days

Interactions

DRUGS

anticholinergics, epinephrine, norepinephrine: Increased effects of these drugs
barbiturates: Decreased amitriptyline level
carbamazepine: Decreased serum amitriptyline level and increased serum

Mechanism of Action

Normally, when an impulse reaches adrenergic nerves, the nerves release serotonin and norepinephrine from their storage sites. Most of this is taken back into the nerves and stored by the reuptake mechanism, as shown below on the left.

Amitriptyline blocks serotonin and norepinephrine reuptake by adrenergic nerves. By doing so, it raises serotonin and norepinephrine levels at nerve synapses. This action may elevate mood and reduce depression.

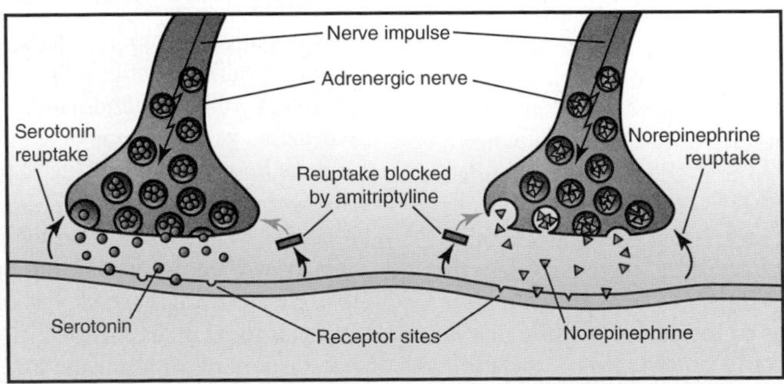

carbamazepine level, which increases therapeutic and toxic effects of carbamazepine
cimetidine, disulfiram, fluoxetine, fluvoxamine, haloperidol, H_2-receptor antagonists, methylphenidate, oral contraceptives, paroxetine, phenothiazines, sertraline: Increased serum amitriptyline level
cisapride: Possibly prolonged QT interval and increased risk of arrhythmias
clonidine, guanethidine, and other antihypertensives: Decreased antihypertensive effects
dicumarol: Increased anticoagulant effect
levodopa: Decreased levodopa absorption; sympathetic hyperactivity, sinus tachycardia, hypertension, agitation
MAO inhibitors: Possibly seizures and death
thyroid replacement drugs: Arrhythmias and increased antidepressant effects

ACTIVITIES

alcohol use: Enhanced CNS depression
smoking: Decreased amitriptyline effects

Adverse Reactions

CNS: Anxiety, ataxia, **coma**, chills, delusions, disorientation, drowsiness, extrapyramidal reactions, fatigue, fever, headache, insomnia, nightmares, peripheral neuropathy, **suicidal ideation**, tremor
CV: Arrhythmias (including prolonged AV conduction, **heart block**, and tachycardia), **cardiomyopathy**, hypertension, **MI**, nonspecific ECG changes, orthostatic hypotension, palpitations
EENT: Abnormal taste, black tongue, blurred vision, dry mouth, increased salivation, nasal congestion, tinnitus
ENDO: Gynecomastia, **hyperglycemia**, **hypoglycemia**, increased prolactin level, syndrome of inappropriate ADH secretion
GI: Abdominal cramps, constipation, diarrhea, flatulence, ileus, increased appetite, nausea, vomiting
GU: Impotence, libido changes, menstrual irregularities, testicular swelling, urinary hesitancy, urine retention
HEME: Agranulocytosis, **bone marrow depression**, eosinophilia, **leukopenia**, **thrombocytopenia**
SKIN: Alopecia, flushing, purpura
Other: Weight gain

Nursing Considerations

- Use caution if patient has a history of seizures, urine retention, or angle-closure glaucoma because of amitriptyline's atropine-like effects.

WARNING **Don't give an MAO inhibitor within 14 days of amitriptyline because of the risk of seizures and death.**

- Closely monitor patient with CV disorder because amitriptyline may cause arrhythmias, such as sinus tachycardia.
- Watch patients closely (especially adolescents and young adults), for suicidal tendencies, particularly when therapy starts and dosage changes. Depression may worsen temporarily during these times.
- Monitor blood pressure for hypotension or hypertension.
- Stay alert for behavior changes, such as hallucinations and decreased interest in personal appearance. Be aware that psychosis may develop in schizophrenic patients, and symptoms may increase in paranoid patients.
- Avoid abrupt withdrawal after long use because nausea, headache, vertigo, and nightmares may occur.

PATIENT TEACHING

- Instruct patient to avoid using alcohol or OTC drugs that contain alcohol during amitriptyline therapy because alcohol enhances CNS depressant effects.
- Urge family or caregiver to watch patient closely for suicidal tendencies, especially when therapy starts or dosage changes and particularly if patient is a teenager or young adult.

amlodipine besylate

Norvasc

Class and Category

Pharmacologic class: Calcium channel blocker
Therapeutic class: Antianginal, antihypertensive
Pregnancy category: Not classified

Indications and Dosages

➤ *To control hypertension*

TABLETS

Adults. *Initial:* 5 mg daily, increased gradually over 10 to 14 days, as needed. *Maximum:* 10 mg daily.

Children age 6 to 17 years. 2.5 to 5 mg once daily. Maximum: 5 mg once daily.

DOSAGE ADJUSTMENT Initially 2.5 mg daily for elderly, fragile, or small patients or patients with impaired hepatic function. Increased gradually over 7 to 14 days based on response.

➤ *To treat chronic stable angina and vasospastic angina (Prinzmetal's or Variant angina); to treat angiographically documented coronary artery disease (CAD) in patients without heart failure or an ejection fraction less than 40%*

TABLETS

Adults. 5 to 10 mg daily.

DOSAGE ADJUSTMENT 2.5 to 5 mg daily for elderly patients and those with impaired hepatic function.

Route	Onset	Peak	Duration
P.O.	Unknown	6–12 hr	24 hr

Mechanism of Action

Binds to dihydropyridine and nondihydropyridine cell membrane receptor sites on myocardial and vascular smooth-muscle cells and inhibits influx of extracellular calcium ions across slow calcium channels. This decreases intracellular calcium level, inhibiting smooth-muscle cell contractions and relaxing coronary and vascular smooth muscles, decreasing peripheral vascular resistance, and reducing systolic and diastolic blood pressure. Decreased peripheral vascular resistance also decreases myocardial workload, oxygen demand, and possibly angina. Also, by inhibiting coronary artery muscle cell contractions and restoring blood flow, drug may relieve Prinzmetal's angina.

Contraindications

Hypersensitivity to amlodipine or its components

Interactions

DRUGS

ACE inhibitors, aliskiren (in patients with diabetes or renal impairment): Increased risk of hyperkalemia, hypotension, and renal dysfunction

cyclosporine, simvastatin, tacrolimus: Possibly increased blood levels of these drugs

CYP3A4 inhibitors such as diltiazem, ketoconazole, itraconazole, and ritonavir: Possibly increased blood amlodipine level

sildenafil: Possibly excessive hypotension

Adverse Reactions

CNS: Anxiety, dizziness, extrapyramidal disorder, fatigue, headache, lethargy, lightheadedness, paresthesia, somnolence, syncope, tremor

CV: Arrhythmias, chest pain, **hypotension**, palpitations, peripheral edema

EENT: Dry mouth, gingival hyperplasia, pharyngitis

ENDO: Hot flashes

GI: Abdominal cramps or pain, anorexia, constipation, diarrhea, dysphagia, elevated liver enzymes, esophagitis, flatulence, indigestion, jaundice, nausea, **pancreatitis**, vomiting

GU: Decreased libido, impotence, urinary frequency

MS: Myalgia

RESP: Dyspnea

SKIN: Dermatitis, flushing, rash

Other: Weight loss

Nursing Considerations

- Use amlodipine cautiously in patients with heart block, heart failure, impaired renal function, hepatic disorder, or severe aortic stenosis.
- Monitor patient with impaired hepatic function closely because amlodipine is extensively metabolized by the liver, and expect to titrate dosage slowly when administering drug to patients with severe hepatic impairment.
- Monitor blood pressure while adjusting dosage, especially in patients with heart failure or severe aortic stenosis because symptomatic hypotension may occur.
- Assess patient frequently for chest pain when starting or increasing the dose of amlodipine, because worsening of angina or an acute myocardial infarction can occur, especially in patients with severe obstructive coronary artery disease.

PATIENT TEACHING

- Tell patient to take missed dose as soon as remembered and next dose in 24 hours.
- Tell patient to immediately notify prescriber of dizziness, arm or leg swelling, difficulty breathing, hives, or rash.
- Suggest taking amlodipine with food to reduce GI upset.
- Advise patient to have blood pressure checked routinely for possible hypotension.
- Tell mothers interested in breastfeeding to discuss with prescriber, because amlodipine is present in human milk.

amoxicillin trihydrate

(amoxycillin)

Amoxil, Apo-Amoxi (CAN), Larotid, Moxatag, Novamoxin (CAN)

Class and Category

Pharmacologic class: Aminopenicillin
Therapeutic class: Antibiotic
Pregnancy category: B

Indications and Dosages

➤ *To treat ear, nose, throat, GU tract, skin, and soft-tissue infections caused by susceptible gram-positive and gram-negative organisms*

CAPSULES, CHEWABLE TABLETS, ORAL SUSPENSION, TABLETS

Adults and children weighing 40 kg (88 lb) or more. 250 mg every 8 hr; for severe infections, 500 mg or 875 mg every 12 hr.

Children age 12 wk and over weighing less than 40 kg. 20 mg/kg daily in divided doses every 8 hr; for severe infections, 40 to 45 mg/kg/day in divided doses every 12 hr.

Children under age 12 wk. Up to 30 mg/kg/day in divided doses every 12 hr.

➤ *To treat tonsillitis or pharyngitis caused by* Streptococcus pyogenes

E.R. TABLETS (MOXATAG)

Adults and children age 12 and over. 775 mg once daily for 10 days, taken within 1 hr of finishing a meal.

➤ *To treat lower respiratory tract infections caused by susceptible gram-positive and gram-negative organisms*

CAPSULES, CHEWABLE TABLETS, ORAL SUSPENSION, TABLETS

Adults and children weighing 40 kg (88 lb) or more. 875 mg every 12 hr; for severe infections, 500 mg every 8 hr.

Children age 12 wk and over weighing less than 40 kg. 40 mg/kg in divided doses every 8 hr or 45 mg/kg in divided doses every 12 hr.

Children under age 12 wk. Up to 30 mg/kg daily in divided doses every 12 hr.

➤ *To treat gonorrhea and acute uncomplicated anogenital and urethral infections caused by susceptible strains of gram-positive and gram-negative organisms*

CAPSULES, CHEWABLE TABLETS, ORAL SUSPENSION, TABLETS

Adults and postpubertal children. 3 g as a single dose.

Prepubertal children age 2 and over. 50 mg/kg of amoxicillin plus 25 mg/kg of probenecid as a single dose.

➤ *As adjunct to eradicate* Helicobacter pylori *to reduce risk of duodenal ulcer recurrence*

CAPSULES, CHEWABLE TABLETS, ORAL SUSPENSION, TABLETS

Adults. 1 g every 12 hr with 500 mg of clarithromycin every 12 hr and 30 mg of lansoprazole every 12 hr for 14 days, or 1 g every 8 hr with 30 mg of lansoprazole every 8 hr for 14 days.

➤ *To prevent bacterial endocarditis before dental, oral, or upper respiratory tract procedures*

CAPSULES, CHEWABLE TABLETS, ORAL SUSPENSION, TABLETS

Adults and children weighing 40 kg (88 lb) or more. 2 g 1 hr before procedure.

Children weighing less than 40 kg. 50 mg/kg 1 hr before procedure.

DOSAGE ADJUSTMENT For patients with impaired renal function with a glomerular filtration rate less than 30 ml/min, dosage reduced to less than 875 mg; for a glomerular filtration rate of 10 to 30 ml/min dosage reduced to 500 mg or 250 mg every 12 hr; for a glomerular filtration rate less than 10 ml/min dosage reduced to 500 mg or 250 mg and frequency reduced to every 24 hr.

Route	Onset	Peak	Duration
P.O.	Unknown	Unknown	6–8 hr

Mechanism of Action
Kills bacteria by binding to and inactivating penicillin-binding proteins on the inner bacterial cell wall, weakening the bacterial cell wall and causing lysis.

Contraindications
Hypersensitivity including severe reactions (anaphylaxis or Stevens–Johnson syndrome) to amoxicillin, other beta-lactam antibiotics, or their components

Interactions
DRUGS

allopurinol: Increased risk of rash
chloramphenicol, erythromycins, sulfonamides, tetracyclines: Reduced bactericidal effect of amoxicillin
methotrexate: Increased risk of methotrexate toxicity
oral anticoagulants: Possible prolonged prothrombin time (increased international normalized ratio)
oral contraceptives with estrogen: Possibly reduced effectiveness of contraceptive
probenecid: Increased amoxicillin effects

Adverse Reactions
CNS: Agitation, anxiety, behavior changes, confusion, dizziness, insomnia, reversible hyperactivity, **seizures**
CV: Hypersensitivity vasculitis
EENT: Black, hairy tongue; mucocutaneous candidiasis; tooth discoloration
GI: ***Clostridium difficile***-associated diarrhea, diarrhea, elevated liver enzymes, **hemorrhagic or pseudomembranous colitis**, **hepatic dysfunction**, jaundice, nausea, vomiting
GU: Crystalluria, vaginal mycosis
HEME: **Agranulocytosis**, anemia (including **hemolytic anemia**), eosinophilia, granulocytosis, **leukopenia**, **thrombocytopenia**, **thrombocytopenic purpura**
SKIN: **Erythema multiforme**, erythematous maculopapular rash, generalized exanthematous pustulosis, **Stevens–Johnson syndrome**, **toxic epidermal necrolysis**, urticaria
Other: **Allergic reactions**, **anaphylaxis**, serum sickness-like reaction (such as arthralgia, arthritis, fever, myalgia, rash, and urticaria)

Nursing Considerations
- Know that patients with mononucleosis shouldn't receive amoxicillin because this class of drugs may cause an erythematous rash.
- Use drug cautiously in patients with hepatic impairment. Monitor hepatic and renal function and CBC, as ordered, in patients on prolonged therapy. Also use cautiously in breastfeeding and elderly patients.
- Expect to start therapy before culture and sensitivity test results are known.
- Be aware that chewable tablets and tablets for oral suspension contain phenylalanine.

WARNING **Stop amoxicillin immediately and provide emergency care as indicated and ordered if an allergic reaction occurs.**

- Monitor patient closely for diarrhea, which may indicate pseudomembranous colitis caused by *Clostridium difficile.* If diarrhea occurs, notify prescriber, expect to withhold amoxicillin, and treat with fluids, electrolytes, protein, and an antibiotic effective against *C. difficile.*
- Expect treatment that lasts at least 10 days for hemolytic streptococcal infections.
- Monitor patient for superinfection. If it occurs, expect to discontinue drug and provide treatment as ordered.

PATIENT TEACHING

- Tell patient to refrigerate reconstituted suspension and to shake well before each use.
- Know that when amoxicillin suspension is prescribed for a child, instruct parents to place it directly on child's tongue to swallow. If this doesn't work, tell parents to mix dose of suspension with formula or cold drink (milk, fruit juice, ginger ale, water) and have child drink it immediately.
- Tell patient to chew or crush chewable tablets and not to swallow them whole.
- Urge patient to take amoxicillin for full length of time prescribed, even if he feels better.

- Teach patient to report adverse reactions and notify prescriber if infection worsens or doesn't improve after 72 hours.
- Urge patient to tell prescriber about diarrhea that's severe or lasts longer than 3 days. Remind patient that watery or bloody stools can occur 2 or more months after antibiotic therapy and may be serious, requiring prompt treatment.

amphetamine

Adzenys ER, Adzenys XR-ODT, Dyanavel XR

amphetamine sulfate

dextroamphetamine sulfate

Dexedrine ER, Liquadd, ProCentra, Zenzedi

Class and Category

Pharmacologic class: Phenethylamine
Therapeutic class: CNS stimulant
Pregnancy category: C
Controlled substance schedule: II

Indications and Dosages

➤ *To treat attention deficit hyperactivity disorder (ADHD)*

ORAL SOLUTION (LIQUADD, PROCENTRA), TABLETS (ZENZEDI)

Children age 6 and over. *Initial:* 5 mg daily or twice daily. Increased by 5 mg daily at 1-wk intervals until desired response occurs.
Children ages 3 to 6. *Initial:* 2.5 mg daily. Increased by 2.5 mg daily at 1-wk intervals until desired response occurs.

ER CAPSULES (DEXEDRINE ER)

Children age 6 and over. *Initial:* 5 mg daily or twice daily. Increased by 5 mg daily at 1-wk intervals until desired response occurs.

ER ORAL SOLUTION (DYANAVEL XR)

Children age 6 and over. *Initial:* 2.5 or 5 mg once daily in the morning. Increased by 2.5 to 10 mg every 4 to 7 days. *Maximum:* 20 mg daily.

ER ORALLY DISINTEGRATING TABLETS (ADZENYS XR-ODT), ER ORAL SUSPENSION (ADZENYS ER)

Adults. 12.5 mg daily.
Children age 6 and over. *Initial:* 6.3 mg once daily in the morning. Increased by 3.1 or 6.3 mg at weekly intervals. *Maximum:* 18.8 mg daily (children 6 to 12 years); 12.5 mg daily (children 13 to 17 years).

➤ *To treat narcolepsy*

ER CAPSULES (DEXEDRINE ER), ORAL SOLUTION (LIQUADD, PROCENTRA), TABLETS (ZENZEDI)

Adults. 5 to 60 mg daily in divided doses, depending on response.
Children age 12 and over. *Initial:* 10 mg daily. Increased by 10 mg daily at 1-wk intervals until desired response occurs.
Children ages 6 to 12. *Initial:* 5 mg daily. Increased by 5 mg daily at 1-wk intervals until desired response occurs.

Mechanism of Action

May produce its CNS stimulant effects by facilitating release and blocking reuptake of norepinephrine at adrenergic nerve terminals and by direct stimulation of alpha and beta receptors in the peripheral nervous system. It also releases and blocks reuptake of dopamine in limbic regions of the brain. The drug's main action appears to be in the cerebral cortex and, possibly, the reticular activating system. These actions cause decreased motor restlessness, increased alertness, and diminished drowsiness and fatigue. Its peripheral actions include increased blood pressure and mild bronchodilation and respiratory stimulation.

Contraindications

Advanced arteriosclerosis, agitation (for narcolepsy treatment), glaucoma, history of drug abuse, hypersensitivity or idiosyncratic reaction to sympathomimetic amines, hyperthyroidism, MAO inhibitor therapy including I.V. methylene blue or linezolid within 14 days, moderate to severe hypertension, symptomatic cardiovascular disease

Interactions

DRUGS

acetazolamide, alkalinizers (such as sodium bicarbonate), some thiazides: Increased blood level and effects of amphetamine
adrenergic blockers: Inhibited adrenergic blockade
antihistamines: Possibly reduced sedation from antihistamine
antihypertensives: Possibly decreased antihypertensive effects

buspirone, CYP 206 inhibitors, fentanyl, lithium, MAO inhibitors, selective serotonin reuptake inhibitors, serotonin norepinephrine reuptake inhibitors, St. John's wort, tramadol, tricyclic antidepressants, triptans: Increased risk of serotonin syndrome
chlorpromazine: Inhibited CNS stimulant effects of amphetamine
ethosuximide: Possibly delayed ethosuximide absorption
GI acidifiers (such as ascorbic acid), reserpine: Decreased amphetamine absorption
guanethidine: Decreased antihypertensive effect and decreased amphetamine absorption
haloperidol: Decreased CNS stimulation
lithium carbonate: Possibly decreased anorectic and stimulant effects of amphetamine
MAO inhibitors: Potentiated effects of amphetamine; possibly hypertensive crisis
meperidine: Increased analgesia
methenamine: Increased urine excretion and decreased effects of amphetamine
norepinephrine: Possibly increased adrenergic effect of norepinephrine
phenobarbital, phenytoin: Synergistic anticonvulsant action
propoxyphene: Increased CNS stimulation, potentially fatal seizures
proton pump inhibitors: Possibly decreased effectiveness of amphetamines
tricyclic antidepressants: Possibly enhanced antidepressant effects and decreased effects of amphetamine
urinary acidifiers (such as ammonium chloride and sodium acid phosphate): Increased amphetamine excretion and decreased amphetamine blood level and effects
veratrum alkaloids: Decreased hypotensive effect

FOODS

acidic fruit juices: Decreased amphetamine absorption

Adverse Reactions

CNS: Aggression, anger, anxiety, depression, dizziness, dyskinesia, dysphoria, euphoria, exacerbation of motor and phonic tics and Tourette's syndrome, excessive talkativeness, hallucinations, headache, insomnia, irritability, over-stimulation, paranoia, psychotic episodes, restlessness, **serotonin syndrome**, tremor
CV: **Cardiomyopathy**, hypertension, **MI**, palpitations, tachycardia
EENT: Blurred vision, dry mouth, mydriasis, unpleasant taste
GI: Anorexia, constipation, diarrhea
GU: Frequent or prolonged erections, impotence, libido changes
MS: Rhabdomyolysis
SKIN: Alopecia, excessive skin picking, rash, **Stevens–Johnson syndrome**, **toxic epidermal necrolysis**, urticaria
Other: **Anaphylaxis**, **angioedema**, weight loss

Nursing Considerations

- Keep in mind that when symptoms of ADHD occur with acute stress reactions, treatment with amphetamines usually isn't indicated.

WARNING Don't give amphetamine during or for up to 14 days after MAO therapy, to prevent hypertensive crisis.

- Be aware that 5 ml of oral solution contains 5 mg of dexamphetamine.
- Expect to decrease dosage if patient has bothersome adverse reactions, such as insomnia and anorexia. To minimize insomnia, administer drug earlier in day.
- Be alert for evidence of long-term amphetamine abuse, such as hyperactivity, irritability, marked insomnia, personality changes, and severe dermatoses. If patient suddenly stops drug after long-term, high-dose regimen, watch for extreme fatigue and depression.

WARNING Monitor patient closely for evidence of serotonin syndrome, such as agitation, coma, diarrhea, hallucinations, hyperreflexia, hyperthermia, incoordination, labile blood pressure, nausea, tachycardia, and vomiting. Notify prescriber immediately because serotonin syndrome reactions may be life-threatening. Expect to discontinue amphetamine therapy and any other serotonergic agents patient may be taking. Be prepared to provide supportive care.

PATIENT TEACHING

- Instruct breastfeeding patient to avoid breastfeeding during amphetamine therapy because drug is excreted in breast milk.
- Teach patient to take first dose on awakening and subsequent doses as prescribed. Tell him not to take last dose

late in evening because insomnia may occur.

- Inform patient or caregiver that each 5 ml of oral solution contains 5 mg of dexamphetamine. Advise patient to use a calibrated measuring device for accurate dose.
- Instruct patient prescribed orally disintegrating tablets how to remove tablets from package and to avoid pushing tablets through the foil. Tablet should be immediately placed on the tongue and allowed to dissolve without chewing or crushing.
- Urge patient to avoid hazardous activities until drug's effects are known.
- Advise patient not to take amphetamine with acidic fruit juice because doing so decreases drug absorption.
- Explain drug's abuse potential, and caution against altering dosage unless prescribed.
- Instruct patient to notify prescriber before taking any new drugs, including over-the-counter preparations.
- Tell patient to report any new or worsening behavior and thought problems; new or worsening bipolar illness; new manic symptoms; or new psychotic symptoms such as believing things that are not true, feeling suspicious, or hearing voices.

amphotericin B

Fungizone Intravenous

amphotericin B lipid complex

Abelcet

amphotericin B liposomal complex

AmBisome

Class and Category

Pharmacologic class: Amphoteric polyene
Therapeutic class: Antifungal
Pregnancy category: B

Indications and Dosages

➤ *To treat severe fungal infections*

I.V. INFUSION (FUNGIZONE)

Adults and adolescents. *Initial:* 1-mg test dose in 20 ml of D_5W infused over 20 to 30 min; if test dose is tolerated, then 0.25 to 0.3 mg/kg daily prepared as a 0.1 mg/ml infusion, given over 2 to 6 hr. Increased in 5- to 10-mg increments up to 50 mg daily, based on patient tolerance and infection severity, not to exceed a total daily dose of 1.5 mg/kg. *Maximum:* 1 mg/kg daily or 1.5 mg/kg every other day.

Children. *Initial:* 0.25 mg/kg daily in D_5W infused over 6 hr; then increased in 0.125- to 0.25-mg/kg increments daily or every other day as tolerated. *Maximum:* 1 mg/kg or 30 mg/m^2 of body surface daily.

➤ *To treat oral candidiasis*

ORAL SUSPENSION (AMPHOTERICIN B)

Adults and children. 1 ml (100 mg) four times daily for 14 days.

➤ *To treat invasive amphotericin B-resistant fungal infections*

I.V. INFUSION (ABELCET)

Adults and children. 5 mg/kg daily infused at 2.5 mg/kg/hr.

➤ *To treat severe aspergillosis, candidiasis, or cryptococcosis*

I.V. INFUSION (AMBISOME)

Adults and children. 3 to 5 mg/kg daily infused over 2 hr. Infusion time may be decreased to 1 hr if tolerated or increased if patient experiences discomfort.

➤ *To treat leishmaniasis*

I.V. INFUSION (AMBISOME)

Immunocompetent adults and children. 3 mg/kg daily on days 1 through 5 and on days 14 and 21, infused over 2 hr. Infusion time may be decreased to 1 hr if tolerated or increased if patient has discomfort.

Immunocompromised adults and children. 4 mg/kg daily on days 1 through 5 and days 10, 17, 24, 31, and 38 infused over 2 hr. Infusion time may be decreased to 1 hr if tolerated or increased if patient has discomfort.

Route	Onset	Peak	Duration
P.O.	Unknown	Unknown	Unknown
I.V.	Immediate	Unknown	Unknown

Mechanism of Action

Binds to sterols in fungal cell plasma membranes, which changes membrane permeability and allows loss of potassium and small molecules from cells. This action results in fungal cell impairment or death.

Incompatibilities

Don't reconstitute amphotericin B with diluents other than those recommended because solutions with sodium chloride or bacteriostatic agents (such as benzyl alcohol) may cause drug precipitation.

Contraindications

Hypersensitivity to amphotericin B or its components

Interactions

DRUGS

antineoplastics: Increased risk of bronchospasm, hypotension, and nephrotoxicity
corticosteroids, corticotropin: Increased risk of hypokalemia and cardiac dysfunction
cyclosporine, nephrotoxic drugs: Increased risk of nephrotoxicity
digitalis glycosides: Possibly hypokalemia and more severe digitalis toxicity
flucytosine: Possibly increased flucytosine toxicity
leukocyte transfusion: Possibly dyspnea, hypoxemia, and pulmonary infiltrates
skeletal muscle relaxants: Possibly hypokalemia and increased muscle relaxation
zidovudine: Possibly myelotoxicity and nephrotoxicity

Adverse Reactions

CNS: Fever, headache, shaking chills, tiredness, weakness
CV: Chest pain, **hypotension**, irregular heartbeat
EENT: Difficulty swallowing, pharyngitis
GI: Abdominal pain, anorexia, diarrhea, **hepatic failure**, indigestion, Jaundice, nausea, vomiting
GU: Decreased or increased urine output, hemorrhagic cystitis, impaired renal function
HEME: Agranulocytosis, anemia, **leukopenia**, **thrombocytopenia**, **unusual bleeding** or bruising
MS: Arthralgia, muscle spasms, myalgia, **rhabdomyolysis**
RESP: Apnea, **bronchospasm**, **cyanosis**, dyspnea, **hypoventilation**, **hypoxia**, **pulmonary edema**, tachypnea
SKIN: Erythemia, flushing, maculopapular rash, pruritus and redness especially around ears, urticaria
Other: Anaphylaxis, **angioedema**, **hypocalcemia**, **hypokalemia**, **hypomagnesemia**, infusion-site pain, and thrombophlebitis

Nursing Considerations

- Prepare amphotericin B by adding 10 ml of sterile water for injection without a bacteriostatic agent to vial containing 50 mg of amphotericin B. For I.V. infusion, dilute solution containing 5 mg/ml to 0.1 mg/ml by adding 1 ml (5 mg) of solution to 49 ml of D_5W with a pH above 4.2.
- Know that before using D_5W to dilute amphotericin B solution, determine the injection's pH aseptically. If pH is below 4.2, follow manufacturer's instructions for buffering it.
- Avoid using in-line membrane filter or use one with a mean pore diameter of more than 1 micron to prevent significant drug removal because reconstituted amphotericin B is a colloidal suspension.
- Prepare amphotericin B cholesteryl sulfate complex by reconstituting with sterile water for injection. Using a sterile syringe and 20G needle, rapidly add 10- or 20-ml sterile water for injection to a 50- or 100-mg vial, respectively, to obtain a solution containing 5 mg of amphotericin B per milliliter. Shake gently by hand, rotating vial until solids are dissolved; fluid may be clear or opalescent. For infusion, further dilute reconstituted solution to about 0.6 mg/ml. Don't filter solution or use an in-line filter. Flush existing line with D_5W or use a separate line.
- Prepare amphotericin B lipid complex by shaking vial gently until no yellow sediment is seen. Using an 18G needle, withdraw prescribed dose from required number of vials into one or more 20-ml syringes. Replace needle with 5-micron filter needle supplied with each vial. Empty syringe contents into bag of D_5W

so that final concentration is 1 mg/ml. Expect to use a concentration of 2 mg/ml for children and patients with cardiovascular disease. Before infusion, shake bag until contents are mixed thoroughly. Flush existing line with D_5W, or use a separate line. Don't use an in-line filter. If infusion exceeds 2 hours, shake infusion bag every 2 hours.

- Prepare amphotericin B liposomal complex by adding 12 ml sterile water for injection (without bacteriostatic agent) to each 50-mg vial to achieve a concentration of 4 mg amphotericin B per milliliter. Immediately shake vial vigorously for at least 30 seconds until all particles completely disperse. Withdraw prescribed dose of amphotericin B liposomal complex suspension. Then use a 5-micron filter to inject it into D_5W to provide a final concentration of 1 to 2 mg/ml. Expect to use a lower concentration (0.2 to 0.5 mg/ml) for infants and young children. Flush existing line with D_5W, or use a separate line. An in-line filter with a mean pore diameter of at least 1 micron may be used.
- Expect to give an antihistamine, antipyretic, or corticosteroid just before infusing amphotericin B to help minimize fever and shaking chills.
- Shake well before giving amphotericin B oral suspension. Drop suspension on tongue with calibrated dropper. Then tell patient to swish suspension in mouth for as long as possible before swallowing. If drug must be swabbed on, use a nonabsorbent swab.
- Give amphotericin B oral suspension between meals to permit prolonged contact with oral lesions.
- Assess I.V. insertion site regularly to detect extravasation of amphotericin B, which may cause severe local irritation. To minimize local thrombophlebitis, plan to add heparin to infusion or expect to administer amphotericin on alternate days, which also may help prevent anorexia. Alternate-day dose shouldn't exceed 1.5 mg/kg.
- Monitor renal function because of the risk of renal impairment. Plan to obtain serum creatinine level every other day while amphotericin B dosage is increasing and then at least twice weekly during therapy. If serum creatinine or BUN level increases significantly, expect to stop amphotericin B until renal function improves. Know that a cumulative dose of more than 4 g may cause irreversible renal dysfunction.
- Expect to monitor CBC and platelet count weekly during therapy to detect adverse hematologic effects. Also monitor serum calcium, magnesium, and potassium levels twice weekly to detect abnormalities.
- Use reconstituted amphotericin B within 24 hours if stored at room temperature, 1 week if refrigerated. Use reconstituted amphotericin B cholesteryl sulfate complex within 24 hours. Use amphotericin B lipid complex within 6 hours if stored at room temperature, 48 hours if refrigerated. Use diluted amphotericin B liposomal complex within 24 hours if refrigerated, but begin infusion within 6 hours.
- Be aware that false elevations of serum phosphate may occur when samples are analyzed using the PHOSm assay.

PATIENT TEACHING

- Instruct patient to shake bottle of oral suspension well before each dose; to drop suspension directly on his tongue using calibrated dropper; and then to swish suspension in his mouth for as long as possible before swallowing. If prescriber orders drug to be swabbed onto oral lesions, tell patient to use nonabsorbent swab. Instruct him to take drug four times a day (between meals and at bedtime).
- Tell patient to notify prescriber if he develops local irritation, if existing symptoms worsen or return, or if new symptoms arise.

ampicillin

ampicillin sodium

ampicillin trihydrate

Class and Category

Pharmacologic class: Aminopenicillin
Therapeutic class: Antibiotic
Pregnancy category: B

Indications and Dosages

➤ *To treat GI infections and genitourinary infections (other than gonorrhea) caused by susceptible strains of* Shigella, Salmonella typhi *and other species,* Escherichia coli, Proteus mirabilis, *and enterococci*

CAPSULES, ORAL SUSPENSION

Adults and children weighing 20 kg (44 lb) or more. 500 mg every 6 hr.
Children weighing less than 20 kg (44 lb). 100 mg/kg daily in divided doses every 6 hr.

I.M. INJECTION, I.V. INFUSION, I.V. INJECTION

Adults and children weighing 40 kg (88 lb) or more. 500 mg every 6 hr. For I.V. infusion, infuse over 15 to 30 min. For I.V. injection, inject slowly over 10 to 15 min and do not exceed 100 mg/ml.
Children weighing less than 40 kg. 50 mg/kg daily in divided doses every 6 to 8 hr. For I.V. infusion, infuse over 15 to 30 min. For I.V. injection, inject slowly over 10 to 15 min and do not exceed 100 mg/ml.

➤ *To treat uncomplicated gonorrhea caused by susceptible strains of non–penicillinase-producing* Neisseria gonorrhoeae

CAPSULES, ORAL SUSPENSION

Adults and children. 3.5 g as a single dose with 1 g of probenecid.

➤ *To treat respiratory tract infections caused by susceptible strains of non–penicillinase-producing* Haemophilus influenzae, *staphylococci, and streptococci, including* Streptococcus pneumoniae

CAPSULES, ORAL SUSPENSION

Adults and children weighing 20 kg (44 lb) or more. 250 mg every 6 hr.
Children weighing less than 20 kg (44 lb). 50 mg/kg daily in divided doses every 6 hr.

I.M. INJECTION, I.V. INFUSION, I.V. INJECTION

Adults and children weighing 40 kg (88 lb) or more. 250 to 500 mg every 6 to 8 hr. For I.V. infusion, infuse over 15 to 30 min. For I.V. injection, inject slowly over 10 to 15 min and do not exceed 100 mg/ml.
Children weighing less than 40 kg. 25 to 50 mg/kg daily in divided doses every 6 to 8 hr. For I.V. infusion, infuse over 15 to 30 min. For I.V. injection, inject slowly over 10 to 15 min and do not exceed 100 mg/ml.

➤ *To treat septicemia; to treat bacterial meningitis caused by susceptible strains of* Neisseria meningitidis

I.M. INJECTION, I.V. INFUSION, I.V. INJECTION

Adults and children. 150 to 200 mg/kg daily I.V. in divided doses every 3 to 4 hr for at least 3 days; then continued I.M. For I.V. infusion, infuse over 15 to 30 min. For I.V. injection, inject slowly over 10 to 15 min and do not exceed 100 mg/ml.

➤ *To treat urethritis in males due to* N. gonorrhoeae

I.M. INJECTION, I.V. INFUSION, I.V. INJECTION

Adult men. Two doses of 500 mg at 8- or 12-hr intervals. May repeat or extend treatment, if needed. For I.V. infusion, infuse over 15 to 30 min. For I.V. injection, inject slowly over 10 to 15 min and do not exceed 100 mg/ml.

➤ To treat soft tissue infections caused by susceptible strains of staphylococci and streptococci organisms

I.M. INJECTION, I.V. INFUSION, I.V. INJECTION

Adults and children weighing 40 kg (88 lb) or more. 250 to 500 mg every 6 or 8 hr. For I.V. infusion, infuse over 15 to 30 min. For I.V. injection, inject slowly over 10 to 15 min and do not exceed 100 mg/ml.
Adults and children weighing less than 40 kg (88 lb). 25 to 50 mg/kg daily in divided doses every 6 to 8 hr. For I.V. infusion, infuse over 15 to 30 min. For I.V. injection, inject slowly over 10 to 15 min and do not exceed 100 mg/ml.

Route	Onset	Peak	Duration
P.O.	Unknown	Unknown	Unknown
I.V.	Immediate	Unknown	Unknown

Mechanism of Action

Inhibits bacterial cell wall synthesis. The rigid, cross-linked cell wall is assembled in several steps. Ampicillin exerts its effects on susceptible bacteria in the final stage of the cross-linking process by binding with and inactivating penicillin-binding proteins (enzymes responsible for linking the cell wall strands). This action causes bacterial cell lysis and death.

Incompatibilities

Don't mix ampicillin and any amino-glycoside in the same I.V. bag, bottle, or tubing; otherwise, both drugs will be inactivated. If patient must receive both drugs, administer them in separate sites at least 1 hour apart.

Contraindications

Hypersensitivity to ampicillin, other pencillins, or their components; infection caused by penicillinase-producing organism

Interactions

DRUGS

allopurinol: Increased risk of rash, particularly in hyperuricemic patient
aminoglycosides: Possibly inactivated action
bacteriostatic antibiotics such as chlorampheicol, erythromycins, sulfonamides, tetracyclines: Possibly impaired action of ampicillin
live-virus vaccines such as BCG (intravesical) and typhoid: May decrease effectiveness of vaccine *oral anticoagulants:* Increased risk of bleeding
oral contraceptives: Possibly reduced contraceptive effectiveness and breakthrough bleeding
probenecid: Possibly increased serum ampicillin level and ampicillin toxicity

Adverse Reactions

CNS: Chills, fatigue, fever, headache, malaise
CV: Chest pain, edema, thrombophlebitis
EENT: Epistaxis, glossitis, **laryngeal stridor**, mucocutaneous candidiasis, stomatitis, **throat tightness**
GI: Abdominal distention, ***Clostridium difficile***-associated diarrhea, diarrhea, enterocolitis, flatulence, gastritis, nausea, **pseudomembranous colitis**, vomiting
GU: Dysuria, urine retention, vaginal candidiasis
HEME: Agranulocytosis, anemia, eosinophilia, **leukopenia**, **thrombocytopenia**, **thrombocytoenic purpura**
SKIN: Erythema multiforme; erythematous, mildly pruritic maculopapular rash or other types of rash; **exfoliative dermatitis**; pruritus; urticaria
Other: Anaphylaxis, **angioedema**, injection-site pain

Nursing Considerations

- Avoid giving ampicillin to patients with mononucleosis because of increased risk of rash.
- Expect to give ampicillin for 48 to 72 hours after patient becomes asymptomatic. For streptococcal infection, expect to give ampicillin for at least 10 days after cultures show streptococcal eradication to reduce risk of rheumatic fever or glomerulonephritis.
- Dilute ampicillin for I.M. use by adding (depending on manufacturer) 1.2 ml of sterile water or bacteriostatic water for injection to each 125-mg vial, 1 ml of diluent to each 250-mg vial, 1.8 ml of diluent to each 500-mg vial, 3.5 ml of diluent to each 1-g vial, or 6.8 ml of diluent to each 2-g vial.
- Dilute ampicillin for intermittent infusion by adding 5 ml of sterile water or bacteriostatic water for injection to each 125-, 250-, or 500-mg vial or 7.4 to 10 ml of diluent to each 1- or 2-g vial. Infuse in suitable diluent at less than 30 mg/ml.

WARNING For I.V. infusion, infuse over 15 to 30 min. For I.V. injection, inject slowly over 10 to 15 min and do not exceed 100 mg/ml. More rapid infusion may cause seizures.

- Monitor patient closely for anaphylaxis, which may be life-threatening. Patients at greatest risk are those with a history of multiple allergies, hypersensitivity to cephalosporins, or a history of asthma, hay fever, or urticaria.

WARNING Stop drug in an anaphylactic reaction, notify prescriber immediately, and provide immediate treatment with epinephrine, airway management, oxygen, and I.V. corticosteroids, as needed.

- Notify prescriber if patient has evidence of superinfection; expect to stop drug and provide appropriate treatment.
- Closely monitor results of renal and liver function tests and CBCs if long-term or high-dose ampicillin therapy is required.
- Monitor patient closely for diarrhea, which may be pseudomembranous colitis caused by *Clostridium difficile.* If diarrhea occurs, notify prescriber and expect to withhold ampicillin and administer fluids,

electrolytes, protein, and an antibiotic effective against *C. difficile.*

PATIENT TEACHING

- Emphasize the importance of taking the full course of ampicillin exactly as prescribed.
- Tell patient to take oral dose with 8 ounces of water 30 minutes before or 2 hours after meals.
- Instruct patient to shake suspension well before each use, keep bottle tightly closed between uses, and discard unused portion after 14 days if refrigerated or 7 days if stored at room temperature.
- Review signs of allergic reaction; if they occur, tell patient to hold next ampicillin dose and contact prescriber immediately.
- Urge patient to tell prescriber about diarrhea that's severe or lasts longer than 3 days. Remind patient that watery or bloody stools may occur 2 or more months after antibiotic therapy and may be serious, requiring prompt treatment.

anakinra

Kineret

Class and Category

Pharmacologic class: Interleukin-1 receptor blocker
Therapeutic class: Immunologic (antirheumatic, anti-inflammatory)
Pregnancy category: B

Indications and Dosages

➤ *To reduce signs and symptoms and slow structural damage in moderate to severe active rheumatoid arthritis in patients who have not responded to disease-modifying antirheumatics*

SUBCUTANEOUS INJECTION

Adults. 100 mg daily.

➤ *To treat Neonatal-Onset Multisystem Inflammatory Disease (NOMID) in patients with Cryopyrin-Associated Periodic Syndrome (CAPS)*

SUBCUTANEOUS INJECTION

Children. *Initial:* 1 to 2 mg/kg daily or dosage split into twice daily administration followed by dosage adjustments in 0.5 to 1.0 mg/kg increments, as needed.
Maximum: 8 mg/kg daily

DOSAGE ADJUSTMENT Interval reduced to every other day in severe renal insufficiency or end-stage renal disease (creatinine clearance less than 30 ml/min).

Mechanism of Action

Inhibits the binding of interleukin-1 (IL-1) to its type 1 receptor, blocking its activity. Inflammatory stimuli prompt T cells to release IL-1, a mediator of inflammation.

Contraindications

Active infection; hypersensitivity to anakinra, its components, or *Escherichia coli*–derived proteins

Interactions

DRUGS

etanercept and other drugs that block tumor necrosis factor: Increased risk of serious infection
live-virus vaccines: Possibly decreased antibody response to vaccine, potential for infection with live virus

Adverse Reactions

CNS: Fever, headache
CV: Elevated cholesterol levels
EENT: Nasopharyngitis, sinusitis
GI: Abdominal pain, diarrhea, elevated liver enzmes, nausea, **noninfectious hepatitis**, vomiting
HEME: Neutropenia, thrombocytopenia
MS: Arthralgia, bone and joint infections
RESP: Pneumonia, upper respiratory tract infection
SKIN: Cellulitis, pruritus, rash, urticaria
Other: Anaphylaxis; **angioedema**; flu-like symptoms; **hypersensitivity reactions**; injection-site ecchymosis, erythema, inflammation, pain, and pruritus; **malignancies**; positive results for anti-anakinra antibodies; serious infections

Nursing Considerations

- Expect to obtain baseline neutrophil count before therapy and to monitor neutrophil count every month for 3 months and every 3 months for up to 1 year.
- Discard solution if it contains particles or is discolored. Use prefilled syringe and needles to administer drug. Don't shake

syringe; allow time for solution to clear if it becomes foamy.
- Give drug about the same time each day.

WARNING Be aware that anakinra isn't recommended for patients with active infections. Monitor patient for evidence of infection, such as fever, chills, sore throat, and mouth sores, before and during therapy because drug increases the risk of infections, such as cellulitis, pneumonia, and bone and joint infections. Notify prescriber if signs are present. Patients with asthma and those receiving etanercept or infliximab are at increased risk for serious infections. Expect anakinra to be stopped if serious infection develops.

- Know that anakinra may possibly increase risk of reactivation of tuberculosis or development of other atypical or opportunistic infections. Follow current Center for Disease Control (CDC) guidelines to evaluate patients and, if needed, treat a possible latent tubercuolosis infection, as ordered, before starting anakinra therapy.
- Be aware that live-virus vaccines shouldn't be given to patients receiving anakinra because drug decreases immune response.
- Monitor patients with impaired renal function for signs of anakinra toxicity; they're at increased risk because drug is excreted primarily by the kidneys.
- Store anakinra at 2° to 8°C (36° to 46°F). Protect from freezing and light.

PATIENT TEACHING
- Teach proper injection technique if patient will self-administer drug. Make sure patient understands the process and can correctly prepare and inject doses.
- Instruct patient to rotate injection sites among thighs, stomach, and upper arms and to avoid areas that are tender, hard, red, or bruised. Advise him to make sure that each injection site is at least 1 inch away from the previous site.
- Urge patient to discard used needles and syringes in a puncture-resistant container and not to reuse them.
- Review evidence of allergic reaction, including rash and shortness of breath.
- Urge patient to immediately report signs of infection, such as cough, fever, chills, dyspnea, or headache, to prescriber.

angiotensin II

Giapreza

Class and Category

Pharmacologic class: Peptide hormone of the renin–angiotensin–aldosterone system
Therapeutic class: Antihypertensive
Pregnancy category: Not classified

Indications and Dosages

➤ *To increase blood pressure in patients with septic or other distributive shock*

I.V. INFUSION

Adults. *Initial:* 20 ng/kg/min continuously then increased in increments of up to 15 ng/kg/min every 5 minutes, as needed, to achieve or maintain target blood pressure but not to exceed 80 ng/kg/min during first 3 hr and not to exceed 40 ng/kg/min for remainder of treatment. When no longer needed, dosage decreased in increments of up to 15 ng/kg/min every 5 to 15 minutes, with adjustments made based upon blood pressure.

DOSAGE ADJUSTMENT Dosage may be decreased to as low as 1.25 ng/kg/min in patients sensitive to angiotension II effects.

Route	Onset	Peak	Duration
I.V.	Within 1 min	Unknown	Unknown

Mechanism of Action

Binds to the G-protein-coupled angiotensin II receptor type I on vascular smooth muscle cells, which stimulates myosin and causes smooth muscle contraction. These actions raise blood pressure by increasing aldosterone release and causing vasoconstriction.

Contraindications

Hypersensitivity to angiotensin II components

Interactions

DRUGS

angiotensin-converting enzyme (ACE) inhibitors: Possibly increased response to angiotensin II
angiotensin II receptor blockers (ARBs): Possibly decreased response to angiotensin II

Adverse Reactions

CNS: Delirium
CV: Arterial and venous thrombotic events, deep vein thrombosis, peripheral ischemia, tachycardia
ENDO: Hyperglycemia
HEME: Thrombocytopenia
Other: Acidosis, fungal infection

Nursing Considerations

- Administer angiotensin II only as an intravenous infusion, adjusting dosage every 5 minutes as needed. Do not exceed a dosage of 80 ng/kg/min during first 3 hours of treatment or 40 ng/kg/min for remainder of treatment.
- Dilute angiotensin II in 0.9% sodium chloride solution prior to use to achieve a final concentration of 5,000 ng/ml or 10,000 ng/ml. To prepare a 5,000 ng/ml solution, use angiotensin II vial strength of 2.5 mg/ml, withdraw 1 ml from vial, and add to 500-ml infusion bag of 0.9% sodium chloride. To prepare a 10,000 ng/ml solution, use angiotensin II vial strength of 2.5 mg/ml, withdraw 1 ml from vial, and add to a 250-ml infusion bag of 0.9% sodium chloride or use angiotensin II vial strength 5 mg/2 ml, withdraw 2 ml of angiotensin II, and add to 500-ml infusion bag of 0.9% sodium chloride.
- Know that diluted solution may be stored at room temperature or in refrigerator. Discard unused prepared solution after 24 hours regardless of how it was stored.
- Monitor patient closely for thrombotic events. Take precautions to prevent these events, especially deep venous thromboses.

PATIENT TEACHING

- Instruct patient on angiotensin II use, if patient is able to understand.
- Tell patient to report any abnormal symptoms, if patient is able to understand.

anidulafungin

Eraxis

Class and Category

Pharmacologic class: Echinocandin
Therapeutic class: Antifungal
Pregnancy category: Not classified

Indications and Dosages

➤ *To treat Candidemia and other forms of* Candida *infections (intra-abdominal abscess and peritonitis)*

I.V. INFUSION

Adults. 200 mg on day 1 infused over 3 hr, followed by 100 mg daily infused over 90 min and continued for a minimum of 14 days and for at least 14 days following last positive culture.

➤ *To treat esophageal candidiasis*

I.V. INFUSION

Adults. 100 mg on day 1 infused over 90 min, followed by 50 mg daily infused over 45 min for a minimum of 14 days and continued for at least 7 days following resolution of symptoms.

Mechanism of Action

Inhibits glucan synthase, an enzyme present in fungal cells. This results in inhibition of the formation of an essential D-glucan component of the fungal cell wall, thereby eliminating the fungal infection.

Incompatibilities

Do not use with other intravenous substances, additives, or medications other than 5% Dextrose Injection and normal saline because compatibility is unknown.

Contraindications

Hypersensitivity to anidulafungin, its components, or other echinocandins

Adverse Reactions

CNS: Confusion, depression, dizziness, fever, headache, insomnia, rigors, **seizures**
CV: Atrial fibrillation, chest pain, **deep vein thrombosis**, hypertension **hypotension**, peripheral edema, **QT prolongation**, right bundle branch block, sinus arrhythmia, superficial thrombophlebitis, **ventricular extrasystoles**
EENT: Blurred vision, eye pain, oral candidiasis, visual disturbance
ENDO: Hot flashes, hyperglycemia, **hypoglycemia**
GI: Abdominal pain, cholestasis, constipation, diarrhea, dyspepsia, elevated liver enzymes, **hepatic necrosis**, nausea, vomiting
GU: Elevated blood creatinine levels, UTI
HEME: Anemia, **leukocytosis, prolonged prothrombin time, thrombocytopenia**

MS: Back pain
RESP: **Bronchospasm**, cough, dyspnea, pleural effusion, pneumonia, **respiratory distress**
SKIN: Diaphoresis, erythema, flushing, pruritus, rash, ulceration, urticaria
Other: **Anaphylaxis**, **angioedema**, **bacteremia**, **clostridial infection**, dehydration, **hyperkalemia**, **hypokalemia**, **hypomagnesemia**, infusion-related reactions, **multiorgan failure**, **sepsis**, systemic *Candida* infection in the arm used for infusion

Nursing Considerations

- Reconstitute each 50-mg vial with 15 ml of sterile water for injection and each 100-mg vial with 30 ml of sterile water for injection to provide a concentration of 3.33 mg/ml. The reconstituted solution can be stored for up to 24 hours at temperatures up to 25°C (77°F) prior to dilution into the infusion solution.
- Transfer the contents of the reconstituted vial(s) aseptically into the appropriately sized I.V. bag or bottle containing either 5% Dextrose Injection or normal saline following the manufacturer guidelines for the amount of infusion volume to use.
- Infuse at 1.4 ml/min (which is equivalent to 1.1 mg/min). Do not infuse at a higher rate because infusion-related adverse reactions that are possibly histamine-mediated may occur. If total infusion volume is 65 ml, infuse at least over 45 minutes; if total infusion volume is 130 ml, infuse over at least 90 minutes; and, if total infusion volume is 260 ml, infuse over at least 180 minutes. The infusion solution may be stored up to 48 hours at temperatures up to 25°C (77°F).
- Monitor patient's liver function and enzyme levels closely during anidulafungin therapy because significant hepatic dysfunction, hepatitis, or hepatic failure have been reported, although a causal relationship has not been established. If patient begins to complain of fatigue and shows signs of jaundice or his liver enzymes become abnormal, notify prescriber, as drug may be discontinued.

WARNING Monitor patient closely for hypersensitivity reactions that could lead to anaphylactic reactions, including shock. If present, withhold drug, notify prescriber, and be prepared to provide emergency treatment.

PATIENT TEACHING

- Instruct patient to promptly report any hypersensitivity reaction such as flushing, hives, itching, rash, difficulty breathing, or dizziness.
- Advise patient to comply with blood tests that may be ordered to monitor reaction to anidulafungin.
- Tell women of childbearing age that anidulafungin may cause fetal harm. If pregnancy is suspected or confirmed, or patient is planning to breastfeed, advise patient to alert prescriber.

antihemophilic factor (recombinant) PEGylated-aucl

Jivi

Class and Category

Pharmacologic class: Coagulation Factor VIII
Therapeutic class: Coagulant
Pregnancy category: Not classified

Indications and Dosages

➤ *To treat on-demand and control of bleeding episodes in previously treated patients with hemophilia A*

I.V. INFUSION

Adults and adolescents. *For minor bleeding:* 10 to 20 international units and repeated every 24 to 48 hr until bleeding resolved. *For moderate bleeding:* 15 to 30 international units and repeated every 24 to 48 hr until bleeding resolved. For major bleeding: 30 to 50 international units and repeated every 8 to 24 hr until bleeding is resolved. Infused over 1 to 15 min, with rate of administration adapted to patient's response. *Maximum:* 2.5 ml/min infusion rate.

➤ *To manage perioperative bleeding in previously treated patients with hemophilia A*

I.V. INFUSION

Adults and adolescents. *For minor surgery:* 15 to 30 international units and repeated every 24 hr for at least 1 day and until healing is achieved. *For major surgery:* 40 to 50 international units and repeated every 12 to 24 hr until adequate wound healing is complete, then therapy continued for at least another 7 days to maintain Factor VIII activity of 30% to 60%. Infused over 1 to 15 min, with rate of administration adapted to patient's response. *Maximum:* 2.5 ml/min infusion rate.

➤ *To reduce frequency of bleeding episodes in previously treated patients with hemophilia A*

I.V. INFUSION

Adults and adolescents. *Initial:* 30 to 40 international units twice weekly with regimen adjusted to 45 to 60 international units every 5 days based on bleeding episodes. Dosing then adjusted to less or more frequent dosing as needed. Infused over 1 to 15 min, with rate of administration adapted to patient's response. *Maximum:* 2.5 ml/min infusion rate.

Mechanism of Action

Temporarily replaces the missing coagulation Factor VIII.

Contraindications

Hypersensitivity to antihemophilic factor (recombinant) PEGylated-aucl or to hamster or mouse proteins, polyethylene glycol, or their components

Interactions

DRUGS

None reported

Adverse Reactions

CNS: Dizziness, fever, headache, insomnia
CV: Chest tightness, hypotension (mild)
EENT: Distorted sense of taste, **throat tightness**
GI: Abdominal pain, nausea, vomiting
RESP: Cough
SKIN: Erythema, **erythema multiforme**, flushing, pruritus, rash
Other: Anaphylaxis, anti-PEG antibody formation, injection-site reactions (pruritus, rash), neutralizing antibodies

Nursing Considerations

- Know that dosage and duration of treatment depends on the severity of the Factor VIII deficiency, the location and extent of bleeding, and the patient's clinical condition.
- Be aware that potency assignment for the drug is determined using a chromogenic substrate assay.
- Monitor the Factor VIII activity of the drug in plasma, as ordered, knowing that the activity will be assessed using either a validated chromogenic substrate assay or a validated one-stage clotting assay.
- Know that calculation of the required dose of Factor VIII is based on one international unit of Factor VIII/kilogram ability to increase the plasma Factor VIII level by 2 international units/dl.
- Expect to adjust dose and frequency according to patient's clinical response, as ordered.
- Prepare antihemophilic factor (recombinant) PEGylated-aucl by first warming both the unopened vial and prefilled diluent syringe in your hands to a comfortable temperature (not to exceed 37°C [99°F]). Then remove the protective cap from the vial and cleanse the rubber stopper with a sterile alcohol swab, being careful not to handle the rubber stopper. Place the vial on a firm, nonskid surface. Peel off the paper cover on the vial adapter plastic housing. Do not remove the adapter from the plastic housing. Holding the adapter housing, place it over the product vial and firmly press down. The adapter will snap over the vial cap. Do not remove the adapter housing at this step. Holding the syringe by the barrel, snap the syringe cap off the tip. Do not touch the syringe tip with your hand or any surface. Set the syringe aside. Now remove and discard the adapter plastic housing. Attach the prefilled syringe to the vial adapter thread by turning clockwise. Remove the clear plastic plunger rod from the carton. Grasp the plunger rod by the top plate. Avoid touching the sides and threads of the plunger rod. Attach the plunger rod by turning it clockwise into the threaded rubber stopper of the

prefilled syringe. Inject the diluent slowly by pushing down on the plunger rod. Swirl vial gently until all powder on all sides of the vial is dissolved. Do not shake vial. Be sure that all powder is completely dissolved. Do not use if solution contains visible particles or is cloudy. Push down on the plunger to push all air back into the vial. Then, while holding the plunger down, turn the vial with syringe upside-down (inverted) so the vial is now above the syringe.

- Know that if the dose requires more than one vial, each vial must be reconstituted as described in the preceding bullet with the diluent syringe provided. Use a larger plastic syringe (not supplied) to combine the contents of the vials into one syringe. Filter the reconstituted product to remove potential particulate matter in the solution. Filtering is achieved by using the vial adapter. Withdraw all the solution through the vial adapter into the syringe by pulling the plunger rod back slowly and smoothly. Tilt the vial to the side and back to make sure all the solution has been drawn toward the large opening in the rubber stopper and into the syringe. Remove as much air as possible before removing the syringe from the vial by slowly and carefully pushing the air back into the vial. Detach the syringe with the plunger rod from the vial adapter by turning counter-clockwise. Attach the syringe to the infusion set provided and inject the reconstituted product intravenously.
- Administer the reconstituted drug as soon as possible after preparation. If unable to do so, store at room temperature for no longer than 3 hours. Infuse intravenously over 1 to 15 minutes, adapting the rate of administration to patient's response. Do not exceed the maximum infusion rate of 2.5 ml/min.
- Monitor patient for hypersensitivity reactions that could progress to anaphylaxis. If any signs or symptoms of an allergic reaction occur, immediately discontinue administration of the drug, notify prescriber, and initiate treatment according to institutional protocol.
- Be aware that neutralizing antibodies may form following the administration of antihemophilic factor (recombinant) PEGylated-aucl. If plasma Factor VIII activity levels are not attained or if bleeding is not controlled as expected with the administered dose, suspect the presence of a neutralizing antibody and notify prescriber. Expect testing for Factor VIII inhibitors and Factor VIII recovery. A low postinfusion Factor VIII level in the absence of detectable Factor VIII inhibitors indicates that the loss of drug effect is likely due to anti-PEG antibodies. In this situation, expect drug to be discontinued and know that patient will need to be switched to a previously effective Factor VIII product.

PATIENT TEACHING

- Instruct patient to report early signs of an allergic reaction such as dizziness, nausea, and tightness of his chest or throat during or after the infusion. If patient is home, stress importance of seeking immediate emergency attention, as the reaction can progress to a life-threatening situation.
- Tell patient to notify prescriber or treatment center if he experiences a lack of response to the drug.
- Advise patient to consult his prescriber prior to traveling.

apixaban

Eliquis

Class and Category

Pharmacologic class: Factor Xa inhibitor
Therapeutic class: Anticoagulant
Pregnancy category: B

Indications and Dosages

➤ *To reduce the risk of stroke and systemic embolism in patients with nonvalvular atrial fibrillation*

TABLETS

Adults. 5 mg twice daily.
DOSAGE ADJUSTMENT For patients with at least two of the following characteristics: 80 years or older, body weight of 60 kg (132 lbs) or less, or a serum creatinine

of 1.5 mg/dl or greater; dosage decreased to 2.5 mg twice daily.

➤ *To prevent deep vein thrombosis following hip or knee replacement surgery*

TABLETS

Adults. 2.5 mg twice daily beginning 12 to 24 hours after surgery and lasting 12 days for knee replacement and 35 days for hip replacement.

➤ *To treat deep vein thrombosis and pulmonary embolism*

TABLETS

Adults. 10 mg twice daily for 7 days followed by 5 mg twice daily.

➤ *To reduce risk of recurrence of deep vein thrombosis and pulmonary embolism*

TABLETS

Adults. 2.5 mg twice daily following 6 months of treatment for deep vein thrombosis or pulmonary embolism.

DOSAGE ADJUSTMENT For patients receiving 5 mg or 10 mg dosage twice daily, dosage reduced by 50% if patient also receiving combined strong dual inhibitors of cytochrome P450 3A4 (CYP3A4) and P-glycoprotein (P-gp) such as itraconazole, ketoconazole, or ritonavir. For patients receiving 2.5 mg dosage twice daily, coadministration with combined strong CYP3A4 and P-gp inhibitors are avoided.

Mechanism of Action

Inhibits free and clot-bound factor Xa and prothrombinase activity. Although apixaban has no direct effect on platelet aggregation, it does indirectly inhibit platelet aggregation induced by thrombin. By inhibiting factor Xa, apixaban decreases thrombin generation and thrombus development.

Contraindications

Active pathological bleeding, severe hypersensitivity to apixaban or its components

Interactions

DRUGS

antiplatelets, aspirin, fibrinolytics, heparin NSAIDs (chronic use): Possibly increased risk of bleeding

strong dual inducers of CYP3A4 and P-gp such as carbamazepine, phenytoin, rifampin, St. John's wort: Decreased effectiveness of apixaban

strong dual inhibitors of CYP3A4 and P-gp such as itraconazole, ketoconazole, ritonavir: Increased effects of apixaban

Adverse Reactions

CNS: Hemorrhagic stroke, syncope

GI: GI bleeding

HEME: Excessive bleeding, including hemorrhage

SKIN: Rash

Other: Anaphylaxis, angioedema

Nursing Considerations

- Know that apixaban should not be given to patients with severe hepatic dysfunction.
- Crush tablet and mix with apple juice or water or put in applesauce and administer immediately for patient unable to swallow whole tablets. For patient with a nasogastric tube, crush tablet and suspend in 60 ml of 5% dextrose and water or plain water and immediately administer through the nasogastric tube.
- Expect apixaban to be discontinued 48 hours before an invasive procedure or surgery if patient has a moderate or high risk of hemorrhage and 24 hours before an invasive procedure or surgery if patient has a mild risk of hemorrhage.
- Be aware that manufacturer guidelines should be followed when patient is switching from or to other anticoagulants. For example, when patient is switching from warfarin to apixaban therapy, expect warfarin to be discontinued and apixaban started when the International Normalized Ratio (INR) is below 2. When switching from apixaban to warfarin, expect apixaban to be discontinued and both a parenteral anticoagulant and warfarin given at the time the next dose of apixaban would have been given. Then the parenteral anticoagulant is discontinued when INR reaches an acceptable range. When switching between apixaban and anticoagulants other than warfarin, expect to discontinue the one being taken and begin the other at the next scheduled dose.
- Be aware that if apixaban is discontinued prematurely and adequate alternative anticoagulation is not present, the risk of thrombosis increases.

WARNING Monitor patient closely for bleeding, as apixaban may cause life-threatening bleeding. Expect drug to be discontinued with active pathological hemorrhage and expect to give the antidote, coagulation factor Xa (recombinant), inactivated-zhzo (Andexxa) to reverse effects of anticoagulation. Know that effects of apixaban may persist for at least 24 hours after the last dose.

PATIENT TEACHING

- Emphasize the importance of taking apixaban exactly as prescribed.
- Tell patient unable to swallow whole tablets to crush tablet and mix with apple juice or water or mix with applesauce and take immediately.
- Tell patient not to stop taking apixaban without first consulting prescriber. If patient misses a dose, instruct him to take it as soon as possible on the same day and resume the dosing schedule the next day. Caution patient not to double dose to make up for the missed dose the day before.
- Advise patient to report any unusual bleeding or bruising to the prescriber. Inform patient that it may take longer for her to stop bleeding and to take bleeding precautions, such as avoiding the use of a razor and using a soft-bristle toothbrush.
- Tell patient to alert all prescribers to use of apixaban therapy before any invasive procedure, including dental work, is scheduled.
- Advise female patient to notify prescriber immediately if pregnancy is suspected or known.

apomorphine hydrochloride

Apokyn

Class and Category

Pharmacologic class: Dopamine agonist (non-ergot)
Therapeutic class: Antiparkinsonian
Pregnancy category: Not classified

Indications and Dosages

➤ *To treat hypomobility "off" episodes (end-of-dose wearing off and unpredictable on/off episodes) in advanced Parkinson's disease as acute, intermittent treatment*

SUBCUTANEOUS INJECTION

Adults. *Initial when patient is in an "off" state:* 0.2 ml (2 mg) as a test dose. If tolerated, a second 0.2 ml (2 mg) dose given at least 2 hr after test dose and adjusted as needed in 0.1-ml (1-mg) increments every few days. *Maximum:* 0.6 ml (6 mg) as a single dose, 2 ml (20 mg) total daily dose, and no more than 5 doses per day.

DOSAGE ADJUSTMENT For patients who tolerate 0.2 ml (2 mg) but have no response, a 0.4-ml (4-mg) dose may be given under medical supervision, with standing and supine blood pressure checked every 20 min for 1 hr at the next observed "off" period, as long as it is at least 2 hr after the initial 0.2-ml (2-mg) test dose. If tolerated, a dose 0.1 ml (1 mg) lower may be given as needed and increased in 0.1-ml (1-mg) increments every few days as needed to a maximum dose of 0.6 ml (6 mg).
If patient doesn't tolerate a 0.4-ml (4-mg) test dose, a 0.3-ml (3-mg) test dose may be given under medical supervision, with standing and supine blood pressure checked every 20 min for 1 hr at the next observed "off" period, as long as it is at least 2 hr after the initial 0.4-ml (4-mg) test dose. If tolerated, a 0.2-ml (2-mg) dose can be started as needed and increased to no more than 0.3 ml (3 mg) if needed after a few days. For patients with mild to moderate renal impairment, the initial dose should be reduced to 0.1 ml (1 mg).

Route	Onset	Peak	Duration
SubQ	10–60 min	Unknown	Unknown

Mechanism of Action

May stimulate postsynaptic dopamine D_2 receptors in the caudate–putamen of the brain. As a result, apomorphine improves motor function and activity levels in patients with Parkinson's disease.

Contraindications

Concurrent use of 5-HT_3 antagonists including antiemetics, such as alosetron, dolasetron, granisetron, ondansetron, and palonosetron; hypersensitivity to apomorphine, sulfites such as sodium metabisulfite, or their components

Interactions

DRUGS

5-HT_3 antagonists: Increased risk of profound hypotension and loss of consciousness
antihypertensives, vasodilators: Increased risk of serious adverse reactions, such as bone or joint injuries, hypotension, and MI
dopamine antagonists (such as butyrophenones, metoclopramide, phenothiazines, thioxanthenes): Decreased apomorphine effectiveness
drugs that prolong QT interval: Increased risk of torsades de pointes

ACTIVITIES

alcohol use: Increased risk of hypotension

Adverse Reactions

CNS: Aggravated Parkinson's disease, anxiety, confusion, depression, dizziness, drowsiness, dyskinesia, euphoria, fatigue, hallucinations, headache, insomnia, psychotic-like behavior, somnolence, weakness, yawning
CV: Angina, chest pain, **congestive heart failure**, edema, **MI**, orthostatic hypotension, **prolonged QT interval**
EENT: Rhinorrhea
GI: Constipation, diarrhea, nausea, vomiting
GU: UTI
MS: Arthralgia, back or limb pain
RESP: Dyspnea, pneumonia, tachypnea
SKIN: Contact dermatitis, diaphoresis, ecchymosis, flushing, pallor
Other: Dehydration; injection-site bruising, granuloma, or pruritus; intense urges to perform certain activities, such as gambling and sexual acts

Nursing Considerations

- Be aware that apomorphine therapy is usually not recommended in a patient with a major psychotic disorder because of the risk of exacerbating psychosis.
- Use apomorphine cautiously in patients with hepatic or renal insufficiency.
- Be aware that an antiemetic, such as trimethobenzamide 300 mg three times daily, should be started 3 days before apomorphine starts and continue for at least the first 2 months of therapy. Apomorphine may cause severe nausea and vomiting, even with an antiemetic.
- Monitor patient's blood pressure closely because drug can cause severe orthostatic hypotension.
- Give a 0.2-ml (2-mg) test dose of apomorphine, as prescribed, and then check patient's supine and standing blood pressure 20, 40, and 60 minutes later.
- Monitor patient closely if he has an increased risk of prolonged QT interval, as from bradycardia, genetic predisposition, hypokalemia, hypomagnesemia, or use of certain drugs. QT-interval prolongation may lead to torsades de pointes.
- Monitor patient for evidence of apomorphine abuse. Although rare, drug may cause psychosexual stimulation and increased libido, which may cause patient to use apomorphine more often than needed.

PATIENT TEACHING

- Explain that an antiemetic will be prescribed starting 3 days before first apomorphine dose. Urge patient to take the antiemetic exactly as prescribed. Explain that it will be needed for 2 months or longer during apomorphine therapy.
- Explain that a test dose will determine response and drug's effects on blood pressure before patient goes home with drug.
- Teach caregiver how to use dosing pen and how to give drug subcutaneously.
- Emphasize that apomorphine doses are expressed as milliliters, not milligrams. Tell caregiver to draw up each dose carefully to reduce the chance of dosage error.
- Instruct caregiver to rotate injection sites in a systematic manner.
- Stress importance of taking apomorphine only as prescribed because serious adverse reactions may occur.
- Advise patient to avoid hazardous activities until drug's CNS effects are known. In particular, caution patient that apomorphine increases the risk of falling asleep suddenly, without feeling sleepy.
- Instruct patient to notify prescriber about intense urges, such as for gambling or sex, because dosage may need to be reduced or drug discontinued.

- Advise patient or caregiver to report immediately any psychotic-like behavior, such as seeing or hearing things that are not real, confusion, excessive suspicion, aggressive behavior, agitation, believing things that are not real, or disorganized thinking.

apremilast

Otezla

Class and Category

Pharmacologic class: Phosphodiesterase 4 inhibitor
Therapeutic class: Antirheumatic
Pregnancy category: C

Indications and Dosages

➤ *To treat active psoriatic arthritis; to treat moderate to severe plaque psoriasis in patients who are candidates for phototherapy or systemic therapy*

TABLETS

Adults. *Initial:* 10 mg in a.m. on day 1; 10 mg in a.m. and p.m. on day 2; 10 mg in a.m. and 20 mg in p.m. on day 3; 20 mg in a.m. and p.m. on day 4; 20 mg in a.m. and 30 mg in p.m. on day 5; and 30 mg in a.m. and p.m. on day 6 and thereafter. *Maintenance:* 30 mg in a.m. and p.m.

DOSAGE ADJUSTMENT For patients with severe renal impairment (creatinine clearance less than 30 ml/min), dosage titration decreased to once daily using only the a.m. titration schedule and maintenance dosage kept at 30 mg once daily in a.m.

Mechanism of Action

Inhibits phosphodiesterase 4, which is specific for cyclic adenosine monophosphate (cAMP). This action results in increased intracellular cAMP levels, which are thought to help relieve symptoms of psoriatic arthritis.

Contraindications

Hypersensitivity to apremilast or its components

Interactions

DRUGS

rifampin: Decreased apremilast exposure with loss of effectiveness

strong CYP450 inducers such as carbamazepine, phenobarbital, phenytoin

Adverse Reactions

CNS: Depression, fatigue, headache, insomnia, migraine, **suicidal ideation**
EENT: Nasopharyngitis
GI: Anorexia, diarrhea, dyspepsia, gastroesophageal reflux disease, nausea, upper abdominal pain, vomiting
MS: Back pain
RESP: Bronchitis, cough, upper respiratory infection
SKIN: Rash
Other: Weight loss

Nursing Considerations

- Watch patient closely for evidence of depression, especially when apremilast therapy begins, because apremilast therapy may increase risk of depression and possibly lead to suicidal thinking or behavior.
- Monitor patient's weight regularly because apremilast may cause weight loss. Notify prescriber if weight loss occurs that is unexplained or is significant.

PATIENT TEACHING

- Tell patient to follow titration schedule exactly, as this will help reduce the incidence and severity of gastrointestinal symptoms associated with initial therapy.
- Instruct patient to swallow the tablets whole and not to crush, split, or chew the tablets.
- Instruct caregivers to watch patient closely for evidence of suicidal tendencies, especially when therapy starts, and to report concerns to prescriber immediately.

aprepitant

Cinvanti, Emend

fosaprepitant dimeglumine

Emend for Injection

Class and Category

Pharmacologic class: Substance P/neurokinin 1 (NK1) receptor antagonist
Therapeutic class: Antiemetic
Pregnancy category: Not classified

Indications and Dosages

➤ *As adjunct to prevent acute and delayed nausea and vomiting associated with moderately to highly emetogenic chemotherapy, including high-dose cisplatin*

CAPSULES (EMEND)

Adults and children age 12 and over. 125 mg 1 hr before chemotherapy treatment, followed by 80 mg daily 1 hr before chemotherapy or if no chemotherapy in morning on next 2 days.

I.V. INFUSION (EMEND FOR INJECTION)

Adults. 150 mg infused over 20 to 30 min before chemotherapy begins on day 1 only.

I.V. INFUSION (CINVANTI)

Adults receiving highly emetogenic cancer chemotherapy. 130 mg as a single dose infused over 30 min about 30 min prior to chemotherapy on day 1 only.

I.V. INFUSION (CINVANTI) FOLLOWED BY CAPSULES (EMEND)

Adults receiving moderately emetogenic cancer chemotherapy. 100 mg as a single dose infused over 30 min about 30 min prior to chemotherapy on day 1, followed by 80 mg of oral aprepitant on days 2 and 3.

ORAL SUSPENSION (EMEND)

Adults and children age 12 and over who cannot swallow oral capsules: 125 mg 1 hr before chemotherapy treatment, followed by 80 mg daily 1 hr before chemotherapy or if no chemotherapy in morning on next 2 days.

Children 6 months to less than 12 years: 3 mg/kg (maximum 125 mg) on day 1, followed by 2 mg/kg (maximum 80 mg) 1 hr before chemotherapy or if no chemotherapy in morning on next 2 days.

➤ *To prevent nausea and vomiting associated with moderately to highly emetogenic chemotherapy with single-day pediatric chemotherapy regimens*

I.V. INFUSION (EMEND FOR INJECTION)

Adolescents age 12 to 17. 150 mg as a single dose infused over 30 min about 30 min prior to chemotherapy on day 1 only.

Children age 2 to less than 12. 4 mg/kg (maximum 150 mg) as a single dose infused over 60 min and completed about 30 min prior to chemotherapy on day 1 only.

Children 6 months to less than 2 years. 5 mg/kg (maximum 150 mg) as a single dose infused over 60 min and completed about 30 min prior to chemotherapy on day 1 only.

➤ To prevent nausea and vomiting associated with moderately to highly emetogenic chemotherapy with multi-day pediatric chemotherapy regimens

I.V. INFUSION (EMEND FOR INJECTION), CAPSULES (EMEND), ORAL SUSPENSION (EMEND)

Adolescents age 12 to 17. 115 mg as a single dose infused over 30 min about 30 min prior to chemotherapy on day 1 only followed by 80 mg daily of oral aprepitant on days 2 and 3.

Children age 6 months to less than 12 years. 3 mg/kg (maximum 115 mg) as a single dose infused over 60 min and completed about 30 min prior to chemotherapy on day 1 only followed by 80 mg daily of oral aprepitant in suspension form on days 2 and 3.

➤ *As adjunct to prevent postoperative nausea and vomiting*

CAPSULES (EMEND)

Adults. 40 mg within 3 hr before induction of anesthesia

Route	Onset	Peak	Duration
P.O., I.V.	Unknown	4 hr	Unknown

Mechanism of Action

Crosses the blood–brain barrier to occupy brain NK1 receptors, which prevents nerve transmission of signals that cause nausea and vomiting.

Incompatibilities

Do not mix aprepitant with any solutions containing divalent cations (e.g., calcium, magnesium), including Lactated Ringer's solution and Hartmann's solution.

Contraindications

Concurrent use of primozide, hypersensitivity to aprepitant or its components

Interactions

DRUGS

carbamazepine, other CYP3A4 inducers, phenytoin, rifampin: Possibly decreased blood aprepitant level

CYP3A4 inhibitors (such as clarithromycin, diltiazem, itraconazole, ketoconazole, nefazodone, nelfinavir, ritonavir, and

troleandomycin): Increased blood aprepitant level
CYP3A4 substrates (such as astemizole, benzodiazepines, cisapride, docetaxel, etoposide, imatinib, irinotecan, paclitaxel, pimozide, terfenadine, vinblastine, vincristine, and vinorelbine): Increased level of CYP3A4 substrates, resulting in possibly serious or life-threatening adverse reactions
dexamethasone, methylprednisolone: Increased effects of these drugs and risk of adverse reactions
ifosfamide: Increased risk of neurotoxicity and possibly other serious or life threatening adverse reactions
oral contraceptives: Possibly decreased effectiveness of hormonal contraceptives
paroxetine: Possibly decreased blood level of both drugs
warfarin: Decreased effectiveness of warfarin and increased prothrombin time

Adverse Reactions

CNS: Anxiety, asthenia, confusion, depression, dizziness, fatigue, fever, headache, hypoesthesia, hypothermia, insomnia, malaise, peripheral or sensory neuropathy, rigors, somnolence, syncope, tremor
CV: Bradycardia, **deep vein thrombosis**, edema, hypertension, **hypotension**, **MI**, palpitations, peripheral edema, tachycardia
EENT: Conjunctivitis, dry mouth, increased salivation, mucous membrane alteration, nasal discharge, oral candidiasis, oropharyngeal pain, pharyngitis, stomatitis, taste perversion, tinnitus, vocal disturbance
ENDO: Hot flashes, hyperglycemia
GI: Abdominal pain, anorexia, constipation, diarrhea, dysphagia, elevated liver enzymes, epigastric discomfort, flatulence, gastritis, gastroesophageal reflux, heartburn, hiccups, nausea, obstipation (intractable constipation), vomiting
GU: Dysuria, elevated BUN and serum creatinine levels, hematuria, leukocyturia, proteinuria, **renal insufficiency**, UTI
HEME: Anemia, **febrile neutropenia**, hematoma, leukocytosis, **leukopenia**, **neutropenia**, **thrombocytopenia**
MS: Arthralgia, back pain, muscle weakness, musculoskeletal pain, myalgia, pelvic pain
RESP: Cough, dyspnea, **hypoxia**, **non-small-cell lung carcinoma**, **pneumonitis**, **pulmonary emboism**, **respiratory depression or insufficiency**, respiratory tract infection
SKIN: Acne, alopecia, diaphoresis, flushing, pruritus, rash, **Stevens–Johnson syndrome**, **toxic epidermal necrolysis**, urticaria
Other: Anaphylaxis, **angioedema**, candidiasis, dehydration, elevated alkaline phosphatase, herpes simplex, **hypokalemia**, **hyponatremia**, infusion-site pain or induration, **malignant neoplasm**, **septic shock**, weight loss

Nursing Considerations

- Use caution when giving aprepitant to patients with severe hepatic insufficiency because drug's effects on such patients aren't known.
- Expect to administer aprepitant with dexamethasone and a 5-HT_3 antagonist, such as dolasetron, granisetron, or ondansetron for maximum antiemetic effects.
- Administer capsule form only to children age 12 and over. Suspension form should be administered to children under 12 or to an older patient who cannot swallow capsules.
- Know that when drug is administered intravenously, it is given only as the first dose 30 minutes before chemotherapy.
- Reconstitute parenteral aprepitant (Cinvanti brand) by aseptically filling an infusion bag with 130 ml for 130-mg dose or 100 ml for 100-mg dose with 0.9% sodium chloride injection, USP, or 5% Dextrose for Injection, USP. Then withdraw 18 ml for 130-mg dose or 14 ml for 100-mg dose from drug vial and transfer it into the infusion bag. Gently invert the bag four or five times. Avoid shaking. Before administration, inspect bag for particulate matter and discoloration.
- Reconstitute parental aprepitant (Emend brand) by injecting 5 ml normal saline for injection along vial wall to prevent foaming. Swirl vial gently. Withdraw contents from vial and add to an infusion bag containing 110 ml normal saline solution. Gently invert the bag two or three times. Administer over

15 minutes. Reconstituted solution may be stored at room temperature for 24 hours.

WARNING Monitor patient closely for hypersensitivity reactions, which could include anaphylaxis and anaphylactic shock during or soon after infusion of drug. Symptoms to be alert for include dyspnea, erythema, flushing, hypotension, and syncope. If a hypersensitivity reaction occurs, stop infusion if still being given, notify prescriber, expect drug to be discontinued, and be prepared to provide supportive care.

- Be aware that ifosfamide-induced neurotoxicity may occur after aprepitant and ifosfamide have been coadministered.

PATIENT TEACHING

- Instruct patient to take 125-mg dose of oral aprepitant 1 hour before chemotherapy, 80-mg dose in the morning for 2 days after chemotherapy, or 40-mg dose within 3 hours before induction of anesthesia.
- Instruct patient to report an allergic reaction such as difficulty breathing, dizziness, fainting, or flushing, and seek immediate medical attention.
- Tell female patients taking hormonal contraceptives to use an alternative or backup method of contraception during aprepitant therapy and for 1 month after last dose because drug reduces effectiveness of hormonal contraceptives.
- Tell patient taking warfarin to have clotting status monitored closely for 2 weeks after first aprepitant dose, especially every 7 to 10 days during each chemotherapy cycle in which the drug is used.
- Caution patient to inform prescriber of any drugs he's taking, including OTC drugs and herbal preparations, because they may interact with aprepitant.

arformoterol

Brovana

Class and Category

Pharmacologic class: Long-acting selective beta$_2$-agonist
Therapeutic class: Bronchodilator
Pregnancy category: C

Indications and Dosages

➤ *To provide maintenance treatment of bronchoconstriction in patients with COPD, including chronic bronchitis and emphysema*

INHALATION SOLUTION

Adults. 15 mcg (contents of one 2-ml vial) twice daily (morning and evening) via nebulization. *Maximum:* 30 mcg daily.

Mechanism of Action

Attaches to beta$_2$ receptors on bronchial cell membranes, stimulating the intracellular enzyme adenylate cyclase to convert adenosine triphosphate to cyclic adenosine monophosphate (cAMP). The resulting increase in intracellular cAMP level relaxes bronchial smooth-muscle cells, stabilizes mast cells, and inhibits histamine release.

Contraindications

Acute bronchospasm; acute deterioration of COPD condition; hypersensitivity to arformoterol, racemic formoterol, or their components; symptoms of COPD; use to treat asthma without use of a long-term asthma control medication

Interactions

DRUGS

adrenergics: Potentiated sympathetic effects
beta blockers: Decreased effectiveness of either drug
corticosteroids, methylxanthines such as aminophylline or theophylline, non–potassium-sparing (such as loop and thiazide) diuretics: Increased risk of hypokalemia
drugs known to prolong the QT interval, MAO inhibitors, tricyclic antidepressants: Increased risk of life-threatening ventricular arrhythmias

Adverse Reactions

CNS: Agitation, asthenia, circumoral paresthesia, CVA, dizziness, fatigue, fever, headache, hypokinesia, insomnia, malaise, nervousness, paralysis, somnolence, tremor
CV: **Angina**, **arrhythmias**, **atrial flutter**, chest pain, **congestive heart failure**, **heart block**, hyperlipemia, hypertension, **MI**, palpitations, peripheral edema, **prolonged QT interval**

EENT: Abnormal vision, dry mouth, glaucoma, herpes simplex or zoster, oral candidiasis, sinusitis, voice alteration
ENDO: Hyperglycemia, **hypoglycemia**
GI: Constipation, diarrhea, gastritis, melena, nausea, pelvic pain, **rectal hemorrhage**, **retroperitoneal hemorrhage**, vomiting
GU: Cystitis, hematuria, nocturia, PSA elevation, pyuria, renal calculi
HEME: Leukocytosis
MS: Arthralgia, arthritis, back pain, leg or muscle cramps, neck rigidity
RESP: Bronchitis, **bronchospasm**, dyspnea, pulmonary congestion
SKIN: Discoloration, dryness, hypertrophy, photosensitivity, rash, urticaria
Other: Anaphylaxis, **angioedema**, dehydration, flu-like syndrome, gout, **hyperkalemia**, **hypokalemia**, **metabolic acidosis**

Nursing Considerations

- Know that arformoterol should not be initiated in patients with acutely deteriorating COPD, which may be a life-threatening condition because arformoterol's onset of action is too prolonged.
- Use cautiously in patients with cardiovascular disorders, especially insufficiency, cardiac arrhythmias, and hypertension; convulsive disorders; thyrotoxicosis; and unusual sensitivity to sympathomimetic amines because arformoterol may cause significant adverse effects.
- Be aware that arformoterol shouldn't be used to relieve bronchospasm quickly because of its prolonged onset of action. Patients already taking the drug twice daily shouldn't take additional doses for exercise-induced bronchospasm.
- Know that drug should not be used with other inhaled, long-acting beta$_2$-agonists or with other medications containing long-acting beta$_2$-agonists.

WARNING Be aware that asthma-related deaths have increased in patients receiving salmeterol, a drug in the same class as arformoterol. Use of long-acting beta$_2$-adrenergic agonists, such as arformoterol, is contraindicated in patients with asthma without the use of a long-term asthma control medication, such as an inhaled corticosteroid. Monitor patient closely, and notify prescriber immediately of any changes in patient's respiratory status.

- Watch for arrhythmias and changes in heart rate or blood pressure after use in patients with cardiovascular disorders because of drug's beta-adrenergic effects.

WARNING Stop arformoterol immediately and notify prescriber if patient develops paradoxical bronchospasm or an allergic reaction.

- Monitor patient's blood glucose level, especially if diabetic, and plasma potassium level, as ordered, because arformoterol may cause significant changes.

PATIENT TEACHING

- Advise patient to take doses 12 hours apart, morning and evening, for optimum effect. Caution against using drug more than every 12 hours.
- Teach patient to self-administer drug with a standard jet nebulizer connected to an air compressor and to use vial immediately after removing from foil package.
- Caution patient not to swallow solution.
- Tell patient to return unused vials to pouch and store arformoterol in the refrigerator.
- Instruct patient taking inhaled, short-acting beta$_2$-agonists on a regular basis to discontinue regular use of these drugs as ordered, and to use them only for symptomatic relief of acute respiratory symptoms as prescribed.
- Instruct patient to notify prescriber if he needs four or more oral inhalations of rapid-acting inhaled bronchodilator a day for 2 or more consecutive days, or if he uses more than one canister of rapid-acting bronchodilator in an 8-week period.
- Emphasize importance of seeking emergency medical attention immediately if his breathing problems worsen or if he used his rescue inhaler but it did not relieve his breathing problem.

argatroban

Acova

Class and Category

Pharmacologic class: Direct thrombin inhibitor
Therapeutic class: Anticoagulant
Pregnancy category: B

Indications and Dosages

➤ *To prevent or treat thrombosis in patients with heparin-induced thrombocytopenia (HIT)*

I.V. INFUSION

Adults without hepatic impairment. 2 mcg/kg/min as a continuous infusion. *Maximum:* 10 mcg/kg/min.

DOSAGE ADJUSTMENT Dosage adjusted as prescribed to maintain patient's APTT at 1.5 to 3 times the initial baseline value, not to exceed 100 sec. Initial dosage reduced to 0.5 mcg/kg/min for patients with moderate or severe hepatic impairment.

➤ *To prevent or treat thrombosis in patients with or at risk for HIT when undergoing percutaneous coronary intervention (PCI)*

I.V. INFUSION

Adults without hepatic impairment. *Initial:* 350 mcg/kg over 3 to 5 min followed by continuous infusion of 25 mcg/kg/min.

DOSAGE ADJUSTMENT Dosage adjusted as prescribed to keep activated clotting time (ACT) at 300 to 450 sec. If ACT is less than 300 sec, additional I.V. bolus dose of 150 mcg/kg given and infusion increased to 30 mcg/kg/min; if ACT exceeds 450 sec, dosage reduced to 15 mcg/kg/min. For dissection, impending abrupt closure, thrombus formation during PCI, or inability to reach or keep ACT above 300 sec, additional bolus dose of 150 mcg/kg given and infusion increased to 40 mcg/kg/min.

Route	Onset	Peak	Duration
I.V.	Immediate	3–4 hr	Unknown

Mechanism of Action

Forms a tight bond with thrombin, neutralizing this enzyme's actions, even when the enzyme is trapped within clots. Thrombin causes fibrinogen to convert to fibrin, which is essential for clot formation.

Contraindications

Active major bleeding, hypersensitivity to argatroban or its components

Interactions

DRUGS

heparin, oral anticogulants: Increased risk of bleeding

Adverse Reactions

CNS: **Cerebrovascular bleeding**, fever, headache
CV: **Atrial fibrillation**, **cardiac arrest**, **hypotension**, **unstable angina**, **ventricular tachycardia**
GI: Abdominal pain, anorexia, diarrhea, elevated liver enzymes, **GI bleeding**, **melena**, nausea, vomiting
GU: Elevated BUN and serum creatinine levels, hematuria (microscopic), UTI
HEME: **Hemorrhage**, **hypoprothrombinemia**, **usual bleeding** or bruising
RESP: Cough, dyspnea, **hemoptysis**, pneumonia
SKIN: Bleeding at puncture site, rash
Other: Sepsis

Nursing Considerations

WARNING Know that argatroban isn't recommended for PCI patients with significant hepatic disease or AST/ALT levels three times or more the upper limits of normal.

- Reconstitute drug to 1 mg/ml before giving.
- Protect solution from direct sunlight.

WARNING Monitor patients with thrombocytopenia or those receiving daily doses of salicylates greater than 6 g for signs and symptoms of bleeding; these patients are at increased risk of bleeding from hypoprothrombinemia.

WARNING Expect to perform blood coagulation tests before and 2 hours after start of therapy because of the major risk of bleeding associated with argatroban. Be aware that coagulopathy must be ruled out before therapy starts. When giving drug to a patient undergoing PCI, expect to check ACT 5 to 10 minutes after each bolus and each infusion rate change and every 20 to 30 minutes during the PCI.

- Monitor the following patients for signs and symptoms of bleeding which may become severe and occur at any site in the body because they're at increased risk during argatroban therapy: patients who have recently had a large vessel puncture or organ biopsy, lumbar puncture, major bleeding (including intracranial, GI, intraocular, retroperitoneal, or pulmonary bleeding), major surgery (including brain, eye, or spinal cord surgery), spinal anesthesia, or stroke; patients with vascular or organ abnormalities, such as advanced renal disease, dissecting aortic aneurysm, diverticulitis, hemophilia, hepatic disease (especially if associated with a deficiency of vitamin K-dependent clotting factors), infective endocarditis inflammatory bowel disease, or peptic ulcer disease such as severe uncontrolled hypertension; and women with active menstruation. Risk of bleeding, especially hemorrhage, is also increased with concomitant use with other anticoagulants, antiplatelets, and thrombolytics.
- Avoid I.M. injections, whenever possible, in patients receiving argatroban to decrease the risk of bleeding.
- Be aware that thrombin times may not be helpful for monitoring argatroban activity because the drug affects all thrombin-dependent coagulation tests.
- Monitor pregnant women during labor and delivery for excessive bleeding or unexpected changes in coagulation parameters. Know that exposure to argatroban may increase the risk of bleeding in the fetus and neonate. Monitor closely.
- Expect dosage to be tapered before stopping to prevent the risk of rebound hypercoagulopathy; drug's effects last only a short time once drug is discontinued.

PATIENT TEACHING

- Inform patient that argatroban is a blood thinner that's given in the hospital by infusion into a vein. If he needs long-term anticoagulation, he'll be switched to another drug before discharge.
- Advise patient to report immediately any unusual or unexplained bleeding, such as blood in urine, easy bruising, nosebleeds, tarry stools, and vaginal bleeding.
- Instruct patient to avoid injury while receiving argatroban. For example, suggest that he brush his teeth gently, using a soft-bristled toothbrush, and take special care when flossing.

aripiprazole

Abilify, Abilify Maintena

aripiprazole lauroxil

Aristada, Aristada Initio

Class and Category

Pharmacologic class: Atypical antipsychotic
Therapeutic class: Antipsychotic
Pregnancy category: Not classified

Indications and Dosages

➤ *To treat acute schizophrenia; to maintain stability in patients with schizophrenia*

SOLUTION, ORALLY DISINTEGRATING TABLETS, TABLETS

Adults. *Initial:* 10 or 15 mg daily. Increased to 30 mg daily, as needed, with dosage adjustments at 2-wk intervals.
Adolescents. *Initial:* 2 mg daily for 2 days, then increased to 5 mg daily for 2 days, then increased to 10 mg daily

I.M. INJECTION (ABILIFY MAINTENA)

Adults. 400 mg monthly (no sooner than 26 days after last dose). Dosage reduced to 300 mg monthly if adverse reactions occur.

I.M. INJECTION (ARISTADA)

Adults. 441, 662, or 882 mg monthly. Alternatively, 882 mg every 6 wk or 1064 mg every 2 months. Early dosing should not be given sooner than 14 days after the previous injection.

TABLET (ABILIFY MYCITE)

Adults. *Initial:* 10 to 15 mg daily, with dosage increased no sooner than every 2 wk. *Maximum:* 30 mg daily.

➤ As adjunct with oral aripiprazole to initiate Aristada treatment for patients with schizophrenia

I.M. INJECTION (ARISTADA INITIO)

Adults. 675 mg as a single dose given at the same time as a 30 mg oral dose of aripiprazole. First dose of Aristada is then administered on the same day or up to 10 days thereafter.

➤ *To re-initiate treatment with Aristada following a missed dose of Aristada in patients with schizophrenia*

I.M. INJECTION (ARISTADA INITIO)

Adults taking 441 mg of Aristada. If time lapse from last dose of Aristada is greater than 6 weeks but less than 7 weeks, 675 mg as a single dose of Aristada Initio.

Adults taking 662 mg or 882 mg of Aristada. If time lapse from last dose of Aristada is greater than 8 wks but 12 wks or less, 675 mg as a single dose of Aristada Initio.

Adults taking 1064 mg of Aristada. If time lapse from last dose of Aristada is greater than 10 wks but 12 weeks or less, 675 mg as a single dose of Aristada Initio.

I.M. INJECTION (ARISTADA INITIO) PLUS ORAL SOLUTION, ORALLY DISINTEGRATING TABLETS, OR TABLETS

Adults taking 441 mg of Aristada. If time lapse from last dose of Aristada is greater than 7 wks, 675 mg as a single dose of Aristada Initio plus a single 30 mg oral dose of aripiprazole.

Adults taking 662 mg, 882 mg, or 1064 mg of Aristada. If time lapse from last dose of Aristada is greater than 12 wks, 675 mg as a single dose of Aristada Initio plus a single 30 mg oral dose of aripiprazole.

➤ *To treat acute manic and mixed episodes in bipolar I disorder with or without psychotic features; to maintain stability in patients with bipolar I disorder; as adjunct with lithium or valproate in patients with bipolar I disorder*

ORAL SOLUTION, ORALLY DISINTEGRATING TABLETS, TABLETS

Adults. *Initial:* 15 mg daily, increased to 30 mg daily, as needed. *Maintenance:* 15 to 30 mg daily. *Maximum:* 30 mg daily.

Children ages 10 to 17. *Initial:* 2 mg daily, increased after 2 days to 5 mg daily and then after 2 days to 10 mg daily. Increased in 5-mg increments, as needed, at 2-wk intervals. *Maintenance:* Lowest dose possible to maintain remission. *Maximum:* 30 mg daily.

TABLETS (ABILIFY MYCITE)

Adults with acute and mixed episodes of bipolar I disorder. *Initial:* 15 mg once daily. *Maximum:* 30 mg daily.

Adults with bipolar I disorder receiving adjunct treatment with lithium or valproate. *Initial:* 10 to 15 mg once daily. *Maximum:* 30 mg daily.

➤ *To maintain stability with monotherapy treatment of bipolar I disorder*

I.M. INJECTION (ABILIFY MAINTENA)

Adults. 400 mg monthly (no sooner than 26 days after the previous injection). Dosage reduced to 300 mg monthly if adverse reactions occur.

➤ *As adjunct to treat depression in patients already taking an antidepressant*

ORAL SOLUTION, ORALLY DISINTEGRATING TABLETS, TABLETS

Adults. *Initial:* 2 to 5 mg daily, with dosage increased by 5 mg daily at 1-wk intervals. *Maximum:* 15 mg daily.

TABLETS (ABILIFY MYCITE)

Adults. *Initial:* 2 to 5 mg daily, increased as needed, no less than once a wk. *Maximum:* 15 mg daily.

➤ *To treat irritability associated with autistic disorder*

ORAL SOLUTION, ORALLY DISINTEGRATING TABLETS, TABLETS

Children ages 6 to 17. *Initial:* 2 mg daily, with dosage increased after 1 wk to 5 mg daily and then after 1 wk to 10 mg daily and then after 1 wk to 15 mg daily, as needed.

➤ *To treat Tourette's disorder*

ORAL SOLUTION, ORALLY DISINTEGRATING TABLETS, TABLETS

Children ages 6 to 18 weighing 50 kg (110 lb) or more. *Initial:* 2 mg daily for 2 days, then 5 mg daily for 5 days, followed by dosage increased to 10 mg daily on day 8. Dosage increased 5 mg daily at weekly intervals, as needed, to control tics. *Maximum:* 20 mg daily.

Children age 6 to 18 weighing less than 50 kg (110 lb). *Initial:* 2 mg daily for 2 days, with dosage increased to 5 mg daily on day 3. Dosage increased gradually weekly, as needed, to control tics. *Maximum:* 10 mg daily.

➤ *To treat agitation associated with bipolar mania or schizophrenia*

I.M. INJECTION (ABILIFY)

Adults. 5.25 to 9.75 mg, repeated, as needed, after 2 or more hr. *Maximum:* Cumulative daily doses up to 30 mg with dosing intervals of 2 hr or more.

DOSAGE ADJUSTMENT Aristada Initio administration avoided in patients who are known CYP2D6 poor metabolizers or in patients taking strong CYP2D6 or CYP3A4 inhibitors or strong CYP3A4 inducers because dosage adjustment cannot be made as product is only available in a single strength. For other aripiprazole products, dosage reductions made for patients who are known CYP2D6 poor metabolizers and patients taking concomitant CYP2D6 inhibitors, CYP3A4 inhibitors, and/or CYP3A4 inducers for more than 14 days. Dosage reduction individualized taking into account current dosage prescribed and type of aripiprazole formulation being used. Dosage of Abilify formulation doubled over 1 to 2 weeks for patients taking strong CYP3A4 inducers such as carbamazepine or rifampin.

Mechanism of Action

May produce antipsychotic effects through partial agonist and antagonist actions. Aripiprazole acts as a partial agonist at dopamine (especially D_2) receptors and serotonin (especially 5-HT_{1A}) receptors. The drug acts as an antagonist at 5-HT_{2A} serotonin receptor sites.

Contraindications

Hypersensitivity to aripiprazole or its components

Interactions

DRUGS

antihypertensives: Possibly enhanced antihypertensive effects
benzodiazepines such as lorazepam: Increased risk of othostatic hypotension and sedation
carbamazepine and other strong CYP3A4 inducers: Possibly increased clearance and decreased blood level of aripiprazole

ACTIVITIES

alcohol use: Increased CNS depression

Adverse Reactions

CNS: Abnormal gait, aggression, agitation, akathisia, anxiety, asthenia, catatonia, cognitive and motor impairment, confusion, **CVA (elderly)**, delusions, depression, dizziness, dream disturbances, dystonia, extrapyramidal reactions, fatigue, fever, hallucinations, headache, **homicidal ideation**, hostility, insomnia, **intracranial hemorrhage**, lethargy, light-headedness, mania, nervousness, **neuroleptic malignant syndrome**, paranoia, Parkinsonism, restlessness, schizophrenic reaction, **seizures**, sleep walking, somnolence, **suicidal ideation**, tardive dyskinesia, transient ischemic attack (elderly), tremor
CV: Angina pectoris, **arrhythmias**, **bradycardia**, **cardiopulmonary arrest**, chest pain, **circulatory collapse**, **deep vein thrombosis**, dyslipidemia, elevated serum CK levels, **heart failure**, hyperlipidemia, hypertension, **MI**, orthostatic hypotension, palpitations, peripheral edema, **prolonged QT interval**, tachycardia
EENT: Blurred vision, conjunctivitis, diplopia, dry mouth, increased salivation, **laryngospasm**, nasal congestion, nasopharyngitis, **oropharyngeal spasm**, pharyngitis, photophobia, rhinitis, sinusitis
ENDO: Breast pain, gynecomastia, hyperglycemia, diabetes mellitus
GI: Abdominal discomfort, constipation, decreased appetite, diarrhea, difficulty swallowing, **GI bleeding**, gastroesophageal reflux disease, **hepatitis**, hiccups, indigestion, jaundice, nausea, vomiting
GU: Decreased or increased libido, erectile dysfunction, menstrual disorders, nocturia, priapism, **renal failure**, urinary incontinence or retention
HEME: Agranulocytosis, anemia, **leukopenia**, **neutropenia**, **thrombocytopenia**
MS: Arthralgia, joint stiffness, muscle spasms or weakness, musculoskeletal pain, myalgia, neck and limb rigidity, **rhabdomyolysis**, trismus
RESP: Apnea, **aspiration**, **asthma**, cough, dyspnea, pneumonia, **pulmonary edema or embolism**, **respiratory failure**
SKIN: Alopecia, diaphoresis, dry skin, ecchymosis, photosensitivity, pruritus, rash, ulceration, urticaria
Other: Anaphylaxis; **angioedema**; dehydration; elevated blood creatine phosphokinase (Aristada); flu-like symptoms; **heat stroke**; injection-site induration, pain, redness, swelling (Aristada); **hypokalemia**; **hyponatremia**; intense uncontrollable urges to perform certain activities, such as gambling and sexual acts; weight gain

Nursing Considerations

- Know that aripiprazole shouldn't be used to treat dementia-related psychosis in the elderly because of an increased risk of death.
- Use cautiously in patients with cardiovascular disease, cerebrovascular disease, or conditions that would predispose them to hypotension. Also use cautiously in those with a history of seizures or with conditions that lower the seizure threshold, such as Alzheimer's disease.
- Use cautiously in elderly patients because of increased risk of serious adverse cerebrovascular effects, such as stroke and transient ischemic attack.
- Know that you may give oral solution on a milligram-per-milligram basis in place of tablets up to 25 mg.
- Be aware that for patients who have never taken aripiprazole, tolerability must be established with oral form prior to initiating parenteral therapy. After first dose of Abilify Maintena, expect to continue to administer oral aripiprazole (10 to 20 mg) for 14 consecutive days to achieve a therapeutic level during the initiation of the intramuscular injection.
- Be aware that Abilify Maintena comes in two types of kits: prefilled chamber syringe or single-use vials.
- Reconstitute Abilify Maintena lyophilized powder in prefilled dual-chamber syringe by pushing plunger rod slightly to engage threads. Then rotate plunger rod until the rod stops rotating to release diluent. After plunger rod is at a complete stop, middle stopper will be at the indicator line. Vertically shake the syringe vigorously for 20 seconds until drug is uniformly milky white.
- Reconstitute Abilify Maintena using single-use vials by using the syringe with the preattached needle to withdraw the predetermined volume from the vial of into the syringe. Slowly inject the into the vial containing the lyophilized powder. Withdraw air to equalize the pressure, then remove the needle from the vial. Engage the needle safety device by using the one-handed technique. Gently press the sheath against a flat surface until the needle is firmly engaged in the needle protection sheath and discard appropriately. Shake the vial vigorously for 30 seconds until the reconstituted suspension appears uniform. It should be opaque and milky-white in color. If the injection is not given immediately after reconstitution, keep the vial at room temperature and shake the vial vigorously for at least 60 seconds to resuspend prior to administration. Do not store the reconstituted suspension in a syringe.
- Prepare Abilify Maintena prior to injection after reconstituting from a single-use vial by removing cover from the vial adapter package but do not remove the vial adapter from the package. Using the vial adapter package to handle the vial adapter, attach the prepackaged BD Luer-Lok syringe to the vial adapter. Use the syringe to remove the vial adapter from the package and discard the vial adapter package. Do not touch the spike tip of the adapter at any time. Determine the recommended volume for injection using the manufacturer chart for size vial being used and dosage prescribed. After wiping top of vial with a sterile alcohol swab, place and hold the vial of the reconstituted suspension on a hard surface. Attach the adapter-syringe assembly to the vial by holding the outside of the adapter and pushing the adapter's spike firmly through the rubber stopper until the adapter snaps in place. Slowly withdraw the recommended volume from the vial into the syringe.
- Inject Abilify Maintena form slowly, deep into the gluteal muscle, and never I.V. or subcutaneously. Do not massage the injection site.
- Use the following guide for determining when to administer missed doses of the long-acting formulation, Abilify Maintena. If a second or third dose is missed and it's been more than 4 weeks but less than 5 weeks since the last injection, administer the injection as soon as possible. If more than 5 weeks have elapsed since the last injection, restart concomitant oral aripiprazole, as ordered, for 14 days with the next administered injection. If a fourth or subsequent doses are missed and it's been more than 4 weeks but less than 6 weeks since the last injection, administer the injection as soon as possible. If more than 6 weeks have elapsed since the last injection, restart concomitant oral aripiprazole, as ordered, for 14 days with the next administered injection.

- Prepare Aristada for injection by first tapping the syringe at least 10 times and then shaking syringe vigorously for 30 seconds to ensure a uniform suspension. If pen is not used within 15 minutes, shake again for 30 seconds. Select needle length based on injection site and attach to syringe. Prime the syringe to remove air.
- Administer Aristada formulation into the gluteal muscle by I.M. injection only for all dosages except the 441-mg dose, which may also be administered into the deltoid muscle. Inject in a rapid and continuous manner in less than 10 seconds.
- Follow manufacturer guidelines when a dose of Aristada is missed which is based upon the dosage missed and length of time that has elapsed. However, be aware that Aristada Initio may be used to re-initiate treatment with Aristada.
- Prepare Aristada Initio for injection in the same manner as Aristada. Administer Aristada Initio into the deltoid muscle using a 21-gauge, 1-inch or 20-gauge, 1½-inch needle or into the gluteal muscle using a 20-gauge, 1½-inch or 20-gauge, 2-inch needle. Avoid overtightening the needle when attaching to syringe because needle hub may crack. Inject in a rapid and continuous manner intramuscularly. Do not inject by any other route.
- Be aware that Abilify Mycite is a drug-device combination product comprised of aripiprazole tablets embedded with an ingestible event marker (IEM) sensor intended to track drug ingestion. Other ways used to track ingestion of aripiprazole include a Mycite patch, which is a wearable sensor that detects signals from the IEM sensor after ingestion of aripiprazole and transmits data to a smartphone. Alternatively, there is a Mycite app, which is a smartphone application, which is used with a compatible smartphone to display information for the patient and web-based portal for healthcare professionals and caregivers to track compliance.
- Know that most ingestions can be tracked with Abilify Mycite within 30 minutes, but it may take up to 2 hours for the smartphone app and web portal to detect that the tablet has been taken.
- When administering Abilify Mycite in tablet form, have patient swallow tablets whole; do not have him chew tablets and do not crush or divide tablets.
- Apply the Abilify Mycite patch to the left side of the body just above the lower edge of the rib cage. Do not place it in areas where the skin is cracked, inflamed, irritated, or scraped or in a location that overlaps the area of the most recently removed patch. Be aware that the patch must be removed before patient undergoes an MRI.
- Monitor patient for difficulty swallowing or excessive somnolence, which could predispose to accidental injury or aspiration. For patients with medical conditions or who are taking medications that could exacerbate CNS effects, complete a fall risk assessment and institute safety measures.

WARNING Be aware that aripiprazole rarely may cause neuroleptic malignant syndrome, seizures, and tardive dyskinesia. Monitor patient closely throughout therapy, and take safety precautions as needed. Be aware that tardive dyskinesia may resolve, partially or completely, if aripiprazole is discontinued.

- Watch patients closely (especially children, adolescents, and young adults) for suicidal tendencies, particularly when therapy starts and dosage changes, because depression may worsen temporarily during these times.
- Monitor patient's CBC, as ordered, because serious adverse hematologic reactions may occur, such as agranulocytosis, leukopenia, and neutropenia. Assess more often during first few months of therapy if patient has a history of drug-induced leukopenia or neutropenia or a significantly low WBC count. If abnormalities occur during therapy, watch for fever or other signs of infection, notify prescriber and, if severe, expect drug to be stopped.
- Monitor patient's weight, blood glucose level, and lipid levels, as ordered, because atypical antipsychotic drugs such as aripiprazole may cause metabolic changes.

If patient is already a diabetic, monitor blood glucose levels more closely.

PATIENT TEACHING

- Instruct patient prescribed orally disintegrating tablets to open the blister pack only when ready to take the tablet. Tell him to peel back the foil carefully and not to push tablet through the foil because doing so could damage the tablet. Tell him to place the tablet on his tongue without breaking it and let it dissolve. If needed, he may take a drink.
- Instruct patient how to use the Abilify Mycite system. If taking drug orally, tell patient to swallow tablets whole and not to chew, crush, or divide them. If using the patch, tell patient to keep patch on when exercising, showering, and swimming. Tell patient the patch will have to be changed at least weekly. Inform patient that the app will prompt patient to change the patch and will direct patient on how to apply and remove the patch correctly. Inform patient that if undergoing an MRI, the patch must be removed and a new one applied after the test. Advise patient that if skin irritation occurs, he should remove the patch and notify prescriber.
- Advise patient to get up slowly from a lying or sitting position during aripiprazole therapy to minimize orthostatic hypotension.
- Urge patient to avoid alcohol during aripiprazole therapy.
- Instruct patient to avoid hazardous activities until drug's effects are known. Also, alert patient and family of increased risk for falls, especially if patient has other medical conditions or takes medication that may affect the nervous system.
- Urge patient to avoid activities that raise body temperature suddenly, such as strenuous exercise and exposure to extreme heat, and to compensate for situations that cause dehydration, such as vomiting or diarrhea.
- Instruct patient and caregivers to notify prescriber about intense urges, such as for gambling or sex, because dosage may need to be reduced or drug discontinued.
- Instruct patient to inform all prescribers of any drugs he's taking, including OTC drugs, because of risk of interactions.
- Advise female patient of childbearing age to notify prescriber if she intends to become or suspects that she is pregnant during therapy.
- Instruct diabetic patient to monitor blood glucose levels closely, especially if taking the oral solution form because each milliliter of solution contains 400 mg of sucrose and 200 mg of fructose.
- Urge family or caregiver to watch patient closely for suicidal tendencies, especially when therapy starts or dosage changes, and particularly if patient is a child, teenager, or young adult.

armodafinil

Nuvigil

Class and Category

Pharmacologic class: Analeptic modafinil derivative
Therapeutic class: CNS stimulant
Pregnancy category: Not classifed
Controlled substance schedule: IV

Indications and Dosages

➤ *To treat narcolepsy or as adjunct to standard therapy for excessive daytime sleepiness in obstructive sleep apnea/hypopnea syndrome*

TABLETS

Adults. 150 or 250 mg once daily in the morning.

➤ *To improve daytime wakefulness in patients with excessive sleepiness from circadian rhythm disruption (shift-work sleep disorder)*

TABLETS

Adults. 150 mg once daily about 1 hr before start of work shift.

DOSAGE ADJUSTMENT Dosage decreased for patients who are elderly or have severe hepatic impairment.

Route	Onset	Peak	Duration
P.O.	Unknown	2 hr (fasting) 4–6 hr (with food)	Unknown

Mechanism of Action

May produce CNS-stimulant effects by binding to dopamine transporter in the brain and inhibiting dopamine reuptake in limbic regions. These actions increase alertness and reduce drowsiness and fatigue.

Contraindications

Hypersensitivity to armodafinil, modafinil, or their components

Interactions

DRUGS

cyclosporine: Possibly decreased blood cyclosporine level and increased risk of organ transplant rejection
CYP2C19 substrates such as clomipramine, diazepam, omeprazole, and propranolol: Possibly prolonged elimination time and increased blood levels of these drugs
fosphenytoin, mephenytoin, phenytoin: Possibly decreased effectiveness of armodafinil, increased blood phenytoin level, and increased risk of phenytoin toxicity
MAO inhibitors: Increased risk of serious adverse reactions
midazolam, triazolam: Possibly decreased effectiveness of triazolam or midazolam
oral steroidal contraceptives: Possibly decreased effectiveness of oral contraceptive
warfarin: Possibly decreased warfarin metabolism and increased risk of bleeding

FOODS

ACTIVITIES

alcohol use: Possibly adverse CNS effects
all foods: 2- to 4-hr delay for armodafinil to reach peak levels and possibly delayed onset of action
caffeine: Increased CNS stimulation

Adverse Reactions

CNS: Aggression, agitation, anxiety, attention disturbance, delusions, depression, dizziness, drowsiness, excessive sleepiness, fatigue, fever, hallucinations, headache (including migraine), insomnia, irritability, mania, nervousness, paresthesia, **suicidal ideation**, thirst, tremor
CV: Increased heart rate, palpitations
EENT: Dry mouth, mouth sores
GI: Abdominal pain (upper), anorexia, constipation, diarrhea, dyspepsia, loose stools, nausea, vomiting
GU: Polyuria
RESP: Bronchospasm, dyspnea
SKIN: Contact dermatitis, **Stevens–Johnson syndrome, toxic epidermal necrolysis**
Other: Anaphylaxis, angioedema, drug reaction with eosinophilia and system symptoms (DRESS), flu-like illness

Nursing Considerations

- Know that armodafinil shouldn't be given to patients with mitral valve prolapse syndrome or a history of left ventricular hypertrophy because drug may cause ischemic changes.

WARNING **Know whether patient has a history of alcoholism, stimulant abuse, or other substance abuse, and ensure compliance with armodafinil therapy. Watch for signs of misuse or abuse, including frequent prescription refill requests, increased frequency of dosing, and drug-seeking behavior. Also watch for evidence of excessive armodafinil use, including agitation, anxiety, diarrhea, nausea, nervousness, palpitations, sleep disturbances, and tremor.**

- Know that armodafinil, like other CNS stimulants, may alter mood, perception, thinking, judgment, feelings, and motor skills and may produce signs that patient needs sleep.
- Giving drug to patient with a history of psychosis, emotional instability, or psychological illness with psychotic features may require a baseline behavioral assessment or frequent clinical observation.
- Stop drug at first sign of rash, and notify prescriber. Although rare, rash may indicate a potentially life-threatening event.
- Monitor patient for signs and symptoms of multisystem organ hypersensitivity, such as may require a fever, hematologic abnormalities, hepatitis, myocarditis, pruritus, rash, or any other serious abnormality because multiorgan hypersensitivity may vary in its presentation. While multisystem organ hypersensitivity has only occurred with modafinil, the possibility that it may occur with armodafinil cannot be ruled out because the two drugs are very closely related. Therefore, if suspected, notify prescriber immediately, expect to discontinue drug, and provide supportive care, as ordered.

- Watch closely for suicidal tendencies, especially in patients with a psychiatric history.

PATIENT TEACHING

- Inform patient that armodafinil can help, but not cure, narcolepsy and that drug's full effects may not be seen right away.
- Advise patient to avoid taking armodafinil within 2 hours of eating because food may delay time to peak drug effect and onset of action. If patient drinks grapefruit juice, encourage him to drink a consistent amount daily.

WARNING Tell patient to stop taking armodafinil immediately and seek emergency medical treatment if he experiences an allergic reaction such as difficulty breathing or swallowing; hives; or swelling of eyes, face, lips, or tongue.

- Inform patient that drug can affect his concentration and ability to function and can hide signs of fatigue. Urge him not to drive or perform activities that require mental alertness until drug's full CNS effects are known.
- Instruct patient to continue previously prescribed treatments such as CPAP and not to stop without consulting prescriber first.
- Tell patient to contact prescriber immediately if she begins to experience psychiatric symptoms such as anxiety, depression, or signs of mania or psychosis.
- Advise patient to avoid alcohol with armodafinil because drug may decrease alertness.
- Encourage a regular sleeping pattern.
- Caution patient to avoid excessive intake of foods, beverages, and OTC drugs that contain caffeine because caffeine may lead to increased CNS stimulation.
- Advise patient to report the presence of blisters, mouth sores, peeling, or rash immediately to prescriber and to stop taking armodafinil. Also encourage patient to report any unusual or persistent signs and symptoms to prescriber.
- Inform woman that armodafinil can decrease effectiveness of certain contraceptives, including birth control pills and implantable hormonal contraceptives. If she uses such contraceptives, urge her to use an alternate birth control method during armodafinil therapy and for up to 1 month after it stops. Tell patient to notify prescriber if pregnancy is suspected or occurs and encourage her to notify the pregnancy exposure registry.
- Instruct patient to notify prescriber before taking any new medication, including over-the-counter preparations.
- Urge family or caregiver to watch patient closely for abnormal behaviors, including suicidal tendencies, especially if patient has a psychiatric history.
- Advise patient to keep follow-up appointments with prescriber so that her progress can be monitored.

asenapine

Saphris

Class and Category

Pharmacologic class: Dopamine-serotonin antagonist
Therapeutic: Atypical antipsychotic
Pregnancy category: Not classified

Indications and Dosages

➤ *To treat schizophrenia*

SUBLINGUAL TABLETS

Adults. *Initial:* 5 mg twice daily, increased to 10 mg twice daily after 1 wk, if needed and tolerated. *Maximum:* 10 mg twice daily.

➤ *To treat manic or mixed episodes associated with bipolar I disorder as monotherapy*

SUBLINGUAL TABLETS

Adults. 5 to 10 mg twice daily for monotherapy and 5 mg twice daily for adjunct therapy and then increased to 10 mg, if needed and tolerated. *Maintenance:* 10 mg twice daily. *Maximum:* 10 mg twice daily.

Children age 10 and over. *Initial:* 2.5 mg twice daily increased after 3 days to 5 mg twice daily and after an additional 3 days to 10 mg twice daily, as needed and tolerated. *Maximum:* 10 mg twice daily.

➤ *To provide maintenance monotherapy in adults in the treatment of bipolar I disorder*

A

SUBLINGUAL TABLETS
Adults. 5 or 10 mg twice daily, whichever dosage patient was stabilized on. Then dosage decreased, if needed. *Maximum:* 10 mg twice daily.

➤ *As adjunct therapy with lithium or valproate to treat bipolar I disorder*
Adults. *Initial:* 5 mg twice daily, increased to 10 mg twice daily, as needed. *Maximum:* 10 mg twice daily.
DOSAGE ADJUSTMENT Dosage may be decreased to 5 mg twice daily if adverse reactions occur.

Route	Onset	Peak	Duration
P.O.	Unknown	30–90 min	Unknown

Mechanism of Action
May produce antipsychotic effects through antagonist actions at dopamine receptors, especially D_2, and serotonin receptors, especially 5-HT_{2A}.

Contraindications
Hypersensitivity to asenapine or its components, severe hepatic impairment

Interactions
DRUGS
antihypertensives, CNS depressants: Possibly enhanced effects
class I A and III antiarrhythmics, gatifloxacin, moxifloxacin, other antipsychotic drugs: Increased risk of prolonged QT interval
paroxetine: Possibly increased paroxetine effect
ACTIVITIES
alcohol use: Possibly enhanced effect

Adverse Reactions
CNS: Agitation, akathisia, anger, anxiety, depression, dizziness, dyskinesia, dystonia, extrapyramidal symptoms, fatigue, fever, gait disturbance, headache, hyperkinesia, insomnia, irritability, mania, masked facies, **neuroleptic malignant syndrome**, Parkinsonism, **seizures**, somnolence, **suicidal ideation**, syncope, tardive dyskinesia, torticollis, tremor
CV: Hyperlipidemia, hypertension, orthostatic hypotension, peripheral edema, **prolonged QT interval**, tachycardia, temporary bundle branch block
EENT: Accommodation disorder; blepharospasm; blurred vision; **choking**; diplopia; dry mouth; nasopharyngitis; nasal congestion; oral hypoesthesia or paraesthesia; salivary hypersecretion; sublingual application-site reactions such as blisters, inflammation, oral ulcers, peeling, or sloughing; oropharyngeal pain; swollen tongue; taste perversion; toothache
ENDO: Hyperglycemia, diabetes mellitus, hyperprolactinemia
GI: Abdominal pain, constipation, dyspepsia, dysphagia, elevated liver enzymes, gastroesophageal reflux disease, increased appetite, stomach discomfort, vomiting
GU: Dysmenorrhea, enuresis (children)
HEME: Anemia, **leukopenia**, **neutropenia**, **thrombocytopenia**
MS: Arthralgia, dysarthria, extremity pain, muscle rigidity, myalgia
RESP: Dyspnea
SKIN: Photosensitivity reaction
Other: Anaphylaxis, **angioedema**, dehydration, elevated creatine kinase, **hyponatremia**, weight gain

Nursing Considerations
- Avoid asenapine in patients with a history of cardiac arrhythmias; conditions that might prolong the QT interval, such as bradycardia, hypokalemia, or hypomagnesemia; or congenital QT-interval prolongation because of increased risk of torsades de pointes or sudden death.
- Know that asenapine shouldn't be used for dementia-related psychosis in elderly patients because of an increased risk of death.
- Use cautiously in patients with mild to moderate hepatic impairment.
- Use cautiously in patients with a history of seizures or who have conditions that may lower the seizure threshold, such as Alzheimer's dementia, because drug increases risk of seizures in these patients.

WARNING Monitor patient closely even with the first dose for life-threatening hypersensitivity reactions that may include anaphylaxis and angioedema.

- Monitor elderly patients with psychosis closely for adverse effects because asenapine drug exposure has been found to be higher in these patients than in younger adult patients.
- Monitor patient's blood glucose level, lipid levels and weight, as ordered, because atypical antipsychotic drugs such as asenapine may cause metabolic changes. If patient is already diabetic, monitor blood glucose levels more closely.
- Know that the smallest dose of asenapine and the shortest duration of treatment should be used to minimize the risk of the patient developing tardive dyskinesia, which may become irreversible. If signs and symptoms appear, notify the prescriber, and know that the drug may need to be discontinued.

WARNING **Know that asenapine rarely may cause neuroleptic malignant syndrome or tardive dyskinesia. Monitor patient closely throughout therapy, and take safety precautions as needed. Expect to stop drug if any of these adverse effects occur.**

- Monitor patient's CBC regularly, as ordered. Notify prescriber of any change because drug may need to be stopped.
- Monitor patient for trouble swallowing or excessive somnolence, which could predispose him to aspiration, choking, or injury.

PATIENT TEACHING

- Tell patient to remove tablet from package only when ready to take it and to use dry hands. Tell him to firmly press and hold thumb button, and then pull out tablet pack from case. Then, he should peel back the colored tab, being careful not to push tablet through the tab because doing so could damage tablet. Instruct patient to place tablet under his tongue and let it dissolve completely. Tell him to then slide tablet pack back into case until it clicks.
- Caution patient not to crush, chew, or swallow tablets.
- Advise him not to eat or drink for at least 10 minutes after taking asenapine.
- Inform patient that application-site reactions may occur in the sublingual area, which may include blisters, inflammation, oral ulcers, peeling, or sloughing of tissue. Also inform patient that numbness or tingling of his mouth or throat may occur after administration of asenapine, but that it usually resolves within 1 hour.
- Teach patient the signs and symptoms of a serious allergic reaction and to seek immediate emergency treatment if present. Also inform patient of other serious adverse reactions and tell patient to report any persistent, severe, or unusual effects to prescriber immediately, including abnormal movements.
- Urge patient to avoid alcohol while taking asenapine.
- Instruct diabetic patient taking asenapine to monitor blood glucose levels closely because hyperglycemia may occur.
- Advise patient to get up slowly from lying or sitting position during asenapine therapy to minimize orthostatic hypotension.
- Caution patient to avoid hazardous activities until drug's effects are known. Also, alert patient and family of increased risk for falls, especially if patient has other medical conditions or takes medication that may affect the nervous system.
- Urge patient to avoid activities that raise body temperature suddenly, such as strenuous exercise and exposure to extreme heat, and to compensate for situations that cause dehydration, such as vomiting or diarrhea.
- Tell patient that if he has a preexisting low WBC or a history of drug-induced low WBC, he should have her CBC monitored throughout asenapine therapy.
- Inform prescriber of any new medication being prescribed or use of any over-the-counter drugs.
- Advise female patient of childbearing age to notify prescriber if she intends to become or suspects that she is pregnant during therapy, because drug may affect the fetus. Inform her that if she does become pregnant she should contact the pregnancy registry.

A

aspirin (acetylsalicylic acid, ASA)

Ancasal (CAN), Arthrinol (CAN), Arthrisin (CAN), Aspir-81, Aspirin, Aspir-Low, Atria S.R. (CAN), Bayer, Durlaza, Easprin, Ecotrin, Empirin, Genprin, Miniprin, Norwich, Novasen (CAN), Sal-Adult (CAN), Sal-Infant (CAN), St. Joseph Children's, Supasa (CAN), Zorprin

Class and Category

Pharmacologic class: Salicylate
Therapeutic class: NSAID (anti-inflammatory, antiplatelet, antipyretic, nonopioid analgesic)
Pregnancy category: Not classified

Indications and Dosages

➤ *To relieve mild pain or fever*

CHEWABLE TABLETS, CONTROLLED-RELEASE TABLETS, ENTERIC-COATED TABLETS, SOLUTION, TABLETS, TIMED-RELEASE TABLETS, SUPPOSITORIES

Adults and adolescents. 325 to 650 mg every 4 hr, as needed; or 500 mg every 3 hr, as needed; or 1,000 mg every 6 hr, as needed. *Maximum:* 4,000 mg daily.

Children ages 2 to 14. 10 to 15 mg/kg/dose every 4 hr, as needed, up to 80 mg/kg daily.

➤ *To relieve mild to moderate pain from inflammation, as in rheumatoid arthritis and osteoarthritis*

CHEWABLE TABLETS, CONTROLLED-RELEASE TABLETS, ENTERIC-COATED TABLETS, SOLUTION, TABLETS, TIMED-RELEASE TABLETS, SUPPOSITORIES

Adults and adolescents. 3 g daily in divided doses.

➤ *To treat juvenile rheumatoid arthritis*

CHEWABLE TABLETS, CONTROLLED-RELEASE TABLETS, ENTERIC-COATED TABLETS, SOLUTION, TABLETS, TIMED-RELEASE TABLETS, SUPPOSITORIES

Children. 90 to 130 mg/kg daily in divided doses every 6 to 8 hr.

➤ *To reduce the risk of recurrent transient ischemic attacks or ischemic stroke*

Adults. 50 to 325 mg once daily.

➤ *To reduce the severity of or prevent acute MI*

TABLETS

Adults. *Initial:* 160 to 325 mg as soon as MI is suspected. *Maintenance:* 160 to 325 mg daily for 30 days.

➤ *To reduce risk of MI in patients with previous MI or unstable angina*

TABLETS

Adults. 75 to 325 mg daily.

➤ *To reduce the risk of death and MI in patients with chronic coronary artery disease; to reduce risk of death and recurrent stroke in patients who have had an ischemic stroke or transient ischemic attack*

E.R. CAPSULES (DURLAZA)

Adults. 162.5 mg once daily.

➤ *To prepare patient for carotid endarterectomy*

TABLETS

Adults. 80 mg once daily to 650 mg twice daily, started presurgery.

➤ *Adjunct therapy with coronary artery bypass graft*

TABLETS

Adults. 75 to 325 mg daily starting 6 hr after procedure and continued for 1 yr.

➤ *Adjuct treatment for percutaneous transluminal coronary angioplasty*

Route	Onset	Peak	Duration
P.O. (chewable tablets)	Rapid	Unknown	1–4 hr
P.O. (controlled-release)	5–30 min	1–4 hr	4–6 hr
P.O. (enteric-coated)	5–30 min	Unknown	1–4 hr
P.O. (solution)	5–30 min	15–40 min	1–4 hr
P.O. (tablets)	15–30 min	1–2 hr	4–6 hr
P.O. (timed-release)	5–30 min	1–4 hr	4–6 hr
P.R.	Unknown	Unknown	4–6 hr

TABLETS

Adults. 325 mg 2 to 3 hr before procedure, then 160 to 325 mg daily.

➤ *To treat spondyloarthropathies*

TABLETS

Adults. Up to 4 g daily in divided doses.

Mechanism of Action

Blocks the activity of cyclooxygenase, the enzyme needed for prostaglandin synthesis. Prostaglandins, important mediators in the inflammatory response, cause local vasodilation with swelling and pain. With blocking of cyclooxygenase and inhibition of prostaglandins, inflammatory symptoms subside. Pain is also relieved because prostaglandins play a role in pain transmission from the periphery to the spinal cord. Aspirin inhibits platelet aggregation by interfering with production of thromboxane A2, a substance that stimulates platelet aggregation. Aspirin acts on the heat-regulating center in the hypothalamus and causes peripheral vasodilation, diaphoresis, and heat loss.

Contraindications

Active bleeding or coagulation disorders; breastfeeding; current or recent GI bleed or ulcers; hypersensitivity to aspirin, aspirin products, other NSAIDs, tartazine dye, or their components; third trimester of pregnancy

Interactions

DRUGS

ACE inhibitors: beta blockers: Decreased antihypertensive effect
acetazolamide: Possibly acetazolamide toxicity
activated charcoal: Decreased aspirin absorption
antacids, urine alkalinizers: Decreased aspirin effectiveness
anticoagulants, antiplatelets: Increased risk of bleeding; prolonged bleeding time
carbonic anhydrase inhibitors: Salicylism
corticosteroids: Increased excretion and decreased blood level of aspirin
diuretics: Possibly decreased diuretic effectiveness, especially in patients with renal impairment
heparin: Increased risk of bleeding
ibuprofen: Possibly reduced cardioprotective and stroke preventive effects of aspirin
methotrexate: Increased blood level and decreased excretion of methotrexate, causing toxicity
nizatidine: Increased blood aspirin level
other NSAIDs: Possibly decreased blood NSAID level and increased risk of adverse GI effects
oral antidiabetic agents: Possibly enhanced hypoglycemic effects, *probenecid, sulfinpyrazone:* Possibly decreased uriocosuric effect
sulfonylureas: Possibly enhanced effect of sulfonylureas with large doses of aspirin
urine acidifiers (such as ammonium chloride, ascorbic acid): Decreased aspirin excretion
valproic acid: Possibly increased valproic acid level and incidence of adverse reactions
vancomycin: Increased risk of ototoxicity

ACTIVITIES

alcohol use: Increased risk of ulcers

Adverse Reactions

CNS: Confusion, **CNS depression**
EENT: Hearing loss, tinnitus
GI: Diarrhea, **GI bleeding**, heartburn, **hepatotoxicity**, nausea, stomach pain, vomiting
HEME: Decreased blood iron level, **leukopenia**, **prolonged bleeding time**, shortened life span of RBCs, **thrombocytopenia**
RESP: Bronchospasm
SKIN: Ecchymosis, rash, urticaria
Other: Angioedema, **Reye's syndrome**, salicylism (CNS depression, confusion, diaphoresis, diarrhea, difficulty hearing, dizziness, headache, hyperventilation, lassitude, tinnitis, and vomiting) with regular use of large doses

Nursing Considerations

- Don't crush timed-release or controlled-release aspirin tablets unless directed.

WARNING Use an immediate-release aspirin in situations where a rapid onset of action is required such as in the acute treatment of myocardial infarction or before percutaneous coronary intervention.

- Ask about tinnitus. This reaction usually occurs when blood aspirin level reaches or exceeds maximum dosage for therapeutic effect.

PATIENT TEACHING

WARNING Advise parents not to give aspirin to a child or adolescent with chickenpox or flu symptoms because of risk of Reye's syndrome (rare life-threatening reaction). Tell them to consult prescriber for alternative drugs.

- Advise adult patient taking low-dose aspirin not to also take ibuprofen because it may reduce the cardioprotective and stroke preventive effects of aspirin.
- Instruct patient to take aspirin with food or after meals because it may cause GI upset if taken on an empty stomach.
- Caution patient not to take Durlaza 2 hours before or 1 hour after consuming alcohol. Also advise him to take the capsule with a full glass of water at the same time every day and to swallow the capsule whole.
- Instruct patient to stop taking aspirin and notify prescriber if any symptoms of stomach or intestinal bleeding occur such as passage of bloody or tarry stools or if patient is coughing up blood or vomit that looks like coffee grounds.
- Advise patient with tartrazine allergy not to take aspirin.
- Tell patient to consult prescriber before taking aspirin with any prescription drug for blood disorder, diabetes, gout, or arthritis.
- Tell patient not to use aspirin if it has a strong vinegar-like odor.

atazanavir

Reyataz

Class and Category

Pharmacologic class: Protease inhibitor
Therapeutic class: Antiretroviral
Pregnancy category: Not classified

Indications and Dosages

➤ *As adjunct to treat HIV-1 infection*

CAPSULES, ORAL POWDER

Adults. 300 mg once daily with food in combination with ritonavir 100 mg once daily.
Adults who are HIV treatment-naïve and cannot tolerate ritonavir. 400 mg once daily with food.
Adults who are HIV treatment-naïve and also taking efavirenz, adults who are treatment-experienced and also taking both H2RA and tenofovir DF. 400 mg once daily with food in combination with ritonavir 100 mg once daily.
Children ages 13 to 18 who weigh at least 40 kg (88 lb) and are HIV treatment-naïve and cannot tolerate ritonavir. 400 mg once daily with food.
Children ages 6 to 18 who weigh at least 35 kg (77 lb). 300 mg once daily with food in combination with ritonavir 100 mg once daily.
Children ages 6 to 18 who weigh less than 35 kg (77 lb) but at least 15 kg (33 lb). 200 mg once daily with food in combination with ritonavir 100 mg once daily.

ORAL POWDER

Children up to age 6 who weigh less than 25 kg (55 lb) but at least 15 kg (33 lb). 250 mg once daily with food in combination with ritonavir 80 mg once daily.
Infants 3 months of age and over who weigh less than 15 kg (33 lb) but at least 5 kg (11 lb). 200 mg once daily with food in combination with ritonavir 80 mg once daily.

DOSAGE ADJUSTMENT For HIV treatment-experienced pregnant patients who are in the second or third trimester and also being treated with either H2RA or tenofovir DF, atazanavir dosage increased to 400 mg once daily with food and given with ritonavir 100 mg once daily. For HIV treatment-naïve adults with mild hepatic impairment, atazanavir dosage increased to 400 mg once daily and given without ritonavir. For HIV treatment-naïve adults with moderate hepatic impairment, atazanavir dosage kept at 300 mg once daily but given without ritonavir.

Mechanism of Action

Selectively inhibits the virus-specific processing of specific polyproteins in HIV-1-infected cells to prevent formation of mature virions.

Contraindications

Concurrent therapy with alfuzosin, cisapride, dihydroergotamine, elbasvir/grazoprevir, ergonovine, ergotamine, glecaprevir/pibrentasvir, indinavir, irinotecan, lovastatin, lurasidone, methylergonovine, midazolam (oral), nevirapine, pimozide, rifampin, sildenafil (when used for treatment of pulmonary arterial hypertension), simvastatin, St. John's wort, triazolam; hypersensitivity to atazanavir or any of its components

Interactions

DRUGS

amiodarone, atorvastatin, bepridil, buprenorphine, colchicine, diltiazem, ethinyl and norethindrone, felodipine, fluticasone, ketoconazole, itraconazole, immunosuppressants, lidocaine (systemic) lurasidone, midazolam, nicardipine, nifedipine, norbuprenorphine, PDE5 inhibitors (sildenafil, tadalafil, vardenafil), quetiapine, rifabutin, quinidine, rosuvastatin, salmeterol, trazodone, tricyclic antidepressants, verapamil, voxilaprevir: Increased plasma concentrations of these drugs with possible increased risk of adverse effects that could be serious or life-threatening
antacids, buffered medications, efavirenz, H2-receptor antagonists, proton pump inhibitors: Decreased plasma concentration of atazanavir, decreasing effectiveness
boceprevir: Decreased plasma concentrations of both atazanavir and ritonavir when administered together, decreasing effectiveness of both drugs
bosentan: Decreased plasma concentration of atazanavir and increased plasma concentration of bosentan
carbamazepine: Decreased plasma concentration of atazanavir and increased plasma concentration of carbamazepine, increasing risk of serious carbamazepine-induced adverse reactions
clarithromycin: Increased plasma concentration of both atazanavir and clarithromycin, increasing risk of QT prolongation
didanosine: Decreased plasma concentration of both atazanavir and didanosine, with decreased effectiveness
ethinyl estradiol and norgestimate: Decreased plasma concentration of ethinyl estradiol and increased plasma concentration of norgestimate, possibly affecting contraceptive effectiveness
lamotrigine: Possibly decreased plasma concentration of lamotrigine, with increased risk of seizure activity
other protease inhibitors such as saquinavir: Possibly increased plasma concentration of protease inhibitor
phenobarbital, phenytoin: Decreased plasma concentration of atazanavir, phenobarbital, and phenytoin, decreasing effectiveness and increasing risk of seizures
ritonavir: Increased plasma concentration of atazanavir and risk of serious adverse reactions
tenofovir disoproxil fumarate: Decreased plasma concentration of atazanavir; increased plasma concentration of tenofovir
voriconazole: Decreased plasma concentrations of both atazanavir and voriconazole in patients with a functional CYP2C19 allele; decreased plasma concentration of atazanavir and increased plasma concentration of voriconazole in patients without a functional CYP2C19 allele
warfarin: Increased plasma concentration of warfarin, increasing risk of serious or life-threatening bleeding

Adverse Reactions

CNS: Depression, dizziness, fever, headache, insomnia, peripheral nervous system abnormalities
CV: Cardiac conduction abnormalities (second- or third-degree AV block, left bundle branch block), edema, elevated cholesterol and triglyceride levels, peripheral edema **QT prolongation**
EENT: Nasal congestion (children), oropharyngeal pain (children), rhinorrhea (children), scleral icterus
ENDO: Diabetes mellitus, fat redistribution, hyperglycemia, **hypoglycemia (children)**
GI: Abdominal pain, cholecystitis, cholelithiasis, cholestasis, diarrhea, elevated liver enzymes, **hepatic dysfunction**, hyperbilirubinemia, jaundice, nausea, **pancreatitis**, vomiting
GU: Chronic kidney disease, granulomatous interstitial nephritis, interstitial nephritis, nephrolithiasis
HEME: Decreased hemoglobin or platelet count, **neutropenia**

MS: Arthralgia, extremity pain (children), myalgia
RESP: Cough (children), wheezing (children)
SKIN: Alopecia, **erythema multiforme**, pruritus, rash, **Stevens–Johnson syndrome**
Other: Angioedema, drug reaction with eosinophilia and systemic symptoms (DRESS), immune reconstitution syndrome

Nursing Considerations

- Be aware that atazanavir is not recommended for HIV treatment-experienced patients with end-stage renal disease managed with hemodialysis. Expect all patients to have renal laboratory testing prior to atazanavir being initiated and periodically throughout drug therapy. Testing should include estimated creatinine clearance, serum creatinine, and urinalysis with miroscopic examination. If kidney disease occurs and becomes progressive, expect that atazanavir may be discontinued.
- Expect patients with underlying hepatitis B or C viral infections or marked elevations in transaminases that have occurred before atazanavir treatment to have hepatic function evaluated prior to start of therapy and periodically during treatment, because these patients may experience further transaminase elevations or hepatic decompensation while taking atazanavir.
- Be aware that patients with preexisting conduction system disease should be monitored by ECG.
- Administer atazanavir with food.
- Mix oral powder as follows: Determine number of packets needed and tap each packet to settle powder. Using a clean pair of scissors, cut each packet along the dotted line. Mix with food such as applesauce or yogurt using a minimum of 1 tablespoon of food mixed in a container and then administered to patient. Follow with mixing second tablespoon in container and administering the residual mixture. For infants, oral powder may be mixed with 30 ml of infant formula, milk, or water if infant can drink from a cup. After administering drug in this way, add 15 ml of liquid to the cup and have child drink the residual mixture. Know that if water was used to mix the drug, the child should immediately be given something to eat. For infants less than 6 months old who cannot drink from a cup or eat solid food, mix with 10 ml of infant formula and give using an oral dosing syringe and administer into either inner cheek of infant. Add an additional 10 ml of formula to cup used to mix drug and formula, draw up residual mixture, and administer to infant. Do not use an infant bottle to administer drug, because full dose may not be delivered. Know that when drug is mixed with food or liquid, it must be administered within 1 hr of preparation. Mixture may remain at room temperature during this time.
- Administer ritonavir, if prescribed, immediately after atazanavir.
- Monitor patient closely for the appearance of a rash. Although common and usually not affecting the use of atazanavir, some rashes may become severe and life-threatening. Report all rashes to prescriber and expect drug to be discontinued if rash becomes severe.
- Report signs or symptoms suggestive of cholelithiasis or nephrolithiasis to prescriber, as drug may have to be temporarily interrupted or discontinued if confirmed.
- Monitor patient's blood glucose level throughout atazanavir therapy, because drug has been associated with new-onset diabetes mellitus and exacerbation of preexisting diabetes mellitus. Treat hyperglycemia as prescribed.
- Be aware that immune reconstitution syndrome has occurred in patients treated with combination antiretroviral therapy, including atazanavir. The inflammatory response predisposes susceptible patients to opportunistic infections such as cytomegalovirus infection, *Mycobacterium avium* infection, *Pneumocystis jiroveci* pneumonia, or tuberculosis. Autoimmune disorders such as Graves' disease, Guillain–Barré syndrome, or polymyositis have also occurred. Report sudden or unusual adverse reactions to prescriber.
- Monitor patients with hemophilia for increased bleeding, because spontaneous skin hemarthrosis and hematomas have

occurred in these patients while taking atazanavir. Provide supportive care as prescribed.

PATIENT TEACHING

- Instruct patient prescribed capsule form of atazanavir not to open capsule and to ingest it whole.
- Instruct patient, parent, or caregiver how to mix oral powder form, if prescribed. Tell parent/caregiver of an infant younger than 6 months who cannot drink from a cup or eat solid food to mix with infant formula but to administer it with an oral dosing syringe. The drug should not be delivered using an infant bottle.
- Tell patient prescribed both atazanavir and ritonavir to take atazanavir first and then immediately take ritonavir.
- Alert patient that atazanavir may redistribute or cause accumulation of body fat which may include breast enlargement, a buffalo hump on the back of the neck, central obesity, and wasting appearance of extremities and face.
- Advise patient to report the appearance of a rash to prescriber. Inform patient that severe skin reactions may occur that begin with a rash and caution patient to report any rash immediately to prescriber.
- Advise patient to report dizziness or lightheadedness to prescriber because drug may causes changes in how the heart functions. Also tell patient to report any yellowing of the skin or whites of the eyes.
- Stress importance of maintaining adequate hydration throughout therapy as drug may cause chronic kidney disease.
- Alert patient, parent, or caregiver using the oral powder form of atazanavir that it contains 35 mg of phenylalanine, which can be harmful if patient has phenylketonuria. The capsule form of drug contains no phenylalanine.
- Review signs and symptoms of the presence of gallbladder or kidney stones with patient and advise patient to notify prescriber if any such signs and symptoms develop, as drug may have to be temporarily withheld or discontinued.
- Stress importance of informing all prescribers of atazanavir therapy, because drug interacts with many other drugs. Tell patient not to take any over-the-counter medication, including herbals, without consulting prescriber first.
- Tell patient with diabetes mellitus to monitor glucose levels during atazanavir therapy, as adjustments in her diabetes treatment regimen may be needed. Also review signs and symptoms of diabetes mellitus with all patients, because new-onset diabetes mellitus has occurred during atazanavir therapy.
- Instruct patient to report any signs and symptoms of infection or persistent or unusual adverse effects to prescriber.
- Encourage women who become pregnant to register on the pregnancy exposure registry through their prescriber.
- Instruct women not to breastfeed while taking atazanavir as drug may pass through breast milk to the infant.

atenolol

Tenormin

Class and Category

Pharmacologic class: Beta-adrenergic blocker ($beta_1$ and at high doses $beta_2$)
Therapeutic class: Antianginal, antihypertensive
Pregnancy category: D

Indications and Dosages

➤ *To treat angina pectoris; to treat hypertension*

TABLETS

Adults. 50 mg daily increased, as needed, after 1 to 2 wk to 100 mg daily. *Maximum:* 100 mg for treatment of hypertension; 200 mg for treatment of angina pectoris.

➤ *To treat acute myocardial infarction in hemodynamically stable patients*

I.V. INJECTION

Adults. 5 mg given over 5 min followed in 10 min by 5 mg given over 5 min.

TABLETS

Adults. *Initial:* 50 mg following last I.V. dose, then 50 mg 12 hr later. *Maintenance:* 100 mg once daily or 50 mg twice daily for 6 to 9 days or until discharge.

DOSAGE ADJUSTMENT Dosage usually not increased above 50 mg daily P.O. for the elderly and for patients with a creatinine clearance, of 15 to 35 ml/min. For patients with creatinine clearance less than 15 ml/min, dosage reduced to 25 mg daily.

Route	Onset	Peak	Duration
P.O.	1 hr	2–4 hr	24 hr

Mechanism of Action

Inhibits stimulation of $beta_1$-receptor sites, located mainly in the heart, decreasing cardiac excitability, cardiac output, and myocardial oxygen demand. Atenolol also acts to decrease release of renin from the kidneys, aiding in reducing blood pressure. At high doses, it inhibits stimulation of $beta_2$ receptors in the lungs, which may cause bronchoconstriction.

Contraindications

Cardiogenic shock, heart block greater than first degree, hypersensitivity to atenolol, other beta blockers or their components, overt heart failure, sinus bradycardia

Interactions

DRUGS

amiodarone: Additive atenolol effects
calcium channel blockers, such as verapamil and diltiazem: Possibly symptomatic bradycardia and conduction abnormalities
catecholamine-depleting drugs, such as reserpine: Additive antihypertensive effect
clonidine: Possible rebound hypertension following discontinuation of clonidine
disopyramide: Increased risk of severe bradycardia, asystole, and heart failure

Adverse Reactions

CNS: Depression, disorientation, dizziness, drowsiness, emotional lability, fatigue, fever, lethargy, light-headedness, short-term memory loss, vertigo
CV: Arrhythmias, including bradycardia and heart block; **cardiogenic shock**; cold arms and legs; **mitral insufficiency**; **myocardial reinfarction**; orthostatic hypotension; Raynaud's phenomenon
EENT: Dry eyes, **laryngospasm**, pharyngitis
GI: Diarrhea, **ischemic colitis**, **mesenteric artery thrombosis**, nausea
GU: Renal failure
HEME: Agranulocytosis
MS: Leg pain
RESP: Bronchospasm, dyspnea, **pulmonary emboli**, **respiratory distress**, wheezing
SKIN: Erythematous rash
Other: Allergic reaction

Nursing Considerations

- Use atenolol cautiously in patients with heart failure controlled by digitalis glycosides or diuretics, patients with conduction abnormalities or left ventricular dysfunction who take verapamil or diltiazem, patients with arterial circulatory disorders, and patients with impaired renal function.
- Use atenolol cautiously in diabetic patients because it may mask tachycardia caused by hypoglycemia. Unlike other beta-adrenergic blockers, it doesn't mask other signs of hypoglycemia, cause hypoglycemia, or delay the return of blood glucose to a normal level.
- Monitor patient for heart failure. At first sign of heart failure, expect patient to receive a digitalis glycoside, a diuretic, or both and to be monitored closely. If failure continues, expect to stop atenolol.
- Closely monitor patient with hyperthyroidism because atenolol may mask some signs of thyrotoxicosis. Abrupt withdrawal of atenolol may precipitate thyrotoxicosis.
- Know that if patient also receives clonidine, expect to stop atenolol several days before gradually withdrawing clonidine. Then expect to restart atenolol therapy several days after clonidine has been discontinued.
- Stop atenolol and notify prescriber if patient develops bradycardia, hypotension, or other serious adverse reaction.
- Be aware that chronic beta blocker therapy such as atenolol is not routinely withheld prior to major surgery because the benefits outweigh the risks associated with its use with general anesthesia and surgical procedures.

PATIENT TEACHING

- Instruct patient not to stop taking atenolol abruptly. Otherwise, angina may worsen, and an MI or arrhythmia may occur.

- Tell him to perform minimal physical activity to prevent chest pain when he is being weaned from atenolol therapy.
- Instruct patient to take a missed dose as soon as possible. However, if it's within 8 hours of the next scheduled dose, tell him to skip the missed dose and return to his regular schedule.
- Explain that atenolol may alter serum glucose level and mask hypoglycemia.
- Inform the patient that he may experience fatigue and reduced tolerance to exercise and that he should notify his prescriber if this interferes with his normal lifestyle.

atomoxetine hydrochloride

Strattera

Class and Category

Pharmacologic class: Selective norepinephrine reuptake inhibitor
Therapeutic class: Anti–ADHD agent
Pregnancy category: C

Indications and Dosages

➤ *To treat attention deficit hyperactivity disorder (ADHD)*

CAPSULES

Adults and children weighing more than 70 kg (154 lb). *Initial:* 40 mg daily, increased after at least 3 days to 80 mg daily given either as a single dose in the morning or in evenly divided doses morning and late afternoon or early evening. After 2 to 4 additional wk, dosage may be increased to 100 mg daily if optimal response hasn't been achieved. *Maximum:* 100 mg daily.
Adults and children weighing 70 kg (154 lb) or less. *Initial:* 0.5 mg/kg daily, increased after at least 3 days to 1.2 mg/kg daily given either as a single dose in the morning or in evenly divided doses morning and late afternoon or early evening, as needed. *Maximum:* 1.4 mg/kg or 100 mg daily, whichever is less.

DOSAGE ADJUSTMENT For patients with moderate (Child-Pugh Class B) hepatic impairment, dosage reduced by 50%. For patients with severe (Child-Pugh Class C) hepatic impairment, dosage reduced by 75%. For patients weighing more than 70 kg and taking strong CYP2D6 inhibitors (fluoxetine, paroxetine, or quinidine), initial dosage of 40 mg daily increased to 80 mg daily only if symptoms fail to improve after 4 wk. For patients weighing 70 kg or less and taking strong CYP2D6 inhibitors, initial dosage of 0.5 mg/kg daily increased to 1.2 mg/kg daily only if symptoms fail to improve after 4 wk.

Mechanism of Action

Selectively inhibits presynaptic norepinephrine transport in the nervous system to increase attention span and produce a calming effect.

Contraindications

Angle-closure glaucoma, hypersensitivity to atomoxetine or its components, pheochromocytoma, severe cardiovascular disorders, use within 14 days of MAO inhibitor therapy

Interactions

DRUGS

albuterol and other beta$_2$ agonists: May potentiate action of albuterol and other beta$_2$ agonists on cardiovascular system
CYP2D6 inhibitors (such as fluoxetine, paroxetine, and quinidine): Increased blood atomoxetine level
MAO inhibitors: Possibly induced hypertensive crisis
pressor agents: Possibly altered blood pressure

Adverse Reactions

CNS: Aggressiveness, anxiety, chills, crying **CVA**, depression, dizziness, early morning awakening, fatigue, headache, hostility, hypoaesthesia, insomnia, irritability, jittery feeling, lethargy, mood changes, paresthesia (children and adolescents), peripheral coldness, pyrexia, rigors, sedation, **seizures**, sensory disturbances, sleep disturbance, somnolence, **suicidal ideation**, syncope, tics, tremor, unusual dreams
CV: Chest pain, hypertension, orthostatic hypotension, **MI**, palpitations, **QT-interval prolongation**, Raynaud's phenomenon, tachycardia
EENT: Blurred vision, conjunctivitis, dry mouth, ear infection, mydriasis, nasal congestion, nasopharyngitis, pharyngitis, rhinorrhea, sinus congestion

ENDO: Hot flashes
GI: Abdominal pain (upper), anorexia, constipation, diarrhea, dyspepsia, elevated liver enzymes, flatulence, gastroenteritis (viral), indigestion, nausea, **severe hepatic dysfunction**, vomiting
GU: Decreased libido, dysmenorrhea, dysuria, ejaculation disorders, erectile dysfunction, impotence, male pelvic pain, menstrual irregularities, orgasm abnormality, priapism, prostatitis, urinary hesitancy (children and adolescents), urine retention (children and adolescents)
MS: Arthralgia, back pain, myalgia, **rhabdomyolysis**
RESP: Cough, upper respiratory tract infection
SKIN: Alopecia, dermatitis, diaphoresis, hyperhidrosis, pruritus, rash, urticaria
Other: Anaphylaxis, **angioedema**, flu-like symptoms, weight loss

Nursing Considerations

- Use atomoxetine cautiously in patients with cerebrovascular or CV disease (especially hypertension or tachycardia) because drug may increase blood pressure and heart rate. Also use cautiously in those prone to orthostatic hypotension and those with serious structural cardiac abnormalities, cardiomyopathy, serious heart rhythm abnormalities, or other serious cardiac problems because drug may increase risk of sudden death from these conditions.

WARNING Monitor patient closely for evidence of suicidal thinking and behavior as well as for psychotic or manic symptoms such as hallucinations, delusional thinking, or mania because atomoxetine increases the risk of suicidal ideation and the onset of psychotic or manic symptoms. In addition, monitor patients, especially children and adolescents with ADHD, for the appearance or worsening of aggressive behavior or hostility. Notify prescriber if psychiatric adverse reactions are observed during atomoxetine therapy.

- Obtain baseline blood pressure and heart rate before starting therapy. Monitor patient's vital signs after dosage increases and periodically during therapy.
- Monitor patient closely for allergic reactions. If these occur, notify prescriber.
- Monitor child's or adolescent's growth and weight. Expect to interrupt therapy, as prescribed, if patient isn't growing or gaining weight appropriately.
- Monitor patient's liver function studies, as ordered. Notify prescriber immediately if enzyme levels are elevated or patient has evidence of hepatic dysfunction. Expect to stop drug permanently.

PATIENT TEACHING

- Caution patient not to open capsules. If a capsule opens, urge patient to promptly wash his hands and any surface drug touches. If drug gets in his eyes, tell him to flush immediately with water and seek medical care.
- Instruct patient or parent to immediately report to prescriber any adverse reactions to atomoxetine therapy, such as facial swelling, itching, or rash.

WARNING Urge parents to watch their child or adolescent closely for evidence of abnormal thinking or behavior, or increased aggression or hostility. Emphasize need to notify prescriber about unusual changes.

- Urge patient to tell prescriber immediately about dark urine, flu-like symptoms, itchiness, right upper abdominal pain, or yellowing of his skin or eyes. Also tell patient to notify prescriber immediately if he experiences exertional chest pain, unexplained syncope, or other symptoms suggestive of heart disease.
- Caution patient to assume sitting or standing position slowly because of drug's potential effect on blood pressure.
- Urge male patient to seek immediate medical attention for a penile erection that becomes prolonged or painful.
- Advise patient to report urinary hesitancy or urine retention to prescriber.
- Remind patient of the importance of alerting all prescribers to any OTC drugs, dietary supplements, or herbal remedies he's taking.
- Caution patient to avoid hazardous activities until drug's CNS effects are known.
- Reassure patient or parent that drug doesn't cause physical or psychological dependence.
- Instruct patient or parent to monitor weight during therapy.

atorvastatin calcium

Lipitor

Class and Category

Pharmacologic class: HMG-CoA reductase inhibitor
Therapeutic class: Antihyperlipidemic
Pregnancy category: Not classified

Indications and Dosages

➤ *To control lipid levels as adjunct to diet in primary (heterozygous familial and nonfamilial) hypercholesterolemia and mixed dyslipidemia*

TABLETS

Adults. *Initial:* 10 or 20 mg once daily; then increased according to lipid level. *Maintenance:* 10 to 80 mg once daily.

DOSAGE ADJUSTMENT Initial dose may be increased to 40 mg once daily for patients who need cholesterol level reduced more than 45%.

➤ *To control lipid levels in homozygous familial hypercholesterolemia*

TABLETS

Adults. 10 to 80 mg daily.

➤ *To control lipid levels in pediatric heterozygous familial hypercholesterolemia*

TABLETS

Adolescents and children ages 10 to 17. *Initial:* 10 mg daily, adjusted at intervals of 4 wk or more, as needed. *Maximum:* 20 mg daily.

➤ *To reduce risk of acute cardiovascular events such as angina, CVA, or MI and to reduce risk for revascularization procedures or hospitalization for congestive heart failure in patients with coronary heart disease*

TABLETS

Adults. 10 to 80 mg once daily.

DOSAGE ADJUSTMENT **FOR ALL INDICATIONS**
For patient taking lopinavir plus ritonavir dosage decreased. For patient taking clarithromycin, darunavir plus ritonavir, fosamprenavir, forsamprenavir plus ritonavir, itraconazole, or saquinavir plus ritonavir, dosage should not exceed 20 mg daily. For patient taking boceprevir or nelfinavir, dosage should not exceed 40 mg daily.

Mechanism of Action

Reduces plasma cholesterol and lipoprotein levels by inhibiting HMG-CoA reductase and cholesterol synthesis in the liver and by increasing the number of LDL receptors on liver cells to enhance LDL uptake and breakdown.

Contraindications

Active hepatic disease, breastfeeding, hypersensitivity to atorvastatin or its components, pregnancy, unexplained persistent rise in serum transaminase level

Interactions

DRUGS

colchicine, gemfibrozil, niacin, other fibrates: Increased risk of myopathy and rhabdomyolysis
cyclosporine, CYP3A4 strong inhibitors such as clarithromycin, HIV protease inhibitors including combination drugs, itraconazole: Possibly increased plasma concentrations of atorvastatin and adverse reactions
digoxin: Increased digoxin level and increased risk of toxicity
efavirenz, rifampin, other CYP450 3A4 inducers: Possible decreased plasma atorvastatin level and effectiveness
oral contraceptives such as ethinyl estradiol and norethindrone: Increased hormone levels

FOODS

grapefruit juice: Increased blood atorvastatin level

Adverse Reactions

CNS: Abnormal dreams, amnesia, asthenia, cognitive impairment, depression, dizziness, emotional lability, facial paralysis, fatigue, fever, headache, hyperkinesia, lack of coordination, malaise, paresthesia, peripheral neuropathy, somnolence, syncope, weakness
CV: Arrhythmias, elevated serum CK level, orthostatic hypotension, palpitations, phlebitis, vasodilation
EENT: Amblyopia, altered refraction, dry eyes, dry mouth, epistaxis, eye hemorrhage, gingival hemorrhage, glaucoma, glossitis, hearing loss, lip swelling, loss of taste, pharyngitis, sinusitis, stomatitis, taste perversion, tinnitus
ENDO: Hyperglycemia, **hypoglycemia**

GI: Abdominal or biliary pain, anorexia, colitis, constipation, diarrhea, duodenal or stomach ulcers, dysphagia, elevated liver enzymes, eructation, esophagitis, flatulence, gastroenteritis, **hepatic failure, hepatitis,** increased appetite, indigestion, jaundice, melena, **pancreatitis, rectal hemorrhage,** vomiting
GU: Abnormal ejaculation; cystitis; decreased libido; dysuria; epididymitis; hematuria; impotence; nephritis; nocturia; renal calculi; urinary frequency, incontinence, or urgency; urine retention; vaginal hemorrhage
HEME: Anemia, **thrombocytopenia**
MS: Arthralgia, back or muscle pain, bursitis, gout, **immune-mediated necrotizing myopathy**, leg cramps, myalgia, myasthenia gravis, myopathy, myositis, neck rigidity, **rhabdomyolysis,** tendon contracture or rupture, tenosynovitis, torticollis
RESP: Dyspnea, pneumonia
SKIN: Acne, alopecia, contact dermatitis, diaphoresis, dry skin, ecchymosis, eczema, **erythema multiforme**, petechiae, photosensitivity, pruritus, rash, seborrhea, **Stevens-Johnson, toxic epidermal necrolysis**, ulceration, urticaria
Other: Anaphylaxis, angioedema, flu-like symptoms, infection, lymphadenopathy, weight gain

Nursing Considerations

- Know that atorvastatin is used in patients with homozygous familial hypercholesterolemia as an adjunct to other lipid-lowering treatments or alone only if other treatments aren't available.
- Know that treatment of heterozygous familial hypercholesterolemia, in children who have failed an adequate trial of diet therapy, may include atorvastatin therapy if their LDL-C is 190 mg/dl or greater, or their LDL-C is 160 mg/dl or greater and they have a positive family history of familial hypercholesterolemia or premature cardiovascular disease in a first- or second-degree relative, or two or more other cardiovascular risk factors are present.
- Be aware that atorvastatin may be used with colestipol or cholestyramine for additive antihyperlipidemic effects.
- Know that atorvastatin should not be used in patients taking cyclosporine, gemfibrozil, tipranavir plus ritonavir, or telaprevir because of high risk for rhabdomyolysis with acute renal failure.
- Use atorvastatin cautiously in patients who consume substantial quantities of alcohol or have a history of liver disease because atorvastatin use increases risk of liver dysfunction.
- Expect atorvastatin to be used in patients without obvious coronary artery disease (CAD) but with multiple risk factors (such as age 55 or over, family history of early CAD, history of hypertension or low HDL level, or smoker).
- Expect liver function tests to be performed before atorvastatin therapy starts and then thereafter as clinically necessary. If clinical symptoms such as hyperbilirubinemia and jaundice occurs, notify prescriber and expect atorvastatin therapy to be discontinued until cause of liver dysfunction has been identified. If no cause can be found, expect the drug to be discontinued permanently.
- Expect to measure lipid levels 2 to 4 weeks after therapy starts, to adjust dosage as directed, and to repeat periodically until lipid levels are within desired range.
- Monitor diabetic patient's blood glucose levels because atorvastatin therapy can affect blood glucose control.

WARNING Notify prescriber immediately and expect to withhold atorvastatin therapy if patient develops an acute condition suggestive of a myopathy (unexplained muscle pain, tenderness or weakness, especially if accompanied by elevated CPK level, fever, or malaise) or has a risk factor predisposing to the development of renal failure secondary to rhabdomyolysis, such as an acute severe infection; hypotension; major surgery; severe electrolyte, endocrine, or metabolic disorder; or uncontrolled seizures.

PATIENT TEACHING

- Emphasize that atorvastatin is an adjunct to—not a substitute for—a low-cholesterol diet.
- Tell patient to take drug at the same time each day to maintain its effects.

- Instruct patient to take a missed dose as soon as possible. If it's almost time for his next dose, he should skip the missed dose. Tell him not to double the dose.
- Instruct patient to consult prescriber before taking OTC niacin because of increased risk of rhabdomyolysis.
- Advise patient to notify prescriber immediately if he develops unexplained muscle pain, tenderness, or weakness, especially if accompanied by fatigue or fever.
- Reinforce the benefits of therapy, and urge patient to comply if possible.
- Advise patient with diabetes to monitor blood glucose levels closely.
- Inform women of childbearing age to use effective contraception while taking atorvastatin because atorvastatin is contraindicated in pregnancy. Tell female patient to notify prescriber immediately if pregnancy is suspected or known, as drug will have to be discontinued. Also tell mothers that breastfeeding is contraindicated during atorvastatin therapy.

atovaquone

Mepron

Class and Category

Pharmacologic class: Ubiquinone analogue
Therapeutic class: Antiprotozoal
Pregnancy category: C

Indications and Dosages

➤ *To prevent* Pneumocystis jiroveci *pneumonia in patients who can't tolerate trimethoprim-sulfamethoxazole*

SUSPENSION, TABLETS

Adults and adolescents. 1,500 mg (10 ml) once daily with meals.

➤ *To treat mild to moderate* P. jiroveci *pneumonia in patients who can't tolerate trimethoprim-sulfamethoxazole*

SUSPENSION, TABLETS

Adults and adolescents. 750 mg (5 ml) twice daily with meals for 21 days. *Maximum:* 1,500 mg/day.

Mechanism of Action

May destroy *P. jiroveci* organisms by inhibiting the enzymes needed to synthesize nucleic acid and adenosine triphosphate.

Contraindications

Hypersensitivity to atovaquone or its components

Interactions

DRUGS

indinavir: Possible loss of efficacy of indinavir
metoclopramide, rifabutin, rifampin, tetracycline: Possibly decreased blood atovaquone level

Adverse Reactions

CNS: Fever, headache, insomnia
EENT: Rhinitis, throat tightness, vortex keratopathy
GI: Abdominal pain, diarrhea, elevated liver enzymes, **hepatic failure**, **hepatitis**, nausea, **pancreatitis**, vomiting
GU: Acute renal dysfunction
HEME: Anemia, **thrombocytopenia**
RESP: Bronchospasm, cough, dyspnea
SKIN: Desquamation, **erythema multiforme**, **Stevens-Johnson syndrome**, rash, urticaria
Other: Allergic reaction, **angioedema**, **methemoglobinemia**

Nursing Considerations

- Use atovaquone cautiously in patient with severe hepatic impairment because, although rare, serious adverse reactions affecting liver function may occur.
- Monitor blood test results because atovaquone may decrease serum sodium, hemoglobin levels, and neutrophil count; and may increase AST, ALT, alkaline phosphatase, and serum amylase levels.
- Crush atovaquone tablets, if needed.
- Don't use tablets and oral suspension interchangeably; they aren't bioequivalent.

PATIENT TEACHING

- Instruct patient to take atovaquone with meals for maximum effectiveness.
- Remind patient taking suspension form to shake the suspension gently before using each time.
- Instruct patient to take a missed dose as soon as possible. If it's almost time for the next dose, tell him to skip the missed dose. Tell him not to double the next dose.
- Tell patient to notify prescriber if his condition doesn't improve in a few days or if he develops signs of an allergic reaction, such as fever or rash.

A

atropine
AtroPen
atropine sulfate

Class and Category
Pharmacologic class: Anticholinergic
Therapeutic class: Antiarrhythmic, antimuscarinic
Pregnancy category: C

Indications and Dosages
➤ *To reduce secretions and block vagal effects preoperatively*

I.V., I.M., OR SUBCUTANEOUS INJECTION

Adults. 0.5 to 1 mg given 30 to 60 min before surgery, repeated in 1 to 2 hr, if needed.

Children. 0.01 to 0.03 mg/kg given 30 to 60 min before surgery, repeated in 4 to 6 hr, as needed.

To reverse adverse muscarinic anticholinesterase effects

I.V. INJECTION (ATROPINE SULFATE)

Adults. 0.6 to 1.2 mg for each 0.5 to 2.5 mg of neostigmine methylsulfate or 10 to 20 mg of pyridostigmine bromide.

➤ *As an anidote for organophosphorus or muscarinic mushroom poisoning*

I.M. INJECTION, I.V. INJECTION, SUBCUTENOUS INJECTION (ATROPINE SULFATE)

Adults. 2 to 3 mg, repeated every 20 to 30 min, as needed, until signs of poisoning are significantly lessened or signs of atropine toxicity occur.

ENDOTRACHEAL INSTILLATION (ATROPINE SULFATE)

Adults. 1 to 2 mg diluted in no more than 10 ml of sterile water or normal saline.

➤ *To treat bradyasystolic cardiac arrest*

I.V. INJECTION (ATROPINE SULFATE)

Adults. 1 mg, repeated in 3 to 5 min, and repeated again in 3 to 5 min, as needed. *Maximum:* 3 mg total dose.

ENDOTRACHEAL INSTILLATION (ATROPINE SULFATE)

Adults. 1 to 2 mg diluted in no more than 10 ml of sterile water or normal saline.

➤ *To treat known or suspected exposure to chemical nerve agent or insecticide*

I.M. INJECTION (ATROPEN)

Adults and children weighing over 41 kg (90 lb) with two or more mild symptoms. 2 mg, if severe symptoms develop after injection, two or more 2-mg injections given in rapid succession 10 min after initial injection.

Adults and children weighing over 41 kg (90 lb) who are unconscious or have other severe symptoms. 2 mg given immediately 3 times in rapid succession.

Children weighing 18 to 41 kg (40 to 90 lb) with two or more mild symptoms. 1 mg, if severe symptoms develop after injection, two more 1-mg injections given in rapid succession 10 min after initial injection.

Children weighing 18 to 41 kg (40 to 90 lb) who are unconscious or exhibit any other severe symptoms. 1 mg given immediately 3 times in rapid succession.

Children weighing 7 to 18 kg (15 to 40 lb) with two or more mild symptoms. 0.5 mg. If severe symptoms develop after injection, two more 0.5-mg injections given in rapid succession 10 min after initial injection.

Children weighing 7 to 18 kg (15 to 40 lb) who are unconscious or exhibit any other severe symptoms. 0.5 mg given immediately three times in rapid succession.

Route	Onset	Peak	Duration
I.V.	Immediate	2–4 min	Brief
I.M.	5–40 min	20–60 min	Brief
SubQ	Unknown	Unknown	Brief

Mechanism of Action
Inhibits acetylcholine's muscarinic action at the neuroeffector junctions of smooth muscles, cardiac muscles, exocrine glands, SA and AV nodes, and the urinary bladder. In small doses, atropine inhibits salivary and bronchial secretions and diaphoresis. In moderate doses, it increases impulse conduction through the AV node and increases heart rate. In large doses, it decreases GI and urinary tract motility and gastric acid secretion.

Contraindications
Angle-closure glaucoma, GI obstructive disease (achalasia, pyloric obstruction,

pyloroduodenal stenosis), hypersensitivity to atropine or its components, ileus, intestinal atony, myasthenia gravis, obstructive uropathy, severe ulcerative colitis, tachycardia secondary to cardiac insufficiency or thyrotoxicosis, toxic megacolon, unstable cardiovascular status in acute hemorrhage

Interactions

DRUGS

amantadine, anticholinergics, antidyskinetics, glutethimide, meperidine, muscle relaxants, phenothiazines, tricyclic antidepressants and other drugs with anticholinergic properties, including antiarrhythmics (disopyramide, procainamide, quinidine), antihistamines, buclizine, meclizine: Increased atropine effects
ketoconazole: Decreased ketoconazole absorption
levodopa: Decreased plasma levodopa concentration and effectiveness
opioid analgesics: Increased risk of ileus, severe constipation, and urine retention
potassium chloride, especially wax-matrix forms: Possibly GI ulcers
urinary alkalizers (calcium or magnesium antacids, carbonic anhydrase inhibitors, citrates, sodium bicarbonate): Delayed excretion, increased risk of adverse atropine effects

Adverse Reactions

CNS: Agitation, amnesia, anxiety, ataxia, Babinski's or Chaddock's reflex, behavioral changes, CNS stimulation (at high doses), **coma**, confusion, decreased concentration, decreased tendon reflexes, delirium, dizziness, drowsiness, fever, hallucinations, headache, hyperreflexia, insomnia, lethargy, mania, mental disorders, nervousness, paranoia, restlessness, **seizures**, somnolence, stupor, syncope, vertigo, weakness
CV: Arrhythmias, bradycardia (at low doses), cardiac dilation, chest pain, hypertension, **hypotension, left ventricular failure, MI**, palpitations, tachycardia (at high doses), **weak or impalpable peripheral pulses**
EENT: Acute angle-closure glaucoma, altered taste, blepharitis, blindness, blurred vision, conjunctivitis, cyclophoria, cycloplegia, decreased visual acuity or accommodation, dry eyes or conjunctiva, dry mucous membranes, dry mouth, eye irritation, eyelid crusting, heterophoria, increased intraocular pressure, keratoconjunctivitis, lacrimation, laryngitis, **laryngospasm**, mydriasis, nasal congestion, oral lesions, photophobia, pupils poorly reactive to light, strabismus, tongue chewing
GI: Abdominal distention, abdominal pain, bloating, constipation, decreased bowel sounds or food absorption, delayed gastric emptying, dysphagia, heartburn, ileus, nausea, vomiting
GU: Bladder distention, enuresis, impotence, polydipsia, urinary hesitancy, urinary urgency, urine retention
MS: Dysarthria, hypertonia, muscle twitching
RESP: Bradypnea, dyspnea, **inspiratory stridor, pulmonary edema, respiratory failure, shallow breathing, subcostal recession**, tachypnea
SKIN: Cold skin, cyanosis, decreased sweating, dermatitis, flushing, rash, urticaria
Other: Anaphyaxis, dehydration, injection-site reaction, sensations of warmth

Nursing Considerations

WARNING Know that for patient prescribed AtroPen for suspected nerve gas or insecticide exposure, dosage is determined by severity of symptoms. Mild symptoms include acute onset of stomach cramps, blurred vision, bradycardia, chest tightness, difficulty breathing, excessive unexplained teary eyes or runny nose, increased salivation, miosis, muscle twitching, nausea, tachycardia, unexplained wheezing or coughing, and vomiting. Severe symptoms include confusion or other strange behavior, extreme secretions from airway or lungs, involuntary urination and defecation, seizures, severe difficulty breathing, severe muscle twitching and general weakness, tremors, and unconsciousness.

- Be aware that high-dose atropine sulfate should not be used in patients with ulcerative colitis because of risk of toxic megacolon or in patients with hiatal hernia and reflux esophagitis because of risk of esophagitis.

- Know that AtroPen has no absolute contraindications when used to treat life-threatening nerve gas or insecticide exposure.

WARNING Assess for symptoms of toxic doses of atropine, such as agitation, confusion, drowsiness, and excitement, which are likely to affect elderly patients even with low doses. If symptoms occur, take safety precautions to prevent injury.

- Assess bowel and bladder elimination. Notify prescriber of constipation, diarrhea, urinary hesitancy, or urine retention.

PATIENT TEACHING

- Teach patient prescribed an AtroPen because of risk of nerve gas or insecticide exposure, when and how to self-administer the drug.
- Advise patient to notify prescriber if he has constipation, difficulty urinating, or persistent or severe diarrhea.

auranofin

Ridaura

Class and Category

Pharmacologic class: Gold salt
Therapeutic class: Anti-inflammatory (antiarthritic)
Pregnancy category: C

Indications and Dosages

➤ *To treat active rheumatoid arthritis in patients that are intolerant to or unresponsive to nonsteroidal anti-inflammatory drugs (NSAIDs)*

CAPSULES

Adults. *Initial:* 6 mg daily or 3 mg twice daily. *Maintenance:* Up to 9 mg daily in 3 divided doses after 3 mo of treatment, if needed.

Route	Onset	Peak	Duration
P.O.	3–6 mo	1–2 hr	Up to 26 days

Mechanism of Action

Decreases rheumatoid factor and humoral antibody (immunoglobulin) levels. Although exact anti-inflammatory action is unknown, drug may suppress the increased phagocytic activity of macrophages and polymorphonuclear leukocytes that occur with rheumatoid arthritis and thereby inhibit release of destructive enzymes that cause joint inflammation.

Contraindications

Bone marrow aplasia, exfoliative dermatitis, hypersensitivity to auranofin or its components, necrotizing enterocolitis, pulmonary fibrosis, severe hematologic disorders

Interactions

DRUGS

phenytoin: Possibly increased phenytoin level

Adverse Reactions

CNS: Confusion, dizziness, EEG abnormalities, hallucinations, **seizures**
EENT: Gingivitis, glossitis, iritis or corneal ulcers from gold deposits in ocular tissue, metallic taste, stomatitis
GI: Abdominal cramps, anorexia, constipation, diarrhea, enterocolitis, flatulence, indigestion, jaundice, **melena**, nausea, vomiting
GU: Hematuria, elevated BUN and serum creatinine levels, proteinuria, vaginitis
HEME: Agranulocytosis, **aplastic anemia**, eosinophilia, **leukopenia**, **neutropenia**, **thrombocytopenia**
RESP: Cough, dyspnea, **fibrosis**, **interstitial pneumonitis**
SKIN: Alopecia, dermatitis, **exfoliative dermatitis**, photosensitivity, pruritus, rash, urticaria

Nursing Considerations

- Monitor blood and urine tests for signs of gold toxicity during auranofin therapy.

WARNING Know that gold toxicity may occur during treatment or several months afterward. It usually occurs with a cumulative dose of 400 to 800 mg and may cause decreased hemoglobin level, WBC count less than 4,000/mm^3, granulocyte count less than 1,500/mm^3, platelet count less than 150,000/mm^3, severe diarrhea, stomatitis, hematuria, proteinuria, pruritus, rash, severe diarrhea, and stomatitis.

- Monitor fluid intake and output imbalance. If urine output decreases, assess BUN and serum creatinine levels for signs of renal impairment.

- Notify prescriber about possible allergic reaction (dermatitis, pruritus, or rash). Drug may need to be discontinued.

PATIENT TEACHING

- Advise patient that diarrhea is common but that he should notify prescriber immediately if it becomes severe.
- Tell patient to take drug exactly as prescribed and to have monthly blood tests.
- Inform patient that drug may take 3 to 4 months to reach a therapeutic level.
- Urge patient to report fatigue, skin problems, or stomatitis (possible blood dyscrasias).
- Tell patient to report bleeding gums, blood in stool or urine, and easy bruising.

avanafil

Stendra

Class and Category

Pharmacologic class: Phosphodiesterase 5 (PDE5) inhibitor
Therapeutic class: Erectile dysfunction
Pregnancy category: C

Indications and Dosages

➤ *To treat erectile dysfunction*

TABLETS

Adults. 100 mg as early as 15 min before sexual activity, as needed. *Maximum:* Once daily.

DOSAGE ADJUSTMENT Dosage may be decreased to 50 mg 30 min before sexual activity or dosage may be increased to 200 mg as early as 15 min before sexual activity, as needed. For patient who is stable on alpha-blocker therapy or who is taking a moderate CYP3A4 inhibitor such as amprenavir, aprepitant, diltiazem, erythromycin, fluconazole, fosamprenavir, or verapamil, dosage is limited to 50 mg.

Mechanism of Action

Enhances the effect of nitric oxide released in the penis through stimulation. Nitric oxide increases cGMP level, relaxes smooth muscle, and increases blood flow to the corpus cavernosum, thus producing an erection.

Contraindications

Concomitant therapy with strong CYP3A4 inhibitors (including atazanavir, clarithromycin, indinavir, itraconazole, ketoconazole, nefazodone, nelfinavir, ritonavir, saquinavir, and telithromycin) or riociguat, hypersensitivity to avanafil or its components, nitrate therapy

Interactions

DRUGS

alpha blockers and other antihypertensives: Increased risk of hypotension
CYP3A4 inhibitors: Possibly increased plasma levels of avanafil
desipramine, omeprazole, rosiglitazone: Possibly increased effect of these drugs
guanylate cyclase stimulators such as riociguat: Possibly increased risk of hypotension
nitrates: Profound hypotension
sodium nitroprusside: Possibly potentiation of antiaggregatory effect of sodium nitroprusside

ACTIVITIES

alcohol use: Increased risk of orthostatic hypotension

Adverse Reactions

CNS: Depression, dizziness, fatigue, headache, insomnia, somnolence, vertigo
CV: **Abnormal ECG**, angina, **deep vein thrombosis**, hypertension, palpitations, peripheral edema
EENT: Epistaxis, eyelid swelling, hearing or vision loss, nasal or sinus congestion, nasopharyngitis, nonarteritic anterior ischemic optic neuropathy, oropharyngeal pain, sinusitis, tinnitus
ENDO: Hyperglycemia, **hypoglycemia**
GI: Constipation, diarrhea, dyspepsia, elevated liver enzymes, gastric pain, gastritis, gastroesophageal reflux disease, nausea, vomiting
GU: Hematuria, nephrolithiasis, pollakiuria, prolonged erection, urinary tract infection
MS: Arthralgia, back or musculoskeletal pain, muscle spasms, myalgia
RESP: Bronchitis, cough, exertional dyspnea, upper respiratory infection, wheezing
SKIN: Flushing, pruritus, rash
Other: Flu-like symptoms

Nursing Considerations

- Be aware that avanafil should not be used in a patient taking a strong CYP3A4 inhibitor (such as atanazavir, clarithromycin, indinavir, itraconazole, ketoconazole, nefazadone, nelfinavir, ritonavir, saquinavir, telithromycin) because of increased risk of elevated avanafil levels that could cause serious adverse effects.

- Know that although nitrate therapy is a contraindication to avanafil therapy, in a life-threatening situation, at least 12 hours should elapse after the last dose of avanafil before nitrate administration is given. In this situation, be prepared to hemodynamically monitor the patient and expect hypotension to be treated, if it occurs.
- Use avanafil cautiously in a patient with preexisting cardiovascular disease because of the potential for increased cardiac adverse effects during sexual activity. Patient with left ventricular outflow obstruction or severely impaired autonomic control of blood pressure may be especially sensitive to the vasodilatation effect of avanafil.
- Use avanafil cautiously in the elderly and patients with mild to moderate renal or hepatic dysfunction. The effects of avanafil in the presence of severe renal or hepatic dysfunction is unknown.
- Monitor the patient's vision, especially in patients over age 50; who have diabetes, hypertension, coronary artery disease, or hyperlipidemia; or who smoke, because avanafil rarely may cause nonarteritic anterior ischemic optic neuropathy that may lead to decreased vision or permanent vision loss.

PATIENT TEACHING

- Explain to patient that avanafil should be taken as early as 15 minutes before sexual activity and that sexual stimulation is required for drug to be effective.
- Remind patient that avanafil should not be taken more than once a day.

WARNING Warn patient not to take avanafil if he also takes any form of organic nitrate, either continuously or intermittently or other PDE5 inhibitors, because profound hypotension and death could result.

- Tell patient to stop taking drug and contact prescriber immediately if vision decreases suddenly in one or both eyes, or if he has a sudden loss of hearing, possibly with dizziness and tinnitus.
- Advise patient taking avanafil to seek sexual counseling to enhance the drug's effects.
- Instruct patient to notify prescriber immediately if erection is painful or lasts longer than 4 hours.
- Warn patient that alcohol ingestion may increase risk of low blood pressure, accompanied by dizziness when changing position, increased heart rate, and headache.

azathioprine

Azasan, Imuran

azathioprine sodium

Imuran I.V.

Class and Category

Pharmacologic class: Purine antagonist
Therapeutic class: Immunosuppressant, antirheumatic
Pregnancy category: D

Indications and Dosages

➤ *To prevent kidney rejection after transplantation*

TABLETS

Adults and children. *Initial:* 3 to 5 mg/kg daily P.O. as a single dose on, or 1 to 3 days before, day of transplantation then decreased according to patient's response and tolerance to 1 to 3 mg/kg daily following surgery. *Maintenance:* 1 to 3 mg/kg daily.

I.V. INFUSION (IMURAN I.V.)

Adults unable to tolerate oral dosage. *Initial:* 3 to 5 mg/kg as a single dose on, or 1 to 3 days daily before day of transplantation infused over 30 to 60 min, then decreased according to patient's response and tolerance to 1 to 3 mg/kg infused over 30 to 60 min daily following surgery until P.O. dose is tolerated (usually 1 to 4 days.)

DOSAGE ADJUSTMENT Dosage reduced for patients with oliguria (as from tubular necrosis) after transplantation because drug or metabolite excretion may be delayed.

➤ *To reduce signs and symptoms of acute rheumatoid arthritis*

TABLETS

Adults. *Initial:* 1 mg/kg (50 to 100 mg) daily as a single dose or twice daily for 6 to 8 wk. *Maintenance:* If initial therapy doesn't produce therapeutic effects or serious adverse effects, dosage increased every 4 wk by 0.5 up to 2.5 mg/kg.

DOSAGE ADJUSTMENT Dosage reduced to 25% to 33% of usual dosage for patients who also take allopurinol.

Route	Onset	Peak	Duration
P.O., I.V.	4–8 wk	Unknown	Several days

Mechanism of Action

May prevent proliferation and differentiation of activated B and T cells by interfering with purine (protein) and nucleic acid (DNA and RNA) synthesis.

Contraindications

Hypersensitivity to azathioprine or its components

Interactions

DRUGS

ACE inhibitors and drugs that affect bone marrow and cell development in bone marrow, such as trimethoprim-sulfamethoxazole: Possibly severe leukopenia

cyclosporine: Possibly decreased plasma cyclosporine level

ribavirin: Possibly induced severe pancytopenia and possibly increase risk of azathioprine related myelotoxicity

xanthine oxidase inhibitors such as allopurinol, febuxostat: Increased plasma azathioprine levels possibly leading to azathioprine toxicity

Adverse Reactions

CNS: Fever, malaise, **progressive multifocal leukoencephalopathy**

GI: Abdominal pain, diarrhea, **hepatotoxicity**, nausea, **pancreatitis**, steatorrhea, vomiting

HEME: Immunosuppression (severe), leukopenia, macrocytic anemia, **pancytopenia**, **thrombocytopenia**

MS: Arthralgia, myalgia

SKIN: Acute febrile neutrophilic dermatosis (Sweet's syndrome), alopecia, **cancer**, rash

RESP: Interstitial pneumonitis

Other: Infection, **lymphomas and other neoplasms**, negative nitrogen balance

Nursing Considerations

- Obtain results of baseline laboratory tests, including WBC, RBC, and platelet counts. Expect to monitor results once a week during first month of therapy, twice a month during second and third months, and once a month or more thereafter.
- Know that hematologic reactions typically are dose-related and may occur late in therapy, especially in patients with transplant rejection.

WARNING Expect to reduce dosage or discontinue azathioprine, if WBC count decreases rapidly or remains significantly and consistently low.

WARNING Monitor patient closely for abnormal signs and symptoms suggestive of lymphomas, especially in adolescent and young adult males who have a history of inflammatory bowel disease, in patients who have received a renal transplant, or in patients with rheumatoid arthritis, because the majority of patients who develop a lymphoma fall into one of these categories.

- Monitor liver enzymes, as ordered, for early signs of hepatotoxicity.
- Take action if patient develops thrombocytopenia, such as bleeding precautions, such as avoiding I.M. injections and venipunctures, applying ice to areas of trauma, and checking I.V. infusion sites every 2 hours for bleeding.
- Be aware that patients with low or absent thiopurine S-methyl transferase (TPMT) or nucleutide diphoshatase (NUDT15) levels are at risk for developing severe and life-threatening myelosuppression. Expect patient to be tested for these disorders if significant myelosuppression occurs. If confirmed, expect dosage to be decreased in the presence of heterozygous deficiency and drug discontinued in the presence of homozygous deficiency.
- Monitor the patient's prothrombin time if he also receives an oral anticoagulant.

- Be aware that azathioprine therapy increases risk of bacterial, fungal, protozoal, and viral infections. Watch for evidence of infection, such as fever, chills, sore throat, and mouth sores. Expect to administer aggressive antibiotic, antiviral, or other drug therapy and reduce azathioprine dosage.
- Minimize the risk of infection. If patient has severe leukopenia, take neutropenic precautions, such as placing him in a private room and limiting visitors.
- Know that rheumatoid arthritis requires at least 12 weeks of azathioprine therapy. During this time, continue other pain-relief measures, such as physical therapy, rest, and other drugs, such as salicylates and corticosteroids if it causes GI upset.
- Give oral azathioprine in divided doses or with meals if GI upset occurs.
- Expect to use lowest possible maintenance dosage for rheumatoid arthritis, reducing it gradually in 0.5-mg/kg (about 25-mg) increments at 4-week intervals, as ordered.
- Know that drug can be stopped abruptly, but its effects may persist several days.

PATIENT TEACHING

- Advise patient to take oral drug with food or meals to minimize GI upset.

WARNING Teach patient to recognize and report signs of infection, such as sore throat and fever and to seek medical attention for any abnormal signs and symptoms that might be suggestive of a malignancy.

- Teach patient how to reduce the risk of bleeding and falling.

azelastine hydrochloride

Astelin, Astepro

Class and Category

Pharmacologic class: H_1-receptor antagonist
Therapeutic class: Antihistamine
Pregnancy category: C

Indications and Dosages

➤ *To treat symptoms of seasonal allergic rhinitis*

NASAL SPRAY (ASTELIN)

Adults and children age 12 and over. 1 or 2 sprays in each nostril twice daily. Alternatively, 2 sprays in each nostril once daily.
Children age 5 to 11 years. 1 spray in each nostril twice daily.

NASAL SPRAY (ASTEPRO)

Adults and children age 12 and over. 1 or 2 sprays (0.1% or 0.15%) in each nostril twice daily. Alternatively, 0.15% solution may be administered as 2 sprays in each nostril once daily.
Children age 6 to 11 years. 1 spray (0.1% or 0.15%) in each nostril twice daily.
Children age 2 to 5 years: 1 spray (0.1%) in each nostril twice daily.

➤ *To treat symptoms of perennial allergic rhinitis*

NASAL SPRAY (ASTEPRO)

Adults and children age 12 and over. 2 sprays (0.15%) in each nostril twice daily.
Children age 6 to 11. 1 spray (0.1% or 0.15%) in each nostril twice daily.
Children age 6 months to 5 years: 1 spray (0.1%) in each nostril twice daily.

➤ To treat symptoms of vasomotor rhinitis

NASAL SPRAY (ASTEPRO)

Adults and children age 12 and over. 2 sprays in each nostril twice daily.

Route	Onset	Peak	Duration
Nasal	In 3 hr	Unknown	12 hr

Mechanism of Action

Binds nonselectively to central and peripheral H_1 receptors, preventing histamine from reaching its site of action, which reduces or prevents most of histamine's physiologic effects. By blocking histamine at its site of action, azelastine inhibits GI, respiratory, and vascular smooth-muscle contraction; decreases capillary permeability, which reduces flares, itching, and wheals; and decreases lacrimal and salivary gland secretions.

Contraindications

Hypersensitivity to azelastine or its components

Interactions

DRUGS

cimetidine: Possibly increased blood azelastine level
CNS depressants: Possibly increased sedative effects and reduced mental alertness

ACTIVITIES

alcohol use: Possibly increased sedative effects and reduced mental alertness

Adverse Reactions

CNS: Dizziness, fatigue, headache, somnolence
CV: Atrial fibrillation, palpitations
EENT: Bitter taste, dry mouth, epistaxis, nasal burning, paroxysmal sneezing, pharyngitis, rhinitis
GI: Nausea
Other: Weight gain

Nursing Considerations

- Assess for changes in alertness, and take safety precautions, if needed.

PATIENT TEACHING

- Teach patient how to use azelastine nasal spray properly to achieve maximum therapeutic effects.
- Instruct patient to prime pump before using for first time by placing his thumb on base and his index and middle fingers on shoulder area of bottle and then pressing thumb firmly and quickly against bottle four times, or until fine mist appears.
- Tell patient if he hasn't used spray in more than 3 days, he will need to reprime pump with two sprays or until fine mist appears.
- Advise patient to clear nostrils gently, if needed, before using spray.
- Teach patient to inhale deeply after each spray and then exhale through his mouth and tilt his head back so drug can spread over nasopharynx.
- Advise patient to store bottle upright and keep it tightly closed.

WARNING **Emphasize that patient must consult prescriber before taking any OTC drug, such as cough syrup or a cold remedy, because of the risk of extreme CNS depression.**

- Inform patient that decreased alertness may occur. Advise him to avoid hazardous activities or those that require alertness, such as driving or operating machinery, until drug's effects are known.
- Inform breastfeeding mothers to monitor infant for milk rejection because drug may cause a bitter taste in breast milk.

azilsartan medoxomil

Edarbi

Class and Category

Pharmacologic class: Angiotensin II receptor blocker
Therapeutic class: Antihypertensive
Pregnancy category: D

Indications and Dosages

➤ *To manage hypertension, alone or with other antihypertensives*

TABLETS

Adults. 80 mg once daily.
DOSAGE ADJUSTMENT For patients who are receiving high doses of diuretics, initial dosage is decreased to 40 mg once daily.

Mechanism of Action

Selectively blocks binding of angiotensin (AT) II to AT_1 receptor sites in many tissues, including vascular smooth muscle and adrenal glands. This inhibits vasoconstrictive and aldosterone-secreting effects of AT II, which reduces blood pressure.

Contraindications

Concurrent aliskiren use in patients with diabetes, hypersensitivity to azilsartan or its components

Interactions

DRUGS

ACE inhibitors, aliskiren, other angiotensin receptor blockers: Increased risk of hyperkalemia, hypotension, and renal dysfunction
lithium: Possibly increased risk of serum lithium concentrations resulting in lithium toxicity
NSAIDs: Possible decreased renal function in patients who are elderly, volume-depleted, or have existing compromised renal function

Adverse Reactions

CNS: Asthenia, dizziness, fatigue
CV: **Hypotension**, orthostatic hypotension
GI: Diarrhea, nausea
GU: Elevated BUN and serum creatinine levels
MS: Muscle spasm
RESP: Cough
SKIN: Pruritus, rash
Other: **Angioedema**

Nursing Considerations

- Expect to provide treatment for hypovolemia before starting azilsartan therapy.
- Monitor patient for hypotension. If it occurs, place patient in a supine position, and if needed, give an I.V. infusion of normal saline, as ordered. Be aware that a transient hypotensive episode does not require the drug to be discontinued.
- Watch for elevated BUN and serum creatinine levels, especially if patient has congestive heart failure, renal artery stenosis, or volume depletion. Report significant or persistent increases immediately.

PATIENT TEACHING

- Instruct patient to take azilsartan exactly as prescribed and to monitor his blood pressure for effectiveness.
- Advise female patient to report known or suspected pregnancy immediately. Explain that if she becomes pregnant, prescriber may replace azilsartan with another antihypertensive that's safe to use during pregnancy.

azithromycin

Zithromax, Zmax

Class and Category

Pharmacologic class: Macrolide
Therapeutic class: Antibiotic
Pregnancy category: B

Indications and Dosages

➤ *To treat mild community-acquired pneumonia, otitis media, pharyngitis, tonsillitis, and uncomplicated skin and soft-tissue infections caused by susceptible bacteria*

ORAL SUSPENSION, TABLETS (ZITHROMAX)

Adults. 500 mg as a single dose on day 1, followed by 250 mg daily on days 2 through 5.
Children age 6 months or over with community-acquired pneumonia. 10 mg/kg as a single dose (not to exceed 500 mg daily) on day 1, followed by 5 mg/kg (not to exceed 250 mg daily) daily on days 2 through 5.
Children age 6 months or over with acute otitis media. 30 mg/kg as a single dose. Alternatively, 10 mg/kg once daily for 3 days, or 10 mg/kg as a single dose on day 1 followed by 5 mg/kg on days 2 through 5.

➤ *To treat community-acquired pneumonia caused by* Chlamydophila pneumoniae, Haemophilus influenzae, Legionella pneumophila, Moraxella catarrhalis, Mycoplasma pneumoniae, Staphylococcus aureus, *or* Streptococcus pneumoniae *and requiring initial I.V. therapy*

ORAL SUSPENSION, TABLETS, I.V. INFUSION (ZITHROMAX)

Adults and adolescents age 16 or over. 500 mg I.V. (1 mg/ml concentration given over 3 hrs; 2 mg/ml concentration given over 1 hr) as a single dose daily for at least 2 days, followed by 500 mg P.O. as a single dose daily until patient completes 7 to 10 days of therapy.

➤ *To treat community-acquired pneumonia caused by* C. pneumoniae, H. influenzae, M. pneumoniae, *or* S. pneumoniae using extended release form

E.R. ORAL SUSPENSION (ZMAX)

Adults. 2 g as a single dose on an empty stomach.
Children age 6 months and over. 60 mg/kg as a single dose on an empty stomach.

➤ *To treat acute bacterial exacerbations of COPD including chronic bronchitis caused by* H. influenzae, M. catarrhalis, *or* S. pneumoniae

ORAL SUSPENSION, TABLETS (ZITHROMAX)

Adults. 500 mg daily for 3 days. Or, 500 mg as a single dose on day 1, followed by 250 mg daily on days 2 through 5.

➤ *To treat chancroid in men caused by* Haemophilus ducreyi; *urethritis or cervicitis, caused by* Chlamydia trachomatis

ORAL SUSPENSION, TABLETS (ZITHROMAX)

Adults. 1 g as a one-time dose.

➤ *To treat urethritis or cervicitis caused by* Neisseria gonorrhoeae

ORAL SUSPENSION, TABLETS (ZITHROMAX)

Adults. 2 g as a one-time dose.

➤ *To prevent* Mycobacterium avium *complex in patients with advanced HIV infection*

ORAL SUSPENSION, TABLETS (AZITHROMYCIN)

Adults. 1.2 g once weekly, as indicated.

➤ *To treat pelvic inflammatory disease*

ORAL SUSPENSION, TABLETS, I.V. INFUSION (ZITHROMAX)

Adults. 500 mg I.V. (1 mg/ml concentration given over 3 hrs; 2 mg/ml concentration given over 1 hr) as a single dose daily for 1 to 2 days, followed by 250 mg P.O. as a single dose daily until patient completes 7 days of therapy.

ORAL SUSPENSION, TABLETS (ZITHROMAX)

Adults. 500 mg daily for 3 days.

Children. 10 mg/kg daily for 3 days.

E.R. ORAL (SUSPENSION) (ZMAX)

Adults. 2 g as a single dose on an empty stomach.

Children age 6 months and over. 60 mg/kg as a single dose on an empty stomach.

Route	Onset	Peak	Duration
P.O., I.V.	Varies	Unknown	Unknown

Mechanism of Action

Binds to a ribosomal subunit of susceptible bacteria, blocking peptide translocation and inhibiting RNA-dependent protein synthesis. Drug concentrates in phagocytes, macrophages, and fibroblasts, which release it slowly and may help move it to infection sites.

Incompatibilities

Don't add I.V. substances, additives, or drugs to azithromycin I.V. solution, and don't infuse through the same I.V. line.

Contraindications

History of cholestatic jaundice or hepatic dysfunction associated with prior use of azithromycin; hypersensitivity to azithromycin, erythromycin, ketolide antibiotics, other macrolide antibiotics or their components

Interactions

DRUGS

antacids that contain aluminum or magnesium: Possibly decreased peak blood azithromycin level

dihydroergotamine, ergotamine: Possibly severe peripheral vasospasm and abnormal sensations (acute ergot toxicity)

HMG-CoA reductase inhibitors: Increased risk of severe myopathy or rhabdomyolysis

nelfinavir, theophylline: Possibly increased blood levels of these drugs

pimozide: Increased risk of prolonged QT interval and subsequent ventricular tachycardia

oral anticoagulants such as warfarin: Possibly potentiated effects of oral anticoagulants

triazolam: Possibly decreased excretion and increased therapeutic effects of triazolam

FOODS

any food: Altered absorption rate of azithromycin

Adverse Reactions

CNS: Aggressiveness, agitation, anxiety, asthenia, dizziness, fatigue, headache, hyperactivity, malaise, nervousness, paresthesia, **seizures**, somnolence, syncope, vertigo

CV: Arrhythmias, chest pain, edema, elevated serum CK level, **hypotension**, palpitations, **prolonged QT interval, torsades de pointes**, **ventricular tachycardia**

EENT: Hearing loss, oral candidiasis, perversion or loss of taste or smell, tinnitus, tongue discoloration

ENDO: Hyperglycemia

GI: Abdominal pain, anorexia, cholestatic jaundice, constipation, diarrhea, dyspepsia, elevated liver enzymes, flatulence, **hepatic necrosis or failure, hepatitis**, nausea, **pancreatitis**, pyloric stenosis, **pseudomembranous colitis**, vomiting

GU: Acute renal failure, elevated BUN and serum creatinine levels, nephritis, vaginal candidiasis

HEME: Leukopenia, neutropenia, thrombocytopenia

MS: Arthralgia
SKIN: Acute generalized exanthematous pustulosis, **erythema multiforme**, photosensitivity, pruritus, rash, **Stevens–Johnson syndrome, toxic epidermal necrolysis**, urticaria
Other: Allergic reaction, anaphylaxis, angioedema, drug reaction with eosinophilia and systemic symptoms (DRESS), elevated serum phosphorus level, **hyperkalemia**, infusion-site reaction (such as pain and redness), new or worsening myasthenia syndrome, superinfection

Nursing Considerations

- Be aware that azithromycin should not be used in patients with known QT prolongation, bradyarrhythmias, congenital long QT syndrome, uncompensated heart failure, or history of torsades de pointes; patients with ongoing proarrhythmic conditions such as uncorrected hypokalemia or hypomagnesemia, or significant bradycardia; or patients receiving drugs known to prolong the QT interval such as class IA (procainamide, quinidine) or class III (amiodarone, dofetilide, sotalol) antiarrhythmic agents because of increased risk of life-threatening arrhythmias such as torsades de pointes.
- Know that azithromycin should not be used in patients who have undergone donor stem cell transplant for cancer of the blood or lymph nodes because of an increased risk for cancer relapse and possibly death.
- Monitor elderly patients closely for arrhythmias because they are more susceptible to drug effects on the QT interval.
- Obtain culture and sensitivity test results, if possible, before starting therapy.
- Use azithromycin cautiously in patients with hepatic dysfunction not associated with prior use of azithromycin (drug is metabolized in the liver) or renal dysfunction (effects are unknown in this group).
- Give azithromycin capsules 1 hour before or 2 to 3 hours after food. Give tablets or suspension without regard to food.

WARNING Don't give azithromycin by I.V. bolus or I.M. injection because it may cause erythema, pain, swelling, tenderness, or other reaction at the site. Infuse it over 60 minutes or longer, as prescribed (typically 1 mg/ml over 3 hours or 2 mg/ml over 1 hour).

- Monitor liver enzymes closely in patients with impaired liver function and expect to discontinue the drug immediately if signs and symptoms of hepatitis occur.
- Assess patient for bacterial or fungal superinfection, which may occur with prolonged or repeated therapy. If it occurs, expect to give another antibiotic or antifungal.
- Monitor bowel elimination; if needed, obtain stool culture to rule out pseudomembranous colitis. If it occurs, expect to stop azithromycin and give fluid, electrolytes, and antibiotics effective with *Clostridium difficile.*
- Be aware that laboratory abnormalities may occur during azithromycin therapy. If present, alert prescriber, as changes can be reversible.

PATIENT TEACHING

- Tell patient to take azithromycin capsules 1 hour before or 2 to 3 hours after food. Instruct patient to take tablets or suspension without regard to food.

WARNING Urge patient to consult prescriber before taking OTC drugs, including antacids. If they're prescribed, tell patient to take azithromycin 1 hour before or 2 to 3 hours after taking antacids.

- Tell patient to report signs and symptoms of allergic reaction (such as rash, itching, hives, chest tightness, and trouble breathing) immediately.
- Warn patient that abdominal pain and loose, watery stools may occur. If diarrhea persists or becomes severe, urge him to contact prescriber and replace fluids.
- Teach patient to watch for and immediately report signs of superinfection, such as white patches in the mouth.

aztreonam

Azactam, Cayston

Class and Category

Pharmacologic class: Monobactam
Therapeutic class: Antibiotic
Pregnancy category: B

Indications and Dosages

➤ *To improve respiratory symptoms in cystic fibrosis patients with* Pseudomonas aeruginosa

INHALATION (CAYSTON)

Adults and children age 7 and over. 75 mg (1 vial) 3 times a day with doses at least 4 hr apart for 28 days (followed by 28 days off therapy).

➤ *To treat infections of the female reproductive tract; lower respiratory tract, skin, soft tissue, or urinary tract; intra-abdominal infections; septicemia; and surgical abscesses caused by susceptible strains of gram-negative bacteria*

I.V. INFUSION, I.V. OR I.M. INJECTION (AZACTAM)

Adults with a urinary tract infection. 500 mg or 1 g every 8 or 12 hours. I.V. bolus given slowly over 3 to 5 min. I.V. infusion given over 20 to 60 min.

Adults with moderately severe systemic infections. 1 or 2 g given every 8 to 12 hrs. I.V. bolus given slowly over 3 to 5 min. I.V. infusion given over 20 to 60 min.

Adults with severe systemic or life-threatening infections. 2 g every 6 or 8 hrs. I.V. bolus given slowly over 3 to 5 min. I.V. infusion given over 20 to 60 min. *Maximum:* 8 g daily.

I.V. INFUSION OR INJECTION

Children ages 9 months and over. 30 mg/kg every 6 to 8 hr up to 120 mg/kg daily.

DOSAGE ADJUSTMENT If creatinine clearance is 10 to 30 ml/min, initial dose is 1 to 2 g; then 50% of usual dose at usual interval. If creatinine clearance is less than 10 ml/min, initial dose is 500 mg to 2 g; then 25% of the usual dose every 6, 8, or 12 hr. For hemodialysis patients with serious or life-threatening infections, in addition to the maintenance doses, one-eighth of the initial dose given after each hemodialysis session.

Route	Onset	Peak	Duration
I.V. infusion	Immediate	Immediate	Unknown
I.V. injection	Immediate	Immediate	Unknown
I.M.	Variable	60 min	Unknown
Inhalation	Variable	60 min	Unknown

Mechanism of Action

Inhibits bacterial cell wall synthesis in susceptible aerobic gram-negative bacteria. These bacteria assemble rigid, cross-linked cell walls in several steps. Aztreonam affects the final cross-linking step by inactivating penicillin-binding protein 3 (the enzyme that links cell wall strands), which causes cell lysis and death.

Incompatibilities

Don't mix aztreonam in same I.V. solution as cephradine, metronidazole, or nafcillin sodium. Don't mix it in same I.M. injection solution as local anesthetic.

Contraindications

Hypersensitivity to aztreonam or its components

Interactions

DRUGS

aminoglycosides (prolonged or high-dose therapy): Increased risk of nephrotoxicity and ototoxicity
cefoxitin, imipenem: Possibly antagonized action of aztreonam
furosemide, probenecid: Possibly increased blood aztreonam level

Adverse Reactions

CNS: Confusion, dizziness, **encephalopathy**, fever, headache, insomnia, malaise, paresthesia, **seizures**, vertigo
CV: Chest pain, **hypotension**, transient ECG changes
EENT: Altered taste, diplopia, halitosis, mouth ulcers, mucocutaneous candidiasis, nasal congestion, sneezing, tinnitus, tongue numbness
GI: Abdominal cramps, diarrhea, elevated enzymes, **GI bleeding**, **hepatitis**, jaundice, nausea, **pseudomembranous colitis**, vomiting
GU: Breast tenderness, elevated serum creatinine level, vaginal candidiasis
HEME: Anemia, eosinophilia, leukocytosis, **neutropenia**, **pancytopenia**, positive Coombs' test, **prolonged PT and APTT**, **thrombocytopenia**, thrombocytosis
MS: Arthralgia, joint swelling, myalgia
RESP: **Bronchospasm**, dyspnea, wheezing
SKIN: Diaphoresis, **erythema multiforme**, **exfoliative dermatitis**, flushing, petechiae,

pruritus, purpura, rash, **toxic epidermal necrolysis**, urticaria
Other: Allergic reaction; injection-site pain, phlebitis, swelling, or thrombophlebitis

Nursing Considerations

- Obtain culture and sensitivity test results, if possible, before starting aztreonam therapy. If patient is acutely ill, expect to begin therapy before results are available.
- Keep in mind that other antimicrobials may be used with aztreonam in seriously ill patients at risk for gram-positive infection.
- Expect to use I.V. route for patients who need single doses over 1 g and those with life-threatening systemic infections, such as septicemia or peritonitis.
- Reconstitute aztreonam for I.V. bolus injection by using sterile water for injection. Immediately after adding diluent to vial, shake it vigorously to mix. After obtaining correct dose, discard unused solution. Reconstituted solution may turn light pink on standing at room temperature. This doesn't affect drug potency.
- Give I.V. bolus injection directly into I.V. tubing over 3 to 5 minutes.

WARNING Prepare aztreonam for I.V. infusion by using at least 50 ml of appropriate infusion solution per gram of aztreonam. Further dilute drug in I.V. solution, such as normal saline solution, D_5W, dextrose 5% in normal saline solution, lactated Ringer's solution, or Ringer's solution.

- Know that I.V. infusion may be administered over 20 to 60 minutes.
- Flush I.V. tubing with a solution, such as normal saline solution, before and after administering I.V. infusion to reduce risk of incompatibilities.
- Know that if prescribed, mix aztreonam in same I.V. solution with other antibiotics (such as ampicillin sodium, cefazolin sodium, clindamycin phosphate, gentamicin sulfate, or tobramycin sulfate), or mix it with cloxacillin sodium and vancomycin hydrochloride in peritoneal dialysis solution.
- Prepare solution for I.M. injection using sterile or bacteriostatic water or sodium chloride for injection. Administer injection deep into large muscle, such as in dorsogluteal or ventrogluteal area.
- Dilute each vial of inhalation solution with 1 ampule of diluent that comes with the drug. To do so, open the glass medication vial carefully, remove metal ring by pulling the tab, and remove the gray rubber stopper. Twist the tip off the diluent ampule and squeeze the liquid into the glass medication vial. Replace the rubber stopper, then gently swirl the vial until contents have been completely dissolved. Administer immediately.
- Administer diluted inhalation solution using only an Altera Nebulizer System.
- Be aware that patient should use a bronchodilator prior to aztreonam inhalation therapy. A short-acting bronchodilator should be used at least 15 minutes before but no longer than 4 hours prior to aztreonam inhalation therapy, or a long-acting bronchodilator at least 30 minutes before but no longer than 12 hours prior to aztreonam inhalation therapy. If patient is receiving multiple inhaled therapies, administer the bronchodilator first, followed by mucolytics, and last of all aztreonam.
- Assess for signs of bacterial or fungal superinfection, which may occur with prolonged or repeated therapy. If superinfection occurs, treat it as prescribed.
- Monitor bowel elimination; if needed, obtain stool culture to rule out pseudomembranous colitis. If it occurs, expect to discontinue aztreonam and administer fluid, electrolytes, and antibiotics effective against *Clostridium difficile*.
- Evaluate patient's renal and liver function test results, as ordered, if patient has renal or hepatic impairment.
- Monitor renal function if patient is receiving an aminoglycoside because of the increased risk of nephrotoxicity.

PATIENT TEACHING

- Emphasize the need to take full course of aztreonam exactly as prescribed, even if patient feels better before finishing it.

- Instruct patient how to dilute and administer inhalation form of drug, if ordered.
- Teach patient to recognize and immediately report signs and symptoms of allergic reactions, such as chest tightness, difficulty breathing, hives, itching, and rash.
- Warn patient that abdominal pain and loose, watery stools may occur 2 months or more after aztreonam therapy stops. If diarrhea persists or becomes severe, urge him to contact prescriber and replace fluids.
- Teach patient to watch for and immediately report signs of superinfection, such as white patches in mouth.

B

baloxavir marboxil

Xofluza

Class and Category

Pharmacologic class: Polymerase acidic endonuclease inhibitor
Therapeutic class: Influenza antiviral
Pregnancy category: Not classified

Indications and Dosages

➤ *To treat acute uncomplicated influenza in patients who have been symptomatic for no more than 48 hours*

TABLETS

Adults and children 12 years and over weighing at least 80 kg (176 lb). 80 mg as a single dose.
Adults and children 12 years and over weighing 40 kg (88 lb) to less than 80 kg (176 lb). 40 mg as a single dose.

Mechanism of Action

Inhibits the endonuclease activity of the polymerase acidic protein, an influenza virus-specific enzyme required for viral gene transcription. This action prevents the influenza virus from being replicated.

Contraindications

Hypersensitivity to baloxavir marboxil or its components

Interactions

DRUGS

antacids, laxatives, oral supplements, and other polyvalent cation-containing products (e.g., calcium, iron, magnesium, selenium, or zinc): Possibly decreased plasma concentrations of baloxavir which may reduce its effectiveness
live attenuated intranasal influenza vaccine: Possibly decreased effectiveness of vaccination

FOODS

calcium-fortified beverages, dairy products: Possibly decreased effectiveness of baloxavir

Adverse Reactions

CNS: Headache
EENT: Nasopharyngitis
GI: Diarrhea, nausea
RESP: Bronchitis

Nursing Considerations

- Be aware that baloxavir is not effective in treating infections other than influenza.
- Know that baloxavir should be administered to patients who have had flu symptoms for no more than 48 hours.
- Do not administer baloxavir with calcium-fortified beverages, dairy products, or drugs that contain cation-containing products such as calcium, iron, magnesium, selenium, or zinc.

PATIENT TEACHING

- Inform patient that baloxavir will be administered only once.
- Instruct patient that drug must not be taken with a calcium-fortified beverage or a meal containing dairy products. Also, tell patient to alert prescriber if he is taking any drugs that contain calcium, iron, magnesium, selenium, or zinc, because baloxavir may not be as effective when taken with such drugs.

balsalazide disodium

Colazal, Giazo

Class and Category

Pharmacologic class: Salicylate
Therapeutic class: Anti-inflammatory
Pregnancy category: B

Indications and Dosages

➤ *To treat mildly to moderately active ulcerative colitis*

CAPSULES (COLAZAL)

Adults. 2.25 g three times daily for 8 to 12 wk. *Maximum:* 6.75 g daily for 12 wk.
Children ages 5 to 17. 750 mg or 2.25 g three times daily for up to 8 wk.

TABLETS (GIAZO)
Adults. 3.3 g twice daily for up to 8 wk.

Mechanism of Action

After it has been metabolized to 5-ASA, balsalazide may reduce inflammation by inhibiting the enzyme cyclooxygenase and decreasing production of arachidonic acid metabolites, which may be increased in patients with inflammatory bowel disease.

Cyclooxygenase is needed to form prostaglandin from arachidonic acid. Prostaglandin mediates inflammatory activity and produces signs and symptoms of inflammation. By inhibiting prostaglandin synthesis, balsalazide may reduce signs and symptoms of inflammation in inflammatory bowel disease.

Balsalazide also interferes with leukotriene synthesis and inhibits the enzyme lipoxygenase. These substances are involved in the inflammatory response.

Contraindications

Hypersensitivity to balsalazide, salicylates, or their components

Interactions

DRUGS
None reported

Adverse Reactions

CNS: Fatigue, fever, headache, insomnia
CV: **Myocarditis**, **pericarditis**, vasculitis
EENT: Dry mouth, nasopharyngitis, pharyngitis, rhinitis, stomatitis
GI: Abdominal cramps or pain, anorexia, cirrhosis, constipation, diarrhea, dyspepsia, elevated liver enzyme levels, exacerbation of colitis, flatulence, **hepatotoxicity**, jaundice, nausea, **pancreatitis**, vomiting
GU: Dysmenorrhea, interstitial nephritis, **renal failure**, UTI
MS: Arthralgia, myalgia
RESP: Alveolitis, cough, pleural effusion, pneumonia, respiratory tract infection
SKIN: Alopecia, pruritus
Other: **Anaphylaxis**, flu-like syndrome

Nursing Considerations

WARNING Monitor patients who are sensitive to olsalazine or sulfasalazine for possible cross-sensitivity to balsalazide.

- Monitor patients with pyloric stenosis for decreased or delayed drug effects due to prolonged gastric retention of balsalazide capsules.
- Monitor patient for possible exacerbation of colitis symptoms.

PATIENT TEACHING

- Inform patient that balsalazide is used to reduce bowel inflammation and pain in ulcerative colitis and to minimize recurring inflammation.
- Instruct patient to swallow capsules whole, with a full glass of water, and not to chew or crush them.
- Advise patient to notify prescriber of any other drugs she may be taking, including herbal products, nutritional supplements, and OTC drugs, because they may interact with balsalazide.
- Instruct patient to notify prescriber immediately if colitis symptoms worsen.
- Inform patient that she can expect some improvement in symptoms in 3 to 21 days but that optimal results may take up to 6 weeks of treatment.

baricitinib

Olumiant

Class and Category

Pharmacologic class: Janus kinase inhibitor
Therapeutic class: Antirheumatic
Pregnancy category: Not classified

Indications and Dosages

➤ *To treat moderate to severe active rheumatoid arthritis in patients who have had an inadequate response to one or more tumor necrosis factor (TNF) antagonist therapies*

TABLETS
Adults. 2 mg once daily.
DOSAGE ADJUSTMENT For patients who develop an absolute lymphocyte count (ALC) less than 500 cells/mm^3, drug withheld until ALC is 500 cells/mm^3 or greater. For patients who develop an absolute neutrophil count (ANC) less than 1,000 cells/mm^3, drug withheld until ANC is 1,000 cells/mm^3 or greater. For patients who develop a hemoglobin value less than

8 g/dl, drug withheld until hemoglobin is 8 g/dl or greater.

Mechanism of Action

Janus kinases are intracellular enzymes that influence cellular processes of hematopoiesis and immune cell function. Janus kinase inhibitors interfere with these actions, thereby reducing the signs and symptoms of rheumatoid arthritis, which is thought to be an autoimmune disorder.

Contraindications

Hypersensitivity to baricitinib or its components

Interactions

DRUGS

Strong organic anion transporter 3 inhibitors, such as probenecid: Increased baricitinib exposure, increasing risk of adverse reactions

Live vaccines: Decreased effectiveness of vaccine

Adverse Reactions

CV: Elevated lipid levels, **thrombosis (including arterial and deep vein thrombosis)**

GI: Elevated liver enzymes, **gastrointestinal perforation**, nausea

GU: UTI

HEME: Anemia, **elevated platelet count, lymphopenia, neutropenia**

MS: Elevated creatine phosphokinase (CPK) levels

RESP: Bronchitis, pneumonia, **pulmonary embolus,** upper respiratory infections

SKIN: Acne, **non-melanoma skin cancers**

Other: Infections such as bacterial, fungal (invasive), mycobacterial, viral, or other opportunistic infections; **lymphomas and other malignancies**

Nursing Considerations

- Be aware that baricitinib should not be used in patients with an ALC less than 500 cells/mm^3, ANC less than 1,000 cells/mm^3, or hemoglobin level less than 8 g/dl.
- Know that baricitinib therapy should also be avoided in patients with an active, serious infection, including localized infections. In addition, drug is not recommended in patients with a glomerular filtration rate less than 60 ml/min, patients who have severe hepatic impairment, or patients who are taking strong organic anion transporter 3 inhibitors such as probenecid.
- Test patients for latent tuberculosis, as ordered, prior to initiating baricitinib therapy. If positive, expect patient to receive treatment. Monitor all patients for signs and symptoms of tuberculosis throughout therapy, including patients who were negative for latent tuberculosis infection prior to initiating therapy. Know that tuberculosis therapy also may be prescribed for patients with a history of active or latent tuberculosis in whom an adequate course of treatment cannot be confirmed and for patients with a negative test for latent tuberculosis but who have risk factors for tuberculosis.
- Expect liver enzymes to be determined prior to baricitinib therapy and periodically throughout therapy, because drug can affect liver function. Know that if increases in liver enzymes occur and liver injury is suspected, drug therapy should be stopped until liver dysfunction is ruled out.
- Be aware that viral reactivation, including herpes zoster, may occur. If patient develops herpes zoster during therapy with baricitinib, expect drug therapy to be interrupted until the episode has been resolved. Know that patients should be screened for viral hepatitis before initiating therapy with baricitinib.
- Use baricitinib cautiously in patients who may be at increased risk for gastrointestinal perforation or thrombosis, as drug use may increase the risk for these life-threatening disorders.

WARNING Monitor patient's complete blood count closely, as drug may cause anemia, lymphopenia, or neutropenia. Expect drug to be withheld if patient develops an ALC less than 500 cells/mm^3 until ALC is 500 cells/mm^3 or greater; an ANC less than 1,000 cells/mm^3 until ANC is 1,000 cells/mm^3 or greater; or a hemoglobin value becomes less than 8 g/dl until the hemoglobin level is 8 g/dl or greater.

- Assess patient regularly for signs and symptoms of infection, because serious and sometimes fatal infections due to bacterial, invasive fungal, mycobacterial, viral, or other opportunistic pathogens may occur. Patients at higher risk are those who are taking immunosuppressants such as corticosteroids or methotrexate. Notify prescriber if infection is suspected and expect antibiotic therapy to be prescribed, if confirmed. Know that baricitinib may be temporarily stopped if patient is not responding to antibiotic therapy and not restarted until the infection is under control.
- Be aware that baricitinib increases the risk of cancer. Assess the patient regularly, especially for non-melanoma skin cancers.

WARNING Assess patient regularly for thrombosis, including arterial, deep venous thrombosis, and pulmonary embolism, as drug increases risk of thrombus formation.

- Monitor patient for new-onset abdominal symptoms, especially patients with a history of diverticulitis, because baricitinib increases the risk for gastrointestinal perforation.
- Monitor patient's lipid profile periodically, as ordered, during baricitinib therapy. Know that a lipid profile should be performed about 12 weeks into baricitinib therapy to determine if management of hyperlipidemia is needed.
- Avoid giving patient live vaccines during baricitinib therapy because drug may reduce effectiveness of the vaccination.

PATIENT TEACHING

- Instruct patient to take baricitinib exactly as prescribed.
- Inform patient of her risk for infections. Review signs and symptoms of infection and stress importance of notifying prescriber if an infection is suspected or develops. Also tell patient that herpes zoster may also occur. Because it could become quite serious, it should be reported.
- Tell patient that baricitinib therapy increases the risk of certain cancers. Encourage her to report any unusual, persistent, or severe signs or symptoms to prescriber. Also instruct patient to periodically examine her skin for signs of skin cancer.
- Review signs and symptoms of a blood clot with patient and stress importance of seeking immediate medical attention if suspected.
- Alert patient that laboratory abnormalities such as an elevated lipid profile or liver enzymes may occur during baricitinib therapy and may require treatment. Stress importance of complying with ordered laboratory tests.
- Advise mothers not to breastfeed during treatment with baricitinib. Instruct women of childbearing age to report suspected or known pregnancy to prescriber, as fetal effects of baricitinib are unknown.
- Instruct patient not to receive vaccinations containing live virus during baricitinib therapy.

beclomethasone dipropionate

Beconase AQ, QVAR REDIHALER

Class and Category

Pharmacologic class: Corticosteroid
Therapeutic class: Antiasthmatic, anti-inflammatory
Pregnancy category: Not classified

Indications and Dosages

➤ *To maintain treatment of asthma as prophylactic therapy*

ORAL INHALATION AEROSOL (QVAR)

Adults and adolescents who are not on an inhaled corticosteroid. *Initial:* 1 to 2 inhalations (40 to 80 mcg) twice daily, depending on strength used, approximately 12 hr apart. *Maximum:* 4 to 8 inhalations (up to 320 mcg) twice daily approximately 12 hr apart, depending on strength used.

Adults and adolescents switching from another inhaled corticosteroid. *Initial:* 1 to 4 inhalations (160 mcg) twice daily approximately 12 hr apart, depending on strength used previously. *Maximum:* 4 to 8 inhalations (up to 320 mcg) twice daily.
Children ages 4 to 11. 1 inhalation (40 mcg) twice daily, approximately 12 hr apart, increased after 2 wk to 2 inhalations (80 mcg) twice daily, approximately 12 hr apart, as needed. *Maximum:* 1 to 2 inhalations (80 mcg) twice daily.

➤ *To relieve symptoms of seasonal or perennial allergic and nonallergic (vasomotor) rhinitis; to prevent recurrence of nasal polyps after surgical removal*

NASAL SPRAY (BECONASE AQ)
Adults and children age 12 and over. 1 or 2 inhalations (42 or 84 mcg) in each nostril twice daily for total dose of 168 or 336 mcg daily.
Children ages 6 to 12. *Initial:* 1 inhalation (42 mcg) in each nostril twice daily, increased to 2 inhalations (84 mcg) in each nostril twice daily, as needed with further increases in strength but no more than 2 inhalations per nostril, as needed. Once control is achieved, dosage decreased to 1 spray (42 mcg) in each nostril twice daily. *Maximum:* 336 mcg (2 inhalations in each nostril) daily given in two divided doses 12 hr apart.

Mechanism of Action

May decrease number and activity of cells involved in the inflammatory response of allergies, asthma, and rhinitis, such as basophils, eosinophils, lymphocytes, macrophages, mast cells, and neutrophils. Also may inhibit production or secretion of chemical mediators, such as cytokines, eicosanoids, histamine, and leukotrienes. May produce direct smooth-muscle cell relaxation and decrease airway hyperresponsiveness.

Contraindications

Hypersensitivity to beclomethasone or its components, relief of acute bronchospasm or of asthma controlled by bronchodilators or other nonsteroidal drugs, treatment of nonasthmatic bronchial disorders, status asthmaticus

Interactions

DRUGS
None reported

Adverse Reactions

CNS: Aggression, depression, fatigue, fever, headache, insomnia, light-headedness, mania, psychomotor hyperactivity, sleep disorders, **suicidal ideation**
CV: Chest pain, tachycardia
EENT: Blurred vision, burning sensation in nasal passages, cataracts, central serous chorioretinopathy, dry mouth, dysphonia, earache, elevated intraocular pressure, epistaxis, glaucoma, hoarseness, lacrimation, loss of smell and taste, nasal congestion or ulceration, nasal septal perforation, nose and throat dryness and irritation, nose and oral candidiasis, pharyngitis, rhinorrhea, sinusitis, sneezing, unpleasant smell and taste
ENDO: Adrenal insufficiency, cushingoid symptoms
GI: Diarrhea, indigestion, nausea, **rectal hemorrhage**
GU: Dysmenorrhea, UTI
MS: Arthralgia, growth suppression in children (nasal aerosol)
RESP: Bronchitis, **bronchospasm**, chest congestion, cough, **pulmonary infiltrates**, upper respiratory tract infection, wheezing
SKIN: Acne, eczema, pruritus, rash, skin discoloration, urticaria
Other: Anaphylaxis, **angioedema**, flu-like symptoms, impaired wound healing, lymphadenopathy, weight gain

Nursing Considerations

- Be aware that beclomethasone should not be used with patients who have experienced recent nasal septal ulcers, nasal surgery, or nasal trauma because of corticosteroids' adverse effects on wound healing.
- Know that if patient also takes an oral corticosteroid, expect to taper dosage slowly (by decreasing daily dosage or taking drug every other day, as ordered)

about 1 week after beclomethasone therapy begins.

WARNING Be aware that when gradually switching patient from oral corticosteroid to inhaled beclomethasone, watch for signs of life-threatening adrenal insufficiency, such as fatigue, hypotension, lassitude, nausea, vomiting, and weakness, during transition period and when exposed to infection, surgery, trauma, or other stressor. If signs occur, notify prescriber immediately.

- Expect to resume oral corticosteroid during a stressful period or severe asthma attack.
- Watch for signs of adrenal insufficiency during periods of stress because beclomethasone may be absorbed systemically.
- Be prepared, if patient has acute asthma attack or increased wheezing after receiving beclomethasone, to give a fast-acting bronchodilator, as prescribed. Expect to discontinue beclomethasone.
- Assess for signs of candidiasis, such as thick white coating or plaques on tongue and sides of mouth. Tell patient to rinse mouth with water without swallowing after inhalation; this may help to prevent oral candidiasis. If present, notify prescriber and expect to reduce dose or frequency or to stop beclomethasone. Also anticipate treatment with antifungal drug.
- Assess nasal discharge regularly when patient is prescribed nasal spray. Look for color or consistency changes, which may indicate infection when patient is using beclomethasone nasal spray.
- Monitor the growth of children receiving beclomethasone nasally.
- Monitor patients with a change in vision or a history of blurred vision, cataracts, glaucoma, or intraocular pressure because use of intranasal and inhaled corticosteroids may cause eye abnormalities.
- Monitor patient closely for altered thinking such as suicidal thoughts. If present, notify prescriber because drug will have to be discontinued.

PATIENT TEACHING

- Advise patient not to abruptly stop taking beclomethasone because adrenal insufficiency may occur. Urge her to notify prescriber if she develops signs of adrenal insufficiency, such as anorexia, dizziness, dyspnea, fainting, fatigue, fever, hypotension, malaise, or nausea.
- Instruct her to prime pump before using nasal spray for first time by placing her thumb on its base, and her index and middle fingers on its shoulder area (the canister should be on top, pointing down), and then pressing her thumb firmly and quickly against the bottle four times into the air away from eyes and face. If nasal spray has not been used for 7 consecutive days, remind patient that container needs to be primed by spraying two times prior to use. Before patient uses nasal inhalation canister for first time, instruct her to shake it and check that it's working properly by spraying it once in the air while looking for fine mist.
- Teach patient to inhale deeply after each nasal spray or inhalation, exhaling through mouth and tilting head back to let drug spread over the nasopharynx.
- Teach patient how to properly use oral inhalation aerosol, shaking canister well before using. If patient has trouble using device and coordinating inhalation with it, suggest using a spacer device.
- Advise patient prescribed two inhalations to wait a minute between them.
- Tell patient prescribed an inhaled bronchodilator with beclomethasone oral inhalation to use bronchodilator first, wait for 5 minutes, and then use beclomethasone.

WARNING Warn patient that beclomethasone isn't intended to relieve acute bronchospasm. Urge patient to notify prescriber if asthma symptoms don't respond.

- Advise patient to wear medical identification that states need for supplemental oral corticosteroids during severe asthma attack or stress. Inform patient that prescriber may order high-dose oral corticosteroid therapy.

- Warn patient and caretakers to report any abnormal thinking such as suicidal thoughts immediately to prescriber.

WARNING Caution patient to avoid exposure to chickenpox and measles because drug may cause immunosuppression. If she's exposed to these disorders, urge her to notify prescriber immediately.

- Tell patient to report any changes in vision to prescriber.

belimumab

Benlysta

Class and Category

Pharmacologic class: Monoclonal antibody
Therapeutic class: Immunosuppressant
Pregnancy category: Not classified

Indications and Dosages

➤ *To treat active, autoantibody-positive systemic lupus erythematosus (SLE) in patients who are receiving standard therapy*

I.V. INFUSION

Adults. 10 mg/kg infused over 1 hr every 2 wk for first 3 doses followed by 10 mg/kg infused over 1 hr every 4 wk.

SUBCUTANEOUS INJECTION

Adults. 200 mg once wk injected into the abdomen or thigh.
Adults transitioning from intravenous therapy. 200 mg once wk injected into the abdomen or thigh, with first dose given 1 to 4 wk after the last I.V. dose.

Mechanism of Action

Blocks the binding of soluble B-cell lymphocyte stimulator protein, a B-cell survival factor, to its receptors on B cells. This action causes cell death, which helps to relieve the signs and symptoms of active, autoantibody-positive, systemic lupus erythematosus.

Incompatibilities

Dextrose intravenous solutions are incompatible with belimumab.

Contraindications

Hypersensitivity to belimumab or its components

Interactions

DRUGS

Live virus vaccines: Possibly suppressed immune response and increased adverse effects of vaccine

Adverse Reactions

CNS: Anxiety, depression, fatigue, fever, headache, insomnia, migraines, myalgia, **progressive multifocal leukoencephalopathy**, **suicidal ideation**
CV: Bradycardia, **hypotension**
EENT: Nasopharyngitis, pharyngitis, sinusitis
GI: Diarrhea, nausea
GU: Cystitis, lupus nephritis, UTI
HEME: Leukopenia
MS: Extremity pain, myalgia
RESP: Bronchitis, dyspnea, pneumonia, upper respiratory tract infection
SKIN: Cellulitis, pruritus, rash, urticaria
Other: Anaphylaxis, **angioedema**, anti-belimumab antibody formation, flu-like symptoms, infusion reactions, injection site reactions (erythema, hematoma, induration, pain, pruritus), **malignancies**, serious infections

Nursing Considerations

- Know that belimumab should not be used to treat patients who are receiving drug therapy to treat a chronic infection. Monitor patient closely for signs and symptoms of infections during belimumab therapy. If present, notify prescriber. If the infection is determined to be new, belimumab therapy may have to be interrupted until infection is resolved.
- Be aware that patient should be premedicated prior to receiving belimumab intravenously, to prevent hypersensitivity and infusion reactions before each dose of belimumab. Patients with a history of multiple drug allergies or significant hypersensitivity may be at increased risk. If an infusion reaction still occurs, slow or temporarily stop the infusion, as ordered. If a serious hypersensitivity reaction occurs, discontinue drug immediately and notify prescriber. Know that a nonacute hypersensitivity reaction that may be evident as facial edema, fatigue, headache,

myalgia, nausea, and rash may occur up to a week after an infusion.
- Remove vial for intravenous use from refrigerator and allow to stand 10 to 15 minutes prior to reconstitution. Use aseptic technique when reconstituting with 1.5 ml of sterile water for injection, USP for a 120-mg vial and 4.8 ml of sterile water for injection, USP when reconstituting a 400-mg vial. When injecting diluent solution into the vial, direct stream of sterile water toward the side of the vial to minimize foaming. Gently swirl the vial for 60 seconds every 5 minutes until the powder is dissolved. Do not shake or refrigerate during this process. It typically takes 10 to 15 minutes for powder to dissolve but may take as long as 30 minutes. Once reconstituted, protect from sunlight. When using a mechanical reconstitution device (swirler), do not exceed 500 rpm, and swirl no longer than 30 minutes.
- Use only 0.9% sodium chloride injection, USP (normal saline) to further dilute the drug being prepared for intravenous administration. Withdraw amount of normal saline from the infusion bag or bottle equivalent to the vial contents of reconstituted drug required for the patient's dose. Then add the required volume of the reconstituted solution of the drug into the infusion bag or bottle. Gently invert the bag or bottle to mix the solution. Discard any unused solution left in the vial(s). The solution should be stored in the refrigerator protected from direct sunlight, if not used immediately. Know that the total time from the drug being reconstituted to completion of infusion should not exceed 8 hours.
- Infuse belimumab intravenously over 1 hour separately from any other medication given concomitantly intravenously.
- Be aware that vials containing belimumab are intended for intravenous use only and autoinjectors and prefilled syringes are intended for subcutaneous use only.
- Know that the first subcutaneous injection of belimumab should be given under the supervision of a healthcare professional.
- Remove the autoinjector or prefilled syringe from the refrigerator and allow it to sit at room temperature for 30 minutes prior to administering. Do not warm the drug any other way. The solution should appear clear to opalescent and colorless to pale yellow. Discard if product exhibits discoloration or particulate matter or if the autoinjector or prefilled syringe is accidentally dropped on a hard surface. Use a different injection site each week; do not give the injection into areas where the skin is bruised, hard, red, or tender.

WARNING **Monitor patient for a hypersensitivity reaction following administration of belimumab because hypersensitivity reactions, including anaphylaxis, may occur on the same day of infusion. Notify prescriber immediately if a reaction occurs, because death has occurred with some patients experiencing hypersensitivity reactions. Expect to provide emergency medical treatment as ordered and indicated by severity of reaction.**

- Monitor African-American patients closely during belimumab therapy for decreased effectiveness, because clinical trials have shown the response rate may be lower in these patients.
- Watch for evidence of infection (such as cough, fever, malaise, pain) because patients receiving immunosuppressants such as belimumab are at increased risk for serious infections such as bronchitis, cellulitis, pneumonia, and urinary tract infection. If patient develops an infection, notify prescriber, monitor patient closely, and know that drug therapy may be interrupted until infection is gone.
- Be aware that other biologic therapies, such as B-cell targeted therapies or intravenous cyclophosphamide therapy, are not recommended during belimumab therapy because potential drug interactions are unknown.

PATIENT TEACHING

- Instruct patient who will be self-injecting belimumab, as a subcutaneous injection, how to administer the injection and dispose of needle and syringe after injection.

- Tell patient to remove the autoinjector or prefilled syringe from the refrigerator and allow it to sit at room temperature for 30 minutes prior to administering. Tell patient not to warm the drug in any other way. Have patient inspect the solution. The solution should appear clear to opalescent and colorless to pale yellow. Instruct patient to discard if product exhibits discoloration or particulate matter or if the autoinjector or prefilled syringe is accidentally dropped on a hard surface. Tell patient to use a different injection site each week and not to give the injection into areas where the skin is bruised, hard, red, or tender.
- Advise patient that if a subcutaneous dose is missed, she should administer a dose as soon as she remembers. Then patient can resume dosing on the usual day of administration or start a new weekly schedule from the day that the missed dose was administered. Tell patient not to administer two doses on the same day.
- Instruct patient to report any signs of a hypersensitivity reaction such as difficulty breathing, hives, itching, or a rash to prescriber, and to seek medical attention immediately.
- Caution patient to report new or worsening depression, suicidal thoughts, or other mood changes.
- Tell patient to contact the prescriber if he develops new or worsening neurologic symptoms such as confusion, difficulty talking or walking, dizziness, loss of balance, memory loss, or vision problems.
- Advise patient not to receive any immunization with live vaccines for 30 days before or concurrently with belimumab and to avoid contact with anyone who has an infection.
- Tell female patient of childbearing age to use effective contraception during treatment and for at least 4 months after the final treatment because of potential adverse effects to infants exposed to drug in utero. Advise her to notify prescriber if pregnancy occurs and encourage her to enroll in the belimumab pregnancy registry by calling 1-877-681-6296.
- Encourage patient to report any persistent, severe, or unusual signs and symptoms to prescriber because drug may increase risk for cancer.

benazepril hydrochloride

Lotensin

Class and Category

Pharmacologic class: Angiotensin-converting enzyme (ACE) inhibitor
Therapeutic class: Antihypertensive
Pregnancy category: D

Indications and Dosages

➤ *To control hypertension alone or with a thiazide diuretic*

SUSPENSION, TABLETS

Adults who aren't receiving a diuretic. *Initial:* 10 mg daily. *Maintenance:* 20 to 40 mg daily as a single dose or in two equally divided doses.

Adults who are receiving a diuretic. 5 mg daily.

DOSAGE ADJUSTMENT Initial dosage of 5 mg/day for adult patients with impaired renal function and creatinine clearance less than 30 ml/min; then increased gradually until blood pressure is controlled or dosage reaches maximum of 40 mg daily.

TABLETS, SUSPENSION

Children age 6 and over with glomerular filtration rate of 30 ml/min or higher. *Initial:* 0.2 mg/kg daily. *Maximum:* 0.6 mg/kg daily or 40 mg daily.

Route	Onset	Peak	Duration
P.O.	1 hr	2–4 hr	24 hr

Mechanism of Action

May reduce blood pressure by affecting renin–angiotensin–aldosterone system. By inhibiting angiotensin-converting enzyme, benazepril:

- prevents conversion of angiotensin I to angiotensin II, a potent vasoconstrictor that also stimulates aldosterone release

- may inhibit renal and vascular production of angiotensin II
- decreases serum angiotensin II level and increases serum renin activity. This decreases aldosterone secretion, slightly increasing serum potassium level and fluid loss.
- decreases vascular tone and blood pressure
- inhibits aldosterone release, which reduces sodium and water resorption, increases their excretion, and reduces blood pressure.

Contraindications

Aliskiren therapy in patients with diabetes; concurrent therapy with a neprilysin inhibitor (e.g., sacubitril) or within 36 hours of switching to or from sacubitril/valsartan combination; history of angioedema; hypersensitivity to benazepril, other ACE inhibitors, or their components

Interactions

DRUGS

aliskiren (in patients with diabetes or renal impairment), angiotensin receptor blockers, other ACE inhibitors: Increased risk of hyperkalemia, hypotension, and renal dysfunction
antidiabetics (oral), insulin: Possibly increased risk of hypoglycemia
diuretics: Possibly excessive hypotension
gold salts: Possibly nitritoid reaction including facial flushing, hypotension, nausea, and vomiting
lithium: Increased serum lithium level and risk of lithium toxicity
mTOR inhibitors (everolimus, sirolimus, temsirolimus), neprilysin inhibitors: Increased risk for angioedema
NSAIDs: Possible decreased renal function in patients who are elderly, volume-depleted, or have a compromised renal function; may increase antihypertensive effect of benazepril
potassium preparations, potassium-sparing diuretics: Possibly increased serum potassium level

Adverse Reactions

CNS: Anxiety, asthenia, dizziness, drowsiness, fatigue, headache, hypertonia, insomnia, nervousness, paresthesia, sleep disturbance, somnolence, syncope, weakness
CV: Angina, **ECG changes**, **hypotension**, orthostatic hypotension, palpitations, peripheral edema
EENT: Sinusitis
ENDO: Hyperglycemia
GI: Abdominal pain, **acute liver failure**, **cholestatic hepatitis**, constipation, elevated liver enzymes, gastritis, **hepatic necrosis**, **melena**, nausea, **pancreatitis**, small bowel angioedema, vomiting
GU: Acute renal failure, decreased libido, elevated BUN and serum creatinine levels, frequent urination, impotence, **nephrotic syndrome**, oliguria, **progressive azotemia**, proteinuria, **renal insufficiency**, UTI
HEME: Agranulocytosis, decreased hemoglobin level, **hemolytic anemia**, **leukopenia**, **neutropenia**, **thrombocytopenia**
MS: Arthralgia, arthritis, myalgia
RESP: ACE cough, **asthma**, bronchitis, **bronchospasm**, dyspnea
SKIN: Alopecia, dermatitis, diaphoresis, flushing, pemphigus, photosensitivity, pruritus, rash, **Stevens–Johnson syndrome**
Other: Anaphylaxis, **angioedema**, **hyperkalemia**, **hyponatremia**

Nursing Considerations

- Evaluate blood pressure with patient lying down, sitting, and standing before starting benazepril and then regularly, as appropriate, to monitor effectiveness.
- Monitor urine output and BUN and serum creatinine levels, as needed, before therapy and then during therapy, especially in patients with renal artery stenosis, severe heart failure, postmyocardial infarction or in patients who are volume depleted. Also monitor patients closely who are also receiving NSAID or angiotensin receptor blocker therapy because these patients may be at increased risk for developing acute renal failure.

WARNING Monitor patient closely during dialysis because sudden and potentially life-threatening anaphylactoid reactions have occurred in some patients dialyzed with high-flux membranes while receiving an ACE inhibitor like benazepril. If anaphylaxis occurs, institute emergency measures, as ordered, and stop dialysis.

• Monitor liver enzymes regularly, as ordered. Assess patient routinely for signs and symptoms of liver dysfunction, such as jaundice and fatigue. Notify prescriber if patient develops jaundice or exhibits elevated liver enzyme levels, as drug will need to be discontinued.

WARNING Be alert for angioedema, especially after first dose. If it extends to larynx and patient has laryngeal stridor or signs of airway obstruction, prepare to give epinephrine subcutaneously immediately, as prescribed, and discontinue benazepril. Be aware that black patients have a higher incidence of angioedema compared to nonblacks.

• Monitor WBC count periodically to detect neutropenia and agranulocytosis.
• Check serum potassium and other electrolyte levels to detect electrolyte imbalances.
• Take safety precautions, such as having patient change positions slowly and sit on edge of bed before arising to prevent injury caused by orthostatic hypotension.

PATIENT TEACHING

• Teach patient how to monitor blood pressure, if appropriate, and how to recognize signs of hypertension and hypotension.

WARNING Urge patient to contact prescriber before using any OTC salt substitutes, which may contain potassium, or potassium supplements. These substances increase the risk of hyperkalemia.

• Explain that a persistent dry cough may develop and may not subside unless benazepril is stopped. If cough becomes bothersome or interferes with sleep or activities, patient should notify prescriber.

WARNING Instruct patient to contact prescriber immediately if she has signs of angioedema, such as swelling of the face, eyes, lips, or tongue.

• Caution patient to avoid sudden position changes and to rise slowly from sitting or lying to minimize orthostatic hypotension.

WARNING Advise patient to stop benazepril and notify prescriber as soon as possible if she experiences syncope.

WARNING Caution women of childbearing age to use reliable contraception and to notify prescriber immediately if pregnancy is suspected. Benazepril may cause fetal harm and should be discontinued.

benralizumab

Fasenra

Class and Category

Pharmacologic class: Monoclonal antibody
Therapeutic class: Antiasthmatic
Pregnancy category: Not classified

Indications and Dosages

➤ *To treat severe asthma as an add-on maintenance treatment in patients with eosinophilic phenotype*

SUBCUTANEOUS INJECTION

Adults. 30 mg once every 4 wk for the first 3 doses, then once every 8 wk.

Mechanism of Action

Binds to the alpha subunit of the human interleukin-5 receptor, which is expressed on the surface of basophils and eosinophils. Eosinophils play a part in the inflammatory process, which is present in the pathogenesis of asthma. When binding to the interleukin-5 receptor occurs, eosinophils are reduced through an antibody-dependent cell-mediated cytotoxicity to help relieve inflammation found in asthma.

Contraindications

Hypersensitivity to benralizumab or its components

Interactions

DRUGS

None

Adverse Reactions

CNS: Fever, headache
EENT: Pharyngitis
SKIN: Rash, urticaria
Other: Anaphylaxis, **angioedema**, benralizumab antibody formation, injection-site reactions (erythema, pain, papule, pruritus)

Nursing Considerations

• Expect to treat patients with preexisting parasitic (helminth) infections before benralizumab therapy is begun, because it is not known if the drug will influence a patient's response to treatment for such an infection. If patient develops a parasitic infection while taking benralizumab and does not respond to treatment, expect benralizumab to be discontinued until the infection is resolved.

WARNING Know that benralizumab should never be used to treat acute asthma symptoms, acute bronchospasms, acute exacerbations of asthma, or status asthmaticus.

- Warm benralizumab by leaving carton at room temperature for about 30 minutes before administration. Grasp the syringe body, not the plunger, to remove the prefilled syringe from the tray. Inspect the solution, which should appear clear to opalescent, colorless to slightly yellow, and may contain a few translucent or white to off-white particles. The syringe may contain a small air bubble, which is normal. If present, do not expel the air bubble prior to administration. Do not remove needle cover until ready to give the injection subcutaneously. When ready, hold the syringe body and remove the needle cover by pulling straight off. Do not hold the plunger or plunger head while removing the needle cover or the plunger may move.
- Inject benralizumab subcutaneously into the abdomen, thigh, or upper arm. Inject all the drug by pushing in the plunger all the way until the plunger head is completely between the needle guard activation clips. This is necessary to activate the needle guard. After injection, maintain pressure on the plunger head and remove the needle from the skin. Release pressure on the plunger head to allow the needle guard to cover the needle. Do not recap the syringe. Discard the used syringe into a sharps container.
- Monitor patient closely for hypersensitivity reactions that may occur within hours after benralizumab has been administered. If present, notify prescriber, provide supportive emergency care, and expect drug to be discontinued.
- Expect inhaled or systemic corticosteroids used to treat asthma to be gradually withdrawn, if no longer needed. Corticosteroid therapy should never be withdrawn abruptly.

PATIENT TEACHING

- Instruct patient that benralizumab is not effective in treating acute asthma symptoms or acute exacerbations. If asthma remains uncontrolled or worsens after benralizumab therapy is begun, tell patient to notify prescriber or seek emergency medical care.

WARNING Tell patient to report any signs of an allergic reaction such as difficulty breathing, hives, or rash immediately. Remind patient that although an allergic reaction usually occurs within hours after benralizumab is administered, a delayed reaction could occur even days later.

- Emphasize importance of not decreasing any prescribed inhaled or systemic corticosteroid dosage without prescriber knowledge.

benztropine mesylate

Cogentin

Class and Category

Pharmacologic class: Antichlolinergic
Therapeutic class: Antiparkinsonian, central-acting anticholinergic
Pregnancy category: C

Indications and Dosages

➤ *As adjunct, to treat all forms of Parkinson's disease*

TABLETS, I.M. OR I.V. INJECTION

Adults with Parkinson's disease. *Initial:* 0.5 to 1 mg daily, increased gradually in increments of 0.5 mg as needed. *Maximum:* 6 mg daily.

Adults with idiopathic Parkinson's disease. *Initial:* 0.5 to 1 mg at bedtime. *Maximum:* 4 to 6 mg daily.

Adults with postencephalitic Parkinson's disease. *Initial:* 0.5 mg to 2 mg at bedtime and then increased as needed. *Maximum:* 6 mg daily.

➤ *To control extrapyramidal symptoms (except tardive dyskinesia) caused by phenothiazines and other neuroleptics*

TABLETS, I.M. OR I.V. INJECTION

Adults. 1 to 4 mg once or twice daily.

➤ *To treat acute dystonic reactions*

TABLETS, I.M. OR I.V. INJECTION

Adults. *Initial:* 1 to 2 ml (1 to 2 mg total dose) I.V. or I.M. *Maintenance:* 1 to 2 mg P.O. twice daily to prevent recurrence.

Route	Onset	Peak	Duration
P.O.	1–2 hr	Unknown	24 hr
I.V., I.M.	15 min	Unknown	24 hr

Mechanism of Action

Blocks acetylcholine's action at cholinergic receptor sites. This restores the brain's normal dopamine and acetylcholine balance, which relaxes muscle movement and decreases drooling, rigidity, and tremor. Benztropine also may inhibit dopamine reuptake and storage, which prolongs dopamine's action.

Contraindications

Angle-closure glaucoma, children younger than age 3, hypersensitivity to benztropine mesylate or its components, presence of tardive dyskinesia

Interactions

DRUGS

amantadine, phenothiazines, tricyclic antidepressants: Possibly increased adverse anticholinergic effects
haloperidol: Possibly increased schizophrenic symptoms, decreased serum haloperidol level, and development of tardive dyskinesia

Adverse Reactions

CNS: Agitation, confusion, delirium, delusions, depression, disorientation, dizziness, drowsiness, euphoria, excitement, fever, hallucinations, headache, lightheadedness, listlessness, memory loss, nervousness, paranoia, psychosis, weakness
CV: Hypotension, mild bradycardia, orthostatic hypotension, palpitations, tachycardia
EENT: Blurred vision, diplopia, dry mouth, increased intraocular pressure, mydriasis, narrow-angle glaucoma, suppurative parotitis
GI: Constipation, duodenal ulcer, epigastric distress, ileus, nausea, vomiting
GU: Dysuria, urinary hesitancy, urine retention
MS: Muscle spasms, muscle weakness
SKIN: Decreased sweating, dermatoses, flushing, rash, urticaria

Nursing Considerations

- Expect to administer I.V. or I.M. benztropine when patient needs more rapid response than oral drug can provide. Be aware that I.M. route is commonly used because it provides effects in about the same time as I.V. route. Watch for improvement a few minutes after administration. If parkinsonian symptoms reappear, expect to repeat dose, as ordered.
- Know that therapy typically begins with a low dose followed by gradual increases of 0.5 mg every 5 or 6 days because benztropine has a cumulative action.
- Assess muscle rigidity and tremor at baseline. Then monitor them often for improvement, which indicates drug's effectiveness.
- Give drug before or after meals based on patient's need and response. If patient has increased salivary secretions, expect to administer benztropine after meals. If patient has dry mouth, plan to give drug before meals unless nausea develops.

WARNING Know that when giving drug to patient with drug-induced extrapyramidal reactions, watch for worsening psychiatric symptoms.

- Monitor patient's movements closely. High-dose benztropine therapy may cause weakness and inability to move specific muscle groups. If this occurs, expect to reduce benztropine dosage.

PATIENT TEACHING

- Warn patient that drug has a cumulative effect, increasing risk of adverse reactions and overdose.
- Caution against driving and similar activities until benztropine's effects are known because it may cause blurred vision, dizziness, or drowsiness.

WARNING Know that because benztropine decreases sweating, urge patient to avoid extremely hot or humid conditions to reduce risk of heatstroke and severe hyperthermia. This is especially important for elderly patients and those who abuse alcohol or have chronic illness or CNS disease.

- Stress need for periodic eye examinations and intraocular pressure measurements because drug may cause narrow-angle glaucoma and increase intraocular pressure.

betamethasone
Celestone
betamethasone acetate–betamethasone sodium phosphate
Celestone Soluspan
betamethasone sodium phosphate
Betnesol (CAN), Celestone Phosphate, Selestoject

Class and Category
Pharmacologic class: Glucocorticoid
Therapeutic class: Immunosuppressant (anti-inflammatory)
Pregnancy category: C

Indications and Dosages
➤ *To treat conditions with severe inflammation and conditions requiring immunosuppression*

ORAL SOLUTION, SYRUP, TABLETS (BETAMETHASONE)
Adults. 0.6 to 7.2 mg daily divided in 2 to 4 doses.
Children. Variable ranging from 0.02 to 0.25 mg/kg/day divided in 3 or 4 doses.

I.M. INJECTION (BETAMETHASONE ACETATE–BETAMETHASONE SODIUM PHOSPHATE)
Adults. 0.5 to 9 mg I.M. daily divided in 2 doses, or one-third to one-half of P.O. dose every 12 hr.
Children. Highly variable ranging from 0.02 to 0.125 mg/kg/day divided in 2 to 4 doses.

I.M. OR I.V. INJECTION (BETAMETHASONE SODIUM PHOSPHATE)
Adults. *Initial:* Variable (given in emergency situations or when oral therapy isn't possible). *Maximum:* 9 mg daily.

➤ *To treat bursitis, gouty arthritis, osteoarthritis, periostitis of cuboid, peritendinitis, rheumatoid arthritis, skin lesions, tenosynovitis*

INTRA-ARTICULAR, INTRABURSAL, OR INTRADERMAL INJECTION (BETAMETHASONE ACETATE–BETAMETHASONE SODIUM PHOSPHATE)
Adults with bursitis, peritendinitis, or tenosynovitis. 1 ml by intrabursal or intra-articular injection. Three or four injections given every 1 to 2 wk.
Adults with osteoarthritis or rheumatoid arthritis. 0.25 to 2 ml, based on joint size.
Adults with foot bursitis. 0.25 to 0.5 ml every 3 to 7 days.
Adults with foot tenosynovitis or periostitis of cuboid. 0.5 ml every 3 to 7 days.
Adults with acute gouty arthritis. 0.5 to 1 ml every 3 to 7 days.
Adults with skin lesions. 0.2 ml/cm^2 intradermally, up to 1 ml weekly.
DOSAGE ADJUSTMENT Dosage reduced for elderly patients and accompanied by periodic monitoring of blood pressure and blood glucose and electrolyte levels.

Route	Onset	Peak	Duration
P.O.	Unknown	1–2 hr	3.25 days
I.V., I.M.*	Rapid	Unknown	Unknown
I.M.†	1–3 hr	Unknown	1 wk
Other†	Unknown	Unknown	1–2 wk‡

* Sodium phosphate.
† Acetate–sodium phosphate.
‡ For intra-arterial or intrasynovial injection; 1 wk for intralesional injection in soft tissue.

Mechanism of Action
Binds to intracellular glucocorticoid receptors and suppresses inflammatory and immune responses by:
- inhibiting neutrophil and monocyte accumulation at inflammation site and suppressing their phagocytic and bactericidal activity
- stabilizing lysosomal membranes
- suppressing antigen response of macrophages and helper T cells
- inhibiting synthesis of inflammatory response mediators, such as cytokines, interleukins, and prostaglandins.

Contraindications

Hypersensitivity to betamethasone or its components, idiopathic thrombocytopenic purpura (I.M. injection), live virus vaccination, systemic fungal infection

Interactions

DRUGS

amphotericin B (injection), potassium-depleting diuretics: Increased risk of hypokalemia
anticholinesterase drugs: Possibly antagonized anticholinesterase effects in myasthenia gravis with possible development of severe weakness
barbiturates: Possibly decreased effects of betamethasone
cholestyramine: Possibly increased clearance of betamethasone
cyclosporine: Possibly increased effects of both drugs resulting possibly in seizures
digitalis glycosides: Possibly increased risk of arrhythmias
estrogens: Possibly decreased excretion of betamethasone
insulin, oral antidiabetic agents: Possibly decreased effects of these agents
isoniazid: Possibly decreased serum isoniazid level
ketoconazole: Possibly decreased excretion of betamethasone
macrolide antibiotics: Possibly significant decrease in betamethasone clearance
NSAIDs: Increased risk of gastrointestinal adverse effects; possibly increased clearance of salicylates
oral anticoagulants: Possibly increased or decreased action of anticoagulants, requiring adjusted anticoagulant dosage
oral contraceptives: Possibly increased half-life and concentration and decreased excretion of betamethasone
toxoids, vaccines: Possibly diminished response to toxoids and vaccines with prolonged betamethasone therapy

Adverse Reactions

CNS: Fatigue, headache, **increased intracranial pressure with papilledema**, insomnia, malaise, neuritis, paresthesia, **seizures**, steroid psychosis, syncope, vertigo
CV: **Arrhythmias**, **ECG changes**, edema, **fat embolism**, **heart failure**, hypertension, **thromboembolism**, thrombophlebitis
EENT: Cataracts, exophthalmos, glaucoma, increased intraocular pressure
ENDO: Cushingoid symptoms (buffalo hump, central obesity, decreased carbohydrate tolerance, fat pad enlargement, moon face), growth suppression in children, hyperglycemia, masked signs of infection, negative nitrogen balance, **secondary adrenocortical and pituitary unresponsiveness (in times of stress)**
GI: Abdominal distention, increased appetite, nausea, **pancreatitis**, peptic ulcer **possibly with perforation**, ulcerative esophagitis, vomiting
GU: Amenorrhea, glycosuria, menstrual irregularities
HEME: Leukocytosis
MS: Aseptic necrosis of femoral and humeral heads, loss of muscle mass, muscle weakness, osteoporosis, spontaneous pathologic and vertebral compression fractures, tendon rupture
SKIN: Acneiform lesions, allergic dermatitis, ecchymosis, facial erythema, hirsutism, impaired wound healing, increased sweating, petechiae, lupus-like lesions, purpura, subcutaneous fat atrophy, thin and fragile skin, urticaria
Other: Angioedema, **hypernatremia**, **hypocalcemia**, **hypokalemia**, suppressed reaction to skin tests, weight gain

Nursing Considerations

- Expect prescriber to order baseline ophthalmologic examination before starting therapy because prolonged betamethasone use may lead to glaucoma, increased intraocular pressure, and optic nerve damage. Use betamethasone cautiously in patients with ocular herpes simplex because corneal perforation may occur.
- Determine if latent or active amebiasis has been ruled out in patients who have spent time in the tropics, or who have unexplained diarrhea, before betamethasone therapy starts because drug may worsen it.

WARNING Give betamethasone with extreme care in patients with known or suspected Strongyloides (threadworm) infestation because corticosteroids such as betamethasone may result in immunosuppression, Strongyloides hyperinfection and dissemination, and widespread larval migration, resulting in severe enterocolitis and potentially life-threatening gram-negative septicemia.

- Assess for signs of infection before administering betamethasone because drug may mask those signs. Because drug may cause immunosuppression, new infection may develop during therapy. If so, expect to administer appropriate antibiotic.
- Review serum electrolyte levels, as ordered, before starting therapy. Monitor these levels often during therapy to detect imbalances. Sodium and water retention and potassium and calcium depletion may occur with high-dose betamethasone therapy. If so, expect to restrict sodium intake and provide potassium and calcium supplements.
- Administer oral betamethasone with an antacid or H2-receptor blocker because it is linked to peptic ulcer formation.

WARNING Monitor ECG tracings for arrhythmias, and evaluate patient for anaphylactic reactions, such as angioedema and seizures, which have been associated with rapid I.V. administration of high-dose corticosteroids.

WARNING Assess for signs of adrenal suppression and insufficiency (fatigue, hypotension, lassitude, nausea, vomiting, and weakness) when patient is exposed to stress during long-term betamethasone therapy. If she exhibits these signs, notify prescriber at once.

- Watch for signs of steroid psychosis, such as clouded sensorium, delirium, euphoria, insomnia, mood swings, personality changes, and severe depression, which may develop 15 to 30 days after therapy begins. Expect to stop therapy. If this isn't possible, expect to give psychotropic drugs.
- Rotate I.M. injection sites. To prevent muscle atrophy, avoid subcutaneous injection, injection in deltoid site, and repeated I.M. injections into same site.
- Administer oral betamethasone before 9 a.m., if appropriate, to mimic body's natural release of corticosteroids.
- Assess joint for marked increase in local swelling, pain, and more restricted movement after intra-articular injection. If patient also develops fever and malaise, suspect septic arthritis and notify prescriber immediately. Expect to assist with joint fluid aspiration to confirm septic arthritis.
- Monitor patient for cushingoid signs and symptoms, such as acne, buffalo hump, central obesity, ecchymosis, moon face, striae, and weight gain. Notify prescriber if you detect these symptoms.
- Expect to slowly taper oral betamethasone dosage to prevent adrenal insufficiency.

PATIENT TEACHING

- Instruct patient to take oral betamethasone with food if GI upset occurs.
- Review signs of adrenal insufficiency and possible need for dosage increases during stress. Advise patient to notify prescriber immediately if signs of insufficiency occur or if she's exposed to stress.
- Instruct patient to avoid exposure to infections because drug can cause immunosuppression. Also teach patient to recognize and immediately report signs of infection.
- Advise patient not to overuse joint after intra-articular use, and to continue other treatments such as physical therapy.

bethanechol chloride

Duvoid, Urecholine

Class and Category

Pharmacologic class: Cholinergic agonist
Therapeutic class: Urinary tract stimulant
Pregnancy category: C

Indications and Dosages

➤ *To treat acute postoperative and postpartum nonobstructive urine retention and retention caused by neurogenic atony of bladder*

TABLETS

Adults. 10 to 50 mg three times daily or four times daily. *To determine minimum effective dose:* 5 to 10 mg repeated every hour until response is obtained or maximum of 50 mg is reached.

SUBCUTANEOUS INJECTION

Adults. 2.5 to 5 mg three times daily or four times daily. *To determine minimum* *effective dose:* 2.5 mg repeated every 15 to 30 min until response is obtained or maximum of four doses is reached. Minimum effective dose may be repeated three times daily or four times daily, as needed.

Route	Onset	Peak	Duration
P.O.	30–90 min	60 min	6 hr
SubQ	5–15 min	15–30 min	2 hr

Mechanism of Action
Acts directly on muscarinic receptors of the parasympathetic nervous system, increasing detrusor muscle tone in the bladder and allowing contraction strong enough to start voiding. Like natural neurotransmitter acetylcholine, bethanechol stimulates gastric motility, increases gastric tone, and enhances peristalsis.

Contraindications
Acute inflammatory lesions of GI tract, bronchial asthma, coronary artery disease, epilepsy, hypersensitivity to bethanechol or its components, hyperthyroidism, hypotension, marked vagotonia, mechanical obstruction of GI or GU tract, Parkinson's disease, peptic ulcer disease, peritonitis, pronounced bradycardia, questionable integrity of GI or GU mucosa, spastic GI disorders, vasomotor instability

Interactions
DRUGS
cholinergic drugs: Possibly increased effects of bethanechol
ganglionic blockers: Possibly severe hypotension, usually first manifested by severe adverse GI reactions
procainamide, quinidine: Possibly decreased effects of bethanechol

Adverse Reactions
CNS: Headache, malaise
CV: Hypotension with reflex tachycardia, vasomotor response
EENT: Excessive salivation, lacrimation, miosis
GI: Abdominal cramps, colicky pain, diarrhea, eructation, nausea, vomiting
GU: Urinary urgency
RESP: Asthma attack, bronchoconstriction

Nursing Considerations
- Assess urine elimination before starting bethanechol therapy.

WARNING Be aware that patient must have functioning urinary sphincter because a sphincter that doesn't relax when bladder contracts can push urine upward into renal pelvis and cause reflux infection.

- Give oral bethanechol 1 hour before or 2 hours after meals to reduce risk of nausea and vomiting.

WARNING Don't give bethanechol I.M. or I.V. because of risk of cholinergic overstimulation, which can cause abdominal cramps, bloody diarrhea, hypotension, shock, or sudden cardiac arrest. Always keep atropine nearby during subcutaneous administration.

PATIENT TEACHING
- Advise patient to take bethanechol on an empty stomach 1 hour before or 2 hours after meals to reduce risk of nausea and vomiting.

betrixaban
Bevyxxa

Class and Category
Pharmacologic class: Factor Xa inhibitor
Therapeutic class: Antithrombotic
Pregnancy category: Not classified

Indications and Dosages
➤ *To prevent venous thromboembolism (VTE) in patients hospitalized for an acute medical illness who are at risk for thromboembolic complications due to moderate or severe restricted mobility and other risk factors for VTE*

CAPSULES
Adults. *Initial:* 160 mg, followed by 80 mg once daily for 35 to 42 days.
DOSAGE ADJUSTMENT For patient with severe renal impairment who has a creatinine clearance less than 30 ml/min but greater than 15 ml/min or who is starting or receiving concomitant P-gp

inhibitors, initial dose is reduced to 80 mg, followed by 40 mg once daily.

Route	Onset	Peak	Duration
P.O.	Unknown	3–4 hr	72 hr or more

Mechanism of Action

Selectively blocks the active site of FXa to inhibit free FXa and prothrombinase activity. This decreases thrombin formation.

Contraindications

Active pathological bleeding, hypersensitivity to betrixaban or its components

Interactions

DRUGS

anticoagulants, antiplatelets, thrombolytics: Possibly increased risk of bleeding
P-gp inhibitors such as amiodarone, azithromycin, clarithromycin, ketoconazole, verapamil: Increased effects of betrixaban with possible increased adverse reactions

Adverse Reactions

CNS: Headache, **intracranial hemorrhage**, intraspinal bleeding
CV: Hypertension, **pericardial bleeding**
EENT: Epistaxis, intraocular bleeding
GI: Constipation, diarrhea, **gastrointestinal bleeding**, nausea, **retroperitoneal bleeding**
GU: Hematuria, UTI
HEME: Major and minor **bleeding events**
MS: Intra-articular bleeding, intramuscular bleeding with compartment syndrome
Other: Hypersensitivity reaction, hypokalemia

Nursing Considerations

- Be aware that patients with severe renal impairment taking P-gp inhibitors should not receive betrixaban.
- Monitor patient closely for bleeding, which can range from minor bleeding to hemorrhage. Be aware that use of drugs that affect hemostasis, such as anticoagulants, antiplatelets like aspirin, heparin, nonsteroidal anti-inflammatory drugs, other anticoagulants, selective serotonin reuptake inhibitors, serotonin norepinephrine reuptake inhibitors, and thrombolytics, increase the risk of bleeding. Notify prescriber immediately if bleeding occurs and expect drug to be discontinued if bleeding is significant. Be aware that there is no treatment to stop the anticoagulant effect of betrixaban and that its effect can persist for at least 72 hours after the last dose.

WARNING **Know that an epidural catheter should not be removed earlier than 72 hours after betrixaban has been administered because of the risk of intraspinal bleeding, which can result in long-term or permanent paralysis. Monitor patient receiving epidural or spinal anesthesia or puncture frequently for signs and symptoms of neurological impairment, such as bladder or bowel dysfunction, numbness, or weakness in legs. Be aware that prompt diagnosis and treatment are crucial if any neurological abnormalities occur.**

- Monitor patient with severe renal dysfunction closely because of increased risk of bleeding and report any bleeding immediately.

PATIENT TEACHING

- Tell patient if he misses a dose, to take it as soon as possible on the same day. Remind him that the dose should not be doubled to make up for a missed dose.
- Instruct patient to watch for any signs and symptoms of bleeding and to report them immediately and seek emergency care.
- Tell patient to notify prescriber of any new medication, including over-the-counter drugs, before taking them.
- Stress importance of telling all doctors about betrixaban use, especially prior to procedures or surgery in which epidural or spinal anesthesia will be used.

bezlotoxumab

Zinplava

Class and Category

Pharmacologic class: Monoclonal antibody
Therapeutic class: Clostridium difficile recurrence inhibitor
Pregnancy category: Not classified

Indications and Dosages

➤ *To reduce recurrence of* Clostridium difficile *infection (CDI) in patients who are receiving antibacterial drug treatment for CDI and are at a high risk for CDI recurrence*

I.V. INFUSION

Adults. 10 mg/kg given over 60 min as a single dose.

Mechanism of Action

Binds to *C. difficile* toxin B and neutralizes its effects.

Incompatibilities

Do not administer simultaneously through the same I.V. line with any other drugs.

Contraindications

Hypersensitivity to bezlotoxumab or its components

Interactions

DRUGS

None reported

Adverse Reactions

CNS: Dizziness, fatigue, fever, headache
CV: Heart failure, hypertension, **ventricular tachyarrhythmia**
GI: Nausea
RESP: Dyspnea
Other: Antibezlotoxumab antibodies, infusion-related reactions

Nursing Considerations

- Be aware that bezlotoxumab alone is not to be used to treat *C. difficile* infection (CDI), as it is not an antibacterial drug. It should only be used in conjunction with antibacterial drug treatment of CDI.
- Use with extreme caution in patients with a history of congestive heart failure, as drug may exacerbate congestive heart failure and may become severe enough to cause death.
- Dilute bezlotoxumab prior to administering. Withdraw the required volume from the drug vial based on the patient's weight in kg and transfer into an intravenous bag containing either 0.9% sodium chloride injection USP or 5% dextrose injection USP to prepare a diluted solution with a final concentration ranging from 1 to 10 mg/ml. Mix diluted solution by gentle inversion. Do not shake.
- Store diluted solution at room temperature up to 15 hours or under refrigeration for up to 23 hours prior to administration. If refrigerated, allow the intravenous bag to come to room temperature before administering but do not allow total time following mixture and including administration to exceed 16 hours if kept at room temperature or 24 hours if refrigerated.
- Administer as an intravenous infusion over 60 minutes using a sterile, nonpyrogenic, low-protein binding 0.2 to 5 micron in-line or add-on filter.
- Know that the diluted solution can be infused via a central line or peripheral catheter. The drug should never be administered as an intravenous bolus or push.
- Monitor patient for adverse reactions, especially infusion reactions that may include dizziness, dyspnea, fatigue, fever, hypertension, and nausea. Know that these reactions usually resolve within 24 hours.

WARNING Monitor patient closely for signs and symptoms of congestive heart failure, especially in patients with a history of the disorder. Notify prescriber immediately if such signs or symptoms are present, and expect to provide supportive care.

PATIENT TEACHING

- Remind patient that bezlotoxumab does not take the place of the prescribed antibacterial therapy. Reinforce need to continue taking the antibacterial agent as prescribed.
- Reassure patient that although infusion reactions may occur, they usually resolve within 24 hours and are not usually serious.

WARNING Urge patient to seek immediate medical attention if signs and symptoms of congestive heart failure occur.

bisoprolol fumarate

Class and Category

Pharmacologic class: Beta$_1$-adrenergic blocker
Therapeutic class: Antihypertensive
Pregnancy category: C

Indications and Dosages

➤ *To treat hypertension, alone or with other antihypertensives*

TABLETS

Adults. 2.5 to 5 mg daily, increased to 10 to 20 mg daily if blood pressure doesn't respond to lower dosage.

DOSAGE ADJUSTMENT Dosage reduced to 2.5 mg daily initially and then increased gradually for patients with impaired renal function and creatinine clearance less than 40 ml/min or who have impaired hepatic function, as from cirrhosis or hepatitis.

Mechanism of Action

Inhibits stimulation of beta$_1$-receptors primarily in the heart, which decreases cardiac excitability, cardiac output, and myocardial oxygen demand. Bisoprolol also decreases renin release from kidneys, which helps reduce blood pressure.

Contraindications

Cardiogenic shock, hypersensitivity to bisoprolol or its components, overt heart failure, second- or third-degree heart block, sinus bradycardia

Interactions

DRUGS

antiarrhythmics such as disopyramide; calcium channel blockers such as diltiazem, verapamil: Increased risk of conduction delay and decreased heart rate

beta blockers, digoxin: Increased risk of bradycardia

catecholamine-depleting drugs such as guanethidine, reserpine: Increased risk of bradycardia or hypotension

clonidine: Possibly severe hypertension from withdrawal of clonidine or both drugs

rifampin: Possibly increased bisoprolol metabolism with decreased bisoprolol effects

Adverse Reactions

CNS: Anxiety, confusion, depression, dizziness, emotional lability, fatigue, fever, hallucinations, headache, insomnia, malaise, nightmares, paresthesia, sleep disturbances, syncope, tremor, unsteadiness, vertigo

CV: Bradycardia, heart block, and other arrhythmias; chest pain; claudication; cold arms and legs; edema; **heart failure**; hypercholesterolemia; hyperlipidemia; **hypotension; MI**; orthostatic hypotension; palpitations; peripheral vascular insufficiency

EENT: Altered taste, blurred vision, dry mouth, eye pain or pressure, hearing loss, increased salivation, laryngospasm, pharyngitis, rhinitis, sinusitis, tinnitus

GI: Constipation, diarrhea, epigastric pain, gastritis, indigestion, **ischemic colitis, mesenteric artery thrombosis**, nausea, vomiting

GU: Cystitis, decreased libido, impotence, Peyronie's disease **renal artery thrombosis**, renal colic

HEME: Agranulocytosis, eosinophilia, **leukopenia, thrombocytopenia, thrombocytopenic purpura**

MS: Arthralgia, gout, muscle twitching, neck pain

RESP: Asthma, bronchitis, **bronchospasm**, cough, dyspnea, **respiratory distress**, upper respiratory tract infection

SKIN: Alopecia, dermatitis, diaphoresis, eczema, **exfoliative dermatitis**, flushing, pruritus, psoriasis, rash

Other: Angioedema, hyperkalemia, hyperuricemia, weight gain

Nursing Considerations

- Administer bisoprolol cautiously in patients with peripheral vascular disease because reduced cardiac output can cause or worsen arterial insufficiency. Assess patient's arms and legs for changes in color, temperature, and pulses; ask about numbness, tingling, and pain.
- Be aware that chronic beta blocker therapy such as bisoprolol is not routinely witheld prior to major surgery because the benefits outweigh the risks associated with its use with general anesthesia and surgical procedures.
- Measure blood pressure with patient lying, sitting, and standing before starting bisoprolol and then every 4 to 8 hours, as appropriate, to evaluate effectiveness.
- Know that if patient has diabetes, patient should be monitored closely for signs of hypoglycemia, which drug may mask.
- Be aware that if patient has hyperthyroidism, she should be watched for tachycardia and hypertension, which may be masked by bisoprolol.

WARNING Keep in mind that abrupt withdrawal of bisoprolol may cause or worsen thyroid storm. During drug withdrawal, monitor patient closely.

- Expect to stop bisoprolol over 1 to 2 weeks to prevent MI, ventricular arrhythmias, and, possibly, death from catecholamine hypersensitivity caused by beta blocker therapy.

- Monitor patient's blood pressure. If systolic blood pressure falls to less than 90 mm Hg, expect to discontinue drug. Prepare for hemodynamic monitoring, if needed.

WARNING **Expect to discontinue bisoprolol about 48 hours beforehand if patient is scheduled for surgery with general anesthesia, to reduce risk of excessive myocardial depression during anesthesia.**

PATIENT TEACHING

- Teach patient how to monitor her blood pressure, if appropriate, and to recognize signs of hypertension and hypotension.
- Instruct patient to avoid sudden position changes and to rise slowly from a lying or sitting position to minimize the effects of orthostatic hypotension.
- Advise patient to avoid driving and other activities that require mental alertness until bisoprolol's CNS effects are known.
- Instruct patient to contact prescriber before using any OTC product, such as a cold remedy or nasal decongestant.

bivalirudin

Angiomax

Class and Category

Pharmacologic class: Direct thrombin inhibitor
Therapeutic class: Anticoagulant
Pregnancy category: B

Indications and Dosages

➤ *As adjunct to provide anticoagulation and prevent thrombosis in patients with unstable angina who are having percutaneous transluminal coronary angioplasty; to provide anticoagulation in patients undergoing percutaneous coronary intervention (PCI); to treat patients with or at risk of heparin-induced thrombocytopenia (HIT) or heparin-induced thrombocytopenia and thrombosis syndrome (HITTS) undergoing PCI*

I.V. INFUSION

Adults who do not have heparin-induced thrombocytopenia (HIT) or heparin-induced thrombocytopenia and thrombosis syndrome (HITTS). *Initial:* Immediately before procedure, 0.75-mg/kg bolus; then 1.75 mg/kg/hr as continuous infusion for duration of procedure. Five minutes after bolus dose and with continuous infusion running, another 0.3-mg/kg dose may be given, if needed, and patient does not have HIT or HITTS. After procedure, 1.75 mg/kg/hr given for up to 4 hr by continuous infusion, followed by 0.2 mg/kg/hr for up to 20 hr, if needed for patients with ST segment elevation myocardial infarction (STEMI) to prevent stent thrombosis and may be considered for patients without STEMI, if clinically indicated.

DOSAGE ADJUSTMENT Infusion dosage possibly reduced to 1 mg/kg/hr for patients with severe renal impairment (glomerular filtration rate less than 30 ml/min) and to 0.25 mg/kg/hr for patients having hemodialysis.

Route	Onset	Peak	Duration
I.V.	Immediate	Unknown	1 hr after end of infusion

Mechanism of Action

Selectively binds to thrombin, including thrombin trapped in established clots. Without thrombin, fibrinogen can't convert to fibrin and clots can't form.

Incompatibilities

Don't mix other drugs in same I.V. line before or during bivalirudin administration. Mixing with alteplase, amiodarone, amphotericin B, chlorpromazine HCl, diazepam, prochlorperazine edisylate, reteplase, streptokinase, or vancomycin HCl can result in haze, particulate formation, or precipitation.

Contraindications

Active major bleeding, hypersensitivity to bivalirudin or its components

Interactions

DRUGS

glycoprotein IIb/IIIa inhibitors such as abciximab, heparin, warfarin: Risk of bleeding

Adverse Reactions

CNS: Headache, **intracranial hemorrhage**
CV: **Acute stent thrombosis (patients with ST segment elevation myocardial infarction), cardiac tamponade, hypotension, thrombosis during PCI**
EENT: Epistaxis, gingival bleeding
GI: Abdominal cramps, diarrhea, GI or **retroperitoneal bleeding**, nausea, vomiting
GU: Hematuria, vaginal bleeding
HEME: **Absence of anticoagulant effect**, decreased hemoglobin, **increased INR, severe bleeding**
MS: Back pain
RESP: Hemoptysis, **hemothorax, pulmonary hemorrhage**
SKIN: Ecchymosis
Other: **Anaphylaxis**, antibody formation to bivalirudin, injection-site bleeding, hematoma, or pain

Nursing Considerations

- Reconstitute bivalirudin by adding 5 ml sterile water for injection to 250-mg vial and swirl gently until dissolved. For initial infusion, dilute reconstituted vial in 50 ml D_5W or normal saline solution to yield 5 mg/ml.
- Know that for subsequent low-rate infusion, further dilute reconstituted drug in 500 ml D_5W or normal saline solution to final concentration of 0.5 mg/ml.
- Expect to give 300 to 325 mg of aspirin P.O. daily during bivalirudin therapy.

WARNING Monitor blood coagulation tests before and regularly during therapy; bleeding is a major bivalirudin risk. Be aware that drug affects International Normalized Ratio (INR), so INR may not be useful for determining an appropriate warfarin dose.

WARNING Monitor patient often for bleeding because there's no antidote for bivalirudin. All patients with unexplained drop in blood pressure or hematocrit should be evaluated for bleeding. If life-threatening bleeding occurs, notify prescriber immediately, stop drug, and monitor APTT and other coagulation tests as ordered. Blood transfusions may be needed. Patients with increased bleeding risk include menstruating women; patients with large vessel or lumbar puncture, major surgery (including brain, eye, or spinal cord), major bleeding (including GI, intracranial, intraocular, pulmonary bleeding, or retroperitoneal), organ biopsy, recent stroke, or spinal anesthesia; and patients with organ or vascular abnormalities, such as advanced renal disease, dissecting aortic aneurysm, diverticulitis, hemophilia, hepatic disease (especially from deficient vitamin K–dependent clotting factors), infective endocarditis, inflammatory bowel disease, peptic ulcer disease, or severe uncontrolled hypertension. These patients should be monitored more frequently for bleeding.

- Know that if patient is receiving gamma brachytherapy, watch closely for evidence of thrombosis (weak or absent pulse, pallor, pain); use of bivalirudin may increase the risk in these patients.
- Avoid I.M. injections of any kind, if possible, to decrease the risk of bleeding.
- Discard any unused portion of drug.

PATIENT TEACHING

- Inform patient that bivalirudin is a blood thinner administered only in the hospital.
- Urge patient to check her skin for bruising or red spots and to immediately report back for stomach pain, dizziness, fainting, trouble breathing, and unusual bleeding (black, tarry stool; blood in urine; coughing blood; heavy menses; nosebleeds). Drug may need to be stopped.
- Encourage patient to reduce the risk of injury while receiving bivalirudin, such as by brushing her teeth gently with a soft-bristled toothbrush.
- Caution patient not to take anti-inflammatories, such as aspirin or aspirin-like products, ibuprofen, ketoprofen, and naproxen, or other blood thinners, such as warfarin, while receiving bivalirudin unless directed.

brexpiprazole

Rexulti

Class and Category

Pharmacologic class: Atypical antipsychotic
Therapeutic class: Antipsychotic
Pregnancy category: Not classified

Indications and Dosages

➤ *Adjunct treatment of major depressive disorder*

TABLETS

Adults. *Initial:* 0.5 or 1 mg once daily, then increased to 1 or 2 mg once daily after 1 wk. Further increases in 1 mg increments made weekly, as needed. *Maximum:* 3 mg once daily.

➤ *To treat schizophrenia*

TABLETS

Adults. *Initial:* 1 mg once daily for 4 days, followed by 2 mg once daily for 3 days, then increased to 4 mg once daily. *Maximum:* 4 mg once daily.

DOSAGE ADJUSTMENT For patients with moderate to severe hepatic impairment or moderate to severe or end-stage renal impairment (creatinine clearance less than 60 ml/min), maximum dosage should not exceed 2 mg once daily for patients with major depressive disorder and 3 mg for patients with schizophrenia. For patient who is a CYP2D6 poor metabolizer or patient is taking strong CYP2D6 or CYP3A4 inhibitors, dosage reduced by 50%. For patient who is a CYP2D6 poor metabolizer or patient who is taking strong CYP2D6 or CYP3A4 inhibitors, dosage reduced by 50%. For patient who is a CYP2D6 poor metabolizer who is also taking moderate to strong CYP3A4 inhibitors or patient taking both a moderate to strong CYP2D6 inhibitor and a moderate to strong CYP3A4 inhibitor, dosage reduced by 75%. For patient taking strong CYP3A4 inducers, dosage doubled over 1 to 2 wk.

Mechanism of Action

May produce antipsychotic effects through partial agonist and antagonist actions. Brexpiprazole acts as a partial agonist at dopamine (especially D_2) receptors and serotonin (especially 5-HT1A) receptors. The drug acts as an antagonist at 5-HT2A serotonin receptor sites.

Contraindications

Hypersensitivity to brexpiprazole or its components

Interactions

DRUGS

clarithyromycin, itraconazole, ketoconazole, and other strong CYP3A4 inhibitors; fluoxetine, paroxetine, quinidine, and other strong CYP2D6 inhibitors: Increased brexpiprazole exposure and possibly increased adverse brexpiprazole-related reactions

rifampin, St. John's wort, and other strong CYP3A4 inducers: Decreased brexpiprazole exposure and effectiveness

Adverse Reactions

CNS: Abnormal dreams, akathisia, anxiety, body temperature dysregulation, **CVA**, dizziness, dyskinesia, dystonia, fatigue, headache, impaired cognitive and motor skills, insomnia, restlessness, **seizures**, somnolence, **suicidal ideation**, syncope, tardive dyskinesia, tremor

CV: Dyslipidemia, orthostatic hypotension

EENT: Blurred vision, dry mouth, excessive salivation, nasopharyngitis

ENDO: Decreased blood cortisol levels, hyperglycemia

GI: Abdominal pain, constipation, diarrhea, dyspepsia, flatulence, increased appetite, nausea

GU: UTI

HEME: Agranulocytosis, **leukopenia**, **neutropenia**

MS: Myalgia

SKIN: Hyperhidrosis

Other: Increased blood creatine phosphokinase level, pathological gambling and other compulsive behaviors, weight gain

Nursing Considerations

- Be aware that brexpiprazole shouldn't be used to treat dementia-related psychosis in the elderly because of an increased risk of death.
- Use brexpiprazole cautiously in patients with a history of seizures or with conditions that lower the seizure threshold. Also use cautiously in patients at risk for aspiration pneumonia because esophageal dysphagia has been associated with antipsychotic drug use.
- Monitor patient's CBC, as ordered, because serious adverse hematologic reactions, such as agranulocytosis, leukopenia, and neutropenia may occur with atypical antipsychotic therapy. Assess more often during first few months of therapy if patient has a history of drug-induced leukopenia or neutropenia or a significantly low WBC count. If abnormalities occur during therapy, watch for fever or other signs of infection, notify

prescriber and, if severe, expect drug to be stopped.

- Monitor patient for tardive dyskinesia, especially in elderly women. Know that it has the potential to be irreversible and the risk for developing tardive dyskinesia increases the longer brexpiprazole is used and the higher the total cumulative dose. If it occurs, notify prescriber and expect drug to be discontinued, if possible.
- Monitor patient's blood glucose level, lipid levels, and weight, as ordered, because atypical antipsychotic drugs such as brexpiprazole may cause metabolic changes. If patient is already a diabetic, monitor blood glucose levels more closely.

WARNING **Know that antipsychotic drugs may cause neuroleptic malignant syndrome. Monitor patient closely throughout brexpiprazole therapy. If suspected, notify prescriber immediately, be prepared to provide emergency supportive care, and expect drug to be discontinued.**

- Watch patients closely for suicidal tendencies, particularly when therapy starts and dosage changes, because depression may worsen temporarily during these times.

PATIENT TEACHING

- Advise patient to get up slowly from a lying or sitting position during brexpiprazole therapy to minimize a drop in blood pressure.
- Instruct patient to avoid hazardous activities until drug's effects are known. Also, alert patient and family of increased risk for falls, especially if patient has other medical conditions or takes medication that may affect the nervous system.
- Urge patient to avoid activities that raise body temperature suddenly, such as strenuous exercise and exposure to extreme heat, and to compensate for situations that cause dehydration, such as vomiting or diarrhea.
- Instruct patient to inform all prescribers of any drugs he's taking, including OTC drugs, because of risk of interactions.
- Advise female patient of childbearing age to notify prescriber if she intends to become or suspects that she is pregnant during therapy.
- Instruct diabetic patient to monitor blood glucose levels closely.
- Tell family or caregiver to watch patient closely for suicidal tendencies, especially when therapy starts or dosage changes.
- Inform patient and family or caregiver that drug may cause intense urges, particularly for gambling, but may also cause sexual urges, uncontrollable shopping, binge eating, and other impulsive or compulsive behaviors. These behaviors may not be recognized as abnormal by patient. Urge the reporting of such behaviors as a dosage reduction or discontinuation of the drug may be required to protect patient from these harmful effects.

brivaracetam

Briviact

Class, Category, Schedule

Pharmacologic class: Anticonvulsant
Therapeutic class: Anticonvulsant
Pregnancy category: Not classified
Controlled substance schedule: V

Indications and Dosages

➤ *To treat partial-onset seizures in patients with epilepsy*

ORAL SOLUTION, TABLETS

Adults and adolescents age 16 and over. *Initial:* 50 mg twice daily followed by dosage reduction to 25 mg twice daily or dosage increase to 100 mg twice daily depending on therapeutic response and patient tolerance.

Children age 4 to 16 weighing 50 kg (110 lb) or more. *Initial:* 25 to 50 mg twice daily followed by dosage adjustment depending on patient tolerance and therapeutic response. Dosage maybe be reduced to 25 mg twice daily if dose started at 50 mg twice daily or dosage increased to 100 mg twice daily, if needed.

Children age 4 to 16 weighing 20 kg (44 lb) to less than 50 kg (110 lb). *Initial:* 0.5 mg/kg to 1 mg/kg twice daily followed by dosage increase up to 4 mg/kg twice daily depending on therapeutic response and patient tolerance.

Children age 4 to 16 weighing 11 kg (24.2 lb) to less than 20 kg (44 lb). *Initial:* 0.5 mg/kg to 1.25 mg/kg twice daily followed by dosage increase up to 2.5 mg/kg twice daily depending on therapeutic response and patient tolerance.

I.V. INJECTION

Adults and adolescents age 16 and over. *Initial:* 50 mg injected over 2 to 15 min twice daily followed by dosage reduction to 25 mg twice daily or dosage increase to 100 mg twice daily depending on therapeutic response and patient tolerance.

DOSAGE ADJUSTMENT For adult patient and pediatric patient weighing 50 kg (110 lb) or more with hepatic impairment of any severity, initial dosage reduced to 25 mg twice daily, with maximum dosage not to exceed 75 mg twice daily. For pediatric patient with hepatic impairment weighing 11 kg (24.2 lb) to less than 50 kg (110 lb), initial dosage not to exceed 0.5 mg/kg twice daily. For pediatric patient with hepatic impairment weighing 20 kg (44 lb) to less than 50 kg (110 lb), maximum dosage not to exceed 1.5 mg/kg twice daily and for pediatric patient with hepatic impairment weighing 11 kg (24.2 lb) to less than 20 kg (44 lb), maximum dosage not to exceed 2 mg/kg. For patient receiving rifampin concurrently, dosage of brivaracetam doubled.

Route	Onset	Peak	Duration
P.O., I.V.	1 hr	Unknown	Unknown

Mechanism of Action

Displays a high and selective affinity for synaptic vesicle protein 2A (SV2A) in the brain, which may contribute to the anticonvulsant effect, although the exact mechanism is unknown.

Incompatibilities

Do not mix with solutions other than 0.9% sodium chloride injection USP; 5% Dextrose Injection, USP; or Lactated Ringer's injection and do not administer with other drugs in same intravenous line because incompatibilities are unknown.

Contraindications

Hypersensitivity to brivaracetam or its components

Interactions

DRUGS

carbamazepine: Possibly increased exposure of carbamazepine that may lead to adverse reactions

phenytoin: Increased plasma concentrations of phenytoin that may lead to adverse reactions

rifampin: Decreased plasma concentrations of brivaracetam significantly interfering with its effectiveness and requiring a dosage increase to compensate

Adverse Reactions

CNS: Abnormal behavior, acute psychosis, adjustment disorder, affect lability, aggression, agitation, altered mood, anger, anxiety, apathy, balance and cerebellar coordination disturbances, belligerence, depression, dizziness, euphoria (parenteral form), fatigue, feeling drunk (parenteral form), hallucinations, irritability, mood swings, nervousness, paranoia, psychomotor hyperactivity, psychotic behavior or disorder, restlessness, sedation, somnolence, **suicidal ideation**

EENT: Taste disturbance (parenteral form)

GI: Constipation, nausea, vomiting

HEME: Leukopenia, neutropenia

RESP: Bronchospasm

Other: Angioedema, infusion-site pain

Nursing Considerations

- Be aware that brivaracetam oral solution may be administered via a gastrostomy or nasogastric tube.
- Administer parenteral form of brivaracetam only as an intravenous injection. It may be given without further dilution or it may be mixed with any of the following solutions: 0.9% sodium chloride injection, USP, 5% Dextrose Injection, USP, or Lactated Ringer's injection. Administer over 2 to 15 minutes. If diluted, the solution should not be stored for more than 4 hours at room temperature and may be stored in polyvinyl chloride bags. Discard any unused portion of the parenteral solution remaining in the vial.
- Know that oral dosage and parenteral dosage are interchangeable. However, be aware that the parenteral form should not be used in children under the age of 16 because safety as not been established.

WARNING Monitor patient closely for abnormal behavior or thoughts, because brivaracetam may increase risk of suicidal thoughts or behavior.

WARNING Monitor patient for hypersensitivity reactions, especially angioedema and bronchospasm. If present, notify prescriber, expect brivaracetam to be discontinued, and be prepared to provide supportive care.

- Take safety measures to prevent patient from falling, because brivaracetam may cause dizziness and disturbances in coordination and gait.
- Know that brivaracetam may cause psychiatric adverse reactions. Notify prescriber, if present, and take measures to keep patient calm and safe.
- Be aware that brivaracetam should not be discontinued abruptly, because of increased risk of seizure frequency and the potential for status epilepticus.

PATIENT TEACHING

- Inform patient prescribed tablet form to swallow tablets whole with a beverage. Tell patient tablets should not be chewed or crushed.
- Inform patient prescribed oral solution form to use a calibrated measuring device to measure and deliver the prescribed dose. Remind patient that a household tablespoon or teaspoon is not an adequate measuring device. Tell patient the oral solution need not be diluted. Have patient discard any unused oral solution after 5 months of first opening the bottle.

WARNING Have family or caregiver monitor patient closely for abnormal behavior or thoughts, because drug may increase risk of suicidal thoughts and behavior.

- Advise patient to avoid performing hazardous activities such as driving or operating machinery until central nervous system effects of brivaracetam are known and have abated.
- Remind patient to be careful and use safety precautions when walking or performing physical activities because brivaracetam may cause disturbances in coordination and gait and dizziness.
- Advise patient and family or caregiver that brivaracetam may cause changes in behavior such as aggression, agitation, anger, anxiety, and irritability along with psychotic symptoms. Instruct patient or family/caregiver to report these changes immediately to the prescriber.
- Tell women of childbearing age to notify prescriber if pregnancy is suspected or known. If confirmed, encourage patient to enroll in the pregnancy exposure registry by calling 1-888-233-2334.

brodalumab

Siliq

Class and Category

Pharmacologic class: Monoclonal IgG2 antibody
Therapeutic class: Antipsoriatic
Pregnancy category: Not classified

Indications and Dosages

➤ *To treat moderate to severe plaque psoriasis in patients who are candidates for systemic therapy or phototherapy and have failed to respond or have lost response to other systemic therapies*

SUBCUTANEOUS INJECTION

Adults. *Initial:* 210 mg followed by 210 mg repeated at day 7 and 14, and then 210 mg every 2 wk.

Mechanism of Action

Binds to human IL-17RA and inhibits its interactions with selective cytokines. This inhibits the release of pro-inflammatory chemokines and cytokines, which are thought to be part of the pathogenesis of plaque psoriasis.

Contraindications

Crohn's disease, hypersensitivity to brodalumab or its components

Interactions

DRUGS

CYP450 substrates such as cyclosporine or warfarin: Possibly altered effectiveness of these drugs
live vaccines: Failure to produce an adequate immune response

Adverse Reactions

CNS: Headache, fatigue, **suicidal ideation**
EENT: Nasopharyngitis, oropharyngeal pain, pharyngitis
GI: Crohn's disease, diarrhea, nausea
GU: UTI
HEME: Neutropenia
MS: Arthralgia, myalgia

RESP: Bronchitis, upper respiratory infections
SKIN: Tinea infections, urticaria
Other: Anti-brodalumab antibody formation, flu-like symptoms, injection-site reactions (bruisng, erythema, hemorrhage, pain, pruritus)

Nursing Considerations

- Expect patient to be evaluated for tuberculosis before brodalumab therapy is begun. If present, know that brodalumab should not be initiated until treatment for latent tuberculosis has been given. Monitor all patients for signs and symptoms of tuberculosis during and after brodalumab therapy.
- Use cautiously in patients with a chronic infection or who have a history of recurrent infections, because brodalumab increases the risk of infections, especially fungal infections. If an infection occurs and does not respond to standard therapy for the infection, expect brodalumab to be withheld until the infection is resolved.

WARNING Know that brodalumab is only available through a restricted program because of its potential to cause suicidal behavior and thoughts. Monitor patient closely and expect drug to be discontinued if suicidal ideation is present.

- Allow prefilled syringe to reach room temperature before administering, which is about 30 minutes. Administer only as a subcutaneous injection. Do not inject into an area that is affected by psoriasis or is bruised, hard, red, scaly, tender, or thick. Know that the solution in the pen should appear clear to slightly opalescent, colorless to slightly yellow, and may have a few translucent to white particles. Do not use if cloudy or discolored or if foreign matter is present. Inject the full amount in the syringe to provide the correct dosage.
- Monitor patient for Crohn's disease and know that brodalumab must be discontinued if patient develops this disease while taking the drug.
- Avoid administering live vaccines while patient is receiving brodalumab because vaccines may not be effective.

PATIENT TEACHING

- Instruct patient self-administering brodalumab how to properly administer a subcutaneous injection. Tell patient not to inject the drug in an area that is affected by psoriasis or is bruised, hard, scaly, tender, or thick.
- Tell patient to allow the prefilled syringe to reach room temperature (which takes about 30 minutes) before injecting the drug. Remind patient not to remove the gray needle cap on the syringe while allowing it to reach room temperature. Prior to injection, tell patient to look at solution inside the syringe. It should be clear to slightly opalescent, colorless to slightly yellow. A few translucent to white particles may be present. If solution appears cloudy or discolored or if foreign matter is present, the syringe should be discarded and a replacement obtained. Tell patient to inject the full amount of solution contained in the prefilled syringe. Advise patient to rotate sites.
- Advise patient to seek medical attention if signs or symptoms of infection occur.
- Tell patient to notify prescriber if persistent or severe bowel problems develop. If Crohn's disease is diagnosed, inform patient that brodalumab therapy must be discontinued.

WARNING Alert patient or family that drug may produce suicidal behavior or thoughts. If present, suicide precautions should be undertaken, prescriber notified, and drug discontinued.

bromocriptine mesylate

Alti-Bromocriptine (CAN), Apo-Bromocriptine (CAN), Cycloset, Parlodel, Parlodel SnapTabs

Class and Category

Pharmacologic class: Dopamine receptor agonist
Therapeutic class: Antidiabetic, antidyskinetic, antihyperprolactinemic, dopamine-receptor agonist, growth hormone suppressant, infertility therapy adjunct
Pregnancy category: B

Indications and Dosages

➤ *To treat amenorrhea, galactorrhea, male hypogonadism, and infertility from hyperprolactinemia*

CAPSULES, TABLETS (PARLODEL)
Adults and adolescents age 15 and over. *Initial:* 1.25 to 2.5 mg daily with snack. Increased by 2.5 mg every 2 to 7 days as needed. *Maintenance:* 2.5 to 15 mg daily.
Children ages 11 to 15 years with a prolactin-secreting pituitary adenoma. 1.25 to 2.5 mg daily with snack. Increased as needed and tolerated. *Maintenance:* 2.5 to 10 mg daily.

➤ *To treat Parkinson's disease*

CAPSULES, TABLETS (PARLODEL)
Adults. *Initial:* 1.25 mg twice daily with meals. Increased by 2.5 mg every 14 to 28 days, as needed. *Maximum:* 100 mg daily.

➤ *To treat acromegaly*

CAPSULES, TABLETS (PARLODEL)
Adults and children age 15 and over. *Initial:* 1.25 to 2.5 mg at bedtime with snack for 3 days. Then increased by 1.25 to 2.5 mg every 3 to 7 days, if needed. *Maintenance:* Usually 20 to 30 mg daily. *Maximum:* 100 mg daily.

➤ *To control blood glucose level in type 2 diabetes mellitus, with diet and exercise*

TABLETS (CYCLOSET)
Adults. *Initial:* 0.8 mg once daily within 2 hr after waking up in morning. Increased weekly in increments of 0.8 mg, as needed. *Maximum:* 4.8 mg daily.

DOSAGE ADJUSTMENT For patients taking Cycloset and a moderate CYP3A4 inhibitor such as erythromycin, dosage not to exceed beyond 1.6 mg once daily.

Route	Onset	Peak	Duration
P.O.*	2 hr	8 hr	24 hr
P.O.†	30–90 min	2 hr	Unknown
P.O.‡	1–2 hr	4–8 wk	4–8 hr

* For amenorrhea, galactorrhea, male hypogonadism, infertility from hyperprolactinemia, and prolactin-secreting adenoma.
† For Parkinson's disease.
‡ For acromegaly.

Mechanism of Action

Inhibits release of growth and prolactin hormones from the anterior pituitary gland, thus restoring ovarian or testicular function and suppressing lactation. Bromocriptine decreases dopamine turnover in the CNS, depleting dopamine or blocking its receptors in the brain, alleviating dyskinesia.

Contraindications

Breastfeeding; hypersensitivity to bromocriptine, other ergot alkaloids, or their components; hypertensive disorders of pregnancy; severe ischemic heart disease or peripheral vascular disease; syncopal migraine; uncontrolled hypertension

Interactions

DRUGS
antihypertensives: Increased hypotensive effects
CYP3A4 inducers: Decreased bromocriptine level
CYP3A4 inhibitors: Increased bromocriptine level
dopamine receptor antagonists, including neuroleptic drugs (such as butyrophenones, phenothiazines, or thioxanthenes), metoclopramide: Possibly decreased effectiveness of both drugs
ergot alkaloids or derivatives: Increased risk of hypertension
highly protein bound drugs such as chloramphenicol, probenecid, salicylates, sulfonamides: Possibly altered effectiveness of these drugs and increased risk of adverse reactions
levodopa: Additive effects requiring reduced levodopa dose
macrolide antibiotics such as erythromycin: Increased plasma bromocriptine levels
sympathomimetic drugs: Possibly increased risk of hypertension and tachycardia

ACTIVITIES
alcohol use: Possibly increased risk of adverse effects of bromocriptine

Adverse Reactions

CNS: Asthenia, confusion, dizziness, drowsiness, fatigue, hallucinations, headache, light-headedness, syncope
CV: Hypertension, **hypotension**, orthostatic hypotension, pericardial effusion, pericarditis, Raynaud's phenomenon
EENT: Amblyopia, dry mouth, nasal congestion, rhinitis, sinusitis
ENDO: Hypoglycemia

GI: Abdominal cramps, anorexia, constipation, diarrhea, **GI bleeding**, indigestion, nausea, vomiting
RESP: Pleural effusion or thickening, **pulmonary firbosis**
Other: Intense urge to gamble, engage in sexual activity, or spend money uncontrollably

Nursing Considerations

- Use bromocriptine cautiously if patient has a history of psychosis or cardiovascular disease, especially after MI with residual arrhythmia. In severe psychotic disorder, bromocriptine isn't recommended because it may worsen the disorder or reduce the effects of drugs used to treat it.
- Use bromocriptine cautiously in patients with Parkinson's disease because high doses of the drug may cause confusion and mental disturbances in these patients. Drug should not be discontinued abruptly, as a symptom complex resembling the neuroleptic malignant syndrome has occurred with rapid dose reduction, withdrawal, or changes in antiparkinsonian therapy.
- Expect to perform a pregnancy test every 4 weeks during the amenorrheic period. Once menses resume, test whenever a period is missed, as ordered.
- Plan to withhold bromocriptine if patient becomes pregnant.
- Know that if rapidly expanding adenoma needs continued therapy, watch closely for hypertensive crisis.
- Be aware that bromocriptine shouldn't be given postpartum if patient has a history of coronary artery disease or other severe cardiovascular problem unless risk of withdrawing drug is greater than risk of use. If so, monitor closely for signs and symptoms of CV dysfunction, such as chest pain.
- Expect to give drug with levodopa if patient is being treated for Parkinson's disease.
- Assess for hypotension when bromocriptine therapy starts and hypertension (typically during second week). Monitor blood pressure often if patient takes other antihypertensives.
- Assess patient who has a history of peptic ulcer or GI bleeding for new bleeding.
- Take safety precautions, such as keeping bed in low position with side rails up, because drug can cause dizziness, drowsiness, light-headedness, and syncope.

PATIENT TEACHING

- Tell patient to take each dose with a meal, milk, or a snack to minimize nausea.
- Caution patient about possible dizziness, drowsiness, and light-headedness. Urge patient to avoid hazardous activities until drug effects are known.
- Advise against sudden position changes to minimize orthostatic hypotension.
- Warn patient to avoid alcohol while taking bromocriptine because it may cause disulfiram-like reactions, such as blurred vision, chest pain, confusion, diaphoresis, a fast or pounding heartbeat, facial flushing, nausea, severe weakness, throbbing headache, or vomiting.
- Tell patient to take a missed dose as soon as she remembers it, unless it's almost time for the next dose. In that case, tell her to wait until the next scheduled dose. Warn her not to double the dose. Advise her to contact prescriber if she misses more than one dose.
- Urge patient to report adverse reactions, such as nausea, unremitting headache, vomiting, or other signs of CNS toxicity.
- Tell patient who takes large doses of bromocriptine to schedule regular dental checkups because the drug can decrease saliva flow, which may encourage dental caries, oral candidiasis, oral discomfort, or periodontal disease.
- Tell patient with acromegaly to keep her fingers warm to prevent cold-sensitive digital vasospasm.
- Teach patient with type 2 diabetes about diet, exercise, effects of hyperglycemia and hypoglycemia, hygiene, foot care, and ways to avoid infection.
- Warn patient to report intense urges to gamble, engage in sexual activity, or spend money uncontrollably.

budesonide

Entocort EC, Pulmicort Flexhaler, Pulmicort Respules, Rhinocort Aqua, Uceris

Class and Category

Pharmacologic class: Corticosteroid
Therapeutic class: Antiasthmatic, anti-inflammatory

Pregnancy category: B (Pulmicort, Rhinocort), C (Uceris), not classified (Entocort EC)

Indications and Dosages

➤ *To manage symptoms of seasonal or perennial allergic rhinitis*

NASAL SPRAY (RHINOCORT AQUA)

Adults and children age 6 and over. 32 mcg in each nostril daily. *Maximum:* 256 mcg daily (adults and adolescents); 128 mcg daily (children age 6 and over). *Maintenance:* Lowest dosage that controls symptoms.

➤ *To provide maintenance therapy in asthma*

ORAL INHALATION (PULMICORT FLEXHALER)

Adults and adolescents age 18 and over. *Initial:* 180 or 360 mcg twice daily, increased as needed. *Maximum:* 720 mcg twice daily.
Children ages 6 to 17. *Initial:* 180 or 360 mcg twice daily. *Maximum:* 360 mcg twice daily.

NEBULIZED INHALATION (PULMICORT RESPULES)

Children ages 1 to 8 previously on bronchodilators alone. 0.25 mg twice daily. or 0.5 mg daily by jet nebulizer. *Maximum:* 0.5 mg/day.
Children ages 1 to 8 previously on inhaled steroids. 0.25 mg twice daily or 0.5 mg daily inhaled by jet nebulizer. *Maximum:* 1 mg/day.
Children ages 1 to 8 previously on systemic corticosteroids. 0.5 mg twice daily or 1 mg daily inhaled by jet nebulizer. *Maximum:* 1 mg/day.

➤ *To treat mild to moderate active Crohn's disease involving the ileum, the ascending colon, or both*

CAPSULES (ENTOCORT EC)

Adults. 9 mg daily in the morning for up to 8 wk.
Children age 8 to 17 weighing more than 25 kg (55 lb). 9 mg once daily for 8 wk, followed by 6 mg once daily for 2 wk.

➤ *To maintain clinical remission of mild to moderate Crohn's disease involving the ileum, the ascending colon, or both*

CAPSULES (ENTOCORT EC)

Adults. 6 mg daily in the morning for up to 3 mo.

DOSAGE ADJUSTMENT *For Entocort EC:* For adult patients with moderate hepatic impairment, dosage reduced to 3 mg once daily for duration of treatment.

➤ *To induce remission in patients with active, mild to moderate ulcerative colitis*

E.R. TABLETS (UCERIS)

Adults. 9 mg daily in the morning for up to 8 wk.

DOSAGE ADJUSTMENT *For Uceris:* Dosage reduced for patients with hepatic insufficiency and those taking ketoconazole or other CYP3A4 inhibitor.

➤ *To induce remission in patients with active, mild to moderate distal ulcerative colitis extending up to 40 cm from the anal verge*

RECTAL FOAM (UCERIS)

Adults. 1 metered dose (2 mg) twice daily for 2 wk followed by 1 metered dose (2 mg) once daily for 4 wk.

Route	Onset	Peak	Duration
Nasal suspension	In 4 wk	Unknown	Unknown
Oral inhalation	In 4 wk	Unknown	Unknown
Nebulized inhalation	2–8 days	4–6 wk	Unknown
P.O. (capsules)	Unknown	30 min–10 hr	Unknown
P.O. (ER tablets)	Unknown	13 hr	Unknown
Rectal foam	Unknown	Unknown	Unknown

Mechanism of Action

Inhibits inflammatory cells and mediators, possibly by decreasing influx into nasal passages, bronchial walls, or the intestines. As a result, nasal or airway inflammation decreases. Oral inhalation form also inhibits mucus secretion in airways, decreasing the amount and viscosity of sputum.

Contraindications

Hypersensitivity to budesonide or its components, recent septal ulcers or nasal surgery or trauma (nasal spray); status asthmaticus or other acute asthma episodes (oral inhalation)

Interactions

DRUGS

clarithromycin, erythromycin, itraconazole, katoconazole and other strong CYP3A4 inhibitors such as atazanavir, clarithromycin, indinavir, itraconazole, nefazodone, nelfinavir, ritonavir, saquinavir, telithromycin: Possibly increased blood budesonide level

FOOD

grapefruit juice: Possibly increased blood budesonide level

Adverse Reactions

CNS: Amnesia, asthenia, **benign intracranial hypertension**, changes in mood, dizziness, fatigue, fever, headache
CV: Hypertension, peripheral edema
EENT: Bad taste, cataracts, dry mouth, epistaxis, glaucoma, nasal irritation, oral or pharyngeal candidiasis, pharyngitis, rhinitis, sinusitis
ENDO: Adrenal insufficiency, growth suppression in children, hypercorticism
GI: Abdominal pain, diarrhea, dyspepsia, flatulence, indigestion, nausea, **pancreatitis**, **rectal bleeding**, vomiting
GU: UTI
MS: Arthralgia, back pain, muscle cramps and spasms
RESP: Bronchospasm, increased cough, respiratory tract infection
SKIN: Allergic or contact dermatitis, maculo-papular rash, pruritus, purpura, rash, urticaria
Other: Anaphylaxis, **angioedema**, increased risk of infection

Nursing Considerations

- Use budesonide cautiously if patient has ocular herpes simplex; tubercular infection; or untreated fungal, bacterial, or systemic viral infection.
- Closely monitor a child's growth pattern; budesonide may stunt growth.

WARNING Assess patient who switches from a systemic corticosteroid to inhaled budesonide for adrenal insufficiency (fatigue, hypotension, lassitude, nausea, vomiting, weakness), which may be life-threatening. Hypothalamic–pituitary–adrenal axis function may take several months to recover after stopping systemic corticosteroids. Stopping budesonide abruptly may cause adrenal insufficiency.

- Administer Respules by jet nebulizer connected to an air compressor.
- Monitor patient exposed to chickenpox. Know that he may receive varicella zoster immune globulin or pooled I.V. immunoglobulin. If chickenpox develops, give antiviral as ordered. A patient exposed to measles may need pooled I.M. immunoglobulin.
- Assess patient for effectiveness of budesonide therapy, especially if being weaned from a systemic corticosteroid. If patient has increased asthma or an immunologic condition previously suppressed by systemic corticosteroid—such as arthritis, conjunctivitis, an eosinophilic condition, eczema, or rhinitis—notify prescriber.
- Determine if patient has a milk allergy. Pulmicort Flexhaler contains small amounts of lactose, which may trigger coughing, wheezing, or bronchospasm in a patient with a severe milk-protein allergy.
- Monitor patient for evidence of hypersensitivity. If present, notify prescriber immediately. Expect to stop budesonide and provide emergency supportive care.
- Monitor patients with conditions such as diabetes mellitus, glaucoma or cataracts, hypertension, osteoporosis, or peptic ulcer, as glucocorticosteroid therapy may increase adverse effects. Also monitor patients with a family history of diabetes or glaucoma.

PATIENT TEACHING

- Urge patient taking oral capsules or E.R. tablets to swallow them whole and not to chew or break them.
- Instruct patient who uses nasal spray to shake container before each use. Instruct her to blow her nose, tilt her head slightly forward, and insert tube into a nostril, pointing toward inner corner of eye, away from nasal septum. Tell her to hold the other nostril closed and spray while inhaling gently. Then have her repeat in the other nostril.
- Instruct patient to prime oral inhaler before using it for first time by holding canister upright with mouthpiece on top and twisting base of device fully to right and then fully to left until it clicks. Teach her to load each dose just before use in the same way. After loading a dose,

caution patient not to shake device or blow into it. Tell patient to turn her head away from device and exhale. Then have her hold device upright, place her lips around mouthpiece, and inhale deeply. Device will discharge a dose. Tell patient to remove her lips from mouthpiece to exhale.
- Instruct patient to empty her bowels before using rectal foam. Although product is lubricated, tell patient she may use petroleum jelly or petrolatum if more lubrication is needed. Tell her to warm the canister in her hands while shaking it vigorously for 10 to 15 seconds prior to use. Inform her that she may apply the rectal foam while standing, lying, or sitting. When applied in the evening, instruct her to do so immediately before bedtime and advise her to try not to empty her bowels again until morning. Warn patient to keep canister away from heat sources, as its contents are flammable.
- Caution patient not to use an oral inhaler with a spacer device.
- Advise patient to rinse her mouth with water after each orally inhaled dose and to spit the water out. Tell her to contact her prescriber if she develops a mouth or throat infection.
- Instruct patient not to use budesonide as a rescue inhaler.
- Tell patient to contact prescriber if symptoms persist or have worsened after 3 weeks. Caution against increasing the dose on her own.
- Inform parents of small children using nebulized Respules that improvement may begin within 2 to 8 days but that full effect may not be evident for 4 to 6 weeks.
- Caution patient to avoid exposure to chickenpox and measles and, if exposed, to contact prescriber immediately.
- Caution against stopping drug abruptly.
- Instruct patient on long-term therapy to have regular eye examinations.
- Urge female patient to notify prescriber if she is or could be pregnant.
- Strongly encourage mothers who wish to breastfeed an infant to discuss breastfeeding with prescriber before doing so.

bumetanide

Bumex

Class and Category

Pharmacologic class: Loop diuretic as sulfonamide derivative
Therapeutic class: Diuretic
Pregnancy category: Not classified

Indications and Dosages

➤ *To treat edema caused by heart failure, hepatic disease, and renal disease, including nephrotic syndrome*

TABLETS

Adults. 0.5 to 2 mg daily, increased as needed, with a second or third dose every 4 to 5 hr or 0.5 to 2 mg every other day or daily for 3 or 4 days each week. *Maximum:* 10 mg daily.

I.M. INJECTION, I.V. INFUSION, I.V. INJECTION

Adults. 0.5 to 1 mg daily, increased as needed with a second or third dose every 2 to 3 hr. I.V. infusion given at 0.1 mg/hr to 1 mg/hr. I.V. injection given over 1 to 2 min. *Maximum:* 10 mg daily.

DOSAGE ADJUSTMENT In patients with severe chronic renal insufficiency, continuous infusion (12 mg over 12 hr) may be more effective and less toxic than intermittent infusion.

Route	Onset	Peak	Duration
P.O.	30–60 min	1–2 hr	4–6 hr
I.V.	In min	15–30 min	3.5–4 hr

Mechanism of Action

Inhibits reabsorption of sodium, chloride, and water in the ascending limb of the loop of Henle, which promotes their excretion and reduces fluid volume.

Contraindications

Anuria, hepatic coma, hypersensitivity to bumetanide or its components, severe electrolyte depletion

Interactions

DRUGS

aminoglycosides: Increased risk of ototoxicity
antihypertensives: Increased hypotensive effect

indomethacin: Slowed increase in urine and sodium excretion, inhibited plasma renin activity
lithium: Reduced lithium renal clearance, increased risk of lithium toxicity
probenecid: Reduced sodium excretion

Adverse Reactions

CNS: Dizziness, **encephalopathy**, headache
CV: Hypotension
EENT: Ototoxicity
ENDO: Hyperglycemia
GI: Nausea
GU: Azotemia, elevated serum creatinine level
MS: Muscle spasms
SKIN: Stevens–Johnson syndrome, toxic epidermal necrolysis
Other: Hyperuricemia, **hypocalcemia**, hypochloremia, **hypokalemia**, **hyponatremia**, hypovolemia

Nursing Considerations

WARNING Know that a patient hypersensitive to sulfonamides may be hypersensitive to bumetanide. Monitor such a patient closely when starting therapy.

- Expect to use parenteral route for patients with impaired GI absorption or in whom the oral route isn't practical. Switch to oral route, as prescribed, as soon as possible.
- Discard unused parenteral solution 24 hours after preparation.
- Assess fluid and electrolyte balance closely because bumetanide is a potent diuretic (40 to 60 times more potent than furosemide). Monitor fluid intake and output once every 8 hours, evaluate serum electrolyte levels when ordered, and assess for imbalances.

WARNING Be aware that high-dose or too-frequent administration can cause profound diuresis and water and electrolyte depletion, especially in elderly patients.

- Monitor serum potassium level regularly to check for hypokalemia, especially if patient takes a digitalis glycoside for heart failure or has aldosteronism, ascites, diarrhea, hepatic cirrhosis, potassium-losing nephropathy, or a history of ventricular arrhythmias.
- Assess for evidence of ototoxicity, such as tinnitus, daily. Rarely, drug may cause ototoxicity, especially with I.V. use, high doses, and increased frequency of dosing in a patient with renal impairment.
- Monitor results of renal function tests during therapy to detect adverse reactions.

PATIENT TEACHING

- Advise patient to avoid hazardous activities until drug's CNS effects are known.
- Stress importance of monitoring fluid intake and output and watching for evidence of electrolyte imbalance, such as dizziness, headache, and muscle spasms.
- Review adverse reactions, and tell patient to report severe or persistent reactions.
- Review potassium-rich foods, and urge patient to include them in her daily diet.
- Urge patient to return for appropriate follow-up care, especially if she's receiving bumetanide for a chronic condition.
- Tell diabetic patient to monitor blood glucose level regularly and to notify prescriber about persistent hyperglycemia.
- Advise patient to report any changes in skin that are new, unusual, persistent, or severe.

buprenorphine

Butrans, Sublocade, Subutex

buprenorphine hydrochloride

Belbuca, Buprenex

Class, Category, and Schedule

Pharmacologic class: Opioid
Therapeutic class: Opioid analgesic
Pregnancy category: C (Buprenex), not classified (Belbuca, Butrans, Sublocade)
Controlled substance schedule: III

Indications and Dosages

➤ *To control pain severe enough to require opioid treatment and for which alternative treatment options (i.e., nonopioid analgesics or opioid combination products) are inadequate or not tolerated*

I.V. OR I.M. INJECTION (BUPRENEX)

Adults and children age 13 and over. 0.3 mg every 6 hr or more, as needed. A second 0.3-mg dose may be given 30 to 60 min after first dose, if needed. I.V. injection given over at least 2 min.

DOSAGE ADJUSTMENT For patients not at high risk for opioid toxicity, I.M. dose increased to 0.6 mg or frequency increased to every 4 hr, if needed, depending on pain severity and patient response. For elderly or debilitated patients and patients who have respiratory disease or also use another CNS depressant, I.V. or I.M. dose reduced by half.

Children ages 2 to 12. 0.002 to 0.006 mg/kg every 4 to 6 hr, as needed.

➤ *To control severe chronic pain in patients requiring a continuous, around-the-clock opioid analgesic for an extended period of time for which alternative treatment options are inadequate*

TRANSDERMAL PATCH (BUTRANS)

Opioid-naïve adults and adults whose daily dose of oral morphine or equivalent was less than 30 mg. *Initial:* 5 mcg/hr, increased after 72 hr, as needed, to 10 mcg/hr. *Maximum:* 20 mcg/hr.

Adults whose daily dose of oral morphine or equivalent was between 30 and 80 mg.
Initial: Current around-the-clock opioid use tapered for up to 7 days to no more than 30 mg of morphine or equivalent per day. Then a 10 mcg/hr patch applied, increased after 72 hr, as needed, to 20 mcg/hr. *Maximum:* 20 mcg/hr.

BUCCAL FILM (BELBUCA)

Opioid-naïve adults and adults whose daily dose of oral morphine or equivalent was less than 30 mg. *Initial:* 75 mcg once daily, or if tolerated, every 12 hr for at least 4 days, then increased to 150 mcg every 12 hr. Then, dosage increased in increments of 150 mcg every 4 or more days, as needed. *Maximum:* 900 mcg every 12 hr.

Adults whose daily dose of oral morphine or equivalent was between 30 and 89 mg. *Initial:* 150 mcg every 12 hr, then increased in increments of 150 mcg every 4 or more days, as needed. *Maximum:* 900 mcg every 12 hr.

Adults whose daily dose of oral morphine or equivalent was between 90 and 160 mg. *Initial:* 300 mcg every 12 hr, then increased in increments of 150 mcg every 4 or more days, as needed. *Maximum:* 900 mcg every 12 hr.

DOSAGE ADJUSTMENT For patients with oral mucositis or severe hepatic impairment, initial dose and subsequent titrations, dosage decreased by half.

➤ *To treat opioid dependence*

SUBLINGUAL TABLETS (BUPRENORPHINE)

Adults. *Induction:* 8 mg daily on day 1 followed by 16 mg daily on days 2 to 4. *Maintenance:* 4 to 24 mg daily, with increases or decreases in 2- to 4-mg increments, as needed. *Maximum:* 24 mg daily.

➤ *To treat moderate to severe opioid use disorder in patients who have initiated treatment with a transmucosal buprenorphine-containing product, followed by dose adjustment for a minimum of seven days*

SUBCUTANEOUS INJECTION (SUBLOCADE)

Adults. 300 mg monthly for first 2 months followed by maintenance dose. *Maintenance:* 100 mg monthly. Maintenance dose may be increased to 300 mg monthly, if needed.

Route	Onset	Peak	Duration
I.V.	Under 15 min	Under 1 hr	6–10 hr*
I.M.	15 min	1 hr	6–10 hr*
Transdermal	Unknown	17 hr	Unknown
Sublingual	Unknown	1.40 hr	Unknown

* 4 to 5 hr in children ages 2 to 12.

Mechanism of Action

May bind with CNS receptors to alter the perception of and emotional response to pain. Buprenorphine may act by displacing narcotic agonists from their binding sites and competitively inhibiting their actions.

Incompatibilities

Don't give I.V. buprenorphine through the same I.V. line as diazepam or lorazepam.

Contraindications

Acute or severe bronchial asthma in an unmonitored setting or in the absence of resuscitative equipment, hypersensitivity to buprenorphine or its components, known or suspected GI obstruction including paralytic ileus, significant respiratory depression

Interactions

DRUGS

anticholinergic drugs: Increased risk of urinary retention and/or severe constipation that could lead to paralytic ileus
antimigraine agents, cyclobenzaprine; dextromethorphan; dolasetron; granisetron; linezolid; MAO inhibitors; methylene blue; ondansetron; palonosetron; selected psychiatric drugs such as amoxapine, buspirone, lithium, maprotiline, mirtazapine, nefazodone, trazodone, vilazodone; selective serotonin reuptake inhibitors; serotonin-norepinephrine reuptake inhibitors; St. John's wort; tricyclic antidepressants; tryptophan: Increased risk of serotonin syndrome
benzodiazepines, CNS depressants, other opioids, sedating antihistamines, tricyclic antidepressants: Increased risk of significant respiratory depression and other life-threatening adverse effects
CNS depressants, MAO inhibitors: Additive hypotensive and respiratory and CNS depressant effects of these drugs that may be life-threatening
opioid analgesics: Reduced therapeutic effects if buprenorphine is given before another opioid analgesic; possibly life-threatening adverse effects
serotonergic drugs: Increased risk of serotonin syndrome

Activities

alcohol use: Increased serum buprenorphine levels possibly resulting in fatal overdose owing to CNS and respiratory depression

Adverse Reactions

CNS: CNS depression, dizziness, headache, sedation, **seizures**, vertigo
CV: Bradycardia, hypertension, **hypotension**, **QT prolongation**
EENT: Miosis; *Sublingual form:* Burning mouth syndrome, glossitis, mucosal erythema, oral hypoesthesia, stomatitis
ENDO: Adrenal insufficiency (rare)
GI: Elevated liver enzymes or serum amylase level, **hepatitis**, **hepatotoxicity**, jaundice, nausea, spasm of the sphincter of Oddi, vomiting
GU: Androgen deficiency with chronic use, decreased libido, erectile dysfunction, impotency, infertility, lack of menstruation
RESP: Bronchospasm, **hypoventilation**, **respiratory depression**
SKIN: Diaphoresis, pruritus, rash, urticaria
Other: Anaphylaxis; angioedema; application-site inflammation, burns, discharge and vesicle occurrence; injection-site pain, redness, and swelling; physical and psychological dependence

Nursing Considerations

- Evaluate patient's risk for abuse and addiction prior to the start of buprenorphine therapy, as excessive use of drug may lead to abuse, addiction, misuse, overdose, and possibly death. Be prepared to monitor patient's intake throughout therapy. Because of the potential risks associated with buprenorphine therapy, be aware that the FDA now requires a Risk Evaluation and Mitigation Strategy (REMS) for buprenorphine use.
- Know that the transdermal patch should not be used in patients whose prior total daily dose of opioid use is greater than 80 mg of oral morphine equivalents per day because the maximum 20 mcg/hr dosage may not provide adequate analgesia. An alternate analgesic should be considered.
- Be aware that opioids like buprenorphine should not be given to women during pregnancy and labor and while breast feeding, as the newborn or infant may experience neonatal opioid withdrawal syndrome (NOWS). This syndrome may exhibit as excessive or high-pitched crying, poor feeding, rapid breathing, or trembling.

WARNING Be aware that opioid therapy like buprenorphine should only be used concomitantly with benzodiazepine therapy in patients for whom other treatment options are inadequate. If prescribed together, expect dosing and duration of the opioid to be limited. Monitor patient closely for signs and symptoms of decrease in consciousness, including coma, profound sedation, and significant respiratory depression. Notify prescriber immediately and provide emergency supportive care, as death may occur.

- Use buprenorphine cautiously in patients with adrenal insufficiency, alcohol withdrawal syndrome, acute alcoholism, biliary tract dysfunction, CNS depression, coma, hypothyroidism, kyphoscoliosis, myxedema, prostatic hypertrophy, psychosis, severe hepatic or renal impairment, toxic psychosis, or urethral stricture. Also use cautiously in patients who take a drug that decreases hepatic clearance, are known drug abusers, or have been addicted to opioids.
- Use drug cautiously in patients with head injury, intracranial lesions, or other conditions that could increase CSF pressure. Be particularly cautious when administering drug to patients with chronic obstructive pulmonary disease or cor pulmonale and in patients who have decreased respiratory reserve, hypoxia, hypercapnia, or preexisting respiratory depression.
- Be aware that Subutex trade name of buprenorphine should not be used to treat pain because of the risk of overdose in opioid-naïve patients.
- Know that to avoid causing withdrawal, drug shouldn't be given for opioid dependence until signs of withdrawal occur.
- Expect to obtain liver function tests prior to initiation of buprenorphine therapy and periodically throughout therapy because drug may cause hepatic dysfunction ranging from transient asymptomatic elevations in liver enzymes to hepatic failure and death. Acute hepatitis may also occur and, in some cases, require the drug to be discontinued, although in other cases even a dosage reduction of buprenorphine may not be needed. Monitor patient closely and report any signs and symptoms of hepatic dysfunction to prescriber.
- Know that an extended-release formulation (Sublocade) given as a subcutaneous injection monthly is available for patients who have initiated treatment with a transmucosal buprenorphine-containing product, followed by dose adjustment for a minimum of seven days. Administer drug subcutaneously into the abdomen. Administer only using the syringe and safety needle included with the product. Administer monthly with a minimum of 26 days between doses. If Sublocade is discontinued, monitor patient for several months for signs and symptoms of withdrawal and treat as prescribed.
- Remove subcutaneous form (Sublocade) from refrigerator at least 15 minutes prior to administration to allow drug to reach room temperature. Then remove the foil pouch and safety needle from the carton. Open pouch and remove the syringe. Check the solution, which should be colorless to yellow to amber. Attach the safety needle. Do not remove the plastic cover from the needle at this time. Choose an injection site on the patient's abdomen between the transpyloric and transtubercular planes that has adequate subcutaneous tissue that is free of excessive pigment, lesions, or nodules. Also, do not inject into an area where the skin is bruised, infected, irritated, reddened, or scarred in any way. Have patient assume a supine position. Clean injection site with an alcohol swab. To avoid irritation, rotate injection sites, which requires keeping a monthly log of sites used. Remove excess air from syringe and administer drug. Use a slow, steady push to inject the drug until all of the drug is given. Withdraw the needle, lock the needle guard, and discard the syringe.
- Know that the drug (Sublocade) may be removed from a subcutaneous site surgically under local anesthesia within 14 days of the injection. If removed, monitor patient for signs and symptoms of withdrawal and treat appropriately, as prescribed.
- Be aware that an implantable form of the drug (Probuphine) may be prescribed for a patient who has achieved and sustained prolonged clinical stability on low-to-moderate doses of a transmucosal buprenorphine-containing product (i.e., doses of no more than 8 mg/day). It is not appropriate for patients new to a

treatment program nor for those who have not achieved clinical stability. Because of the risks related to insertion and removal of the implant, the implant has restricted use.

- Give I.V. form over at least 2 minutes.
- Inspect injection site for local reactions; don't use the same site twice.
- Monitor vital signs and response to drug often, especially after giving first dose and if patient develops a fever. Be aware that drug may cause severe hypotension, including orthostatic hypotension and syncope in ambulatory patients.

WARNING **Monitor patient closely for respiratory depression, especially in cachectic, debilitated, or elderly patients; when initiating and titrating dosages; or when other drugs that depress respiration are given together. Report respiratory depression immediately, because respiratory arrest may occur. Be prepared to provide emergency supportive care.**

- Monitor patient with a seizure disorder, as buprenorphine may worsen seizure control.
- Assess elderly patients for signs and symptoms of toxicity or overdose, as these patients may be at increased risk because of decreased cardiac, hepatic, or renal function and the presence of concomitant disease and other drug therapy.

WARNING **Know that many drugs may interact with opioids like buprenorphine to cause serotonin syndrome. Monitor patient closely for signs and symptoms such as agitation, diaphoresis, diarrhea, fever, hallucinations, labile blood pressure, muscle twitching or stiffness, nausea, shakiness, shivering, tachycardia, trouble with coordination, or vomiting. Notify prescriber at once because serotonin syndrome may be life-threatening. Be prepared to discontinue drug, if possible and ordered, and provide supportive care.**

- Monitor patient for adrenal insufficiency. Although rare, this can be life-threatening. Monitor patient for anorexia, dizziness, fatigue, hypotension, nausea, vomiting, or weakness. Notify prescriber if adrenal insufficiency is suspected and expect diagnostic testing to be done to determine if present. If diagnosis is confirmed, expect to administer corticosteroids and wean patient off buprenorphine, if possible.
- Do not discontinue therapy abruptly when buprenorphine therapy is no longer needed. Instead, expect a gradual downward titration of the dose to prevent signs and symptoms of withdrawal.
- Be aware that dosage adjustments of buprenorpine may be required during pregnancy even if patient was stable prior to pregnancy. Monitor pregnant patient closely for signs and symptoms of withdrawal and expect dosage to be adjusted as needed.

PATIENT TEACHING

- Warn patient not to take more drug than prescribed and not to take it longer than absolutely needed, because excessive or prolonged use can lead to abuse, addiction, misuse, overdose, and possibly death.
- Advise patient that if a dose is missed, patient should take it as soon as it is remembered but if it is almost time for the next dose, the missed dose should be skipped and the next dose taken at the regular time. Dose should never be doubled to make up for a missed dose.

WARNING **Warn patient not to consume alcohol or take benzodiazepines or other CNS depressants including other opioids, during buprenorphine therapy without prescriber knowledge, as severe respiratory depression can occur that may lead to death.**

WARNING **Inform patient about potentially fatal additive effects of combining buprenorphine with benzodiazepines or other opioids. Instruct patient to inform all prescribers of buprenorphine use.**

- Explain that buprenorphine may be habit forming. Urge her to notify prescriber if she develops any unusual or persistent symptoms.
- Instruct patient taking sublingual form to place tablets under her tongue until they dissolve. If patient takes more than two tablets per dose, tell her to place all tablets under her tongue at the same time. If they won't fit, tell her to place two at a time under her tongue until full dose has dissolved. Caution against swallowing tablets.
- Instruct patient prescribed the transdermal patch to place patch only on intact skin that is hairless and clean (washed with water only) and dry. If a hairless site is not

available, instruct patient to clip, not shave, area prior to application. Emphasize importance of not applying patch to irritated skin. Inform patient patch must be applied immediately after its removal from pouch and placed on her upper outer arm, upper back, upper chest, or the side of her chest. Tell patient patch is to be worn for 7 days and that she should not cut the patch. If problems with adhesion occur, she may tape the edges of the patch with first-aid tape. If the patch should fall off during the 7-day interval, tell her to dispose of the patch and apply a new one at a different skin site. When removing the patch, tell patient to fold it over on itself and flush it down the toilet or seal it in the patch disposal unit provided and dispose of in the trash.

- Instruct patient prescribed the buccal film form to first use his tongue to wet the inside of his cheek or rinse his mouth with water to wet the area. Then, he should place the yellow side of the film against the inside of his cheek after immediately removing it from the package and using clean, dry fingers, hold it in place for 5 seconds following which the film should be left in place until fully dissolved, usually within 30 minutes. Doing this time he should not manipulate the film with his tongue or fingers nor should he eat or drink anything until the film has dissolved. Remind patient to dispose of unused film by removing from the foil packages and flush down the toilet. Discard foil packaging in the trash. He should not flush the drug down the toilet in the foil package.
- Tell patient receiving the drug as an extended-release subcutaneous injection that a lump may appear at injection site and last for several weeks. Tell patient not to massage or rub the injection site and to be careful of the placement of any belts or clothing waistbands so as not to irritate the site.
- Caution patient to keep drug, including patch form, out of the reach of others, especially children, as exposure to even one dose or patch could be fatal.
- Inform patient wearing a buprenorphine patch not to expose it to any external heat source such as heating pads, electric blankets, heat lamps, saunas, heated water beds or hot tubs, as absorption may be affected.
- Warn patient not to stop taking drug abruptly.
- Advise patient to get up slowly from a lying or sitting position to avoid a sudden drop in blood pressure.
- Caution patient to avoid hazardous activities while receiving buprenorphine.
- Instruct patient not to drink alcohol or take CNS depressants or sleep aids without checking with prescriber first.
- Inform patient that long-term use of opioids like buprenorphine may decrease sex hormone levels causing decreased libido, erectile dysfunction, impotence, infertility, or lack of menstruation. Encourage patient to report any such symptoms.
- Advise patient to report any persistent, severe, or unusual signs and symptoms to prescriber.
- Advise patient to keep buprenorphine in a safe place and to protect it from theft because of it being an opioid.
- Advise patient to notify prescriber if she becomes pregnant or is breastfeeding, as drug may have to be discontinued or dosage altered. Also tell mothers who are taking buprenorphine while breastfeeding to monitor their infant for breathing difficulties and increased drowsiness. If present, tell patient to stop breastfeeding and notify prescriber.
- Alert patient that chronic use of opioids such as buprenorphine may result in reduced fertility.

bupropion hydrobromide

Aplenzin

bupropion hydrochloride

Forfivo XL, Wellbutrin, Wellbutrin SR, Wellbutrin XL, Zyban

Class and Category

Pharmacologic class: Aminoketone
Therapeutic class: Antidepressant, smoking cessation adjunct
Pregnancy category: C

Indications and Dosages

➤ *To treat depression*

E.R. TABLETS (WELLBUTRIN SR)

Adults. *Initial:* 150 mg daily in morning for 3 days; then 150 mg twice daily with at least 8 hr between successive doses and, after several wk, 200 mg twice daily, as needed and tolerated. *Maximum:* 400 mg daily, given as 200 mg twice daily. Single doses should not exceed 200 mg/dose.

E.R. TABLETS (WELLBUTRIN XL)

Adults. *Initial:* 150 mg daily in morning for 4 days; then 300 mg daily and, after 4 wk, 450 mg daily, as needed and tolerated. *Maximum:* 450 mg daily.

E.R. TABLETS (APLENZIN)

Adults. *Initial:* 174 mg daily in the morning for 4 days. Then, if tolerated well, dosage increased to 348 mg daily in the morning. After 4 wk of therapy, dosage increased to 522 mg daily in the morning, if needed.

E.R. TABLETS (FORFIVO XL)

Adults already treated with a bupropion product. 450 mg once daily.

TABLETS (WELLBUTRIN)

Adults. *Initial:* 100 mg twice daily, increased after 3 or more days to 100 mg three times daily with at least 6 hr between successive doses, as needed. *Maximum:* 450 mg daily or 150 mg/dose.

➤ *To aid in smoking cessation*

E.R. TABLETS (ZYBAN)

Adults. *Initial:* 150 mg daily for 3 days and then 150 mg twice daily with at least 8 hr between each dose for 7 to 12 wk. *Maximum:* 300 mg daily or 150 mg/dose.

➤ *To prevent seasonal major depressive episodes in patient with seasonal affective disorder*

E.R. TABLETS (WELLBUTRIN XL)

Adults. *Initial:* 150 mg once daily in morning starting in autumn, increased after 1 wk to 300 mg once daily in morning, if tolerated and needed. Decreased to 150 mg once daily 2 wk before stopping in early spring.

E.R. TABLETS (APLENZIN)

Adults. *Initial:* 174 mg once daily in morning starting in autumn, increased after 1 wk to 348 mg once daily in morning, if tolerated and needed. Decreased to 174 mg once daily 2 wk before stopping in early spring.

DOSAGE ADJUSTMENT For patients with severe hepatic cirrhosis, no more than 75 mg daily of Wellbutrin, 100 mg daily or 150 mg every other day of Wellbutrin SR, 150 mg every other day of Wellbutrin XL or Zyban, and 174 mg every other day of Aplenzin. In renal impairment, dosage or frequency decreased on an individual basis.

Route	Onset	Peak	Duration
P.O.	1–3 wk	Unknown	Unknown

Mechanism of Action

May inhibit dopamine, norepinephrine, and serotonin uptake by neurons, which significantly relieves evidence of depression.

Contraindications

Hypersensitivity to bupropion or its components, seizure disorder or conditions that increase risk of seizures (i.e., abrupt discontinuation of alcohol, antiepileptic drugs, barbiturates or benzodiazepines; anorexia nervosa; bulimia; use within 14 days of a MAO inhibitor (MAOI) including reversible MAOIs such as linezolid or intravenous methylene blue; use of another form of bupropion concurrently

Interactions

DRUGS

amantadine, levodopa: Increased CNS adverse reactions to bupropion, antidepressants, antipsychotics, *concurrent use of other bupropion products, systemic corticosteroids, theophylline:* Increased risk of seizures

carbamazepine, phenobarbital, phenytoin: Increased bupropion metabolism

CYP2B6 inducers such as efavirenz, lopinavir, ritonavir: Possibly decreased bupropion exposure and subsequent effectiveness

CYP2B6 inhibitors such as clopidogrel, ticlopidine: Possibly increased bupropion exposure and risk of adverse reactions

drugs metabolized by CYP2D6 such as certain antidepressants (i.e. desipramine, fluoxetine, imipramine, nortriptyline, paroxetine, sertraline, venlafaxine). antipsychotics (i.e. haloperidol, risperidone, thioridazine), beta blockers (i.e. metoprolol), type IC antiarrhythmics (i.e. flecainide, propafenone): Increased blood exposure of these drugs and risk of adverse reactions

MAO inhibitors including reversible MAOIs such as linezolid and intravenous methylene blue: Increased risk of acute bupropion toxicity and serious hypertensive reactions
nicotine: Possibly increased blood pressure
tamoxifen: Possibly reduced effectiveness of tamoxifen

ACTIVITIES

alcohol use, recreational drug abuse: Possible rare adverse neuropsychiatric events; reduced alcohol tolerance

Adverse Reactions

CNS: Abnormal coordination, abnormal EEG, aggression, agitation, akathisia, akinesia, anxiety, aphasia, asthenia, CNS stimulation, **coma**, confusion, **CVA**, decreased concentration or memory, delirium, delusions, depersonalization, depression, dizziness, dream abnormalities, emotional lability, euphoria, extrapyramidal syndrome, fever, general or migraine headache, hallucinations, **homicidal ideation**, hostility, hyperkinesia, hypertonia, hyperesthesia, insomnia, irritability, mania, nervousness, neuralgia, neuropathy, panic, paranoia, paresthesia, parkinsonism, psychosis and other neuropsychiatric reactions, restlessness, **seizures**, sleep disorder, somnolence, **suicidal ideation**, syncope, tremor, unmasking tardive dyskinesia, vertigo
CV: **Arrhythmias**, chest pain, **complete AV block**, **extrasystoles**, hypertension, **MI**, orthostatic hypotension, palpitations, phlebitis, tachycardia, vasodilation
EENT: Acute-angle glaucoma, altered taste, amblyopia, blurred vision, dry mouth, gum hemorrhage, hearing loss, increased ocular pressure, increased salivation, mydriasis, pharyngitis, sinusitis, taste perversion, tinnitus
ENDO: Hyperglycemia, **hypoglycemia**, syndrome of inappropriate ADH secretion
GI: Abdominal pain, anorexia, colitis, constipation, diarrhea, dysphagia, esophagitis, flatulence, **GI hemorrhage**, GI ulceration, **hepatic dysfunction**, **hepatitis**, increased appetite, **intestinal perforation**, nausea, **pancreatitis**, vomiting
GU: Abnormal ejaculation, cystitis, decreased or increased libido, dyspareunia, dysuria, incontinence, painful erection, prostate disorder, salpingitis, urinary frequency and urgency, UTI, vaginal hemorrhage, vaginitis
HEME: Anemia, leukocytosis, **leukopenia**, lymphadenopathy, **pancytopenia**, **thrombocytopenia**
MS: Arthralgia; arthritis; muscle rigidity, twitching, and weakness; myalgia; **rhabdomyolysis**
RESP: **Bronchospasm**, cough, dyspnea, pneumonia, **pulmonary embolism**
SKIN: Alopecia, diaphoresis, **erythema multiforme**, **exfoliative dermatitis**, flushing, hirsutism, pruritus, rash, **Stevens–Johnson syndrome**, urticaria
Other: **Anaphylaxis**, **angioedema**, generalized pain, hot flashes, **hyponatremia**, infection, serum sickness–like reaction, weight loss

Nursing Considerations

- Know that certain forms of bupropion are not approved for smoking cessation treatment, such as Aplenzin, Forfivo XL, Wellbutrin SR, and Wellbutrin XL
- Be aware that Forfivo XL should not be used in patients with hepatic or renal impairment because the only dosage available for Forfivo XL is 450 mg once daily, which may be too high a dose for the liver or kidneys to handle.
- Use cautiously in patients with renal impairment (all other brands); drug is excreted by kidneys.
- Know that Forfivo XL should never be used to initiate treatment of depression because the dose is too high. Only after the patient has received other bupropion products first and then requires a 450-mg dose should Forfivo XL be used.
- Assess patient's blood pressure before bupropion therapy begins and monitor periodically during therapy because bupropion may cause hypertension.
- Monitor depressed patients closely for worsened depression and increased suicide risk, especially when therapy starts or dosage changes.
- Monitor patient taking bupropion to stop smoking for neuropsychiatric symptoms. If present, notify prescriber immediately, begin safety measures, and expect to discontinue drug.

WARNING **Monitor patient for seizures. To reduce seizure risk, allow at least 4 hours (tablets) or 8 hours (E.R. tablets) between doses. Know that maximum dosage should not be exceeded and dosage reduction should be gradual because risk of seizures is dose-related.**

- Use seizure precautions, especially in patients who are addicted to cocaine, opioids, or stimulants; have a history of CNS tumors, head trauma, or seizures; have hyponatremia, hypoxia, or severe hepatic cirrhosis; take drugs that lower the seizure threshold; take insulin or an oral antidiabetic; take OTC stimulants or anorectics; or use excessive alcohol, benzodiazepines, hypnotics, or sedatives.
- Know that using transdermal nicotine with bupropion may cause hypertension. Watch closely.

PATIENT TEACHING

- Advise patient to take bupropion for 7 or more days before stopping smoking.
- Tell patient to swallow E.R. tablets whole and not to cut, crush, or chew them.
- Tell patient to take bupropion with food and to store tablets at room temperature while keeping tablets dry and out of the light.
- Urge patient to avoid or minimize consuming alcohol and sedatives during therapy and not to stop drug abruptly or exceed dosage prescribed because seizures may occur.

WARNING **Advise patient to seek medical help immediately and stop taking drug if signs of rash, itching, hives, chest pain, shortness of breath, or swelling, especially of face, occurs.**

- Urge caregivers to monitor depressed patient closely for worsened depression, especially when therapy starts or dosage changes. Also inform caregiver that drug may cause a variety of neuropsychiatric adverse events that could be serious. If changes in behavior or thought patterns emerge with bupropion use, instruct caregiver to notify prescriber immediately.
- Alert patient that drug may cause mild pupillary dilation, which can lead to an episode of acute-closure glaucoma. Encourage him to have an eye exam to determine if he is susceptible to angle closure.
- Warn patient taking bupropion for smoking cessation by explaining that it may cause serious adverse effects, including suicidal thoughts and behavior. If present, patient should notify prescriber immediately and expect to discontinue drug.
- Alert patient that bupropion therapy may produce a false-positive urine screening test for amphetamines even after drug has been discontinued. Other tests may be required to distinguish bupropion from amphetamines.

buspirone hydrochloride

Bustab (CAN)

Class and Category

Pharmacologic class: Azaspirone
Therapeutic class: Anxiolytic
Pregnancy category: B

Indications and Dosages

➤ *To manage anxiety*

TABLETS

Adults. *Initial:* 7.5 mg twice daily increased by 5 mg daily at 2- to 3-day intervals until desired response occurs. *Maintenance:* 20 to 30 mg daily (usual therapeutic range). *Maximum:* 60 mg daily.

DOSAGE ADJUSTMENT When used with nefazodone, dosage decreased to 2.5 mg daily.

Route	Onset	Peak	Duration
P.O.	1–4 wk	3–6 wk	Unknown

Mechanism of Action

May act as a partial agonist at serotonin 5-hydroxytryptamine$_{1A}$ receptors in the brain, producing antianxiety effects.

Contraindications

Hypersensitivity to buspirone or its components, severe hepatic or renal impairment

Interactions

DRUGS

CYP3A4 inducers, such as certain anticonvulsants (carbamazepine, phenobarbital, phenytoin) and

dexamethasone: Possibly increased rate of buspirone metabolism and decreased effectiveness of buspirone
CYP3A4 inhibitors, such as ketoconazole and ritonavir: Possibly inhibited buspirone metabolism and increased blood level of buspirone
diltiazem, erythromycin, itraconazole, nefazodone, nordiazepam, verapamil: Increased blood level and adverse effects of buspirone
haloperidol: Increased haloperidol level
MAO inhibitors: Increased risk of hypertension
rifampin: Decreased blood buspirone level and pharmacodynamic effects

FOODS

any food: Possibly decreased buspirone clearance
grapefruit juice: Increased blood buspirone level

Adverse Reactions

CNS: Akathisia, anger, ataxia, cogwheel rigidity, confusion, decreased concentration, depression, dizziness, dream disturbances, drowsiness, dyskinesias, dystonia, excitement, extrapyramidal symptoms, fatigue, headache, hostility, insomnia, lack of coordination, light-headedness, mood swings, nervousness, paresthesia, Parkinsonism, restless leg syndrome, restlessness, **serotonin syndrome**, transient recall impairment, tremor, weakness
CV: Chest pain, palpitations, tachycardia
EENT: Blurred vision, dry mouth, nasal congestion, pharyngitis, tinnitus, tunnel vision
GI: Abdominal or gastric distress, constipation, diarrhea, nausea, vomiting
GU: Urine retention
MS: Myalgia
SKIN: Diaphoresis, ecchymosis, rash, urticaria
Other: Angioedema

Nursing Considerations

- Use buspirone cautiously in patients with hepatic or renal impairment.
- Institute safety precautions because of possible adverse CNS reactions.
- Follow closely if patient is being withdrawn from long-term therapy with benzodiazepines or other sedative-hypnotic drugs while starting buspirone because buspirone won't prevent withdrawal symptoms.

PATIENT TEACHING

- Advise patient to take buspirone consistently, either always with or always without food.
- Caution patient to avoid drinking large amounts of grapefruit juice.
- Inform patient that 1 to 2 weeks of therapy may be needed before she notices drug's antianxiety effect.
- Emphasize the importance of not taking more buspirone than prescribed.
- Advise patient to avoid hazardous activities until drug's CNS effects are known.

butorphanol tartrate

Class, Category, and Schedule

Pharmacologic class: Opioid agonist-antagonist
Therapeutic class: Anesthesia adjunct, opioid analgesic
Pregnancy category: C
Controlled substance schedule: IV

Indications and Dosages

➤ *To manage pain*

I.V. INJECTION

Adults. 0.5 to 2 mg (usually 1 mg) every 3 to 4 hr, as needed.

I.M. INJECTION

Adults. 1 to 4 mg (usually 2 mg) every 3 to 4 hr, as needed. *Maximum:* 4 mg/single dose.

NASAL INHALATION

Adults. 1 spray (1 mg) in one nostril. Dose repeated after 60 to 90 min, as needed; two-dose sequence repeated every 3 to 4 hr, as needed. For severe pain, 2 sprays (1 in each nostril) every 3 to 4 hr, as needed.

DOSAGE ADJUSTMENT Dose reduced to 1 spray in one nostril for elderly patients and those with impaired hepatic or renal function. Dose repeated after 90 to 120 min, as needed; two-dose sequence repeated every 6 hr or more, as needed.

➤ *As adjunct to provide preoperative anesthesia*

I.M. INJECTION
Adults. Individualized. *Usual:* 2 mg 60 to 90 min before surgery.
➤ *As adjunct to provide anesthesia*
I.V. INJECTION
Adults. Individualized. *Usual:* 1 to 4 mg and then supplemental doses of 0.5 to 1 mg, as needed. Total usually required during surgery is 60 to 180 mcg/kg.
DOSAGE ADJUSTMENT For elderly patients and patients with impaired hepatic or renal function, initial parenteral dose kept at 1 mg followed, if needed, by 1 mg in 90 to 120 min and dosage interval for subsequent doses increased to at least 6 hr or more.

Route	Onset	Peak	Duration
I.V.	2–3 min	30 min	2–4 hr
I.M.	10–30 min	30–60 min	3–4 hr
Inhalation	In 15 min	1–2 hr	4–5 hr

Mechanism of Action
Binds with specific CNS receptors to alter the perception of and emotional response to pain.

Contraindications
Acute or severe bronchial asthma in an unmonitored setting or in the absence of resuscitative equipment; GI obstruction, including paralytic ileus; hypersensitivity to butorphanol or its components (including the preservative benzethonium chloride)

Interactions
DRUGS
CNS depressants: Additive CNS depression that can be significant, causing coma, prolonged sedation, or significant respiratory depression
Nasal vasoconstrictors, such as oxymetazoline: Decreased absorption rate and delayed onset of butorphanol
serotonergic drugs: Increased risk of serotonin syndrome
ACTIVITIES
alcohol use: Additive CNS depression that could be significant

Adverse Reactions
CNS: Anxiety, confusion, difficulty making purposeful movements, difficulty speaking, dizziness, euphoria, floating feeling, headache, insomnia (with nasal form), lethargy, nervousness, paresthesia, sensation of heat, somnolence, syncope, tremor, vertigo
CV: Chest pain, **hypotension**, palpitations, tachycardia, vasodilation
EENT: Blurred vision, dry mouth, ear pain, epistaxis, nasal congestion or irritation (with nasal form), pharyngitis, rhinitis, sinus congestion, sinusitis, tinnitus, unpleasant taste
GI: Anorexia, constipation, epigastric pain, nausea, vomiting
RESP: **Apnea**, bronchitis, cough, dyspnea, **respiratory depression**, **shallow breathing**, upper respiratory tract infection
SKIN: Clammy skin, pruritus

Nursing Considerations
- Know that butorphanol should be used cautiously, if at all, in patients with depression, suicidal tendency, history of drug abuse, or hepatic or renal dysfunction.
- Use it cautiously, if at all, in patients with head injury because drug can raise CSF pressure. Because it can increase cardiac workload, use with extreme caution in patients with acute MI, ventricular dysfunction, or coronary insufficiency.
- Be aware that butorphanol has a high potential for abuse.
- Monitor patient after first dose of nasal form; hypotension and syncope may occur.
- Take safety precautions because butorphanol causes CNS depression.
- Assess respiratory status closely because drug causes respiratory depression.
- Monitor blood pressure often after giving drug. If severe hypertension develops (rare), stop drug at once and notify prescriber. If patient isn't narcotic-dependent, expect to administer naloxone to reverse butorphanol's effects.

PATIENT TEACHING
- Emphasize the importance of taking butorphanol exactly as prescribed because it can be addictive. Warn patient not to increase the dose or decrease the dosage interval without consulting prescriber.
- Advise patient to avoid hazardous activities until drug's CNS effects are known.
- Tell patient to avoid alcohol and other CNS depressants, including OTC drugs,

while taking butorphanol because of additive adverse CNS reactions.

- Teach patient how to use nasal form properly by giving these instructions: After blowing nose to clear the nostrils, pull clear cover from the pump unit and remove protective clip from its neck. Prime pump unit by placing the nozzle between first and second fingers with thumb on the bottom of the bottle. Then pump sprayer unit firmly and quickly until a fine spray appears (7 or 8 strokes). Insert spray tip about 1 cm (one-third inch) into one nostril, pointing tip toward the back of the nose. Close other nostril with one finger and tilt head slightly forward. Then pump sprayer firmly and quickly by pushing down on the pump unit's finger grips and against the thumb at the bottom of the bottle. Sniff gently with mouth closed. After spraying, remove pump from nose, tilt head back, and sniff gently for a few more seconds. Then replace protective clip and clear cover.

C

cabergoline

Class and Category
Pharmacologic class: Dopamine agonist
Therapeutic class: Antihyperprolactinemic
Pregnancy category: B

Indications and Dosages
➤ ***To treat idiopathic or pituitary adenoma-induced hyperprolactinemic disorders***

TABLETS

Adults. 0.25 mg twice/wk. Increased by 0.25 mg/wk at 4-wk intervals, if needed, up to 1 mg twice/wk.

Route	Onset	Peak	Duration
P.O.	Unknown	48 hr	Up to 14 days

Mechanism of Action
Binds with dopamine D_2 receptors to block prolactin synthesis and secretion by the anterior pituitary gland, thereby reducing the serum prolactin level.

Contraindications
History of cardiac valvular, pericardial, pulmonary, or retroperitoneal fibrotic disorders; hypersensitivity to cabergoline, ergot derivatives, or their components; uncontrolled hypertension

Interactions
DRUGS

antihypertensives: Increased risk of hypotension
dopamine antagonists (butyrophenones, metoclopramide, phenothiazines, or thioxanthenes): Decreased cabergoline effectiveness

Adverse Reactions
CNS: Aggression, asthenia, depression, fatigue, headache, nervousness, paresthesia, somnolence, psychotic disorder, vertigo
CV: Orthostatic hypotension, **valvulopathy**
EENT: Dry mouth
ENDO: Breast pain
GI: Abdominal pain, constipation, diarrhea, flatulence, indigestion, nausea, vomiting
GU: Dysmenorrhea, increased libido
RESP: Pulmonary effusion, **pulmonary fibrosis**
SKIN: Alopecia
Other: Extracardiac fibrotic reactions, pathological gambling behavior

Nursing Considerations
- Ensure that patient has undergone a cardiovascular evaluation, including an echocardiogram to determine the presence of valvular disease prior to administering cabergoline because the presence of valvular disease is a contraindication to the use of cabergoline therapy.
- Obtain a chest x-ray, an erythrocyte sedimentation rate, and serum creatinine measurement, as ordered, prior to initiating cabergoline therapy and repeat during therapy if the patient develops any signs and symptoms of an extracardiac fibrotic reaction.
- Check serum prolactin level to assess cabergoline's effectiveness before each dose increase.
- Know that if patient has moderate to severe hepatic impairment, monitor closely for adverse reactions because of decreased cabergoline metabolism.
- Expect patient who takes cabergoline long term to undergo periodic reassessment of cardiac status, including echocardiography, because valvulopathy can occur with prolonged cabergoline use.
- Monitor erythrocyte sedimentation rate, as it may increase in a patient with pleural effusion or pleural fibrosis.

WARNING **Monitor patient for evidence of overdose, such as hallucinations, light-headedness, nasal congestion, syncope, and tachycardia. If present, prescribe and treat as ordered.**

PATIENT TEACHING

- Urge patient to read and follow printed information that explains how to use cabergoline for best therapeutic results.
- Advise patient to take drug with meals to help decrease GI distress.
- Tell patient to take a missed dose as soon as possible within 1 to 2 days. If missed dose isn't remembered until it's time for the next dose, instruct him to double the

dose if drug is generally well tolerated and doesn't cause nausea. If drug isn't well tolerated, instruct patient to consult prescriber before taking the missed dose.

- Urge patient to change positions slowly to avoid orthostatic hypotension. Tell him to notify prescriber if it occurs.
- Urge patient to keep regular appointments to monitor drug effectiveness.
- Advise patient that drug therapy will end when serum prolactin level is normal for 6 months. Explain that he'll need periodic monitoring to determine whether therapy should resume.
- Tell female patient of childbearing age to notify prescriber if she is, could be, or plans to become pregnant during therapy; drug may need to be discontinued.
- Caution patient to avoid gambling during therapy because drug may increase the risk of pathological gambling behaviors.

calcitonin, salmon

Calcimar (CAN), Fortical, Miacalcin

Class and Category

Pharmacologic class: Hormone
Therapeutic class: Antihypercalcemic, anti-osteoporitic
Pregnancy category: C

Indications and Dosages

➤ *To treat an early hypercalcemic emergency*

I.M. OR SUBCUTANEOUS INJECTION (MIACALCIN)
Adults. *Initial:* 4 international units/kg every 12 hr. Increased after 1 or 2 days, if needed, to 8 international units/kg every 12 hr. *Maximum:* 8 international units/kg every 6 hr.

➤ *To treat postmenopausal osteoporosis in women who are at least 5 years postmenopausal*

I.M. OR SUBCUTANEOUS INJECTION (MIACALCIN)
Adults. *Initial:* 100 international units daily.

NASAL SPRAY (FORTICAL)
Adults. 200 international units (1 spray) daily, alternating nostrils.

➤ *To treat Paget's disease of the bone*

I.M. OR SUBCUTANEOUS INJECTION (MIACALCIN)
Adults. *Initial:* 100 international units daily.

Route	Onset	Peak	Duration
I.M., SubQ	In 15 min*	2 hr†	6–8 hr†
Nasal spray	10 min	Unknown	Unknown

* For hypercalcemia; 6 to 24 mo for Paget's disease.
† For hypercalcemia; unknown for other indications.

Mechanism of Action

Directly inhibits bone resorption. Besides reducing the serum calcium level, this action slows bone metabolism (a major factor in the development of Paget's disease) and calcium loss from the bone (a major factor in the development of osteoporosis).

Contraindications

Hypersensitivity to calcitonin salmon or its components

Interactions

DRUGS
lithium: Possibly decreased lithium level

Adverse Reactions

CNS: Agitation, anxiety, **CVA**, dizziness, fatigue, headache, insomnia, neuralgia, paresthesia, tremor, vertigo
CV: Bundle branch block, hypertension, **MI**, palpitations, peripheral edema, tachycardia, thrombophlebitis
EENT: Blurred vision; dry mouth; earache; epistaxis; eye pain; hearing loss; nasal irritation or ulceration (nasal spray), lesions, or redness; pharyngitis; rhinitis; salty taste; sinusitis; taste perversion; tinnitus; vitreous floaters
ENDO: Goiter, hyperthyroidism
GI: Abdominal pain, anorexia, cholelithiasis, diarrhea, epigastric discomfort, flatulence, gastritis, **hepatitis**, increased appetite, nausea, thirst, vomiting
GU: Hematuria, nocturia, polyuria, **pyelonephritis**, renal calculi
HEME: Anemia
MS: Arthralgia, arthrosis, back or muscloskeletal pain, joint stiffness, polymyalgia rheumatica
RESP: Bronchitis, **bronchospasm**, cough, dyspnea, pneumonia, upper respiratory tract infection

SKIN: Alopecia, diaphoresis, eczema, flushing of face or hands, pruritus of earlobes, rash, ulceration, urticaria
Other: **Anaphylaxis**, **anaphylactic shock**, **angioedema**, antibody formation, feverish sensation, **hypocalcemia**, influenza-like symptoms, injection-site inflammation, lymphadenopathy, **malignancies**, mild tetanic symptoms

Nursing Considerations

- Expect to perform a skin test before giving drug if sensitivity to drug is suspected. Prepare a mixture of 10 international units/ml by withdrawing 0.05 ml from a 200-international unit solution in a tuberculin syringe and filling the syringe to 1 ml with sodium chloride for injection. Mix well, discard 0.9 ml, and inject 0.1 ml intradermally on the inner forearm. Observe the site for 15 minutes after injection. If you detect evidence of sensitivity, such as more than mild erythema or a wheal, notify prescriber.

WARNING Monitor all patients for hypersensitivity reactions, which could be severe. Have appropriate equipment and drugs present to treat a hypersensitivity reaction if it occurs. Notify prescriber, expect drug to be discontinued, and provide supportive care, as directed by prescriber.

- Monitor serum calcium level, as ordered, if patient receives calcitonin for hypercalcemia. During first several doses, keep parenteral calcium available in case the calcium level is inadvertently overcorrected.
- Know that if prescribed calcitonin dose exceeds 2 ml, expect to use I.M. route and multiple injection sites.
- Know that for patient receiving calcitonin for postmenopausal osteoporosis, know that hypocalcemia and other mineral metabolism disorders, such as vitamin D deficiency, must be corrected before calcitonin therapy begins. These patients should also be monitored during therapy for signs and symptoms of hypocalcemia such as muscle cramps, twitching, and seizures. Also, expect to give 1.5 g of supplemental calcium carbonate and at least 400 units of vitamin D daily. Plan to provide a balanced diet that includes foods high in calcium and vitamin D.
- Periodically examine patient using nasal spray for nasal ulcers. If severe ulceration of the nasal mucosa occurs (ulcers greater than 1.5 mm, ulcers penetrating below the mucosa, or ulcers causing heavy bleeding), notify prescriber and expect nasal spray form to be discontinued. Also, know that nasal spray should be discontinued for smaller or less severe ulcers until healing occurs.
- Assess for nausea, especially with the first dose. Nausea tends to decrease or disappear with continued use.
- Be aware if patient with Paget's disease relapses after treatment, check for antibody formation, as ordered.

PATIENT TEACHING

- Tell patient to refrigerate injection or unopened nasal spray container.
- Teach patient to self-administer injections.
- Be aware that if patient has postmenopausal osteoporosis, teach her about dietary needs, including foods rich in calcium and vitamin D.
- Teach patient how to administer nasal spray, if ordered. Explain how to activate nasal pump by holding the bottle upright and depressing two white side arms toward the bottle six times. When bottle emits a faint spray, pump is activated. Tell patient to store activated nasal pump upright at room temperature and to discard it after 30 days.
- Instruct patient to place nozzle firmly into one nostril while holding head upright. Tell her to then depress the pump toward the bottle.
- Remind patient that she doesn't need to reactivate the pump before each dose.
- Instruct patient to report nasal symptoms to prescriber.

calcitriol (1,25-dihydroxy-cholecalciferol)

Calcijex, Rocaltrol

Class and Category

Pharmacologic class: Vitamin D analogue
Therapeutic class: Antihypocalcemic
Pregnancy category: C

Indications and Dosages

➤ *To treat hypocalcemia in dialysis patients*

CAPSULES, ORAL SOLUTION (ROCALTROL)

Adults. *Initial:* 0.25 mcg daily. Increased by 0.25 mcg daily every 4 to 8 wk, if needed to achieve normal serum calcium level. *Maintenance:* 0.5 to 1 mcg daily.

I.V. INJECTION (CALCIJEX)

Adults. *Initial:* 0.5 mcg every other day, 3 times wk given rapidly at end of dialysis. Increased by 0.25 mcg to 0.5 mcg at 2- to 4-wk intervals, if needed. *Usual:* 0.5 mcg to 3 mcg 3 times a wk.

➤ *To treat hypocalcemia in predialysis patients*

CAPSULES, ORAL SOLUTION (ROCALTROL)

Adults and children age 3 and over. *Initial:* 0.25 mcg daily. Increased after 4 to 8 wk, if needed, to 0.5 mcg daily.

ORAL SOLUTION

Children up to age 3. 10 to 15 ng/kg daily.

➤ *To treat hypoparathyroidism*

CAPSULES, ORAL SOLUTION (ROCALTROL)

Adults and children age 6 and over. *Initial:* 0.25 mcg daily in the morning. Increased every 2 to 4 wk, if needed, to achieve normal serum calcium level. *Usual:* 0.5 to 2 mcg daily.
Children ages 1 to 5. 0.25 to 0.75 mcg daily in the morning.

Route	Onset	Peak	Duration
I.V.	Unknown	Unknown	3–5 days
P.O.	2–6 hr	10 hr	3–5 days

Mechanism of Action

Binds to specific receptors on intestinal mucosa to increase calcium absorption from intestine. Drug may also regulate calcium ion transfer from bone to blood and stimulate calcium reabsorption in the distal renal tubules, making more calcium available in the body.

Contraindications

Hypercalcemia, hypersensitivity to calcitriol or its components, vitamin D toxicity

Interactions

DRUGS

calcium supplements: Increased risk of hypercalcemia
cholestyramine: Decreased calcitriol absorption
corticosteroids: Possibly inhibits calcium absorption
digitalis glycosides: Possibly arrhythmias
ketoconazole: Decreased calcitriol level
magnesium-containing antacids (I.V. form): Hypermagnesemia
mineral oil: Decreased blood calcitriol level (with prolonged use of mineral oil)
phenobarbital, phenytoin: Decreased synthesis and blood level of calcitriol
phosphate-binding agents: Possibly altered phosphate transport in bone, intestine, and kidneys
thiazide diuretics: Hypercalcemia
vitamin D: Additive effects, including possible hypercalcemia

Adverse Reactions

SKIN: **Erythema multiforme**, lip swelling, pruritus, rash, urticaria
Other: Anaphylaxis

Nursing Considerations

- Check to be sure patient receives enough calcium.
- Store drug at room temperature, and protect from heat and direct light.
- Monitor patient closely. In high-dose or long-term calcitriol therapy, be alert for vitamin D toxicity. Early evidence includes abdominal or bone pain, constipation, dry mouth, headache, metallic taste, myalgia, nausea, somnolence, vomiting, and weakness. Late evidence includes albuminuria, anorexia, arrhythmias, azotemia, conjunctivitis (calcific), decreased libido, elevated AST and ALT levels, elevated BUN level, vascular calcification, hypercholesterolemia, hypertension, hyperthermia, irritability, mild acidosis, nephrocalcinosis, nocturia, pancreatitis, photophobia, polydipsia, polyuria, pruritus, rhinorrhea, and weight loss.

PATIENT TEACHING

- Warn patient not to take other forms of vitamin D while taking calcitriol.
- Instruct patient to take a missed dose as soon as possible.
- Advise patient to notify prescriber immediately about possible toxicity, such as headache, irritability, nausea, photophobia, vomiting, weakness, and weight loss.

calcium acetate

Calphron, Eliphos, PhosLo, Phoslyra

calcium carbonate

Apo-Cal (CAN), Calci-Mix, Calsan (CAN), Liqui-Cal, Liquid Cal-600, Titralac

calcium chloride

Calciject (CAN)

calcium citrate

Cal-C Cap, Cal-Cee, Citracal

calcium gluconate

calcium lactate

Cal-Lac

Class and Category

Pharmacologic class: Calcium salts
Therapeutic class: Antacid, antihypermagnesemic, antihyperphosphatemic, antihypocalcemic, calcium replacement, cardiotonic
Pregnancy category: C (Not classified for calcium carbonate, citrate, and lactate)

Indications and Dosages

➤ ***To treat hyperphosphatemia***

CAPSULES, TABLETS (CALCIUM ACETATE)

Adults. *Initial:* 2 capsules or tablets three times daily with meals. Dosage increased to reduce serum phosphorus level below 6 mg/dl as long as hypercalcemia doesn't develop. *Usual:* 3 or 4 capsules or tablets three times daily with each meal.

ORAL SOLUTION (CALCIUM ACETATE)

Adults. *Initial:* 10 ml with each meal. Dosage increased every 2 to 3 wk to reduce serum phosphorus levels to the target range, as long as hypercalcemia doesn't develop. *Usual:* 15 to 20 ml with each meal.

➤ ***To prevent hypocalcemia with oral supplementation***

CAPSULES, ORAL SUSPENSION, TABLETS (CALCIUM CARBONATE); EFFERVESCENT TABLETS, TABLETS (CALCIUM CITRATE); TABLETS (CALCIUM GLUCONATE OR LACTATE)

Adults. 1,000 to 1,200 mg daily.
Pregnant and breastfeeding women. 1,000 to 1,300 mg daily.
Children ages 9 to 18. 1,300 mg daily.
Children ages 4 to 8. 1,000 mg daily.
Children ages 1 to 4. 700 mg daily.
Children ages 7 to 12 months. 260 mg daily.
Infants up to 6 months. 200 mg daily.

➤ ***To provide antacid effects***

CHEWABLE TABLETS, ORAL SUSPENSION, TABLETS (CALCIUM CARBONATE)

Adults and children age 12 and over. 350 to 1,500 mg 1 hr after meals and at bedtime, as needed.

➤ ***To provide emergency treatment for hypocalcemia***

I.V. INJECTION (CALCIUM CHLORIDE)

Adults. 500 to 1,000 mg given slowly over 5 to 10 min, repeated as needed.

I.V. INFUSION (CALCIUM GLUCONATE)

Adults with mild hypocalcemia. 1,000 to 2,000 mg infused over 2 hr.
Adults with severe hypocalcemia but without seizure or tetany. 0.5 mg/kg/hr, increased up to 2 mg/kg/hr, as needed. *Maximum:* 4,000 mg over 4 hr.
Infants and children with severe hypocalcemia but without tetany. 200 to 500 mg/kg/day as continuous infusion or divided every 6 hr as intermittent infusions.
Neonates with severe hypocalcemia but without tetany. 200 to 800 mg/kg/day by continuous infusion or divided every 6 hr as intermittent infusions.

I.V. INJECTION, I.V. INFUSION (CALCIUM GLUCONATE)

Adults with tetany. 100 to 300 mg elemental calcium given as a bolus over 5 to 10 min, not to exceed 200 mg/min, followed by continuous infusion at 0.5 mg/kg/hr, increased to 2 mg/kg/hr, as needed, with rate adjusted, as needed, based on serum calcium levels.
Children with tetany. 100 to 200 mg/kg given as bolus over 10 min, not to exceed 100 mg/min, repeated after 6 hr, as needed. Alternatively, up to 500 mg/kg/day as continuous infusion with rate adjusted, as needed, based on serum calcium levels.

➤ ***As adjunct to treat magnesium intoxication***

I.V. INJECTION (CALCIUM CHLORIDE)
Adults. 500 to 1,000 mg given over 2 to 5 min and repeated if CNS depression persists.

➤ *To treat arrhythmias associated with hyperkalemia, hypermagnesemia, or hypocalcemia*

I.V. INJECTION (CALCIUM CHLORIDE)
Adults. 500 to 1,000 mg given slowly over 5 to 10 min.

➤ *To treat beta-blocker overdose that is refractory to glucagon and high-dose vasopressor treatment*

I.V. INJECTION (CALCIUM CHLORIDE)
Adults. 1,000 mg given via a central line.

➤ *To treat calcium channel blocker overdose*

I.V. INFUSION (CALCIUM CHLORIDE)
Adults. 1,000 to 2,000 mg infused over 10 to 20 min, repeated every 20 min, as needed, up to 5 doses.

Mechanism of Action

Increases levels of intracellular and extracellular calcium, which is needed to maintain homeostasis, especially in the nervous and musculoskeletal systems. Also plays a role in normal cardiac and renal function, respiration, coagulation, and cell membrane and capillary permeability. Helps regulate the release and storage of neurotransmitters and hormones. Oral forms also neutralize or buffer stomach acid to relieve discomfort caused by hyperacidity.

Contraindications

Hypercalcemia, hypersensitivity to calcium salts or their components, hypophosphatemia, renal calculi, ventricular fibrillation

Incompatibilities

To avoid precipitation, don't give I.V. calcium chloride, or gluconate through same I.V. line as bicarbonates, carbonates, phosphates, sulfates, or tartrates.

Interactions

DRUGS

bisphosphonates (alendronate, etidronate, ibandronate, risedronate): Possibly decreased absorption of bisphosphonates
calcium supplements, magnesium-containing preparations: Increased serum calcium or magnesium level, especially in patients with impaired renal function
digitalis glycosides: Increased risk of arrhythmias
fluoroquinolones: Reduced fluoroquinolone absorption by calcium carbonate
iron salts: Decreased gastric iron absorption
levothyroxine: Decreased absorption of levothyroxine
tetracyclines: Decreased tetracycline absorption and blood level, leading to decreased anti-infective response
thiazide diuretics: Possibly hypercalcemia
verapamil: Reversed verapamil effects
vitamin D (high doses): Excessively increased calcium absorption

FOODS

caffeine, high-fiber food: Possibly decreased calcium absorption

ACTIVITIES

alcohol use (excessive), smoking: Possibly decreased calcium absorption

Adverse Reactions

CNS: Paresthesia (parenteral form)
CV: Hypotension, irregular heartbeat (parenteral form)
GI: Nausea or vomiting (parenteral form)
SKIN: Diaphoresis, flushing, or sensation of warmth (parenteral form)
Other: Hypercalcemia; injection-site burning, pain, rash, or redness (parenteral form)

Nursing Considerations

- Store at room temperature, and protect from heat, moisture, and direct light. Don't freeze.
- Warm solution to room temperature before parenteral administration.
- Keep patient in a recumbent position for 30 minutes after parenteral administration to prevent dizziness from hypotension.
- Administer I.V. calcium through an infusing I.V. solution using a small-bore needle inserted into a large vein to minimize irritation. Give calcium slowly to prevent excess calcium from reaching the heart and causing adverse cardiovascular reactions. Adverse reactions often result from too-rapid

administration. If ECG tracings are abnormal or patient reports injection-site discomfort, expect to temporarily discontinue administration.

- Check regularly for infiltration because calcium causes necrosis. If infiltration occurs, stop infusion and tell prescriber immediately.
- Monitor serum calcium level, as ordered, and evaluate therapeutic response by assessing for Chvostek's and Trousseau's signs, which shouldn't appear.
- Be aware that calcium chloride injection contains three times as much calcium per milliliter as calcium gluconate injection.

PATIENT TEACHING

- Urge patient to chew chewable tablets thoroughly before swallowing and to drink a glass of water afterward.
- Tell patient to shake bottle well before each use if suspension form is prescribed.
- Tell patient to dissolve calcium citrate effervescent tablets in water and drink immediately.
- Instruct patient to take calcium carbonate tablets 1 to 2 hours after meals and other forms with meals.
- Advise storing calcium at room temperature away from heat, moisture, and light. Warn against freezing suspension or syrup.
- Instruct patient to avoid taking calcium within 2 hours of another oral drug because of risk of interactions.
- Urge patient to ask prescriber before taking OTC drugs because of risk of interactions.
- Tell patient to avoid excessive use of tobacco and excessive consumption of alcoholic beverages, caffeine-containing products, and high-fiber foods because these substances may decrease calcium absorption.
- Remind patient to take calcium separate from other prescribed drugs. For example, tell the patient to take fluoroquinolone at least 2 hours before or 6 hours after calcium; if prescribed levothyroxine to take it at least 4 hours before or after calcium; if prescribed a tetracycline to take it at least 1 hour before calcium.

canagliflozin

Invokana

Class and Category

Pharmacologic class: Sodium-glucose co-transporter 2 (SGLT2) inhibitor
Therapeutic class: Antidiabetic
Pregnancy category: Not classified

Indications and Dosages

➤ *To control blood glucose level in type 2 diabetes mellitus; to reduce the risk of major adverse cardiovascular events such as nonfatal myocardial infarction and nonfatal stroke in patients with type 2 diabetes mellitus and established cardiovascular disease*

TABLETS

Adults. 100 mg once daily before first meal of the day, followed by dosage increase to 300 mg once daily before first meal of the day, if needed, and patient has a glomerular filtration rate of 60 ml/min or greater. *Maximum:* 300 mg once daily before first meal of the day.

DOSAGE ADJUSTMENT For patients with moderate renal impairment (glomerular filtration rate less than 60 ml/min but at least 45 ml/min), dosage limited to 100 mg once daily. For patients receiving an UDP-glucuronosyltransferase (UGT) enzyme inducer such as phenobarbital, phenytoin, rifampin, or ritonavir, dosage may be increased to 300 mg once daily before first meal of the day if glomerular filtration rate is 60 ml/min or greater.

Mechanism of Action

Inhibits sodium-glucose co-transporter 2 (SGLT2) responsible for the majority of the reabsorption of filtered glucose from the tubular lumen in the kidneys. By inhibiting SGLT2, reabsorption of filtered glucose is reduced along with a lowering of the renal threshold for glucose, which increases urinary glucose excretion.

Contraindications

End-stage renal disease, hypersensitivity to canagliflozin or its components, severe renal impairment (glomerular filtration rate less than 30 ml/min), use of dialysis

Interactions

DRUGS

digoxin: Possibly increased serum digoxin levels and digitalis toxicity
insulin, insulin secretagogues: Possibly increased risk of hypoglycemia
phenobarbital, phenytoin, rifampin, ritonavir: Decreased effectiveness of canaglifoxin

Adverse Reactions

CNS: Asthenia, fatigue, postural dizziness, syncope
CV: Elevation of low-density lipoprotein cholesterol (LDL-C) and non-high-density lipoprotein cholesterol (non-HDL-C), **hypotension**
ENDO: Hypoglycemia, ketoacidosis
GI: Abdominal pain, constipation, nausea, **pancreatitis**
GU: Acute renal failure, decreased glomerular filtration rate, elevated serum creatinine levels, genital mycotic infections, **necrotizing fasciitis of the perineum (Fournier's gangrene), pyelonephritis**, renal impairment, UTIs, vulvovaginal pruritus, **urosepsis**
HEME: Elevated hemoglobin
MS: Bone fracture (upper extremity), decreased bone density, lower limb amputation
SKIN: Erythema, photosensitivity, pruritus, rash, urticaria
Other: Anaphylaxis, angioedema, dehydration, elevated phosphate levels, **hyperkalemia, hypermagnesemia**, thirst

Nursing Considerations

- Use drug cautiously in patients with chronic kidney insufficiency, congestive heart failure, decreased blood volume, and in patients taking medications such as angiotensin-converting enzyme inhibitors and angiotensin receptor blockers, diuretics, and NSAIDs because these conditions and treatments may predispose the patient to acute kidney injury while receiving canagliflozin. Ensure that kidney function has been assessed prior to start of canagliflozin therapy and then periodically thereafter.
- Know that patients with volume depletion should have the condition corrected before canagliflozin therapy is begun because drug causes intravascular volume contraction. Patients especially at risk for symptomatic hypotension caused by volume depletion include patients with impaired renal function, the elderly, patients taking either diuretics or drugs that interfere with the renin–angiotensin–aldosterone system, or patients with low systolic blood pressure.
- Expect drug to be temporarily discontinued in patients who develop a reduced oral intake, such as in an acute illness or fasting, or who experience excessive fluid losses because of significant heat exposure or gastrointestinal illness, to reduce risk of acute kidney injury.
- Be aware that canagliflozin dosage should only be increased in patients who have at least a glomerular filtration rate of 45 ml/min and need greater glucose control.
- Assess renal function, as ordered prior to starting canagliflozin therapy and then periodically thereafter, because canagliflozin may cause renal impairment, especially in patients with hypovolemia. Expect drug to be discontinued if the patient's glomerular filtration rate becomes persistently less than 45 ml/min. Also monitor patient for a UTI, because canagliflozin increases risk of UTIs. Report promptly and expect to treat because the UTI can quickly become serious, developing into pyelonephritis and urosepsis.
- Monitor serum potassium levels regularly, as ordered, during canagliflozin therapy in patients with impaired renal function and in patients predisposed to hyperkalemia due to medications or other medical conditions.
- Monitor patient's blood glucose levels to determine effectiveness of canagliflozin therapy. Be aware that canagliflozin can increase urinary glucose excretion, leading to positive urine glucose tests, and should not be used to monitor glucose levels in patients with diabetes mellitus. Assess patient also receiving insulin or insulin secretagogues for hypoglycemia.

WARNING **Monitor patient closely for ketoacidosis that may occur despite the patient having type 2 diabetes and even may be present even if a blood glucose level is less than 250 mg/dl. If signs and symptoms occur such as dehydration, fruity odor to breath, malaise, nausea, shortness**

of breath, and vomiting, notify prescriber and expect drug to be discontinued. Provide supportive care, as ordered.

- Be aware that patients with a history of genital mycotic infections, as well as uncircumcised males, are at greater risk for developing genital mycotic infections.

WARNING **Report immediately signs and symptoms of necrotizing fasciitis of the perineum (Fournier's gangrene), a rare but serious and life-threatening necrotizing infection that has been linked to canagliflozin therapy. Report patient's complaints of erythema, pain or tenderness, or swelling in the genital or perineal area, along with fever or malaise, as treatment requires urgent surgical intervention along with immediate broad-spectrum antibiotic therapy. If confirmed, expect canagliflozin to be discontinued and an alternative treatment for glycemic control prescribed.**

- Monitor patient's lipid levels and expect to treat if an elevation occurs.

WARNING **Assess patient for hypersensitivity reactions such as angioedema and generalized urticaria, especially within hours to days after canagliflozin therapy is begun. The hypersensitivity reaction can become severe, causing anaphylaxis. If hypersensitivity to canagliflozin occurs, expect drug to be discontinued and provide supportive care as ordered.**

- Institute safety precautions to prevent falls because drug may increase risk of falls leading to bone fracture. The risk of bone fracture may occur as early as 12 weeks after therapy is begun.
- Be aware that canagliflozin has been linked to an increase in foot and leg amputations in patients receiving the drug. Assess patient's feet and legs regularly for any abnormalities and notify prescriber immediately if present. Be aware that patients may be at higher risk of lower-limb amputation if they have had diabetic foot sores or ulcers, have had blocked or narrowed blood vessels (usually in leg), have had damage to the nerves (neuropathy) in the leg, or have a history of amputation, heart disease, or are at risk for heart disease. Know that canagliflozin may be discontinued if abnormalities develop.

PATIENT TEACHING

- Instruct patient to take canagliflozin before the first meal of the day. Tell her that if a dose is missed, she should take it as soon as she remembers unless it is almost time for the next dose. Then patient should skip the missed dose and take her normal dose of canagliflozin at the regular time. She should never double the dose.
- Urge patient not to skip doses or increase dosage without consulting prescriber. However, tell patient to notify prescriber if he is unable to take a normal amount of daily fluids due to illness or fasting or experiences an excessive loss of fluids from excessive perspiration or gastrointestinal illnesses, as drug may need to be temporarily withheld.
- Emphasize importance of reporting signs of hypoglycemia, such as anxiety, confusion, dizziness, excessive sweating, headache, and nausea.
- Tell patient to carry identification indicating that he has diabetes.
- Teach patient how to monitor his blood glucose level. Advise patient with diabetes mellitus not to use urine glucose tests to monitor her glycemic control, as drug will cause a false positive result. Review signs and symptoms of ketoacidosis with patient and urge her to seek immediate medical attention, if present, even if blood glucose level is less than 250 mg/dl.
- Inform patient that canagliflozin is not a substitute for diet and exercise management.
- Inform patient that drug may increase his risk for bone fractures and to take safety precautions to prevent falls.
- Advise patient to avoid direct sunlight and to wear sunscreen when outdoors.
- Instruct patient to notify prescriber right away if she notices any new pain or tenderness, sores or ulcers, or symptoms of infections in her feet or legs. Tell patient this is very important, because canagliflozin therapy increases the risk of lower-limb amputations.
- Advise patient to seek medical care promptly if pain or tenderness, redness, or swelling of the genitals or the area from the genitals back to the rectum occurs, along with a fever above 38°C (100.4°F) or malaise develops.

candesartan cilexetil

Atacand

Class and Category

Pharmacologic class: Angiotensin receptor blocker
Therapeutic class: Antihypertensive
Pregnancy category: D

Indications and Dosages

➤ *To manage, or as adjunct in managing, hypertension*

ORAL SUSPENSION, TABLETS

Adults.
Initial: 16 mg daily. *Maintenance:* 8 to 32 mg daily or 4 to 16 mg every 12 hr. *Maximum:* 32 mg daily.
Children ages 6 to 17 weighing more than 50 kg (110 lb). *Initial:* 8 to 16 mg daily. *Maintenance:* 4 to 32 mg daily. *Maximum:* 32 mg daily.
Children ages 6 to 17 weighing 50 kg (110 lb) or less. *Initial:* 4 to 8 mg daily. *Maintenance:* 2 to 16 mg. *Maximum:* 16 mg daily.
Children ages 1 to 6. *Initial:* 0.20 mg/kg daily. *Maintenance:* 0.05 to 0.4 mg/kg daily. *Maximum:* 0.4 mg/kg daily.
DOSAGE ADJUSTMENT For adult patients with moderate hepatic impairment, initial dosage reduced to 8 mg daily.

➤ *To treat heart failure in patients with an ejection fraction of 40% or less and NYHA class II–IV to reduce the risk of death from cardiovascular causes and reduce hospitalizations for heart failure*

ORAL SUSPENSION, TABLETS

Adults. *Initial:* 4 mg daily for 2 wk; then doubled every 2 wk as tolerated until reaching target dose of 32 mg daily.

Route	Onset	Peak	Duration
P.O.	In 2 wk	4–5 wk	Unknown

Mechanism of Action

Selectively blocks binding of angiotensin (AT) II to AT_1 receptor sites in many tissues, including adrenal glands and vascular smooth muscle. This inhibits vasoconstrictive and aldosterone-secreting effects of AT II, which reduces blood pressure.

Contraindications

Concurrent aliskiren therapy in presence of diabetes, hypersensitivity to candesartan or its components

Interactions

DRUGS

aliskiren, angiotensin-converting enzyme inhibitors, angiotensin receptor blockers: Increased risk of hypotension, hyperkalemia, and renal dysfunction in presence of diabetes or existing renal dysfunction
diuretics, other antihypertensives: Possibly increased risk of hypotension
lithium: Increased blood lithium level
NSAIDs: Possible decreased renal function in patients who are elderly, volume-depleted, or have a compromised renal function
potassium-sparing diuretics, potassium supplements, potassium-containing salt substitutes: Possibly increased risk of hyperkalemia

Adverse Reactions

CNS: Dizziness, headache
CV: Hypotension
EENT: Pharyngitis, rhinitis
GI: Elevated liver enzymes, **hepatitis**, impaired liver function
GU: Elevated BUN and serum creatinine levels
HEME: Agranulocytosis, leukopenia, neutropenia
MS: Back pain, **rhabdomyolysis**
RESP: Cough, upper respiratory tract infection
SKIN: Pruritus, rash, urticaria
Other: Angioedema, hyperkalemia, hyponatremia

Nursing Considerations

- Determine if patient has fluid or salt depletion prior to starting candesartan. If patient has known or suspected hypovolemia and/or salt depletion such as may occur with prolonged diuretic therapy, dietary salt restriction, dialysis, diarrhea or vomiting, expect to provide treatment, such as I.V. normal saline solution, as prescribed, to correct it

before starting candesartan. Continue to monitor blood pressure throughout candesartan therapy, especially after a dosage increase.
- Monitor patient closely during major surgery and anesthesia because candesartan increases risk of hypotension by blocking renin–angiotensin system.
- Watch for elevated BUN and serum creatinine levels, especially if patient has heart failure or impaired renal function; drug may cause acute renal failure. Report significant or persistent increases immediately.

WARNING **Know that if patient receives a diuretic or antihypertensive with candesartan, has heart failure, or is elderly, assess blood pressure often because of added risk of hypotension.**

- Monitor patient for hypotension. If patient develops hypotension, expect to stop drug temporarily. Immediately place patient in supine position and prepare to give I.V. normal saline solution, as prescribed. Expect to resume therapy after blood pressure stabilizes.
- Monitor patient for fluid deficit. If patient receives a diuretic, provide hydration, as ordered, to help prevent hypovolemia. Watch for evidence, such as hypotension with dizziness and fainting. If patient has heart failure and develops hypotension, dosage of diuretic, candesartan, or both may be reduced when blood pressure stabilizes and therapy resumes.
- Check CBC for decreases in hemoglobin and hematocrit. If they're significant or persistent, notify prescriber immediately.

PATIENT TEACHING
- Advise patient that full effects of candesartan may not occur for 4 to 5 weeks.
- Explain importance of lifestyle choices in controlling hypertension.
- Advise female patient of childbearing age to immediately report known or suspected pregnancy. Explain that if she becomes pregnant, candesartan will need to be discontinued as soon as possible and treatment started with another antihypertensive that's safe to use during pregnancy.

cangrelor

Kengreal

Class and Category

Pharmacologic class: $P2Y_{12}$ platelet inhibitor
Therapeutic class: Antiplatelet
Pregnancy category: C

Indications and Dosages

➤ *Adjunct to percutaneous coronary intervention (PCI) to reduce risk of periprocedural myocardial infarction, repeat coronary revascularization and stent thrombosis in patients who have not been treated with a $P2Y_{12}$ platelet inhibitor and are not being given a glycoprotein IIb/IIIa inhibitor*

I.V. INFUSION, I.V. INJECTION
Adults. 30 mcg/kg IV bolus before the PCI followed immediately by a 4 mcg/kg/min infusion for at least 2 hr or for the duration of PCI, whichever is longer.

Mechanism of Action

Blocks ADP-induced platelet activation and aggregation by binding selectively and reversibly to the $P2Y_{12}$ receptor to prevent further signaling and platelet activation.

Contraindications

Hypersensitivity to cangrelor or its components, significant active bleeding

Interactions

DRUGS
clopidogrel, prasugrel: Increased antiplatelet effect when next dose of either of these drugs are administered

Adverse Reactions

CNS: Intracranial bleeding or hemorrhage
CV: Coronary artery dissection or perforation
EENT: Stridor
GU: Decreased renal function
HEME: Bleeding events
RESP: Bronchospasm, dyspnea
Other: Anaphylaxis including shock, angioedema

Nursing Considerations

- Reconstitute each 50 mg vial by adding 5 ml of sterile water for injection. Swirl

gently until all material is dissolved. Avoid vigorous mixing. Allow any foam to settle. Ensure that the contents are fully dissolved and the reconstituted material is clear and colorless to pale yellow.
- Dilute reconstituted solution immediately with normal saline or 5% dextrose injection. For example, withdraw the contents from one reconstituted vial and add to one 250-ml saline bag. Mix the bag thoroughly. Know that patients weighing 100 kg or more will require a minimum of two bags. Diluted cangrelor is stable for 12 hr if diluted in 5% dextrose injection and 24 hr if diluted in normal saline and kept at room temperature.
- Administer via a dedicated I.V. line. Administer the bolus rapidly in less than 1 minute from the diluted bag via manual IV push or pump. Make sure the bolus is completely administered before the start of PCI and then start infusion immediately after administration of the bolus.
- Be aware that after cangrelor is discontinued, an oral $P2Y_{12}$ platelet inhibitor should be administered such as clopidogrel 600 mg after discontinuation of cangrelor, prasugrel 60 mg immediately after discontinuation of cangrelor, or ticagrelor 180 mg at any time during cangrelor infusion or immediately after discontinuation.
- Monitor patient closely for bleeding that can range from being minor to severe. Be prepared to treat bleeding events immediately and notify prescriber. Know that once cangrelor is discontinued, there is no antiplatelet effect after an hour.

WARNING **Monitor patient closely for allergic reactions following administration. Alert prescriber immediately, if present, and be prepared to discontinue drug and provide supportive emergency care, as ordered.**

PATIENT TEACHING
- Tell patient to alert medical staff immediately if difficulty breathing occurs.
- Inform patient that the effects of cangrelor are gone after 1 hour of the drug being discontinued.

captopril

Class and Category

Pharmacologic class: Angiotensin-converting enzyme (ACE) inhibitor
Therapeutic class: Antihypertensive, vasodilator
Pregnancy category: D

Indications and Dosages

➤ *To control hypertension*

TABLETS

Adults and adolescents. *Initial:* 25 mg twice daily or three times daily. Increased to 50 mg twice daily or three times daily after 1 to 2 wk, if needed. If blood pressure isn't well controlled at this dosage and with the addition of a diuretic, dosage increased to 100 mg twice daily or three times daily and then, if needed, to 150 mg twice daily or three times daily while continuing diuretic. *Maximum:* 450 mg daily.

➤ ***To control accelerated or malignant hypertension when temporary discontinuation of current antihypertensive therapy isn't practical or when prompt titration of blood pressure is needed***

TABLETS

Adults and adolescents. *Initial:* 25 mg twice daily or three times daily while continuing diuretic but discontinuing current antihypertensive drug. Increased every 24 hr as needed until satisfactory response is obtained or maximum dosage is reached. *Maximum:* 450 mg daily.

➤ *To treat congestive heart failure*

TABLETS

Adults and adolescents with normal or low blood pressure, who have been vigorously treated with diuretics. *Initial:* 6.25 mg or 12.5 mg three times daily, increased gradually over several days to 50 mg three times daily. Further increases done in 2 wk intervals, as needed. *Maximum:* 450 mg daily.

Adults and adolescents. *Initial:* 6.25 mg, 12.5 mg, or 25 mg three times daily. Increased to 50 mg three times daily, as needed. After 14 days, increased to 100 mg three times daily and then to 150 mg three times daily, if needed. *Maximum:* 450 mg daily.

➤ *To treat left ventricular dysfunction after MI*

TABLETS

Adults and adolescents. *Initial:* 6.25 mg as single dose starting 3 days after MI and then 12.5 mg three times daily. Increased to 25 mg three times daily for several days and then again to maintenance dosage. *Maintenance:* 50 mg three times daily.

➤ *To treat diabetic nephropathy*

TABLETS

Adults and adolescents. 25 mg three times daily.

DOSAGE ADJUSTMENT For patient with renal impairment, initial dosage reduced and smaller increments utilized for titration.

Route	Onset	Peak	Duration
P.O.	15–60 min	60–90 min	6–12 hr

Mechanism of Action

By inhibiting angiotensin-converting enzyme, captopril:

- prevents conversion of angiotensin I to angiotensin II, a potent vasoconstrictor that also stimulates the adrenal cortex to secrete aldosterone. Inhibiting aldosterone increases sodium and water excretion, reducing blood pressure and water retention.
- may inhibit renal and vascular production of angiotensin II.
- decreases serum angiotensin II level and increases renin activity. This decreases aldosterone secretion, slightly increasing serum potassium level and fluid loss.
- decreases vascular tone and blood pressure.

Contraindications

Combination therapy with a neprilysin inhibitor (e.g., sacubitril) or within 36 hours of switching to or from sacubitril/valsartan; concurrent aliskiren use in patients with diabetes or patients with renal impairment (GFR less than 60 ml/min); hypersensitivity to captopril, other ACE inhibitors, or their components

Interactions

DRUGS

adrenergic neuron-blocking drugs, beta adrenergic drugs, ganglionic blocking drugs: Possibly increased risk of hypotension

aliskiren in patients with diabetes, other ACE inhibitors, angiotension receptor blockers: Increased risk of hypotension, hyperkalemia, and renal impairment

antacids: Possibly impaired captopril absorption

capsaicin: Possibly cause or worsening of cough from ACE inhibitor

cyclosporine, potassium-containing drugs, potassium-sparing diuretics, potassium supplements: Increased risk of hyperkalemia

diuretics; hypotension-producing drugs, such as hydralazine: Additive hypotensive effects

gold: Increased risk of nitritoid reaction, including facial flushing, hypotension, nausea, and vomiting.

lithium: Increased risk of lithium toxicity

mTOR (everolimus, sirolimus, temsirolimus), neprilysin inhibitor such as sacubitril: Increased risk for angioedema

nitrates, other vasodilators: Possibly potentiated effects

NSAIDs: Decreased antihypertensive response to ACE inhibition; possible decreased renal function in elderly patients or those who are volume-depleted or already have existing impaired renal function

ACTIVITIES

alcohol use: Additive hypotensive effects

FOOD

moderate to high potassium-containing foods: Possibly increased risk of hyperkalemia

Adverse Reactions

CNS: Fever
CV: Chest pain, **hypotension**, orthostatic hypotension, palpitations, tachycardia
EENT: Loss of taste
GU: Dysuria, impotence, **nephrotic syndrome**, nocturia, oliguria, polyuria, proteinuria, urinary frequency
HEME: Eosinophilia
MS: Arthralgia
RESP: Cough
SKIN: Photosensitivity, pruritus, rash
Other: **Angioedema**, **hyperkalemia**, **hyponatremia**, positive ANA titer

Nursing Considerations

- Monitor closely patient's blood pressure, especially when therapy starts and dosage increases. Also know that excessive hypotension, although rare, may occur in hypertensive patients when captopril is used in patients with heart failure or those who are undergoing renal dialysis or in

patients with salt/volume depletion (such as occurs with vigorous treatment with diuretics). Keep patient supine if hypotension occurs.
- Monitor patient's blood pressure and electrolytes routinely if patient is receiving other drugs that also affect the renin–angiotensin system because hypotension and hyperkalemia may occur.
- Monitor renal function tests for signs of nephrotic syndrome, such as proteinuria and increased BUN and serum creatinine levels. Also watch for such renal evidence as oliguria, polyuria, and urinary frequency or other signs of impaired renal function, especially in patients who are receiving other drugs that also affect the renin–angiotensin system.
- Monitor WBC regularly, as ordered, especially if patient has collagen vascular disease or renal disease.

PATIENT TEACHING
- Instruct patient to take captopril 1 hour before meals.
- Tell patient to rise slowly from sitting or lying to minimize orthostatic hypotension.
- Tell patient to avoid sunlight or wear sunscreen in direct sunlight because photosensitivity may occur.
- Warn patient not to stop taking drug abruptly.
- Urge patient not to use salt substitutes that contain potassium and to consult prescriber before increasing potassium intake to avoid increasing risk of hyperkalemia.
- Urge patient to tell prescriber about signs and symptoms of infection, such as sore throat or fever.
- Advise female patient of childbearing age to notify prescriber immediately if pregnancy occurs.

carbamazepine

Apo-Carbamazepine (CAN), Carbatrol, Carnexiv, Epitol, Equetro, Novo-Carbamaz (CAN), Tegretol, Tegretol-XR

Class and Category

Pharmacologic class: Iminostilbene derivative
Therapeutic class: Analgesic, anticonvulsant
Pregnancy category: D

Indications and Dosages

➤ *To treat epilepsy*

E.R. CAPSULES (CARBATROL), E.R. TABLETS (TEGRETOL-XR)

Adults and children age 12 and over. *Initial:* 200 mg twice daily. Increased weekly by 200 mg daily, if needed, and given in divided doses twice daily. *Maximum:* 1,600 mg daily in adults, 1,200 mg daily in children age 16 and over, and 1,000 mg daily in children ages 12 to 16.
Children ages 6 to 12. *Initial:* 100 mg twice daily. Increased weekly by 100 mg daily, if needed, and given in divided doses twice daily. *Maximum:* 1,000 mg daily.

ORAL SUSPENSION

Adults and children age 12 and over. *Initial:* 100 mg four times daily. Increased weekly by 200 mg daily, if needed, given in divided doses three times daily or four times daily. *Maximum:* 1,600 mg daily in

Mechanism of Action

Normally, sodium moves into a neuronal cell by passing through a gated sodium channel in the cell membrane. Carbamazepine may prevent or halt seizures by closing or blocking sodium channels, as shown here, thus preventing sodium from entering the cell. Keeping sodium out of the cell may slow nerve impulse transmission, thus slowing the rate at which neurons fire.

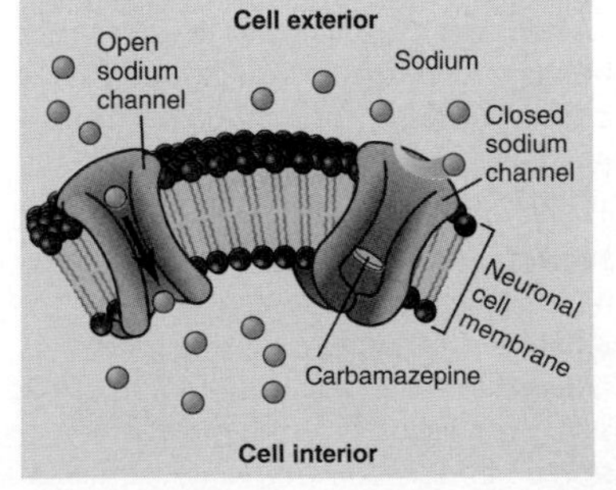

adults, 1,200 mg daily in children age 16 and over, and 1,000 mg daily in children ages 12 to 16.
Children ages 6 to 12. *Initial:* 50 mg four times daily. Increased weekly by 100 mg daily, if needed, given in divided doses three times daily or four times daily. *Maximum:* 1,000 mg daily.
Children up to age 6. *Initial:* 10 to 20 mg/kg/day in divided doses four times daily. *Maximum:* 35 mg/kg daily.

TABLETS

Adults and children age 12 and over. *Initial:* 200 mg twice daily. Increased weekly by 200 mg/day, if needed, given in divided doses three times daily or four times daily *Maximum:* 1,600 mg daily in adults, 1,200 mg daily in children age 16 and over, and 1,000 mg daily in children ages 12 to 16.
Children ages 6 to 12. *Initial:* 100 mg twice daily. Increased weekly by 100 mg daily, if needed, given in divided doses three times daily or four times daily. *Maximum:* 1,000 mg daily.
Children up to age 6. *Initial:* 10 to 20 mg/kg daily in divided doses twice daily or three times daily. Increased weekly, if needed, divided and given three times daily or four times daily. *Maximum:* 35 mg/kg/day.

I.V. INFUSION (CARNEXIV)

Adults. 70% of total daily oral carbamazepine dose divided equally into four 30-minute infusions with each infusion separated by 6 hr.

➤ ***To relieve pain in trigeminal neuralgia***

E.R. CAPSULES (CARBATROL), E.R. TABLETS (TEGRETOL-XR), TABLETS

Adults. *Initial:* 100 mg twice daily. Increased by up to 200 mg daily, if needed, in increments of 100 mg every 12 hr. *Maintenance:* 400 to 800 mg/day. *Maximum:* 1,200 mg daily.

ORAL SUSPENSION

Adults. 50 mg four times daily. Increased by up to 200 mg daily, if needed, in increments of 50 mg four times daily. *Maintenance:* 400 to 800 mg daily. *Maximum:* 1,200 mg daily.

➤ ***To treat acute manic and mixed episodes in bipolar disorder***

E.R. CAPSULES (EQUETRO)

Adults. *Initial:* 200 mg twice daily, increased as needed in 200-mg increments. *Maximum:* 1,600 mg daily.

Route	Onset	Peak	Duration
P.O. (all forms)	In 1 mo*	Unknown	Unknown

* For anticonvulsant use; 8 to 72 hr for use in trigeminal neuralgia.

Contraindications

Concurrent therapy with delavirdine or other non-nucleoside reverse transcriptase inhibitors, or nefazodone; history of bone marrow depression; hypersensitivity to carbamazepine, tricyclic compounds, or their components; MAO inhibitor therapy within 14 days

Interactions

DRUGS

acetaminophen (long-term use): Increased metabolism, leading to acetaminophen-induced hepatotoxicity or decreased acetaminophen effectiveness
acetazolamide, aprepitant, cimetidine, ciprofloxacin, clarithromycin, danazol, dantrolene, delavirdine or other non-nucleoside reverse transcriptase inhibitors, diltiazem, erythromycin, fluconazole, fluoxetine, fluvoxamine, ibuprofen, isoniazid, itraconazole, ketoconazole, loratadine, loxapine, macrolides, niacinamide, nicotinamide, olanzapine, omeprazole, oxybutynin, propoxyphene, protease inhibitors, quetiapine, terfenadine, ticlopidine, trazodone, troleandomycin, valproate, valproic acid, verapamil, voriconazole: Increased blood carbamazepine level
albendazole, alprazolam, amitriptyline, aprepitant, aripiprazole, buprenorphine, bupropion, buspirone, citalopram, clobazam, clonazepam, clozapine, corticosteroids, cyclosporine, delavirdine, desipramine, diazepam, dicumarol, doxycycline, ethosuximide, everolimus, felodipine, glucocorticoids, haloperidol, imatinib, imipramine, itraconazole, lamotrigine, levothyroxine, lorazepam, methadone, methsuximide, mianserin, midazolam, mirtazapine, nortriptyline, olanzapine, oral contraceptives, oxcarbazepine, paliperidone, phensuximide, phenytoin, praziquantel, protease inhibitors, quetiapine, risperidone, sertraline, sirolimus, tacrolimus, tadalafil, theophylline, tiagabine, topiramate,

tramadol, triazolam, trazodone, valproate, warfarin, ziprasidone, zonisamide: Decreased blood levels of these drugs
aminophylline, cisplatin, doxorubicin, felbamate, methsuximide, phenobarbital, phenytoin, primidone, rifampin, theophylline: Decreased blood carbamazepine level
clomipramine, phenytoin, primidone: Increased blood levels of these drugs
cyclophosphamide: Possibly increased cyclophosphamide toxicity
felbamate: Decreased blood level of felbamate or carbamazepine
furosemide, hydrochlorothiazide: Possibly increased risk of symptomatic hyponatremia
isoniazid: Increased risk of carbamazepine toxicity and isoniazid hepatotoxicity
lamotrigine, phenobarbital, primidone, tricyclic antidepressants, valproic acid: Decreased blood levels of these drugs, increased blood level of carbamazepine
lapatinib, temsirolimus: Altered effectiveness of these drugs
lithium: Increased risk of CNS toxicity
MAO inhibitors: Increased risk of serotonin syndrome
nefazodone: Decreased nefazodone effectiveness and increased carbamazepine level
nondepolarizing neuromuscular blockers: Possibly reduced duration or decreased effectiveness of neuromuscular blocker
oral anticoagulants: Increased metabolism and decreased effectiveness of anticoagulant

FOODS

grapefruit juice: Increased blood carbamazepine level

ACTIVITIES

alcohol use: Increased sedative effect

Adverse Reactions

CNS: Chills, confusion, dizziness, drowsiness, fatigue, fever, headache, **suicidal ideation**, syncope, talkativeness, unsteadiness, visual hallucinations
CV: **Arrhythmias**, **including AV block**; edema; **heart failure**; hypertension; **hypotension**; **thromboembolism**; thrombophlebitis; worsened coronary artery disease
EENT: Blurred vision, conjunctivitis, dry mouth, glossitis, nystagmus, oculomotor disturbances, stomatitis, tinnitus, transient diplopia
ENDO: Syndrome of inappropriate ADH secretion, water intoxication
GI: Abdominal pain, anorexia, constipation, diarrhea, dyspepsia, elevated liver enzymes, **hepatitis**, jaundice, nausea, **pancreatitis**, vanishing bile duct syndrome, vomiting
GU: Acute urine retention, albuminuria, **azotemia**, glycosuria, impotence, oliguria, **renal failure**, urinary frequency
HEME: Acute intermittent porphyria, **agranulocytosis**, **aplastic anemia**, **bone marrow depression**, eosinophilia, leukocytosis, **leukopenia**, **pancytopenia**, **thrombocytopenia**
MS: Arthralgia, leg cramps, myalgia, osteoporosis
RESP: Pulmonary hypersensitivity (dyspnea, fever, pneumonia, or pneumonitis)
SKIN: Aggravation of disseminated lupus erythematosus, alopecia, altered skin pigmentation, diaphoresis, **erythema multiforme**, erythema nodosum, **exfoliative dermatitis**, nail shedding (onychomadesis), photosensitivity reactions, pruritic and erythematous rash, purpura, **Stevens–Johnson syndrome**, **toxic epidermal necrolysis**, urticaria
Other: Adenopathy, **drug reaction with eosinophilia and systemic symptoms (DRESS) multiorgan hypersensitivity or other hypersensitivity**, **hypocalcemia**, **hypogammaglobulinemia**, **hyponatremia**, lymphadenopathy

Nursing Considerations

- Avoid using carbamazepine in patients with a history of hepatic porphyria because it may prompt an acute attack. Also, be aware that the Tegretol brand suspension contains sorbitol and should not be given to a patient with fructose intolerance.

WARNING **Note patient's ancestry. If patient has Asian ancestry, make sure he has been evaluated for the genetic allelic variant HLA-B 1502 before starting carbamazepine therapy. If patient has African-American, Chinese, European, Indian including Native American, Japanese, Korean, Latin American, Taiwanese or Thai ancestry, make sure he has been evaluated for the genetic allelic variant HLA-A 3101 before starting carbamazepine therapy. Patients positive for**

HLA-A 3101 or HLA-B 1502 shouldn't take carbamazepine because of the risk of serious, sometimes fatal, dermatologic reactions. The risk is between 5% and 15% in patients with these variants.

- Use carbamazepine cautiously in patients with impaired hepatic function because it's mainly metabolized in the liver. Monitor liver function tests, as directed.
- Prepare intravenous form by transferring the single dose volume to 100 ml of diluent solution such as 0.9% sodium chloride, 5% dextrose and water, or lactated Ringer's solution and mixing gently. Prepared solution may be stored up to 4 hours at room temperature or 24 hours refrigerated. Administer each infusion over 30 minutes.

WARNING **Be aware that anaphylaxis and angioedema may occur in patients after taking the first or subsequent doses of carbamazepine. Monitor patient closely.**

- Monitor patient closely for other adverse reactions because many of them are serious and some can become life-threatening, such as DRESS multiorgan hypersensitivity.
- Periodically monitor blood carbamazepine level, as ordered, to assess for therapeutic and toxic levels; a blood level of 6 to 12 mcg/ml is optimal for anticonvulsant effects.
- Monitor patient's electrolytes, especially sodium level, as ordered. Hyponatremia may occur as an adverse reaction to carbamazepine therapy, especially in the elderly and patients treated with diuretics. Assess patient regularly for signs and symptoms of hyponatremia such as confusion, difficulty concentrating, headache, memory impairment, unsteadiness, and weakness. If present, notify prescriber and expect drug to be discontinued.

WARNING **Monitor WBC and platelet counts monthly for first 2 months. Decreased counts may indicate bone marrow depression. Monitor patient closely, especially for agranulocytosis or aplastic anemia.**

- Monitor patient closely for evidence of suicidal thinking or behavior, especially when therapy starts or dosage changes.
- Withdraw carbamazepine gradually to minimize risk of seizures.
- Monitor renal function in patients who are receiving carbamazepine intravenously, as they may be at greater risk of developing adverse effects on the renal system. Know that intravenous form should not be used in patients with moderate or severe renal impairment.

PATIENT TEACHING

- Tell patient to take carbamazepine with food (except the oral suspension form, which shouldn't be taken with other liquid drugs or diluents).
- Warn patient about possible dizziness, blurred vision, and unsteadiness.
- Inform patient that coating of E.R. tablets isn't absorbed and may appear in stool.
- Advise patient not to crush or chew E.R. capsules or tablets. If he can't swallow capsules whole, have him open them and sprinkle contents on food.

WARNING **Instruct patient to seek immediate medical care and to stop taking carbamazepine if difficulty in breathing or swallowing occurs or swelling of eyes, face, lips, or tongue develops.**

- Urge patient to wear sunscreen and protective clothing to reduce photosensitivity.
- Tell patient to report bruising, fever, mouth ulcers, rash, or unusual bleeding or bruising.
- Tell female patient of childbearing age that drug decreases oral contraceptive effectiveness, and urge her to use different contraception. Because drug may cause fetal harm, tell her to notify prescriber about possible pregnancy.
- Be aware that if she becomes pregnant during therapy, urge her to enroll in the antiepileptic drug pregnancy registry by calling 1-888-233-2334. Explain that the registry is collecting information about the safety of antiepileptic drugs during pregnancy.
- Instruct caregivers to watch patient closely for evidence of suicidal tendencies, especially when therapy starts or dosage changes, and to report such tendencies to prescriber immediately.
- Advise patient to inform all prescribers of carbamazepine therapy. This is especially important if patient has had a hypersensitivity reaction to carbamazepine because about one-third of such patients will also experience hypersensitivity to oxcarbazepine.

C

cariprazine

Vraylar

Class and Category

Pharmacologic class: Atypical antipsychotic
Therapeutic class: Antipsychotic
Pregnancy category: Not classified

Indications and Dosages

➤ *To treat schizophrenia*

CAPSULES

Adults. *Initial:* 1.5 mg once daily, then increased to 3 mg once daily on day 2, as needed, with further increases in 1.5 mg to 3 mg increments, as needed. *Usual:* 1.5 mg to 6 mg once daily. *Maximum:* 6 mg once daily.

➤ *To treat acute manic or mixed episodes associated with bipolar I disorder*

CAPSULES

Adults. *Initial:* 1.5 mg once daily, then increased to 3 mg once daily on day 2, with further increases in 1.5 to 3 mg increments, as needed. *Usual:* 3 mg to 6 mg once daily. *Maximum:* 6 mg once daily.

DOSAGE ADJUSTMENT For patient initiating cariprazine therapy while already taking a strong CYP3A4 inhibitor, a dose of 1.5 mg given on day 1 and day 3 with no dose on day 2. From day 4 onward, 1.5 mg daily given with possible increase to a maximum dose of 3 mg daily, as needed. For patient prescribed a strong CYP3A4 inhibitor after being on a stable dose of cariprazine, dosage reduced by half; if patient is taking 4.5 mg daily, dosage decreased to 1.5 or 3 mg daily; if patient is taking 1.5 mg, dosing frequency reduced to every other day.

Mechanism of Action

May produce antipsychotic effects through partial agonist and antagonist actions. Cariprazine acts as a partial agonist at dopamine (especially D2) receptors and serotonin (especially 5-HT1A) receptors. The drug acts as an antagonist at 5-HT2A serotonin receptor sites.

Contraindications

Hypersensitivity to cariprazine or its components

Interactions

DRUGS

CYP3A4 inducers such as carbamazepine, rifampin: Possibly decreased effectiveness of cariprazine

CYP3A4 strong inhibitors such as itraconazole, ketoconazole: Increased exposure of cariprazine and risks of adverse reactions

Adverse Reactions

CNS: Agitation, akathisia, anxiety, body temperature dysregulation, **CVA**, dystonia, dizziness, extrapyramidal symptoms, fatigue, fever, headache, insomnia, **neuroleptic malignant syndrome**, Parkinsonism, restlessness, **seizures**, somnolence, syncope, tardive dyskinesia

CV: Hyperlipidemia, hypertension, orthostatic hypotension, tachycardia

EENT: Diabetic ketoacidosis, hyperglycemia, **hyperosmolar coma**

ENDO: Blurred vision, dry mouth, nasopharyngitis, oropharyngeal pain

GI: Abdominal pain, anorexia, constipation, diarrhea, dyspepsia, dysphagia, elevated liver enzymes, nausea, vomiting

GU: UTI

HEME: Agranulocytosis, **leukopenia**, **neutropenia**

MS: Arthralgia, back or extremity pain, elevated creatine phosphokinase, musculoskeletal stiffness, **rhabdomyolysis**

RESP: Cough

SKIN: Rash, **Stevens-Johnson syndrome**

Other: Hyponatremia, weight gain

Nursing Considerations

- Know that cariprazine should not be given to patients with severe hepatic or renal impairment nor to patients receiving a CYP3A4 inducer.
- Be aware that cariprazine should not be used to treat dementia-related psychosis in the elderly because of an increased risk of death.
- Use cautiously in patients with CV disease, cerebrovascular disease, seizure disorders, or conditions that would predispose them to hypotension. Also use cautiously in elderly patients because of increased risk of serious adverse effects such as MI or stroke.
- Monitor patient for difficulty swallowing or excessive somnolence, which could predispose to accidental injury or aspiration.

- Watch patient closely for suicidal tendencies, particularly when therapy starts and with dosage changes.

WARNING **Know that atypical antipsychotics such as cariprazine rarely may cause neuroleptic malignant syndrome, seizures, or tardive dyskinesia. Monitor patient closely throughout therapy, and take safety precautions as needed.**

- Monitor patient's CBC, as ordered, because serious adverse hematologic reactions may occur, such as agranulocytosis, leukopenia, and neutropenia. Assess more often during first few months of therapy if patient has a history of drug-induced leukopenia or neutropenia or a significantly low WBC count. If abnormalities occur during therapy, watch for fever or other signs of infection, notify prescriber, and, if severe, expect drug to be discontinued.
- Monitor patient's blood glucose level, lipid levels, and weight, as ordered, because atypical antipsychotic drugs such as cariprazine may cause metabolic changes. If patient is already a diabetic, monitor blood glucose levels more closely.
- Assess patient for late-occurring adverse reactions, especially akathisia or extrapyramidal symptoms that may first appear several weeks after cariprazine therapy begins. Also be on the alert for an increase in adverse reactions after each dosage increase. If late-effect adverse reactions occur, notify prescriber, and expect dosage to be reduced or drug discontinued.

PATIENT TEACHING

- Advise patient to get up slowly from a lying or sitting position during cariprazine therapy to minimize orthostatic hypotension and syncope.
- Instruct patient to avoid hazardous activities until drug's effects are known. Also, alert patient and family of increased risk for falls, especially if patient has other medical conditions or takes medication that may affect the nervous system.
- Urge patient to avoid activities that raise body temperature suddenly, such as strenuous exercise and exposure to situations that cause dehydration.
- Instruct patient to inform all prescribers of any drugs she's taking, including OTC drugs, because of risk of interactions.
- Advise female patient of childbearing age to notify prescriber if she intends to become or suspects that she is pregnant during therapy.
- Instruct diabetic patient to monitor blood glucose levels closely.
- Urge family or caregiver to watch patient closely for suicidal tendencies, especially when therapy is started and dosage changes are made.

carisoprodol

Soma, Vanadom

Class and Category

Pharmacologic class: Carbamate derivative
Therapeutic class: Skeletal muscle relaxant
Pregnancy category: C
Controlled substance schedule: IV

Indications and Dosages

➤ ***As adjunct to relieve acute musculoskeletal pain and stiffness***

TABLETS

Adults and children over age 16. 250 to 350 mg three times daily and at bedtime. *Maximum:* 3 weeks duration of therapy.

Route	Onset	Peak	Duration
P.O.	30 min	Unknown	4–6 hr

Mechanism of Action

Blocks interneuronal activity in descending reticular formation and spinal cord, producing muscle relaxation and sedation.

Contraindications

Hypersensitivity or idiosyncratic reactions to carisoprodol, to its components, or to meprobamate-related compounds; intermittent porphyria

Interactions

DRUGS

CNS depressants, psychotropic drugs: Additive CNS depression
fluvoxamine, omeprazole: Increased blood carisoprodol level
rifampin, St. John's wort: Decreased blood carisoprodol level

ACTIVITIES

alcohol use: Additive CNS depression

Adverse Reactions

CNS: Agitation, ataxia, depression, dizziness, drowsiness, fever, headache, insomnia, irritability, **seizures**, somnolence, syncope, tremor, vertigo
CV: Orthostatic hypotension, tachycardia
EENT: Diplopia, transient vision loss
GI: Epigastric discomfort, hiccups, nausea, vomiting
HEME: Eosinophilia
SKIN: Erythema multiforme, **Erythema multiforme**, facial flushing, pruritus, rash
Other: Drug dependence or withdrawal

Nursing Considerations

- Use carisoprodol cautiously in patients with history of drug addiction and in patients taking other CNS depressants, including alcohol.
- Know that carisoprodol therapy should last no longer than 3 weeks.
- Monitor patient closely for hypersensitivity or idiosyncratic reactions. They typically occur before the fourth dose in patients who have no previous carisoprodol exposure.
- Provide rest and other pain-relief measures.
- Expect to taper therapy as prescribed, rather than stopping it abruptly in order to avoid mild withdrawal symptoms.

PATIENT TEACHING

- Tell patient to take carisoprodol with meals if GI distress occurs.
- Caution patient that drug dependence and withdrawal may occur, especially if therapy lasts a long time or patient changes dosage without consulting prescriber.
- Warn patient about possible dizziness, drowsiness, syncope, and vertigo. Discourage hazardous activities, such as driving, until effects of drug are known.
- Inform patient that abruptly stopping drug can cause headache, insomnia, nausea, and other adverse reactions.
- Instruct patient to avoid alcohol and other CNS depressants while taking drug.
- Explain that saliva, sweat, and urine may appear darker (red, brown, or black). Reassure him that this discoloration is harmless but may stain garments.
- Tell patient to store drug in a tightly capped container at room temperature.
- Tell patient not to store drug in bathroom, near kitchen sink, or in other damp places to protect it from heat and moisture.
- Advise mothers who are breastfeeding while taking carisoprodol to monitor the infant for sedation.

carvedilol

Coreg

carvedilol phosphate

Coreg CR

Class and Category

Pharmacologic class: Nonselective beta blocker and alpha-1 blocker
Therapeutic class: Antihypertensive, heart failure treatment adjunct
Pregnancy category: C

Indications and Dosages

➤ *To control hypertension*

TABLETS

Adults. 6.25 mg twice daily with food for 7 to 14 days, if tolerated. Then dosage increased to 12.5 mg twice daily with food for 7 to 14 days, and then up to 25 mg twice daily with food, if tolerated and needed. *Maximum:* 50 mg daily with food.

E.R. CAPSULES

Adults. *Initial:* 20 mg once daily with food in morning. After 7 to 14 days, increased to 40 mg once daily with food in morning. After another 7 to 14 days, increased to 80 mg once daily with food in morning. *Maximum:* 80 mg once daily with food in morning.

➤ *As adjunct to treat mild to severe chronic heart failure of ischemic or cardiomyopathic origin*

TABLETS

Adults. 3.125 mg twice daily with food for 2 wk; then increased to 6.25, 12.5, and 25 mg twice daily with food at successive 2-wk intervals, as tolerated. *Maximum (for patients with mild to moderate heart failure):* 50 mg twice daily with food if patient weighs more than 85 kg (187 lb).

E.R. CAPSULES

Adults. *Initial:* 10 mg once daily with food in morning for 2 wk. Then increased to

20 mg once daily with food in morning, as needed. Subsequent dosage increased by 20 mg every 2 wk with food in morning, as needed. *Maximum:* 80 mg once daily.

➤ ***To reduce CV mortality after acute phase of MI in patients with left ventricular ejection fraction of 40% or less***

TABLETS

Adults. 6.25 mg twice daily with food with food for 3 to 10 days, if tolerated. Then dosage increased to 12.5 mg twice daily for 3 to 10 days and up to 25 mg twice daily with food, if needed and tolerated.

E.R. CAPSULES

Adults. *Initial:* 10 to 20 mg once daily with food in morning. After 3 to 10 days, increased to 20 to 40 mg once daily with food in morning. Increased again as needed every 3 to 10 days until reaching tolerance or target dose of 80 mg once daily with food in morning. *Maximum:* 80 mg once daily.

DOSAGE ADJUSTMENT For patient with fluid retention or low blood pressure or heart rate, starting dosage may be decreased, titration may be slowed, or both.

Route	Onset	Peak	Duration
P.O.	In 30 min	1.5–7 hr	Unknown

Mechanism of Action

Reduces cardiac output and tachycardia, causes vasodilation, and decreases peripheral vascular resistance, which reduces blood pressure and cardiac workload. When given for at least 4 weeks, carvedilol reduces plasma renin activity.

Contraindications

Asthma or related bronchospastic conditions; cardiogenic shock; decompensated heart failure that requires I.V. inotropics; history of serious hypersensitivity reactions, such as anaphylaxis, angioedema, or Stevens–Johnson syndrome; hypersensitivity to carvedilol or its components; second- or third-degree AV block, severe bradycardia, or sick sinus syndrome unless pacemaker is in place; severe hepatic impairment

Interactions

DRUGS

amiodarone; other CYP2C9 drugs, such as fluconazole: Increased risk of bradycardia or heart block
anesthetic agents that depress myocardial function (such as cyclopropane, trichloroethylene): Increased risk of depressed myocardial function
beta blockers, digoxin: Increased risk of bradycardia
calcium channel blockers (especially diltiazem and verapamil): Abnormal cardiac conduction and, possibly, increased adverse effects of calcium channel blockers
catecholamine-depleting drugs (such as MAO inhibitors, reserpine): Additive effects, increased risk of bradycardia and hypotension
cimetidine: Increased blood carvedilol level
clonidine: Risk of hypertension and tachycardia when clonidine is discontinued
cyclosporine, digoxin: Increased blood levels of these drugs
digoxin: Possibly increased digoxin level
insulin, oral antidiabetics: Increased risk of hypoglycemia
potent CYP2D6 inhibitors such as fluoxetine, paroxetine, propafenone, quinidine: Possibly increased blood carvedilol levels
rifampin: Decreased blood carvedilol level

Adverse Reactions

CNS: Asthenia, CVA, depression, dizziness, fatigue, fever, headache, hypesthesia, hypotonia, insomnia, light-headedness, malaise, paresthesia, somnolence, syncope, vertigo
CV: **Angina**, **AV block**, **bradycardia**, edema, **heart failure**, hypertension, hypertriglyceridemia, orthostatic hypotension, palpitations, peripheral vascular disorder
EENT: Blurred vision, dry eyes, periodontitis, pharyngitis, rhinitis
ENDO: hyperglycemia, **hypoglycemia**
GI: Abdominal pain, diarrhea, elevated liver enzymes, jaundice, **melena**, nausea, vomiting
GU: Albuminuria, hematuria, elevated BUN and creatinine levels, impotence, incontinence, **renal insufficiency**, UTI
HEME: **Aplastic anemia**, **decreased PT**, **thrombocytopenia**, **unusual bleeding** or bruising
MS: Arthralgia, arthritis, back pain, muscle cramps
RESP: Dyspnea, increased cough, **interstitial pneumonitis**
SKIN: **Erythema multiforme**, pruritus, purpura, **Stevens–Johnson syndrome**, **toxic**

C

epidermal necrolysis, Stevens–Johnson syndrome, toxic epidermal necrolysis, urticaria
Other: Anaphylaxis, angioedema, gout, **hyperkalemia,** hyperuricemia, **hyponatremia,** hypovolemia, viral infection, weight gain or loss

Nursing Considerations

- Use carvedilol cautiously in patients with peripheral vascular disease because it may aggravate symptoms of arterial insufficiency. In patients with diabetes mellitus it may mask signs of hypoglycemia, such as tachycardia, and may delay recovery.
- Monitor patient's blood glucose level, as ordered, during carvedilol therapy because drug may alter blood glucose level.

WARNING **Avoid stopping drug abruptly in patients with hyperthyroidism because thyroid storm may occur, and in patients with angina because it may worsen or MI may occur.**

- Know that if patient has heart failure, expect to also give digoxin, a diuretic, and an ACE inhibitor.
- Be aware that chronic beta blocker therapy such as carvedilol is not routinely withheld prior to major surgery because the benefits outweigh the risks associated with its use with general anesthesia and surgical procedures.

PATIENT TEACHING

- Instruct patient to swallow extended-release capsules whole. If swallowing capsules is difficult, tell patient he may open capsule and sprinkle beads on a spoonful of cold applesauce and then eat the applesauce immediately without chewing.
- Warn patient that drug may cause dizziness, light-headedness, and orthostatic hypotension; advise him to take precautions.
- Tell patient with heart failure to notify prescriber if he gains 5 lb or more in 2 days or if shortness of breath increases, which may signal worsening heart failure.
- Alert patient with diabetes to monitor his glycemic control closely because drug may increase blood glucose level or mask symptoms of hypoglycemia.
- Emphasize the need to seek emergency care if patient develops hives or swelling of the face, lips, tongue, or throat that causes trouble swallowing or breathing.
- Advise patient to notify ophthalmologist of carvedilol therapy because if cataract surgery is required, modifications of the surgical technique may be necessary.
- Tell patient to notify prescriber of all medications taken, including over-the-counter preparations, before using them.
- Tell women of childbearing age to inform prescriber if pregnancy is known or suspected, as safety in pregnancy is unknown. Also, tell mothers wishing to breastfeed to discuss this decision with prescriber before doing so.

caspofungin acetate

Cancidas

Class and Category

Pharmacologic class: Echinocandins
Therapeutic class: Antifungal
Pregnancy category: C

Indications and Dosages

➤ *To treat invasive aspergillosis in patients refractory to or intolerant of other therapies; to treat candidemia and candidal infections in intra-abdominal abscesses, peritonitis, and pleural space infections*

I.V. INFUSION

Adults. *Initial:* 70 mg infused over 1 hr on day 1, followed by 50 mg infused over 1 hr once daily. *Maximum:* 70 mg once daily.
Children ages 3 months to 17 years. *Initial:* 70 mg/m^2 infused over 1 hr on day 1, followed by 50 mg/m^2 infused over 1 hr once daily and increased to 70 mg/m^2 once daily and given over 1 hr, if needed and tolerated. *Maximum:* 70 mg once daily regardless of dose calculated based on patient's body surface area.

➤ *To treat presumed fungal infections in febrile, neutropenic patients*

I.V. INFUSION

Adults. *Initial:* 70 mg infused over 1 hr on day 1, followed by 50 mg infused over 1 hr once daily for at least 14 days, including at least 7 days after neutropenia and symptoms have resolved. Increased to 70 mg infused over 1 hr once daily as needed. *Maximum:* 70 mg once daily.
Children ages 3 months to 17 years.

Mechanism of Action

Caspofungin acetate interferes with fungal cell membrane synthesis by inhibiting the synthesis of β (1, 3)-D-glucan. A polypeptide, β (1, 3)-D-glucan is the essential component of the fungal cell membrane that makes it rigid and protective. Without it, fungal cells rupture and die. This mechanism of action is most effective against susceptible filamentous fungi, such as *Aspergillus*.

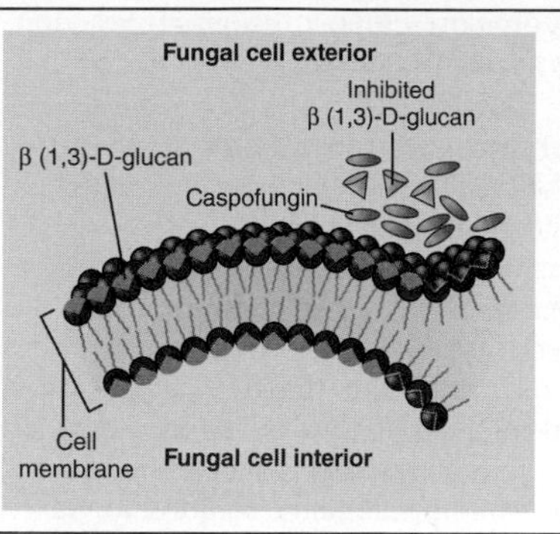

Initial: 70 mg/m^2 infused over 1 hr on day 1, followed by 50 mg/m^2 infused over 1 hr once daily for at least 14 days, including at least 7 days after neutropenia and symptoms have resolved. *Maximum:* 70 mg once daily regardless of dose calculated based on patient's body surface area.

➤ *To treat esophageal candidiasis*

I.V. INFUSION

Adults. 50 mg infused over 1 hr once daily for 7 to 14 days after symptoms have resolved.

Children ages 3 months to 17 years. *Initial:* 70 mg/m^2 infused over 1 hr on day 1, followed by 50 mg/m^2 infused over 1 hr once daily. *Maximum:* 70 mg once daily regardless of dose calculated based on patient's body surface area.

DOSAGE ADJUSTMENT For patients with moderate hepatic insufficiency, dosage reduced to 35 mg daily after initial 70-mg loading dose, if a loading dose is required. For patients receiving carbamazepine, dexamethasone, efavirenz, nevirapine, phenytoin, or rifampin, dosage may be increased to 70 mg once daily for adults and 70 mg/m^2 once daily for children (not to exceed 70 mg daily).

Incompatibilities

Don't mix or infuse with other drugs. Don't admix with diluents that contain dextrose.

Contraindications

Hypersensitivity to caspofungin acetate or its components

Interactions

DRUGS

carbamazepine, dexamethasone, efavirenz, nelfinavir, nevirapine, phenytoin, rifampin: Possibly decreased blood caspofungin level

cyclosporine: Transient increases in ALT and AST levels

tacrolimus: Possibly decreased blood tacrolimus level

Adverse Reactions

CNS: Asthenia, anxiety, chills, confusion, depression, dizziness, fatigue, fever, headache, insomnia, paresthesia, **seizures**, somnolence, tremor, warmth sensation

CV: Edema, hypertension, **hypotension**, phlebitis, tachycardia, thrombophlebitis

EENT: Epistaxis, mucosal inflammation, **stridor**

ENDO: Hyperglycemia

GI: Abdominal distention or pain, anorexia, constipation, diarrhea, dyspepsia, elevated liver enzymes, **hepatic dysfunction or necrosis**, hepatomegaly, hyperbilirubinemia, jaundice, nausea, **pancreatitis**, vomiting

GU: Elevated BUN or serum creatinine level, hematuria, proteinuria, **renal failure or insufficiency**, UTI

HEME: Decreased hemoglobin and hematocrit

MS: Arthralgia, back or extremity pain, myalgia

RESP: Bronchospasm, cough, crackles, dyspnea, **hypoxia**, pleural effusion, pneumonia, **respiratory failure**, tachypnea

SKIN: Diaphoresis, erythema, **erythema multiforme**, flushing, petechiae, pruritus, rash, sensation of warmth, skin exfoliation, **Stevens–Johnson syndrome**, **toxic epidermal necrolysis**, urticaria

Other: Anaphylaxis, **angioedema**, **bacteremia**, **decreased serum bicarbonate level**, elevated gamma-glutamyltransferase level, **hypercalcemia**, **hyperkalemia**, hyperphosphatemia, **hypokalemia**,

hypomagnesemia, infusion-site reaction, **sepsis**, **septic shock**

Nursing Considerations

- Use cautiously in patients with a history of allergic skin reactions because caspofungin may cause serious skin reactions such as Stevens–Johnson syndrome and toxic epidermal necrolysis, which can be life-threatening. Prepare a 70-mg loading dose by letting vial reach room temperature. Reconstitute by adding 10.5 ml normal saline solution to vial. Dilute for administration by transferring 10 ml of reconstituted drug to 250 ml normal saline solution.
- Prepare a 70-mg loading dose from two 50-mg vials by adding 10.5 ml normal saline solution to each vial; then transfer 14 ml of prepared solution to 250 ml normal saline solution.
- Prepare a daily 50-mg infusion by letting vial reach room temperature. Reconstitute by adding 10.5 ml normal saline solution to vial. Dilute for administration by transferring only 10 ml of reconstituted drug to 250 ml normal saline solution.
- Prepare a daily 50-mg infusion at reduced volume by adding 10 ml of reconstituted drug to 100 ml normal saline solution.
- Prepare a 35-mg daily dose for patient with moderate hepatic insufficiency, by reconstituting 50-mg vial with 10.5 ml normal saline solution. To dilute, transfer only 7 ml of reconstituted drug to 250 ml normal saline solution or, if needed, to 100 ml normal saline solution.
- Mix powder gently to obtain clear solution. Don't use if solution is cloudy or contains precipitate. Discard unused solution after 24 hours.
- Infuse drug slowly over about 1 hour.
- Watch for flushed skin, and assess patient often for unexplained temperature elevation.
- Monitor patient for possible histamine-mediated adverse reactions such as angioedema, bronchospasm, facial swelling, pruritus, rash, or warmth sensation. Report these symptoms immediately and expect caspofungin therapy to be discontinued.

WARNING **Assess for airway patency if patient develops excessive facial edema or respiratory stridor. Provide emergency airway management if complete obstruction occurs.**

- Monitor patient's liver function test results, as ordered, and report abnormalities.

PATIENT TEACHING

- Urge patient to notify prescriber immediately if he has difficulty talking, swallowing, or breathing during drug administration.

cefaclor

Ceclor (CAN)

Class and Category

Pharmacologic class: Second-generation cephalosporin
Therapeutic class: Antibiotic
Pregnancy category: B

Indications and Dosages

➤ ***To treat otitis media caused by*** **Haemophilus influenzae,** ***staphylococci,*** **Streptococcus pneumoniae,** ***or*** **Streptococcus pyogenes;** ***lower respiratory tract infections, including pneumonia caused by*** **H. influenzae, S. pneumoniae,** ***or*** **S. pyogenes;** ***pharyngitis and tonsillitis caused by*** **S. pyogenes;** ***UTI, including cystitis and pyelonephritis, caused by*** **Escherichia coli, Klebsiella** ***species,*** **Proteus mirabilis,** ***or coagulase-negative staphylococci; and skin and soft-tissue infections caused by*** **S. pyogenes** ***or*** **Staphylococcus aureus**

CAPSULES

Adults and adolescents. 250 mg every 8 hr. For severe infections, such as pneumonia, or those caused by less susceptible organisms, 500 mg every 8 hr. *Maximum:* 4 g daily.

CHEWABLE TABLETS, ORAL SUSPENSION

Adults and adolescents. 250 mg every 8 hr. For severe infections, such as pneumonia, or those caused by less susceptible organisms, 500 mg every 8 hr. *Maximum:* 4 g daily.

Children. 20 mg/kg daily in divided doses every 8 hr. For serious infections, such as otitis media, and infections caused by less susceptible organisms, 40 mg/kg daily in divided doses every 8 hr. For otitis media and pharyngitis, total daily dosage divided and given every 12 hr, if needed. *Maximum:* 1 g daily.

➤ ***To treat acute bacterial infection in chronic bronchitis or secondary bacterial infection in acute bronchitis caused by* H. influenzae, Moraxella catarrhalis, *or* S. pneumoniae**

E.R. TABLETS

Adults and adolescents age 16 and over. 500 mg with food every 12 hr for 7 days.

➤ ***To treat pharyngitis and tonsillitis caused by* S. pyogenes**

E.R. TABLETS

Adults and adolescents age 16 and over. 375 mg with food every 12 hr for 10 days.

➤ ***To treat uncomplicated skin and soft-tissue infections caused by* S. aureus**

E.R. TABLETS

Adults and adolescents age 16 and over. 375 mg with food every 12 hr for 7 to 10 days.

Mechanism of Action

Interferes with bacterial cell wall synthesis by inhibiting cross-linking of peptidoglycan strands, which stiffen cell membranes. As a result, bacterial cells rupture.

Contraindications

Hypersensitivity to cefaclor, other cephalosporins, or their components

Interactions

DRUGS

aminoglycosides, loop diuretics: Increased risk of nephrotoxicity
antacids: Decreased blood cefaclor level (E.R. tablets)
oral anticoagulants: Increased anticoagulation

Adverse Reactions

CNS: Chills, fever, headache, **seizures**
CV: Edema
EENT: Hearing loss, oral candidiasis
GI: Abdominal cramps, diarrhea, elevated liver enzymes, **hepatic failure**, hepatomegaly, nausea, **pseudomembranous colitis**, vomiting
GU: Elevated BUN level, **nephrotoxicity**, **renal failure**, vaginal candidiasis
HEME: Eosinophilia, **hemolytic anemia**, **hypoprothrombinemia**, **neutropenia**, **thrombocytopenia**, **unusual bleeding**
MS: Arthralgia
RESP: Dyspnea
SKIN: Ecchymosis, erythema, **erythema multiforme**, pruritus, rash, **Stevens–Johnson syndrome**
Other: **Anaphylaxis**, superinfection

Nursing Considerations

- Use cefaclor cautiously in patients with impaired renal function or a history of GI disease, particularly colitis, and in patients who are hypersensitive to penicillin; about 10% of them have cross-sensitivity.
- Obtain culture and sensitivity test results, if possible and as ordered, before giving drug.
- Monitor BUN and serum creatinine levels for early signs of nephrotoxicity. Also monitor fluid intake and output; decreasing urine output may indicate nephrotoxicity.
- Be aware that an allergic reaction may occur a few days after therapy starts.
- Assess bowel pattern daily; severe diarrhea may indicate pseudomembranous colitis.
- Assess patient for superinfection: cough or sputum changes, diarrhea, drainage, fever, malaise, pain, perineal itching, rash, redness, and swelling.

PATIENT TEACHING

- Instruct patient to complete the prescribed course of therapy, even if he feels better.
- Tell patient to swallow E.R. tablets whole and not to break, chew, or crush them.
- Advise patient to take E.R. tablets with food to enhance absorption.
- Instruct patient to take capsules or E.R. tablets with a full glass of water.
- Tell patient to shake oral suspension well before measuring and to use a calibrated measuring device to ensure accurate dose.
- Tell patient to refrigerate oral suspension and to discard unused portion after 14 days.
- Instruct patient to report severe diarrhea to prescriber immediately.
- Explain that buttermilk and yogurt protect intestinal flora and decrease diarrhea.
- Urge patient to report evidence of superinfection.

cefadroxil

Class and Category

Pharmacologic class: First-generation cephalosporin
Therapeutic class: Antibiotic
Pregnancy category: B

Indications and Dosages

➤ *To treat UTI caused by* Escherichia coli, Klebsiella *species, or* Proteus mirabilis

CAPSULES, TABLETS

Adults. For uncomplicated lower UTI, 1 to 2 g once daily or in divided doses every 12 hr. For all other UTIs, 2 g daily in divided doses every 12 hr.

ORAL SUSPENSION

Adults. For uncomplicated lower UTI, 1 to 2 g once daily or in divided doses every 12 hr. For all other UTIs, 2 g daily in divided doses every 12 hr.

Children. 30 mg/kg daily in divided doses every 12 hr. *Maximum:* Adult dosage.

➤ *To treat skin and soft-tissue infections caused by staphylococci or streptococci*

CAPSULES, TABLETS

Adults. 1 g daily or 500 mg every 12 hr.

ORAL SUSPENSION

Adults. 1 g daily or 500 mg every 12 hr.

Children. 30 mg/kg daily in divided doses every 12 hr. *Maximum:* Adult dosage.

➤ *To treat pharyngitis and tonsillitis caused by group A beta-hemolytic streptococci*

CAPSULES, TABLETS

Adults. 1 g daily or 500 mg twice daily for 10 days.

ORAL SUSPENSION

Adults. 1 g daily or 500 mg twice daily for 10 days.

Children. 30 mg/kg daily as a single dose or in equally divided doses every 12 hr for 10 days. *Maximum:* 1 g daily or 500 mg twice daily for 10 days.

DOSAGE ADJUSTMENT For adult patients with renal impairment, initial dose of 1 g; then maintenance of 0.5 g every 12 hr if creatinine clearance is 25 to 50 ml/min; 0.5 g every 24 hr if creatinine clearance is 10 to 25 ml/min; and every 36 hr if creatinine clearance is 0 to 10 ml/min.

Mechanism of Action

Interferes with bacterial cell wall synthesis by inhibiting the final step in the cross-linking of peptidoglycan strands. Peptidoglycan makes cell membranes rigid and protective. Without it, bacterial cells rupture and die.

Contraindications

Hypersensitivity to cefadroxil, other cephalosporins or their components

Interactions

DRUGS

aminoglycosides, loop diuretics: Increased toxicity of these drugs

Adverse Reactions

CNS: Chills, fever, headache, **seizures**
CV: Edema
EENT: Hearing loss, oral candidiasis
GI: Abdominal cramps, diarrhea, elevated liver enzymes, **hepatic failure**, hepatomegaly, nausea, **pseudomembranous colitis**, vomiting
GU: Elevated BUN level, **nephrotoxicity**, **renal failure**, vaginal candidiasis
HEME: Eosinophilia, **hemolytic anemia**, **hypoprothrombinemia**, **neutropenia**, **thrombocytopenia**, **unusual bleeding**
MS: Arthralgia
RESP: Dyspnea
SKIN: Ecchymosis, erythema, **erythema multiforme**, pruritus, rash, **Stevens–Johnson syndrome**
Other: Anaphylaxis, superinfection

Nursing Considerations

- Use cefadroxil cautiously in patients with impaired renal function or a history of GI disease, particularly colitis. Also use drug cautiously in patients who are hypersensitive to penicillin because cross-sensitivity has occurred in about 10% of such patients.
- Obtain culture and sensitivity test results, if possible and as ordered, before giving drug.
- Be aware that an allergic reaction may occur a few days after therapy starts.
- Monitor BUN and serum creatinine levels for early signs of nephrotoxicity. Also monitor fluid intake and output; decreasing urine output may indicate nephrotoxicity.
- Assess bowel pattern daily; severe diarrhea may indicate pseudomembranous colitis.
- Assess patient for superinfection: cough or sputum changes, diarrhea, drainage, fever, malaise, pain, perineal itching, rash, redness, and swelling.

PATIENT TEACHING

- Instruct patient to complete the prescribed course of therapy.
- Tell patient to shake oral suspension before measuring and to use a liquid-measuring device to ensure accurate doses.

- Tell patient to refrigerate oral suspension and to discard the unused portion after 14 days.
- Urge patient to report watery, bloody stools to prescriber immediately, even up to 2 months after drug therapy has ended.
- Inform patient that buttermilk and yogurt can help maintain intestinal flora and decrease diarrhea.
- Teach patient to recognize and report evidence of superinfection, such as furry tongue, perineal itching, and loose, foul-smelling stools.

cefazolin sodium

Ancef, Kefzol

Class and Category

Pharmacologic class: First-generation cephalosporin
Therapeutic class: Antibiotic
Pregnancy category: B

Indications and Dosages

➤ *To treat respiratory tract infections caused by* Staphylococcus aureus, Streptococcus pneumoniae, *or* S. pyogenes; *skin and soft-tissue infections caused by* S. aureus, *group A beta-hemolytic,* S. pyogenes, *or other strains of streptococci; biliary or urinary tract infections caused by* Escherichia coli, Proteus mirabilis, S. aureus, *or various strains of streptococci; bone and joint infections caused by* S. aureus; *genital infections, such as epididymitis and prostatitis, caused by* E. coli, Klebsiella *species, or* P. mirabilis; *septicemia caused by* E. coli, P. mirabilis; *and endocarditis caused by* S. aureus *or* S. pyogenes

I.V. INFUSION, I.V. OR I.M. INJECTION

Adults. For mild infections, 250 to 500 mg every 8 hr; for moderate to severe infections, 500 to 1,000 mg every 6 to 8 hr; and for severe life-threatening infections, 1,000 to 1,500 mg every 6 hr. I.V. injection given as a bolus slowly over 3 to 5 min. I.V. infusion given over 30 min. *Maximum:* 6 g daily.

Children. For mild to moderate infections, 25 to 50 mg/kg daily divided equally and given three times daily or four times daily; for severe infections, 100 mg/kg daily divided equally and given three times daily or four times daily. I.V. injection given as a bolus slowly over 3 to 5 min. I.V. infusion given over 30 min.

➤ *To treat pneumococcal pneumonia*

I.V. INFUSION, I.V. OR I.M. INJECTION

Adults. 500 mg every 12 hr. I.V. injection given as bolus slowly over 3 to 5 min. I.V. infusion given over 30 min.

➤ *To treat acute uncomplicated UTI caused by* E. coli, Klebsiella *species, or* P. mirabilis, *and some strains of* Enterobacter *and* Enterococcus

I.V. INFUSION, I.V. OR I.M. INJECTION

Adults. 1 g every 12 hr. I.V. injection given as a bolus slowly over 3 to 5 min. I.V. infusion given over 30 min.

➤ *To provide surgical prophylaxis*

I.V. INFUSION, I.V. OR I.M. INJECTION

Adults. 1 to 2 g 30 to 60 min before surgery; 0.5 to 1 g during surgery if it lasts 2 hr or longer; 0.5 to 1 g every 6 to 8 hr for 24 hr after surgery. I.V. injection given as a bolus slowly over 3 to 5 min. I.V. infusion given over 30 min.

DOSAGE ADJUSTMENT After initial loading dose appropriate to infection's severity, dosage interval restricted to at least 8 hr for adults with creatinine clearance of 35 to 54 ml/min; dosage reduced by 50% and given every 12 hr for adults with creatinine clearance of 11 to 34 ml/min; and dosage reduced by 50% and given every 18 to 24 hr for adults with creatinine clearance of 10 ml/min or less. Dosage reduced to 60% and given every 12 hr for children with creatinine clearance of 40 to 70 ml/min; dosage reduced to 25% and given every 12 hr for children with creatinine clearance of 20 to 40 ml/min; and dosage reduced to 10% and given every 24 hr for children with creatinine clearance of 5 to 20 ml/min.

Mechanism of Action

Interferes with bacterial cell wall synthesis by inhibiting the final step in the cross-linking of peptidoglycan strands. Peptidoglycan makes cell membranes rigid and protective. Without it, bacterial cells rupture and die.

Incompatibilities

To prevent mutual inactivation, don't mix cefazolin with aminoglycosides. Also avoid mixing cefazolin with other drugs, including pentamidine isethionate.

Contraindications

Hypersensitivity to cefazolin, other cephalosporins or their components

Interactions

DRUGS

aminoglycosides, loop diuretics: Additive nephrotoxicity
probenecid: Increased and prolonged blood cefazolin level

Adverse Reactions

CNS: Chills, fever, headache, **seizures**
CV: Edema
EENT: Hearing loss, oral candidiasis
GI: Abdominal cramps, diarrhea, elevated liver enzymes, **hepatic failure**, **hepatitis**, hepatomegaly, nausea, **pseudomembranous colitis**, vomiting
GU: Elevated BUN and serum creatinine levels, **nephrotoxicity**, **renal failure**, vaginal candidiasis
HEME: Eosinophilia, **hemolytic anemia**, **hypoprothrombinemia**, **neutropenia**, **thrombocytopenia**, **unusual bleeding**
MS: Arthralgia
RESP: Dyspnea
SKIN: Ecchymosis, erythema, **erythema multiforme**, pruritus, rash, **Stevens–Johnson syndrome**
Other: Anaphylaxis; injection-site pain, redness, and swelling; superinfection

Nursing Considerations

- Use cefazolin cautiously in patients with impaired renal function or a history of GI disease, particularly colitis. Also use cautiously in patients hypersensitive to penicillin because cross-sensitivity has occurred in about 10% of such patients.
- Obtain culture and sensitivity test results, if possible and as ordered, before giving drug.

WARNING Know that to prevent unintentional overdose, the 2-g dose container of cefazolin for injection USP and dextrose injection USP shouldn't be used in children who require less than the full adult dose. Instead, use only the 1-g container of cefazolin for injection USP and dextrose injection USP for children when the individual dose is the entire contents of the 1-g container and not any fraction of it.

- Reconstitute 500-mg drug vial with 2 ml of sterile water for injection (or 1-g vial with 2.5 ml). Shake well until dissolved.
- For direct I.V. injection, further dilute reconstituted solution with at least 5 ml sterile water for injection. Inject slowly over 3 to 5 minutes through tubing of a flowing compatible I.V. solution.
- For intermittent I.V. infusion, reconstitute 500 to 1,000 mg in 50 to 100 ml normal saline solution, D_5W, $D_{10}W$, dextrose 5% in lactated Ringer's solution, dextrose 5% in quarter-normal (0.2) saline solution, dextrose 5% in half-normal (0.45) saline solution, dextrose 5% in normal saline solution, lactated Ringer's injection, 5% or 10% invert sugar in sterile water for injection, 5% sodium bicarbonate (Ancef), or Ringer's injection.
- Administer I.M. injection deep into large muscle mass, such as the gluteus maximus.
- Store reconstituted drug up to 24 hours at room temperature or 10 days refrigerated.
- Monitor I.V. site for irritation, phlebitis, and extravasation.
- Monitor BUN and serum creatinine for early signs of nephrotoxicity. Also monitor fluid intake and output; decreasing urine output may indicate nephrotoxicity.
- Be aware that an allergic reaction may occur a few days after therapy starts.
- Assess bowel pattern daily; severe diarrhea may indicate pseudomembranous colitis.
- Watch for evidence of superinfection: cough, diarrhea, drainage, fever, malaise, pain, perineal itching, rash, redness, swelling.
- Assess for arthralgia, bleeding, ecchymosis, and pharyngitis; they may indicate a blood dyscrasia.

PATIENT TEACHING

- Instruct patient to complete the prescribed course of therapy.
- Reassure patient that I.M. injection doesn't typically cause pain.
- Tell patient to report watery, bloody stools to prescriber immediately, even up to 2 months after drug therapy has ended.

cefdinir

Class and Category

Pharmacologic class: Third-generation cephalosporin
Therapeutic class: Antibiotic
Pregnancy category: B

Indications and Dosages

➤ *To treat community-acquired pneumonia caused by* Haemophilus influenzae *(including beta-lactamase–producing strains),* Haemophilus parainfluenzae *(including beta-lactamase–producing strains),* Streptococcus pneumoniae *(penicillin-susceptible strains only), and* Moraxella catarrhalis *(including beta-lactamase–producing strains)*

CAPSULES

Adults and adolescents. 300 mg every 12 hr for 10 to 14 days. *Maximum:* 600 mg daily.

➤ *To treat pharyngitis or tonsillitis caused by* Streptococcus pyogenes *and acute exacerbations of chronic bronchitis caused by* H. influenzae *(including beta-lactamase–producing strains),* H. parainfluenzae *(including beta-lactamase–producing strains),* S. pneumoniae *(penicillin-susceptible strains only), and* M. catarrhalis *(including beta-lactamase–producing strains)*

CAPSULES

Adults and adolescents. 300 mg every 12 hr for 5 to 10 days or 600 mg every 24 hr for 10 days. *Maximum:* 600 mg daily.

ORAL SUSPENSION

Children ages 6 months to 12 years. 7 mg/kg every 12 hr for 5 to 10 days or 14 mg/kg every 24 hr for 10 days (for pharyngitis or tonsillitis).

➤ *To treat acute maxillary sinusitis caused by* H. influenzae *(including beta-lactamase–producing strains),* S. pneumoniae *(penicillin-susceptible strains only), and* M. catarrhalis *(including beta-lactamase–producing strains)*

CAPSULES

Adults and adolescents. 300 mg every 12 hr or 600 mg every 24 hr for 10 days. *Maximum:* 600 mg daily.

ORAL SUSPENSION

Children ages 6 months to 12 years. 7 mg/kg every 12 hr or 14 mg/kg every 24 hr for 10 days.

➤ *To treat uncomplicated skin and soft-tissue infections caused by* Staphylococcus aureus *(including beta-lactamase–producing strains) and* Streptococcus pyogenes

CAPSULES

Adults and adolescents. 300 mg every 12 hr for 10 days. *Maximum:* 600 mg daily.

ORAL SUSPENSION

Children ages 6 months to 12 years. 7 mg/kg every 12 hr for 10 days.

➤ *To treat acute bacterial otitis media caused by* H. influenzae *(including beta-lactamase–producing strains),* S. pneumoniae *(penicillin-susceptible strains only), and* M. catarrhalis *(including beta-lactamase–producing strains)*

ORAL SUSPENSION

Children ages 6 months to 12 years. 7 mg/kg every 12 hr for 5 to 10 days or 14 mg/kg every 24 hr for 10 days.

DOSAGE ADJUSTMENT For adults with creatinine clearance less than 30 ml/min, dosage not to exceed 300 mg daily; for children with creatinine clearance less than 30 ml/min, dosage not to exceed 7 mg/kg (up to 300 mg) daily. For patients undergoing intermittent hemodialysis, dosage is 300 mg or 7 mg/kg every other day, beginning at the end of each hemodialysis session, as prescribed.

Mechanism of Action

Interferes with bacterial cell wall synthesis by inhibiting the final step in the cross-linking of peptidoglycan strands. Peptido-glycan makes cell membranes rigid and protective. Withoutit, bacterial cells rupture and die. Because cefdinir is not degraded by some bacterial beta-lactamase enzymes, it's effective against many organisms that are resistant to both penicillins and some cephalosporins.

Contraindications

Hypersensitivity to cefdinir, other cephalosporins, or their components

Interactions

DRUGS

antacids that contain aluminum or magnesium: Decreased cefdinir absorption if given within 2 hours of antacid
iron salts: Reduced cefdinir absorption if given within 2 hours of iron
probenecid: Increased blood level and prolonged half-life of cefdinir

Adverse Reactions

CNS: Asthenia, dizziness, drowsiness, headache, insomnia, somnolence
EENT: Dry mouth, pharyngitis, rhinitis
GI: Abdominal pain, anorexia, constipation, diarrhea, flatulence, indigestion, nausea, **pseudomembranous colitis**, stool discoloration, vomiting
GU: Leukorrhea, vaginal candidiasis, vaginitis
HEME: Leukopenia
SKIN: Pruritus, rash
Other: Anaphylaxis, serum sickness–like reaction

Nursing Considerations

- Reconstitute cefdinir powder for oral suspension by tapping bottle to loosen powder, and then dilute with water to 125 mg/5 ml. Shake well before each use. Discard any unused portion after 10 days. Keep suspension bottle tightly closed, and store it at room temperature.
- Give antacids that contain aluminum or magnesium and iron salts at least 2 hours before or after cefdinir because they may interfere with cefdinir absorption.
- Monitor patient allergic to penicillin for evidence of hypersensitivity reaction, from a mild rash to fatal anaphylaxis, because cross-sensitivity can occur.
- Monitor patient with a chronic GI condition, such as colitis, for signs and symptoms of a drug-related exacerbation.
- Know that because all cephalosporins have the potential to cause bleeding, monitor elderly patients and patients with a preexisting coagulopathy, including vitamin K deficiency, for elevated PT or APTT.
- Monitor patient closely for diarrhea, which may indicate pseudomembranous colitis caused by *Clostridium difficile.* If diarrhea occurs, notify prescriber and expect to withhold cefdinir and treat with fluids, electrolytes, protein, and an antibiotic effective against *C. difficile.*
- Assess for other evidence of superinfection, including perineal itching; loose, foul-smelling stools; and vaginal drainage.

PATIENT TEACHING

- Advise patient taking cefdinir oral suspension to shake bottle well before use and to use a liquid-measuring device to ensure accurate dose.
- Inform patient that tablet coating may cause stools to become a reddish color.
- Instruct patient to complete entire course of therapy, even if he feels better.
- Advise patient to take iron salts and aluminum- or magnesium-containing antacids at least 2 hours before or after taking cefdinir.
- Inform patient with history of colitis that cefdinir may worsen it; urge him to notify prescriber promptly if symptoms develop.
- Inform patient with diabetes mellitus that oral suspension contains 2.86 g of sucrose per teaspoon; advise him to monitor his blood glucose levels as appropriate.
- Teach patient to recognize and report evidence of superinfection, such as perineal itching; loose, foul-smelling stools; and vaginal drainage.
- Inform patient that buttermilk and yogurt can help prevent superinfection and may decrease diarrhea.
- Urge patient to tell prescriber about diarrhea that's severe or lasts longer than 3 days. Remind patient that watery or bloody stools can occur 2 or more months after antibiotic therapy and can be serious, requiring prompt treatment.

cefditoren pivoxil

Spectracef

Class and Category

Pharmacologic class: Third-generation cephalosporin
Therapeutic class: Antibiotic
Pregnancy category: B

Indications and Dosages

➤ *To treat mild to moderate acute bacterial exacerbation of chronic bronchitis or community-acquired pneumonia caused by* Haemophilus influenzae *(including beta-lactamase–producing strains),* Haemophilus parainfluenzae *(including beta-lactamase–producing strains),* Streptococcus pneumoniae *(penicillin-susceptible strains), or* Moraxella catarrhalis *(including beta-lactamase–producing strains)*

TABLETS

Adults and children age 12 and over. 400 mg twice daily for 10 days or for 14 days for community-acquired pneumonia.

➤ *To treat mild to moderate pharyngitis and tonsillitis caused by* Streptococcus pyogenes

TABLETS

Adults and children age 12 and over. 200 mg twice daily for 10 days.

➤ *To treat mild to moderate uncomplicated skin and soft-tissue infections caused by* Staphylococcus aureus *(including beta-lactamase–producing strains) or* S. pyogenes

TABLETS

Adults and children age 12 and over. 200 mg twice daily for 10 days.

DOSAGE ADJUSTMENT For patient with a creatinine clearance of 30 to 49 ml/min, maximum dosage reduced to 200 mg twice daily. For patient with a creatinine clearance less than 30 ml/min, maximum dosage reduced to 200 mg daily.

Mechanism of Action

Interferes with bacterial cell wall synthesis by inhibiting the final step in the cross-linking of peptidoglycan strands. Peptidoglycan makes the cell membrane rigid and protective. Without it, bacterial cells rupture and die. This mechanism of action is most effective against bacteria that divide rapidly, including many gram-positive and gram-negative bacteria. Cefditoren isn't inactivated by beta lactamase produced by some bacteria.

Contraindications

Carnitine deficiency or inborn metabolic disorder that causes it; hypersensitivity to cefditoren, other cephalosporins or their components, or to milk

Interactions

DRUGS

aluminum- and magnesium-containing antacids, H_2-receptor antagonists: Reduced cefditoren absorption

H_2-receptor antagonists such as famotidine: Possibly reduced absorption of cefditoren

probenecid: Increased and prolonged blood cefditoren level

FOODS

any food: Increased cefditoren absorption

Adverse Reactions

CNS: Headache, hyperactivity, hypertonia, **seizures**

GI: Abdominal pain, diarrhea, dyspepsia, **hepatic dysfunction**, nausea, **pseudomembranous colitis**, vomiting

GU: Acute renal failure, **renal dysfunction**, **toxic nephropathy**

HEME: Aplastic anemia, **hemolytic anemia**, **hemorrhage**, **thrombocytopenia**

MS: Arthralgia

RESP: Pneumonia

SKIN: Erythema multiforme, **Stevens–Johnson syndrome**, **toxic epidermal necrolysis**

Other: Allergic reaction, **anaphylaxis**, carnitine deficiency, drug fever, serum sickness–like reaction, superinfection

Nursing Considerations

WARNING Be aware that before starting cefditoren therapy, determine if patient is hypersensitive to milk protein because cefditoren contains sodium caseinate, a milk protein. Drug should not be given to patient with this hypersensitivity. Also determine if patient has had a hypersensitivity reaction to cefditoren or other cephalosporins (because drug is contraindicated in these patients) or to penicillin (because cross-sensitivity has occurred in about 10% of such patients).

- Know that cefditoren shouldn't be used for prolonged treatment because of the risk of carnitine deficiency.
- Obtain culture and sensitivity test results before giving cefditoren, if possible and as ordered.
- Assess patient for evidence of *Clostridium difficile* infection and pseudomembranous colitis, such as profuse, watery diarrhea. For mild cases, expect to discontinue cefditoren.

For moderate to severe cases, expect to also give fluids and electrolytes, protein supplementation, and an antibacterial drug effective against *C. difficile.*

- Monitor patient for an allergic reaction. If an allergic reaction occurs, expect to discontinue drug, as prescribed. For serious acute hypersensitivity reactions, expect to also give antihistamines, corticosteroids, epinephrine, I.V. fluids, oxygen, and vasopressors, as prescribed.
- Monitor BUN and serum creatinine levels to detect early signs of renal dysfunction. Also monitor fluid intake and output.
- Watch for a decreased PT, as ordered, in at-risk patients, such as those with renal or hepatic impairment, those with a poor nutritional state, and those receiving anticoagulant or prolonged antibiotic therapy. Notify prescriber if a decrease occurs, and give vitamin K as ordered.

PATIENT TEACHING

- Urge patient to complete prescribed course of therapy.
- Instruct patient to take cefditoren with meals to enhance drug absorption.
- Advise patient not to take cefditoren with aluminum- or magnesium-containing antacids or other drugs used to reduce stomach acids because these drugs may interfere with cefditoren absorption.
- Explain that buttermilk and yogurt help maintain normal intestinal flora and can decrease diarrhea during therapy.
- Instruct patient to report severe diarrhea to prescriber immediately.

cefepime hydrochloride

Maxipime

Class and Category

Pharmacologic class: Fourth-generation cephalosporin
Therapeutic class: Antibiotic
Pregnancy category: B

Indications and Dosages

➤ *To treat mild to moderate UTI caused by* Escherichia coli, Klebsiella pneumoniae, *or* Proteus mirabilis

I.V. INFUSION, I.M. INJECTION (ONLY FOR UTI CAUSED BY *E. COLI*)

Adults and children age 16 and over. 500 to 1,000 mg every 12 hr for 7 to 10 days. I.V. infusion given over 30 min.
Children ages 2 months to 16 years weighing up to 40 kg (88 lb). 50 mg/kg/dose every 12 hr for 7 to 10 days. I.V. infusion given over 30 min.
Maximum: Not to exceed adult dose.

➤ *To treat severe UTI caused by* E. coli *or* K. pneumoniae, *moderate to severe skin and soft-tissue infections caused by* Staphylococcus aureus *or* Streptococcus pyogenes

I.V. INFUSION

Adults and children age 16 and over. 2 g given over 30 min every 12 hr for 10 days.

I.V. INFUSION

Children ages 2 months to 16 years weighing up to 40 kg (88 lb). 50 mg/kg/dose given over 30 min every 12 hr for 10 days.
Maximum: Not to exceed adult dose.

➤ *To treat moderate to severe pneumonia caused by* Enterobacter *species,* K. pneumoniae, Pseudomonas aeruginosa, *or* Streptococcus pneumoniae

I.V. INFUSION

Adults and children age 16 and over. 1 to 2 g given over 30 min every 8 hr if caused by *P. aeruginosa* or every 12 hr for other infections for 10 days.

➤ *To treat moderate to severe pneumonia caused by* P. aeruginosa

I.V. INFUSION

Children ages 2 months to 16 years weighing up to 40 kg (88 lb). 50 mg/kg/dose infused over 30 min every 8 hr for 10 days. *Maximum:* Not to exceed adult dose.

➤ *To treat febrile neutropenia*

I.V. INFUSION

Adults and children age 16 and over. 2 g infused over 30 min every 8 hr for 7 days or until neutropenia resolves.
Children ages 2 months to 16 years weighing up to 40 kg (88 lb). 50 mg/kg/dose infused over 30 min every 8 hr for 7 days or until neutropenia resolves.
Maximum: Not to exceed adult dose.

➤ *To treat complicated intra-abdominal infections (together with metronidazole) caused by alpha-hemolytic streptococci,*

Bacteroides fragilis, E. coli, Enterobacter *species,* K. pneumoniae, *or* P. aeruginosa

I.V. INFUSION

Adults and children age 16 and over. 2 g infused over 30 min every 8 to 12 hr for 7 to 10 days.

DOSAGE ADJUSTMENT For adult patient with creatinine clearance between 30 and 60 ml/min, dosing interval increased to every 24 hr if dosing interval had been every 12 hr, and dosing interval increased to every 12 hr if dosing interval had been every 8 hr. For adult patient with creatinine clearance between 11 and 29 ml/min, dosage decreased to 500 mg every 24 hr if dosage had been 1 g every 24 hr; dosage decreased to 1 g every 24 hr if dosage had been 2 g every 24 hr; and dosing interval decreased to 24 hr if dosing interval had been every 12 hr while maintaining a dosage of 2 g. For adult patient with creatinine clearance less than 11 ml/min, dosage decreased to 250 mg every 24 hr if dosage had been 500 mg every 24 hr; dosage decreased to 500 mg every 24 hr if dosage had been 1 g every 24 hr; and dosage decreased to 1 g every 24 hr if dosage had been 2 g every 24 hr. For adult patient on continuous abdominal peritoneal dialysis or hemodialysis, dosage interval and dosage further altered. For pediatric patient, dosage decreased and dosage interval increased in similar proportion as adults.

Mechanism of Action

Interferes with bacterial cell wall synthesis by inhibiting the final step in the cross-linking of peptidoglycan strands. Peptidoglycan makes cell membranes rigid and protective. Without it, bacterial cells rupture and die.

Incompatibilities

Don't add cefepime to solutions that contain ampicillin in a concentration of more than 40 mg/ml. Don't add drug to solutions that contain aminophylline, gentamycin, metronidazole, netilmicin sulfate, tobramycin, or vancomycin.

Contraindications

Hypersensitivity to cefepime, other beta-lactam antibiotics, other cephalosporins, penicillins, or their components

Interactions

DRUGS

aminoglycosides: Increased risk of nephrotoxicity and ototoxicity

potent diuretics: Increased risk of nephrotoxicity

Adverse Reactions

CNS: Aphasia, chills, **coma**, confusion, **encephalopathy**, fever, hallucinations, headache, myoclonus, **neurotoxicity**, **nonconvulsive status epilepticus**, **seizures**, stupor

CV: Edema

EENT: Hearing loss, oral candidiasis

GI: Abdominal cramps, diarrhea, elevated liver enzymes, **hepatic failure**, hepatomegaly, nausea, **pseudomembranous colitis**, vomiting

GU: Elevated BUN level, **nephrotoxicity**, **renal failure**, vaginal candidiasis

HEME: Agranulocytosis, eosinophilia, **hemolytic anemia**, **hypoprothrombinemia**, **leukopenia**, **neutropenia**, positive direct Coombs' tests, **thrombocytopenia**, **unusual bleeding**

MS: Arthralgia

RESP: Dyspnea

SKIN: Ecchymosis, erythema, **erythema multiforme**, pruritus, rash, **Stevens–Johnson syndrome**

Other: Anaphylaxis; injection-site pain, redness, and swelling; superinfection

Nursing Considerations

- Use cefepime cautiously in patients with impaired renal function or a history of GI disease, particularly colitis. Also use cautiously in patients hypersensitive to other cephalosporins, other drugs, or penicillins because cross-sensitivity has occurred.
- Obtain culture and sensitivity test results, if possible and as ordered, before giving drug.
- For I.V. infusion, reconstitute using manufacturer's guidelines. Give over 30 minutes.
- For I.M. injection, reconstitute 500-mg vial of drug with 1.3 ml of diluent, such as sterile water for injection (or 1-g vial with 2.4 ml of diluent). See drug guidelines for complete list of appropriate diluents.

WARNING Monitor patient closely for hypersensitivity reactions. Be aware that an allergic reaction may occur even up to a few

C

days after therapy starts. Notify prescriber immediately and expect cefepime to be discontinued. Be prepared to administer treatment with corticosteroids, epinephrine, intravenous fluids, intravenous antihistamines, oxygen, pressor amines and airway management, if reaction is severe.

- Monitor BUN and serum creatinine levels for early signs of nephrotoxicity. Also monitor fluid intake and output; decreasing urine output may indicate nephrotoxicity.
- Be aware that in renally impaired patients, neurotoxicity may occur, especially if dosage has not been adjusted for their degree of renal impairment. If neurotoxicity occurs, notify prescriber and expect dosage to be modified or drug discontinued.
- Assess bowel pattern daily; severe diarrhea may indicate pseudomembranous colitis.
- Assess for signs of superinfection, such as cough or sputum changes, diarrhea, drainage, fever, malaise, pain, perineal itching, rash, redness, and swelling.
- Assess for arthralgia, bleeding, ecchymosis, and pharyngitis; they may indicate a blood dyscrasia. Be aware that positive direct Coombs' tests may occur with cefepime use. Expect drug to be discontinued and appropriate therapy instituted if patient develops hemolytic anemia.
- Monitor patient for evidence of neurotoxicity such as aphasia, encephalopathy, myoclonus, nonconvulsive status epilepticus, or seizures. Be prepared to provide immediate treatment, as ordered. Be aware that although most cases occurred in patients with renal impairment who did not receive appropriate dosage adjustment, some did not.

PATIENT TEACHING

- Tell patient to immediately report severe diarrhea to prescriber, even if it occurs as late as 2 or more months after the last dose was taken.
- Instruct patient and caregiver to immediately seek emergency care for any change in mental status, development of seizure activity, difficulty speaking or understanding spoken or written words, or sudden jerking movements. Cefepime should be stopped until patient is evaluated.
- Alert patients with diabetes that cefepime therapy may result in a false-positive reaction for glucose in the urine when using some methods such as Clinitest tablets.

cefixime

Suprax

Class and Category

Pharmacologic class: Third-generation cephalosporin
Therapeutic class: Antibiotic
Pregnancy category: B

Indications and Dosages

➤ *To treat uncomplicated UTI caused by* Escherichia coli *or* Proteus mirabilis; *pharyngitis and tonsillitis caused by* S. pyogenes; *acute bronchitis and acute exacerbations of chronic bronchitis caused by* H. influenzae *or* Streptococcus pneumoniae

CAPSULES, CHEWABLE TABLETS, ORAL SUSPENSION, TABLETS

Adults and children weighing 45 kg (99 lb) or more or age 12. 400 mg once daily or 200 mg every 12 hr.

➤ *To treat otitis media caused by* Haemophilus influenzae, Moraxella catarrhalis, *or* Streptococcus pyogenes

CHEWABLE TABLETS, ORAL SUSPENSION

Adults and children weighing 45 kg (99 lb) and over or age 12 and over. 400 mg once daily or 200 mg every 12 hr.
Children age 6 months to 12 years weighing less than 45 kg (99 lb). 8 mg/kg once daily or 4 mg/kg every 12 hr.

➤ *To treat uncomplicated gonorrhea caused by* Neisseria gonorrhoeae

TABLETS

Adults. 400 mg as a single dose.

DOSAGE ADJUSTMENT Dosage reduced to 75% for patients who have creatinine clearance of 21 to 60 ml/min or receive hemodialysis. Dosage reduced to 50% for patients who have creatinine clearance of 20 ml/min or less.

ORAL SUSPENSION

Children age 6 months to 12 years weighing less than 45 kg (99 lb). 8 mg/kg once daily or 4 mg/kg every 12 hr.

Mechanism of Action

Interferes with bacterial cell wall synthesis by inhibiting the final step in the cross-linking of peptidoglycan strands. Peptidoglycan makes cell membranes rigid and protective. Without it, bacterial cells rupture and die.

Contraindications

Hypersensitivity to cephalosporins or their components

Interactions

DRUGS

aminoglycosides, loop diuretics: Increased risk of nephrotoxicity
carbamazepine: Increased blood carbamazepine level

Adverse Reactions

CNS: Chills, dizziness, fever, headache, **seizures**
CV: Edema, elevated LDH level
EENT: Hearing loss, oral candidiasis
GI: Abdominal cramps, diarrhea, elevated liver enzymes, **hepatic failure**, **hepatitis**, hepatomegaly, hyperbilirubinemia, jaundice, nausea, **pseudomembranous colitis**, vomiting
GU: Elevated BUN or creatinine levels, genital pruritus, **nephrotoxicity**, **renal failure**, vaginal candidiasis
HEME: Agranulocytosis, eosinophilia, **hemolytic anemia**, **hypoprothrombinemia**, **leukopenia**, **neutropenia**, **pancytopenia**, **prolonged prothrombin time**, **thrombocytopenia**, **unusual bleeding**
MS: Arthralgia
RESP: Dyspnea
SKIN: Ecchymosis, erythema, **erythema multiforme**, pruritus, rash, **Stevens–Johnson syndrome**, **toxic epidermal necrolysis**, urticaria
Other: Anaphylaxis, **angioedema**, drug fever, serum sickness-like reactions, superinfection

Nursing Considerations

- Use cefixime cautiously in patients with impaired renal function or a history of GI disease, especially colitis. Also use cautiously in patients hypersensitive to penicillin because cross-sensitivity has occurred in about 10% of such patients.
- Obtain culture and sensitivity test results, if possible and as ordered, before giving drug.
- Know that tablets shouldn't be substituted for oral suspension to treat otitis media because cefixime suspension produces a higher peak blood level than do tablets when administered at the same dose.
- Monitor BUN and serum creatinine for early signs of nephrotoxicity. Also monitor fluid intake and output; decreasing urine output may indicate nephrotoxicity.
- Be aware that an allergic reaction may occur a few days after therapy starts.
- Assess bowel pattern daily; severe diarrhea may indicate pseudomembranous colitis.
- Assess for signs of superinfection, such as cough or sputum changes, diarrhea, drainage, fever, malaise, pain, perineal itching, rash, redness, and swelling.
- Assess for arthralgia, bleeding, ecchymosis, and pharyngitis; they may indicate a blood dyscrasia.

PATIENT TEACHING

- Instruct patient to complete the prescribed course of therapy.
- Advise patient to shake oral suspension well before pouring dose and to use a calibrated device to obtain an accurate dose.
- Instruct patient to store oral suspension at room temperature and to discard unused portion after 14 days.
- Alert patient that chewable tablets contain aspartame, a source of phenylalanine, which can be harmful to patients with phenylketonuria (PKU).
- Tell patient to report severe diarrhea to prescriber immediately; this may occur even up to 2 months after cefixime therapy has been discontinued.
- Inform patient that buttermilk and yogurt can help maintain intestinal flora and decrease diarrhea.
- Teach patient to recognize and report signs of superinfection, such as furry tongue, perineal itching, and loose, foul-smelling stools.

cefotaxime sodium

Claforan

Class and Category

Pharmacologic class: Third-generation cephalosporin
Therapeutic class: Antibiotic
Pregnancy category: B

Indications and Dosages

➤ *To provide perioperative prophylaxis*

I.V. INFUSION, I.V. OR I.M. INJECTION

Adults and children weighing more than 50 kg (110 lb). 1 g 30 to 90 min before surgery. I.V. administration given over at least 3 to 5 min.

➤ *To provide perioperative prophylaxis related to cesarean section*

I.V. INFUSION, I.V. OR I.M. INJECTION

Adults. 1 g as soon as cord is clamped, then 1 g every 6 hr for up to two doses. I.V. administration given over at least 3 to 5 min.

➤ *To treat gonococcal urethritis and cervicitis in men and women*

I.M. INJECTION

Adults weighing more than 50 kg. 500 mg as a single dose.

➤ *To treat rectal gonorrhea in women*

I.M. INJECTION

Adults weighing more than 50 kg. 500 mg as a single dose.

➤ *To treat rectal gonorrhea in men*

I.M. INJECTION

Adults weighing more than 50 kg. 1 g as a single dose.

➤ *To treat uncomplicated infections caused by susceptible organisms*

I.V. INFUSION, I.V. OR I.M. INJECTION

Adults and children weighing more than 50 kg. 1 g every 12 hr. I.V. administration given over at least 3 to 5 min.
Children ages 1 month to 12 years weighing less than 50 kg. 50 to 180 mg/kg daily in four to six divided doses. I.V. administration given over at least 3 to 5 min.
Children ages 1 to 4 weeks. 50 mg/kg I.V. every 8 hr. I.V. administration given over at least 3 to 5 min.
Children age 1 week and under. 50 mg/kg I.V. every 12 hr. I.V. administration given over at least 3 to 5 min.

➤ *To treat moderate to severe infections caused by susceptible organisms*

I.V. INFUSION, I.V. OR I.M. INJECTION

Adults and children weighing more than 50 kg. 1 to 2 g every 8 hr. I.V. administration given over at least 3 to 5 min.
Children ages 1 month to 12 years weighing less than 50 kg. 50 to 180 mg/kg daily in four to six divided doses. For more serious infections, including meningitis, the higher dosages are used. I.V. administration given over at least 3 to 5 min.
Children ages 1 to 4 weeks. 50 mg/kg I.V. every 8 hr. I.V. administration given over at least 3 to 5 min.
Children age 1 week and younger. 50 mg/kg I.V. every 12 hr. I.V. administration given over at least 3 to 5 min.

➤ *To treat septicemia and other infections that commonly require antibiotics in higher doses than those used to treat moderate to severe infections*

I.V. INFUSION OR INJECTION

Adults and children weighing more than 50 kg. 2 g every 6 to 8 hr. I.V. administration given over at least 3 to 5 min.

➤ *To treat life-threatening infections caused by susceptible organisms*

I.V. INFUSION OR INJECTION

Adults and children weighing more than 50 kg. 2 g every 4 hr. I.V. administration given over at least 3 to 5 min. *Maximum:* 12 g daily.
Children ages 1 month to 12 years weighing less than 50 kg. 50 to 180 mg/kg daily in four to six divided doses. I.V. administration given over at least 3 to 5 min.
Children ages 1 to 4 weeks. 50 mg/kg every 8 hr. I.V. administration given over at least 3 to 5 min.
Children age 1 week and younger. 50 mg/kg every 12 hr. I.V. administration given over at least 3 to 5 min.

DOSAGE ADJUSTMENT Dosage reduced by 50% for patients with estimated creatinine clearance below 20 ml/min.

Mechanism of Action

Interferes with bacterial cell wall synthesis by inhibiting cross-linking of peptidoglycan strands. Peptidoglycan makes cell membranes rigid and protective. Without it, bacterial cells rupture and die.

Incompatibilities

To prevent mutual inactivation, don't mix cefotaxime with aminoglycosides. Also avoid mixing cefotaxime with other drugs, including pentamidine isethionate.

Contraindications

Hypersensitivity to cefotaxime, other cephalosporins, or their components

Interactions

DRUGS

aminoglycosides, loop diuretics, NSAIDs: Increased risk of nephrotoxicity
probenecid: Increased and prolonged blood cefotaxime level

Adverse Reactions

CNS: Chills, fever, headache, **seizures**
CV: Edema
EENT: Hearing loss, oral candidiasis
GI: Abdominal cramps, cholestasis, diarrhea, elevated enzymes, **hepatic failure**, **hepatitis**, hepatomegaly, jaundice, nausea, **pseudeomembranous colitis**, vomiting
GU: Elevated BUN level, **nephrotoxicity**, **renal failure**, vaginal candidiasis
HEME: Eosinophilia, **hemolytic anemia**, **hypoprothrombinemia**, **neutropenia**, **thrombocytopenia**, **unusual bleeding**
MS: Arthralgia
RESP: Dyspnea
SKIN: Ecchymosis, erythema, **erythema multiforme**, pruritus, rash, **Stevens–Johnson syndrome**, **toxic epidermal necrolysis**
Other: Anaphylaxis; injection-site pain, redness, and swelling; superinfection

Nursing Considerations

- Use cefotaxime cautiously in patients with impaired renal function, a history of GI disease (especially colitis), or hypersensitivity to penicillin because cross-sensitivity has occurred in about 10% of such patients.
- Obtain culture and sensitivity test results, if possible and as ordered, before giving drug.
- For I.V. use, reconstitute each 0.5-, 1-, or 2-g vial with 10 ml of sterile water for injection. Shake to dissolve.
- For intermittent I.V. infusion, further dilute in 50 to 100 ml of D_5W or normal saline solution.
- For I.M. use, reconstitute each 500-mg vial with 2 ml sterile water for injection or bacteriostatic water for injection; each 1-g vial with 3 ml diluent; and each 2-g vial with 5 ml diluent. Shake to dissolve.

WARNING Don't use diluent that contains benzyl alcohol when preparing drug for a neonate; it could cause a fatal toxic syndrome.

- Give cefotaxime by I.V. injection over 3 to 5 minutes through tubing of a free-flowing compatible I.V. solution. Temporarily stop other solutions being given through same I.V. site.
- Discard unused drug after 24 hours if stored at room temperature, 5 days if refrigerated.
- Protect cefotaxime powder and solution from light and heat.
- Monitor I.V. sites for signs of phlebitis or extravasation. Rotate I.V. sites every 72 hours.
- Monitor BUN and serum creatinine levels and fluid intake and output for signs of nephrotoxicity.
- Be aware that allergic reaction may occur a few days after cefotaxime therapy starts.
- Assess bowel pattern daily; severe diarrhea may indicate pseudomembranous colitis caused by *Clostridium difficile.* If diarrhea occurs, notify prescriber and expect to withhold cefotaxime and treat with fluids, electrolytes, protein, and an antibiotic effective against *C. difficile.*
- Assess patient for arthralgia, bleeding, ecchymosis, and pharyngitis, which may indicate a blood dyscrasia. Monitor bleeding time, CBC, and PT, as ordered.
- Monitor patient closely for superinfection. If evidence appears, notify prescriber and expect to stop drug and provide care.
- Be aware that cephalosporins, such as cefotaxime, may produce a positive direct Coombs' test.

PATIENT TEACHING

- Explain that I.M. injection may be painful.
- Instruct patient to report watery, bloody stools to prescriber immediately, even up to 2 months after drug therapy has ended.

cefotetan disodium

Cefotan

Class and Category

Pharmacologic class: Second-generation cephalosporin
Therapeutic class: Antibiotic
Pregnancy category: B

Indications and Dosages

➤ *To provide surgical prophylaxis*

I.V. INJECTION

Adults. 1 to 2 g given over 3 to 5 min 30 to 60 min before surgery or, in cesarean section, as soon as cord is clamped.

➤ *To treat lower respiratory tract infections caused by* Escherichia coli, Haemophilus influenzae, Klebsiella *species,* Proteus mirabilis, Serratia marcescens, Staphylococcus aureus, *or* Streptococcus pneumoniae; *gynecologic infections caused by* Bacteroides *species (excluding* B. distasonis, B. ovatus, *or* B. thetaiotaomicron*),* E. coli, Fusobacterium *species, gram-positive anaerobic cocci,* Neisseria gonorrhoeae, P. mirabilis, S. aureus, Staphylococcus epidermidis, *or* Streptococcus *species (excluding enterococci); intra-abdominal infections caused by* Bacteroides *species (excluding* B. distasonis, B. ovatus, *or* B. thetaiotaomicron*),* Clostridium *species,* E. coli, Klebsiella *species, or* Streptococcus *species (excluding enterococci); and bone and joint infections caused by* S. aureus

I.V. INFUSION, I.V. OR I.M. INJECTION

Adults. For mild to moderate infections, 1 to 2 g every 12 hr. For I.V injection, given over 3 to 5 min; for I.V. infusion, given over more than 5 min.

I.V. INFUSION OR INJECTION

Adults. For severe infections, 2 g every 12 hr; for life-threatening infections, 3 g every 12 hr. For I.V. injection, given over 3 to 5 min; for I.V. infusion, given over more than 5 min.

➤ *To treat UTI caused by* E. coli, Klebsiella *species, or* Proteus *species*

I.V. INFUSION, I.V. OR I.M. INJECTION

Adults. 0.5 to 2 g every 12 hr or 1 to 2 g every 24 hr. For I.V. injection, given over 3 to 5 min; for I.V. infusion, given over more than 5 min.

➤ *To treat skin and soft-tissue infections caused by* E. coli, Klebsiella pneumoniae, Peptostreptococcus *species,* S. aureus, S. epidermidis, Streptococcus pyogenes, *and* Streptococcus *species (excluding enterococci)*

I.V. INFUSION, I.V. OR I.M. INJECTION

Adults. For mild to moderate infections due to *K. pneumoniae,* 1 or 2 g every 12 hr. For mild to moderate infections caused by other organisms, 1 g I.M. or I.V. every 12 hr or 2 g I.V. every 24 hr; for severe infections, 2 g I.V. every 12 hr. For I.V injection, given over 3 to 5 min; for I.V. infusion, given over more than 5 min.

DOSAGE ADJUSTMENT Dosing interval reduced to 24 hr if creatinine clearance is 10 to 30 ml/min and to 48 hr if creatinine clearance is less than 10 ml/min.

Mechanism of Action

Interferes with bacterial cell wall synthesis by inhibiting the final step in the cross-linking of peptidoglycan strands. Peptidoglycan makes cell membranes rigid and protective. Without it, bacterial cells rupture and die.

Incompatibilities

To prevent mutual inactivation, don't mix cefotetan with aminoglycosides.

Contraindications

History of cephalosporin-induced hemolytic anemia; hypersensitivity to cefotetan, other cephalosporins, or their components

Interactions

DRUGS

aminoglycosides, loop diuretics: Increased risk of nephrotoxicity
probenecid: Increased and prolonged blood cefotetan level

ACTIVITIES

alcohol use: Disulfiram-like reaction

Adverse Reactions

CNS: Chills, fever, headache, **seizures**
CV: Edema
EENT: Hearing loss, oral candidiasis
GI: Abdominal cramps, diarrhea, elevated liver enzymes, **hepatic failure**, hepatomegaly, nausea, **pseudomembranous colitis**, vomiting

GU: Elevated BUN level, **nephrotoxicity**, **renal failure**, vaginal candidiasis
HEME: Eosinophilia, **hemolytic anemia**, **hypoprothrombinemia**, **neutropenia**, **thrombocytopenia**, **unusual bleeding**
MS: Arthralgia
RESP: Dyspnea
SKIN: Ecchymosis, erythema, **erythema multiforme**, pruritus, rash, **Stevens–Johnson syndrome**
Other: Anaphylaxis; injection-site pain, redness, and swelling; superinfection

Nursing Considerations

- Use cefotetan cautiously in patients with impaired renal function or a history of GI disease, especially colitis. Also use cautiously in patients hypersensitive to penicillin because cross-sensitivity has occurred in about 10% of such patients.
- Obtain culture and sensitivity test results, if possible and as ordered, before giving drug.
- For I.V. use, reconstitute each 1-g vial of drug with 10 ml sterile water for injection. For each 2-g vial, use 10 to 20 ml diluent. For I.V. infusion, further dilute solution in 50 to 100 ml D_5W or normal saline solution.
- For direct I.V. injection, give drug slowly over 3 to 5 minutes through tubing of a flowing compatible I.V. solution.
- For I.M. use, reconstitute each 1-g vial of drug with 2 ml of sterile or bacteriostatic water for injection, or sodium chloride for injection. For a 2-g vial, use 3 ml diluent.
- Monitor I.V. site for signs and symptoms of phlebitis and extravasation; rotate sites every 72 hours.
- Protect reconstituted solution from light, and store for up to 24 hours at room temperature or 96 hours under refrigeration.
- Be aware that an allergic reaction may occur a few days after therapy starts.
- Monitor BUN and serum creatinine levels and fluid intake and output for signs of nephrotoxicity.
- Monitor patient receiving even short-term cefotetan therapy for signs and symptoms of hemolytic anemia, such as marked pallor and fatigue.
- Monitor ALT, AST, bilirubin, CBC, LD, and serum alkaline phosphatase levels if patient receives long-term therapy.
- Assess patient's bowel pattern daily; severe diarrhea may indicate pseudomembranous colitis.
- Watch for arthralgia, bleeding, ecchymosis, and pharyngitis which may indicate a blood dyscrasia. Monitor PT and bleeding time, as ordered. Be prepared to give vitamin K, if ordered, to treat hypoprothrombinemia.

PATIENT TEACHING

- Explain that I.M. injection may be painful.
- Tell patient to immediately report severe diarrhea to prescriber even up to 2 months after therapy has stopped.
- Urge patient to avoid alcohol during and for at least 3 days after cefotetan therapy.

cefoxitin sodium

Mefoxin

Class and Category

Pharmacologic class: Second-generation cephalosporin
Therapeutic class: Antibiotic
Pregnancy category: B

Indications and Dosages

➤ *To provide surgical prophylaxis in patients undergoing uncontaminated abdominal or vaginal hysterectomy or gastrointestinal surgery*

I.V. INFUSION OR INJECTION

Adults. 2 g given over at least 3 to 5 min 30 to 60 min before surgery and then 2 g given over at least 3 to 5 min every 6 hr after first dose for up to 24 hr.
Children age 3 months or over. 30 to 40 mg/kg given over at least 3 to 5 min 30 to 60 min before surgery and every 6 hr after first dose for up to 24 hr.

➤ *To provide surgical prophylaxis for cesarean section*

I.V. INFUSION OR INJECTION

Adults. 2 g given over at least 3 to 5 min as a single dose as soon as cord is clamped; or 2 g given over at least 3 to 5 min as soon as cord is clamped, followed by 2 g given over at least 3 to 5 min 4 and 8 hr after initial dose.

➤ *To treat bone and joint infections caused by* Staphlococcus aureus; *gynecological infections, including endometritis and pelvic cellulitis or inflammatory disease caused by* Bacteroides *species,* Clostridium *species,* E. coli, Neisseria gonorrhoeae, Peptococcus niger, Peptostreptococcus *species, or* Streptococcus agalactiae; *intra-abdominal infections including intra-abdominal abscess and peritonitis caused by* Bacteroides *or* Clostridium *species,* E. coli, *or* Klebsiella *species; lower respiratory infections, including lung abscess and pneumonia caused by* Bacteroides *species,* E. coli, Haemophilus influenzae, Klebsiella *species,* S. aureus, Streptococcus pneumoniae, *and other streptococci (excluding* enterococci); *skin and skin structure infections caused by* Bacteroides *and* Clostridium *species,* Enterococcus faecalis, E. coli, P. niger, Peptostreptococcus *species,* Proteus mirabilis, S. aureus, S. epidermidis, S. pyogenes, *and other streptococci (excluding* enterococci*);* septicemia caused by *Bacteroides* species, E. coli, Klebsiella *species,* S. aureus or S. pneumoniae; *and urinary tract infections caused by* E. coli, Klebsiella *species,* Morganella morganii, P. mirabilis, P. vulgaris, *or Providencia species*

I.V. INFUSION OR INJECTION

Adults. For uncomplicated infections, 1 g given over at least 3 to 5 min every 6 to 8 hr; for moderate to severe infections, 1 g given over at least 3 to 5 min every 4 hr or 2 g given over at least 3 to 5 min every 6 to 8 hr. For infections that commonly require high-dose antibiotics (such as gas gangrene), 2 g every 4 hr, or 3 g every 6 hr. I.V. injection given over at least 3 to 5 min. I.V. infusion given continuously.

Children age 3 months or over. 80 to 160 mg/kg daily in equally divided doses given every 4 to 6 hr (higher dosages used for more severe infections). *Maximum:* 12 g daily given over at least 3 to 5 min.

DOSAGE ADJUSTMENT Dosage reduced to 1 to 2 g every 8 to 12 hr if creatinine clearance is 30 to 50 ml/min; 1 to 2 g every 12 to 24 hr if clearance is 10 to 29 ml/min; 0.5 to 1 g every 12 to 24 hr if clearance is 5 to 9 ml/min; and 0.5 to 1 g every 24 to 48 hr if clearance is less than 5 ml/min.

Mechanism of Action

Interferes with bacterial cell wall synthesis by inhibiting the final step in the cross-linking of peptidoglycan strands. Peptidoglycan makes cell membranes rigid and protective. Without it, bacterial cells rupture and die.

Incompatibilities

To prevent mutual inactivation, don't mix cefoxitin with aminoglycosides. Also avoid mixing cefoxitin with other drugs, including pentamidine isethionate.

Contraindications

Hypersensitivity to cefoxitin, other cephalosporins, or their components

Interactions

DRUGS

aminoglycosides, loop diuretics: Increased risk of nephrotoxicity

Adverse Reactions

CNS: Chills, fever, headache, **seizures**
CV: Edema
EENT: Hearing loss, oral candidiasis
GI: Abdominal cramps, diarrhea, elevated liver enzymes, **hepatic failure**, hepatomegaly, nausea, **pseudomembranous colitis**, vomiting
GU: Elevated BUN level, **nephrotoxicity**, **renal failure**, vaginal candidiasis
HEME: Eosinophilia, **hemolytic anemia**, **hypoprothrombinemia**, **neutropenia**, **thrombocytopenia**, **unusual bleeding**
MS: Arthralgia
RESP: Dyspnea
SKIN: Ecchymosis, erythema, **erythema multiforme**, flushing, pruritus, rash, **Stevens–Johnson syndrome**, urticaria
Other: **Anaphylaxis**; injection-site pain, redness, and swelling; superinfection

Nursing Considerations

- Use cefoxitin cautiously in patients hypersensitive to penicillin; cross-sensitivity has occurred in about 10% of such patients.
- Use cautiously in patients with a history of GI disease, particularly colitis, because of an increased risk of pseudomembranous colitis.
- Obtain culture and sensitivity test results, if possible and as ordered, before giving drug.
- For I.V. use, reconstitute 1 g with 10 ml sterile water for injection, or 2 g with 10 to 20 ml diluent.

- For I.V. injection, give slowly over 3 to 5 minutes through tubing of a flowing compatible I.V. solution.
- For intermittent infusion, further dilute with 50 to 100 ml D_5W or normal saline solution.
- For continuous high-dose infusion, add cefoxitin to I.V. solutions of D_5W, normal saline solution, or dextrose 5% in normal saline solution.
- Discard unused drug after 24 hours if stored at room temperature, or after 1 week if refrigerated.
- Be aware that powder or solution may darken during storage, which doesn't reflect altered potency.
- Be aware that an allergic reaction may occur a few days after therapy starts.
- Monitor BUN and serum creatinine for early signs of nephrotoxicity. Also monitor fluid intake and output; decreasing urine output may indicate nephrotoxicity.
- Assess patient's bowel pattern daily; severe diarrhea may indicate pseudomembranous colitis.
- Assess for arthralgia, bleeding, ecchymosis, and pharyngitis; they may indicate a blood dyscrasia.

PATIENT TEACHING

- Tell patient to report severe diarrhea to prescriber immediately.
- Instruct patient to complete the course of therapy as prescribed.

cefpodoxime proxetil

Class and Category

Pharmacologic class: Third-generation cephalosporin
Therapeutic class: Antibiotic
Pregnancy category: B

Indications and Dosages

➤ *To treat acute community-acquired pneumonia caused by* Haemophilus influenzae *or* Streptococcus pneumoniae

ORAL SUSPENSION, TABLETS

Adults and adolescents. 200 mg every 12 hr for 14 days.

➤ *To treat acute bacterial exacerbation of chronic bronchitis caused by* H. influenzae, Moraxella catarrhalis, *or* S. pneumoniae

TABLETS

Adults and adolescents. 200 mg every 12 hr for 10 days.

➤ *To treat uncomplicated gonorrhea in men and women and rectal gonococcal infections in women caused by* Neisseria gonorrhoeae

ORAL SUSPENSION, TABLETS

Adults. 200 mg as a single dose.

➤ *To treat uncomplicated UTI caused by* Escherichia coli, Klebsiella pneumoniae, Proteus mirabilis, *or* Staphylococcus saprophyticus

ORAL SUSPENSION, TABLETS

Adults. 100 mg every 12 hr for 7 days.

➤ *To treat skin and soft-tissue infections caused by* S. aureus *or* S. pyogenes

ORAL SUSPENSION, TABLETS

Adults and adolescents. 400 mg every 12 hr for 7 to 14 days.

➤ *To treat acute otitis media caused by* H. influenzae, M. catarrhalis, S. pneumoniae, *or* S. pyogenes

ORAL SUSPENSION, TABLETS

Children ages 2 months through 12 years. 5 mg/kg every 12 hr for 5 days. *Maximum:* 200 mg/dose.

➤ *To treat pharyngitis and tonsillitis caused by* S. pyogenes

ORAL SUSPENSION, TABLETS

Adults and adolescents. 100 mg every 12 hr for 5 to 10 days.
Children ages 2 months through 12 years. 5 mg/kg every 12 hr for 5 to 10 days. *Maximum:* 100 mg/dose.

➤ *To treat acute maxillary sinusitis caused by* H. influenzae, M. catarrhalis, *or* S. pneumoniae

ORAL SUSPENSION, TABLETS

Adults. 200 mg every 12 hr for 10 days.
Children ages 2 months through 12 years. 5 mg/kg every 12 hr for 10 days. *Maximum:* 200 mg/dose.

DOSAGE ADJUSTMENT Dosing interval increased to 24 hr in patients with creatinine clearance less than 30 ml/min.

Mechanism of Action

Interferes with bacterial cell wall synthesis by inhibiting the final step in the cross-linking of peptidoglycan strands. Peptidoglycan makes cell membranes rigid and protective. Without it, bacterial cells rupture and die.

Contraindications

Hypersensitivity to cefpodoxime, other cephalosporins, or their components

Interactions

DRUGS

aminoglycosides, loop diuretics: Increased risk of nephrotoxicity
antacids, H_2-receptor antagonists: Reduced bioavailability and blood level of cefpodoxime
oral anticholinergics: Delayed peak blood level of cefpodoxime
probenecid: Possibly increased and prolonged blood cefpodoxime level

Adverse Reactions

CNS: Chills, fever, headache, **seizures**
CV: Edema
EENT: Hearing loss, oral candidiasis
GI: Abdominal cramps, diarrhea, elevated liver enzymes, **hepatic failure**, hepatomegaly, nausea, **pseudomembranous colitis**, vomiting
GU: Elevated BUN level, **nephrotoxicity**, **renal failure**, vaginal candidiasis
HEME: Eosinophilia, **hemolytic anemia**, **hypoprothrombinemia**, **neutropenia**, **thrombocytopenia**, **unusual bleeding**
MS: Arthralgia
RESP: Dyspnea
SKIN: Ecchymosis, erythema, **erythema multiforme**, pruritus, rash, **Stevens–Johnson syndrome**
Other: **Anaphylaxis**, superinfection

Nursing Considerations

- Use cefpodoxime cautiously in patients who have impaired renal function or are receiving potent diuretics. Also use drug cautiously in patients hypersensitive to penicillin because cross-sensitivity has occurred in about 10% of such patients.
- Obtain culture and sensitivity test results, if possible and as ordered, before giving cefpodoxime.
- Assess patient's bowel pattern daily; severe diarrhea may indicate pseudomembranous colitis.
- Be aware that an allergic reaction may occur a few days after therapy starts.

PATIENT TEACHING

- Urge patient to complete the prescribed course of therapy.
- Tell patient to take tablets with food to enhance absorption.
- Advise patient to refrigerate oral suspension and discard after 14 days.
- Instruct patient to shake oral suspension bottle well before pouring dose and to use a calibrated liquid-measuring device to ensure accurate doses.
- Inform patient that buttermilk and yogurt can help maintain intestinal flora and decrease diarrhea.
- Warn patient not to take an antacid within 2 hours before or after taking cefpodoxime.
- Tell patient to report watery, bloody stools to prescriber immediately, even up to 2 months after drug therapy has ended.

cefprozil

Class and Category

Pharmacologic class: Second-generation cephalosporin
Therapeutic class: Antibiotic
Pregnancy category: B

Indications and Dosages

➤ *To treat secondary bacterial infections in patients with acute bronchitis and acute bacterial exacerbations of chronic bronchitis caused by* Haemophilus influenzae, Moraxella catarrhalis, *and* Streptococcus pneumoniae

ORAL SUSPENSION, TABLETS

Adults and adolescents. 500 mg every 12 hr for 10 days.

➤ *To treat uncomplicated skin and soft-tissue infections caused by* Staphylococcus aureus *and* Streptococcus pyogenes

ORAL SUSPENSION, TABLETS

Adults and adolescents. 250 mg every 12 hr or 500 mg every 12 to 24 hr for 10 days.
Children ages 2 to 12. 20 mg/kg every 24 hr for 10 days. *Maximum:* Not to exceed adult dose.

➤ *To treat pharyngitis and tonsillitis caused by* S. pyogenes

ORAL SUSPENSION, TABLETS
Adults and adolescents. 500 mg every 24 hr for 10 days.
Children ages 2 to 12. 7.5 mg/kg every 12 hr for 10 days. *Maximum:* Not to exceed adult dose.

➤ *To treat otitis media caused by* H. influenzae, M. catarrhalis, *and* S. pneumoniae

ORAL SUSPENSION, TABLETS
Children ages 6 months to 12 years. 15 mg/kg every 12 hr for 10 days.

➤ *To treat acute sinusitis caused by* H. influenzae, M. catarrhalis, *and* S. pneumoniae

ORAL SUSPENSION, TABLETS
Adults and adolescents. 250 to 500 mg every 12 hr for 10 days.
Children ages 6 months to 12 years. 7.5 or 15 mg/kg every 12 hr for 10 days. *Maximum:* Not to exceed adult dose.
DOSAGE ADJUSTMENT Dosage reduced by half and given at usual intervals in patients with creatinine clearance less than 30 ml/min.

Mechanism of Action

Interferes with bacterial cell wall synthesis by inhibiting the final step in the cross-linking of peptidoglycan strands. Peptidoglycan makes the cell membrane rigid and protective. Without it, bacterial cells rupture and die.

Contraindications

Hypersensitivity to cefprozil, other cephalosporins, or their components

Interactions

DRUGS
aminoglycosides, loop diuretics: Increased risk of nephrotoxicity
probenecid: Increased blood cefprozil level

Adverse Reactions

CNS: Chills, fever, headache, **seizures**
CV: Edema
EENT: Hearing loss, oral candidiasis
GI: Abdominal cramps, diarrhea, elevated liver enzymes, **hepatic failure**, hepatomegaly, nausea, **pseudomembranous colitis**, vomiting
GU: Elevated BUN level, **nephrotoxicity**, **renal failure**, vaginal candidiasis
HEME: Eosinophilia, **hemolytic anemia**, **hypoprothrombinemia**, **neutropenia**, **thrombocytopenia**, **unusual bleeding**
MS: Arthralgia
RESP: Dyspnea
SKIN: Ecchymosis, erythema, **erythema multiforme**, pruritus, rash, **Stevens–Johnson syndrome**
Other: **Anaphylaxis**, superinfection

Nursing Considerations

- Use cefprozil cautiously in patients who have impaired renal function or a history of GI disease, especially colitis. Also use drug cautiously in patients who are hypersensitive to penicillin because cross-sensitivity has occurred in about 10% of such patients.
- Obtain culture and sensitivity test results, if possible and as ordered, before giving drug.

WARNING **Don't administer oral suspension to patients with phenylketonuria because it contains phenylalanine 28 mg/5 ml.**

- Monitor BUN and serum creatinine levels to detect early signs of nephrotoxicity. Also monitor fluid intake and output; decreasing urine output may indicate nephrotoxicity.
- Be aware that an allergic reaction may occur a few days after therapy starts.
- Assess patient's bowel pattern daily; severe diarrhea may indicate pseudomembranous colitis.

PATIENT TEACHING

- Urge patient to complete the prescribed course of therapy.
- Tell patient to refrigerate oral suspension and discard after 14 days.
- Instruct patient to shake oral suspension well before pouring and to use a calibrated measuring device to ensure accurate doses.
- Inform patient that buttermilk and yogurt can help maintain intestinal flora and decrease diarrhea.
- Tell patient to report watery, bloody stools to prescriber immediately, even up to 2 months after drug therapy has ended.

ceftaroline fosamil

Teflaro

Class and Category

Pharmacologic class: Fifth-generation cephalosporin

Therapeutic class: Antibiotic
Pregnancy category: B

Indications and Dosages

➤ *To treat acute bacterial skin and skin structure infection caused by* Escherichia coli, Klebsiella oxytoca, K. pneumoniae, Staphylococcus aureus, Streptococcus agalactiae, *or* S. pyogenes

I.V. INFUSION

Adults. 600 mg administered over 5 to 60 min every 12 hr for 5 to 14 days.
Children ages 2 to 18 years weighing more than 33 kg (72.5 lb). 400 mg every 8 hr or 600 mg every 12 hr administered over 5 to 60 min for 5 to 14 days.
Children ages 2 to 18 years weighing 33 kg (72.5 lb) or less. 12 mg/kg every 8 hr administered over 5 to 60 min for 5 to 14 days.
Children 2 months to less than 2 years. 8 mg/kg every 8 hr administered 5 to 60 min for 5 to 14 days.

➤ *To treat community-acquired bacterial pneumonia caused by* E. coli, Haemophilus influenzae, K. oxytoca, K. pneumoniae, S. aureus, *or* S. pneumoniae

I.V. INFUSION

Adults. 600 mg administered over 5 to 60 min every 12 hr for 5 to 7 days.
Children ages 2 to 18 years weighing more than 33 kg (72.5 lb). 400 mg every 8 hr or 600 mg every 12 hr administered over 5 to 60 min for 5 to 14 days.
Children ages 2 to 18 years weighing 33 kg (72.5 lb) or less. 12 mg/kg every 8 hr administered over 5 to 60 min for 5 to 14 days.
Children 2 months to less than 2 years. 8 mg/kg every 8 hr administered 5 to 60 min for 5 to 14 days

DOSAGE ADJUSTMENT For adult patients with a creatinine clearance above 30 ml/min but no higher than 50 ml/min, dosage reduced to 400 mg every 12 hr; for adult patients with a creatinine clearance above 15 ml/min but no higher than 30 ml/min, dosage reduced to 300 mg every 12 hr; for adult patients with a creatinine clearance of less than 15 ml/min including those on hemodialysis, dosage reduced to 200 mg every 12 hr. For pediatric patients, dosage adjustment is unclear if creatinine clearance is below 50 ml/min.

Mechanism of Action

Interferes with bacterial cell wall synthesis by inhibiting the final step in the cross-linking of peptidoglycan strands. Peptidoglycan makes the cell membrane rigid and protective. Without it, bacterial cells rupture and die. Ceftaroline is unique in that it is effective against methicillin-resistant *S. aureus*, unlike other cephalosporins.

Incompatibilities

Don't mix parenteral ceftaroline with any other drug because compatibility is not known.

Contraindications

Hypersensitivity to ceftaroline, other cephalosporins, or their components

Drug Reactions

None reported

Adverse Reactions

CNS: Dizziness, fever, headache, **seizures**
CV: Bradycardia, palpitations, phlebitis
ENDO: Hyperglycemia
GI: Abdominal pain, ***Clostridium difficile*–associated diarrhea**, constipation, diarrhea, elevated liver enzymes, **hepatitis**, nausea, vomiting
GU: Renal failure
HEME: Agranulocytosis, anemia, **hemolytic anemia**, eosinophilia, **leukopenia**, **neutropenia**, **thrombocytopenia**
SKIN: Pruritus, rash, urticaria
Other: Anaphylaxis, direct Coombs' test seroconversion, **hyperkalemia**, **hypokalemia**, **hypersensitivity reactions**

Nursing Considerations

- Use ceftaroline cautiously in patients hypersensitive to penicillins or carbapenems because cross-sensitivity may occur.
- Obtain culture and sensitivity results, if possible and as ordered, before giving drug.
- Reconstitute each drug vial with 20 ml of sterile water for injection. Mix gently to ensure drug is completely dissolved. Color may range from clear to light to dark yellow, depending on the concentration and storage conditions. Then further dilute in 250 ml of appropriate solution such as dextrose in water, half normal

saline, lactated Ringer's solution, or normal saline solution.

- Infuse reconstituted solution within 6 hours of mixing if stored at room temperature or within 24 hours if refrigerated.
- Administer as an I.V. infusion over 5 minutes to 1 hour.
- Monitor patient for hypersensitivity to ceftaroline. If present, discontinue ceftaroline, as ordered, and prepare to provide emergency supportive care.
- Assess bowel pattern daily; severe diarrhea may indicate pseudomembranous colitis caused by *C. difficile*. If diarrhea occurs, notify prescriber and expect to withhold drug and treat with electrolytes, fluids, protein, and an antibiotic effective against *C. difficile*.
- Be aware that seroconversion from a negative to a positive direct Coombs' test result may occur. If anemia develops during or after ceftaroline therapy, expect a direct Coombs' test to be ordered. If drug-induced hemolytic anemia is suspected, expect to discontinue the drug and provide supportive care, as indicated.

PATIENT TEACHING

- Urge patient to report hypersensitivity reactions, such as a rash, immediately.
- Instruct patient to report watery, bloody stools to prescriber immediately, even up to 2 months after drug therapy has ended.

ceftazidime

Fortaz, Tazicef

Class and Category

Pharmacologic class: Third-generation cephalosporin
Therapeutic class: Antibiotic
Pregnancy category: B

Indications and Dosages

➤ *To treat infections caused by gram-negative organisms (including* Acinetobacter, Citrobacter, Enterobacter, Escherichia coli, Haemophilus influenzae, Klebsiella, Neisseria, Proteus mirabilis, Proteus vulgaris, Pseudomonas aeruginosa, Salmonella, Serratia, *and* Shigella*), gram-positive organisms (including* Streptococcus agalactiae, Streptococcus pneumoniae, *and* Streptococcus pyogenes *[group B streptococci]), as well as* Staphylococcus aureus *(penicillinase- and non–penicillinase-producing strains)*

I.V. INFUSION, I.V. INJECTION, I.M. INJECTION

Adults and children age 12 and over. 1 g every 8 to 12 hr. I.V. given over at least 3 to 5 min.

I.V. INFUSION, I.V. INJECTION

Children ages 1 month to 12 years. 30 to 50 mg/kg given over at least 3 to 5 min every 8 hr. *Maximum:* 6 g daily.

Neonates up to age 1 month. 30 mg/kg given over at least 3 to 5 min every 12 hr.

➤ *To treat uncomplicated UTI*

I.V. INFUSION, I.V. INJECTION, I.M. INJECTION

Adults and children age 12 and over. 250 mg every 12 hr. I.V. given over at least 3 to 5 min.

➤ *To treat complicated UTI*

I.V. INFUSION, I.V. INJECTION, I.M. INJECTION

Adults and children age 12 and over. 500 mg every 8 to 12 hr. I.V. given over at least 3 to 5 min.

➤ *To treat uncomplicated pneumonia and mild skin and soft-tissue infections*

I.V. INFUSION, I.V. INJECTION, I.M. INJECTION

Adults and children age 12 and over. 0.5 to 1 g every 8 hr. I.V. given over at least 3 to 5 min.

➤ *To treat bone and joint infections*

I.V. INFUSION, I.V. INJECTION

Adults and children age 12 and over. 2 g, given over at least 3 to 5 min, every 12 hr.

➤ *To treat serious gynecologic and intra-abdominal infections, meningitis, and life-threatening infections, especially in immunocompromised patients*

I.V. INFUSION, I.V. INJECTION

Adults and children age 12 and over. 2 g, given over 3 to 5 min, every 8 hr.

➤ *To treat pseudomonal lung infection in patients with cystic fibrosis and normal renal function*

I.V. INFUSION, I.V. INJECTION

Adults. 30 to 50 mg/kg, given over at least 3 to 5 min, every 8 hr. *Maximum:* 6 g daily.

DOSAGE ADJUSTMENT Dosage reduced to 1 g every 12 hr if creatinine clearance is 31 to 50 ml/min; to 1 g every 24 hr if 16 to 30 ml/min; to 0.5 g every 24 hr if 6 to 15 ml/min; and to 0.5 g every 48 hr if less than 6 ml/min.

Mechanism of Action

Interferes with bacterial cell wall synthesis by inhibiting the cross-linking of peptidoglycan strands. Peptidoglycan makes the cell membrane rigid and protective. Without it, bacterial cells rupture and die.

Incompatibilities

Don't mix ceftazidime with aminoglycosides to prevent mutual inactivation. Vancomycin is physically incompatible with ceftazidime (precipitate may form); flush I.V. line between these drugs if given through same tubing. Avoid mixing ceftazidime with other drugs, including pentamidine isethionate.

Contraindications

Hypersensitivity to ceftazidime, other cephalosporins, or their components

Interactions

DRUGS

aminoglycosides, loop diuretics: Increased risk of nephrotoxicity
chloramphenicol: Antagonistic effect on ceftazidime
oral combined estrogen-progesterone contraceptives: Decreased effectiveness of oral contraceptive

Adverse Reactions

CNS: Chills, fever, headache, **seizures**
CV: Edema
EENT: Hearing loss, oral candidiasis
GI: Abdominal cramps, diarrhea, elevated liver enzymes, **hepatic failure**, hepatomegaly, nausea, **pseudomembranous colitis**, vomiting
GU: Elevated BUN level, **nephrotoxicity**, **renal failure**, vaginal candidiasis
HEME: Eosinophilia, **hemolytic anemia**, **hypoprothrombinemia**, **neutropenia**, **thrombocytopenia**, **unusual bleeding**
MS: Arthralgia
RESP: Dyspnea
SKIN: Ecchymosis, erythema, **erythema multiforme**, pruritus, rash, **Stevens–Johnson syndrome**
Other: **Anaphylaxis**; injection-site pain, redness, and swelling; superinfection

Nursing Considerations

- Use ceftazidime cautiously in patients hypersensitive to penicillin because cross-sensitivity occurs in about 10% of such patients. Watch for allergic reactions a few days after therapy starts.
- Use cautiously in patients with a history of GI disease, particularly colitis, because risk of pseudomembranous colitis is increased.
- Use cautiously in patients with renal insufficiency, because high and prolonged serum ceftazidime concentrations can occur from usual dosages. This can lead to asterixis, coma, encephalopathy, myoclonia, neuromuscular excitability, nonconvulsive status epilepticus, and seizures. Ensure that patients with significant renal insufficiency are receiving reduced dosage based on their creatinine clearance.
- Obtain culture and sensitivity test results, if possible and as ordered, before giving drug.
- Protect ceftazidime powder and reconstituted drug from heat and light; both tend to darken during storage.
- Thaw frozen solution at room temperature, not in water bath or microwave. Store thawed solution for up to 12 hours at room temperature or 7 days in refrigerator; don't refreeze.

WARNING **Know that when preparing drug for neonates or immature infants, don't use diluents containing benzyl alcohol because they are linked to a fatal toxic syndrome.**

- For I.V. bolus, reconstitute 1 to 2 g with 10 ml sterile water for injection, D_5W, or sodium chloride for injection. Shake to dissolve. Administer I.V. injection slowly over 3 to 5 minutes through tubing of a flowing compatible I.V. fluid.
- For intermittent infusion, further dilute in 50 to 100 ml D_5W or normal saline solution. Avoid using sodium bicarbonate injection as a diluent because drug is least stable in it. During ceftazidime administration, temporarily stop other solutions being given at the same I.V. site.
- For I.M. use, reconstitute each gram with 3 ml sterile water for injection or bacteriostatic water for injection.
- Give I.M. injection deep into large muscle mass, such as gluteus maximus.
- Rotate I.V. sites every 72 hours. Assess for extravasation and phlebitis.
- Assess patient's bowel pattern daily; severe diarrhea may indicate pseudomembranous colitis.

- Monitor ALT, AST, bilirubin, CBC, hematocrit, LD, and serum alkaline phosphatase, levels during long-term therapy.
- Monitor PT, as ordered, in at-risk patients, such as those with hepatic or renal impairment or poor nutritional state and those receiving anticoagulant or prolonged antibiotic therapy. Notify prescriber if PT decreases, and expect to give vitamin K.
- Assess for signs of superinfection, such as cough or sputum changes, diarrhea, drainage, fever, malaise, pain, perineal itching, rash, redness, and swelling.
- Watch for arthralgia, bleeding, ecchymosis, and pharyngitis (possible blood dyscrasia). Monitor PT and bleeding time.

PATIENT TEACHING

- Tell patient to take ceftazidime exactly as prescribed.
- Tell patient to report evidence of blood dyscrasia or superinfection to prescriber immediately.
- Urge patient to report watery, bloody stools to prescriber immediately, even up to 2 months after drug therapy has ended.

ceftibuten

Cedax

Class and Category

Pharmacologic class: Third-generation cephalosporin
Therapeutic class: Antibiotic
Pregnancy category: B

Indications and Dosages

➤ *To treat acute bacterial exacerbations of chronic bronchitis caused by* Haemophilus influenzae, *or* Moraxella catarrhalis, *or* Streptococcus pneumoniae; *pharyngitis and tonsillitis caused by* Streptococcus pyogenes; *and acute bacterial otitis media caused by* H. influenzae, M. catarrhalis, *or* S. pneumoniae

CAPSULES, ORAL SUSPENSION

Adults and children weighing more than 45 kg (99 lb). 400 mg daily for 10 days. Oral suspension administered 2 hr before or 1 hr after a meal.

➤ *To treat pharyngitis and tonsillitis caused by* S. pyogenes *and acute bacterial otitis media caused by* H. influenzae, M. catarrhalis, *or* S. pyogenes

ORAL SUSPENSION

Children weighing 45 kg (99 lb) or less. 9 mg/kg daily 2 hr before or 1 hr after a meal for 10 days. *Maximum:* 400 mg daily.

DOSAGE ADJUSTMENT Dosage reduced to 4.5 mg/kg (children weighing 45 kg [99 lb] or less) or 200 mg (adults and children weighing more than 45 kg [99 lb]) every 24 hr if creatinine clearance is 30 to 49 ml/min; dosage reduced to 2.25 mg/kg (children weighing 45 kg [99 lb] or less) or 100 mg (adults and children weighing more than 45 kg [99 lb]) every 24 hr if it's 5 to 29 ml/min. For patients receiving hemodialysis at least 2 times a week, a single dose of 9 mg/kg (children weighing 45 kg [99 lb] or less) or 400 mg (adult and children weighing more than 45 kg [99 lb]) given as oral suspension at end of each dialysis session.

Mechanism of Action

Interferes with bacterial cell wall synthesis by inhibiting the cross-linking of peptidoglycan strands. Peptidoglycan makes the cell membrane rigid and protective. Without it, bacterial cells rupture and die.

Contraindications

Hypersensitivity to ceftibuten, other cephalosporins, or their components

Interactions

DRUGS

aminoglycosides, loop diuretics: Increased risk of nephrotoxicity

Adverse Reactions

CNS: Aphasia, chills, fever, headache, psychosis, **seizures**
CV: Edema
EENT: Hearing loss, oral candidiasis
GI: Abdominal cramps, diarrhea, elevated liver enzymes, **hepatic failure**, hepatomegaly, jaundice, **melena**, nausea, **pseudomembranous colitis**, vomiting
GU: Elevated BUN level, **nephrotoxicity**, **renal failure**, vaginal candidiasis

HEME: Eosinophilia, **hemolytic anemia**, **hypoprothrombinemia**, **neutropenia**, **thrombocytopenia**, **unusual bleeding**
MS: Arthralgia
RESP: Dyspnea
SKIN: Ecchymosis, erythema, **erythema multiforme**, pruritus, rash, **Stevens–Johnson syndrome**, **toxic epidermal necrolysis**
Other: **Anaphylaxis**, serum sickness, superinfection

Nursing Considerations

- Use ceftibuten cautiously in patients hypersensitive to penicillins because cross-sensitivity occurs in up to 10% of such patients.
- Obtain culture and sensitivity test results, if possible and as ordered, before giving drug.
- Refrigerate oral suspension; shake well before using. Discard after 14 days.
- Monitor BUN and serum creatinine levels to detect early signs of nephrotoxicity. Also monitor fluid intake and output; decreasing urine output may indicate nephrotoxicity.
- Be aware that an allergic reaction may occur a few days after therapy starts.
- Assess bowel pattern daily; severe diarrhea may indicate pseudomembranous colitis.
- Assess for signs of superinfection, such as cough or sputum changes, diarrhea, drainage, fever, malaise, pain, perineal itching, rash, redness, and swelling.
- Assess for arthralgia, bleeding, ecchymosis, and pharyngitis; they may indicate a blood dyscrasia.

PATIENT TEACHING

- Urge patient to complete the drug therapy as prescribed.
- Instruct patient to take drug on an empty stomach at least 2 hours before or 1 hour after meals.
- Inform patient that unflavored oral suspension has a bitter taste. Suggest having a flavor added when prescription is filled.
- Advise patient that buttermilk and yogurt can help maintain intestinal flora and decrease diarrhea during therapy.
- Tell patient to immediately report hypersensitivity reactions, severe diarrhea, and evidence of blood dyscrasia or superinfection.

ceftriaxone sodium

Rocephin

Class and Category

Pharmacologic class: Third-generation cephalosporin
Therapeutic class: Antibiotic
Pregnancy category: B

Indications and Dosages

➤ *To treat infections such as bacterial septicemia caused by* Escherichia coli, Haemophilus influenzae, Klebsiella pneumoniae, Staphylococcus aureus, *or* Streptococcus pneumoniae; *bone and joint infections caused by* Enterobacter *species,* E. coli, K. pneumoniae, Proteus mirabilis, S. aureus, *or* S. pneumoniae; *intra-abdominal infections caused by* Bacteroides fragilis, Clostridium *species,* E. coli, *or* K. pneumoniae; *lower respiratory tract infections caused by* Enterobacter aerogenes, E. coli, H. influenzae, H. parainfluenzae, K. pneumoniae, P. mirabilis, Serratia marcescens, S. aureus, *or* S. pneumoniae; *skin and soft tissue infections caused by* Acinetobacter calcoaceticus, B. fragilis, E. cloacae, E. coli, K. pneumoniae, K. oxytoca, Morganella morganii, Peptostreptococcus *species,* P. mirabilis, Pseudomonas aeruginosa, Serratia marcescens, S. aureus, S. epidermidis, S. pyogenes, *or* Viridans *group streptococci; and urinary tract infections caused by* E. coli, K. pneumoniae, M. morganii, P. mirabilis, *or* P. vularis

I.V. INFUSION, I.M. INJECTION

Adults. 1 to 2 g daily or in equally divided doses twice daily I.V. infusion given over 30 min. *Maximum:* 4 g daily.
Children. 50 to 75 mg/kg daily or in equally divided doses every 12 hr. I.V. infusion given over 30 min for children and 60 min for neonates. *Maximum:* 2 g daily.

➤ *To treat meningitis caused by* H. influenzae, Neisseria meningitidis, *or* S. pneumoniae

I.V. INFUSION

Adults. 1 to 2 g infused over 30 min daily or in equally divided doses twice daily. *Maximum:* 4 g daily.

Children. *Initial:* 100 mg/kg infused over 30 min for children and 60 min for neonates on first day, then 100 mg/kg infused over 30 min for children and 60 min for neonates daily or in divided doses every 12 hr for 7 to 14 days. *Maximum:* 4 g daily.

➤ *To treat acute bacterial otitis media caused by* H. influenzae, Moraxella catarrhalis, *or* S. pneumoniae

I.M. INJECTION

Children. 50 mg/kg as a single dose. *Maximum:* 1 g.

➤ *To treat uncomplicated gonorrhea (cervical/urethral, pharyngeal, or rectal) caused by* Neisseria gonorrhoeae

I.M. INJECTION

Adults. 250 mg as a single dose.

➤ *To provide surgical prophylaxis*

I.V. INFUSION

Adults. 1 g given over 30 min, 30 min to 2 hr before surgery.

Mechanism of Action

Interferes with bacterial cell wall synthesis by inhibiting cross-linking of peptidoglycan strands. Peptidoglycan makes the cell membrane rigid and protective. Without it, bacterial cells rupture and die.

Incompatibilities

Don't admix ceftriaxone with labetalol, pentamidine isethionate, or other antibiotics, such as aminoglycosides, because of potential for incompatibility, such as substantial mutual inactivation. Also don't mix with calcium-containing solutions or products because a ceftriaxone-calcium salt may precipitate in the kidneys and lungs and may be fatal, especially in newborns.

Contraindications

Calcium-containing I.V. solutions; hyperbilirubinemic or premature neonates; hypersensitivity to ceftriaxone, other beta-lactam antibacterials or cephalosporins, penicillins, or their components; intravenous administration of ceftriaxone solutions containing lidocaine; neonates who are 28 days old or less if they're expected to need calcium-containing solutions, including parenteral nutrition.

Interactions

DRUGS

aminoglycosides, loop diuretics: Increased risk of nephrotoxicity

Adverse Reactions

CNS: Chills, fever, headache, hypertonia, reversible hyperactivity, **seizures**

CV: Edema

EENT: Glossitis, hearing loss, stomatitis

GI: Abdominal cramps, cholestasis, ***Clostridium difficile*-associated diarrhea**, diarrhea, elevated liver enzymes, gallbladder dysfunction, **hepatic failure**, **hepatitis**, hepatomegaly, nausea, oral candidiasis, **pancreatitis**, pseudolithiasis, **pseudomembranous colitis**, vomiting

GU: **Acute renal failure**, elevated BUN level, **nephrotoxicity**, oliguria, vaginal candidiasis, ureteric obstruction, urolithiasis

HEME: **Agranulocytosis**, **aplastic anemia**, eosinophilia, **hemolytic anemia**, **hemorrhage**, **hypoprothrombinemia**, **leukopenia**, **neutropenia**, **thrombocytopenia**

MS: Arthralgia

RESP: **Allergic pneumonitis**, dyspnea

SKIN: Allergic dermatitis, ecchymosis, erythema, **erythema multiforme**, exanthema, pruritus, rash, **Stevens–Johnson syndrome**, **toxic epidermal necrolysis**, urticaria

Other: **Anaphylaxis**; drug fever; injection-site pain, redness, and swelling; serum sickness; superinfection

Nursing Considerations

WARNING Be aware that calcium-containing products must not be given I.V. within 48 hours of ceftriaxone, including solutions given through a different I.V. line and at a different site, because a ceftriaxone-calcium salt may precipitate in the lungs and kidneys and could be fatal.

- Use ceftriaxone cautiously in patients who are hypersensitive to penicillins because cross-sensitivity has occurred in about 1% to 3% of such patients.

WARNING Ask patient if an allergic reaction was ever experienced when given other antibiotics. Patients who have had previous hypersensitivity reactions to carbapenems, other cephalosporins, penicillins, or other drugs may be at high risk for developing a serious reaction that may be fatal. Monitor all patients closely for a hypersensitivity reaction. If present, discontinue ceftriaxone immediately, notify prescriber, and be prepared to provide emergency supportive care, as prescribed.

- Obtain culture and sensitivity results, if possible and as ordered, before giving drug.
- Protect powder from light.
- For I.V. use, reconstitute with an appropriate diluent, such as sterile water for injection or sodium chloride for injection, as follows: for 250-mg vial, add 2.4 ml; for 500-mg vial, add 4.8 ml; for 1-g vial, add 9.6 ml; and for 2-g vial, add 19.2 ml to yield 100 mg/ml. For piggyback bottles, reconstitute with 10 ml of diluent indicated above for 1-g bottle and 20 ml for 2-g bottle. After reconstitution, further dilute to 50 to 100 ml with diluent indicated above and infuse over 30 minutes. Never use a diluent that contains calcium, such as Ringer's solution or Hartmann's solution, because a precipitate can form and may be fatal if injected.

WARNING **Never give ceftriaxone by I.V. infusion and calcium-containing I.V. solutions at the same time, including such continuous calcium-containing infusions as parenteral nutrition via Y-site. For patients other than neonates, ceftriaxone and calcium-containing solutions may be given sequentially if infusion lines are thoroughly flushed with a compatible fluid between infusions.**

- For I.M. administration, reconstitute with an appropriate diluent, such as sterile water for injection or sodium chloride for injection, as follows: for 250-mg vial, add 0.9 ml; for 500-mg vial, add 1.8 ml; for 1-g vial, add 3.6 ml; and for 2-g vial, add 7.2 ml to make a 250-mg/ml concentration. Shake well. Inject deep into large muscle mass, such as the gluteus maximus.
- Know that lidocaine can be used instead of sterile water as a diluent to lessen the pain of an I.M injection of ceftriaxone (follow manufacturer instructions when doing so). However, be aware that local anesthetics such as lidocaine may cause methemoglobinemia as late as several hours after the injection. Monitor patient closely.
- Monitor BUN and serum creatinine levels to detect early signs of nephrotoxicity. Also monitor fluid intake and output; decreasing urine output may indicate nephrotoxicity. Also be alert for precipitates in the patient's urine, especially children. If any signs of renal dysfunction occurs, notify prescriber, expect ceftriaxone to be discontinued, and provide supportive care, as prescribed.
- Assess ALT, AST, bilirubin, CBC, hematocrit, LD, and serum alkaline phosphatase levels during long-term therapy. If abnormalities occur, notify prescriber. Drug may have to be discontinued.
- Assess bowel pattern daily; severe diarrhea may indicate pseudomembranous colitis caused by *C. difficile.* If diarrhea occurs, notify prescriber and expect to treat with electrolytes, fluids, protein, and an antibiotic effective against *C. difficile.* Ceftriaxone therapy may be withheld also.
- Monitor patient for evidence of gallbladder disease (abdominal pain, nausea, vomiting) because drug may cause ceftriaxone-calcium salt to deposit in the gallbladder, which may mimic gallstones. Expect drug to be discontinued if gallbladder disorders arise.
- Assess for signs of superinfection, such as cough or sputum changes, diarrhea, drainage, fever, malaise, pain, perineal itching, rash, redness, and swelling.
- Assess for arthralgia, bleeding, ecchymosis, and pharyngitis; they may indicate a blood dyscrasia.

PATIENT TEACHING

- Tell patient to report evidence of blood dyscrasia or superinfection to prescriber immediately.
- Urge patient to report watery, bloody stools to prescriber immediately, even up to 2 months after drug therapy has ended.
- Advise patient to report any hypersensitivity reactions, such as a rash, itching skin, or hives, to prescriber immediately and to stop taking the drug.
- Tell patient that if he received drug as an I.M. injection that used lidocaine as the diluent, he should watch for signs and symptoms such as fatigue; headache; light-headedness; skin color change of blue, gray, or pale; rapid heart rate; or shortness of breath. If present, patient should seek immediate medical attention.

cefuroxime axetil

Ceftin

cefuroxime sodium

Zinacef

Class and Category

Pharmacologic class: Second-generation cephalosporin
Therapeutic class: Antibiotic
Pregnancy category: B

Indications and Dosages

➤ *To treat pharyngitis and tonsillitis*
ORAL SUSPENSION (CEFTIN)
Adults, adolescents, and children ages 3 months to 12 years. 10 mg/kg daily every 12 hr for 10 days. *Maximum:* 500 mg daily.
TABLETS (CEFTIN)
Adults and adolescents. 250 mg every 12 hr for 10 days.
➤ *To treat acute otitis media*
ORAL SUSPENSION (CEFTIN)
Children ages 3 months to 12 years. 15 mg/kg every 12 hr for 10 days. *Maximum:* 1,000 mg daily.
TABLETS (CEFTIN)
Children under age 13 who can swallow tablets. 250 mg every 12 hr for 10 days.
➤ *To treat impetigo*
ORAL SUSPENSION (CEFTIN)
Children ages 3 months to 12 years. 15 mg/kg every 12 hr for 10 days. *Maximum:* 1,000 mg daily.
➤ *To treat acute bacterial maxillary sinusitis*
ORAL SUSPENSION (CEFTIN)
Children ages 3 months to 12 years. 15 mg/kg every 12 hr for 10 days. *Maximum:* 1,000 mg daily.
TABLETS (CEFTIN)
Adults, adolescents, and children under age 13 who can swallow tablets. 250 mg every 12 hr for 10 days.
➤ *To treat acute bacterial exacerbations of chronic bronchitis and uncomplicated skin and soft-tissue infections*
TABLETS (CEFTIN)
Adults and adolescents. 250 to 500 mg twice daily (12 hr apart) for 10 days.
I.V. INFUSION, I.V. OR I.M. INJECTION (ZINACEF)
Adults. 750 mg every 8 hr for 5 to 10 days. I.V. given over at least 3 to 5 min.
➤ *To treat early Lyme disease*
TABLETS (CEFTIN)
Adults and adolescents. 500 mg every 12 hr for 20 days.
➤ *To treat uncomplicated UTI*
TABLETS (CEFTIN)
Adults. 250 mg every 12 hr for 7 to 10 days.
I.V. INFUSION, I.V. OR I.M. INJECTION
Adults. 750 mg every 8 hr. I.V. given over at least 3 to 5 min.
➤ *To treat uncomplicated gonorrhea*
TABLETS (CEFTIN)
Adults. 1 g as a single dose.
I.M. INJECTION (ZINACEF)
Adults. 1.5 g as a single dose divided equally and injected into two different sites; given with oral probenecid 1 g.
➤ *To treat disseminated gonococcal infection and uncomplicated pneumonia*
I.V. INFUSION, I.V. OR I.M. INJECTION (ZINACEF)
Adults. 750 mg every 8 hr. I.V. given over at least 3 to 5 min.
➤ *To treat bone and joint infections*
I.V. INFUSION, I.V. OR I.M. INJECTION (ZINACEF)
Adults. 1.5 g every 8 hr. I.V. given over at least 3 to 5 min.
Children over age 3 months. 150 mg/kg daily in divided doses every 8 hr. I.V. given over at least 3 to 5 min. *Maximum:* Adult dose.
➤ *To treat bacterial meningitis*
I.V. INFUSION
Adults. 1.5 to 3 g, given over at least 3 to 5 min, every 8 hr.
Children over age 1 month. 50 to 80 mg/kg, given over at least 3 to 5 min, every 6 to 8 hr.
➤ *To treat moderate infections other than those listed above*
I.V. INFUSION, I.V. OR I.M. INJECTION (ZINACEF)
Adults. 750 mg every 8 hr for 5 to 10 days. I.V. given over at least 3 to 5 min.
I.V. INFUSION OR INJECTION (ZINACEF)
Children over age 3 months. 50 mg/kg, given over at least 3 to 5 min, daily in equally divided doses every 6 to 8 hr.
➤ *To treat severe or complicated infections other than those listed above*
I.V. INFUSION OR INJECTION (ZINACEF)
Adults. 1.5 g, given over at least 3 to 5 min, every 8 hr.
Children over age 3 months. 100 mg/kg, given over at least 3 to 5 min, daily in equally divided doses every 6 to 8 hr.
➤ *To treat life-threatening infections other than those listed above*

I.V. INFUSION OR INJECTION (ZINACEF)
Adults. 1.5 g, given over at least 3 to 5 min, every 6 hr.

➤ *To provide perioperative prophylaxis*
I.V. INFUSION OR INJECTION (ZINACEF)
Adults. 1.5 g, given over at least 3 to 5 min, 30 to 60 min before surgery (at induction of anesthesia for open-heart surgery), and then 0.75 g, given over at least 3 to 5 min, every 8 hr for prolonged procedures (1.5 g, given over at least 3 to 5 min, every 12 hr for total of 6 g with open-heart surgery).
DOSAGE ADJUSTMENT Parenteral dosage reduced to 0.75 g every 12 hr if creatinine clearance is 10 to 20 ml/min or to 0.75 g every 24 hr if creatinine clearance less than 10 ml/min.

Mechanism of Action

Interferes with bacterial cell wall synthesis by inhibiting the final step in the cross-linking of peptidoglycan strands. Peptidoglycan makes the cell membrane rigid and protective. Without it, bacterial cells rupture and die.

Incompatibilities

Don't admix parenteral cefuroxime with other antibiotics, such as aminoglycosides, because of potential for incompatibility, such as substantial mutual inactivation. If they're administered concurrently, don't mix them in the same I.V. bag or bottle.

Contraindications

Hypersensitivity to cefuroxime, other cephalosporins, or their components

Interactions

DRUGS
aminoglycosides, loop diuretics: Increased risk of nephrotoxicity
oral combined estrogen–progesterone contraceptives: Decreased effectiveness of oral contraceptive

Adverse Reactions

CNS: Chills, fever, headache, **seizures**
CV: Edema
EENT: Hearing loss, oral candidiasis
GI: Abdominal cramps, diarrhea, elevated liver enzymes, **hepatic failure**, hepatomegaly, nausea, **pseudomembranous colitis**, vomiting
GU: Elevated BUN level, **nephrotoxicity**, **renal failure**, vaginal candidiasis
HEME: Eosinophilia, **hemolytic anemia**, **hypoprothrombinemia**, **neutropenia**, **thrombocytopenia**, **unusual bleeding**
MS: Arthralgia
RESP: Dyspnea
SKIN: Ecchymosis, erythema, **erythema multiforme**, pruritus, rash, **Stevens–Johnson syndrome**
Other: **Anaphylaxis**; injection-site edema, pain, and redness; superinfection

Nursing Considerations

- Use cefuroxime cautiously in patients hypersensitive to penicillin because cross-sensitivity has occurred in about 10% of such patients.
- Obtain culture and sensitivity results, if possible and as ordered, before giving drug.
- Give oral form with food to decrease GI distress, as needed.
- Remember that oral forms—tablets and suspension—aren't bioequivalent.
- For I.V. use, reconstitute using manufacturer's instructions according to type of preparation available. Solution ranges in color from light yellow to amber.
- For I.M. use, add 3 or 3.6 ml sterile water for injection to each 750-mg vial to yield 220 mg/ml.
- Thaw frozen parenteral solution at room temperature or under refrigeration before administration; make sure all ice crystals have melted. Don't force thawing by microwaving.
- Store reconstituted parenteral drug for up to 24 hours at room temperature or 96 hours in refrigerator. (Thawed solutions may be stable 24 hours at room temperature or 28 days if refrigerated.) Store reconstituted oral suspension in refrigerator or at room temperature up to 10 days.
- Give I.V. injection over 3 to 5 minutes through tubing of a flowing compatible I.V. fluid.
- Monitor I.V. site for extravasation and phlebitis.
- Monitor BUN and serum creatinine levels and fluid intake and output to detect signs of nephrotoxicity. Monitor patients with renal impairment closely because they may have greater toxic reactions to cefuroxime.
- Monitor patient for allergic reactions continuing up to a few days after therapy starts. Patients with a history of some

form of allergy, especially to drugs, are at increased risk for an allergic reaction.

- Assess bowel pattern daily; severe diarrhea may indicate pseudomembranous colitis. If it's suspected, stop drug, as ordered, and provide treatment as prescribed.
- Assess patient for arthralgia, bleeding, ecchymosis, and pharyngitis, which may indicate a blood dyscrasia.
- Monitor bleeding time and PT, as ordered. Be prepared to administer vitamin K, if ordered, to treat hypothrombinemia.

PATIENT TEACHING

- Instruct patient to shake oral suspension well before measuring each dose and to use a calibrated liquid-measuring device.
- Advise patient using single-dose packets of oral suspension to empty contents of one packet into a glass and add at least 10 ml (2 tsp) of cold water; apple, grape, or orange juice; or lemonade. Tell him to stir well and consume entire mixture at once.
- Inform patient that buttermilk and yogurt help maintain intestinal flora and can decrease diarrhea during therapy.
- Instruct patient to report evidence of blood dyscrasia to prescriber immediately.
- Urge patient to report watery, bloody stools to prescriber immediately, even up to 2 months after drug therapy has ended.

celecoxib

Celebrex

Class and Category

Pharmacologic class: NSAID
Therapeutic class: Analgesic, anti-inflammatory, antirheumatic
Pregnancy category: C changing to D from 30 weeks gestation onward

Indications and Dosages

➤ *To relieve signs and symptoms of osteoarthritis*

CAPSULES

Adults. 200 mg daily or 100 mg twice daily.

➤ *To relieve signs and symptoms of rheumatoid arthritis*

CAPSULES

Adults. 100 to 200 mg twice daily.

➤ *To relieve signs and symptoms of juvenile rheumatoid arthritis*

CAPSULES

Children age 2 and over weighing more than 25 kg (55 lb). 100 mg twice daily.
Children age 2 and over weighing 10 to 25 kg (22 to 55 lb). 50 mg twice daily.

➤ *To relieve pain from ankylosing spondylitis*

CAPSULES

Adults. 200 mg daily or 100 mg twice daily. Dosage increased to 400 mg daily or 200 mg twice daily after 6 weeks if needed.

➤ *To manage acute pain, to treat primary dysmenorrhea*

CAPSULES

Adults. 400 mg, followed by 200 mg if needed, on 1st day. On subsequent days, 200 mg twice daily as needed.

DOSAGE ADJUSTMENT Daily dosage reduced by 50% for patients with moderate hepatic impairment. For those weighing less than 50 kg (110 lb), expect to start with lowest recommended dose. For patients who are poor CYP2C9 metabolizers, starting dosage should be half the lowest recommended dose.

Mechanism of Action

Selectively inhibits the enzymatic activity of cyclooxygenase-2 (COX-2), the enzyme needed to convert arachidonic acid to prostaglandin. Prostaglandins are responsible for mediating the inflammatory response and causing local vasodilation, swelling, and pain. Prostaglandins also play a role in peripheral pain transmission to the spinal cord. By inhibiting COX-2 activity and prostaglandin production, this reduces inflammatory symptoms and relieves pain.

Contraindications

Allergic reaction (such as anaphylaxis or angioedema) to aspirin, other NSAIDs, or sulfonamide derivatives or history of aspirin-induced nasal polyps with bronchospasm; hypersensitivity to celecoxib or its components; treatment of pain after coronary artery bypass graft surgery

Interactions

DRUGS

ACE inhibitors, angiotensin II receptor antagonists, beta blockers: Decreased antihypertensive effect of these drugs, increased risk of renal failure

aspirin and other salicylates, corticosteroids: Increased risk of GI ulceration and other GI complications, increased risk of bleeding
cyclosporine: Increased risk of cyclosporine-induced nephrotoxicity
CYP2C9 inducers such as rifampin: Possibly decreased effectiveness of celecoxib
CYP2C9 inhibitors such as fluconazole: Possibly increased risk of celecoxib toxicity
digoxin: Increased risk of digitalis toxicity
fluconazole: Increased blood celecoxib level
furosemide, thiazide diuretics: Reduced diuretic effects of these drugs, increased risk of renal failure
lithium: Possibly elevated blood lithium level
methotrexate: Increased risk of methotrexate toxicity (neutropenia, renal dysfunction, thrombocytopenia)
pemetrexed: Increased risk of myelosuppression, GI and renal toxicity
warfarin and other anticoagulants: Possibly increased PT and risk of bleeding

Adverse Reactions

CNS: **Aseptic meningitis**, **cerebral hemorrhage**, **CVA**, depression, dizziness, fever, headache, insomnia, **suicidal ideation**, syncope, transient ischemic attacks, vertigo
CV: **Aortic valve incompetence**, **bradycardia**, chest pain, **congestive heart failure**, **deep vein thrombosis**, fluid retention, hypertension, **MI**, palpitations, peripheral edema, tachycardia, **thrombosis**, **unstable angina**, vasculitis, **ventricular fibrillation**, **ventricular hypertrophy**
EENT: Conjunctival hemorrhage, deafness, labyrinthitis, nasopharyngitis, pharyngitis, rhinitis, sinusitis, vitreous floaters
ENDO: Hyperglycemia, **hypoglycemia**
GI: Abdominal pain, diarrhea, elevated liver enzymes, **esophageal perforation**, flatulence, **GI bleeding** or ulceration, **hepatic failure**, ileus, indigestion, jaundice, nausea, **pancreatitis**, **perforation of intestines or stomach**, vomiting
GU: **Acute renal failure**, interstitial nephritis, ovarian cyst, proteinuria, urinary incontinence, UTI
HEME: **Agranulocytosis**, **aplastic anemia**, decreased hematocrit and hemoglobin, **leukopenia**, **pancytopenia**, **prolonged APTT**, **thrombocytopenia**
MS: Arthralgia, back pain, elevated serum CK level, epicondylitis, tendon rupture
RESP: **Bronchospasm**, cough, dyspnea, pneumonia, **pulmonary embolism**, upper respiratory tract infection
SKIN: **Erythema multiforme**, **exfoliative dermatitis**, phototoxicity, rash, **Stevens–Johnson syndrome**, **toxic epidermal necrolysis**, urticaria
Other: **Anaphylaxis**, **angioedema**, **hyperkalemia**, **hypernatremia**, **hyponatremia**, **sepsis**

Nursing Considerations

- Know that NSAIDs like celecoxib should be avoided in patients with a recent MI because risk of reinfarction increases with NSAID therapy. If therapy is unavoidable, monitor patient closely for signs of cardiac ischemia.
- Be aware that NSAIDs such as celecoxib should not be given to patients with severe heart failure because risk of heart failure increases with NSAID use. If use is unavoidable, monitor patient for worsening of heart failure.
- Use celecoxib with extreme caution in patients who have a history of GI bleeding or ulcer disease because NSAIDs, such as celecoxib, increase the risk of GI bleeding and ulceration. In these patients, drug should be used for shortest time possible.
- Be aware that serious GI tract ulceration and bleeding, as well as perforation of intestine or stomach, can occur without warning or symptoms. Elderly patients are at greatest risk. To minimize risk, give celecoxib with food. If patient develops GI distress, withhold celecoxib and notify prescriber immediately.
- Use celecoxib cautiously in patients with hypertension, and monitor blood pressure closely throughout therapy because drug can start or worsen hypertension.
- Use celecoxib cautiously in children with systemic onset juvenile rheumatoid arthritis because serious adverse reactions can occur, including disseminated intravascular coagulation.
- Use celecoxib cautiously in patients known to be poor CYP2C9 metabolizers

based on history or experience with other CYP2C9 substrates, such as phenytoin or warfarin. Dosage should start at half the lowest recommended amount. For patients with juvenile rheumatoid arthritis who are also poor CYP2C9 metabolizers, alternative management should be considered.

WARNING Know that use of NSAIDs like celecoxib increases risk of serious cardiovascular thrombotic events, including MI and stroke, which can be life-threatening. These events may occur early in treatment and risk increases with duration of use. Be aware that these events have occurred even in patients who do not have a history or known risk factors for cardiovascular disease. Monitor patient for warning signs such as chest pain, shortness of breath, slurring of speech, or weakness. If any signs and symptoms develop, withhold celecoxib, alert prescriber immediately, and provide supportive care, as prescribed.

WARNING Expect to monitor laboratory results (including WBC) and assess for infection in patient who has bone marrow suppression such as occurs with antineoplastic therapy because celecoxib's anti-inflammatory and antipyretic actions may mask signs and symptoms, such as fever and pain.

- Monitor patient—especially if elderly or receiving long-term celecoxib therapy—for less common but serious adverse GI reactions, including anorexia, constipation, diverticulitis, dysphagia, esophagitis, gastritis, gastroenteritis, gastroesophageal reflux disease, hemorrhoids, hiatal hernia, melena, stomatitis, and vomiting.
- Monitor liver enzymes because, in rare cases, elevation may progress to severe hepatic reaction, including fatal hepatitis, or hepatic failure or necrosis.
- Monitor BUN and serum creatinine levels in elderly patients; patients taking ACE inhibitors, angiotensin II receptor antagonists, or diuretics; and patients with heart failure, impaired hepatic dysfunction or renal function because drug may cause renal failure.
- Monitor CBC for decreased hemoglobin level and hematocrit because drug may worsen anemia.
- Assess patient's skin regularly for signs of rash or other hypersensitivity reaction because celecoxib is a sulfur drug and may cause serious skin reactions without warning, even in patients with no history of sensitivity to sulfur. At first sign of reaction, stop drug and notify prescriber.
- Avoid using celecoxib with a nonaspirin NSAID, regardless of the dose, because celecoxib reduces inflammation and fever, which may mask signs of infection.

PATIENT TEACHING

- Instruct patient to swallow celecoxib capsules whole with a full glass of water and with food or milk to prevent stomach upset.
- Tell patient to take celecoxib exactly as prescribed and not to increase dosage or take drug longer than prescribed because serious adverse reactions can occur.
- Advise patient to notify prescriber if pain continues or is poorly controlled.
- Explain that celecoxib may increase the risk of serious adverse CV events; urge patient to seek immediate medical attention if signs or symptoms arise, such as chest pain, shortness of breath, slurred speech, and weakness.
- Inform patient that the risk of congestive heart failure increases with NSAID use. Instruct patient to promptly report any evidence of edema, shortness of breath, or unexplained weight gain.
- Tell patient that celecoxib may increase the risk of serious adverse GI reactions. Stress the need to seek immediate medical attention if signs or symptoms develop, such as abdominal or epigastric, black or tarry stools, indigestion, and vomiting blood or material that resembles coffee grounds.
- Alert patient that celecoxib may cause serious skin reactions. Advise immediate medical attention if signs or symptoms develop, such as rash, blisters, fever, itching, or other evidence of hypersensitivity.
- Urge patient to avoid alcohol consumption and smoking during celecoxib therapy because they may increase the risk of adverse GI reactions.

cephalexin hydrochloride

cephalexin monohydrate

Keflex

Class and Category

Pharmacologic class: First-generation cephalosporin
Therapeutic class: Antibiotic
Pregnancy category: B

Indications and Dosages

➤ *To treat bone infections caused by* Proteus mirabilis *or* Staphylococcus aureus; *genitourinary tract infections caused by* Escherichia coli, Klebsiella pneumoniae, *or* P. mirabilis; *respiratory infections caused by* Streptococcus pneumoniae *or* S. pyogenes; *and skin and skin structure infections caused by* S. aureus *or* S. pyogenes

CAPSULES, ORAL SUSPENSION, TABLETS

Adults and adolescents age 15 and over. 250 mg every 6 hr or 500 mg every 12 hr for 7 to 14 days. *For severe infections:* Up to 4 g daily in 2 to 4 equally divided doses.

Children ages 1 to 15. 25 to 50 mg/kg daily given in equally divided doses for 7 to 14 days. *For severe infections:* 50 to 100 mg/kg daily given in equally divided doses.

➤ *To treat otitis media caused by* Haemophilus influenzae, Moraxella catarrhalis, S. aureus, *or* S. pneumoniae

ORAL SUSPENSION

Children. 75 to 100 mg/kg daily in equally divided doses four times daily.

DOSAGE ADJUSTMENT For patients with a creatinine clearance of 30 to 59 ml/min, maximum dosage not to exceed 1 g; for creatinine clearance of 15 to 29 ml/min, dosage reduced to 250 mg every 8 or 12 hr; for creatinine clearance of 5 to 14 ml/min and patient not yet on dialysis, dosage reduced to 250 mg every 24 hr; and for creatinine clearance of 1 to 4 ml/min and patient not yet on dialysis, dosage reduced to 250 mg every 48 or 60 hr.

Contraindications

Hypersensitivity to cephalexin, other cephalosporins, or their components

Interactions

DRUGS

aminoglycosides, loop diuretics: Increased risk of nephrotoxicity
probenecid: Increased and prolonged blood cephalexin level

Adverse Reactions

CNS: Chills, fever, headache, **seizures**
CV: Edema
EENT: Hearing loss, oral candidiasis
GI: Abdominal cramps, diarrhea, elevated liver enzymes, **hepatic failure**, hepatomegaly, nausea, **pseudomembranous colitis**, vomiting
GU: Elevated BUN level, **nephrotoxicity**, **renal failure**, vaginal candidiasis

Mechanism of Action

Like all cephalosporins, cephalexin interferes with bacterial cell wall synthesis by inhibiting the final step in the cross-linking of peptidoglycan strands. Peptidoglycan makes the cell membrane rigid and protective. Without it, bacterial cells rupture and die. This mechanism of action is most effective against bacteria that divide rapidly, including many gram-positive and gram-negative bacteria.

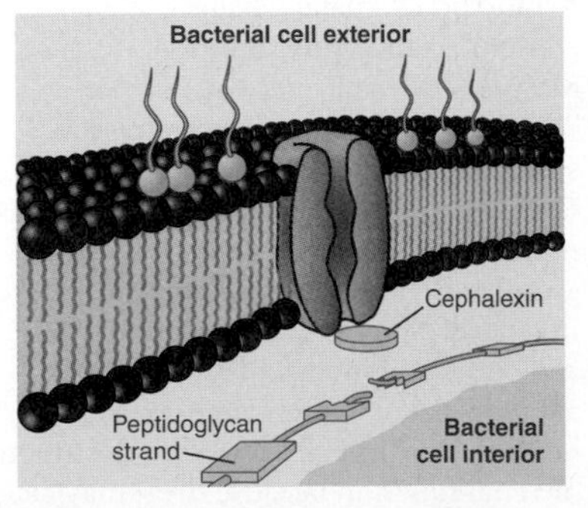

HEME: Eosinophilia, **hemolytic anemia, hypoprothrombinemia, neutropenia, thrombocytopenia, unusual bleeding**
MS: Arthralgia
RESP: Dyspnea
SKIN: Ecchymosis, erythema, **erythema multiforme**, pruritus, rash, **Stevens–Johnson syndrome**
Other: Anaphylaxis, superinfection

Nursing Considerations

- Use cephalexin cautiously in patients hypersensitive to penicillin because cross-sensitivity occurs in about 10% of them.
- Obtain culture and sensitivity test results, if possible and as ordered, before giving drug.
- Monitor patient's BUN and serum creatinine levels to detect early signs of nephrotoxicity. Also monitor fluid intake and output; decreasing urine output may indicate nephrotoxicity. Expect to monitor a patient who already has renal impairment longer for nephrotoxicity, because drug clearance is slowed.
- Monitor for allergic reactions a few days after therapy starts.
- Assess ALT, AST, bilirubin, CBC, hematocrit, LD, and serum alkaline phosphatase, levels during long-term therapy.
- Assess patient's bowel pattern daily; severe diarrhea may indicate pseudomembranous colitis caused by *Clostridium difficile.* If diarrhea occurs, notify prescriber and expect to withhold cefotaxime and treat with electrolytes, fluids, protein, and an antibiotic effective against *C. difficile.*
- Assess patient for arthralgia, bleeding, ecchymosis, and pharyngitis; they may indicate a blood dyscrasia.

PATIENT TEACHING

- Advise patient to complete prescribed course of therapy.
- Instruct patient to shake oral suspension well before measuring each dose and to use a calibrated liquid-measuring device to ensure an accurate dose.
- Tell patient that buttermilk and yogurt can help maintain intestinal flora and decrease diarrhea during therapy.
- Urge patient to report watery, bloody stools to prescriber immediately, even if they occur up to 2 months after cephalexin therapy has ended.

certolizumab pegol

Cimzia

Class and Category

Pharmacologic class: Tumor necrosis factor (TNF) blocker
Therapeutic class: Immunomodulator, disease modifying antirheumatic drug (DMARD)
Pregnancy category: Not classified

Indications and Dosages

➤ *To reduce signs and symptoms of Crohn's disease and maintain clinical response in patients with moderately to severely active disease who have had an inadequate response to conventional therapy*

SUBCUTANEOUS INJECTION

Adults. *Initial:* 400 mg (given as two 200-mg injections) and repeated at wk 2 and 4. *Maintenance:* 400 mg (given as two 200-mg injections) every 4 wk if clinical response occurs.

➤ *To treat active ankylosing spondylitis, active psoriatic arthritis, or moderate to severe active rheumatoid arthritis*

SUBCUTANEOUS INJECTION

Adults. *Initial:* 400 mg (given as two 200-mg injections) and repeated at wk 2 and 4. *Maintenance:* 200 mg every other wk, or 400 mg (given as two 200-mg injections) every 4 wk if clinical response occurs.

➤ To treat moderate to severe plaque psoriasis

SUBCUTANEOUS INJECTION

Adults. 400 mg (given as two 200-mg injections) every other wk.

DOSAGE ADJUSTMENT For patient with plaque psoriasis who weighs 90 kg (198 lb), dosage may be changed to 400 mg (given as two 200-mg injections) and repeated at wk 2 and 4, followed by 200 mg every other week.

Route	Onset	Peak	Duration
SubQ	Unknown	54–171 hr	Unknown

Mechanism of Action

Binds to human tumor necrosis factor (TNF) alpha, inhibiting it. TNF alpha stimulates production of inflammatory mediators, including interleukin-1, nitric oxide, platelet activating factor, and prostaglandins. TNF alpha level is increased in patients with Crohn's disease and rheumatoid arthritis. Inhibition of TNF alpha causes C-reactive protein level to decline in patients with Crohn's disease, and the disease improves.

Contraindications

Active infection, concurrent therapy with disease modifying antirheumatic drugs or other tumor necrosis factor blocker therapy, hypersensitivity to certolizumab or its components

Interactions

DRUGS

abatacept, anakinra, natalizumab, rituximab: Possibly increased risk of serious infection and neutropenia
immunosuppressants: Possibly increased risk of infection
live-virus vaccines: Increased risk of adverse vaccine effects

Adverse Reactions

CNS: Anxiety, bipolar disorder, dizziness, fever, headache, malaise, **suicidal ideation**, syncope
CV: Angina, **arrhythmias**, **heart failure**, hypertension, **hypotension**, **MI**, **pericardial effusion**, **pericarditis**, peripheral edema, vasculitis
EENT: Optic neuritis, retinal hemorrhage, uveitis
ENDO: Hot flashes
GI: Abdominal pain, diarrhea, elevated liver enzymes, **hepatitis**, **intestinal obstruction**
GU: Menstrual dysfunction, **nephrotic syndrome**, pyelonephritis, **renal failure**, UTI
HEME: Anemia, **leukemia**, **leukopenia**, lymphadenopathy, **pancytopenia**, thrombophilia
MS: Arthralgia, extremity pain
RESP: **Cough**, **dyspnea**, pneumonia, upper respiratory infection
SKIN: Allergic dermatitis, alopecia, change of plaque psoriasis into a different psoriasis subtype, **erythema multiforme**, erythema nodosum, **melanoma**, **Merkel cell carcinoma**, new or worsening psoriasis, rash, **Stevens–Johnson syndrome**, **toxic epidermal necrolysis**, urticaria
Other: Anaphylaxis; **angioedema**; antibody formation to certolizumab; bacterial, invasive fungal, mycobacterial, parasitic, viral or other opportunistic infections including aspergillosis, blastomycosis, candidiasis, coccidioidomycosis, histoplasmosis, legionellosis, listeriosis, pneumocystosis, and tuberculosis; herpes infections; injection-site reactions (bruising, discoloration, pain, redness, swelling); **lymphomas and other malignancies**; lupus-like syndrome; sarcoidosis, serum sickness

Nursing Considerations

- Be aware that certolizumab should not be initiated in a patient with an active infection, including serious localized infections.
- Use certolizumab cautiously in patients with recurrent or increased risk of infection, patients who live in regions where histoplasmosis and tuberculosis are endemic, and patients with a history of CNS demyelinating disorders because any of these disorders can occur, rarely, during certolizumab therapy. Be aware that a falsely negative antigen and antibody test for histoplasmosis may occur in some patients during certolizumab therapy, even when an active infection is present. Patient should be monitored closely throughout therapy.
- Use cautiously in patients who are chronic carriers of hepatitis B virus because drug may reactivate the virus. Assess patient for evidence of hepatitis B viral infection before starting and periodically throughout certolizumab therapy. If HBV reactivation occurs, notify prescriber, stop drug, and start appropriate therapy, as ordered.
- Make sure patient has a tuberculin skin test before therapy starts. If skin test is positive (induration 5 mm or greater), treatment of latent tuberculosis must start before certolizumab is given, as prescribed. In addition, expect antituberculosis therapy to be given to a patient with a past history of latent or active tuberculosis in whom an adequate course of treatment cannot be confirmed, and for patients with a negative test for latent tuberculosis but having risk

factors for tuberculosis infection. Be aware that a falsely negative test for latent tuberculosis may occur during certolizumab therapy, so any signs and symptoms suggestive of tuberculosis should be carefully evaluated.

WARNING **Monitor all patients for infection during therapy, especially those who are at higher risk for infection, such as patients receiving immunosuppressants, those who are over 65 years of age, or who have comorbid conditions. If serious infection develops, expect prescriber to stop drug.**

- Reconstitute two 200-mg certolizumab vials for each dose after drug has reached room temperature. Inject 1 ml sterile water for injection using a 20G needle into each vial. Gently swirl each vial without shaking. Continue swirling every 5 minutes as long as undissolved particles are observed, which may take as long as 30 minutes. Do not leave at room temperature, once reconstituted, for more than 2 hours before administration. If administration will be delayed, reconstituted drug can be refrigerated up to 24 hours. Do not let drug freeze.
- Administer drug only when solution has reached room temperature. Using a 20G needle, withdraw drug from vial using a separate syringe and needle for each vial. Switch to a 23G needle and administer subcutaneously into two separate areas on patient's abdomen or thigh.

WARNING **Stop drug immediately and notify prescriber if patient has an allergic reaction. Expect to provide supportive care.**

- Monitor patient closely for evidence of congestive heart failure (anxiety; crackles; dyspnea; sudden, unexplained weight gain), and notify prescriber if they occur.
- Monitor patient's CBC, as ordered, because certolizumab may have adverse hematologic effects. Notify prescriber about persistent bleeding, bruising, fever, or pallor.
- Be aware that certolizumab is a TNF inhibitor. Although rare, malignancies (especially lymphomas and leukemias) have been reported in patients receiving these drugs, including children. Patients with rheumatoid arthritis, especially those with very active disease, and patients with disorders that certolizumab treats are at greatest risk. Monitor these patients closely.
- Assess patient's skin regularly, especially for patients who are at risk for skin cancer, as drug may cause melanomas and Merkel cell carcinoma as well as other life-threatening disorders such as Stevens–Johnson syndrome. At the first sign of a rash, notify prescriber.

PATIENT TEACHING

- Instruct patient on how to administer a subcutaneous injection using the prefilled syringe. Tell patient to keep drug in refrigerator until about 30 min before administering to allow it to warm up to room temperature. Caution him not to warm up the drug any other way. Tell him to inject the drug either into his abdomen or thigh and to make sure he injects the full amount. Review how to safely discard the needle and syringe after the injection.
- Inform the patient that he may receive vaccinations, except for live or live attenuated vaccines.
- Review signs and symptoms of allergic reaction (rash, swollen face, trouble breathing), and tell patient to seek emergency care immediately if these occur.
- Inform patient that injection-site reactions such as pain or redness may occur and usually are mild and transient. Instruct him to apply a towel soaked in cold water to the site if it hurts. Tell patient to call prescriber if reaction persists or worsens.
- Inform patient that drug may lower the ability of the immune system to fight infections. Tell patient to report any signs and symptoms of infection, including tuberculosis or reactivation of hepatitis B virus infections, that may occur during therapy. Instruct him to report fever, including a low-grade fever, persistent cough, or wasting or weight loss to prescriber.
- Tell patient to report evidence of bleeding disorders and infections to prescriber; drug may have to be stopped. Advise patient to avoid people with infections and to comply with all prescribed tests.
- Inform patient that certain kinds of cancer, especially leukemias and lymphomas are more likely in patients taking certolizumab but still rare. Emphasize need to keep follow-up visits

C

and to report sudden or unusual signs or symptoms. Also advise patient to have periodic skin examinations, especially if they are at risk for skin cancer.
- Instruct patient to report lupus-like signs and symptoms that, although rare, may occur during therapy, such as chest pain that doesn't go away, joint pain, rash on cheeks or arms that's sensitive to the sun, or shortness of breath. Explain that drug may need to be discontinued if these occur.
- Advise patient to inform all healthcare providers about certolizumab use and to inform prescriber about any herbal remedies vitamin and mineral supplements, and OTC medications being taken.
- Advise patient to report any signs of new or worsening health issues such as autoimmune disorders, heart disease, or neurological disease, especially bleeding, bruising, or a persistent fever.
- Tell women of childbearing age to notify prescriber if pregnancy occurs or is suspected, because drug's effects on the fetus are unknown. If pregnancy is confirmed, encourage patient to enroll in the pregnancy exposure registry by calling 1-877-311-8972. Also tell mothers wishing to breastfeed their infant to discuss breastfeeding with prescriber before doing so.

cevimeline hydrochloride

Evoxac

Class and Category

Pharmacologic class: Cholinergic agonist
Therapeutic class: Parasympathomimetic
Pregnancy category: C

Indications and Dosages

➤ *To treat dry mouth associated with Sjögren's syndrome*

CAPSULES

Adults. 30 mg three times daily. *Maximum:* 90 mg daily.

Mechanism of Action

As a cholinergic agonist, binds to and activates muscarinic receptors of the parasympathetic nervous system and increases secretions of the exocrine glands, such as salivary glands.

Contraindications

Acute iritis, angle-closure glaucoma, hypersensitivity to cevimeline or its components, uncontrolled asthma

Interactions

DRUGS

amiodarone, cimetidine, clarithromycin, diltiazem, erythromycin, fluconazole, haloperidol, itraconazole, ketoconazole, metoclopramide, mibefradil, nefazodone, propafenone, quinidine, ritonavir, selective serotonin reuptake inhibitors, thioridazine, tricyclic antidepressants, troleandomycin, verapamil: Possibly inhibited metabolism and increased blood level of cevimeline
anticholinergics: Decreased effectiveness of anticholinergics
antimuscarinics: Altered effects of antimuscarinics and decreased therapeutic action of cevimeline
beta blockers: Possibly cardiac conduction disturbances
parasympathomimetics: Additive effects of either drug

Adverse Reactions

CNS: Depression, fatigue, fever, hypoesthesia, insomnia, migraine headache, tremor
CV: Edema, palpitations
EENT: Abnormal vision, conjunctivitis, dry mouth, earache, epistaxis, excessive salivation, eye pain, rhinitis, salivary gland pain
GI: Abdominal pain, anorexia, cholecystitis, constipation, eructation, heartburn, hiccups, nausea, vomiting
HEME: Anemia
MS: Arthralgia, leg cramps, myalgia
RESP: Cough, dyspnea
SKIN: Diaphoresis, pruritus
Other: Flu-like symptoms, hot flashes

Nursing Considerations

- Give cevimeline on an empty stomach because food may decrease rate and extent of absorption, delaying peak concentration.
- Assess patient with a pulmonary disorder for wheezing and increased respiratory secretions because drug may cause airway resistance, increased bronchiolar smooth-muscle contractions, and respiratory secretions.

- Monitor patient with known or suspected gallbladder disease for abdominal pain and other warnings of biliary obstruction, cholangitis, or cholecystitis; each of these conditions may be precipitated by cevimeline.

PATIENT TEACHING

- Instruct patient to take cevimeline on an empty stomach.
- Inform patient that cevimeline may cause vision changes; advise him to avoid driving at night or performing hazardous activities until drug's adverse effects are known.
- Urge patient to drink plenty of fluids during hot weather and while exercising because drug may cause excessive sweating and dehydration.

chlordiazepoxide hydrochloride

Librium

Class, Category, and Schedule

Pharmacologic class: Benzodiazepine
Therapeutic class: Anxiolytic
Pregnancy category: Not classified
Controlled substance schedule: IV

Indications and Dosages

➤ *To provide short-term management of mild anxiety*

CAPSULES

Adults. 5 to 10 mg three or four times daily.
Children over age 6. 5 mg two to four times daily increased as needed to 10 mg two or three times daily, or 0.5 mg/kg daily in equally divided doses every 6 to 8 hr.

➤ *To provide short-term management of severe anxiety*

CAPSULES

Adults. 20 to 25 mg three or four times daily.

I.V. OR I.M. INJECTION

Adults. *Initial:* 50 to 100 mg. Then, 25 to 50 mg three or four times daily, as needed. I.V. given slowly over 1 min. *Maximum:* 300 mg daily.

I.M. INJECTION

Children age 12 and over. 0.5 mg/kg daily in equally divided doses every 6 to 8 hr.

➤ *To provide short-term treatment of acute alcohol withdrawal*

CAPSULES, I.V. OR I.M. INJECTION

Adults. *Initial:* 50 to 100 mg, usually given I.V. or I.M. Repeated in 2 to 4 hr followed by individualized oral dosage if needed to control symptoms. I.V. given slowly over 1 min. *Maximum:* 300 mg daily.

➤ *To provide perioperative relaxation and reduce apprehension and anxiety*

CAPSULES, I.M. INJECTION

Adults. 5 to 10 mg P.O. three or four times daily several days before surgery; 50 to 100 mg I.M. 1 hr before surgery.

DOSAGE ADJUSTMENT Dosage reduced to 5 mg P.O. two to four times daily, as needed, for elderly or debilitated patients. For patients with a creatinine clearance less than 10 ml/min, dosage reduced by 50%.

Mechanism of Action

May potentiate the effects of gamma-aminobutyric acid (GABA) and other inhibitory neurotransmitters by binding to specific benzodiazepine receptors in cortical and limbic areas of the CNS. By binding to these receptors, chlordiazepoxide increases GABA's inhibitory effects and blocks cortical and limbic arousal, which helps control emotional behavior. It also helps relieve symptoms of alcohol withdrawal by causing CNS depression.

Contraindications

Hypersensitivity to chlordiazepoxide or its components

Interactions

DRUGS

antacids: Altered rate of chlordiazepoxide absorption
cimetidine, disulfiram, fluoxetine, isoniazid, ketoconazole, metoprolol, oral contraceptives, propoxyphene, propranolol, valproic acid: Increased blood chlordiazepoxide level
CNS depressants, opioids, other benzodiazepines, sedating antihistamines, tricyclic antidepressants: Increased risk of sedation and somnolence and other CNS effects
digoxin: Increased blood digoxin level and risk of digitalis toxicity
levodopa: Decreased efficacy of levodopa's antiparkinsonian effects
neuromuscular blockers: Potentiated, counteracted, or diminished effects of neuromuscular blockers

opioids: Increased risk of significant respiratory depression
phenytoin: Possibly increased phenytoin toxicity
probenecid: Shortened onset of action or prolonged effect of chlordiazepoxide
rifampin: Decreased chlordiazepoxide effect
theophyllines: Antagonized sedative effects of chlordiazepoxide

ACTIVITIES

alcohol use: Increased CNS effects, including severe respiratory depression and significant sedation and somnolence

Adverse Reactions

CNS: Ataxia, confusion, depression, drowsiness, **suicidal ideation**
CV: ECG changes, hypotension,
GI: Elevated liver enzymes, **hepatic dysfunction**, jaundice
HEME: Agranulocytosis
Other: Injection-site pain, redness, and swelling

Nursing Considerations

- Use chlordiazepoxide cautiously in patients with hepatic or renal impairment or porphyria.

WARNING Be aware that benzodiazepine therapy such as chlordiazepoxide should only be used concomitantly with opioid therapy in patients for whom other treatment options are inadequate. If prescribed together, expect dosing and duration of the opioid to be limited. Monitor patient closely for signs and symptoms of decrease in consciousness, including coma, profound sedation, and significant respiratory depression. Notify prescriber immediately and provide emergency supportive care, as death may occur.

WARNING Be aware that prolonged use of chlordiazepoxide at therapeutic doses can lead to dependence.

- For I.V. use, reconstitute ampule contents with 5 ml sterile water for injection or sodium chloride for injection. Agitate gently until completely dissolved. Give slowly over 1 minute.
- For I.M. use, reconstitute only with diluent provided by manufacturer.

WARNING Don't use supplied diluent to prepare drug for I.V. use because air bubbles form on the surface.

- Don't give opalescent or hazy solution.
- Monitor patient for evidence of phlebitis or thrombophlebitis after I.V. chlordiazepoxide administration.
- Monitor liver enzymes during therapy.
- Know that if patient is an aggressive, hyperactive child or has a history of psychiatric disorders, watch for paradoxical reactions, such as acute rage excitement, and stimulation, during first 2 weeks of therapy.
- Watch patients closely (especially children, adolescents, and young adults) for suicidal tendencies, particularly when chlordiazepoxide therapy starts and dosage changes.

PATIENT TEACHING

- Warn that drug may cause drowsiness.

WARNING Warn patient not to consume alcohol or take an opioid during chlordiazepoxide therapy without prescriber knowledge, as severe respiratory depression can occur that may lead to death.

WARNING Inform patient about potentially fatal additive effects of combining a benzodiazepine like chlordiazepoxide with an opioid. Instruct patient to inform all prescribers of chlordiazepoxide use, especially if pain medication may be prescribed.

- Advise patient to avoid other CNS depressants during therapy.
- Warn patient not to take antacids with chlordiazepoxide.
- Urge family or caregiver to watch patient closely for suicidal tendencies, especially when therapy starts or dosage changes and particularly if patient is a child, teenager, or young adult.

chlorothiazide

Diuril

chlorothiazide sodium

Diuril

Class and Category

Pharmacologic class: Thiazide diuretic
Therapeutic class: Antihypertensive, diuretic
Pregnancy category: Not classified

Indications and Dosages

➤ *To treat hypertension*

ORAL SUSPENSION, TABLETS

Adults. 250 to 1,000 mg daily in a single dose or divided doses twice daily. *Maximum:* 2,000 mg daily in divided doses.
Children age 6 months and over. 10 to 20 mg/kg daily in a single dose or divided doses twice daily. *Maximum:* 1,000 mg daily for ages 2 to 12; 375 mg daily for ages 6 months to 2 years.
Children under age 6 months. Up to 30 mg/kg daily in divided doses given twice daily.

➤ *To produce diuresis in patients with edema associated with corticosteroid and estrogen therapy, congestive heart failure, hepatic cirrhosis, and renal dysfunction*

ORAL SUSPENSION, TABLETS

Adults. 250 mg every 6 to 12 hr. Administered on an intermittent schedule, if needed, such as alternate days or 3 to 5 days/wk.
Children age 6 months and over. 10 to 20 mg/kg daily in a single dose or divided doses twice daily. *Maximum:* 1,000 mg daily for children ages 2 to 12; 375 mg daily for children ages 6 months to 2 years.
Children under age 6 months. Up to 33 mg/kg daily in divided doses twice daily.

I.V. INFUSION OR INJECTION

Adults. 500 mg to 1 g given slowly over at least 5 min for I.V. injection and 30 min for I.V. infusion once or twice daily.

Route	Onset	Peak	Duration
P.O.	2 hr	4 hr	6–12 hr
I.V.	15 min	4 hr	6–12 hr

Mechanism of Action

May promote chloride, sodium, and water excretion by inhibiting sodium reabsorption in the kidneys' distal tubules. Initially, chlorothiazide may reduce blood pressure by decreasing cardiac output, extracellular fluid volume, and plasma volume. It also may dilate arteries directly, reducing peripheral vascular resistance. After several weeks, cardiac output, extracellular fluid and plasma volume return to normal, but peripheral vascular resistance remains decreased.

Contraindications

Hypersensitivity to chlorothiazide, sulfonamides, or their components

Interactions

DRUGS

ACTH, barbiturates, narcotics: Possibly increased risk of orthostatic hypotension
corticosteroids, ACTH: Intensified electrolyte depletion, especially hypokalemia
cholestyramine, colestipol: Decreased chlorothiazide absorption
diazoxide: Hyperglycemia, hypotension
insulin, oral hypoglycemics: Possible alteration in blood glucose control
lithium: Increased risk of lithium toxicity
nondepolarizing skeletal muscle relaxants: Possibly increased effects of muscle relaxants
NSAIDs: Possibly reduced diuretic effect of chlorothiazide; increased risk of renal failure if patient has compromised renal function
other antihypertensives: Increased antihypertensive effect

ACTIVITIES

alcohol: Increased risk of orthostatic hypotension

Adverse Reactions

CNS: Dizziness, headache, paresthesia, restlessness, vertigo, weakness
CV: Orthostatic hypotension
ENDO: Hyperglycemia
GI: Abdominal cramps, anorexia, constipation, diarrhea, gastric irritation, jaundice, nausea, **pancreatitis**, vomiting
GU: Glycosuria, hematuria (I.V. form), impotence, interstitial nephritis, renal dysfunction, **renal failure**
HEME: Agranulocytosis, aplastic anemia, hemolytic anemia, leukopenia, thrombocytopenia
MS: Muscle spasms
SKIN: Photosensitivity, purpura, rash, urticaria
Other: Anaphylactic reactions, hypercalcemia, hyperuricemia, hypochloremic alkalosis, **hypokalemia**, **hypomagnesemia**, **hyponatremia**, hypovolemia

Nursing Considerations

- Don't give parenteral form of chlorothiazide by I.M. or subcutaneous route.
- For I.V. use, reconstitute with at least 18 ml of sterile water for injection. Discard unused solution after 24 hours. Reconstituted solution is compatible with

dextrose solution or normal saline solution for infusion.

- Watch I.V. site closely. If extravasation occurs, stop infusion and tell prescriber at once.
- Weigh patient daily to assess fluid loss and drug effectiveness. If used to treat hypertension, check blood pressure often; antihypertensive effect may not appear for days.
- Assess patient for electrolyte imbalances.
- Monitor renal function closely, especially in elderly patients, because risk of toxicity increases with renal impairment.

PATIENT TEACHING

- Tell patient to take chlorothiazide early in the day to avoid nocturia and to take it with food or milk if GI distress occurs.
- Urge patient to eat a high-potassium diet.
- Instruct patient to rise slowly to minimize effects of orthostatic hypotension.
- Urge patient to weigh himself at least weekly and to notify prescriber if weight rises or falls by 5 lb (2.25 kg) or more in 2 days.
- Tell patient to immediately notify prescriber if he develops cramps, diarrhea, dizziness, drowsiness, excessive thirst, increased heart rate, nausea, restlessness, sudden joint pain, tiredness, vomiting, or weakness.
- Know that if patient has diabetes mellitus, tell him to check blood glucose level often. Insulin or oral antidiabetic dosage may have to be increased.
- Tell patient to avoid prolonged exposure to sun, use sunscreen, and wear protective clothing.
- Advise patient to consult prescriber or pharmacist before using alcohol and such OTC drugs as those used for appetite control, colds, cough, hay fever, and sinus problems.

chlorpromazine

chlorpromazine hydrochloride

Class and Category

Pharmacologic class: Phenothiazine
Therapeutic class: Antiemetic, antipsychotic, tranquilizer
Pregnancy category: Not classified

Indications and Dosages

➤ *To manage symptoms of psychotic disorders or control manic manifestations of manic-depression in outpatients*

E.R. CAPSULES

Adults. 30 to 300 mg 1 to 3 times daily, with dosage adjusted as needed. *Maximum:* 1 g daily.

ORAL CONCENTRATE, SYRUP, TABLETS

Adults. 10 mg three times daily or four times daily, or 25 mg twice daily or three times daily. After 1 or 2 days, dose increased by 20 to 50 mg semiweekly until patient is calm. After 2 wk of calmness, dosage gradually reduced to maintenance level of 200 to 800 mg daily in equally divided doses.

➤ *To control acutely disturbed or manic hospitalized patients*

I.M. INJECTION

Adults. 25 mg. Repeated 25 to 50 mg in 1 hr, if needed. Increased gradually over several days up to 400 mg every 4 to 6 hr for severe cases until behavior is controlled. Then, regimen switched to oral form and outpatient dosage.

➤ *To treat severe behavioral problems in children*

ORAL CONCENTRATE, SYRUP, TABLETS

Children ages 6 months to 12 years. 0.5 mg/kg every 4 to 6 hr, as needed.

SUPPOSITORIES

Children ages 6 months to 12 years. 1 mg/kg every 6 to 8 hr, as needed.

I.M. INJECTION

Children ages 6 months to 12 years. 0.5 to 1 mg/kg every 6 to 8 hr. *Maximum:* 75 mg daily for children ages 5 to 12 years or weighing 50 to 100 lb (23 to 45 kg), except in unmanageable cases; 40 mg daily for children up to age 5 or weighing up to 50 lb.

➤ *To treat nausea and vomiting*

ORAL CONCENTRATE, SYRUP, TABLETS

Adults and adolescents. 10 to 25 mg every 4 to 6 hr, as needed.
Children ages 6 months to 12 years. 0.5 mg/kg every 4 to 6 hr, as needed.

I.M. INJECTION

Adults. 25 mg. If no hypotension occurs, 25 to 50 mg every 3 to 4 hr, as needed, until vomiting stops; then drug switched to oral form.
Children age 6 months and over. 0.5 to 1 mg/kg every 6 to 8 hr, as needed.

Maximum: 75 mg daily for children ages 5 to 12 or weighing 50 to 100 lb; 40 mg daily for children up to age 5 or weighing up to 50 lb.

SUPPOSITORIES

Adults and adolescents. 50 to 100 mg every 6 to 8 hr, as needed.

Children ages 6 months to 12 years. 1 mg/kg every 6 to 8 hr, as needed.

➤ *To provide intraoperative control of nausea and vomiting*

I.V. INJECTION

Adults. 25 mg diluted to 1 mg/ml with sodium chloride for injection and given at no more than 2 mg every 2 min. *Maximum:* 25 mg.

Children age 6 months and over. 0.275 mg/kg diluted to at least 1 mg/ml with sodium chloride for injection and given at no more than 1 mg every 2 min. *Maximum:* 75 mg/day for children ages 5 to 12 or weighing 50 to 100 lb; 40 mg daily for children up to age 5 years or weighing up to 50 lb.

I.M. INJECTION

Adults. 12.5 mg. Repeated in 30 min if needed and no hypotension occurs.

Children age 6 months and over. 0.275 mg/kg. Repeated in 30 min if needed and tolerated.

➤ *To treat intractable hiccups*

TABLETS

Adults. 25 to 50 mg three times daily or four times daily. If hiccups last longer than 2 days, route switched to I.M., as prescribed.

I.V. INFUSION

Adults. 25 to 50 mg diluted in 500 to 1,000 ml of normal saline solution and given at 1 mg/min with patient supine.

I.M. INJECTION

Adults. 25 to 50 mg given only if oral route is ineffective. If symptoms persist, route switched to I.V., as prescribed.

➤ *To provide preoperative relaxation*

ORAL CONCENTRATE, SYRUP, TABLETS

Adults and adolescents. 25 to 50 mg 2 to 3 hr before surgery.

Children ages 6 months to 12 years. 0.5 mg/kg 2 to 3 hr before surgery.

I.M. INJECTION

Adults. 12.5 to 25 mg 1 to 2 hr before surgery.

Children age 6 months and over. 0.5 mg/kg 1 to 2 hr before surgery.

➤ *To treat acute intermittent porphyria*

ORAL CONCENTRATE, SYRUP, TABLETS

Adults and adolescents. 25 to 50 mg three times daily or four times daily.

I.M. INJECTION

Adults. 25 mg three times daily or four times daily until oral route is possible.

➤ *To treat tetanus (usually as adjunct with barbiturates)*

I.V. INFUSION

Adults. 25 to 50 mg diluted to at least 1 mg/ml and given at no more than 1 mg/min.

Children age 6 months and over. 0.5 mg/kg every 6 to 8 hr, diluted to at least 1 mg/ml and given at no more than 1 mg/2 min. *Maximum:* 75 mg daily for children ages 5 to 12 years or weighing 50 to 100 lb; 40 mg daily for children up to age 5 years or weighing up to 50 lb.

I.M. INJECTION

Adults. 25 to 50 mg three times daily or four times daily.

Children age 6 months and over. 0.5 mg/kg every 6 to 8 hr. *Maximum:* 75 mg daily for children ages 5 to 12 or weighing 50 to 100 lb; 40 mg daily for children up to age 5 years or weighing up to 50 lb.

DOSAGE ADJUSTMENT Dosage possibly reduced for patients with hepatic dysfunction. Dosage reduced to one-third to one-half the normal adult dosage for elderly or debilitated patients.

Mechanism of Action

Depresses brain areas that control activity and aggression, including the cerebral cortex, hypothalamus, and limbic system, by an unknown mechanism. Prevents nausea and vomiting by inhibiting or blocking dopamine receptors in the medullary chemoreceptor trigger zone and peripherally by blocking the vagus nerve in the GI tract. May relieve anxiety by indirect reduction in arousal and increased filtering of internal stimuli to the reticular activating system in the brain stem.

Incompatibilities

Don't mix chlorpromazine with atropine, thiopental, or solutions that don't have a pH of 4 to 5 because a precipitate will form. Don't mix chlorpromazine injection with other drugs in a syringe.

Contraindications

Comatose states; hypersensitivity to chlorpromazine, phenothiazines, or their components; use of large amounts of CNS depressants

Interactions

DRUGS

amphetamines: Decreased amphetamine effectiveness, decreased antipsychotic effectiveness of chlorpromazine
antacids (aluminum hydroxide or magnesium trisilicate gel): Decreased chlorpromazine absorption and effectiveness
barbiturates: Decreased plasma level and, possibly, effectiveness of chlorpromazine
CNS depressants: Prolonged and intensified CNS depression
metrizamide: Possibly lowered seizure threshold
oral anticoagulants: Decreased anti-coagulation
phenytoin: Interference with phenytoin metabolism, increased risk of phenytoin toxicity
propranolol: Increased plasma levels of both drugs
thiazide diuretics: Possibly increased orthostatic hypotension

ACTIVITIES

alcohol use: Prolonged and intensified CNS depression

Adverse Reactions

CNS: Drowsiness, extrapyramidal reactions (such as dystonia, fever, motor restlessness, pseudoparkinsonism, and tardive dyskinesia), **neuroleptic malignant syndrome, seizures**
CV: ECG changes, such as nonspecific, usually reversible Q- and T-wave changes; orthostatic hypotension; tachycardia
EENT: Blurred vision, dry mouth, nasal congestion, ocular changes (fine particle deposits in lens and cornea) with long-term therapy
ENDO: Gynecomastia, hyperglycemia, **hypoglycemia**, lactation, moderate breast engorgement
GI: Constipation, ileus, nausea
GU: Amenorrhea, ejaculation disorders, impotence, priapism, urine retention
HEME: Agranulocytosis, aplastic anemia, eosinophilia, **hemolytic anemia, leukopenia, pancytopenia, thrombocytopenic purpura**
SKIN: Exfoliative dermatitis, photosensitivity, tissue necrosis, urticaria

Nursing Considerations

- Don't open or crush E.R. capsules.
- Know that chlorpromazine shouldn't be used to treat dementia-related psychosis in the elderly because of an increased risk of death.
- Use chlorpromazine cautiously in patients (especially children) with chronic respiratory disorders (such as severe asthma or emphysema) or acute respiratory tract infections because drug has CNS depressant effect. Also use cautiously in patients with cardiovascular, hepatic, or renal disease because of increased risk of developing arrhythmias, heart failure, and hypotension.
- Know that because of chlorpromazine's anticholinergic effects, use it cautiously in patients with glaucoma. Also use it cautiously in those who are exposed to extreme heat or organophosphate insecticides and those receiving atropine or related drugs.
- Protect concentrate from light. Refrigeration isn't required.
- Dilute concentrate in at least 60 ml of diluent just before administering it. Use a carbonated beverage, coffee, milk, orange syrup, pudding and soup, semisolid food, simple syrup, tea, tomato or fruit juice, or water.
- Protect parenteral solution from light. Solution should be clear and colorless to pale yellow. Discard markedly discolored solution.
- Don't inject drug by subcutaneous route because it can cause severe tissue necrosis.
- Wear gloves when working with liquid or injectable form because parenteral solution may cause contact dermatitis.
- For I.V. injection, dilute chlorpromazine with sodium chloride to a concentration of 1 mg/ml.
- Give I.M. injection slowly and deep into upper outer quadrant of buttocks, such as in the gluteus maximus. To minimize hypotensive effects, keep patient lying flat and monitor blood pressure for 30 minutes after injection.

WARNING Stay alert for possible suppressed cough reflex, which increases the risk of the patient's aspirating vomitus.
- Monitor patient for increased sensitivity to drug's CNS effects if patient has a history of hepatic encephalopathy from cirrhosis.

WARNING Notify prescriber immediately if neuroleptic malignant syndrome (altered mental status, autonomic instability hyperpyrexia, muscle rigidity) develops, and expect to stop drug and start intensive treatment. Watch for recurrence if patient resumes antipsychotic therapy.

PATIENT TEACHING
- Instruct patient to swallow E.R. capsules whole and not to crush, break, or chew them.
- Tell patient not to take drug within 2 hours of an antacid. Allow him to take drug with food or a full glass of milk or water.
- Tell patient using suppository form to chill the suppository, moisten it with cold water, and insert it well into rectum.
- Tell patient to store oral concentrate at room temperature, away from light, to measure it with the dropper provided, and to dilute it in 4 ounces of fluid just before use.
- Know that because of possible blurred vision, dizziness, and drowsiness (especially during the first few days of therapy), advise patient to avoid hazardous activities until drug's CNS effects are known.
- Tell patient to avoid alcohol because of possible additive effects and hypotension.
- Advise patient, especially if elderly, to rise slowly from a supine or seated position to avoid dizziness, fainting, and light-headedness.
- Tell patient to inform doctors and dentists that he's taking chlorpromazine before he has dental work, medical tests, or surgery.
- Explain that drug may reduce the body's response to cold and heat; tell patient to avoid temperature extremes, as in a hot tub, sauna, or very cold or hot shower. Remind patient to dress warmly in cold weather.
- Warn patient not to take OTC drugs for an allergy or a cold because they can increase the risk of heatstroke and other unwanted effects.
- Inform patient that drug increases sensitivity to sunlight; tell him to stay out of the sun as much as possible and to protect his skin.
- Suggest fluids, hard candy, or sugarless gum for patient who is experiencing a dry mouth.
- Urge patient to report sudden sore throat or other signs of infection.
- Advise female patient of childbearing age to notify prescriber if she intends to become or suspects that she is pregnant during therapy.

chlorthalidone

Hygroton, Thalitone, Uridon (CAN)

Class and Category

Pharmacologic class: Thiazide-like diuretic
Therapeutic class: Antihypertensive, diuretic
Pregnancy category: B

Indications and Dosages

➤ *As adjunct to reduce edema caused by heart failure, corticosteroid or estrogen therapy, hepatic cirrhosis, or renal dysfunction*

TABLETS

Adults. *Initial:* 50 to 100 mg (Thalitone, 30 to 60 mg) daily, 100 mg (Thalitone, 60 mg) every other day, or 150 to 200 mg (Thalitone, 90 to 120 mg) daily or every other day. *Maintenance:* Individualized; may be lower than initial dosage.

➤ *To treat hypertension*

TABLETS

Adults. *Initial:* 12.5 to 25 mg daily (Thalitone, 15 mg daily). If response is insufficient, dosage increased to 50 mg daily (Thalitone, 30 to 50 mg daily). If additional control is required, dosage increased to 100 mg daily (except Thalitone) or a second antihypertensive added. *Maintenance:* Individualized; may be lower than initial dosage.

Route	Onset	Peak	Duration
P.O.	2–3 hr	2–6 hr	24–72 hr

Mechanism of Action

May promote chloride, sodium, and water excretion by inhibiting sodium reabsorption in the distal tubules of the kidneys. Initially, chlorthalidone may decrease cardiac output, extracellular fluid volume, and plasma volume, which helps explain how it reduces blood pressure. It may also dilate arteries directly, which helps reduce peripheral vascular resistance and blood pressure. After several weeks, cardiac output, extracellular fluid, and plasma volume return to normal, but peripheral vascular resistance remains decreased.

Contraindications

Anuria; hypersensitivity to chlorthalidone, other sulfonamides, or their components

Interactions

DRUGS

antihypertensives: Potentiated action of antihypertensives and chlorthalidone
insulin, oral hypoglycemics: Possibly altered blood glucose control
lithium: Decreased renal lithium clearance and increased risk of lithium toxicity
loop diuretics: Increased synergistic effects, resulting in profound diuresis and serious electrolyte imbalances
tubocurine: Increased response to tubocurine

Adverse Reactions

CNS: Dizziness, headache, insomnia, lightheadedness, paresthesia, restlessness, vertigo, weakness
CV: Orthostatic hypotension, vasculitis
EENT: Yellow vision
ENDO: Hyperglycemia
GI: Abdominal cramps or pain, anorexia, bloating, constipation, diarrhea, gastric irritation, nausea, **pancreatitis**, vomiting
GU: Decreased libido, impotence
HEME: Agranulocytosis, aplastic anemia, hypoplastic anemia, leukopenia, thrombocytopenia
MS: Gout attacks, muscle spasms
SKIN: Cutaneous vasculitis, **exfoliative dermatitis**, necrotizing vasculitis, photosensitivity, purpura, rash, urticaria
Other: Hyperuricemia

Nursing Considerations

- Use chlorthalidone cautiously in patients with impaired hepatic function or progressive hepatic disease because minor changes in fluid and electrolyte balance may cause hepatic coma.
- Assess blood glucose levels, BUN, serum electrolyte, and uric acid levels before therapy and periodically throughout therapy. Monitor patient for signs of fluid and electrolyte imbalance.

WARNING Monitor renal function periodically to detect cumulative drug effects, which may cause azotemia in patients with impaired renal function.

PATIENT TEACHING

- Stress the importance of taking chlorthalidone even when feeling well.
- Tell patient to store drug at room temperature in tightly closed container.
- Tell patient to take drug in the morning with food or milk.
- Instruct patient to rise slowly from a seated or lying position to minimize effects of orthostatic hypotension.
- Advise patient to check blood pressure regularly.
- Instruct patient to report signs of low potassium level, such as fatigue and muscle weakness.
- Advise patient to protect his skin from the sun.
- Urge patient to immediately report sudden joint pain to prescriber because drug can cause sudden gout attacks.
- Instruct patient to take a missed dose as soon as he remembers it. If he misses one day in an every-other-day schedule, tell him to take the dose on the off day and then resume usual dosing schedule. Warn against taking double or extra doses.

chlorzoxazone

Lorzone, Parafon Forte DSC

Class and Category

Pharmacologic class: Benzoxazole derivative
Therapeutic class: Skeletal muscle relaxant
Pregnancy category: Not classified

Indications and Dosages

➤ *As adjunct to relieve acute musculoskeletal pain and stiffness*

TABLETS

Adults. 250 to 750 mg three times daily or four times daily, usually 500 mg three times daily or four times daily, increased or decreased according to response.

Route	Onset	Peak	Duration
P.O.	In 1 hr	Unknown	3–4 hr

Mechanism of Action

Reduces muscle spasm by inhibiting multisynaptic reflex arcs at the level of the spinal cord and subcortical areas of the brain that are active in producing and maintaining skeletal muscle spasm.

Contraindications

Hypersensitivity to chlorzoxazone or any of its components

Interactions

DRUGS

CNS depressants: Additive CNS depression

ACTIVITIES

alcohol use: Additive CNS depression

Adverse Reactions

CNS: Dizziness, drowsiness, headache, light-headedness, malaise, paradoxical stimulation
GI: Abdominal cramps or pain, constipation, diarrhea, **GI bleeding**, heartburn, **hepatotoxicity**, nausea, vomiting
GU: Urine discoloration
HEME: **Agranulocytosis**, anemia
SKIN: Allergic dermatitis, ecchymosis, petechiae
Other: **Anaphylaxis, angioedema**

Nursing Considerations

- Crush chlorzoxazone tablets and mix with food or liquid for easier swallowing, if needed.
- Assess patients, especially those who have a history of allergies, for evidence of hypersensitivity, such as hives, itching, and rash.

WARNING Monitor patient for signs of hepatotoxicity, including darkened urine, fever, jaundice, and rash. Notify prescriber immediately and expect to discontinue drug if any of these signs or symptoms occur. Monitor patient for abnormal liver function test results, such as elevated ALT, AST, alkaline phosphatase, and bilirubin levels, and expect to discontinue drug, as ordered, if any of these occurs.

- Ensure adequate rest, and provide other pain-relief measures as needed.
- Institute safety measures to prevent falls or injury until drug's full CNS effects are known.

PATIENT TEACHING

- Advise patient to take a missed dose of chlorzoxazone as soon as possible unless it's almost time for the next dose.
- Advise patient to avoid hazardous activities until drug's CNS effects are known.
- Instruct patient to avoid alcohol and other CNS depressants during therapy.
- Inform patient that, in rare instances, urine may turn orange or reddish purple during therapy.
- Advise patient to store drug in a tightly capped container at room temperature.

cholestyramine

Locholest, Locholest Light, Prevalite, Questran, Questran Light

Class and Category

Pharmacologic class: Bile acid sequestrant
Therapeutic class: Antihyperlipidemic, antipruritic (cholestasis)
Pregnancy category: Not rated

Indications and Dosages

➤ *As adjunct to reduce serum cholesterol level in patients with primary hypercholesterolemia, to reduce LDL cholesterol in patients who also have hypertriglyceridemia when hypertriglyceridemia is not the abnormality of most concern, to relieve pruritus associated with partial biliary obstruction*

ORAL SUSPENSION

Adults. *Initial:* 4 g once or twice daily before meals. *Maintenance:* 8 to 24 g equally divided and given 2 to 6 times a day. *Maximum:* 24 g daily when used as antihyperlipidemic and 16 g daily when used as antipruritic.

Route	Onset	Peak	Duration
P.O.	In 1–2 wk*	Unknown	2–4 wk†

* For hypercholesterolemia; in 1 to 3 wk for pruritus.

† For hypercholesterolemia; 1 to 2 wk for pruritus.

Mechanism of Action

Increases bile acid excretion in feces. The resulting decreased bile acid level increases the activity of the enzyme that regulates cholesterol synthesis in the liver. As a result, the liver increases its cholesterol synthesis to produce more bile acids. However, the liver's synthesis of cholesterol typically can't match the amount needed to synthesize bile acids, which reduces the cholesterol level. Also, a decreased cholesterol level causes liver cells to increase their uptake of LDLs, which further reduces the cholesterol level. Cholestyramine may relieve pruritus by decreasing the body's bile acid level. This reduces the amount of excess bile acids that are deposited in the dermis and that typically cause pruritus in patients with cholestasis.

Contraindications

Complete biliary obstruction (when bile isn't excreted into intestine), hypersensitivity to cholestyramine or its components

Interactions

DRUGS

oral drugs such as chenodiol, digitalis glycosides, estrogens, fat-soluble vitamins, folic acid, gemfibrozil, penicillin G (oral), phenobarbital (oral), phenylbutazone, progestins, propranolol (oral), tetracyclines (oral), thiazide diuretics (oral), thyroid hormones, ursodiol, vancomycin (oral), warfarin: Decreased absorption and effects of these drugs

Adverse Reactions

CNS: Dizziness, headache

GI: Bloating, constipation, diarrhea, epigastric pain, eructation, fecal impaction, flatulence, indigestion, nausea, vomiting

Nursing Considerations

- Store cholestyramine at room temperature.
- Don't give dry powder because it may cause esophageal distress; mix it in a beverage.

WARNING Be aware that long-term use may increase bleeding tendency from hyperprothrombinemia caused by vitamin K deficiency. If this occurs, patient will require treatment with vitamin K_1.

- Monitor for deficiencies of fat-soluble vitamins, such as A and D. If long-term therapy prevents absorption of these vitamins, expect to provide supplementation.

PATIENT TEACHING

- Urge patient to follow a low-cholesterol, low-fat diet and regular exercise program.
- Tell patient to take drug before meals.
- Instruct patient to mix dry powder as follows: Place amount of powder needed for dose in any beverage and stir vigorously. Then, vigorously stir in another 2 to 4 ounces of beverage. After drinking mixture, rinse glass with more liquid, and swallow it to make sure full dose is taken. Patient also may mix drug in thin soups or moist, pulpy fruits, such as applesauce or crushed pineapple.
- Tell patient to drink plenty of fluids and increase bulk in his diet to minimize constipation; remind him to notify prescriber if constipation, nausea, or other adverse GI reactions develop.
- Explain that serum cholesterol level will need to be measured often for first few months of therapy and periodically thereafter.
- Advise patient to take other drugs at least 1 hour before or 4 to 6 hours after cholestyramine to avoid interference with their absorption.
- Tell patient to take a missed dose as soon as he remembers but not to take double or extra doses.

ciclesonide

Alvesco, Omnaris, Zetonna

Class and Category

Pharmacologic class: Corticosteroid
Therapeutic class: Antiasthmatic, anti-inflammatory
Pregnancy category: C

Indications and Dosages

➤ *To prevent asthma attacks as part of maintenance therapy*

INHALATION AEROSOL (ALVESCO)

Adults and children age 12 and over using bronchodilator therapy. *Initial:* 80 mcg twice daily. *Maximum:* 160 mcg twice daily.

Adults and children age 12 and over switching from another inhaled corticosteroid. *Initial:* 80 mcg twice daily, adjusted to lowest effective dose when stabilized. *Maximum:* 320 mg twice daily.
Adults and children age 12 and over using oral corticosteroid therapy. *Initial and maximum:* 320 mcg twice daily, adjusted to lowest effective dose when stabilized.

➤ *To treat nasal congestion in seasonal allergic rhinitis*

NASAL AEROSOL (OMNARIS)
Adults and children age 6 and over. 200 mcg daily as 2 sprays in each nostril.
NASAL AEROSOL (ZETONNA)
Adults and children age 12 and over. 74 mcg daily as 1 spray in each nostril.

➤ *To treat nasal congestion in perennial allergic rhinitis*

NASAL AEROSOL (OMNARIS)
Adults and children age 12 and over. 200 mcg daily as 2 sprays in each nostril.
NASAL AEROSOL (ZETONNA)
Adults and children age 12 and over. 74 mcg daily as 1 spray (37 mcg) in each nostril.

Route	Onset	Peak	Duration
Inhalation	Unknown	4 wk or longer	Several days
Nasal aerosol	Unknown	Unknown	Unknown

Mechanism of Action
Inhibits cells involved in the asthma inflammatory response, such as basophils, eosinophils, lymphocytes, macrophages, mast cells, and neutrophils. Ciclesonide also inhibits production or secretion of chemical mediators, such as cytokines, eicosanoids, histamine, and leukotrienes.

Contraindications
Hypersensitivity to ciclesonide or its components, primary treatment of status asthmaticus or other acute asthma episodes that require intensive measures

Interactions
DRUGS
ketoconazole: Increased exposure time of ciclesonide

Adverse Reactions
CNS: Dizziness, fatigue, headache
EENT: Cataracts, conjunctivitis, dry mouth or throat, dysphonia, epistaxis, glaucoma, hoarseness, nasal congestion or ulceration, nasal septal perforation, nasopharyngitis, oral candidiasis, pharyngolaryngeal pain, sinusitis
ENDO: Adrenal insufficiency, cushingoid symptoms, decreased bone mineral density, hyperglycemia, slower growth in children
GI: Nausea
MS: Arthralgia, back or limb pain, musculoskeletal chest pain
RESP: Bronchospasm, cough, pneumonia, upper respiratory tract infection
SKIN: Urticaria
Other: Angioedema, flu-like symptoms, infections

Nursing Considerations
- Know that ciclesonide should not be used in patients with recent nasal septal ulcers, nasal surgery, or nasal trauma until healing has occurred.
- Use cautiously in patients with tuberculosis; bacterial, fungal, parasitic, or viral infection; ocular herpes simplex; or chickenpox or measles because these conditions may worsen with ciclesonide therapy.
- Also use cautiously in patients with a history of cataracts, glaucoma, or increased intraocular pressure because ciclesonide may increase intraocular pressure or cause cataract formation; and in patients with major risk factors for decreased bone mineral content, such as family history of osteoporosis, prolonged immobilization, or long-term use of drugs that can reduce bone mass, such as anticonvulsants and oral corticosteroids.
- Inspect patient's oral cavity if using inhaler form, or nasal cavity if using nasal spray regularly for abnormalities. Have patient rinse mouth following inhalation of ciclesonide to reduce risk of oral candidiasis. If nasal or oral candidiasis occurs, expect to continue ciclesonide therapy, unless severe. If nasal erosion, ulceration, or perforation occurs, notify prescriber and expect nasal spray to be discontinued.

- Be aware that if patient takes a systemic corticosteroid, expect to taper dosage by no more than 2.5 mg/day at weekly intervals, starting 1 week after ciclesonide therapy begins.

WARNING Know that if patient is switched from systemic corticosteroid to ciclesonide, assess for adrenal insufficiency (fatigue, hypotension, lassitude, nausea, vomiting, weakness) early in therapy and whenever patient has infection, stress, surgery, or trauma, or other steroid-depleting conditions or procedures. Notify prescriber immediately if signs or symptoms develop.

- Administer a fast-acting inhaled bronchodilator, as prescribed, if an acute asthma attack occurs. Ciclesonide inhalation is not a bronchodilator and its action takes longer than needed to abort acute asthma symptoms. If bronchospasm occurs immediately after ciclesonide use, expect to stop drug and start another drug regimen.
- Monitor growth in children because ciclesonide may suppress growth.

PATIENT TEACHING

- Urge patient to use ciclesonide regularly, as prescribed, but not for acute bronchospasm. Also tell her never to increase or decrease the dosage without consulting prescriber.
- Tell patient to use inhalation form only with the actuator supplied with the product. Explain that when the dose indicator shows a red zone in the window, about 20 inhalations are left, indicating a need for a refill. When the indicator shows zero, she should discard the inhaler. Advise against relying solely on the dose indicator, especially if inhaler has been dropped, but to keep track of number of inhalations used.
- Instruct patient to use inhaler form according to package instructions. Emphasize need to make sure canister is firmly seated in the plastic mouthpiece adapter before each use and to press inhaler slowly but firmly until it can go no further in the adapter for each spray. Inform patient that she doesn't need to shake inhaler before use.
- Advise her on first use, to spray three times into the air (away from her eyes), looking for a fine mist. If inhaler or spray hasn't been used for more than 4 days (Omnaris) or 10 days (Alvesco, Zetonna), it should be primed again.
- Advise patient using nasal spray form to avoid spraying the drug directly onto the nasal septum.
- Instruct patient to gargle and rinse her mouth after each dose of inhaler to help prevent dry mouth and throat, relieve throat irritation, and prevent oral yeast infection.
- Tell patient to always replace cap on inhaler after use, to keep mouthpiece clean, and to clean mouthpiece once a week with a clean, dry tissue or cloth.
- Explain that the full effect of drug may not occur for 4 weeks or more.
- Stress importance of notifying prescriber if symptoms continue or worsen.
- Instruct patient to notify prescriber immediately if asthma attacks don't respond to bronchodilators during ciclesonide inhaler use.
- Make patient aware that if she is switching from an oral corticosteroid to inhaled ciclesonide, she should carry medical identification indicating the need for supplemental systemic corticosteroids during a severe asthma attack or stress.
- Caution patient to avoid contact with people who have infections because drug suppresses the immune system, increasing the risk of infection. Instruct patient to notify prescriber about exposure to chickenpox, measles, or other infections because additional treatment may be needed.

cilostazol

Pletal

Class and Category

Pharmacologic class: Phosphodiesterase 3 (PDE 3) inhibitor
Therapeutic class: Antiplatelet
Pregnancy category: C

Indications and Dosages

➤ *To reduce symptoms of intermittent claudication*

TABLETS

Adults. 100 mg twice daily taken at least 30 min before or 2 hr after breakfast and dinner.

DOSAGE ADJUSTMENT For patient taking a moderate or strong CYP3A4 inhibitor (diltiazem, erythromycin, itraconazole, ketoconazole) or taking a CYP2C19 inhibitor (fluconazole, omeprazole, ticlopidine), dosage reduced to 50 mg twice daily.

Mechanism of Action

May inhibit phosphodiesterase, decreasing phosphodiesterase activity and suppressing cyclic adenosine monophosphate (cAMP) degradation. This action increases cAMP in platelets and blood vessels, which inhibits platelet aggregation and causes vasodilation. This in turn relieves symptoms of claudication.

Contraindications

Heart failure, hypersensitivity to cilostazol or its components

Interactions

DRUGS

CYP2C19 inhibitors (e.g., fluconazole, omeprazole, ticlopidine) or CYP3A4 inhibitors (e.g., diltiazem, erythromycin, omeprazole, ticlopidine): Increased plasma cilostazol level

FOODS

grapefruit: Increased risk of adverse reactions

high-fat foods: Faster cilostazol absorption and increased risk of adverse reactions

ACTIVITIES

smoking: Decreased cilostazol effects by about 20%

Adverse Reactions

CNS: Cerebral hemorrhage, dizziness, headache, paresthesia

CV: Angina, chest pain, hypertension, **hypotension**, **left ventricular outflow tract obstruction** (patients with sigmoid-shaped interventricular septum), palpitations, peripheral edema, **prolonged OT interval**, **supraventricular or ventricular tachycardia**, **thrombosis**, **torsades de pointes**

EENT: Pharyngitis, rhinitis

ENDO: Diabetes mellitus, hot flashes, hyperglycemia

GI: Abdominal pain, abnormal stool, diarrhea, elevated liver enzymes, flatulence, **GI hemorrhage**, **hepatic dysfunction**, indigestion, jaundice, vomiting

GU: Elevated BUN level, hematuria

HEME: Agranulocytosis, **aplastic anemia**, **bleeding tendency**, **decreased platelet count**, **granulocytopenia**, **leukopenia**, **pancytopenia**, **thrombocytopenia**

MS: Back pain, myalgia

RESP: Cough, **interstitial pneumonia**, **pulmonary hemorrhage**

SKIN: Eruptions, pruritus, rash, **Stevens–Johnson syndrome**

Other: Infection, increased blood uric acid level

Nursing Considerations

- Monitor patient's vital signs and cardiovascular status closely because cilostazol may cause cardiovascular lesions, which could lead to problems, such as endocardial hemorrhage.
- Be aware that left ventricular outflow tract obstruction has been reported in patients with sigmoid-shaped interventricular septum. Monitor patients for development of new cardiac symptoms, including a systolic murmur, after starting cilostazol.
- Monitor blood glucose level to detect hyperglycemia. Also assess for signs of type 2 diabetes mellitus, such as fatigue, polydipsia, polyphagia, and polyuria.

PATIENT TEACHING

- Instruct patient to take cilostazol on an empty stomach because high-fat foods can increase the risk of adverse reactions.
- Warn patent to avoid grapefruit juice during therapy because it can increase the risk of adverse reactions.
- Urge patient not to smoke because it decreases drug's effects.
- Explain that assessment of drug effectiveness is based on ability to walk increased distances. Stress that drug effects won't appear until 2 to 4 weeks after therapy starts and that full effects may take up to 12 weeks.

cimetidine

Tagamet, Tagamet HB

cimetidine hydrochloride

Class and Category

Pharmacologic class: Histamine H_2 antagonist
Therapeutic class: Antiulcer agent
Pregnancy category: B

Indications and Dosages

➤ *To treat and prevent recurrence of duodenal ulcer*

ORAL SOLUTION, TABLETS

Adults and adolescents age 16 and over. *Initial:* 800 mg (or 1,600 mg if ulcer is greater than 1.0 cm and patient is heavy smoker) at bedtime, 300 mg four times daily with meals and at bedtime, or 400 to 600 mg in morning and at bedtime for 4 to 6 wk. *Maintenance:* 400 mg at bedtime.

I.V. OR I.M. INJECTION

Adults. *Initial:* 300 mg every 6 to 8 hr. I.V. given slowly over 5 min.

I.V. INFUSION

Adults. 37.5 mg/hr if continuous or infused over 15 to 20 min if given intermittently. *Maximum:* 100 mg/hr (2,400 mg daily).

➤ *To treat active, benign gastric ulcer*

ORAL SOLUTION, TABLETS

Adults and adolescents age 16 and over. 800 mg at bedtime or 300 mg four times daily with meals and at bedtime for up to 8 wk.

I.V. OR I.M. INJECTION

Adults and adolescents age 16 and over. 300 mg every 6 to 8 hr. I.V. given slowly over at least 5 min.

I.V. INFUSION

Adults and adolescents age 16 and over. *Initial:* 37.5 mg/hr if given continuously or infused over 15 to 20 min if given intermittently, increased as needed. *Maximum:* 2,400 mg daily.

➤ *To manage erosive gastroesophageal reflux disease*

ORAL SOLUTION, TABLETS

Adults. 1,600 mg daily in divided doses (800 mg twice daily or 400 mg four times daily) for up to 12 wk.
Children. 40 to 80 mg/kg daily in divided doses four times daily.

➤ *To treat pathological hypersecretory conditions, such as Zollinger–Ellison syndrome*

ORAL SOLUTION, TABLETS

Adults and adolescents age 16 and over. 300 mg four times daily with meals and at bedtime. Given more often, if needed. *Maximum:* 2,400 mg daily.

I.V. OR I.M. INJECTION

Adults and adolescents age 16 and over. 300 mg every 6 to 8 hr. I.V. given slowly over at least 5 min.

I.V. INFUSION

Adults. *Initial:* 37.5 mg/hr if given continuously or infused over 15 to 20 min if given inermittently, increased as needed. *Maximum:* 2,400 mg daily.

➤ *To treat heartburn and acid indigestion*

ORAL SOLUTION, TABLETS

Adults and children age 12 and over. *Initial:* 200 mg with water at onset of symptoms or up to 30 minutes before eating. *Maximum:* 400 mg every 24 hr for no more than 2 wk unless prescribed.

➤ *To prevent stress-related upper GI bleeding during hospitalization*

I.V. INFUSION

Adults. 50 mg/hr by continuous infusion for 7 days.

DOSAGE ADJUSTMENT For patient with severe renal impairment, dosage reduced to 300 mg and frequency lengthened to every 12 hr (and increased to every 8 hr with caution, if needed). For patient with a creatinine clearance less than 30 ml/min and being treated to prevent stress-related upper GI bleeding during hospitalization, dosage reduced by 50%.

Route	Onset	Peak	Duration
P.O.	Unknown	1–2 hr	4–5 hr
I.V., I.M.	Unknown	Unknown	4–5 hr

Mechanism of Action

Blocks histamine's action at H_2-receptor sites on stomach's parietal cells. This action reduces gastric fluid volume and acidity. Cimetidine also decreases the amount of gastric acid secreted in response to betazole, caffeine, food, insulin, or pentagastrin.

Incompatibilities

Don't mix cimetidine with aminophylline or barbiturates in I.V. solution. Don't mix drug with pentobarbital sodium in the same syringe.

Contraindications

Hypersensitivity to cimetidine or its components

Interactions

DRUGS

antacids, metoclopramide: Decreased cimetidine absorption
chlordiazepoxide, diazepam, lidocaine, metronidazole, nifedipine, phenytoin, propranolol, quinidine, theophylline, tricyclic antidepressants, warfarin: Reduced metabolism and increased blood levels and effects of these drugs, possibly toxicity from these drugs
drugs with narrow therapeutic range, such as digoxin, lidocaine, phenytoin, theophylline, warfarin: Increased risk of altered blood levels of these drugs, requiring close monitoring and possible dosage adjustments, especially when cimetidine is begun or discontinued

FOODS

caffeine: Reduced metabolism and increased blood level and effects of caffeine

ACTIVITIES

alcohol use: Possibly increased blood alcohol level

Adverse Reactions

CNS: Confusion, dizziness, hallucinations, headache, peripheral neuropathy, somnolence
ENDO: Mild gynecomastia if used longer than 1 month
GI: Mild and transient diarrhea
GU: Impotence, transiently elevated serum creatinine level
SKIN: Rash
Other: Pain at I.M. injection site

Nursing Considerations

WARNING Be aware that rapid administration of cimetidine can increase risk of arrhythmias and hypotension.

- For I.V. injection, dilute cimetidine in normal saline solution to a total volume of 20 ml. Inject over 5 minutes or more.
- For intermittent I.V. infusion, dilute cimetidine in at least 50 ml of D_5W or other compatible I.V. solution. Infuse over 15 to 20 minutes.
- For I.M. injection, don't dilute cimetidine before administering it.
- Be alert for confusion in debilitated or elderly patients who receive cimetidine.

PATIENT TEACHING

- Tell patient to use a liquid-measuring device to ensure accurate dose of solution.
- Advise patient to avoid alcohol while taking cimetidine to prevent interactions.
- Instruct patient to avoid taking antacids within 1 hour of taking cimetidine.
- Warn patient that cigarette smoking increases gastric acid secretion and can worsen gastric disease.
- Caution patient not to take drug for more than 14 days, unless prescribed.

cinacalcet hydrochloride

Sensipar

Class and Category

Pharmacologic class: Calcimimetic
Therapeutic class: Calcium reducer
Pregnancy category: Not classified

Indications and Dosages

➤ *To treat secondary hyperparathyroidism in patients with chronic renal disease who are on dialysis*

TABLETS

Adults. *Initial:* 30 mg daily, increased by 30 mg every 2 to 4 wk daily, as needed. *Maximum:* 180 mg daily.

➤ *To treat hypercalcemia in patients with parathyroid carcinoma; to treat primary hyperparathyroidism in patients who are unable to undergo parathyroidectomy*

TABLETS

Adults. *Initial:* 30 mg twice daily, increased in 2 to 4 wk to 60 mg twice daily, then in 2 to 4 wk to 90 mg twice daily, and then in 2 to 4 wk to 90 mg three times daily or four times daily, as needed to normalize serum calcium level.

Route	Onset	Peak	Duration
P.O.	Unknown	2–6 hr	Unknown

Mechanism of Action

Increases sensitivity of calcium-sensing receptors on the surface of parathyroid cells to extracellular calcium. This sensitivity directly reduces parathyroid hormone (PTH) level, which in turn decreases serum calcium level.

Contraindications

Hypersensitivity to cinacalcet or its components, hypocalcemia

Interactions

DRUGS

CYP2D6 substrates, such as carvedilol, desipramine, metoprolol; drugs that have a narrow therapeutic index, such as flecainide, tricyclic antidepressants (most): Possibly increased blood level of these drugs

strong CYP3A4 inhibitors such as itraconazole, ketoconazole: Possibly increased blood cinacalcet level due to drug being partially metabolized

Adverse Reactions

CNS: Asthenia, dizziness, **seizures**

CV: Arrhythmias, hypertension, **hypotension** (in the presence of impaired cardiac function), **worsening heart failure** (in the presence of impaired cardiac function)

GI: Anorexia, diarrhea, **gastrointestinal bleeding**, nausea, vomiting

MS: Adynamic bone disease, myalgia

SKIN: Rash, urticaria

Other: Allergic reaction, **angioedema**, **hypocalcemia**, noncardiac chest pain

Nursing Considerations

- Be aware that cinacalcet is not recommended for use in patients with chronic kidney disease who are not on dialysis because of an increased risk of hypocalcemia.
- Use cinacalcet cautiously in patients with a history of seizures because reduced blood calcium level may lower seizure threshold. Also use cautiously in patients with hepatic insufficiency because cinacalcet metabolism may be reduced.

WARNING Monitor patient for hypocalcemia exhibited by cramping, myalgia, paresthesia, prolonged QT interval that may cause ventricular arrhythmias, seizures, and tetany. Also monitor patient's blood calcium and phosphorus levels within 1 week after starting therapy or adjusting dosage, and every month or two once maintenance dose is established, as ordered. If hypocalcemia develops, notify prescriber immediately because treatment to raise calcium level will be needed. Treatment may include giving supplemental calcium, starting or increasing dosage of calcium-based phosphate binder or vitamin D sterols, or temporarily withholding cinacalcet.

- Be aware that if patient starts or stops therapy with a strong CYP3A4 inhibitor, such as itraconazole, or ketoconazole, cinacalcet dosage may have to be adjusted.
- Monitor dialysis patient's intact PTH levels 1 to 4 weeks after therapy starts or dose is adjusted and then every 1 to 3 months thereafter, as ordered. Keep in mind that adynamic bone disease may develop if iPTH levels drop below 100 pg/ml. Expect to reduce dosage or discontinue cinacalcet, as ordered, in a patient whose intact PTH level falls below the target range of 150 to 300 pg/ml.
- Monitor patient for worsening of common gastrointestinal adverse reactions of nausea and vomiting associated with cinacalcet therapy and for signs and symptoms of GI bleeding and ulcerations. Risk factors include esophagitis, gastritis, severe vomiting, or ulcers. Notify prescriber if such symptoms present, and provide supportive care, as ordered.

PATIENT TEACHING

- Instruct patient to take cinacalcet with food or shortly after a meal.
- Caution patient to take tablet whole and not divide it or crush it.
- Review signs and symptoms of hypocalcemia with patient and urge him to notify prescriber of changes.
- Advise patient to report any symptoms of gastrointestinal bleeding, nausea, or vomiting to prescriber.
- Alert patient with heart failure that cinacalcet may worsen the heart failure.
- Inform patient that regular blood tests will be ordered to monitor the safe use of cinacalcet and the importance of actually having the tests done.

ciprofloxacin

Cipro, Cipro I.V., Cipro XR, Otiprio

Class and Category

Pharmacologic class: Fluoroquinolone derivative
Therapeutic class: Antibiotic
Pregnancy category: C

Indications and Dosages

➤ *To prevent inhalation anthrax after exposure or to treat inhalation anthrax*

ORAL SUSPENSION, TABLETS

Adults. 500 to 750 mg every 12 hr for 14 days.
Children. 15 mg/kg/dose (maximum 500 mg/dose) every 8 to 12 hr for 10 to 21 days.

ORAL SUSPENSION, TABLETS

Adults and adolescents. 500 mg infused over 60 min every 12 hr for 60 days.
Children. 15 mg/kg every 12 hr for 60 days. *Maximum:* 500 mg/dose.

I.V. INFUSION

Adults and adolescents. 400 mg infused over 60 min every 12 hr for 60 days.
Children. 10 mg/kg every 12 hr for 60 days. *Maximum:* 400 mg per dose.

➤ *To treat acute sinusitis caused by susceptible organisms*

ORAL SUSPENSION, TABLETS

Adults. 500 mg every 12 hr for 10 days.

I.V. INFUSION

Adults. For mild to moderate infections, 400 mg infused over 60 min every 12 hr for 10 days.

➤ *To treat bone and joint infections caused by susceptible organisms*

ORAL SUSPENSION, TABLETS

Adults. For mild to moderate infections, 500 mg every 12 hr for 4 to 8 wk. For severe or complicated infections, 750 mg every 12 hr for 4 to 8 wk.

I.V. INFUSION

Adults. For mild to moderate infections, 400 mg infused over 60 min every 12 hr for 4 to 8 wk. For severe or complicated infections, 400 mg infused over 60 min every 8 hr for 4 to 8 wk.

➤ *To treat skin and soft-tissue infections caused by susceptible organisms*

ORAL SUSPENSION, TABLETS

Adults. For mild to moderate infections, 500 mg every 12 hr for 7 to 14 days. For severe or complicated infections, 750 mg every 12 hr for 7 to 14 days.

I.V. INFUSION

Adults. For mild to moderate infections, 400 mg infused over 60 min every 12 hr for 7 to 14 days. For severe or complicated infections, 400 mg infused over 60 min every 8 hr for 7 to 14 days.

➤ *To treat chronic bacterial prostatitis caused by susceptible organisms*

ORAL SUSPENSION, TABLETS

Adults. 500 mg every 12 hr for 28 days.

I.V. INFUSION

Adults. 400 mg infused over 60 min every 12 hr for 28 days.

➤ *To treat infectious diarrhea caused by susceptible organisms*

ORAL SUSPENSION, TABLETS

Adults. 500 mg every 12 hr for 5 to 7 days.

➤ *To treat UTI caused by susceptible organisms*

ORAL SUSPENSION, TABLETS

Adults. For acute uncomplicated infections, 100 mg every 12 hr for 3 days. For mild to moderate infections, 250 mg every 12 hr for 7 to 14 days. For severe or complicated infections, 500 mg every 12 hr for 7 to 14 days.

I.V. INFUSION

Adults. For mild to moderate infections, 200 mg infused over 60 min every 12 hr for 7 to 14 days. For severe or complicated infections, 400 mg infused over 60 min every 12 hr for 7 to 14 days.

➤ *To treat plague, including pneumonic and septicemic plague, due to* Yersinia pestis

I.V. INFUSION

ORAL SUSPENSION, TABLETS

Adults. 400 mg infused over 60 min every 8 to 12 hr for 14 days.
Children. 10 mg/kg (maximum 400 mg/dose) infused over 60 min every 8 to 12 hr for 10 to 21 days.

➤ *To prevent plague postexposure*

ORAL SUSPENSION, TABLETS

Adults. 500 mg twice daily for 7 days.
Children. 15 mg/kg twice daily for 7 days. *Maximum:* 1 g daily.

E.R. TABLETS

Adults. 1,000 mg daily for 7 to 14 days.

➤ *To treat acute uncomplicated cystitis*

ORAL SUSPENSION, TABLETS

Adults. 250 mg every 12 hr for 3 days.

E.R. TABLETS

Adults. 500 mg daily for 3 days.

➤ *To treat lower respiratory tract infections caused by susceptible organisms*

ORAL SUSPENSION, TABLETS

Adults. For mild to moderate infections, 500 mg every 12 hr for 7 to 14 days. For severe or complicated infections, 750 mg every 12 hr for 7 to 14 days.

I.V. INFUSION

Adults. For mild to moderate infections, 400 mg infused over 60 min every 12 hr for 7 to 14 days. For severe or complicated infections, 400 mg infused over 60 min every 8 hr for 7 to 14 days.

➤ *To treat complicated intra-abdominal infections caused by susceptible organisms*

ORAL SUSPENSION, TABLETS

Adults. 500 mg every 12 hr for 7 to 14 days.

I.V. INFUSION

Adults. 400 mg infused over 60 min every 12 hr for 7 to 14 days.

➤ *To treat nosocomial pneumonia caused by susceptible organisms*

I.V. INFUSION

Adults. 400 mg infused over 60 min every 8 hr for 10 to 14 days.

➤ *To treat typhoid fever caused by susceptible organisms*

ORAL SUSPENSION, TABLETS

Adults. 500 mg every 12 hr for 10 days.

➤ *To treat uncomplicated urethral or cervical gonococcal infections caused by* N. gonorrhoeae

ORAL SUSPENSION, TABLETS

Adults. 250 mg as a single dose.

➤ *To provide empirical therapy in febrile neutropenic patients*

I.V. INFUSION

Adults. 400 mg infused over 60 min every 8 hr for 7 to 14 days.

➤ *To treat acute otitis externa caused by* Pseudomonas aeruginosa *or* Staphylococcus aureus

OTIC SUSPENSION

Children age 6 months and over. 0.2 ml (12 mg) as a single dose to the external ear canal of each affected ear.

DOSAGE ADJUSTMENT For patients taking oral suspension or tablets, dosage reduced to 250 to 500 mg every 12 hour if creatinine clearance is 30 to 50 ml/min; and to 250 to 500 mg every 18 hr if creatinine clearance is 5 to 29 ml/min. For patient on dialysis, dosage reduced to 250 mg to 500 mg every 24 hr and given after dialysis. For patient with a creatinine clearance of 30 ml/min or less taking E.R. tablets, dosage reduced to 500 mg daily and drug administered after dialysis, if patient is receiving dialysis. For patient receiving drug intravenously and who has a creatinine clearance between 5 to 29 ml/min, dosage reduced to 200 to 400 mg every 18 to 24 hr.

Mechanism of Action

Inhibits the enzyme DNA gyrase, which is responsible for the unwinding and supercoiling of bacterial DNA before it replicates. By inhibiting this enzyme, ciprofloxacin causes bacterial cells to die.

Incompatibilities

Don't administer parenteral ciprofloxacin with aminophylline, amoxicillin, cefepime, clindamycin, dexamethasone, floxacillin, furosemide, heparin, or phenytoin.

Contraindications

Concurrent therapy with tizanidine; hypersensitivity to ciprofloxacin, quinolones, or their components

Interactions

DRUGS

antacids, didanosine, iron supplements, multivitamins that contain iron or zinc sucralfate: Decreased ciprofloxacin absorption
caffeine, clozapine, methotrexate, methylxanthines, olanzapine, ropinirole, theophylline, tizanidine, zolpidem: Increased plasma levels of these drugs and increased risk of serious adverse reactions including toxicity
cyclosporine: Elevated serum creatinine and blood cyclosporine levels
NSAIDs (except acetylsalicylic acid): Increased risk of seizures with high doses of ciprofloxacin
oral anticoagulants: Enhanced anticoagulant effects
oral hypoglycemics: Possibly increased risk of hypoglycemia that may be severe (especially with glyburide)
phenytoin: Increased or decreased blood phenytoin level
probenecid: Increased blood ciprofloxacin level and, possibly, toxicity

FOODS

caffeine: Increased caffeine effects
dairy products: Delayed drug absorption

Adverse Reactions

CNS: Abnormal gait, agitation, anxiety, ataxia, **cerebral thrombosis**, confusion delirium, depersonalization, depression, disorientation,

disturbance in attention, dizziness, drowsiness, fever, hallucinations, headache, **increased intracranial pressure including pseudotumor cerebri**, insomnia, irritability, lethargy, light-headedness, malaise, manic reaction, memory impairment, migraine, nervousness, nightmares, paranoia, paresthesia, peripheral neuropathy, phobia, restlessness, **seizures**, **status epilepticus**, **suicidal ideation**, syncope, tremor, toxic psychosis, unresponsiveness, weakness
CV: Angina, **atrial flutter**, **cardiopulmonary arrest**, **cardiovascular collapse**, hypertension, **MI**, orthostatic hypotension, palpitations, phlebitis, tachycardia, **torsades de pointes**, vasculitis, **ventricular ectopy**
EENT: Oral candidiasis
ENDO: Hyperglycemia, **hypoglycemia**
GI: Abdominal pain, anorexia, constipation, diarrhea, dysphagia, elevated liver enzymes, flatulence, **GI bleeding**, **hepatic failure or necrosis**, **hepatitis**, indigestion, **intestinal perforation**, jaundice, nausea, **pancreatitis**, **pseudomembranous colitis**, vomiting
GU: Acute renal failure or insufficiency, crystalluria, hematuria, increased serum creatinine level, interstitial nephritis, **nephrotoxicity**, renal calculi, urine retention, vaginal candidiasis
HEME: Agranulocytosis, **aplastic or hemolytic anemia**, **bone marrow depression**, **leukopenia**, lymphadenopathy, **pancytopenia**, **thrombocytopenia**
MS: Arthralgia, myalgia, tendinitis, tendon rupture
RESP: Allergic pneumonitis, **bronchospasm**, **pulmonary embolism**, **respiratory arrest**
SKIN: Acute generalized exanthematous pustulosis (AGEP), **erythema multiforme**, **exfoliative dermatitis**, photosensitivity, rash, **Stevens–Johnson syndrome**, **toxic epidermal necrolysis**, urticaria
Other: Acidosis, **anaphylaxis**, **angioedema**, serum sickness–like reaction

Nursing Considerations

- Obtain culture and sensitivity test results, as ordered, before giving ciprofloxacin.
- Know that ciprofloxacin should not be used in a patient with myasthenia gravis as it may exacerbate muscle weakness.
- Use drug cautiously in patients with CNS disorders and disorders that may predispose patient to seizures, such as history of epilepsy or conditions that may lower the seizure threshold, such as history of altered brain structure, reduced cerebral blood flow, severe cerebral arteriosclerosis, or stroke. Take seizure precautions. If a seizure occurs, expect ciprofloxacin to be discontinued immediately.
- Use drug cautiously in patients who may be more susceptible to drug's effect on QT interval, such as those taking Class IA or III antiarrhythmics; those with uncorrected hypokalemia or hypomagnesemia; or in the presence of a history of cardiac disease such as heart failure, QT-interval prolongation, or torsades de pointes.
- Know that E.R. and immediate-release tablets aren't interchangeable.
- Be aware that during preparation of otic suspension (Otiprio) for each ear, the product must be kept cold. If solution thickens during preparation, the vial should be placed back in refrigeration. Shake vial for 5 to 8 seconds to mix well until a visually homogenous suspension is obtained. Hold vial by the aluminum seal to prevent gelation when shaking vial. Using an 18- to 21-gauge needle, withdraw 0.3 ml of the suspension into the 1-ml syringe. Replace the needle with a 20- to 24-gauge, 1.5-inch blunt, flexible catheter. Prime the syringe after the administration catheter has been attached by leaving a dose of 0.2 ml in the syringe. Know that the syringes can be kept at room temperature or in the refrigerator prior to administration, but the syringes must be kept on their sides. Discard syringes if not administered in 3 hours.
- Be aware that patient should be well hydrated during therapy to help prevent alkaline urine, which may lead to crystalluria and nephrotoxicity.
- Assess patient's hematologic, hepatic, and renal functions periodically, as ordered. Report any abnormalities, including signs and symptoms of dysfunction, to prescriber. For example, severe liver toxicity has occurred with ciprofloxacin use (within 1 to 39 days of therapy) and has been associated more frequently with hypersensitivity reactions. If dysfunction occurs, expect drug to be discontinued and provide supportive care, as ordered and needed.
- Assess patient routinely for signs of rash or other hypersensitivity reactions, even after patient has received multiple doses.

C

Stop drug at first sign of rash, or other sign of hypersensitivity, and notify prescriber immediately. Be prepared to provide supportive emergency care.
- Monitor patient closely for diarrhea, which may reflect pseudomembranous colitis. If it occurs, notify prescriber and expect to withhold drug and treat diarrhea.
- Assess patient for evidence of peripheral neuropathy. Notify prescriber and expect to stop drug if patient complains of burning, numbness, pain, tingling, or weakness in extremities or if physical examination reveals deficits in light touch, motor strength, pain, position sense, temperature, or vibratory sensation.
- Monitor patients (especially children, elderly patients, patients receiving corticosteroids, and patients who have renal failure or who have had a heart, kidney, or lung transplant) for evidence of tendon rupture, such as inflammation, pain, and swelling at the site. Be aware that tendon rupture may occur within the first 48 hours of therapy, throughout therapy, or months after ciprofloxacin therapy. Notify prescriber about suspected tendon rupture, and have patient rest and refrain from exercise until tendon rupture has been ruled out. If present, expect to provide supportive care as ordered.
- Monitor patient closely for changes in behavior or mood that may be caused by ciprofloxacin-induced depression or worsening psychotic reactions potentially resulting in self-injurious behavior, such as suicide. Be aware these reactions may occur even after just one dose. Notify prescriber immediately and expect to discontinue ciprofloxacin therapy, if present, and institute precautions to keep patient safe until adverse effects have disappeared.
- Monitor patient's blood glucose levels, especially diabetic patients, and for signs and symptoms of changes in blood glucose levels. Both symptomatic hyperglycemia and hypoglycemia may occur as a result of ciprofloxacin therapy. If present, alert prescriber and initiate appropriate treatment, as prescribed. Also be aware that severe hypoglycemia has occurred when drug has been administered intravenously. If a hypoglycemic reaction occurs in a patient receiving drug intravenously, discontinue administration immediately and initiate appropriate emergency treatment for hypoglycemia.

PATIENT TEACHING
- Urge patient to complete the prescribed course of therapy, even if he feels better before it's finished.
- Tell patient not to take drug with calcium-fortified juices or dairy products.
- Advise patient to take ciprofloxacin 2 hours before or 6 hours after antacids, iron supplements, or multivitamins that contain iron or zinc. Tell him to shake oral suspension for 15 seconds, not to chew microcapsules, and not to chew, crush, or split E.R. tablets. Advise patient to take drug about the same time every day and if prescribed a twice-daily dose to take first dose in the morning and second dose in the evening about 12 hours apart.
- Encourage patient to drink plenty of fluids during therapy to help prevent crystalluria.
- Urge patient to avoid caffeinated products because caffeine may accumulate in the body during ciprofloxacin therapy and cause excessive stimulation.
- Caution patient to avoid excessive exposure to sunlight or artificial ultraviolet light because severe sunburn may result. Tell patient to notify prescriber if sunburn develops; drug will need to be stopped.
- Urge patient to avoid hazardous activities until CNS effects of drug are known.
- Advise patient to notify prescriber about changes in limb movement or sensation and about inflammation, pain, or swelling over a joint. Urge patient to rest the affected limb at the first sign of discomfort.
- Tell patient to stop taking drug and to notify prescriber at first sign of rash or other hypersensitivity reaction.
- Urge patient to report bloody, watery stools to prescriber immediately, even up to 2 months after drug therapy has ended.
- Urge caregivers to monitor him closely for suicidal tendencies if patient develops depression or worsening of psychotic behavior and to notify prescriber.
- Warn patient, especially diabetic patient, that ciprofloxacin may alter blood glucose levels. Review signs and symptoms of hyperglycemia and hypoglycemia. Tell patient to report symptomatic changes in blood glucose levels immediately to prescriber and review how to treat hypoglycemia.

citalopram hydrobromide

Celexa

Class and Category

Pharmacologic class: Selective serotonin reuptake inhibitor (SSRI)
Therapeutic class: Antidepressant
Pregnancy category: C

Indications and Dosages

➤ *To treat depression*

ORAL SOLUTION, TABLETS

Adults. *Initial:* 20 mg daily. Increased to 40 mg daily, after 1 wk as needed. *Maximum:* 40 mg daily.

DOSAGE ADJUSTMENT Dosage should not exceed 20 mg daily in patients taking concomitant cimetidine or CYP2C19 inhibitors, who are poor CYP2C19 metabolizers, who have hepatic impairment, or who are older than 60 years of age.

Route	Onset	Peak	Duration
P.O.	1 wk	Unknown	Unknown

Mechanism of Action

Blocks serotonin reuptake by adrenergic nerves, which normally release this neurotransmitter from their storage sites when activated by a nerve impulse. This blocked reuptake increases serotonin levels at nerve synapses, which may elevate mood and reduce depression.

Contraindications

Hypersensitivity to citalopram or its components, pimozide therapy, use within 14 days of MAO inhibitor therapy

Interactions

DRUGS

amitriptyline, bromocriptine, buspirone, clomipramine, dextromethorphan, fluoxetine, fluvoxamine, furazolidone, imipramine, levodopa, lithium, meperidine, naratriptan, nefazodone, paroxetine, pentazocine, phenelzine, procarbazine, selegiline, sertraline, sibutramine, sumatriptan, tramadol, tranylcypromine, trazodone, venlafaxine, zolmitriptan: Possibly enhanced serotonergic effects of citalopram, resulting in agitation, chills, confusion, diaphoresis, diarrhea, fever, hyperreflexia, hypomania, incoordination, myoclonus, or tremor
antipsychotics, Class IA and Class III antiarrhythmics, CYP2C19 inhibitors, gatifloxacin, moxifloxacin, pimozide: Increased risk of QT prolongation and torsades de pointes
aspirin, NSAIDs, warfarin: Increased risk of bleeding ranging from ecchymoses to life-threatening hemorrhage
carbamazepine: Possibly increased clearance of citalopram
cimetidine: Possibly increased blood citalopram level and increased risk of QT prolongation
CNS depressants: Possible potentiated CNS effect
MAO inhibitors: Increased risk of life-threatening serotonin syndrome or neuroleptic malignant syndrome
metoprolol, tricyclic antidepressants such as desipramine: Possibly increased blood levels of these drugs

Adverse Reactions

CNS: Agitation, akathisia, amnesia, anxiety, apathy, asthenia, confusion, **CVA**, delirium, depression, dizziness, drowsiness, dyskinesia, fatigue, fever, impaired concentration, insomnia, migraine, myoclonus, **neuroleptic malignant syndrome**, paresthesia, **seizures**, **serotonin syndrome**, **suicidal ideation**, tremor
CV: Angina, bundle branch block, chest pain, **heart failure**, **MI**, orthostatic hypotension, **prolonged QT interval**, tachycardia, **thrombosis**, **ventricular arrhythmias**
EENT: Abnormal accommodation, acute-angle glaucoma, blurred vision, dry mouth, rhinitis, sinusitis, taste perversion
GI: Abdominal pain, anorexia, diarrhea, flatulence, **GI bleeding**, **hepatic necrosis**, indigestion, nausea, **pancreatitis**, vomiting
GU: **Acute renal failure**, amenorrhea, anorgasmia, decreased libido, dysmenorrhea, ejaculation disorders, impotence, polyuria, priapism
HEME: Abnormal bleeding, **decreased PT**, **hemolytic anemia**, **thrombocytopenia**

MS: Arthralgia, myalgia, **rhabdomyolysis**
RESP: Cough, upper respiratory tract infection
SKIN: Diaphoresis, ecchymosis, **erythema multiforme**, pruritus, rash
Other: Anaphylaxis, angioedema, hyponatremia, weight gain or loss

Nursing Considerations

WARNING Monitor patient for possible serotonin syndrome, when dosage increases and which may include agitation, chills, confusion, diaphoresis, diarrhea, fever, hyperactive reflexes, poor coordination, restlessness, shaking, talking or acting with uncontrolled excitement, tremor, and twitching. In its most severe form, serotonin syndrome can resemble neuroleptic malignant syndrome, which includes a high fever, muscle rigidity, or autonomic instability with possible changes in vital signs, and mental status changes.

- Be aware that citalopram should not be given to patients with congenital long QT syndrome, bradycardia, hypokalemia or hypomagnesemia, recent acute myocardial infarction, or uncompensated heart failure because of increased risk of prolonged QT interval and torsades de pointes. It should also not be given to patients who are taking other drugs that prolong the QT interval. Expect hypokalemia and hypomagnesemia to be corrected before citalopram therapy is begun.
- Use citalopram cautiously in patients with other cardiac conditions. ECG monitoring may be ordered to monitor the patient's QT interval and detect the development of serious arrhythmias.
- Use citalopram cautiously in patients with hepatic impairment because citalopram clearance is affected and can lead to increased plasma citalopram levels.
- Be aware that effective antidepressant therapy may convert depression into mania in predisposed people. If patient develops symptoms of mania, notify prescriber immediately and expect to discontinue citalopram.
- Assess elderly patients and those taking diuretics for signs suggesting syndrome of inappropriate secretion of antidiuretic hormone, including hyponatremia and increased serum and urine osmolarity.
- Monitor patient closely for suicidal tendencies, especially when therapy starts or dosage changes, because depression may worsen at these times.
- Expect to reduce dosage gradually when drug is no longer needed to avoid serious adverse reactions.

PATIENT TEACHING

- Inform patient that citalopram's full effects may take up to 4 weeks.
- Advise patient not to self-medicate for allergies colds, or coughs without consulting prescriber because these preparations can increase the risk of adverse reactions.
- Caution patient not to stop citalopram abruptly because doing so may lead to serious adverse reactions.
- Urge caregivers to monitor patient closely for suicidal tendencies, especially when therapy starts or dosage changes.
- Caution against taking OTC aspirin, NSAIDs, or other remedies (including herbal products, such as St. John's wort) while taking citalopram because they may increase the risk of bleeding.
- Advise patient that drug may cause mild pupillary dilation, which may lead to an episode of acute closure glaucoma. Encourage patient to have an eye exam before starting therapy to see if he is at risk.
- Urge patient to report sudden, severe, or unusual adverse reactions promptly to prescriber. Although uncommon, life-threatening adverse effects may occur.

clarithromycin

Biaxin, Biaxin XL

Class and Category

Pharmacologic class: Macrolide
Therapeutic class: Antibiotic
Pregnancy category: C

Indications and Dosages

➤ *To treat pharyngitis and tonsillitis caused by* Streptococcus pyogenes

ORAL SUSPENSION, TABLETS
Adults. 250 mg every 12 hr for 10 days.
Children. 15 mg/kg daily in divided doses every 12 hr for 10 days. *Maximum:* 250 mg every 12 hr.

➤ *To treat acute maxillary sinusitis caused by* Haemophilus influenzae, Moraxella catarrhalis, *or* Streptococcus pneumoniae

ORAL SUSPENSION, TABLETS
Adults. 500 mg every 12 hr for 14 days.
Children. 15 mg/kg daily in divided doses every 12 hr for 10 days. *Maximum:* 500 mg every 12 hr.

E.R. TABLETS
Adults. 1,000 mg every 24 hr for 14 days.

➤ *To treat acute exacerbations of chronic bronchitis caused by* H. influenzae, H. parainfluenzae, M. catarrhalis, *or* S. pneumoniae

ORAL SUSPENSION, TABLETS
Adults. 250 to 500 mg every 12 hr for 7 to 14 days (7 days for *H. parainfluenzae*).
Children. 15 mg/kg daily in divided doses every 12 hr for 10 days. *Maximum:* 500 mg every 12 hr.

E.R. TABLETS
Adults. 1,000 mg every 24 hr for 7 days.

➤ *To treat uncomplicated skin and soft-tissue infections caused by* Staphylococcus aureus *or* S. pyogenes

ORAL SUSPENSION, TABLETS
Adults. 250 mg every 12 hr for 7 to 14 days.
Children. 15 mg/kg daily in divided doses every 12 hr for 10 days. *Maximum:* 250 mg every 12 hr.

➤ *To treat community-acquired pneumonia caused by* Chlamydia pneumoniae, Mycoplasma pneumoniae, *or* S. pneumoniae

ORAL SUSPENSION, TABLETS
Adults. 250 mg every 12 hr for 7 to 14 days.
Children. 15 mg/kg daily in divided doses every 12 hr for 10 days. *Maximum:* 250 mg every 12 hr.

➤ *To treat community-acquired pneumonia caused by* H. influenzae

ORAL SUSPENSION, TABLETS
Adults. 250 mg every 12 hr for 7 days.
Children. 15 mg/kg daily in divided doses every 12 hr for 10 days. *Maximum:* 250 mg every 12 hr.

E.R. TABLETS
Adults and adolescents. 1,000 mg every 24 hr for 7 days.

➤ *To treat community-acquired pneumonia caused by* H. parainfluenzae *or* M. catarrhalis

E.R. TABLETS
Adults and adolescents. 1,000 mg every 24 hr for 7 days.

➤ *To treat acute otitis media caused by* H. influenzae, M. catarrhalis, *or* S. pneumoniae

ORAL SUSPENSION, TABLETS
Children. 15 mg/kg daily in divided doses every 12 hr for 10 days. *Maximum:* 250 mg every 12 hr.

➤ *To treat active duodenal ulcer caused by* Helicobacter pylori

ORAL SUSPENSION, TABLETS
Adults. 500 mg every 8 hr for 14 days with omeprazole 40 mg daily in the morning. Then, omeprazole continued at 20 mg daily in the morning days 15 through 28. Or, 500 mg every 12 hr for 14 days with lansoprazole 30 mg and amoxicillin 1 g every 12 hr for 14 days. Alternatively, 500 mg every 12 hr with omeprazole 20 mg and amoxicillin 1 g every 12 hr for 10 days.

➤ *To prevent or treat* Mycobacterium avium *complex in patients with HIV infection*

ORAL SUSPENSION, TABLETS
Adults. 500 mg every 12 hr for 7 to 14 days.
Children. 7.5 mg/kg every 12 hr. *Maximum:* 500 mg twice daily.

DOSAGE ADJUSTMENT For patient with severe renal impairment (creatinine clearance less than 30 ml/min), dosage reduced by 50%. For patient with moderate renal impairment (creatinine clearance 30 to 60 ml/min) who is also taking atazanavir or ritonavir, dosage reduced by 50%. For patient with severe renal impairment (creatinine clearance less than 30 ml/min) who is also taking atazanavir or ritonavir, dosage reduced by 75%.

Mechanism of Action

Inhibits RNA-dependent protein synthesis in many types of aerobic, anaerobic, gram-negative, and gram-positive bacteria. By binding with the 50S ribosomal subunit of the bacterial 70S ribosome, clarithromycin causes bacterial cells to die.

Contraindications

Concurrent therapy with cisapride, colchicine (in patients with renal or hepatic impairment), dihydroergotamine, ergotamine, lovastatin, pimozide, or simvastatin; history of cholestatic jaundice, hepatic dysfunction, QT prolongation or ventricular cardiac arrhythmias, including torsades de pointes; hypersensitivity to clarithromycin, erythromycin, or any macrolide antibiotic or their components

Interactions

DRUGS

alfentanil, bromocriptine, cilostazol, cyclosporine, methylprednisolone, phenobarbital, St. John's wort, tacrolimus, vinblastine: Possibly increased risk of adverse reactions
alprazolam, midazolam (oral), triazolam: Possibly increased effects of these triazolobenzodiazepines, including increased and/or prolonged sedation
amiodarone, dofetilide, procainamide, quinidine, sotalol: Increased risk of prolonged QT interval, torsades de pointes, or other life-threatening arrhythmias
amlodipine, diltiazem, nifedipine, verapamil: Increased risk of acute kidney dysfunction and hypotension, especially in patients 65 years or older
atazanavir, efavirenz, etravirine, nevirapine, rifampicin, rifapentine, ritonavir, saquinavir: Decreased concentration of clarithromycin with decreased effectiveness
carbamazepine, other drugs metabolized by cytochrome P450 enzyme system, tolterodine: Increased blood levels of these drugs
cisapride, pimozide: Increased risk of cardiac arrhythmias
colchicine: Increased risk of colchicine toxicity
colchicine: Increased risk of life-threatening colchicine toxicity
digoxin: Increased serum digoxin level, increasing risk of toxicity
dihydroergotamine, ergotamine: Risk of acute ergot toxicity
disopyramide: Hypoglycemia, increased risk of torsades de pointes
hexobarbital, phenytoin, valproate: Increased risk of adverse reactions
insulin, oral hypoglycemics such as nateglinide, pioglitazone, repaglinide, rosiglitazone: Increased risk of severe hypoglycemia
itraconazole: Increased plasma concentration of clarithromycin and itraconazole with increased risk of adverse reactions that may become prolonged
maraviroc: Possibly increased maraviroc exposure, resulting in increased risk of adverse reactions
omeprazole: Increased clarithromycin concentrations in gastric tissue and mucus
oral anticoagulants: Potentiated anticoagulant effects
quetiapine: Increased quetiapine exposure and related toxicity
rifabutin: Decreased clarithromycin serum levels, increased rifabutin serum levels, increased risk of uveitis
sildenafil, tadalafil, vardenafil: Possibly increased exposure of these phosphodiesterase inhibitors
statins such as atorvastatin, lovastatin, pravastatin, simvastatin: Increased risk of rhabdomyolysis
theophylline: Increased blood theophylline level
zidovudine: Decreased blood zidovudine level

Adverse Reactions

CNS: Anxiety, confusion, disorientation, dizziness, fatigue, hallucinations, headache, insomnia, mania, nightmares, **seizures**, somnolence, tremor, vertigo
CV: Prolonged QT interval, **ventricular arrhythmias**
EENT: Altered smell, altered taste, glossitis, hearing loss, oral moniliasis, stomatitis, tinnitus, tongue or tooth discoloration
ENDO: Hypoglycemia
GI: Abdominal pain, anorexia, **cholestatic hepatitis**, diarrhea, elevated liver enzymes, **hepatic dysfunction**, **hepatitis**, **hepatotoxicity**, indigestion, jaundice, nausea, **pancreatitis**, **pseudomembranous colitis**, vomiting
GU: Elevated BUN level
HEME: Increased prothrombin time, **leukopenia**, **neutropenia**, **thrombocytopenia**
MS: Rhabdomyolysis
SKIN: Acute generalized exanthematous pustulosis, Henoch–Schönlein purpura, pruritus, rash, **Stevens–Johnson syndrome**, **toxic epidermal necrolysis**, urticaria

Other: Anaphylaxis, angioedema, drug reaction with eosinophilia and systemic symptoms (DRESS), new or worsening myasthenia gravis symptoms, superinfection

Nursing Considerations

- Expect to obtain a specimen for culture and sensitivity tests before giving first dose.
- Know that clarithromycin therapy should be avoided in patients at risk for QT prolongation such as uncorrected hypokalemia or hypomagnesemia or significant bradycardia, and in patients receiving Class IA or Class III antiarrhythmias. Elderly patients are more susceptible to clarithromycin's effect on the QT interval, as well.

WARNING Be aware that use of clarithromycin in patients with coronary artery disease is not recommended because of an increased risk of heart problems or death that may occur even years after exposure to drug.

- Use clarithromycin cautiously in patients with renal impairment. Be aware that patients with severe renal impairment may need decreased dosage.
- Monitor patient closely for acute hypersensitivity reactions such as anaphylaxis and serious skin disorders. If present, expect clarithromycin therapy to be discontinued immediately and appropriate emergency treatment initiated.
- Monitor patient for signs and symptoms of liver dysfunction, especially hepatitis (anorexia, dark urine, jaundice, pruritus, or tender abdomen). Notify prescriber immediately if present, and expect clarithromycin to be discontinued.
- Monitor patients with diabetes who are also receiving insulin or oral hypoglycemics closely for hypoglycemia, which could be severe.
- Be watchful for an elevated INR and prothrombin time in patients who are also taking warfarin, as serious bleeding may occur.
- Assess patient's bowel pattern daily; severe diarrhea may indicate pseudomembranous colitis caused by *Clostridium difficile.* If diarrhea occurs, notify prescriber and expect to withhold clarithromycin and treat with fluids, electrolytes, protein, and an antibiotic effective against *C. difficile.*

PATIENT TEACHING

- Emphasize importance of taking the full course of clarithromycin exactly as prescribed, even after feeling better, because skipped doses or not completing the full course prescribed may hinder drug from eliminating the bacterial infection and increases risk of bacterial resistance.
- Caution patient not to chew or crush E.R. tablets.
- Advise patient to take drug with food if he takes E.R. tablets or has GI distress.
- Instruct patient taking suspension form not to refrigerate it.
- Tell patient to report itching, rash, severe nausea, or any other persistent, severe, or unusual reaction to prescriber immediately.
- Instruct patient not to take OTC or prescription drugs without consulting prescriber of clarithromycin.
- Urge patient to report bloody, watery stools to prescriber immediately, even if they occur 2 months or more after therapy has ended.
- Advise patient to report signs and symptoms of liver dysfunction immediately to prescriber.
- Instruct patient not to perform hazardous activities such as driving until effects on the nervous system such as confusion and dizziness are known.
- Instruct patient with diabetes who is also taking insulin or an oral hypoglycemic agent to monitor his blood glucose level closely.

WARNING Advise patient who has coronary artery disease to continue lifestyle modifications and medications for the heart condition, because clarithromycin may be associated with increased risk for worsening heart problems or mortality years after the end of clarithromycin therapy. Review signs and symptoms of heart disease with all patients, because some patients may not know coronary artery disease is present. Emphasize importance of reporting such signs and symptoms to prescriber even if it is years after exposure to clarithomycin.

- Advise women of childbearing age to use contraception throughout clarithromycin therapy, because drug may cause fetal harm.

clindamycin hydrochloride

Cleocin, Dalacin C (CAN)

clindamycin palmitate hydrochloride

Cleocin Pediatric, Dalacin C Flavored Granules (CAN)

clindamycin phosphate

Cleocin, Clindesse 2%, Dalacin C Phosphate (CAN), Evoclin

Class and Category

Pharmacologic class: Lincosamide
Therapeutic class: Antibiotic
Pregnancy category: B

Indications and Dosages

➤ *To treat serious respiratory tract infections caused by anaerobes such as occur with anaerobic pneumonitis, empyema, and lung abscess and those caused by pneumococci, staphylococci, and streptococci; serious skin and soft-tissue infections caused by anaerobes, staphylococci, and streptococci; septicemia caused by anaerobes; intra-abdominal infections caused by anaerobes such as occur with intra-abdominal abscess and peritonitis; infections of the female pelvis and genital tract caused by anaerobes such as occur with endometritis, nongonococcal tubo-ovarian abscess, pelvic cellulitis, and postsurgical vaginal cuff infection; bone and joint infections caused by* Staphylococcus aureus; *as adjunct therapy in chronic bone and joint infections*

CAPSULES, ORAL SOLUTION

Adults and adolescents. For serious infections, 150 to 300 mg every 6 hr; for severe infections, 300 to 450 mg every 6 hr.
Children. For serious infections, 8 to 16 mg/kg daily in equally divided doses three times daily or four times daily; for severe infections, 16 to 20 mg/kg/day in equally divided doses three times daily or four times daily.

I.V. INFUSION, I.M. INJECTION

Adults and adolescents age 16 and over. For serious infections, 600 to 1,200 mg daily in equally divided doses twice daily to four times daily; for severe infections, 1,200 to 2,700 mg daily in equally divided doses twice daily to four times daily; for life-threatening infections, 4,800 mg daily in equally divided doses twice daily to four times daily. I.V. infusion not to exceed 30 mg/min
Children ages 1 month to 16 years. 20 to 40 mg/kg daily in equally divided doses three times daily or four times daily, depending on severity of infection. I.V. infusion not to exceed 30 mg/min.
Neonates less than age 1 month. 15 to 20 mg/kg daily in equally divided doses three times daily or four times daily, depending on severity of infection. I.V. infusion not to exceed 30 mg/min.

➤ *To treat bone and joint infections caused by* Staphylococcus aureus; *as adjunct therapy in chronic bone and joint infections*

I.V. INFUSION, I.M. INJECTION

Adults and adolescents age 16 and over. *For serious infections:* 600 to 1,200 mg daily in equally divided doses twice daily to four times daily. *For severe infections:* 1,200 to 2,700 mg daily in equally divided doses twice daily to four times daily. *For life-threatening infections:* 4,800 mg daily in equally divided doses twice daily to four times daily. I.V. infusion not to exceed 30 mg/min.

➤ *To treat vaginal infections caused by anaerobes,* Corynebacterium, Gardnerella *or* Haemophilus

VAGINAL CREAM

Nonpregnant females. 100 mg (1 applicatorful) into vagina daily, preferably at bedtime, for 3 to 7 consecutive days.
Pregnant females in second or third trimester. 100 mg (1 applicatorful) into vagina daily, preferably at bedtime, for 7 consecutive days.

VAGINAL CREAM (CLINDESSE 2%)

Nonpregnant females. 5 g (1 applicatorful) into vagina as a single dose.

➤ *To treat acne vulgaris*

FOAM (EVOCLIN)
Adults and adolescents. Apply to affected area daily, using enough to cover the entire affected area(s).

Mechanism of Action
Inhibits protein synthesis in susceptible bacteria by binding to the 50S subunits of bacterial ribosomes and preventing peptide bond formation, which causes bacterial cells to die.

Incompatibilities
To prevent physical incompatibility, don't administer with aminophylline, ampicillin, barbiturates, calcium gluconate, magnesium sulfate, or phenytoin.

Contraindications
Hypersensitivity to clindamycin or lincomycin or any of their components

Interactions
DRUGS
CYP3A4 and CYP3A5 inducers: Possibly decreased plasma concentrations of clindamycin decreasing its effectiveness
CYP3A4 and CYP3A5 inhibitors: Possibly increase plasma concentrations of clindamycin with potential for adverse reactions
erythromycin: Possibly blocked access of clindamycin to its site of action
kaolin-pectin antidiarrheals: Decreased absorption of oral clindamycin
neuromuscular blockers: Increased neuromuscular blockade

Adverse Reactions
CNS: Fatigue, headache
CV: **Hypotension**, thrombophlebitis (after I.V. injection)
EENT: Eye pain (topical), glossitis, metallic or unpleasant taste (with high I.V. doses), stomatitis
GI: Abdominal pain, ***Clostridium difficile*-associated diarrhea**, diarrhea, elevated liver enzymes, esophagitis, jaundice, nausea, **pseudomembranous colitis**, vomiting
GU: Cervicitis, renal dysfunction, vaginitis, and vulvar irritation (with vaginal form)
HEME: **Agranulocytosis**, eosinophilia, **leukopenia**, **neutropenia**, **thrombocytopenic purpura**
MS: Polyarthritis
SKIN: Acute generalized exanthematous pustulosis, contact dermatitis (topical), **erythema multiforme**, **exfoliative dermatitis**, irritation, maculopapular rash, pruritus, rash, **Stevens–Johnson syndrome**, **toxic epidermal necrolysis**, urticaria
Other: **Anaphylaxis**; **angioedema**; **drug reaction with eosinophilia and systemic symptoms (DRESS)**; induration, pain, or sterile abscess after injection; superinfection

Nursing Considerations
- Expect to obtain a specimen for culture and sensitivity testing before giving first dose.
- Use clindamycin cautiously in patients who have a history of asthma, GI disease, or significant allergies; in those with hepatic or renal dysfunction; and in atopic or elderly patients.

WARNING Don't give 75- and 150-mg capsules to tartrazine-sensitive patients.

- Store oral solution for up to 2 weeks at room temperature or reconstituted parenteral solution for up to 24 hours at room temperature.
- Give I.V. dose by infusion only; don't give bolus dose. Dilute 300 mg of clindamycin in 50 ml of diluent and give over 10 minutes. Dilute 600 mg of clindamycin in 50 ml of diluent and give over 20 minutes. Dilute 900 mg of clindamycin in 50 to 100 ml of diluent and give over 30 minutes. Dilute 1,200 mg of clindamycin in 100 ml of diluent and give over 40 minutes.

WARNING Don't use diluents that contain benzyl alcohol when clindamycin is to be administered to neonates because a fatal toxic syndrome may occur.

- Do not dilute clindamycin phosphate prior to administering I.M. Give I.M. injection deep into large muscle mass, such as the gluteus maximus. Rotate injection sites, and avoid giving more than 600 mg in a single I.M. injection.
- Check I.V. site often for phlebitis and irritation.
- For topical foam, wash the affected area with mild soap, let it dry fully, and then apply foam to entire affected area. Be aware that if dermatitis or irritation develops, notify prescriber as foam will need to be discontinued.
- Monitor results of CBC, liver enzymes, and platelet counts during prolonged therapy.
- Observe patient for signs and symptoms of superinfection, such as sore mouth and

vaginal itching, which may occur 2 to 9 days after therapy begins.

- Assess patient's skin regularly for abnormalities because clindamycin may cause severe skin reactions. If present, notify prescriber, expect drug to be discontinued, and be prepared to administer supportive treatment, as prescribed.
- Assess patient's bowel pattern daily; severe diarrhea may indicate pseudomembranous colitis caused by *C. difficile*. If diarrhea occurs, notify prescriber and expect to withhold clindamycin and treat with fluids, electrolytes, protein, and an antibiotic effective against *C. difficile*.

PATIENT TEACHING

- Tell patient to complete the prescribed course of therapy, even if he feels better before it's finished.
- Instruct patient to take clindamycin capsule with at least 8 ounces of water to prevent esophageal irritation.
- Advise patient to take oral drug with food, if needed, to reduce GI distress.
- Tell patient not to refrigerate reconstituted oral solution because it may become thick and difficult to pour and to discard unused drug after 14 days.
- Tell patient using topical foam to wash affected area with mild soap, let it dry fully, and then apply foam to entire area. Caution against dispensing foam directly onto hands or face because foam will melt when it contacts warm skin. Instead, patient should dispense amount to be used into the cap or onto a cool surface. Tell patient to pick up a small amount with fingertips and gently massage into affected area until foam disappears. If foam feels warm or looks runny, tell patient to run the can under cold water before dispensing.
- Advise patient using topical foam to avoid contact with eyes, lips, mouth, other mucous membranes or areas of broken skin. If contact occurs, tell patient to rinse area thoroughly with water.
- Warn patient not to rely on latex or rubber condoms and diaphragms for 72 hours after vaginal treatment because mineral oil in vaginal cream may weaken these items.
- Explain that having sexual intercourse after using vaginal cream can increase irritation.
- Inform patient that I.M. injection may be painful.
- Tell patient to immediately report an inflamed mouth or vagina, and lesions or rash. Also tell patient to immediately report any skin abnormalities such as rash, pruritus, or urticaria.
- Urge patient to report bloody, watery stools to prescriber immediately, even up to 2 months after drug therapy has ended.
- Advise mothers not to breastfeed because drug does appear in breast milk and cause adverse gastrointestinal effects for infant.

clobazam

Onfi, Sympazan

Class and Category

Pharmacologic class: Benzodiazepine
Therapeutic class: Anticonvulsant
Pregnancy category: Not classified
Controlled substance schedule: IV

Indications and Dosages

➤ *Adjunct treatment of seizures associated with Lennox-Gastaut syndrome*

ORAL DISSOLVING FILM STRIPS, ORAL SUSPENSION, TABLETS

Adults and children age 2 and over weighing more than 30 kg (66 lb). *Initial:* 5 mg twice daily increased to 10 mg twice daily on day 7 and further increased to 20 mg twice daily on day 14. *Maximum:* 40 mg daily.

Adults and children age 2 and over weighing less than or equal to 30 kg (66 lb). *Initial:* 5 mg once daily increased to 5 mg twice daily on day 7 and further increased to 10 mg twice daily on day 14. *Maximum:* 20 mg daily.

DOSAGE ADJUSTMENT For elderly patients and patients who are CYP2C19 poor metabolizers or those with hepatic dysfunction, initial dose begun at 5 mg once daily regardless of weight and then titrated according to weight, but only to half the dose normally given for weight category. If needed, an additional titration to the maximum dose for the patient's weight may be started on day 21.

Mechanism of Action

May possibly involve potentiation of GABAergic neurotransmission, which causes binding at the benzodiazepine site of the $GABA_A$ receptor to stop seizure activity.

Contraindications

Hypersensitivity to clobazam or its components

Interactions

DRUGS

CNS depressants, opioids, other benzodiazepines, sedating antihistamines, tricyclic antidepressants: Increased risk of significant sedation and somnolence
fluconazole, fluvoxamine, ticlopidine and other strong inhibitors of CYP2C19 and omeprazole, a moderate inhibitor of CYP2C19: Increased action of clobazam and adverse effects
midazolam: Decreased effect of midazolam
opioids: Increased risk of significant respiratory depression
oral contraceptives: Possible diminished effectiveness of oral contraceptive

ACTIVITIES

alcohol use: Additive CNS effect including severe respiratory depression and significant sedation and somnolence; increased effect of clobazam

Adverse Reactions

CNS: Aggression, agitation, anxiety, apathy, ataxia, confusion, depression, delirium, delusion, fatigue, hallucination, insomnia, irritability, lethargy, psychomotor hyperactivity, pyrexia, sedation, somnolence, **suicidal ideation**
EENT: Blurred vision, diplopia, drooling
GI: Abdominal distention, change in appetite, constipation, dysphagia, elevated liver enzymes, vomiting
GU: UTI
HEME: Anemia, eosinophilia, **leukopenia, thrombocytopenia**
MS: Dysarthria, muscle spasms
RESP: Bronchitis, cough, pneumonia, **respiratory depression**, upper respiratory infection
SKIN: Rash, **Stevens–Johnson syndrome, toxic epidermal necrolysis**, urticaria
Other: Physical and psychological dependence

Nursing Considerations

- Watch for signs of physical and psychological dependence (strong desire or need to increase dose to maintain drug effects), especially in patients with a history of substance abuse. Alert prescriber, if present.

WARNING Be aware that benzodiazepine therapy like clobazam should only be used concomitantly with opioids in patients for whom other treatment options are inadequate. If prescribed together, expect dosing and duration of the opioid to be limited. Monitor patient closely for signs and symptoms of decrease in consciousness, including coma, profound sedation, and significant respiratory depression. Notify prescriber immediately and provide emergency supportive care, as death may occur.

- Monitor patient closely for skin reactions, especially during the first 8 weeks of therapy or when reintroducing clobazam therapy. If the patient develops a rash, notify prescriber immediately and expect drug to be discontinued, as serious dermatological adverse reactions have occurred with clobazam therapy.
- Monitor patient for suicidal tendencies, particularly when therapy starts and dosage changes.
- Expect to withdraw clobazam therapy gradually when the drug is discontinued by decreasing total daily dose by 5 to 10 mg/day on a weekly basis until discontinued, as ordered, to avoid withdrawal symptoms such as anxiety, dysphoria, and insomnia.

PATIENT TEACHING

- Advise patient or parents that clobazam prescribed as a tablet may be given as a whole tablet or crushed and mixed in applesauce.
- Instruct patient prescribed oral suspension form to shake container well before every administration. The oral dosing syringe provided with the product should be the only device used to measure dosage. Tell patient to firmly insert adapter into the neck of the bottle before the first use and keep it there. To withdraw the dose, she should pull back on dosing syringe to dosage amount that will be withdrawn from bottle, insert the dosing syringe into

the adapter, invert bottle, slowly push the air from the syringe into the bottle and then slowly pull back the plunger to the prescribed dose. After removing the syringe from the bottle adapter, the patient should be told to slowly squirt the suspension into the corner of her mouth. Then she should replace the cap over the adapter until next dose is due and rinse syringe well with warm water.

- Tell patient prescribed the oral dissolving film strip form to place the film on top of the tongue and allow it to dissolve. As the film dissolves, saliva should be swallowed in a normal manner, but tell patient to refrain from chewing, spitting, or talking. Although it can be taken with or without food, it should not be taken with liquids. Remind patient that only one film strip should be taken at a time. If more than one film strip is needed, patient should wait until the first film strip is dissolved before placing the second film strip on the tongue.
- Tell patient not to take more drug or more often, or for a longer time than prescribed. Warn her that physical and psychological dependence can occur and teach her to recognize the signs.

WARNING Warn patient not to consume alcohol or take an opioid during clobazam therapy without prescriber knowledge, as severe respiratory depression can occur and may lead to death.

WARNING Inform patient about potentially fatal additive effects of combining clobazam with an opioid. Instruct patient to inform all prescribers of clobazam use, especially if an opioid pain medication may be prescribed.

- Warn patient to stop taking drug at the first sign of a rash and to notify prescriber immediately.
- Instruct patient to avoid performing hazardous activities such as driving until the effects of clobazam are known.
- Tell patient not to stop taking clobazam abruptly, as withdrawal symptoms may occur.
- Urge family or caregiver to watch patient closely for suicidal tendencies, especially when therapy starts or dosage changes.
- Inform female patient of childbearing age to discuss clobazam therapy with her prescriber because drug could interfere with the effectiveness of oral contraceptives. Additional nonhormonal forms of contraception should be used during clobazam therapy if pregnancy is not desired.
- Encourage women of childbearing age who become pregnant while taking clobazam to register with the pregnancy exposure registry by calling 1-888-233-2334. Also advise them that clobazam therapy may pose a potential risk to the fetus. Infants born to mothers who have taken benzodiazepines such clobazam during the later stages of pregnancy can develop dependence, and subsequently withdrawal, during the postnatal period.
- Advise mothers not to breastfeed while taking clobazam, because the drug is found in breast milk. If breastfeeding does occur, tell mothers to monitor the infant for poor sucking and possible sedation. If present, breastfeeding should be discontinued.

clomipramine hydrochloride

Anafranil

Class and Category

Pharmacologic class: Tricyclic antidepressant
Therapeutic class: Antiobsessional agent
Pregnancy category: C

Indications and Dosages

➤ *To treat obsessive-compulsive disorder*

CAPSULES, TABLETS

Adults. *Initial:* 25 mg daily with a meal. Gradually increased to 100 mg daily in divided doses over 2 wk, then to maximum of 250 mg daily in divided doses with meals over next few weeks. At maximum dose, total daily amount may be given at bedtime.
Children age 10 and over. *Initial:* 25 mg daily with a meal. Gradually increased to the lesser of 3 mg/kg daily or 100 mg daily in divided doses over 2 wk, then to maximum of 3 mg/kg daily or 200 mg daily with meals, whichever is less. At maximum dose, total daily amount may be given at bedtime.

Route	Onset	Peak	Duration
P.O.	Unknown	2–4 wk	Unknown

Mechanism of Action

May inhibit neuronal reuptake of norepinephrine and serotonin, which may be a factor in normalizing neurotransmission in obsessive–compulsive behavior.

Contraindications

Acute recovery period after MI, hypersensitivity to clomipramine or its components, linezolid or methylene blue (I.V.) administration, use of an MAO inhibitor within 14 days

Interactions

DRUGS

barbiturates, phenytoin: Possibly decreased level and effects of clomipramine; additive CNS depression; possibly increased barbiturate effect
cimetidine, flecainide, fluoxetine, haloperidol, methylphenidate, other antidepressants, phenothiazines, propafenone, quinidine, H_2-receptor antagonists, selective serotonin reuptake inhibitors: Possibly increased blood level and therapeutic and adverse effects of clomipramine; possibly altered plasma concentrations of these drugs
clonidine: Antagonized antihypertensive effect of clonidine, possibly causing increased blood pressure and risk of hypertensive crisis
CNS depressants: Increased CNS depression dicumarol: Increased anticoagulant effect
guanethidine: Antagonized antihypertensive effect of guanethidine
MAO inhibitors: Increased risk of coma, seizures, or death
phenobarbital: Increased plasma concentration of phenobarbital

ACTIVITIES

alcohol use: Increased CNS depression

Adverse Reactions

CNS: Anxiety, confusion, depersonalization, depression, dizziness, drowsiness, emotional lability, fatigue, headache, insomnia, panic reaction, paresthesia, **serotonin syndrome**, somnolence, **suicidal ideation (children and teens)**, syncope, tremor, unusual dreams, yawning
CV: Orthostatic hypotension, palpitations, tachycardia
EENT: Acute-angle glaucoma, blurred vision, dry mouth, epistaxis, pharyngitis, rhinitis, sinusitis, unpleasant taste
GI: Abdominal pain, anorexia, constipation, diarrhea, flatulence, increased appetite, indigestion, nausea, vomiting
GU: Dysmenorrhea, ejaculation failure, impotence, urinary hesitancy, urine retention
RESP: Bronchospasm
SKIN: Abnormal skin odor, acne, dermatitis, dry skin, photosensitivity, rash, urticaria
Other: Drug reaction with eosinophilia and systemic symptoms (DRESS), weight gain

Nursing Considerations

- Be aware that stopping clomipramine abruptly may cause withdrawal symptoms and worsen disorder.

WARNING Don't give drug within 14 days of an MAO inhibitor to avoid possible coma, seizures, or possibly death.

WARNING Monitor patient closely for evidence of suicidal ideation; clomipramine increases the risk.

WARNING Monitor patient closely for evidence of serotonin syndrome, such as agitation, coma, diarrhea, hallucinations, hyperreflexia, hyperthermia, incoordination, labile blood pressure, nausea, tachycardia, or vomiting. Notify prescriber at once because serotonin syndrome maybe life-threatening. Be prepared to discontinue drug and provide supportive care.

PATIENT TEACHING

- Tell patient not to use alcohol, barbiturates, or other CNS depressants; clomipramine increases their effects.

WARNING Urge families to watch patient closely for abnormal thinking or behavior, or increased aggression or hostility. Emphasize the need to notify prescriber if they occur.

- Inform male patients about risk of sexual dysfunction while taking drug.

C

- Caution patient that drug may cause drowsiness, especially during initial dosage adjustment.
- Warn patient not to stop taking drug abruptly.
- Instruct patient to take a missed dose as soon as he remembers unless it's almost time for the next scheduled dose, in which case he should skip the missed dose. Warn against doubling the next dose.
- Teach patient how to prevent photosensitivity reactions.
- Tell patient to report difficulty urinating, dizziness, dry mouth, mental changes, or sedation.
- Advise patient that drug may cause mild pupillary dilation, which may lead to an episode of acute-angle glaucoma. Encourage patient to have an eye exam before starting therapy to see if he is at risk.
- Caution patient to avoid hazardous activities until CNS effects of drug are known.

clonazepam

Clonapam (CAN), Klonopin, Rivotril (CAN)

Class, Category, and Schedule

Pharmacologic class: Benzodiazepine
Therapeutic class: Anticonvulsant, antipanic
Pregnancy category: Not classified
Controlled substance schedule: IV

Indications and Dosages

➤ *As adjunct or to treat Lennox–Gastaut syndrome (type of absence seizure disorder) and akinetic and myoclonic seizures*

ORAL DISINTEGRATING TABLETS, TABLETS

Adults and children over age 10. 1.5 mg daily in divided doses three times daily. Increased by 0.5 to 1 mg every 3 days, if needed, until seizures are controlled. *Maximum:* 20 mg daily.
Children age 10 and under or weighing less than 30 kg (66 lb). 0.01 to 0.03 mg/kg daily in divided doses twice daily or three times daily. Increased by 0.25 to 0.5 mg every third day up to maintenance dosage. *Maintenance:* 0.1 to 0.2 mg/kg daily, preferably in three equal doses, or if unequal, largest dose given at bedtime.

➤ *To treat panic disorder*

ORALLY DISINTEGRATING TABLETS, TABLETS

Adults. *Initial:* 0.25 mg twice daily. Increased, if needed, to 1 mg daily after 3 days. If more than 1 mg daily is required, dosage increased in increments of 0.125 to 0.25 mg twice daily every 3 days until panic disorder is controlled or adverse reactions make further increases undesirable. This maintenance dosage may be given as a single dose at bedtime. *Maximum:* 4 mg daily.

Mechanism of Action

Although unknown, drug is thought to prevent panic and seizures by potentiating the effects of gamma-aminobutyric acid (GABA), which is an inhibitory neurotransmitter. This action is also thought to suppress the spread of seizure activity caused by seizure-producing foci in the cortex, limbic, and thalamus structures.

Contraindications

Acute–narrow-angle glaucoma; hepatic disease; hypersensitivity to clonazepam, other benzodiazepines, or their components

Interactions

DRUGS

antianxiety drugs, barbiturates, CNS depressants, MAO inhibitors, other benzodiazepines, phenothiazines, sedating antihistamines, tricyclic antidepressants: Increased risk of CNS depression including significant sedation and somnolence
carbamazepine, lamotrigine, phenobarbital, phenytoin: Possibly decreased plasma clonazepam levels with potential for interference with its effectiveness
fluconazole: Possibly impaired clonazepam metabolism with potential for exaggerated concentrations and effects
opioids: Increased risk of severe respiratory depression
phenytoin: Possibly altered plasma concentrations of phenytoin

ACTIVITIES

alcohol use: Increased CNS depression, including severe respiratory depression and significant sedation and somnolence

Adverse Reactions

CNS: Abnormal dreams, aggression, agitation, amnesia, anxiety, apathy, ataxia, attention disturbance, confusion, depersonalization, depression, dizziness, drowsiness, emotional lability, excessive dreaming, fatigue, hallucinations, headache, hostility, hysteria, insomnia, irritability, memory loss, nervousness, nightmares, organic disinhibition, psychosis, reduced intellectual ability, sleep disturbances, **suicidal ideation**
CV: Palpitations
EENT: Blurred vision, eyelid spasm, increased salivation, loss of taste, pharyngitis, rhinitis, sinusitis, yawning
GI: Abdominal pain, anorexia, constipation, increased appetite
GU: Altered libido, difficult ejaculation, dysmenorrhea, dysuria, enuresis, impotence, nocturia, urine retention, UTI
HEME: Anemia, eosinophilia, **leukopenia, thrombocytopenia**
MS: Dysarthria, myalgia
RESP: Bronchitis, cough, **respiratory depression**
Other: Allergic reaction

Nursing Considerations

- Use clonazepam cautiously in patients with mixed seizure disorder (because drug can increase the risk of generalized tonic–clonic seizures), renal failure, or troublesome secretions (because clonazepam increases salivation) and in elderly patients (because they're more sensitive to drug's CNS effects). Also use cautiously in patients with compromised respiratory function and porphyria.
- Monitor blood drug level, CBC, and liver enzymes during long-term or high-dose therapy, as ordered.
- Monitor patient closely for signs of loss of effectiveness of anticonvulsant activity, especially within the first 3 months of administration. Notify prescriber if noted, because a dosage adjustment may reestablish effectiveness.

WARNING Know that the drug should not be stopped abruptly. Instead, expect to taper dosage gradually by 0.125 mg twice daily every 3 days, until the drug is completely discontinued, to avoid withdrawal symptoms and seizures.

- Monitor patient closely for evidence of suicidal thinking or behavior, especially when therapy starts or dosage changes.
- Be aware that paradoxical and psychiatric reactions have occurred with benzodiazepines. Because clonazepam is a benzodiazepine, monitor patient for aggression, agitation, anger, anxiety, hallucinations, irritability, nightmares, and psychoses. Children and elderly patients are at greater risk of developing paradoxical reactions. If noted, notify prescriber and expect drug to be discontinued gradually.

WARNING Be aware that benzodiazepine therapy like clonazepam should only be used concomitantly with opioids in patients for whom other treatment options are inadequate. If prescribed together, expect dosing and duration of the opioid to be limited. Monitor patient closely for signs and symptoms of decrease in consciousness, including coma, profound sedation, and significant respiratory depression. Notify prescriber immediately and provide emergency supportive care, as death may occur.

- Know that although the risk of teratogenicity is inconclusive, administration of benzodiazepines like clonazepam immediately before or during childbirth can cause a syndrome of difficulty feeding, hypothermia, hypotonia, and respiratory depression in the infant after birth. Also know that if mothers have taken clonazepam during the later stages of pregnancy, their infants may develop a dependency on the drug and experience withdrawal after birth.

PATIENT TEACHING

- Tell patient to take drug exactly as prescribed. Explain that stopping abruptly can cause seizures and withdrawal symptoms.
- Urge patient to carry medical identification of his seizure disorder and drug therapy.
- Warn patient about possible drowsiness.
- Instruct patient to report, difficulty urinating, palpitations, persistent drowsiness, seizure activity, severe dizziness, and other disruptive adverse reactions.
- Suggest that parents monitor child's performance in school because

clonazepam can cause drowsiness or inattentiveness.
- Urge caregivers to watch patient closely for evidence of suicidal tendencies, especially when therapy starts or dosage changes, and to report concerns to prescriber immediately.

WARNING Warn patient not to consume alcohol or take an opioid during clonazepam therapy without prescriber knowledge, as severe respiratory depression can occur and may lead to death.

WARNING Inform patient about potentially fatal additive effects of combining clonazepam with an opioid. Instruct patient to inform all prescribers of clonazepam use, especially if pain medication may be prescribed.

- Warn women of childbearing age who become pregnant while taking clonazepam to notify prescriber of pregnancy. Tell them not to take clonazepam during later part of pregnancy because of potential adverse effects on infant and to discuss alternative therapy with prescriber while pregnant. Urge female patient who becomes pregnant while taking clonazepam to enroll in the Antiepileptic Drug Pregnancy Registry by calling 1-888-233-2334. Explain that the registry is studying the safety of antiepileptic drugs during pregnancy.
- Encourage mothers to discuss breastfeeding with prescriber before doing so.
- Tell patient to let prescriber know about any new drug prescribed by another healthcare provider or before using any new over-the-counter preparations.

clonidine

Catapres-TTS

clonidine hydrochloride

Catapres, Dixarit (CAN), Duraclon, Kapvay

Class and Category

Pharmacologic class: Centrally acting alpha agonist
Therapeutic class: Analgesic, antihypertensive, behavior modifier
Pregnancy category: C

Indications and Dosages

➤ *To manage hypertension*

TABLETS

Adults. *Initial:* 0.1 mg twice daily, increased by 0.1 mg/wk to produce desired response. *Maintenance:* 0.2 to 0.6 mg daily in divided doses twice daily or three times daily. *Maximum:* 2.4 mg daily.

TRANSDERMAL PATCH (CATAPRES-TTS)

Adults. *Initial:* 0.1-mg patch applied to hairless area of intact skin on upper arm or torso every 7 days. After 1 to 2 wk, if blood pressure isn't controlled, two 0.1-mg patches or one 0.2-mg patch applied to skin. Dosage adjusted, as needed, every 7 days. *Maximum:* Two 0.3-mg patches worn at same time.

DOSAGE ADJUSTMENT Dosage individualized for patients with renal failure.

➤ *To treat attention deficit hyperactivity disorder (ADHD) alone or as adjunct therapy with stimulant drugs*

E.R. TABLETS (KAPVAY)

Children age 6 to 17. *Initial:* 0.1 mg at bedtime, increased in increments of 0.1 mg daily at weekly intervals, as needed, with total daily dosage equally divided and given twice a day with the second dose of an equal or higher split dosage given at bedtime as soon as dosage begins to be increased. *Maximum:* 0.4 mg/day.

➤ *As adjunct to relieve severe pain (in cancer patients) that isn't adequately relieved by opioid analgesics alone*

CONTINUOUS EPIDURAL INFUSION (DURACLON)

Adults. *Initial:* 30 mcg/hr. Titrated up or down, if needed, depending on comfort. *Maximum:* 40 mcg/hr.

Route	Onset	Peak	Duration
P.O.	30–60 min	2–4 hr	8 hr
Transdermal	2–3 days	Unknown	7 days

Mechanism of Action

Stimulates peripheral alpha-adrenergic receptors in the CNS to produce transient vasoconstriction and then stimulates central alpha-adrenergic receptors in the brain stem to reduce heart rate, peripheral vascular resistance, heart rate, and systolic and diastolic blood pressure. Although $alpha_2$ adrenergic receptors in the brain are stimulated, the precise action that calms children with ADHD is unknown. May produce analgesia by preventing transmission of pain signals to the brain at presynaptic and postjunctional $alpha_2$-adrenoreceptors in the spinal cord. With epidural administration, clonidine produces analgesia in body areas innervated by the spinal cord segments in which the drug concentrates.

Contraindications

Anticoagulant therapy (epidural infusion); bleeding diathesis; (epidural infusion); hypersensitivity to clonidine or its components, including adhesive used in transdermal patch; injection-site infection (epidural infusion)

Interactions

DRUGS

barbiturates, other CNS depressants: Increased depressant effects of these drugs
beta blockers, calcium channel blockers, digoxin: Additive effects, such as bradycardia and AV block; increased risk of worsened hypertensive response when clonidine is withdrawn (beta blockers only)
diuretics, other antihypertensive drugs: Increased hypotensive effect
epidural local anesthetics: Prolonged effects of epidural local anesthetics when used with epidural clonidine
neuroleptics: Increased risk of dizziness, fatigue, and orthostatic hypotension
sympatholytics: Increased risk of worsening sinus node dysfunction and AV block, if present
tricyclic antidepressants: Decreased antihypertensive effect of clonidine

ACTIVITIES

alcohol use: Enhanced CNS depressant effects of alcohol

Adverse Reactions

CNS: Agitation, delusional perception, depression, dizziness, drowsiness, fatigue, hallucinations, headache, malaise, nervousness, paresthesia, sedation, syncope, weakness, tremor
CV: Arrhythmias, **AV block**, **bradycardia (severe)**, chest pain, **congestive heart failure**, orthostatic hypotension, Raynaud's phenomenon
EENT: Accommodation disorder, blurred vision, burning eyes, decreased lacrimation, dry eyes and mouth, salivary gland pain
GI: Constipation, **hepatitis**, mildly elevated liver enzymes, nausea, vomiting
GU: Decreased libido, erectile dysfunction, nocturia
HEME: Thrombocytopenia
SKIN: Pruritus, rash, urticaria
Other: Angioedema, weight gain, withdrawal symptoms

Nursing Considerations

- Be aware that clonidine should not be used in most patients with severe cardiovascular disease or in those who are not hemodynamically stable because of the potential for severe hypotension.
- Use clonidine cautiously in elderly patients, who may be more sensitive to its hypotensive effect.
- Monitor blood pressure and heart rate often during clonidine therapy because clonidine may worsen AV block and sinus node dysfunction, especially if patient is taking another sympatholytic drug. If severe bradycardia occurs, be prepared to administer IV atropine or isoproterenol and assist with insertion of temporary cardiac pacing.
- Be aware that extended-release tablets are not interchangeable with immediate-release tablets.
- Expect transdermal clonidine to take 2 to 3 days to lower blood pressure.
- Remove patch before patient has an MRI to avoid possible burns at the patch site.
- Be aware that stopping drug abruptly can elevate serum catecholamine levels and cause such withdrawal symptoms as agitation, confusion headache, nervousness, rebound hypertension, and tremor. Be aware that when drug has been used to treat ADHD, dosage should be decreased by 0.1 mg every 3 to 7 days when it is being discontinued.
- Monitor patient with AV block and sinus node dysfunction closely if patient is taking sympatholytics concurrently with clonidine

because these conditions may worsen, causing severe bradycardia, requiring treatment with IV atropine or isoproterenol therapy and temporary cardiac pacing.
- Expect hypertension to return within 48 hours after drug is discontinued.

PATIENT TEACHING
- Advise patient to take drug exactly as prescribed and not to stop abruptly because severe hypertension and withdrawal symptoms may occur.
- Instruct patient to consult prescriber if dry mouth or drowsiness becomes a problem during oral clonidine therapy. To minimize these effects, prescriber may suggest taking most of dosage at bedtime.
- Know that if a transdermal patch loosens during 7-day application period, tell patient to place adhesive overlay directly over patch to ensure adhesion.
- Tell patient to rotate transdermal sites.
- Instruct patient to remove patch and place a fresh one on another site if skin irritation, rash, or redness develops at patch site.
- Advise patient to fold used transdermal patch in half with adhesive sides together and discard it out of the reach of children.
- Instruct patient to swallow E.R. tablets whole and never chew, crush, or cut the tablets.
- Advise patient to avoid hazardous activities until drug's CNS effects are known. Caution patient that these effects are increased by concomitant use of alcohol, barbiturates, or other sedating drugs.
- Advise men that libido may decrease.
- Instruct patient to report chest pain, dizziness with position changes, excessive drowsiness, rash, urine retention, and vision changes. As needed, tell patient to rise slowly to avoid hypotensive effects.
- Inform patient who wears contact lenses that clonidine may cause dry eyes.

clopidogrel bisulfate

Plavix

Class and Category

Pharmacologic class: $P2Y_{12}$ platelet inhibitor
Therapeutic class: Platelet aggregation inhibitor
Pregnancy category: B

Indications and Dosages

➤ *To reduce thrombotic events, such as MI and stroke, in patients with atherosclerosis documented by recent MI, peripheral artery disease, or stroke*

TABLETS

Adults. 75 mg daily.

➤ *To reduce thrombotic events, such as MI and stroke, in patients with acute coronary syndrome*

TABLETS

Adults. *Loading dose:* 300 mg as a single dose. *Maintenance:* 75 mg daily.

Route	Onset	Peak	Duration
P.O.	2 hr	3–7 days*	5 days

*With repeated doses.

Mechanism of Action

Binds to adenosine diphosphate (ADP) receptors on the surface of activated platelets. This action blocks ADP, which deactivates nearby glycoprotein IIb/IIIa receptors and prevents fibrinogen from attaching to receptors. Without fibrinogen, platelets can't aggregate and form thrombi.

Contraindications

Active pathological bleeding, including peptic ulcer and intracranial hemorrhage; hypersensitivity to clopidogrel or its components

Interactions

DRUGS

aspirin: Increased risk of bleeding
CYP2C19 inhibitors, such as cimetidine, esomeprazole, etravirine, felbamate, fluconazole, fluoxetine, fluvoxamine, ketoconazole, omeprazole, ticlopidine, voriconazole: Decreased plasma clopidogrel level, decreased platelet inhibition
fluvastatin, phenytoin, tamoxifen, tolbutamide, torsemide: Interference with metabolism of these drugs
NSAIDs: Increased risk of GI bleeding, interference with NSAID metabolism

opioids: Delayed and reduced absorption of clopidogrel
repaglinide: Increased repaglinide exposure possibly increasing risk of adverse reactions, especially hypoglycemia
warfarin: Prolonged bleeding time, interference with warfarin metabolism

Adverse Reactions

CNS: Confusion, depression, dizziness, **fatal intracranial bleeding**, fatigue, fever, hallucinations, headache
CV: Chest pain, edema, hypercholesterolemia, hypertension, **hypotension**, vasculitis
EENT: Altered or loss of taste; conjunctival, ocular, or retinal bleeding; epistaxis; rhinitis; stomatitis; taste disorders
GI: Abdominal pain; **acute liver failure**; colitis; diarrhea; duodenal, gastric, or peptic ulcer; elevated liver enzymes; gastritis; **gastrointestinal and retroperitoneal hemorrhage**; indigestion; nausea; **noninfectious hepatitis**, **pancreatitis**
GU: Elevated serum creatinine level, **glomerulopathy**, UTI
HEME: Acquired hemophilia A, **agranulocytosis**, **aplastic anemia**, **neutropenia**, **pancytopenia**, **prolonged bleeding time**, **thrombocytopenic purpura**, **thrombotic thrombocytopenic purpura**, **unusual bleeding** or bruising
MS: Arthralgia, back pain, musculoskeletal bleeding, myalgia
RESP: Bronchitis, **bronchospasm**, cough, dyspnea, **eosinophilic pneumonia**, **interstitial pneumonitis**, **respiratory tract bleeding**, upper respiratory tract infection
SKIN: Acute generalized exanthematous pustulosis, bullous dermatitis, **erythema multiforme**, **exfoliative dermatitis**, skin bleeding, **Stevens–Johnson syndrome**, **toxic epidermal necrolysis**, urticaria
Other: Anaphylaxis, **angioedema**, **drug reaction with eosinophilia and systemic symptoms (DRESS)**, flu-like symptoms, serum sickness

Nursing Considerations

- Avoid clopidogrel in patients who have a genetic variation in CYP2C19 or are receiving CYP2C19 inhibitors. Platelet inhibition may decline, increasing the risk of adverse cardiovascular effects after MI.
- Determine if patient has a history of hypersensitivity that may have included a hematologic reaction to any other thienopyridine drug, such as prasugrel or ticlopidine, because allergic cross-reactivity has been reported.
- Use clopidogrel cautiously in patients with severe hepatic or renal disease, risk of bleeding from surgery or trauma, or conditions that predispose to bleeding (such as peptic ulcer disease or thrombotic thrombocytopenic purpura).
- Expect to give aspirin with clopidogrel in patient with acute coronary syndrome.

WARNING Be aware that clopidogrel prolongs bleeding time; expect to stop it 5 days before elective surgery.

- Obtain blood cell count, as ordered, whenever signs and symptoms suggest a hematologic problem.
- Monitor patient who takes aspirin closely because risk of bleeding is increased.

PATIENT TEACHING

- Discourage use of NSAIDs, including OTC preparations, during clopidogrel therapy because of potential for bleeding.
- Caution patient that bleeding may continue longer than usual. Instruct him to report unusual bleeding or bruising.
- Urge patient to inform all other healthcare providers, including dentists, that he takes clopidogrel before having surgery or other procedures or taking a new drug because he has an increased risk of bleeding.
- Advise patient to notify prescriber promptly if he experiences extreme skin paleness, fever, neurologic changes, purple skin patches, weakness, or yellowing of his skin or eyes.
- Instruct patient not to discontinue clopidogrel abruptly or without first consulting prescriber.
- Advise female patients of childbearing age to notify prescriber immediately if pregnancy is suspected or has occurred. Also advise women who are breastfeeding that it is not known if drug passes into breast milk, so they should discuss wisdom of breastfeeding with prescriber.

clozapine

Clozaril, Fazaclo, FazaClo ODT, Versacloz

Class and Category

Pharmacologic class: Atypical antipsychotic
Therapeutic class: Atypical antipsychotic
Pregnancy category: B

Indications and Dosages

➤ *To treat severe schizophrenia unresponsive to standard drugs; to reduce risk of recurrent suicidal behavior in schizophrenia or schizoaffective disorders*

ORALLY DISINTEGRATING TABLETS, ORAL SUSPENSION, TABLETS

Adults. *Initial:* 12.5 mg once or twice daily. Increased by 25 to 50 mg daily to 300 to 450 mg daily in divided doses by the end of 2 wk. Subsequently, dosage titration shouldn't exceed 100 mg twice per wk. *Maximum:* 900 mg daily in divided doses.

DOSAGE ADJUSTMENT If patient is receiving a strong CYP1A2 inhibitor such as ciprofloxacin, enoxacin, or fluvoxamine concurrently, dosage decreased by two-thirds and then adjusted according to clinical response. If a patient is receiving a strong CYP1A2 inducer such as carbamazepine, phenytoin, rifampin, or St. John's wort concurrently, clozapine dosage may need to be increased if clinical response is ineffective. If patient has significant renal or hepatic impairment or is a CYP2D6 poor metabolizer, clozapine dosage may be decreased if patient develops significant adverse reactions.

Route	Onset	Peak	Duration
P.O.	1–6 hr	Unknown	4–12 hr

Mechanism of Action

May produce antipsychotic effects by interfering with dopamine binding to dopamine—especially D_4—receptors in the limbic region of the brain and by antagonizing adrenergic, cholinergic, histaminic, and serotoninergic receptors.

Contraindications

Absolute neutrophil count (ANC) below 1,500/mm^3, history of clozapine-induced agranulocytosis or severe granulocytopenia, hypersensitivity to clozapine or its components that may have been serious, myeloproliferative disorders, severe CNS depression, uncontrolled epilepsy

Interactions

DRUGS

anticholinergics: Potentiated anticholinergic effects
benzodiazepines, psychotropics: Additive hypotensive effects; increased risk of cardiopulmonary collapse
bone marrow depressants: Potentiated myelosuppressive effects
bupropion, cimetidine, citalopram, ciprofloxacin, duloxetine, enoxacin, erythromycin, escitalopram, fluoxetine, fluvoxamine, oral contraceptives, paroxetine, quinidine, sertraline, terbinafine: Possibly increased blood clozapine level and increased risk of adverse reactions
carbamazepine, phenytoin, rifampin, St. John's wort: Decreased blood clozapine level
chlorpromazine, class 1Aa antiarrhythmias such as quinidine or procainamide, class III antiarrhythmias such as amiodarone or sotalol, dolasetron, droperidol, erythromycin, gatifloxacin, halofantrine, iloperidone, levomethadyl, mesoridazine, mefloquine, methadone, moxifloxacin, pentamidine, pimozide, probucol, sparfloxacin, tacrolimus, thioridazine: Possible increased risk of prolonged QT interval
CNS depressants: Increased CNS depression
digoxin, warfarin: Increased blood level of digoxin and warfarin; displacement of clozapine from its binding site
lithium: Increased risk of confusion, dyskinesia, neuroleptic malignant syndrome, and seizures
selective serotonin reuptake inhibitors: Markedly increased blood clozapine level; increased risk of adverse effects and leukocytosis

ACTIVITIES

alcohol use: Increased CNS depression
caffeine: Increased blood clozapine level
smoking: Decreased blood clozapine level

Adverse Reactions

CNS: Agitation, akinesia, anxiety, ataxia, cholinergic rebound adverse reactions

postdiscontinuation, confusion, delirium, depression, dizziness, drowsiness, dystonia, EEG abnormality, fatigue, fever, headache, hyperkinesia, hypokinesia, insomnia, lethargy, myoclonic jerks, **neuroleptic malignant syndrome**, nightmares, obsessive–compulsive symptoms, paresthesia, possible cataplexy, restlessness, rigidity, sedation, **seizures**, sleep disturbance including **sleep apnea**, slurred speech, **status epilepticus**, syncope, tardive dyskinesia, tremor, vertigo, weakness
CV: Atrial or ventricular fibrillation, **bradycardia**, **cardiac arrest**, **cardiomyopathy**, chest pain, **deep vein thrombosis**, **ECG changes**, hypercholesterolemia, **hypertension**, hypertriglyceridemia, hypotension, leukocytoclastic vasculitis, **MI**, **mitral valve incompetence**, **myocarditis**, orthostatic hypotension, palpitations, **QT-interval prolongation**, tachycardia, **torsades de pointes**, vasculitis, **ventricular tachycardia**
EENT: Blurred vision, dry mouth, increased nasal congestion, increased salivation, narrow-angle glaucoma, periorbital edema, pharyngitis, salivary gland swelling, tongue numbness or soreness
ENDO: Ketoacidosis, **pseudopheochromocytoma**, **severe hyperglycemia**
GI: Abdominal discomfort, **acute pancreatitis**, anorexia, cholestasis, colitis, constipation, diarrhea, dysphagia, elevated liver enzymes, heartburn, **hepatic cirrhosis or fibrosis**, **hepatitis**, **hepatotoxicity**, jaundice, **liver failure or injury**, nausea, vomiting
GU: Abnormal ejaculation including retrograde; acute interstitial nephritis; nocturnal enuresis; priapism; **renal failure**; urinary frequency, urgency, and incontinence; urine retention
HEME: Agranulocytosis; elevated hemoglobin, hematocrit and erythrocyte sedimentation rate; eosinophilia; **granulocytopenia**; **leukopenia**; **neutropenia (may become severe)**; **thrombocytopenia**; thrombocytosis
MS: Back or leg pain, elevated creatine phosphokinase, muscle spasm or weakness, myalgia, myasthenic syndrome, **rhabdomyolysis**
RESP: Aspiration, dyspnea, lower respiratory tract infection, pleural effusion, pneumonia, **pulmonary embolism**, **respiratory arrest**
SKIN: Erythema multiforme, photosensitivity, pigmentation disorder, pruritus, rash, **Stevens–Johnson syndrome**, urticaria
Other: Angioedema, **hypersensitivity reactions**, hyperuricemia, **hyponatremia**, **sepsis**, systemic lupus erythematosus, weight gain

C

Nursing Considerations

- Use clozapine cautiously in patients with cardiovascular, hepatic, or renal disease because they have increased risk of serious or fatal adverse reactions. Also use cautiously in patients with risk factors for a stroke because drug use may increase risk of cerebrovascular adverse events.
- Be aware that clozapine should not be given to elderly patients with dementia-related psychosis.
- Use cautiously in patients with a history of prolonged QT syndrome or who have existing conditions that might prolong the QT interval such as a recent MI, serious cardiac arrhythmia, or uncompensated heart failure. Drug should also be used cautiously in patients with cardiovascular disease or a family history of prolonged QT syndrome because clozapine therapy may increase the QT interval enough to cause life-threatening arrhythmias such as torsades de pointes, especially in patients who are hypokalemic. Know that hypokalemia should be corrected, if present, before clozapine therapy begins and the serum potassium level monitored closely throughout therapy. If QT prolongation occurs, notify prescriber and expect drug to be discontinued if the QT interval exceeds 500 msec.

WARNING Know that, rarely, clozapine causes severe or life-threatening adverse reactions, such as agranulocytosis, cardiac or respiratory arrest, deep vein thrombosis, myocarditis (especially in first month), neuroleptic malignant syndrome, and severe hyperglycemia with ketoacidosis in nondiabetic patients. It also may cause seizures and tardive dyskinesia. Monitor patient closely. Know that these risks are often dose-related.

Expect therapy to begin with a dose as low as 12.5 mg with titration done slowly and divided daily dosing used.

WARNING Check patient's baseline complete blood count (CBC), including differential before therapy and weekly for first 6 months, as ordered. Know that the baseline absolute neutrophil count (ANC) must be at least 1,500/µl for the general population; and must be at least 1,000/µl for patients with documented Benign Ethnic Neutropenia (BEN) before therapy can begin. If ANC remains equal to or greater than 1,500/µl during the first 6 months, expect to check the patient's ANC to check every 2 weeks for next 6 months, as ordered. If counts remain stable, expect to continue checking every 4 weeks thereafter. Also, know that laboratory monitoring may be reduced for hospice patients with an estimated life expectancy of 6 months or less. Be aware that because of the risk for severe neutropenia, clozapine is only available through a restricted program.

- Be aware that because of the risk of severe neutropenia, clozapine is available only through a restricted program called the Clozapine REMS Program. If patient develops mild neutropenia (1,000 to 1,499/µl), treatment should be expected to continue but ANC monitoring should be increased to three times weekly until level reaches 1,500/µl. If patient develops moderate neutropenia (500 to 999/µl), expect treatment to be interrupted and daily monitoring of the patient's ANC done until the level reaches 1,000/µl, then three times a week monitoring until level reaches 1,500/µl. Expect therapy to be resumed once ANC reaches 1,000/µl. If patient develops severe neutropenia (less than 500/µl) expect drug to be discontinued, and daily monitoring of ANC until it reaches 1,000/µl, then three times weekly until it is normal. Be aware that clozapine therapy should not be restarted unless the benefits outweigh future risks and if restarted, the patient should resume treatment as a new patient receiving drug for the first time.
- Monitor temperature. Expect to withhold clozapine if patient develops a fever of 38.5°C (101.3°F) or higher and obtain an ANC level immediately as fever is often the first sign of neutropenic infection.
- Expect to check ANC weekly for at least 4 weeks after therapy ends or until ANC is 1,500/µl or more.
- Monitor patients, especially male patients and younger patients, for dystonia, particularly during the first few days of treatment. Be alert for complaints of neck spasms, which sometimes may progress to throat tightness, trouble swallowing or breathing, and tongue protrusion.
- Monitor patient for signs and symptoms of cardiomyopathy, mitral valve incompetence, or myocarditis such as chest pain, dyspnea, ECG changes, fever, flu-like symptoms, hypotension, palpitations, or tachycardia. If present, notify prescriber immediately and expect drug to be discontinued and a cardiac evaluation done promptly.
- Monitor patient's liver enzymes, as ordered. Report any signs of liver dysfunction such as anorexia, fatigue, jaundice, malaise, or nausea to prescriber. Expect clozapine to be discontinued if liver enzymes become elevated in combination with symptoms or patient develops hepatitis.

PATIENT TEACHING

- Tell patient that he'll receive only a 1-week supply at a time.
- Instruct patient taking orally disintegrating tablets (Fazaclo) to leave tablet in blister pack until ready to take it. Tell him to peel foil back to remove tablet (rather than pushing tablet through foil) and then to immediately place tablet in mouth and let it dissolve before swallowing. Explain that no water is needed.
- Instruct patient prescribed oral suspension form to shake container for 10 seconds before every administration. The oral dosing syringe provided with the product should be the only device used to measure dosage. Tell patient to firmly insert adapter into the neck of the bottle before the first use and keep it there. Instruct patient to first fill the syringe with air equivalent to the dose being withdrawn from the bottle.To withdraw the dose, he should insert the dosing syringe into the adapter and push air from syringe into the

bottle. Then he should invert bottle and slowly pull back the plunger to the prescribed dose. After removing the syringe from the bottle adapter, the patient should be told to slowly squirt the suspension into his mouth. Then he should replace the cap over the adapter until next dose is due and rinse syringe well with warm water and dry.
- Inform patient that he'll need weekly blood tests. Review evidence of dyscrasias (fatigue, fever, sore throat, weakness); urge patient to report them to prescriber if they occur.
- Instruct patient to avoid hazardous activities until drug's CNS effects are known.
- Alert patient and family of increased risk for falls, especially if patient has other medical conditions or takes medication that may affect the nervous system.
- Tell patient to report any persistent, severe, or unusual adverse effects to prescriber immediately.
- Advise patient to rise slowly from lying or sitting position to minimize orthostatic hypotension.
- Warn patient that if he stops drug for more than 2 days, he will need to contact prescriber for instructions; dosage will need to be changed.
- Tell patient to consult prescriber before using alcohol or taking OTC drugs.
- Advise female patients of childbearing age to notify prescriber if pregnancy occurs or is suspected. Alert her that breastfeeding is not recommended while on clozapine therapy.

coagulation factor Xa, inactivated-zhzo

Andexxa

Class and Category

Pharmacologic class: Human coagulation factor Xa, recombinant
Therapeutic class: Factor Xa inhibitor antidote
Pregnancy category: Not classified

Indications and Dosages

➤ *To reverse life-threatening or uncontrolled bleeding induced by apixaban or rivaroxaban therapy*

I.V INFUSION, I.V. INJECTION

Adults. *For low dose (used if last dose of apixaban was less than 5 mg, rivaroxaban was 10 mg or less, or last dose of either drug was taken within 8 hr or less):* 400 mg infused at 30 mg/min given as an I.V. bolus, followed by 4 mg/min for up to 120 min given as an I.V. infusion. *For high dose (used if last dose of apixaban was greater than 5 mg or unknown or rivaroxaban was greater than 10 mg or unknown):* 800 mg infused at 30 mg/min given as an I.V. bolus, followed by 8 mg/min for up to 120 min given as an I.V. infusion.

Route	Onset	Peak	Duration
I.V.	2–5 min (bolus)	4 hr	2 hr (following infusion)

Mechanism of Action

Binds and sequesters the factor Xa inhibitors apixaban and rivaroxaban, thereby exerting its procoagulant effect.

Contraindications

Hypersensitivity to coagulation factor Xa, inactivated-zhzo or its components

Interactions

DRUGS

None reported

Adverse Reactions

CV: Thromboembolic events
EENT: Altered sense of taste
GU: UTI
RESP: Cough, dyspnea, pneumonia
SKIN: Flushing, urticaria
Other: Anticoagulation factor Xa, inactivated-zhzo antibodies; feeling hot

Nursing Considerations

- Be aware that the dosing of coagulation factor Xa, inactivated-zhzo is based on the specific drug that had been administered (apixaban or rivaroxaban), dose of the drug taken, and the time since the patient's last dose of the drug.

- Prepare I.V. bolus by reconstituting each 100-mg vial of coagulation factor Xa, inactivated-zhzo by slowly injecting 10 ml of sterile water for injection using a 20-gauge needle or higher and directing the solution onto the inside wall of the vial to minimize foaming. Gently swirl each vial until powder is completely dissolved. Do not shake, to avoid foaming. This takes about 3 to 5 minutes. Use a 60-ml syringe or larger with a 20-gauge needle to withdraw the reconstituted solution from each of the vials until the required dosing volume is achieved. Transfer the solution from the syringe into an empty polyolefin or polyvinyl chloride I.V. bag with a volume of 250 ml or less. Administer the bolus at a rate of 30 mg/min.
- Prepare I.V. infusion following the same procedure for I.V. bolus preparation. Use a 0.2- or 0.22-micron in-line polyethersulfone or equivalent low protein-binding filter. Within 2 minutes following the bolus dose, administer the continuous I.V. infusion for up to 120 minutes, as prescribed.
- Know that vials that have been reconstituted are stable at room temperature for up to 8 hours, or may be stored for up to 24 hours if refrigerated. Reconstituted solution in I.V. bags is stable at room temperature for up to 8 hours and may be stored for up to 16 hours if refrigerated.

WARNING **Monitor patient closely for thrombosis, because patients treated with coagulation factor Xa, inactivated-zhzo have underlying disease states that predispose them to thromboembolic events that can occur up to 30 days after drug has been administered. Expect patient to resume anticoagulant therapy as soon as possible following use of coagulation factor Xa, inactivated-zhzo to reduce the risk of thrombosis.**

PATIENT TEACHING

- Inform patient that coagulation factor Xa, inactivated-zhzo is administered in two steps: first, as an intravenous bolus; then followed by a continuous intravenous infusion that may last up to 2 hours after the bolus has been given.

WARNING **Inform patient that reversing the effects of the prescribed apixaban or rivaroxaban increases the risk of thromboembolic events for up to 30 days following the administration of coagulation factor Xa, inactivated-zhzo. Review the signs and symptoms of a blood clot that may occur in various areas of the body. Urge patient to seek immediate medical attention if a blood clot is suspected.**

codeine phosphate
codeine sulfate

Class, Category, and Schedule

Pharmacologic class: Opioid
Therapeutic class: Antitussive, opioid analgesic
Pregnancy category: C
Controlled substance schedule: II

Indications and Dosages

➤ *To treat pain severe enough to require opioid treatment and for which alternative treatment options (e.g., nonopioid analgesics or opioid combination products) are inadequate or not tolerated*

ORAL SOLUTION, TABLETS, I.M. OR SUBCUTANEOUS INJECTION

Adults. 15 to 60 mg (usual, 30 mg) every 4 to 6 hr, as needed.

➤ *To treat cough from chemical or mechanical irritation of respiratory system*

ORAL SOLUTION, TABLETS

Adults. 10 to 20 mg every 4 to 6 hr. *Maximum:* 120 mg daily.

Route	Onset	Peak	Duration
P.O.	30–45 min	1–2 hr	4 hr*
I.M.	10–30 min	30–60 min	4 hr*
SubQ	10–30 min	Unknown	4 hr*

* For pain; 4 to 6 hr for cough.

Mechanism of Action

May produce analgesia through partial metabolism to morphine. Drug binds with delta, kappa, and mu receptors in the spinal cord and with kappa$_3$ and mu$_1$ receptors higher in the CNS, decreasing intracellular cAMP, which inhibits adenylate cyclase activity and prevents release of pain neurotransmitters, such as dopamine and substance P, and altering perception of and emotional response to pain. Drug also suppresses cough by acting on opiate receptors in the cough center.

Contraindications

Acute or severe bronchial asthma in an unmonitored setting or absence of resuscitative equipment, children under the age of 12 for all uses and adolescents under the age of 18 for use with cold and cough medications; hypersensitivity to codeine, other opioids, or their components; significant respiratory depression; use for postoperative pain management in adolescents under the age of 18 who have undergone adenoidectomy and/or tonsillectomy

Interactions

DRUGS

anticholinergics, paregoric: Increased risk of severe constipation
antihypertensives, diuretics: Potentiated hypotensive effects
antimigraine agents, cyclobenzaprine; dextromethorphan; dolasetron; granisetron; linezolid; MAO inhibitors; methylene blue; ondansetron; palonosetron; selected psychiatric drugs such as amoxapine, buspirone, lithium, maprotiline, mirtazapine, nefazodone, trazodone, vilazodone; selective serotonin reuptake inhibitors; serontonin-norepinephrine reuptake inhibitors; St. John's wort; tricyclic antidepressants; tryptophan: Increased risk of serotonin syndrome
benzodiazepines, CNS depressants, sedating antihistamines, tricyclic antidepressants: Increased risk of severe respiratory depression and significant sedation and somnolence
CYP2D6 inhibitors (such as amiodarone, quinidine): Possibly increased plasma codeine concentrations but decreased active metabolite morphine plasma concentration with possible decreased effectiveness of codeine that may cause some patients to experience opioid withdrawal
CYP2D6 inhibitor that is being discontinued: Possibly decreased plasma codeine concentration but increased active metabolite morphine plasma concentration, which could increase or prolong adverse reactions and cause potentially fatal respiratory depression
CYP3A4 inducers (such as carbamazepine, phenytoin, rifampin) or discontinuation of a CYP3A4 inhibitor (such as azole antifungals, macrolide antibiotics, protease inhibitors): Decreased plasma codeine concentration with possible decreased effectiveness, causing some patients to experience opioid withdrawal
CYP3A4 inhibitors or discontinuation of a CYP3A4 inducer: Increased plasma codeine concentration leading to increased or prolonged adverse reactions and potentially fatal respiratory depression
hydroxyzine: Increased analgesia; increased CNS depressant and hypotensive effects
MAO inhibitors: Increased risk of unpredictable, severe, and sometimes fatal reactions
naloxone: Antagonized codeine effect
naltrexone: Precipitated withdrawal symptoms in codeine-dependent patients
neuromuscular blockers: Additive respiratory depressant effects
other opioids: Additive CNS and respiratory depressant, and hypotensive effects

ACTIVITIES

alcohol use: Additive CNS effects, including severe respiratory depression and significant sedation and somnolence

Adverse Reactions

CNS: Coma, delirium, depression, disorientation, dizziness, drowsiness, euphoria, hallucinations, headache, lack of coordination, lethargy, light-headedness, mental and physical impairment, mood changes, restlessness, sedation, **seizures**, tremor
CV: Bradycardia, heart block, hypertension, orthostatic hypotension, palpitations, tachycardia
EENT: Altered taste, blurred vision, diplopia, dry mouth, **laryngeal edema, laryngospasm**, miosis
ENDO: Adrenal insufficiency (rare)

C

GI: Abdominal cramps and pain, anorexia, constipation, flatulence, gastroesophageal reflux, ileus, indigestion, nausea, vomiting
GU: Decreased libido, difficult ejaculation, dysuria, erectile dysfunction, impotence, infertility with prolonged use, lack of menstruation, oliguria, ureteral spasm, urinary incontinence, urine retention
MS: Muscle rigidity
RESP: Apnea, bronchoconstriction, bronchospasm, depressed cough reflex, respiratory depression
SKIN: Diaphoresis, flushing, pallor, pruritus, rash, urticaria
Other: Anaphylaxis, angioedema, physical and psychological dependence

Nursing Considerations

- Evaluate patient's risk for abuse and addiction prior to the start of codeine therapy as excessive use of the drug may lead to abuse, addiction, misuse, overdose, and possibly death. Be prepared to monitor patient's intake throughout therapy. Because of the potential risks associated with codeine therapy, be aware that the FDA now requires a Risk Evaluation and Mitigation Strategy (REMS) for codeine use to educate the patient.

WARNING Know that codeine should not be given to children under the age of 12 for any reason and for adolescents under the age of 18 when used in cold or cough preparations, as well as following adenoidectomy and/or tonsillectomy. Also know that codeine should not be given to children age 12 to 18 if they have other risk factors that may increase their sensitivity to the respiratory depressant effects of codeine. Risk factors include conditions associated with hypoventilation such as concomitant use of other medications that cause respiratory depression or the presence of neuromuscular disease, obesity, obstructive sleep apnea, or severe pulmonary disease. In addition, codeine should not be given to patients who are known ultrarapid metabolizers of codeine, including mothers who are breastfeeding, as breast-fed infants have died when exposed to high levels of morphine (codeine converts to morphine) in breast milk. Monitor any patient receiving codeine closely, especially the patient who has never received a narcotic like codeine or morphine, for signs of overdose such as confusion, extreme sleepiness, or shallow breathing because patient may not know he is an ultrarapid metabolizer. Some patients are ultrarapid metabolizers because of a CYP2D6 polymorphism. How prevalent this phenotype is varies widely. It is estimated that 0.5% to 1% Chinese, Hispanics, and Japanese; 1% to 10% Caucasians; 3% African Americans; and 16% to 28% of Arabs, Ethiopians, and North Africans may carry the CYP2D6 genotype.

- Evaluate patient for therapeutic response, including decreased cough, facial grimacing, and pain.

WARNING Be aware that opioid therapy like codeine should only be used concomitantly with benzodiazepine therapy in patients for whom other treatment options are inadequate. If prescribed together, expect dosing and duration of the opioid to be limited. Monitor patient closely for signs and symptoms of decrease in consciousness, including coma, profound sedation, and significant respiratory depression. Notify prescriber immediately and provide emergency supportive care, as death may occur.

- Take safety precautions, if needed.
- Monitor respiratory depth, effort, and rate, because codeine can cause respiratory depression that could become life-threatening. Notify prescriber immediately if respiratory rate drops below 10 breaths/min.
- Assess urine output to detect retention.
- Repeated injection in same site may cause tissue irritation, pain, and induration.
- Rotate sites for subcutaneous delivery.

WARNING Know that many drugs may interact with opioids like codeine to cause serotonin syndrome. Monitor patient closely for signs and symptoms such as agitation, diaphoresis, diarrhea, fever, hallucinations, labile blood pressure, muscle twitching or stiffness, nausea, shakiness, shivering, tachycardia, trouble with coordination, or vomiting. Notify prescriber at once because serotonin syndrome may be life-threatening. Be prepared to discontinue drug, if possible, and provide supportive care.

- Monitor patient for adrenal insufficiency. Although rare, it can be life-threatening. Monitor patient for anorexia, dizziness, fatigue, hypotension, nausea, vomiting, or weakness. Notify prescriber if adrenal insufficiency is suspected and expect diagnostic testing to be done to determine if present. If diagnosis is confirmed, expect to administer corticosteroids and wean patient off codeine, if possible.
- Be aware that drug therapy should not be stopped abruptly in a physically dependent patient.
- Know that chronic maternal use of codeine during pregnancy can result in neonatal opioid withdrawal syndrome (NOWS), which may be life-threatening, if not recognized and treated appropriately. NOWS occurs when a newborn was exposed to opioid drugs like codeine for a prolonged period while in utero.

PATIENT TEACHING

- Instruct patient to take codeine exactly as prescribed and not to adjust dose or frequency without consulting prescriber, because misuse increases risk of addiction.
- Suggest that patient take drug with food to minimize nausea.
- Advise patient to avoid hazardous activities until drug's CNS effects are known.
- Caution patient to get up slowly from a sitting or lying position.
- Urge patient to consume plenty of fluids and high-fiber foods, if not contraindicated, to prevent constipation.

WARNING Warn patient not to consume alcohol or take a benzodiazepine during codeine therapy without prescriber knowledge, as severe respiratory depression can occur and may lead to death.

WARNING Inform patient about potentially fatal additive effects of combining codeine with a benzodiazepine. Instruct patient to inform all prescribers of codeine use.

- Advise patient to report difficulty breathing or shortness of breath.
- Urge breastfeeding women to notify prescriber before taking codeine because drug appears in breast milk and could lead to overdose in infant.
- Inform patient that long-term use of opioids like codeine may decrease sex hormone levels, causing decreased libido, erectile dysfunction, impotence, infertility, or lack of menstruation. Encourage patient to report any such symptoms.
- Caution pregnant patient not to increase dosage or take codeine for a prolonged period, because infant may experience withdrawal when born.
- Warn patient to keep codeine out of the reach of children to prevent accidental ingestion that could be life-threatening.
- Instruct patient to tell all prescribers of codeine use and not to take any over-the-counter medication, including herbal medicines, without prescriber knowledge.

colchicine

Colcrys, Mitigare

Class and Category

Pharmacologic class: Colchicum alkaloid derivative
Therapeutic class: Antigout
Pregnancy category: C

Indications and Dosages

➤ *To prevent gouty arthritis attacks*

TABLETS

Adults and adolescents age 16 and over. 0.6 mg once or twice daily. *Maximum:* 1.2 mg daily.

➤ *To treat acute gouty arthritis*

TABLETS

Adults. *Initial:* 1.2 mg at first sign of flare; then 0.6 mg 1 hr later. *Maximum:* 1.8 mg over a 1-hr period.

DOSAGE ADJUSTMENT For elderly patients, maximum dosage reduced to 2 mg/24 hr. If treatment of a gout flare occurs during prophylactic treatment, dosage shouldn't exceed 1.2 mg at the first sign of flare, followed by 0.6 mg 1 hr later, and then prophylactic dose resumed 12 hr later. For patient taking strong CYP3A4 inhibitor (atazanavir, clarithromycin, indinavir, itraconazole, ketoconazole, nefazodone, nelfinavir, ritonavir, saquinavir, telithromycin), moderate CYP3A4 inhibitor (amprenavir, aprepitant, diltiazem, erythromycin, fluconazole, fosamprenavir, grapefruit juice, verapamil), or P-gp inhibitor (cyclosporine,

ranolazine), dosage usually halved and not repeated for 3 days.
For patient with moderate to severe renal impairment, dosage adjusted on individual basis. For patient with severe hepatic impairment receiving colchicine prophylactically, dosage decreased on individual basis. For patient with severe hepatic impairment receiving colchicine treatment for acute gout flare but not prophylaxis, dosage not adjusted but treatment course shouldn't be repeated more than once every 2 weeks.

➤ *To treat familial Mediterranean fever (FMF)*

TABLETS

Adults and adolescents ages 12 and over. 1.2 mg to 2.4 mg daily, with daily total divided into two doses, if desired.
Children ages 6 to 12. 0.9 to 1.8 mg daily, with daily total divided into two doses, if desired.
Children ages 4 to 6. 0.3 to 1.8 mg daily, with daily total divided into two doses, if desired.

DOSAGE ADJUSTMENT For adults needing control of FMF, dosage increased in increments of 0.3 mg daily to a maximum of 2.4 mg daily.
For adults with intolerable adverse effects, dosage decreased in increments of 0.3 mg daily to tolerable level.
For patients taking strong CYP3A4 inhibitor (atazanavir, clarithromycin, indinavir, itraconazole, ketoconazole, nefazodone, nelfinavir, ritonavir, saquinavir, telithromycin), moderate CYP3A4 inhibitor (amprenavir, aprepitant, diltiazem, erythromycin, fluconazole, fosamprenavir, grapefruit juice, verapamil), or P-gp inhibitor (cyclosporine, ranolazine), dosage usually halved and not repeated for 3 days.
For patient with moderate to severe renal impairment or severe hepatic impairment, dosage adjusted on individual basis.

Route	Onset	Peak	Duration
P.O.	In 12 hr	In 24–48 hr	Unknown

Mechanism of Action

In gouty arthritis, leukocytes phagocytose urate crystals in affected joints, a process that releases chemotactic factors, degradation enzymes, and other inflammatory substances. Colchicine helps stop this process, probably by disrupting microtubules in leukocytes. Normally, microtubules contribute to cell structure and movement. When colchicine binds to tubulin (protein from which microtubules are made), the microtubule falls apart, as shown. This process disrupts cell function and prevents leukocytes from invading joints and causing inflammation.

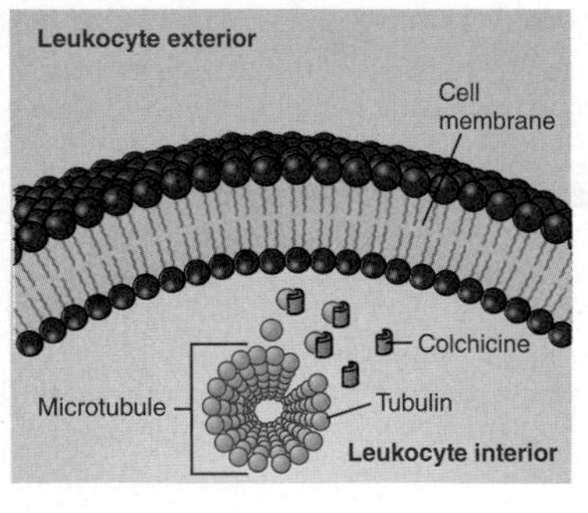

Contraindications

Concurrent use with strong CYP3A4 inhibitors or P-glycoprotein inhibitors in patients with hepatic or renal impairment; hypersensitivity to colchicine or its components; serious cardiovascular, GI, hepatic, or renal disorders

Interactions

DRUGS

digoxin; HMG-CoA reductase inhibitors, such as atorvastatin, fluvastatin, lovastatin, pravastatin, simvastatin; other lipid-lowering drugs, such as fibrates, gemfibrozil: Increased risk of myopathy and rhabdomyolysis
moderate CYP3A4 inhibitors, such as amprenavir, aprepitant, diltiazem, erythromycin, fluconazole, fosamprenavir, grapefruit juice, verapamil: Increased risk of colchicine toxicity

ACTIVITIES

alcohol use: Increased risk of adverse GI effects

Adverse Reactions

CNS: Peripheral neuropathy

GI: Abdominal pain, anorexia, diarrhea, nausea, vomiting
HEME: Agranulocytosis, aplastic anemia, thrombocytopenia
MS: Myopathy
SKIN: Alopecia, rash

Nursing Considerations

- Know that debilitated or elderly patients and those with a history of cardiac disease or impaired hepatic or renal function are at increased risk for cumulative toxicity.
- Expect to monitor CBC and platelet and reticulocyte counts at baseline and every 3 months after therapy starts.
- Notify prescriber immediately and expect to stop colchicine if patient develops evidence of toxicity, such as abdominal pain, diarrhea, nausea, or vomiting.

PATIENT TEACHING

- Instruct patient to have blood tests every 3 months, as ordered, during therapy.
- Explain that gouty arthritis pain and swelling typically subside in 24 to 48 hours after therapy begins.
- Advise patient to notify prescriber immediately if abdominal pain, diarrhea, nausea, or vomiting occurs.
- Tell patient to inform all prescribers of colchicine therapy, especially if patient has kidney or liver dysfunction because of potential drug interactions.

colesevelam hydrochloride

Welchol

Class and Category

Pharmacologic class: Bile acid sequestrant
Therapeutic class: Antilipemic, hypoglycemic
Pregnancy category: B

Indications and Dosages

➤ *As adjunct to diet and exercise to improve glycemic control in type 2 diabetes mellitus*

ORAL SUSPENSION, TABLETS

Adults. 3.75 g once daily or 1.875 g twice daily with a meal and a beverage.

➤ *As adjunct to diet and exercise to reduce elevated LDL cholesterol levels in patients with primary hypercholesterolemia as monotherapy or in combination with an HMG CoA reductase inhibitor*

ORAL SUSPENSION, TABLETS

Adults and children age 10 to 17: 3.75 g once daily or 1.875 g twice daily with a meal and a beverage.

Mechanism of Action

Binds with bile acids in intestine, preventing their absorption and forming an insoluble complex that's excreted in feces. This action decreases amount of bile acids returning through enterohepatic circulation to the liver. As a result, the liver must convert more cholesterol to bile acids, which increases liver's demand for cholesterol. This, in turn, causes increase in production and activity of the hepatic enzyme hydroxymethyl-glutaryl-coenzyme A (HMG-CoA) reductase, which is needed for cholesterol production. However, synthesis of cholesterol in the liver typically can't match the amount needed to synthesize bile acids. Because cholesterol levels can't be sustained, LDLs, lipoproteins composed mostly of cholesterol, are increasingly removed from the blood, thereby decreasing the LDL level in the blood.

How glycemic control is improved in patients with type 2 diabetes mellitus is unknown.

Contraindications

History of bowel obstruction or pancreatitis induced by hypertriglyceridemia, hypersensitivity to colesevelam or its components, serum triglyceride level greater than 500 mg/dl

Interactions

DRUGS

cyclosporine, drugs with narrow therapeutic index, glimepiride, glipizide, glyburide, olmesartan, oral contraceptives containing ethinyl estradiol and norethindrone, thyroid hormone replacement: Possibly altered effectiveness of these drugs
metformin E.R.: Increased blood metformin level, increasing risk of hypoglycemia
phenytoin: Decreased plasma phenytoin levels increasing risk of seizures
warfarin: Reduced INR, increasing risk of clotting

Adverse Reactions

CNS: Asthenia
CV: Hypertension, hypertriglyceridemia
EENT: Oral blistering, pharyngitis, rhinitis
ENDO: Hypertriglyceridemia, **hypoglycemia**
GI: Abdominal distention or pain, bowel or esophageal obstruction, constipation, dyspepsia, dysphagia, elevated liver enzymes, fecal impaction, indigestion, nausea, **pancreatitis**, worsening of hemorrhoids
MS: Myalgia
SKIN: Rash
Other: Flu-like syndrome

Nursing Considerations

- Know that colesevelam shouldn't be given to patients with gastroparesis or other GI motility disorders or to patients who had major GI tract surgery and are at risk for bowel obstruction from constipating effects.
- Use cautiously in patients with dysphagia or esophageal obstruction because size of tablet can cause dysphagia or esophageal obstruction.
- Use colesevelam cautiously in patients whose total triglycerides exceed 300 mg/dl; bile acid sequestrants can increase it.
- Evaluate patient's lipid levels before starting therapy for primary hyperlipidemia, again in 4 to 6 weeks, and then periodically, as ordered, during therapy. Expect drug to be discontinued if patient develops hypertriglyceridemia-induced pancreatitis or triglyceride level exceeds 500 mg/dl.
- Monitor diabetic patient's blood glucose level regularly, as ordered, to assess effectiveness of colesevelam therapy.
- Mix one packet of oral suspension with 4 to 8 ounces of water, fruit juice, or diet soft drinks. Stir well and have patient drink immediately.
- Know that when giving colesevelam with a drug that has a narrow therapeutic index, expect to give that drug at least 4 hours before colesevelam to prevent reduced effectiveness.
- Administer colesevelam separately from other oral drugs because colesevelam may decrease or delay absorption of other drugs.
- Make sure that patient drinks enough fluid when taking drug.

WARNING Monitor patients with preexisting constipation, who are at increased risk for developing fecal impaction.

- Monitor frequency of bowel movements and consistency of stools in patients with coronary artery disease or hemorrhoids because constipation may aggravate these conditions.

PATIENT TEACHING

- Instruct patient to take drug with meals and drink plenty of liquids when taking it.
- Tell patient to protect tablets from moisture.

WARNING Alert patient or caregiver prescribed oral suspension form that it contains phenylalanine and should not be taken by anyone who has a PKU diagnosis. If PKU is present, instruct patient not to take oral suspension and notify prescriber to get a different form of the drug.

- Instruct patient prescribed the oral suspension form to mix 1 packet with 4 to 8 ounces of diet soft drinks, fruit juice, or water; stir well; and then drink immediately. Caution patient never to ingest the contents of the packet dry.
- Caution patient against changing prescribed dosage or stopping colesevelam abruptly because serum lipid level may increase significantly.
- Remind patient that drug therapy doesn't reduce the need for dietary changes.
- Urge patient to keep regularly scheduled appointments for follow-up blood tests.
- Instruct patient to take colesevelam separately from other drugs, as it may decrease or delay absorption of other drugs.

colestipol hydrochloride

Colestid

Class and Category

Pharmacologic class: Bile acid sequestrant
Therapeutic class: Antihyperlipidemic
Pregnancy category: Not classified

Indications and Dosages

➤ *As adjunct to diet and exercise to reduce elevated serum total and LDL-C in patients with primary hypercholesterolemia*

GRANULES

Adults. *Initial:* 5 g once daily. Then, increased, as needed, by 5 g per day at 1 to 2 month intervals. *Maximum:* 30 g daily.

TABLETS

Adults.
Initial: 2 g once daily or in divided doses twice daily, increased every 1 to 2 months in 2-g increments once or twice daily. *Maximum:* 16 g daily.

Mechanism of Action

Combines with bile acids in the intestine, preventing their absorption and forming an insoluble complex that's excreted in feces. Loss of bile acids increases hepatic production of cholesterol to form new bile acids and increases oxidation of cholesterol to bile acids. Depletion of cholesterol increases hepatic LDL receptor activity, which removes LDLs from the blood.

Contraindications

Complete biliary obstruction, hypersensitivity to colestipol or its components

Interactions

DRUGS

chenodiol, ursodiol: Possibly reduced therapeutic effects of colestipol
mycophenolic acid: Possibly reduced effectiveness of mycophenolic acid
oral drugs: Possibly decreased absorption of oral drugs
penicillin G, propranolol, tetracyclines (oral), thiazide diuretics: Decreased absorption of these drugs
vancomycin (oral): Possibly marked decrease in vancomycin antibacterial action
vitamins (fat-soluble): Possibly interference with vitamin absorption

Adverse Reactions

CNS: Headache
GI: Abdominal distention and pain, constipation, diarrhea, eructation, esophageal reaction, fecal impaction, heartburn, nausea, vomiting

Nursing Considerations

- Mix colestipol granules with at least 90 ml of fluid before giving it to prevent accidental inhalation or esophageal distress.
- Give colestipol on a separate schedule from other oral drugs when possible because it may interact with various drugs.
- Make sure patient has adequate fluid intake, and obtain an order for a stool softener or laxative to prevent constipation. To prevent impaction, expect to decrease dosage or discontinue drug if constipation occurs or worsens.
- Expect to discontinue drug if no response occurs after 3 months.
- Monitor patient's serum cholesterol level as appropriate, usually at baseline, 4 to 6 weeks after starting therapy, and then every 3 months. Expect to reduce monitoring frequency to every 4 months if response is adequate.
- Be aware that HDL and serum triglyceride levels may increase or remain unchanged during colestipol therapy.
- Keep in mind that adverse GI reactions are more common in patients over age 60.

PATIENT TEACHING

- Advise patient to mix granules thoroughly in at least 90 ml of fluid so they're completely wet before drinking.
- Remind patient that colestipol doesn't reduce the importance of dietary changes.
- Caution patient not to decrease or increase prescribed dosage or to stop taking drug suddenly. Explain that stopping drug abruptly may significantly increase serum lipid levels.
- Instruct patient to keep appointments for follow-up blood tests.
- Teach patient how to prevent constipation, and advise him to contact prescriber if constipation occurs or worsens.

conivaptan hydrochloride

Vaprisol

Class and Category

Pharmacologic class: Arginine vasopressin antagonist
Therapeutic class: Aquaretic (sodium/water stabilizer)
Pregnancy category: Not classified

Indications and Dosages

➤ *To treat euvolemic and hypervolemic hyponatremia in hospitalized patients*

I.V. INFUSION

Adults. *Loading dose:* 20 mg over 30 minutes followed by 20 mg as a continuous infusion over 24 hours. Additional 20 mg daily given by continuous infusion for 1 to 3 days. *Maximum:* 40 mg daily with total duration of therapy, including loading dose, not to exceed 4 days.
DOSAGE ADJUSTMENT For patient with moderate hepatic impairment, loading dose decreased to 10 mg over 30 minutes followed by a decrease in daily dose to 10 mg/day as a continuous infusion for 2 to 4 days. If serum sodium level does not rise, dosage may be titrated up to 20 mg/day.

Route	Onset	Peak	Duration
I.V.	Unknown	24 hr	Unknown

Mechanism of Action

Binds with arginine vasopressin V2 receptor sites in collecting ducts of kidneys. By doing so, drug blocks action of arginine vasopressin on V2 receptor, decreases water resorption in collecting ducts, increases excretion of free water (urine output), and increases serum sodium concentration, thus correcting water and sodium imbalance.

Incompatibilities

Don't mix with lactated Ringer's solution, normal saline solution, or other drugs.

Contraindications

Anuria; hypersensitivity to conivaptan or its components or to corn or corn products; patients with hypovolemic hyponatremia; use with potent CYP3A4 inhibitors such as clarithromycin, indinavir, itraconazole, ketoconazole, and ritonavir

Interactions

DRUGS

clarithromycin, indinavir, itraconazole, ketoconazole, ritonavir, and other strong CYP3A inhibitors; CYP3A substrates: Increased blood conivaptan level
digoxin: Possibly increased digoxin level and risk of digoxin toxicity
drugs metabolized by CYP3A, such as HMG-CoA reductase inhibitors; CYP3A substrates: Possibly increased risk of rhabdomyolysis

Adverse Reactions

CNS: Confusion, fever, headache, insomnia
CV: **Atrial fibrillation**, hypertension, **hypotension**, orthostatic hypotension, peripheral edema
EENT: Dry mouth, oral candidiasis, pharyngeal pain
ENDO: Hyperglycemia, **hypoglycemia**
GI: Constipation, diarrhea, nausea, thirst, vomiting
GU: Hematuria, pollakiuria, polyuria, UTI
HEME: Anemia
RESP: Pneumonia
SKIN: Erythema, pruritus
Other: Dehydration, **hypokalemia**, **hypomagnesemia**, **hyponatremia**, infusion-site reactions (erythema, pain, phlebitis, swelling)

Nursing Considerations

- Know that conivaptan shouldn't be used to treat patients with heart failure nor is it recommended in patients with severe renal impairment because of a high incidence of infusion-site phlebitis, which can reduce potential vascular access sites.
- Use cautiously in patients with hepatic or mild to moderate renal dysfunction because levels remain elevated longer in these patients.
- Give drug only through large veins, and change infusion site every 24 hours. Drug may cause serious infusion-site reactions even when diluted and infused correctly. Inspect site regularly; change immediately if reactions occur.
- Dilute 20-mg (4-ml) loading dose with 100 ml of 5% dextrose injection before administration. Gently invert bag several

times to mix thoroughly. Use mixture within 24 hours, infusing over 30 minutes.
- Dilute 20-mg (4-ml) or 40-mg (8-ml) continuous infusion dose with 250 ml of D_5W before use. Gently invert the bag several times to mix thoroughly. Infuse immediately over 24 hours. If infusion is interrupted for any reason, discard any remaining solution 24 hours after mixing.
- Monitor neurologic status and serum sodium level closely during therapy because rapid increase in serum sodium level (more than 12 mEq/L/24 hr) may result in serious neurologic impairment. If serum sodium level rises faster than expected, stop infusion temporarily and notify prescriber. If it keeps rising, expect conivaptan to be discontinued. If hyponatremia persists or recurs and patient has no neurologic abnormalities, drug may be resumed at a reduced rate.
- Monitor vital signs, and assess patient regularly for hypovolemia. If patient develops hypotension or hypovolemia while receiving conivaptan, stop infusion, notify prescriber, and provide supportive care, as prescribed. After hypotension and hypovolemia have been corrected, drug may be resumed at a reduced rate.
- Store ampules in cardboard container, protected from light, until ready for use.

PATIENT TEACHING
- Instruct patient to report any infusion-site discomfort immediately.
- Tell patient that frequent laboratory tests will be performed to monitor his serum sodium level and volume status.
- Advise female patient of childbearing age not to breastfeed during conivaptan therapy.

cortisone acetate

Cortisone Acetate-ICN (CAN), Cortone (CAN), Cortone Acetate

Class and Category

Pharmacologic class: Glucocorticoid
Therapeutic class: Anti-inflammatory, corticosteroid replacement, immunosuppressant
Pregnancy category: Not classified

Indications and Dosages

➤ *To treat allergic and inflammatory disorders, collagen disorders, congenital adrenal hyperplasia, dermatologic disorders, edema (from nephrotic syndrome or systemic lupus erythematosus), GI disorders, hematologic disorders, multiple sclerosis (acute exacerbations), neoplastic diseases, primary or secondary adrenocortical insufficiency, respiratory disorders, rheumatic disorders, trichinosis with myocardial or neurologic involvement, and tuberculous meningitis*

TABLETS
Adults and adolescents. *Initial:* 25 to 300 mg once daily or equally divided and given twice. *Maintenance:* Dosage adjusted based on patient response.
Children. 2.5 to 10 mg/kg daily divided into equal doses and given every 6 to 8 hr. For adrenocortical insufficiency, 0.5 to 0.75 mg/kg/daily divided into equal doses and given every 8 hr.

I.M. INJECTION
Adults and adolescents. *Initial:* 25 to 300 mg daily. *Maintenance:* Dosage adjusted based on patient response.
Children. Highly individualized. For adrenocortical insufficiency, 0.25 to 0.35 mg/kg once daily.

Route	Onset	Peak	Duration
P.O.	Rapid	2 hr	1.25–1.5 days
I.M.	Slow	20–48 hr	1.25–1.5 days

Mechanism of Action

Binds to intracellular glucocorticoid receptors and suppresses inflammatory and immune responses by:
- inhibiting neutrophil and monocyte accumulation at the inflammation site and suppressing their phagocytic and bactericidal activity
- stabilizing lysosomal membranes
- suppressing the antigen response of macrophages and helper T cells
- inhibiting synthesis of cellular mediators of inflammatory response, such as cytokines, interleukins, and prostaglandins

Contraindications

Hypersensitivity to cortisone or its components, idiopathic thrombocytopenic purpura (parenteral form), live-virus vaccine administration, systemic fungal infection

Interactions

DRUGS

barbiturates: Decreased cortisone effectiveness, increased cortisol clearance
digitalis glycosides: Possibly digitalis toxicity
estrogens, oral contraceptives: Increased cortisone effects and risk of toxicity
hydantoins, rifampin: Increased metabolism and decreased effects of cortisone
isoniazid: Decreased blood isoniazid level
oral anticoagulants: Possibly obstructed anticoagulant effects
potassium-wasting diuretics: Possibly hypokalemia
salicylates: Decreased effectiveness and blood level of salicylates

Adverse Reactions

CNS: Ataxia, behavior changes, depression, dizziness, euphoria, fatigue, headache, **increased intracranial pressure with papilledema**, insomnia, lassitude, malaise, mood swings, paresthesia, **seizures**, steroid psychosis, syncope, vertigo
CV: Arrhythmias, fat embolism, heart failure, hypertension, **hypotension**, thrombophlebitis
EENT: Exophthalmos, glaucoma, increased intraocular pressure, nystagmus, posterior subcapsular cataracts
ENDO: Adrenal insufficiency during, Cushing's syndrome, diabetes mellitus, growth suppression in children, hyperglycemia, negative nitrogen balance from protein catabolism
GI: Abdominal distention, hiccups, increased appetite, nausea, **pancreatitis**, peptic ulcer, ulcerative esophagitis, vomiting
GU: Glycosuria, menstrual irregularities, perineal burning or tingling
HEME: Leukocytosis
MS: Arthralgia; aseptic necrosis of femoral and humeral heads; compression fractures; muscle atrophy, twitching, and weakness; myalgia; osteoporosis; spontaneous fractures; steroid myopathy; tendon rupture
SKIN: Acne; diaphoresis; ecchymosis; erythema; hirsutism; hyperpigmentation; hypopigmentation; necrotizing vasculitis; petechiae; purpura; rash; scarring; sterile abscesses; striae; subcutaneous fat atrophy; thin, fragile skin; urticaria
Other: Anaphylaxis, hypocalcemia, hypokalemia, hypokalemic alkalosis, impaired wound healing, masking of infection, **metabolic alkalosis**, suppressed skin test reaction, weight gain

Nursing Considerations

- Use cortisone cautiously in patients with ocular herpes simplex because corneal perforation may occur.
- Expect prescriber to order baseline ophthalmologic examination before therapy starts because prolonged use of cortisone may result in glaucoma, increased intraocular pressure, and damage to optic nerve.
- Assess patient for signs and symptoms of infection before giving cortisone because drug may mask them. Be aware that new infections may develop during therapy because of risk of immunosuppression. If a new infection develops, expect to administer appropriate antibiotics.
- Obtain serum electrolyte levels before therapy, as ordered, and monitor results often during therapy to detect electrolyte imbalances. Increased calcium excretion, potassium depletion, and sodium and water retention may occur with large doses of cortisone. Anticipate the need for calcium and potassium supplementation and sodium restriction, if indicated.
- Keep in mind that prescriber will order lowest effective dose.
- Expect patient to receive concurrent antacid or antihistamine therapy to prevent peptic ulcer from cortisone.

WARNING Be aware that live-virus vaccines shouldn't be given during cortisone therapy because patient may become immunosuppressed and develop the viral infection.

WARNING Assess for adrenal suppression or insufficiency (fatigue, hypotension, lassitude, nausea, vomiting, and weakness) in patient exposed to stress or receiving prolonged cortisone therapy. Notify prescriber

immediately if patient has evidence of this life-threatening adverse reaction.
- Watch for signs and symptoms of steroid psychosis (confusion, delirium, euphoria, insomnia, mood swings, personality changes, severe depression), which may develop 15 to 30 days after starting drug. Be prepared to stop drug if such signs occur. If stopping isn't possible, expect to administer a psychotropic drug.
- Watch for cushingoid signs, such as acne, buffalo hump, central obesity, ecchymosis, moon face, striae, and weight gain. Notify prescriber at once if they occur.
- Expect to taper oral cortisone dosage slowly to prevent withdrawal syndrome (abdominal or back pain, anorexia, dizziness, fever, headache, and syncope).

PATIENT TEACHING
- Instruct patient to take oral cortisone exactly as prescribed. Advise him to take it with food to prevent GI distress.
- Caution patient not to stop drug abruptly because doing so may lead to adrenal insufficiency, withdrawal symptoms, or both.
- Inform patient about adrenal insufficiency and need for possible dosage increases during stress. Advise him to notify prescriber immediately if signs or symptoms develop or if he's exposed to stress.
- Caution patient to avoid exposure to people with infections because cortisone can cause immunosuppression. Also, teach him to recognize and immediately report signs and symptoms of infection.
- Teach patient to recognize and report adverse reactions, including Cushing's syndrome.
- Urge patient receiving long-term cortisone therapy to carry medical identification.
- Recommend regular eye examinations.
- Urge patient to keep follow-up appointments with prescriber, which may include laboratory tests, to evaluate effects of therapy.

crofelemer

Mytesi

Class and Category

Pharmacologic class: Botanical
Therapeutic class: Antidiarrheal
Pregnancy category: C

Indications and Dosages

➤ *To provide symptomatic relief of non-infectious diarrhea in patients with HIV/AIDS on antiretroviral therapy*

E.R. TABLETS
Adults. 125 mg twice daily.

Mechanism of Action

Inhibits both the cyclic adenosine monophosphate (cAMP)-stimulated cystic fibrosis transmembrane conductance regulator (CFTR) chloride ion channel, and the calcium-activated chloride channel (CaCC) at the luminal membrane of enterocytes. By blocking chloride secretion and accompanying high-volume water loss in diarrhea, the flow of chloride and water in the GI tract becomes normalized.

Contraindications

Hypersensitivity to crofelemer or its components

Adverse Reactions

CNS: Anxiety, depression, dizziness
EENT: Dry mouth, nasopharyngitis, sinusitis
GI: Abdominal distention or pain, constipation, dyspepsia, elevated bilirubin or liver enzymes, flatulence, gastroenteritis, giardiasis (intestinal parasitic infection), nausea
GU: Frequent daytime urination syndrome, nephrolithiasis, UTI
HEME: Leukopenia
MS: Arthralgia: back, extremity, or musculoskeletal pain
RESP: Bronchitis, cough, upper respiratory infection
SKIN: Acne, dermatitis
Other: Herpes zoster

Nursing Considerations

- Be aware that crofelemer is used only to treat noninfectious diarrhea in patients with HIV/AIDS on antiretroviral. Infectious etiologies should be ruled out before drug is started because crofelemer is not effective against infectious causes of diarrhea.
- Know that no dosage adjustment is needed related to the patient's CD4 cell count and HIV viral load.

PATIENT TEACHING

- Instruct patient to swallow tablet whole, avoiding chewing or crushing tablet.
- Inform patient that crofelemer may be taken with or without food.
- Advise patient to inform prescriber if no improvement in diarrhea is noted.

cyclobenzaprine hydrochloride

Amrix

Class and Category

Pharmacologic class: Tricyclic antidepressant-like agent (TCA)
Therapeutic class: Skeletal muscle relaxant
Pregnancy category: B

➤ *As adjunct to rest and physical therapy for relief of muscle spasm associated with acute, painful musculoskeletal conditions*

TABLETS

Adults and adolescents age 15 and over. 5 mg three times daily, increased as needed to 10 mg three times daily. *Maximum:* 30 mg daily for no more than 3 wk.

DOSAGE ADJUSTMENT Dosage frequency reduced in elderly patients and those with hepatic impairment.

E.R. CAPSULES (AMRIX)

Adults. 15 mg once daily, increased to 30 mg once daily, as needed. *Maximum:* 30 mg once daily for no longer than 3 weeks.

Route	Onset	Peak	Duration
P.O.	1 hr	1–2 wk	12–24 hr

Mechanism of Action

Acts in the brain stem to reduce or abolish tonic muscle hyperactivity. Because cyclobenzaprine doesn't act at the neuromuscular junction or directly on skeletal muscle, it relieves muscle spasm without disrupting muscle function.

Contraindications

Acute recovery phase of MI; age less than 12; arrhythmias, including heart block and other conduction disturbances; heart failure; hypersensitivity to cyclobenzaprine or its components; hyperthyroidism; MAO inhibitor use within 14 days

Interactions

DRUGS

anticholinergics, antidyskinetics: Possibly potentiated anticholinergic effects of these drugs
bupropion, meperidine, MAO inhibitors, selective serotonin reuptake inhibitors (SSRIs), serotonin norepinephrine reuptake inhibitors (SNRIs), tramadol, tricyclic antidepressants: Possibly increased risk of serotonin syndrome
CNS depressants, tricyclic antidepressants: Possibly additive CNS depressant effects of these drugs, increased risk of adverse effects of antidepressants and cyclobenzaprine
guanadrel, guanethidine: Possibly decreased or blocked antihypertensive effects of these drugs
MAO inhibitors: Possibly hyperpyretic crisis, severe seizures, and death
tricyclic antidepressants: Increased risk of MI or stroke

ACTIVITIES

alcohol use: Possibly additive CNS depression

Adverse Reactions

CNS: Asthenia, confusion, depression, dizziness, drowsiness, fatigue, fever, headache, insomnia, irritability, nervousness, paresthesia, **seizures**, tremor, weakness
CV: Arrhythmias, including tachycardia; orthostatic hypotension; palpitations; vasodilation
EENT: Blurred vision, diplopia, dry mouth, transient vision loss, unpleasant taste
GI: Constipation, hiccups, indigestion, nausea, vomiting
GU: Libido changes, urinary frequency, urine retention
SKIN: Diaphoresis, facial flushing, pruritus, rash

Nursing Considerations

- Use cyclobenzaprine cautiously in patients with history of low seizure threshold.

- Avoid giving drug to elderly patients, if possible, because of its anticholinergic effects.

WARNING Monitor patient closely if cyclobenzaprine is being given with other serotonergic drug, especially when treatment is started and during dosage increases, because of the potential for life-threatening serotonin syndrome to develop. Assess patient for autonomic instability, mental status changes, and nervous system abnormalities. If present, stop both cyclobenzaprine and other serotonergic drugs immediately and notify prescriber. Provide supportive care, as ordered.

- Take safety precautions to prevent falls if patient is confused, dizzy, or weak.

PATIENT TEACHING

- Urge patient to avoid alcohol and other CNS depressants during therapy.
- Inform patient about possible lack of alertness and dexterity.
- Advise patient to ask for assistance with walking, driving, or hazardous activities if he experiences dizziness or weakness.

cyclosporine
(cyclosporin A)
Gengraf, Neoral, Sandimmune

Class and Category
Pharmacologic class: Polypeptide
Therapeutic class: Antipsoriatic, antirheumatic, immunosuppressant
Pregnancy category: C

Indications and Dosages
➤ *To prevent or treat organ rejection in heart, kidney, and liver allogenic transplantation*

CAPSULES, MODIFIED CAPSULES, MODIFIED ORAL SOLUTION, ORAL SOLUTION

Adults and children. *Initial:* 12 to 15 mg/kg daily in divided doses every 12 hr starting 4 to 12 hr before surgery and continuing 1 to 2 wk afterward. Then, dosage reduced by 5% every wk to maintenance dose. *Maintenance:* 5 to 10 mg/kg daily in divided doses every 12 hr.

I.V. INFUSION

Adults. 5 to 6 mg/kg daily and infused over 2 to 6 hr starting 4 to 12 hr before surgery and continuing afterward until patient can tolerate oral form of drug.

➤ *To treat severe rheumatoid arthritis*

MODIFIED CAPSULES, MODIFIED ORAL SOLUTION

Adults. 2.5 mg/kg daily in divided doses every 12 hr, increased by 0.5 to 0.75 mg/kg daily after 8 wk and again after 12 wk. *Maximum:* 4 mg/kg daily.

➤ *To treat severe plaque psoriasis in non-immunocompromised patients who have failed to respond to at least one systemic therapy or in patients for whom other systemic therapies are contraindicated, or cannot be tolerated*

MODIFIED CAPSULES, MODIFIED ORAL SOLUTION

Adults. *Initial:* 2.5 mg/kg daily in divided doses twice daily, increased by 0.5 mg/kg daily after 4 wk. Then dosage increased every 2 wk, if needed. *Maximum:* 4 mg/kg daily.

DOSAGE ADJUSTMENT For patients with severe liver dysfunction, dosage reduced. For patients receiving cyclosporine to treat psoriasis or rheumatoid arthritis and experiencing serious adverse reactions, dosage reduced 25% to 50% in effort to bring adverse reactions under control.

Mechanism of Action
Causes immunosuppression by inhibiting the proliferation of T lymphocytes, the production and release of lymphokines, and the release of interleukin-2, responsible for organ rejection and in disease processes such as psoriasis and rheumatoid arthritis.

Contraindications
Abnormal renal function, neoplastic diseases, and uncontrolled hypertension in patients with psoriasis or rheumatoid arthritis (modified capsules and oral solution); hypersensitivity to cyclosporine, its components, or polyoxyethylated castor oil (all indications; I.V. infusion for castor oil)

Interactions
DRUGS

ACE inhibitors, angiotensin II receptor antagonists, potassium-sparing diuretics, potassium supplements: Increased risk of hyperkalemia

aliskiren, ambrisentan, bosentan, colchicine, CYP3A4 substrates, dabigatran, digoxin, daunorubicin, doxorubicin, etoposide, HMG-CoA reductase inhibitors (statins), methotrexate, mitoxantrone, NSAIDs, organic anion transporter protein substrates, P-glycoprotein substrates, prednisolone, repaglinide, sirolimus: Increased blood concentrations of these drugs and possible toxicity
allopurinol, amiodarone, azithromycin, bromocriptine, clarithromycin, colchicine, danazol, diltiazem, erythromycin, fluconazole, HIV protease inhibitors, imatinib, itraconazole, ketoconazole, methylprednisolone, metoclopramide, nefazodone, nicardipine, oral contraceptives, quinupristin and dalfopristin, verapamil, voriconazole: Increased cyclosporine level
amphotericin B, azapropazone, cimetidine, ciprofloxacin, colchicine, co-trimoxazole, diclofenac, fibric acid derivatives (bezafibrate, fenofibrate), gentamicin, ketoconazole, melphalan, naproxen, NSAIDs, ranitidine, sulindac, tacrolimus, tobramycin, vancomycin: Increased risk of nephrotoxicity
atorvastatin, fluvastatin, lovastatin, pravastatin, simvastatin: Risk of myotoxicity
bosentan, carbamazepine, nafcillin, octreotide, orlistat, oxcarbazepine, phenobarbital, phenytoin, rifampin, St. John's wort, sulfinpyrazone, terbinafine, ticlopidine: Decreased blood cyclosporine level and therapeutic response
methotrexate: Increased blood methotrexate level and risk of renal dysfunction
methylprednisolone (high dose): Increased risk of seizures
nifedipine: Increased risk of gingival hyperplasia
other immunosuppressants: Possibly excessive immunosuppression
repaglinide: Possibly increased repaglinide level and risk of hypoglycemia
vaccines (killed or live virus): Possibly suppressed immune response and increased adverse effects of vaccine

FOODS

grapefruit, grapefruit juice: Increased risk of nephrotoxicity; increased plasma concentration of cyclosporine
potassium-rich foods: Increased risk of hyperkalemia

Adverse Reactions

CNS: Altered level of consciousness, confusion, **encephalopathy**, headache, **intracranial hypertension**, lethargy, loss of motor function, migraine, **neurotoxicity**, paresthesia, **progressive multifocal leukoencephalopathy**, **posterior reversible encephalopathy syndrome (PRES)**, psychiatric disturbances, **seizures**, tremor
CV: Chest pain, hypertension, **MI**
EENT: Gingival hyperplasia, optic disc edema, oral candidiasis, sinusitis, visual impairment including blindness
ENDO: Gynecomastia
GI: Cholestasis, diarrhea, **hepatitis**, **hepatotoxicity**, jaundice, **liver failure**, nausea, **pancreatitis**, vomiting
GU: Albuminuria, elevated serum creatinine and blood urea nitrogen levels, glomerular capillary thrombosis, hematuria, **nephropathy associated with BK virus**, **nephrotoxicity**, proteinuria, **renal failure**
HEME: Anemia, **leukopenia**, **thrombocytopenia**
MS: Lower extremity pain
SKIN: Acne, **cancer**, flushing, hirsutism, pruritus, rash
Other: Anaphylaxis; bacterial, fungal, protozoal, and viral infections including opportunistic infections such as polyomavirus; hyperkalemia; **hypomagnesemia**; **life-threatening infections**; **lymphoma and other malignancies**

Nursing Considerations

- Be aware that capsules and oral solution aren't interchangeable with modified capsules and modified oral solution. Modified forms have greater bioavailability. Also know that Neoral is not bioequivalent to Sandimmune and requires close monitoring of blood concentration to avoid the potential of underdosing if a conversion from Neoral to Sandimmune is ordered.
- Prepare I.V. infusion by diluting each milliliter of concentrate in 20 to 100 ml of normal saline solution or D_5W. Use glass containers because of possible leaching of diethylhexyphthalate from polyvinyl chloride bags into cyclosporine solution.

- Administer I.V. infusion over 2 to 6 hr. If needed, drug may be infused over 24 hr.

WARNING Be aware that rapid I.V. infusion may cause acute nephrotoxicity.

- Don't draw blood to measure cyclosporine level through same I.V. tubing used to administer drug, even if line was flushed after administration. Blood level may be falsely elevated.
- Discard diluted solution after 24 hours.
- Be aware that intravenous and oral solutions contain alcohol and shouldn't be administered to patient who drinks heavily or has a history of alcohol dependence. In addition, these forms of cyclosporine should not used in patients in whom alcohol intake should be avoided or minimized, such as breastfeeding or pregnant women, patients with epilepsy or liver disease, and children. Be aware that for an adult weighing 70 kg or 150 pounds, the maximum daily oral dose would deliver about 6% and a daily intravenous dose would deliver about 15% of the amount of alcohol contained in a standard drink.
- Don't add water to oral solution because it will alter drug's effectiveness.
- Avoid giving oral cyclosporine with grapefruit juice, which may raise trough level, increasing risk of nephrotoxicity.

WARNING Monitor patient closely for hypersensitivity reactions, especially at the beginning of cyclosporine therapy and for at least the first 30 minutes following the start of an intravenous dose and then frequently thereafter. Know that while anaphylaxis may rarely occur, anaphylactic reactions have not occurred with the use of soft gelatin capsules or oral solution that did not contain Cremophor EL (polyoxyethylated castor oil). If anaphylaxis occurs, stop drug immediately and be prepared to administer epinephrine and oxygen, as ordered.

- Monitor blood pressure, especially in patients with a history of hypertension, because drug can worsen this condition. Expect to decrease dosage if hypertension develops.
- Monitor liver and renal function tests, as ordered, to detect decreased function. Be aware that it is not unusual for serum creatinine and BUN levels to be elevated during cyclosporine therapy. These elevations warrant investigation but do not always reflect kidney transplant rejection. If not related to rejection, a dosage reduction of cyclosporine often helps to decrease these levels.
- Be aware that an association between the development of interstitial fibrosis and higher cumulative doses or persistently high circulating trough concentrations of cyclosporine, especially during first 6 months post-transplant, may increase the risk of chronic nephrotoxicity.
- Be aware that although uncommon, cyclosporine may cause neurotoxicity, especially after liver transplantation. Watch for evidence of encephalopathy (impaired consciousness, loss of motor function, psychiatric disturbance, seizures, visual disturbance). Notify prescriber immediately if present, and expect cyclosporine dosage to be decreased or the drug discontinued to increase possibility of a reversible or improvement of encephalopathy. Also monitor patients closely for seizures, especially if they are also receiving high-dose methylprednisolone therapy.
- Be aware that cyclosporine use may result in increased serum cholesterol levels.
- Be aware that St. John's wort may decrease blood cyclosporine level.
- Store capsules at 25°C (77°F) in prepackaged foil wrap to protect them from light.
- Expect about 50% of patients treated for psoriasis to relapse about 4 months after therapy stops. Know that patients with chronic plaque psoriasis may develop erythrodermic psoriasis or generalized pustular psoriasis when cyclosporine dose is reduced or drug is discontinued.

WARNING Watch for evidence of infection (such as cough, fever, malaise, pain) because patients receiving immunosuppressants such as cyclosporine are at increased risk for bacterial, fungal, parasitic, and viral infection. Watch for both generalized and localized infections, including worsening of preexisting infections, and be aware that these infections may become life-threatening.

Activation of latent viral infections may also occur and include BK virus–associated nephropathy that can lead to decreased renal function and renal graft loss.

PATIENT TEACHING

- Instruct patient to take drug at same time each day and in same relation to type and timing of food intake to help increase compliance and maintain steady blood level.
- Advise patient to mix oral solution in a glass—not plastic—container with room-temperature orange or apple juice to improve flavor. Caution him to avoid grapefruit juice because it alters drug metabolism.
- Instruct patient to use syringe supplied by manufacturer to ensure accurate measurement of oral solution dose and to wipe—not rinse—syringe after use to prevent cloudiness.
- Advise patient not to stop taking drug without consulting prescriber.
- Instruct patient to avoid virus vaccines during therapy and people who have received such vaccines. Or, suggest wearing a protective mask when he's around them.
- Caution patient to avoid people who have infections during therapy because cyclosporine causes immunosuppression.
- Advise good dental hygiene because of risk of gingival hyperplasia.
- Advise patient to discard oral solution after it has been opened for 2 months.
- Inform patient with rheumatoid arthritis that drug effects may not appear for 4 to 6 weeks.
- Caution patient to avoid excessive exposure to ultraviolet light.

D

dabigatran etexilate

Pradaxa

Class and Category

Pharmacologic class: Direct thrombin inhibitor
Therapeutic class: Anticoagulant
Pregnancy category: Not classified

Indications and Dosages

➤ *To reduce the risk of stroke and systemic embolism in patients with nonvalvular atrial fibrillation*

CAPSULES

Adults with creatinine clearance greater than 30 ml/min. 150 mg twice daily.
Adults with creatinine clearance between 15 and 30 ml/min. 75 mg twice daily.
DOSAGE ADJUSTMENT For patient with a creatinine level between 30 and 50 ml/min and taking dronedarone or systemic ketoconazole concomitantly, dosage decreased to 75 mg twice daily.

➤ *To treat deep vein thrombosis and pulmonary emboli; to reduce risk of recurrence of deep vein thrombosis and pulmonary emboli*

CAPSULES

Adults with creatinine clearance greater than 30 ml/min. 150 mg twice daily after 5 to 10 days of parenteral anticoagulation.

➤ *To prevent deep vein thrombosis and pulmonary embolism following a hip replacement*

CAPSULES

Adults with creatinine clearance greater than 30 ml/min. 110 mg 1 to 4 hr after surgery and after hemostasis has been achieved on first day, then 220 mg once daily for 28 to 35 days.
DOSAGE ADJUSTMENT For patient with creatinine clearance less than 50 ml/min and prescribed a P-gp inhibitor, dabigatran discontinued.

Route	Onset	Peak	Duration
P.O.	Unknown	1 hr (fasting) 2 hr (after high-fat meal)	Unknown

Mechanism of Action

Directly inhibits thrombin from converting fibrinogen into fibrin during the coagulation cascade. Inhibition of this activity prevents the development of a blood clot.

Contraindications

Active pathologic bleeding, hypersensitivity to dabigatran or its components, presence of mechanical prosthetic heart valve

Interactions

DRUGS

dronedarone, ketoconazole: Increased dabigatran exposure
P-gp inducers such as rifampin: Decreased exposure to dabigatran
P-gp inhibitors: Increased exposure to dabigatran in patients with renal impairment
rifampin: Reduced effectiveness of rifampin

Adverse Reactions

CNS: Intracranial or intraspinal hemorrhage
CV: Pericardial bleeding
EENT: Intraocular bleeding
GI: Diarrhea, dyspepsia, esophageal ulcer, gastritis-like symptoms, **gastrointestinal hemorrhage**, nausea, **retroperitoneal bleeding**, upper abdominal pain
HEME: Bleeding (serious), **thrombocytopenia**
MS: Intra-articular bleeding, intramuscular bleeding with compartment syndrome
SKIN: Pruritus, rash, urticaria
Other: Anaphylactic reaction or shock, **angioedema**

Nursing Considerations

- Assess renal function, as ordered, prior to beginning dabigatran therapy because dose is based on the patient's creatinine level. Continue to monitor the patient's serum creatinine level throughout therapy, as ordered, and expect frequency of serum creatinine tests to increase if patient develops a condition that affects renal function because a dosing adjustment may be required. Know that the drug should be discontinued if the patient develops acute renal failure.

- Be aware that patients converting from warfarin to dabigatran therapy should begin dabigatran therapy when their international normalized ratio (INR) is below 2.0.
- Expect patients converting from dabigatran to warfarin therapy to do so based on their creatinine clearance level. For patients who have a creatinine clearance level greater than 50 ml/min, expect warfarin to be started 3 days before dabigatran is discontinued. For patients who have a creatinine clearance level of 31 to 50 ml/min, expect warfarin to be started 2 days before dabigatran is discontinued. For patients who have a creatinine clearance level of 15 to 30 ml/min, expect warfarin to be started 1 day before dabigatran is discontinued. No recommendations are available for patients who have a creatinine clearance level of less than 15 ml/min.
- Be aware that degree of anticoagulation does not need to be assessed by routine laboratory testing with dabigatran use. However, when necessary, expect the prescriber to use activated partial thromboplastin time (aPTT) or ecarin clotting time (ECT), and not INR, to assess for anticoagulant activity for the patient receiving dabigatran therapy.
- Know that dabigatran can elevate the patient's INR. Therefore, when patients are transitioned, dabigatran must be stopped for at least 2 days before the most accurate effects of warfarin can be known.
- Begin dabigatran therapy, as ordered, for a patient currently receiving a parenteral anticoagulant, such as heparin, within 2 hours before the next dose of the parenteral drug was to have been administered. If the parenteral anticoagulant being used is continuous in nature, expect to begin dabigatran therapy upon discontinuation of the continuously administered parenteral anticoagulant.
- Expect to begin treatment with a parenteral anticoagulant, if ordered, 12 hours after the patient's final dabigatran dose if the patient has a creatinine clearance of 30 ml/min or greater, and 24 hours after the patient's final dabigatran dose if the patient's creatinine clearance is less than 30 ml/min.
- Know that dabigatran therapy should be discontinued, if possible, 1 to 2 days before invasive or surgical procedures for patients with a creatinine clearance of 50 ml/min or more, and 3 to 5 days for patients whose creatinine clearance is less than 50 ml/min because of the increased risk for bleeding. Longer times may be required for patients undergoing major surgery, spinal puncture, or placement of a spinal or epidural catheter or port, in whom complete hemostasis is required. If surgery cannot be postponed, monitor patient closely for bleeding and assess bleeding risk with the ECT. If an ECT measurement is not possible, know that the aPTT can provide an approximation of dabigatran's anticoagulant activity.

WARNING Monitor patient closely for bleeding because dabigatran increases risk for bleeding, which can become severe. Bleeding risk increases in patients taking concurrent antiplatelet drugs, fibrinolytic therapy, heparin, or with chronic use of NSAIDs. It also increases during labor and delivery. Monitor patient very closely. Promptly report any signs or symptoms of bleeding such as a drop in hemoglobin and/or hematocrit or the development of hypotension or overt bleeding. Expect to discontinue drug if active bleeding occurs and is persistent or serious. Know that protamine sulfate and vitamin K will not affect the anticoagulant activity of dabigatran. Instead, the prescriber may prescribe platelet concentrates if thrombocytopenia is present or the patient has been exposed to long-acting antiplatelet drugs. If bleeding is life-threatening or uncontrolled or emergency surgery or urgent procedures are necessary, expect to administer idarucizumab to reverse the anticoagulant effect of dabigatran.

- Know that premature discontinuation of dabigatran increases the risk of thrombotic events. Be aware that patients receiving spinal/epidural anesthesia or a spinal puncture are at risk of developing an epidural or spinal hematoma, which can result in long-term or permanent paralysis. Monitor patient frequently for signs or symptoms of neurologic impairment. Notify prescriber immediately if patient complains of bladder or bowel dysfunction, midline back pain, or numbness, tingling, or weakness in the lower extremities.
- Assess patient closely for stroke if dabigatran therapy must be discontinued temporarily because of an active bleed, elective surgery, or an invasive procedure. Also, be aware that premature discontinuation of the drug increases risk of thrombotic events. Know that therapy should be restarted as soon as possible. If the drug must be discontinued for reasons other than pathological bleeding, expect patient to receive coverage with another anticoagulant to decrease the risk of thrombotic events, such as stroke.

WARNING Be on the alert for an epidural or spinal hematoma formation in patients receiving dabigatran and neuraxial anesthesia or undergoing spinal puncture. This hematoma may result in long-term or permanent paralysis. Assess patient frequently for signs and symptoms of neurological impairment. If present, notify prescriber immediately as urgent treatment is necessary.

PATIENT TEACHING

- Tell patient to take dabigatran exactly as prescribed.
- Instruct patient to swallow capsule whole without breaking, chewing, or emptying the contents of the capsule prior to ingestion.
- Tell patient that if she misses a dose, she should take it as soon as she remembers on the same day she missed the dose, unless it is within 6 hours of the next dose. She should never double a dose to make up for a missed dose.
- Instruct patient to keep bottle tightly closed when not in use and store in the original package to protect from moisture. Have patient date bottle when opened and tell her to discard any remaining drug if not used within 4 months of initially opening the bottle.
- Urge patient to take precautions against bleeding, such as using an electric shaver and a soft-bristled toothbrush.
- Caution patient to avoid activities that could cause traumatic injury and bleeding.
- Urge patient to notify prescriber immediately about unusual bleeding and any unexplained symptoms, such as abnormal vaginal bleeding; dizziness; easy bruising; gum bleeding; red or dark brown urine; stools that are black or tarry; vomiting blood or vomit that looks like coffee grounds; and weakness.
- Caution patient not to stop taking dabigatran abruptly.
- Urge patient to carry medical identification that reveals she is taking dabigatran.
- Tell patient to inform all healthcare providers that she is taking dabigatran and not to take any medication, including OTC drugs, without first consulting the prescriber.
- Warn mothers not to breastfeed while taking dabigatran because of increased risk of bleeding in the infant.

daclatasvir

Daklinza

Class and Category

Pharmacologic class: Hepatitis C virus NS5A inhibitor
Therapeutic class: Antiviral
Pregnancy category: Not classified

Indications and Dosages

➤ *As adjunct to treat chronic hepatitis C virus (HCV) genotype 1 or genotype 3 infection concomitantly with sofosbuvir therapy and with or without ribavirin therapy*

TABLETS

Adults. 60 mg once daily for 12 wk.

DOSAGE ADJUSTMENT For patients taking certain HIV antiviral agents such as atazanavir with ritonavir, indinavir, nelfinavir, or saquinavir and strong CYP3A inhibitors, dosage reduced to 30 mg once daily. For patients taking moderate CYP3A inducers or nevirapine, dosage increased to 90 mg once daily.

Mechanism of Action

Inhibits both viral RNA replication and virion assembly against the hepatitis C virus to destroy it.

Contraindications

Concurrent therapy with drugs that strongly induce CYP3A, such as carbamazepine, phenytoin, rifampin, or St. John's wort; hypersensitivity to daclatasvir or its components

Interactions

DRUGS

amiodarone, sofosbuvir: Increased risk of significant bradycardia
buprenorphine, buprenorphine/naloxone: Possible increased risk of buprenorphine-associated adverse reactions
dabigatran etexilate mesylate: Increased plasma dabigatran level with increased risk of adverse reactions
digoxin: Increased risk of digitalis toxicity
HMG-CoA reductase inhibitors such as atorvastatin, fluvastatin, pitavastatin, pravastatin, rosuvastatin, simvastatin: Increased plasma concentration of HMG-CoA reductase inhibitors with increased risk of adverse reactions.
moderate CYP3A inducers such as bosentan, dexamethasone, modafinil, nafcillin, rifapentine; non-nucleoside reverse transcriptase inhibitors (NNRTI) such as efavirenz, etravirine, nevirapine: Possibly decreased plasma daclatasvir level with possible decreased effectiveness
other antiretrovirals such as atazanavir/cobicistat, elvitegravir/cobicistat/emtricitabine/tenofovir disoproxil fumarate; protease inhibitors such as atazanavir with ritonavir, indinavir, nelfinavir, saquinavir; strong CYP3A inhibitors such as clarithromycin, itraconazole, ketoconazole, nefazodone, posaconazole, telithromycin, voriconazole: Possibly increased plasma daclatasvir level with possible increased risk of adverse reactions

Adverse Reactions

CNS: Dizziness, fatigue, headache, insomnia, somnolence
CV: Bradycardia
GI: Diarrhea, elevated liver and pancreatic enzymes, hyperbilirubinemia, nausea
HEME: Anemia
SKIN: Rash

Nursing Considerations

- Know that patient should be tested for hepatitis B before starting daclatasvir therapy, because HBV reactivation has occurred in HCV/HBV co-infected patients when given treatment with HCV direct-acting antivirals such as daclatasvir who were not receiving HBV antiviral therapy. Fulminant hepatitis, hepatic failure, and even death have occurred. Monitor co-infected patients for HBV reactivation or hepatitis flare during daclatasvir therapy. If HBV infection is detected, expect treatment to be given.
- Be aware that daclatasvir must be given with sofosbuvir, with or without ribavirin, in the treatment of chronic hepatitis C. If sofosbuvir is discontinued, know that daclatasvir should also be discontinued.

WARNING Monitor patient's heart rate closely, as serious symptomatic bradycardia may occur because of coadministration with sofosbuvir and amiodarone. Bradycardia most often occurs during the first 2 weeks of daclatasvir therapy. Expect patient to have cardiac monitoring in an inpatient setting for the first 48 hr of daclatasvir therapy, followed by patient monitoring of pulse for the first 2 weeks of therapy. Know that patients at greater risk for bradycardia include patients receiving amiodarone or beta blocker therapy or patients who have advanced liver disease or underlying cardiac disease.

PATIENT TEACHING

- Tell patient that daclatasvir is never prescribed alone to treat hepatitis C and will be combined with another drug called sofosbuvir and possibly a third drug called ribavirin.
- Instruct patient to take daclatasvir once daily at the same time every day after taking pulse.
- Stress importance of not stopping daclatasvir therapy without prescriber knowledge.
- Inform patient that HBV reactivation can occur in patients co-infected with HBV during or after treatment of HCV infection. Tell patient to inform prescriber if she has a history of hepatitis B.

- Tell patient to notify all prescribers of daclatasvir therapy, because significant drug interactions can occur between daclatasvir and many other drugs.

WARNING Instruct patient how to take pulse. Stress importance of patient seeking immediate medical attention if she develops signs or symptoms of bradycardia such as chest pain, confusion, dizziness, excessive tiredness, fainting, lightheadedness, malaise, shortness of breath, or weakness.

- Instruct female patient of childbearing age to avoid pregnancy during therapy and for 6 months after completion of treatment. Tell her to notify prescriber if pregnancy occurs or is suspected.
- Advise mothers who wish to breastfeed to discuss the benefits and risks with prescriber before doing so.

dalbavancin

Dalvance

Class and Category

Pharmacologic class: Lipoglycopeptide
Therapeutic class: Antibacterial antibiotic
Pregnancy category: C

Indications and Dosages

➤ *To treat acute bacterial skin and skin structure infections caused by* Staphylococcus aureus *(including methicillin-susceptible and methicillin-resistant strains),* Streptococcus agalactiae, S. anginosus *group (including* S. anginosus, S. constellatus, *and* S. intermedius*) and* S. pyogenes

I.V. INFUSION

Adults. 1,500 mg infused as a single dose over 30 min. Alternatively, 1,000 mg infused over 30 min, followed by 500 mg infused over 30 min 1 wk later.

DOSAGE ADJUSTMENT For patients with renal impairment (creatinine clearance less than 30 ml/min) and who are not receiving hemodialysis, initial dosage reduced to 1,125 mg as a single dose or 750 mg, followed by 375 mg 1 wk later.

Mechanism of Action

Interferes with bacterial cell wall synthesis, which leads to impaired bacterial cell growth or cell death.

Incompatibilities

Do not co-infuse with other medications or electrolytes. Also, do not mix or infuse with saline-based infusion solutions because a precipitation may occur.

Contraindications

Hypersensitivity to dalbavancin or its components

Adverse Reactions

CNS: Dizziness, headache
EENT: Oral candidiasis
ENDO: **Hypoglycemia**
GI: Abdominal pain, ***Clostridium difficile*-associated colitis**, diarrhea, elevated liver enzymes, **gastrointestinal hemorrhage**, **hepatotoxicity**, **melena**, nausea, passage of bright red blood through anus
GU: Vulvovaginal mycotic infection
HEME: Anemia, **elevated international normalized ratio (INR)**, eosinophilia, **hemorrhagic anemia**, **leukopenia**, **neutropenia**, spontaneous hematoma, thrombocytosis, **thrombocytopenia**
MS: Back pain
RESP: **Bronchospasm**
SKIN: Flushing of upper body, petechiae, pruritus, rash, urticaria
Other: **Anaphylaxis**, phlebitis, red man syndrome (with rapid infusion), **wound hemorrhage**

Nursing Considerations

- Use cautiously in patients with a history of glycopeptides allergy because of a possibility of cross-sensitivity.
- Use cautiously in patients with a history of hepatic impairment because dosing adjustments for dalbavancin in patients with moderate to severe hepatic impairment are not known. Dosage adjustment is not required for patients with mild hepatic impairment.
- Reconstitute with 25 ml of sterile water for injection, USP for each 500-mg vial. Avoid foaming by alternating between gently

swirling and inverting the vial until contents are completely dissolved. Do not shake. Solution should appear clear and colorless to yellow. Once reconstituted, the vial may be refrigerated for up to 48 hours. Do not freeze. Prior to administration, further dilute reconstituted vial by aseptically transferring the required dose from the vial to an intravenous bag or bottle containing enough solution of 5% dextrose injection, USP to provide a final dalbavancin concentration of 1 to 5 mg/ml. Discard any unused portion of the reconstituted solution. Once diluted, the intravenous bag or bottle may be refrigerated until administration as long as the total time from the vial being reconstituted until administration does not exceed 48 hours. Never freeze the diluted solution.

- Administer as an intravenous infusion over 30 minutes to minimize the risk of infusion-related reactions that resemble red man syndrome, such as flushing of the upper body, pruritus, rash, or urticaria. Monitor patient for back pain, which also has been identified as an infusion-related reaction. If present, stopping or slowing the infusion may cause these reactions to disappear. Always flush intravenous line with 5% dextrose injection, USP before and after administration if the line is used to administer other drugs.
- Assess patient for signs of secondary infection, such as profuse, watery diarrhea. If such diarrhea develops, contact prescriber and expect to obtain a stool specimen to rule out pseudomembranous colitis caused by *C. difficile*. If diarrhea occurs, notify prescriber and expect to withhold dalbavancin and treat patient with an antibiotic effective against *C. difficile* along with electrolytes, fluids, and protein.

PATIENT TEACHING

- Emphasize importance of obtaining second dose of dalbavancin if patient was prescribed the two-dose regimen.
- Tell patient to immediately report any signs and symptoms of an allergic reaction.
- Advise patient to report severe diarrhea to prescriber immediately.

dalteparin sodium (tedelparin)

Fragmin

Class and Category

Pharmacologic class: Low-molecular-weight heparin
Therapeutic class: Anticoagulant
Pregnancy category: Not classified

Indications and Dosages

➤ *To prevent ischemic complications in patients who receive aspirin as part of treatment for unstable angina and non-Q-wave MI*

SUBCUTANEOUS INJECTION

Adults. 120 international units/kg every 12 hr with aspirin (75 to 165 mg daily) until patient is stable, usually 5 to 8 days. *Maximum:* 10,000 international units/dose.

➤ *To prevent blood clots in patients undergoing hip replacement surgery*

SUBCUTANEOUS INJECTION

Adults. *Initial:* 2,500 international units 4 to 8 hr after surgery (or later if hemostasis has not been achieved) and then 5,000 international units once daily for 5 to 10 days postoperatively or 2,500 international units 1 to 2 hr before surgery, repeated in 4 to 8 hr after surgery and then 5,000 international units once daily for 5 to 10 days postoperatively. Alternatively, 5,000 international units the evening before surgery followed by 5,000 international units 4 to 8 hr after surgery and then 5,000 international units once daily for 5 to 10 days postoperatively.

➤ *To prevent blood clots in patients undergoing abdominal surgery who are at risk for thromboembolic complications*

SUBCUTANEOUS INJECTION

Adults. 2,500 international units daily, starting 1 to 2 hr before surgery and repeated once daily for 5 to 10 days. For patients at high risk (i.e., those with cancer), 5,000 international units the evening before surgery, repeated once daily for 5 to 10 days; or alternatively for patients with cancer, 2,500 international units 1 to 2 hr before surgery followed by 2,500 international units 12 hr later and then 5,000 international units once daily for 5 to 10 days.

➤ *To prevent blood clots in patients with severe mobility restrictions during acute illness*

SUBCUTANEOUS INJECTION

Adults. 5,000 international units once daily for 12 to 14 days.

➤ *To provide extended treatment of symptomatic venous thromboembolism in patients with cancer*

SUBCUTANEOUS INJECTION

Adults. 200 international units/kg once daily for 30 days. Then 150 international units/kg once daily for 5 more months. *Maximum:* 18,000 international units daily.

DOSAGE ADJUSTMENT For patient who experiences a platelet count between 50,000 and 100,000/mm^3, dosage reduced by 2,500 international units until platelet count recovers to or above 100,000 mm^3. For patient who experiences a platelet count less than 50,000 mm^3, dalteparin withheld until platelet count is above 50,000 mm^3. For patient with severely impaired renal function (creatinine clearance below 30 ml/min), anti-Xa levels monitored to determine appropriate dose. Target anti-Xa range is 0.5 to 1.5 international units/ml.

Mechanism of Action

Binds to and accelerates the activity of antithrombin III, thus inhibiting thrombin and blocking the formation of fibrin clots.

Incompatibilities

Don't mix dalteparin with other drugs.

Contraindications

Active major bleeding; history of heparin-induced thrombocytopenia or heparin-induced thrombocytopenia with thrombosis; hypersensitivity to dalteparin, other low-molecular-weight heparins, heparin, or pork products; treatment for unstable angina and non-Q-wave MI or for prolonged venous thromboembolism prophylaxis while undergoing epidural/neuraxial anesthesia

Interactions

DRUGS

NSAIDs, oral anticoagulants, platelet aggregation inhibitors, thrombolytics: Possibly increased risk of hemorrhage and spinal or epidural hematoma

Adverse Reactions

GI: Elevated liver enzymes
HEME: **Hemorrhage**, **thrombocytopenia**
SKIN: Alopecia, bullous eruption, necrosis, pruritus, rash
Other: **Anaphylaxis**, injection-site hematoma and pain

Nursing Considerations

- Use dalteparin with extreme caution in patients with a history of heparin-induced thrombocytopenia; those at increased risk for hemorrhage (such as those who use a platelet inhibitor or have active ulcerative GI disorder, bacterial endocarditis, bleeding disorders, hemorrhagic stroke, or uncontrolled hypertension); and those with recent brain, eye, or spinal surgery.
- Use drug cautiously in patients with bleeding diathesis, diabetic retinopathy, platelet defects, recent GI bleeding, severe hepatic or renal insufficiency, or thrombocytopenia.
- Inform Jewish or Islamic patients that drug comes from porcine intestine before giving first dose.

WARNING Question patient regarding use of aspirin and other NSAIDs, platelet inhibitors or other anticoagulants prior to dalteparin therapy that may increase risk of bleeding.

- Be aware that risk factors for thromboembolic events include age over 40, cancer, history of deep vein thrombosis or pulmonary embolism, obesity, and planned use of anesthesia for more than 30 minutes.

D

- Don't give drug by I.M. or I.V. injection.
- Administer drug deep into subcutaneous tissue in U-shaped area around navel, upper outer thigh, or upper outer quadrant of buttocks with patient seated. If using area around navel or on thigh, lift skin fold with thumb and forefinger while giving injection. Insert entire length of needle at a 45- to 90-degree angle. Rotate sites daily.
- Know that routine coagulation tests and dosage adjustments usually aren't required.

WARNING Monitor patient receiving dalteparin and epidural or spinal anesthesia or spinal puncture because spinal hematomas can occur, causing long-term or permanent paralysis. Watch for evidence of neurologic impairment, such as changes in motor or sensory. If present, notify prescriber immediately; patient needs urgent care to minimize effect of hematoma. Use of indwelling epidural catheters; concurrent use of other drugs that affect hemostasis such as nonsteroidal anti-inflammatory drugs, platelet inhibitors, and other anticoagulants; a history of traumatic or repeated epidural or spinal punctures; or a history of spinal deformity or spinal surgery increase the risk of spinal or epidural hematoma in patients receiving dalteparin.

PATIENT TEACHING

- Teach patient or caregiver administering drug at home how to select injection sites, give subcutaneous injections, and rotate sites daily. Tell patient to discard drug if it's discolored or contains particles. Review safe handling and disposal of syringes and needles.
- Teach patient to store drug at room temperature, away from moisture and heat.
- Urge patient to report adverse reactions, especially bleeding, and to seek help immediately if signs of blood clots develop, such as severe difficulty breathing or changes in mental status or motor or sensory abnormalities.
- Instruct patient to inform all dentists and prescribers of dalteparin therapy. Tell patient who is receiving spinal anesthesia or a spinal puncture to alert medical staff immediately if he experiences muscular weakness, numbness (especially in his legs), or tingling following the procedure.
- Emphasize the importance of follow-up visits.

dantrolene sodium

Dantrium, Dantrium Intravenous, Revonto, Ryanodex

Class and Category

Pharmacologic class: Skeletal muscle relaxant
Therapeutic class: Antispastic, malignant hyperthermia therapy adjunct
Pregnancy category: C

Indications and Dosages

➤ *To treat chronic spastic conditions caused by severe chronic disorders, such as cerebral palsy, multiple sclerosis, spinal cord injury, and stroke*

CAPSULES

Adults. *Initial:* 25 mg daily for 7 days. Then dosage increased to 25 mg three times a day for 7 days followed by 50 mg three times a day for 7 days, to 100 mg three to four times a day. *Maximum:* 400 mg daily.
Children. *Initial:* 0.5 mg/kg once daily for 7 days. Then dosage increased to 0.5 mg/kg three times daily for 7 days followed by 1 mg/kg three times daily for 7 days and then 2 mg/kg three or four times daily.

➤ *To prevent malignant hyperthermia before surgery*

CAPSULES

Adults and children. 4 to 8 mg/kg daily in divided doses three times daily or four times daily 1 or 2 days before surgery, with last dose given 3 to 4 hr before surgery.

I.V. INFUSION (DANTRIUM INTRAVENOUS, REVONTO)

Adults and children. *Initial:* 2.5 mg/kg 60 to 75 min before anesthesia and infused over 1 hr (Dantrium Intravenous). Additional individualized doses given as needed during surgery.

I.V. INJECTION (RYANODEX)

Adults and children. 2.5 mg/kg about 75 min before anesthesia and injected over 1 min. Additional individualized doses given as needed during surgery.

➤ *To treat malignant hyperthermic crisis*

I.V. INJECTION

Adults and children. *Initial:* 1 mg/kg by rapid bolus; repeated, as needed, until symptoms subside or cumulative dose of 10 mg/kg has been reached and if symptoms reappear.

➤ *To treat postmalignant hyperthermic crisis*

CAPSULES

Adults and children. 4 to 8 mg/kg daily in divided doses four times daily for 1 to 3 days.

I.V. INFUSION

Adults and children. *Initial:* Individualized dosage beginning with 1 mg/kg or more as needed if oral therapy can't be used. *Maximum:* 10 mg/kg total dose.

Route	Onset	Peak	Duration
P.O.	1 wk*	Unknown	Unknown

* For spasticity; unknown for malignant hyperthermia.

Mechanism of Action

Acts directly on skeletal muscle to reduce the force of reflex muscle contraction. This in turn reduces hyperreflexia, spasticity, involuntary movements, and clonus, probably by preventing calcium release from the sarcoplasmic reticulum of skeletal muscle cells. Blocked calcium release also inhibits the activation of acute catabolism associated with malignant hyperthermic crisis syndrome.

Incompatibilities

Don't administer parenteral dantrolene with acidic solutions, including D_5W and normal saline solution.

Contraindications

For oral drug only: Active hepatic disease (such as cirrhosis and hepatitis), conditions in which spasticity helps maintain upright posture and improve balance or function, hypersensitivity to dantrolene or its components

Interactions

DRUGS

calcium channel blockers (especially verapamil): Possibly hyperkalemia, life-threatening arrhythmias, shock
CNS depressants: Possibly profound sedation
estrogens: Possibly increased risk of hepatotoxicity
hepatotoxic drugs: Increased risk of hepatotoxicity with long-term oral dantrolene use
vecuronium: Possibly potentiated vecuronium-induced neuromuscular block

ACTIVITIES

alcohol use: Possibly increased CNS depression

Adverse Reactions

CNS: Chills, confusion, depression, dizziness, drowsiness, fatigue, fever, headache, insomnia, light-headedness, malaise, nervousness, **seizures**, slurred speech or other speech problems, weakness
CV: Heart failure (I.V.), labile blood pressure, **pericarditis**, phlebitis, tachycardia
EENT: Abnormal vision, altered taste, diplopia, drooling, excessive tearing, lacrimation
GI: Abdominal cramps, anorexia, constipation, diarrhea, dysphagia, gastric irritation, **GI bleeding**, **hepatitis**, **hepatotoxicity**, **intestinal obstruction**, nausea, vomiting
GU: Crystalluria, dysuria, erectile dysfunction, hematuria, nocturia, urinary frequency, urinary incontinence, urine retention
HEME: Aplastic anemia, anemia, **leukopenia**, **thrombocytopenia**
MS: Backache, myalgia
RESP: Feeling of suffocation, pleural effusion, **respiratory depression**
SKIN: Acne, diaphoresis, eczematoid eruption, erythema (I.V.), extravasation with tissue damage, hirsutism, pruritus, rash, urticaria
Other: Anaphylaxis, **lymphocytic lymphoma**

Nursing Considerations

- Use dantrolene cautiously in patients with impaired pulmonary function, especially those with COPD, and in those with severe cardiac or hepatic dysfunction.
- Reconstitute drug with 60 ml sterile water for injection. Shake vial until clear. Store reconstituted solution at room temperature, protected from direct sunlight. Discard after 6 hours.

- Transfer reconstituted drug to a plastic I.V. bag, rather than a glass bottle, for infusion to prevent precipitation.
- Infuse into a central vein, if possible, to avoid tissue damage from extravasation.
- Monitor blood pressure and heart rate often during administration to detect tachycardia and blood pressure changes.
- Notify prescriber about persistent diarrhea with oral therapy; drug may need to be stopped.
- Monitor results of liver function tests—especially alkaline phosphatase, ALT, AST, and total bilirubin levels—to detect hepatotoxicity. Expect to stop drug after 45 days if benefits aren't sufficient because risk of hepatotoxicity increases with dose and time, especially for women and patients over age 35.

PATIENT TEACHING

- Advise patient to take dantrolene capsules with food if gastric irritation develops.
- Tell patient that drug may weaken muscles used for walking and climbing stairs.
- Explain drug's sedating effects. Caution patient to avoid sedatives (unless prescribed), including alcohol.
- Advise patient to report yellow skin or anorexia, fatigue, itching, and sclerae.
- Advise patient who has missed a dose to wait until the next scheduled dose if more than 2 hours have passed since the missed dose. Instruct her not to double the dose.
- Caution patient not to stop taking drug without consulting prescriber. Gradual dosage reduction may be required, especially after long-term use.

dapagliflozin

Farxiga

Class and Category

Pharmacologic class: Sodium glucose co-transporter 2 inhibitor
Therapeutic class: Antidiabetic
Pregnancy category: Not classified

Indications and Dosages

➤ *Adjunct to diet and exercise to improve glycemic control in patients with type 2 diabetes mellitus*

TABLETS

Adults. 5 mg once daily in morning, increased to 10 mg once daily in morning, as needed.

Mechanism of Action

Inhibits sodium glucose co-transporter 2 in the kidneys, which prevents glucose reabsorption. This decreases blood glucose levels.

Contraindications

Dialysis therapy, end-stage renal disease, hypersensitivity to dapagliflozin or its components, severe renal impairment (glomerular filtration rate less than 30 ml/min)

Interactions

DRUGS

exenatide extended-release: Possibly decreased serum bicarbonate level of 13 mEq/L or less
insulin, insulin secretagogues: Increased risk of hypoglycemia

Adverse Reactions

CNS: Syncope
CV: Dyslipidemia, elevated low-density lipoprotein cholesterol, **hypotension**
EENT: Nasopharyngitis
ENDO: **Hypoglycemia**, **ketoacidosis**
GI: Constipation, nausea
GU: **Acute kidney injury**, decreased glomerular filtration rate, dysuria, elevated serum creatinine levels, genital mycotic infections, impaired renal function, increased urination, **necrotizing fasciitis of the perineum (Fournier's gangrene)**, osmotic diuresis, **potential bladder cancer**, pyelonephritis, **urosepsis**, UTI
HEME: Elevated hematocrit level
MS: Back or extremity pain
SKIN: **Severe cutaneous reactions**, rash, urticaria
Other: **Anaphylaxis**, **angioedema**, dehydration, elevated serum phosphorus levels

Nursing Considerations

- Use drug cautiously in patients with chronic kidney insufficiency, congestive heart failure, decreased blood volume, and patients taking medications such as angiotensin-converting enzyme inhibitors, angiotensin receptor blockers, diuretics, and NSAIDs because these conditions and treatments may predispose the patient to acute kidney injury while receiving dapagliflozin. Ensure that kidney function has been assessed prior to starting dapagliflozin therapy and then periodically thereafter.

- Know that dapagliflozin should not be given to patients with active bladder cancer, as it is not known if the drug has an effect on preexisting bladder tumors. Use cautiously in patients with a history of bladder cancer. Monitor patient throughout therapy for hematuria, as this is a potential indicator for the presence of bladder tumor.
- Assess patient's volume status and correct, if needed and as prescribed, prior to starting dapagliflozin therapy, because drug can cause intravascular volume contraction leading to acute kidney injury or symptomatic hypotension. Patients at highest risk include elderly patients, patients receiving loop diuretic therapy or drugs that interfere with the renin–angiotensin–aldosterone system, and patients who have low systolic blood pressure or impaired renal function.
- Expect drug to be temporarily discontinued in patients who experience a reduced oral intake, such as with an acute illness or fasting, or who experience excessive fluid losses because of significant gastrointestinal illness or heat exposure, to reduce risk of acute kidney injury.
- Monitor patient's blood pressure and cholesterol level throughout dapagliflozin therapy.

WARNING Monitor patient for hypersensitivity reactions. Although rare, anaphylaxis, angioedema, and severe cutaneous adverse reactions have occurred. If present, stop drug immediately and notify prescriber. Provide care, as prescribed, according to the standard of care until signs and symptoms subside.

- Be aware that patients receiving insulin or insulin secretagogues may require a lower dose of these agents because dapagliflozin in combination increases risk of hypoglycemia. Monitor patient closely for hypoglycemia. If present, treat according to standard of care and notify prescriber.

WARNING Monitor patient for a rare but serious and life-threatening necrotizing infection of the perineum called Fournier's gangrene. Notify prescriber immediately if patient develops erythema, pain, swelling, or tenderness in the genital or perineal area, along with fever or malaise. Expect treatment with broad-spectrum antibiotics and, if needed, surgical debridement of the area. Know that dapagliflozin will be discontinued if this occurs. Monitor patient's blood glucose levels closely and expect an alternative treatment for glycemic control.

- Monitor patients for genital mycotic infections, especially those with a history of such infections. If present, notify prescriber and treat, as prescribed.

WARNING Monitor patient closely for ketoacidosis that may occur despite the patient having type 2 diabetes and may be present even if a blood glucose level is less than 250 mg/dl. If signs and symptoms occur such as dehydration, fruity odor to breath, malaise, nausea, shortness of breath, and vomiting notify prescriber and expect drug to be discontinued. Provide supportive care, as ordered.

PATIENT TEACHING

- Inform patient that dapagliflozin therapy is not a replacement for diet and exercise therapy.
- Instruct patient on the signs and symptoms of hypoglycemia and how to treat it. Inform patient who is also receiving a sulfonylurea or insulin that the risk of hypoglycemia is greater. Tell patient to notify prescriber if hypoglycemia occurs frequently or is severe.
- Inform patient that dapagliflozin may have an adverse effect on the bladder, increasing the risk for bladder cancer. Tell patient to report blood in the urine immediately to the prescriber.
- Tell patient to monitor the blood glucose level using blood tests instead of urine tests because the drug increases urinary glucose excretion and will lead to positive urine glucose tests. Review signs and symptoms of ketoacidosis with patient and urge her to seek immediate medical attention, if present, even if blood glucose level is less than 250 mg/dl.

- Instruct patient to stop taking drug and seek immediate medical attention if an allergic reaction such as hives or facial or throat swelling occurs while taking dapagliflozin.
- Advise female patients to notify prescriber if pregnancy occurs or is suspected because the drug may cause fetal harm if taken in the second or third trimester. Also, inform female patients that drug may cause harm to infants who are breastfed. Mothers should discuss desire to breastfeed with prescriber prior to breastfeeding.
- Advise patient to maintain adequate fluid intake throughout dapagliflozin therapy. However, tell patient to notify prescriber if he is unable to take a normal amount of daily fluids due to illness or fasting or experiences an excessive loss of fluids from excessive perspiration or gastrointestinal illnesses, as drug may need to be temporarily withheld.

WARNING Warn patient to stop dapagliflozin and seek immediate medical attention if pain, redness, swelling, or tenderness occur in the genital or perineal area, along with fever or malaise because, although rare, this cluster of symptoms may become life-threatening.

daptomycin

Cubicin, Cubicin RF

Class and Category

Pharmacologic class: Cyclic lipopeptide
Therapeutic class: Antibiotic
Pregnancy category: Not classified

Indications and Dosages

➤ *To treat complicated skin and skin structure infections caused by* Staphylococcus aureus *(including methicillin-resistant isolates),* Streptococcus agalactiae, S. dysgalactiae *subspecies* Enterococcus faecalis *(vancomycin-susceptible isolates only) and* equisimilis, S. pyogenes

I.V. INFUSION, I.V. INJECTION (CUBICIN, CUBICIN RF)

Adults. 4 mg/kg administered over 2 min as an I.V. injection or over 30 min as an I.V. infusion once daily for 7 to 14 days.

I.V. INFUSION (CUBICIN, CUBICIN RF)

Children ages 12 to 17. 5 mg/kg once every 24 hr infused over 30 min and given for up to 14 days.

Children ages 7 to 11. 7 mg/kg once every 24 hr infused over 30 min and given for up to 14 days.

Children ages 2 to 6. 9 mg/kg every 24 hr infused over 60 min and given for up to 14 days.

Children ages 1 to less than 2 years. 10 mg/kg once every 24 hr infused over 60 min and given for up to 14 days.

➤ *To treat* Staphylococcus aureus *bloodstream infections (bacteremia), including right-sided infective endocarditis, caused by methicillin-susceptible and methicillin-resistant isolates*

I.V. INFUSION, I.V. INJECTION

Adults. 6 mg/kg administered over 2 min as an I.V. injection or over 30 min as an I.V. infusion once daily for 2 to 6 wk.

➤ *To treat pediatric patients with* S. aureus *bloodstream infections (bacteremia)*

I.V. INFUSION (CUBICIN)

Children ages 12 to 17. 7 mg/kg infused over 30 min once daily for up to 42 days.

Children ages 7 to 11. 9 mg/kg infused over 30 min once daily for up to 42 days.

Children ages 1 to 6. 12 mg/kg infused over 60 min once daily for up to 42 days.

DOSAGE ADJUSTMENT For adult patients with creatinine clearance less than 30 ml/min, dosage is 4 mg/kg for complicated skin or skin-structure infections or 6 mg/kg for bacteremia once every 48 hr. No dosage adjustment has been established for children with renal impairment.

Mechanism of Action

Binds to bacterial membranes to cause rapid depolarization of membrane potential. This loss of membrane potential inhibits protein, DNA, and RNA synthesis, which results in bacterial cell death.

Incompatibilities

Don't mix daptomycin with dextrose-containing diluents and with other intravenously administered drugs or infusions.

Contraindications

Hypersensitivity to daptomycin or its components

Interactions

DRUGS

HMG-CoA reductase inhibitors: Possibly increased CPK level and increased risk of myopathy

Adverse Reactions

CNS: Anxiety, asthenia, confusion, dizziness, dyskinesia, fatigue, fever, hallucination, headache, insomnia, mental status changes, paresthesia, peripheral neuropathy, rigors, weakness
CV: **Atrial fibrillation or flutter**, **cardiac arrest or failure**, chest pain, hypertension, **hypotension**, peripheral edema, **supraventricular tachycardia**
EENT: Blurred vision, dry mouth, eye irritation, gingival pain, hypoesthesia of mouth, pharyngolaryngeal pain, oral candidiasis, sore throat, stomatitis, taste disturbance, tinnitus, visual disturbances
ENDO: Hyperglycemia, **hypoglycemia**
GI: Abdominal distention or pain, anorexia, ***Clostridium difficile*-associated diarrhea**, constipation, diarrhea, dyspepsia, dysphagia, elevated liver enzymes or serum lactate dehydrogenase, **GI hemorrhage**, jaundice, nausea, vomiting
GU: **Acute kidney injury**, **renal failure or insufficiency**; proteinuria; UTI; vaginal candidiasis
HEME: Anemia, **decreased platelet count**, eosinophilia, **increased international normalized ratio (INR)**, leukocytosis, **prolonged prothrombin time**, **thrombocythemia**, **thrombocytopenia**, thrombocytosis
MS: Arthralgia, back or limb pain, elevated myoglobin level, muscle cramps or weakness, myalgia, myopathy, osteomyelitis, **rhabdomyolysis**
RESP: Cough, dyspnea, **eosinophilic pneumonia**, pleural effusion, pneumonia, shortness of breath
SKIN: Acute generalized exanthematous pustulosis, cellulitis, diaphoresis, eczema, erythema, flushing, pruritus, rash, **Stevens–Johnson syndrome**, truncal erythema, urticaria, vesiculobullous rash
Other: **Anaphylaxis**, **angioedema**, **bacteremia**, **drug reaction with eosinophilia and systemic symptoms (DRESS)**, **electrolyte disturbance**, elevated alkaline phosphatase or creatine phosphokinase levels, **elevated serum sodium bicarbonate level**, fungal infection, **hyperkalemia**, **hypokalemia**, **hypomagnesemia**, injection-site reactions, lymphadenopathy, **sepsis**

Nursing Considerations

- Use cautiously in patients with moderate to severe renal impairment and monitor drug effectiveness closely, as daptomycin may not be as effective in this patient population.
- Obtain blood samples for culture and sensitivity testing before starting daptomycin.
- Reconstitute daptomycin powder (Cubicin formulation) by slowly transferring 10 ml normal saline for injection into vial and pointing needle toward wall of vial to minimize foaming. Then gently rotate vial until all powder is wet. Don't agitate or shake vial. Let vial stand undisturbed for 10 minutes, and then gently rotate or swirl contents for a few minutes, as needed, to obtain a completely reconstituted solution.
- Reconstitute daptomycin powder (Cubicin RF formulation) within the vial with 10 ml of either sterile water for injection or bacteriostatic water for injection using a beveled sterile transfer needle that is 21 gauge or smaller in diameter. Saline-based diluents should not be used because this will result in a hyperosmotic solution that may cause infusion-site reactions if the reconstituted product is administered as an intravenous injection. Rotate or swirl vial contents for a few minutes, as needed, to obtain a completely reconstituted solution.
- Administer as an I.V. injection over a period of 2 minutes. If the drug is to be administered as an I.V. infusion, further dilute either formulation of reconstituted

daptomycin solution with normal saline for injection, and administer over 30 minutes for adults and children age 7 and older and 60 minutes for children 6 and under. Reconstituted drug is stable in infusion bag for 12 hours at room temperature or 48 hours refrigerated. Do not infuse with the ReadyMED elastomeric infusion pumps, as daptomycin is not as stable when stored in these pumps.

- Monitor results of the patient's bleeding studies, as ordered. Daptomycin may cause a significant false increase in PT and INR with some brands of laboratory assays. If this occurs during daptomycin therapy, draw blood sample just before next daptomycin dose and evaluate other causes of the increase.
- Monitor patient closely for diarrhea, which may herald pseudomembranous colitis caused by *C. difficile*. If diarrhea occurs, notify prescriber. If pseudomembranous colitis develops, expect to discontinue drug and give fluids, electrolytes, protein, and antibiotic effective against *C. difficile*.
- Monitor patient for evidence of super-infection, and inform prescriber if present. Expect to stop drug and provide care.
- Assess patient for muscle pain or weakness, especially of distal limbs. Expect to monitor creatine phosphokinase (CPK) level weekly or more often in patients recently or currently taking an HMG-CoA reductase inhibitor. Expect to stop daptomycin, as ordered, if patient has myopathy or marked rise in CPK level.
- Monitor patient's BUN and serum creatinine levels and patient's response to drug closely, especially if renal insufficiency is already present because daptomycin may not be as effective in the presence of renal insufficiency.
- Expect to discontinue daptomycin therapy immediately if patient develops signs and symptoms of eosinophilic pneumonia, such as dyspnea with hypoxic respiratory insufficiency and diffuse pulmonary infiltrates or fever, and prepare to administer systemic steroids, as ordered.

PATIENT TEACHING

- Inform patient that diarrhea may occur 2 months or more after daptomycin therapy stops. If severe or prolonged, advise patient to notify prescriber as soon as possible; additional treatment may be needed.
- Urge patient to report muscle pain, tenderness, or weakness, and other symptoms of myopathy immediately.
- Instruct patient to notify prescriber immediately if skin reactions occur, because drug may need to be discontinued.

darbepoetin alfa

Aranesp

Class and Category

Pharmacologic class: Recombinant human erythropoietin
Therapeutic class: Antianemic
Pregnancy category: C

Indications and Dosages

➤ *To treat anemia from chronic renal failure*

I.V. OR SUBCUTANEOUS INJECTION

Adults on dialysis other than hemodialysis. *Initial:* 0.45 mcg/kg as a single dose every wk. Alternatively, 0.75 mcg/kg once every 2 wk. *Maintenance:* Dosage individualized and increased monthly to maintain a hemoglobin level not to exceed 11 g/dl.
Adults not on dialysis. *Initial:* 0.45 mcg/kg as a single dose every 4 wk, as needed.
Children age 1 month and over on dialysis. 0.45 mcg/kg once every wk.
Children age 1 month and over not on dialysis. 0.45 mcg/kg once every wk. Alternatively, 0.75 mcg/kg once every 2 wk.

I.V. INJECTION

Adults on hemodialysis. *Initial:* 0.45 mcg/kg as a single dose every wk. *Alternatively,* 0.75 mcg/kg once every 2 wk. *Maintenance:* Dosage individualized and increased monthly to maintain a hemoglobin level not to exceed 11 g/dl.

DOSAGE ADJUSTMENT Dosage reduced or therapy interrupted if hemoglobin level increases and approaches 12 g/dl for children, 11 g/dl for adults on dialysis, and 10 g/dl for adults not on dialysis. Dosage reduced by about 25% if hemoglobin level increases by more than 1 g/dl in a 2-wk period. Dosage increased by about 25% of previous dose if hemoglobin level increases less than 1 g/dl over 4 wk but only if serum ferritin level is 100 mcg/L or greater and serum transferrin saturation is 20% or greater. Further increases made at 4-wk intervals until specified hemoglobin level is obtained.

DOSAGE ADJUSTMENT For conversion from epoetin alfa to darbepoetin alfa, dosage administered every wk for patient who previously received epoetin alfa 2 to 3 times/wk and once every 2 wk for patient who previously received epoetin alfa once/wk. For conversion from epoetin alfa, 6.25 mcg/wk darbepoetin alfa given every wk for adult patients who received less than 1,500 units/wk of epoetin alfa; 6.25 mcg/week darbepoetin alfa given every wk for adult and pediatric patients who received 1,500 to 2,499 units/wk of epoetin alfa; 12.5 mcg/wk (10 mcg/wk for children) darbepoetin alfa every wk for patients who received 2,500 to 4,999 units/wk of epoetin alfa; 25 mcg/wk (20 mcg/wk for children) darbepoetin alfa every wk for adult and pediatric patients who received 5,000 to 10,999 units/wk of epoetin alfa; 40 mcg/wk darbepoetin alfa every wk for adult and pediatric patients who received 11,000 to 17,999 units/wk of epoetin alfa; 60 mcg/wk darbepoetin alfa every wk for adult and pediatric patients who received 18,000 to 33,999 units/wk of epoetin alfa; 100 mcg/wk darbepoetin alfa every wk for adult and pediatric patients who received 34,000 to 89,999 units/wk of epoetin alfa; 200 mcg/wk darbepoetin alfa every wk for adult and pediatric patients who received 90,000 or more units/wk of epoetin alfa.

➤ *To treat chemotherapy-induced anemia in patients with nonmyeloid malignancies and hemoglobin level less than 10 g/dl and if there is a minimum of 2 additional months of planned chemotherapy*

SUBCUTANEOUS INJECTION

Adults. *Initial:* 2.25 mcg/kg as a single dose every wk until completion of a chemotherapy course. Alternatively, 500 mcg every 3 wk until completion of a chemotherapy course. *Maintenance:* Dosage individualized to maintain a target hemoglobin level.

DOSAGE ADJUSTMENT Dosage increased to 4.5 mcg/kg/wk (no dosage adjustment if patient is already receiving 500 mcg every 3 wk) if hemoglobin level increases less than 1.0 g/dl after 6 wk of therapy. If it increases more than 1.0 g/dl over 2 wk, dosage reduced by about 40%. If hemoglobin level exceeds a level needed to avoid RBC transfusion, dose withheld until hemoglobin approaches level when RBC transfusion may be required. Then, therapy is restarted at a dose about 40% less than last dose given.

Route	Onset	Peak	Duration
I.V., SubQ	2–6 wk	Unknown	Unknown

Mechanism of Action

Stimulates release of reticulocytes from the bone marrow into the bloodstream, where they develop into mature RBCs.

Incompatibilities

Don't mix darbepoetin alfa with any other drug.

Contraindications

History of pure red cell aplasia that began after treatment with darbepoetin alpha or other erythropoietin protein drugs, hypersensitivity to darbepoetin alpha or its components, uncontrolled hypertension

Interactions

DRUGS

None reported

Adverse Reactions

CNS: Asthenia, **CVA**, dizziness, fatigue, fever, headache, **seizures**, transient ischemic attack

CV: **Acute MI**, angina, **arrhythmias**, **cardiac arrest or death**, chest pain, **congestive heart failure**, edema, hypertension, **hypotension**, peripheral edema, vascular access thrombosis, **thromboembolic events**

GI: Abdominal pain, constipation, diarrhea, nausea, vomiting

MS: Arthralgia, back pain, limb pain, muscle spasm, myalgia

D

RESP: Bronchitis, cough, dyspnea, pneumonia, **pulmonary embolism**, upper respiratory tract infection
SKIN: Erythema multiforme, pruritus, rash, **Stevens–Johnson syndrome**, urticaria
Other: Dehydration, infection, flu-like symptoms, injection-site pain, **sepsis**

Nursing Considerations

- Know that before starting darbepoetin alfa therapy, expect to correct folic acid or vitamin B_{12} deficiencies because these conditions may interfere with drug's effectiveness.
- Ensure that patient has received the medication guide and patient instructions for darbepoetin alpha and that a written acknowledgment of a discussion of the risks involved with this type of therapy has been obtained before first dose is given.
- Be aware that darbepoetin alfa shouldn't be given to cancer patients when a cure is anticipated because drug may decrease survival rate and increase tumor progression in patients with certain types of cancers, such as breast, cervical, head and neck, lymphoid, and non-small-cell lung cancers. Be aware that all prescribers and hospitals must enroll in and comply with the ESA APPRISE oncology program to be able to prescribe and dispense the drug.
- Use extreme caution with darbepoetin alfa therapy in patients undergoing coronary artery bypass graft surgery because of increased risk of death, and in patients undergoing orthopedic procedures because of increased risk of deep venous thrombosis.
- Be aware that to ensure effective drug response, expect to obtain serum ferritin level and transferrin saturation before and during therapy, as ordered. If serum ferritin level is less than 100 mcg/L or serum transferrin saturation is less than 20%, expect to begin supplemental iron therapy.
- Don't shake vial during preparation to avoid denaturing drug and rendering it biologically inactive.
- Discard drug if discoloration or particulate matter is present.
- Don't dilute drug before giving it.
- Know that needle cover on prefilled syringe contains dry natural rubber and may cause allergic reaction in those with latex sensitivity.
- Discard unused portion of drug because it contains no preservatives.
- Monitor patient closely for hypertension during therapy. Expect to reduce dosage or withhold drug if blood pressure is poorly controlled with antihypertensive and dietary measures.
- Monitor hemoglobin level weekly, as ordered, until hemoglobin stabilizes and maintenance dosage has been achieved. Then monitor hemoglobin level regularly, as ordered. After each dosage adjustment, expect to check hemoglobin level weekly for 4 weeks until it stabilizes in response to dosage change.

WARNING **Know that if hemoglobin level increases more than about 1 g/dl during any 2-week period or it exceeds 12 g/dl for children, 11 g/dl for adult patient on dialysis, 10 g/dl for adult patient not on dialysis, or target range for cancer patient, the risk of acute MI, cardiac arrest, congestive heart failure, fluid overload with peripheral edema, seizures, shortened survival, stroke, tumor progression, vascular infarction, vascular ischemia, vascular thrombosis, and worsened hypertension increases. Expect to decrease dosage if this occurs.**

- Expect to discontinue darbepoetin in cancer patients if hemoglobin level hasn't increased after 8 weeks or if patient continues to need transfusions despite therapy.
- Institute seizure precautions according to facility policy.
- Monitor patient for severe skin reactions that may include blistering and skin exfoliation. Notify prescriber immediately, if noted, and expect darbepoetin therapy to be discontinued. Prepare to provide supportive care, as ordered.
- Monitor renal function test results and fluid and electrolyte balance for signs of declining renal function in patients with renal impairment. If patient starts dialysis, monitor hemoglobin and blood pressure closely and expect dosage and route of administration to be adjusted, as needed, for type of dialysis.

- Store drug at 2° to 8° C (36° to 46° F). Don't freeze, and do protect from light.

PATIENT TEACHING

- Instruct patient how to administer a subcutaneous injection, rotate sites, and properly dispose of needles, syringes, or unused portions of single-dose vials.
- Advise patient that the risk of seizures is highest during the first 90 days of therapy. Discourage her from engaging in hazardous activities during this time.
- Emphasize the importance of complying with the dosage regimen and keeping follow-up medical and laboratory appointments.
- Advise patient to follow up with her prescriber for blood pressure monitoring.
- Encourage patient to eat adequate quantities of iron-rich foods.
- Teach patient and her caregiver the proper administration technique if darbepoetin alpha will be administered at home.
- Caution patient and her caregiver not to reuse needles, syringes, or drug product. Thoroughly instruct them in proper needle and syringe disposal using a puncture-resistant container.
- Explain that needle cover on prefilled syringe contains dry natural rubber and may cause allergic reaction in those with latex sensitivity.
- Review possible adverse reactions, and urge patient to notify prescriber if she experiences chest pain, headache, rash, seizures, shortness of breath, or swelling.

darifenacin

Enablex

Class and Category

Pharmacologic class: Anticholinergic
Therapeutic class: Bladder antispasmodic
Pregnancy category: C

Indications and Dosages

➤ *To treat overactive bladder with symptoms of frequency, urge incontinence, or urgency*

E.R. TABLETS

Adults. *Initial:* 7.5 mg daily, increased to 15 mg daily after 2 wk as needed.

DOSAGE ADJUSTMENT For patients with moderate hepatic impairment and those taking potent CYP3A4 inhibitors (such as clarithromycin, itraconazole, ketoconazole, nefazodone, nelfinavir, and ritonavir) daily dosage should not exceed 7.5 mg.

Route	Onset	Peak	Duration
P.O.	Unknown	7 hr	Unknown

Mechanism of Action

Antagonizes effect of acetylcholine on muscarinic receptors in detrusor muscle, decreasing muscle spasms that cause inappropriate bladder emptying. This action increases bladder capacity and volume, which relieves sensations of frequency and urgency and enhances bladder control.

Contraindications

Gastric retention, hypersensitivity to darifenacin or its components, uncontrolled narrow-angle glaucoma, urine retention, and patients at risk for these conditions

Interactions

DRUGS

anticholinergics: Increased frequency and severity of anticholinergic adverse reactions
CYP2D6 substrates such as flecainide, thioridazine, tricyclic antidepressants: Risk of toxicity with these drugs
potent CYP3A4 inhibitors (such as clarithromycin, itraconazole, ketoconazole, nefazodone, nelfinavir, and ritonavir): Decreased metabolism and increased effects of darifenacin, possibly increasing the risk of adverse reactions

Adverse Reactions

CNS: Asthenia, confusion, dizziness, hallucinations, headache, somnolence
CV: Hypertension, palpitations, peripheral edema
EENT: Abnormal vision, dry eyes or mouth, pharyngitis, rhinitis, sinusitis
GI: Abdominal pain, constipation, diarrhea, indigestion, nausea, vomiting
GU: Urine retention, UTI, vaginitis
MS: Arthralgia, back pain
RESP: **Airway obstruction**, bronchitis
SKIN: Dry skin, **erythema multiforme**, interstitial granuloma annulare, pruritus, rash

Other: Anaphylaxis, angioedema, flu-like symptoms, **hypersensitivity reactions**, weight gain

Nursing Considerations

- Use darifenacin cautiously in patients with significant bladder outflow obstruction; they have increased risk of urine retention. Also use cautiously in patients with controlled narrow-angle glaucoma, as darifenacin therapy may worsen this condition.
- Use darifenacin cautiously in patients with myasthenia gravis, severe constipation, or ulcerative colitis, because it may decrease GI motility. Also use drug cautiously in obstructive GI disorders because it increases the risk of gastric retention.
- Monitor patient for signs of anticholinergic CNS effects such as confusion, hallucinations, headache, and somnolence, especially at beginning of therapy and with dosage increases.

WARNING **Monitor patient closely for serious adverse reactions that may become life-threatening, such as anaphylaxis and angioedema of the face, larynx, lips, and/or tongue that may occur even after just one dose. If present, withhold drug, notify prescriber immediately, and provide emergency supportive care, as indicated.**

PATIENT TEACHING

- Tell patient to swallow tablets with liquid and not to break, crush, or split them.
- Advise patient to avoid exercising in hot weather because darifenacin decreases sweating, increasing the risk of heatstroke.
- Caution patient to avoid hazardous activities until drug's CNS effects are known.
- Warn patient to seek immediate medical attention if he experiences any signs of a serious drug reaction, including swelling of his face, lips, throat, and/or tongue.

darunavir

Prezista

Class and Category

Pharmacologic class: Protease inhibitor
Therapeutic class: Antiretroviral
Pregnancy category: Not classified

Indications and Dosages

➤ *As adjunct to treat human immunodeficiency virus (HIV) infection*

ORAL SUSPENSION, TABLETS

Adults who are treatment-naïve or who are treatment-experienced with no darunavir-resistance-associated substitutions. 800 mg once daily with ritonavir 100 mg once daily with food.
Adults who are treatment-experienced with at least one darunavir-resistance-associated substitution, adults with no baseline resistance information, and pregnant women. 600 mg twice daily with ritonavir 100 mg twice daily with food.
Children ages 3 to 17 weighing 40 kg (88 lb) or more who are treatment-naïve or who are treatment-experienced with no darunavir-resistance-associated substitutions. 800 mg once daily with ritonavir 100 mg once daily with food.
Children ages 3 to 17 weighing 40 kg (88 lb) or more who are treatment-experienced with at least one darunavir-resistance-associated substitution. 600 mg twice daily with ritonavir 100 mg twice daily with food.
Children ages 3 to 17 weighing 30 kg (66 lb) to less than 40 kg (88 lb) who are treatment-naïve or who are treatment-experienced with no darunavir-resistance-associated substitutions. 675 mg once daily with ritonavir 100 mg once daily with food.
Children ages 3 to 17 weighing 30 kg (66 lb) to less than 40 kg (88 lb) who are treatment-experienced with at least one darunavir-resistance-associated substitution. 450 mg twice daily with ritonavir 60 mg twice daily with food.
Children ages 3 to 17 weighing 15 kg (33 lb) to less than 30 kg (66 lb) who are treatment-naïve or who are treatment-experienced with no darunavir-resistance-associated substitutions. 600 mg once daily with ritonavir 100 mg once daily with food.
Children ages 3 to 17 weighing 15 kg (33 lb) to less than 30 kg (66 lb) who are treatment-experienced with at least one darunavir-resistance-associated substitution. 375 mg twice daily with ritonavir 48 mg twice daily with food.

Children age 3 and over weighing at least 10 kg (22 lb) but less than 15 kg (33 lb) who are treatment-naïve or who are treatment-experienced with no darunavir-resistance-associated substitutions. 35 mg/kg once daily with ritonavir 7 mg/kg once daily with food.
Children age 3 and over weighing at least 10 kg (22 lb) but less than 15 kg (33 lb) who are treatment-experienced with at least one darunavir-resistance-associated substitution. 20 mg/kg twice daily with ritonavir 3 mg/kg twice daily with food.

Mechanism of Action
Inhibits HIV-1 protease by selectively inhibiting cleavage of the HIV-1 encoded Gag-Pol polyproteins in infected cells. This prevents the formation of mature virus particles.

Contraindications
Children under age of 3: concurrent therapy with alfuzosin, cisapride, colchicine (in presence of hepatic or renal impairment), dihydroergotamine, dronedarone, elbasvir/grazoprevir, ergotamine, lomitapide, lovastatin, lurasidone, methylergonovine, midazolam (oral), pimozide, ranolazine, rifampin, sildenafil (for treatment of pulmonary arterial hypertension), simvastatin, St. John's wort, triazolam; hypersensitivity to darunavir or its components; severe hepatic impairment

Interactions
DRUGS
alfuzosin, amiodarone, amitriptyline, antipsychotics, apixaban, atorvastatin, bepridil, beta blockers, calcium channel blockers, carbamazepine, cisapride, clarithromycin, clonazepam, colchicine, corticosteroids (inhaled, nasal, ophthalmic, systemic), dabigatran, dasatinib, desipramine, digoxin, disopyramide, dronedarone, elbasvir/grazoprevir, ergot derivatives, fentanyl, flecainide, HMG-CoA reductase inhibitors, hypnotics, imipramine, immunosuppressants, lidocaine (systemic), lomitapide, lurasidone, lumefantrine, maraviroc, mexiletine, midazolam, nilotinib, norbuprenorphine, nortriptyline, oxycodone, PDE-5 inhibitors, perphenazine, pimozide, pravastatin, propafenone, quetiapine, quinidine, ranolazine, risperidone, rivaroxaban, rosuvastatin, salmeterol, sedatives, thioridazine, ticagrelor, tramadol, trazodone, triazolam, vinblastine, vincristine, warfarin: Increased plasma concentration of these drugs, increasing risk of adverse effects
artemether, dihydroartemisinin, ethinyl estradiol, methadone, norethindrone, omeprazole, paroxetine, phenobarbital, phenytoin, sertraline, voriconazole, warfarin: Decreased plasma concentration of these drugs, with decreased effectiveness
boceprevir: Decreased plasma concentration of both drugs and their effectiveness
corticosteroids (inhaled, nasal, ophthalmic, systemic), lopinavir, lopinavir/ritonavir, rifampin, rifapentine, saquinavir, St. John'swort: Decreased plasma concentration of darunavir and its effectiveness
didanosine: Altered absorption of didanosine
drospirenone: Increased risk of hyperkalemia
HMG-CoA reductase inhibitors: Possibly increased risk of rhabdomyolysis
indinavir, itraconazole, ketoconazole, rifabutin, simeprevir: Increased plasma concentrations of both drugs, increasing risk of adverse effects

Adverse Reactions
CNS: Abnormal dreams, asthenia, fatigue, fever, headache
CV: Elevated cholesterol and triglyceride levels
ENDO: Cushingoid appearance, fat redistribution, hyperglycemia, new-onset diabetes mellitus
GI: Abdominal distention or pain, **acute hepatitis or pancreatitis**, anorexia, diarrhea, dyspepsia, elevated liver or pancreatic enzymes, flatulence, **hepatotoxicity**, hyperbilirubinemia, nausea, vomiting
MS: Myalgia, osteonecrosis
SKIN: Acute generalized exanthematous pustulosis, pruritus, rash, **Stevens–Johnson syndrome**, **toxic epidermal necrolysis**, urticaria
Other: Angioedema, **drug reaction with eosinophilia and systemic symptoms (DRESS)**, immune reconstitution syndrome

Nursing Considerations
- Know that prior to initiating therapy with darunavir, serum liver biochemistry

should be performed. In patients who are treatment-experienced, a history plus genotypic and/or phenotypic testing are recommended to assess drug susceptibility of the HIV-1 virus. Depending on outcome, dosage may have to be altered.

- Be aware that darunavir must be coadministered with ritonavir and food to have a therapeutic effect.
- Use darunavir cautiously in patient with known sulfonamide allergy, because drug contains a sulfonamide moiety.

WARNING **Be aware that patient is at risk for serious adverse reactions if taking other drugs, due to multiple drug interactions associated with darunavir therapy. Take a complete drug history and alert prescriber of any potential interactions that could occur. These drug interactions can be potentially severe, life-threatening, or fatal.**

- Monitor patient's transaminase levels periodically, as ordered. Patients with underlying chronic hepatitis, cirrhosis, or patients who have pretreatment elevations of transaminases may develop an elevation in serum liver biochemistry, especially during the first several months of darunavir therapy. Report any evidence of liver dysfunction (anorexia, dark urine, elevated liver enzymes, fatigue, jaundice, liver tenderness), because drug-induced hepatitis has occurred during therapy and drug may have to be temporarily withheld or discontinued.
- Monitor patient for changes in skin. Be alert for a rash that often occurs within the first month of therapy but usually resolves. However, other severe skin reactions, accompanied by elevations of transaminases and fever in some cases, have occurred. Report abnormal signs and symptoms, especially the appearance of blisters, conjunctivitis, elevated liver enzymes, fatigue, fever, general malaise, joint or muscle aches, and oral lesions.
- Monitor patient's blood glucose level during therapy, as ordered. New-onset diabetes mellitus, exacerbation of preexisting diabetes mellitus and hyperglycemia may occur with darunavir use. Notify prescriber about any abnormalities that are persistent or severe.
- Be aware that immune reconstitution syndrome has occurred in patients treated with combination antiretroviral therapy, including darunavir. The inflammatory response predisposes susceptible patients to opportunistic infections such as cytomegalovirus, *Mycobacterium avium* infection, *Pneumocystis jiroveci* pneumonia, or tuberculosis. Autoimmune disorders such as Graves' disease, Guillain–Barré syndrome, or polymyositis have also occurred. Report sudden or unusual adverse reactions to prescriber.
- Monitor patients with hemophilia type A and B because of the risk of increased bleeding, including spontaneous hemarthrosis and skin hematomas.

PATIENT TEACHING

- Instruct patient to take darunavir with ritonavir and food to obtain full effectiveness.
- Tell patient to report all drugs being taken, including over-the-counter medications and herbals, as serious drug interactions may occur. Advise patient not to begin any new drug therapy without first checking with prescriber.
- Inform patient that periodic blood tests may be needed to check the drug's susceptibility to the HIV-1 virus and to monitor his liver function. Review signs and symptoms of liver dysfunction and stress importance of reporting these to prescriber.
- Encourage patient to examine his skin regularly. Reassure him that although a rash most often occurs within the first month of therapy, it is usually harmless and disappears without treatment. However, review other skin changes such as the appearance of blisters and oral ulcers, as well as other signs and symptoms associated with more severe skin reactions. These should be reported immediately.
- Alert diabetic patient that darunavir may increase the risk of hyperglycemia. For patient who does not have diabetes, review

signs and symptoms of hyperglycemia and stress the importance of reporting any such signs and symptoms so that his blood glucose level can be checked and treatment provided, if necessary.
- Inform patient that darunavir therapy may cause changes in his body appearance because of fat redistribution. Prepare him for the possibility of developing breast enlargement, central obesity, dorsocervical fat enlargement (buffalo hump), facial wasting, and peripheral wasting.
- Instruct patient to report any persistent, severe, or unusual signs and symptoms.
- Encourage women of childbearing age to report known or suspected pregnancy. Tell patient using a combined hormonal contraceptive that darunavir may reduce its effectiveness. Instead, she should use an effective alternative (nonhormonal) contraceptive method or add a barrier method of contraception. Also inform patients of childbearing age that the progestin-only pill may be less effective during darunavir therapy.
- Alert mothers that breastfeeding is not recommended during darunavir therapy, because drug is present in human breast milk.

deferoxamine mesylate

Desferal

Class and Category

Pharmacologic class: Iron chelator
Therapeutic class: Heavy metal chelator
Pregnancy category: C

Indications and Dosages

➤ *To treat acute iron intoxication*

I.M. INJECTION

Adults and children age 3 and over who are not in shock. *Initial:* 1,000 mg, followed by 500 mg every 4 hr for 2 doses, if needed. Additional doses of 500 mg may be administered every 4 to 12 hr, as needed. *Maximum:* 6,000 mg in 24 hr.

I.V. INFUSION

Adults and children age 3 and over who are in shock. *Initial:* 1,000 mg administered at a rate not to exceed 15 mg/kg/hr, followed by 500 mg administered at a rate not to exceed 125 mg/hr every 4 hr for 2 doses, if needed. Additional doses of 500 mg may be administered at a rate not to exceed 125 mg/hr every 4 to 12 hr, as needed. *Maximum:* 6,000 mg in 24 hr.

➤ *To treat chronic iron overload due to transfusion-dependent anemias*

I.M. INJECTION

Adults and children age 3 and over. 500 to 1,000 mg daily. *Maximum:* 1,000 mg daily in absence of transfusion.

I.V. INFUSION

Adults. 40 to 50 mg/kg/day infused at a rate no greater than 15 mg/kg/hr and given over 8 to 12 hr for 5 to 7 days per week. *Maximum:* 60 mg/kg/day.

Children age 3 and over. 20 to 40 mg/kg/day infused at a rate no greater than 15 mg/kg/hr and given over 8 to 12 hr. *Maximum:* 40 mg/kg/day.

SUBCUTANEOUS INFUSION

Adults and children age 3 and over. 20 to 40 mg/kg/day administered over 8 to 24 hr.

Mechanism of Action

Binds iron by forming a stable complex with it. This prevents iron from entering into further chemical reactions. The chelate then passes through the kidneys and out of the body in urine, thereby decreasing the iron level in the body.

Contraindications

Anuria, hypersensitivity to deferoxamine or its components, severe renal disease

Interactions

DRUGS

prochlorperazine: Possibly impaired consciousness
vitamin C: Increased availability of iron for chelation by deferoxamine

Adverse Reactions

CNS: Dizziness, **exacerbation or precipitation of aluminum-related**

dialysis encephalopathy, fever, headache, paresthesias, peripheral neuropathy, **seizures**
CV: **Hypotension**, **shock**, tachycardia
EENT: Blurred vision, cataracts, decreased acuity, dyschromatopsia, high-frequency sensorineural hearing loss, loss of vision, night blindness, optic neuritis, retinopathy, scotoma, tinnitus, visual field defects
GI: Abdominal discomfort, diarrhea, **hepatic dysfunction**, increased liver enzymes, nausea, vomiting
GU: **Acute renal failure**, dysuria, increased serum creatinine, renal tubular disorder
HEME: **Leukopenia**, **thrombocytopenia**
MS: Arthralgia, growth retardation, metaphyseal dysplasia, myalgia
RESP: **Acute respiratory distress syndrome**, **asthma**
SKIN: Rash, urticaria
Other: **Anaphylaxis**; **angioedema**; infections with *Yersinia* or *Mucormycosis;* injection-site reactions such as localized irritation, pain, burning, swelling, induration, infiltration, pruritus, erythema, wheal formation, eschar, crust, vesicles, or local edema

Nursing Considerations

- Expect to administer other supportive measures, as ordered, when treating acute iron intoxication with deferoxamine because acute respiratory distress syndrome may occur. Supportive measures include control of shock with blood transfusions, intravenous fluids, oxygen, and vasopressors; correction of acidosis; gastric lavage; induction of emesis with syrup of ipecac; and suction and maintenance of a clear airway.
- Know that patients with thalassemia inadvertently given a high dose or rapid intravenous infusion of deferoxamine may develop acute respiratory distress syndrome and other life-threatening disorders such as hypotension, CNS depression, and acute renal failure. Symptomatic treatment is required, as there is no specific antidote for deferoxamine, although the drug is readily dialyzable.
- Reconstitute drug according to how the drug will be administered. For intramuscular administration, add 2 ml of diluent (sterile water for injection) to a 500-mg vial or 8 ml of diluent to a 2-g vial. For intravenous or subcutaneous administration, add 5 ml of diluent (sterile water for injection) to a 500-mg vial or 20 ml of diluent to a 2-g vial. Make sure drug is completely dissolved before the solution is withdrawn. Discard unused portion.
- Further dilute reconstituted solution with normal or half normal saline, glucose in water, or Ringer's lactate solution if drug will be administered intravenously.
- Follow infusion rates exactly as ordered when drug is administered intravenously because flushing, urticaria, hypotension, and shock have occurred in a few patients when deferoxamine was administered by rapid intravenous injection.
- Use a portable pump capable of providing continuous mini-infusion when administering drug by subcutaneous infusion. Be aware that the duration of infusion must be individualized as some patients excrete more iron after a short infusion of 8 to 12 hours, while another patient may need a 24-hour infusion to excrete the same amount.
- Monitor patient closely for changes in hearing or vision, especially in patients receiving deferoxamine at high doses or over prolonged periods of time, or in patients who have low ferritin levels. If present, notify prescriber immediately and expect drug to be discontinued. Expect audiometry, fundoscopy, slit-lamp examinations, and visual acuity tests to be performed periodically in patients treated for prolonged periods of time. Early detection improves the possibility of reversal of these symptoms or test abnormalities.
- Monitor patient's serum creatinine level, and assess patient for symptoms of renal dysfunction, because deferoxamine has been associated with renal dysfunction.
- Assess children regularly for growth retardation, especially if high doses of the drug are being administered in the presence of low ferritin levels. Monitor the child's body weight and growth every 3 months. If abnormalities are detected, notify the prescriber because growth velocity may partially resume to

pretreatment rates after a reduction of deferoxamine dosage occurs.

- Monitor patient, especially children, closely for signs and symptoms of respiratory distress, especially following treatment with excessively high intravenous doses of deferoxamine.

WARNING **Assess patient regularly for infections because either deferoxamine therapy or iron overload may enhance susceptibility to generalized infections. Some cases of mucormycosis have been fatal. If signs and symptoms occur, notify prescriber immediately and expect drug to be discontinued and appropriate treatment instituted.**

- Expect to administer vitamin C with deferoxamine therapy because iron overload usually causes a vitamin C deficiency. However, be aware that high doses (more than 500 mg daily in adults, 100 mg in children age 10 and older, and 50 mg in children under age 10) may cause cardiac dysfunction. Therefore, make sure patient is not receiving vitamin C if he has cardiac failure, expect supplemental vitamin C therapy to begin only after an initial month of regular treatment with deferoxamine, and make sure the daily dose of vitamin C does not exceed 200 mg in adults, given in divided doses. Monitor all patients receiving deferoxamine and vitamin C therapy concomitantly for cardiac dysfunction and report any dysfunction immediately to prescriber.
- Be aware that patients with aluminum-related encephalopathy who are receiving dialysis may develop seizures as a result of deferoxamine therapy. Deferoxamine therapy may also precipitate the onset of dialysis dementia in these patients, as well as cause a decrease in the patient's serum calcium levels and aggravate hyperparathyroidism, if present.
- Discontinue deferoxamine therapy, as ordered, 48 hours prior to scintigraphy because imaging results may be distorted as a result of the rapid urinary excretion of deferoxamine-bound gallium-67.

PATIENT TEACHING

- Inform patient that deferoxamine therapy is an adjunct to, and not a substitute for, standard measures used to treat acute iron intoxication.
- Advise patient not to exceed the recommended dose of daily vitamin C therapy prescribed.
- Caution patient not to perform hazardous activities such as driving until CNS, visual, and auditory adverse effects are known.
- Inform patient that his urine may have a reddish discoloration because of deferoxamine therapy.

delafloxacin

Baxdela

Class and Category

Pharmacologic class: Fluoroquinolone
Therapeutic class: Antibacterial
Pregnancy category: Not classified

Indications and Dosages

➤ *To treat acute bacterial skin and skin structure infections caused by gram-negative organisms* (Enterobacter cloacae, Escherichia coli, Klebsiella pneumoniae, Pseudomonas aeruginosa) *and gram-positive organisms* (Enterococcus faecalis, Staphylococcus aureus, S. haemolyticus, S. lugdunensis, Streptococcus agalactiae, S. anginosus, S. pyogenes)

TABLETS

Adults. 450 mg every 12 hr for 5 to 14 days.

I.V. INFUSION

Adults. 300 mg every 12 hr over 60 min for 5 to 14 days. Alternatively, 300 mg every 12 hr by I.V. infusion over 60 min, switched to 450 mg orally every 12 hr at the discretion of the prescriber for 5 to 14 days.

DOSAGE ADJUSTMENT For patients with an estimated glomerular filtration rate (eGFR) between 15 and 29 ml/min who are receiving the drug intravenously, dosage reduced to 200 mg every 12 hr or dosage reduced to 200 mg every 12 hr, then switched to 450 mg orally every 12 hr at the discretion of the prescriber.

Route	Onset	Peak	Duration
P.O.	Unknown	1 hr	Unknown
I.V.	Unknown	Unknown	Unknown

Mechanism of Action

Inhibits both bacterial topoisomerase IV and DNA gyrase enzymes, which are required for bacterial DNA recombination, repair, replication, and transcription.

Incompatibilities

Do not administer with other additives, medications, or substances other than 0.9% sodium chloride injection or D5W because incompatibilities are unknown.

Contraindications

Hypersensitivity to delafloxacin, other fluoroquinolones, or any of its components

Interactions

DRUGS

antacids containing aluminum or magnesium, didanosine, iron preparations, multivitamins containing iron or zinc, sucralfate: Significantly decreased absorption of oral delafloxacin

Adverse Reactions

CNS: Abnormal dreams, agitation, anxiety, confusion, delirium, depression, disorientation, disturbances in attention, dizziness, hallucinations, headache, hypoesthesia, **increased intracranial pressure**, insomnia, memory impairment, nervousness, nightmares, paresthesia, paranoia, peripheral neuropathy, **seizures**, **suicidal ideation**, syncope, tremors, toxic psychosis, vertigo
CV: Bradycardia, hypertension, **hypotension**, palpitations, phlebitis, tachycardia
EENT: Blurred vision, oral candidiasis, taste alteration, tinnitus
ENDO: Hyperglycemia, **hypoglycemia**
GI: Abdominal pain, ***Clostridium difficile*-associated diarrhea**, diarrhea, dyspepsia, elevated liver enzymes, nausea, vomiting
GU: Elevated blood creatinine levels, **renal failure**, renal impairment, vulvovaginal candidiasis
MS: Myalgia, tendinitis, tendon rupture
RESP: Dyspnea
SKIN: Dermatitis, flushing, pruritus, rash, urticaria
Other: Anaphylaxis, **angioedema**, elevated alkaline phosphatase and creatine phosphokinase levels, fungal infection, infusion-site reactions (bruising, discomfort, edema, erythema, irritation, pain, phlebitis, swelling, thrombosis)

Nursing Considerations

- Know that fluoroquinolones, including delafloxacin, may exacerbate muscle weakness in patients with myasthenia gravis and should not be given to patients with a history of myasthenia gravis.
- Administer delafloxacin tablets at least 2 hours before or 6 hours after antacids containing aluminum or magnesium, didanosine, iron preparations, multivitamins containing iron or zinc, or sucralfate, because absorption is affected by these drugs.
- Reconstitute powder for intravenous administration by using 10.5 ml of 0.9% sodium chloride injection or 5% Dextrose Injection (D5W) for each 300-mg vial. Shake the vial vigorously until contents are completely dissolved. The reconstituted vial will contain 300 mg per 12 ml of clear yellow to amber-colored solution. Further dilute to a total volume of 250 ml, using either 0.9% Sodium Chloride or D5W to achieve a concentration of 1.2 mg/ml. To do so, withdraw 12 ml for a 300-mg dose and 8 ml for a 200-mg dose from the vial and transfer to an intravenous bag to achieve a 250-ml volume of infusion solution. Discard any unused portion of the reconstituted solution. Reconstituted vials or diluted solution already added to an intravenous bag may be stored either in the refrigerator or at room temperature for up to 24 hours. The solution should not be frozen.
- Administer delafloxacin intravenously over 60 minutes. If a common intravenous line is being used to administer other drugs in addition to delafloxacin, the line should be flushed before and after each delafloxacin infusion with 0.9% sodium chloride injection or D5W.

WARNING Know that fluoroquinolones like delafloxacin have been associated with disabling and potentially irreversible serious adverse reactions that have occurred together, including central nervous system effects, peripheral neuropathy, tendinitis, and tendon rupture. Fluoroquinolones also have been

associated with an increased risk of increased intracranial pressure and seizures. At the first sign or symptom of any serious adverse reaction, withhold delafloxacin and notify prescriber. Expect delafloxacin to be discontinued.

- Monitor patients with severe renal impairment receiving intravenous delafloxacin by obtaining serum creatinine levels and eGFR values, as ordered. Know that if serum creatinine level increases, prescriber should be notified; expect patient to be switched to oral form. Notify prescriber if patient's eGFR decreases to less than 15 ml/min and expect drug to be discontinued.
- Assess patient for evidence of peripheral neuropathy. Notify prescriber and expect to stop drug if patient complains of burning, numbness, pain, tingling, or weakness in extremities or if physical examination reveals deficits in light touch, motor strength, pain, position sense, temperature, or vibratory sensation.
- Monitor patients (especially patients over 60 years of age, patients receiving corticosteroids, and patients who have renal failure or who have had a heart, kidney, or lung transplant) for evidence of tendon rupture, such as inflammation, pain, and swelling at the site. Be aware that tendon rupture may occur within the first 48 hours of therapy, throughout therapy, or months after delafloxacin therapy. Notify prescriber about suspected tendon rupture, and have patient rest and refrain from exercise until tendon rupture has been ruled out. If present, expect to provide supportive care, as ordered.
- Monitor patient closely for changes in behavior or mood that may be caused by delafloxacin-induced depression or worsening psychotic reactions potentially resulting in self-injurious behavior, such as suicide. Be aware that these reactions may occur even after just one dose. Notify prescriber immediately and expect to discontinue delafloxacin therapy, if present, and institute precautions to keep patient safe until adverse effects have disappeared.
- Assess patient routinely for signs of rash or other hypersensitivity reactions, even after patient has received multiple doses. Stop drug at first sign of rash or other sign of hypersensitivity, and notify prescriber immediately. Be prepared to provide supportive emergency care.
- Monitor patient closely for diarrhea, which may reflect pseudomembranous colitis caused by *Clostridium difficile* infection. If it occurs, notify prescriber and expect to withhold drug and treat diarrhea.
- Monitor patient's blood glucose levels, especially in diabetic patients, and for signs and symptoms of changes in blood glucose levels. Both symptomatic hyperglycemia and hypoglycemia may occur as a result of delafloxacin therapy. If present, alert prescriber and initiate appropriate treatment, as prescribed. Also be aware that severe hypoglycemia has occurred with other fluoroquinolones. If a hypoglycemic reaction occurs, discontinue administration immediately and initiate appropriate treatment for hypoglycemia.

PATIENT TEACHING

- Urge patient to complete the prescribed course of therapy, even if he feels better before it's finished.
- Tell patient that if he misses a dose, he should take it as soon as possible anytime up to 8 hours prior to the next dose. If less than 8 hours remain before the next dose, he should wait until the next scheduled dose.
- Instruct patient to take tablets at least 2 hours before or 6 hours after antacids containing aluminum or magnesium, didanosine, iron preparations, multivitamins containing iron or zinc, or sucralfate.
- Urge patient to avoid hazardous activities until CNS effects of drug are known.
- Advise patient to notify prescriber about changes in limb movement or sensation and about inflammation, pain, or swelling over a joint. Urge patient to rest the affected limb at the first sign of discomfort.
- Tell patient to stop taking drug and to notify prescriber at first sign of rash or other hypersensitivity reaction.
- Urge patient to report bloody, watery stools to prescriber immediately, even up to 2 months after drug therapy has ended.
- Urge caregivers to monitor patient closely for suicidal tendencies if patient develops depression or worsening of psychotic behavior during therapy and to notify prescriber.

D

- Instruct patient to report any persistent, severe, or unusual signs and symptoms to prescriber.
- Warn patients, especially diabetics, that delafloxacin may alter blood glucose levels. Review signs and symptoms of hyperglycemia and hypoglycemia. Tell patient to immediately report symptomatic changes in blood glucose levels to prescriber and review how to treat hypoglycemia.

denosumab

Prolia, Xgeva

Class and Category

Pharmacologic class: Monoclonal antibody
Therapeutic class: Antiresorptive, anti-osteoporotic
Pregnancy category: Not classified

Indications and Dosages

➤ *To treat men and postmenopausal women with osteoporosis at high risk for fracture; to treat bone loss in men receiving androgen deprivation therapy for prostate cancer; to treat bone loss in women receiving adjuvant aromatase inhibitor therapy for breast cancer to treat glucocorticoid-induced osteoporosis in men and women at high risk of fracture who are either initiating or continuing systemic glucocorticoids in a daily dosage equivalent to 7.5 mg or greater of prednisone and expected to remain on glucocorticoids for at least 6 months*

SUBCUTANEOUS INJECTION (PROLIA)

Adult. 60 mg once every 6 months.

➤ *To prevent skeletal-related events in patients with multiple myeloma and in patients with bone metastasis from solid tumors*

SUBCUTANEOUS INJECTION (XGEVA)

Adult. 120 mg every 4 wk.

➤ *To treat giant cell tumor of bone; to treat hypercalcemia of malignancy refractory to bisphosphonate therapy*

SUBCUTANEOUS INJECTION (XGEVA)

Adult. 120 mg every 4 wk with additional 120 mg doses on days 8 and 15 of the first month of therapy.

Route	Onset	Peak	Duration
SubQ	Unknown	10 days	Unknown

Mechanism of Action

Binds to RANKL, a transmembrane or soluble protein required for the formation, function, and survival of osteoclasts, the cells responsible for bone resorption. By preventing RANKL from activating its receptor, RANK, on the surface of osteoclasts, osteoclast formation, function, and survival are inhibited. This action decreases bone resorption and increases bone mass and strength in both cortical and trabecular bone.

Contraindications

Hypersensitivity to denosumab and its components, hypocalcemia

Interactions

DRUGS

other calcium-lowering drugs: Augmentation of calcium-lowering effect with possible severe hypocalcemia

Adverse Reactions

CNS: Asthenia, headache, insomnia, sciatica, vertigo
CV: Angina pectoris, **atrial fibrillation**, **endocarditis**, hypercholesterolemia, peripheral edema
EENT: Ear infection, nasopharyngitis
ENDO: Increased serum parathyroid hormone levels (presence of severe renal impairment or dialysis)
GI: Abdominal pain, constipation, diarrhea, flatulence, gastroesophageal reflux disease, nausea, **pancreatitis**, upper abdominal pain
GU: Cystitis, UTI
HEME: Anemia, **thrombocytopenia**
MS: Arthralgia; atypical subtrochanteric and diaphyseal femoral fractures; back, bone, extremity including joint, or musculoskeletal pain; jaw osteonecrosis; myalgia; spinal osteoarthritis
RESP: Pneumonia, upper respiratory infection
SKIN: Cellulitis, dermatitis, eczema, erysipelas (infection of upper dermis and superficial lymphatics), erythema, pruritus, rash, urticaria
Other: Anaphylaxis, **angioedema**, antibodies to denosumab, herpes zoster, **hypercalcemia of malignancy**,

hypocalcemia, hypophosphatemia, **malignancies (breast, gastrointestinal, reproductive)**, serious infections

Nursing Considerations

- Know that preexisting hypocalcemia must be corrected prior to denosumab therapy.
- Ensure that a pregnancy test has been performed and is negative for all childbearing women before denosumab therapy is begun, because the drug can be toxic to the fetus.
- Be aware that the drug solution may contain trace amounts of translucent to white proteinaceous particles. However, do not use if the solution is discolored or cloudy, or if the solution contains many particles or foreign particulate matter.
- Do not handle the gray needle cap on the prefilled syringe if allergic to latex.
- Prior to administration, remove drug from refrigerator and bring to room temperature, which generally takes 15 to 30 minutes. Do not warm the drug any other way.
- Know that when preparing to administer drug using the single prefilled syringe, do not slide the green safety guard forward over the needle, as it will lock in place and prevent injection. Do so only after the injection to prevent an accidental needle stick.
- Withdraw solution from a single-use vial using a 27G needle. Also administer the drug using a 27G needle.
- Administer denosumab in the upper arm, thigh, or abdomen.

WARNING Monitor patient closely for hypersensitivity reactions that may be severe such as dyspnea, hypotension, lip swelling, pruritus rash, upper airway edema, and urticaria. If present, stop denosumab therapy immediately, notify prescriber, and provide supportive care, as needed and ordered.

WARNING Monitor patient's calcium level, as ordered, especially in patients predisposed to hypocalcemia or disturbances of mineral metabolism, such as a history of excision of the small intestine, hypoparathyroidism, parathyroid or thyroid surgery, malabsorption syndromes, or severe renal impairment. Know that severe hypocalcemia has occurred with denosumab therapy resulting, in some cases, in death. Monitor patient closely for signs and symptoms of hypocalcemia such as neuromuscular irritability, and notify prescriber immediately if present. Expect drug to be discontinued, administer calcium replacement therapy, as ordered, and provide supportive care.

- Be aware that significant hypercalcemia has also occurred in patients with growing skeletons and patients with a giant cell tumor of the bone weeks to months after drug was discontinued. Monitor patient for signs of hypercalcemia (abdominal or bone pain, confusion, constipation, fatigue, frequent urination, muscle weakness, nausea, thirst, vomiting) and if present, notify prescriber and expect to treat, as prescribed.
- Know that fracture risk increases, including the risk of multiple vertebral fractures, when denosumab is discontinued. New vertebral fractures may occur as early as 7 months after the last dose. If denosumab therapy is discontinued, discuss possibility of patient transitioning to an alternative antiresorptive therapy with prescriber.
- Monitor patient for signs and symptoms of infection, because denosumab increases risk, especially if patient is receiving immunosuppressant therapy or has an impaired immune sytem. Serious skin infections as well as infections of the abdomen, ear, and urinary tract have occurred. There has also been increased incidence of endocarditis in patients receiving denosumab. Notify prescriber if an infection is suspected.

PATIENT TEACHING

- Tell patient that if a dose of denosumab is missed, injection should be administered as soon as convenient. Thereafter, future injections should be scheduled from the date of the actual injection.
- Instruct patient to take a calcium supplement of 1,000 mg and at least 400 international units of vitamin D daily. Review signs and symptoms of hypocalcemia and instruct patient to seek medical care promptly, if present.

- Tell patient to stop taking denosumab and seek immediate emergency care if allergic reactions occur.
- Advise patient to notify prescriber if signs and symptoms of infection occur, such as drainage, fever, pain, redness, or swelling.
- Inform patient to report bone, joint, and/or muscle pain as drug may need to be discontinued depending on the severity.
- Tell patient to notify prescriber if severe adverse skin reactions occur, as drug may need to be discontinued.
- Instruct patient on proper oral hygiene and on the need to notify dentist of denosumab therapy before invasive dental procedures are performed.
- Instruct women of childbearing age to use effective contraception during treatment and for at least 5 months after the last dose of denosumab. Also tell patient to report suspected or confirmed pregnancy immediately, as drug may cause fetal harm and have to be discontinued. Also inform her that breastfeeding is not recommended while taking denosumab.
- Advise patient to report new or unusual groin, hip, or thigh pain or tingling or numbness in fingers and toes.
- Advise patient not to interrupt denosumab therapy without talking with prescriber, because of increased risk for multiple vertebral fractures.
- Advise patients with growing skeletons to report decreased alertness, headache, nausea, or vomiting following discontinuation of drug, as this could indicate a higher than normal calcium level requiring prompt treatment.

desipramine hydrochloride

Norpramin

Class and Category

Pharmacologic class: Tricyclic antidepressant
Therapeutic class: Antidepressant
Pregnancy category: Not classified

Indications and Dosages

➤ *To treat depression*

TABLETS

Adults. *Initial:* 100 to 200 mg daily as single dose or divided doses. Increased gradually to 300 mg daily, if needed. *Maximum:* 300 mg daily.
Adolescents and elderly patients. *Initial:* 25 to 50 mg daily in divided doses. Increased gradually, if needed. *Maximum:* 150 mg daily.

Route	Onset	Peak	Duration
P.O.	2–3 wk	Unknown	Unknown

Mechanism of Action

Blocks norepinephrine and serotonin reuptake by adrenergic nerves, which normally release these neurotransmitters from their storage sites when activated by a nerve impulse. By blocking reuptake, this tricyclic antidepressant increases norepinephrine and serotonin levels at nerve synapses, which may elevate mood and reduce depression.

Contraindications

Acute recovery phase of MI; hypersensitivity to desipramine, other tricyclic antidepressants, or their components; linezolid or I.V. methylene blue; MAO inhibitor therapy within 14 days

Interactions

DRUGS

anticholinergics, sympathomimetics: Altered effectiveness of these drugs
barbiturates: Increased CNS depression
clonidine: Increased risk of hypertensive crisis
MAO inhibitors: Increased risk of life-threatening adverse effects, such as hyperpyretic or hypertensive crisis and severe seizures
P450 2D6 inhibitors (cimetidine, quinidine), class 1C antiarrhythmics (flecainide, propafenone), many other antidepressants, phenothiazines, selective serotonin reuptake inhibitors: Increased blood level and adverse effects of desipramine; potential increased blood levels of and adverse reactions to these drugs
quinolones: Increased risk of arrhythmias, including torsades de pointes

ACTIVITIES

alcohol use: Possibly increased alcohol effects

Adverse Reactions

CNS: Agitation, akathisia, anxiety, ataxia, confusion, **CVA**, delusions, disorientation, dizziness, drowsiness, extrapyramidal reactions, fatigue, headache, hypomania, insomnia, lack of coordination, nervousness, nightmares, paresthesia, peripheral neuropathy, psychosis exacerbation, restlessness, **seizures**, **serotonin syndrome**, sleep disturbance, **suicidal ideation**, tremor, weakness
CV: **Arrhythmias, including heart block**; hypertension; **hypotension**; palpitations
EENT: Acute-angle glaucoma, black tongue, blurred vision, dry mouth, mydriasis, stomatitis, taste perversion, tinnitus
ENDO: Breast enlargement and galactorrhea (women), gynecomastia (men), hyperglycemia, **hypoglycemia**, syndrome of inappropriate ADH secretion
GI: Abdominal cramps, anorexia, constipation, diarrhea, elevated liver enzymes, elevated pancreatic enzyme levels, epigastric distress, **hepatitis**, ileus, increased appetite, nausea, vomiting
GU: **Acute renal failure**, impotence, libido changes, nocturia, painful ejaculation, testicular swelling, urinary frequency and hesitancy, urine retention
HEME: **Agranulocytosis**, eosinophilia, **thrombocytopenia**
SKIN: Acne, alopecia, dermatitis, diaphoresis, dry skin, flushing, petechiae, photosensitivity, pruritus, purpura, rash, urticaria
Other: **Angioedema**, drug fever, weight gain

Nursing Considerations

- Use desipramine with extreme caution in patients with cardiovascular disease, glaucoma, seizure disorder, thyroid disease, or urine retention or with a family history of sudden death, cardiac arrhythmias, or conduction disturbances.

WARNING Be aware that desipramine increases risk of suicidal ideation in teens; monitor them closely for evidence.

WARNING Expect drug to produce sedation and possibly to lower seizure threshold. Take safety and seizure precautions. Seizures may precede arrhythmias and death in some patients. Alert prescriber immediately if seizure activity occurs.

- Monitor blood glucose level often.
- Be prepared to obtain blood sample for leukocyte and differential counts if patient develops fever during therapy.
- Expect to discontinue drug as soon as possible before elective surgery because of its possible adverse cardiovascular effects.

WARNING Monitor patient closely for evidence of serotonin syndrome, such as agitation, coma, diarrhea, hallucinations, hyperreflexia, hyperthermia, incoordination, labile blood pressure, nausea, tachycardia, or vomiting. Notify prescriber at once because serotonin syndrome maybe life-threatening. Be prepared to discontinue drug and provide supportive care.

PATIENT TEACHING

WARNING Urge parents to watch teen closely and to report abnormal thinking or behavior, aggression, or hostility.

- Urge patient to use sunscreen outdoors and to avoid sunlamps and tanning beds.
- Instruct patient to notify prescriber immediately about fainting, a fast and pounding heartbeat, restlessness, severe agitation, and strange behavior or thoughts.
- Caution patient not to stop drug abruptly; doing so may cause dizziness, headache, hyperthermia, irritability, malaise, nausea, sleep disturbances, and vomiting.
- Advise against drinking alcohol because of increased risk of adverse CNS reactions.
- Advise patient to avoid hazardous activities until drug's CNS effects are known.
- Advise patient that drug may cause mild pupillary dilation, which may lead to an episode of acute-angle glaucoma. Encourage patient to have an eye exam before starting therapy to see if she is at risk.
- Urge diabetic patient to monitor blood glucose level often.

desmopressin acetate

DDAVP, Minirin, Nocdurna, Noctiva, Stimate

Class and Category

Pharmacologic class: Posterior pituitary hormone
Therapeutic class: Antidiuretic, hemostatic
Pregnancy category: B (DDAVP, Stimate); not classified (Minirin)

Indications and Dosages

➤ *To manage primary nocturnal enuresis*

TABLETS

Adults and children age 4 and over. *Initial:* 0.2 mg at bedtime, increased as needed. *Maximum:* 0.6 mg daily.

➤ *To treat nocturia due to nocturnal polyuria in patients who awaken at least 2 times per night to void*

NASAL SPRAY (NOCTIVA)

Adults younger than 65 years who are not at increased risk for hyponatremia. 1 spray (1.66 mcg) in either the left or right nostril about 30 min before bedtime.

Adults 65 years or older who are not at increased risk for hyponatremia. 1 spray (0.83 mcg) in either the left or right nostril about 30 min before bedtime.

SUBLINGUAL TABLETS (NOCDURNA)

Women. 27.7 mcg once daily, 1 hr before bedtime.

Men. 55.3 mcg once daily, 1 hr before bedtime.

➤ *To control symptoms of central diabetes insipidus*

TABLETS

Adults and children age 4 and over. *Initial:* 0.05 mg twice daily, increased as needed. *Usual:* 0.1 to 0.8 mg in divided doses twice daily or three times daily. *Maximum:* 1.2 mg daily.

I.V. INFUSION, SUBCUTANEOUS INJECTION

Adults. 2 to 4 mcg daily in divided doses twice daily. Dosage adjusted as needed.

NASAL SPRAY (DDAVP)

Adults and adolescents. 0.1 to 0.4 ml daily (10 to 40 mcg daily) as a single dose or in divided doses twice daily or three times daily. Dosage adjusted as needed. If daily dose is divided, each dose adjusted separately.

Children ages 3 months to 12 years. 0.05 to 0.3 ml daily (5 to 30 mcg daily) as a single dose or in divided doses twice daily. Dosage adjusted as needed. If daily dose is divided, each dose adjusted separately.

NASAL SPRAY (MINIRIN)

Adults. 10 mcg once daily into one nostril, increased as needed up to 40 mcg once daily. 40-mcg doses may be divided into two or three daily doses.

Children age 4 and over. 10 mcg once daily into one nostril, increased as needed up to 30 mcg once daily. 30-mcg dose may be divided into two daily doses, usually with 20 mcg given in morning and 10 mcg given in evening.

➤ *To prevent or manage bleeding episodes in hemophilia A or mild to moderate type I von Willebrand's disease*

I.V. INFUSION

Adults and children age 3 months and over weighing more than 10 kg (22 lb). 0.3 mcg/kg diluted in 50 ml of normal saline solution and infused over 15 to 30 min. If used preoperatively, given 30 min before procedure.

Children age 3 months and over weighing 10 kg (22 lb) or less. 0.3 mcg/kg diluted in 10 ml normal saline solution and infused over 15 to 30 min. If used preoperatively, given 30 min before procedure.

NASAL SOLUTION (STIMATE)

Adults and children weighing more than 50 kg (110 lb). 150 mcg in each nostril. If used preoperatively, given 2 hr before procedure.

Adults and children weighing 50 kg or less. 150 mcg in one nostril. If used preoperatively, given 2 hr before procedure.

Route	Onset	Peak	Duration
P.O.	1 hr*	4–7 hr*	8–12 hr*
I.V.	15–30 min†	30–60 min†	3 hr‡
Nasal	In 1 hr*	1–5 hr*	8–20 hr*

* For antidiuretic effect.

† For antihemorrhagic effect.

‡ For von Willebrand disease; 4 to 20 hr for mild hemophilia A.

Mechanism of Action

Exerts an antidiuretic effect similar to that of vasopressin by increasing cellular permeability of renal collecting ducts and distal tubules, thus enhancing water reabsorption, reducing urine flow, and increasing osmolality. As a hemostatic, drug increases blood level of clotting factor VIII (antihemophilic factor) and activity of von Willebrand factor (factor VII_{VWF}). It also may increase platelet aggregation and adhesion at injury sites by directly affecting blood vessel walls.

Contraindications

All forms: History or presence of hyponatremia, hypersensitivity to desmopressin or its components, moderate to severe renal impairment (creatinine clearance below 50 ml/min)
DDVAP, Minirin, and Noctiva only: Primary nocturnal enuresis
Intranasal and sublingual forms: Concurrent therapy with inhaled or systemic glucocorticoids or loop diuretics, during illnesses that can cause fluid and electrolyte imbalance, polydipsia, syndrome of inappropriate antidiuretic hormone (SIADH) secretion
Nocdurna: Heart failure
Noctiva only: New York Heart Association Class II–IV congestive heart failure
Nocdurna and Noctiva: Uncontrolled hypertension

Interactions

DRUGS

carbamazepine, chlorpromazine, lamotrigine, NSAIDs, opioid analgesics, selective serotonin reuptake inhibitors, tricyclic antidepressants: Possibly increased risk of water intoxication with hyponatremia
vasopressor drugs: Possibly potentiated vasopressor effect of desmopressin

Adverse Reactions

CNS: Asthenia, chills, **CVA**, dizziness, headache
CV: Hypertension (with high doses), **MI**, **thrombosis**, transient hypotension
EENT: Conjunctivitis, epistaxis, lacrimation, nasal congestion (nasal form), ocular edema, pharyngitis, rhinitis, sore throat
GI: Abdominal cramps, nausea
GU: Vulvar pain (parenteral form)
RESP: Cough, upper respiratory infections
SKIN: Flushing
Other: **Anaphylaxis**, **hyponatremia**, injection-site pain and redness, water intoxication

Nursing Considerations

- Use desmopressin cautiously in patients with conditions associated with fluid and electrolyte imbalance, such as cystic fibrosis, heart failure, and renal disorders; these patients are prone to hyponatremia.
- Also use cautiously in patients with habitual or psychogenic polydipsia; they may be more likely to drink excessive water, raising the risk of hyponatremia.
- Be aware that nasal cavity scarring, edema, and other abnormalities may cause erratic absorption and require a different administration route.
- Do not shake bottle of Noctiva before administering. Prime the bottle when using for the first time by pumping 5 actuations into the air away from the face. Re-prime by pumping 2 actuations into the air if the product has not been used for more than 3 days. Be aware that 2 sprays of 0.83 mcg are not interchangeable with one spray of 1.66-mcg dose.
- Know that the recommended dose for women using the sublingual form of the drug is lower than for men because women are more sensitive to the effects of the sublingual form and have a higher risk of hyponatremia with the 55.3-mcg dose.
- Check blood pressure often during therapy.

WARNING **Monitor patient closely for evidence of hyponatremia, such as changes in mental status, depressed reflexes, fatigue, headache, lethargy, nausea, restlessness, and vomiting. If left undetected, coma, respiratory arrest, and seizures may occur. Monitor patient's serum sodium level, and notify prescriber of abnormalities.**

- Be aware that the nasal spray formulation is not used for the treatment of primary nocturnal enuresis due to a higher risk of hyponatremia and hyponatremic seizures.

PATIENT TEACHING

- Be aware that to prevent hyponatremia and water intoxication in a child or an elderly patient, family should be urged to restrict patient's fluids as prescribed.
- Tell patient to refrigerate nasal solution.
- Instruct patient who uses nasal spray to prime pump before first use by pressing down four times. Advise her to discard pump after 25 or 50 doses (Stimate) or 50 doses (DDAVP, Minirin), depending on bottle, because delivery of an accurate dose can't be assured.
- Teach patient who uses Noctiva nasal spray not to shake container before administering.

Tell patient to prime the container when using for the first time by pumping 5 actuations into the air away from the face. Re-prime by pumping 2 actuations into the air if the product has not been used for more than 3 days. Emphasize to patient that 2 sprays of 0.83 mcg are not interchangeable with one spray of 1.66 mcg.
- Instruct patient taking sublingual tablets to keep tablet under the tongue until it is fully dissolved. Also instruct patient to empty the bladder immediately before bedtime and to limit fluids to a minimum from 1 hour before until 8 hours after taking drug.
- Teach patient or caregiver how to administer subcutaneous injection, if appropriate.
- Urge patient to report adverse reactions.

dexamethasone

Dexamethasone Intensol

dexamethasone acetate

dexamethasone sodium phosphate

Class and Category

Pharmacologic class: Glucocorticoid
Therapeutic class: Anti-inflammatory, diagnostic aid, immunosuppressant
Pregnancy category: Not classified

Indications and Dosages

➤ *To treat inflammatory or neoplastic conditions*

ELIXIR, ORAL SOLUTION, TABLETS

Adults. Highly individualized dosage based on severity of disorder. *Usual:* 0.75 to 9 mg/day in divided doses.
Children. Highly individualized, based on severity of disorder. 0.02 to 0.3 mg/kg/day in three or four divided doses.

➤ *To manage adrenocortical insufficiency*

ELIXIR, ORAL SOLUTION, TABLETS, I.V. OR I.M. INJECTION

Adults. 0.5 to 9 mg daily as a single dose or in divided doses.

ELIXIR, ORAL SOLUTION, TABLETS

Children. 0.024 to 0.34 mg/kg/day in four divided doses.

➤ *To test for Cushing's syndrome*

ELIXIR, ORAL SOLUTION, TABLETS

Adults. 0.5 mg every 6 hr for 48 hr, followed by collection of 24-hr urine specimen to determine 17-hydroxycorticosteroid level. Or, 1 mg at 11 p.m., followed by plasma cortisol test performed at 8 a.m. the next day.

➤ *To distinguish Cushing's syndrome related to pituitary corticotropin excess from Cushing's syndrome from other causes*

ELIXIR, ORAL SOLUTION, TABLETS

Adults. 2 mg every 6 hr for 48 hr, followed by collection of 24-hr urine specimen to determine 17-hydroxycorticosteroid level.

➤ *To decrease cerebral edema*

ELIXIR, ORAL SOLUTION, TABLETS

Adults. 2 mg every 8 to 12 hr as maintenance after parenteral form has controlled initial symptoms.

I.V. INFUSION AND INJECTION

Adults. 10 mg I.V. followed by 4 mg I.M. every 6 hr. Decreased after 2 to 4 days, if needed, gradually tapering off over 5 to 7 days unless inoperable or recurring brain tumor is present. If such a tumor is present, dosage gradually decreased after 2 to 4 days to maintenance dosage of 2 mg I.M. every 8 to 12 hr and switched to P.O. regimen as soon as possible.

➤ *To treat unresponsive shock*

I.V. INFUSION AND INJECTION

Adults. 20 mg as a single dose, followed by 3 mg/kg over 24 hr as a continuous infusion; 40 mg as a single dose, followed by 40 mg every 2 to 6 hr, as needed; or 1 mg/kg to 6 mg/kg as a single dose. All regimens used no more than 3 days.

➤ To treat acute exacerbation of multiple sclerosis

ELIXIR, ORAL SOLUTION, TABLETS

Adults. 30 mg/day for 1 wk, followed by 4 to 12 mg/day for 1 month.

➤ To control incapacitating or severe allergic conditions unresponsive to conventional treatment

ELIXIR, I.M INJECTION, ORAL SOLUTION, TABLETS

Adults. *Day 1:* 4 to 8 mg I.M. *Days 2 and 3:* 3 mg/day P.O. divided every 12 hr.

Day 4: 1.5 mg/day P.O. divided every 12 hr.
Days 5 and 6: 0.75 mg/day P.O. as a single dose.

➤ *To decrease localized inflammation*

INTRA-ARTICULAR INJECTION

Adults. 2 to 4 mg for large joint; 0.8 to 1 mg for small joint; 2 to 3 mg for bursae; 0.4 to 1 mg for tendon sheaths.

SOFT-TISSUE INJECTION

Adults. 2 to 6 mg; 1 to 2 mg for ganglia.

INTRALESIONAL INJECTION

Adults. 0.8 to 1.6 mg/injection site.

Mechanism of Action

Binds to intracellular glucocorticoid receptors and suppresses inflammatory and immune responses by:

- inhibiting monocyte and neutrophil accumulation at inflammation site and suppressing bactericidal and phagocytic action
- stabilizing lysosomal membranes
- suppressing antigen response of helper T cells and macrophages
- inhibiting synthesis of inflammatory response mediators, such as cytokines, interleukins, and prostaglandins.

Contraindications

Administration of live-virus vaccine to patient or family member, hypersensitivity to dexamethasone or its components (including sulfites), idiopathic thrombocytopenic purpura (I.M. administration), systemic fungal infections

Interactions

DRUGS

aminoglutethimide, amphotericin B (parenteral), antacids, barbiturates, potassium-depleting drugs: Risk of hypokalemia
anticholinesterases: Decreased anticholinesterase effectiveness in myasthenia gravis
aspirin, NSAIDs: Increased risk of adverse GI effects
barbiturates, carbamazepine, rifampin: Decreased dexamethasone effects
cholestyramine: Increased dexamethasone clearance
cyclosporine: Increased activity of both drugs, possibly resulting in seizures
digoxin: Increased risk of digitalis toxicity related to hypokalemia
ephedrine: Decreased half-life and increased clearance of dexamethasone
erythromycin, indinavir: Increased clearance and decreased levels of these drugs
estrogens, ketoconazole, macrolide antibiotics: Decreased dexamethasone clearance and increased dexamethasone effects
isoniazid: Decreased blood isoniazid level
neuromuscular blockers: Possibly potentiated or counteracted neuromuscular blockade
oral anticoagulants: Possibly altered coagulation times, requiring reduced anticoagulant dosage
phenytoin: Increased risk of seizures
potassium-wasting diuretics: Increased potassium loss and risk of hypokalemia
salicylates: Decreased blood level and effectiveness of salicylates
thalidomide: Increased risk of toxic epidermal necrolysis
theophyllines: Altered effects of either drug
toxoids, vaccines: Decreased antibody response

ACTIVITIES

alcohol use: Increased risk of GI bleeding

Adverse Reactions

CNS: Depression, emotional lability, euphoria, fever, headache, **increased intracranial pressure (ICP) with papilledema**, insomnia, light-headedness, malaise, neuritis, neuropathy, paresthesia, psychosis, **seizures**, syncope, tiredness, vertigo, weakness
CV: Arrhythmias, bradycardia, edema, **fat embolism, heart failure**, hypercholesterolemia, hyperlipidemia, hypertension, **myocardial rupture**, tachycardia, **thromboembolism**, thrombophlebitis, vasculitis
EENT: Blurred vision, cataracts, exophthalmos, glaucoma, ocular infections, *All forms:* Epistaxis, loss of smell and taste, nasal burning and dryness, oral candidiasis, perforated nasal septum, pharyngitis, rebound nasal congestion, rhinorrhea
ENDO: Cushingoid symptoms, decreased iodine uptake, growth suppression in children, hyperglycemia, menstrual irregularities, **secondary adrenocortical and pituitary unresponsiveness**
GI: Abdominal distention, bloody stools, elevated liver enzymes, heartburn, hepato-

megaly, increased appetite, indigestion, **intestinal perforation**, **melena**, nausea, **pancreatitis**, peptic ulcer **with possible perforation**, ulcerative esophagitis, vomiting
GU: Glycosuria, increased or decreased number and motility of spermatozoa, perineal irritation, urinary frequency
HEME: Leukocytosis, **leukopenia**
MS: Aseptic necrosis of femoral and humeral heads; muscle atrophy, spasms, or weakness; myalgia; osteoporosis; pathologic fracture of long bones; tendon rupture (intra-articular injection); vertebral compression fracture
RESP: Bronchospasm
SKIN: Acne, allergic dermatitis, diaphoresis, ecchymosis, erythema, hirsutism, necrotizing vasculitis, petechiae, subcutaneous fat atrophy, striae, thin and fragile skin, urticaria
Other: Aggravated or masked signs of infection, **anaphylaxis**, **angioedema**, **hypernatremia**, **hypocalcemia**, **hypokalemia**, **hypokalemic alkalosis**, impaired wound healing, **metabolic acidosis**, suppressed skin test reaction, **tumor lysis syndrome**, weight gain

Nursing Considerations

- Use dexamethasone cautiously in patients with congestive heart failure, hypertension, or renal insufficiency because drug can cause sodium retention, which may lead to edema and hypokalemia.
- Also use cautiously in patients who have had intestinal surgery and in those with diverticulitis, peptic ulcer, or ulcerative colitis because of the risk of perforation.
- Give once-daily dose of dexamethasone in the morning to coincide with the body's natural cortisol secretion.
- Give oral drug with food to decrease GI distress.
- Be aware that dosage forms with a concentration of 24 mg/ml are for I.V. use only.
- Shake I.M. solution before injecting deep into large muscle mass.

WARNING Avoid subcutaneous injection; it may cause atrophy and sterile abscess.

- Inject undiluted I.V. dose directly into I.V. tubing of infusing compatible solution over 30 seconds or less, as prescribed.

WARNING Don't give acetate form by I.V. injection.

- Expect to taper drug rather than stopping it abruptly; prolonged use can cause adrenal suppression.
- Monitor fluid intake and output and daily weight, and watch for crackles, dyspnea, peripheral edema, and steady weight gain.
- Evaluate growth if patient is a child.
- Test stool for occult blood.
- Monitor results of hematology studies and blood glucose, cholesterol, lipids levels, and serum electrolyte. Dexamethasone may cause hyperglycemia, hypernatremia, hypocalcemia, hypokalemia, or leukopenia. It also may increase serum cholesterol and lipid levels, and it may decrease iodine uptake by the thyroid.
- Assess patient for evidence of Cushing's syndrome, osteoporosis, and other systemic effects during long-term use.
- Monitor neonate for signs of hypoadrenocorticism if mother received dexamethasone during pregnancy. Be aware that some preparations contain benzyl alcohol, which may cause a fatal toxic syndrome in neonates and immature infants.
- Watch for hypersensitivity reactions after giving acetate or sodium phosphate form; both may contain bisulfites or parabens, to which some people are allergic.
- Be aware that the use of corticosteroids such dexamethasone, especially for longer than 6 weeks, increases the risk of development of eye disorders, including cataracts and glaucoma, which can possibly damage the optic nerves, and ocular infections due to bacteria, fungi, or viruses. Know that patient should be referred to an ophthalmologist if patient develops ocular symptoms while taking dexamethasone.

PATIENT TEACHING

- Instruct patient not to store drug in damp or hot places and to protect liquid form from freezing.
- Instruct patient to take once-daily oral dose in the morning with food to help prevent GI distress.
- Caution against consuming alcohol during dexamethasone therapy because it increases the risk of GI bleeding.
- Advise patient to follow a low-sodium, high-potassium, high-protein diet, if prescribed, to help minimize weight gain, which is common with dexamethasone

therapy. Instruct her to inform prescriber if she's on a special diet.

- Instruct patient not to stop drug abruptly.
- Advise patient to notify prescriber if condition recurs or worsens after dosage is reduced or therapy stops.
- Urge patient to have regular eye examinations during long-term use and to report any eye abnormalities to prescriber.
- Advise patient on long-term therapy to carry medical identification and to notify all healthcare providers that she takes dexamethasone.
- Instruct patient (especially a child) to avoid close contact with anyone who has chickenpox or measles and to notify prescriber immediately if exposure occurs.
- Advise patient and family members to avoid live-virus vaccinations during therapy unless prescriber approves.
- Inform diabetic patient that drug may affect her blood glucose level.
- Instruct patient having drug injected into a joint to avoid putting excessive pressure on it and to notify prescriber if it becomes red or swollen.
- Tell patient to notify prescriber about anorexia, depression, lightheadedness, malaise, muscle pain, nausea, vomiting, and early hyperadrenocorticism (abdominal distention, amenorrhea, easy bruising, extreme weakness, facial hair, increased appetite, moon face, weight gain). Tell patient and family about possible changes in appearance.
- Urge patient to notify prescriber about illness, surgery, or changes in stress level.

dexchlorpheniramine maleate

Dexgen-SR, Polaramine, Polaramine Repetabs, Polmon

Class and Category

Pharmacologic class: Propylamine derivative
Therapeutic class: Antihistamine
Pregnancy category: B

Indications and Dosages

➤ *To treat allergic conjunctivitis; transfusion reaction; dermographism; mild, uncomplicated allergic skin reactions, such as urticaria and angioedema; perennial and seasonal allergic rhinitis; and vasomotor rhinitis and as adjunct to treat anaphylaxis*

E.R. TABLETS

Adults and adolescents. 4 to 6 mg daily at bedtime or every 8 to 10 hr, as needed.

SYRUP, TABLETS

Adults and adolescents. 2 mg every 4 to 6 hr, as needed.

Children ages 6 to 12. 1 mg every 4 to 6 hr or 150 mcg/kg in divided doses four times daily, as needed.

Children ages 2 to 6. 0.5 mg every 4 to 6 hr, as needed.

Route	Onset	Peak	Duration
P.O.	15–60 min*	Unknown*	4–8 hr*

* For syrup and tablets; unknown for E.R. tablets.

Mechanism of Action

Binds to central and peripheral H_1 receptors, competing with histamine for these sites and preventing histamine from reaching its site of action. By blocking histamine, dexchlorpheniramine:

- inhibits GI, respiratory, and vascular smooth-muscle contraction, which prevents wheezing
- decreases capillary permeability, which reduces flares, itching, and wheals
- decreases lacrimal and salivary gland secretions, reducing nasal secretions, itching, sneezing, and watery eyes.

Contraindications

Breastfeeding; hypersensitivity to dexchlorpheniramine, other antihistamines, or their components; lower respiratory tract disorders, such as asthma; MAO inhibitor use within 14 days

Interactions

DRUGS

anticholinergics: Potentiated anticholinergic effects
CNS depressants: Increased CNS depression

MAO inhibitors: Possibly severe hypotension and prolonged and intensified anticholinergic and sedative effects of dexchlorpheniramine

ACTIVITIES

alcohol use: Increased CNS depression

Adverse Reactions

CNS: Ataxia, confusion, dizziness, drowsiness, euphoria, excitement, headache, insomnia, irritability, nervousness, neuritis, nightmares, paresthesia, restlessness, vertigo, weakness
CV: **Hypotension**, palpitations, tachycardia
EENT: Acute labyrinthitis, blurred vision, dry mouth, tinnitus, vision changes
GI: Anorexia, constipation, diarrhea, indigestion, nausea, vomiting
GU: Urinary hesitancy, urine retention
RESP: Tenacious bronchial secretions
SKIN: Diaphoresis, photosensitivity, rash

Nursing Considerations

- Use dexchlorpheniramine cautiously in elderly patients and those with CV disease, hyperthyroidism, increased intraocular pressure, prostatic hypertrophy, or renal disease.
- Monitor patient for adverse reactions, especially in elderly patients and children.
- Watch for evidence of overdose, including clumsiness; drowsiness; dry mouth, nose, or throat; dyspnea; flushed or red face; hallucinations; insomnia; lightheadedness; seizures; and unsteadiness.

PATIENT TEACHING

- Inform patient that drug provides temporary relief of symptoms.
- Advise patient to take drug with food, milk, or water to reduce GI irritation. Inform her that she can crush regular (not E.R.) tablets and mix with food or fluid.
- For E.R. tablets, tell patient not to break, chew, or crush them before swallowing.
- Urge patient to take missed dose as soon as possible unless it's almost time for next dose.
- Caution patient to avoid hazardous activities until its CNS effects are known, because drug may cause drowsiness.
- Instruct her to avoid prolonged sun exposure and to use a sunscreen.
- Suggest the patient to use sugarless candy or gum, ice chips, or saliva substitute to relieve dry mouth. If dryness lasts longer than 2 weeks, urge her to notify prescriber.
- Caution patient to avoid alcohol and CNS depressants, such as sedatives, sleeping pills, and tranquilizers, during therapy.
- Urge patient to inform prescriber if she takes high doses of aspirin, because antihistamines may mask adverse reactions to aspirin overdose, such as tinnitus.
- Inform patient that drug needs to be discontinued 3 to 4 days before skin tests for allergies are performed.

dexmethylphenidate hydrochloride

Focalin, Focalin XR

Class, Category, and Schedule

Pharmacologic class: Methylphenidate derivative
Therapeutic class: CNS stimulant
Pregnancy category: C
Controlled substance schedule: II

Indications and Dosages

➤ *To treat attention deficit hyperactivity disorder (ADHD)*

TABLETS

Adults and children age 6 and over who are new to methylphenidate. 2.5 mg twice daily at least 4 hr apart, increased weekly by 2.5 to 5 mg. *Maximum:* 10 mg twice daily.
Adults and children age 6 and over who take methylphenidate. Half of racemic methylphenidate dosage. *Maximum:* 10 mg twice daily at least 4 hr apart.

DOSAGE ADJUSTMENT Dosage decreased for paradoxical aggravation of symptoms or adverse reactions.

E.R. CAPSULES
Adults who are new to methylphenidate. 10 mg daily, increased weekly by 10 mg daily, as needed. *Maximum:* 40 mg daily.
Children age 6 and over who are new to methylphenidate. 5 mg daily, increased weekly as needed by 5-mg increments. *Maximum:* 30 mg daily.
Adults and children age 6 and over who take methylphenidate. Half of racemic methylphenidate dosage. *Maximum:* 20 mg daily.

Mechanism of Action

May block reuptake of dopamine and norepinephrine into presynaptic neurons in cerebral cortex, which increases availability of dopamine and norepinephrine in extraneuronal space.

Contraindications

Diagnosis or family history of Tourette syndrome; glaucoma; hypersensitivity to dexmethylphenidate, methylphenidate, or their components; marked agitation, anxiety, and tension; motor tics; use within 14 days of MAO inhibitor

Interactions

DRUGS
anticoagulants (selected, oral), anticonvulsants, antidepressants (selected, tricyclic and selective serotonin reuptake inhibitors): Possibly decreased metabolism of these drugs
antihypertensives: Decreased therapeutic effect of these drugs
dopamine and other vasopressors: Altered effect on blood pressure
MAO inhibitors: Increased adverse effects, risk of hypertensive crisis
serotonergic drugs: Increased risk of serotonin syndrome

Adverse Reactions

CNS: Aggression, **cerebral arteritis or occlusion**, depression, dizziness, drowsiness, dyskinesia, fever, headache, insomnia, motor or vocal tics, nervousness, **seizures**, Tourette syndrome, toxic psychosis
CV: Angina, **arrhythmias**, decreased or increased pulse rate, hypertension, **hypotension**, palpitations, peripheral vasculopathy including Raynaud's phenomenon, tachycardia
EENT: Accommodation abnormality, blurred vision
GI: Abdominal pain, anorexia, elevated liver enzymes, **hepatic dysfunction**, nausea
GU: Libido changes, priapism
HEME: Anemia, **leukopenia**, **thrombocytopenic purpura**
MS: Arthralgia, **rhabdomyolysis**
SKIN: Alopecia, **erythema multiforme**, **exfoliative dermatitis**, necrotizing vasculitis, rash, urticaria
Other: Anaphylaxis, **angioedema**, weight loss (prolonged therapy)

Nursing Considerations

WARNING Be aware that dexmethylphenidate may induce CNS stimulation, mania, and psychosis and may worsen behavior disturbances and thought disorders. Use drug cautiously in children with mania or psychosis. Be aware that withdrawal symptoms may occur with long-term use.

- Also know that dexmethylphenidate should be used cautiously in patients with serious cardiac abnormalities (structural), cardiomyopathy, serious heart rhythm abnormalities, or other serious cardiac problems because drug may increase risk of sudden death from these conditions.
- Monitor blood pressure and pulse rate to detect hypertension and excessive stimulation. Notify prescriber if signs appear.

WARNING Monitor patient for signs of physical or psychological dependence. Use drug cautiously in patients with a history of drug abuse, including alcoholism.

- Monitor CBC and differential and platelet counts, as ordered, during prolonged therapy.
- Expect to stop drug if seizures occur. Drug may lower seizure threshold, especially in patients with a history of seizures or EEG abnormalities.
- Assess patient for signs and symptoms of peripheral vasculopathy, including Raynaud's phenomenon. Although mild

and intermittent, know that digital ulceration and/or soft tissue breakdown has occurred. Notify prescriber if present, as drug dosage may need to be reduced or drug discontinued.

WARNING Question male patients, including male children, about painful and prolonged erections, especially after a dosage increase or during a period of drug withdrawal. Know that presence of priapism has sometimes required emergency surgical intervention, so report any findings to prescriber immediately.

- Monitor children on long-term dexmethylphenidate therapy for signs of growth suppression, which has been noted during long-term use of stimulants.

PATIENT TEACHING

- Tell patient that extended-release capsules should either be taken whole, without being chewed, crushed, or divided, or capsule contents should be sprinkled on a small amount of applesauce.
- Urge patient to notify prescriber if she has excessive nervousness, fever, insomnia, nausea, palpitations, or rash while taking dexmethylphenidate.
- Caution patient with seizure disorder that drug may cause seizures.
- Advise patient to protect drug from light and moisture.
- Teach patient (or parent) to watch for improvement in signs and symptoms of ADHD, such as decreased impulsiveness and increased attention. Stress the need for continued follow-up care, and suggest participation in an ADHD program.

WARNING Inform male patients and parents or caregivers of male children that dexmethylphenidate may cause abnormally sustained or frequent and painful erections, especially when a dosage increase occurs or during a period of drug withdrawal. Advise immediate emergency care if this should occur.

- Instruct patient to inspect his fingers and toes daily for changes such as skin breakdown or ulcer formation. Although usually intermittent and mild, patient should contact prescriber if abnormalities occur, as drug may have to be discontinued or dosage reduced.

dextrose
(d-glucose)

B-D Glucose, Glutose, Insta-Glucose, Insulin Reaction

glucose

2.5% Dextrose Injection, 5% Dextrose Injection, 10% Dextrose Injection, 20% Dextrose Injection, 25% Dextrose Injection, 50% Dextrose Injection, 60% Dextrose Injection, 70% Dextrose Injection

Class and Category

Pharmacologic class: Carbohydrate
Therapeutic class: Glucose-elevating agent, nutritional supplement
Pregnancy category: C

Indications and Dosages

➤ *To treat insulin-induced hypoglycemia*

CHEWABLE TABLETS, ORAL GEL

Adults and children. *Initial:* 10 to 20 g. Repeated in 10 to 20 min, if needed, based on serum glucose level.

I.V. INFUSION OR INJECTION

Adults and adolescents. *Initial:* 20 to 50 ml of 50% solution given at 3 ml/min. *Maintenance:* 10% to 15% solution by continuous infusion until blood glucose level reaches therapeutic range.
Children older than 6 months. *Initial:* 0.5 to 1 g/kg/dose of 25% solution. *Maximum:* 25 g/dose.
Infants less than 6 months of age and neonates. *Initial:* 0.25 to 0.5 g/kg/dose of 25% solution. *Maximum:* 25 g/dose.

➤ *To replace calories*

I.V. INFUSION

Adults and children. Individualized dosage of 2.5%, 5%, or 10% solution, based on need for fluids or calories and given by peripheral I.V. line. Or 10% to 70% solution given by central vein, if needed, typically with amino acids or other solutions.

Route	Onset	Peak	Duration
P.O.	10–20 min	40 min	Unknown
I.V.	2–3 min	Unknown	Unknown

Mechanism of Action

Prevents nitrogen and protein loss, promotes glycogen deposition, prevents or decreases ketosis, and, in large amounts, acts as an osmotic diuretic. Dextrose is readily metabolized and undergoes oxidation to carbon dioxide and water. The oral form—glucose—is absorbed directly into the bloodstream from the intestines and is distributed, stored, or used in the liver.

Incompatibilities

Don't give dextrose through same infusion set as blood or blood products because pseudoagglutination of RBCs may occur.

Contraindications

For all solutions: Diabetic coma with excessively elevated blood glucose level
For concentrated solutions: Anuria, alcohol withdrawal syndrome in dehydrated patient, glucose-galactose malabsorption syndrome, hepatic coma, hypersensitivity to corn or corn products, intracranial or intraspinal hemorrhage, overhydration, severe dehydration

Interactions

DRUGS

corticosteroids, corticotropin: Increased risk of fluid and electrolyte imbalance if dextrose solution contains sodium ions

Adverse Reactions

CNS: Chills, confusion, fever
CV: Hypotension
ENDO: Hyperglycemic hyperosmolar coma
GI: *For concentrated solutions:* Cholecystitis; cholelithiasis; cholestasis; **cirrhosis**; **hepatic failure**, **fibrosis**, **or steatosis**
GU: Glycosuria
RESP: Bronchospasm, **cyanosis**
Concentrated forms: **pulmonary embolism**, **respiratory distress**
SKIN: Pruritis, rash
Other: Anaphylaxis; **angioedema**; dehydration; **electrolyte deficits**; hypervolemia; hypovolemia; injection-site extravasation with tissue necrosis, infection, phlebitis, and **venous thrombosis**

Nursing Considerations

- Use dextrose cautiously in patients with renal impairment because solutions contain aluminum that could be toxic in prolonged parenteral therapy. Also, premature infants receiving prolonged treatment with concentrated forms of dextrose are at risk for aluminum toxicity because of immature renal function.
- Give highly concentrated dextrose solution by central venous catheter—not by I.M. or subcutaneous route.

WARNING **Know that excessive or rapid delivery of dextrose solution in a very low-birth-weight infant may increase serum osmolality and cause intracerebral hemorrhage.**

- Assess infusion site regularly for signs of infiltration, such as pain or swelling.

WARNING **Monitor patient closely for a hypersensitivity reaction. Stop infusion immediately and treat patient according to institutional protocol if patient develops angioedema, bronchospasm, chills, cyanosis, hypotension, pruritis, pyrexia, or rash.**

- Monitor patient's liver function including ammonia levels regularly, as ordered, because concentrated solutions of dextrose may cause hepatic dysfunction. If hepatic dysfunction occurs, expect dosage to be decreased or solution discontinued.
- Assess patient's blood glucose level frequently to determine effectiveness and detect hyperglycemia, which can result in an increase in serum osmolality, causing dehydration, electrolyte loss, and osmotic diuresis. Know that patients with CNS disease and renal impairment may be at higher risk. Also assess patient and monitor patient's electrolytes and fluid balance, as ordered, to detect electrolyte imbalances and fluid overload as early as possible. Patients at increased risk for hyponatremic encephalopathy include children, the elderly, patients with underlying CNS disease or hypoxemia, and premenopausal women.
- Expect to give a 5% to 10% dextrose infusion to avoid rebound hypoglycemia when discontinuing a concentrated solution.
- Monitor patient for signs of hypervolemia, such as jugular vein distention and crackles.
- Know that concentrated solutions of dextrose pose a risk of pulmonary vascular precipitates passing through an in-line filter that can result in a pulmonary embolism.

D

Always inspect the catheter, infusion set, and solution for precipitates. If patient develops respiratory distress, stop the infusion and notify prescriber immediately.
- Assess patient for signs and symptoms, including chills and fever, when administering concentrated forms of dextrose. This is because the nutritional components of these solutions can support microbial growth. Monitor patient's parenteral access device and insertion site for discharge, edema, or redness and laboratory test results that may reveal hyperglycemia and leukocytosis.

PATIENT TEACHING
- Advise patient to swallow oral dextrose; it isn't absorbed from the buccal cavity.
- Instruct patient to monitor her blood glucose level as directed.
- Emphasize importance of reporting discomfort, pain, or signs of infection at I.V. site.

diazepam

Diastat, Diazepam Intensol, Dizac, Valium

Class, Category, and Schedule

Pharmacologic class: Benzodiazepine
Therapeutic class: Anticonvulsant, anxiolytic, sedative-hypnotic, skeletal muscle relaxant
Pregnancy category: D
Controlled substance schedule: IV

Indications and Dosages

➤ *To relieve anxiety*

ORAL SOLUTION, TABLETS

Adults. 2 to 10 mg twice daily to four times daily.
DOSAGE ADJUSTMENT Dosage reduced to 2 to 2.5 mg daily or twice daily and increased gradually as needed and tolerated for debilitated or elderly patients.
Children age 6 months and over. *Initial:* 1 to 2.5 mg three times daily or four times daily. Increased gradually as needed and tolerated.

I.V. OR I.M. INJECTION

Adults. 2 to 5 mg every 3 to 4 hr, as needed, for moderate anxiety; 5 to 10 mg every 3 to 4 hr, as needed, for severe anxiety. I.V. injection given slowly, not exceeding 5 mg/min.

➤ *To treat symptoms of acute alcohol withdrawal*

ORAL SOLUTION, TABLETS

Adults. 10 mg three times daily or four times daily during first 24 hr. Then 5 mg three times daily or four times daily, if needed.

I.V. OR I.M. INJECTION

Adults. 10 mg and then 5 to 10 mg in 3 to 4 hr, if needed. I.V. injection given slowly, not exceeding 5 mg/min.

➤ *To provide muscle relaxation; to provide sedation*

ORAL SOLUTION, TABLETS

Adults. 2 to 10 mg three times daily or four times daily.
DOSAGE ADJUSTMENT Dosage reduced to 2 to 2.5 mg once or twice daily and increased gradually as needed and tolerated for debilitated or elderly patients.
Children age 6 months and over. *Initial:* 1 to 2.5 mg t.i.d. or q.i.d. Increased gradually as needed and tolerated.

I.V. OR I.M. INJECTION

Adults. *Initial:* 5 to 10 mg, then repeated every 3 to 4 hr, as needed. I.V. injection given slowly, not exceeding 5 mg/min.

➤ *To treat seizures*

ORAL SOLUTION, TABLETS

Adults. 2 to 10 mg twice daily to four times daily.
DOSAGE ADJUSTMENT Dosage reduced to 2 to 2.5 mg once or twice daily and increased gradually as needed and tolerated for debilitated or elderly patients.
Children age 6 months and over. *Initial:* 1 to 2.5 mg three times daily or four times daily. Increased gradually as needed and tolerated.

➤ *To treat status epilepticus and severe recurrent seizures*

I.V. INJECTION

Adults. 5 to 10 mg given slowly, not exceeding 5 mg/min, repeated every 10 to 15 min, as needed, up to a cumulative dose of 30 mg. Regimen repeated, if needed, in 2 to 4 hr. (Use I.M. route if I.V. access is impossible.)
Children age 5 and over. 1 mg given slowly over 3 min, not exceeding 0.25 mg/kg, repeated every 2 to 5 min, as needed, up to a cumulative dose of 10 mg. Regimen repeated, if needed, in 2 to 4 hr.
Children ages 1 month to 5 years. 0.2 to 0.5 mg given slowly over 3 min, not

exceeding 0.25 mg/kg, repeated every 2 to 5 min, as needed, up to a cumulative dose of 5 mg. Regimen repeated, if needed, in 2 to 4 hr.

RECTAL GEL

Adults and adolescents. 0.2 mg/kg rounded up to next available unit dose (or rounded down for debilitated or elderly patient). Repeated in 4 to 12 hr, if needed.

Children ages 6 to 12. 0.3 mg/kg rounded up to next available unit dose. Repeated in 4 to 12 hr, if needed.

Children ages 2 to 6. 0.5 mg/kg rounded up to next available unit dose. Repeated in 4 to 12 hr, if needed.

➤ *To provide preoperative sedation*

I.V. OR I.M. INJECTION

Adults. 5 to 10 mg 30 min before surgery. I.V. injection given slowly, not exceeding 5 mg/min.

➤ *To reduce anxiety before cardioversion*

I.V. INJECTION

Adults. 5 to 15 mg given slowly, not exceeding 5 mg/min, 5 to 10 min before procedure.

➤ *To reduce anxiety before endoscopic procedures*

I.V. INJECTION

Adults. Up to 20 mg given slowly, not exceeding 5 mg/min, titrated to desired sedation and given immediately before procedure.

I.M. INJECTION

Adults. 5 to 10 mg 30 min before procedure.

➤ *To treat tetanus*

I.V. OR I.M. INJECTION

Adults and children age 5 and over. *Initial:* 5 to 10 mg repeated every 3 to 4 hr, if needed. I.V. injection given slowly, not exceeding 5 mg/min for adults, and given slowly over 3 min and not exceeding 0.25 mg/kg for children. Sometimes larger doses are needed for adults.

DOSAGE ADJUSTMENT Initial dose reduced to 2 to 5 mg and increased gradually as needed and tolerated for debilitated patients.

Children ages 1 month to 5 years. 1 to 2 mg repeated every 3 to 4 hr, as needed. I.V. injection given slowly over 3 min, not exceeding 0.25 mg/kg.

Mechanism of Action

May potentiate effects of gamma-aminobutyric acid (GABA) and other inhibitory neurotransmitters by binding to specific benzodiazepine receptors in cortical and limbic areas of CNS. GABA inhibits excitatory stimulation, which helps control emotional behavior. Limbic system contains a dense area of benzodiazepine receptors, which may explain drug's antianxiety effects. Diazepam suppresses spread of seizure activity caused by seizure-producing foci in cortex, limbic, and thalamus structures.

Incompatibilities

Don't mix diazepam injection with aqueous solutions. Don't mix diazepam emulsion for I.M. injection with glycopyrrolate or morphine or administer it through an infusion set that contains polyvinyl chloride.

Contraindications

For all forms: Acute angle-closure glaucoma, hypersensitivity to diazepam or its components, untreated open-angle glaucoma
For oral forms: Children under 6 months of age, myasthenia gravis, severe hepatic impairment, severe respiratory insufficiency, sleep apnea

Interactions

DRUGS

antacids: Altered rate of diazepam absorption
cimetidine, disulfiram, fluoxetine, fluvoxamine, isoniazid, itraconazole, ketoconazole, metoprolol, omeprazole, oral contraceptives, propranolol, valproic acid: Decreased diazepam metabolism, increased blood level and risk of adverse effects including prolonged sedation
CNS depressants including anesthetics, anticonvulsants, antipsychotics, anxiolytics, barbiturates, hypnotics, MAO inhibitors, narcotics, phenothiazines, sedatives including sedative antihistamines, and other antidepressants: Increased CNS depression and risk of falls and fractures
digoxin: Increased serum digoxin level and risk of digitalis toxicity
levodopa: Decreased antidyskinetic effect of levodopa
opioids: Increased risk of severe respiratory depression

phenytoin: Decreased metabolic elimination of phenytoin, increased risk of adverse reactions

ACTIVITIES

alcohol use: Increased CNS depression, including severe respiratory depression, significant sedation and somnolence, and increased risk of falls and fractures

Adverse Reactions

CNS: Anterograde amnesia, anxiety, ataxia, confusion, depression, dizziness, drowsiness, fatigue, headache, insomnia, lethargy, light-headedness, paradoxical reactions, psychiatric effects, sedation, sleepiness, slurred speech, **suicidal ideation**, tremor, vertigo
CV: Hypotension, palpitations, tachycardia
EENT: Blurred vision, diplopia, dry mouth, increased salivation
GI: Anorexia, constipation, diarrhea, elevated liver enzymes, jaundice, nausea, vomiting
GU: Libido changes, urinary incontinence, urine retention
HEME: Neutropenia
MS: Dysarthria, muscle weakness
RESP: Respiratory depression
SKIN: Dermatitis
Other: Physical and psychological dependence

Nursing Considerations

- Use diazepam with extreme caution in patients with a history of alcohol or drug abuse because it can cause physical and psychological dependence, and in patients with hepatic disorders such as hepatic fibrosis and hepatitis because of potentially significant increase in drug's half-life.
- Use diazepam cautiously in patients with hepatic or renal impairment.
- Expect to give a lower diazepam dose to patient with chronic respiratory insufficiency because of the risk of respiratory depression.
- Mix concentrated oral solution (Intensol) with liquid or semisolid food. Use supplied calibrated dropper to measure doses.
- Protect diazepam injection from light. Don't use solution that's more than slightly yellow or that contains precipitate.
- Give I.M. injection into deltoid muscle for rapid, complete absorption. Using other sites may cause slow, erratic absorption.
- Know that for an infant or a child, administer I.V. injection slowly over 3 minutes in a dose not to exceed 0.25 mg/kg. For an adult, administer I.V. injection no more than 5 mg/minute and if possible into a large vein or, if not possible, inject through infusion tubing as close to the insertion site as possible.
- Monitor patient for adverse reactions, especially if she has hypoalbuminemia, which increases the risk of sedation.

WARNING **Watch for signs of physical and psychological dependence (strong desire or need to continue taking diazepam, need to increase dose to maintain drug effects, and posttherapy withdrawal symptoms, such as abdominal cramps, insomnia, irritability, nervousness, and tremor).**

- Monitor patient closely for increase in frequency or severity of grand mal seizures when diazepam is used with standard anticonvulsant therapy. Dosage of other anticonvulsants may have to be increased.
- Avoid abrupt withdrawal of diazepam, as ordered, when used as part of the patient's seizure control regimen because a transient increase in frequency or severity of seizures may occur.
- Monitor severely depressed patient or one with depression-related anxiety for suicidal tendencies, particularly when therapy starts and dosage changes; depression may worsen temporarily during these times.
- Watch for paradoxical and psychiatric reactions to diazepam, especially in children and the elderly. If reactions occur, notify prescriber and expect drug to be discontinued.
- Monitor patient for decreased drug effectiveness, especially with prolonged use.

WARNING **Be aware that benzodiazepine therapy like diazepam should only be used concomitantly with opioids in patients for whom other treatment options are inadequate. If prescribed together, expect dosing and duration of the opioid to be limited. Monitor patient closely for signs and symptoms of decrease in**

consciousness, including coma, profound sedation, and significant respiratory depression. Notify prescriber immediately and provide emergency supportive care, as death may occur.
- Check patient's blood counts and liver function periodically, as ordered, because prolonged diazepam therapy rarely causes jaundice and neutropenia.

PATIENT TEACHING
- Instruct patient not to take more drug, more often, or for a longer time than prescribed. Warn her that physical and psychological dependence can occur, and teach her to recognize the signs.
- Advise patient not to take drug to relieve everyday stress.
- Instruct patient to avoid hazardous activities until drug's CNS effects are known. Warn her that risk of falls and fractures increases when diazepam is taken with other sedatives or alcohol and to avoid this combination.
- Advise patient to avoid CNS depressants during therapy.

WARNING Warn patient not to consume alcohol or take an opioid during diazepam therapy without prescriber knowledge, as severe respiratory depression can occur and may lead to death.

WARNING Inform patient about potentially fatal additive effects of combining diazepam with an opioid. Instruct patient to inform all prescribers of diazepam use, especially if pain medication may be prescribed.
- Instruct patient not to stop taking drug abruptly without prescriber's supervision. If patient has a history of seizures, warn that abrupt withdrawal may trigger them.
- Instruct patient to mix Diazepam Intensol with water, soda, or a similar beverage; applesauce; or pudding just before taking it. Caution her not to save the mixture for later. Tell her to use calibrated dropper that's provided to measure each dose.
- Teach patient how to self-administer a rectal form, if prescribed.
- Instruct female patient of childbearing age to notify prescriber immediately if she is or could be pregnant because diazepam therapy will need to be discontinued.
- Urge family or caregiver to watch patient closely for suicidal tendencies, especially when therapy starts or dosage changes.

diazoxide

Hyperstat, Proglycem

Class and Category

Pharmacologic class: Benzothiadiazine derivative
Therapeutic class: Antihypertensive, antihypoglycemic
Pregnancy category: C

Indications and Dosages

➤ *To manage hypoglycemia caused by hyperinsulinism*

CAPSULES, ORAL SUSPENSION (PROGLYCEM)

Adults and children. *Initial:* 1 mg/kg every 8 hr. *Maintenance:* 3 to 8 mg/kg daily in 2 or 3 equal doses given every 8 or 12 hr. *Maximum:* 15 mg/kg daily.
Infants and neonates. *Initial:* 3.3 mg/kg every 8 hr. *Maintenance:* 8 to 15 mg/kg daily in 2 or 3 equal doses given every 8 or 12 hr.

➤ *To treat severe hypertension in hospitalized patients*

I.V. INJECTION (HYPERSTAT)

Adults. *Initial:* 1 to 3 mg/kg by rapid bolus, repeated every 5 to 15 min until diastolic pressure falls below 100 mm Hg. Repeated in 4 to 24 hr, if needed, until oral antihypertensive therapy begins. *Maximum:* 150 mg/dose, 1.2 g daily.

Route	Onset	Peak	Duration
P.O.	In 1 hr	Unknown	8 hr
I.V.	1 min	2–5 min	2–12 hr

Mechanism of Action

Directly affects smooth muscle cells of peripheral arteries and arterioles, causing them to dilate. This action decreases peripheral resistance, which helps reduce blood pressure. Diazoxide also inhibits insulin release from the pancreas, stimulates catecholamine release, and increases hepatic glucose release.

D

Contraindications

Acute aortic dissection; functional hypoglycemia; hypersensitivity to diazoxide, thiazides, other sulfonamide derivatives, or their components; treatment of compensatory hypertension, as occurs with aortic coarctation or arteriovenous shunt

Interactions

DRUGS

antihypertensives, beta blockers, nitrates: Additive hypotensive effects
beta blockers: Increased hypotensive effects of diazoxide
diuretics, especially thiazides: Potentiated hyperglycemic, hyperuricemic, and antihypertensive effects of diazoxide
oral anticoagulants: Increased anticoagulation
peripheral vasodilators: Additive, possibly severe, hypotensive effects

Adverse Reactions

CNS: Anxiety, apprehension, **cerebral ischemia**, dizziness, euphoria, headache, insomnia, light-headedness, malaise, somnolence, weakness
CV: **Bradycardia**, chest pain, edema, **hypotension**, palpitations, tachycardia, transient hypertension
EENT: Blurred vision, dry mouth, increased salivation, taste perversion, tinnitus, transient hearing loss
ENDO: Transient hyperglycemia
GI: Abdominal pain, anorexia, constipation, diarrhea, ileus, nausea, vomiting
MS: Gout
RESP: **Pulmonary hypertension**
SKIN: Diaphoresis, flushing, pruritus, rash, sensation of warmth
Other: Extravasation with injection-site cellulitis and pain; **hypernatremia**

Nursing Considerations

- Use diazoxide cautiously in patients with uncompensated heart failure (can cause fluid retention and heart failure) and patients with impaired cardiac or cerebral circulation in whom abrupt blood pressure drop, mild tachycardia, and decreased blood perfusion may be harmful.
- Give I.V. drug undiluted over 10 to 30 seconds. Don't give it I.M. or subcutaneously.
- Keep patient supine during I.V. injection and for 1 hour afterward.
- Monitor blood pressure throughout treatment to check for changes. Know that risk for hypotension is increased in patients taking thiazide diuretics. Before monitoring ends, measure patient's standing blood pressure if she's ambulatory.
- Assess I.V. site often for extravasation; drug is alkaline and can irritate tissue.
- Expect to adjust dosage if patient switches from oral suspension to capsules; suspension causes a higher blood diazoxide level.
- Know that if diabetic patient receives I.V. diazoxide to treat hypertension, patient should be watched for evidence of hyperglycemia, because parenteral form commonly causes transient hyperglycemia.
- Monitor blood glucose level of all patients who receive oral diazoxide to see if drug has raised blood glucose level to normal.

WARNING Monitor infants and neonates closely for pulmonary hypertension exhibited by respiratory distress. If present, notify prescriber immediately and expect drug to be discontinued because condition can be reversed when drug therapy is stopped.

PATIENT TEACHING

- Tell patient who receives I.V. diazoxide that she'll be on bed rest until taking oral drug.
- Advise patient to protect oral suspension from light.
- Tell patient to take oral drug on a regular schedule and not to skip or double doses.
- Urge patient to monitor blood glucose level if she takes oral drug for hypoglycemia.
- Caution patient not to take antidiabetic drugs unless prescribed.
- Advise patient to notify prescriber if she has signs of hyperglycemia, such as fatigue, or increased hunger, thirst, or urinary frequency.

diclofenac

Zorvolex

diclofenac potassium

Cambia, Voltaren Rapide (CAN), Zipsor

diclofenac sodium

Apo-Diclo (CAN), Dyloject, Voltaren, Voltaren SR (CAN)

Class and Category

Pharmacologic class: NSAID
Therapeutic class: Analgesic, anti-inflammatory
Pregnancy category: C prior to 30 weeks' gestation; D starting at 30 weeks' gestation

Indications and Dosages

➤ *To manage signs and symptoms of rheumatoid arthritis*

TABLETS
Adults. 50 mg three or four times daily or 75 mg twice daily.

DELAYED-RELEASE TABLETS
Adults. *Initial:* 150 to 200 mg daily in divided doses three times daily or four times daily.

E.R. TABLETS
Adults. *Initial:* 100 mg daily, increased to 200 mg daily and divided into two equal doses, morning or evening as needed.

➤ *To manage signs and symptoms of osteoarthritis*

APSULES (ZORVOLEX)
Adults. 35 mg three times daily.

TABLETS
Adults. 50 mg two or three times daily or 75 mg twice daily.

DELAYED-RELEASE TABLETS
Adults. 100 to 150 mg daily in divided doses twice daily or three times daily. *Maximum:* 150 mg daily.

E.R. TABLETS
Adults. 100 mg daily.

➤ *To relieve pain in patients with ankylosing spondylitis*

DELAYED-RELEASE TABLETS, TABLETS
Adults. 100 to 125 mg daily in 4 or 5 divided doses.

➤ *To relieve pain and dysmenorrhea*

TABLETS
Adults. 50 mg three times daily, as needed; if needed, 100 mg for first dose only.

➤ *To manage mild to moderate pain; to manage moderate to severe pain alone or in combination with opioid analgesics*

I.V. INJECTION (DYLOJECT)
Adults. 37.5 mg given over 15 seconds every 6 hours, as needed. *Maximum:* 150 mg daily.

➤ *To relieve mild to moderate acute pain*

CAPSULES (ZIPSOR)
Adults. 25 mg four times daily.

CAPSULES (ZORVOLEX)
Adults. 18 mg or 35 mg three times daily.

➤ *To treat acute migraine attacks*

ORAL SOLUTION (CAMBIA)
Adults. 50 mg (1 packet) per attack.

DOSAGE ADJUSTMENT For patient prescribed Zorvolex with hepatic impairment, dosage no higher than 18 mg three times daily. For elderly patients and those with hepatic or renal dysfunction, dosage may have to be reduced.

Route	Onset	Peak	Duration
P.O.*	30 min	Unknown	8 hr

* For tablets; unknown for delayed-release and E.R. tablets.

Mechanism of Action

Blocks the activity of cyclooxygenase, the enzyme needed to synthesize prostaglandins, which mediate inflammatory response and cause local pain, swelling, and vasodilation. By blocking cyclooxygenase and inhibiting prostaglandins, diclofenac reduces inflammatory symptoms. This mechanism also relieves pain because prostaglandins promote pain transmission from periphery to spinal cord.

Contraindications
Active GI bleeding or ulcers; history of asthma attacks, rhinitis, or urticaria from aspirin or other NSAIDs; hypersensitivity to diclofenac, NSAIDs, or their components; moderate to severe renal insufficiency in perioperative period with patients at risk for volume depletion (I.V. form); pain management following coronary artery bypass graft (CABG) surgery

Interactions
DRUGS

angiotensin-converting enzyme (ACE) inhibitors, angiotensin receptor blockers (ARBs): Decreased antihypertensive effects of these drugs; decreased renal function in elderly patients or those with existing renal impairment or volume depletion
anticoagulants, antiplatelets, selective serotonin reuptake inhibitors (SSRIs), serotonin norepinephrine reuptake inhibitors (SNRIs), thrombolytics: Prolonged PT, increased risk of bleeding
aspirin, other NSAIDs, salicylates: Increased GI irritability and bleeding, decreased diclofenac effectiveness with aspirin use
beta blockers: Impaired antihypertensive effect
cyclosporine, nephrotoxic drugs: Increased risk of nephrotoxicity
CYP2C9 inducers such as rifampin: Decreased effectiveness of diclofenac
CYP2C9 inhibitors such as voriconazole: Increased risk of diclofenac adverse reactions and toxicity
digoxin: Increased blood digoxin level
lithium: Increased risk of lithium toxicity
loop or thiazide diuretics: Decreased diuretic effects
methotrexate: Increased risk of methotrexate toxicity
serotonin norepinephrine reuptake inhibitors, serotonin reuptake inhibitors: Possibly increased risk of bleeding events

FOODS

any food: Delayed absorption of delayed-release tablets

ACTIVITIES

alcohol use: Increased risk of GI irritability and bleeding

Adverse Reactions
CNS: **Aseptic meningitis, cerebral hemorrhage, CVA,** dizziness, drowsiness, headache
CV: **Bradycardia and other arrhythmias,** edema, **heart failure, hypotension, MI, thrombotic events,** vasculitis
EENT: Glaucoma, hearing loss, tinnitus
ENDO: **Hypoglycemia**
GI: Abdominal pain, constipation, diarrhea, dysphagia, elevated liver enzymes, esophageal ulceration, flatulence, **GI bleeding** or ulceration, **hepatic failure, hepatitis,** indigestion, jaundice, nausea, **perforation of intestine or stomach**
GU: **Acute renal failure,** interstitial nephritis
HEME: **Agranulocytosis,** anemia including **aplastic anemia, bleeding events,** eosinophilia, leukocytosis, **leukopenia, pancytopenia,** porphyria, **thrombocytopenia**
SKIN: **Erythema multiforme, exfoliative dermatitis,** pruritus, rash, **Stevens–Johnson syndrome, toxic epidermal necrolysis**
Other: **Anaphylaxis, angioedema, hyperkalemia,** hyperuricemia, **hyponatremia,** lymphadenopathy

Nursing Considerations
- Be aware that NSAIDs like diclofenac should be avoided in patients with a recent MI because risk of reinfarction increases with NSAID therapy. If therapy is unavoidable, monitor patient closely for signs of cardiac ischemia.
- Be aware that the risk of heart failure increases with use of NSAIDs such as diclofenac. Diclofenac should not be given to patients with severe heart failure, but if unavoidable, monitor patient for worsening of heart failure.
- Use diclofenac with extreme caution and for shortest possible time in patients with a history of GI bleeding or ulcer disease because NSAIDs increase risk of GI bleeding and ulceration.
- Don't substitute one form of oral diclofenac for another. Different formulations aren't bioequivalent.
- Assess patient's hydration status before administering diclofenac intravenously because the patient must be well hydrated to reduce the risk of renal adverse reactions.
- Be aware that serious GI tract bleeding and ulceration, as well as perforation of

intestine or stomach, can occur without warning or symptoms. Elderly patients are at greater risk. Monitor patient for signs of GI irritation and ulceration, especially if patient has a predisposing condition (such as a history of GI bleeding); takes an anticoagulant, NSAID (long-term), or oral corticosteroid; or has other factors such as being an alcoholic or smoker, has poor health, is over the age of 60; or tests positive for *Helicobacter pylori.* To minimize risk, give diclofenac with food. If patient develops GI distress, withhold drug and notify prescriber immediately.

- Use diclofenac cautiously in patients with hypertension, and monitor blood pressure closely; drug can cause or worsen hypertension.

WARNING **Know that use of NSAIDs like diclofenac increases risk of serious cardiovascular thrombotic events, including MI and stroke, which can be life-threatening. These events may occur early in treatment and risk increases with duration of use. Be aware that these events have occurred even in patients who do not have a history of or risk factors for cardiovascular disease. Monitor patient for warning signs such as chest pain, shortness of breath, slurring of speech, or weakness. If any signs and symptoms develop, withhold diclofenac, alert prescriber immediately, and provide supportive care as prescribed.**

- Report signs of bleeding, such as bleeding gums, bloody or cloudy urine, ecchymoses, melena, and petechiae. Know that risk of bleeding is increased when patient is taking certain drugs like anticoagulants such as warfarin, antiplatelet agents such as aspirin, serotonin norepinephrine reuptake inhibitors, and serotonin reuptake inhibitors.
- Monitor BUN and serum creatinine levels in elderly patients, patients taking ACE inhibitors, ARDs, or diuretics, and patients with heart failure or impaired hepatic or renal function. These patients may have an increased risk of renal failure.
- Assess patient's skin routinely for rash or other signs of hypersensitivity reaction; drug may cause serious skin reactions without warning. At first sign of reaction, stop drug and notify prescriber.
- Know that because severe hepatic reactions may occur during diclofenac therapy, monitor liver enzymes and serum uric acid level as ordered. Liver enzyme elevations usually occur within 2 months of starting drug and should be reported promptly because dosage may need adjustment. Also monitor patient for evidence of hepatic dysfunction (diarrhea, fatigue, flu-like symptoms, jaundice, lethargy, nausea, pruritus, right upper quadrant tenderness).
- Report weight gain of more than 1 kg (2 lb) in 24 hours because it suggests fluid retention.

PATIENT TEACHING

- Advise patient not to chew, crush, or dissolve tablet, but to swallow it whole.
- Tell patient prescribed Cambia brand to mix packet in 1 to 2 ounces of water, mix well, and drink immediately. Caution patient not to use any other liquids to mix the drug. Remind patient taking this form of diclofenac that taking it with food may decrease its effectiveness.
- Instruct patient to take diclofenac with food to minimize GI distress unless he is prescribed Zorvolex, which should be taken on an empty stomach.
- Instruct patient not to lie down for 15 to 30 minutes after taking drug to decrease risk of esophageal ulceration.
- Warn patient to avoid hazardous activities until diclofenac's CNS effects are known.
- Urge patient to notify prescriber about dizziness, edema, impaired hearing, ringing or buzzing in ears, or unexplained weight gain.
- Advise patient to consult prescriber before taking aspirin or other OTC analgesics or drinking alcohol.
- Explain that diclofenac may increase risk of serious adverse cardiovascular reactions; urge patient to seek immediate medical attention for signs and symptoms such as chest pain, shortness of breath, slurred speech, and weakness.
- Inform patient that diclofenac therapy may increase risk of congestive heart failure. Instruct patient to promptly report to prescriber if edema, shortness of breath, or unexplained weight gain occurs.

- Tell patient that diclofenac also may increase risk of serious adverse GI reactions; stress need to seek immediate medical attention for such evidence as abdominal or epigastric pain, black or tarry stools, indigestion, and vomiting blood or material that looks like coffee grounds.
- Alert patient about possibly serious skin reactions and need to seek immediate medial attention for problems such as blisters, fever, itching, rash, and other signs of hypersensitivity such as difficulty breathing or swelling of face or throat.
- Urge patient to promptly report adverse liver effects (diarrhea, fatigue, flu-like symptoms, jaundice, lethargy, nausea, pruritus, right upper quadrant discomfort).
- Advise female patients to notify prescriber if pregnancy occurs or is suspected.
- Tell patient prescribed drug to treat migraine headaches not to overuse drug. Explain that this is because overuse, defined as using 10 or more days per month, may lead to exacerbation of headache. Inform patient that overuse headache may appear as migraine-like daily headaches or as a marked increase in frequency of migraine attacks. If this occurs, tell patient to notify prescriber, as a withdrawal period may be needed.

dicloxacillin sodium

Class and Category

Pharmacologic class: Penicillinase-resistant penicillin
Therapeutic class: Antibiotic
Pregnancy category: B

Indications and Dosages

➤ *To treat mild to moderate upper respiratory tract and localized skin and soft-tissue infections caused by penicillinase-producing staphylococci*

CAPSULES, ORAL SOLUTION

Adults and children weighing 40 kg (88 lb) or more. 125 mg every 6 hr.
Children weighing less than 40 kg. 12.5 mg/kg daily divided into four equal doses and given every 6 hr.

➤ *To treat severe infections, such as lower respiratory tract or disseminated infections, caused by penicillinase-producing staphylococci*

CAPSULES, ORAL SOLUTION

Adults and children weighing 40 kg or more. 250 mg every 6 hr, or higher doses, if needed. *Maximum:* 6 g daily.
Children over age 1 month weighing less than 40 kg. 25 mg/kg daily divided into 4 equal doses and given every 6 hr, or higher doses if needed.

Mechanism of Action

Inhibits cell wall synthesis in susceptible bacteria, which assemble rigid, cross-linked cell walls in several steps. Dicloxacillin affects final cross-linking by inactivating penicillin-binding protein (the enzyme needed to link cell wall strands). This action inhibits cell wall synthesis and causes cell lysis and death.

Contraindications

Clostridium difficile infection; hypersensitivity to dicloxacillin, other penicillins, beta-lactamase inhibitors or their components

Interactions

DRUGS

hepatotoxic drugs: Increased risk of hepatotoxicity
methotrexate: Decreased methotrexate clearance and increased risk of toxicity
oral contraceptives: Decreased contraceptive action
probenecid: Increased and prolonged blood dicloxacillin level
tetracyclines: Decreased dicloxacillin effectiveness

FOODS

all foods: Possibly delayed absorption

Adverse Reactions

CNS: Dizziness, fatigue, fever, insomnia
EENT: Black "hairy" tongue, dry mouth, glossitis, **laryngeal edema**, **laryngospasm**, stomatitis, taste perversion
GI: Abdominal pain, anorexia, diarrhea, flatulence, nausea, **pseudomembranous colitis**, transient hepatitis, vomiting
GU: Nephropathy, vaginitis
MS: Prolonged muscle relaxation
SKIN: Dermatitis, **erythema multiforme**, pruritus, rash, urticaria, vesicular eruptions
Other: **Anaphylaxis**, serum sickness-like reaction, superinfection

Nursing Considerations

- Expect to obtain body fluid and tissue samples for culture and sensitivity tests, as ordered, and review the results, if possible, before dicloxacillin therapy begins. Also check for history of sensitivity to cephalosporins, penicillins, and other substances.
- Notify prescriber if diarrhea develops; it could be the development of pseudomembranous colitis.

PATIENT TEACHING

- Instruct patient to take drug 1 hour before or 2 hours after meals.
- Instruct patient to take drug around the clock, not to miss a dose, and to complete the entire prescription unless directed otherwise by prescriber.
- Advise patient to take oral solution with a cold beverage but not acidic juice, such as orange juice. Explain that solution is effective for 7 days at room temperature and for 14 days if refrigerated.
- Caution patient not to open capsules and mix contents with food or liquids because an unpleasant taste and decreased drug absorption will result.
- Instruct patient to shake oral solution thoroughly and measure doses with a calibrated device for accuracy.
- Advise patient to notify prescriber if she experiences adverse GI reactions or signs of hypersensitivity or superinfection.
- Be aware that if patient takes an oral contraceptive, she should be advised to use an additional form of contraception during therapy.
- Instruct patient to store drug away from direct light, heat, and moisture and to refrigerate—but not freeze—oral solution.

dicyclomine hydrochloride

Bentyl, Bentylol (CAN)

Class and Category

Pharmacologic class: Anticholinergic
Therapeutic class: Antispasmodic
Pregnancy category: Not classified

Indications and Dosages

➤ *To treat functional or irritable bowel syndrome*

CAPSULES, SYRUP, TABLETS

Adults. 20 mg four times daily, increased as needed and tolerated after 1 wk to 40 mg four times daily. *Maximum:* 160 mg daily.

I.M. INJECTION

Adults. 10 to 20 mg every 6 hr. Dosage adjusted as needed and tolerated but not given longer than 2 days.

D

Mechanism of Action

Inhibits acetylcholine's muscarinic actions at postganglionic parasympathetic receptors in CNS, secretory glands, and smooth muscles. These actions relax smooth muscles and diminish and biliary, GI, and GU tract secretions.

Contraindications

Angle-closure glaucoma; GI obstruction; hemorrhagic shock; hypersensitivity to dicyclomine, other anticholinergic, or their components; ileus; myasthenia gravis; obstructive uropathy; severe ulcerative colitis; toxic megacolon

Interactions

DRUGS

adsorbent antidiarrheals, antacids: Decreased dicyclomine absorption
amantadine, antihistamines, antipsychotics such as phenothiazines, benzodiazepines, Class 1 antiarrhythmics such as quinidine, MAO inhibitors, narcotic analgesics such as meperidine, nitrates and nitrites, other anticholinergics, tricyclic antidepressants: Increased dicyclomine effects
digoxin: Increased risk of digitalis toxicity
metoclopramide: Decreased effect of metoclopramide on GI motility
opioid analgesics: Increased risk of ileus, severe constipation, and urine retention

Adverse Reactions

CNS: Agitation, delirium, dizziness, drowsiness, dyskinesia, excitement, fever, insomnia, lethargy, light-headedness (I.M.

use), nervousness, paresthesia, psychosis, syncope
CV: Palpitations, tachycardia
EENT: Blurred vision, cycloplegia, dry mouth, loss of taste, mydriasis, nasal congestion, photophobia
GI: Constipation, dysphagia, heartburn, ileus, vomiting
GU: Impotence, urine retention
SKIN: Decreased sweating, flushing, pruritus
Other: Heatstroke; injection-site pain, redness, and swelling

Nursing Considerations

- Assess patient for tachycardia before giving dicyclomine; heart rate may increase.
- Don't give drug by I.V. route because major adverse reactions may occur.
- Watch for symptoms of hypersensitivity, such as agitation and pruritus. They usually resolve within 48 hours of stopping drug.
- Assess patient during long-term use for chronic constipation and fecal impaction, and take corrective measures, as prescribed.
- Monitor patient, especially the elderly and/or patients with mental illness, for delirium and psychosis. If present, notify prescriber and expect drug to be discontinued and symptoms to disappear within 12 to 24 hours.

PATIENT TEACHING

- Instruct patient to store dicyclomine in a tightly sealed container at room temperature, protected from moisture and direct light. Advise her not to refrigerate syrup.
- Inform patient that dicyclomine relieves symptoms but doesn't cure the disorder.
- Instruct patient to take drug 30 to 60 minutes before eating.
- Advise patient not to take an antacid or an antidiarrheal within 2 hours of dicyclomine.
- Inform patient that blurred vision, dizziness, or drowsiness may occur.
- Advise patient to eat high-fiber foods and drink at least eight glasses of water daily to prevent constipation.

WARNING Urge patient to avoid getting overheated during exercise or in hot weather because heatstroke may result. Inform patient that hot baths or saunas may cause dizziness or fainting.

- Instruct patient to change position slowly to avoid light-headedness.
- Inform patient that stopping drug abruptly may cause dizziness and vomiting.
- Tell patient to take a missed dose as soon as she remembers, unless it's nearly time for the next dose. Caution against doubling the dose.
- Urge patient and family that if delirium or psychosis occurs, stop the drug and notify the prescriber. Inform them that these symptoms usually resolve within 12 to 24 hours after drug is discontinued.

didanosine

Videx, Videx EC

Class and Category

Pharmacologic class: Nucleoside reverse transcriptase inhibitor (NRTI)
Therapeutic class: Antiretroviral
Pregnancy category: Not classified

Indications and Dosages

➤ *As adjunct to treat human immunodeficiency virus (HIV) infection*

ORAL SOLUTION

Adults weighing at least 60 kg (132 lb). 200 mg twice daily. Alternative (but less preferred) dosing, 400 mg once daily.
Adults weighing less than 60 kg (132 lb). 125 mg twice daily. Alternative (but less preferred) dosing, 250 mg once daily.
Children older than 8 months. 120 mg/m^2 twice daily. *Maximum:* Not to exceed adult dosage.
Children 2 weeks to 8 months old. 100 mg/m^2 twice daily. *Maximum:* Not to exceed adult dosage.

D.R. CAPSULES

Adults and children weighing at least 60 kg (132 lb). 400 mg once daily.
Adults and children weighing 25 kg (55 lb) to less than 60 kg (132 lb). 250 mg once daily.
Children weighing 20 kg (44 lb) to less than 25 kg (55 lb). 200 mg once daily.

DOSAGE ADJUSTMENT

For oral solution: For adult patient with a creatinine clearance between 30 and 59 ml/min and weighing at least 60 kg (132 lb), dosage decreased to 100 mg twice daily or

200 mg once daily; for adult patient weighing less than 60 kg (132 lb), dosage decreased to 75 mg twice daily or 150 mg once daily. For adult patient with a creatinine clearance between 10 and 29 ml/min and weighing at least 60 kg (132 lb), dosage decreased to 150 mg once daily; for adult patient weighing less than 60 kg (132 lb), dosage decreased to 100 mg once daily. For adult patient with a creatinine clearance less than 10 ml/min and weighing at least 60 kg (132 lb), dosage decreased to 100 mg once daily; for adult patient weighing less than 60 kg (132 lb), dosage decreased to 75 mg once daily. For pediatric patients with renal insufficiency, dosage reduced, but specific dose adjustment is unknown due to insufficient data.
For D.R. capsules: For adult patient with a creatinine clearance of 30 ml/min or below and weighing at least 60 kg (132 lb), dosage decreased to 200 mg once daily; for adult patient weighing less than 60 kg (132 lb), dosage decreased to 125 mg once daily. For adult patient with a creatinine clearance between 10 and 29 ml/min regardless of weight, dosage decreased to 125 mg once daily. For adult patient with a creatinine clearance less than 10 ml/min and weighing at least 60 kg, dosage also reduced to 125 mg once daily. Drug discontinued for patient with a creatinine clearance less than 10 ml/min and weighing less than 60 kg (132 lb). For pediatric patients with renal insufficiency, dosage reduced, but specific dose adjustment is unknown due to insufficient data.
For adult patients taking tenofovir disoproxil fumarate concomitantly with either oral didanosine solution or D.R. didanosine capsules: For patient with a creatinine clearance of at least 60 ml/min and weighing at least 60 kg (132 lb), dosage reduced to 250 mg once daily; for patient weighing less than 60 kg (132 lb), dosage reduced to 200 mg once daily. The appropriate dosage reduction for patients taking tenofovir disoproxil with creatinine clearance levels less than 60 ml/min is not established.

Mechanism of Action

Inhibits the activity of HIV-1 reverse transcriptase in two ways. It competes with the natural substrate in the virus and it incorporates itself into the viral DNA causing termination of viral DNA chain elongation.

Contraindications

Concomitant therapy with allopurinol, ribavirin, and stavudine; hypersensitivity to didanosine or its components

Interactions

DRUGS

allopurinol, ganciclovir, ribavirin, tenofovir disoproxil fumarate: Increased plasma didanosine concentration increasing risk for serious didanosine adverse reactions such as pancreatitis, peripheral neuropathy, and symptomatic hyperlactatemia/lactic acidosis
antacids containing aluminum or magnesium: Increased adverse reactions associated with antacids, such as constipation and diarrhea
ciprofloxacin, delavirdine, indinavir: Decreased plasma levels of these drugs with potential for decreased effectiveness
drugs that may cause pancreatic toxicity: Increased risk of pancreatitis
hydroxyurea: Increased risk of fatal hepatotoxicity, pancreatitis, or severe peripheral neuropathy
methadone: Decreased plasma didanosine concentrations with potential for decreased effectiveness
neurotoxic drugs: Increased risk of neuropathy
stavudine: Increased risk of fatal lactic acidosis in pregnant women

ACTIVITIES

alcohol use: Possibly increased risk of liver dysfunction

Adverse Reactions

CNS: Asthenia, chills, fever, headache, peripheral neuropathy
EENT: Dry eyes or mouth, inflamed salivary glands, optic neuritis, parotid gland enlargement, retinal changes
ENDO: Hyperglycemia, **hypoglycemia**
GI: Abdominal pain, anorexia, diarrhea, dyspepsia, elevated liver or pancreatic enzymes, flatulence, **hepatic toxicity, hepatitis, liver failure,** nausea, **non-cirrhotic portal hypertension,**

pancreatitis, severe hepatomegaly with steatosis, vomiting
GU: **Acute renal failure**
HEME: Anemia, **leukopenia, thrombocytopenia**
MS: Arthralgia, myalgia, myopathy, **rhabdomyolysis**
SKIN: Alopecia, rash
Other: Anaphylaxis, generalized pain, **hyperlactatemia,** hyperuricemia, **lactic acidosis**

Nursing Considerations

- Use didanosine with extreme caution in patients with risk factors for pancreatitis such as advanced HIV infection or renal impairment and in the elderly. Be aware that the use of didanosine with stavudine is contraindicated because the combination increases risk of pancreatitis. Know that the frequency of pancreatitis is dose related. Monitor patient for signs and symptoms of pancreatitis throughout therapy. Be aware that drug must be discontinued if pancreatitis is confirmed.
- Use didanosine cautiously in patients with known risk factors for liver disease. Be aware that the combined use of didanosine with hydroxyurea and stavudine is contraindicated because this combination has resulted in the highest number of fatal hepatic events. Monitor patient and liver enzymes for evidence of liver disease throughout therapy. If liver disease develops or becomes worse, expect drug to be discontinued and supportive care given.
- Administer didanosine on an empty stomach at least 30 minutes before or 2 hours after patient has eaten.

WARNING Know that lactic acidosis and severe hepatomegaly with steatosis have occurred with didanosine therapy, and death has occurred in some patients. Fatal lactic acidosis has been reported in pregnant women who received the combination of didanosine and stavudine with other antiretrovirals. Risk factors include presence of obesity, prolonged nucleoside exposure, and being female. However, know that lactic acidosis and severe hepatomegaly with steatosis have also occurred in patients with no known risk factors. Expect drug to be discontinued in any patient who develops clinical or laboratory findings suggestive of lactic acidosis or pronounced hepatotoxicity, even in the absence of marked transaminase elevations.

- Monitor patient for early signs of portal hypertension such as the presence of splenomegaly accompanied by thrombocytopenia, because didanosine has been linked to non-cirrhotic portal hypertension. Expect to monitor the patient with the following laboratory tests: complete blood count, international normalized ratio, liver enzymes, and serum albumin and bilirubin levels. Ultrasonography may be warranted as well. If confirmed, expect didanosine therapy to be discontinued.
- Assess patient for signs and symptoms of peripheral neuropathy such as complaints of numbness, pain, or tingling in the feet or hands. Risk factors for developing didanosine-related peripheral neuropathy include advanced HIV disease, history of neuropathy, or being treated with neurotoxic therapy. Report such complaints to prescriber, as drug may have to be discontinued.
- Ensure that patient has periodic retinal examinations while receiving didanosine, because drug may cause optic neuritis and retinal changes.
- Be aware that immune reconstitution syndrome has occurred in patients treated with combination antiretroviral therapy, including didanosine. The inflammatory response predisposes susceptible patients to opportunistic infections such as cytomegalovirus, *Mycobacterium avium* infection, *Pneumocystis jiroveci* pneumonia, or tuberculosis. Autoimmune disorders such as Graves' disease, Guillain–Barré syndrome, or polymyositis have also occurred. Report sudden or unusual adverse reactions to prescriber.

PATIENT TEACHING

- Instruct patient to take didanosine exactly as prescribed. If a dose is missed, instruct patient to take it as soon as possible. Stress importance of taking drug on a regular schedule and not missing doses, if possible, to avoid the development of resistance to the drug.

- Tell patient to take drug on an empty stomach, at least 30 minutes before or 2 hours after eating.
- Warn patient to alert all prescribers of didanosine therapy, because drug may cause serious interactions with some other drugs. Also tell patient not to take any over-the-counter preparations, including herbal products, without consulting prescriber first.
- Stress importance of reporting persistent, severe, or unusual signs and symptoms to prescriber, because serious adverse reactions can occur with didanosine, especially affecting the liver and pancreas. Also stress the need to report any numbness, pain, or tingling in patient's feet or hands.
- Caution patient to be compliant with laboratory monitoring for early detection of adverse reactions associated with didanosine use.
- Inform patient to report any changes in vision, especially blurred vision, to prescriber. Stress importance of having regular eye examinations when taking didanosine.
- Tell patient to immediately report any symptoms of infections to prescriber.
- Inform patient that loss of body fat from his arms, face, or legs may occur while taking didanosine.
- Instruct patient to avoid alcohol while taking didanosine.
- Tell women of childbearing age to alert prescriber if pregnancy is suspected or known. If confirmed, encourage patient to register with the antiretroviral pregnancy registry that monitors fetal outcomes of pregnant women exposed to didanosine.
- Warn mothers with HIV infection not to breastfeed the infant, because the HIV-1 virus can be passed to the baby in breast milk.

diflunisal

Class and Category

Pharmacologic class: NSAID
Therapeutic class: Analgesic, anti-inflammatory
Pregnancy category: C (first trimester), not classified (later trimesters)

Indications and Dosages

➤ *To relieve mild to moderate pain*

TABLETS

Adults. 1 g followed by 0.5 g every 8 to 12 hr. Alternatively, 500 mg followed by 250 mg every 8 to 12 hr. *Maximum:* 1.5 g daily.

➤ *To reduce inflammation in osteoarthritis or rheumatoid arthritis*

TABLETS

Adults. 0.5 to 1 g daily in divided doses twice daily. *Maximum:* 1.5 g daily.

DOSAGE ADJUSTMENT Dosage reduced for elderly patients and those who use diuretics; who could be harmed by prolonged bleeding time; or who have compromised cardiac function, conditions that cause fluid retention, hepatic or renal impairment, hypertension, or upper GI disease.

Route	Onset	Peak	Duration
P.O.*	1 hr	2–3 hr	8–12 hr

Mechanism of Action

Blocks the activity of cyclooxygenase, the enzyme needed to synthesize prostaglandins, which mediate the inflammatory response and cause local vasodilation, swelling, and pain. By blocking cyclooxygenase and inhibiting prostaglandins, this NSAID reduces inflammatory symptoms. This mechanism also relieves pain because prostaglandins promote pain transmission from the periphery to the spinal cord.

Contraindications

Asthma attacks, rhinitis, or urticaria precipitated by aspirin or other NSAIDs; hypersensitivity to diflunisal or its components; treatment of perioperative pain after coronary artery bypass graft surgery

Interactions

DRUGS

acetaminophen: Increased plasma levels of acetaminophen; risk of adverse hepatic effects with long-term use
angiotensin-converting enzyme (ACE) inhibitors, angiotensin II antagonists: Decreased effectiveness of antihypertensive effect of these drugs

antacids: Decreased blood diflunisal level
antihypertensives: Decreased antihypertensive effects
aspirin, other NSAIDs, salicylates: Increased GI irritability and bleeding, possible decreased diflunisal effectiveness with aspirin
cyclosporine, nephrotoxic drugs: Increased risk of nephrotoxicity
digoxin: Increased blood digoxin level
indomethacin: Significantly increased plasma levels of indomethacin
lithium: Increased risk of lithium toxicity
loop and thiazide diuretics: Decreased diuretic effectiveness
methotrexate: Increased risk of methotrexate toxicity
naproxen: Decreased urinary excretion of naproxen increasing risk of adverse reactions
oral anticogulants: Increased risk of serious GI bleeding; prolonged prothrombin time
sulindac: Decreased plasma levels of sulindac

ACTIVITIES

alcohol use: Increased GI irritability and bleeding

Adverse Reactions

CNS: Aseptic meningitis, **cerebral hemorrhage**, dizziness, drowsiness, headache, insomnia
CV: Vasculitis
EENT: Tinnitus
ENDO: Hypoglycemia
GI: Abdominal pain, constipation, diarrhea, esophageal irritation, **GI bleeding** or ulceration, **hepatic failure**, **hepatitis**, indigestion, jaundice, nausea, **perforation of intestine or stomach**, vomiting
GU: Acute renal failure, interstitial nephritis
HEME: Agranulocytosis, **aplastic anemia**, **leukopenia**, **pancytopenia**, **thrombocytopenia**
SKIN: Erythema multiforme, **exfoliative dermatitis**, rash, **Stevens-Johnson syndrome**, **toxic epidermal necrolysis**
Other: Anaphylaxis, **angioedema**, **hyponatremia**

Nursing Considerations

- Use diflunisal with extreme caution and for shortest time possible in patients with a history of GI bleeding or ulcer disease because NSAIDs such as diflunisal increase the risk.
- Be aware that serious GI tract bleeding and ulceration, as well as perforation of intestine or stomach, can occur without warning or symptoms. Elderly patients are at greater risk. To minimize risk, give diflunisal with food. If patient has GI distress, withhold drug and notify prescriber immediately.
- Use diflunisal cautiously in patients with hypertension, and monitor blood pressure closely during therapy; drug can cause or worsen hypertension.
- Use drug cautiously in elderly patients, those with renal dysfunction, and those who should avoid prolonged bleeding time.

WARNING **Monitor patient closely for thrombotic events, including MI and stroke, because NSAIDs such as diflunisal increase the risk of these events.**

- Monitor BUN and serum creatinine levels in elderly patients, patients taking ACE inhibitors or diuretics, and patients with heart failure or impaired hepatic or renal function. These patients may have an increased risk of renal failure.
- Assess patient's skin routinely for rash or other signs of hypersensitivity reaction; drug may cause serious skin reactions without warning. At first sign of reaction, stop drug and notify prescriber.
- Assess intensity, location, and type of pain before and 1 to 2 hours after giving drug.
- Assess patient carefully because high-dose or long-term therapy may mask fever.

PATIENT TEACHING

- Teach patient not to chew or crush diflunisal tablets.
- Instruct patient to take tablet with a full glass of water and not to lie down for 30 minutes afterward to avoid esophageal irritation.
- Inform patient that drug will start working in about 1 week but that full effects may not occur for several weeks.
- Explain that diflunisal may increase the risk of serious adverse cardiovascular reactions; urge patient to seek immediate medical attention for such signs and symptoms as chest pain, shortness of breath, slurred speech, and weakness.

- Tell patient that diflunisal also may increase risk of serious adverse GI reactions; stress need to seek immediate medical attention for signs and symptoms such as abdominal or epigastric pain, black or tarry stools, indigestion, and vomiting blood or material that resembles coffee grounds.
- Alert patient about possibly serious skin reactions and the need to seek immediate medial attention for problems such as blisters, fever, itching, rash, and other signs of hypersensitivity.
- Caution patient to avoid acetaminophen, alcohol, aspirin, and other salicylates during diflunisal therapy, unless directed otherwise by prescriber.
- Advise patient to avoid hazardous activities until drug's CNS effects are known.
- Advise patient to tell healthcare providers about diflunisal therapy before surgery, including dental surgery. Therapy should stop for 1 week before procedure.

digoxin

Cardoxin, Digitek, Lanoxicaps, Lanoxin, Lanoxin Pediatric

Class and Category

Pharmacologic class: Cardiac glycoside
Therapeutic class: Antiarrhythmic, cardiotonic
Pregnancy category: C

Indications and Dosages

➤ *To treat mild to moderate heart failure with rapid digitalization*

CAPSULES, I.V. INJECTION

Adults and children over age 10. *Loading:* 8 to 12 mcg/kg in 3 divided doses, with first dose equal to 50% of total dose and 25% of the total loading dose every 6 to 8 hr for two doses. I.V. injection given slowly over 5 min or longer. Subsequent doses given every 6 to 8 hr. *Maintenance:* 2.4 to 3.6 mcg/kg once daily.
Children ages 5 to 10. *Loading:* 15 to 30 mcg/kg in 3 divided doses, with first dose equal to 50% of total dose and 25% of the total loading dose given every 6 to 8 hr for two doses. I.V. injection given over 5 min or longer. *Maintenance:* 2.3 to 4.5 mcg/kg twice daily.
Children ages 2 to 5. *Loading:* 25 to 35 mcg/kg in 3 divided doses, with first dose equal to 50% of total dose and 25% of the total loading dose given every 6 to 8 hr for two doses. I.V. injection given slowly over 5 min or longer. *Maintenance:* 3.8 to 5.3 mcg/kg twice daily.
Infants ages 1 to 24 months. *Loading:* 30 to 50 mcg/kg in 3 divided doses, with first dose equal to 50% of total dose and 25% of the total loading dose given every 6 to 8 hr for two doses. I.V. injection given slowly over 5 min or longer. *Maintenance:* 4.5 to 7.5 mcg/kg twice daily.
Full-term neonates. *Loading:* 20 to 30 mcg/kg in 3 divided doses, with first dose equal to 50% of total dose and 25% of total loading dose given every 6 to 8 hr for two doses. I.V. injection given slowly over 5 min or longer. *Maintenance:* 3 to 4.5 mcg/kg twice daily.
Premature neonates. *Loading:* 15 to 25 mcg/kg in 3 divided doses, with first dose equal to 50% of total dose and 25% of the total loading dose given every 6 to 8 hr for two doses. I.V. injection given slowly over 5 min or longer. *Maintenance:* 1.9 to 3.1 mcg/kg twice daily.

TABLETS

Adults and children over age 10. *Loading:* 10 to 15 mcg/kg total given in 3 divided doses every 6 to 8 hr, with first dose equal to 50% of total dose and subsequent two doses given each as 25% of the total loading dose. *Maintenance:* 3.4 to 5.1 mcg/kg once daily.
Children ages 5 to 10. *Loading:* 20 to 45 mcg/kg in 3 divided doses every 6 to 8 hr and subsequent two doses given each as 25% of the total loading dose. *Maintenance:* 3.2 to 6.4 mcg/kg daily in 2 divided doses.

ELIXIR

Adults and children over age 10. *Loading:* 10 to 15 mcg/kg total given in 3 divided doses every 6 to 8 hr, with first dose equal to 50% of total dose and each of remaining two doses given as 25% of total dose. *Maintenance:* 3.4 to 5.1 mcg/kg once daily.

Children ages 5 to 10. *Loading:* 20 to 45 mcg/kg in 3 divided doses every 6 to 8 hr, with first dose equal to 50% of total dose and each of remaining two doses given as 25% of total dose. *Maintenance:* 3.2 to 6.4 mcg/kg twice daily.
Children ages 2 to 5. *Loading:* 30 to 40 mcg/kg in 3 divided doses every 6 to 8 hr, with first dose equal to 50% of total dose and each of remaining two doses equal to 25% of total dose. *Maintenance:* 7.5 to 10 mcg/kg daily in 2 divided doses.
Infants ages 1 to 24 months. *Loading:* 35 to 60 mcg/kg in 3 divided doses every 6 to 8 hr, with first dose equal to 50% of total dose and each of remaining two doses equal to 25% of total dose. *Maintenance:* 10 to 15 mcg/kg daily in 2 divided doses.
Full-term neonates. *Loading:* 25 to 35 mcg/kg in 3 divided doses every 6 to 8 hr, with first dose equal to 50% of total dose and each of remaining two doses equal to 25% of total dose. *Maintenance:* 6 to 10 mcg/kg daily in 2 divided doses.
Premature neonates. *Loading:* 20 to 30 mcg/kg in 3 divided doses every 6 to 8hr, with first dose equal to 50% of total dose and each of remaining two doses equal to 25% of total dose. *Maintenance:* 5 to 7.5 mcg/kg daily in 2 divided doses.

➤ ***To control ventricular response rate in chronic atrial fibrillation***

ELIXIR, TABLETS
Adults. *Loading:* 10 to 15 mcg/kg in 3 divided doses every 6 to 8 hr, with first dose equal to 50% of total loading dose and each of remaining two doses given as 25% of total loading dose. *Maintenance:* 3.4 to 5.1 mcg/kg once daily for tablets and 3.0 to 4.5 mcg/kg once daily for elixir.

I.V. INJECTION
Adults. *Initial:* 8 to 12 mcg/kg every 6 to 8 hr, with first dose equal to 50% of total loading dose and each of remaining two doses given as 25% of total loading dose. *Maintenance:* 2.4 to 3.6 mcg/kg once daily. I.V. injection given slowly over 5 min or longer.

CAPSULES, ELIXIR, I.V. INJECTION, TABLETS
DOSAGE ADJUSTMENT Dosage carefully adjusted for patients who are debilitated or elderly or have implanted pacemakers because toxicity may develop at doses tolerated by most patients.

Route	Onset	Peak	Duration
P.O.	30–120 min	6–8 hr	3–4 days
I.V.	5–30 min	1–5 hr	3–4 days

Mechanism of Action

Increases the force and velocity of myocardial contraction, resulting in positive inotropic effects. Digoxin produces antiarrhythmic effects by decreasing the conduction rate and increasing the effective refractory period of the AV node.

Contraindications

History or presence of digitalis toxicity or idiosyncratic reaction to digoxin, hypersensitivity to digoxin or its components, ventricular fibrillation, ventricular tachycardia unless heart failure occurs unrelated to digoxin therapy

Interactions

DRUGS

acarbose, activated charcoal, albuterol, antacids, certain chemotherapy drugs, cholestyramine, colestipol, exenatide, kaolin-pectin, metoclopramide, miglitol, neomycin, penicillamine, phenytoin, rifampin, St. John's wort, sucralfate, sulfasalazine: Decreased digoxin concentrations with decreased effectiveness
alprazolam, azithromycin, cyclosporine, diclofenac, diphenoxylate, epoprostenol, esomeprazole, ibuprofen, ketoconazole, lansoprazole, metformin, omeprazole, reabeprazole: Increased digoxin concentration, but magnitude unclear with potential risk of digitalis toxicity
amiodarone, captopril, clarithromycin, dronedarone, gentamicin, erythromycin, itraconazole, nitrendipine, propafenone, quinidine, ranolazine, ritonavir, tetracycline, verapamil: Increased digoxin concentration by more than 50%, significantly increasing risk of digitalis toxicity
atorvastatin, carvedilol, diltiazem, indomethacin, nefazodone, nifedipine, propantheline, quinine, saquinavir, spironolactone, telmisartan, tolvaptan, trimethoprim: Increased digoxin

concentrations up to 50%, increasing risk of digitalis toxicity
beta blockers, calcium channel blockers: Increased additive effects of slowing heart rate, possibly producing bradycardia
calcium supplements given rapidly I.V.: Increased risk of serious arrhythmias
dofetilide: Increased risk for torsades de pointes
dronedarone: Increased risk of sudden death
nephrotoxic drugs: Increased risk of digitalis toxicity
neuromuscular blocking agents: Possibly sudden release of potassium from muscle cells increasing risk of arrhythmias
sotalol: Increased risk of proarrhythmias
sympathomimetics: Increased risk of arrhythmias
thyroid hormone: Decreased plasma digoxin level, requiring an increase in dosage

FOODS

high-fiber food: Decreased oral digoxin absorption

Adverse Reactions

CNS: Confusion, depression, drowsiness, extreme weakness, headache, syncope
CV: **Arrhythmias, heart block**
EENT: Blurred vision, colored halos around objects
GI: Abdominal discomfort or pain, anorexia, diarrhea, nausea, vomiting
Other: **Electrolyte imbalances**

Nursing Considerations

- Be aware that digoxin therapy is not recommended in patients with acute cor pulmonale involving heart failure associated with amyloid heart disease, constrictive pericarditis, preserved left ventricular ejection fraction, or restrictive cardiomyopathy because of increased susceptibility to digoxin toxicity. The drug is also not recommended in patients with idiopathic hypertrophic subaortic stenosis because outflow obstruction may worsen because of the inotropic effects of digoxin.
- Expect to treat underlying thiamine deficiency in patients with beri-beri heart disease because if left untreated, digoxin therapy may be ineffective.
- Give parenteral digoxin undiluted, or dilute with a fourfold or greater volume of sterile water for injection, normal saline solution, or D_5W for I.V. administration. Once diluted, give immediately over 5 minutes or longer. Discard if solution is markedly discolored or contains precipitate.
- Take patient's apical pulse before giving each dose and notify prescriber if it's below 60 beats/minute (or other specified level).
- Monitor patient closely for signs of digitalis toxicity, such as altered mental status, arrhythmias, heart block, nausea, vision disturbances, and vomiting. If they appear, notify prescriber, check serum digoxin level as ordered, and expect to withhold drug until level is known. Monitor ECG tracing continuously.
- Be aware that because digoxin has a narrow therapeutic index and interacts with many different drugs, monitoring of serum digoxin levels is important when other drugs are prescribed or discontinued or dosages adjusted.
- Assess for drug effectiveness if patient has acute or unstable chronic atrial fibrillation. Ventricular rate may not normalize even when serum drug level falls within therapeutic range; raising the dosage probably won't produce a therapeutic effect and may lead to toxicity.
- Obtain frequent ECG tracings as ordered in elderly patients because of their smaller body mass and reduced renal clearance. Elderly patients, especially those with coronary insufficiency, are more susceptible to arrhythmias—particularly ventricular fibrillation—if digitalis toxicity occurs.
- Monitor patient's serum potassium level regularly because hypokalemia predisposes to digitalis toxicity and serious arrhythmias. Also monitor potassium level often when giving potassium salts because hyperkalemia in patients receiving digoxin can be fatal.
- Be aware that digoxin requirements may increase during pregnancy and decrease in the postpartum period. Expect digoxin levels to be monitored closely during pregnancy and the postpartum period. Also be aware that digoxin does cross the placenta. Monitor neonates of mothers taking digoxin during pregnancy for signs and symptoms of digoxin toxicity, including arrhythmias and vomiting.

PATIENT TEACHING

- Emphasize importance of taking digoxin exactly as prescribed. Warn about possible toxicity from taking too much and decreased effectiveness from taking too little.
- Instruct patient to take digoxin at same time each day to help increase compliance.
- Teach patient how to take her pulse, and instruct her to do so before each dose. Urge her to notify prescriber if pulse falls below 60 beats/minute or suddenly increases.
- Inform patient that small, white 0.25-mg tablets can easily be confused with other drugs. Caution against carrying digoxin in anything other than its original labeled container.
- Emphasize need to use special dropper supplied with elixir to ensure accurate dose measurement.
- Instruct patient to take a missed dose as soon as she remembers if within 12 hours of scheduled dose. If not, urge her to notify prescriber immediately.
- Urge patient to notify prescriber if she experiences adverse reactions, such as GI distress or pulse changes.
- Instruct patient to carry medical identification that indicates her need for digoxin.
- Advise patient to consult prescriber before using other drugs, including OTC products.

digoxin immune Fab (ovine)

DigiFab

Class and Category

Pharmacologic class: Antibody fragment
Therapeutic class: Cardiac glycoside antidote
Pregnancy category: C

Indications and Dosages

➤ *To treat acute digoxin or digitoxin toxicity*

I.V. INJECTION

Adults. Individualized dosage based on amount ingested. *Usual:* 240 mg (6 vials) to 800 mg (20 vials). I.V. infusion given slowly over at least 30 minutes, with I.V. injection reserved for use if cardiac arrest is imminent and given as a bolus.
Children weighing more than 20 kg (44 lb). Individualized dosage based on amount ingested. *Usual:* 40 mg (1 vial) to 240 mg (6 vials). I.V. infusion given slowly over at least 30 minutes with I.V. injection reserved for use if cardiac arrest is imminent and given as a bolus.
Infants and children weighing 20 kg (44 lb) or less. Individualized dosage based on amount ingested. *Usual:* 40 mg (1 vial) usually is effective. I.V. infusion given slowly over at least 30 minutes, with I.V. injection reserved for use if cardiac arrest is imminent and given as a bolus.
DOSAGE ADJUSTMENT Higher dose administered, as prescribed, if the dose based on ingested amount differs substantially from the dose based on serum digoxin or digitoxin level. Dose repeated after several hours, if needed.

Route	Onset	Peak	Duration
I.V.	15–30 min	Unknown	8–12 hr

Mechanism of Action

Binds with digoxin or digitoxin molecules. The resulting complex is excreted through the kidneys. As the free-serum digoxin level declines, tissue-bound digoxin enters the serum and also is bound and excreted.

Contraindications

Hypersensitivity to digoxin immune Fab or its components

Adverse Reactions

CV: **Increased ventricular rate (in atrial fibrillation), worsening of heart failure or low cardiac output**
Other: **Allergic reaction**, febrile reaction, **hypokalemia**

Nursing Considerations

- Expect each 38-mg vial of purified digoxin immune Fab to bind about 0.5 mg of digoxin or digitoxin.
- Reconstitute for I.V. use by dissolving 40 mg in 4 ml of sterile water for injection to yield 10 mg/ml. Mix gently. Further dilute with normal saline solution to proper volume for I.V. infusion. For very small doses, reconstituted 40-mg vial may

be diluted with 36 ml of normal saline solution to yield 1 mg/ml.

WARNING Monitor patient for an acute allergic reaction (angioedema, bronchospasm with cough or wheezing, erythema, hypotension, laryngeal edema, pruritus, stridor, tachycardia, or urticaria). If an anaphylactic reaction occurs during infusion, stop administration. Expect to treat all allergic reactions according to protocol. Be aware that patients with a history of hypersensitivity to papaya or papain are at high risk for an allergic reaction; digoxin immune Fab should be administered to this patient only if the benefits outweigh the risks. Also know that prior treatment with digoxin-specific Fab might increase the risk of diminished effects of the drug.

- Know that for an infant, reconstitute digoxin immune Fab as ordered and administer with a tuberculin syringe.
- Watch for fluid volume overload when administering drug to an infant or small child.
- Be aware that when giving a large dose, expect a faster onset but watch closely for febrile reaction.
- Give I.V. infusion through a 0.22-micron membrane filter slowly over at least 30 minutes. Keep in mind that drug may be given by rapid I.V. injection if cardiac arrest is imminent.
- Monitor serum potassium level often, especially during first few hours of therapy. Potassium level may drop rapidly.

PATIENT TEACHING

- Inform patient of the purpose of digoxin immune Fab and how it will be given.
- Advise patient to immediately report any signs and symptoms associated with an allergic reaction.

dihydroergotamine mesylate

D.H.E. 45, Dihydroergotamine-Sandoz (CAN), Migranal

Class and Category

Pharmacologic class: Ergot alkaloid
Therapeutic class: Antimigraine
Pregnancy category: X

Indications and Dosages

➤ *To treat acute migraine with or without aura*

I.M. INJECTION, SUBCUTANEOUS INJECTION

Adults. 1 mg at first sign of headache, repeated every hour up to 3 mg, if needed. *Maximum:* 3 mg/24 hr, 6 mg/wk.

I.V. INJECTION

Adults. 1 mg, repeated in 1 hr, if needed. *Maximum:* 2 mg/24 hr, 6 mg/wk.

NASAL SPRAY

Adults. 1 spray (0.5 mg) in each nostril, repeated in 15 min for a total dose of 2 sprays in each nostril or 2 mg. *Maximum:* 3 mg/24 hr, 4 mg/wk.

➤ *To treat acute episodes of cluster headaches*

I.M. INJECTION, SUBCUTANEOUS INJECTION

Adults. 1 mg at first sign of headache, repeated every hour up to 3 mg, if needed. *Maximum:* 3 mg/24 hr, 6 mg/wk.

I.V. INJECTION

Adults. 1 mg at first sign of headache, repeated in 1 hr, if needed. *Maximum:* 2 mg/24 hr, 6 mg/wk.

Route	Onset	Peak	Duration
I.V.	In 5 min	15 min–2 hr	About 8 hr
I.M., SubQ	15–30 min	15 min–2 hr	3–4 hr
Nasal	In 30 min	30–60 min	Unknown

Mechanism of Action

Produces intracranial and peripheral vasoconstriction by binding to all known 5-hydroxytryptamine$_1$ (5-HT$_1$) receptors, alpha$_1$- and alpha$_2$-adrenergic receptors, and dopaminergic receptors. Activation of 5-HT$_1$ receptors on intracranial blood vessels probably constricts large intracranial arteries and closes arteriovenous anastomoses to relieve cluster and migraine headaches. Activation of 5-HT$_1$ receptors on sensory nerves in the trigeminal system also may inhibit the release of proinflammatory neuropeptides.

Peripherally, dihydroergotamine causes vasoconstriction by stimulating alpha-adrenergic receptors. At therapeutic doses, it inhibits norepinephrine reuptake, increasing vasoconstriction. Drug constricts veins more than arteries, increasing venous return while decreasing venous stasis and pooling.

Contraindications

Basilar or hemiplegic headaches; coronary artery disease, including vasospasm; hypersensitivity to dihydroergotamine, other ergot alkaloids, or their components; ischemic heart disease; malnutrition; peripheral vascular disease or after vascular surgery; pregnancy; sepsis; severe hepatic or renal impairment; uncontrolled hypertension; use of macrolide antibiotics or protease inhibitors; use within 24 hours of 5-HT_1 agonist, ergotamine-containing or ergot-type drug, or methysergide

Interactions

DRUGS

beta blockers: Possibly peripheral vasoconstriction and peripheral ischemia, increased risk of gangrene
macrolides, protease inhibitors: Possibly increased risk of vasospasm, acute ergotism with peripheral ischemia
other ergot drugs, including ergoloid mesylates, ergonovine, methylergonovine, methysergide, and sumatriptan: Increased risk of serious adverse effects including coronary artery vasospasm
peripheral vasoconstrictors: Risk of severe hypertension

ACTIVITIES

smoking: Possibly increased ischemic response to ergot therapy

Adverse Reactions

CNS: Anxiety, confusion, dizziness, fatigue, headache, paresthesia, somnolence, weakness
CV: **Bradycardia**, chest pain, peripheral vasospasm, tachycardia
EENT: Abnormal vision; dry mouth; epistaxis, nasal congestion or rhinitis, and sore nose (nasal spray); miosis; pharyngitis; sinusitis; taste perversion
GI: Diarrhea, nausea, vomiting
MS: Muscle stiffness
SKIN: Localized edema of face, feet, fingers, and lower legs; sensation of heat or warmth; sudden diaphoresis

Nursing Considerations

WARNING **Monitor patient for signs of dihydroergotamine overdose, such as abdominal pain, confusion, delirium, dizziness, dyspnea, headache, nausea, pain in legs or arms, paresthesia, seizures, and vomiting.**

- Assess patient's capillary refill, peripheral pulses, and skin sensation and warmth. After giving nasal dihydroergotamine, monitor patient for signs of widespread blood vessel constriction and adverse reactions caused by decreased circulation to many body areas.

PATIENT TEACHING

- Instruct patient to use nasal spray or give self a subcutaneous injection, if prescribed, when headache pain—not aura—begins.
- Teach her to prime spray pump by squeezing it four times.
- Advise patient to wait 15 minutes between each set of nasal sprays.
- Teach patient prescribed drug via subcutaneous route how to administer injection and how to properly dispose of needles.
- Encourage patient to lie down in a quiet, dark room after using drug.
- Instruct patient to use more dihydroergotamine if headache returns or worsens but not to exceed maximum prescribed amount or frequency.
- Remind patient to take drug only as needed, not on a daily basis.
- Instruct patient to discard residual nasal spray in an open ampule after 8 hours.
- Caution her not to use dihydroergotamine and to notify prescriber if she experiences a different type of headache than drug prescribed to treat.
- Inform patient that nasal drug won't relieve pain other than throbbing headaches.
- Advise patient to avoid alcohol, which can cause or worsen headaches, and to avoid smoking, which may cause an ischemic response.

diltiazem hydrochloride

Apo-Diltiaz (CAN), Cardizem, Cardizem CD, Cardizem LA, Cartia XL, Dilacor XR, Dilt-CD, Diltzac, Taztia XT, Tiazac ER

Class and Category

Pharmacologic class: Calcium channel blocker
Therapeutic class: Antianginal, antiarrhythmic, antihypertensive
Pregnancy category: C

Indications and Dosages

➤ *To treat Prinzmetal's (variant) angina and to improve exercise tolerance in patients with chronic stable angina*

TABLETS

Adults and adolescents. *Initial:* 30 mg three times daily or four times daily before meals and at bedtime, increased every 1 or 2 days as appropriate. *Maximum:* 360 mg daily in divided doses three times daily or four times daily.

E.R. TABLETS

Adults and adolescents. *Initial:* 120 mg or 180 mg daily, increased every 7 to 14 days as needed. *Maximum:* 360 mg daily (Cardizem LA), 480 mg (Cardizem CD, Cartia XT, or Dilacor XR), and 540 mg (Taztia XT, Tiazac).

➤ *To improve exercise tolerance in patients with chronic stable angina*

E.R. TABLETS (CARDIZEM LA)

Adults. *Initial:* 180 mg once daily, increased in 7 to 14 days, as needed. *Maximum:* 360 mg daily.

➤ *To control hypertension*

E.R. CAPSULES

Adults and adolescents. *Initial:* 120 to 240 mg daily, increased in 7 to 14 days. *Maximum:* 540 mg daily.

E.R. TABLETS

Adults. *Initial:* 180 to 240 mg daily, increased after 14 days, as needed. *Maximum:* 540 mg daily.

➤ *To treat atrial fibrillation, atrial flutter, and paroxysmal supraventricular tachycardia*

I.V. INFUSION OR INJECTION

Adults and adolescents. 0.25 mg/kg given by bolus over 2 min. If response is inadequate after 15 min, 0.35 mg/kg given by bolus over 2 min. Then 5 or 10 mg/hr for continued reduction of heart rate after bolus, increased by 5 mg/hr, as needed. *Maximum:* 15 mg/hr for up to 24 hr.

Route	Onset	Peak	Duration
P.O.	30–60 min	In 2 wk	Unknown
P.O. (E.R.)	2–3 hr	In 2 wk	Unknown
I.V.	In 3 min	2–7 min	30 min–10 hr*

* For infusion; 1 to 3 hr for injection.

Mechanism of Action

Diltiazem inhibits calcium movement into coronary and vascular smooth-muscle cells by blocking slow calcium channels in cell membranes, as shown. This action decreases intracellular calcium, which:

- inhibits smooth-muscle cell contractions
- decreases myocardial oxygen demand by relaxing coronary and vascular smooth muscle, reducing peripheral vascular resistance and systolic and diastolic blood pressures
- slows AV conduction time and prolongs AV nodal refractoriness
- interrupts the reentry circuit in AV nodal reentrant tachycardias.

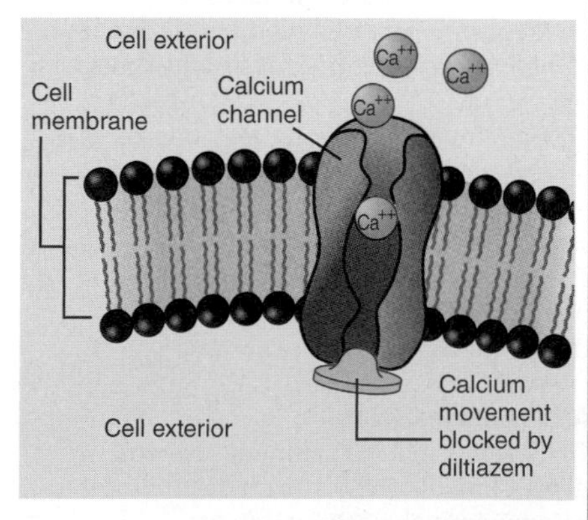

D

Incompatibilities

Don't give diltiazem through same I.V. line as acetazolamide, acyclovir, aminophylline, ampicillin sodium/sulbactam sodium, cefamandole, cefoperazone, diazepam, furosemide, heparin, hydrocortisone sodium succinate, methylprednisolone sodium succinate, mezlocillin, nafcillin, phenytoin, rifampin, or sodium bicarbonate.

Contraindications

Acute MI; cardiogenic shock; Lown–Ganong–Levine or Wolff–Parkinson–White syndrome, second- or third-degree AV block, or sick sinus syndrome, unless artificial pacemaker is in place; pulmonary edema; systolic blood pressure below 90 mm Hg; ventricular tachycardia (wide complex)

Interactions

DRUGS

anesthetic: Additive hypotension; possibly decreased cardiac contractility, conductivity, and automaticity
benzodiazepines: Increased risk of prolonged sedation
beta blockers: Possibly increased risk of adverse cardiovascular effects, especially AV block and bradycardia
buspirone: Increased effects and risk of buspirone toxicity
carbamazepine, quinidine: Decreased hepatic clearance and increased serum levels of these drugs, leading to toxicity
cimetidine: Decreased diltiazem metabolism, increased blood diltiazem level
clonidine: Increased risk of serious sinus bradycardia
digoxin: Increased blood digoxin level; increased risk of AV block or bradycardia
rifampin: Decreased blood diltiazem level to undetectable amounts
statins: Increased blood statin level with increased risk of myopathy and rhabdomyolysis

Adverse Reactions

CNS: Abnormal gait, amnesia, asthenia, depression, dizziness, dream disturbances, extrapyramidal reactions, fatigue, hallucinations, headache, insomnia, nervousness, paresthesia, personality change, somnolence, syncope, tremor, weakness
CV: Angina, **atrial flutter**, **AV block**, **bradycardia**, bundle-branch block, **ECG abnormalities**, **heart failure**, **hypotension**, palpitations, peripheral edema, **PVCs**, **sinus arrest**, sinus tachycardia, **ventricular fibrillation**, **ventricular tachycardia**
EENT: Amblyopia, dry mouth, epistaxis, eye irritation, gingival bleeding and hyperplasia, gingivitis, nasal congestion, retinopathy, taste perversion, tinnitus
ENDO: Hyperglycemia
GI: Anorexia, constipation, diarrhea, elevated liver enzymes, indigestion, nausea, thirst, vomiting
GU: **Acute renal failure**, impotence, nocturia, polyuria, sexual dysfunction
HEME: **Hemolytic anemia**, **leukopenia**, **prolonged bleeding time**, **thrombocytopenia**
MS: Arthralgia, muscle spasms, myalgia
RESP: Cough, dyspnea
SKIN: Acute generalized exanthematous pustulosis, alopecia, diaphoresis, **erythema multiforme**, **exfoliative dermatitis**, flushing, leukocytoclastic vasculitis, petechiae, photosensitivity, pruritus, purpura, rash, **Stevens–Johnson syndrome**, **toxic epidermal necrolysis**, urticaria
Other: **Angioedema**, hyperuricemia, weight gain

Nursing Considerations

- Use diltiazem cautiously in patients with impaired hepatic or renal function, and monitor liver and renal function, as appropriate; drug is metabolized mainly in the liver and excreted by the kidneys.

WARNING Monitor patient's blood pressure, heart rate and rhythm by continuous ECG, and pulse rate as appropriate during therapy. Keep emergency equipment and drugs available.

- Assess patient for signs and symptoms of heart failure.
- Watch for digitalis toxicity (nausea, vomiting, and visual color distortion) if patient takes digoxin and has an elevated serum digoxin level.
- Administer sublingual nitroglycerin, as prescribed, during diltiazem therapy.

- Expect to discontinue drug if adverse skin reactions, usually transient, persist although some may be severe.

PATIENT TEACHING

- Explain that capsules and E.R. tablets must be swallowed whole.

WARNING **Tell patient that stopping drug suddenly may have life-threatening effects.**

- Advise patient to monitor blood pressure and pulse rate regularly and to report significant changes to prescriber.
- Urge patient to report chest pain, difficulty breathing, dizziness, fainting, irregular heartbeat, rash, or swollen ankles.
- Instruct patient to maintain good oral hygiene, perform gum massage, and see a dentist every 6 months to prevent gingival bleeding and hyperplasia and gingivitis.
- Inform all prescribers of diltiazem therapy. Tell patient to consult prescriber before taking any OTC medication.
- Tell patient to inform prescriber if pregnancy occurs or is suspected.

dimenhydrinate

Dinate, Dramamine, Gravol (CAN), Hydrate

Class and Category

Pharmacologic class: Antihistamine
Therapeutic class: Antiemetic, antivertigo
Pregnancy category: B

Indications and Dosages

➤ ***To treat dizziness, nausea, vertigo, or vomiting associated with motion sickness***

CHEWABLE TABLETS, ORAL SOLUTION, SYRUP, TABLETS

Adults and adolescents. 50 to 100 mg every 4 to 6 hr, as needed. *Maximum:* 400 mg/24 hr.
Children ages 6 to 12. 25 to 50 mg every 6 to 8 hr, as needed. *Maximum:* 150 mg/24 hr.
Children ages 2 to 6. 12.5 to 25 mg every 6 to 8 hr, as needed. *Maximum:* 75 mg/24 hr.

I.M. INJECTION

Adults and adolescents. 50 mg every 4 hr, as needed.
Children. 1.25 mg/kg or 37.5 mg/m^2 every 6 hr, as needed. *Maximum:* 300 mg daily.

I.V. INFUSION OR INJECTION

Adults and adolescents. 50 mg in 10 ml of normal saline solution administered slowly, over at least 2 min, every 4 hr, as needed.

Route	Onset	Peak	Duration
P.O.	Unknown	Unknown	3–6 hr
I.M.	20–30 min	Unknown	3–6 hr
I.V.	Immediate	Unknown	3–6 hr

Mechanism of Action

May inhibit labyrinthine and vestibular stimulation and function by acting on the otolith system and, with larger doses, on the semicircular canals.

D

Contraindications

Age less than 1 month, hypersensitivity to dimenhydrinate or its components

Interactions

DRUGS

aminoglycosides, other ototoxic drugs: Masked symptoms of ototoxicity
anticholinergics, drugs with anticholinergic activity: Potentiated anticholinergic effects of dimenhydrinate
barbiturates, other CNS depressants: Possibly increased CNS depression
MAO inhibitors: Increased anticholinergic and CNS depressant effects of dimenhydrinate

ACTIVITIES

alcohol use: Possibly increased CNS depression

Adverse Reactions

CNS: Confusion, drowsiness, hallucinations, nervousness, paradoxical stimulation
CV: **Hypotension**, palpitations, tachycardia
EENT: Blurred vision, diplopia, dry eyes, dry mouth, nasal congestion
GI: Anorexia, constipation, diarrhea, epigastric discomfort, nausea, vomiting
GU: Dysuria
HEME: **Hemolytic anemia**
RESP: Thickening of bronchial secretions, wheezing
SKIN: Photosensitivity, rash, urticaria
Other: **Anaphylaxis**

Nursing Considerations

WARNING Be aware that the 50-mg/ml concentration of dimenhydrinate is intended for I.M. use. For I.V. use,

the solution must be diluted further with at least 10 ml normal saline solution, for each milliliter of dimenhydrinate.

- Monitor patients with angle-closure glaucoma, bladder neck obstruction, bronchial asthma, cardiac arrhythmias, prostatic hyperplasia, pyloroduodenal obstruction, or stenosing peptic ulcer for worsening of these conditions caused by anticholinergic effects.
- Monitor elderly patients for increased sensitivity to dimenhydrinate, such as confusion, excessive drowsiness, and restlessness.
- Assess patients, especially children and elderly patients, for evidence of paradoxical stimulation, such as irritability, nervousness, nightmares, restlessness, or unusual excitement.
- Store parenteral drug at 15° to 30° C (59° to 86° F); don't freeze.

PATIENT TEACHING

- Instruct patient to avoid hazardous activities until drug's CNS effects are known.
- Advise patient to inform healthcare providers about dimenhydrinate therapy, especially if she's being evaluated for medical conditions that are affected by this drug, such as appendicitis.
- Instruct patient to avoid alcohol, sedatives, and tranquilizers while taking dimenhydrinate.
- Encourage patient to use sunscreen to prevent photosensitivity reactions.

dimethyl fumarate

Tecfidera

Class and Category

Pharmacologic class: Nuclear factor-like 2 (Nrf2) activator
Therapeutic class: Immunomodulatory agent
Pregnancy category: C

Indications and Dosages

➤ To treat relapsing forms of multiple sclerosis

DELAYED RELEASE CAPSULES

Adults. *Initial:* 120 mg twice daily for 7 days; then increased to 240 mg twice daily. *Maintenance*: 240 mg twice daily.
DOSAGE ADJUSTMENT Dosage decreased to 120 mg twice daily for up to 4 weeks for patients who cannot initially tolerate maintenance dose.

Mechanism of Action

Possibly activates the nuclear factor (erythroid-derived 2)-like 2 (Nrf2) pathway, which is involved in the cellular response to oxidative stress thought to be a factor in multiple sclerosis.

Contraindications

Hypersensitivity to dimethyl fumarate or its components

Interactions

DRUGS

None reported

Adverse Reactions

CNS: Progressive multifocal leukoencephalopathy
GI: Abdominal pain, diarrhea, dyspepsia, elevated liver enzymes, **liver injury**, nausea, vomiting
GU: Albuminuria
HEME: Eosinophilia, **lymphopenia**
SKIN: Erythema, flushing, pruritus, rash
Other: Anaphylaxis, **angioedema**

Nursing Considerations

- Check to be sure patient has had a complete blood cell count (CBC) within the past 6 months prior to starting dimethyl fumarate therapy to identify patients with preexisting low lymphocyte counts. Know that a CBC should be obtained 6 months after therapy begins and then repeated every 6 to 12 months thereafter, and as needed.
- Obtain alkaline phosphatase, aminotransferase, and total bilirubin levels, as ordered, as a baseline prior to treatment with dimethyl fumarate, because drug may cause liver injury. If liver function abnormalities occur during treatment, expect drug to be discontinued.
- Know that dimethyl fumarate may decrease patient's lymphocyte counts as much as 30% during the first year of treatment but

then stabilizes but that therapy should be temporarily stopped if lymphocyte counts fall below 0.5×10^9/L for more than 6 months or if patient develops a serious infection until it is resolved.

WARNING **Be aware that progressive multifocal leukoencephalopathy (PML) has occurred with dimethyl fumarate use, especially in patients who develop lymphopenia. The majority of cases occurred in patients with lymphocyte counts less than 0.5×10^9/L. Notify prescriber at the first sign of PML, withhold drug, and expect patient to undergo a diagnostic workup to confirm diagnosis. Signs and symptoms to be alert for include changes in thinking, memory, and orientation that lead to confusion; disturbances of vision; personality changes; and progressive clumsiness or weakness on one side of the body. Be aware that these changes can gradually occur over days to weeks.**

- Notify prescriber if patient is suspected of having an infection, as dimethyl fumarate may need to be withheld if confirmed until it is resolved.

PATIENT TEACHING

- Instruct patient to swallow capsule whole, avoiding crushing or chewing it.
- Remind patient that drug should not be sprinkled on food.
- Warn patient that dimethyl fumarate may cause flushing but that it is generally not severe, nor is it life-threatening. Advise patient that taking dimethyl fumarate with food or taking up to 325 mg of non-enteric-coated aspirin, if prescribed, 30 minutes prior to taking drug may reduce flushing. Tell her that it generally begins soon after drug therapy has begun and usually improves or resolves over time.

WARNING **Instruct patient to seek immediate emergency medical attention if a severe allergic reaction occurs, such as difficulty breathing, hives, or swelling of throat and tongue. Tell patient that an allergic reaction can occur after the first dose or at any time during treatment.**

- Inform patient that dimethyl fumarate may cause liver injury. Tell patient to promptly report any of the following: dark urine, fatigue, loss of appetite, right upper abdominal discomfort, or yellowing of the skin or whites of the eyes.
- Advise patient to report any signs and symptoms of infection to prescriber immediately. Also, advise patient to report persistent, severe, or unusual signs and symptoms.
- Inform women of childbearing age to alert prescriber if pregnancy is suspected or known, as effects of drug on the fetus is unknown and drug may need to be discontinued. Also, if pregnancy occurs while taking drug, encourage patient to enroll in the pregnancy registry by calling 1-866-810-1462 or visiting the online site: www.tecfiderapregnancyregistry.com.
- Warn patient to protect capsules from light and to discard any unused capsules if container has been opened for 90 days.

diphenhydramine hydrochloride

Allerdryl (CAN), Banophen, Benadryl, Benadryl Allergy, Diphenhist CapTabs, Genahist, Nytol QuickCaps, Siladryl, Sleep-Eze D Extra Strength, Unisom SleepGels Maximum Strength

Class and Category

Pharmacologic class: Antihistamine
Therapeutic class: Antianaphylactic adjunct, antidyskinetic, antiemetic, antihistamine, antitussive (syrup), antivertigo, sedative-hypnotic
Pregnancy category: B

Indications and Dosages

➤ *To treat hypersensitivity reactions, such as perennial and seasonal allergic rhinitis, vasomotor rhinitis, allergic conjunctivitis, uncomplicated allergic skin eruptions, and transfusion reactions*

CAPSULES, TABLETS

Adults and adolescents. 25 to 50 mg every 4 to 6 hr, as needed. *Maximum:* 300 mg daily.
Children ages 6 to 12. 12.5 to 25 mg every 4 to 6 hr. *Maximum:* 150 mg daily.
Children up to age 6. 6.25 to 12.5 mg every 4 to 6 hr.

ELIXIR

Adults and adolescents. 25 to 50 mg every 4 to 6 hr, as needed. *Maximum:* 300 mg daily.

Children. 1.25 mg/kg every 4 to 6 hr. *Maximum:* 300 mg daily.

I.V. OR I.M. INJECTION

Adults and adolescents. 10 to 50 mg every 4 to 6 hr, not to exceed 25 mg/min I.V. or per I.M. site, up to 100 mg/dose, as needed. *Maximum:* 400 mg daily.

Children. 1.25 mg/kg, not to exceed 25 mg/min I.V. or per I.M. site, every 4 to 6 hr. *Maximum:* 300 mg daily.

➤ *To treat sleep disorders*

CAPSULES, TABLETS

Adults and adolescents. 50 mg 20 to 30 min before bedtime.

➤ *To provide antitussive effects*

ELIXIR

Adults and adolescents. 25 mg every 4 hr. *Maximum:* 150 mg/24 hr.

Children ages 6 to 12. 12.5 mg every 4 to 6 hr. *Maximum:* 75 mg daily.

Children ages 2 to 6. 6.25 mg every 4 to 6 hr. *Maximum:* 25 mg daily.

➤ *To prevent motion sickness or treat vertigo*

CAPSULES, ELIXIR, TABLETS

Adults and adolescents. 25 to 50 mg every 4 to 6 hr, as needed. *Maximum:* 300 mg daily.

Children. 1 to 1.5 mg/kg every 4 to 6 hr, as needed. *Maximum:* 300 mg daily.

I.V. OR I.M. INJECTION

Adults and adolescents.
Initial: 10 mg. Increased to 20 to 50 mg not to exceed 25 mg/min I.V. or per I.M. site every 4 to 6 hr, if needed. *Maximum:* 100 mg/dose, 400 mg daily.

Children. 1 to 1.5 mg/kg not to exceed 25 mg/min I.V. or per I.M. site every 6 hr, as needed. *Maximum:* 300 mg daily.

➤ *To treat symptoms of Parkinson's disease and drug-induced extrapyramidal reactions in elderly patients who can't tolerate more potent antidyskinetic drugs*

CAPSULES, ELIXIR, TABLETS

Adults. 25 mg three times daily, increased gradually to 50 mg four times daily, as needed. *Maximum:* 300 mg daily.

I.V. OR I.M. INJECTION

Adults and adolescents. 10 to 50 mg, not to exceed 25 mg/min I.V. or per I.M. site, four times daily, as needed. *Maximum:* 100 mg/dose, 400 mg daily.

Route	Onset	Peak	Duration
P.O.	15–60 min	1–3 hr	6–8 hr
I.V.	Immediate	1–3 hr	6–8 hr
I.M.	30 min	1–3 hr	6–8 hr

Mechanism of Action

Binds to central and peripheral H_1 receptors, competing with histamine for these sites and preventing it from reaching its site of action. By blocking histamine, diphenhydramine produces antihistamine effects, inhibiting GI, respiratory, and vascular smooth-muscle contraction; decreasing capillary permeability, which reduces flares, itching, and wheals; and decreasing lacrimal and salivary gland secretions.

Diphenhydramine produces antidyskinetic effects, possibly by inhibiting acetylcholine in the CNS. It also produces antitussive effects by directly suppressing the cough center in the medulla oblongata in the brain. Diphenhydramine's antiemetic and antivertigo effects may be related to its ability to bind to CNS muscarinic receptors and depress vestibular stimulation and labyrinthine function. Its sedative effects are related to its CNS depressant action.

Contraindications

Breastfeeding; hypersensitivity to diphenhydramine, similiar antihistamines, or their components; use in newborns or premature infants

Interactions

DRUGS

barbiturates, other CNS depressants: Possibly increased CNS depression

MAO inhibitors: Increased anticholinergic and CNS depressant effects of diphenhydramine

ACTIVITIES

alcohol use: Possibly increased CNS depression

Adverse Reactions

CNS: Confusion, dizziness, drowsiness
CV: **Arrhythmias**, palpitations, tachycardia
EENT: Blurred vision, diplopia
GI: Epigastric distress, nausea
HEME: **Agranulocytosis, hemolytic anemia, thrombocytopenia**
RESP: Thickened bronchial secretions
SKIN: Photosensitivity

Nursing Considerations

- Expect to give parenteral form of diphenhydramine only when oral ingestion isn't possible.
- Keep elixir container tightly closed. Protect elixir and parenteral forms from light.
- Expect to discontinue drug at least 72 hours before skin tests for allergies because drug may inhibit cutaneous histamine response, thus producing false-negative results.

PATIENT TEACHING

- Instruct patient to take diphenhydramine at least 30 minutes before exposure to situations that may cause motion sickness.
- Advise her to take drug with food to minimize GI distress.
- Urge patient to avoid alcohol while taking diphenhydramine.
- Caution patient to avoid hazardous activities until drug's CNS effects are known.
- Instruct her to use sunscreen to prevent photosensitivity reactions.
- Advise patient to avoid taking other OTC drugs that contain diphenhydramine to prevent additive effects.

dipyridamole

Persantine

Class and Category

Pharmacologic class: Pyrimidine analogue
Therapeutic class: Antiplatelet
Pregnancy category: B

Indications and Dosages

➤ *To prevent thromboembolic complications of cardiac valve replacement*

TABLETS

Adults. 75 to 100 mg four times daily with warfarin.

➤ *To aid diagnosis during thallium perfusion imaging of myocardium*

I.V. INFUSION

Adults. 0.57 mg/kg in 50 ml of D_5W infused over 4 min. *Maximum:* 60 mg.

Route	Onset	Peak	Duration
I.V.	Unknown	Unknown	8.7 min*

* After start of infusion, for increased velocity of coronary artery blood flow.

Mechanism of Action

May increase the intraplatelet level of adenosine, which causes coronary vasodilation and inhibits platelet aggregation. Dipyridamole also may increase the intraplatelet level of cyclic adenosine monophosphate (cAMP) and may inhibit formation of the potent platelet activator stimulant thromboxane A_2, which decreases platelet activation. Vasodilation and increased blood flow occur preferentially in nondiseased coronary vessels, which results in redistribution of blood away from significantly diseased vessels. These changes in perfusion are observed during thallium imaging studies.

Contraindications

Hypersensitivity to dipyridamole or its components

Interactions

DRUGS

adenosine: Potentiated effects of adenosine
cholinesterase inhibitors: Decreased anticholinesterase effect, possibly aggravating myasthenia gravis
heparin, NSAIDs, thrombolytics: Possibly increased risk of bleeding
theophylline: Reversal of coronary vasodilation caused by dipyridamole, possibly false-negative thallium imaging result

Adverse Reactions

CNS: Dizziness, headache
CV: Angina, **arrhythmias**, **ECG changes (specifically ST-segment and T-wave changes)**
GI: Abdominal pain, diarrhea, nausea, vomiting
RESP: Dyspnea
SKIN: Flushing, pruritus, rash

Nursing Considerations

- Protect I.V. form of dipyridamole from direct light and freezing.
- Monitor blood pressure, pulse rate and rhythm, and breath sounds every 10 to 15 minutes during I.V. infusion.
- Keep parenteral aminophylline available to relieve adverse reactions to dipyridamole infusion.
- Expect adverse reactions to be minimal and transient at therapeutic doses. They typically resolve with long-term use.

PATIENT TEACHING

- Urge patient to take dipyridamole at least 1 hour before or 2 hours after meals for faster absorption. If she experiences GI distress, advise her to take drug with meals or milk.
- Advise patient to take drug at evenly spaced intervals.
- Inform patient that drug commonly is taken with warfarin. Tell patient that aspirin should not be administered concomitantly with warfarin.
- Urge her to keep appointments for coagulation tests.
- Instruct patient to seek immediate emergency treatment if chest pain occurs.
- Caution patient to consult prescriber before taking over-the-counter NSAIDs because of the possible increased risk of bleeding.
- Advise patient to notify all healthcare providers about dipyridamole use.

disulfiram

Antabuse

Class and Category

Pharmacologic class: Aldehyde dehydrogenase inhibitor
Therapeutic class: Alcohol deterrent
Pregnancy category: Not classified

Indications and Dosages

➤ *As adjunct to maintain sobriety in treatment of chronic alcoholism*

TABLETS

Adults. *Initial:* Up to 500 mg daily for 1 to 2 wk. *Maintenance:* 125 to 500 mg daily. *Maximum:* 500 mg daily.

Route	Onset	Peak	Duration
P.O.	1–2 hr	Unknown	Up to 14 days

Mechanism of Action

Interferes with the enzyme responsible for hepatic oxidation of acetaldehyde to acetate, which occurs during alcohol catabolism. Ingestion of even a small amount of alcohol after taking disulfiram raises the blood acetaldehyde level to 5 to 10 times normal. Disulfiram doesn't alter the rate of alcohol elimination. Its major metabolite, diethyldithiocarbamate, inhibits norepinephrine synthesis and may be responsible for the drug's hypotensive effect.

Contraindications

Alcohol intoxication; coronary artery occlusion; hypersensitivity to disulfiram, its components, rubber, pesticides, or fungicides; psychosis; recent use of alcohol, alcohol-containing preparations, metronidazole, or paraldehyde; severe myocardial disease

Interactions

DRUGS

isoniazid: Increased risk of additive neurotoxic effect of disulfiram; possibly increased adverse CNS effects
metronidazole: Risk of CNS toxicity, resulting in confusion and psychosis
oral anticoagulants: Possibly increased anticoagulant effects
paraldehyde: Decreased paraldehyde metabolism, increased blood paraldehyde level
phenytoin: Possibly increased blood phenytoin level and risk of phenytoin toxicity

ACTIVITIES

alcohol use: Disulfiram–alcohol reaction (if within 14 days of disulfiram therapy)

Adverse Reactions

CNS: Drowsiness, headache, peripheral neuropathy, psychotic reaction, tiredness
EENT: Blurred vision, garlic or metallic taste, optic atrophy, optic neuritis
GU: Impotence
SKIN: Rash

Nursing Considerations

- Keep in mind that disulfiram is given only to patients who are highly motivated to stop drinking and who are receiving psychotherapy or substance abuse counseling.
- Know that the alcohol content of patient's other drugs should be checked before starting therapy.

WARNING **Never give drug to patient without her knowledge or if she is intoxicated.**

- Crush tablet and mix with fluids before administration, if needed.
- Don't give drug within 14 days of patient's ingestion of alcohol-containing substance.
- Expect alcohol ingestion during disulfiram therapy to produce a severe reaction that lasts from 30 minutes to several hours. Symptoms may include angina, anxiety, blurred vision, confusion, diaphoresis, dyspnea, heart failure, hypotension, nausea, palpitations, sinus tachycardia, syncope, thirst, throbbing headache, throbbing in neck, vertigo, vomiting, and weakness. A deep sleep usually follows.

WARNING **Be aware that the ingestion of three or more alcoholic beverages with a disulfiram dose greater than 500 mg daily may cause respiratory depression, arrhythmias, and cardiac arrest.**

- Know that if patient takes phenytoin, monitor blood phenytoin level before and during disulfiram therapy, and adjust dosage of either drug as prescribed. Interactions may not occur if disulfiram therapy starts before phenytoin therapy. A subtherapeutic phenytoin level may result if disulfiram therapy stops.
- Be aware that if patient takes an oral anticoagulant, monitor PT before and during disulfiram therapy, and adjust anticoagulant dosage as prescribed. Drug interactions may not occur if disulfiram therapy starts before warfarin therapy. If disulfiram therapy stops, be prepared to adjust warfarin dosage to avoid loss of hypoprothrombinemic effects.
- Expect some adverse reactions, such as drowsiness, headache, and impotence, to subside over time or with a brief dosage reduction.
- Know that because one-fifth of a disulfiram dose may stay in the body for 1 week or longer, alcohol ingestion may continue to produce unpleasant symptoms for up to 2 weeks after therapy stops.
- Expect therapy to last months to years, depending on patient's ability to abstain from alcohol.

PATIENT TEACHING

- Teach patient's household and family members about precautions needed and risks associated with disulfiram therapy.
- Explain that drug doesn't cure alcoholism but does help deter alcohol consumption.
- Advise her to take drug in the evening if she reports daytime drowsiness.
- Warn patient to avoid alcohol-containing substances, such as cough syrup, sauces, and vinegar during therapy because a disulfiram–alcohol reaction may occur after ingesting as little as 15 ml of 100-proof alcohol. Urge her to avoid alcohol-containing liniments and lotions as well.
- Teach patient what to expect if disulfiram alcohol reaction occurs. Inform her that a deep sleep usually follows the reaction.
- Advise patient that a reaction can occur up to 14 days after therapy stops and that a severe reaction may cause arrhythmias, cardiac arrest, and respiratory depression.
- Instruct patient to carry medical identification that indicates drug, describes possible reactions, and lists someone to notify in case of emergency.

dobutamine hydrochloride

Class and Category

Pharmacologic class: Sympathomimetic
Therapeutic class: Inotropic
Pregnancy category: Not classified

Indications and Dosages

➤ *To treat low cardiac output and heart failure short term*

I.V. INFUSION

Adults and children. *Initial:* 0.5 to 1.0 mcg/kg/min as continuous infusion adjusted every couple of minutes according to hemodynamic response. *Usual maintenance:* 2 to 20 mcg/kg/min. *Maximum:* 40 mcg/kg/min.

Route	Onset	Peak	Duration
I.V.	1–2 min	Unknown	Under 5 min

Mechanism of Action

Mainly stimulates $beta_1$-adrenergic receptors, and mildly stimulates $beta_2$- and $alpha_1$-adrenergic receptors. $Beta_1$-receptor stimulation produces a positive inotropic effect on the myocardium, increasing cardiac output by boosting myocardial contractility and stroke volume. Increased myocardial contractility raises coronary blood flow and myocardial oxygen consumption. Systolic blood pressure typically rises as a result of increased stroke volume. Other hemodynamic effects include decreased systemic vascular resistance, which reduces afterload, and decreased ventricular filling pressure, which reduces preload.

Incompatibilities

Don't combine dobutamine with cefamandole, cefazolin, hydrocortisone sodium succinate, cephalothin, penicillin, sodium ethacrynate, and sodium heparin because of incompatibility. Don't mix dobutamine with alkaline solutions, such as sodium bicarbonate, because of possible physical incompatibility. Don't use diluents that contain sodium bisulfite or ethanol.

Contraindications

Hypersensitivity to dobutamine or its components, idiopathic hypertrophic subaortic stenosis

Interactions

DRUGS

beta blockers: Possibly increased alpha-adrenergic activity and peripheral resistance

nitroprusside: Increased cardiac output and lowered pulmonary wedge pressure

Adverse Reactions

CNS: Fever, headache, nervousness, restlessness
CV: Angina, **bradycardia**, hypertension, **hypotension**, nonspecific chest pain, palpitations, **PVCs**, tachycardia
GI: Nausea, vomiting
RESP: Dyspnea, shortness of breath
SKIN: Extravasation with tissue necrosis and sloughing, rash
Other: Hypokalemia

Nursing Considerations

- Avoid giving dobutamine to patients with uncorrected hypovolemia. Expect prescriber to order whole blood or plasma volume expanders to correct hypovolemia. Also avoid giving dobutamine to patients with acute MI because it can intensify or extend myocardial ischemia.
- Use drug cautiously in patients allergic to sulfites because drug may cause anaphylactic-like signs and symptoms; commercially available dobutamine injections contain sodium bisulfite. Also use drug cautiously in patients with atrial fibrillation because drug increases AV conduction. Keep in mind that patient should be adequately digitalized before administration.
- Dilute concentrate with at least 50 ml compatible I.V. solution. A common dilution is 500 mg (40 ml from 250-ml bag) in 210 ml D_5W or normal saline solution to yield 2,000 mcg/ml. Or dilute 1,000 mg (80 ml from 250-ml bag) in 170 ml D_5W or normal saline solution to yield 4,000 mcg/ml. Adjust maximum concentration according to patient's fluid requirements as prescribed. Don't exceed 5,000 mcg/ml. Discard solution after 24 hours.
- Inspect parenteral solution for particles and discoloration before administering it.
- Give I.V. drug using an infusion pump.
- Monitor blood pressure continuously during therapy, preferably by continuous intra-arterial monitoring; systolic increase of 10 to 20 mm Hg may indicate dobutamine-induced increase in cardiac output.

- Expect to reduce dosage or discontinue drug if hypotension develops.
- Monitor heart rate and rhythm via ECG recordings continuously for PVCs, which may result from drug's stimulatory effect on heart's conduction system, and sinus tachycardia, which results from positive chronotropic effect of beta stimulation and may increase heart rate by 5 to 15 beats/minute.
- Monitor hemodynamic parameters, such as cardiac output, central venous pressure, and pulmonary artery wedge pressure, as indicated, to assess drug's effectiveness.

WARNING Monitor serum potassium level to check for hypokalemia, a rare result of $beta_2$ stimulation that causes electrolyte imbalance.

- Monitor urine output hourly, as appropriate, to check for improved renal blood flow.
- Know that dobutamine isn't indicated for long-term treatment of heart failure because it may not be effective and may increase the risk of hospitalization and death.

PATIENT TEACHING

- Explain the need for frequent hemodynamic monitoring.

docusate calcium

(dioctyl calcium sulfosuccinate)

Doxidan (CAN), Surfak

docusate potassium

(dioctyl potassium sulfosuccinate)

Kasof

docusate sodium

(dioctyl sodium sulfosuccinate)

Colace, Colax, Correctol, Dialose, Diocto, DOK, D.O.S., Silace

Class and Category

Pharmacologic class: Surfactant
Therapeutic class: Laxative, stool softener
Pregnancy category: C

Indications and Dosages

➤ *To treat constipation*

CAPSULES, LIQUID, SYRUP, TABLETS (ALL SALTS)

Adults and adolescents. 50 to 500 mg in 1 to 4 divided doses.
Children ages 6 to 12. 40 to 150 mg in 1 to 4 divided doses.
Children ages 3 to 6. 20 to 60 mg in 1 to 4 divided doses.
Children under age 3. 10 to 40 mg in 1 to 4 divided doses.

RECTAL ENEMA (DOCUSATE SODIUM)

Adults. 200 to 283 mg once or twice.
Children age 3 and over. 200 to 283 mg once daily, as needed.

CAPSULES, TABLETS (DOCUSATE POTASSIUM)

Adults and adolescents. 100 mg three times daily until bowel movements are normal.
Children age 6 and over. 100 mg at bedtime.

Route	Onset	Peak	Duration
P.O.	24–72 hr	Unknown	Unknown
Rectal	within 24 hr	Unknown	Unknown

Mechanism of Action

Acts as a surfactant that softens stool by decreasing surface tension between oil and water in feces. This action lets more fluid penetrate stool, forming a softer fecal mass.

Contraindications

Fecal impaction; hypersensitivity to docusate salts or their components; intestinal obstruction; nausea, vomiting, or other symptoms of appendicitis; undiagnosed abdominal pain

Interactions

DRUGS

mineral oil: Increased mineral oil absorption, increased risk of toxicity

Adverse Reactions

CNS: Dizziness, syncope
CV: Palpitations
GI: Abdominal cramps and distention, diarrhea, nausea, perianal irritation, vomiting
MS: Muscle weakness

Nursing Considerations

WARNING Expect excessive or long-term use of docusate to cause dependence on

D

laxatives for bowel movements, electrolyte imbalances, osteomalacia, steatorrhea, and vitamin and mineral deficiencies.
- Assess for laxative abuse syndrome, especially in women with anorexia nervosa, depression, or personality disorders.

PATIENT TEACHING
- Tell patient not to use docusate when she has abdominal pain, nausea, or vomiting.
- Advise patient to take docusate with a full glass of milk or water.
- Encourage patient to increase fiber intake, exercise regularly, and drink 6 to 8 glasses (240 ml/glass) of water daily to help prevent constipation.
- Instruct patient to notify prescriber about rectal bleeding; symptoms of electrolyte imbalances, such as dizziness, light-headedness, muscle cramping, and weakness; and unrelieved constipation.

dofetilide

Tikosyn

Class and Category

Pharmacologic class: Class III antiarrhythmic
Therapeutic class: Antiarrhythmic
Pregnancy category: Not classified

Indications and Dosages

➤ *To convert symptomatic atrial fibrillation or flutter to normal sinus rhythm or to maintain normal sinus rhythm in patients converted from symptomatic atrial fibrillation or flutter*

CAPSULES

Adults. Highly individualized based on creatinine clearance and QTc (QT interval used if heart rate is below 60 beats per min). *Usual:* 500 mcg twice daily for patients with creatinine clearance above 60 ml/min. *Maximum:* 500 mcg twice daily.
DOSAGE ADJUSTMENT For patient with renal impairment, initial dose reduced to 250 mcg twice daily if creatinine clearance is 40 to 60 ml/min and to 125 mcg twice daily if clearance is 20 to 39 ml/min, as prescribed. If, 2 to 3 hr after initial dose, QTc interval has increased by at least 15% or is more than 500 milliseconds (msec) (550 msec in patients with ventricular conduction abnormalities), dosage decreased by 50%, as prescribed. However, for patients receiving lowest initial dose of 125 mcg twice daily, dosage reduced to 125 mcg daily, as prescribed. If at any time after second dose, QTc interval increases to more than 500 msec (550 msec in patients with ventricular conduction abnormalities), expect to discontinue drug, as prescribed.

Route	Onset	Peak	Duration
P.O.	Unknown	2 hr	4 hr

Mechanism of Action

Selectively blocks potassium channels in myocardial cell membranes involved in cardiac repolarization. By blocking potassium channels, dofetilide prolongs action potential duration, effective refractory period, and ventricular refractoriness (widens QT interval). These actions terminate or prevent reentrant tachyarrhythmias, such as atrial fibrillation, atrial flutter, and ventricular tachycardia.

Contraindications

Acquired or congenital QT prolongation syndrome; concurrent therapy with cimetidine, dolutegravir, hydrochlorothiazide, ketoconazole, megestrol, prochlorperazine, trimethoprim, or verapamil; hypersensitivity to dofetilide or its components; severe renal impairment (creatinine clearance less than 20 ml/min)

Interactions

DRUGS

amiloride, cimetidine, cotrimoxazole, ketoconazole, megestrol, metformin, sulfamethoxazole-trimethoprim, triamterene, trimethoprim: Possibly increased blood dofetilide level
azole antifungals, cannabinoids, diltiazem, nefazodone, norfloxacin, protease inhibitors, quinine, selective serotonin reuptake inhibitors, zafirlukast: Possibly increased blood dofetilide level and risk of dofetilide toxicity
bepridil, cisapride, macrolide antibiotics, phenothiazines, selected fluoroquinolones,

tricyclic antidepressants: Possibly prolonged QT interval
class I and III antiarrhythmics, especially amiodarone: Possibly prolonged QT interval and increased risk of dofetilide-induced proarrhythmias
diuretics (potassium-depleting): Increased risk of torsades de pointes in patients with hypokalemia or hypomagnesemia
hydrochlorothiazide, verapamil: Possibly increased blood dofetilide level and increased risk of torsades de pointes

FOODS

grapefruit juice: Increased dofetilide level

Adverse Reactions

CNS: Cerebral ischemia, **CVA**, dizziness, facial or flaccid paralysis, headache, insomnia, paresthesia, slurred speech, syncope
CV: AV block, **bradycardia**, **cardiac arrest**, chest pain, edema, **MI**, tachycardia, **ventricular arrhythmias (including torsades de pointes and ventricular tachycardia)**
GI: Abdominal pain, diarrhea, **hepatic dysfunction**, jaundice, nausea
MS: Back pain, muscle weakness
RESP: Cough, dyspnea, respiratory tract infection
SKIN: Rash
Other: Angioedema, flu-like symptoms, weight gain

Nursing Considerations

WARNING **Be aware that dofetilide shouldn't be started if patient has previously received amiodarone until blood amiodarone level is less than 0.3 mcg/ml or until amiodarone has been withdrawn for at least 3 months.**

- Evaluate and document QTc interval before and during dofetilide therapy.
- Place patient on continuous ECG monitoring for at least 3 days, as ordered, during dofetilide therapy.

WARNING **Know that if patient does not convert to normal sinus rhythm within 24 hours of starting dofetilide, expect possible synchronized electrical cardioversion.**

- Be prepared to reevaluate renal function and QTc interval every 3 months, as ordered, during dofetilide therapy.
- Monitor continuous ECG for at least 30 hours, as ordered when switching to dofetilide from class I or class III antiarrhythmics, or after withdrawing antiarrhythmic treatment.
- Be aware that if patient requires a drug that may interact with dofetilide, expect to discontinue dofetilide, as prescribed, for 2 or more days before starting the other drug.

WARNING **Monitor laboratory test results for hypokalemia or hypomagnesemia, especially in patients taking diuretics, because of the increased risk of dofetilide-induced torsades de pointes.**

- Monitor women often for adverse reactions, including prolonged QTc interval and torsades de pointes; they have 12% to 18% lower renal clearance of drug than men and therefore a greater risk of adverse reactions.

PATIENT TEACHING

- Advise patient to swallow dofetilide capsules with water.
- Instruct patient to avoid drinking grapefruit juice while taking this drug.
- Inform patient that she may be hospitalized for at least 3 days if dofetilide dosage is increased.
- Teach patient to measure blood pressure and pulse rate during dofetilide therapy.
- Urge patient to report chest discomfort, fluttering, or palpitations immediately.
- Tell patient to notify prescriber immediately if she experiences loss of appetite, severe diarrhea, unusual sweating, or vomiting, or if she develops excessive thirst that may occur as a result of certain drug interactions that cause an electrolyte imbalance.
- Advise patient to consult prescriber before using any OTC drugs, nutritional supplements, or herbal products.
- Instruct patient to keep follow-up appointments to monitor heart rhythm.

dolasetron mesylate

Anzemet

Class and Category

Pharmacologic class: Selective serotonin receptor antagonist
Therapeutic class: Antiemetic
Pregnancy category: B

Indications and Dosages

➤ *To prevent nausea and vomiting due to chemotherapy*

ORAL SOLUTION, TABLETS

Adults and children over age 16. 100 mg within 1 hr before chemotherapy.
Children ages 2 to 16. 1.8 mg/kg within 1 hr before chemotherapy. *Maximum:* 100 mg/dose.

➤ *To prevent postoperative nausea and vomiting*

I.V. INFUSION, I.V. INJECTION

Adults and children over age 16. 12.5 mg 15 min before end of anesthesia.
I.V. injection given rapidly, at 100 mg per 30 seconds, or I.V. infusion diluted to 50 ml and infused up to 15 min.
Children ages 2 to 16. 0.35 mg/kg 15 min before end of anesthesia. *Maximum:* 12.5 mg/dose.

➤ *To treat postoperative nausea and vomiting*

I.V. INFUSION, I.V. INJECTION

Adults and children over age 16. 12.5 mg as single dose as soon as symptoms develop. I.V. injection given rapidly, at 100 mg per 30 seconds, or I.V. infusion diluted to 50 ml and infused up to 15 min.
Children ages 2 to 16. 0.35 mg/kg as single dose as soon as symptoms develop. *Maximum:* 12.5 mg/dose.

Mechanism of Action

With its active metabolite hydrodolasetron, prevents activation of serotonin 5-HT_3 receptors located centrally in chemoreceptor trigger zone and peripherally on vagal nerve terminals thereby decreasing the vomiting reflex.

Contraindications

Congenital long-QT syndrome, hypersensitivity to dolasetron or its components, intravenous administration to prevent nausea and vomiting associated with cancer chemotherapy, use with apomorphine

Interactions

DRUGS

apomorphine: Increased risk of loss of consciousness and profound hypotension
atenolol: Possibly decreased dolasetron clearance
cimetidine: Possibly increased blood dolasetron level
drugs that prolong ECG intervals or cause hypokalemia or hypomagnesemia: Increased risk of serious arrhythmia
fentanyl, I.V. methylene blue, lithium, mirtazapine, MAO inhibitors, selective serotonin reuptake inhibitors, serotonin and norepinephrine reuptake inhibitors: Increased risk of serotonin syndrome
rifampin: Possibly decreased blood dolasetron level

Adverse Reactions

CNS: Headache, **serotonin syndrome**
CV: **Cardiac arrest**; hypertension; **hypotension**; **MI**; **prolongation of QT**, **PR**, **and QRS intervals in ECG**; **torsades de pointes**; **ventricular fibrillation and tachycardia**; **wide-complex tachycardia**
GI: Diarrhea
SKIN: Rash
Other: injection-site pain

Nursing Considerations

- Correct hypokalemia and hypomagnesemia, if present and as ordered, prior to administering dolasetron intravenously as serious arrhythmias may result.
- Expect to give up to 100 mg of dolasetron I.V. in 30 seconds or to dilute it in normal saline solution, D_5W, dextrose 5% in half-normal (0.45) saline solution, or lactated Ringer's solution and infuse for up to 15 minutes, as prescribed.
- Flush I.V. line with compatible solution before and after drug administration.
- Expect to prepare an oral solution of dolasetron for patients unable to swallow tablets by diluting injection solution with apple or apple-grape juice.

WARNING Assess patient for ECG changes, including prolonged PR, QTc, and QT intervals and widened QRS complex, especially in patients with bradycardia or underlying heart disease, congestive heart failure, the elderly, and patients with renal impairment during intravenous dolasetron therapy.

WARNING Monitor patient for serotonin syndrome, which is characterized by agitation, chills, confusion, diaphoresis, diarrhea, fever, hyperactive reflexes, poor coordination, restlessness, shaking, talking or acting with uncontrolled excitement, tremor, and twitching. In its most severe form, serotonin syndrome can resemble neuroleptic malignant syndrome, which includes a high fever, muscle rigidity, autonomic instability with possible fluctuations in vital signs, mental status changes, and mental status changes.

PATIENT TEACHING

- Explain that oral solution can be prepared by diluting injection form of drug with apple or apple-grape juice for children or patients who have trouble swallowing.
- Inform patient that oral solution may be refrigerated for up to 48 hours but should be discarded after 2 hours at room temperature.
- Advise patient to notify prescriber immediately if he experiences dizziness, palpitations, or an abnormally slow or irregular pulse after receiving dolasetron intravenously.

WARNING Instruct patient to seek immediate medical attention if he experiences erratic changes in his blood pressure, heart beat, or temperature; changes in his mental status; adverse gastrointestinal symptoms; or neuromuscular symptoms.

dolutegravir

Tivicay

Class and Category

Pharmacologic class: Integrase stand transfer inhibitor (INSTI)
Therapeutic class: Antiretroviral
Pregnancy category: Not classified

Indications and Dosages

➤ *As adjunct to treat human immunodeficiency virus type 1 (HIV-1) in combination with other antiretroviral agents*

TABLETS

Adults who are treatment-naïve, treatment-experienced INSTI-naïve, or virologically suppressed and switching to dolutegravir plus rilpivirine. 50 mg once daily.
Adults who are treatment-naïve or treatment-experienced INSTI-naïve who are currently receiving carbamazepine, efavirenz, fosamprenavir/ritonavir, rifampin, or tipranavir/ritonavir; adults who are INSTI-experienced who have certain INSTI-associated resistance substitutions or clinically suspected INSTI resistance. 50 mg twice daily.
Children who are treatment-naïve or treatment-experienced INSTI-naïve and weigh at least 40 kg (88 lb) or more. 50 mg once daily.
Children who are treatment-naïve or treatment-experienced INSTI-naïve and weigh at least 30 kg (66 lb) but less than 40 kg (88 lb). 35 mg once daily.

Mechanism of Action

Inhibits HIV integrase by binding to the integrase active site and blocking the strand transfer step of retroviral DNA integration, which is needed for the HIV replication cycle.

Contraindications

Concurrent therapy with dofetilide, hypersensitivity to dolutegravir or its components

Interactions

DRUGS

buffered medications, calcium- or iron-containing products, carbamazepine, cation-containing antacids or laxatives, efavirenz, etravirine, fosamprenavir/ritonavir, nevirapine, oxcarbazepine, phenobarbital, phenytoin, rifampin, St. John's wort, sucralfate, tipranavir/ritonavir: Decreased plasma dolutegravir levels leading to decreased effectiveness
dofetilide: Possibly increased plasma dolutegravir levels leading to potential toxicity
metformin: Increased plasma metformin levels increasing risk of adverse reactions

Adverse Reactions

CNS: Abnormal dreams, depression, dizziness, fatigue, fever, general malaise, headache, insomnia, **suicidal ideation**, vertigo
CV: Elevated cholesterol or triglycerides
EENT: Conjunctivitis, oral blisters or lesions
ENDO: Cushingoid appearance, fat redistribution, hyperglycemia
GI: Abdominal discomfort or pain, **acute liver failure**, diarrhea, elevated bilirubin or liver enzymes, flatulence, **hepatitis**, **hepatitis B reactivation**, **hepatotoxicity**, **liver injury**, nausea, vomiting
GU: Elevated creatinine level, renal impairment

D

HEME: Eosinophilia
MS: Arthralgia, elevated creatine kinase, joint or muscle aches, myalgia, myositis
RESP: Difficulty breathing
SKIN: Blisters, peeling of skin, pruritus, rash
Other: Angioedema, elevated lipase, immune reconstitution syndrome, weight gain

Nursing Considerations

- Expect to perform a pregnancy test in women of childbearing age before dolutegravir therapy is begun, because drug increases risk of neural tube defects in the fetus if administered at the time of conception and in early pregnancy.

WARNING Monitor patient closely for hypersensitivity reactions that may include a severe rash or a rash accompanied by angioedema, conjunctivitis, difficulty breathing, eosinophilia, facial edema, fatigue, fever, general malaise, hepatitis, joint or muscle aches, oral blisters or lesions, and skin blisters or peeling. Report any such signs and symptoms to prescriber immediately. Expect liver enzymes to be checked, as ordered. Provide supportive care as ordered and expect dolutegravir therapy to be discontinued if hypersensitivity is thought to be drug induced, because a life-threatening reaction may occur if therapy is continued.

- Monitor patients with hepatitis B or C for development or worsening of elevated transaminase levels.
- Be aware that immune reconstitution syndrome has occurred in patients treated with combination antiretroviral therapy, including dolutegravir. The inflammatory response predisposes susceptible patients to opportunistic infections such as cytomegalovirus, *Mycobacterium avium* infection, *Pneumocystis jiroveci* pneumonia, or tuberculosis. Autoimmune disorders such as Graves' disease, Guillain–Barré syndrome, or polymyositis have also occurred. Report sudden or unusual adverse reactions to prescriber.
- Watch closely for suicidal tendencies, as dolutegravir may cause suicidal ideation.

PATIENT TEACHING

- Tell women of childbearing age that a pregnancy test will be done before dolutegravir therapy is begun, because drug can be toxic to the fetus if taken at time of conception and early in pregnancy. Warn patient to use effective contraceptive measures while taking drug. If pregnancy occurs during dolutegravir therapy, tell patient to contact prescriber immediately. If confirmed, encourage patient to register with the Antiretroviral Pregnancy Registry at 1-800-258-4263. Expect patient to be switched to a different drug during the first trimester of pregnancy.
- Inform patient that dolutegravir will be prescribed along with other antiviral drugs.

WARNING Review signs and symptoms of a hypersensitivity reaction with patient. Stress importance of reporting blistering or peeling of skin, difficulty breathing, facial swelling, feelings of fatigue, fever, joint or muscle aches, liver problems (dark urine, nausea, pale-colored stools, vomiting, or yellowing of skin or whites of eyes), rash, or any other unusual sign or symptoms immediately, as drug therapy may have to be discontinued to prevent a life-threatening reaction.

- Inform patient that dolutegravir therapy may cause changes in his body appearance because of fat redistribution. Prepare him for the possibility of developing breast enlargement, central obesity, dorsocervical fat enlargement (buffalo hump), facial wasting, and peripheral wasting.
- Instruct patient to report any persistent, severe, or unusual signs and symptoms.
- Warn family or caregiver to watch patient closely for evidence of suicidal behavior or thinking.
- Alert mothers that breastfeeding is not recommended during dolutegravir therapy, because drug is present in human breast milk.

donepezil hydrochloride

Aricept, Aricept ODT

Class and Category

Pharmacologic class: Acetylcholinesterase inhibitor
Therapeutic class: Antidementia
Pregnancy category: C

Indications and Dosages

➤ *To treat mild to moderate Alzheimer's disease*

ORAL SOLUTION, ORALLY DISINTEGRATING TABLETS, TABLETS

Adults. *Initial:* 5 mg at bedtime. After 4 to 6 wk, dosage increased to 10 mg at bedtime, as indicated. *Maximum:* 10 mg daily.

➤ *To treat moderate to severe Alzheimer's disease*

ORAL SOLUTION, ORALLY DISINTEGRATING TABLETS, TABLETS

Adults. *Initial:* 5 mg at bedtime. After 4 to 6 wk, dosage increased to 10 mg at bedtime, as indicated. Dosage may be further increased, as needed, after 3 months to 23 mg daily at bedtime if using tablet form. *Maximum:* 23 mg daily.

Mechanism of Action

Reversibly inhibits acetylcholinesterase and improves acetylcholine's concentration at cholinergic synapses. Raising acetylcholine level in the cerebral cortex may improve cognition. Donepezil becomes less effective as Alzheimer's disease progresses and number of intact cholinergic neurons declines.

Contraindications

Hypersensitivity to donepezil, piperidine derivatives, or their components

Interactions

DRUGS

anticholinergics: Possibly interference with activity of these drugs

cholinergic agonists, succinylcholine and similiar neuromuscular blockers: Possibly synergistic effects of these drugs

Adverse Reactions

CNS: Abnormal gait, agitation, aggression, anxiety, asthenia, confusion, depression, dizziness, dream disturbances, fatigue, fever, hallucinations, headache, hostility, insomnia, nervousness, **neuroleptic malignant syndrome**, **seizures**, somnolence, syncope, tremor

CV: Abnormal ECG, **AV block**, **bradycardia**, chest pain, edema, **heart failure**, hypertension, **hypotension**, **prolonged QT interval**, **torsades de pointes**

EENT: Pharyngitis

ENDO: Hyperglycemia

GI: Abdominal pain, anorexia, cholecystitis, constipation, diarrhea, dyspepsia, fecal incontinence, gastroenteritis, **hepatitis**, nausea, **pancreatitis**, vomiting

GU: Cystitis, glycosuria, hematuria, urinary frequency or incontinence, UTI

HEME: Anemia, **hemolytic hemorrhage**

MS: Arthralgia, back pain, elevated creatine kinase level, muscle cramps or spasms, **rhabdomyolysis**

RESP: Bronchitis, increased cough, pneumonia

SKIN: Ecchymosis, eczema, pruritus, rash, ulceration

Other: Angioedema, dehydration, elevated alkaline phosphatase or lactate dehydrogenase level, flu-like syndrome, **hyponatremia**, weight loss

D

Nursing Considerations

- Use donepezil cautiously in patients with bladder obstruction because drug's weak peripheral cholinergic effect could obstruct outflow.
- Use drug cautiously in patients with asthma, COPD, or other pulmonary disorders because it has weak affinity for peripheral cholinesterase, which may increase bronchoconstriction and bronchial secretions.
- Know that if patient has cardiac disease, monitor heart rate and rhythm for bradycardia, which may result from increased vagal tone caused by drug's inhibition of peripheral cholinesterase. Reduced heart rate may be especially significant if patient has bradycardia, sick sinus syndrome, or other supraventricular arrhythmia.
- Take safety precautions if patient is dizzy or has other adverse CNS reactions.

PATIENT TEACHING

- Advise patient to take donepezil only once per day just before going to bed.
- Inform her that drug may be taken with or without food.
- Tell patient prescribed oral disintegrating tablets not to swallow the tablet whole but to allow it to dissolve on the tongue and follow with a drink of water.
- Instruct patient to avoid hazardous activities, such as driving, until drug's CNS effects are known. Urge her to take safety precautions to prevent falling if she has adverse reactions, such as dizziness.

- Tell patient who has a history of gastric irritation or peptic ulcer disease that drug may aggravate these conditions by increasing gastric acid secretion.
- Advise women of childbearing age to notify prescriber if pregnancy is suspected or occurs.
- Alert patient that drug may cause decreased appetite, diarrhea, fatigue, insomnia, muscle cramps or spasms, nausea, or vomiting as some of the adverse reactions associated with drug use. Tell patient to notify prescriber if signs or symptoms are bothersome, persistent, or severe.

dopamine hydrochloride

Class and Category

Pharmacologic class: Adrenergic
Therapeutic class: Vasopressor
Pregnancy category: Not classified

Indications and Dosages

➤ *To correct hypotension that's unresponsive to adequate fluid volume replacement or occurs as part of shock syndrome caused by bacteremia, chronic cardiac decompensation, drug overdose, MI, open-heart surgery, renal failure, trauma, or other major systemic illnesses; to improve low cardiac output*

I.V. INFUSION

Adults. *Initial:* 2 to 5 mcg/kg/min, increased gradually, as needed. *Usual:* Less than 20 mcg/kg/min.

Adults who are more seriously ill. *Initial:* 5 mcg/kg/min, increased gradually by 5 to 10 mcg/kg/min up to a rate of 20 to 50 mcg/kg/min, as needed.

DOSAGE ADJUSTMENT Initial dosage reduced to 10% of usual amount if patient has taken MAO inhibitor in previous 2 to 3 wk.

Route	Onset	Peak	Duration
I.V.	In 5 min	Unknown	Up to 10 min

Mechanism of Action

Stimulates dopamine$_1$ (D_1) and dopamine$_2$ (D_2) postsynaptic receptors. D_1 receptors causing vasodilation in cerebral, coronary, mesenteric, and renal blood vessels. D_2 receptors inhibit norepinephrine release. In higher doses, dopamine also stimulates alpha$_1$ and alpha$_2$ receptors, causing vascular smooth-muscle contraction.

It also causes increased renal blood flow, improved GFR, and increased urine output. At doses of 2 to 10 mcg/kg/min, dopamine stimulates beta$_1$-adrenergic receptors, increasing cardiac output while maintaining dopaminergic-induced vasodilation. At doses of 10 mcg/kg/min or more, alpha-adrenergic agonism takes over, causing increased peripheral vascular resistance and renal vasoconstriction.

Incompatibilities

Don't add dopamine to 5% sodium bicarbonate, alkaline I.V. solutions, iron salts or oxidizing agents.

Contraindications

Hypersensitivity to dopamine or its components, pheochromocytoma, uncorrected ventricular fibrillation, ventricular tachycardia, and other tachyarrhythmias

Interactions

DRUGS

alpha blockers, haloperidol: Antagonized peripheral vasoconstriction with high doses of dopamine
anesthetics, such as chloroform, enflurane, halothane, isoflurane, and methoxyflurane: Increased risk of severe atrial and ventricular arrhythmias
beta blockers: Antagonized beta receptor–mediated inotropic effects of dopamine
cyclopropane, halogenated hydrocarbon anesthetics: Increased cardiac autonomic irritability with possible increased risk of severe arrhythmias
diuretics: Possibly increased diuretic effects of dopamine or diuretic
ergot alkaloids: Enhanced peripheral vasoconstriction
MAO inhibitors: Prolonged and intensified cardiac stimulation and vasopressor effect

oxytocic drugs, other vasopressors, vasoconstricting agents: Possibly severe hypertension
phenoxybenzamine: Possibly antagonized peripheral vasoconstriction of dopamine, causing hypotension and tachycardia
phenytoin: Possibly sudden bradycardia and hypotension
tricyclic antidepressants: Possibly potentiated pressor response to dopamine

Adverse Reactions

CNS: Anxiety, headache
CV: Angina, **atrial fibrillation**, **bradycardia**, **cardiac conduction abnormalities**, **ectopic beats**, hypertension, **hypotension**, palpitations, peripheral vasoconstriction, sinus tachycardia, **ventricular arrhythmias**, **widened QRS complex**
GI: Nausea, vomiting
GU: **Azotemia**
RESP: Dyspnea
SKIN: Extravasation with tissue necrosis, piloerection

Nursing Considerations

- Avoid, if possible, giving dopamine to patients with occlusive vascular disease, such as atherosclerosis, Buerger's disease, diabetic endarteritis, or Raynaud's disease, because of risk of decreased peripheral circulation. Also, be aware that high doses of dopamine given for a prolonged period of time increase the risk of decreased peripheral circulation and could lead to gangrene in the patient's extremities.
- Use drug cautiously in patients with cardiac disease, particularly coronary artery disease, because dopamine increases myocardial oxygen demand. Also use drug cautiously in patients allergic to sulfites, which are contained in some forms of dopamine.
- Inspect parenteral solution for particles and discoloration before administration.
- Know that, when using the Viaflex Plus plastic container, the overwrap is a moisture and oxygen barrier. Do not remove unit from overwrap until ready for use. Be aware that a sulfur dioxide odor may occur upon removal of drug from the overwrap container. This does not pose a risk to the patient. Visually inspect the container. If the administration port protector is damaged, detached, or not present, discard container, because solution path sterility may be impaired.
- Dilute dopamine concentrate with a compatible I.V. solution before administering. Typical dilution is 400 mg in 250 ml to yield 1.6 mg/ml. Don't exceed 3.2 mg/ml.
- Ensure adequate fluid resuscitation before giving drug.
- Give drug by I.V. infusion using an infusion pump.

WARNING Know that when infusion rate exceeds 20 mcg/kg/min, monitor patient for excessive vasoconstriction and loss of renal vasodilating effects.

- Administer infusion through a central catheter to avoid extravasation and tissue necrosis. If drug must be given via peripheral line, inspect site often for signs of extravasation and necrosis. If such signs are detected, start a new I.V. line for dopamine infusion, discontinue previous I.V. line, and notify prescriber immediately.
- Expect to give 5 to 10 mg phentolamine diluted in 10 to 15 ml normal saline solution, as prescribed, if drug extravasates. Phentolamine infiltrates directly into area to antagonize vasoconstriction and minimize sloughing and tissue necrosis.
- Titrate dopamine gradually to minimize hypotension, especially after a high infusion rate.
- Monitor blood pressure continuously with an intra-arterial line, as indicated.
- Place patient on continuous ECG monitoring, and assess heart rate and rhythm for arrhythmias.
- Monitor patient's hemodynamic parameters, such as cardiac output, central venous pressure, and pulmonary artery wedge pressure, as indicated, to assess effectiveness of dopamine therapy.
- Monitor urine output hourly as appropriate to assess patient for improved renal blood flow.

PATIENT TEACHING

- Explain the need for frequent hemodynamic monitoring.

doravirine

Pifeltro

Class and Category

Pharmacologic class: Non-nucleoside reverse transcriptase inhibitor (NRTI)
Therapeutic class: Antiretroviral
Pregnancy category: Not classified

Indications and Dosages

➤ *As adjunct to treat human immunodeficiency virus (HIV-1) infection in patients with no prior antiretroviral treatment history*

TABLETS

Adults. 100 mg once daily.

DOSAGE ADJUSTMENT For patient taking rifabutin concomitantly, dosage increased to 100 mg twice daily and given about 12 hours apart.

Mechanism of Action

Inhibits HIV-1 replication by noncompetitive inhibition of HIV-1 reverse transcriptase.

Contraindications

Co-administration with carbamazepine, enzalutamide, mitotane, oxcarbazepine, phenobarbital, phenytoin, rifampin, rifapentine, or St. John's wort; hypersensitivity to doravirine or its components

Interactions

DRUGS

CYP3A inducers such as carbamazepine, efavirenz, etravirine, enzalutamide, mitotane, nevirapine, oxcarbazepine, phenobarbital, phenytoin, rifabutin, rifampin, rifapentine, St. John's wort: Possibly decreased concentration of doravirine with decreased effectiveness
CYP3A inhibitors: Possibly increased concentration of doravirine, increasing risk of adverse reactions

Adverse Reactions

CNS: Abnormal dreams, depression, dizziness, fatigue, headache, insomnia, somnolence, **suicidal ideation**
CV: Elevated lipid levels
GI: Abdominal pain, diarrhea, elevated lipase and liver enzymes, nausea
GU: Elevated bilirubin and creatinine levels
MS: Elevated creatine kinase level
SKIN: Rash
Other: Elevated alkaline phosphatase, immune reconstitution syndrome

Nursing Considerations

- Obtain cholesterol and triglyceride levels before doravirine therapy is begun and periodically throughout therapy, because drug may cause an increase in lipid levels.
- Monitor patient's mood and emotional status, as doravirine may cause significant depression, mood changes, and suicidal ideation. Report any changes to prescriber.
- Be aware that immune reconstitution syndrome has occurred in patients treated with combination antiretroviral therapy, including doravirine. The inflammatory response predisposes susceptible patients to opportunistic infections such as cytomegalovirus, *Mycobacterium avium* infection, *Pneumocystis jiroveci* pneumonia, or tuberculosis. Autoimmune disorders such as Graves' disease, Guillain–Barré syndrome, or polymyositis have also occurred. Report sudden or unusual adverse reactions to prescriber.

PATIENT TEACHING

- Advise patient to avoid missing doses of doravirine. If she misses a dose, she should take it as soon as she remembers, but should not double the next dose or take more than prescribed.
- Instruct patient to alert prescriber of all medications taken, including over-the-counter products and any newly prescribed medication from other prescribers.
- Encourage women of childbearing age to report known or suspected pregnancy. If pregnancy occurs, encourage patient to enroll in the pregnancy exposure registry by calling 1-800-258-4263.
- Alert mothers that breastfeeding is not recommended during doravirine therapy.
- Instruct patient to report any persistent, severe, or unusual signs and symptoms.
- Tell patient or caregiver to report any signs of depression, mood changes, sleep disorders, or suicidal thoughts to prescriber.

doripenem

Doribax

Class and Category

Pharmacologic class: Carbapenem
Therapeutic class: Antibiotic
Pregnancy category: B

Indications and Dosages

➤ *To treat complicated intra-abdominal infections caused by* Bacteroides caccae, B. fragilis, B. thetaiotaomicron, B. uniformis, B. vulgatus, Escherichia coli, Klebsiella pneumoniae, Peptostreptococcus micros, Pseudomonas, aeruginosa, Streptococcus constellatus, *or* S. intermedius *and complicated UTIs, including pyelonephritis caused by* Acinetobacter baumannii, E. coli, K. pneumoniae, Proteus mirabilis, *or* P. aeruginosa

I.V. INFUSION

Adults. 500 mg infused over 1 hr every 8 hr for 5 to 14 days for complicated intra-abdominal infection and 10 days (possibly up to 14 days) for complicated UTI, including pyelonephritis. May switch to oral therapy if improvement after 3 days.

DOSAGE ADJUSTMENT For patients with impaired renal function or creatinine clearance of 30 to 50 ml/min, dosage reduced to 250 mg infused over 1 hr every 8 hr. For creatinine clearance of 10 to 30 ml/min, dosage reduced to 250 mg infused over 1 hr every 12 hr.

Route	Onset	Peak	Duration
I.V.	Unknown	1 hr	8 hr

Mechanism of Action

Inhibits cell wall synthesis in susceptible bacteria. Doripenem inactivates multiple penicillin-binding proteins essential in cell wall synthesis to cause cell death.

Incompatibilities

Don't mix doripenem with other drugs or add to solutions containing other drugs because of potential for incompatibility.

Contraindications

History of anaphylactic reactions to beta-lactams; hypersensitivity to doripenem, its components or other carbapenems

Interactions

DRUGS

divalproex sodium, valproic acid: Decreased effectiveness of valproic acid with possible loss of seizure control
probenecid: Increased plasma concentrations of doripenem

Adverse Reactions

CNS: Headache, seizures
CV: Phlebitis
EENT: Oral candidiasis
GI: Diarrhea, elevated liver enzyme, nausea
GU: Renal failure or impairment, vaginitis
HEME: Leukopenia, neutropenia, thrombocytopenia
RESP: Interstitial pneumonia
SKIN: Dermatitis, erythema, **erythema multiforme**, macular or papular eruptions, pruritus, rash, **Stevens–Johnson syndrome**, **toxic epidermal necrolysis**, urticaria
Other: Anaphylaxis

Nursing Considerations

- Use cautiously in patients with a history of hypersensitivity to cephalosporins or penicillins because cross-sensitivity may occur.
- Constitute vial with 10 ml sterile water for injection or normal saline solution, and gently shake to form a suspension. Withdraw suspension using a syringe with a 21G needle and add it to an infusion bag containing 100 ml normal saline solution or 5% dextrose. Gently shake until clear. If administering reduced dosage of 250 mg, remove 55 ml of prepared solution from infusion bag and discard before infusion.
- Be aware that upon constitution, suspension in the vial must be diluted within 1 hour. Once drug is diluted in infusion solution, drug stored at room temperature must be used within 8 hours if mixed in normal saline solution and within 4 hours if mixed in 5% dextrose. If infusion solution is refrigerated, it must be used within 24 hours or discarded.

- Monitor patient closely for evidence of hypersensitivity, especially if patient has multiple allergies, because serious and occasionally fatal hypersensitivity reactions have occurred in patients receiving beta-lactam antibiotics. If an allergic reaction occurs, discontinue drug immediately, notify prescriber, and expect to administer emergency treatment as ordered, and provide airway management.
- Assess patient's bowel pattern daily; severe diarrhea may be caused by *Clostridium difficile.* If suspected, expect to stop drug and provide treatment as prescribed.

PATIENT TEACHING

- Instruct patient to report any evidence of allergic reaction, such as hives, itching, rash, or trouble breathing.
- Advise patient to report diarrhea if severe or persistent.

doxazosin mesylate

Apo-Doxazosin (CAN), Cardura, Cardura XL

Class and Category

Pharmacologic class: Alpha blocker
Therapeutic class: Antihypertensive, benign prostatic hyperplasia therapeutic agent
Pregnancy category: Not classified

Indications and Dosages

➤ *To manage hypertension*

TABLETS

Adults. *Initial:* 1 mg daily. Doubled every 1 to 2 wk, if needed to achieve desired blood pressure. *Maximum:* 16 mg daily.

➤ *To treat benign prostatic hyperplasia (BPH)*

TABLETS

Adults. *Initial:* 1 mg daily. Doubled every 1 to 2 wk, if needed, based on signs and symptoms. *Maximum:* 8 mg daily

E.R. TABLETS

Adults. *Initial:* 4 mg daily, increased to 8 mg after 3 to 4 wk, as needed.

Route	Onset	Peak	Duration
P.O.	1–2 hr*	2–6 hr†	24 hr†

* For hypertension; in 2 wk for BPH.
† For hypertension; unknown for BPH.

Mechanism of Action

Competitively inhibits $alpha_1$-adrenergic receptors in the sympathetic nervous system, causing peripheral vasodilation and reduced peripheral vascular resistance. This action decreases blood pressure, especially when the patient stands. Doxazosin also relaxes smooth muscle of the bladder neck, prostate, and prostate capsule, which reduces urethral resistance and pressure and urinary outflow resistance.

Contraindications

Hypersensitivity to doxazosin, prazosin, terazosin, or their components

Interactions

DRUGS

antihypertensives, diuretics, phosphodiesterase-5 inhibitors, strong CYP3A4 inhibitors: Enhanced hypotensive effects

Adverse Reactions

CNS: Dizziness, drowsiness, headache, nervousness, restlessness, vertigo
CV: Arrhythmias, first-dose orthostatic hypotension, palpitations, peripheral edema, sinus tachycardia
EENT: Intraoperative floppy iris syndrome, rhinitis
GI: GI obstruction, nausea
GU: Priapism
RESP: Dyspnea

Nursing Considerations

- Know that drug should not be given to hypotensive patients.
- Be aware that Cardura XL is not for use in female patients and is not to be used to treat hypertension.
- Use doxazosin cautiously in patients with hepatic disease (because normal dosage may cause exaggerated effects)

and in elderly patients (because hypotensive response may be more pronounced).

WARNING Monitor patient for orthostatic hypotension (which may cause syncope) early in therapy, especially after exercise and in patients with hypovolemia.

- Monitor blood pressure for 2 to 6 hours after first dose and with each increase because orthostatic hypotension commonly occurs at this time. Adjust dose as prescribed, based on standing blood pressure.
- Carefully monitor patients with renal disease for exaggerated effects, such as first-dose orthostatic hypotension.
- Monitor urination, checking for difficulty urinating and urine retention, to assess drug's effects on BPH.

PATIENT TEACHING

- Inform patient that he may take doxazosin in the morning or evening and with food, if desired.
- Instruct patient to change position slowly to minimize orthostatic hypotension.
- Advise patient to avoid exercising, going outside in hot weather, standing for long periods, and using alcohol; these activities may worsen orthostatic hypotension.
- Advise patient to avoid hazardous activities until drug's CNS effects are known.
- Tell patient to inform surgeon that he is taking doxazosin therapy if cataract surgery is required because drug may cause intraoperative floppy iris syndrome with this procedure.
- Inform the patient taking drug for benign prostatic hyperplasia that he may become dizzy or faint if he takes an oral erectile dysfunction medicine during doxazosin therapy. Therefore, he should not use an oral erectile dysfunction medicine until he has discussed its use with the prescriber. Also alert him to the rare possibility of developing a painful penile erection caused by doxazosin therapy that could last for hours and requires immediate medical attention, if it occurs.

doxepin hydrochloride

Silenor

Class and Category

Pharmacologic class: Tricyclic antidepressant
Therapeutic class: Antidepressant
Pregnancy category: C

Indications and Dosages

➤ *To treat mild to moderate depression or anxiety*

CAPSULES, ORAL SOLUTION

Adults. 75 to 150 mg in divided doses daily or once daily at which could be bedtime. *Maximum:* 150 mg daily.

➤ *To treat mild to moderate depression or anxiety with organic disease*

CAPSULES, ORAL SOLUTION

Adults. 25 to 50 mg daily in divided doses daily or once daily and could be at bedtime. *Maximum:* 150 mg daily.

➤ *To treat severe depression or anxiety*

CAPSULES, ORAL SOLUTION

Adults. 50 mg three times daily, gradually increased to 300 mg daily, as needed. *Maximum:* 300 mg daily.

➤ *To treat insomnia characterized by difficulty with sleep maintenance*

TABLET (SILENOR)

Adults. 3 to 6 mg within 30 min of bedtime. *Maximum:* 6 mg daily.

DOSAGE ADJUSTMENT For elderly patients age 65 and over taking Silenor, dosage reduced to 3 mg within 30 min of bedtime but may be increased to 6 mg daily, as needed.

Route	Onset	Peak	Duration
P.O.	2–3 wk	Unknown	Unknown

Mechanism of Action

May block norepinephrine and serotonin reuptake by adrenergic nerves. In this way, the tricyclic antidepressant raises norepinephrine and serotonin levels at nerve synapses, which may elevate mood and reduce depression. It is unknown how doxepin maintains sleep, but is thought to be due to its antagonism of the H1 receptor.

Incompatibilities

Don't mix doxepin solution with carbonated beverages or grape juice.

Contraindications

Hypersensitivity to doxepin, other tricyclic antidepressants, or their components; severe urinary retention; untreated narrow-angle glaucoma; use of MAO inhibitor within 14 days

Interactions

DRUGS

cimetidine, flecainide, other tricyclic antidepressants, phenothiazines, propafenone, quinidine, selective serotonin reuptake inhibitors: Increased blood doxepin level from inhibited systemic clearance, resulting in increased risk of toxicity
CNS depressants, sedating antihistamines: Possibly potentiated CNS depression, hypotension, and respiratory depression
MAO inhibitors: Possibly hyperpyrexia, hypertension, seizures, and death
tolazamide: Possibly severe hypoglycemia

ACTIVITIES

alcohol use: Possibly enhanced CNS depression, hypotension, and respiratory depression

Adverse Reactions

CNS: Confusion, delirium, dream disturbances, drowsiness, fatigue, hallucinations, headache, nervousness, Parkinsonism, restlessness, sedation, **seizures, suicidal ideation (especially teens)**, tremor
CV: **ECG changes**, orthostatic hypotension, palpitations
EENT: Blurred vision, dry mouth, taste perversion
ENDO: Hyperglycemia, **hypoglycemia**
GI: Constipation, diarrhea, heartburn, ileus, increased appetite, jaundice, nausea, vomiting,
GU: Decreased libido, ejaculation disorders
SKIN: Diaphoresis
Other: Weight gain

Nursing Considerations

- Mix oral solution in 120 ml of juice such as grapefruit, orange, pineapple, or tomato; milk; or water, if desired.
- Expect to observe adverse reactions within a few hours after giving drug.
- Evaluate patient for therapeutic response, such as decreased anxiety, apprehension, depression, fear, guilt, somatic symptoms, and worry; increased energy; and more restful sleep.

WARNING **Monitor patients, especially young adults, closely for evidence of suicidal thinking and behavior because doxepin increases the risk in this group of suicidal thinking.**

- Keep in mind that abrupt withdrawal of doxepin after prolonged therapy can cause cholinergic rebound effects, including diarrhea, nausea, and vomiting.
- Plan to discontinue drug, as prescribed, several days before elective surgery to avoid hypertension.
- Monitor elderly patients for Parkinsonism, especially with high-dose therapy.
- Be alert for seizures. Patients with seizure disorder may need increased anticonvulsant dosage to maintain seizure control.
- Know that for patients with asthma or sulfite sensitivity, doxepin tablets may aggravate asthma or cause allergic reactions because they contain sulfites.
- Follow diabetic patient's serum glucose level closely; drug may alter glucose metabolism.

PATIENT TEACHING

WARNING **Alert parents of young adults to watch them closely for abnormal thinking or behavior and increased aggression or hostility. Emphasize importance of notifying prescriber about unusual changes.**

- Instruct patient to avoid alcohol during doxepin therapy because mental alertness may decrease.
- Advise diabetic patient to measure serum glucose level more often than usual.

doxycycline

Oracea

doxycycline calcium

(contains 50 mg of base per 5 ml of oral suspension)
Vibramycin

doxycycline hyclate

(contains 50 or 100 mg of base per capsule, 100 mg of base per delayed-release capsule, 100 mg of base per tablet, and 100 or 200 mg of base per injection vial)
Acticlate, Alti-Doxycycline (CAN), Apo-Doxy (CAN), Atridox, Doryx, Doryx MPC, Doxycin (CAN), Vibramycin

doxycycline monohydrate

(contains 50 or 100 mg of base per capsule and 25 mg of base per 5 ml of oral suspension)
Monodox

Class and Category

Pharmacologic class: Tetracycline
Therapeutic class: Antibiotic
Pregnancy category: D

➤ *To treat inhalation anthrax post exposure*

CAPSULES, ORAL SUSPENSION, SYRUP, TABLETS

Adults and children age 8 and over weighing 45 kg (99 lb) or more. 100 mg (120 mg Doryx MPC) twice daily for 60 days.
Children age 8 and over weighing less than 45 kg (99 lb). 2.2 mg/kg (2.6 mg/kg Doryx MPC) twice daily for 60 days.

➤ *To treat inflammatory lesions (papules and pustules) of rosacea*

E.R. CAPSULES (ORACEA)

Adults. 40 mg once daily in morning

➤ *To treat endocervical, rectal, and urethral infections caused by* Chlamydia trachomatis

CAPSULES, DELAYED-RELEASE TABLETS, ORAL SUSPENSION, SYRUP, TABLETS

Adults. 100 mg (120 mg Doryx MPC) twice daily for 7 days.

➤ *To treat uncomplicated gonococcal infections except anorectal infections in men*

CAPSULES, DELAYED-RELEASE TABLETS, ORAL SUSPENSION, SYRUP, TABLETS

Adults. 100 mg (120 mg Doryx MPC) twice a day for 7 days. Alternatively, 300 mg (360 mg Doryx MPC) followed in 1 hr by a second 300 mg (360 mg Doryx MPC) dose.

➤ *To treat epididymoorchitis caused by* C. trachomatis *or* Neisseria gonorrhoeae

CAPSULES, DELAYED-RELEASE TABLETS, ORAL SUSPENSION, SYRUP, TABLETS

Adults. 100 mg (120 mg Doryx MPC) twice daily for at least 10 days.

➤ *To prevent malaria*

CAPSULES, DELAYED-RELEASE TABLETS, ORAL SUSPENSION, SYRUP, TABLETS

Adults. 100 mg (120 mg Doryx MPC) daily starting 1 to 2 days before travel, continued daily during travel, and then daily for 4 wk after travel ends.
Children over age 8. 2 mg/kg (2.4 mg/kg Doryx MPC) daily starting 1 to 2 days before travel, continued daily during travel, and daily for 4 wk after travel ends.

➤ *To treat early syphilis in penicillin-allergic patients*

CAPSULES, DELAYED-RELEASE TABLETS, ORAL SUSPENSION, SYRUP, TABLETS

Adults. 100 mg (120 mg Doryx MPC) twice daily for 2 wk.

➤ *To treat syphilis of more than 1 year duration in penicillin-allergic patients*

CAPSULES, DELAYED-RELEASE TABLETS, ORAL SUSPENSION, SYRUP, TABLETS

Adults. 100 mg (120 mg Doryx MPC) twice daily for 4 wk.

➤ *To treat all other infections caused by susceptible organisms*

CAPSULES, DELAYED-RELEASE TABLETS, ORAL SUSPENSION, SYRUP, TABLETS

Adults and children over age 8 weighing 45 kg (99 lb) or more. 100 mg (120 mg Doryx MPC) every 12 hr on day 1 and then 100 mg (120 mg Doryx MPC) once daily or 50 mg (base) twice daily. For

severe infections, 100 mg continued every 12 hr.
Children over age 8 weighing less than 45 kg (99 lb). 2.2 mg/kg (2.6 mg/kg Doryx MPC) twice daily on day 1 and then 2.2 to 4.4 mg/kg (2.6 mg/kg Doryx MPC) once daily or 1.1 to 2.2 mg/kg (1.3 mg/kg Doryx MPC) twice daily.

I.V. INFUSION
Adults and children over age 8 weighing more than 45 kg. 200 mg once daily or 100 mg every 12 hr on day 1 and then 100 to 200 mg once daily or 50 to 100 mg every 12 hr. I.V. infused slowly over 1 hr.
Children weighing 45 kg (99 lb) or less. 4.4 mg/kg once daily or 2.2 mg/kg every 12 hr on day 1 and then 2.2 to 4.4 mg/kg once daily or 1.1 to 2.2 mg/kg every 12 hr. I.V. infused slowly over 1 hr.

Mechanism of Action

Exerts a bacteriostatic effect against a wide variety of gram-positive and gram-negative organisms. Doxycycline is more lipophilic than other tetracyclines, which allows it to pass more easily through the bacterial lipid bilayer, where it binds reversibly to 30S ribosomal subunits. Bound doxycycline blocks the binding of aminoacyl transfer RNA to messenger RNA, thus inhibiting bacterial protein synthesis.

Contraindications

Hypersensitivity to doxycycline, other tetracyclines, or their components

Interactions

DRUGS
antacids that contain aluminum, calcium, magnesium, or zinc; calcium supplements; choline and magnesium salicylates; laxatives that contain magnesium: Decreased doxycycline absorption and effects
barbiturates, carbamazepine, phenytoin: Increased clearance and decreased effects of doxycycline
methoxyflurane: Increased risk of severe renal toxicity
oral anticoagulants: Possibly increased hypoprothrombinemic effects of these drugs
oral contraceptives: Decreased effectiveness of estrogen-containing oral contraceptives, increased risk of breakthrough bleeding

Adverse Reactions

CNS: Headache, **intracranial hypertension**, paresthesia
CV: Pericarditis, phlebitis
EENT: Black "hairy" tongue, glossitis, hoarseness, oral candidiasis, pharyngitis, stomatitis, tooth discoloration, visual disturbances
GI: Anorexia; bulky, loose stools; diarrhea; dysphagia; enterocolitis; epigastric distress; esophageal ulceration; esophagitis; **hepatotoxicity**, inflammatory lesions in anogenital region; nausea; **pancreatitis**; **pseudomembranous colitis**; rectal candidiasis; vomiting
GU: Anogenital lesions, dark yellow or brown urine, elevated BUN level, vaginal candidiasis
HEME: Eosinophilia, **hemolytic anemia**, **neutropenia**, **thrombocytopenia**, **thrombocytopenic purpura**
SKIN: Dermatitis, **erythema multiforme**, erythematous and maculopapular rashes, **exfoliative dermatitis**, photosensitivity, rash, skin hyperpigmentation, **Stevens–Johnson syndrome**, **toxic epidermal necrolysis**, urticaria
Other: Anaphylaxis, **angioedema**, **drug reaction with eosinophilia and systemic symptoms (DRESS)**, exacerbation of systemic lupus erythematosus, injection-site phlebitis, Jarisch–Herxheimer (systemic inflammatory response) reaction in presence of spirochete infections, serum sickness

Nursing Considerations

- Avoid giving doxycycline to breastfeeding women because of the risk of enamel hypoplasia, inhibited linear skeletal growth, oral and vaginal candidiasis, photosensitivity reactions, and tooth discoloration in breastfeeding infant.
- Avoid giving drug to children age 8 and under, if possible; it may cause

discoloration and enamel hypoplasia of developing teeth that may be permanent.

- Be aware that Doryx and Doryx MPC are not interchangeable. Doryx 100 mg equals 120 mg of Doryx MPC.
- Use oral suspension cautiously in patients allergic to sulfites because it contains sodium metabisulfite.
- Expect to adjust dosage for patients who have hepatic disease to avoid drug accumulation.

WARNING Don't give doxycycline by I.M. or subcutaneous route.

- Give doxycycline without regard to meals. Food and milk may delay absorption, but they don't significantly reduce it.
- Observe patient often for injection-site phlebitis, a common adverse reaction to I.V. administration.
- Monitor liver function test results as appropriate to detect hepatotoxicity.
- Expect oral or parenteral doxycycline to increase risk of oral, rectal, or vaginal candidiasis—especially in debilitated or elderly patients and those on prolonged therapy—by changing the normal balance of microbial flora.

WARNING Monitor patient for signs and symptoms of intracranial hypertension, such as blurred vision, diplopia, headache, and vision loss; papilledema may be seen on fundoscopy. Patients at greater risk include women of childbearing age who are overweight or have a history of intracranial hypertension. If patient complains of visual changes, notify prescriber to obtain an immediate ophthalmologic evaluation because permanent visual loss can occur. Be aware that intracranial pressure may remain elevated for weeks after doxycycline therapy has been discontinued and warrants close follow-up.

- Monitor patient closely for diarrhea, which may indicate pseudomembranous colitis. If diarrhea occurs, notify prescriber and expect to withhold doxycycline. Expect to treat pseudomembranous colitis with electrolytes, fluids, protein, and an antibiotic effective against *Clostridium difficile.*
- Monitor patient for adverse skin reactions, because doxycycline has caused severe skin reactions that could be life-threatening. Notify prescriber as soon as possible if skin adverse reactions occur, provide supportive care, as ordered, and expect drug to be discontinued.

PATIENT TEACHING

- Instruct patient not to take doxycycline just before bed because it may not dissolve properly when she's recumbent and may cause esophageal burning and ulceration.
- Instruct patient taking doxycycline for rosacea to take the capsule in the morning on an empty stomach with a full glass of water. However, if gastric irritation occurs, tell patient to take with food.
- Advise patient to avoid antacids containing aluminum, calcium, or magnesium
- Instruct patient to drink plenty of fluids while taking doxycycline to reduce the risk of esophageal burning and ulceration.
- Inform patient that her urine may become dark yellow or brown during therapy.
- Urge patient to avoid sun exposure and ultraviolet light as much as possible during therapy and to use sunscreen or sunblock as needed. If patient develops phototoxicity, such as skin eruption, tell her to stop drug and notify prescriber.
- Tell patient to notify prescriber if skin adverse reactions occur, because reactions may become severe and drug may have to be discontinued.
- Advise patients who take an oral contraceptive to use an additional contraceptive method during therapy. Also advise all women of childbearing age to notify prescriber immediately if pregnancy occurs or is suspected, as drug may cause retardation of skeletal development in the fetus.
- Know that if patient is being treated for a sexually transmitted disease, her partner may need treatment as well.

- Tell patient to notify prescriber immediately about anorexia, epigastric distress, nausea, or vomiting as well as any visual changes during therapy.
- Urge patient to report bloody, watery stools to prescriber immediately, even up to 2 months after drug therapy has ended.
- Alert female patients that doxycycline may increase risk of vaginal candidiasis. Tell her to notify prescriber if she develops vaginal discharge or itching.
- Inform mothers wishing to breastfeed their infant during doxycycline therapy that it is not recommended because effects are unknown.

dronabinol
(delta-9-tetrahydro-cannabinol, THC)

Marinol, Syndros

Class, Category, and Schedule

Pharmacologic class: Cannabinoid
Therapeutic class: Antiemetic, appetite stimulant
Pregnancy category: Not classified
Controlled substance schedule: II (Syndros), III (Marinol)

Indications and Dosages

➤ *To prevent nausea and vomiting caused by chemotherapy and unresponsive to other antiemetics*

CAPSULES (MARINOL)

Adults. 5 mg/m^2 1 to 3 hr before chemotherapy on an empty stomach and then every 2 to 4 hr after chemotherapy for a total of 4 to 6 doses daily, increased by 2.5 g/m^2 increments, as needed. *Maximum:* 15 mg/m^2/dose or a total of 4 to 6 doses daily.

ORAL SOLUTION (SYNDROS)

Adults. 4.2 mg/m^2 1 to 3 hr before chemotherapy on an empty stomach and then every 2 to 4 hr after chemotherapy for a total of 4 to 6 doses daily, increased, as needed, in increments of 2.1 mg/m^2. *Maximum:* 12.6 mg/m^2 per dose for 4 to 6 doses daily.

DOSAGE ADJUSTMENT For elderly patients prescribed Marinol, initial dosage may be reduced to 2.5 mg/m^2 1 to 3 hr before chemotherapy to reduce CNS adverse reactions. For elderly patients prescribed Syndros and all patients who experience persistent or severe adverse reactions, dosage reduced to 2.1 mg/m^2 1 to 3 hr before chemotherapy.

➤ *To stimulate appetite in AIDS patients*

CAPSULES (MARINOL)

Adults. *Initial:* 2.5 mg twice daily 1 hr before lunch and dinner, increased as needed. *Maximum:* 10 mg daily in divided doses.

ORAL SOLUTION (SYNDROS)

Adults. 2.1 mg twice daily, 1 hr before lunch and 1 hr before dinner.

DOSAGE ADJUSTMENT Dosage for capsule form (Marinol) reduced to 2.5 mg before supper or at bedtime for the elderly and patients who can't tolerate 5 mg daily. Dosage maintained for oral solution form (Syndros) at 2.1 mg, but dosage frequency reduced to once daily 1 hr before dinner or bedtime in the elderly and patients who can't tolerate a twice-daily dosage.

Route	Onset	Peak	Duration
P.O.	Unknown	Unknown	24 hr or longer*

* For appetite stimulant effects; unknown for antiemetic effects.

Mechanism of Action

May exert antiemetic effect by inhibiting the vomiting control mechanism in the medulla oblongata. As the main psychoactive substance in marijuana (*Cannabis sativa* L.), dronabinol's effects may be mediated by cannabinoid receptors in neural tissues.

Contraindications

For Marinol: Hypersensitivity to dronabinol, its components, alcohol, cannabinoids, or sesame oil; *For Syndros:* Hypersensitivity reaction to dronabinol, its components, or alcohol; use of disulfiram- or metronidazole-containing products within past 14 days

Interactions

DRUGS

amitriptyline; amoxapine; amphetamines; antihistamines; atropine; desipramine; other anticholinergic, sympathomimetic, and tricyclic antidepressants; scopolamine: Possibly increased risk of hypertension, hypotension, tachycardia, and syncope
amphotericin B, cyclosporine, warfarin, other drugs highly bound to plasma proteins with a narrow therapeutic index: Possibly increased risk of adverse reactions associated with these drugs
apomorphine: Possibly potentiated CNS depression, possibly decreased emetic response with prior use of dronabinol
CNS stimulants (such as amphetamines), and CNS depressants (such as benzodiazepines): Additive CNS effects
CYP2C9 inhibitors such as amiodarone, fluconazole; CYP3A4 inhibitors such as clarithromycin, erythromycin, itraconazole, ketoconazole, ritonavir: Possibly increased dronabinol-related adverse reactions
disulfiram, metronidazole: Possible disulfiram-like reaction

ACTIVITIES

alcohol use: Additive CNS depressant effects

Adverse Reactions

CNS: Altered mental state, amnesia, asthenia, anxiety, ataxia, chills, cognitive impairment, confusion, delirium, delusions, depersonalization, depression, disorientation, dizziness, drowsiness, euphoria, exacerbation of mania or schizophrenia, fatigue, hallucinations, headache, insomnia, irritability, loss of consciousness, malaise, mood changes, movement disorder, nervousness, nightmares, panic attack, paranoid reaction, **seizures**, sleep disturbance, speech difficulties, somnolence, syncope
CV: Orthostatic hypotension, palpitations, sinus tachycardia, vasodilation
EENT: Lip swelling, oral lesions, rhinitis, sinusitis, throat tightness, tinnitus, vision difficulties
GI: Abdominal pain, anorexia, diarrhea, elevated liver enzymes, fecal incontinence, nausea, vomiting
MS: Myalgias
RESP: Cough
SKIN: Diaphoresis, disseminated rash, facial flushing, skin burning, urticaria
Other: Physical and psychological dependence

Nursing Considerations

WARNING Know that dronabinol shouldn't be discontinued abruptly; if it is, withdrawal syndrome may occur.

- Be aware that patients should be screened for depression, mania, and schizophrenia prior to treatment, because dronabinol can exacerbate these conditions. Use with extreme caution, if usage cannot be avoided, in these patients. Monitor patient for new or worsening psychiatric symptoms during therapy. Also know that concomitant use with other drugs associated with similar psychiatric effects should be avoided.
- Be aware that oral solution contains alcohol, which can produce disulfiram-like reactions when co-administered with disulfiram or other drugs that produce this reaction. Know that these products should be discontinued at least 14 days before starting oral solution form of dronabinol and not administered for at least 7 days after therapy with dronabinol has ceased.
- Use cautiously in patients with history of seizures because drug may lower seizure threshold. Notify prescriber of seizures immediately, and expect to stop drug.
- Be aware that patients with a history of substance abuse or dependence are at higher risk for abusing dronabinol. Assess patient's risk for abuse or misuse prior to dronabinol therapy and monitor patient throughout for evidence of abuse or misuse.
- Be aware that patients under age 45 may tolerate drug better than those over age 45.
- Be aware that liquid solution of dronabinol may be administered by a feeding tube that is silicone only and equal to or greater than a 14 French. Tubes consisting of polyurethane should not be used. Draw up the prescribed dose of drug using the calibrated dosing syringe packaged with drug. If dose is greater than 5 mg, divide the total dose into 2 or more portions using oral syringe. After administering drug via feeding tube, flush feeding tube

with 30 ml of water using a catheter-tip syringe.
- Anticipate higher risk of cardiovascular reactions, such as blood pressure changes (especially orthostatic hypotension) and increased heart rate, at higher doses and in patients with cardiac conditions. Monitor patient's vital signs closely, especially when drug is initiated or when dosage is increased.

WARNING Expect tolerance to drug to develop over time, especially if patient has smoked marijuana.

- Be aware that short-term, low-dose therapy doesn't typically lead to physical and psychological dependence, which may occur with long-term, high-dose therapy.
- Alert prescriber if patient experiences changes in mental state or cognitive impairment, because dosage will have to be reduced or drug discontinued. Know that elderly patients may be more sensitive to the neurological and psychoactive effects of dronabinol.
- Expect drug to alter REM sleep pattern, even after therapy stops.
- Be aware that oral solution contains alcohol, which can produce disulfiram-like reactions when co-administered with disulfiram or other drugs that produce this reaction. Know that these products should be discontinued at least 14 days before starting oral solution form of dronabinol and not administered for at least 7 days after therapy with dronabinol has ceased.
- Be aware that paradoxical abdominal pain, nausea, and vomiting can occur with chronic, long-term use of dronabinol.

PATIENT TEACHING

- Caution patient not to stop drug abruptly because withdrawal symptoms may occur.
- Instruct patient to take dronabinol with a full glass of water (6 to 8 ounces).
- Urge patient not to use alcohol while taking dronabinol because it may enhance CNS depression.
- Instruct patient to rise slowly to sitting or standing position to minimize effects of orthostatic hypotension.
- Advise patient to avoid hazardous activities until drug's CNS effects are known.
- Inform patient that sleep pattern may be adversely affected during therapy and for sometime afterward.
- Inform women of childbearing age to notify prescriber if pregnancy is known or suspected, because dronabinol may cause fetal harm. Also advise mothers not to breastfeed.
- Monitor elderly patients closely, especially if dementia is present, because they may be more sensitive to the neuropsychiatric and postural hypotensive effects of the drug and be at increased risk of falls.

dronedarone

Multaq

Class and Category

Pharmacologic class: Benzofuran derivative
Therapeutic class: Antiarrhythmic
Pregnancy category: X

Indications and Dosages

➤ *To reduce risk of hospitalization for atrial fibrillation in patients in sinus rhythm with a history of paroxysmal or persistent atrial fibrillation*

TABLETS

Adults. 400 mg twice daily, with morning and evening meals

Route	Onset	Peak	Duration
P.O.	Unknown	3–6 hr	Unknown

Mechanism of Action

Although specific effect on heart rhythm is unknown, dronedarone possesses properties of all four Vaughn–Williams antiarrhythmic classes.

Contraindications

Bradycardia less than 50 beats/minute; concurrent use of drugs or herbal products that prolong QT interval, such as class I and III antiarrhythmics, phenothiazine antipsychotics, oral macrolide antibiotics (selected), and tricyclic antidepressants or strong CYP3A inhibitors, such as clarithromycin, cyclosporine, ketoconazole, itraconazole, nefazodone, ritonavir, telithromycin, and voriconazole; hypersensitivity to dronedarone or its components; liver or lung toxicity related to previous use of amiodarone; nursing mothers; pregnancy; PR interval greater than 280 msec or QTc Bazett interval of 500 msec; permanent atrial fibrillation; second- or third-degree atrioventricular block or sick-sinus syndrome (except when used with a functioning pacemaker); severe hepatic impairment (Child-Pugh class C); symptomatic heart failure with recent decompensation requiring hospitalization or NYHA Class IV symptoms

Interactions

DRUGS

beta blockers: Increased risk of bradycardia
calcium channel blockers: Possibly increased dronedarone effects on conduction
calcium channel blockers, such as diltiazem, nifedipine, and verapamil; CYP3A substrates with narrow therapeutic range such as sirolimus and tacrolimus; CYP2D6 substrates, such as beta blockers, selective serotonin reuptake agents, and tricyclic antidepressant; statins, such as simvastatin: Increased effects of these drugs with possibly increased risk of adverse reactions
class I and III antiarrhythmics, macrolide antibiotics, phenothiazines, tricyclic antidepressants: Possibly increased QT interval
CYP3A inducers, such as carbamazepine, phenobarbital, phenytoin, rifampin, St. John's wort: Decreased dronedarone effects
CYP3A inhibitors, such as clarithromycin, cyclosporine, ketoconazole, itraconazole, nefazodone, ritonavir, telithromycin, and voriconazole: Increased dronedarone effects
digoxin and other P-gp substrates such as dabigatran: Increased effect of these drugs with risk of toxicity; increased risk of adverse GI reactions
warfarin: Possible increased risk of bleeding and INR

FOODS

grapefruit juice: Increased dronedarone effects

Adverse Reactions

CNS: Asthenia
CV: **Bradycardia, heart failure, prolonged QT interval**, vasculitis
GI: Abdominal pain, diarrhea, dyspepsia, **liver injury**, nausea, vomiting
GU: Increased serum creatinine levels
RESP: Dyspnea, **interstitial lung disease such as pneumonitis and pulmonary fibrosis**, nonproductive cough, **pulmonary toxicity**
SKIN: Allergic dermatitis, dermatitis, eczema, photosensitivity, pruritus, rash
Other: Anaphylaxis, angioedema, hypokalemia, hypomagnesemia

Nursing Considerations

- Check that patient has stopped taking any drug contraindicated with dronedarone, as prescribed, before giving first dose. Also check that patient is receiving appropriate antithrombotic therapy prior to giving first dose because patients are at increased risk for stroke, especially in the first 2 weeks of therapy. In addition, check patient's serum potassium and magnesium levels prior to initiating therapy and throughout therapy because of increased risk of deficiency and arrhythmias, especially if patient is also taking a potassium-depleting diuretic.
- Assess patient for evidence of heart failure, such as dependent edema, increasing shortness of breath, or weight gain. If present, notify prescriber; dronedarone may need to be discontinued.
- Review patient's electrocardiogram at least once every 3 months, as ordered to determine patient's rhythm. If atrial fibrillation is found, prepare patient for cardioversion, as ordered or expect dronedarone therapy to be discontinued. Monitor patient's PR and QT interval, as ordered, to see if conduction is delayed. If so, notify prescriber immediately. Dronedarone will have to be stopped.
- Monitor patient's serum creatinine levels, as ordered. Elevation may occur rapidly, plateau after 7 days, and usually is reversible after therapy stops.
- Monitor patient's liver function, as ordered, because severe liver injury may occur with dronedarone therapy. If liver enzymes become elevated or the patient develops symptoms of liver dysfunction such as anorexia, dark urine, fatigue, fever, itching, jaundice, malaise, nausea, right upper quadrant pain, or vomiting, notify prescriber and expect drug to be discontinued immediately.

- Monitor patient for dyspnea or nonproductive cough as possible development of pulmonary toxicity. If confirmed, expect drug to be discontinued.

PATIENT TEACHING

- Inform patient that dronedarone must be taken with a meal.
- Warn patient that dronedarone should not be taken with grapefruit juice.
- Urge patient to contact prescriber if he develops evidence of heart failure, such as dependent edema, increasing shortness of breath or weight gain, because dronedarone may need to be discontinued.
- Inform women of childbearing age of need for contraception if sexually active because drug is contraindicated during pregnancy and breastfeeding. If pregnancy occurs, she should notify prescriber immediately.
- Tell patient to inform all prescribers that she is taking dronedarone and to check with prescriber before taking any herbal product with dronedarone, newly prescribed drug, or OTC product.
- Review symptoms of liver dysfunction with patient and urge her to seek immediate medical attention, if present, and to stop taking dronedarone.

droxidopa

Northera

Class and Category

Pharmacologic class: Norepinephrine prodrug
Therapeutic class: Vasoconstrictor
Pregnancy category: Not classified

Indications and Dosages

➤ *To treat symptomatic neurogenic orthostatic hypotension caused by dopamine beta-hydroxylase deficiency, nondiabetic autonomic neuropathy, and primary autonomic failure seen in multiple-system atrophy, Parkinson's disease, and pure autonomic failure*

CAPSULES

Adults. *Initial:* 100 mg three times daily: upon arising in the morning, at midday, and in the late afternoon at least 3 hr before bedtime. Dosage then titrated to symptomatic response in increments of 100 mg three times daily every 24 to 48 hr to maximum dosage. *Maximum:* 600 mg three times daily.

Mechanism of Action

Produces peripheral arterial and venous vasoconstriction, which increases blood pressure.

Contraindications

Hypersensitivity to droxidopa or its components

Interactions

DRUGS

dopa-decarboxylase inhibitors: Possibly altered plasma droxidopa levels
ephedrine, midodrine, norepinephrine, triptans: Increased risk of supine hypertension
nonselective MAO inhibitors such as rasagiline, selegiline: Possibly increased blood pressure

Adverse Reactions

CNS: Agitation, confusion, **CVA**, delirium, dizziness, fatigue, fever, hallucination, headache, memory disorder, **neuroleptic malignant syndrome-like complex**, psychosis, syncope
CV: Chest pain, **exacerbation of arrhythmias, congestive heart failure, ischemic heart disease**, hypertension, supine hypertension
EENT: Blurred vision
GI: Abdominal pain, diarrhea, nausea, **pancreatitis**, vomiting
GU: UTI
RESP: **Bronchospasm**
SKIN: Rash, urticaria
Other: **Anaphylaxis**, **angioedema**, falls

Nursing Considerations

- Check supine blood pressure prior to initiating droxidopa and after increasing the dose to determine effectiveness and detect hypertension.

WARNING Elevate head of patient's bed when patient is resting or sleeping to minimize effects of supine hypertension, which droxidopa can cause or exacerbate. Monitor blood pressure in both the supine position and head-elevated sleeping position. Notify prescriber if supine hypertension occurs and expect dosage to be reduced or drug discontinued, because it can increase the risk of cardiovascular events, especially stroke.

- Know that, although rare, droxidopa may cause a symptom complex resembling neuroleptic malignant syndrome (NMS). Observe patients carefully when dosage is changed or when concomitant levodopa is reduced abruptly or discontinued, especially if patient is receiving neuroleptics. Monitor patient for signs and symptoms such as altered consciousness, fever, hyperthermia, involuntary movements, mental status changes, and muscle rigidity. Notify prescriber immediately; an early diagnosis is important because NMS can be life-threatening.

WARNING **Monitor patient for hypersensitivity reactions that may include anaphylaxis, angioedema, bronchospasm, rash, and urticaria. If present, withhold droxidopa, notify prescriber, provide emergency supportive care as ordered, and expect drug to be discontinued.**

- Be aware that droxidopa contains FD&C Yellow No. 5 (tartrazine), which may cause an allergic-type reaction such as bronchial asthma. Risk is higher in patients who also have an aspirin hypersensitivity.

PATIENT TEACHING

- Tell patient to take droxidopa three times a day: upon arising in the morning, at midday, and in the late afternoon at least 3 hours prior to bedtime to reduce the potential for supine hypotension during sleep.
- Instruct patient to swallow capsules whole. Advise her that if a dose is missed to wait and take the next scheduled dose. Tell her doses should never be doubled to make up for a missed dose.
- Advise patient to elevate the head of her bed when resting or sleeping to minimize effects of supine hypertension.
- Tell patient to inform prescriber of all new medications, including over-the-counter preparations, prior to taking them.

WARNING **Instruct patient to stop taking droxidopa and seek emergency medical attention if signs and symptoms of an allergic reaction occur, such as difficulty breathing, hives, rash, or swelling.**

- Inform mothers that they should not breastfeed while taking droxidopa.

dulaglutide

Trulicity

Class and Category

Pharmacologic class: Glucagon-like peptide-1 receptor agonist
Therapeutic class: Antidiabetic
Pregnancy category: Not classified

Indications and Dosages

➤ *Adjunct to diet and exercise to improve glycemic control in patients with type 2 diabetes mellitus*

SUBCUTANEOUS INJECTION

Adults. 0.75 mg once weekly, increased to 1.5 mg once weekly, as needed. *Maximum:* 1.5 mg once weekly.

Mechanism of Action

Activates the GLP-1 receptor to increase intracellular cyclic AMP (cAMP) in beta cells, causing a glucose-dependent insulin release. Insulin then lowers blood glucose levels. Dulaglutide also decreases glucagon secretion and slows gastric emptying to further decrease blood glucose levels.

Contraindications

Hypersensitivity to dulaglutide or its components, personal or family history of medullary thyroid carcinoma or multiple endocrine neoplasia syndrome type 2, preexisting severe gastrointestinal disease

Interactions

DRUGS

insulin, insulin secretagogues: Increased risk of hypoglycemia
orally administered drugs: Possibly decreased absorption of the orally administered drugs

Adverse Reactions

CNS: Asthenia, fatigue, malaise
CV: First-degree AV block, sinus tachycardia
ENDO: Hypoglycemia
GI: Abdominal distention or pain, constipation, diarrhea, dyspepsia, elevated

liver enzymes, flatulence, gastroesophageal reflux disease, nausea, **pancreatitis**, vomiting
GU: Acute renal failure, elevated creatinine level, **worsening chronic renal failure**
SKIN: Pruritus, rash, urticaria
Other: Angioedema, injection-site reactions such as erythema and rash

Nursing Considerations

- Know that dulaglutide should not be used as first-line therapy for patients who have inadequately controlled their blood glucose levels on diet and exercise alone.
- Use caution when beginning dulaglutide therapy or titrating dose in patients with renal impairment. Monitor renal function in these patients if they experience severe adverse gastrointestinal reactions. Also use cautiously in patients with hepatic impairment because the effect of dulaglutide therapy on the liver is unknown.
- Be aware that dulaglutide may potentially be linked to the development of thyroid C-cell tumors. While elevated serum calcitonin is a biological marker, its value in routine monitoring is unclear. If an elevated serum calcitonin level is found at any time during therapy, expect patient to be referred to an endocrinologist for further evaluation.
- Monitor patient for signs and symptoms of pancreatitis, such as persistent severe abdominal pain, sometimes radiating to the back, which may or may not be accompanied by vomiting. If confirmed, expect dulaglutide to be discontinued.
- Monitor patient also receiving insulin or insulin secretagogue therapy concomitantly for hypoglycemia. The dosage of insulin or insulin secretagogue may need to be lowered to reduce the risk of hypoglycemia. If hypoglycemia occurs, treat it according to policy and notify prescriber.
- Monitor patient for signs of hypersensitivity such as pruritus, rash, or urticaria. If present, withhold drug, notify prescriber. and expect drug to be discontinued.
- Monitor patient for signs of diarrhea, dehydration, nausea or vomiting, which may suggest renal impairment. If present, notify prescriber because the frequency of these gastrointestinal symptoms may increase as renal function declines.

PATIENT TEACHING

- Inform patient that drug may be administered at any time of day without regard to meals but that it should be administered on the same day each week. However, if the day of the week needs to be changed, that change may be made, as long as the last dose was administered 4 or more days earlier.
- Instruct patient that if a dose is missed and it is within 1 to 2 days of his next regularly scheduled dose, he should administer at the regularly scheduled time.
- Teach patient to administer the injection into the abdomen, thigh, or upper arm region. Instruct patient that if the same body region is being used each week, the sites of injection should be rotated within that region. Tell patient how to safely dispose of the used pen and needle.

WARNING Instruct patient to stop taking dulaglutide and seek immediate emergency care if any of the following allergic reactions occurs: difficulty breathing or swallowing; dizziness, fainting; feeling itching; rapid heartbeat; severe rash; or swelling of face, lips, tongue, or throat.

- Teach female patients to alert prescriber if pregnancy occurs or is suspected.
- Ensure that patient has been informed of the potential risk for developing thyroid tumors before starting dulaglutide therapy. Tell patient to report any symptoms of thyroid tumors such as a mass in the neck, difficulty swallowing or breathing, or persistent hoarseness.
- Instruct patient on the signs and symptoms of hypoglycemia and how to treat it. Inform patient who is also receiving an insulin secretagogue or insulin that the risk of hypoglycemia is greater. Tell patient to notify prescriber if hypoglycemia occurs frequently or is severe.
- Tell patient to notify prescriber if any orally administered drugs appear to be losing their effectiveness, as dulaglutide causes a delay of gastric emptying and has the potential to affect the absorption of drugs taken by mouth. Also tell prescriber about any new prescribed medication or over-the-counter preparation before using.

duloxetine hydrochloride

Cymbalta

Class and Category

Pharmacologic class: Selective serotonin and norepinephrine reuptake inhibitor
Therapeutic: Antidepressant, neuropathic and musculoskeletal pain reliever
Pregnancy category: C

Indications and Dosages

➤ *To treat major depressive disorder*

E.R. CAPSULES

Adults. 20 mg twice daily. Alternatively, 60 mg once daily or 30 mg twice daily.

➤ *To relieve neuropathic pain associated with diabetic peripheral neuropathy*

DOSAGE ADJUSTMENT For patients with renal disease, initial dosage may be lower and increased more gradually as needed.

E.R. CAPSULES

Adults. 60 mg daily.

➤ *To treat generalized anxiety disorder*

E.R. CAPSULES

Adults. *Initial:* 30 or 60 mg once daily, increased in 30-mg increments weekly, as needed. *Maximum:* 120 mg once daily.
Children age 7 to 17 years of age. *Initial*: 30 mg once daily for 2 wk, then increased in 30-mg increments weekly, as needed. *Maximum*: 120 mg daily.

DOSAGE ADJUSTMENT For elderly patients, dosage initiated at 30 mg once daily for 2 weeks, before dosage increased to 60 mg once daily. Further increases in dosage made in 30-mg increments weekly, as needed, to maximum dosage of 120 mg once daily.

➤ *To treat fibromyalgia; to treat chronic musculoskeletal pain*

E.R. CAPSULES

Adults. *Initial:* 30 mg daily for 1 wk; then increased to 60 mg daily.

Route	Onset	Peak	Duration
P.O.	Unknown	6 hr	Unknown

Mechanism of Action

Inhibits dopamine, neuronal serotonin, and norepinephrine reuptake to potentiate noradrengeric and serotonergic activity in the CNS. These activities may elevate mood and inhibit pain signals stemming from peripheral nerves adversely affected by chronically elevated serum glucose level.

Contraindications

Chronic liver disease including cirrhosis, hypersensitivity to duloxetine or its components severe renal impairment (glomerular filtration rate less than 30 ml/min)

D

Interactions

DRUGS

aspirin, NSAIDs, warfarin: Possibly increased risk of bleeding
cimetidine, fluoxetine, fluvoxamine, paroxetine, quinidine, quinolones: Increased blood duloxetine level
CNS drugs: Increased effect of duloxetine
linezolid, methylene blue (I.V.), serotonergic drugs: Increased risk of serotonin syndrome
MAO inhibitors: Serious, sometimes fatal, autonomic instability, hyperthermia, myoclonus, rigidity
plasma protein binders (phenytoin, warfarin): Increased free concentration of these drugs and increased risk of adverse reactions

ACTIVITIES

alcohol use: Increased risk of hepatotoxicity

Adverse Reactions

CNS: Abnormal dreams, aggression, agitation, anger, anxiety, asthenia, chills, dizziness, extrapyramidal disorder, fatigue, fever, hallucinations, headache, insomnia, migraine, nervousness, **neuroleptic malignant syndrome**, parasthesia, restless legs syndrome, **seizures**, **serotonin syndrome**, somnolence, **suicidal ideation**, syncope, tremor, vertigo
CV: Hypertension, **hypertensive crisis**, **MI**, orthostatic hypotension, palpitations, paresthesia, peripheral edema or coldness, **supraventricular arrhythmia**, tachycardia, **Takotsubo cardiomyopathy**
EENT: Acute-angle glaucoma, blurred vision, dry mouth, glaucoma, nasopharyngitis, pharyngitis, taste alteration, tinnitus

ENDO: Galactorrhea, hot flashes, hyperglycemia, hyperprolactinemia
GI: **Acute pancreatitis**, abdominal pain, anorexia, cholestatic jaundice, colitis, constipation, diarrhea, elevated liver enzymes, flatulence, **hepatitis**, **hepatotoxicity**, indigestion, jaundice, nausea, upper abdominal pain, vomiting
GU: Abnormal orgasm; decreased libido; erectile or ejaculatory dysfunction; **gynecological bleeding**; urinary frequency, hesitancy, or retention; UTI
HEME: **Bleeding episodes**, **leukopenia**, **thrombocytopenia**
MS: Arthralgia, back pain, extremity pain, muscle cramp or spasm, myalgia
RESP: Cough, upper respiratory tract infection
SKIN: Cutaneous vasculitis, diaphoresis, **erythema multiforme**, pruritus, rash, **Stevens–Johnson syndrome**, urticaria
Other: **Anaphylaxis**, **angioedema**, **hyponatremia**, weight loss

Nursing Considerations

- Know that duloxetine should not be given to patients with severe renal impairment or end-stage renal disease that requires hemodialysis because blood drug levels increase significantly in these patients. Also know that duloxetine should be avoided in patients with hepatic insufficiency or who use alcohol excessively because drug is metabolized by the liver.
- Use duloxetine cautiously in patients with delayed gastric emptying because drug's enteric coating resists dissolution until it reaches an area where pH exceeds 5.5.
- Give duloxetine cautiously to patients with a history of mania, which it may activate. Also give cautiously to patients with a seizure disorder because drug effects aren't known in these patients.
- Obtain patient's baseline blood pressure before duloxetine therapy starts, and assess it periodically thereafter for changes. If orthostatic hypotension occurs during therapy, notify prescriber and anticipate that drug may need to be discontinued.
- Monitor patient's serum sodium level, as ordered, especially if patient is elderly, is taking a diuretic, or has volume depletion, because drug may lower serum sodium level.
- Monitor patient's hepatic function, as ordered, because drug may increase the risk of hepatotoxicity. Expect to discontinue duloxetine, as ordered, if patient develops jaundice or other serious liver dysfunction manifestation.
- Watch closely for evidence of suicidal thinking or behavior, especially when therapy starts or dosage changes.
- Avoid stopping duloxetine therapy abruptly, if possible, because withdrawal symptoms such as anxiety, diarrhea, dizziness, fatigue, headache, hyperhidrosis, insomnia, irritability, nausea, nightmares, paresthesia, vertigo, and vomiting, may occur. Taper dosage gradually, as ordered.

WARNING **Monitor patient for serotonin syndrome, characterized by agitation, chills, confusion, diaphoresis, diarrhea, fever, hyperactive reflexes, poor coordination, restlessness, shaking, talking or acting with uncontrolled excitement, tremor, and twitching. In its most severe form, serotonin syndrome can resemble neuroleptic malignant syndrome, which includes autonomic instability with possible fluctuations in vital signs, high fever, mental status changes, and muscle rigidity.**

WARNING **Know that treatment with linezolid or I.V. methylene blue is not recommended while patient is taking duloxetine because of increased risk of serotonin syndrome. However, if prescriber feels benefits outweigh the risks, expect duloxetine to be discontinued promptly if serotonin syndrome occurs. Monitor patient closely for serotonin syndrome for 5 days or until 24 hours after the last dose of linezolid or I.V. methylene blue, whichever comes first. Know that therapy with duloxetine may be resumed 24 hours after the last dose of linezolid or I.V. methylene blue.**

PATIENT TEACHING

- Tell patient to take capsule whole and not to chew it, crush it, or sprinkle contents on food or liquids, because doing so alters enteric coating and may affect drug absorption.
- Inform patient that full effect of duloxetine may take weeks to occur; emphasize the importance of continuing to take the drug as directed.

- Caution patient against excessive alcohol consumption while taking duloxetine because it may increase risk of hepatic dysfunction. Also tell him to report a yellowing of skin immediately, as drug may have to be discontinued.
- Advise patient not to stop duloxetine abruptly because adverse reactions may occur. Explain that drug will be stopped gradually.
- Instruct patient to notify prescriber if any serious or troublesome adverse effects develop, especially if they are persistent, severe, or unusual.
- Advise patient to avoid hazardous activities until drug's CNS effects are known.
- Advise patient that drug may cause mild pupillary dilation, which may lead to an episode of acute-angle glaucoma. Encourage him to have an eye exam before starting therapy to see if he is at risk.
- Instruct patient to rise from a lying or sitting position slowly to minimize drug's effect on lowering blood pressure, which may possibly lead to falls or cause patient to faint.
- Urge caregivers to watch closely for evidence of suicidal tendencies, especially when therapy starts or dosage changes.
- Instruct female patients of childbearing age to notify prescriber if they are, could be, or wish to become pregnant; duloxetine therapy may cause adverse reactions in neonates exposed to it during the third trimester. If patient becomes pregnant while taking duloxetine, urge her to enroll in the Pregnancy Registry by calling 1-866-814-6975 or visiting www.cymbaltapregnancyregistry.com.
- Tell patient to stop taking duloxetine and notify prescriber immediately at the first sign of blisters, mucosal erosions, peeling rash, or any other sign of hypersensitivity, as drug will need to be discontinued.
- Advise patient that drug may cause mild pupillary dilation, which may lead to an episode of acute-angle glaucoma. Encourage him to have an eye exam before starting therapy to see if he is at risk.
- Instruct patient with diabetes to monitor his blood glucose levels more closely, as duloxetine therapy can alter control.
- Tell patient to notify prescriber of any new medication, including over-the-counter preparations, before using.

dupilumab

Dupixent

Class and Category

Pharmacologic class: Monoclonal antibody
Therapeutic class: Antidermatitis agent
Pregnancy category: Not classified

Indications and Dosages

➤ *To treat moderate-to-severe atopic dermatitis when disease is not adequately controlled with topical prescription therapies or when those therapies are not advisable*

SUBCUTANEOUS INJECTION

Adults. Initial: 600 mg (given as two 300-mg injections), followed by 300 mg every other wk.

➤ *As add-on maintenance treatment of moderate to severe asthma*

SUBCUTANEOUS INJECTION

Adults and children age 12 and over with an eosinophilic phenotype. 400 mg (two 200-mg injections) followed by 200 mg every other wk. Alternatively, 600 mg (two 300-mg injections) followed by 300 mg every other wk.

Adults and children age 12 and over who are oral corticosteroids-dependent or also have co-morbid moderate to severe atopic dermatitis. 600 mg followed by 300 mg every other wk.

Mechanism of Action

Inhibits signaling from Type I and Type II receptors, which inhibits interleukin-4 and interleukin-13 cytokine-induced responses, including the release of proinflammatory cytokines, chemokines, and IgE.

Contraindications

Hypersensitivity to dupilumab or its components

Interactions

DRUGS

CYP450 enzymes: Altered plasma concentrations of CYP450 enzymes
live vaccines: Decreased effectiveness

Adverse Reactions

EENT: Blepharitis, conjunctivitis, dry eye, eye pruritus, keratitis, oral herpes, oropharyngeal pain
GU: Genital herpes
HEME: Eosinophilia
SKIN: Atopic or exfoliative dermatitis, erythema nodosum, rash, urticaria
Other: Anaphylaxis, anti-dupilumab antibodies, herpes simplex virus infections, injection-site reactions, serum sickness

Nursing Considerations

- Expect to treat patients with preexisting helminth infections before dupilumab therapy is begun, because drug's effect on the immune system's response against helminth infections is unknown. If patient becomes infected while receiving dupilumab therapy and does not respond to the anti-helminth treatment, expect dupilumab to be discontinued until infection is resolved.
- Remove prefilled syringe from refrigerator and allow it to warm to room temperature, which will take about 45 minutes for the 300-mg syringe and 30 minutes for the 200-mg syringe, before administering drug. Know that the solution should be clear to slightly opalescent, colorless to pale yellow.
- Inject the initial two 300-mg injections at two different sites such as the abdomen (except for the 2 inches around the navel), thigh, or upper arm. Rotate injection sites with each subsequent injection.
- Monitor patient for hypersensitivity reactions. If noted, notify prescriber, provide supportive care, and expect dupilumab to be discontinued.
- Know that corticosteroid therapy should not be discontinued abruptly when dupilumab therapy is initiated, but instead should be discontinued gradually.

PATIENT TEACHING

- Instruct patient on how to administer a subcutaneous injection and how to properly dispose of needle and syringe after use.
- Tell patient injection may be given in the abdomen, except for the 2 inches around the navel; thigh; or if caregiver is giving injections, upper arm. The site should be rotated with each injection. Warn patient not to inject dupilumab into skin that is bruised, damaged, scarred, or tender.
- Instruct patient to remove the prefilled syringe from the refrigerator and allow it to reach room temperature (which takes about 45 minutes for 300-mg syringe and 30 minutes for 200-mg syringe) and not to remove the needle cap while drug is warming. After inspecting the solution in the syringe, which should be clear to slightly opalescent, colorless to pale yellow, patient should administer the drug.
- Tell patient that if a dose is missed, he should administer the injection within 7 days and then resume original schedule. However, if the missed dose is not administered within 7 days, tell patient to wait until the next dose on the original schedule.
- Advise patient to stop drug and notify prescriber if an allergic reaction occurs.
- Instruct patient to report new-onset or worsening eye symptoms to prescriber.
- Tell patient with atopic dermatitis and asthma together not to adjust or stop her asthma treatments without consulting prescriber. Also remind patient with asthma that dupilumab should not be used to treat acute asthma exacerbations or symptoms.

dutasteride

Avodart

Class and Category

Pharmacologic class: 5-alpha-reductase enzyme inhibitor
Therapeutic class: Benign prostatic hyperplasia agent
Pregnancy category: X

Indications and Dosages

➤ *To treat symptomatic benign prostatic hyperplasia (BPH); as adjunct with tamsulosin therapy to treat symptomatic BPH*

CAPSULES

Adult men. 0.5 mg daily.

Contraindications

Children; hypersensitivity to dutasteride, its components, or other 5-alpha reductase inhibitors; women

Mechanism of Action

Dutasteride reduces prostate gland enlargement by inhibiting conversion of testosterone to its active metabolite, 5-alpha dihydrotestosterone (DHT). DHT is the main hormone that stimulates prostate cells to grow. As men age, they may become more sensitive to DHT, resulting in excessive growth of prostatic cells and enlargement of the prostate. This condition, benign prostatic hyperplasia, may cause nocturia, urinary hesitancy, and urinary urgency.

Two forms of the intracellular enzyme 5-alpha-reductase (5α-R types 1 and 2) in liver, prostate, and skin, convert testosterone to DHT, as shown below left. Dutasteride, a dual 5α-R inhibitor, deactivates both forms. When 5α-R is inhibited by dutasteride, production of DHT is suppressed, as shown below right. With less circulating DHT, the prostate gland shrinks and symptoms improve.

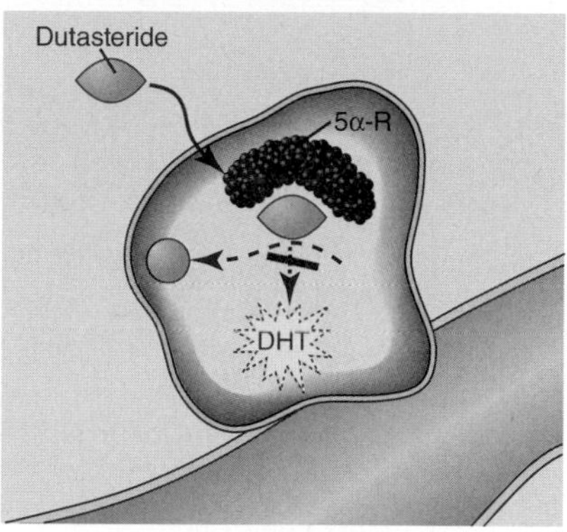

Interactions

DRUGS

cimetidine, ciprofloxacin, diltiazem, ketoconazole, ritonavir, verapamil, and other CYP3A4 inhibitors: Risk of decreased dutasteride metabolism and enhanced effects

Adverse Reactions

CNS: Depression, dizziness
ENDO: Gynecomastia, increased serum testosterone and thyroid-stimulating hormone levels, **male breast cancer**
GU: Decreased ejaculatory volume, decreased libido, **high-grade prostate cancer**, impotence, testicular pain and swelling
SKIN: Localized edema, pruritus, rash, serious skin reactions, urticaria
Other: Angioedema

Nursing Considerations

WARNING Be aware that dutasteride is absorbed through the skin, so female healthcare workers should not handle dutasteride capsules, especially if of childbearing age or pregnant.

- Know that patient should be evaluated for other urologic conditions, including prostate cancer, before dutasteride therapy starts because dutasteride therapy increases risk of patient developing high-grade prostate cancer.
- Expect patient to undergo a digital rectal examination of the prostate before and periodically during dutasteride therapy.
- Anticipate need to obtain a new baseline prostate-specific antigen (PSA) value after 3 to 6 months of dutasteride treatment because drug can decrease PSA concentration by 40% to 50%. Dutasteride also can decrease serum PSA level in the presence of prostate cancer. Any PSA reading in a patient receiving dutasteride should be doubled for comparison with normal values in untreated men. If value still falls within the normal range for men not taking a 5-alpha-reductase inhibitor,

further evaluation should still be done to rule out prostate cancer.

PATIENT TEACHING

WARNING Urge patient and female partners to use reliable contraceptive method during dutasteride therapy because semen of men who take drug can harm male fetuses. Caution women and children against handling capsules.

- Advise patient to inform prescriber if he has liver disease.
- Explain how to take drug properly, and advise patient to follow instructions that accompany drug. Instruct him to swallow capsule whole and to notify pharmacist if capsules are cracked or leaking.
- Inform patient that drug may decrease ejaculatory volume and libido and may cause impotence.
- Instruct patient to postpone blood donations for 6 months after final dose to avoid transmitting dutasteride to a pregnant woman during a blood transfusion.
- Urge patient to have periodic follow-up appointments.

E F

edoxaban

Savaysa

Class and Category

Pharmacologic class: Factor Xa inhibitor
Therapeutic class: Anticoagulant
Pregnancy category: Not classified

Indications and Dosages

➤ *To reduce risk of stroke and systemic embolism in nonvalvular atrial fibrillation*

TABLETS

Adults. 60 mg once daily.

➤ *To treat deep vein thrombosis and pulmonary embolism*

TABLETS

Adults. 60 mg once daily following 5 to 10 days of initial therapy with a parenteral anticoagulant.

DOSAGE ADJUSTMENT For patients with impaired renal failure (creatinine clearance between 15 and 50 ml/min), patients who weigh less than or equal to 60 kg (132 lb), or patients who are taking concomitant P-gp inhibitors, dosage reduced to 30 mg once daily.

Mechanism of Action

Inhibits free FXa and prothrombinase activity and inhibits thrombin-induced platelet aggregation. By inhibiting FXa in the coagulation cascade, thrombin generation and formation is reduced.

Contraindications

Active pathological bleeding, hypersensitivity to edoxaban or its components

Interactions

DRUGS

anticoagulants, antiplatelets, aspirin or aspirin-containing products, NSAIDs (long-term use), selective serotonin reuptake inhibitors, serotonin norepinephrine reuptake inhibitors, thrombolytics: Increased risk of bleeding
rifampin: Decreased effectiveness of edoxaban

Adverse Reactions

CNS: Intracranial bleeding
EENT: Epistaxis, intraocular bleeding
GI: Elevated liver enzymes, **GI bleeding**
GU: Hematuria, vaginal bleeding
HEME: Anemia, **bleeding**
RESP: Interstitial lung disease
SKIN: Rash

Nursing Considerations

- Know that edoxaban should not be administered to a patient who has a creatinine clearance greater than 95 ml/min because of an increased risk ischemic stroke.
- Keep in mind that edoxaban is not recommended for use in patients with a mechanical heart valve or who have moderate to severe mitral stenosis because the effects of edoxaban in these patients are unknown.
- Know that for a patient unable to swallow tablets, tablet should be crushed and mixed with 2 to 3 ounces of water and immediately administered by mouth or through a gastric tube. Crushed tablet can also be mixed with applesauce and immediately given by mouth.
- Be aware that edoxaban should be withheld for at least 24 hours before invasive or surgical procedures are performed to reduce the risk of bleeding. If it is not possible to delay the procedure, monitor patient closely for bleeding. If edoxaban was withheld, know that it may be restarted after the invasive or surgical procedure as soon as the patient has achieved adequate hemostasis. Be prepared to administer a parenteral anticoagulant if oral medication cannot be initially taken and then when oral medication can be taken, the patient may be switched to edoxaban.
- Know that when a patient is being transitioned to edoxaban from warfarin or other vitamin K antagonist, warfarin should be discontinued and edoxaban started when the INR is 2.5 or less; transitioned from oral anticoagulants other than warfarin or other vitamin K antagonists, the current oral anticoagulant should be discontinued and edoxaban started at the time of the next scheduled dose of the other oral anticoagulant;

transitioned from low-molecular-weight heparin, the low-molecular-weight heparin should be discontinued and edoxaban started at the time of the next scheduled administration of the low-molecular-weight heparin; or transitioned from unfractionated heparin, the unfractionated heparin infusion should be discontinued and edoxaban started 4 hours later.

- Be aware that when a patient is being transitioned from edoxaban (60 mg dose) to warfarin, the dose of edoxaban should be reduced to 30 mg and warfarin begun concomitantly. When a patient is being transitioned from edoxaban (30 mg dose) to warfarin, the dose of edoxaban should be reduced to 15 mg and warfarin begun concomitantly. When a stable INR of 2 or greater is achieved in either situation, edoxaban should be discontinued. Know that a second method of transitioning a patient from edoxaban to warfarin may be used. In this method, edoxaban should be discontinued and a parenteral anticoagulant and warfarin administered, as ordered, at the same time of the next scheduled edoxaban dose. Once a stable INR of 2 or greater is achieved, the parenteral anticoagulant should be discontinued and warfarin therapy continued. Be aware that when a patient is being transitioned from edoxaban to a non-vitamin K dependent oral anticoagulant, edoxaban should be discontinued and the other oral anticoagulant started at the time of the next dose of edoxaban. Know that when a patient is being transitioned from edoxaban to a parenteral anticoagulant, edoxaban should be discontinued and the parenteral anticoagulant should be started at the time of the next dose of edoxaban.

WARNING Monitor patient receiving edoxaban and epidural or spinal anesthesia or spinal puncture because spinal hematomas can occur, causing long-term or permanent paralysis. Watch for evidence of neurologic impairment, such as changes in motor or sensory function. If present, notify prescriber immediately; patient needs urgent care to minimize effect of hematoma. Use of indwelling epidural catheters; concurrent use of other drugs that affect hemostasis such as nonsteroidal anti-inflammatory drugs, platelet inhibitors, and other anticoagulants; a history of traumatic or repeated epidural or spinal punctures; or a history of spinal deformity or spinal surgery increases the risk of epidural or spinal hematoma in patients receiving edoxaban.

- Expect to receive another anticoagulant, as ordered, if edoxaban must be discontinued for reasons other than the presence of active bleeding or therapy is no longer needed. This is because premature discontinuation of edoxaban increases the risk of ischemic events.
- Monitor patient closely for bleeding. If present, notify prescriber immediately because there is no antidote to reverse the anticoagulation effects of edoxaban, which may last for up to 24 hours after the last dose. Know that patients who take other drugs that affect hemostasis, such as aspirin and other antiplatelet agents, chronic use of nonsteroidal anti-inflammatory drugs, fibrinolytic therapy, or other antithrombotic drugs, are at increased risk for bleeding.
- Know that the use of anticoagulants, including edoxaban, may increase the risk of bleeding in the fetus and neonate. Monitor neonate for bleeding if mother was taking edoxaban prior to birth.

PATIENT TEACHING

- Tell patient that if she misses a dose of edoxaban, she should take the dose as soon as possible on the same day and resume the dosing for the next day at the normal time. However, if she forgets the dose until the next day, she should not double the dose to make up for the missed dose.
- Inform patient unable to swallow tablets that edoxaban may be crushed and mixed with 2 to 3 ounces of water or mixed in applesauce and immediately taken by mouth.
- Instruct patient on bleeding precautions. If bleeding occurs, tell her to report any unusual bleeding immediately to the prescriber.
- Caution patient not to stop taking edoxaban without talking to her prescriber first.

- Tell patient to alert all healthcare providers and dentists that she is taking edoxaban and to consult the prescriber before taking any new drugs, including OTC drugs.
- Stress importance for females of child-bearing age to notify prescriber if pregnancy occurs or is suspected. This is because anticoagulants, including edoxaban, may increase the risk of bleeding in the fetus and neonate. Tell mother who took edoxaban during late pregnancy to watch neonate for bleeding.
- Advise mothers that breastfeeding is not recommended during edoxaban therapy because of the potential risk of serious adverse reactions.

WARNING Alert patient who is having neuraxial anesthesia or spinal puncture to immediately report signs and symptoms suggestive of epidural or spinal hematomas such as back pain, muscle weakness, numbness (especially in the lower limbs), stool or urine incontinence, and tingling.

efavirenz

Sustiva

Class and Category

Pharmacologic class: Non-nucleoside reverse transcriptase inhibitor
Therapeutic class: Antiretroviral
Pregnancy category: Not classified

Indications and Dosages

➤ *As adjunct to treat human immunodeficiency virus type 1 (HIV-1) in combination with a nucleoside analogue reverse transcriptase inhibitor and/or protease inhibitor*

CAPSULES, TABLETS

Adults and children weighing 40 kg (88 lb) or more. 600 mg once daily at bedtime on an empty stomach.
Children weighing 32.5 kg (71.5 lb) to less than 40 kg (88 lb). 400 mg once daily at bedtime on an empty stomach.
Children weighing 25 kg (55 lb) to less than 32.5 kg (71.5 lb). 350 mg once daily at bedtime on an empty stomach.
Children weighing 20 kg (44 lb) to less than 25 kg (55 lb). 300 mg once daily at bedtime on an empty stomach.
Children weighing 15 kg (33 lb) to less than 20 kg (44 lb). 250 mg once daily at bedtime on an empty stomach.
Children weighing 7.5 kg (16.5 lb) to less than 15 kg (33 lb). 200 mg once daily at bedtime on an empty stomach.
Children weighing 5 kg (11 lb) to less than 7.5 kg (16.5 lb). 150 mg once daily at bedtime on an empty stomach.
Children weighing 3.5 kg (7.7 lb) to less than 5 kg (11 lb). 100 mg once daily at bedtime on an empty stomach.

DOSAGE ADJUSTMENT For adult patients weighing 50 kg (110 lb) and also receiving rifampin, dosage increased to 800 mg once daily. For adult patients receiving voriconazole concurrently, dosage decreased to 300 mg once daily.

Mechanism of Action

Inhibits HIV integrase by binding to the integrase active site and blocking the strand transfer step of retroviral DNA integration, which is needed for the HIV replication cycle.

Contraindications

Concurrent therapy with elbasvir and grazoprevir, hypersensitivity to efavirenz or its components

Interactions

DRUGS

artemether, atazanavir, atorvastatin, atovaquone, boceprevir, bupropion, clarithromycin, dihydroatemisinin, diltiazem, ethinyl estradiol/norgestimate, etonogestrel implant, felodipine, fosamprenavir, hydroxyitraconazole, immunosuppressants, indinavir, ketoconazole, itraconazole, lopinavir, lumefantrine, maraviroc, methadone, nicardipine, nifedipine, posaconazole, pravastatin, proguanil, saquinavir, sertraline, simeprevir, simvastatin, verapamil: Decreased effectiveness of these drugs
other non-nucleoside reverse transcriptase inhibitors: Increased plasma levels of both drugs without added efficacy
psychoactive drugs: Possibly additive central nervous system effects
rifabutin: Decreased plasma levels of both drugs decreasing effectiveness
ritonavir: Increased plasma levels of both efavirenz and ritonavir, possibly leading to

elevated liver enzymes and other adverse reactions
voriconazole: Decreased voriconazole level and increased plasma efavirenz
warfarin: Decreased or increased warfarin levels, requiring close monitoring of INR and adjustment of warfarin dosage as needed
ACTIVITIES
alcohol use: Possibly increased additive central nervous system effects

Adverse Reactions

CNS: Abnormal dreams, aggression, agitation, amnesia, anxiety, ataxia, catatonia, cerebellar balance and coordination disturbances, confusion, delusions, depersonalization, depression (severe), dizziness, emotional lability, euphoria, fatigue, fever, hallucinations, headache, hypoesthesia, impaired concentration, insomnia, paranoid behavior, manic reactions, nervousness, neuropathy, neurosis, paranoia, paresthesia, psychosis-like behavior, **seizures**, somnolence, stupor, **suicidal ideation**, tremor, vertigo
CV: Elevated cholesterol and triglyceride levels, palpitations, **QT prolongation**
EENT: Abnormal vision, tinnitus
ENDO: Cushingoid appearance, fat redistribution, gynecomastia, hyperglycemia
GI: Abdominal pain, anorexia, constipation, diarrhea, dyspepsia, elevated amylase or liver enzymes, **hepatic failure**, **hepatitis, hepatotoxicity**, malabsorption, nausea, **pancreatitis**, vomiting
HEME: Neutropenia
MS: Arthralgia, myalgia, myopathy
RESP: Dyspnea
SKIN: Blisters, **erythema multiforme**, flushing, moist desquamation, photoallergic dermatitis, pruritus, rash, **Stevens–Johnson syndrome**, ulcerations
Other: Allergic reactions, nonspecific pain, immune reconstitution syndrome

Nursing Considerations

- Be aware that efavirenz should not be used as a single agent in treating HIV infection, because resistant virus emerges quickly when drug is used alone.
- Know that efavirenz therapy is not recommended with the combination drug Atripla, which contains efavirenz, unless needed for dose adjustment when coadministered with rifampin.
- Know that drug should not be used in patients taking other medications with a known risk of torsades de pointes or in patients at higher risk of torsades de pointes, because efavirenz may cause QT prolongation.
- Obtain liver enzymes before therapy begins, as ordered, in patients with marked transaminase elevations, patients treated with other medications associated with liver toxicity, and patients with underlying hepatic disease, including hepatitis B or C infections. Also monitor liver enzymes throughout therapy, as ordered, on all patients, because efavirenz may cause hepatotoxicity. Know that persistent elevations of serum transaminase levels greater than five times the upper limit of the normal range may require efavirenz therapy to be discontinued.
- Obtain cholesterol and triglyceride levels before efavirenz is begun and periodically throughout therapy, because drug may cause an increase in total cholesterol and triglycerides.
- Use efavirenz cautiously in patients with a history of seizures, as drug may increase risk of seizures. Know that if patient is also taking anticonvulsant medications metabolized by the liver, such as phenobarbital or phenytoin, periodic monitoring of plasma levels of these drugs may be required.

WARNING Monitor patient for rash. While usually mild to moderate, occurring within the first 2 weeks of therapy, and resolving within a month, a rash rarely may evolve into more serious skin conditions that could become life-threatening and should be reported. Know that it is recommended that children be given antihistamines and/or corticosteroids before initiating therapy, as a prophylactic measure.

- Monitor patient for serious psychiatric adverse reactions such as aggressive behavior, manic reactions, paranoia, severe depression, or suicidal ideation. Patients at increased risk include patients with drug addiction (injected) or psychiatric history including use of psychiatric drugs.

- Monitor patient for nervous system symptoms that commonly occur with efavirenz use. Be especially watchful for abnormal dreams, dizziness, hallucinations, impaired concentration, insomnia, and somnolence. Be aware that these symptoms usually occur within a day or two of starting therapy and usually resolve in the first 2 to 4 weeks.
- Be aware that immune reconstitution syndrome has occurred in patients treated with combination antiretroviral therapy, including efavirenz. The inflammatory response predisposes susceptible patients to opportunistic infections such as cytomegalovirus, *Mycobacterium avium* infection, *Pneumocystis jiroveci* pneumonia, or tuberculosis. Autoimmune disorders such as Graves' disease, Guillain–Barré syndrome, or polymyositis have also occurred. Report sudden or unusual adverse reactions to prescriber.

PATIENT TEACHING

- Inform patient that efavirenz is not to be taken alone and to follow administration instructions as ordered, noting that drug should be taken on an empty stomach at bedtime.
- Instruct patient or parent that if patient is unable to swallow capsule form, it may be opened and sprinkled on 1 to 2 teaspoonfuls of food such as applesauce, grape jelly, or yogurt. The capsule should be opened carefully so as not to spill any of the contents or disperse drug into the air. To accomplish this, tell patient to hold capsule horizontally over a small container and carefully twist open. If child is unable to consume food, the entire capsule contents may be gently mixed into 2 teaspoons of reconstituted room-temperature infant formula, stirred gently with a small spoon, and then drawn up into a 10-ml oral dosing syringe for administration. After administration, an additional 2 teaspoons of formula should be added to the empty mixing container, stirred, and administered. Caution that the food or formula mixture should be administered within 30 minutes of mixing and no additional food should be consumed for 2 hours after the drug is given.
- Inform patient that efavirenz therapy may cause changes in his body appearance because of fat redistribution. Prepare him for the possibility of developing breast enlargement, central obesity, dorsocervical fat enlargement (buffalo hump), facial wasting, and peripheral wasting.
- Instruct patient to report a rash. Also alert patient that drug may cause nervous system symptoms or psychiatric symptoms. Review these symptoms with patient and urge patient to report to prescriber if present. Advise him also to report any persistent, severe, or unusual signs and symptoms.
- Warn family or caregiver to watch patient closely for evidence of suicidal behavior or thinking.
- Advise patient to contact prescriber before taking any new drugs, including over-the-counter preparations and herbals.
- Caution patient to avoid hazardous activities such as driving until nervous system effects are known and abated.
- Warn women of childbearing age that efavirenz may cause fetal harm when administered during the first trimester of pregnancy. Stress importance of using reliable birth control and tell patient to alert prescriber immediately if pregnancy occurs or is suspected.
- Inform mothers that breastfeeding should not be done while taking efavirenz, because drug does appear in human breast milk.

eletriptan hydrobromide

Relpax

Class and Category

Pharmacologic class: Triptan
Therapeutic class: Antimigraine agent
Pregnancy category: C

Indications and Dosages

➤ *To relieve acute migraine attacks with or without aura*

TABLETS

Adults. *Initial:* 20 or 40 mg as a single dose. Repeated in 2 hr, as needed and ordered. *Maximum:* 40 mg as single dose, 80 mg daily.

E F

Mechanism of Action

May stimulate 5-HT_1 receptors, causing selective vasoconstriction of dilated and inflamed cranial blood vessels in carotid circulation, which decreases carotid arterial blood flow and relieves acute migraines.

Contraindications

Bibasilar or hemiplegic migraine, cardiovascular disease (significant), cerebrovascular syndromes (stroke, transient ischemic attack), hepatic impairment (severe), hypersensitivity to eletriptan or components, ischemic bowel disease, ischemic or vasospastic coronary artery disease (CAD), peripheral vascular disease, uncontrolled hypertension, use within 24 hours of another serotonin 5-HT_1 receptor agonist or ergot-type drug, use within 72 hours of a potent CYP3A4 inhibitor (clarithromycin, itraconazole, ketoconazole, nefazodone, nelfinavir, ritonavir, troleandomycin), Wolff–Parkinson–White syndrome or arrhythmias associated with other cardiac accessory conduction pathway disorders

Interactions

DRUGS

clarithromycin, ketoconazole, itraconazole, nefazodone, nelfinavir, ritonavir, troleandomycin, and other potent CYP3A4 inhibitors: Increased blood eletriptan level
ergot-containing drugs, 5-HT_1 receptor agonists: Possibly additive or prolonged vasoconstrictive effects
MAO inhibitors, selective serotonin norepinephrine reuptake inhibitors, selective serotonin reuptake inhibitors, tricyclic antidepressants: Increased risk of serotonin syndrome

Adverse Reactions

CNS: Asthenia, chills, dizziness, headache, hypertonia, hypesthesia, paresthesia, **seizures**, somnolence, tiredness, weakness, vertigo
CV: Chest tightness, pain, or pressure; **coronary artery vasospasm**; hypertension, **MI**, or myocardial ischemia (transient); palpitations; **shock**; **ventricular fibrillation or tachycardia**
EENT: Dry mouth, pharyngitis, **throat tightness**
GI: Abdominal pain, cramps, discomfort, or pressure; dysphagia; indigestion; nausea, vomiting
MS: Back pain
SKIN: Diaphoresis, flushing
Other: Allergic reaction; **angioedema**; feeling of warmth, pain, or pressure

Nursing Considerations

- Ensure that patients who are at risk for CAD undergo a satisfactory CV evaluation before administering the first dose of eletriptan and that they have a periodic reevaluation of their cardiac status during intermittent long-term therapy.
- Obtain an ECG immediately after first dose of drug in patients who have CV risk factors but who have had a satisfactory CV evaluation because of the drug's potential to cause coronary vasospasm.
- Evaluate patient for CV signs and symptoms after administration of eletriptan and notify prescriber if they occur. Expect drug to be withheld, as ordered, while patient undergoes an extensive CV workup, and discontinued if abnormalities are detected.
- Monitor patient's blood pressure during therapy because of drug's potential to increase blood pressure.

PATIENT TEACHING

- Advise patient to take eletriptan as soon as possible after onset of migraine symptoms.
- Urge patient to contact prescriber and avoid taking drug if headache symptoms aren't typical.
- Advise against exceeding prescribed dose.
- Instruct patient to seek emergency care for chest, jaw, or neck tightness after taking drug because these may indicate adverse CV reactions; subsequent doses may require ECG monitoring.
- Urge patient to report palpitations.
- Advise patient to avoid hazardous activities until drug's CNS effects are known.
- Advise yearly ophthalmic examinations during prolonged eletriptan therapy.
- Instruct patient to inform prescriber of all drugs he's taking, including OTC products and herbal remedies.

eltrombopag olamine

Promacta

Class and Category

Pharmacologic class: Thrombopoietin receptor agonist
Therapeutic class: Thrombopoietin agonist
Pregnancy category: Not classified

Indications and Dosages

➤ *To treat thrombocytopenia in patients with chronic immune (idiopathic) thrombocytopenic purpura and who have had an insufficient response to corticosteroids, immunoglobulins, or splenectomy*

ORAL SUSPENSION, TABLETS

Adults and children ages 6 yr and older. *Initial:* 50 mg daily, increased as needed to maintain a platelet count of 50×10^9/L. *Maximum:* 75 mg daily.
Children ages 1 to 5. *Initial:* 25 mg once daily, increased as needed to maintain a platelet count of 50×10^9/L.
DOSAGE ADJUSTMENT For adult and pediatric patients 6 years and older of East Asian ancestry or patients with moderate to severe hepatic impairment, starting dose of 25 mg daily. For patients of East Asian ancestry who also have hepatic impairment, starting dose of 12.5 mg daily. For patients with a platelet count less than 50×10^9/L following at least 2 weeks of therapy, dosage increased by 25 mg daily to maximum of 75 mg/day unless patient started therapy at 12.5 mg daily, then dosage increased to 25 mg daily before increasing the dose amount by 25 mg, as needed. For patients with a platelet count equal to or greater than 200×10^9/L but equal to or less than 400×10^9/L, dosage decreased by 25 mg daily for at least 2 weeks before further dosage adjustment made. For patient with a platelet count greater than 400×10^9/L, drug should be withheld until platelet count is less than 150×10^9/L and then restarted at a daily dose reduced by 25 mg, unless patient had been taking 25 mg daily, then dosage restarted at 12.5 mg daily.

➤ *To treat thrombocytopenia in patients with chronic hepatitis C infection to allow the initiation and maintenance of interferon-based therapy*

TABLETS

Adults. *Initial:* 25 mg daily, increased in increments of 25 mg daily every 2 wk, as needed, to achieve the target platelet count required to initiate antiviral therapy. *Maximum:* 100 mg daily.
DOSAGE ADJUSTMENT For patients with a platelet count equal to or greater than 200×10^9/L but equal to or less than 400×10^9/L, dosage decreased by 25 mg for at least 2 weeks before further dosage adjustment made. For patient with a platelet count greater than 400×10^9/L, drug should be withheld until platelet count is less than 150×10^9/L and then restarted at a daily dose reduced by 25 mg, unless patient had been taking 25 mg daily, then dosage restarted at 12.5 mg daily. For patient receiving antiviral therapy, dosage adjusted, as needed, to avoid dose reductions of peginterferon.

➤ *As adjunct with immunosuppressive therapy for first-line treatment of severe aplastic anemia*

ORAL SUSPENSION, TABLETS

Adults and children 12 years and over. *Initial:* 150 mg once daily for 6 months.
Children age 6 to 11 years. *Initial:* 75 mg once daily for 6 months.
Children age 2 to 5 years. *Initial:* 2.5 mg/kg once daily for 6 months.
DOSAGE ADJUSTMENT For patients of Asian ancestry or patients with hepatic impairment, initial dosage decreased by 50%. For patients with a platelet count greater than 400×10^9/L, drug withheld for 1 week. Once platelet count is less than 200×10^9/L, drug restarted at a daily dosage reduced by 25 mg for adults and and 12.5 mg for children under age 12. For patients with a platelet count greater than 200×10^9 but equal to or less than 400×10^9, daily adult dose decreased by 25 mg every 2 weeks to lowest dose that maintains platelet count equal to or greater than 50×10^9/L, and for children under the age of 12, dosage decreased by 12.5 mg.

➤ *To treat refractory severe aplastic anemia in patients who have had an insufficient response to immunosuppressive therapy*

ORAL SUSPENSION, TABLETS

Adults. *Initial*: 50 mg once daily, increased as needed in 50-mg increments every 2 wk. *Maximum*: 150 mg daily.

DOSAGE ADJUSTMENT For patients of East Asian ancestry or patients with any degree of hepatic impairment, initial dosage decreased to 25 mg daily. For patients with a platelet count less than 50 × 10^9/L following at least 2 weeks of therapy, dosage increased by 50 mg daily to maximum of 150 mg daily. For patients taking 25 mg once daily, dosage increased to 50 mg once daily before dosage increased by 50 mg. For patients with a platelet count equal to or greater than 200 × 10^9/L but equal to or less than 400 × 10^9/L, dosage decreased by 50 mg daily for at least 2 weeks before further dosage adjustment made. For patient with a platelet count greater than 400 × 10^9/L, drug should be withheld for 1 week and until platelet count is less than 150 × 10^9/L and then drug restarted at a daily dose reduced by 50 mg.

Route	Onset	Peak	Duration
P.O.	Unknown	2–6 hr	Unknown

Mechanism of Action

Interacts with the transmembrane domain of the thrombopoietin receptor to signal cascades that induce differentiation and proliferation of megakaryocytes from bone marrow progenitor cells. This action increases platelet production, which is abnormally low in patients with thrombocytopenic purpura.

Contraindications

Hypersensitivity to eltrombopag or its components

Interactions

DRUGS

antacids and mineral supplements containing aluminum, calcium, iron, magnesium, selenium, or zinc: Decreased eltrombopag absorption

BCRP substrates (imatinib, irinotecan, lapatinib, methotrexate, mitoxantrone, rosuvastatin, sulfasalazine, topotecan), OATP1B1 substrates (atorvastatin, bosentan, ezetimibe, fluvastatin, glyburide, olmesartan, pitavastain, pravastatin, rosuvastatin, repaglinide, rifampin, simvastatin acid, valsartan): Possibly increased risk of adverse reactions related to excessive exposure to these drugs

FOODS

all foods, especially dairy: Decreased absorption of eltrombopag

Adverse Reactions

CNS: Asthenia, chills, dizziness, fatigue, fever, headache, insomnia, paresthesia

CV: Arterial and venous thromboembolism, peripheral edema, **primary portal venous system thromboses** (in presence of chronic liver disease)

EENT: Cataract, conjunctival hemorrhage, nasopharyngitis, oropharyngeal pain, pharyngitis, rhinitis, rhinorrhea, toothache

GI: Abdominal pain, anorexia, diarrhea, dyspepsia, elevated bilirubin or liver enzymes, **hepatic decompensation** with antiviral and interferon therapy, **hepatotoxicity**, indirect hyperbilirubinemia (with antiviral and interferon therapy), nausea, vomiting

GU: Acute renal failure with thrombotic microangiopathy, menorrhagia, UTI

HEME: Anemia, **aplastic anemia**, **febrile neutropenia**, **hemorrhage**, **thrombocytopenia**

MS: Arthralgia, back or extremity pain, muscle spasm, myalgia

RESP: Cough, dyspnea, upper respiratory tract infection

SKIN: Alopecia, ecchymosis, pruritus, rash, skin discoloration including hyperpigmentation and skin yellowing

Other: Flu-like symptoms

Nursing Considerations

- Know that eltrombopag should not be used to treat any other kind of thrombocytopenia because of the risk of hematologic malignancies or portal venous system thromboses in patients with chronic liver disease. Also, know the drug should not be used to treat myelodysplastic syndromes because of an increased risk of progression to acute myeloid leukemia which could be fatal.
- Be aware that eltrombopag can be used only through a restricted distribution program called *Promacta Cares*. Patient,

pharmacy, and prescriber must all be enrolled before therapy begins.
- Use cautiously in patients with hepatic impairment because drug may cause hepatotoxicity and arterial and venous thrombosis, although most are portal venous system thromboses. This is especially important if patient with hepatic impairment also has risk factors present for thromboembolism.
- Monitor bilirubin level and liver enzymes, as ordered, before starting eltrombopag, every 2 weeks during dosage adjustment, and monthly once dose is stable. If abnormalities occur, repeat testing within 3 to 5 days and then weekly until liver enzymes return to baseline. Expect to discontinue drug if alanine aminotransferase level (ALT) increases to 3 or more times the upper normal limit, progresses or persists for 4 or more weeks, or is accompanied by an increase in direct bilirubin or clinical symptoms of liver injury.
- Know that there is an increased risk of hepatic decomposition when eltrombopag is used in combination with interferon and ribavirin in patients with chronic hepatitis C. Monitor these patients closely for evidence of hepatic dysfunction.
- Expect to monitor platelet counts every week prior to starting antiviral therapy, as ordered, for patient with hepatitis C. Once antiviral therapy has started, expect to monitor CBCs with differentials including platelet counts weekly during antiviral therapy until a stable platelet count is achieved. Thereafter, monitor platelet counts monthly, as ordered.
- Know that patient should have a baseline eye examination, as ordered, before starting eltrombopag and periodically throughout therapy, because drug may cause cataracts.
- Be aware that dosage adjustments are based on platelet count response and are not used to normalize platelet counts in order to prevent or minimize thrombotic complications.
- Give eltrombopag 1 hour before or 2 hours after the patient has eaten. Separate doses of other drugs by at least 4 hours to prevent drug interactions.
- Do not administer more than one dose of eltrombopag within any 24-hour period because too much drug increases the patient's risk of thrombotic events.
- Expect to discontinue drug for patient with chronic thrombocytopenia if improvement doesn't occur within 4 weeks at maximum dose of 75 mg daily or if the platelet count remains greater than 400×10^9/L after 2 weeks of therapy at the lowest dose of eltrombopag. Expect to discontinue drug for patient with hepatitis C if the platelet count remains greater than 400×10^9/L after 2 weeks of therapy at the lowest dose of eltrombopag or when antiviral therapy is discontinued. Expect to discontinue drug for patient with severe aplastic anemia if improvement doesn't occur after 16 weeks of therapy.
- Monitor patient for hematologic malignancies because eltrombopag stimulates thrombopoietin receptor on the surface of hematopoietic cells, which increases risk of malignancies.
- Monitor patient for increased bleeding after stopping eltrombopag because thrombocytopenia may worsen, increasing bleeding risk, especially if patient is on anticoagulants or antiplatelet therapy. If bleeding occurs, obtain weekly CBC, including platelet count, for at least 4 weeks after therapy stops, and provide supportive care, as indicated and ordered.

PATIENT TEACHING

- Inform patient that before eltrombopag therapy can begin, he must be enrolled in the *Promacta Cares* program, which provides comprehensive education about the drug.
- Urge patient to tell prescriber about all health conditions and all prescribed drugs, OTC drugs, herbs, and supplements taken.
- Tell patient to prepare the prescribed oral suspension using water only, but not hot water, and to ingest immediately after preparation. Any suspension not used should be discarded within 30 minutes. Remind patient that a new oral dosing syringe should be used to prepare every dose of oral suspension.
- Instruct patient to take eltrombopag on an empty stomach with a full glass of water

1 hour before or 2 hours after a meal and to separate use of other drugs by at least 4 hours because food and certain drugs (such as antacids and iron and vitamin supplements) may interfere with eltrombopag absorption.

- Instruct patient to take drug at the same time every day because no more than one dose should be taken within any 24-hour period because too much of the drug may cause blood clots.
- Encourage patient to have regular eye exams because drug may increase the development of cataracts.
- Urge patient to report any adverse reactions, especially signs and symptoms of liver problems such as confusion, right upper stomach area pain or swelling, tiredness or unusual darkening of the urine, or yellowing of the skin or the whites of the eyes, to prescriber. In addition, tell patient to keep all appointments for blood work and follow-up.
- Review bleeding precautions with patient. Tell him that he may be at increased risk for bleeding and should follow bleeding precautions even after drug is discontinued, especially if he is also taking a drug that affects the ability to clot. He should seek medical attention if serious bleeding occurs.
- Inform women of childbearing age to use effective contraception throughout eltrombopag therapy and for at least 7 days after drug is discontinued, because drug may cause fetal harm. If pregnancy is suspected or occurs, prescriber should be notified immediately.
- Tell mothers wishing to breastfeed that breastfeeding is not recommended during eltrombopag therapy, because drug may transfer to infant during breastfeeding and has the potential to cause serious adverse reactions in the breastfed child.

eluxadoline

Viberzi

Class, Category, and Schedule

Pharmacologic class: Mu-opioid receptor agonist
Therapeutic class: Antidiarrheal
Pregnancy category: Not classified
Controlled substance schedule: IV

Indications and Dosages

➤ *To treat irritable bowel syndrome with diarrhea (IBS-D)*

TABLETS

Adults. 100 mg twice daily with food.
DOSAGE ADJUSTMENT For patients who are unable to tolerate the 100-mg dose, who are receiving concomitant OATP1B1 inhibitors, or who have mild to moderate hepatic impairment, dosage reduced to 75 mg twice daily.

Mechanism of Action

Interacts with opioid receptors in the intestines to relieve diarrhea.

Contraindications

Absence of a gallbladder, alcoholism, or patients who drink more than three alcoholic beverages daily, biliary duct obstruction, history of pancreatitis or structural disease of the pancreas, history of chronic or severe constipation, hypersensitivity to eluxadoline or its components, known or suspected mechanical gastrointestinal obstruction, severe hepatic impairment, sphincter of Oddi disease, or dysfunction

Interactions

DRUGS

alosetron, anticholinergics, opioids or other drugs that cause constipation: Increased risk of constipation and constipation-related adverse reactions
OATP1B1 inhibitors such as antivirals, cyclosporine, eltrombopag, gemfibrozil, rifampin: Increased exposure to eluxadoline increasing risk of adverse reactions
rosuvastatin: Increased exposure to rosuvastatin with increased risk for myopathy and rhabdomyolysis

ACTIVITIES

alcohol use: Increased risk for acute pancreatitis

Adverse Reactions

CNS: Dizziness, euphoria, fatigue, sedation, sensation of feeling drunk, somnolence
CV: Chest pain or tightness
EENT: Nasopharyngitis, **throat tightness**

GI: Abdominal distention or pain, constipation (which may become severe), elevated liver enzymes, flatulence, gastroesophageal reflux disease, nausea, **pancreatitis**, sphincter of Oddi spasm, vomiting
RESP: **Asthma**, bronchitis, **bronchospasm**, dyspnea, **respiratory failure**, upper respiratory infection, wheezing
SKIN: Pruritus, rash, urticaria
Other: Anaphylaxis, angioedema

Nursing Considerations

- Assess patient's alcohol intake prior to starting eluxadoline therapy. Also, question patient about gallbladder removal surgery, as drug is contraindicated in patients without a gallbladder.

WARNING Monitor patient closely for hypersensitivity reactions that could include anaphylaxis, angioedema, difficulty breathing or swallowing, and skin reactions such as itching, rash, or urticaria. If present, notify prescriber immediately, stop administering drug, and provide emergency supportive care, as ordered.

- Monitor patient closely for acute abdominal pain, especially during the first few weeks of therapy, because mu-opioid receptor agonism increases risk for sphincter of Oddi spasm, which could result in elevated liver enzymes or pancreatitis. If present, notify prescriber and expect eluxadoline to be discontinued.
- Monitor patient's liver enzymes, as ordered and report any elevations to prescriber.
- Notify prescriber if patient develops severe constipation and expect drug to be discontinued. Severe cases of fecal impaction or intestinal obstruction or perforation have occurred with severe constipation, requiring emergency intervention.

PATIENT TEACHING

- Tell patient that if she misses a dose to take the next dose at the regular time and not to double up the dose to make up for a missed dose.
- Warn patient against acute excessive or chronic alcohol intake while taking eluxadoline.
- Instruct patient to stop taking eluxadoline and immediately seek medical attention if she experiences acute epigastric or right, upper quadrant abdominal pain that may radiate to the back or shoulder and may be accompanied by nausea and vomiting.
- Tell patient to notify prescriber immediately if she develops severe constipation and not to use other drugs that may cause constipation during eluxadoline therapy.
- Advise patient to inform all prescribers of eluxadoline therapy.
- Tell patient not to take other drugs to treat diarrheal symptoms unless prescribed and the prescriber is aware of eluxadoline use.

E F

elvitegravir

Vitekta

Class and Category

Pharmacologic class: Integrase inhibitor
Therapeutic class: Antiretroviral
Pregnancy category: B

Indications and Dosages

➤ *As adjunct to treat human immunodeficiency virus type 1 (HIV-1) in antiretroviral treatment-experienced patients*

TABLETS

Adults taking atazanavir and ritonavir concurrently. 85 mg once daily with food with atazanavir 300 mg once daily and ritonavir 100 mg once daily.
Adults taking lopinavir and ritonavir concurrently. 85 mg once daily with food with lopinavir 400 mg twice daily and ritonavir 100 mg twice daily.
Adults taking darunavir and ritonavir concurrently. 85 mg once daily with food with darunavir 600 mg twice daily and ritonavir 100 mg twice daily.
Adults taking fosamprenavir and ritonavir concurrently. 150 mg once daily with food with fosamprenavir 700 mg twice daily and ritonavir 100 mg twice daily.

Adults taking tipranavir and ritonavir concurrently. 150 mg once daily with food with tipranavir 500 mg twice daily and ritonavir 200 mg twice daily.

Mechanism of Action

Inhibits HIV integrase by binding to the integrase active site and blocking the strand transfer step of retroviral DNA integration, which is needed for the HIV replication cycle.

Contraindications

Concurrent use with cobicistat or the combination drug Stribild, hypersensitivity to elvitegravir or its components

Interactions

DRUGS

antacids, carbamazepine, dexamethasone, efavirenz, nevirapine, oxcarbazepine, phenobarbital, phenytoin, rifampin, rifapentine, St. John's wort: Decreased plasma elvitegravir concentrations, lowering drug's effectiveness
atazanavir, lopinavir/ritonavir: Increased plasma elvitegravir levels, increasing risk of serious adverse reactions
boceprevir, methadone, naloxone, telaprevir: Decreased plasma concentrations of these drugs, reducing effectiveness
bosentan: Increased plasma concentration of bosentan, possibly increasing risk of serious adverse reactions and decreased plasma concentration of elvitegravir that decreases its effectiveness
cobicistat: Possibly decreased effectiveness of elvitegravir
ethinyl estradiol: Decreased plasma concentration of ethinyl estradiol, leading to decreased contraception effectiveness
HIV protease inhibitors: Decreased or increased plasma concentrations of these drugs, which can reduce effectiveness and possibly lead to development of resistance
ketoconazole: Increased plasma concentrations of both drugs, increasing risk of serious adverse reactions
rifabutin: Increased plasma concentration of rifabutin, possibly increasing risk of serious adverse reactions and decreased plasma concentration of elvitegravir that decreases its effectiveness

Adverse Reactions

CNS: Depression, fatigue, headache, insomnia, **suicidal ideation**
CV: Elevated cholesterol and triglycerides
ENDO: Hyperglycemia
GI: Abdominal pain; diarrhea; dyspepsia; elevated amylase, bilirubin, or liver enzymes; nausea; vomiting
GU: Hematuria, glycosuria
HEME: Neutropenia
MS: Elevated creatine kinase
SKIN: Rash
Other: Immune reconstitution syndrome

Nursing Considerations

- Know that the fixed-dose combination drug, Stribild, should not be administered with elvitegravir because elvitegravir is a component of the combination, which could increase the risk of serious adverse reactions.
- Be aware that cobicistat should not be given to patients receiving elvitegravir, because it may cause elvitegravir to be less effective.

WARNING Take a complete drug history, because risk of adverse reactions that may result in serious adverse reactions from greater exposures of concomitant drugs or elvitegravir may occur. Some drug interactions may also cause elvitegravir to become less effective. Make all prescribers aware of patient's use of elvitegravir.

- Monitor patient closely for suicidal ideation.
- Be aware that immune reconstitution syndrome has occurred in patients treated with combination antiretroviral therapy, including elvitegravir. The inflammatory response predisposes susceptible patients to opportunistic infections such as cytomegalovirus, *Mycobacterium avium* infection, *Pneumocystis jiroveci* pneumonia, or tuberculosis. Autoimmune disorders such as Graves' disease, Guillain–Barré syndrome, or polymyositis have also occurred. Report sudden or unusual adverse reactions to prescriber.

PATIENT TEACHING

- Instruct patient to take elvitegravir exactly as prescribed and with food. Tell patient that other drugs will have to be taken with elvitegravir to enhance its effectiveness.
- Warn patient to check with prescriber before taking any new medications,

including over-the-counter and herbal preparations.
- Instruct family or caregiver to watch patient closely for evidence of suicidal behavior or thinking.
- Tell patient to report any persistent, severe, or unusual signs and symptoms to prescriber, including signs of infection.
- Stress importance of alerting prescriber if pregnancy occurs or is suspected.
- Inform mothers that breastfeeding should not be done while taking elvitegravir, because drug does appear in human breast milk.

empagliflozin

Jardiance

Class and Category

Pharmacologic class: Sodium glucose co-transporter 2 inhibitor
Therapeutic class: Antidiabetic
Pregnancy category: C

Indications and Dosages

➤ *Adjunct to diet and exercise to improve glycemic control in patients with type 2 diabetes mellitus; to reduce risk of cardiovascular death in patients with type 2 diabetes mellitus who have established cardiovascular disease*

TABLETS

Adults. 10 mg once daily in morning, increased to 25 mg once daily in morning, as needed.

Mechanism of Action

Inhibits sodium glucose co-transporter 2 in the kidneys, which prevents glucose reabsorption. This decreases blood glucose levels.

Contraindications

Dialysis, therapy, end-stage renal disease, hypersensitivity to empagliflozin or its components, severe renal impairment

Interactions

DRUGS

diuretics: Increased risk of acute kidney injury and renal impairment in presence of dehydration
insulin, insulin secretagogues: Increased risk of hypoglycemia

Adverse Reactions

CNS: Syncope
CV: Dyslipidemia, elevated low-density lipoprotein cholesterol, **hypotension**
ENDO: Ketoacidosis
GI: Nausea
GU: Acute kidney injury, decreased glomerular filtration rate, dysuria, elevated serum creatinine levels, genital mycotic infections, impaired renal function, increased urination, osmotic diuresis, pyelonephritis, **urosepsis**, UTI
MS: Arthralgia, increased risk of bone fracture
RESP: Upper respiratory tract infection
SKIN: Rash, urticaria
Other: Angioedema, dehydration

Nursing Considerations

- Assess patient's volume status and correct, if needed and as prescribed, prior to starting empagliflozin therapy because drug can cause intravascular volume contraction leading to symptomatic hypotension and acute kidney injury. Continue to monitor patient throughout therapy for dehydration and renal dysfunction. Patients at highest risk include the elderly and patients with chronic renal insufficiency, congestive heart failure, and hypovolemia or patients who take diuretics. Notify prescriber immediately if patient has fluid losses or reduced oral intake, as acute kidney injury may occur. Expect that drug may be temporarily withheld until fluid balance can be restored.
- Obtain serum creatinine level, as ordered, prior to starting empagliflozin therapy because empagliflozin can cause adverse renal effects. Be aware that the elderly and patients with existing impaired renal function are at higher risk for these adverse effects. Monitor renal function throughout therapy.
- Monitor patient for hypersensitivity reactions that could be serious, such as the development of angioedema. If present, withhold drug, notify prescriber immediately, and be prepared to provide emergency supportive care, as ordered.
- Monitor patient's blood pressure and cholesterol level throughout empagliflozin therapy.

- Be aware that patients receiving insulin or insulin secretagogues may require a lower dose of these agents because empagliflozin in combination increases risk of hypoglycemia. Monitor patient closely for hypoglycemia. If present, treat according to standard of care and notify prescriber.

WARNING Monitor patient closely for ketoacidosis that have occurred in patients with type 2 diabetes being treated with empagliflozin. Be aware that ketoacidosis can become life-threatening quickly even when blood glucose levels are less than 250 mg/dl. Notify prescriber immediately if ketoacidosis is suspected and expect drug to be discontinued. Be prepared to treat patient's ketoacidosis, as ordered. Be aware that patients at higher risk include patients with a history of alcohol abuse or who have a pancreatic insulin deficiency from any cause or have reduced caloric intake. Expect drug to be temporarily discontinued if patient must undergo prolonged fasting due to acute illness or surgery.

- Monitor patients for genital mycotic infections or urinary tract infections, especially those with a history of such. If present, notify prescriber and treat, as prescribed.

WARNING Monitor patient for a rare but serious and life-threatening necrotizing infection of the perineum called Fournier's gangrene. Notify prescriber immediately if patient develops erythema, pain, swelling, or tenderness in the genital or perineal area, along with fever or malaise. Expect treatment with broad-spectrum antibiotics and, if needed, surgical debridement of the area. Know that empagliflozin will be discontinued if this occurs. Monitor patient's blood glucose levels closely and expect an alternative treatment for glycemic control.

PATIENT TEACHING

- Inform patient that empagliflozin therapy is not a replacement for diet and exercise therapy.
- Tell patient that drug may cause an allergic reaction such as swelling of the eyes, face, throat, and tongue. It may also cause skin reactions such as a rash or hives. If present, stress importance of stopping drug and seeking immediate emergency medical treatment.
- Instruct patient on the signs and symptoms of hypoglycemia and how to treat it. Inform patient who is also receiving insulin or a sulfonylurea that the risk of hypoglycemia is greater. Tell patient to notify prescriber if hypoglycemia occurs frequently or is severe.
- Tell patient to monitor the blood glucose level using blood tests instead of urine tests because drug increases urinary glucose excretion and will lead to positive urine glucose tests.
- Review signs and symptoms of ketoacidosis with patient and urge her to seek immediate medical attention, if present, even if blood glucose level is less than 250 mg/dl.
- Advise female patients to notify prescriber if pregnancy occurs or is suspected. Also advise women that breastfeeding is not recommended while taking empagliflozin.
- Advise patient to maintain adequate fluid intake throughout empagliflozin therapy. However, tell patient to notify prescriber if she is unable to take a normal amount of daily fluids due to fasting or illness or experiences an excessive loss of fluids from excessive perspiration or gastrointestinal illnesses. Drug may have to be temporarily withheld.
- Stress importance of notifying prescriber if patient develops dehyrdration, has onset of hunger or thirst, or notices a sudden change in mental status. Tell patient not to belittle these symptoms and seek medical attention quickly.

WARNING Warn patient to stop empagliflozin and seek immediate medical attention if pain, redness, swelling, or tenderness occurs in the genital or perineal area, along with fever or malaise because, although rare, this cluster of symptoms may become life-threatening.

- Teach patient to take fall precautions and other safety measures because drug may increase risk of bone fracture as early as 12 weeks after empagliflozin therapy is begun.

emtricitabine

Emtriva

Class and Category

Pharmacologic class: Nucleoside analogue
Therapeutic class: Antiretroviral
Pregnancy category: B

Indications and Dosages

➤ *As adjunct to treat human immunodeficiency virus type 1 (HIV-1) infection*

CAPSULES, ORAL SOLUTION

Adults. 200 mg (capsule) or 240 mg (oral solution) once daily.
Children ages 3 months to 18 years who weigh more than 33 kg (72.6 lb) and can swallow an intact capsule. 200 mg once daily.
Children ages 3 months to 18 years prescribed oral solution. 6 mg/kg up to maximum of 240 mg once daily.
Newborns and infants up to 3 months. 3 mg/kg (oral solution) once daily.

DOSAGE ADJUSTMENT For adult patients with a creatinine clearance of 30 to 49 ml/min, dosage interval increased to every 48 hr if using capsules or dosage reduced to 120 mg once daily if using oral solution. For adult patients with a creatinine clearance of 15 to 29 ml/min, dosage interval increased to every 72 hr if using capsules or dosage reduced to 80 mg once daily if using oral solution. For adult patients with a creatinine clearance of less than 15 ml/min or who are on hemodialysis, dosage interval increased to every 96 hr if using capsules or dosage reduced to 60 mg once daily if using oral solution. For pediatric patients with renal impairment, there is insufficient data to recommend a specific dose adjustment, but a reduction in dose and/or an increase in dosing interval similar to adults may be considered.

Mechanism of Action

Phosphorylated by cellular enzymes, emtricitabine then inhibits the activity of the HIV-1 reverse transcriptase by competing with the natural substrate and by being incorporated into the nascent viral DNA, which leads to chain termination of the HIV virus.

Contraindications

Hypersensitivity to emtricitabine or its components

Interactions

DRUGS

None significant

Adverse Reactions

CNS: Abnormal dreams, asthenia, depression, dizziness, fatigue, fever, headache, insomnia, neuropathy, paresthesia, peripheral neuritis
CV: Elevated cholesterol and triglycerides
EENT: Nasopharyngitis, otitis media, rhinitis, sinusitis
ENDO: Cushingoid appearance, fat redistribution, hyperglycemia
GI: Abdominal pain; diarrhea; dyspepsia; elevated amylase, bilirubin, lipase, and liver enzymes; gastroenteritis; nausea; **severe acute exacerbations of hepatitis B**; **severe hepatomegaly with steatosis**; vomiting
GU: Glycosuria, hematuria, new onset or worsening of renal impairment
HEME: Anemia, decreased hemoglobin, **neutropenia**
MS: Arthralgia, elevated creatine kinase, myalgia
RESP: Increased cough, pneumonia, upper respiratory infections
SKIN: Hyperpigmentation on palms and/or soles, pruritus, rash, urticaria
Other: Elevated alkaline phosphatase, immune reconstitution syndrome, infection, **lactic acidosis**

Nursing Considerations

- Expect to test patient for hepatitis B virus (HBV) prior to starting emtricitabine, as ordered. This is because acute exacerbations of hepatitis B have occurred after patient has discontinued the drug. Know that in some cases the exacerbation resulted in liver failure.
- Monitor patient's liver enzymes throughout therapy and for several months after drug is discontinued, because lactic acidosis and severe hepatomegaly with steatosis have occurred with emtricitabine therapy, as have acute exacerbations of hepatitis B. Know that most cases of lactic acidosis and severe hepatomegaly with steatosis have occurred in women with prolonged

nucleoside exposure and obesity. Report abnormal liver function signs and symptoms to prescriber, such as abdominal discomfort, jaundice, nausea, vomiting, or weakness.

- Perform a complete drug history on patient, because combination drugs containing emtricitabine (Atripla, Complera, Truvada) should not be given concurrently with emtricitabine therapy. Also, expect not to coadminister drugs containing lamivudine (Cobivir, Epivir, Epivir-HBV, Epzicom, Trizivir) because of the similarities between emtricitabine and lamivudine.
- Monitor patient's renal function, because drug is primarily eliminated by the kidney and dosage alterations are necessary for those with impaired kidney function.
- Be aware that immune reconstitution syndrome has occurred in patients treated with combination antiretroviral therapy, including emtricitabine. The inflammatory response predisposes susceptible patients to opportunistic infections such as cytomegalovirus, *Mycobacterium avium* infection, *Pneumocystis jiroveci* pneumonia, or tuberculosis. Autoimmune disorders such as Graves' disease, Guillain–Barré syndrome, or polymyositis have also occurred. Report sudden or unusual adverse reactions to prescriber.

PATIENT TEACHING

- Inform patient that emtricitabine will be prescribed along with other antiviral drugs.
- Review signs and symptoms of liver dysfunction (belly discomfort, nausea, vomiting, weakness, yellowing of skin or whites of eyes) and stress importance of reporting any occurrence to prescriber.
- Instruct patient to remind all prescribers of emtricitabine therapy.
- Inform patient that emtricitabine therapy may cause changes in his body appearance because of fat redistribution. Prepare him for the possibility of developing breast enlargement, central obesity, dorsocervical fat enlargement (buffalo hump), facial wasting, and peripheral wasting.
- Instruct patient to report any persistent, severe, or unusual signs and symptoms.
- Encourage women of childbearing age to report known or suspected pregnancy.
- Alert mothers that breastfeeding is not recommended during emtricitabine therapy, because drug is present in human breast milk.

enalapril maleate

Epaned, Vasotec

enalaprilat

Class and Category

Pharmacologic class: Angiotensin converting enzyme (ACE) inhibitor
Therapeutic class: Antihypertensive, vasodilator
Pregnancy category: Not classified

Indications and Dosages

➤ *To control hypertension*

ORAL SOLUTION, TABLETS

Adults. *Initial:* 5 mg daily, increased after 1 to 2 wk, as needed. *Maintenance:* 10 to 40 mg once daily or in divided doses twice daily.

Children older than 1 month. 0.08 mg/kg daily, titrated according to blood pressure response up to 5 mg daily. *Maximum:* 0.58 mg/kg/dose or 40 mg/dose.

I.V. INFUSION

Adults. 1.25 mg over 5 min every 6 hr.

DOSAGE ADJUSTMENT Initial dose reduced to 2.5 mg P.O. or 0.625 mg I.V. for patients who have sodium and water depletion from diuretic therapy, are receiving diuretics, or adults who have a creatinine clearance below 30 ml/min (not used in children who have a glomerular filtration rate below 30 ml/min). For patient who is receiving a diuretic, if response to I.V. dose is inadequate after 1 hr, I.V. dose of 0.625 mg repeated and therapy continued at 1.25 mg every 6 hr.

➤ *To treat heart failure*

TABLETS

Adults. *Initial:* 2.5 mg twice daily, increased after 1 to 2 wk, as needed.
Maintenance: 5 to 40 mg daily in 2 divided doses.

DOSAGE ADJUSTMENT For patients with hyponatremia (serum sodium less than 130 mEq/L) or serum creatinine greater than 1.6 mg/dl, initial dosage reduced to 2.5 mg once daily.

➤ *To treat asymptomatic left ventricular dysfunction*

TABLETS

Adults. *Initial:* 2.5 mg twice daily, increased to 20 mg daily in 2 divided doses.

DOSAGE ADJUSTMENT Initial dosage reduced to 2.5 mg daily and, if possible, diuretic dosage reduced in patients who have a creatinine clearance of 30 ml/min or below.

Route	Onset	Peak	Duration
P.O.	1 hr	4–6 hr	About 24 hr
I.V.	15 min	1–4 hr	About 6 hr

Mechanism of Action

May reduce blood pressure and development of heart failure by affecting the renin–angiotensin–aldosterone system. By inhibiting angiotensin-converting enzyme (ACE), enalapril:

- prevents conversion of angiotensin I to angiotensin II, a potent vasoconstrictor that also stimulates the adrenal cortex to secrete aldosterone
- may inhibit renal and vascular production of angiotensin II
- decreases the serum angiotensin II level and increases serum renin activity, which decreases aldosterone secretion and slightly increases serum potassium level and fluid loss
- decreases vascular tone and blood pressure
- inhibits aldosterone release, which reduces sodium and water reabsorption and increases their excretion, further reducing blood pressure and development of heart failure.

Contraindications

Aliskiren use in patients with diabetes; concurrent therapy with a neprilysin inhibitor such as sacubitril, history of hereditary or idiopathic angioedema; hypersensitivity to enalapril, enalaprilat, other ACE inhibitors, or their components; use within 36 hours of sacubitril/valsartan therapy

Interactions

DRUGS

aliskiren (in patients with diabetes or renal impairment), angiotensin receptor blockers, other ACE inhibitors: Increased risk of hyperkalemia, hypotension, and renal dysfunction

cyclosporine, potassium-sparing diuretics, potassium supplements: Increased risk of hyperkalemia

diuretics, other antihypertensives: Additive hypotensive effects

lithium: Increased blood lithium level and lithium toxicity

mTOR inhibitors (everolimus, sirolimus, temsirolimus); neprilysin inhibitor (sacubitril): Increased risk of angioedema

NSAIDs including selective cyclooxygenase-2 inhibitors: Possibly reduced antihypertensive effects of enalapril and enalaprilat; possibly increased risk of renal dysfunction, especially in the elderly or who are volume-depleted or already have compromised renal function

sodium aurothiomalate: Increased risk of nitritoid reactions, such as facial flushing, nausea, vomiting, and hypotension

thiazide diuretics: Increased loss of potassium

FOODS

potassium-containing salt substitutes: Increased risk of hyperkalemia

Adverse Reactions

CNS: Ataxia, confusion, CVA, depression, dizziness, dream disturbances, fatigue, headache, insomnia, nervousness, peripheral neuropathy, somnolence, syncope, vertigo, weakness

CV: Angina, **arrhythmias**, **cardiac arrest**, **hypotension**, **MI**, orthostatic hypotension, palpitations, Raynaud's phenomenon

EENT: Blurred vision, conjunctivitis, dry eyes and mouth, glossitis, hoarseness, lacrimation, loss of smell, pharyngitis, rhinorrhea, stomatitis, taste perversion, tinnitus

ENDO: Gynecomastia

GI: Abdominal pain, anorexia, constipation, diarrhea, **hepatic failure**, **hepatitis**, ileus, indigestion, **melena**, nausea, **pancreatitis**, vomiting

GU: Flank pain, impotence, oliguria, **renal failure**, UTI
MS: Muscle spasms
RESP: Asthma, bronchitis, **bronchospasm**, cough, dyspnea, pneumonia, **pulmonary edema**, **pulmonary embolism and infarction**, **pulmonary infiltrates**, upper respiratory tract infection
SKIN: Alopecia, diaphoresis, **erythema multiforme**, **exfoliative dermatitis**, flushing, pemphigus, photosensitivity, pruritus, rash, **Stevens–Johnson syndrome**, **toxic epidermal necrolysis**, urticaria
Other: **Anaphylaxis**, **angioedema**, herpes zoster, **hyperkalemia**

Nursing Considerations

- Use enalapril and enalaprilat cautiously in patients with impaired renal function. Avoid giving drug to children with a GFR less than 30 ml/min.
- For adults or children who can't swallow tablets, consult with prescriber and pharmacist about preparing an oral suspension from tablets as directed by manufacturer. Alternatively, have prescriber order the oral solution form (Epaned).
- Reconstitute oral solution by tapping bottle containing the drug powder on a hard surface 5 times to loosen powder. Add about half (75 ml) of the Ora-Sweet SF diluent that comes with the drug to the powder bottle. Replace cap and shake well for 30 seconds. Reopen and add remainer diluent to the drug powder bottle. Replace cap and shake well again for 30 seconds. Calculate 60 days from the date of reconstitution and write this date as the discard date on the front of the label.
- Administer each I.V. dose over at least 5 minutes.
- Measure patient's blood pressure immediately after first dose and frequently for at least 2 hours thereafter. If hypotension requires a dosage reduction, monitor blood pressure frequently for 2 hours after reduced dosage is administered and for another hour after blood pressure has stabilized.
- Monitor blood pressure regularly during therapy. If hypotension develops, place patient in a supine position and expect to give I.V. normal saline solution or other volume expander as prescribed.
- Monitor patient's heart rate and rhythm. Expect to obtain repeated 12-lead ECG tracings.
- Monitor laboratory test results to check hepatic and renal function, leukocyte count, and serum potassium level.
- Monitor patient closely for angioedema of the face, glottis, larynx, limbs, lips, and tongue. Notify prescriber and stop drug administration immediately. Expect to give an antihistamine, as prescribed. If glottis, larynx, or tongue is involved, assess patient for airway obstruction and prepare to give epinephrine 1:1,000 (0.3 to 0.5 ml) subcutaneously and maintain a patent airway.

PATIENT TEACHING

- Advise patient to take drug at the same time each day.
- Instruct patient not to chew, crush, or split tablets.
- Teach patient how to mix oral solution, if prescribed.
- Inform patient that fainting and lightheadedness may occur, especially during first few days of therapy. Advise him to change position slowly and avoid hazardous activities until drug's CNS effects are known.
- Inform patient that diarrhea, excessive sweating, vomiting, and other conditions may cause dehydration, which can lead to dizziness, fainting, and very low blood pressure during therapy. Urge sufficient fluid intake to prevent dehydration and related adverse reactions. If diarrhea or vomiting is severe or prolonged, instruct patient to notify prescriber.
- Urge patient to stop taking drug and immediately seek emergency care if swelling of extremities, face, lips, throat, or tongue occurs. Also tell patient to notify prescriber if other adverse reactions, including persistent dry cough, occur.
- Advise patient to consult prescriber before using potassium supplements, salt substitutes, or other drugs (including OTC drugs) while taking drug.

WARNING Caution women of childbearing age that they should use a reliable form of contraception and should notify prescriber immediately if pregnancy is suspected because enalapril may cause fetal harm and should be discontinued.

enfuvirtide

Fuzeon

Class and Category

Pharmacologic class: Fusion inhibitor
Therapeutic class: Antiretroviral
Pregnancy category: B

Indications and Dosages

➤ *As adjunct to treat human immunodeficiency virus type 1 (HIV-1) infection*

SUBCUTANEOUS INJECTION

Adults and adolescents ages 17 and over. 90 mg twice daily.
Children ages 6 to 17 weighing at least 11 kg (24.2 lb). 2 mg/kg twice daily. *Maximum:* 90 mg twice daily.

Mechanism of Action

Interferes with the entry of HIV-1 into cells to inhibit fusion of cellular membranes with the virus. It does this by binding to the viral envelope glycoprotein and preventing the conformational changes required for the fusion.

Contraindications

Hypersensitivity to enfuvirtide or its components

Interactions

DRUGS

None reported

Adverse Reactions

CNS: Anxiety, asthenia, chills, depression, fatigue, fever, **Guillain–Barré syndrome**, insomnia, peripheral neuropathy, rigors, sixth nerve palsy, **suicidal ideation**
CV: Elevated triglycerides, **hypotension**, **unstable angina pectoris**
EENT: Conjunctivitis, dry mouth, sinusitis, taste disturbance
ENDO: Hyperglycemia
GI: Anorexia; constipation; diarrhea; elevated amylase, lipase, and liver enzymes; hepatic steatosis; nausea; **pancreatitis**; **toxic hepatitis**; upper abdominal pain; vomiting
GU: Glomerulonephritis, **renal failure or insufficiency**, **tubular necrosis**
HEME: Eosinophilia, **neutropenia**, **thrombocytopenia**
MS: Elevated creatine phosphokinase, extremity pain, myalgia
RESP: Cough, pneumonia (bacterial), respiratory distress
SKIN: Cutaneous amyloidosis at injection site, folliculitis, pruritus, rash
Other: Formation of anti-enfuvirtide antibodies, flu-like symptoms, herpes simplex infection, immune reconstitution syndrome, local injection site reactions (bruising, cyst formation, discomfort, ecchymosis, erythema, hematomas, **hypersensitivity reaction**, induration, infection, neuralgia, nodule formation, pain, paresthesia, pruritus), lymphadenopathy, post-injection bleeding, **sepsis**, weight loss

Nursing Considerations

- Reconstitute with 1 ml of sterile water for injection provided in the convenience kit. Then gently tap vial for 10 seconds, followed by gently rolling vial between hands to avoid foaming and to ensure that all particles of drug are in contact with the liquid. Let vial stand until powder is completely dissolved, which may take up to 45 minutes. When ready to withdraw the drug from the vial and the solution is foamy or jelled, allow more time for it to dissolve. Once reconstituted, use immediately or keep refrigerated in the original vial for up to 24 hours. If refrigerated, allow reconstituted solution to come to room temperature before administration.
- Administer enfuvirtide subcutaneously into patient's abdomen, anterior thigh, or upper arm using the Biojector 2000 needle-free device or a needle and syringe.
- Rotate site of injections, avoiding injecting into any anatomical areas where large nerves course close to the skin; directly over a blood vessel; or into skin abnormalities such as bruises, burn sites, moles, near the navel, scar tissue, surgical scars, or tattoos.
- Assess patient's injection site for local adverse reactions, because most patients experience at least one local injection-site reaction. Be especially alert for infection such as cellulitis or a local infection. Provide supportive care, as ordered, to manage injection-site reactions.
- Monitor patient's respiratory status closely, as bacterial pneumonia may occur and be

serious enough to warrant hospitalization. Be especially alert for pneumonia in patients with a high initial viral load, history of intravenous drug use, low initial CD4 lymphocyte count, prior history of lung disease, or who are smokers.
- Be alert for systemic hypersensitivity reactions associated with enfuvirtide therapy, which may include chills, fever, hypotension, nausea, rash, rigors, and vomiting. Elevated liver enzymes may also occur.
- Know that enfuvirtide may cause formation of anti-enfuvirtide antibodies, which may result in a false positive HIV test with an ELISA assay.
- Be aware that immune reconstitution syndrome has occurred in patients treated with combination antiretroviral therapy, including enfuvirtide. The inflammatory response predisposes susceptible patients to opportunistic infections such as cytomegalovirus, *Mycobacterium avium* infection, *Pneumocystis jiroveci* pneumonia, or tuberculosis. Autoimmune disorders such as Graves' disease, Guillain–Barré syndrome, or polymyositis have also occurred. Report sudden or unusual adverse reactions to prescriber.
- Watch patient closely for suicidal ideation.

PATIENT TEACHING
- Inform patient that enfuvirtide therapy will be used in conjunction with other antiretroviral agents.
- Review how to reconstitute enfuvirtide and how to properly store it if not used immediately. Remind patient that drug does not contain a preservative and therefore must be refrigerated and used within 24 hours after being reconstituted. If refrigerated, tell patient that drug must be brought naturally to room temperature before administering.
- Instruct patient on how to properly use the Biojector 2000 device used to administer enfuvirtide subcutaneously, if needed. Otherwise, instruct her on how to use a needle and syringe and how to give a subcutaneous injection.
- Tell patient that drug should only be injected into her abdomen, front of her thigh, or in her upper arms. Sites must be rotated and drug should not be injected into any abnormal skin area, including tattoos, not near the navel, and not over blood vessels or large nerves close to the skin such as the back or side of thigh or near the elbow, groin, or knee. Advise patient how to safely discard used equipment such as needles and syringes.
- Advise patient to alert prescriber to persistent or severe local injection-site adverse reactions, including any signs or symptoms of infection. Inform her that almost all patients experience at least one injection-site reaction.
- Review signs and symptoms of an allergic reaction with patient and stress importance of seeking immediate medical attention.
- Alert patient that enfuvirtide may produce antibodies that could give a false positive for HIV testing. Remind her to alert all healthcare professionals of enfuvirtide therapy.
- Instruct patient to report any persistent, severe, or unusual signs and symptoms.
- Encourage women of childbearing age to report known or suspected pregnancy.
- Alert mothers that breastfeeding is not recommended during enfuvirtide therapy.
- Tell patient to seek medical attention if she develops signs or symptoms suggestive of pneumonia, such as cough with fever, rapid breathing, or shortness of breath.
- Caution patient and family that drug may cause suicidal thoughts. If present, prescriber should be notified.

enoxaparin sodium

Lovenox

Class and Category

Pharmacologic class: Low-molecular-weight heparin
Therapeutic class: Anticoagulant
Pregnancy category: B

Indications and Dosages

➤ *To prevent deep vein thrombosis (DVT) after hip or knee replacement and for continued prophylaxis after hospitalization for hip replacement*

SUBCUTANEOUS INJECTION

Adults. 30 mg every 12 hr, starting 12 to 24 hr after surgery for up to 14 days. Or, 40 mg daily, starting 9 to 15 hr after hip replacement surgery. *Prophylaxis:* 40 mg daily for 3 wk.

➤ *To prevent DVT after abdominal surgery for patients with thromboembolic risk factors (cancer, general anesthesia lasting longer than 30 minutes, a history of DVT or pulmonary embolism, obesity, or over age 40)*

SUBCUTANEOUS INJECTION

Adults. 40 mg daily, starting 2 hr before surgery and lasting 7 to 10 days.

➤ *To prevent DVT in medical patients who are at risk for thromboembolic complications due to severely restricted mobility during acute illness*

SUBCUTANEOUS INJECTION

Adults. 40 mg once daily for up to 14 days.

➤ *To treat DVT in patients with or without pulmonary embolism*

SUBCUTANEOUS INJECTION

Adults. *For inpatient:* 1 mg/kg every 12 hr for a minimum of 5 days. Alternatively, 1.5 mg/kg once daily for a minimum of 5 days. *For outpatient:* 1 mg/kg every 12 hr for a minimum of 5 days.

➤ *To prevent ischemic complications of unstable angina and non-Q-wave MI*

SUBCUTANEOUS INJECTION

Adults. 1 mg/kg every 12 hr with 100 to 325 mg of aspirin daily for 2 to 8 days or until condition is stable.

DOSAGE ADJUSTMENT Dosage reduced to 30 mg daily if creatinine clearance is less than 30 ml/min and patient is receiving drug as prophylaxis in abdominal, hip, or knee replacement surgery or is acutely ill. Reduced to 1 mg/kg daily if creatinine clearance is less than 30 ml/min and drug is given with aspirin to prevent ischemic complications of unstable angina and non-Q-wave MI, with warfarin as inpatient treatment for acute DVT with or without pulmonary embolism, or with warfarin as outpatient treatment of acute DVT without pulmonary embolism.

➤ *To treat acute ST-segment–elevation MI (STEMI)*

I.V. INJECTION, THEN SUBCUTANEOUS INJECTION

Adults. 30 mg I.V. as a single dose and 1 mg/kg subcutaneously (maximum, 100 mg for first 2 doses). Then, 1 mg/kg subcutaneously every 12 hr.

DOSAGE ADJUSTMENT For patient with STEMI who is also receiving a thrombolytic, enoxaparin should be given between 15 min before and 30 min after fibrinolytic therapy starts. If STEMI patient has percutaneous coronary intervention, expect to give 0.3-mg/kg I.V. bolus if last enoxaparin dose was given more than 8 hr before balloon inflation. For elderly patients with STEMI who are 75 years of age and older, initial I.V. bolus eliminated and initial subcutaneous injection dosage reduced to 0.75 mg/kg every 12 hr (maximum 75 mg for the first 2 doses only, followed by 0.75 mg/kg for remaining doses).

Route	Onset	Peak	Duration
SubQ	Unknown	3–5 hr	Up to 24 hr

Mechanism of Action

Potentiates the action of antithrombin III, a coagulation inhibitor. By binding with antithrombin III, enoxaparin rapidly binds with and inactivates clotting factors (primarily factor Xa and thrombin). Without thrombin, fibrinogen can't convert to fibrin and clots can't form.

Incompatibilities

Don't mix enoxaparin with other I.V. fluids or drugs.

Contraindications

Active major bleeding; history of heparin-induced thrombocytopenia (HIT) or immune-mediated HIT within past 100 days or in the presence of circulating antibodies, which may persist for several years; hypersensitivity to benzyl alcohol (if only the multidose vial is available), enoxaparin, heparin (including low-molecular-weight heparins), pork products or their components

Interactions

DRUGS

NSAIDs; oral anticoagulants; platelet aggregation inhibitors, such as aspirin, dipyridamole, salicylates, sulfinpyrazone, and ticlopidine; thrombolytics, such as alteplase, anistreplase, streptokinase, and urokinase: Possibly increased risk of bleeding and of spinal or epidural hematoma

Adverse Reactions

CNS: Confusion, **CVA**, epidural or spinal hematoma, fever, headache, paralysis
CV: **Atrial fibrillation**, **congestive heart failure**, hyperlipidemia, peripheral edema, **thrombosis**
EENT: Epistaxis
GI: Bloody stools, **cholestatic and hepatocellular liver injury**, diarrhea, elevated liver enzymes, **hematemesis**, **melena**, nausea, vomiting
GU: Hematuria, menstrual irregularities
HEME: Anemia, eosinophilia, **hemorrhage**, **HIT or immune-mediated thrombocytopenia**, **purpura**, **thrombocytopenia**, purpura, thrombocytopenia, thrombocytosis
MS: Osteoporosis (with long-term therapy)
RESP: Dyspnea, pneumonia, **pulmonary edema**, **or embolism**
SKIN: Alopecia, cutaneous vasculitis, ecchymosis, persistent bleeding or oozing from mucous membranes or surgical wounds, pruritus, skin necrosis at injection site or distant from injection site, urticaria, vesiculobullous rash
Other: Anaphylaxis including shock; **hyperkalemia**; injection-site erythema, hematoma, inflammation, irritation, nodules, oozing, and pain

Nursing Considerations

- Use enoxaparin with extreme caution in patients with a history of heparin-induced thrombocytopenia (HIT). Know that enoxaparin should only be used in these patients if more than 100 days have elapsed since the prior HIT episode and no circulating antibodies are present.
- Use also extreme caution in patients with an increased risk of hemorrhage, as from active ulcerative or angiodysplastic GI disease; bacterial endocarditis; congenital or acquired bleeding disorder; concurrent treatment with a platelet inhibitor; hemorrhagic stroke; or recent brain, ophthalmologic, or spinal surgery.
- Use cautiously in those with bleeding diathesis, diabetic retinopathy, hepatic or renal impairment, recent GI hemorrhage or ulceration, or uncontrolled hypertension. Expect delayed elimination in elderly patients and those with renal insufficiency.
- Be aware that drug isn't recommended for patients with prosthetic heart valves, especially pregnant women, because of risk of prosthetic valve thrombosis. If enoxaparin is needed, monitor peak and trough antifactor Xa levels often and adjust dosage as needed.
- Know that use of multidose vials should be avoided if at all possible in pregnant women because benzyl alcohol may cross the placenta and cause fetal harm.
- Don't give drug by I.M. injection.

WARNING Know that if patient is receiving enoxaparin with epidural or spinal anesthesia or spinal puncture, watch closely for development of spinal hematoma, which may cause long-term or permanent paralysis. If evidence of neurologic impairment, such as changes in sensory or motor function, occurs, notify prescriber immediately because urgent care is needed to minimize hematoma's effect. Risk of epidural or spinal hematoma during enoxaparin therapy is increased by indwelling epidural catheters, concurrent use of other drugs that affect hemostasis, a history of traumatic or repeated epidural or spinal punctures, or a history of spinal deformity or spinal surgery. Know that placement or removal of a catheter should be delayed for at least 12 hours after administration of lower doses of enoxaparin (30 mg once or twice daily or 40 mg once daily) and at least 24 hours after the administration of higher doses. (0.75 mg/kg twice daily, 1 mg/kg twice daily, or 1.5 mg/kg once daily). However, for patients with creatinine clearance of less than 30 ml/min, timing of removal should be doubled because enoxaparin elimination is more prolonged in renal dysfunction.

- Expect to give drug with aspirin to patient with unstable angina, STEMI, and non-Q-wave MI. To minimize risk of bleeding after vascular procedures, give enoxaparin at recommended intervals.
- Know that after a percutaneous revascularization procedure, it is important to achieve hemostasis at the puncture site. A closure device may be removed right away; however, if a manual compression method is used, the sheath should be removed 6 hours after last enoxaparin dose. If enoxaparin therapy

will continue, give next scheduled dose no sooner than 6 to 8 hours after sheath removal.

- Watch closely for bleeding. Notify prescriber immediately if platelet count falls below 100,000/mm^3. Expect to stop drug and start treatment if patient has a thromboembolic event, such as a stroke.
- Test stool for occult blood, as ordered.
- Keep protamine sulfate nearby in case of accidental overdose.
- Check serum potassium level for elevation, especially in patients with renal impairment or who are currently using potassium-sparing diuretics.

PATIENT TEACHING

- Advise patient to notify prescriber about adverse reactions, especially bleeding. Inform patient that taking aspirin or other NSAIDs may increase risk for bleeding.
- Instruct patient to seek immediate help for evidence of thromboembolism, such as neurologic changes and severe shortness of breath. Also tell patient to report any unusual bleeding, bruising, or rash of dark red spots under the skin to prescriber.
- Emphasize the importance of complying with follow-up visits with prescriber.
- Teach patient or family member how to give enoxaparin at home, if needed. Show how to give drug by deep subcutaneous injection while lying down. Instruct him not to expel air bubble from a prefilled syringe to avoid losing some of the drug. Tell him to insert the entire needle into a skin fold held between the thumb and forefinger. Remind him to alternate injection sites between the left and right anterolateral abdominal wall.
- Caution patient not to rub the site after giving the injection to minimize bruising.
- Review safe handling and disposal of syringes and needles.
- Instruct patient to alert all healthcare providers, but especially those administering anesthesia, about enoxaparin therapy. If neuraxial anesthesia or spinal puncture is necessary, and especially if taking other drugs that could affect bleeding, tell patient to watch for signs and symptoms of epidural or spinal bleeding such as muscle weakness or numbness or tingling in lower extremities.
- Inform patient that he may bruise and/or bleed more easily and that it may take longer than usual to stop bleeding while taking enoxaparin. Review bleeding precautions with patient.

entacapone

Comtan

Class and Category

Pharmacologic class: COMT inhibitor
Therapeutic class: Antidyskinetic
Pregnancy category: Not classified

Indications and Dosages

➤ *As adjunct to carbidopa and levodopa to treat end-of-dose "wearing-off" in patients with Parkinson's disease*

TABLETS

Adults. 200 mg with each dose of carbidopa and levodopa. *Maximum:* 1,600 mg daily.

Mechanism of Action

Inhibits peripheral catechol-*O*-methyltransferase (COMT), the major metabolizing enzyme for levodopa. During levodopa metabolism, COMT causes the formation of a levodopa metabolite that reduces the effectiveness of levodopa. By inhibiting COMT, entacapone leads to higher sustained blood levels of levodopa and its increased availability for diffusion into the CNS, where it is converted to dopamine. By replenishing dopamine stores, entacapone increases dopaminergic stimulation in the brain and reduces the symptoms of Parkinson's disease. Carbidopa is given with levodopa because it inhibits the peripheral distribution of levodopa, making more levodopa available for transport to the brain.

Contraindications

Hypersensitivity to entacapone or its components

Interactions

DRUGS

ampicillin, chloramphenicol, cholestyramine, erythromycin, probenecid, rifampicin: Decreased biliary excretion of entacapone

apomorphine, bitolterol, dobutamine, dopamine, epinephrine, isoetharine, isoproterenol, methyldopa, norepinephrine: Possibly arrhythmias, excessive changes in blood pressure, and increased heart rate
nonselective MAO inhibitors such as phenelzine, tranylcypromine: Possibly inhibited entacapone metabolism
warfarin: Possibly significant increase in INR level

Adverse Reactions

CNS: Agitation, anxiety, asthenia, confusion, dizziness, dyskinesia, fatigue, falling asleep during activities of daily living, fever, hallucinations, hyperkinesia, hypokinesia, psychotic-like behavior, somnolence, syncope
CV: Orthostatic hypotension
EENT: Dry mouth, taste perversion
GI: Abdominal pain, constipation, drug-induced microscopic colitis, diarrhea, flatulence, gastritis, **hepatitis**, indigestion, nausea, vomiting
GU: Brown-orange urine
MS: Back pain, **rhabdomyolysis**
RESP: Dyspnea
SKIN: Diaphoresis, purpura
Other: Intense urges to perform certain acts, such as gambling or sex

Nursing Considerations

WARNING Be aware that entacapone should not be discontinued abruptly because doing so may precipitate signs and symptoms resembling those of neuroleptic malignant syndrome, such as fever, muscle rigidity, altered level of consciousness, confusion, and elevated creatine kinase level. Patients may also experience a rapid reemergence of parkinsonian symptoms.

- Know that entacapone should not be given to patients with a major psychotic disorder because the drug can exacerbate psychosis.
- Monitor patient for drug-induced diarrhea during first 4 to 12 weeks of therapy but be aware that in some patients it may appear as early as the first week of therapy and last many months after therapy is begun.
- Help patient with activities as needed because drug may increase risk of orthostatic hypotension or syncope.
- Monitor patient for daytime sleepiness or episodes of falling asleep during activities that require active participation. If present, notify prescriber and expect drug to be discontinued.
- Watch for worsening dyskinesia because entacapone potentiates dopaminergic adverse effects of levodopa.
- Be aware that drug may be taken with selective MAO inhibitors, such as selegiline.
- Assess patient for skin changes regularly because risk of melanoma is increased in those with Parkinson's disease. It isn't clear whether increased risk results from the disease or drugs used to treat it.

PATIENT TEACHING

- Instruct patient to always take entacapone with carbidopa and levodopa because it has no antidyskinetic effect of its own.
- Inform patient that dizziness and sleepiness are more common at beginning of treatment, especially in those with hypotension.
- Advise patient not to participate in potentially hazardous activities until drug's CNS effects are known, especially if he's also taking CNS depressants. Warn patient that drug has been known to cause patients to suddenly fall asleep without prior warning of sleepiness while engaged in activities of daily living.
- Instruct patient scheduled for surgery to inform surgeon and anesthesiologist about entacapone use before the procedure because COMT inhibitors such as entacapone may interact with some drugs used in surgical procedures.
- Caution patient that entacapone may increase adverse effects of carbidopa and levodopa, such as nausea and uncontrolled movements. If these adverse effects do increase, advise him to contact prescriber immediately because carbidopa and levodopa dosage may have to be lowered.
- Inform patient that urine may turn brown-orange while he's taking entacapone but that this is a harmless effect.
- Urge patient to have regular skin examinations by a dermatologist or other qualified health professional.
- Advise patient to notify prescriber about intense urges, including those for gambling or sex. Dosage may have to be reduced or drug discontinued.

- Tell patient to notify prescriber if diarrhea occurs at any time during therapy because diarrhea may become severe requiring drug to be discontinued.

entecavir

Baraclude

Class and Category

Pharmacologic class: Nucleoside analogue
Therapeutic class: Antiviral
Pregnancy category: C

Indications and Dosages

➤ *To treat chronic hepatitis B virus infection in patients with evidence of active viral replication and either evidence of persistent elevations in serum aminotransferases (ALT or AST) or histologically active disease*

ORAL SOLUTION, TABLETS

Adults and adolescents ages 16 and over if treatment-naive. 0.5 mg once daily 2 hr before or after a meal.

Adults and adolescents ages 16 and over who have a history of hepatitis B viremia while receiving lamivudine or have experienced known lamivudine or telbivudine resistance substitutions; adults with decompensated liver disease. 1 mg once daily 2 hr before or after a meal.

Children ages 2 and over weighing more than 30 kg (66 lb). 0.5 mg (10 ml oral solution) once daily if treatment-naïve or 1 mg (20-ml oral solution) once daily if lamivudine-experienced, 2 hr before or after a meal.

Children ages 2 and over weighing more than 26 kg (57.2 lb) but less than 30 kg (66 lb). 9 ml oral solution once daily if treatment-naïve or 18 ml oral solution once daily if lamivudine-experienced, 2 hr before or after a meal.

Children ages 2 and over weighing more than 23 kg (50.6 lb) but less than 26 kg (57.2 lb). 8 ml oral solution once daily if treatment-naïve or 16 ml oral solution once daily if lamivudine-experienced, 2 hr before or after a meal.

Children ages 2 and over weighing more than 20 kg (44 lb) but less than 23 kg (50.6 lb). 7 ml oral solution once daily if treatment-naïve or 14 ml oral solution once daily if lamivudine-experienced, 2 hr before or after a meal.

Children ages 2 and over weighing more than 17 kg (37.4 lb) but less than 20 kg (44 lb). 6 ml oral solution once daily if treatment-naïve or 12 ml oral solution once daily if lamivudine-experienced, 2 hr before or after a meal.

Children ages 2 and over weighing more than 14 kg (30.8 lb) but less than 17 kg (37.4 lb). 5 ml oral solution once daily if treatment-naïve or 10 ml oral solution once daily if lamivudine-experienced, 2 hr before or after a meal.

Children ages 2 and over weighing more than 11 kg (24.2 lb) but less than 14 kg (30.8 lb). 4 ml oral solution once daily if treatment-naïve or 8 ml oral solution once daily if lamivudine-experienced, 2 hr before or after a meal.

Children ages 2 and over weighing at least 10 kg (22 lb) but less than 11 kg (24.2 lb). 3 ml oral solution once daily if treatment-naïve or 6 ml oral solution once daily if lamivudine-experienced, 2 hr before or after a meal.

DOSAGE ADJUSTMENT For adult patient with a creatinine clearance between 30 and less than 50 ml/min, dosage reduced to 0.25 mg once daily or 0.5 mg every 48 hr if treatment-naïve, and dosage reduced to 0.5 mg once daily or 1 mg every 48 hr if lamivudine-refractory or decompensated liver disease is present. For adult patient with a creatinine clearance between 10 and less than 30 ml/min, dosage reduced to 0.15 mg once daily or 0.5 mg every 72 hr if treatment-naïve, and dosage reduced to 0.3 mg once daily or 1 mg every 72 hr if lamivudine-refractory or decompensated liver disease is present. For adult patient with a creatinine clearance less than 10 ml/min or who is on dialysis, dosage reduced to 0.05 mg once daily or 0.5 mg every 7 days (given after hemodialysis) if treatment-naïve, and dosage reduced to 0.1 mg once daily or 1 mg every 7 days (given after hemodialysis) if lamivudine-refractory or decompensated liver disease is present. For pediatric patients with renal impairment, there is insufficient data to recommend a specific dose adjustment but a reduction in dose and/or an increase in dosing interval similar to adults may be considered.

Mechanism of Action

Inhibits all three activities of the hepatitis B virus (HBV) reverse transcriptase which are base priming, reverse transcription of the negative strand from the pregenomic messenger RNA, and synthesis of the positive strand of HBV DNA. This lowers the ability of HBV to multiply and infect new liver cells.

Contraindications

Hypersensitivity to entecavir or its components

Interactions

DRUGS

drugs that reduce renal function or compete for active tubular secretion: Possibly increased serum concentrations of either entecavir or the coadministered drug, increasing risk of adverse reactions

Adverse Reactions

CNS: Dizziness, fatigue, fever, headache, **hepatic encephalopathy**, insomnia, somnolence
CV: Peripheral edema
EENT: Taste abnormality
ENDO: Hyperglycemia
GI: Abdominal pain, ascites, diarrhea, dyspepsia, elevated liver and pancreatic enzymes, **exacerbation of hepatitis** (after discontinuation of therapy), **gastrointestinal hemorrhage**, **hepatic failure**, **hepatorenal syndrome**, hyperalbuminemia, hyperbilirubinemia, nausea, **severe hepatomegaly with steatosis**, vomiting
GU: Elevated creatinine level, glycosuria, hematuria, **renal failure**
HEME: Decreased platelet count
RESP: Upper respiratory infection
SKIN: Alopecia, rash
Other: Anaphylaxis, **decreased serum bicarbonate level**, **lactic acidosis**

Nursing Considerations

- Ensure that patient has been tested for HIV infection before entecavir therapy begins, because resistance to HIV therapy may develop when entecavir is administered to treat chronic hepatitis B virus infection in patients who also have an HIV infection that is not being treated. Know that entecavir therapy is not recommended for co-infected patients who are not receiving treatment.

WARNING Know that lactic acidosis and severe hepatomegaly with steatosis have occurred with entecavir therapy and death has occurred in some patients. Risk factors include the presence of obesity, prolonged nucleoside exposure, and being a woman. However, know that lactic acidosis and severe hepatomegaly with steatosis have also occurred in patients with no known risk factors. Monitor patient's liver enzymes as ordered. Expect entecavir to be discontinued in any patient who develops clinical or laboratory findings suggestive of lactic acidosis or pronounced hepatotoxicity, even in the absence of marked transaminase elevations.

- Expect patient to be closely monitored for at least several months after entecavir has been discontinued, because severe acute exacerbation of hepatitis may occur.

PATIENT TEACHING

- Instruct patient with hepatitis B on the importance of testing for HIV before therapy begins and then periodically throughout therapy to avoid development of resistance to HIV treatment.
- Instruct patient to take entecavir once daily on an empty stomach either 2 hours before a meal or 2 hours after a meal.
- Tell patient that entecavir therapy does not reduce the transmission of HBV to others through blood contamination or sexual contact.
- If patient misses a dose, tell him to take it as soon as he remembers but not to double the next dose or take more than the prescribed dose.
- Instruct patient using the oral solution to hold the dosing spoon in a vertical position and fill it gradually to the mark corresponding to the prescribed dose. The dosing spoon should be rinsed after each daily dose.
- Warn patient with hepatitis B that acute severe exacerbations of hepatitis B may occur following discontinuation of entecavir. He should not discontinue drug without prescriber knowledge. Tell patient to report any reappearance of signs and symptoms of hepatitis B.
- Instruct mothers not to breastfeed while receiving entecavir therapy, as drug is present in human breast milk.

- Advise female patient to notify prescriber if pregnancy occurs or is suspected. If pregnancy occurs, encourage patient to register with the Antiretroviral Pregnancy Registry at 1-800-258-4263.

WARNING Alert patient that severe conditions may develop while taking entecavir. Encourage him to stop taking drug and seek medical attention immediately if he experiences any persistent, severe, or unusual symptoms.

epinephrine

(adrenaline)

Adrenalin, Auvi-Q, EpiPen, EpiPen Jr., Symjepi

Class and Category

Pharmacologic class: Sympathomimetic
Therapeutic class: Antianaphylactic, bronchodilator, cardiac stimulant, vasopressor
Pregnancy category: C

Indications and Dosages

To treat croup

INHALED SOLUTION (RACEPINEPHRINE)

Children. 0.05 ml/kg diluted to 3 ml in normal saline solution and given over 15 min every 2 hr, as needed. *Maximum:* 0.5 ml/dose.

➤ *To treat anaphylaxis*

I.M. OR SUBCUTANEOUS INJECTION

Adults and children weighing 30 kg (66 lb) or more. 0.3 to 0.5 mg, repeated every 5 to 10 min, as needed.

Children weighing less than 30 kg (66 lb). 0.01 mg/kg up to maximum of 0.3 mg per injection, repeated every 5 to 10 min, as needed.

➤ *To provide emergency treatment of allergic reactions (Type I), including anaphylaxis to allergen immunotherapy, biting and stinging insects, diagnostic testing substances, drugs, foods, and other allergens, as well as exercise-induced or idiopathic anaphylaxis*

I.M. INJECTION, SUBCUTANEOUS INJECTION (AUVI-Q, SYMJEPI)

Adults and children weighing 30 kg (66 lb) or more who are at increased risk for anaphylaxis. 0.3 mg immediately upon exposure.

I.M. INJECTION, SUBCUTANEOUS INJECTION (AUVI-Q, SYMJEPI)

Adults and children weighing 15 to 30 kg (33 to 66 lb) who are at increased risk of anaphylaxis. 0.15 mg immediately upon exposure.

Children weighing 7.5 to 15 kg (16.5 to 33 lb) who are at increased risk of anaphylaxis. 0.1 mg immediately upon exposure.

Route	Onset	Peak	Duration
I.M.	Rapid	Unknown	1–2 min
SubQ	5–10 min	In 20 min	Short
Oral inhalation	1–5 min	In 5–15 min	Up to 3 hr

Mechanism of Action

Acts on alpha and beta receptors. This nonselective adrenergic agonist stimulates:

- $alpha_1$ receptors, which constricts arteries and may decrease bronchial secretions
- presynaptic $alpha_2$ receptors, which inhibits norepinephrine release by way of negative feedback
- postsynaptic $alpha_2$ receptors, which constricts arteries
- $beta_1$ receptors, which induces positive chronotropic and inotropic responses
- $beta_2$ receptors, which dilates arteries, relaxes bronchial smooth muscles, increases glycogenolysis, and prevents mast cells from secreting histamine and other substances, thus reversing bronchoconstriction and edema.

Incompatibilities

Don't mix epinephrine with alkalis or oxidizing agents, including bromine, chlorine, chromates, iodine, metal salts (as from iron), nitrites, oxygen, and permanganates, because these substances can destroy epinephrine.

Contraindications

Cerebral arteriosclerosis, coronary insufficiency, dilated cardiomyopathy, general anesthesia with halogenated hydrocarbons or cyclopropane, hypersensitivity to epinephrine or its components, labor,

E F

angle-closure glaucoma, organic brain damage, shock (nonanaphylactic)

Interactions

DRUGS

alpha-adrenergic blockers, drugs with alpha-adrenergic action, rapid-acting vasodilators: Blockage of epinephrine's alpha-adrenergic effect, possibly causing severe hypotension and tachycardia
beta blockers: Mutual inhibition of therapeutic effects
chlorpheniramine, diphenhydramine, levothyroxine, MAO inhibitors, tricyclic antidepressants, tripelennamine: Possibly increased effects of epinephrine
digoxin, diuretics, quinidine and other antiarrhythmics: Increased risk of arrhythmias
dihydroergotamine, ergoloid mesylates, ergonovine, ergotamine, methylergonovine, methysergide, oxytocin: Increased risk of vasoconstriction, causing gangrene, peripheral vascular ischemia, or severe hypertension
ergot alkaloids: Possibly reversed pressor effects of epinephrine
hydrocarbon inhalation anesthetics: Increased risk of severe atrial and ventricular arrhythmias
sympathomimetics: Additive CNS stimulation, increased cardiovascular effects of either drug

Adverse Reactions

CNS: Anxiety, apprehensiveness, chills, **CVA**, disorientation, dizziness, drowsiness, excitability, fever, hallucinations, headache, impaired memory, insomnia, light-headedness, nervousness, panic, psychomotor agitation, restlessness, **seizures**, sleepiness, temporary worsening of Parkinson's disease, tingling, tremor, weakness
CV: Arrhythmias, including ventricular fibrillation; chest discomfort or pain; fast, irregular, or slow heartbeat; palpitations; **severe hypertension**; **stress cardiomyopathy**; tachycardia; vasoconstriction; **ventricular ectopy**
EENT: Blurred vision, dry mouth or throat, miosis
ENDO: Hyperglycemia in diabetics
GI: Anorexia, heartburn, nausea, vomiting
GU: Dysuria
MS: Muscle twitching, severe muscle spasms
RESP: Dyspnea
SKIN: Cold skin, diaphoresis, ecchymosis, flushed or red face or skin, pallor, tissue necrosis
Other: Hyperkalemia; **hypokalemia**; injection-site coldness, hypoesthesia, infections (*Clostridia*), pain, pallor, and stinging

Nursing Considerations

- Use epinephrine with extreme caution in patients with angina, arrhythmias, asthma, degenerative heart disease, or emphysema. Epinephrine's inotropic effect equals that of dopamine and dobutamine; its chronotropic effect exceeds that of both.
- Use drug cautiously in elderly patients and those with cardiovascular disease (other than listed above), diabetes mellitus, hypertension, hyperthyroidism, prostatic hypertrophy, and psychoneurologic disorders.
- Know that if the Adrenalin brand of epinephrine is used during intraocular surgery to induce and maintain mydriasis, the 30-ml multiple-dose vial of the drug should not be used because it contains chlorobutanol, which may be harmful to the corneal endothelium. Also, be aware that the Adrenalin 1-ml single-use vial must be diluted before intraocular use.
- Be aware that some preparations contain sulfites, which may cause allergic-type reactions. However, the presence of sulfites in epinephrine should not deter its use in a patient with anaphylaxis, even if patient is sensitive to sulfites. Monitor patient closely for adverse effects.
- Be aware that the brands, Auvi-Q and Symjepi, are intended for use as emergency supportive therapy only and are not a substitute for immediate medical care.
- Inspect epinephrine solution before use. If it's pink or brown, air has entered a multidose vial. If it's discolored or contains particles, discard it. Also discard unused portions of parenteral epinephrine.
- For injection, inject the drug into the anterolateral aspect of the thigh. Do not use the deltoid muscle because absorption may not be the same. When administering

drug to a child, hold the leg firmly in place and limit movement prior to and during an injection to minimize the risk of injury related to the injection.
- Remember to rotate sites because repeated injections in the same site may cause vasoconstriction and localized necrosis.
- Assess injection site periodically after administration of epinephrine for signs of infection such as persistent redness, swelling, tenderness, or warmth. Report any findings immediately to prescriber because, although rare, serious skin and soft-tissue infections, including myonecrosis and necrotizing fascitis caused by *Clostridia* (gas gangrene), have been reported at the injection site following epinephrine injection.
- Be aware that drug shouldn't be given by intra-arterial injection because marked vasoconstriction may cause gangrene. Also know that accidental injection of the drug into the patient's feet, fingers, or hands may result in loss of blood flow to the affected area.

WARNING **Know that clostridial infections (gas gangrene) have occurred when administered in the buttocks. Know that cleansing the site with alcohol does not kill bacterial spores and therefore does not lower this risk. Also, the drug may be less effective when given there, especially for treating anaphylaxis. Therefore, avoid injecting epinephrine into the buttocks.**

- Monitor patient for potassium imbalances. Initially, hyperkalemia occurs when hepatocytes release potassium. Hypokalemia may quickly follow as skeletal muscles take up potassium.

PATIENT TEACHING

- Teach patient how to use oral inhaler or inhalation solution, as needed.
- Instruct patient using an oral corticosteroid inhaler to use epinephrine inhaler first, wait for 5 minutes, and then use corticosteroid inhaler to increase effectiveness.
- Teach patient and family how to administer epinephrine subcutaneously in an emergency. Tell them to inject drug only into anterolateral aspect of the thigh, through the clothing if necessary. If injecting drug into a child, stress importance of holding the leg firmly in place and limiting movement prior to and during the injection, to prevent injury. Tell them to inspect the site for signs of infection afterward and report if persistent redness, swelling, tenderness, and warmth develop.

WARNING **Instruct patient and family never to give epinephrine in the buttocks, as absorption may be hindered. Also, a serious infection (gas gangrene) may occur if injected in the buttocks. In addition, tell patient and family to inspect the thigh for signs of infection at the injection site and report if persistent redness, swelling, tenderness, and warmth develop.**

- Remind patient or family using the brands Auvi-Q or Symjepi that drug is intended for emergency supportive therapy only. Stress importance of seeking immediate care after drug is administered.
- Explain that solution is light sensitive and should be stored in the carrying case and at room temperature. Tell them not to refrigerate drug and to replace solution if it discolors.
- Caution patient to avoid accidental injecting drug into his fingers, hands, toes, or feet because epinephrine is a strong vasoconstrictor and could cause loss of blood flow to the area, resulting in gangrene. If accidental injection occurs in any of these areas, instruct patient to go immediately to nearest emergency room.
- Advise patient to notify prescriber immediately if he has blurred vision, chest pain, fast or irregular heartbeat, increased sweating, or trouble breathing.
- Inform patient with diabetes that epinephrine may cause hyperglycemia. Inform patient with Parkinson's disease that symptoms may temporarily worsen but this should not deter use of drug.

eplerenone

Inspra

Class and Category

Pharmacologic class: Aldosterone receptor blocker
Therapeutic class: Antihypertensive
Pregnancy category: Not classified

Indications and Dosages

➤ *To improve survival of stable patients with left ventricular systolic dysfunction and congestive heart failure after an acute MI*

TABLETS

Adults. *Initial:* 25 mg daily, increased to 50 mg daily within 4 wk, as needed.

➤ *To treat hypertension alone or with other antihypertensive drugs*

TABLETS

Adults. *Initial:* 50 mg daily, increased to 50 mg twice daily after 4 wk, if needed.

DOSAGE ADJUSTMENT For patients taking moderate CYP450 3A4 inhibitors, such as erythromycin, fluconazole, saquinavir, and verapamil, initial dosage for hypertension reduced to 25 mg daily. If patient's blood pressure is not controlled with this dose, dosing increased to maximum of 25 mg twice daily. For post-MI congestive heart failure patient, maximum dosage is 25 mg once daily. For patients taking eplerenone because of congestive heart failure after an acute MI, dosage adjustment based upon serum potassium levels. If potassium level is less than 5.0 mEq/L and patient is taking 25 mg every other day, dosage interval increased to daily; if patient is taking 25 mg once daily, dosage increased to 50 mg once daily. If potassium level is 5.0 to 5.4 mEq/L, no adjustment needed. If potassium level is between 5.5 and 5.9 mEq/L and patient is taking 50 mg once daily, dosage reduced to 25 mg daily, or if patient is taking 25 mg once daily, dosage interval increased to 25 mg every other day; if already taking 25 mg every other day or potassium level is 6.0 mEq/L or higher, drug withheld until potassium level returns to acceptable level.

Mechanism of Action

Blocks the binding of aldosterone at its mineralocorticoid receptor sites located in the blood vessels, brain, heart, and kidneys. This action decreases blood pressure by preventing aldosterone from inducing sodium reabsorption and possibly other mechanisms that contribute to raising blood pressure.

Contraindications

For all patients: Concurrent therapy with strong CYP3A inhibitors, creatinine clearance 30 ml/min or less, hyperkalemia (greater than 5.5 mEq), hypersensitivity to eplerenone or its components
For patients with hypertension: Concurrent therapy with potassium supplements or potassium-sparing diuretics, creatinine level greater than 2 mg/dl in males and greater than 1.8 mg/dl in females, creatinine clearance greater than 50 ml/min, type 2 diabetes mellitus with microalbuminuria

Interactions

DRUGS

ACE inhibitors, angiotensin II receptor antagonists: Increased risk of hyperkalemia
CYP450 3A4 inhibitors: Increased blood level and effect of eplerenone
lithium: Possibly lithium toxicity
NSAIDs: Possibly reduced antihypertensive effect of eplerenone

FOODS

grapefruit: Possibly increased blood level and effect of eplerenone

Adverse Reactions

CNS: Dizziness, fatigue, headache
CV: Angina pectoris, hypercholesterolemia, hypertriglyceridemia, **MI**
ENDO: Gynecomastia, mastodynia
GI: Abdominal pain, diarrhea, increased liver enzymes
GU: Albuminuria, elevated BUN and serum creatinine levels, vaginal bleeding
RESP: Cough
Other: Flu-like symptoms, **hyperkalemia**, **hyponatremia**, increased uric acid level

Nursing Considerations

- Monitor patient's blood pressure regularly to evaluate eplerenone effectiveness.
- Be aware that patients with diabetes, impaired renal function, or proteinuria or who take an ACE inhibitor or an angiotensin II receptor antagonist during eplerenone therapy have an increased risk of hyperkalemia.
- Monitor patient's serum potassium level every 2 weeks for the first month or two of therapy until the effects of eplerenone are known and monthly thereafter, as ordered. Notify prescriber of abnormalities, as dosage will need to be adjusted.
- Monitor patients over 65 closely, because the risk of hyperkalemia may be increased because of age-related decreases in creatine clearance.

PATIENT TEACHING

- Caution patient not to use potassium salt substitutes or potassium-containing supplements because increased potassium levels can lead to serious adverse reactions to eplerenone.
- Urge patient to tell all prescribers about eplerenone use because of possible interactions.

epoetin alfa

(EPO, erythropoietin alfa, recombinant erythropoietin, r-HuEPO)

Epogen, Eprex (CAN), Procrit

Class and Category

Pharmacologic class: Erythropoietin
Therapeutic class: Antianemic
Pregnancy category: Not classified

Indications and Dosages

➤ *To treat anemia from renal failure*

I.V. OR SUBCUTANEOUS INJECTION

Adults on dialysis but not hemodialysis. *Initial:* 50 to 100 units/kg 3 times/wk, increased as needed by 25% at 4-wk intervals or longer. *Maintenance:* Dosage gradually decreased by 25 units/kg at 4-wk intervals or longer to lowest dose that keeps hemoglobin below 11 g/dl.

Neonates age 1 month and older and children on dialysis. 50 units/kg 3 times/wk; increased as needed by 25% at 4-wk intervals or longer. *Maintenance:* Dosage gradually decreased to lowest dose that keeps hemoglobin below 11 g/dl.

I.V. INJECTION

Adults on hemodialysis. *Initial:* 50 to 100 units/kg 3 times/wk, increased as needed by 25% at 4-wk intervals or longer. *Maintenance:* Dosage gradually decreased by 25 units/kg at 4-wk intervals or longer to lowest dose that keeps hemoglobin below 11 g/dl.

I.V. OR SUBCUTANEOUS INJECTION

Adults not on dialysis. *Initial:* 50 to 100 units/kg 3 times/wk, increased as needed at 4-wk intervals or longer that keeps hemoglobin below 10 g/dl.

Neonates age 1 month and older and children not on dialysis. 50 units/kg 3 times/wk; increased as needed by 25% at 4-wk intervals or longer.

DOSAGE ADJUSTMENT For patients with anemia from renal failure on dialysis, dosage temporarily reduced or drug discontinued if hemoglobin approaches or exceeds 11 g/dl. For patients with anemia from renal failure not on dialysis, dosage temporarily reduced or drug discontinued if hemoglobin exceeds 10 g/dl. For patients with anemia from renal failure with or without dialysis, dosage reduced 25% or more if hemoglobin rises rapidly (more than 1 g/dl in any 2-week period).

➤ *To treat anemia in HIV-infected patients who take zidovudine*

I.V. OR SUBCUTANEOUS INJECTION

Adults with serum erythropoietin level of 500 mU/ml or less who receive 4,200 mg or less of zidovudine/wk. *Initial:* 100 units/kg 3 times/wk, increased by 50 to 100 units/kg every 4 to 8 wk after 8 wk of therapy. *Maintenance:* Dosage gradually titrated to maintain desired response, based on such factors as variations in zidovudine dosage and occurrence of infection or inflammation. If hemoglobin exceeds 12 g/dl, drug withheld and resumed at a dose 25% below the previous dose when hemoglobin has declined to less than 11 g/dl. *Maximum:* 300 units/kg 3 times/wk.

➤ *To treat anemia from chemotherapy*

SUBCUTANEOUS INJECTION

Adults. *Initial:* 150 units/kg 3 times/wk or 40,000 units weekly until completion of a chemotherapy course. Dosage decreased by 25% if hemoglobin level approaches a level needed to avoid RBC transfusion or increases more than 1 g/dl in any 2-wk period. Dose withheld if hemoglobin exceeds a level needed to avoid RBC transfusion and resumed at 25% less than previous dose when hemoglobin approaches a level where RBC transfusions may be required. Dosage increased to 300 units/kg 3 times/wk or 60,000 units weekly after 4 wk if response is inadequate. *Maximum:* 300 units/kg 3 times/wk; or 60,000 units weekly.

I.V. INJECTION

Children ages 5 to 18. 600 units/kg until completion of a chemotherapy course.

Dosage decreased by 25% if hemoglobin level approaches a level needed to avoid RBC transfusion or increases more than 1 g/dl in any 2-wk period. Dose withheld if hemoglobin exceeds a level needed to avoid RBC transfusion, then dose reinitiated at a dose 25% below the previous dose when hemoglobin approaches a level where RBC transfusions may be required. Dosage increased to 900 units/kg weekly after initial 4 wk of therapy if hemoglobin increases by less than 1 g/dl and remains below 10 g/dl. *Maximum:* 60,000 units weekly.

➤ *To reduce the need for blood transfusion in anemic patients having surgery*

SUBCUTANEOUS INJECTION

Adults. 300 units/kg daily for 10 days before surgery, on day of surgery, and 4 days after surgery; or 600 units/kg/wk starting 3 wk before surgery for a total of 3 doses. Dose of 300 units/kg repeated on day of surgery.

Route	Onset	Peak	Duration
I.V., SubQ	In 2–6 wk	In 2 mo	About 2 wk

Mechanism of Action

Stimulates the release of reticulocytes from the bone marrow into the bloodstream, where they develop into mature RBCs.

Incompatibilities

Don't mix epoetin alfa with any other drug.

Contraindications

Breastfeeding (use of multidose vial); hypersensitivity to human albumin or products made from mammal cells or their components; infants or neonates (use of multidose vial); pregnancy (use of multidose vial); uncontrolled hypertension

Interactions

DRUGS

None reported

Adverse Reactions

CNS: Anxiety, asthenia, **CVA**, dizziness, fatigue, fever, headache, insomnia, paresthesia, **seizures**
CV: Chest pain, **congestive heart failure**, **deep vein thrombosis**, edema, hypertension, **MI**, tachycardia, **thromboembolic events**
GI: Constipation, diarrhea, indigestion, nausea, vomiting
GU: UTI
HEME: Polycythemia
MS: Arthralgia, bone pain, muscle weakness
RESP: Cough, dyspnea, **pulmonary congestion**, upper respiratory tract infection
SKIN: **Erythema multiforme**, rash, pruritus, **Stevens–Johnson syndrome**, **toxic epidermal necrolysis**, urticaria
Other: Flu-like symptoms, **hyperkalemia**, injection-site reaction, trunk pain

Nursing Considerations

- Be aware that epoetin alfa shouldn't be given to cancer patients when a cure is anticipated because drug may decrease survival rate and increase tumor progression in patients with certain types of cancers, such as breast, non-small-cell lung, head and neck, lymphoid, and cervical cancers. All prescribers and hospitals must enroll and comply with the ESA APPRISE Oncology program to be able to prescribe and dispense the drug.
- Ensure that patient has received the medication guide and patient instructions for epoetin alfa and that a written acknowledgment of a discussion of the risks involved with this type of therapy has been obtained before first dose is given.
- Evaluate the patient's serum iron level before and during treatment, as ordered. Expect to give an iron supplement (I.V. iron dextran, if needed) because iron requirements rise when erythropoiesis consumes existing iron stores.
- Use epoetin alfa cautiously in patients who have conditions that could decrease or delay response to drug, such as aluminum intoxication, folic acid deficiency, hemolysis, infection, inflammation, iron deficiency, malignant neoplasm, osteitis (fibrosa cystica), or vitamin B_{12} deficiency.
- Also use drug cautiously in patients with cardiovascular disorders caused by hypertension, a history of porphyria or seizures, vascular disease, or a hematologic disorder, such as hypercoagulation, myelodysplastic syndrome, or sickle cell disease.

WARNING Be aware that the multidose vial of epoetin contains benzyl alcohol, which can cause a fatal toxic syndrome in neonates and immature infants characterized by circulatory, CNS, renal, and respiratory impairment and metabolic acidosis. Know that use of multidose vial is contraindicated in infants and neonates and during pregnancy.

- Use lowest possible dose in cancer patients because drug has shortened survival rate and increased tumor progression in patients with certain types of cancers, such as breast, non-small-cell lung, head and neck, and lymphoid cancers. Drug should only be used to treat anemia caused by myelosuppressive chemotherapy in cancer patients.
- Don't shake vial while preparing to avoid denaturing glycoprotein, inactivating drug.
- Discard unused portion of single-dose vial because it contains no preservatives. Discard unused portion of multidose vial after 21 days.
- Be aware that baseline hemoglobin level should be above 10 but below 13 g/dl if drug is given to patient scheduled for surgery. Watch closely throughout surgical period for deep vein thrombosis, especially in patients not receiving prophylactic anticoagulation, because risk increases.
- Evaluate the patient's serum iron level before and during treatment, as ordered. Expect to give an iron supplement (I.V. iron formulation, if needed) because iron requirements rise when erythropoiesis consumes existing iron stores.
- Check hemoglobin levels, as ordered, with twice-weekly measurements recommended for chronic renal failure patients, until stable and then monthly thereafter and weekly measurements recommended for zidovudine-treated HIV-infected and cancer patients.

WARNING Know that hemoglobin shouldn't exceed 11 g/dl when treating anemia in patients with chronic renal failure on dialysis and 10 g/dl for patients not on dialysis. Exceeding these parameters increases risk of life-threatening adverse cardiovascular effects.

- Expect to increase heparin dose if patient receives hemodialysis because epoetin alfa can increase the RBC volume, which could cause clots to form in the dialyzer, hemodialysis vascular access, or both.
- Monitor patient for hypertensive or thrombotic complications, especially if hemoglobin is approaching target goal.
- Monitor patient throughout therapy for skin reactions which may include blistering and skin exfoliation that could be severe. If present, notify prescriber at once and expect drug to be discontinued.

PATIENT TEACHING

- Ensure that patient has been instructed on the serious adverse effects related to epoetin alfa therapy before therapy begins.
- Teach patient how to administer drug and how to dispose of needles properly. Caution him against reusing needles.
- Emphasize the importance of complying with the dosage regimen and keeping follow-up medical appointments and appointments for laboratory tests.
- Encourage patient to eat iron-rich foods.
- Review possible adverse reactions, and urge patient to notify prescriber if he experiences chest pain, headache, hives, rapid heartbeat, rash, seizures, shortness of breath, or swelling. Also inform patient of the possibility of severe skin reactions such as blistering and exfoliation. Stress importance of stopping drug and alerting prescriber immediately if present.
- Advise women of childbearing age to use effective contraception during therapy if pregnancy isn't desired because menses may resume after epoetin alfa therapy.

eprosartan mesylate

Teveten

Class and Category

Pharmacologic class: Angiotensin II receptor blocker (ARB)
Therapeutic class: Antihypertensive
Pregnancy category: D

Indications and Dosages

➤ *To control blood pressure in patients with essential hypertension*

TABLETS

Adults. *Initial:* 600 mg daily. *Usual:* 400 mg to 600 mg once daily or in 2 divided doses. *Maximum:* 800 mg (600 mg in the presence of moderate and severe renal impairment) once daily or in divided doses twice daily.

Mechanism of Action
Blocks the effects of angiotensin II (a potent vasoconstrictor that's part of the renin–angiotensin–aldosterone system) by blocking its binding to angiotensin I receptors in adrenal glands, vascular smooth muscles, and other tissues. This action halts angiotensin II's negative feedback on renin secretion. Thus, circulating renin and angiotensin II levels rise and vascular resistance declines.

Contraindications
Aliskirein use in patients with diabetes or renal impairment (GRF less than 60 ml/min); hypersensitivity to eprosartan or components

Interactions
DRUGS

aliskiren (in patients with diabetes or renal impairment), angiotensin receptor blockers, other ACE inhibitors: Increased risk of hyperkalemia, hypotension, and renal dysfunction
lithium: Possibly increased serum lithium level and lithium toxicity
NSAIDs: Possible decreased renal function in patients who are elderly, volume-depleted, or have a compromised renal function

Adverse Reactions
CNS: Depression, dizziness, drowsiness, fatigue
CV: Angina pectoris, **atrial fibrillation**, **bradycardia**, **extrasystole**, hypertriglyceridemia, **hypotension**, palpitations, tachycardia
EENT: Pharyngitis, rhinitis
GI: Abdominal pain
GU: Oliguria, UTI
MS: Myalgia, **rhabdomyolysis**
RESP: Cough, upper respiratory tract infection

Nursing Considerations
- Watch for excessive hypotension if patient receives other cardiac drugs.
- Expect maximum blood pressure response after about 3 weeks.
- Be aware that, unlike ACE inhibitors, eprosartan doesn't affect bradykinin breakdown and cause the characteristic ACE cough.

PATIENT TEACHING
- Explain that maximum blood pressure response may not occur for 3 to 4 weeks.
- Tell patient that drug may cause dizziness, drowsiness, or very low blood pressure. Urge him to rise slowly to upright position.

WARNING Caution women of childbearing age to use reliable contraception and to notify prescriber immediately if pregnancy is suspected. Eprosartan may cause fetal harm and should be discontinued.

eptifibatide
Integrilin

Class and Category
Pharmacologic class: Glycoprotein IIb/IIIa inhibitor
Therapeutic class: Antiplatelet
Pregnancy category: B

Indications and Dosages
➤ *To treat acute coronary syndrome (unstable angina and non-ST-elevation MI)*

I.V. INFUSION

Adults. *Initial:* 180 mcg/kg over 1 to 2 min as soon as possible after diagnosis. *Maintenance:* 2 mcg/kg/min by continuous infusion starting immediately after initial dose and continuing until discharge or coronary artery bypass grafting, up to 72 hr.

DOSAGE ADJUSTMENT For nondialysis-dependent patient with serum creatinine level less than 50 ml/min, initial bolus remains unchanged at 180 mcg/kg over 1 to 2 minutes as soon as possible after diagnosis but maintenance dosage decreased to 1.0 mcg/kg/min by continuous infusion.

➤ *To treat patients undergoing percutaneous transluminal coronary angioplasty (PTCA), including intracoronary stenting*

I.V. INFUSION

Adults. *Initial:* 180 mcg/kg over 1 to 2 min immediately before procedure followed by second bolus of 180 mcg/kg over 1 to 2 min, 10 min after the first bolus. *Maintenance:* 2 mcg/kg/min by continuous infusion beginning just after initial bolus and continued for at least 12 hr but could be infused up to 24 hr.

DOSAGE ADJUSTMENT For nondialysis-dependent patient with serum creatinine level less than 50 ml/min, initial bolus remains unchanged at 180 mcg/kg over 1 to 2 minutes immediately before procedure, immediately followed by a continuous infusion of 1.0 mcg/kg/min, and a second 180 mcg/kg bolus administered 10 minutes after the first.

Route	Onset	Peak	Duration
I.V.	Immediate	In 15 min	4–8 hr

Mechanism of Action

Reversibly inhibits platelet aggregation by preventing fibrinogen, von Willebrand factor, and other adhesive ligands from binding to glycoprotein IIb/IIIa receptors on activated platelets. As a result, eptifibatide disrupts final cross-linking stage of platelet aggregation—and thrombus formation.

Incompatibilities

Don't administer eptifibatide through the same I.V. line as furosemide.

Contraindications

Active bleeding, bleeding diathesis, or stroke during prior 30 days, dependency on dialysis, history of hemorrhagic stroke, hypersensitivity to eptifibatide or its components, major surgery during previous 4 weeks, severe uncontrolled hypertension (systolic pressure above 200 mm Hg, diastolic pressure above 110 mm Hg), thrombocytopenia (platelet count below 100,000/mm^3)

Interactions

DRUGS

anticoagulants, clopidogrel, dipyridamole, NSAIDs, thrombolytics, ticlopidine: Additive pharmacologic effects, increased risk of bleeding

other platelet aggregation inhibitors (especially inhibitors of platelet receptor glycoprotein IIb/IIIa, such as abciximab): Increased risk of additive pharmacologic effects

Adverse Reactions

CNS: **Intracranial hemorrhage**
CV: **Hypotension**
GI: **GI hemorrhage, hematemesis**
GU: Hematuria
HEME: **Bleeding that may be severe**, decreased hemoglobin level, **immune-mediated thrombocytopenia, thrombocytopenia**
RESP: **Pulmonary hemorrhage**
Other: **Anaphylaxis**

Nursing Considerations

- Expect to obtain APTT and PT as a baseline and hematocrit and hemoglobin, platelet count, and serum creatinine during therapy
- Withdraw bolus dose of eptifibatide from a 10-ml (2 mg/ml) vial into a syringe.
- Using vented I.V. infusion set, give continuous infusion directly from the 100-ml (0.75 mg/ml) vial. Be sure to center the spike in the circle on top of vial stopper.
- Expect to keep APTT between 50 and 70 seconds or per facility protocol during therapy unless patient has PTCA.
- Be aware that if patient has PTCA, expect to maintain activated clotting time between 200 and 250 seconds during the procedure.
- Avoid arterial and venous punctures, I.M. injections, urinary catheters, nasotracheal or nasogastric intubation, and use of noncompressible I.V. sites, such as subclavian and jugular veins during therapy.
- Expect to discontinue eptifibatide and heparin and monitor patient closely if platelet count falls below 100,000/mm^3.
- Plan to stop drug, as prescribed, if patient undergoes coronary artery bypass surgery.

PATIENT TEACHING

- Instruct patient to immediately report bleeding during eptifibatide therapy.
- Reassure patient that he'll be monitored closely throughout therapy.
- Advise patient to avoid activities that may lead to bruising and bleeding.

eravacycline

Xerava

Class and Category

Pharmacologic class: Synthetic tetracycline
Therapeutic class: Antibiotic
Pregnancy category: Not classified

Indications and Dosages

➤ *To treat complicated intra-abdominal infections caused by* Bacteroides *species,* Citrobacter freundii, Clostridium perfringens, Enterobacter cloacae, Enterococcus faecalis, Enterococcus faecium, Escherichia coli, Klebsiella oxytoca, Klebsiella pneumoniae, Parabacteroides distasonis, Staphylococcus aureus, *or* Streptococcus anginosus *group*

I.V. INFUSION

Adults. 1 mg/kg infused over 60 min every 12 hr for 4 to 14 days.

DOSAGE ADJUSTMENT For patient with severe hepatic impairment, 1 mg/kg administered every 12 hr on day 1 followed by 1 mg/kg every 24 hr starting on day 2 for up to 14 days.

Mechanism of Action

Passes through the bacterial lipid bilayer, where it binds reversibly to 30S ribosomal subunits to block the binding of aminoacyl transfer RNA to messenger RNA. This inhibits bacterial protein synthesis.

Incompatibilities

Do not infuse with any other drugs or solutions except for 0.9% sodium chloride injection, USP

Contraindications

Hypersensitivity to eravacycline, tetracycline-class antibacterials, or their components

Interactions

DRUGS

anticoagulants: Possibly depressed plasma prothrombin activity

strong CYP3A inducers: Decreased exposure of eravacycline with possible decreased effectiveness

Adverse Reactions

CNS: Anxiety, depression, dizziness, insomnia

CV: Chest pain, **hypotension**, palpitations

EENT: Distorted sense of taste, tooth discoloration

GI: Acute pancreatitis, *Clostridium difficile*–associated diarrhea, elevated liver enzymes, nausea, **pancreatic necrosis**, vomiting

GU: Elevated creatinine

HEME: Decreased white blood cell count, neutropenia, prolonged activated partial thromboplastin time

MS: Inhibited bone growth

RESP: Dyspnea, pleural effusion

SKIN: Excessive sweating, rash

Other: Anaphylaxis, hypocalcemia, infusion-site reactions

Nursing Considerations

- Be aware that drug may cause permanent tooth discoloration if given during tooth development and therefore should be avoided in pregnant women during the last half of the pregnancy.
- Reconstitute 50-mg vial with 5 ml sterile water for injection. Gently swirl vial until powder is completely dissolved. Do not shake solution, to avoid foaming. Reconstituted solution should appear clear and pale yellow to orange. Further dilute in an 0.9% sodium chloride infusion bag to a target concentration of 0.3 mg/ml. Do not shake the diluted bag. Infuse over 60 min. Infuse within 6 hours of preparation if stored at room temperature or within 24 hours if refrigerated.

WARNING Monitor patient for hypersensitivity reactions, which could become life-threatening. If an allergic reaction occurs, stop eravacycline immediately, notify prescriber, and provide emergency care as prescribed.

- Assess patient for signs of secondary infection, such as profuse, watery diarrhea. If such diarrhea develops, contact prescriber and expect drug to be withheld if pseudomembranous colitis caused by *Clostridium difficile* occurs. Be prepared to treat with electrolyte replacement, fluids, and protein as well as an antibiotic effective against *C. difficile.*

PATIENT TEACHING

- Instruct patient to immediately report any signs of an allergic reaction.
- Urge patient to notify prescriber if diarrhea develops, even 2 months or more after eravacycline therapy has been discontinued.
- Inform pregnant women to notify prescriber if pregnant, because eravacycline may cause permanent tooth

discoloration if given during the second and third trimesters of pregnancy.
- Advise women not to breastfeed during eravacycline therapy and for 4 days after the last dose of eravacycline.

erenumab-aooe

Aimovig

Class and Category

Pharmacologic class: Human monoclonal antibody
Therapeutic class: Antimigraine
Pregnancy category: Not classified

Indications and Dosages

➤ *To prevent migraine headaches*

SUBCUTANEOUS INJECTION

Adults. 70 mg to 140 mg (given as two 70-mg consecutive injections) monthly.

Route	Onset	Peak	Duration
SQ	Unknown	4 to 6 days	Unknown

Mechanism of Action

Binds to the calcitonin gene-related peptide (CGRP) receptor. The CGRP receptor is thought to be responsible for transmitting signals that can cause incapacitating pain. By binding to the CGRP receptor, the drug antagonizes its function, preventing pain signals from being transmitted.

Contraindications

Hypersensitivity to erenumab-aooe or its components

Interactions

DRUGS

None reported

Adverse Reactions

GI: Constipation
MS: Muscle cramps or spasms
Other: Erenumab-aooe antibody formation, injection-site reactions (erythema, pain, pruritus)

Nursing Considerations

- Be aware that the needle shield within the white cap of the prefilled autoinjector and the gray needle cap of the prefilled syringe contain dry natural rubber, a derivative of latex. Handling the caps may cause allergic reactions in individuals sensitive to latex.
- Allow erenumab-aooe to sit at room temperature for at least 30 minutes protected from direct sunlight prior to administration. Drug should not be warmed by using a heat source such as hot water or a microwave. Do not shake the product. Inspect solution for discoloration or particulate matter prior to administration. Do not use if solution is cloudy or discolored or contains flakes or particles.
- Administer in the abdomen, thigh, or upper arm subcutaneously. Do not inject into areas where the skin is bruised, hard, red, or tender.
- Monitor effectiveness of drug to relieve migraine headaches.

PATIENT TEACHING

- Instruct patient how to prepare and administer erenumab-aooe as a subcutaneous injection using the single-dose prefilled autoinjector or single-dose prefilled syringe.
- Warn patient that the needle shield within the white cap of the prefilled autoinjector and the gray needle cap of the prefilled syringe contain dry natural rubber, a derivative of latex. Handling the caps may cause allergic reactions in individuals sensitive to latex.
- Tell patient to allow drug to sit at room temperature for at least 30 minutes protected from direct sunlight. Caution patient not to warm drug by using a heat source such as hot water or a microwave. Also caution patient not to shake the syringe. Instruct patient to inspect solution for discoloration or particulate matter prior to administration. Tell him not to use solution if it is cloudy or discolored or contains flakes or particles. Remind him that both the prefilled autoinjector and prefilled syringe are single-dose and to deliver the entire contents with each injection.
- Inform patient prescribed the 140-mg dose to administer the drug once a month as two separate but consecutive subcutaneous injections of 70 mg each.

- Instruct patient to administer the injection in the abdomen, thigh, or upper arm subcutaneously. Advise patient not to inject into areas where the skin is bruised, hard, red, or tender.
- Inform patient that drug may cause injection-site reactions such as itching, pain, or redness. Also tell patient that muscle cramps or spasms may occur, as well as constipation.
- Instruct patient that if a dose is missed, he should administer drug as soon as possible. Thereafter, drug can be given monthly from the date of that dose.

ertapenem sodium

Invanz

Class and Category

Pharmacologic class: Carbapenem
Therapeutic class: Antibiotic
Pregnancy category: B

Indications and Dosages

➤ *To treat moderate to severe infections, such as acute pelvic infections (including postpartum endomyometritis, postsurgical gynecologic infections, or septic abortion) due to* Bacteroides fragilis, Escherichia coli, Peptostretococcus *species,* Prevotella bivia, Porphyromonas asaccharolytica, *or* Streptococcus agalactiae; *community-acquired pneumonia due to* Haemophilus influenzae *(beta-lactamase-negative strains only),* Moraxella catarrhalis, *or* Streptococcus pneumoniae *(penicillin-susceptible strains only, including cases with concurrent bacteremia); complicated intra-abdominal infections due to* B. distasonis, B. fragilis, B. ovatus, B. thetaiotaomicron, B. uniformis, Clostridium clostridioforme, E. coli, Eubacterium lentum, *or* Peptostreptococcus *species; complicated skin and skin-structure infections, including diabetic foot infections without osteomyelitis, due to* staphylococcus aureus *(methicillin-susceptible strains only),* Streptococcus pyogenes, E. coli, *or* Peptostreptococcus *species; and complicated UTI (including pyelonephritis) due to* E. coli *(including cases with concurrent bacteremia) or* Klebsiella pneumoniae

I.V. INFUSION

Adults and adolescents. 1 g daily, infused over 30 min, for up to 14 days.
Children ages 3 months to 13 years. 15 mg/kg twice daily, infused over 30 min, for up to 14 days. *Maximum:* 1 g daily.

I.M. INJECTION

Adults and adolescents. 1 g daily for up to 7 days.
Children ages 3 months to 13 years. 15 mg/kg twice daily for up to 7 days. *Maximum:* 1 g daily.

➤ *To provide prophylaxis of surgical site infection following elective colorectal surgery*

I.V. INFUSION

Adults. 1 g infused over 30 min, given 1 hr prior to surgical incision.

DOSAGE ADJUSTMENT Dosage decreased to 500 mg daily for patients with advanced renal insufficiency (creatinine clearance less than or equal to 30 ml/min) or end-stage renal insufficiency (creatinine clearance less than or equal to 10 ml/min). For patients on hemodialysis who have received 500 mg of ertapenem within 6 hr of hemodialysis, supplemental dose of 150 mg given after hemodialysis.

Mechanism of Action

Inhibits bacterial cell wall synthesis by binding to specific penicillin-binding proteins inside the cell wall. Penicillin-binding proteins are responsible for various steps in bacterial cell wall synthesis. By binding to these proteins, ertapenem leads to bacterial cell wall lysis.

Incompatibilities

Don't mix ertapenem with other drugs. Don't dilute it with solutions containing dextrose.

Contraindications

Hypersensitivity to ertapenem, beta-lactams, other drugs in the same class, or their components; hypersensitivity to local anesthetics of the amide type

Interactions

DRUGS

probenecid: Increased ertapenem half-life, increased and prolonged blood ertapenem level *valproic acid:* Possibly decreased serum valproic acid level and increased risk of breakthrough seizures

Adverse Reactions

CNS: Abnormal coordination, aggression, agitation, anxiety, asthenia, confusion, delirium, depressed level of consciousness, disorientation, dizziness, dyskinesia, fatigue, fever, gait disturbance, hallucinations, headache, hypothermia, insomnia, mental changes, myoclonus, **seizures**, somnolence, stupor, tremor
CV: Chest pain, edema, hypertension, **hypotension**, tachycardia, thrombophlebitis
EENT: Nasopharyngitis, oral candidiasis, rhinitis, rhinorrhea, teeth staining, viral pharyngitis
ENDO: Hyperglycemia
GI: Abdominal pain, acid regurgitation, anorexia, ***Clostridium difficile*-associated diarrhea**, constipation, diarrhea, elevated liver enzymes, indigestion, nausea, **small intestine obstruction**, vomiting
GU: Dysuria, elevated serum creatinine level, genital rash, proteinuria, RBCs and WBCs in urine, UTI, vaginitis
HEME: Anemia, decreased hematocrit, eosinophilia, leukocytosis, **leukopenia**, **neutropenia**, **prolonged PT**, **thrombocytopenia**, thrombocytosis
MS: Arthralgia, leg pain, muscle weakness
RESP: **Atelectasis**, cough, crackles, dyspnea, pleural effusion, pneumonia, **respiratory distress**, upper respiratory tract infection, wheezing
SKIN: Cellulitis, dermatitis, erythema, extravasation, pruritus, rash
Other: **Anaphylaxis**, **death**, **drug reaction with eosinophilia and systemic symptoms (DRESS)**, **hyperkalemia**, **hypokalemia**, infusion-site induration, pain, phlebitis, pruritus, redness, swelling, or warmth

Nursing Considerations

- Obtain sputum, urine, or other specimens for culture and sensitivity testing, as ordered, before giving ertapenem. Expect to start therapy before results are available.
- For I.V. use, know that when preparing drug for I.V. use, reconstitute 1 g with 10 ml of sterile water for injection, 0.9% sodium chloride injection, or bacteriostatic water for injection. Don't use solutions that contain dextrose. Shake well to dissolve. Immediately transfer reconstituted drug to 50 ml normal saline solution. Use within 6 hours if stored at room temperature, 24 hours if refrigerated at 5° C (41° F). Don't freeze. Give I.V. infusion over 30 minutes.
- Inspect drug for particles and discoloration after reconstitution.
- For I.M. injection, reconstitute 1 g of drug with 3.2 ml of 1% lidocaine hydrochloride injection (without epinephrine). Shake thoroughly to form solution. Use within 1 hour after preparation. Withdraw contents of vial and inject deep into a large muscle mass such as the gluteal muscle.

WARNING **Don't give reconstituted I.M. solution by I.V. route because of possible adverse reaction to lidocaine hydrochloride injection used to reconstitute drug.**

- Monitor patient closely for a life-threatening anaphylactic reaction. Patients with a history of hypersensitivity to cephalosporins, penicillin, other allergens or other beta-lactams are at increased risk.

WARNING **Know that if drug triggers an anaphylactic reaction, stop drug, notify prescriber immediately, and provide appropriate therapy. Anaphylaxis requires immediate treatment with epinephrine as well as airway management and administration of I.V. corticosteroids and oxygen, as needed.**

- Be aware that patients with a history of seizures, other CNS disorders that predispose them to seizures (such as brain lesions), or compromised renal function may be at increased risk for seizures. Administer anticonvulsant, as ordered.
- Monitor patient for diarrhea during and for at least 2 months after drug therapy; diarrhea may signal pseudomembranous colitis caused by *C. difficile*. If diarrhea occurs, notify prescriber and expect to withhold ertapenem and treat with an antibiotic effective against *C. difficile*, electrolytes, fluids, and protein.
- Be aware that because ertapenem is excreted in breast milk, its use by nursing mothers should be carefully evaluated.

PATIENT TEACHING

- Instruct patient receiving ertapenem to immediately report signs of anaphylaxis, such as itching, rash, or shortness of breath; or signs of superinfection, such as

severe diarrhea or white patches on tongue or in mouth.
- Urge patient to tell prescriber about diarrhea that's severe or lasts longer than 3 days. Remind patient that watery or bloody stools can occur 2 or more months after antibiotic therapy and can be serious, requiring prompt treatment.
- Alert patient taking divalproex or valproic acid for seizure control to notify prescriber of this type of concurrent therapy because ertapenem may interfere with these drugs' effectiveness to control seizures.

ertugliflozin

Steglatro

Class and Category

Pharmacologic class: Sodium glucose-dependent cotransporter inhibitor
Therapeutic class: Antidiabetic
Pregnancy category: Not classified

Indications and Dosages

➤ *As adjunct to improve glycemic control in patients with type 2 diabetes mellitus*

TABLETS

Adults. *Initial:* 5 mg once daily in morning, increased as needed. *Maximum:* 15 mg once daily.

Route	Onset	Peak	Duration
P.O.	Unknown	1 hr	Unknown

Mechanism of Action

Inhibits sodium glucose link transporter-2 to reduce renal reabsorption of filtered glucose and lower the renal threshold for glucose. These actions increase urinary glucose excretion and lower blood glucose levels.

Contraindications

Dialysis, end-stage renal disease, hypersensitivity to ertugliflozin or its components, severe renal impairment, type I diabetes mellitus

Interactions

DRUGS

insulin, insulin secretagogues: Increased risk of hypoglycemia

Adverse Reactions

CNS: Headache, thirst
CV: Elevated low-density lipoprotein cholesterol, **hypotension**
EENT: Nasopharyngitis
ENDO: Ketoacidosis
GU: Acute kidney injury and impairment, **acute prerenal failure**, decreased estimated glomerular filtration rate, elevated serum creatinine levels, genital mycotic infections, increased urination, **necrotizing fasciitis of the perineum (Fournier's gangrene)**, pyelonephritis, **urosepsis**, UTI, vaginal pruritus
HEME: Increased hemoglobin level
MS: Back pain
Other: Dehydration, elevated serum phosphate level, **hyperphosphatemia**, weight loss

Nursing Considerations

- Know that volume depletion should be corrected before ertugliflozin therapy is begun.
- Assess patient for factors that may predispose patient to acute kidney injury before ertugliflozin therapy is begun. Risk factors may include presence of chronic renal insufficiency, congestive heart failure, and hypovolemia and use of drugs such as ACE inhibitors, ARBs, diuretics, and NSAIDs.
- Review patient's history for any risk factors that may predispose patient to need a lower-limb amputation, such as presence of diabetic foot ulcers, neuropathy, peripheral vascular disease, or a prior amputation, before ertugliflozin therapy is begun. This is because an increased risk for lower-limb amputation has been found with another drug in the same class as ertugliflozin.
- Monitor patient's blood pressure closely because ertugliflozin causes intravascular volume contraction. Those at greater risk include the elderly and patients with impaired renal function or low systolic blood pressure or with concomitant use of diuretics.

WARNING **Monitor patient for signs and symptoms of metabolic acidosis. If present, also assess patient for ketoacidosis. Know that patient may have ketoacidosis even if her blood glucose level is less than 250 mg/dl. If ketoacidosis is suspected, notify prescriber. If**

confirmed, expect ertugliflozin to be discontinued and treatment with carbohydrate, fluid, and insulin replacement to be given.

- Expect ertugliflozin to be withheld when oral intake is reduced, such as in acute illness or fasting, or when fluid losses occur, such as excessive heat exposure or gastrointestinal illness. This is because dehydration increases risk of kidney impairment that could be quite serious.
- Monitor patient for signs and symptoms of infection, new pain or tenderness, sores, or ulcers involving the lower limbs. If present, notify prescriber and expect drug to be discontinued.
- Monitor patients also receiving insulin or an insulin secretagogue such as a sulfonylurea for hypoglycemia. Dosage of these drugs may have to be reduced to minimize the risk of hypoglycemia.
- Assess both men and women for genital mycotic infections, which may occur with ertugliflozin therapy. Patients at higher risk include those with a history of genital mycotic infections or men who are uncircumcised.

WARNING **Monitor patient for a rare but serious and life-threatening necrotizing infection of the perineum called Fournier's gangrene. Notify prescriber immediately if patient develops erythema, pain, swelling, or tenderness in the genital or perineal area, along with fever or malaise. Expect treatment with broad-spectrum antibiotics and, if needed, surgical debridement of the area. Know that ertugliflozin will be discontinued if this occurs. Monitor patient's blood glucose levels closely and expect an alternative treatment for glycemic control.**

PATIENT TEACHING

- Advise patient to take ertugliflozin exactly as prescribed. Tell her if a dose is missed to take it as soon as it's remembered unless it is close to the next dose. Warn patient never to double the dose.
- Inform patients also prescribed insulin or antidiabetic agents known to cause hypoglycemia to monitor blood glucose level closely, as hypoglycemia may occur. Also review the signs and symptoms of hypoglycemia and how to treat.
- Instruct patient to maintain adequate fluid intake, as dehydration increases the risk of the blood pressure dropping. Advise patient to notify prescriber if he experiences dizziness or light-headedness and weakness.

WARNING **Teach patient how to check urine for ketones and review signs and symptoms of ketoacidosis with patient. Remind patient that ketoacidosis may occur even when her blood glucose is not elevated. Tell patient to seek immediate medical attention if she experiences abdominal pain, labored breathing, nausea, tiredness, and vomiting and ketones are present in urine.**

- Instruct patient to report any persistent, severe, or unusual signs and symptoms to prescriber, especially if changes in kidney function occur.
- Inform patient of the potential for an increased risk of amputations. Review preventative foot care with patient. Tell patient to report any infection, new pain or tenderness, sore, or ulcer involving the foot or leg to prescriber and seek immediate medical attention.
- Tell patient to seek medical care if a urinary tract infection occurs, because it can become serious if left untreated.
- Review signs and symptoms of genital mycotic infection such as itching, rash, or redness in the area. Tell patient to notify prescriber if present.

WARNING Warn patient to stop ertugliflozin and seek immediate medical attention if pain, redness, swelling, or tenderness occurs in the genital or perineal area along with fever or malaise because, although rare, this cluster of symptoms may become life-threatening.

- Remind patient to monitor her diabetes by testing blood glucose, as she will test positive for glucose in the urine while taking ertugliflozin.
- Advise women of childbearing age to notify prescriber if pregnancy occurs, because ertugliflozin therapy is not recommended during the second and third trimesters of pregnancy.
- Tell women considering breastfeeding that it is not recommended during ertugliflozin therapy because of the potential to cause harm to fetus or neonate's developing kidneys.

erythromycin

(contains 250, 333, or 500 mg of base per delayed-release capsule, delayed-release tablet, or tablet)
Apo-Erythro (CAN), E-Mycin, Erybid (CAN), ERYC, Ery-Tab, Ilotycin, Novo-Rythro Encap (CAN), PCE

erythromycin ethylsuccinate

(contains 1 g of base per 1.6 g of oral suspension or tablet)
Apo-Erythro-ES (CAN), E.E.S., EryPed

erythromycin lactobionate

(contains 500 or 1,000 mg of base per vial)
Erythrocin

erythromycin stearate

(contains 125 or 250 mg of base per 5 ml of oral suspension, or 250 or 500 mg of base per tablet)
Erythro-S (CAN), Erythrocin, Stearate

Class and Category

Pharmacologic class: Macrolide
Therapeutic class: Antibiotic
Pregnancy category: B

Indications and Dosages

➤ *To treat mild to moderate respiratory tract infections caused by* Haemophilus influenzae, Streptococcus pneumoniae, *or* Streptococcus pyogenes *(group A beta-hemolytic streptococcus)*

CAPSULES, CHEWABLE TABLETS, DELAYED-RELEASE CAPSULES, DELAYED-RELEASE TABLETS, ORAL SUSPENSION, TABLETS

Adults. 250 to 500 mg (base) or 400 mg to 800 mg (ethylsuccinate) every 6 hr for 10 days.
Children. 30 to 50 mg (base)/kg daily in divided doses every 6 hr for 10 days. For *H. influenzae* infections, erythromycin ethylsuccinate is administered with 150 mg/kg daily of sulfisoxazole.

➤ *To treat severe respiratory tract infections caused by* H. influenzae, S. pneumoniae, *or* S. pyogenes *(group A beta-hemolytic streptococcus)*

I.V. INFUSION

Adults. 1 to 4 g daily continuously or in divided doses infused over 20 to 60 min every 6 hr for 10 days.
Children. 15 to 20 mg/kg daily in divided doses infused over 20 to 60 min every 4 to 6 hr for 10 days.

➤ *To treat respiratory tract infections caused by* Mycoplasma pneumoniae

CAPSULES, CHEWABLE TABLETS, DELAYED-RELEASE CAPSULES, DELAYED-RELEASE TABLETS, ORAL SUSPENSION, TABLETS

Adults with mild to moderate infection. 250 to 500 mg (base) every 6 hr for up to 3 wk.

➤ *To treat skin and soft-tissue infections caused by* S. pyogenes *or* Staphylococcus aureus

CAPSULES, CHEWABLE TABLETS, DELAYED-RELEASE CAPSULES, DELAYED-RELEASE TABLETS, ORAL SUSPENSION, TABLETS

Adults with mild to moderate infection. 250 mg to 500 mg or 400 mg to 800 g (ethylsuccinate) every 6 hr.

I.V. INFUSION

Adults with severe infection. 1 to 4 g daily continuously or in divided doses infused over 20 to 60 min every 6 hr for up to 3 wk.

➤ *To treat pertussis (whooping cough) caused by* Bordetella pertussis

CAPSULES, CHEWABLE TABLETS, DELAYED-RELEASE CAPSULES, DELAYED-RELEASE TABLETS, ORAL SUSPENSION, TABLETS

Children. 40 to 50 mg (base)/kg daily in divided doses every 6 hr for 5 to 14 days.

➤ *To treat intestinal amebiasis caused by* Entamoeba histolytica

CAPSULES, CHEWABLE TABLETS, DELAYED-RELEASE CAPSULES, DELAYED-RELEASE TABLETS, ORAL SUSPENSION, TABLETS

Adults. 250 mg (base) or 400 mg (ethylsuccinate) every 6 hr or 500 mg every 12 hr for 10 to 14 days.

Children. 30 to 50 mg (base or ethylsuccinate)/kg daily in divided doses for 10 to 14 days.

➤ *To treat pelvic inflammatory disease caused by* Neisseria gonorrhoeae

CAPSULES, CHEWABLE TABLETS, DELAYED-RELEASE CAPSULES, DELAYED-RELEASE TABLETS, ORAL SUSPENSION, TABLETS, I.V. INFUSION

Adults. 500 mg (base) I.V. infused over 20 to 60 min every 6 hr for 3 days and then 250 mg to 500 mg (base) P.O. every 6 hr for 7 days.

➤ *To treat conjunctivitis in newborns*

I.V. INFUSION, ORAL SUSPENSION

Neonates. 50 mg (base)/kg daily in 4 divided doses for 14 days.

➤ *To treat pneumonia in neonates*

I.V. INFUSION

Neonates. 15 to 20 mg/kg daily continuously or in divided doses infused over 20 to 60 min every 6 hr.

ORAL SUSPENSION

Neonates. 50 mg/kg daily in 4 divided doses for at least 3 wk.

➤ *To treat urogenital infections caused by* Chlamydia trachomatis *during pregnancy*

CAPSULES, CHEWABLE TABLETS, DELAYED-RELEASE CAPSULES, DELAYED-RELEASE TABLETS, ORAL SUSPENSION, TABLETS

Adults. 500 mg (base) on an empty stomach every 6 hr for 7 days; or 250 mg (base) on an empty stomach every 6 hr for at least 14 days.

➤ *To treat nongonococcal urethritis or uncomplicated urethral, endocervical, or rectal infections caused by* C. trachomatis

CAPSULES, CHEWABLE TABLETS, DELAYED-RELEASE CAPSULES, DELAYED-RELEASE TABLETS, ORAL SUSPENSION, TABLETS

Adults. 500 mg (base) every 6 hr for 7 days. If patient can't tolerate high doses, 250 mg (base) every 6 hr for 14 days.

➤ *To treat Legionnaire's disease*

CAPSULES, CHEWABLE TABLETS, DELAYED-RELEASE CAPSULES, DELAYED-RELEASE TABLETS, ORAL SUSPENSION, TABLETS, I.V. INFUSION

Adults. 1 to 4 g (base) daily in divided doses every 6 hr for 10 to 14 days. I.V. dosage infused continuously or, if dosage is divided, infused over 20 to 60 min for each dose.

➤ *To prevent rheumatic fever*

CAPSULES, CHEWABLE TABLETS, DELAYED-RELEASE CAPSULES, DELAYED-RELEASE TABLETS, ORAL SUSPENSION, TABLETS

Adults. 250 mg (base) every 12 hr.

➤ *To prevent bacterial endocarditis in patients with penicillin allergy who plan dental or upper respiratory tract surgery*

CAPSULES, CHEWABLE TABLETS, DELAYED-RELEASE CAPSULES, DELAYED-RELEASE TABLETS, ORAL SUSPENSION, TABLETS

Adults. 1 g (base) or 800 mg (ethylsuccinate) given 2 hr before procedure and then 500 mg (base) 6 hr after initial dose.

Children. 20 mg (base or ethylsuccinate)/kg given 2 hr before procedure and then 10 mg (base)/kg 6 hr after initial dose.

Mechanism of Action

Binds with the 50S ribosomal subunit of the 70S ribosome in many types of aerobic, anaerobic, gram-negative, and gram-positive. This action inhibits RNA-dependent protein synthesis in bacterial cells, causing them to die.

Contraindications

Astemizole, cisapride, lovastatin, pimozide, simvastatin, or terfenadine therapy; hypersensitivity to erythromycin, other macrolide antibiotics, or their components

Interactions

DRUGS

alfentanil: Decreased alfentanil clearance, prolonged alfentanil action

astemizole, cisapride, terfenadine: Increased risk of cardiotoxicity, torsades de pointes, ventricular tachycardia, and death

carbamazepine, valproic acid: Possibly inhibited metabolism of these drugs, increasing their blood levels and risk of toxicity

chloramphenicol, lincomycins: Antagonized effects of these drugs

colchicine: Possible life-threatening colchicine toxicity

cyclosporine: Increased risk of nephro-toxicity

digoxin: Increased serum digoxin level and risk of digitalis toxicity

dihydroergotamine, ergotamine: Decreased ergotamine metabolism, increased risk of vasospasm from ergotamine use

HMG-CoA reductase inhibitors such as lovastatin, simvastatin: Possibly increased risk of rhabdomyolysis
midazolam, triazolam: Increased pharmacologic effects of these drugs
oral anticoagulants: Increased anticoagulant effects, especially in the elderly
oral contraceptives: Failed contraception
sildenafil: Increased effects of sildenafil
verapamil: Increased risk of bradyarrhythmias, hypotension, and lactic acidosis
xanthines (except dyphylline): Increased serum theophylline level and risk of theophylline toxicity

ACTIVITIES

alcohol use: Increased alcohol level (by 40%) with I.V. erythromycin

Adverse Reactions

CNS: Fatigue, fever, malaise, weakness
CV: **Prolonged QT interval**, **torsades de pointes**, **ventricular arrhythmias**
EENT: Hearing loss, oral candidiasis
GI: Abdominal cramps and pain, diarrhea, **hepatotoxicity**, nausea, **pseudomembranous colitis**, vomiting
GU: Interstitial nephritis, jaundice, vaginal candidiasis
MS: New or aggravated myasthenia gravis syndrome
SKIN: Erythema, pruritus, rash
Other: Fluid overload (from I.V. infusion), injection-site inflammation and phlebitis

Nursing Considerations

- Be aware that erythromycin should not be used in patients with history of QT-interval prolongation or in patients with ongoing proarrhythmic conditions such as uncorrected hypokalemia or hypomagnesemia, serious bradycardia, and in patients receiving Class IA or Class III antiarrhythmic agents. Monitor the elderly closely as well because they are more susceptible to drug effects on the QT interval.
- Use erythromycin cautiously in patients with impaired hepatic function because drug is metabolized by the liver.
- Use erythromycin cautiously in elderly patients, especially those with renal or hepatic dysfunction, because these patients are at increased risk of hearing loss and torsades de pointes. They're also at increased risk of bleeding if taking an oral anticoagulant.
- Expect to obtain body fluid or tissue sample for culture and sensitivity testing before giving first erythromycin dose.
- Reconstitute parenteral form before administration. Add at least 10 ml of preservative-free sterile water for injection to each 500-mg vial or at least 20 ml of diluent to each 1-g vial.
- For prolonged infusion, expect to infuse a buffered solution up to 24 hours after dilution.
- For intermittent infusion, dilute dose in 100 to 250 ml normal saline solution or D_5W if needed; give slowly over 20 to 60 minutes.
- When giving I.V. erythromycin lactobionate, dilute the solution, if needed, to 1 to 5 mg/ml in normal saline solution, lactated Ringer's solution, or other electrolyte solution for slow, continuous infusion. Diluted solution remains potent for 14 days if refrigerated and for 24 hours at room temperature.
- Be aware that infusions prepared in piggyback infusion bottles stay potent for 30 days if frozen, 24 hours if refrigerated, or 8 hours at room temperature. Don't store infusions prepared in the ADD-Vantage system.
- Don't use diluent with benzyl alcohol if parenteral erythromycin is for a neonate. It may cause a fatal toxic syndrome of CNS depression, hypotension, metabolic acidosis, renal failure, respiratory problems, and, possibly, intracranial hemorrhage and seizures.
- Monitor liver enzymes periodically to detect hepatotoxicity, which is most common with erythromycin estolate. Signs typically appear within 2 weeks after continuous therapy starts and resolve when it stops.
- Assess hearing regularly, especially in elderly patients and those who receive 4 g or more daily or have hepatic or renal disease. Hearing impairment begins 36 hours to 8 days after treatment starts and usually begins to improve 1 to 14 days after it stops.
- Watch for evidence of fluid overload, such as acute dyspnea and crackles, during I.V. therapy.
- Monitor infants for vomiting or irritability with feeding because infantile

hypertrophic pyloric stenosis has been reported.
- Assess myasthenia gravis patients for weakness because drug may aggravate it. Keep in mind that myasthenic syndrome may arise in patients previously undiagnosed with myasthenia gravis.
- Watch closely for signs and symptoms of superinfection. If they occur, notify prescriber and expect to stop drug and provide appropriate therapy.
- Monitor patient for diarrhea during and for at least 2 months after erythromycin therapy; diarrhea may signal pseudomembranous colitis caused by *Clostridium difficile.* If diarrhea occurs, notify prescriber and expect to withhold drug and treat with fluids, electrolytes, protein, and an antibiotic effective against *C. difficile.*
- Know that if patient receives an order for urine catecholamine analysis, notify prescriber because erythromycin interferes with fluorometric measurement of urine catecholamines.

PATIENT TEACHING
- Urge patient to complete prescribed therapy, even if he feels better before it's finished.
- Tell patient to notify prescriber if symptoms worsen or don't improve after a few days.
- Teach patient how to administer prescribed form of erythromycin. Instruct him to swallow capsules or tablets whole. For an oral suspension, teach him to use the calibrated measuring device provided to ensure accurate doses. Remind him to shake the suspension before measuring a dose.
- Advise patient to take oral form of erythromycin with a full glass of water on an empty stomach (except erythromycin ethylsuccinate, which is better absorbed with food).
- Instruct patient to take oral form with food if GI distress occurs.
- Instruct patient to promptly notify prescriber if he develops allergic reactions, hearing changes, or signs of hepatic dysfunction.
- Urge patient to tell prescriber about diarrhea that's severe or lasts longer than 3 days. Remind patient that watery or bloody stools can occur 2 or more months after antibiotic therapy and can be serious, requiring prompt treatment.

escitalopram oxalate

Lexapro

Class and Category

Pharmacologic class: Selective serotonin reuptake inhibitor (SSRI)
Therapeutic class: Antidepressant
Pregnancy category: C

Indications and Dosages

➤ *To treat generalized anxiety disorder*

ORAL SOLUTION, TABLETS

Adults. *Initial:* 10 mg daily in morning or evening, increased to 20 mg daily after 1 or more wk, as needed.

➤ *To treat major depression*

ORAL SOLUTION, TABLETS

Adults. *Initial:* 10 mg daily, morning or evening, increased to 20 mg daily after 1 wk, as needed.

Adolescents ages 12 to 17. *Initial:* 10 mg daily, morning or evening, increased to 20 mg daily after 3 wk, as needed.

DOSAGE ADJUSTMENT Dosage shouldn't exceed 10 mg daily for elderly patients and those with hepatic impairment.

Mechanism of Action

Inhibits reuptake of the neurotransmitter serotonin by CNS neurons, thereby increasing the amount of serotonin available in nerve synapses. An elevated serotonin level may result in elevated mood and reduced anxiety or depression.

Contraindications

Concomitant therapy with pimozide, hypersensitivity to escitalopram, citalopram or its components; use within 14 days of MAO inhibitor therapy

Interactions

DRUGS

aspirin, NSAIDs, warfarin: Possibly increased risk of bleeding
carbamazepine: Possibly increased clearance of escitalopram
cimetidine: Possibly increased plasma escitalopram level
CNS drugs: Additive CNS effects

E F

lithium: Possible enhancement of the serotonergic effects of escitalopram
MAO inhibitors: Possibly hyperpyretic episodes, hypertensive crisis, serotonin syndrome, and severe seizures
metoprolol: Increased plasma metoprolol levels with decreased cardioselectivity of metoprolol
sumatriptan: Increased risk of hyperreflexia, incoordination, and weakness
triptans: Increased risk of serotonin syndrome

ACTIVITIES

alcohol use: Possibly increased cognitive and motor effects of alcohol

Adverse Reactions

CNS: Abnormal gait, acute psychosis, aggression, akathisia, delirium, dizziness, dyskinesia, dystonia, extrapyramidal effects, fatigue, headache, hypomania, insomnia, lethargy, mania, myoclonus, **neuroleptic malignant syndrome**, paresthesia, **seizures**, **serotonin syndrome**, somnolence, **suicidal ideation**
CV: **Atrial fibrillation**, **cardiac failure**, **deep vein thrombosis**, **hypotension**, **MI**, **prolonged QT interval**, **torsades de pointes**, **ventricular arrhythmias**
EENT: Acute-angle glaucoma, diplopia, dry mouth, nystagmus, rhinitis, sinusitis, toothache, visual hallucinations
ENDO: Diabetes mellitus, hyperprolactinemia, syndrome of inappropriate ADH secretion
GI: Abdominal pain, constipation, decreased appetite, diarrhea, flatulence, **GI bleeding or hemorrhage**, **hepatic necrosis**, **hepatitis**, indigestion, nausea, **pancreatitis**, **rectal hemorrhage**, vomiting
GU: **Acute renal failure**, anorgasmia, decreased libido, ejaculation disorders, impotence, priapism
HEME: **Bleeding**, **decreased prothrombin time**, **hemolytic anemia**, **leukopenia**, **thrombocytopenia**
MS: Neck or shoulder pain, **rhabdomyolysis**
RESP: **Pulmonary embolism**
SKIN: Ecchymosis, **erythema multiforme**, increased sweating, photosensitivity, **Stevens–Johnson syndrome**, **toxic epidermal necrolysis**, urticaria
Other: **Anaphylaxis**, **angioedema**, flu-like symptoms, **hyponatremia**

Nursing Considerations

- Use escitalopram cautiously in patients with history of mania or seizures, patients with severe renal impairment, and those with diseases or conditions that produce altered metabolism or hemodynamic responses.

WARNING Know that when escitalopram dosage increases, monitor patient for possible serotonin syndrome, which may include agitation, chills, confusion, diaphoresis, diarrhea, fever, hyperactive reflexes, poor coordination, restlessness, shaking, talking or acting with uncontrolled excitement, tremor, and twitching. In its most severe form, serotonin syndrome can resemble neuroleptic malignant syndrome, which includes autonomic instability with possible changes in vital signs, a high fever, muscle rigidity, and mental status changes.

- Be aware that escitalopram should not be given to patients with bradycardia, congenital long QT syndrome, hypokalemia or hypomagnesemia, recent acute myocardial infarction, or uncompensated heart failure because of increased risk of prolonged QT interval and torsades de pointes. It should also not be given to patients who are taking other drugs that prolong the QT interval. Expect hypokalemia and hypomagnesemia to be corrected before escitalopram therapy is begun.
- Monitor patient—especially elderly patient—for hypo-osmolarity of serum and urine and for hyponatremia (headache, impaired memory, trouble concentrating, unsteadiness, weakness) because they may indicate escitalopram-induced syndrome of inappropriate ADH secretion.
- Watch for signs of abuse or misuse; drug's potential for physical and psychological dependence is unknown.
- Monitor patient for bleeding, especially if patient is also taking an anticoagulant, aspirin, or an NSAID. Bleeding can range from ecchymoses, epistaxis, hematomas, and petechiae to life-threatening hemorrhages.
- Expect prescriber to reassess patient periodically to determine the continued need for therapy and evaluate dosage.

- Know that if patient (particularly an adolescent) takes escitalopram for depression, she must be watched closely for suicidal tendencies, especially when therapy starts or dosage changes, because depression may worsen temporarily.
- Expect to taper dosage to avoid serious adverse reactions when therapy is no longer needed.

PATIENT TEACHING

- Inform patient that alcohol use isn't recommended during escitalopram therapy because it may decrease his ability to think clearly and perform motor skills.
- Advise patient to avoid hazardous activities until drug's CNS effects are known.
- Instruct patient that drug shouldn't be taken with citalopram hydrobromide because of potentially additive effects.
- Tell patient that improvement may not be noticed for 1 to 4 weeks after therapy begins. Emphasize the importance of continuing therapy as prescribed.
- Urge caregivers to watch closely for suicidal tendencies, especially when therapy starts or dosage changes.
- Warn patient not to stop taking drug abruptly. Explain that gradual tapering helps to avoid withdrawal symptoms.
- Urge patient to inform prescriber of any OTC drugs he takes because of potential for interactions.
- Review signs and symptoms of hyponatremia, and instruct patient to report them to prescriber.
- Advise patient that drug may cause mild pupillary dilation, which may lead to an episode of acute-angle glaucoma. Encourage patient to have an eye exam before starting therapy to see if he is at risk.
- Warn patient that escitalopram increases bleeding risk if taken with an anticoagulant, aspirin, or an NSAID and that bleeding events could range from mild to severe. Tell patient to seek emergency care for serious or prolonged bleeding.
- Instruct patient to notify prescriber promptly of any persistent, severe, or unusual signs and symptoms.

eslicarbazepine acetate

Aptiom

Class and Category

Pharmacologic class: Carboxamide derivative
Therapeutic class: Anticonvulsant
Pregnancy category: Not classified

Indications and Dosages

➤ *Adjunct or monotherapy to treat partial-onset seizures*

TABLETS

Adults. *Initial*: 400 or 800 mg once daily, increased weekly in increments of 400 to 600 mg, as needed. *Maintenance*: 800 mg once daily when used as monotherapy and patient unable to tolerate a 1,200 mg daily dose; 1,600 mg once daily when used as adjunctive therapy and patient did not achieve a satisfactory response with a 1,200 mg daily dose. *Maximum*: 1,600 mg once daily.
Children age 4 to 17 weighing more than 38 kg (83.6 lb). *Initial:* 400 mg once daily, increased as needed by no more than 400 mg weekly. *Maintenance:* 800 to 1,200 mg daily. *Maximum:* 1,200 mg daily.
Children age 4 to 17 weighing 32 kg (70.4 lb) to 38 kg (83.6 lb). *Initial:* 300 mg once daily, increased as needed by no more than 300 mg weekly. *Maintenance:* 600 to 900 mg daily. *Maximum:* 900 mg daily.
Children age 4 to 17 weighing 22 kg (48.4 lb) to 31 kg (68.2 lb). *Initial:* 300 mg once daily, increased as needed by no more than 300 mg weekly. *Maintenance:* 500 to 800 mg daily. *Maximum:* 800 mg daily.
Children age 4 to 17 weighing 11 kg (24.2 lb) to 21 kg (46.2 lb). *Initial:* 200 mg once daily, increased as needed by no more than 200 mg weekly. *Maintenance:* 400 to 600 mg daily. *Maximum:* 600 mg daily.

DOSAGE ADJUSTMENT For patients with moderate and severe renal impairment (creatinine clearance less than 50 ml/min), dosage decreased by half beginning with initial dosage. For patients receiving carbamazepine, phenobarbital, phenytoin, or primidone concomitantly, dosage may have to be increased.

Mechanism of Action

Possibly inhibits voltage-gated sodium channels to exert anticonvulsant effect.

Contraindications

Hypersensitivity to eslicarbazepine acetate or oxcarbazepine and their components

Interactions

DRUGS

carbamazepine, phenobarbital, phenytoin, primidone: Decreased plasma concentration of eslicarbazepine
clobazam, omeprazole, phenytoin: Increased plasma levels of these drugs
lovastatin, simvastatin: Decreased plasma concentration of these drugs
oral contraceptives: Decreased effectiveness of oral contraceptives

Adverse Reactions

CNS: Amnesia, aphasia, asthenia, ataxia, attention deficits, confusion, coordination abnormality, depression, disorientation, dizziness, fatigue, gait disturbance, headache, insomnia, lethargy, malaise, memory impairment, psychomotor disturbances, somnolence, **suicidal ideation**, tremor, vertigo
CV: Hypertension, peripheral edema
EENT: Blurred vision, diplopia, impaired vision, nystagmus
ENDO: Decreased serum T3 and T4 levels, syndrome of inappropriate antidiuretic hormone secretion
GI: Abdominal pain, constipation, diarrhea, elevated liver enzymes, gastritis, **liver dysfunction**, nausea, vomiting
GU: UTI
HEME: Agranulocytosis, leukopenia, megaloblastic anemia, **pancytopenia, thrombocytopenia**
MS: Dysarthria
RESP: Cough
SKIN: Rash, **Stevens–Johnson syndrome, toxic epidermal necrolysis**
Other: Anaphylaxis, angioedema, drug reaction with eosinophilia and systemic symptoms (DRESS), hypochloremia, **hyponatremia**

Nursing Considerations

WARNING Monitor patient closely for adverse reactions because many of them are serious and some can become life threatening, such as DRESS multi-organ hypersensitivity. Notify prescriber immediately, expect drug to be discontinued, and provide emergency supportive care, as ordered.

- Monitor patient closely for evidence of suicidal thinking or behavior, especially when therapy starts or dosage changes.
- Monitor patient's electrolytes, especially sodium level, as ordered. Hyponatremia may occur as an adverse reaction to eslicarbazepine therapy, especially in the elderly and patients treated with diuretics. Assess patient regularly for signs and symptoms of hyponatremia such as confusion, difficulty concentrating, headache, memory impairment, unsteadiness, and weakness. If present, notify prescriber and expect drug to be discontinued.
- Withdraw eslicarbazepine slowly when discontinued and as ordered to minimize risk of seizures and status epilepticus.

PATIENT TEACHING

- Instruct patient to take eslicarbazepine exactly as prescribed and not to abruptly stop taking drug without consulting prescriber.
- Warn patient about possible dizziness and unsteadiness that may develop while taking eslicarbazepine. Discourage performing hazardous activities such as driving until the neurologic effects of the drug are known.

WARNING Tell patient to discontinue drug immediately and seek emergency medical care if patient develops difficulty breathing, fever, or a rash or experiences facial or throat swelling. Also instruct patient to promptly report other skin reactions such as blistering or exfoliation or other persistent, severe, or unusual signs and symptoms.

- Instruct caregivers to watch patient closely for evidence of suicidal tendencies, especially when therapy starts or dosage changes, and to report such tendencies to prescriber immediately.
- Tell female patients taking oral contraceptives to use additional or alternative nonhormonal birth control. Encourage patient to enroll in the North American Antiepileptic Drug Pregnancy

Registry if pregnancy occurs, by calling 1-888-233-2334.

- Advise patient to report symptoms of low sodium such as confusion, irritability, muscle weakness or spasms, tiredness, or more frequent or severe seizure activity.

esmolol hydrochloride

Brevibloc

Class and Category

Pharmacologic class: Beta blocker
Therapeutic class: Antiarrhythmic, antihypertensive
Pregnancy category: Not classified

Indications and Dosages

➤ *To treat supraventricular tachycardia including atrial fibrillation and atrial flutter; to control heart rate in noncompensatory sinus tachycardia*

I.V. INFUSION

Adults. *Loading:* 500 mcg/kg over 1 min. *Maintenance:* If response to loading dose is adequate after 5 min, 50 mcg/kg/min infused for 4 min. If response is inadequate after 5 min, another 500 mcg/kg may be given over 1 min followed by 100 mcg/kg/min for 4 min. Sequence repeated, as needed, until adequate response occurs, increasing maintenance dosage by 50 mcg/kg/min at each step. *Maximum:* 200 mcg/kg/min for 48 hr.

➤ *To treat intraoperative and postoperative tachycardia and hypertension*

I.V. INFUSION

Adults. *For immediate control:* 1 mg/kg over 30 sec, followed by 150 mcg/kg/min, if needed. *For gradual control:* 500 mcg/kg over 1 min, then 50 mcg/kg/min infused over 4 min. If response is inadequate after 5 min, another 500 mcg/kg may be given over 1 min followed by 100 mcg/kg/min for 4 min. Sequence repeated, as needed, up to 4 times, increasing by 50 mcg/kg/min each time. *Maximum:* 200 mcg/kg/min for tachycardia; 300 mcg/kg/min for hypertension.

DOSAGE ADJUSTMENT Loading doses omitted, increments decreased to 25 mcg/kg/min, and titration intervals increased to 10 min as heart rate approaches desired level or if blood pressure decreases too much.

Route	Onset	Peak	Duration
I.V.	Immediate	Unknown	10–20 min

Mechanism of Action

Inhibits stimulation of beta$_1$ receptors mainly in the heart, which decreases cardiac excitability, cardiac output, and myocardial oxygen demand. Esmolol also decreases renin release from kidneys, which helps reduce blood pressure.

Incompatibilities

Don't mix esmolol with 5% sodium bicarbonate injection.

Contraindications

Cardiogenic shock; decompensated heart failure; hypersensitivity to esmolol, other beta blockers and their components; I.V. administration of cardiodepressant calcium-channel anagonists (i.e., verapamil) and esmolol close together while cardiac effects from other drug are still present; pulmonary hypertension; second- or third-degree heart block; severe sinus bradycardia

Interactions

DRUGS

calcium channel antagonists: Increased risk of fatal cardiac arrest in patients with depressed myocardial function
clonidine, guanfacine, moxonidine: Increased risk of withdrawal rebound hypertension
digitalis glycosides: Increased risk of bradycardia
mivacurium: Increased risk of moderately prolonged duration and recovery of mivacurium index
positive inotropic and vasoconstrictive agents such as dopamine, epinephrine, or norepinephrine: Increased risk of reducing cardiac contractility in presence of high systemic resistance
succinylcholine: Prolonged duration of succinylcholine-induced blockade
sympathomimetics, xanthine derivatives: Possibly inhibited therapeutic effects of both drugs

E F

Adverse Reactions

CNS: Anxiety, confusion, depression, dizziness, fatigue, fever, headache, syncope
CV: **Bradycardia**, chest pain, decreased peripheral circulation, **heart block**, **hypotension**
GI: Nausea, vomiting
RESP: Dyspnea, wheezing
SKIN: Diaphoresis, flushing, pallor
Other: Infusion-site pain, redness, and swelling

Nursing Considerations

- Use esmolol cautiously if patient has supraventricular arrhythmias with decreased cardiac output, hypotension, or other hemodynamic compromise or is taking drugs that decrease contractility, impulse generation, myocardial filling, or peripheral resistance.
- Also use drug cautiously in patients with impaired renal function because drug is excreted by the kidneys. Patients with end-stage renal disease have an increased risk of adverse reactions.
- Be aware that esmolol should not be given for intraoperative or postoperative hypertension caused by hypothermia-induced vasoconstriction.
- Expect to give lowest possible dose to patients with allergies, asthma, bronchitis, or emphysema. If patient develops bronchospasm, expect to discontinue infusion immediately and give a beta$_2$-stimulating drug, as ordered.
- Don't give 250 mg/ml (2,500 mg/10 ml) dosage strength by direct I.V. push. Dilute it to a 10-mg/ml infusion by first removing 20 ml from 500 ml of a compatible I.V. solution, such as D_5W or dextrose 5% in normal saline solution, and then adding 5 g of esmolol to the solution.
- Use diluted solution within 24 hours if stored at room temperature.
- Use 100-mg vial (prediluted to 10 mg/ml) for loading dose. For 70-kg (154-lb) patient, loading dose for 500 mcg/kg/min is 3.5 ml.
- Monitor blood pressure and heart rate often during therapy. Hypotension can occur at any dose but usually is dose related. It typically reverses within 30 minutes after dose is decreased or infusion stopped.
- Inspect site often for thrombophlebitis (pain, redness, swelling at site). Infusion of 20 mg/ml is more likely to cause serious vein irritation than 10 mg/ml. Extravasation of 20 mg/ml may cause a serious local reaction and skin necrosis. Don't give more than 10 mg/ml into a small vein or using a butterfly catheter.

PATIENT TEACHING

- Urge patient to report adverse reactions immediately.
- Reassure patient that his blood pressure, heart rate, and response to therapy will be monitored throughout esmolol therapy.

esomeprazole magnesium

Nexium, Nexium 24 HR

esomeprazole sodium

Nexium I.V.

esomeprazole strontium

Class and Category

Pharmacologic class: Proton pump inhibitor
Therapeutic class: Antiulcerative
Pregnancy category: C

Indications and Dosages

➤ *To treat symptomatic gastroesophageal reflux disease (GERD)*

DELAYED-RELEASE CAPSULES, DELAYED-RELEASE SUSPENSION (NEXIUM)

Adults. 20 mg daily for 4 wk. *Maintenance:* 20 mg daily for up to 6 months.
Adolescents ages 12 to 17. 20 mg once daily for 4 wk.
Children ages 1 to 11. 10 mg once daily for up to 8 wk.

DELAYED-RELEASE CAPSULES (ESOMEPRAZOLE STRONTIUM)

Adults. 24.65 mg once daily for 4 wk.

➤ *To promote healing of erosive esophagitis in patient with GERD*

DELAYED-RELEASE CAPSULES, DELAYED-RELEASE SUSPENSION (NEXIUM)
Adults. 20 or 40 mg once daily for 4 to 8 wk, with cycle repeated once more if healing has not taken place after first 8 wk. *Maintenance:* 20 mg once daily for up to 6 months.
Adolescents ages 12 to 17. 20 or 40 mg once daily for 4 to 8 wk.
Children ages 1 to 11 weighing 20 kg(44 lb) or more. 10 or 20 mg once daily for 8 wk.
Children ages 1 to 11 weighing less than 20 kg (44 lb). 10 mg once daily for 8 wk.
Infants age 1 month to less than 1 year weighing 7.5 (16.5 lb)to 12 kg (26.4 lb). 10 mg once daily for up to 6 wk.
Infants age 1 month to less than 1 year weighing 5 kg (11 lb) to 7.5 kg (16.5 lb). 5 mg once daily for up to 6 wk.
Infants age 1 month to less than 1 year weighing 3 kg (6.6 lb)to 5 kg (11 lb). 2.5 mg once daily for up to 6 wk.
DELAYED-RELEASE CAPSULES (ESOMEPRAZOLE STRONTIUM)
Adults. 24.65 or 49.3 mg once daily for 4 to 8 wk, with cycle repeated once more if healing has not taken place after first 8 wk. *Maintenance*: 24.65 mg once daily for up to 6 months.

➤ *To treat GERD in a patient with erosive esophagitis who can't take the drug by mouth*

I.V. INJECTION
Adults. 20 or 40 mg daily injected over no less than 3 min with switch to oral therapy as soon as possible.
I.V. INFUSION
Adults. 20 or 40 mg daily infused over 10 to 30 min with switch to oral therapy as soon as possible.
Children ages 1 to 17 weighing 55 kg (121 lb) or more. 20 mg daily infused over 10 to 30 min with switch to oral therapy as soon as possible.
Children ages 1 to 17 weighing less than 55 kg (121 lb). 10 mg daily infused over 10 to 30 min with switch to oral therapy as soon as possible.
Children ages 1 month to less than 1 year. 0.5 mg/kg daily infused over 10 to 30 min with switch to oral therapy as soon as possible.
DOSAGE ADJUSTMENT For adult patient with severe liver impairment, dosage should not exceed 20 mg daily.
I.V. INJECTION
Adults. 20 or 40 mg daily given over no less than 3 min.

➤ *As adjunct to treat duodenal ulcer associated with* Helicobacter pylori

DELAYED-RELEASE CAPSULES (NEXIUM), DELAYED-RELEASE SUSPENSION (NEXIUM)
Adults. 40 mg daily with amoxicillin 1,000 mg twice a day and clarithromycin 500 mg twice a day for 10 days.
DELAYED-RELEASE CAPSULES (ESOMEPRAZOLE STRONTIUM)
Adults. 49.3 mg once daily with amoxicillin 1,000 mg twice daily and clarithromycin 500 mg twice daily for 10 days.

➤ *To reduce the risk of gastric ulcer formation in patients who are receiving continuous NSAID therapy and who either are over age 60 or have a history of gastric ulcer*

DELAYED-RELEASE CAPSULES (NEXIUM), DELAYED-RELEASE SUSPENSION (NEXIUM)
Adults. 20 or 40 mg daily for up to 6 months.
DELAYED-RELEASE CAPSULES (ESOMEPRAZOLE STRONTIUM)
Adults. 24.65 or 49.3 mg once daily for up to 6 months.

➤ *To treat pathological hypersecretory conditions, including Zollinger–Ellison syndrome*

DELAYED-RELEASE CAPSULES, DELAYED-RELEASE SUSPENSION
Adults. 40 mg twice daily.
DOSAGE ADJUSTMENT For patients with severe hepatic insufficiency, maximum 20 mg daily.
DELAYED-RELEASE CAPSULES (ESOMEPRAZOLE STRONTIUM)
Adults. 49.3 mg twice daily.

➤ *To reduce risk of rebleeding of duodenal or gastric ulcers following therapeutic endoscopy for acute-bleeding duodenal or gastric ulcers*

I.V. INFUSION
Adults. 80 mg over 30 min followed by 8 mg per hour for 71.5 hr after initial 30-min dose is completed.
DOSAGE ADJUSTMENT For patients with mild to moderate liver impairment, maximum continuous infusion should not exceed 6 mg/hr; for patients with severe liver impairment, maximum continuous infusion should not exceed 4 mg/hr.

Mechanism of Action

Interferes with gastric acid secretion by inhibiting the hydrogen–potassium–adenosine triphosphatase (H^+–K^+–ATPase) enzyme system, or proton pump, in gastric parietal cells. Normally, the proton pump uses energy from hydrolysis of ATPase to drive H^+ and chloride (Cl^-) out of parietal cells and into the stomach lumen in exchange for potassium (K^+), which leaves the stomach lumen and enters parietal cells. After this exchange, H^+ and Cl^- combine in the stomach to form hydrochloric acid (HCl). Esomeprazole irreversibly inhibits the final step in gastric acid production by blocking exchange of intracellular H^+ and extracellular K^+, thus preventing H^+ from entering the stomach and additional HCl from forming.

Incompatibilities

Don't give esomeprazole with any other drug through the same I.V. site or tubing.

Contraindications

Hypersensitivity to esomeprazole, substituted benzimidazoles, or their components

Interactions

DRUGS

atazanavir, erlotinib, ketoconazole, iron salts, mycophenolate mofetil, nelfinavir: Decreased blood levels of these drugs
cilostazol: Possibly increased blood cilostazol levels
clopidogrel: Reduced effectiveness of clopidogrel
diazepam: Possibly increased diazepam level
digoxin: Possibly increased absorption of digoxin
methotrexate: Increased risk of methotrexate toxicities
rifampin, St. John's wort: Decreased blood esomeprazole level
saquinavir: Increased plasma saquinavir level with increased toxicity
tacrolimus: Increased serum tacrolimus level
voriconazole: Increased esomeprazole exposure and risk of adverse effects
warfarin: Possibly increased INR and PT, leading to abnormal bleeding

FOODS

all foods: Decreased bioavailability of esomeprazole

Adverse Reactions

CNS: Agitation, aggression, depression, dizziness, fever, headache, hallucinations, **hepatic encephalopathy**
EENT: Blurred vision, dry mouth, mucosal discoloration, sinusitis, stomatitis, taste disturbance
ENDO: Gynecomastia
GI: Abdominal pain; Barrett's esophagus; benign polyps or nodules; candidiasis; ***Clostridium difficile*-associated diarrhea**; constipation; diarrhea; duodenitis; dyspepsia; esophagitis; esophageal stricture, ulceration, or varices; flatulence; fundic gland polyps; gastric ulcer; gastritis; **hepatic failure**; **hepatitis**; jaundice; microscopic colitis; nausea; **pancreatitis**
GU: Interstitial nephritis
HEME: Agranulocytosis, pancytopenia
MS: Bone fracture, muscle weakness, myalgia
RESP: Bronchospasm, respiratory tract infection
SKIN: Alopecia, cutaneous lupus erythematosus, diaphoresis, **erythema multiforme**, photosensitivity, pruritus, **Stevens–Johnson syndrome**, **toxic epidermal necrolysis**
Other: Anaphylaxis, cyanocobalamin deficiency (prolonged use), **hypocalcemia**, **hypokalemia**, **hypomagnesemia**, infusion-site redness or pruritus, systemic lupus erythematosus, vitamin B_{12} deficiency

Nursing Considerations

- Give oral esomeprazole at least 1 hour before meals because food decreases bioavailability.
- Use delayed-release capsules or oral suspension specific for nasogastric tube administration and delayed-release oral suspension specific for nasogastric or gastric tube administration when administering esomeprazole to a patient with a nasogastric or gastric tube.

WARNING Be aware that if patient takes drug with amoxicillin or clarithromycin for *H. pylori*-related ulcer, severe diarrhea

may indicate pseudomembranous colitis. Obtain stool cultures, as ordered.
- Always flush I.V. line with normal saline solution injection, lactated Ringer's injection, or 5% dextrose injection before and after giving esomeprazole intravenously.
- For I.V. injection used to treat GERD in patients who cannot take oral esomeprazole, reconstitute powder with 5 ml of normal saline solution injection and give as a bolus dose over 3 or more minutes. Once reconstituted, drug may be stored at room temperature for up to 12 hours.
- For I.V. infusion for adults treated for GERD and unable to take esomeprazole by mouth, reconstitute powder with 5 ml of normal saline solution injection, lactated Ringer's injection, or 5% dextrose injection. Further dilute reconstituted solution to make a final volume of 50 ml, and infuse over 10 to 30 minutes. Reconstituted drug may be stored at room temperature up to 6 hours if mixed with 5% dextrose injection or up to 12 hours if mixed with normal saline solution or lactated Ringer's injection.
- For I.V. infusion for children treated for GERD who are unable to take esomeprazole by mouth, reconstitute powder with 5 ml of 0.9% sodium chloride injection. Further dilute reconstituted solution with 0.9% sodium chloride injection to make final volume of 50 ml. Using a 40-mg vial, the final concentration will be 0.8 mg/ml. Using a 20-mg vial, the final concentration will be 0.4 mg/ml. Infuse over 10 to 30 minutes. Reconstituted drug may be stored at room temperature for up to 12 hours.
- For I.V. infusion used for adults to reduce risk of rebleeding of duodenal or gastric ulcers following therapeutic endoscopy, prepare the loading dose of 80 mg by reconstituting two 40-mg vials. Reconstitute each vial with 5 ml of 0.9% sodium chloride injection, then further dilute the contents of the two vials in 100 ml of 0.9% sodium chloride injection. Administer over 30 minutes. Prepare the continuous infusion in the same manner but administer over 71.5 hours at a rate of 8 mg/hr or decrease rate to 6 mg/hr for mild to moderate liver impairment and to 4 mg/hr for severe liver impairment, as ordered.
- Be aware that patient receiving I.V. esomeprazole should be switched to oral form as soon as possible.
- Monitor patients for bone fractures, especially in patients who are receiving multiple daily doses for a year or longer as proton pump inhibitors such as esomeprazole have been associated with an increased risk for osteoporosis-related fractures of the hip, spine, or wrist.
- Monitor patient's magnesium level, as ordered, because hypomagnesemia may occur with esomeprazole therapy that has lasted longer than 3 months, although most cases have occurred after therapy had been given for more than a year. Notify prescriber if magnesium level drops below normal as hypomagnesemia may cause tetany, arrhythmias, and seizures. Expect patient to receive magnesium replacement and esomeprazole to be discontinued.
- Be aware that esomeprazole therapy may need to be temporarily halted for at least 14 days if patient is undergoing testing for neuroendocrine tumors because drug may cause false positive results in diagnostic testing.
- Monitor patient for diarrhea, because esomeprazole therapy may increase the risk of *Clostridium difficile*–associated diarrhea. Know that the lowest dose possible for the shortest amount of time should be used to decrease this risk. If diarrhea occurs, expect to obtain a stool specimen to determine if diarrhea is *C. difficile* so that it may be treated appropriately.
- Monitor patient for signs and symptoms of cutaneous and systemic lupus erythematosus or exacerbation of these conditions if already present. Notify prescriber if present and expect serological testing to be done. If results are positive, expect drug to be discontinued. Symptoms are usually relieved in most patients within 4 to 12 weeks.
- Be aware that patients who take esomeprazole long term, especially after 1

year, are at increased risk for developing fundic gland polyps.

PATIENT TEACHING

- Inform patient that drug should be taken at the lowest dose possible and for the shortest time to decrease risk of adverse effects. Tell him he should never increase dosage or take it long term without consulting prescriber.
- Tell patient that if he has trouble swallowing esomeprazole capsules, tell him to open capsule and sprinkle pellets into a tablespoon of cool applesauce. Tell him not to chew pellets and to discard any unused pellets.
- Remind patient that esomeprazole, including the over-the-counter preparation, is not intended for immediate relief of heartburn; the drug may take up to 4 days before the full effect is experienced.
- Instruct patient to seek immediate medical attention if he experiences an allergic reaction to esomeprazole.
- Urge patient to tell prescriber if he takes antacids or any other OTC or prescription drug.
- Advise patient to contact prescriber if he develops abdominal pain, diarrhea, and fever that does not improve, especially if he has recently taken or is taking an antibiotic. Also advise patient to report any other persistent or serious signs and symptoms that occur while taking esomeprazole. Instruct patient to stop taking drug if he develops joint pain or rash and to see his doctor for an evaluation of these symptoms.
- Advise patient that drug may increase risk for osteoporosis-related fractures of the hip, spine, or wrist. Instruct him to take fall precautions and have bone health evaluated regularly.

estazolam

Class, Category, and Schedule

Pharmacologic class: Benzodiazepine
Therapeutic class: Sedative-hypnotic
Pregnancy category: X
Controlled substance schedule: IV

Indications and Dosages

➤ *To treat insomnia short-term*

TABLETS

Adults. 1 to 2 mg at bedtime.
DOSAGE ADJUSTMENT Starting dose 0.5 mg for small or debilitated elderly patients.

Route	Onset	Peak	Duration
P.O.	Unknown	Unknown	6–8 hr

Mechanism of Action

May potentiate effects of gamma-aminobutyric acid (GABA) and other inhibitory neurotransmitters by binding to specific benzodiazepine receptors in limbic and cortical areas of CNS. By binding to these receptors, estazolam increases GABA's inhibitory effects and blocks cortical and limbic arousal.

Contraindications

Concurrent therapy with itraconazole or ketoconazole; hypersensitivity to estazolam, other benzodiazepines, or their components; pregnancy

Interactions

DRUGS

anticonvulsants, antihistamines, barbiturates, CNS depressants, MAO inhibitors, narcotics, phenothiazines, psychotropics: Possibly potentiated action of estazolam
barbiturates, carbamazepine, phenytoin, rifampin: Possibly decreased estazolam level
carbamazepine: Possibly increased blood carbamazepine level
cimetidine, diltiazem, fluvoxamine, isoniazid, itraconazole, ketoconazole, nefazodone, selected macrolide antibiotics: Possibly increased blood level and impaired hepatic metabolism of estazolam
opioids: Possibly significant respiratory depression and sedation

ACTIVITIES

alcohol use: Possibly potentiated CNS depression, including respiratory depression and sedation
smoking: Increased clearance of estazolam

Adverse Reactions

CNS: Amnesia, anxiety, ataxia, confusion, delusions, depression, dizziness, drowsiness, euphoria, headache, hypokinesia, irritability, malaise, nervousness, slurred speech, tremor
CV: Chest pain, palpitations, tachycardia
EENT: Blurred vision, dry mouth, increased salivation, photophobia
GI: Abdominal pain, constipation, diarrhea, nausea, thirst, vomiting
GU: Libido changes
RESP: **Respiratory depression**
SKIN: Diaphoresis
Other: Physical or psychological dependence

Nursing Considerations

- Use estazolam with extreme caution in patients with a history of alcohol or drug abuse because of risk of addiction. Expect to give drug for no more than 12 weeks.
- Use cautiously in debilitated or elderly patients and those with depression or impaired hepatic, renal, or respiratory function.
- Expect to stop drug gradually to prevent withdrawal symptoms. Avoid stopping abruptly if patient has history of seizures.
- Monitor respiratory status, especially in patients with respiratory compromise, who are at increased risk for respiratory depression.
- Be aware that if patient takes estazolam for depression, watch for suicidal tendencies, especially when therapy starts or dosage changes.

PATIENT TEACHING

- Warn patient not to exceed prescribed time because of risk of addiction.
- Advise patient to avoid hazardous activities until CNS effects of the drug are known.
- Advise patient not to drink alcohol or take other CNS depressants during therapy because of the risk of additive effects.
- Warn debilitated or elderly patients and those with impaired hepatic or renal function about risk of excessive sedation or mental impairment and need to report them.
- Tell patient that if he takes 2-mg dosage for a long time, he should not stop drug abruptly.

estradiol

Divigel 1%, Estrace, Estrasorb, Estring, Estrogel, Evamist, Imvexxy, Vagifem

estradiol acetate

Femring, Femtrace

estradiol cypionate

Depo-Estradiol

estradiol transdermal system

Alora, Climara, Estraderm, Estrasorb, Estrogel, Menostar, Minivelle, Vivelle, Vivelle-Dot

estradiol valerate

Delestrogen, Femogex (CAN)

E F

Class and Category

Pharmacologic class: Estrogen
Therapeutic class: Hormone
Pregnancy category: X

Indications and Dosages

➤ *To treat menopausal symptoms*

TABLETS (ESTRADIOL)
Adult menopausal and postmenopausal women. *Initial:* 0.45 mg daily. May be increased to 0.9 mg daily and then to 1.8 mg daily, as needed.

VAGINAL RING (ESTRADIOL ACETATE [FEMRING])
Adult women. One ring (0.05 or 0.1 mg of estradiol/24 hr) inserted into upper third of vaginal vault and replaced every 3 months.

TABLETS (ESTRADIOL ACETATE [FEMTRACE])
Adult menopausal and postmenopausal women. *Initial:* 0.45 mg daily. May be increased to 0.9 mg daily and then 1.8 mg daily as needed.

DOSAGE ADJUSTMENT Dosage may be reduced to less than 1 mg daily for patients with only vaginal or vulvar symptoms.

I.M. INJECTION (ESTRADIOL CYPIONATE IN OIL)
Adult women. 1 to 5 mg as a single dose every 3 to 4 wk as needed.

I.M. INJECTION (ESTRADIOL VALERATE IN OIL)
Adult women. 10 to 20 mg every 4 wk as needed.

TRANSDERMAL (ALORA, ESTRADERM, VIVELLE, VIVELLE-DOT)

Adult menopausal and postmenopausal women. *Initial:* 0.025 to 0.05 mg daily if uterus is not present or in cycles of 3 wk on, 1 wk off if uterus is intact and Alora is prescribed. One patch applied to trunk or buttocks and replaced twice/wk (every 3 to 4 days). Adjust dosage to control symptoms, as prescribed.

TRANSDERMAL (CLIMARA)

Adult women. *Initial:* 0.025 mg daily. One patch applied to trunk or buttocks, replaced every wk. Titrate dosage to control symptoms, as prescribed. Schedule will be cyclic unless patient has had a hysterectomy.

TRANSDERMAL (ESTRASORB)

Adult women. 3.48 g daily in morning. Half of dose (1 pouchful) applied to one thigh and rubbed over entire thigh and calf for 3 min, repeated with second half of dose (1 pouchful) on other thigh and calf.

TRANSDERMAL (ESTROGEL)

Adult women. 1.25 g daily applied in thin layer from wrist to shoulder on inside and outside of one arm.

TRANSDERMAL MIST (EVAMIST)

Adult women. *Initial:* 1.53 mg (1 spray) once daily in the morning. Dosage may be increased to 3.06 mg (2 sprays) once daily in the morning and then to 4.59 mg (3 sprays) once daily in the morning as needed.

➤ *To treat postmenopausal vaginal and urogenital symptoms*

VAGINAL CREAM (ESTRACE)

Adult women. *Initial:* 2 to 4 g (200 to 400 mcg) daily for 1 to 2 wk. Then, dosage gradually reduced to half of initial dose, as prescribed, for 1 to 2 wk. *Maintenance:* 1 g (100 mcg) daily 1 to 3 times/wk for 3 wk, followed by 1 wk of no drugs. Repeat cyclically as needed.

VAGINAL RING (ESTRING)

Adult women. One ring (7.5 mcg of estradiol/24 hr) inserted into upper third of vaginal vault and replaced every 3 months.

VAGINAL RING (FEMRING)

Adult women. One ring (0.05 or 0.1 mg of estradiol/24 hr) inserted into upper third of vaginal vault and replaced every 3 months.

INTRAVAGINAL TABLETS (VAGIFEM)

Adult women. *Initial:* 10-mcg insert daily for 2 wk, followed by 1 insert twice weekly. Dosage increased to 25 mcg, as needed.

➤ *To treat moderate to severe dyspareunia*

VAGINAL INSERT (IMVEXXY)

Adult women. *Initial:* 4 mcg (1 insert) daily for 2 wk, followed by 4 mcg (1 insert) twice weekly. Dosage increased to 10 mcg (1 insert), as needed.

➤ *To treat moderate to severe vasomotor symptoms*

TRANSDERMAL (MINIVELLE)

Adult women. 0.0375 mg daily continuously. Patch replaced twice weekly.

GEL (DIVIGEL 1%)

Adult women. *Initial:* 0.25 mg once daily to skin of left or right upper thigh and then dosage increased, as needed.

➤ *To prevent osteoporosis secondary to estrogen deficiency due to either natural or surgical menopause*

TABLETS (ESTRADIOL)

Adult women. At least 0.5 mg daily cyclically or continuously, adjusted as needed to control concurrent menopausal symptoms, as prescribed.

TRANSDERMAL (ALORA, MINIVELLE, VIVELLE-DOT)

Adult women. Initial: 0.025 mg daily continuously. One patch applied to lower abdomen or buttocks and replaced twice/wk. Adjust dosage to control symptoms and maintain bone density, as prescribed.

TRANSDERMAL (CLIMARA)

Adult women. *Initial:* 0.025 mg daily. One patch applied to trunk or buttocks and replaced every wk. Adjust dosage to control symptoms, as prescribed. Follow a cyclic schedule, as prescribed, unless patient has had a hysterectomy.

TRANSDERMAL (MENOSTAR)

Adult women. *Initial:* 0.014 mg daily. One patch applied to lower abdomen and replaced every wk. Follow a cyclic schedule, as prescribed, unless patient has had a hysterectomy.

➤ *To treat estrogen deficiency due to oophorectomy, primary ovarian failure, or female hypogonadism*

TABLETS (ESTRADIOL)

Adult women. 0.5 to 2 mg daily continuously or in cycles of 3 wk on, 1 wk off.

I.M. INJECTION (ESTRADIOL CYPIONATE IN OIL)
Adult women. 1.5 to 2 mg every month (for female hypogonadism only).
I.M. INJECTION (ESTRADIOL VALERATE IN OIL)
Adult women. 10 to 20 mg every month as needed.
TRANSDERMAL (ALORA, ESTRADERM, VIVELLE)
Adult women. *Initial:* 0.025 mg daily. One patch applied to trunk or buttocks and replaced twice/wk. Titrate dosage to control symptoms, as prescribed. Follow a cyclic schedule, as prescribed, unless patient has had a hysterectomy.
TRANSDERMAL (CLIMARA)
Adult women. *Initial:* 0.05 mg daily. One patch applied to trunk or buttocks and replaced every wk. Adjust dosage to control symptoms, as prescribed. Follow a cyclic schedule, as prescribed, unless patient has had a hysterectomy.

➤ *To provide palliative treatment for inoperable, progressive breast cancer in selected men and postmenopausal women*

TABLETS (ESTRADIOL)
Adults. 10 mg 3 times daily for at least 3 months.
TABLETS (ETHINYL ESTRADIOL)
Adults. 1 mg 3 times daily for at least 3 months.

➤ *To treat advancing, inoperable prostate cancer*

TABLETS (ESTRADIOL)
Adult men. 1 to 2 mg or 3 times daily, adjusted or continued, as prescribed, according to patient response.
I.M. INJECTION (ESTRADIOL VALERATE)
Adult men. 30 mg every 1 to 2 wk, adjusted or continued, as prescribed, according to patient response.

Mechanism of Action

Increases the rate of DNA and RNA synthesis in cells of female reproductive organs, pituitary gland, hypothalamus, and other target organs. In the hypothalamus, estrogens reduce release of gonadotropin-releasing hormone, which decreases pituitary release of follicle-stimulating hormone and luteinizing hormone. In women, these hormones are required for normal genitourinary and other essential body functions.

At the cellular level, estrogens increase cervical secretions, cause endometrial cell proliferation, and improve uterine tone. Estrogen replacement helps maintain genitourinary function and reduces vasomotor symptoms when estrogen production declines as a result of menopause, surgical removal of ovaries, or other estrogen deficiency states. Estrogen replacement also helps prevent osteoporosis by inhibiting bone resorption.

In men, estrogens inhibit pituitary secretion of luteinizing hormone and decrease testicular secretion of testosterone. These actions may decrease prostate tumor growth and lower the level of prostate-specific antigen (PSA).

Contraindications

Active deep vein thrombosis, pulmonary embolism, or history of these conditions; active or recent (within past year) arterial thromboembolic disease, such as MI or stroke; hepatic dysfunction or disease; history of anaphylactic reaction or angioedema to estradiol; history of jaundice with previous oral contraceptive use; hypersensitivity to estradiol, ethinyl estradiol, or their components; hypersensitivity to tartrazine dye (contained in 0.02-mg estradiol and ethinyl estradiol tablets); known or suspected breast cancer or history of breast cancer except in appropriately selected patients being treated for metastatic disease; known or suspected estrogen-dependent cancer; known protein C, protein S, or antithrombin deficiency, or other known thrombophilic disorders; uncontrolled diabetes mellitus with hypertension or vascular involvement; pregnancy; liver tumors; uncontrolled diabetes mellitus with hypertension or vascular involvement; undiagnosed abnormal genital bleeding

Interactions

DRUGS

aromatase inhibitors: Possible interference with aromatase inhibitor's effectiveness
barbiturates, carbamazepine, hydantoins, rifabutin, rifampin: Possibly reduced activity of estradiol
corticosteroids: Increased therapeutic and toxic effects of corticosteroids
cyclosporine: Increased risk of hepatotoxicity and nephrotoxicity
hepatotoxic drugs, such as isoniazid: Increased risk of hepatitis and hepatotoxicity

insulin, oral antidiabetic drugs: Decreased therapeutic effects of these drugs
tamoxifen: Possibly decreased therapeutic effects of tamoxifen
thyroid hormone replacement: Decreased effectiveness
warfarin: Decreased anticoagulant effect

FOODS

grapefruit juice: Decreased estradiol metabolism and possibly increased adverse effects

ACTIVITIES

smoking: Increased risk of pulmonary embolism, stroke, thrombophlebitis, and transient ischemic attack

Adverse Reactions

CNS: Affect liability, chorea, **CVA**, dementia, depression, dizziness, emotional lability, fatigue, headache, irritability, malaise, migraine headache, mood swings, nervousness, paresthesia
CV: **Deep venous thrombosis**, hypertension, **MI**, palpitations, peripheral edema, **thromboembolism**, thrombophlebitis, **thromboembolism**, **unstable angina**
EENT: Intolerance of contact lenses, oral paresthesia, **pharyngeal edema**, retinal vascular thrombosis, swollen lip or tongue, vision changes
ENDO: Breast enlargement, pain, tenderness, or **tumors**; **breast cancer**, fibrocystic breast changes; gynecomastia; hyperglycemia; nipple discharge or nipple and areola discoloration
GI: Abdominal cramps or pain, anorexia, bloating, **bowel obstruction** (vaginal ring), cholelithiasis, constipation, diarrhea, elevated liver enzymes, enlargement of abdomen or hepatic hemangiomas, gallbladder disease, **gallbladder obstruction**, **GI hemorrhage**, **hepatitis**, increased appetite, jaundice, nausea, **pancreatitis**, **portal vein thrombosis**, vomiting
GU: Amenorrhea, breakthrough bleeding, cervical or vaginal erosion, clear vaginal discharge, decreased libido, dysmenorrhea, **endometrial cancer**, genital edema, impotence, increased libido (females), **ovarian cancer**, pelvic pain, **portal vein thrombosis**, prolonged or heavy menstrual bleeding, ring adherence to vaginal wall, testicular atrophy, urinary frequency, uterine leiomyomata, vaginitis, vaginal abrasion or ulceration (ring), vaginal candidiasis, worsening of endometriosis
MS: Arthralgia, leg cramps, muscle spasms
RESP: Dyspnea, **pulmonary embolism**
SKIN: Acne, alopecia, diaphoresis, discoloration or dry skin, **erythema multiforme**, erythema nodosum, facial pigmentation, hirsutism, melasma, oily skin, pruritus, purpura, rash, seborrhea, urticaria
Other: **Angioedema**, application-site reactions (transdermal), folic acid deficiency, **hypercalcemia** (in metastatic bone disease), **hypersensitivity reactions**, **toxic shock syndrome** (vaginal ring), weight gain or loss

Nursing Considerations

WARNING **Be aware that estradiol (Estrace) and ethinyl estradiol (Estinyl) are distinct and separate products and that their dosing isn't equivalent.**

- Use estradiol cautiously in patients with asthma, chorea, diabetes mellitus, epilepsy, migraine headaches, porphyria, systemic lupus erythematosus, or hepatic hemangiomas because estradiol may worsen these disorders.
- Administer oral preparations with or immediately after food to decrease nausea.
- For I.M. injection of estradiol cypionate or estradiol valerate, roll vial and syringe between palms to evenly disperse drug. Use at least a 21G needle because of viscosity of oil-based solution. Use a dry, sterile syringe. Inject deep into upper outer quadrant of gluteal muscle. Aspirate before injection to avoid injection into a blood vessel.
- Be aware that if patients are converting from oral estrogen to transdermal system, oral estrogen should be stopped 1 week before skin patches are applied.
- Expect to begin prophylaxis treatment against osteoporosis at the start of menopause.
- Be aware that estrogen therapy should be given cyclically or combined with a progestin for 10 to 14 days per month in women with an intact uterus to minimize the risk of endometrial hyperplasia.

WARNING **Be aware that severe hypercalcemia may occur in patients with bone**

metastasis due to breast cancer because estrogens influence the metabolism of calcium and phosphorus. Monitor for toxic effects of increased calcium absorption in patients who are predisposed to hypercalcemia or nephrolithiasis.

WARNING Assess patient for possible contact lens intolerance or changes in vision or visual acuity because estrogens can cause keratoconus, leading to increased curvature of the cornea. Be prepared to discontinue drug immediately, as prescribed, if patient experiences sudden partial or complete loss of vision or sudden onset of diplopia, migraine, or proptosis.

- Monitor PT test results of patients receiving warfarin for loss of anticoagulant effect because estrogens increase production of clotting factors VII, VIII, IX, and X and promote platelet aggregation.
- Watch for elevated liver enzymes because estrogens may worsen such conditions as acute intermittent or variegate hepatic porphyria.
- Closely monitor patient's blood pressure. A few patients may experience a substantial increase in blood pressure as an idiosyncratic reaction to estrogen. Monitor patients who already have hypertension for increases in blood pressure because estrogens may cause fluid retention. Also monitor patients with asthma, heart disease, migraines, renal disease, or seizure disorder for exacerbation of these conditions.
- Watch for peripheral edema or mild weight gain because estrogens can cause sodium and fluid retention.
- Monitor serum glucose level frequently in patients who have diabetes mellitus because estrogens may decrease insulin sensitivity and alter glucose tolerance.

WARNING Expect to stop estrogen therapy in any woman who develops signs or symptoms of cancer; cardiovascular disease, such as MI, pulmonary embolism, stroke; dementia; or venous thrombosis.

- Be aware that women at risk for arterial vascular disease include those with diabetes mellitus, hypercholesterolemia, hypertension, obesity, tobacco use, or venous thromboembolism. Know that these factors, if present, should be addressed and brought under control.
- Be aware that exogenous estradiol and progestins may worsen mood disorders, including depression. Monitor patient for anxiety, depression, dizziness, fatigue, insomnia, or mood changes.
- Assess skin for melasma (tan or brown patches), which may develop on forehead, cheeks, temples, and upper lip. These patches may persist after drug is stopped.
- Check patient's triglyceride level routinely because, in patients with hypertriglyceridemia, estrogen therapy may increase serum triglyceride level enough to cause pancreatitis and other complications.
- Monitor serum PSA level in patients with inoperable prostate cancer to determine if patient is responding to hormone therapy. If patient responds (usually within 3 months), expect therapy to continue until disease is significantly advanced.
- Expect to stop estrogen therapy several weeks before patient undergoes major surgery, as prescribed, because certain procedures are associated with prolonged immobilization and therefore pose a risk of thromboembolism.
- Be aware that if patient takes thyroid hormone replacement therapy, monitor her for increased signs and symptoms of hypothyroidism because estradiol may increase thyroid binding globulin levels, which may make the patient's current dose of thyroid hormone insufficient.

WARNING Monitor patient closely for signs of anaphylaxis, which may occur any time during therapy and may require emergency medical treatment. Monitor patient with history of hereditary angioedema closely because estradiol may exacerbate symptoms of angioedema.

PATIENT TEACHING

- Inform patient of risks involved in estrogen therapy before therapy starts. These risks may include increased risk of breast, endometrial, or ovarian cancer; cardiovascular disease; dementia (if age 65 or over); gallbladder disease; and vision abnormalities.
- Advise patient to remain recumbent for at least 30 minutes after applying estradiol vaginal cream. Inform her that she may use a sanitary napkin (but not a tampon) to protect clothing after application.

- Teach patient proper application and use of transdermal patch. Instruct her not to apply patch to breasts, waistline, or other areas where it may not adhere properly. Advise her to rotate application sites at least weekly and to remove old patch before applying new one. If patch falls off, instruct her to reapply it to another area or to apply a new patch and continue the original treatment schedule. Caution her not to expose patch to sun for long periods. Explain that she may bathe while wearing the patch. Instruct patient to discard used patch in household trash in a way that prevents accidental application or ingestion by children, pets, or others.
- Teach patient to apply Estrogel to clean, dry skin of one arm, using applicator. Emphasize importance of transferring all of the gel from applicator to arm. Tell patient to spread gel as thinly as possible over entire inside and outside of arm from wrist to shoulder. Advise her to wash her hands with soap and water afterward and to avoid fire and smoking until gel has dried because it's flammable. Tell patient never to apply gel to breasts. Warn that gel is alcohol-based and that patient should avoid fire, flame, or smoking until gel has dried.
- Instruct patient to apply Divigel to either the left or right upper thigh once daily, but to rotate to the opposite site on alternating days. Explain that the application surface area should be about 5 to 7 inches (about the size of two palm prints). The entire contents of a unit-dose packet should be applied each day. Remind patient that gel should never be applied to her breasts, face, irritated skin, or in or around her vagina. After application, tell patient to let gel dry before dressing and not to wash the site for 1 hour after application. Instruct patient to wash her hands after applying gel.
- Inform patient that each pouch of Estrasorb contains half of daily dose. Instruct her to apply emulsion to clean, dry skin on top of thigh and to rub it into entire thigh and calf for 3 minutes. Tell her to rub any excess emulsion onto her buttocks. Then, advise her to repeat procedure on her other thigh and calf using the second pouch. Tell her to wash her hands with soap and water after the application and to dress only after affected areas are dry.
- Tell patient using Imvexxy vaginal inserts to insert the smaller end up for a depth of about two inches into the vaginal canal. Each insert should be inserted at about the same time every day.
- Teach patient proper use of estradiol vaginal ring. Instruct her to insert ring in upper third of vagina, to keep it there for 90 days, and then to remove it and insert a new ring. Or she may remove it during the 90-day dosage period, rinse it with lukewarm (not hot or boiling) water, and reinsert it as needed for personal hygiene. Remind patient that she shouldn't be able to feel the ring when it's in place. If she does, she should use a finger to push the ring farther into her vagina. If vaginal wall ulceration or erosion occurs, suggest that patient leave ring out and not replace it until healing is complete to keep ring from adhering to healing tissue.
- Instruct patient using estradiol vaginal ring to remove ring immediately and contact prescriber if she develops fever, nausea, vomiting, diarrhea, muscle pain, dizziness, faintness, or a sunburn rash on face or body that may suggest a rare but serious bacterial infection called toxic shock syndrome. Also urge patient to seek prompt medical care if ring becomes attached to vaginal wall (rare), making removal difficult.
- Instruct patient prescribed transdermal Evamist to prime the pump of a new device before the first dose by holding the container upright with the cover in place and spraying 3 sprays. Then, to deliver a dose, she should spray the mist on the inner aspect of her forearm starting near the elbow. Instruct her to let the mist dry for 2 minutes and not to wash the area for at least 30 minutes. Warn her that secondary exposure may occur if a child or other adult comes into contact with sprayed area. To avoid this, she should cover the area with clothing after the spray dries.
- Inform patient receiving estradiol treatment that she should have an annual pelvic examination to screen for cervical dysplasia and be followed closely for other types of cancers and disorders associated with estradiol use.
- Tell patient who has an intact uterus and is prescribed transdermal Menostar that she will need to receive progestin for 14 days

every 6 to 12 months and have an endometrial biopsy yearly.

- Advise patient that less serious but common side effects of estradiol therapy include abdominal or stomach cramps, bloating, breast pain or tenderness, fluid retention, hair loss, irregular vaginal bleeding or spotting, nausea and vomiting, and vaginal yeast infection.

estrogens (conjugated)

C.E.S. (CAN), Premarin

synthetic estrogens, A (conjugated)

Cenestin

synthetic estrogens, B (conjugated)

Enjuvia

Class and Category

Pharmacologic class: Estrogen
Therapeutic class: Hormone
Pregnancy category: X

Indications and Dosages

➤ *To treat moderate to severe vasomotor menopausal symptoms*

TABLETS

Adults. 0.3 (C.E.S., Enjuvia, Premarin) or 0.45 mg (Cenestin) daily or cyclically 25 days on, 5 days off (C.E.S, Premarin only). Dosage increased as needed to control symptoms. *Maximum:* 1.25 mg daily.

➤ *To treat vaginal and vulvar atrophy*

TABLETS

Adults. 0.3 mg daily or cyclically 25 days on, 5 days off (Premarin only). Dosage increased as needed to control symptoms.

➤ *To treat atrophic vaginitis and vaginal and vulvar atrophy*

VAGINAL CREAM (PREMARIN)

Adults. 0.5 to 2 g daily in cycles of 3 wk on, 1 wk off.

➤ *To treat moderate to severe vaginal dryness and pain with intercourse and symptoms of vulvar and vaginal atrophy in menopause*

TABLETS (ENJUVIA)

Adults. 0.3 mg daily.

VAGINAL CREAM (PREMARIN)

Adults. 0.5 g twice/wk. Or, 0.5 g daily for 21 days followed by 7 days off, with cycle repeated every 28 days.

➤ *To prevent postmenopausal osteoporosis*

TABLETS (PREMARIN)

Adults. 0.3 mg daily continuously or in cycles of 25 days on, 5 days off. Dosage increased as needed to control symptoms.

➤ *To provide palliative treatment for advanced androgen-dependent prostate cancer*

TABLETS (PREMARIN)

Adult men. 1.25 to 2 mg 3 times daily.

➤ *To provide palliative treatment for metastatic breast cancer*

TABLETS (PREMARIN)

Adults. 10 mg 3 times daily for 3 months or longer.

➤ *To treat dysfunctional uterine bleeding*

I.V. INJECTION, I.M. INJECTION (PREMARIN)

Adults. 25 mg, repeated in 6 to 12 hr as needed. I.V. injection preferred route; given slowly.

➤ *To treat estrogen deficiency from oophorectomy or primary ovarian failure*

TABLETS (PREMARIN)

Adults. 1.25 mg daily in cycles of 3 wk on, 1 wk off. Dosage adjusted as needed.

➤ *To treat female hypogonadism*

TABLETS (PREMARIN)

Adults. 0.3 to 0.625 mg daily in cycles of 3 wk on, 1 wk off. Dosage adjusted as needed.

Mechanism of Action

Increase the rate of DNA and RNA synthesis in the cells of female reproductive organs, hypothalamus, pituitary glands, and other target organs. In the hypothalamus, estrogens reduce the release of gonadotropin-releasing hormone, which decreases pituitary release of follicle-stimulating hormone and luteinizing hormone. In women, these hormones are required for normal genitourinary and other essential body functions. At the cellular level, estrogens increase cervical secretions, cause endometrial cell proliferation, and increase uterine tone. Estrogen replacement helps maintain genitourinary function and reduce vasomotor symptoms when estrogen production declines from menopause, surgical removal of ovaries, or other estrogen deficiency. Estrogen also helps prevent osteoporosis by keeping bone resorption from exceeding bone formation.

In men, estrogens inhibit pituitary secretion of luteinizing hormone and decrease testicular secretion of testosterone. These actions may decrease prostate tumor growth and lower the level of prostate-specific antigen.

Contraindications

Active deep vein thrombosis, pulmonary embolism, or history of these conditions; active or recent (within past year) arterial thromboembolic disease such as MI or stroke; history of anaphylactic reaction or angioedema to estradiol; hypersensitivity to estrogens or their components; known or suspected breast cancer or history of breast cancer; known or suspected estrogen-dependent cancer; known protein C, protein S, or antithrombin deficiency or other known thrombophilic disorders; pregnancy; liver impairment or disease; undiagnosed abnormal genital bleeding

Incompatibilities

Don't combine I.V. estrogens with acid solutions, ascorbic acid, and protein hydrolysate because they're incompatible.

Interactions

DRUGS

aromatase inhibitors: Possibly interference with aromatase inhibitor's effectiveness
barbiturates, carbamazepine, hydantoins, rifabutin, rifampin: Possibly reduced activity of estrogen and medroxyprogesterone
corticosteroids: Increased therapeutic and toxic effects of corticosteroids
cyclosporine: Increased risk of hepatotoxicity and nephrotoxicity
hepatotoxic drugs (such as isoniazid): Increased risk of hepatitis and hepatotoxicity
insulin, oral antidiabetic drugs: Decreased therapeutic effects of these drugs
tamoxifen: Possibly interference with tamoxifen's therapeutic effects
thyroid hormone replacement: Decreased effectiveness
warfarin: Decreased anticoagulant effect

ACTIVITIES

smoking: Increased risk of pulmonary embolism, stroke, thrombophlebitis, and transient ischemic attack

Adverse Reactions

CNS: Asthenia, **CVA**, dementia, depression, dizziness, growth benign meningioma, headache, insomnia, migraine headache, mood disturbance, nervousness, paresthesia
CV: Deep vein thrombosis, hypertension, **MI**, peripheral edema, **thromboembolism**, thrombophlebitis, vasodilation
EENT: Intolerance of contact lenses, pharyngitis, retinal vascular thrombosis, rhinitis, sinusitis
ENDO: Breast enlargement, pain, tenderness, or **tumors**; gynecomastia (men); hot flashes; hyperglycemia
GI: Abdominal cramps or pain, abdominal distention, anorexia, cholestatic jaundice, constipation, diarrhea, flatulence, gallbladder disease, **gallbladder obstruction**, hepatic hemangioma enlargement, **hepatitis**, increased appetite, **ischemic colitis**, nausea, **pancreatitis**, vomiting
GU: Amenorrhea, breakthrough bleeding, cervical erosion, clear vaginal discharge, decreased libido (men), dysmenorrhea, **endometrial cancer** or hyperplasia, impotence, increased libido (women), leukorrhea, **ovarian cancer**, prolonged or heavy menstrual bleeding, testicular atrophy, uterine leiomyomata enlargement, vaginal candidiasis, vaginitis, vaginal-site reactions (vaginal administration only) such as burning, irritation, and genital pruritus
MS: Arthralgias, back pain, muscle spasms
RESP: Bronchitis, increased cough, **pulmonary embolism**
SKIN: Acne, alopecia, chloasma, **erythema multiforme**, erythema nodosum, hemorrhagic eruption, hirsutism, melasma, oily skin, pruritus, purpura, rash, seborrhea, urticaria
Other: Anaphylaxis, **angioedema**, flu-like syndrome, folic acid deficiency, **hypercalcemia** (in metastatic bone disease), weight gain

Nursing Considerations

- Use conjugated estrogens cautiously in patients with severe hypocalcemia because a sudden increase in serum calcium level may cause adverse reactions.

- Reconstitute conjugated estrogens with normal saline solution, dextrose, or invert sugar solution and use within a few hours. Discard solution that contains precipitate.

WARNING Monitor serum calcium level to detect severe hypercalcemia in patients with bone metastasis from breast cancer.

WARNING Monitor patient closely, especially within minutes to hours of taking first dose, as anaphylaxis may occur, requiring emergency intervention. Be aware that estrogen therapy may exacerbate symptoms of angioedema in women with hereditary angioedema. Monitor for signs of swelling of the face, lips, throat, or tongue, and provide emergency care, as needed.

- Watch for elevated liver enzymes because estrogen and progestins may worsen such conditions as acute intermittent or variegate hepatic porphyria.
- Assess hypertensive patients for increases in blood pressure because estrogens may cause fluid retention.
- Monitor patients with asthma, diabetes mellitus, endometriosis, heart disease, lupus erythematosus, migraine headaches, renal disease, or seizure disorder for worsening of these conditions.
- Assess PT for loss of anticoagulant effects if patient takes warfarin, because estrogens increase production of clotting factors and promote platelet aggregation.
- Expect to stop drug during periods of immobilization, 4 weeks before elective surgery, and if jaundice develops.

WARNING Expect to stop estrogen therapy in any woman who develops signs or symptoms of cancer; cardiovascular disease, such as MI, pulmonary embolism, stroke, venous thrombosis; or dementia.

- Check triglyceride level routinely because, in hypertriglyceridemia, estrogen therapy may increase triglycerides enough to cause pancreatitis and other complications.
- Know that if patient takes thyroid hormone replacement therapy, monitor her for increased signs and symptoms of hypothyroidism because estrogen may increase thyroid-binding globulin level, which may make the patient's current dose of thyroid hormone insufficient.
- Be aware that estrogen may worsen mood disorders, including depression. Monitor patient for depression, fatigue, insomnia, or mood changes.

PATIENT TEACHING

- Explain the risks of estrogen therapy, including increased risk of breast, endometrial, or ovarian cancer; cardiovascular disease; dementia; and gallbladder disease.
- Instruct patient how to use vaginal cream and to cleanse plunger by removing it from barrel and washing it with mild soap and warm water after each use.
- Urge patient to immediately report breakthrough bleeding to prescriber.
- Instruct patient to perform monthly breast self-examination and to comply with all prescribed follow-up examinations.
- Warn female patient that long-term use may increase risk of breast or endometrial cancer, dementia, gallbladder disease, heart disease, and stroke.
- Inform patient that estrogen vaginal cream may alter effectiveness of cervical caps, condoms, or diaphragms made of latex or rubber.
- Instruct patient to notify prescriber if she sees something that resembles a tablet in her stool.

eszopiclone

Lunesta

Class, Category, and Schedule

Pharmacologic class: Pyrrolopyrazine derivative
Therapeutic class: Sedative-hypnotic
Pregnancy category: C
Controlled substance schedule: IV

Indications and Dosages

➤ *To treat insomnia*

TABLETS

Adults. *Initial:* 1 mg immediately at bedtime. May be increased to 2 or 3 mg at bedtime, as needed. *Maximum:* 3 mg at bedtime.

DOSAGE ADJUSTMENT For patients with severe hepatic impairment, patients who take potent CYP3A4 inhibitors, or patients who are debilitated or elderly, dosage should not exceed 2 mg at bedtime.

Route	Onset	Peak	Duration
P.O.	Unknown	1 hr	Unknown

Mechanism of Action

May potentiate effects of the inhibitory neurotransmitter gamma-aminobutyric acid (GABA) by binding close to or with benzodiazepine receptors in limbic and cortical areas of the CNS. By binding to these receptor sites and areas, eszopiclone increases GABA's inhibitory effects and blocks cortical and limbic arousal, thereby inducing and maintaining sleep.

Contraindications

Hypersensitivity to eszopiclone or its components

Interactions

DRUGS

clarithromycin, itraconazole, ketoconazole, nefazodone, nelfinavir, ritonavir, troleandomycin: Increased eszopiclone level
other CNS depressants: Possibly additive effects
rifampin: Decreased eszopiclone level

ACTIVITIES

alcohol use: Additive effect on psychomotor performance

FOOD

Heavy, high-fat meal: Possibly reduced effectiveness of eszopiclone

Adverse Reactions

CNS: Agitation, anxiety, bizarre behavior such as sleep driving, confusion, depersonalization, depression, dizziness, hallucinations, headache (including migraine), nervousness, neuralgia, somnolence, unusual dreams
CV: Chest pain, peripheral edema
EENT: Dry mouth, smell distortion, taste perversion
ENDO: Gynecomastia
GI: Diarrhea, **hepatitis**, indigestion, nausea, vomiting
GU: Decreased libido, dysmenorrhea, UTI
RESP: **Asthma**, respiratory tract infection
SKIN: Pruritus, rash
Other: Generalized pain, **heatstroke**, viral infection

Nursing Considerations

- Use eszopiclone cautiously in patients with severe mental depression or reduced respiratory function; drug may intensify mental depression and lead to respiratory depression.

PATIENT TEACHING

- Instruct patient not to exceed prescribed eszopiclone dosage and not to stop drug abruptly because withdrawal symptoms may occur.
- Advise patient to take drug immediately before bedtime and to avoid potentially hazardous activities until drug's CNS effects are known.
- Urge patient to avoid alcohol and CNS depressants because of additive effects.
- Advise woman of childbearing age to notify prescriber if she becomes or intends to become pregnant during therapy.
- Explain that sleep may be disturbed for the first few nights after therapy stops.
- Warn patient and caregiver that some patients have performed bizarre activities after taking drug, such as driving the car, preparing and eating food, making phone calls, or having sex while not fully awake and often with no memory of the event. These episodes usually occur in patients who have taken the drug with alcohol or other CNS depressant, who have taken the drug with less than a full night of sleep remaining (7 to 8 hours), or who have exceeded the recommended dose. If such an episode occurs, the prescriber should be notified and eszopiclone therapy discontinued immediately.

etanercept

Enbrel

etanercept-szzs

Erelzi

Class and Category

Pharmacologic class: Tumor necrosis factor (TNF) blocker
Therapeutic class: Immunosuppressant
Pregnancy category: Not classified

Indications and Dosages

➤ *To reduce signs and symptoms of rheumatoid arthritis, slow structural damage in active arthritis, and improve physical function in patients with rheumatoid arthritis, alone or in combination with methotrexate; to reduce signs and symptoms of active ankylosing spondylitis*

SUBCUTANEOUS INJECTION (ENBREL, ERELZI)

Adults. 50 mg once/wk on same day each wk. *Maximum:* 50 mg/wk.

➤ *To treat psoriatic arthritis, alone or in combination with methotrexate*

SUBCUTANEOUS INJECTION (ENBREL)

Adults. 50 mg once/wk on same day eack wk. *Maximum:* 50 mg/wk.

➤ *To treat chronic moderate-to-severe plaque psoriasis in candidates for systemic therapy or phototherapy*

SUBCUTANEOUS INJECTION (ENBREL)

Adults. *Initial:* 50 mg twice/wk 3 to 4 days apart for 3 months; then reduced to 50 mg/wk. Alternatively but less common, 25 mg or 50 mg/wk.

SUBCUTANEOUS INJECTION (ENBREL)

Children ages 4 and older weighing 63 kg (138 lb) or more. 50 mg once/wk on same day each wk.

Children ages 4 and older weighing less than 63 kg (138 lb). 0.8 mg/kg/wk.

➤ *To reduce signs and symptoms of moderately to severely active poly-articular juvenile idiopathic arthritis*

SUBCUTANEOUS INJECTION (ENBREL)

Children ages 2 to 17 weighing 63 kg (138 lb) or more. 50 mg once/wk on same day each wk.

Children ages 2 to 17 weighing less than 63 kg (138 lb). 0.8 mg/kg/wk. *Maximum:* 50 mg/wk.

SUBCUTANEOUS INJECTION (ERELZI)

Children ages 2 to 17 weighing 63 kg (138 lb) or more. 50 mg once/wk on same day each wk.

Incompatibilities

Don't combine etanercept with other drugs.

Contraindications

Hypersensitivity to etanercept or its components, sepsis or risk of it

Interactions

DRUGS

cyclophosphamide: Possibly increased risk of malignancy
live vaccines: Possibly increased risk of secondary transmission of infection from live vaccine
sulfasalazine: Possibly decreased neutrophil count

Adverse Reactions

CNS: Asthenia, chills, demyelination including both central and peripheral nervous systems, dizziness, fever, headache, multiple sclerosis, paresthesias, **seizures**
CV: Chest pain, **congestive heart failure**, hypertension, **hypotension**, peripheral edema, systemic vasculitis
EENT: Optic neuritis, pharyngitis, rhinitis, scleritis, sinusitis, uveitis
GI: Abdominal abscess or pain, **autoimmune hepatitis**, cholecystitis, diarrhea, elevated liver enzymes, gastroenteritis, indigestion, inflammatory bowel disease, nausea, **noninfectious hepatitis**, **reactivation of hepatitis B**, vomiting
GU: Pyelonephritis
HEME: Anemia, **aplastic anemia**, **leukemia**, **leukopenia**, lymphadenopathy, **neutropenia**, **pancytopenia**, **thrombocytopenia**
MS: Osteomyelitis, septic arthritis, transverse myelitis
RESP: Bronchitis, cough, **interstitial lung disease**, pneumonia, upper respiratory tract infection
SKIN: Cellulitis, cutaneous lupus erythematosus or vasculitis, **erythema multiforme**, foot abscess, leg ulceration, **melanoma and nonmelanoma skin cancers**, **Merkel cell carcinoma**, new or worsening psoriasis, pruritus, rash, **Stevens–Johnson syndrome**, **toxic epidermal necrolysis**, urticaria
Other: Angioedema; bacterial, fungal, mycobacterial, parasitic, and viral infections; injection-site bruising, edema, erythema, itching, and pain; etanercept-induced antibodies; lymphadenopathy; lupus-like syndrome, **macrophage activation syndrome**, **malignancy**, **such as lymphoma**; sarcoidosis; **sepsis**

Mechanism of Action

Etanercept reduces joint inflammation from rheumatoid arthritis by binding with tumor necrosis factor (TNF), a cytokine, or protein that plays an important role in normal inflammatory and immune responses.

In rheumatoid arthritis, the immune and inflammatory process triggers release of TNF, mainly from macrophages. TNF then binds to TNF receptors on cell membranes, as shown below left. This action renders TNF biologically active and triggers a cascade of inflammatory events that results in increased inflammation of the synovial membrane, release of destructive lysosomal enzymes, and further joint destruction.

Etanercept binds to TNF and prevents it from binding with TNF receptors on the cell membranes, as shown below right. This action renders bound TNF biologically inactive, prevents TNF-mediated cellular responses, and significantly reduces inflammatory activity.

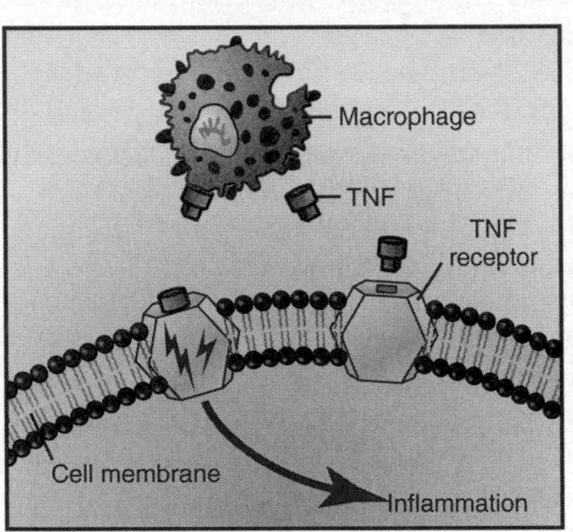

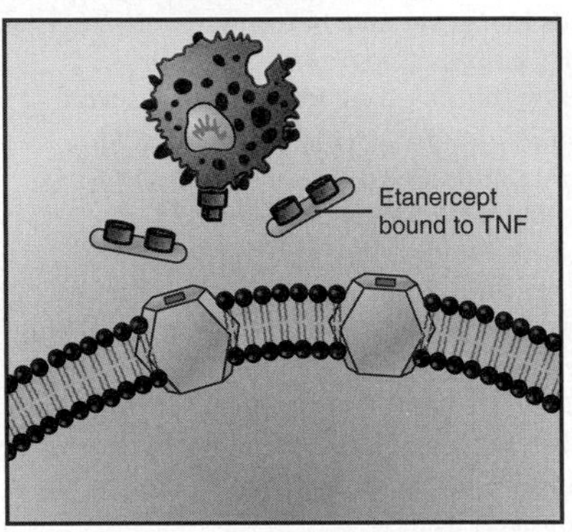

Nursing Considerations

- Screen patient for latent tuberculosis with a tuberculin skin test before starting etanercept therapy. If test is positive, expect to give treatment, as ordered, before starting etanercept. Also screen patient for hepatitis B. If present, expect etanercept therapy to be withdrawn because antirheumatic therapies like etanercept may reactivate hepatitis B.
- Be aware that patients treated with tumor necrosis factor-alpha blockers such as etanercept are at increased risk for developing serious infections due to bacterial (including *Legionella* and *Listeria*), fungal, mycobacterial, parasitic, and viral pathogens. These infections can become life-threatening and involve multiple organ systems. Monitor patient closely throughout therapy.
- Know that tumor necrosis factor antagonists shouldn't be given with etanercept because doing so increases the risk of serious infection.
- Use cautiously in patients with a history of recurrent infection, underlying conditions that may predispose them to infections, or an existing chronic, latent, or localized infection because etanercept increases their risk of infection.
- Use cautiously in patients with COPD, and monitor respiratory status closely because etanercept therapy may increase patient's risk of adverse respiratory reactions.
- Use cautiously in patients with preexisting or recent onset CNS demyelinating disorders because drug may worsen these conditions. Also use cautiously in patients with heart failure or who have a history of serious hematologic abnormalities because drug may worsen these conditions.

WARNING **Don't use the diluent provided with the Enbrel brand of etanercept (bacteriostatic water for injection, USP, with 0.9% benzyl alcohol) for patients who**

have benzyl alcohol hypersensitivity. Instead, use sterile water for injection for these patients.

WARNING **Avoid handling needle cover of diluent syringe for Enbrel brand of drug, the needle cover within the white cap of the SureClick autoinjector, or inside the purple cap of the Enbrel Mini cartridge if latex allergy is present because these components contain dry natural rubber.**

- Know that when giving the Enbrel brand of etanercept to children, don't use the 25-mg prefilled syringe if the child weighs less than 31 kg (68 lb). The 50-mg prefilled syringe or SureClick autoinjector may be used for children who weigh 63 kg (138 lb) or more.
- Know that when giving the Erelzi brand of etanercept using the single-dose prefilled syringe or single-dose prefilled Sensorready pen, it is important to leave drug at room temperature for 15 to 30 minutes before injecting. Do not remove the needle cover while allowing the prefilled syringe to reach room temperature. Be aware that it is normal for small white particles of protein to be present in the solution but that the solution should not be discolored, cloudy, or contain foreign particulate matter.

WARNING **Expect to stop etanercept if patient develops sepsis.**

- Avoid giving live-virus vaccines to patients who are taking etanercept because drug decreases immune response and increases risk of secondary transmission of vaccine virus.
- Monitor immunosuppressed patients for evidence of acute or chronic infection, including chills, fever, and tachycardia, because etanercept decreases defenses against infection. It also increases the risk of developing malignant tumors.
- Continue giving corticosteroids, NSAIDs, and other analgesics, as prescribed, during etanercept therapy.
- Be aware that malignancies, especially leukemias and lymphomas, have been reported rarely in patients taking tumor necrosis factor blockers such as etanercept. Children, adolescents, and patients with rheumatoid arthritis, especially those with very active disease, are at greatest risk. Monitor closely.

PATIENT TEACHING

- Reassure patient or caregiver that other medications such as analgesics, NSAIDs, and steroid therapy may be continued while patient is receiving etanercept.
- Inform patient that etanercept is given by a small injection into the skin, and teach him proper injection technique if needed.
- Tell patient that a prefilled syringe or pen, depending on brand used, is available if the dose prescribed is 50 mg.
- Tell patient that if he will take less than a 50-mg dose or prefers not to use prefilled syringe, he will need to use the Enbrel brand. In this case, advise him to use drug as soon as possible after dissolving powder. Dissolved powder may be kept in refrigerator for up to 6 hours after mixing and then should be discarded.
- Alert patient using Enbrel brand of drug and SureClick autoinjector that the window turns yellow or if using Erelzi the window turns green, when the injection is complete. If after removing the autoinjector the window has not turned yellow or green, respectively, or it appears drug is still injecting, stress that patient has not received the full dose. If this happens, tell patient to notify prescriber.
- Alert patient using the AutoTouch reusable autoinjector with Enbrel Mini single-dose prefilled cartridge that the AutoTouch makes sounds to help guide the injection. If patient wants to turn the sounds off, she should slide the sound switch up (red bar visible). However, remind patient that even when the sound is turned off, she will still hear the noise of the motor during the injection and also error alerts. Instruct her what to do if an error alert occurs and how to reset the AutoTouch.
- Instruct patient to rotate injection sites among abdomen, thigh, and upper arms and to avoid areas that are bruised, hard, red, or tender. Advise him to keep each site at least 1 inch away from a previous site.
- Urge patient to use needles and syringes only once and discard in puncture-proof container.
- Stress importance of seeking immediate medical care if a severe allergic reaction occurs. Also, alert patients who are latex-

sensitive that the needle cover of the prefilled syringe, the needle cover within the white cap of the SureClick autoinjection, and inside the purple cap of the Enbrel Mini cartridge all contain dry natural rubber, which is a derivative of latex.
- Caution patient that the risk of malignancies such as leukemia and lymphoma may be higher in those who take etanercept, especially children and adolescents. Tell him to seek medical attention promptly for any suspicious signs and symptoms.
- Urge patient to consult prescriber immediately if he develops an infection because drug may decrease the body's infection-fighting ability.
- Caution patient who hasn't had chickenpox to contact prescriber right away if he's exposed because he may develop a more serious infection.
- Urge patient to seek immediate emergency care if he develops a bleeding, bruising, persistent fever or pallor while taking drug.
- Instruct patient to seek medical attention promptly for any unusual or persistent adverse signs or symptoms.
- Advise women of childbearing age to alert prescriber if pregnancy occurs or is suspected. Tell mothers that drug does pass into breast milk, so breastfeeding should be discussed with prescriber before doing so.

etelcalcetide

Parsabiv

Class and Category

Pharmacologic class: Parathyroid hormone analogue and modifier
Therapeutic class: Calcimimetic
Pregnancy category: Not classified

Indications and Dosages

➤ *To treat secondary hyperparathyroidism in patients with chronic kidney disease on hemodialysis*

I.V. INJECTION

Adults. *Initial:* 5 mg three times a wk at the end of hemodialysis treatment, followed by titration in 2.5- or 5-mg increments no more frequently than every 4 wk, as indicated by an elevation of PTH levels above the recommended target range. *Maintenance:* Highly individualized, ranging from 2.5 mg to 15 mg three times a wk. *Maximum:* 15 mg three times a wk.

DOSAGE ADJUSTMENT For patients with a corrected serum calcium below the lower limit of normal but at or above 7.5 mg/dl and who do not have symptoms of hypocalcemia, dose possibly decreased or temporarily withheld. If drug temporarily withheld, dose restarted at a lower dose when the PTH is within target range and hypocalcemia has been corrected. For patients with a corrected serum calcium below 7.5 mg/dl or patients who have symptoms of hypocalcemia, dose withheld until corrected serum calcium is within normal limits, symptoms of hypocalcemia have been resolved, and predisposing factors for hypocalcemia have been addressed. Dose restarted at a dose 5 mg lower than the last administered dose. If last administered dose was 2.5 mg or 5 mg, dose restarted at 2.5 mg.

Route	Onset	Peak	Duration
I.V.	Within 30 min	Unknown	Unknown

Mechanism of Action

Binds to the calcium-sensing receptor to enhance activation of the receptor by extracellular calcium. This activation on parathyroid chief cells decreases PTH secretion, which lowers serum calcium levels.

Contraindications

Hypersensitivity to etelcalcetide or its components

Adverse Reactions

CNS: Headache, paresthesia
CV: **Congestive heart failure**, **hypotension**, **prolonged QT interval** (with hypocalcemia)
GI: Diarrhea, **GI bleeding** or ulceration, nausea, vomiting
MS: Adynamic bone, muscle spasms, myalgia
SKIN: Pruritis, rash, urticaria
Other: **Angioedema**, etelcalcetide-induced antibody formation, **hyperkalemia**, **hypocalcemia**, **hypophosphatemia**

Nursing Considerations

- Check to be sure patient's corrected serum calcium is at or above the lower limit of normal prior to beginning etelcalcetide therapy, and when dose is increased, or when drug is reinitiated after a dosing interruption of more than 2 weeks.
- Do not dilute or mix etelcalcetide prior to administration. Know that the solution should be clear and colorless.
- Administer etelcalcetide only at the end of hemodialysis treatment into the venous line of the dialysis circuit at the end of the hemodialysis treatment during rinse-back or intravenously after rinse-back.
- Know that when patient is being switched from cinacalcet to etelcalcetide, cinacalcet should be discontinued for at least 7 days prior to start of etelcalcetide therapy.
- Know that if a regularly scheduled hemodialysis treatment is missed, drug should not be administered to make up for the missed dose. The dosing schedule should be resumed at the end of the next hemodialysis treatment at the prescribed dose.
- Monitor patient's corrected serum calcium levels and parathyroid hormone levels, as ordered. Expect corrected serum calcium levels to be checked 1 week after drug is initiated and when dose is adjusted, and then checked every 4 weeks during maintenance therapy. Expect parathyroid hormone levels to be checked 4 weeks after drug is initiated and when dose is adjusted, and then as prescriber feels is necessary during maintenance therapy. Know that for maintenance therapy, the corrected serum calcium should be within the normal range and the PTH levels should be within the recommended target range.

WARNING Monitor patient's serum calcium level closely because etelcalcetide therapy lowers serum calcium, sometimes severely. Monitor patient for muscle spasms, myalgia, paresthesia, and seizures. Know that ECG changes indicative of hypocalcemia include prolonged QT interval and ventricular arrhythmia. If patient develops hypocalcemia, notify prescriber and expect dosage adjustment to be made or drug temporarily withheld. Expect to start or increase calcium supplementation to treat hypocalcemia.

- Watch patient with heart failure for signs of worsening.
- Monitor patient for signs and symptoms of GI bleeding and ulcerations during etelcalcetide therapy. Know that risk factors include the presence of esophagitis, gastritis, severe vomiting, or ulcers. Be especially alert for worsening of nausea and vomiting. Notify prescriber if GI bleeding is suspected or occurs.
- Be aware that adynamic bone may develop if PTH levels are chronically suppressed.

PATIENT TEACHING

- Review signs and symptoms of hypocalcemia with patient, including muscle spasms, myalgia, paresthesia, and seizures. Stress importance of reporting any such effects to prescriber immediately.
- Tell patient with heart failure that etelcalcetide therapy may worsen his condition, which may require closer monitoring.
- Instruct patient to report any signs of gastrointestinal bleeding, such as vomiting coffee-ground–like material, to prescriber.
- Inform patient that regular blood tests will be needed to monitor the effectiveness of etelcalcetide and to detect adverse effects.
- Inform mothers wishing to breastfeed that etelcalcetide is present in breast milk and that breastfeeding is not recommended during therapy.

ethacrynic acid

Edecrin

ethacrynate sodium

Edecrin

Class and Category

Pharmacologic class: Loop diuretic
Therapeutic class: Diuretic
Pregnancy category: B

Indications and Dosages

➤ *To promote diuresis in heart failure; hepatic cirrhosis; renal disease; ascites of short duration caused by cancer, idiopathic edema, or lymphedema; and edema in hospitalized children (excluding infants with congenital heart disease or nephrotic syndrome)*

ORAL SOLUTION, TABLETS

Adults. *Initial:* 50 to 100 mg daily as a single dose or in divided doses. Dosage increased by 25 to 50 mg daily, as needed. *Maintenance:* 50 to 200 mg daily.

Children (except infants). *Initial:* 25 mg daily. Dosage increased in 25-mg increments daily, as needed.

I.V. INFUSION, I.V. INJECTION

Adults. *Initial:* 50 mg or 0.5 to 1 mg/kg. Dose repeated in 2 to 4 hr, if needed. *Maximum:* 100 mg as single dose. I.V. infusion given slowly over at least 30 min and I.V. injection given slowly over several minutes with a running infusion.

Route	Onset	Peak	Duration
P.O.	30 min	2 hr	6–8 hr
I.V.	5 min	15–30 min	2 hr

Mechanism of Action

Probably inhibits the sulfhydryl-catalyzed enzyme systems that cause sodium and chloride resorption in the proximal and distal tubules and the ascending limb of the loop of Henle. These inhibitory effects increase urinary excretion of sodium, chloride, and water, causing profound diuresis. Drug also increases the ammonium, bicarbonate, calcium, excretion of potassium, hydrogen, magnesium, and phosphate.

Contraindications

Anuria; hypersensitivity to ethacrynic acid, ethacrynate sodium, sulfonylureas, or their components; infancy; severe diarrhea

Interactions

DRUGS

aminoglycosides, some cephalosporins: Increased risk of ototoxicity
amphotericin B: Increased risk of electrolyte imbalances, nephrotoxicity, and ototoxicity
corticosteroids: Increased risk of gastric hemorrhage
digoxin: Increased risk of digitalis toxicity
lithium: Increased risk of lithium toxicity
neuromuscular blockers: Possibly increased neuromuscular blockade
NSAIDs: Possibly decreased effects of ethacrynic acid
warfarin: Increased risk of bleeding

Adverse Reactions

CNS: Confusion, fatigue, headache, malaise, nervousness
CV: Orthostatic hypotension
EENT: Blurred vision, hearing loss, ototoxicity (ringing or buzzing in ears), sensation of fullness in ears, yellow vision
ENDO: Hyperglycemia, **hypoglycemia**
GI: Abdominal pain, anorexia, diarrhea, dysphagia, **GI bleeding (I.V.)**, nausea, vomiting
GU: Hematuria (I.V. form), interstitial nephritis, polyuria
HEME: Agranulocytosis, severe neutropenia, thrombocytopenia
SKIN: Rash
Other: Hyperuricemia, **hypochloremic alkalosis, hypokalemia, hypomagnesemia, hyponatremia**, hypovolemia, infusion-site irritation and pain

Nursing Considerations

WARNING Give ethacrynic acid and ethacrynate sodium cautiously in patients with advanced hepatic cirrhosis, especially those with a history of electrolyte imbalance or hepatic encephalopathy; both forms of drug may lead to lethal hepatic coma.

- Dilute ethacrynate sodium with D_5W or normal saline solution for I.V. infusion. Discard unused portion after 24 hours.
- Don't use diluted ethacrynate sodium that's cloudy or opalescent.
- Infuse I.V. ethacrynate sodium slowly over 30 minutes if given as an infusion or injected directly into a running infusion slowly over several minutes.
- Weigh patient daily, and assess him for signs and symptoms of dehydration and electrolyte imbalances.
- Monitor blood pressure and fluid intake and output, and check laboratory test results.
- Report significant changes. Prescriber may reduce dosage or temporarily stop drug.
- Know that if hypokalemia develops, administer replacement potassium, as ordered.
- Monitor serum glucose level frequently, especially if patient has diabetes mellitus; both forms of drug may cause hyperglycemia or hypoglycemia.

- Notify prescriber if patient experiences hearing loss; buzzing, sense of fullness, or ringing in his ears; or vertigo. Drug may have to be discontinued.

PATIENT TEACHING

- Instruct patient to take the last dose of ethacrynic acid several hours before bedtime to avoid sleep interruption from diuresis. If patient receives once-daily dosing, advise him to take the dose in the morning to avoid sleep disturbance caused by nocturia.
- Suggest that patient take ethacrynic acid with food or milk to reduce the likelihood of GI distress.
- Advise patient to change position slowly to minimize effects of orthostatic hypotension, especially if he also takes an antihypertensive.
- Urge patient to eat more high-potassium foods unless contraindicated and to take a potassium supplement, if prescribed, to prevent hypokalemia.
- Caution patient not to drink alcohol, stand for prolonged periods, or exercise during hot weather because these activities may exacerbate orthostatic hypotension.
- Instruct patient to notify prescriber if he has buzzing, fullness, or ringing in his ears; diarrhea; hearing loss; severe nausea; vertigo; or vomiting. Drug may need to be discontinued.
- Remind diabetic patients to check their serum glucose levels often for changes.

ethambutol hydrochloride

Etibi (CAN), Myambutol

Class and Category

Pharmacologic class: Synthetic antituberculotic
Therapeutic class: Antituberculotic
Pregnancy category: C

Indications and Dosages

➤ *As adjunct to treat pulmonary tuberculosis caused by* Mycobacterium tuberculosis

TABLETS

Adults and adolescents who haven't received previous antituberculotic therapy. 15 mg/kg daily.
Adults and adolescents who have received antituberculotic therapy. 25 mg/kg daily; after 60 days, decreased to 15 mg/kg daily.

Mechanism of Action

May suppress bacterial multiplication by interfering with RNA synthesis in susceptible bacteria that are actively dividing.

Contraindications

Hypersensitivity to ethambutol or its components, inability to report changes in vision, optic neuritis

Interactions

DRUGS

antacids that contain aluminum hydroxide: Decreased absorption of ethambutol

Adverse Reactions

CNS: Burning sensation or weakness in arms and legs, confusion, disorientation, dizziness, fever, headache, malaise, paresthesia, peripheral neuritis
EENT: Blurred vision, decreased visual acuity, eye pain, optic neuritis, red-green color blindness
GI: Abdominal pain, anorexia, **hepatic dysfunction**, nausea, vomiting
HEME: **Leukopenia**, **neutropenia**, **thrombocytopenia**
MS: Arthralgia, gouty arthritis, joint pain
RESP: **Pulmonary infiltrates**
SKIN: Dermatitis, **erythema multiforme**, **exfoliative dermatitis**, pruritus, rash
Other: **Anaphylaxis**, **hypersensitivity syndrome**, lymphadenopathy

Nursing Considerations

- Expect prescriber to refer patient for an ophthalmologic examination that includes tests for acuity, red-green color blindness, and visual fields before taking ethambutol and monthly thereafter. This is especially likely if therapy is prolonged or dosage exceeds 15 mg/kg daily.

WARNING Notify prescriber immediately if patient develops vision changes, and expect ethambutol to be stopped if they occur.

- Expect to give the patient at least one other antituberculotic with ethambutol, as prescribed, because bacteria may become resistant quickly to a single drug.
- Monitor laboratory test results for changes in liver function or for increased serum

uric acid level if patient has gouty arthritis or impaired renal function. Notify prescriber of any abnormalities.
- Obtain a monthly sputum specimen, as ordered, to check bacteriologic response in sputum-positive patient.
- Know that successful ethambutol therapy typically takes 6 to 12 months but may take years.

PATIENT TEACHING
- Teach patient to recognize possible adverse reactions to ethambutol.
- Advise patient to take drug with food if he experiences adverse GI reactions.
- Instruct patient to take a missed dose as soon as he remembers, unless it's nearly time for the next dose, but not to double-dose.
- Explain that ethambutol therapy may last months or years and that compliance is essential.
- Advise patient to notify prescriber if no improvement occurs within 3 weeks of starting ethambutol therapy; if bothersome or severe adverse reactions occur; if his vision changes; or if a fever, joint pain, or rash (possible hypersensitivity) develops.

ethosuximide

Zarontin

Class and Category

Pharmacologic class: Succinimide
Therapeutic class: Anticonvulsant
Pregnancy category: Not classified

Indications and Dosages

➤ *To manage absence seizures*

CAPSULES, SYRUP

Adults and children age 6 and over. *Initial:* 500 mg daily. *Maintenance:* Increased by 250 mg every 4 to 7 days until control is achieved with minimal adverse reactions. *Optimal for children:* 20 mg/kg/day.
Children ages 3 to 6. *Initial:* 250 mg daily. *Maintenance:* Increased by 250 mg every 4 to 7 days until control is achieved with minimal adverse reactions. *Optimal:* 20 mg/kg/day.

Mechanism of Action

Elevates the seizure threshold and reduces the frequency of attacks by depressing the motor cortex and elevating the threshold of CNS response to convulsive stimuli.

Contraindications

Hypersensitivity to ethosuximide, other succinimides, or their components

Interactions

DRUGS

phenytoin: Possibly increased blood phenytoin level
valproic acid: Increased or decreased blood ethosuximide level

Adverse Reactions

CNS: Aggressiveness, ataxia, decreased concentration, depression, dizziness, drowsiness, euphoria, fatigue, headache, hyperactivity, irritability, lethargy, lightheadedness, nightmares, psychosis, sleep disturbance, **suicidal ideation**, unsteadiness when walking
EENT: Gingival hypertrophy, myopia, tongue swelling
GI: Abdominal and epigastric pain, abdominal cramps, anorexia, diarrhea, hiccups, indigestion, nausea, vomiting
GU: Increased libido, microscopic hematuria, vaginal bleeding
HEME: Agranulocytosis, **aplastic anemia**, eosinophilia, **leukopenia**, **pancytopenia**
SKIN: Erythematous and pruritic rashes, hirsutism, **Stevens–Johnson syndrome**, systemic lupus erythematosus, urticaria
Other: Drug reaction with eosinophilia and systemic symptoms (DRESS), **hypersensitivity reaction**, weight loss

Nursing Considerations

- Use ethosuximide with extreme caution in patients with hepatic or renal disease.
- Give other anticonvulsants concurrently, as prescribed, to control generalized tonic–clonic seizures.
- Monitor CBC and platelet count and assess for signs of infection, such as cough, fever, and pharyngitis. Also routinely evaluate liver and renal function test results.
- Take safety precautions because drug may cause adverse CNS reactions, such as dizziness and drowsiness.
- Monitor patient closely for evidence of suicidal thinking or behavior, especially when therapy starts or dosage changes.

- Assess patient regularly for signs of skin adverse effects. Stop ethosuximide immediately at first sign of rash and notify prescriber.

PATIENT TEACHING

- Emphasize the importance of complying with ethosuximide regimen.
- Advise patient to take a missed dose as soon as he remembers, unless it's nearly time for the next dose. Warn him not to double the dose.
- Instruct patient not to engage in potentially hazardous activities until drug's CNS effects are known.
- Caution patient not to stop taking drug abruptly; doing so increases the risk of absence seizures.
- Inform patient that the most common side effects of ethosuximide therapy include diarrhea, dizziness or lightheadedness, fatigue, headache, hiccups, indigestion, loss of concentration or appetite, nausea, stomach pain, unsteadiness when walking, vomiting, and weight loss.
- Urge caregivers to watch patient closely for evidence of suicidal tendencies, especially when therapy starts or dosage changes, and to report any concerns immediately to prescriber.
- Advise patient or caregiver that prescriber should be notified immediately if a skin rash develops. Also tell patient to notify prescriber if persistent or serious adverse effects develop while taking ethosuximide.
- Caution female patient of childbearing age to use effective contraception methods while taking ethosuximide and to alert prescriber if pregnancy is suspected or known, as drug may cause fetal harm. Encourage female patient who becomes pregnant while taking ethosuximide to enroll in the North American antiepileptic drug pregnancy registry by calling 1-888-233-2334. Explain that this registry is collecting information about the safety of antiepileptic drugs during pregnancy.
- Inform female patients desiring to breastfeed an infant that ethosuximide does pass into human breast milk. Advise patient to discuss the benefits against the risks with prescriber before doing so.

ethotoin

Peganone

Class and Category

Pharmacologic class: Hydantoin
Therapeutic class: Anticonvulsant
Pregnancy category: D

Indications and Dosages

➤ *To manage tonic–clonic and complex partial seizures*

TABLETS

Adults and adolescents. *Initial:* 0.5 to 1 g on the first day in 4 to 6 divided doses, increased over several days until desired response is reached. *Maintenance:* 2 to 3 g daily in 4 to 6 divided doses. *Maximum:* 3 g daily.
Children. *Initial:* Up to 750 mg daily, based on weight and age, in 4 to 6 divided doses, adjusted as needed and tolerated. *Maintenance:* 0.5 to 1 g daily in 4 to 6 divided doses. *Maximum:* 3 g daily.

DOSAGE ADJUSTMENT For debilitated patients, initial dosage lowered to reduce the risk of adverse reactions.

Mechanism of Action

Limits the spread of seizure activity and the start of new seizures by:

- regulating voltage-dependent sodium and calcium channels in neurons
- inhibiting calcium movement across neuronal membranes
- enhancing sodium–potassium adenosine triphosphatase activity in neurons and glial cells.

These actions may result from ethotoin's ability to slow the recovery rate of inactivated sodium channels.

Contraindications

Hematologic disorders; hepatic dysfunction; hypersensitivity to ethotoin, phenytoin, other hydantoins, or their components

Interactions

DRUGS

drugs affecting hematopoietic system: Increased risk of hematologic adverse effects
oral anticoagulants: Possibly impaired metabolism of these drugs and increased risk of ethotoin toxicity; possibly increased anticoagulant effect initially, but decreased effect with prolonged therapy

E F

Adverse Reactions

CNS: Clumsiness, confusion, drowsiness, excitement, peripheral neuropathy, sedation, slurred speech, stuttering, **suicidal ideation**, tremor
EENT: Nystagmus
GI: Constipation, diarrhea, nausea, vomiting
HEME: Agranulocytosis, leukopenia, thrombocytopenia
SKIN: Rash, **Stevens-Johnson syndrome, toxic epidermal necrolysis**
Other: Lymphadenopathy, systemic lupus erythematosus

Nursing Considerations

- Obtain CBC and differential before treatment and monthly for first few months of ethotoin therapy, as ordered.

WARNING **Know that ethotoin shouldn't be stopped abruptly because of risk of status epilepticus. Plan to reduce dosage gradually or substitute another drug, as prescribed.**

- Monitor patient for signs and symptoms of infection or unusual bleeding because ethotoin may cause hematologic toxicity.
- Know that because of ethotoin's potential for hepatotoxicity, monitor liver enzymes and expect drug to be discontinued if test results are abnormal.
- Notify prescriber immediately and expect ethotoin to be stopped and replaced with another drug if patient has decreased blood counts, enlarged lymph nodes, or rash.
- Be aware that ethotoin may be substituted for phenytoin without loss of seizure control if patient develops severe gingival hyperplasia or other adverse reactions. Expect ethotoin dosage to be 4 to 6 times greater than phenytoin dosage.
- Institute and maintain seizure precautions according to facility protocol.
- Monitor patient closely for evidence of suicidal thinking or behavior, especially when therapy starts or dosage changes.

PATIENT TEACHING

- Instruct patient to take ethotoin exactly as prescribed and not to stop it abruptly.
- Advise patient to take drug with food to enhance absorption and reduce adverse GI effects.
- Advise patient to report easy bruising, epistaxis, fever, malaise, petechiae, or sore throat to prescriber immediately.
- Instruct patient to keep medical appointments to monitor drug effectiveness and check for adverse reactions. Explain the need for periodic laboratory tests.
- Urge patient to avoid alcohol during ethotoin therapy.
- Caution patient to avoid hazardous activities until drug's adverse effects are known.
- Encourage patient to wear or carry medical identification indicating his diagnosis and drug therapy.
- Urge caregivers to watch patient closely for evidence of suicidal tendencies, especially when therapy starts or dosage changes, and to report any concerns immediately to prescriber.
- Encourage female patient who becomes pregnant while taking ethotoin to enroll in the North American antiepileptic drug pregnancy registry by calling 1-888-233-2334. Explain that this registry is collecting information about the safety of antiepileptic drugs during pregnancy.
- Advise patient to tell all healthcare providers about ethotoin therapy because drug may react with other medication, including herbal supplements, over-the-counter drugs, and vitamins.

etidronate disodium

Didronel

Class and Category

Pharmacologic class: Bisphosphonate
Therapeutic class: Antihypercalcemic agent, bone resorption inhibitor
Pregnancy category: C

Indications and Dosages

➤ *To treat Paget's disease of bone (osteitis deformans)*

TABLETS

Adults. 5 to 10 mg/kg daily for up to 6 months, or 11 to 20 mg/kg daily for up to 3 months.

➤ *To prevent and treat heterotopic ossification after total hip replacement*

TABLETS

Adults. 20 mg/kg daily for 1 month before surgery and then 20 mg/kg daily for 3 months after surgery for a total of 4 mo of treatment.

➤ *To prevent and treat heterotopic ossification after spinal cord injury*

TABLETS

Adults. 20 mg/kg daily for 2 wk and then 10 mg/kg daily for 10 wk for a total of 12 wk of treatment.

Mechanism of Action

Inhibits normal and abnormal bone resorption by reducing bone turnover and slowing the remodeling of pagetic or heterotopic bone. Etidronate also decreases the elevated cardiac output seen in Paget's disease of bone and reduces local increases in skin temperature. It also inhibits the abnormal bone resorption that may occur with cancer and reduces the amount of calcium that enters the blood from resorbed bone.

Contraindications

Esophageal abnormalities that delay gastric emptying, such as achalasia and stricture; hypersensitivity to etidronate, bisphosphonates, or their components

Interactions

DRUGS

antacids that contain aluminum, calcium, or magnesium; vitamin and mineral supplements that contain aluminum, calcium, iron, or magnesium: Decreased etidronate absorption

warfarin: Possibly increased prothrombin time

FOODS

high-calcium food (such as milk and other dairy products): Decreased etidronate absorption

Adverse Reactions

CNS: Amnesia, confusion, depression, hallucination, headache, paresthesias

EENT: Altered taste, glossitis, metallic taste

GI: Diarrhea, elevated liver enzymes, nausea

GU: Nephrotoxicity

HEME: Agranulocytosis, **leukopenia**, **pancytopenia**

MS: Atypical arthralgia, arthritis, atypical subtrochanteric and diaphyseal femoral fractures, bone pain, leg cramps, osteomalacia, osteonecrosis of jaw

SKIN: Alopecia, follicular eruption, macular rash, maculopapular rash, pruritus, **Stevens-Johnson syndrome**, **toxic epidermal necrolysis**, urticaria

Other: Angioedema, **hypocalcemia**

Nursing Considerations

- Use etidronate cautiously in patients with upper GI problems such as Barrett's esophagus, duodenitis, dysphagia, gastritis, other esophageal diseases, or ulcers because drug may cause local irritation of the upper GI mucosa.
- Anticipate starting etidronate as soon as possible after spinal cord injury, preferably before signs of heterotopic ossification.
- Expect etidronate not to inhibit healing of spinal fractures, affect prosthesis, or disrupt trochanter attachment when used after total hip replacement.
- Give 2 hours before meals to prevent decreased absorption.

WARNING Watch for hypocalcemia if patient receives parenteral form for more than 3 days.

- Know that when treating hypercalcemia, you should expect to continue giving drug for up to 90 days if serum calcium level remains within acceptable range.
- Monitor patient for adverse esophageal effects such as esophagitis, esophageal erosions, and esophageal ulcers that may occur with bleeding, as well as duodenal and gastric ulcers, because these adverse effects have occurred with other oral biphosphonates.
- Know that risk of severe adverse esophageal reactions increases in patients who lie down after taking drug, who fail to swallow it with a full glass of water, or who continue to take drug after developing symptoms of esophageal irritation.
- Make sure patient has had a dental checkup before having an invasive dental procedures during etidronate therapy, especially if he has cancer; is receiving chemotherapy, head or neck radiation, or a corticosteroid; or has poor oral hygiene because the risk of osteonecrosis of the jaw is increased in these patients. Be aware that the risk increases the longer the patient takes etidronate.

PATIENT TEACHING

- Instruct patient to take etidronate tablets on an empty stomach—2 hours before meals, antacids, or calcium supplements. Urge him to drink a full glass of water with tablets and to avoid taking drug with milk or other high-calcium foods.

- Tell patient to take a missed dose as soon as he remembers as long as 2 hours have elapsed since his last meal. Instruct him not to eat for another 2 hours. Warn against doubling the dose.
- Inform patient with Paget's disease that his response to etidronate may be slow and may continue for months after treatment.
- Instruct patient to inform prescriber if he develops chest pain, difficulty swallowing or pain when swallowing, or new or worsening heartburn.
- Advise patient to notify prescriber if he develops new or worsening groin or thigh pain.
- Stress importance of patient notifying prescriber if invasive dental procedures are going to be done because etidronate therapy may need to be discontinued as the risk of osteonecrosis of the jaw may be decreased in the absence of etidronate therapy.

etodolac

Class and Category

Pharmacologic class: NSAID
Therapeutic class: Analgesic, anti-inflammatory
Pregnancy category: C

Indications and Dosages

➤ *To manage osteoarthritis and rheumatoid arthritis*

CAPSULES, TABLETS

Adults. 600 to 1,000 mg daily divided and given every 8 to 12 hr. Alternatively, 300 mg every 8 hr. *Maximum:* 1,000 mg daily.

E.R. TABLETS

Adults. 400 to 1,000 mg daily.

➤ *To manage juvenile rheumatoid arthritis*

E.R. TABLETS

Children ages 6 to 16 weighing greater than 60 kg (132 lb). 1,000 mg once daily.
Children ages 6 to 16 weighing 46 kg (101 lb) to 60 kg (132 lb). 800 mg once daily.
Children ages 6 to 16 weighing 31 kg (68 lb) to 45 kg (99 lb). 600 mg once daily.
Children ages 6 to 16 weighing 20 kg (44 lb) to 30 kg (66 lb). 400 mg once daily.

➤ *To relieve mild to moderate pain*

CAPSULES, TABLETS

Adults. *Initial:* 400 mg and then 200 to 400 mg every 6 to 8 hr. *Maximum:* 1,000 mg daily.

Route	Onset	Peak	Duration
P.O.	30 min	1–2 hr	4–12 hr

Mechanism of Action

Blocks the activity of cyclooxygenase, the enzyme needed for prostaglandin synthesis. Prostaglandins, important mediators of the inflammatory response, cause local vasodilation with pain and swelling. By inhibiting cyclooxygenase and prostaglandins, this NSAID causes inflammatory symptoms and pain to subside.

Contraindications

Angioedema, asthma, bronchospasm, nasal polyps, rhinitis, or urticaria induced by aspirin, iodides, or NSAIDs; coronary artery bypass graft surgery; hypersensitivity to etodolac or its components

Interactions

DRUGS

ACE inhibitors: Possibly decreased hypotensive effects of these drugs
antacids: Decreased blood etodolac level
antiplatelets, oral anticoagulants, thrombolytics: Prolonged PT (with warfarin), increased risk of bleeding
cyclosporine: Increased nephrotoxic effects, increased blood cyclosporine level
digoxin: Increased blood digoxin level and risk of digitalis toxicity
diuretics: Possibly increased risk of renal insufficiency with prolonged use
lithium: Increased blood lithium level and, possibly, toxicity
methotrexate: Increased risk of methotrexate toxicity

ACTIVITIES

alcohol use: Increased risk of adverse GI effects

Adverse Reactions

CNS: Asthenia, chills, **CVA**, depression, dizziness, drowsiness, fatigue, fever, insomnia, irritability, malaise, nervousness, **seizures**, somnolence, syncope

CV: Edema, **heart failure**, hypertension, **MI**, palpitations, tachycardia, vasculitis
EENT: Blurred vision, deafness, loss of taste, photophobia, tinnitus
ENDO: Hyperglycemia in diabetics
GI: Abdominal pain or distention, anorexia, constipation, diarrhea, diverticulitis, dyspepsia, dysphagia, elevated liver enzymes, esophagitis, flatulence, gastritis, gastroenteritis, gastroesophageal reflux disease, **GI bleeding** and ulceration, **GI perforation**, hemorrhoids, **hepatic failure**, **hepatitis**, hiatal hernia, indigestion, **melena**, nausea, **pancreatitis**, peptic ulcer, stomatitis, vomiting
GU: Dysuria, elevated serum creatinine level, hematuria, **renal failure or insufficiency**, **renal papillary necrosis**, urinary frequency
HEME: Agranulocytosis, **aplastic anemia**, easy bruising, **hemolytic anemia**, **leukopenia**, **neutropenia**, **pancytopenia**, **thrombocytopenia**
MS: Arthralgia, muscle pain
RESP: Asthma, **bronchospasm**, **pulmonary infiltrate with eosinophilia**, **respiratory depression**
SKIN: Erythema multiforme, **exfoliative dermatitis**, flushing, leukocytoclastic vasculitis, pruritus, **Stevens–Johnson syndrome**, **toxic epidermal necrolysis**, urticaria, vesiculobullous or other rash
Other: Anaphylaxis, **angioedema**, lymphadenopathy, **sepsis**

Nursing Considerations

- Assess patient's hydration status and rehydrate, if needed and as ordered, before starting etodolac therapy.
- Use etodolac with extreme caution in patients with a history of GI bleeding or ulcer disease because NSAIDs increase the risk of GI bleeding and ulceration. Expect to use etodolac for the shortest time possible in these patients. Also use with extreme caution in patients with advanced renal disease because etodolac is eliminated mainly by the kidneys.
- Be aware that serious GI tract bleeding, perforation, and ulceration may occur without warning symptoms. Elderly patents are at greater risk. To minimize risk, give drug with food. If GI distress occurs, withhold drug and notify prescriber immediately.
- Use etodolac cautiously in patients with hypertension, and monitor blood pressure closely throughout therapy. Drug may cause hypertension or worsen it.

WARNING Monitor patient closely for thrombotic events, including MI and stroke, because NSAIDs increase the risk.

- Watch for less common but serious adverse GI reactions, including anorexia, constipation, diverticulitis, dysphagia, esophagitis, gastritis, gastroenteritis, gastroesophageal reflux disease, hemorrhoids, hiatal hernia, melena, stomatitis, and vomiting, especially if patient is elderly or taking etodolac long term.
- Monitor liver enzymes. Rarely, elevated levels may progress to severe hepatic reactions, including fatal hepatitis, hepatic necrosis, and hepatic failure.
- Monitor BUN and serum creatinine levels in patients with heart failure, hepatic dysfunction, or impaired renal function; those taking ACE inhibitors or diuretics; and elderly patients because drug may cause renal failure.
- Monitor CBC for decreased hemoglobin level and hematocrit because drug may worsen anemia.

WARNING Know that if patient has bone marrow suppression or is receiving antineoplastic drug therapy, monitor laboratory results (including WBC count), and watch for evidence of infection because anti-inflammatory and antipyretic actions of etodolac may mask it, such as fever and pain.

- Assess patient's skin routinely for rash or other signs of hypersensitivity reaction because etodolac and other NSAIDs may cause serious skin reactions without warning, even in patients with no history of NSAID hypersensitivity. Stop drug at first sign of reaction and notify prescriber.

PATIENT TEACHING

- Tell patient to take etodolac with food or after meals if adverse GI reactions occur.
- Caution him to avoid aspirin or aspirin-containing products while taking drug.
- Advise patient not to drink alcohol during therapy because this can increase the risk of adverse GI reactions.
- Inform patient that he may experience dizziness or drowsiness.

- Instruct him to notify prescriber immediately about blood in urine, easy bruising, itching, rash, swelling, or yellow eyes or skin.
- Caution pregnant patient not to take etodolac or other NSAIDs during the third trimester because drug may cause premature closure of the ductus arteriosus.
- Explain that etodolac may increase the risk of serious adverse cardiovascular reactions; urge patient to seek immediate medical attention for possible reactions, chest pain, shortness of breath, slurring of speech, or weakness.
- Tell patient that etodolac therapy also may increase the risk of serious adverse GI reactions; stress the importance of seeking immediate medical attention for such signs and symptoms such as abdominal or epigastric pain, black or tarry stools, indigestion, or vomiting blood or material that looks like coffee grounds.
- Explain the possibility of rare but serious skin reactions. Urge patient to seek immediate medical attention for blisters, fever, itching, rash, or other indications of hypersensitivity.

etravirine

Intelence

Class and Category

Pharmacologic class: Non-nucleoside reverse transcriptase inhibitor (NNRTI)
Therapeutic class: Antiretroviral
Pregnancy category: B

Indications and Dosages

➤ *As adjunct to treat HIV-1 infection in patients who are antiretroviral treatment-experienced and have evidence of viral replication and HIV-1 strains resistant to an NNRTI and other antiretroviral agents*

TABLETS

Adults and children ages 6 to 18 weighing 30 kg (66 lb) or more. 200 mg twice daily following a meal.
Children ages 6 to 18 yr weighing 25 kg (55 lb) to less than 30 kg (66 lb). 150 mg twice daily following a meal.
Children ages 6 to 18 yr weighing 20 kg (44 lb) to less than 25 kg (55 lb). 125 mg twice daily following a meal.
Children ages 6 to 18 yr weighing 16 kg (35.2 lb) to less than 20 kg (44 lb). 100 mg twice daily following a meal.

Mechanism of Action

Binds directly to reverse transcriptase and blocks the RNA-dependent and DNA-dependent DNA polymerase activities by causing a disruption of the enzyme's catalytic site.

Contraindications

Hypersensitivity to etravirine or its components

Interactions

DRUGS

amiodarone, artemether, atazanavir, atazanavir/ritonavir, atorvastatin, bepridil, buprenorphine, clopidogrel, cyclosporine, dihydroartemisinin, disopyramide, dolutegravir, dolutegravir/darunavir/ritonavir, dolutegravir/lopinavir/ritonavir, flecainide, indinavir, lidocaine (systemic), lovastatin, lumefantrine, maraviroc, mexiletine, propafenone, quinidine, rilpividine, sildenafil, simvastatin, sirolimus, tacrolimus, telaprevir, warfarin: Decreased plasma concentrations of these drugs with possible decreased effectiveness
boceprevir: Decreased plasma concentration of etravirine with possible decreased effectiveness; increased plasma concentration of boceprevir with possible increased risk of adverse reactions
carbamazepine, darunavir/ritonavir, dexamethasone (systemic), efavirenz, lopinavir/ritonavir, nevirapine, phenobarbital, phenytoin, rifampin, rifapentine, ritonavir, St. John's wort, saquinavir/ritonavir, tipanavir/ritonavir: Decreased plasma concentration of etravirine and its effectiveness
clarithromycin, itraconazole, ketoconazole: Decreased plasma concentrations of these drugs with possible decreased effectiveness; increased plasma concentration of etravirine
delavirdine: Increased plasma concentration of etravirine with possible increased risk of serious adverse reactions
diazepam, digoxin, fluvastatin, fosamprenavir, fosamprenavir/ritonavir, maravirox/darunavir/ritonavir, nelfinavir,

pitavastatin: Increased plasma concentration of these drugs with possible increased risk of serious adverse reactions
rifabutin: Decreased plasma concentration of both etravirine and rifabutin with possible decreased effectiveness of both drugs
voriconazole: Increased plasma concentrations of both etravirine and voriconazole with possible increased risk of serious adverse reactions

Adverse Reactions

CNS: Abnormal dreams, amnesia, anxiety, confusion, **CVA**, difficulty concentrating, disorientation, fatigue, fever, general malaise, hypoesthesia, nervousness, nightmares, paresthesia, peripheral neuropathy, **seizures**, sleep disorders, sluggishness, somnolence, syncope, tremor, vertigo
CV: Angina pectoris, **atrial fibrillation**, dyslipidemia, elevated cholesterol and triglyceride levels, **MI**
EENT: Blurred vision, conjunctivitis, dry mouth, oral lesions, stomatitis
ENDO: Cushingoid appearance, diabetes mellitus, fat redistribution, gynecomastia, hyperglycemia
GI: Abdominal distention, anorexia, constipation, elevated liver or pancreatic enzymes, flatulence, gastroesophageal reflux disease, gastritis, hematemesis, **hepatic failure**, hepatic steatosis, **hepatitis**, hepatomegaly, **pancreatitis**, vomiting
GU: Acute renal failure, elevated creatinine level
HEME: Decreased hemoglobin eosinophilia, **hemolytic anemia**, **leukopenia**, **neutropenia**, **thrombocytopenia**
MS: Joint or muscle aches, **rhabdomyolysis**
RESP: Bronchospasm, exertional dyspnea
SKIN: Blisters, diaphoresis, dry skin, **erythema multiforme**, lipohypertrophy, night sweats, **Stevens–Johnson syndrome**, **toxic epidermal necrolysis**
Other: Angioedema, **drug reaction with eosinophilia and systemic symptoms (DRESS)**, immune reconstitution syndrome, lipodystrophy

Nursing Considerations

- Administer etravirine twice daily following meals.
- Dissolve tablet in 5 ml of water and stir well until the water looks milky for the patient who cannot swallow tablets. If needed, mixture can be further diluted with milk or orange juice (not carbonated beverages, grapefruit juice, or warm liquids). However, water must be used first to dissolve tablet before any other liquid is used. Have patient drink mixture immediately and then add more milk, orange juice, or water to glass and have patient drink it. Do this several times to ensure that patient has received the entire dose.

WARNING Assess patient for skin alterations, especially a rash that may occur anytime but most commonly within the first 6 weeks of treatment because, although uncommon, etravirine has caused severe skin and hypersensitivity reactions. Notify prescriber immediately if rash and other symptoms that may accompany the rash (such as angioedema, blisters, fatigue, jaundice, joint or muscle aches, or oral lesions) occur. Expect to check patient's liver enzymes and drug to be discontinued if rash is serious. Know that symptoms can evolve into a life-threatening reaction if drug is not promptly discontinued.

- Be aware that immune reconstitution syndrome has occurred in patients treated with combination antiretroviral therapy, including etravirine. The inflammatory response predisposes susceptible patients to opportunistic infections such as cytomegalovirus, *Mycobacterium avium* infection, *Pneumocystis jiroveci* pneumonia, or tuberculosis. Autoimmune disorders such as Graves' disease, Guillain–Barré syndrome, or polymyositis have also occurred. Report sudden or unusual adverse reactions to prescriber.
- Observe patient for redistribution of body fat, including breast enlargement, central obesity, development of buffalo hump, facial wasting, and peripheral wasting, which may produce a cushingoid-type appearance.

PATIENT TEACHING

- Tell patient to take etravirine twice daily following a meal. Tell her not to chew the tablets but to swallow them whole.
- Instruct patient to swallow the tablet(s) with a liquid such as water. If patient is

unable to swallow tablet, tell her to do the following: place tablet in a glass containing 1 teaspoon of water; stir well until water is milky looking; add more water or alternatively milk or orange juice, if needed (milk or orange juice should only be used after water has been used first); drink immediately; add milk, orange juice, or water to glass and drink. Repeat this procedure several times to ensure that entire dose has been taken. Caution patient not to use carbonated beverages, grapefruit juice, or warm liquids to dissolve drug.

- Advise patient that if a dose is missed and it is less than 6 hours from the time it is usually taken, she should take the drug following the intake of a meal. However, if it is longer than 6 hours, tell her to skip the dose and resume her normal dosing schedule with the next dose.
- Tell mothers not to breastfeed their infants while receiving etravirine.
- Alert patient to the possibility of fat distribution with the appearance of a buffalo hump, thin extremities and face, and breast enlargement.
- Instruct patient to inform all prescribers of etravirine therapy and not to take any drugs, including over-the-counter drugs and herbal medicines, without prescriber consent, because etravirine interacts with many drugs.

WARNING Tell patient to notify prescriber immediately of any alteration in skin but especially a rash that may be associated with other symptoms. Drug will have to be discontinued if serious.

everolimus

Afinitor, Afinitor Disperz, Zortress

Class and Category

Pharmacologic class: M-TOR kinase inhibitor
Therapeutic class: Immunosuppressant
Pregnancy category: Not classified

Indications and Dosages

➤ *As adjunct to prevent organ rejection in renal transplantation*

TABLETS (ZORTRESS)

Adults. *Initial:* 0.75 mg twice daily in combination with reduced-dose cyclosporine, administered as soon as possible after transplantation.

➤ *As adjunct to prevent organ rejection in liver transplantation*

TABLETS (ZORTRESS)

Adults. *Initial*: 1 mg twice daily in combination with reduced-dose tacrolimus begun 30 days post-transplant.

DOSAGE ADJUSTMENT For patient taking Zortress, dosage adjusted at 4- to 5-day intervals, as needed, according to everolimus blood concentrations, tolerability, change in concomitant medications, the clinical situation, and individual response. For patients with mild hepatic impairment, initial daily dose reduced by one-third, and for patients with moderate or severe hepatic impairment, initial daily dose is reduced by 50% with further adjustments made according to everolimus blood concentration levels.

➤ *To treat advanced hormone receptor-positive, HER2-negative breast cancer in postmenopausal women in combination with exemestane after failure of treatment with anastrozole or letrozole; to treat progressive neuroendocrine tumors of pancreatic origin or are progressive, well-differentiated, nonfunctional tumors of gastrointestinal or lung origin that are locally advanced, metastatic, or unresectable; to treat renal cell carcinoma after failure of treatment with sorafenib or sunitinib; to treat tuberous sclerosis complex-associated renal angiomyolipoma that does not require immediate surgery*

TABLETS (AFINITOR)

Adults. 10 mg once daily. Treatment continued until disease progression or unacceptable toxicity occurs.

➤ *To treat tuberous sclerosis complex-associated subependymal giant cell astrocytoma (SEGA)*

ORAL SUSPENSION (AFINITOR DISPERZ), TABLETS (AFINITOR)

Adults and children age 1 year and over. 4.5 mg/m^2 once daily until disease progresses or unacceptable toxicity occurs.

➤ *As adjunct to treat tuberous sclerosis complex-associated partial-onset seizures*

ORAL SUSPENSION (AFINITOR DISPERZ)

Adults and children age 2 years and over. 5 mg/m^2 once daily until disease progresses or unacceptable toxicity occurs.

DOSAGE ADJUSTMENT For patients taking Afinitor or Afinitor Disperz, dosage adjusted according to degree of adverse reactions present. Also, for patients with breast cancer, neuroendocrine tumors, renal cell carcinoma, or tuberous sclerosis complex-associated renal angiomyolipoma and mild hepatic impairment, dosage reduced to 7.5 mg once daily or 5 mg once daily if higher dose is not tolerated; for moderate hepatic impairment, dosage reduced to 5 mg once daily or 2.5 mg once daily if higher dose is not tolerated; and for patients with severe hepatic impairment, dosage reduced to 2.5 mg once daily. For patients with tuberous sclerosis complex-associated subependymal giant cell astrocytoma or tuberous sclerosis complex-associated partial-onset seizures and severe hepatic impairment, dosage reduced to 2.5 mg/m^2 once daily. For patient taking a P-gp and moderate CYP3A inhibitors and who has breast cancer, neuroendocrine tumor, renal cell carcinoma, or tuberous sclerosis complex-associated renal angiomyolipoma, dosage reduced to 2.5 mg once daily, with dosage then increased to 5 mg once daily, if tolerated. For patients taking P-gp and moderate CYP3A inhibitors and who have tuberous sclerosis complex-associated subependymal giant cell astrocytoma or tuberous sclerosis complex-associated partial-onset seizures, daily dosage reduced by 50%. For patients taking a P-gp and strong CYP3A4 inducers and who have any indication treated by everolimus, dosage doubled.

Mechanism of Action

Causes immunosuppression by inhibiting antigenic and interleukin (IL-2 and IL-15) stimulated activation and proliferation of B and T lymphocytes.

Contraindications

Hypersensitivity to everolimus, other rapamycin derivatives, or their components

Interactions

DRUGS

ACE inhibitors: Possibly increased risk of angioedema

amprenavir, aprepitant, atazanavir, clarithromycin, cyclosporine, digoxin, diltiazem, erythromycin, fluconazole, fosamprenavir, indinavir, itraconazole, ketoconazole, macrolide antibiotics, nefazodone, nelfinavir, nicardipine, ritonavir, saquinavir, telithromycin, verapamil, voriconazle: Possible increased blood everolimus level

anticonvulsants, carbamazepine, efavirenz, nevirapine, phenobarbital, phenytoin, rifabutin, rifampin, rifapentine, St. John's wort: Possibly decreased blood everolimus level

live vaccines: Possibly increased risk of contracting disease from live virus

FOODS

grapefruit, grapefruit juice: Possibly decreased metabolism of everolimus

Adverse Reactions

CNS: Aggression, agitation, anxiety, asthenia, chills, dizziness, fatigue, fever, headache, insomnia, **progressive multiple leukoencephalopathy (PML)**, multiple, paresthesia, reflex sympathetic dystrophy

CV: **Arterial thrombotic events**, chest pain, **congestive heart failure**, **deep vein thrombosis**, hyperlipidemia, hypertension, **pericardial effusion**, peripheral edema, tachycardia

EENT: Conjunctivitis, dry mouth, epistaxis, eyelid pain, oropharyngeal pain, rhinorrhea, stomatitis

ENDO: Hot flashes, hyperglycemia, new-onset diabetes mellitus

GI: Abdominal pain, anorexia, ascites, cholecystitis, cholelithiasis, constipation, diarrhea, elevated bilirubin or liver enzymes, gastroenteritis, **hepatic artery thrombosis** (liver transplant), nausea, **pancreatitis**

GU: **Acute renal failure**, amenorrhea, azospermia, **BK virus-associated nephropathy**, elevated creatinine level, **kidney graft thrombosis**, **nephrotoxicity**, oligospermia, proteinuria, UTI

HEME: Anemia, **bleeding**, **elevated partial thromboplastin time**, **elevated prothrombin time**, **leukopenia**,

lymphopenia, neutropenia, thrombocytopenia
MS: Arthralgia; back, extremity, or jaw pain; muscle spasm; myalgia
RESP: Cough, dyspnea, **interstitial lung disease**, noninfectious pneumonitis, pleural effusion, **pulmonary embolism**, upper respiratory infection
SKIN: Acne, alopecia, dermatitis, erythema, nail disorders, pruritus, rash, **skin cancer**
Other: Angioedema; **decreased bicarbonate level**; delayed wound healing; elevated alkaline phosphatase; **hyperkalemia**; **hypersensitivity reactions**; **hypocalcemia**; **hypokalemia**; **hyponatremia**; **hypophosphatemia**; infections such as bacterial, fungal, protozoal, and viral; **lymphomas and other malignancies**; opportunistic infections including polyoma virus; **sepsis**; **septic shock**; weight loss

Nursing Considerations

- Be aware that Zortress brand of everolimus isn't recommended in transplants other than kidney or liver transplantation. Know that everolimus therapy should not begin until 30 days after liver transplant because of patient's increased risk of developing hepatic artery thrombosis, which may lead to graft loss or death.
- Be aware that another form of everolimus under the trade names of Afinitor and Afinitor Disperz are used only to treat certain cancers. The three brands are not interchangeable. To avoid a medication error, make sure that the Zortress brand is being administered for prevention of kidney or liver transplant rejection and do not interchange Afinitor with Afinitor Disperz.
- Know that patients with galactose intolerance, glucose–galactose malabsorption, or Lapp lactase deficiency should not receive everolimus therapy because this may result in diarrhea and malabsorption.
- Expect female patient of childbearing age to undergo a pregnancy test prior to initiating everolimus therapy, because drug can cause fetal harm.
- Assess patient's renal function before therapy with Afinitor or Afinitor Disperz brand of everolimus is begun, and annually thereafter unless patient has underlying risk factors for renal failure. Renal evaluation in these patients should be done every 6 months.

WARNING Monitor patient closely for hypersensitivity reactions that could be severe. These may include anaphylaxis, angioedema, chest pain, dyspnea, or flushing. At the first sign of a reaction, notify prescriber, expect to administer emergency treatment according to institutional protocol, and expect drug to be discontinued.

- Measure whole blood trough concentrations of both cyclosporine and everolimus in patient with kidney transplant or tacrolimus and everolimus in liver transplant because of increased risk of nephrotoxicity when either combination of drugs are used or when drug is used to treat malignancies or tuberous sclerosis complex-associated partial-onset seizures. Everolimus levels, ideally drawn 4 to 5 days after a previous dosing change, will also reveal if the therapeutic range has been achieved (3 to 8 ng/ml).
- Know that dosage adjustments of everolimus can then be made, as needed. In addition, everolimus levels should be obtained during concomitant administration of CYP3A4 inducers or inhibitors, when switching cyclosporine formulations, and/or when cyclosporine dosing is reduced as well as in patients with hepatic impairment. Know that there is little to no pharmacokinetic interaction of tacrolimus on everolimus. Therefore, there is no need to alter everolimus dosing if tacrolimus dosing is altered.
- Monitor patient's incision as everolimus delays wound healing and increases the occurrence of wound-related complications such as wound dehiscence, wound infection, incisional hernia, lymphocele, and seroma.

WARNING Watch for evidence of infection (such as cough, fever, pain, malaise) because patients receiving immunosuppressants such as everolimus are at increased risk for bacterial, fungal, parasitic, or viral infection. Watch for both generalized and localized infections, including worsening of preexisting infections, and be aware that these infections may become life threatening. Activation of latent viral infections may also occur and include BK-virus-associated nephropathy that can lead to decreased renal function and renal graft loss.

- Be aware that interstitial lung disease may occur in patients with symptoms consistent with infectious pneumonia but usually only becomes apparent when patient does not respond to antibiotic therapy and other causes have been ruled out. If this occurs, expect everolimus therapy to be interrupted until the noninfectious pneumonitis has been resolved. Know that glucocorticoid therapy may also be prescribed to help resolve it.
- Monitor patient, especially within the first 30 days post transplantation, for evidence of kidney arterial and venous thrombosis (kidney transplant) or hepatic artery thrombosis (liver transplant) resulting in graft loss.
- Monitor patient's lipid levels routinely because hyperlipidemia may occur as a result of everolimus therapy. If hyperlipidemia drug therapy is required, be aware that lovastatin or simvastatin should not be used to treat it for patient with a kidney transplant because of a potential interaction with cyclosporine.
- Monitor patient's CBC and platelet count, as ordered, routinely because of increased risk of hemolytic uremic syndrome, thrombotic microangiopathy, or thrombotic thrombocytopenic purpura that may occur with combined everolimus and cyclosporine therapy used with kidney transplantation. Also know that drug causes myelosuppression, which may lead to hematologic disorders such as anemia, lymphopenia, neutropenia, and thrombocytopenia.
- Report abnormalities promptly to prescriber.
- Monitor patient's blood glucose levels regularly because everolimus therapy may increase the risk of new-onset diabetes mellitus after transplant.

PATIENT TEACHING

- Instruct patient to swallow tablets whole with a glass of water and not crushed before ingesting.
- Tell patient that ideally twice daily dosages should be consistently taken approximately 12 hours apart and at the same time as his cyclosporine or tacrolimus dose, if prescribed.
- Instruct patient to report any, persistent, severe, or unusual symptoms to prescriber.
- Caution patient to avoid excessive exposure to ultraviolet light, to wear protective clothing when outdoors, and use a sunscreen with a high protection factor.
- Inform patient that stomatitis most often occurs within the first 8 weeks of treatment. Instruct patient that he will be prescribed a dexamethasone alcohol-free oral solution and to use it as a swish-and-spit mouthwash. Caution him to avoid alcohol-, hydrogen peroxide-, iodine-, or thyme-containing products.
- Advise patient to avoid immunizations that use live vaccines such as BCG, intranasal influenza, measles, mumps, rubella, oral polio, TY21a typhoid, varicella, and yellow fever.
- Emphasize importance of avoiding grapefruit and grapefruit juice while receiving concomitant therapy with everolimus and cyclosporine.
- Urge women of childbearing age to use a highly effective birth control method throughout everolimus therapy and for 8 weeks after the drug has been discontinued.
- Alert both men and women that drug may affect fertility.
- Inform mothers that they should not breastfeed while taking everolimus.

evolocumab

Repatha

Class and Category

Pharmacologic class: Proprotein convertase subtilisin kexin type (PCSK9) antibody inhibitor
Therapeutic class: Antilipemic
Pregnancy category: Not classified

Indications and Dosages

➤ *Adjunct to diet as monotherapy or in combination with other lipid-lowering therapies such as ezetimibe or statins to treat primary hyperlipidemia including heterozygous familial hypercholesterolemia to reduce low-density lipoprotein cholesterol; to reduce the risk of coronary revascularization, myocardial infarction, or stroke in patients with established cardiovascular disease*

SUBCUTANEOUS INJECTION

Adults. 140 mg every 2 wk or 420 mg once a month. The 420-mg dose is administered over 9 min by using the single-use body infusor with prefilled cartridge (Pushtronex system), or by giving 3 injections consecutively within 30 min using the single-use prefilled autoinjector or single-use prefilled syringe.

➤ *Adjunct to diet and other LDL-lowering therapies such as ezetimibe, LDL apheresis, or statins to treat homozygous familial hypercholesterolemia in patients who require additional lowering of LDL-C*

SUBCUTANEOUS INJECTION

Adults. 420 mg once a month administered over 9 min by using the single-use body infusor with prefilled cartridge (the Pushtronex system), or by giving 3 injections consecutively within 30 min using the single-use prefilled autoinjector or single-use prefilled syringe.

Mechanism of Action

Proprotein convertase subtillisin kexin type 9 (PCSK9) binds to low-density lipoprotein receptors on the surface of hepatocytes for the purpose of degrading the receptors within the liver. Evolocumab inhibits the binding of PCSK9 therefore increasing the number of LDL receptors available to clear circulating low-density lipoproteins. This results in a lower LDL-C level.

Contraindications

Hypersensitivity to evolocumab or its components

Adverse Reactions

CNS: Dizziness, fatigue, headache
CV: Hypertension
EENT: Nasopharyngitis, rhinorrhea, sinusitis
ENDO: Diabetes mellitus
GI: Diarrhea, gastroenteritis, nausea
GU: UTI
MS: Arthralgia, back pain, muscle spasms, musculoskeletal pain, myalgia
RESP: Cough, upper respiratory infection
SKIN: Eczema, erythema, rash, urticaria
Other: Angioedema; formation of evolocumab-induced antibodies; flu-like symptoms; injection-site reactions such as bruising, erythema, and pain

Nursing Considerations

- Inject evolocumab in the patient's abdomen, thigh, or upper arm in an area that is not bruised, indurated, red, or tender using a single-use prefilled syringe, single-use prefilled autoinjector, or single-use on-body infusor with prefilled cartridge.
- Avoid touching needle covers on single-use prefilled syringes and within needle caps on single-use prefilled SureClick autoinjectors if latex-sensitive. Know that the Pushtronex system is not made of natural rubber latex.
- Administer the 420-mg dose by giving three evolocumab injections consecutively within 30 minutes using the single-use prefilled autoinjector or single-use prefilled syringe. It may also be given over 9 minutes by using the single-use on-body infusor with prefilled cartridge (Pushtronex system).
- Monitor patient for hypersensitivity. If patient develops a rash or urticaria, notify the prescriber and treat according to the standard of care. Be aware that angioedema has occurred in some patients. Monitor patient until signs and symptoms resolve. Know that if reaction is serious, the prescriber may discontinue the drug.

PATIENT TEACHING

- Advise patient that evolocumab therapy does not replace dietary measures or other prescribed therapies.
- Teach patient how to administer a subcutaneous injection and how to dispose of the prefilled syringe, SureClick autoinjector, or the Pushtronex prefilled cartridge. Remind patient that it may take up to 15 seconds to administer drug if using the single-use prefilled autoinjector or single-use prefilled syringe and about 9 minutes to administer the drug using the Pushtronex system. Tell him to always check the drug label before administration to make sure he has the correct drug and dose prescribed for him.
- Inform patient prescribed the 420-mg dose that he will need to give three injections consecutively within 30 minutes unless he uses the Pushtronex system.

- Remind patient to keep drug in refrigerator but allow it to warm to room temperature for at least 30 minutes before administering it. Caution him not to warm it any other way. Make him aware that if he chooses to keep the drug at room temperature stored in the original carton, the drug must be administered within 30 days.
- Instruct patient to administer the injection into his abdomen, thigh, or upper arm in an area that is not bruised, indurated, red, or tender and to rotate the injection site with each injection. Remind him that injection site reactions such as bruising, pain, or redness may occur and should be reported if severe or does not resolve.
- Tell patient that if he misses a dose, he should administer it as soon as possible if there are more than 7 days until his next scheduled dose. If not, he should omit the missed dose and administer the next dose according to his original schedule.
- Advise patient to notify prescriber if he experiences an allergic reaction to the drug such as the development of hives, rash, or swelling in any part of his body. Advise patient that if symptoms are severe, he should seek immediate emergency treatment. Alert patient who is latex sensitive that needle covers on the single-use prefilled syringes and within needle caps on the single-use prefilled SureClick autoinjectors contain dry natural rubber, a derivative of latex. The single-use Pushtronex system does not.
- Tell women of childbearing age to alert prescriber if pregnancy occurs and encourage her to enroll in the pregnancy exposure registry by calling 877-311-8972, or she can register online at https://mothertobaby.org/ongoing-study/repatha/.Ad

exenatide

Bydureon, Bydureon Bcise, Byetta

Class and Category

Pharmacolgoic class: Glucagon-like peptide-1 (GLP-1) receptor agonist
Therapeutic class: Antidiabetic
Pregnancy category: C

Indications and Dosages

➤ *Adjunct treatment to diet and exercise to improve blood glucose levels in patients with type 2 diabetes mellitus*

SUBCUTANEOUS INJECTION (BYETTA)

Adults. *Initial:* 5 mcg twice daily, given within 60 min before morning and evening meals. After 1 month, increased, as needed, to 10 mcg twice daily, given within 60 min before morning and evening meals.

SUBCUTANEOUS INJECTION (BYDUREON, BYDUREON BCISE)

Adults. 2 mg once every 7 days.

Route	Onset	Peak	Duration
SubQ	Immediate	2.1 hr	Unknown

Contraindications

Hypersensitivity to exenatide or its components, personal or family history of medullary thyroid carcinoma or multiple endocrine neoplasia syndrome type 2 (Bydureon)

Interactions

DRUGS

albiglutide, dulaglutide, liraglutide, lixisenatide, semaglutide: Possibly increased risk of hypersensitivity with history of hypersensitivity to any of these drugs
oral antidiabetics such as meglitinides or sulfonylureas, insulin: Increased risk of hypoglycemia
oral drugs: May decrease rate and extent of absorption of these drugs
warfarin: Possibly increased INR with increased risk of bleeding

Adverse Reactions

CNS: Asthenia, dizziness, headache, jitteriness, somnolence
CV: Chest pain
EENT: Decreased taste
ENDO: Hypoglycemia
GI: Abdominal distention or pain, anorexia, constipation, diarrhea, dyspepsia, flatulence, gastroesophageal reflux, indigestion, nausea, **pancreatitis (including life-threatening hemorrhagic or necrotizing)**, vomiting
GU: Acute renal failure, decreased renal function, elevated serum creatinine level, **kidney transplant dysfunction**, **worsening chronic renal failure**
RESP: Chronic hypersensitivity pneumonitis

Mechanism of Action

Normally, when serum glucose level rises, insulin is secreted within 10 minutes. This first-phase insulin response is absent in patients with type 2 diabetes. Exenatide, an incretin mimetic, restores the first-phase insulin response and improves the second-phase response that immediately follows. It does so by promoting incretins that spur insulin synthesis and release from beta cells by binding and activating human GLP-1 receptors to reduce fasting and postprandial serum glucose levels.

The drug also suppresses inappropriately elevated glucagon secretion. Lower serum glucagon level leads to decreased hepatic glucose output and decreased insulin demand. It also slows gastric emptying and thus the rise of serum glucose level.

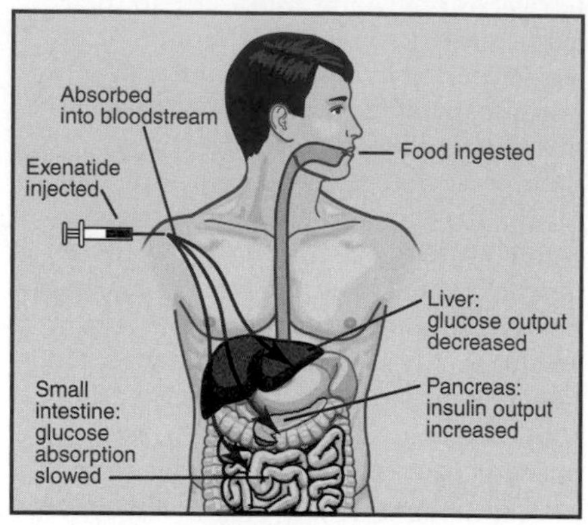

SKIN: Alopecia, diaphoresis, macular or papular rash, pruritus, rash, urticaria
Other: Anaphylaxis, angioedema, dehydration, elevated antiexenatide antibody level, hematoma, injection-site reactions (abscess, cellulitis, necrosis, pruritus, redness, subcutaneous nodules), weight loss

Nursing Considerations

- Know that exenatide isn't recommended for patients with severe GI disease, patients with creatinine clearance less than 30 ml/min, or patients having dialysis because of adverse GI or renal effects.
- Use exenatide cautiously in a renal transplant patient or patient with moderate renal disease when dosage of Byetta is increased from 5 to 10 mcg or the extended-release formulations (Bydureon or Bydureon Bcise) are used. Monitor renal function throughout therapy, and notify prescriber of abnormalities.
- Be aware that if patient also takes a sulfonylurea, the sulfonylurea dosage may need to be decreased to reduce the risk of hypoglycemia. Usually, no dosage adjustment is needed for a patient taking metformin.
- Administer drug into patient's abdomen, thigh, or upper arm.
- Monitor patient's blood glucose level. If control decreases despite the patient's best efforts, drug may have to be discontinued because of the possibility that anti-exenatide antibodies have formed. Be aware that if patient is already taking the rapid-release form of exenatide (Byetta) and is switching to the extended-release form of exenatide (Bydureon or Bydureon Bcise), Byetta must be discontinued first. Also know that he may experience a transient elevation in his blood glucose levels for about 2 weeks as his body adjusts to the extended-release form.
- Monitor patient for evidence of acute pancreatitis, such as persistent, severe abdominal pain accompanied by vomiting, especially when drug is started or dosage increased. Notify prescriber, and expect to stop exenatide and give supportive care.
- Know that the rapid-release form of exenatide (Byetta) may be used concomitantly with insulin glargine (Lantus), which is a long-acting insulin to help improve the patient's blood glucose control. Byetta should not be used with any other type of insulin. If the patient is susceptible to hypoglycemia, expect the insulin glargine dosage to be decreased when used with Byetta.
- Be aware that Bydureon extended-release for injectable suspension can be used as an

add-on to basal insulin in adults with type 2 diabetes who have inadequate glycemic control.

PATIENT TEACHING

- Teach patient how to give a subcutaneous injection and how to use pen injector if prescribed Byetta.
- Teach patient how to mix powder with diluent if prescribed Bydureon and how to give a subcutaneous injection. Remind patient to administer Bydureon immediately after the powder is suspended in the diluent and transferred to the syringe. Also tell him not to substitute needles or any other components in the tray. Alert him that a spare needle has been provided in the tray in the event he needs it.
- Inform patient prescribed Bydureon Bcise of the need to shake hard the autoinjector in an up-and-down motion, until the drug is evenly mixed and no whiteness of the drug is seen along the bottom, sides, or top of device. Tell patient he will need to shake the autoinjector for at least 15 seconds. Remind patient that to get the full dose, the drug must be mixed well. When mixed well, the knob on the device should be turned from lock to unlock position. Patient should hear a click.
- Inform patient that exenatide may be administered in the abdomen, thigh, or upper arm. Stress the need to rotate injection sites.
- Tell patient to inspect injection site daily and to report any adverse effects at site that are persistent or appear serious.
- Emphasize the need to use rapid release form of drug (Byetta) within 60 minutes before morning and evening meals or the two main meals of the day, about 6 hours or more apart, never after a meal.
- Know that if patient misses a dose of Byetta, tell him to resume treatment with the next scheduled dose. If patient is prescribed Bydureon and misses a dose, tell him to administer the drug as soon as he remembers as long as his regularly scheduled dose is at least 3 days later. If the time frame is less than this, tell patient to wait until his next regularly scheduled dose. Make patient aware that he may change the day of weekly administration of Bydureon as long as the last dose was administered 3 or more days before.
- Advise patient that drug should look clear and colorless. Tell him not to use drug solution that looks cloudy or colored or contains particles.
- Instruct patient to check expiration date on the vial and not to use drug if date has passed.
- Advise patient to refrigerate rapid-acting drug (Byetta) before first use and protect it from light. After first use of pen device, drug may be stored at room temperature of 25°C (77° F) or less. Advise patient to refrigerate extended-release drug (Bydureon) in refrigerator and protect from light. A single-use tray of Bydureon may be stored at room temperature for up to 4 weeks.
- Tell patient to discard pen injector 30 days after initial use, even if some drug is left. Caution patient not to share his pen or needles with anyone else.
- Alert patient that pen doesn't come with needles and that he'll need to buy them.
- Warn patient that nausea may occur at the beginning of therapy but usually subsides over time.
- Inform patient taking a sulfonylurea or insulin glargine to be alert for hypoglycemic reactions because risk increases with both drugs. Review ways to treat such reactions, and tell patient to alert prescriber if they occur often or are severe.
- Instruct female patient of childbearing potential to tell her prescriber if she is, could be, or is planning to become pregnant.
- Tell patient to seek emergency care for persistent, severe abdominal pain and vomiting.
- Caution patient that exenatide doesn't replace diet and exercise measures.

WARNING Urge patient to stop taking drug and seek immediate emergency care if signs and symptoms of an allergic reaction occur.

- Alert patient taking extended-release form to report difficulty breathing or swallowing, hoarseness, or a lump in neck.
- Tell patient that kidney function may become impaired and to let prescriber know if dysfunction is noticed.

ezetimibe

Zetia

Class and Category

Pharmacolgic class: Cholesterol absorption inhibitor
Therapeutic class: Antilipemic
Pregnancy category: C

Indications and Dosages

➤ *To treat heterozygous familial and nonfamilial hypercholesterolemia or homozygous sitosterolemia; as adjunct with HMG-CoA reductase inhibitors to treat heterozygous familial and nonfamilial hypercholesterolemia; with fenofibrate to treat mixed hyperlipidemia and with atorvastatin or simvastatin to treat patients with homozygous familial hypercholesterolemia*

TABLETS

Adults. 10 mg daily.

Contraindications

Active liver disease or unexplained persistent elevations in hepatic transaminase levels, breastfeeding, hypersensitivity to ezetimibe or its components, pregnancy

Interactions

DRUGS

cholestyramine: Reduced effects of ezetimibe
cyclosporine: Increased blood cyclosporine and ezetimibe levels
fenofibrate, gemfibrozil: Increased blood ezetimibe level

Adverse Reactions

CNS: Depression, dizziness, fatigue, headache, paresthesia
CV: Chest pain
EENT: Pharyngitis, sinusitis
GI: Abdominal pain, cholelithiasis, cholecystitis, diarrhea, elevated enzymes, **hepatitis**, nausea, **pancreatitis**
HEME: Thrombocytopenia

Mechanism of Action

Reduces blood cholesterol by inhibiting its absorption through the small intestine.

Normally, in the intestinal lumen, lipids break down to cholesterol and other substances that create smaller droplets called micelles, as shown below left. The micelles enter intestinal epithelial cells called enterocytes, where they combine with cholesterol, triglycerides, and other substances to form chylomicrons. Chylomicrons then pass through to the lymphatic system to be carried to the blood.

Ezetimibe blocks cholesterol absorption into enterocytes and keeps cholesterol from moving through the intestinal wall, as shown below right. Reduced cholesterol absorption from the intestine decreases chylomicron and LDL cholesterol content.

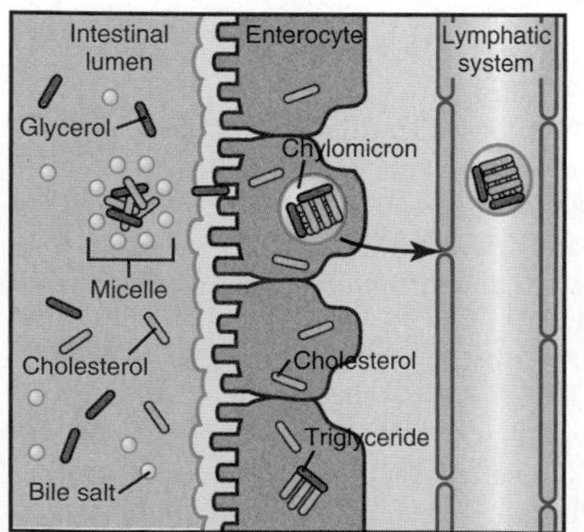

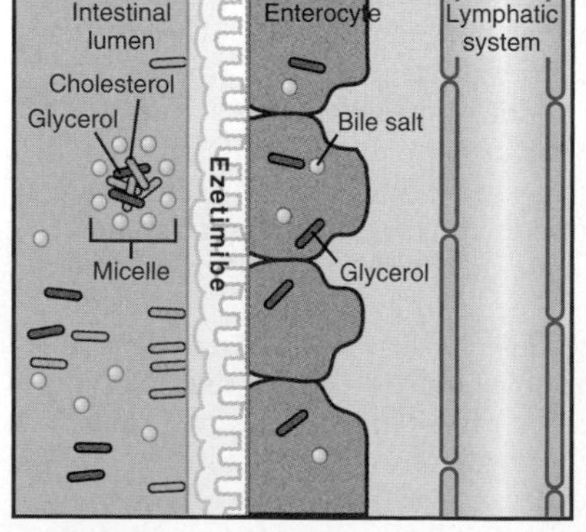

MS: Arthralgia, back or limb pain, elevated CK level, myalgia, myopathy, **rhabdomyolysis**
RESP: Cough, upper respiratory tract infection
SKIN: Erythema multiforme, rash, urticaria
Other: Anaphylaxis, angioedema, flu-like symptoms, viral infection

Nursing Considerations

- Monitor liver enzymes before and during ezetimibe therapy, as ordered.
- Know that ezetimibe should be given 2 hours before or 4 hours after giving bile acid sequestrant or cholestyramine.

PATIENT TEACHING

- Direct patient to follow a low-cholesterol diet as an adjunct to ezetimibe therapy. Recommend weight loss and exercise programs, as appropriate.
- Tell him to take ezetimibe either 2 hours before or at least 4 hours after it if patient also takes a bile acid sequestrant to prevent drug interactions.
- Advise patient to report unexplained muscle pain, tenderness, or weakness.

famciclovir

Famvir

Class and Category

Pharmacologic class: Nucleoside analogue
Therapeutic class: Antiviral
Pregnancy category: B

Indications and Dosages

➤ *To treat recurrent episodes of herpes labialis*

TABLETS

Adults. 1500 mg as a single dose at first sign of burning, itching, lesion formation, pain, or tingling.

➤ *To treat recurrent episodes of genital herpes*

TABLETS

Adults. 1000 mg twice a day for 1 day beginning at the first sign of a recurrent episode (burning, itching, lesion formation, pain, or tingling).

➤ *To suppress chronic recurrent episodes of genital herpes*

TABLETS

Adults. 250 mg twice daily.

➤ *To treat herpes zoster*

TABLETS

Adults. 500 mg every 8 hr for 7 days.

➤ *To treat recurrent episodes of genital or orolabial herpes in HIV-infected patients*

TABLETS

Adults. 500 mg twice daily for 7 days beginning at the first sign of a recurrent episode (burning, itching, lesion formation, pain, tingling).

DOSAGE ADJUSTMENT For patient with renal impairment, dosage decreased and/or dosage interval increased depending on what patient's creatinine clearance level is at the time of treatment and the herpes condition being treated.

Mechanism of Action

Selectively inhibits herpes viral DNA synthesis and replication.

Contraindications

Hypersensitivity to famciclovir or its components

Interactions

DRUGS

drugs eliminated by active renal tubular secretion such as probenecid: Possibly increased plasma concentration of famciclovir, with increased risk of adverse reactions

Adverse Reactions

CNS: Confusion, dizziness, fatigue, hallucinations, headache, migraine, paresthesia, **seizures**, somnolence
CV: Hypersensitivity vasculitis, palpitations
GI: Abdominal pain, cholestatic jaundice, diarrhea, elevated bilirubin or liver or pancreatic enzymes, flatulence, nausea, vomiting
GU: Acute renal failure, dysmenorrhea, elevated serum creatinine
HEME: Anemia, **leukopenia**, **neutropenia**, **thrombocytopenia**
SKIN: Erythema multiforme, pruritus, rash, **Stevens–Johnson syndrome**, **toxic epidermal necrolysis**, urticaria
Other: Anaphylaxis, angioedema

Nursing Considerations

- Use cautiously in patients with renal impairment because of the risk of acute renal failure and hepatic impairment,

E F

because conversion of famciclovir to its active metabolite may be impaired, resulting in a lower plasma concentration and possibly decreased effectiveness of the drug.

WARNING Be aware that dosage adjustment must be made in patients with renal impairment. Acute renal failure has occurred in patients with underlying renal disease who have received inappropriately high doses of famciclovir for their level of renal function.

- Know that famciclovir therapy should be started as soon as possible after the onset of a herpes-related condition. Signs and symptoms to be alert for include patient complaints of burning, itching, pain, or tingling or appearance of a lesion.
- Monitor patient's liver and renal function closely, and laboratory test values as ordered.

PATIENT TEACHING

- Remind patient that famciclovir should be initiated as soon as possible after a recurrent onset of a herpes-related condition exhibited by sensations of burning, itching, pain, or tingling or when a lesion has appeared.

WARNING Tell patient with renal impairment to remind prescriber of this condition when famciclovir is prescribed and when dosage adjustments are made.

WARNING Advise patient to get immediate emergency medical treatment if she develops any signs of an allergic reaction, such as difficulty breathing, hives, or swelling of face, lips, tongue, or throat.

- Inform patient that famciclovir is not a cure for herpes. Because genital herpes is a sexually transmitted disease, instruct patient to avoid contact with lesions or intercourse when lesions and/or symptoms are present, to avoid infecting partners. Remind patient, however, that genital herpes is frequently transmitted in the absence of symptoms and therefore patient should always engage in safe sex practices.
- Instruct patient to notify prescriber at once if she experience serious adverse reactions such as confusion, feeling short of breath, increased thirst, pounding heartbeats, swelling, urinating less than usual or not at all, weakness, or weight gain.
- Alert patient that famciclovir does contain lactose and famciclovir usage should be discussed with patients who experience lactose intolerance or who have galactose intolerance or glucose-galactose malabsorption.
- Inform mothers that breastfeeding is not recommended during famciclovir therapy.

famotidine

Pepcid, Pepcid AC

Class and Category

Pharmacologic class: Histamine-2 blocker
Therapeutic class: Antiulcer agent
Pregnancy category: B

Indications and Dosages

➤ *To provide short-term treatment of active duodenal ulcer*

ORAL SUSPENSION, TABLETS

Adults and adolescents over age 16. 40 mg daily at bedtime or 20 mg twice daily.

Children ages 1 to 16. 0.5 mg/kg daily as a single dose at bedtime or in divided doses twice daily. *Maximum:* 40 mg daily.

I.V. INFUSION OR INJECTION

Adults. 20 mg every 12 hr, infused over 15 to 30 min or injected over at least 2 min.

➤ *To prevent recurrence of duodenal ulcer*

ORAL SUSPENSION, TABLETS (CHEWABLE, ORAL DISINTEGRATING, AND REGULAR)

Adults and adolescents over age 16. 20 mg daily at bedtime.

➤ *To provide short-term treatment for active, benign gastric ulcer*

ORAL SUSPENSION, TABLETS

Adults and adolescents over age 16. 40 mg daily at bedtime.

Children ages 1 to 16. 0.5 mg/kg daily as a single dose at bedtime or in divided doses twice daily.

➤ *To treat gastroesophageal reflux disease (GERD)*

ORAL SUSPENSION, TABLETS

Adults and adolescents over age 16. 20 mg twice daily for up to 6 wk.

Children ages 1 to 16. 1 mg/kg daily in divided doses twice daily. *Maximum:* 40 mg daily.

Mechanism of Action

In normal digestion, parietal cells in the gastric epithelium secrete hydrogen (H^+) ions, which combine with chloride ions (Cl^-) to form hydrochloric acid (HCl), as shown below left. However, HCl can inflame, ulcerate, and perforate gastric and intestinal mucosa normally protected by mucus. Famotidine, an H^2-receptor antagonist, reduces HCl formation by preventing histamine from binding with H^2 receptors on the surface of parietal cells, as shown below right. By doing so, the drug helps prevent peptic ulcers from forming and helps heal existing ones.

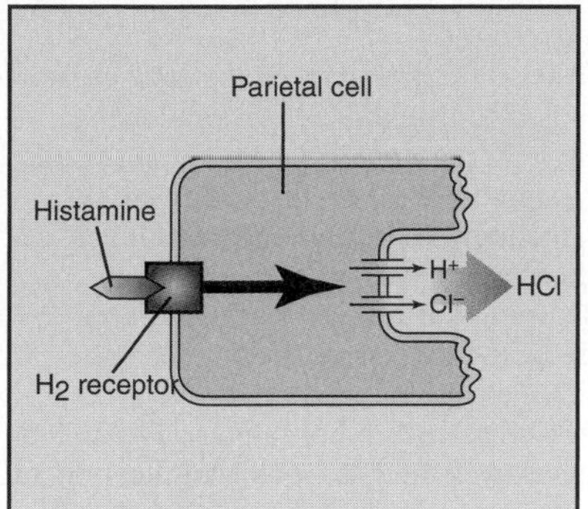

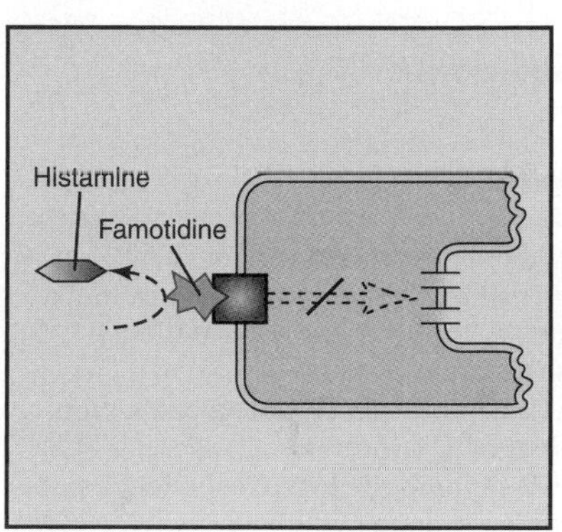

ORAL SUSPENSION

Infants age 4 months to 1 year. 0.5 mg/kg daily in divided doses twice daily for up to 8 wk.

Infants age 3 months or less. 0.5 mg/kg once daily for up to 8 wk.

➤ *To treat esophagitis caused by gastroesophageal reflux*

ORAL SUSPENSION, TABLETS

Adults and adolescents. 20 to 40 mg twice daily for up to 12 wk.

➤ *To treat gastric hypersecretory conditions, such as Zollinger–Ellison syndrome*

ORAL SUSPENSION, TABLETS

Adults and adolescents over age 16. *Initial:* 20 mg every 6 hr. Dosage adjusted, if needed, based on patient response.

➤ *To treat hospitalized patients with intractable ulcers or pathological hypersecretory conditions; to treat patients who are unable to take oral medication*

I.V. INFUSION OR INJECTION

Adults and adolescents over age 16. 20 mg every 12 hr, infused over 15 to 30 min or injected over at least 2 min.

Children ages 1 to 16. *Initial:* 0.25 mg/kg every 12 hr, infused over 15 to 30 min or injected over at least 2 min. *Maximum:* 40 mg daily.

I.V. INFUSION OR INJECTION

Adults. 20 mg every 12 hr infused over 15 to 30 min or injected over at least 2 min. *Maximum:* 160 mg every 6 hr.

➤ *To prevent heartburn and indigestion*

TABLETS

Adults. 10 mg 1 hr before eating. *Maximum:* 20 mg every 24 hr.

➤ *To treat heartburn and indigestion*

TABLETS

Adults. 10 mg at onset of symptoms. *Maximum:* 20 mg every 24 hr for up to 2 wk unless prescribed otherwise.

➤ *To prevent or treat GI bleeding in hospitalized patients who cannot take oral drug*

I.V. INFUSION OR INJECTION

Adults. 20 mg every 12 hr injected over at least 2 min or infused continuously at a rate of 1.7 to 4 mg/hr.

DOSAGE ADJUSTMENT Oral or parenteral dosage reduced or dosing interval increased (to 36 to 48 hr), if needed, in patients with renal insufficiency and creatinine clearance of 49 ml/min or less.

Route	Onset	Peak	Duration
P.O.	1 hr	1–4 hr	10–12 hr
I.V.	In 30 min	0.5–3 hr	10–12 hr

Contraindications
Hypersensitivity to famotidine, other H_2-receptor antagonists, or their components

Interactions
None

Adverse Reactions
CNS: Agitation (infants), anxiety, asthenia, confusion, depression, dizziness, fatigue, fever, hallucinations, headache, insomnia, mental or mood changes, paresthesia, **seizures**, somnolence
CV: **Arrhythmias**, **AV block**, palpitations, **prolonged QT interval**
EENT: Dry mouth, **laryngeal edema**, taste alteration, tinnitus
GI: Abdominal pain, anorexia, cholestatic jaundice, constipation, diarrhea, elevated liver enzymes, **hepatitis**, jaundice, nausea, vomiting
GU: Decreased libido, impotence
HEME: **Agranulocytosis**, **aplastic anemia**, **leukopenia**, **neutropenia**, **pancytopenia**, **thrombocytopenia**
MS: Arthralgia, muscle cramps, musculoskeletal pain, **rhabdomyolysis**
RESP: **Bronchospasm**, dyspnea, **interstitial pneumonia**, wheezing
SKIN: Acne, alopecia, dry skin, **erythema multiforme**, **exfoliative dermatitis**, flushing, pruritus, rash, **Stevens–Johnson syndrome**, **toxic epidermal necrolysis**, urticaria
Other: **Anaphylaxis**, **angioedema**, hyperuricemia

Nursing Considerations
- Shake famotidine oral suspension vigorously for 5 to 10 seconds before administration.
- Dilute injection form (2 ml) with normal saline solution or other solution to 5 to 10 ml; give I.V. injection over at least 2 minutes. Or, dilute in 100 ml of D_5W and infuse over 15 to 30 minutes; or infuse premixed injection (20 mg/50 ml normal saline solution) over 15 to 30 minutes.

WARNING Be aware that Pepcid AC chewable tablets contain aspartame, which can be dangerous for patients who have phenylketonuria.

PATIENT TEACHING
- Instruct patient to store famotidine oral suspension at room temperature (below 86° F [30° C]) and to protect it from freezing. Tell her to shake the bottle vigorously, right before use, for 5 to 10 seconds.
- Instruct patient to carefully chew chewable tablets thoroughly before swallowing.
- Instruct patient who also takes antacids to wait 30 to 60 minutes after taking famotidine, if possible, before taking antacid.
- Caution patient to avoid alcohol and smoking during famotidine therapy because they irritate the stomach and can delay ulcer healing.
- Advise patient to notify prescriber if she develops pain, has trouble swallowing, or if she has bloody vomit or black stools.
- Caution patient not to take famotidine with other acid-reducing products.

febuxostat
Uloric

Class and Category
Pharmacologic class: Xanthine oxidase inhibitor
Therapeutic class: Antigout
Pregnancy category: C

Indications and Dosages
➤ *To treat chronic hyperuricemia in patients with gout*

TABLETS
Adults. *Initial:* 40 mg once daily, increased after 2 wk to 80 mg once daily, if needed.
DOSAGE ADJUSTMENT For patient with severe renal impairment, dosage limited to 40 mg once daily.

Route	Onset	Peak	Duration
P.O.	2–3 days	1–1.5 hr	Unknown

Mechanism of Action
Inhibits the action of xanthine oxidase, the key enzyme responsible for purine break-

down. Xanthine oxidase catalyzes conversion of xanthine to uric acid, thereby increasing uric acid levels. High uric acid levels cause gout attacks. Inhibiting xanthine oxidase causes uric acid levels to drop, decreasing the risk of gout attack.

Contraindications

Concurrent use of azathioprine or mercaptopurine, hypersensitivity to febuxostat or its components

Interactions

DRUGS

azathioprine, mercaptopurine, theophylline: Possibly increased serum levels of these drugs, leading to toxicity

Adverse Reactions

CNS: Aggression, **CVA**, dizziness, hemiparesis, **lacunar infarction**, psychotic behavior, transient ischemic attack
CV: Angina, chest pain or discomfort, **ECG abnormalities**, **MI**
EENT: Blurred vision, deafness, epistaxis, nasal dryness, paranasal sinus hypersecretion, **pharyngeal edema**, sneezing, taste disturbance, throat irritation, tinnitus
ENDO: Breast pain, gynecomastia, hot flashes, **hypoglycemia**
GI: Diarrhea, dyspepsia, elevated liver enzymes, GI discomfort, **hepatic failure**, hepatomegaly, jaundice, nausea, vomiting
GU: Decreased libido, erectile dysfunction, hematuria, nephrolithiasis, pollakiuria, proteinuria, **renal failure or insufficiency**, tubulointerstitial nephritis, urgency
HEME: **Agranulocytosis**, anemia, eosinophilia, **idiopathic thrombocytopenic purpura**, leukocytosis, **leukopenia**, **neutropenia**, **pancytopenia**, splenomegaly, **thrombocytopenia**
MS: Arthralgia, joint stiffness or swelling, **rhabdomyolysis**
RESP: Upper respiratory tract infection
SKIN: Dermatitis, eczema, **erythema multiforme**, flushing, hair color or growth changes, hyperhidrosis, peeling skin, petechiae, photosensitivity, pruritis, rash, **Stevens–Johnson syndrome**, **toxic epidermal necrolysis**, urticaria
Other: **Anaphylaxis**, **drug reaction with eosinophilia and systemic symptoms (DRESS)**, gout flares, **hypersensitivity reactions**

Nursing Considerations

- Know that febuxostat therapy isn't recommended for patients in whom rate of urate formation is greatly increased, as in malignancy and its treatment or Lesch–Nyhan syndrome.
- Obtain a liver test panel, as ordered, prior to initiating febuxostat therapy and then periodically thereafter. Monitor patient for signs and symptoms of liver dysfunction such as anorexia, dark urine, fatigue, jaundice, or right upper abdominal discomfort throughout therapy. If signs and symptoms occur or if abnormal liver tests occur, especially an elevated serum alanine aminotransferase level greater than 3 times the upper normal limit, notify prescriber and expect drug to be withheld until underlying cause is determined. If no other cause can be found other than febuxostat therapy, expect drug to be discontinued permanently.
- Monitor patient's serum uric acid level, as prescribed, to determine drug effectiveness. Expect it to take about 2 weeks for uric acid level to be therapeutically altered. Dose may be increased from 40 to 80 mg daily if target serum uric acid level fails to fall below 6 mg/dl.
- Monitor patient for gout flares, which may occur after therapy is started because of changing serum uric acid levels that result in mobilization of urate from tissue deposits. Expect prescriber to order colchicine or an NSAID when febuxostat therapy starts. If patient has a gout flare-up during treatment, notify prescriber, and expect symptoms to be managed. Know that febuxostat therapy usually isn't discontinued during this time.
- Monitor patient for evidence of cardiovascular thrombosis, such as acute MI or stroke, because drug may increase patient's risk of developing these disorders, which may result in death.
- Assess patient's skin for abnormalities. At first sign of rash or other skin abnormality, notify prescriber and expect drug to be discontinued if serious skin

reactions are suspected or occur, because febuxostat may cause severe skin reactions. Also know that patients who have experienced hypersensitivity reactions to allopurinol may be at increased risk of developing serious skin reactions to febuxostat.

PATIENT TEACHING

- Inform patient that a gout attack may occur when febuxostat therapy starts and that colchicine or an NSAID may be prescribed, usually along with febuxostat, to treat it.
- Instruct patient to seek immediate emergency care for signs or symptoms of a heart attack or stroke.
- Tell patient that periodic blood tests will be needed to determine drug's effectiveness and to detect adverse effects.
- Advise patient to notify prescriber at first sign of a rash or other skin abnormality.

felbamate

Felbatol

Class and Category

Pharmacologic class: Carbamate
Therapeutic class: Anticonvulsant
Pregnancy category: C

Indications and Dosages

➤ *To treat partial seizures as monotherapy in patients who don't respond to other drugs*

ORAL SUSPENSION, TABLETS

Adults and adolescents over age 14. *Initial:* 1,200 mg daily in divided doses 3 times daily or 4 times daily. Dosage increased in 600 mg increments every 2 wks, as needed. *Maximum:* 3,600 mg daily.

➤ *As adjunct to treat partial seizures in patients who respond inadequately to alternative treatments*

ORAL SUSPENSION, TABLETS

Adults and adolescents over age 14. *Week 1:* 1,200 mg daily in 3 or 4 divided doses while other anticonvulsant drugs decreased by 20 to 33%. *Week 2:* Dosage increased to 2,400 mg daily in 3 or 4 divided doses and additional reductions made with other anticonvulsant drugs, as needed. *Week 3:* Dosage increased to 3,600 mg daily in 3 or 4 divided doses with reductions made with other anticonvulsant drugs as needed. *Maximum:* 3,600 mg daily.

➤ *As adjunct to treat generalized or partial seizures associated with Lennox–Gastaut syndrome in children*

ORAL SUSPENSION, TABLETS

Children ages 2 to 14. *Initial:* 15 mg/kg daily in 3 or 4 divided doses while other anticonvulsant drug dosages decreased by 20%. Dosage further increased by 15 mg/kg daily every wk. *Maximum:* 45 mg/kg daily.

DOSAGE ADJUSTMENT Dosage reduced by 50% in patients with renal impairment.

Mechanism of Action

May exert anticonvulsant effects by antagonizing the amino acid glycine. When glycine binds to N-methyl-D-aspartate (NMDA) receptors in the CNS, the frequency at which receptor-gated calcium ion channels open is increased—an important factor in initiating seizures. Felbamate may raise the seizure threshold by blocking NMDA receptors so glycine can't bind to them.

Contraindications

Hepatic dysfunction; history of blood dyscrasias; hypersensitivity to felbamate, other carbamates, or their components

Interactions

DRUGS

carbamazepine: Decreased blood carbamazepine level and increased felbamate clearance, resulting in decreased blood felbamate level
fosphenytoin, phenytoin: Increased blood phenytoin level and increased felbamate clearance, resulting in decreased blood felbamate level
oral contraceptives: Possibly decreased effectiveness of oral contraceptives
phenobarbital: Decreased blood felbamate level, increased blood phenobarbital level and risk of adverse effects
valproic acid: Increased blood valproic acid level and increased risk of adverse effects

Adverse Reactions

CNS: Abnormal gait, aggressiveness, agitation, anxiety, dizziness, drowsiness, fever, headache, insomnia, mood changes, **suicidal ideation**, tremor

EENT: Altered taste, diplopia, rhinitis
GI: Abdominal pain, anorexia, constipation, diarrhea, elevated liver function test results, **hepatic failure**, indigestion, nausea, vomiting
HEME: Aplastic anemia, leukopenia, pancytopenia, thrombocytopenia
RESP: Upper respiratory tract infection
SKIN: Photosensitivity, purpura, rash
Other: Anaphylaxis, lymphadenopathy, weight loss

Nursing Considerations

- Check liver function test results before starting felbamate, and expect to check results every 1 to 2 weeks during treatment. Notify prescriber immediately and expect to stop drug if results are abnormal.

WARNING Assess for signs of aplastic anemia and bone marrow depression. Signs may not appear until several months after therapy begins. Expect to stop felbamate if bone marrow depression develops.

- Know that if patient receives adjunctive therapy, expect adverse reactions may be expected to resolve as other anticonvulsant dosages decrease.
- Monitor patient closely for evidence of suicidal thinking or behavior, especially when therapy starts or dosage changes.

PATIENT TEACHING

- Direct patient to shake suspension before using and to use a calibrated spoon or container to measure each dose.
- Instruct patient to store oral suspension and tablets at room temperature.
- Urge patient to protect skin from sun and to avoid sunlamps and tanning booths.
- Explain that dizziness and drowsiness may occur. Advise her to avoid hazardous activities until drug's CNS effects are known.
- Warn patient not to stop drug abruptly.
- Advise patient to return for ordered liver function tests and to report dark urine and yellow skin or eyes to prescriber.
- Instruct patient to tell prescriber if she experiences bleeding, fatigue, or infection.
- Advise patient to carry medical identification that indicates condition and therapy.
- Discuss alternate contraceptive methods with female patients because felbamate decreases oral contraceptive effectiveness.
- Urge caregivers to watch patient closely for evidence of suicidal tendencies, especially when therapy starts or dosage changes, and to report any concerns immediately.
- Encourage female patient who becomes pregnant while taking felbamate to enroll in the North American antiepileptic drug pregnancy registry by calling 1-888-233-2334. Explain that this registry is collecting information about the safety of antiepileptic drugs during pregnancy.

felodipine

Plendil (CAN)

Class and Category

Pharmacologic class: Calcium channel blocker
Therapeutic class: Antihypertensive
Pregnancy category: C

Indications and Dosages

➤ *To manage essential hypertension alone or with other antihypertensives*

E.R. TABLETS

Adults. *Initial:* 5 mg daily. Dosage adjusted every 2 wk to 2.5 to 10 mg daily based on patient response.

DOSAGE ADJUSTMENT Initial or maintenance dosage reduced, if needed, in patients who are over age 65. For patients with impaired hepatic function, dosage reduced to 2.5 mg daily.

Route	Onset	Peak	Duration
P.O.	2–5 hr	Unknown	16–24 hr

Mechanism of Action

May slow the movement of extracellular calcium into myocardial and vascular smooth-muscle cells by deforming calcium channels in cell membranes, inhibiting ion-controlled gating mechanisms, and interfering with calcium release from the sarcoplasmic reticulum. The effect of these actions is a decrease in intracellular calcium ions, which inhibits contraction of smooth-muscle cells and dilates coronary and systemic arteries. As with other calcium channel blockers, felodipine's actions result in increased oxygen to the myocardium and reduced afterload, blood pressure, and peripheral resistance.

E F

Contraindications

Hypersensitivity to felodipine or its components

Interactions

DRUGS

antihypertensives: Increased risk of hypotension
cimetidine, erythromycin: Increased felodipine bioavailability
NSAIDs, sympathomimetics: Possibly decreased therapeutic effect of felodipine
procainamide, quinidine: Increased risk of prolonged QT interval
tacrolimus: Possibly increased blood tacrolimus level and risk of adverse effects

FOODS

grapefruit juice: Doubled felodipine bioavailability

Adverse Reactions

CNS: Asthenia, dizziness, drowsiness, fatigue, headache, paresthesia, syncope, weakness
CV: Chest pain, **hypotension**, palpitations, peripheral edema, tachycardia
EENT: Gingival hyperplasia, pharyngitis, rhinitis
GI: Abdominal cramps, constipation, diarrhea, indigestion, nausea
HEME: Agranulocytosis
MS: Back pain
RESP: Cough
SKIN: Flushing, rash

Nursing Considerations

- Use felodipine cautiously in patients with heart failure or reduced ventricular function.
- Monitor blood pressure during dosage titration and throughout felodipine therapy, especially in elderly patients.
- Felodipine bioavailability increases up to twofold when taken with grapefruit juice.

WARNING Be aware that felodipine may cause severe hypotension with syncope, which may lead to reflex tachycardia. This can precipitate angina in patients with coronary artery disease or a history of angina.

- Watch for signs of overdose, such as excessive peripheral vasodilation, marked hypotension, and, possibly, bradycardia. If they appear, place patient in supine position with legs elevated and give I.V. fluids, as ordered. Expect to give I.V. atropine for bradycardia.

PATIENT TEACHING

- Instruct patient to swallow tablets whole and not to crush or chew them.
- Caution patient not to alter her intake of grapefruit juice during therapy.
- Advise patient to store felodipine at room temperature and to protect it from light.
- Instruct patient to monitor her pulse rate and blood pressure.
- Teach patient how to minimize gingival hyperplasia.
- Advise patient to notify prescriber immediately if she has palpitations, pronounced dizziness, or swelling of hands or feet.

fenofibrate

Antara, Fenoglide, Lipofen, Lofibra, Tricor, Triglide

fenofibric acid

Fibricor, Trilipix

Class and Category

Pharmacologic class: Fibrate
Therapeutic class: Antilipemic
Pregnancy category: C

Indications and Dosages

➤ *To treat primary hypercholesterolemia or mixed hyperlipidemia*

CAPSULES (LIPOFEN)

Adults. 150 mg daily with food.

CAPSULES (LOFIBRA)

Adults. 160 mg daily with food.

CAPSULES (ANTARA)

Adults. 90 mg daily.

DELAYED-RELEASE CAPSULES (TRILIPIX)

Adults. 135 mg daily.

TABLETS (TRICOR)

Adults. 145 mg daily.

TABLETS (FIBRICOR)

Adults. 105 mg daily.

TABLETS (TRIGLIDE)

Adults. 160 mg daily.

TABLETS (FENOGLIDE)

Adults. 120 mg daily.

➤ *As adjunct to diet to treat severe hypertriglyceridemia*

CAPSULES (ANTARA)
Adults. *Initial:* 30 to 90 mg daily, increased as needed at 4- to 8-wk intervals. *Maximum:* 90 mg daily.
CAPSULES (LIPOFEN)
Adults. *Initial:* 50 to 150 mg daily with food, increased as needed at 4- to 8-wk intervals. *Maximum:* 150 mg daily with food.
DELAYED-RELEASE CAPSULES (TRILIPIX)
Adults. *Initial:* 45 to135 mg once daily, increased as needed at 4- to 8-wk intervals. *Maximum:* 135 mg daily.
TABLETS (FIBRICOR)
Adults. *Initial:* 35 to 105 mg daily, increased as needed at 4- to 8-wk intervals. *Maximum:* 105 mg daily.
TABLETS (TRICOR)
Adults. *Initial:* 48 to 145 mg daily, increased as needed at 4- to 8-wk intervals. *Maximum:* 145 mg daily.
TABLETS (TRIGLIDE)
Adults. *Initial:* 50 to 160 mg daily, increased as needed at 4- to 8-wk intervals. *Maximum:* 160 mg daily.
TABLETS (FENOGLIDE)
Adults. 40 to 120 mg daily, increased as needed at 4- to 8-wk intervals. *Maximum:* 120 mg daily.
TABLETS (LOFIBRA)
Adults. 54 to 160 mg daily with food, increased as needed at 4- to 8-wk intervals. *Maximum:* 160 mg daily.
DOSAGE ADJUSTMENT For patients with mild to moderate renal impairment or elderly patients, dosage limited for all indications to lowest dosage prescribed for treatment of severe hypertriglyceridemia once daily with increase only after drug's therapeutic and renal effects are known.

Route	Onset	Peak	Duration
P.O.	6–8 wk	Unknown	Unknown

Mechanism of Action

May increase the lipolysis of triglyceride-rich lipoproteins and decrease the synthesis of fatty acids and triglycerides by enhancing the activation of lipoprotein lipase and acyl-coenzyme A synthetase. Fenofibrate also may:

- increase hepatic elimination of cholesterol as bile salts
- promote the catabolism of larger, less dense LDLs with a high-binding affinity for cellular LDL receptors.

Contraindications

Breastfeeding; gallbladder disease; hypersensitivity to fenofibrate, fenofibric acid, or their components; hepatic or severe renal impairment

Interactions

DRUGS
bile acid sequestrants: Decreased fenofibrate absorption
colchicine: Increased risk of myopathy and rhabdomyolysis
immunosuppressants such as cyclosporine and tacrolimus: Increased risk of nephrotoxicity
oral anticoagulants: Risk of bleeding
FOODS
all foods: Increased fenofibrate bioavailability when given in capsule form

Adverse Reactions

CNS: Asthenia, fatigue, headache
CV: **Deep vein thrombosis**, severely depressed HDL cholesterol levels
EENT: Rhinitis
GI: Abdominal pain, cholelithiasis, **cirrhosis**, constipation, diarrhea, elevated liver enzymes, **hepatitis**, nausea, **pancreatitis**
GU: Acute renal failure, increased serum creatinine level, **renal failure**
HEME: Agranulocytosis; anemia; decreased hematocrit or hemoglobin, levels; **leukopenia**, **thrombocytopenia**
MS: Arthralgia, back pain, elevated creatinine phosphokinase, muscle spasms, myalgia, myopathy, myositis, **rhabdomyolysis**
RESP: Pulmonary embolus
SKIN: Photosensitivity, rash, **Stevens–Johnson syndrome**, **toxic epidermal necrolysis**, urticaria
Other: Anaphylaxis, **angioedema**, **delayed hypersensitivity reactions**, **drug reaction with eosinophilia and systemic symptoms (DRESS)**, flu-like symptoms

Nursing Considerations

- Be aware that all drugs that increase serum triglycerides, such as beta blockers, estrogens, and thiazides, should be stopped, and baseline lipid levels obtained before starting fenofibrate.

- Be aware that some brands such as Lipofen and Lofibra need to be given with food to enhance absorption.
- Administer drug 1 hour before or 4 hours after bile acid sequestrants.
- Monitor results of liver and renal function tests. If liver enzyme levels rise to more than 3 times the upper limit of normal and persist, or if the patient develops gallstones, expect to stop drug.
- Monitor serum cholesterol and triglyceride levels at 4- to 8-week intervals, as ordered. If levels don't decrease after 2 months at maximum dosage, expect therapy to be discontinued.

WARNING Monitor patient closely for acute hypersensitivity reactions, including severe rash, and notify prescriber if they occur. Patient may need inpatient corticosteroids. Also monitor patient for delayed cutaneous hypersensitivity reactions that may be severe and can occur days to weeks after fenofibrate therapy is initiated.

- Assess blood counts periodically, as ordered, during first 12 months of therapy to detect adverse hematologic effects.
- Watch closely for evidence of deep vein thrombosis (pain, redness in extremity, or swelling) or pulmonary embolus (sudden onset of anxiety, restlessness, or shortness of breath) because risk is higher in patients taking fenofibrate. Notify prescriber immediately, and start emergency treatment, as prescribed.

PATIENT TEACHING

- Emphasize that drug will be effective only if patient carefully follows prescriber's instructions about diet and exercise.
- Instruct patient to take drug with food.
- Instruct patient prescribed tablet form to store the tablets in their original, desiccant-containing bottle and to avoid taking any chipped or broken tablets.
- Advise patient to have laboratory tests, as directed, to determine drug's effectiveness. They typically include liver function tests after 3 to 6 months, hematocrit and hemoglobin levels, and WBC counts periodically during first year.
- Urge patient to notify prescriber immediately about chills, fever, or sore throat, as well as skin changes such as appearance of blisters or a rash. Also urge her to tell prescriber about unexplained muscle pain, tenderness, or weakness, especially if accompanied by fatigue or fever.
- Tell patient to seek emergency treatment if he develops pain, swelling, and redness in his limb or sudden shortness of breath, anxiety, and restlessness.
- Instruct patient to use sunscreen and protective clothing while in sun and to limit time spent in sun because photosensitivity may occur weeks to months after drug is initiated.

fenoprofen calcium

Nalfon

Class and Category

Pharmacologic class: NSAID
Therapeutic class: Analgesic, anti-inflammatory, antirheumatic
Pregnancy category: Not classified

Indications and Dosages

➤ *To manage mild to moderate pain*

CAPSULES

Adults. 200 mg every 4 to 6 hr, as needed.

➤ *To relieve pain, stiffness, and swelling from osteoarthritis or rheumatoid arthritis*

CAPSULES

Adults. 400 to 600 mg 3 times daily or 4 times daily *Maximum:* 3,200 mg daily.

Route	Onset	Peak	Duration
P.O.	15–30 min*	Unknown†	4–6 hr‡

* For analgesia; 2 days for antirheumatic effects.
† For analgesia; 2 to 3 wk for antirheumatic effects.
‡ For analgesia; unknown for antirheumatic effects.

Mechanism of Action

Blocks the activity of cyclooxygenase, the enzyme needed for prostaglandin synthesis. Prostaglandins, important mediators of the inflammatory response, cause local vasodilation with pain and swelling. When cyclooxygenase is blocked and prostaglandins inhibited, inflammatory symptoms subside. Prostaglandin inhibition also relieves pain because prostaglandins play a role in pain transmission from the periphery to the spinal cord.

Contraindications

Angioedema, asthma, bronchospasm, nasal polyps, rhinitis, or urticaria induced by aspirin, iodides, or other NSAIDs; hypersensitivity to fenoprofen or its components; postoperatively after coronary artery bypass graft (CABG) surgery

Interactions

DRUGS

angiotensin converting enzyme (ACE) inhibitors, angiotensin receptor blockers (ARBs): Decreased antihypertensive effects, increased risk of renal dysfunction in the elderly or patients with existing renal impairment or volume depletion
beta blockers: Decreased antihypertensive effects
anticoagulants, antiplatelets (aspirin), selective serotonin norepinephrine reuptake inhibitors: Increased risk of bleeding
cyclosporine: Increased risk of nephrotoxicity
digoxin: Increased risk of digitalis toxicity
diuretics, triamterene: Decreased effectiveness of these drugs
hydantoins, sulfonamides, sulfonylureas: Possibly increased effects and toxicity of these drugs
lithium: Increased risk of lithium toxicity
methotrexate: Increased risk of methotrexate toxicity
pemetrexed: Increased risk of GI and renal toxicity and myelosuppression
phenobarbital: Possibly decreased elimination half-life of fenoprofen
salicylates: Increased risk of GI bleeding

ACTIVITIES

alcohol use, smoking: Increased risk of GI bleeding

Adverse Reactions

CNS: Agitation, confusion, **CVA**, dizziness, drowsiness, headache, **seizures**, sleep disturbance, tremor, weakness
CV: Hypertension, **MI**, palpitations, peripheral edema, tachycardia, vasodilation
EENT: Blurred vision, dry or sore mouth, hearing loss, tinnitus
GI: Abdominal cramps, distention, and pain; anorexia; constipation; diarrhea; diverticulitis; dysphagia; esophagitis; flatulence; gastritis; gastroenteritis; gastroesophageal reflux disease; **GI bleeding**, or ulceration; hemorrhoids; **hepatitis**; hiatal hernia; indigestion; jaundice; **liver failure**; **melena**; nausea; **perforation of intestines or stomach**; vomiting
GU: Acute renal failure, dysuria, interstitial nephritis
HEME: Agranulocytosis, anemia, **hemolytic anemia**, **leukopenia**, **neutropenia**, **pancytopenia**
MS: Muscle spasms and twitching, myalgia
RESP: Dyspnea
SKIN: Diaphoresis, erythema, **erythema multiforme**, **exfoliative dermatitis**, pruritus, **Stevens–Johnson syndrome**, **toxic epidermal necrolysis**, urticaria
Other: Anaphylaxis, **angioedema**

Nursing Considerations

- Be aware that NSAIDs like fenoprofen should be avoided in patients with a recent MI because risk of reinfarction increases with NSAID therapy. If therapy is unavoidable, monitor patient closely for signs of cardiac ischemia.
- Know that the risk of heart failure increases with NSAID use. NSAIDs such as fenoprofen should not be used in patients with severe heart failure; if unavoidable, monitor patient for worsening of heart failure.
- Use fenoprofen with extreme caution in patients with a history of GI bleeding or ulcer disease because NSAIDs such as fenoprofen increase risk of GI bleeding and ulceration. Expect to use fenoprofen for the shortest time possible in these patients.
- Be aware that serious GI tract bleeding, perforation, and ulceration may occur without warning symptoms. Elderly patients are at greater risk. If GI distress occurs, withhold drug and notify prescriber immediately.
- Give drug with antacids, food, or milk to decrease adverse GI reactions.

- Use fenoprofen cautiously in patients with hypertension, and monitor blood pressure closely throughout therapy. Drug may cause hypertension or worsen it.
- Know that patients with rheumatoid arthritis may need higher doses than those with osteoarthritis to control their symptoms.

WARNING Closely monitor patient who is receiving long-term therapy for signs of toxicity, such as agitation; blurred vision; coma; confusion; drowsiness; elevated BUN and serum creatinine levels; indigestion; nausea; rash; seizures; severe headache; slow, labored breathing; tinnitus; and vomiting.

WARNING Monitor patient closely for thrombotic events, including MI and stroke, because NSAIDs increase the risk. These events may occur early in treatment and risk increases with duration of use. Be aware that these events have occurred even in patients who do not have a history or risk factors for cardiovascular disease. Monitor patient for warning signs such as chest pain, slurring of speech, shortness of breath, or weakness. If any signs and symptoms develop, withhold drug, alert prescriber immediately, and provide supportive care, as prescribed.

WARNING If patient has bone marrow suppression or is receiving antineoplastic drug therapy, monitor laboratory results (including WBC count), and watch for evidence of infection because anti-inflammatory and antipyretic actions of fenoprofen may mask signs and symptoms of infection, such as fever and pain.

- Monitor patient—especially if she's elderly or receiving long-term fenoprofen therapy—for less common but serious adverse GI reactions, including anorexia, constipation, diverticulitis, dysphagia, esophagitis, gastritis, gastroenteritis, gastroesophageal reflux disease, hemorrhoids, hiatal hernia, melena, stomatitis, and vomiting.
- Monitor patient's liver function test results because, in rare cases, elevations may progress to severe hepatic reactions, including fatal hepatitis, hepatic failure, and liver necrosis.
- Monitor BUN and serum creatinine levels in elderly patients, patients taking ACE inhibitors or diuretics, and patients with heart failure, hepatic dysfunction, or impaired renal function because drug may predispose these patients to renal failure.
- Monitor CBC for decreased hemoglobin and hematocrit because drug may worsen anemia.
- Assess patient's skin regularly for signs of rash or other hypersensitivity reaction because fenoprofen is an NSAID and may cause serious skin reactions without warning, even in patients with no history of NSAID sensitivity. At first sign of reaction, stop drug and notify prescriber.

PATIENT TEACHING

- Advise patient to take fenoprofen with antacids, food, or milk to minimize GI distress. Also instruct her to take drug with a full glass of water and to stay upright for 30 minutes afterward to decrease the risk of drug lodging in the esophagus and causing irritation.
- Explain that fenoprofen also may increase the risk of serious adverse GI reactions; stress the need to seek immediate medical attention for such signs and symptoms as abdominal or epigastric pain, black or tarry stools, indigestion, or vomiting blood or material that looks like coffee grounds.
- Instruct patient to swallow drug whole and not to break, chew, crush, or open capsules.
- Caution patient to avoid alcohol, aspirin, and other NSAIDs, unless prescribed, while taking fenoprofen.
- Urge patient taking an anticoagulant to immediately report bleeding, including bloody or tarry stools and bloody vomitus.
- Caution patient to avoid hazardous activities until drug's CNS effects are known.
- Explain that NSAIDs may increase the risk of serious adverse cardiovascular reactions; urge patient to seek immediate medical attention if signs or symptoms arise, such as chest pain, shortness of breath, slurring of speech, and weakness, as well as edema and unexplained weight gain.
- Alert patient to the possibility of rare but serious skin reactions. Urge her to seek immediate medical attention for rash, blisters, itching, fever, or other indications of hypersensitivity.

fentanyl citrate

Abstral, Actiq, Fentora, Lazanda, Sublimaze, SUBSYS

fentanyl transdermal system

Duragesic

Class, Category, and Schedule

Pharmacologic class: Opioid
Therapeutic class: Opioid analgesic
Pregnancy category: C (Abstral, Sublimaze), Not classified (Actiq, Duragesic, Fentora, Lazanda, SUBSYS)
Controlled substance schedule: II

Indications and Dosages

➤ *To provide surgical premedication*

I.M. INJECTION (SUBLIMAZE)

Adults. 0.05 to 0.1 mg 30 to 60 min before surgery.

➤ *As adjunct to regional anesthesia*

I.V. OR I.M. INJECTION (SUBLIMAZE)

Adults. 0.05 to 0.1 mg I.M. or slow I.V. over 1 to 2 min.

➤ *To induce and maintain anesthesia*

I.M. INJECTION (SUBLIMAZE)

Children age 2 to 12. 2 to 3 mcg/kg slow I.V. over 1 to 2 min.

➤ *To manage postoperative pain in postanesthesia care unit*

I.M. INJECTION (SUBLIMAZE)

Adults. 0.05 to 0.1 mg. Repeated in 1 to 2 hr, if needed.

➤ *As adjunct to general anesthesia*

I.V. INJECTION (SUBLIMAZE)

Adults. *For low-dose therapy:* 0.002 mg/kg followed by 0.002 mg/kg, as needed. *For moderate-dose therapy:* 0.002 to 0.02 mg/kg, followed by 0.025 to 0.1 mg, as needed. *For high-dose therapy:* 0.02 to 0.05 mg/kg followed by 0.025 mg to one-half initial loading dose, as needed.

➤ *To treat breakthrough pain in cancer patients who are receiving around-the-clock opioid therapy and have developed tolerance to it*

TRANSMUCOSAL LOZENGE (ACTIQ)

Adults. *Initial:* 200 mcg placed between cheek and gum for 15 min followed by second dose 15 min after first dose ends, as needed. Dosage increased according to patient's needs. *Maximum:* 2 doses of same strength per episode with at least 4 hr between episodes treated.

SUBLINGUAL TABLETS (ABSTRAL)

Adults. *Initial:* 100 mcg followed by second dose 30 min after first dose, if needed. Dosage increased in 100-mcg increments until 400-mcg dosage reached, then increased in increments of 200 mcg, as needed, until maximum dosage of 800 mcg per dose is reached. *Maximum: 800 mcg given twice* 30 min apart per episode of breakthrough pain; dosage interval between episodes of breakthrough pain must be at least 2 hr; only four episodes of breakthrough pain treated per day.

BUCCAL TABLETS (FENTORA)

Adults. *Initial:* 100 mcg buccal tablet placed between upper cheek and gum, followed by second dose 30 min after first dose, as needed. Dosage increased to 200 mcg (placing one tablet on each side of mouth in buccal cavity), as needed. Further increased, as needed, to 400 mcg (placing two tablets on each side of mouth in buccal cavity). Further titration done in multiples of 200 mcg, if needed, until maximum dose of 800 mcg per dose is reached. *Maximum:* 800 mcg given twice 30 min apart 4 times daily with at least 4 hr between each episode treated.

NASAL SPRAY (LAZANDA)

Adults. *Initial:* 100 mcg. Increased, as needed, to 200 mcg, then 300 mcg, then 400 mcg, then 600 mcg, and finally to 800 mcg with doses spaced at least 2 hr apart. *Maximum:* 800 mcg 4 times daily with a dosing interval of at least 2 hr between each episode.

SUBLINGUAL SPRAY (SUBSYS)

Adults. *Initial:* 100 mcg followed by 100 mcg 30 minutes later, if needed. Increased, as needed, to 200 mcg, then 400 mcg, then 600 mcg, then 800 mcg, then 1,200 mcg, then 1,600 mcg with doses spaced at least 4 hr apart. A second dose of same strength may be taken 30 minutes after the first dose, as needed and counted as 1 breakthrough episode. *Maximum:* 1,600 mcg given twice 30 minutes apart 4 times daily with doses spaced at least 4 hr apart.

➤ *To relieve severe chronic pain in opioid-tolerant patient who doesn't respond to less potent drugs and requires around-the-clock opioid administration for an extended time*

TRANSDERMAL SYSTEM (DURAGESIC)

Adults and children age 2 and over. *Initial:* Highly individualized and based on current opioid therapy. Each patch may be worn for 48 to 72 hr. Dosage increased after first 72 hr and then every 6 days, as needed. For more than 100 mcg/hr, more than one patch used.

DOSAGE ADJUSTMENT For cachectic, debilitated or elderly patients, initial dosage should not exceed 25 mcg/hr, unless patient is already receiving more of an equivalent dose of another opioid. For patients receiving long-term opioid therapy, dosage adjusted based on previous day's drug requirement. For patients with mild to moderate hepatic or renal failure, initial dosage decreased by 50%.

Route	Onset	Peak	Duration
I.V.	1–2 min	3–5 min	30–60 min
I.M.	7–15 min	20–30 min	1–2 hr
Transdermal	12–24 hr	Unknown	Over 72 hr

Mechanism of Action

Binds to opioid receptor sites in the CNS, altering perception of and emotional response to pain by inhibiting ascending pain pathways. Fentanyl may alter neurotransmitter release from afferent nerves responsive to painful stimuli, and it causes respiratory depression by acting directly on respiratory centers in the brain stem.

Contraindications

All forms: Hypersensitivity to fentanyl, alfentanil, sufentanil or their components; intermittent pain; opioid nontolerance; significant respiratory depression; treatment of mild to moderate pain responsive to nonopioid drugs; upper airway obstruction

Transdermal form: Hypersensitivity to adhesives; management of post-operative pain or pain that may be acute, intermittent, or mild, or pain in patients requiring opioid therapy for a short period of time; patients who are not opioid-tolerant

Transmucosal form: Acute or chronic pain, including postoperative pain

Interactions

anticholinergics: Increased risk of severe constipation and urinary retention

antimigraine agents, cyclobenzaprine; dextromethorphan; dolasetron; granisetron; linezolid; MAO inhibitors; methylene blue; ondansetron; palonosetron; selected psychiatric drugs such as amoxapine, buspirone, lithium, maprotiline, mirtazapine, nefazodone, trazodone, vilazodone; selective serotonin reuptake inhibitors; serontonin-norepinephrine reuptake inhibitors; St. John's wort; tricyclic antidepressants; tryptophan: Increased risk of serotonin syndrome

benzodiazepines, CNS depressants, muscle relaxants, other opioids, sedating antihistamines, tricyclic antidepressants: Increased risk of sedation and somnolence and severe respiratory depression

benzodiazepines: Possibly reduced fentanyl dose required for anesthesia induction

buprenorphine: Possibly decreased therapeutic effects of buprenorphine

CNS depressants: Possibly increased CNS and respiratory depression and hypotension, possibly resulting in life-threatening effects

buprenorphrine, butorphanol, nalbuphine, pentazocin: Decreased analgesic effect of fentanyl and possibly precipitation of withdrawal symptoms

CYP3A4 inducers such as barbiturates, carbamazepine, efavirenz, glucocorticoids, modafinil, nevirapine, oxcarbazepine, phenytoin, pioglitazone, rifabutin, rifampin, St. John's wort, troglitazone: Possibly induced metabolism and increased clearance of fentanyl with decreased effectiveness and potential development of withdrawal syndrome in dependent patients

CYP3A4 inhibitors such as amiodarone, amprenavir, aprepitant, cimetidine, clarithromycin, diltiazem, erythromycin, fluconazole, fosamprenavir, indinavir, itraconazole, ketoconazole, nefazodone, nelfinavir, ritonavir, saquinavir, telithromycin, troleandomycin, verapamil:

Possibly increased opioid effect, leading to increased or prolonged adverse effects, including severe respiratory depression
diuretics: Possibly decreased efficacy of diuretics
MAO inhibitors: Possibly unpredictable or fatal effects if taken within 14 days

FOODS

grapefruit juice: Increased blood fentanyl level

ACTIVITIES

alcohol use: Increased serum fentanyl level, possibly resulting in fatal overdose from CNS and respiratory depression and hypotension

Adverse Reactions

CNS: Agitation, amnesia, anxiety, asthenia, ataxia, confusion, delusions, depression, dizziness, drowsiness, euphoria, fever, hallucinations, headache, lack of coordination, light-headedness, nervousness, paranoia, sedation, **seizures**, sleep disturbance, slurred speech, syncope, tremor, weakness, yawning
CV: Asystole, **bradycardia**, chest pain, edema, **hypotension**, orthostatic hypotension, tachycardia
EENT: Blurred vision, dental caries, dry mouth, gum-line erosion, **laryngospasm**, rhinitis, sneezing, tooth loss
ENDO: Adrenal insufficiency (rare)
GI: Anorexia, constipation, elevated serum amylase levels, ileus, indigestion, nausea, spasm of the sphincter of Oddi, vomiting
GU: Anorgasmia, decreased libido, ejaculatory difficulty, impotence, infertility, lack of menstruation, urinary hesitancy, urine retention
RESP: Apnea, **depressed cough reflex**, dyspnea, **hypoventilation**, **respiratory depression**
SKIN: Diaphoresis, **exfoliative dermatitis**, localized skin redness and swelling (with transdermal form), pruritus, rash
Other: Anaphylaxis, drug tolerance, physical or psychological dependence with long-term use, weight loss

Nursing Considerations

WARNING Know that fentanyl transdermal system should be used only in patients already receiving opioid therapy and with demonstrated opioid tolerance (taking for a week or longer at least 60 mg of morphine daily, 30 mg of oral oxycodone daily, 8 mg of oral hydromorphone daily, or an equianalgesic dose of another opioid), and require at least a fentanyl dosage of 25 mcg/hour to manage their pain.

- Be aware that opioids like fentanyl should not be given to women during pregnancy and labor and while breastfeeding as the newborn or infant may experience neonatal opioid withdrawal syndrome (NOWS) which may be life-threatening and is exhibited as poor feeding, rapid breathing, trembling, and excessive or high-pitched crying.
- Use with extreme caution in patients with significant chronic obstructive pulmonary disease or cor pulmonale, and in patients having a substantially decreased respiratory reserve, hypoxia, hypercapnia, or preexisting respiratory depression, because even therapeutic doses of fentanyl may decrease respiratory drive in these patients to the point of apnea.
- Use with extreme caution in patients who may be susceptible to the intracranial effects of carbon dioxide retention such as those with brain tumors, head injury, increased intracranial pressure, or impaired consciousness. Monitor these patients closely for signs of sedation and respiratory depression.
- Use caution when titrating fentanyl dosage in elderly, cachectic, and debilitated patients, especially when using I.V. route, because these patients are more sensitive to the drug's effects.
- Use cautiously in patients at risk for opioid abuse, such as those with mental illness or personal or family history of substance abuse. Monitor patient throughout therapy for fentanyl abuse or addiction. Be aware that excessive use of fentanyl may lead to abuse, addiction, misuse, overdose, and possibly death. Monitor patient's intake of drug closely.
- Expect the blood fentanyl level to be prolonged if patient chews or swallows the transmucosal form because drug is absorbed slowly from GI tract.

WARNING Never apply a transdermal patch if seal has been broken or patch has been cut, damaged, or changed because excessive exposure could occur, resulting in possibly fatal fentanyl overdose.

- Be aware that 100 mcg of fentanyl is equivalent in potency to 10 mg of morphine.
- Know that to achieve optimum pain control with the lowest possible fentanyl dose, also plan to give a nonopioid analgesic, such as acetaminophen, as prescribed.
- Be aware that fentanyl should only be used concomitantly with benzodiazapines or other CNS depressants in patients for whom other treatment options are inadequate. If prescribed together, expect dosing and duration of opioid to be limited. Monitor patient closely for signs and symptoms of a decrease in consciousness, including coma, profound sedation, and significant respiratory depression. Notify prescriber immediately and provide emergency supportive care, as death may occur.

WARNING Monitor patient's respiratory status closely, especially during the first 24 to 72 hours after therapy starts or with dosage increases, because severe hypoventilation may occur without warning at any time during therapy. Patients at increased risk include the elderly, cachectic, or debilitated patients. Respiratory depression can occur in patients even if the drug is not misused or abused. Be aware that significant amounts of fentanyl can be absorbed from the skin for 24 hours or more after a transdermal patch is removed. Monitor patient for at least 72 hours after patch has been removed for respiratory depression. Have emergency equipment available including an opioid antagonist.

- Monitor cancer patients receiving sublingual spray form of fentanyl closely for oral mucositis because exposure to the drug in this form has been found to be greater than in patients without mucositis. If Grade 1 mucositis is present, the risk of respiratory or CNS depression increases, especially when therapy is initiated. Expect to avoid use of sublingual spray in cancer patients with Grade 2 mucositis or higher.
- Monitor patient closely who is receiving concurrent CYP3A4 inhibitor therapy along with fentanyl because these drugs may result in an increase in plasma fentanyl concentrations, which could increase or prolong adverse drug effects and may cause sedation and potentially fatal respiratory depression. Notify prescriber immediately, if present. Be aware that discontinuation of CYP3A4 inducers can result in a fatal overdose of fentanyl. Monitor these patients closely as well.

WARNING Know that many drugs may interact with opioids like fentanyl to cause serotonin syndrome. Monitor patient closely for signs and symptoms such as agitation, diaphoresis, diarrhea, fever, hallucinations, labile blood pressure, muscle twitching or stiffness, nausea, shakiness, shivering, tachycardia, trouble with coordination, or vomiting. Notify prescriber at once because serotonin syndrome may be life-threatening. Be prepared to discontinue drug, if possible and ordered, and provide supportive care.

- Monitor patient for adrenal insufficiency. Although rare, it can be life-threatening. Monitor patient for anorexia, dizziness, fatigue, hypotension, nausea, vomiting, or weakness. Notify prescriber if adrenal insufficiency is suspected and expect diagnostic testing to be done. If diagnosis is confirmed, expect to administer corticosteroids and wean patient off fentanyl, if possible.
- Know that to prevent withdrawal symptoms after long-term use, expect to taper drug dosage gradually, as prescribed. Assess patient for withdrawal symptoms after dosage reduction or conversion to another opioid analgesic.
- Monitor patient who is receiving the drug via a transdermal system and who develops a fever for opioid adverse effects because a fever may increase fentanyl release from the system and increase skin permeability. If symptoms occur, notify prescriber and anticipate dosage may be decreased.
- Be aware that for a patient with bradycardia, implement cardiac monitoring, as ordered, and assess heart

rate and rhythm frequently during fentanyl therapy because drug may further slow heart rate.

WARNING **Expect respiratory depressant effects to last longer than analgesic effects. Also be prepared for residual drug to potentiate effects of subsequent doses. Residual drug can be detected for at least 6 hours after I.V. dose and 17 hours after other forms. Monitor patient closely for at least 24 hours after therapy ends.**

WARNING **Assess patient for evidence of overdose, such as cardiopulmonary arrest, hypoventilation, pupil constriction, respiratory and CNS depression, seizures, and shock. Give naloxone (possibly in repeated doses), as prescribed. Be prepared to assist with endotracheal intubation and mechanical ventilation and to provide fluids.**

- Monitor blood glucose level of diabetic patient receiving transdermal fentanyl because each unit contains about 2 g of sugar.

WARNING **Do not substitute Actiq, Lazanda, or Subsys for any other fentanyl product, and do not substitute for each other. Do not convert dosage to or from other products on a mcg-per-mcg basis because doing so may result in a fatal overdose.**

PATIENT TEACHING

- Warn patient not to take more drug than prescribed and not to take it longer than absolutely needed because excessive or prolonged use can lead to abuse, addiction, misuse, overdose, and possibly death.
- Instruct patient to avoid alcohol and other CNS depressants including benzodiazepines during fentanyl therapy unless prescribed.
- Advise patient not to stop taking drug unless directed by prescriber because withdrawal symptoms may occur. Warn against increasing dose or frequency without consulting prescriber because drug can cause dependency.
- For transdermal form, instruct patient to choose a site with intact (not irritated or irradiated) skin on a flat surface, such as the chest, back, flank, or upper arm, and, if appropriate, to clip, not shave, hair from the site and clean it with water (no soaps, lotions, oils, or alcohol). After site preparation, instruct patient to press patch firmly in place with palm of hand for 30 seconds, making sure edges are sealed. Tell her to wash her hands immediately after application with soap and water. If patch loosens, tell her to tape edges down but not cover the entire patch. If more than one patch is needed, the edges shouldn't touch or overlap. Instruct patient to remove patch after 72 hours, fold it in half with adhesive sides together, and flush it down the toilet. Remind her not to reuse a site for at least 3 days. Warn patient to avoid accidental secondary exposure to the drug with someone else through contact with unwashed or unclothed application sites. Examples include transfer of a patch from an adult's body to a child while hugging, sharing the same bed as the patient, accidentally sitting on a patch, and possible accidental exposure of a caregiver's skin to the medication in the patch while applying or removing the patch.
- Warn patient never to apply transdermal patch if seal has been broken or the patch has been cut, damaged, or changed in any way because drug may be released too rapidly. Also warn patient not to expose the application site and surrounding area to direct external heat sources, such as heating pads or electric blankets, heat or tanning lamps, saunas, hot tubs, and heated water beds, while wearing the patch. She should also avoid hot baths or sunbathing because increased body temperature may increase fentanyl release, resulting in a possible overdose. If she develops a fever or becomes overheated from strenuous exercise while wearing a patch, she should contact the prescriber immediately.
- For Actiq transmucosal form, instruct patient to open the package just before use and to save plastic cap for discarding the unused part of the lozenge. Tell her to place lozenge between her cheek and gum and to suck, not chew, it for 15 minutes. Show her how to move lozenge from one side of her mouth to the other using the handle provided separately.
- For Abstral sublingual form, instruct patient to place tablet on the floor of the

mouth directly under the tongue immediately after removing tablet from the blister unit. Caution patient not to chew, suck, or swallow the tablet but to allow it to dissolve completely in the mouth. Tell him not to eat or drink anything until the tablet is completely dissolved.
- For transmucosal form, urge patient to see a dentist regularly, to brush teeth and floss after each meal, and to avoid frequent consumption of products high in sugar because of increased risk of dental caries.
- For transmucosal form, inform diabetic patient that each unit contains 2 g of sugar. Instruct her to monitor her blood glucose levels closely.
- For nasal spray (Lazanda), tell patient to prime the device before use by spraying into the pouch 4 sprays in total. To use, insert the nozzle of the Lazanda bottle a short distance (about 1/2 inch or 1 cm) into the nose and point towards the bridge of the nose, tilting the bottle slightly. Have patient press down firmly on the finger grips until he hears a "click" and the number in the counting window advances by 1. Tell patient that the fine mist spray is not always felt on the nasal mucosal membrane and to rely on the audible click and the advancement of the dose counter to confirm a spray has been administered.
- For sublingual spray (Subsys), tell patient to open the blister package with scissors immediately prior to drug use. Tell him never to use a blister package that has been discovered to be open. Instruct him to spray the contents of the unit into his mouth carefully, underneath his tongue.
- Inform patient that long-term use of opioids like fentanyl may decrease sex hormone levels, causing decreased libido, erectile dysfunction, impotence, infertility, or lack of menstruation. Encourage patient to report any such symptoms to prescriber.
- Remind patient to keep used and unused dosage units out of reach of children and to dispose of drug properly. For buccal tablets, patient should flush leftover drug down the toilet when no longer needed. For sublingual spray, remind patient to dispose of any used or unneeded units immediately in the disposal bottle provided with every dispensed carton. For transdermal patch, patient should fold in half and flush down toilet.
- Caution patient that accidentally exposing others to transdermal fentanyl could cause serious adverse reactions that may become life threatening, especially in children, even with one dose. If accidental exposure occurs, the person should remove the patch, wash the area well with water, and seek medical attention.
- Caution patient to avoid hazardous activities until drug's CNS effects are known.
- Inform patient about potentially fatal additive effects of combining fentanyl with a benzodiazepine. Tell patient to inform all prescribers of fentanyl use.
- Tell patient to increase fiber and fluid intake, unless contraindicated, because drug may cause severe constipation. If it persists or becomes severe, urge patient to notify prescriber.
- Advise patient to notify prescriber if she becomes pregnant or is breastfeeding, as drug may need to be discontinued or dosage altered.

ferric citrate

Auryxia

Class and Category

Pharmacologic class: Ferric iron-based phosphate binder
Therapeutic class: Phosphate binder
Pregnancy category: Not classified

Indications and Dosages

➤ *To control serum phosphorus levels in patients with chronic kidney disease on dialysis*

TABLETS

Adults. *Initial*: 2 tablets (420 mg ferric iron, equivalent to 2 g ferric citrate) 3 times a day with meals, increased or decreased by 1 to 2 tablets per day at 1-wk or longer intervals, as needed. *Maximum*: 12 tablets daily.

➤ *To treat iron deficiency anemia in patients with chronic kidney disease not on dialysis*

TABLETS

Adults. 1 tablet (210 ferric iron, equivalent to 1 g ferric citrate) 3 times a day with meals, titrated to achieve and maintain hemoglobin at target levels. *Maximum:* 12 tablets daily (12 g ferric citrate).

Mechanism of Action
Binds dietary phosphate in the gastrointestinal (GI) tract and precipitates as ferric phosphate, which is then excreted in the stool. By binding phosphate in the GI tract and decreasing absorption, serum phosphate levels are reduced.

Contraindications
Hypersensitivity to ferric citrate or its components, iron overload syndromes

Interactions
DRUGS
ciprofloxacin, doxycycline: Decreased effectiveness of these drugs

Adverse Reactions
GI: Abdominal pain, constipation, diarrhea, discolored stools, nausea, vomiting
HEME: Increased serum ferritin and transferrin saturation levels
RESP: Cough
Other: **Hyperkalemia**

Nursing Considerations
- Be aware that ferric citrate produces dark stools because of its iron content, but this effect does not affect laboratory tests for occult bleeding.
- Know that iron absorption from ferric citrate therapy may cause an excessive elevation in iron stores. Assess patients' serum ferritin and transferrin saturation levels before initiating ferric citrate therapy, as ordered, and monitor throughout therapy.
- Expect that patients receiving iron intravenously may need a reduction in dose or discontinuation of I.V. iron therapy.

Patient teaching
- Instruct patient to take ferric citrate exactly as ordered.

WARNING Remind patient that accidental overdose of iron-containing products is a leading cause of death in children under age 6. Stress the importance of keeping ferric citrate tablets out of the reach of children. If accidental overdose occurs, the poison control center should be called and immediate emergency treatment sought for the child.

ferrous salts

ferrous fumarate

(contains 100 mg of elemental iron per capsule or per 5 ml of oral suspension, 33 mg of elemental iron per chewable tablet or per 5 ml of oral suspension, 106 mg of elemental iron per E.R. capsule, 15 mg of elemental iron per 0.6 ml of oral solution, and 20 to 115 mg of elemental iron per tablet)

Femiron, Feostat, Feostat Drops, Ferretts, Fumasorb, Fumerin, Hemocyte, Ircon, Neo-Fer (CAN), Nephro-Fer, Novofumar (CAN), Palafer (CAN), Span-FF

ferrozus carboxymaltose

Injectafer

ferrous gluconate

Apo-Ferrous Gluconate (CAN), FE-40, Ferate, Fergon, Ferralet, Ferralet Slow Release, Fertinic (CAN), Novoferrogluc (CAN), Simron

ferrous sulfate

Feosol, Feratab, Fer-gen-sol, Fer-In-Sol, Fer-Iron, Ferodan, Fero-Grad (CAN), Fero-Gradumet, Ferospace, Ferralyn Lanacaps, Ferra-TD, Feusal Original, Mol-Iron, Novoferrosulfa (CAN), PMS-Ferrous Sulfate (CAN), Slow-Fe

iron, carbonyl

Feosol Natural Release

Class and Category
Pharmacologic class: Hematinic
Therapeutic class: Antianemic, nutritional supplement
Pregnancy category: Not classified

Indications and Dosages
➤ *To prevent iron deficiency based on recommended daily allowances*

CAPLETS, CAPSULES, CHEWABLE TABLETS, DRIED CAPSULES, DRIED E.R. CAPSULES, DRIED E.R. TABLETS, DRIED TABLETS, ELIXIR, ENTERIC-COATED

TABLETS, E.R. CAPSULES, E.R. TABLETS, ORAL SOLUTION, ORAL SUSPENSION, SYRUP, TABLETS
Adults age 51 and over. 8 mg daily.
Adult females age 19 to 50. 18 mg daily.
Adult men age 19 to 50. 8 mg daily.
Pregnant women. 27 mg daily.
Breastfeeding women. 9 to 10 mg daily.
Boys age 14 to 18. 11 mg daily.
Girls age 14 to 18. 15 mg daily.
Children age 9 to 13. 8 mg daily.
Children age 4 to 8. 10 mg daily.
Children age 1 to 3. 7 mg daily.
Infants age 7 to 12 months. 11 mg daily.
Newborns to age 6 months. 0.27 mg daily.

➤ *To replace iron in deficiency states*

CAPLETS, CAPSULES, CHEWABLE TABLETS, DRIED CAPSULES, DRIED E.R. CAPSULES, DRIED E.R. TABLETS, DRIED TABLETS, ELIXIR, ENTERIC-COATED TABLETS, E.R. CAPSULES, E.R. TABLETS, ORAL SOLUTION, ORAL SUSPENSION, SYRUP, TABLETS
Adults and adolescents. 300 to 325 mg daily. *Maintenance:* 325 mg up to 3 times daily for several wk or mo.
Infants and children. *For mild to moderate iron deficiency anemia:* 3 mg elemental iron/kg/day in 1 to 2 divided doses. *For severe iron deficiency anemia:* 4 to 6 mg elemental iron/kg/day in 3 divided doses.
Premature neonates. 2 to 4 mg elemental iron/kg/day divided every 12 to 24 hr. *Maximum:* 15 mg daily.

➤ *To treat iron deficiency in patients who have an intolerance to oral iron, have had unsatisfactory response to oral iron, or who have non-dialysis-dependent chronic kidney disease*

I.V. INFUSION (INJECTAFER), I.V. INJECTION (INJECTAFER)
Adults weighing 50 kg (110 lb) or more. 750 mg followed by second dose of 750 mg given no sooner than 7 days later. I.V. injection given slowly at a rate of 100 mg/min. I.V. infusion given over at least 15 min. *Maximum:* 1,500 mg per course with 2 doses separated by at least 7 days.
Adults weighing less than 50 kg (110 lb). 15 mg/kg followed by second dose of 15 mg/kg given no sooner than 7 days later. I.V. injection given slowly at a rate of 100 mg/min. I.V. infusion given over at least 15 min. *Maximum*: 1,500 mg per course with 2 doses separated by at least 7 days.

➤ *To provide iron supplementation during pregnancy*

CAPLETS, CAPSULES, CHEWABLE TABLETS, DRIED CAPSULES, DRIED E.R. CAPSULES, DRIED E.R. TABLETS, DRIED TABLETS, ELIXIR, ENTERIC-COATED TABLETS, E.R. CAPSULES, E.R. TABLETS, ORAL SOLUTION, ORAL SUSPENSION, SYRUP, TABLETS
Pregnant women. 30 mg elemental iron daily.

DOSAGE ADJUSTMENT Dosage increased if needed for elderly patients, who may not absorb iron as easily as younger adults do.

Mechanism of Action

Acts to normalize RBC production by binding with hemoglobin or by being oxidized and stored as hemosiderin or aggregated ferritin in reticuloendothelial cells of the bone marrow, liver, and spleen. Iron is an essential component of hemoglobin, myoglobin, and several enzymes, including catalase, cytochromes, and peroxidase. Iron is needed for catecholamine metabolism and normal neutrophil function.

Contraindications

Hemochromatosis, hemolytic anemias, hemosiderosis, hypersensitivity to iron salts or their components, other anemic conditions unless accompanied by iron deficiency

Interactions

DRUGS

bisphosphonates, dolutegravir, integrase inhibitors: Decreased absorption of these drugs
dimercaprol: Increased risk of nephrotoxic effect of iron salts
levodopa: Possibly chelation with iron, decreasing levodopa absorption and blood level
levothyroxine: Decreased levothyroxine effectiveness and, possibly, hypothyroidism
methyldopa: Decreased methyldopa absorption and efficacy
mycophenolate mofetil: Possibly decreased effectiveness of mycophenolate mofetil
penicillamine: Decreased penicillamine absorption
quinolones, tetracyclines: Decreased effectiveness of these antibiotics

FOODS

coffee; eggs; foods that contain bicarbonates, carbonates, oxalates, or phosphates; milk and milk products; tea that contains tannic acid; whole-grain breads and cereals and other high-fiber foods: Decreased iron absorption and effectiveness

ACTIVITIES

alcohol abuse (acute or chronic): Increased serum iron level

Adverse Reactions

CNS: Dizziness, fever, headache, paresthesia, syncope

CV: Chest pain, hypertension, **hypotension**, tachycardia

EENT: Metallic taste, tooth discoloration

GI: Abdominal cramps, constipation, epigastric pain, nausea, stool discoloration, vomiting

HEME: Hemochromatosis, **hemolysis**, hemosiderosis

RESP: Dyspnea, wheezing

SKIN: Diaphoresis, flushing, pruritus, rash, urticaria

Other: Anaphylaxis (with I.V. administration), **angioedema**, injection-site discoloration

Nursing Considerations

- Give iron tablets and capsules with a full glass of juice or water. Don't crush enteric-coated tablets or open capsules.
- Dilute and administer with a straw or place drops in back of patient's throat, because iron solutions may stain teeth. Mix the elixir form in water. Fer-In-Sol Drops or Syrup may be mixed with juice or water.
- Know that to maximize absorption, iron salts should be given 1 hour before or 2 hours after meals. If GI irritation occurs, give with or just after meals.
- Protect liquid form from freezing.
- Administer Injectafer intravenously, either as an undiluted slow I.V. push or by infusion. When administering as a slow I.V. push, give at the rate of about 100 mg (2 ml) per minute. When administering via infusion, dilute up to 750 mg of iron in no more than 250 ml of sterile 0.9% sodium chloride injection, USP, such that the concentration of the infusion is not less than 2 mg of iron per ml, and administer over at least 15 minutes. Once diluted, solution is stable for 72 hours at room temperature.
- Avoid extravasation with I.V. administration because brown discoloration of the extravasation site may be long-lasting.

WARNING Monitor patients closely for hypersensitivity reactions for at least 30 minutes after I.V. administration. If present, discontinue drug immediately, notify prescriber, and be prepared to provide supportive care, as needed.

- Monitor patient's blood pressure after each I.V. dose for significant increases, as hypertension may occur immediately after administration but usually resolves within 30 minutes.
- Be aware that at usual dosages, serum hemoglobin level usually normalizes in about 2 months unless blood loss continues. Treatment may last for 3 to 6 months to help replenish iron stores.

WARNING Monitor patient for signs of iron overdose, which may include abdominal pain, diarrhea (possibly bloody), nausea, severe vomiting, and sharp abdominal cramps. In case of iron toxicity or accidental iron overdose (a leading cause of fatal poisoning in children under age 6), give deferoxamine, as prescribed. As few as 3 adult iron tablets can cause serious poisoning in young children.

- Don't give antacids, coffee, dairy products, eggs, tea, or whole-grain breads or cereals within 1 hour before or 2 hours after iron.
- Remember that unabsorbed iron turns stool black or green and can mask blood in stool. Check stool for occult blood, as ordered.

PATIENT TEACHING

- Instruct patient not to chew any solid form of iron except for chewable tablets.
- Caution patient receiving Injectafer to immediately report any signs and symptoms of an allergic reaction such as hives, itching, wheezing, or feeling faint. Also alert patient that Injectafer may raise his blood pressure and to report dizziness, flushing, or nausea to prescriber.
- Urge patient to eat chicken, fish, lean red meat, and turkey, as well as foods rich in vitamin C (such as citrus fruits and fresh vegetables) to improve iron absorption.
- Urge patient to avoid foods that impair iron absorption, including dairy products, eggs, spinach, and high-fiber foods, such as whole-grain breads and cereals and bran. Also advise her to avoid drinking coffee or tea within 1 hour of iron intake.

- Caution patient not to take antacids or calcium supplements within 1 hour before and 2 hours after taking iron supplement.
- Inform patient that stool should become dark green or black during therapy. Advise her to notify prescriber if it doesn't.
- Tell patient to minimize tooth stains from liquid iron, by mixing dose with, fruit juice, tomato juice, or water and to drink it with a straw. If patient must take liquid iron by dropper, direct her to place drops well back on the tongue and to follow with water or juice. Tell her that iron stains can be removed by brushing with baking soda (sodium bicarbonate).
- Advise patient to consult prescriber before taking large amounts of iron for longer than 6 months.
- Warn patient about high risk of accidental poisoning, and urge her to keep iron preparations out of the reach of children.
- Tell mothers who are breastfeeding while receiving Injectafer to monitor their infant for gastrointestinal toxicity such as constipation and diarrhea.

ferumoxytol

Feraheme

Class and Category

Pharmacologic class: Iron agent
Therapeutic class: Hematinic
Pregnancy category: Not classified

Indications and Dosages

➤ *To treat iron deficiency anemia in patients with chronic kidney disease or who are intolerant to oral iron or who have had an unsatisfactory response to oral iron*

I.V. INFUSION

Adults. 510 mg administered over at least 15 min followed by another 510 mg in 3 to 8 days administered over at least 15 min. Dose repeated after 1 or more months, as needed.

Mechanism of Action

Isolates the bioactive iron from plasma components until the iron–carbohydrate complex enters the reticuloendothelial system macrophages of the bone marrow, liver, and the iron is released from the iron–carbohydrate complex within vesicles in the macrophages. Iron then either enters the intracellular storage iron pool (e.g., ferritin) or is transferred to plasma transferrin for transport to erythroid precursor cells for incorporation into hemoglobin.

Contraindications

History of allergic reaction to any I.V. iron product, hypersensitivity to ferumoxytol or its components, iron overload

Interactions

DRUGS

oral iron preparations: Reduced absorption of these preparations

Adverse Reactions

CNS: Dizziness, fatigue, fever, headache, loss of consciousness, **seizures**, syncope, unresponsiveness
CV: Arrhythmias, **cardiac arrest**, chest pain, **congestive heart failure**, hypertension, **hypotension (may be severe)**, **myocardial ischemia**, tachycardia
GI: Abdominal pain, constipation, diarrhea, gastroenteritis, nausea, vomiting
GU: Acute kidney dysfunction, **chronic renal failure**
HEME: Hemorrhagic anemia, increased ferritin level
MS: Arthralgia, back pain, muscle spasms
RESP: Cough, **cyanosis**, dyspnea, pneumonia, **respiratory arrest**
SKIN: Ecchymosis, flushing, pruritus, rash, urticaria
Other: Anaphylaxis, **angioedema**, injection-site swelling

Nursing Considerations

- Question patient about a history of experiencing an allergic reaction to iron or any other medication administered intravenously before administering first dose of ferumoxytol. If present, withhold drug and notify prescriber.
- Do not dilute drug prior to administration. At time of administration, add drug to 50 to 200 ml of 0.9% sodium chloride injection, USP or 5% dextrose injection, USP and infuse immediately over at least 15 minutes. Have patient be

in a recline or semi-reclined position during administration because of risk of hypotension, which may be more pronounced in the elderly patient.

- Administer drug to patient receiving hemodialysis at least 1 hour after hemodialysis has started and once the patient's blood pressure has stabilized. Monitor patient for signs and symptoms of hypotension following each injection.
- Evaluate the hematologic response by measuring the patient's hemoglobin, ferritin, iron, and transferrin saturation at least 1 month following the second injection. Expect to readminister the drug in patients with persistent or recurrent iron deficiency anemia.

WARNING Monitor patient closely for signs and symptoms of hypersensitivity for at least 30 minutes following each injection because anaphylactoid reactions have occurred following administration. Know that a serious allergic reaction may occur even in patients who did not experience a reaction with a previous dose and may be more serious in the elderly patient. Also, do not administer any other drugs that could potentially cause serious hypersensitivity reactions and/or hypotension such as chemotherapeutic agents or monoclonal antibodies for at least 30 minutes after ferumoxytol administration. If a reaction occurs, provide supportive care, as indicated, by severity of reaction and expect drug to be discontinued.

- Monitor patient's blood pressure after administering each dose of ferumoxytol because severe hypotension has occurred with drug use.
- Monitor patient's response to ferumoxytol therapy because excessive therapy with parenteral iron can lead to excess storage of iron with the possibility of iatrogenic hemosiderosis.
- Be aware that ferumoxytol therapy may transiently affect the diagnostic ability of magnetic resonance imaging for up to 3 months after the last dose.

PATIENT TEACHING

- Instruct patient to immediately report any signs and symptoms of hypersensitivity such as hives, itchiness or rash along with breathing problems, dizziness, lightheadedness, and swelling, especially in throat area.
- Advise patient to comply with follow-up visits and laboratory tests required to determine drug effectiveness.

fesoterodine fumarate

Toviaz

Class and Category

Pharmacologic class: Muscarinic receptor antagonist
Therapeutic class: Antispasmodic
Pregnancy category: Not classified

Indications and Dosages

➤ *To treat overactive bladder with symptoms of urinary frequency, incontinence, and urgency*

E.R. TABLETS

Adults. *Initial:* 4 mg daily, increased to 8 mg, as needed. *Maximum:* 8 mg daily.

DOSAGE ADJUSTMENT For patients with severe renal insufficiency or who are taking potent CYP3A4 inhibitors (such as clarithromycin, itraconazole, and ketoconazole), dosage shouldn't exceed 4 mg daily.

Route	Onset	Peak	Duration
P.O.	Unknown	5 hr	Unknown

Mechanism of Action

Exerts antimuscarinic (atropine-like) and potent direct antispasmodic (papaverine-like) actions on smooth muscle in the bladder. The result is increased bladder capacity and a decreased urge to void. Fesoterodine has an active metabolite that inhibits bladder contraction and decreases detrussor pressure.

Contraindications

Gastric retention; hypersensitivity to fesoterodine, tolterodine tartrate extended-release capsules or immediate-release tablets, or their components; uncontrolled narrow-angle glaucoma; urine retention

E
F

Interactions

DRUGS

antimuscarinic agents: Possibly increased anticholinergic effects; possibly altered absorption of oral drugs taken concurrently

potent CYP3A4 inhibitors, such as clarithromycin, itraconazole, ketoconazole: Possibly increased serum fesoterodine level and increased risk of adverse effects

FOODS

caffeine: May aggravate bladder symptoms

ACTIVITIES

alcohol use: Increased drowsiness

Adverse Reactions

CNS: Dizziness, drowsiness, headache, insomnia, somnolence

CV: Angina, chest pain, palpitations, peripheral edema, **QT-interval prolongation**

EENT: Blurred vision; dry eyes, mouth, or throat

GI: Constipation, diverticulitis, dyspepsia, elevated liver enzymes, gastroenteritis, irritable bowel syndrome, nausea, upper abdominal pain

GU: Dysuria, urine retention, UTI

MS: Back pain

RESP: Cough, upper respiratory tract infection

SKIN: Decreased sweating, pruritus, rash, urticaria

Other: **Angioedema**

Nursing Considerations

- Use cautiously in patients with significant bladder outlet obstruction because fesoterodine can cause urine retention.
- Use cautiously in patients with controlled narrow-angle glaucoma, decreased GI motility, or myasthenia gravis because drug can make these conditions worse.
- Use cautiously in patients taking other drugs with anticholinergic effects, such as antihistamines.
- Monitor patient closely for angioedema, which may occur after the first dose. If present, discontinue fesoterodine therapy immediately, as ordered, and provide emergency supportive care, including maintaining a patent airway, as needed.
- Monitor patient for CNS anticholinergic effects, especially after beginning fesoterodine therapy or increasing the dose. If present, notify prescriber, as dosage may need to be reduced or drug discontinued.

PATIENT TEACHING

- Instruct patient to take drug exactly as prescribed.
- Tell patient to take drug with a full glass of water and not to cut, crush, or chew tablets.
- Explain that drug can cause adverse effects such as constipation and urine retention. If they occur and are severe or prolonged, patient should notify prescriber.
- Tell patient to seek immediate emergency medical attention if he experiences difficulty breathing or any swelling of his face, lips, throat, or tongue.
- Advise patient to avoid alcohol consumption during fesoterodine therapy.
- Tell patient to avoid hazardous activities until drug's CNS effects are known.
- Caution patient to avoid strenuous exercise and excessive sun exposure because of increased risk of heatstroke.
- Advise patient to limit caffeine consumption during drug therapy.
- Explain that full benefits of fesoterodine therapy may take 2 to 3 months.
- Inform patient that chewing sugarless gum or sucking hard candy (especially lemon drops) may help ease dry mouth.

fidaxomicin

Dificid

Class and Category

Pharmacologic class: Macrolide
Therapeutic class: Antibiotic
Pregnancy category: B

Indications and Dosages

➤ *To treat* Clostridium difficile*-associated diarrhea (CDAD)*

TABLET

Adults. 200 mg twice daily for 10 days.

Mechanism of Action

Inhibits RNA synthesis in *Clostridium difficile* bacterial cells by RNA polymerases, causing the cells to die.

Contraindications
Hypersensitivity to fidaxomicin or its components

Interactions
DRUGS
cyclosporine: Possible increased blood fidaxomicin level

Adverse Reactions
ENDO: Hyperglycemia
GI: Abdominal distention or pain, dyspepsia, dysphagia, elevated liver enzymes, flatulence, **GI hemorrhage**, **intestinal obstruction**, **megacolon**, nausea, vomiting
HEME: Anemia, **neutropenia**, **thrombocytopenia**
RESP: Dyspnea
SKIN: Drug eruption, pruritus, rash
Other: Angioedema, **decreased blood bicarbonate**, elevated blood alkaline phosphatase, **metabolic acidosis**

Nursing Considerations
- Know that fidaxomicin and other drugs for *C. difficile*–associated diarrhea are most effective when patients are not taking other antibiotics. If other antibiotics can be stopped safely, expect them to be withheld during the 10 days of fidaxomicin therapy.
- Monitor patient for hypersensitivity reactions that may include angioedema, dyspnea, pruritus, or rash. Patients with a history of allergy to other macrolides are at increased risk. If a severe reaction occurs, discontinue fidaxomicin immediately and notify prescriber. Provide supportive care, as needed and ordered.
- Monitor patient for adverse effects and notify prescriber, if present.

PATIENT TEACHING
- Instruct patient to take fidaxomicin exactly as prescribed and for the full 10 days, regardless of how he is feeling.
- Tell patient to seek immediate emergency care if an allergic reaction occurs during fidaxomicin therapy.
- Tell patient to notify prescriber if symptoms worsen at any time or don't improve after a few days.

filgrastim
(granulocyte colony-stimulating factor, rG-CSF)
Grastofil (CAN), Neupogen

filgrastim-aafi
Nivestym

filgrastim-sndz
(granulocyte colony-stimulating factor, G-CSE)
Zarxio

tbo-filgrastim
Granix

Class and Category
Pharmacologic class: Colony-stimulating factor
Therapeutic class: **Hematopoietic**
Pregnancy category: Not classified

Indications and Dosages
➤ *To reduce infection in patients with nonmyelid malignancies after myelosuppressive chemotherapy; to reduce neutrophil recovery time and duration of fever following induction or consolidation chemotherapy in patients with acute myeloid leukemia*

I.V. INFUSION (GRASTOFIL, NEUPOGEN, NIVESTYM, ZARXIO)
Adults and children. 5 mcg/kg daily over 15 to 30 min by short intravenous infusion or as continuous infusion infused over 24 hr given daily for up to 2 wk beginning 24 hr or more after cytotoxic chemotherapy. Increased, as needed, by 5 mcg/kg with each chemotherapy cycle.

SUBCUTANEOUS INJECTION (GRASTOFIL, NEUPOGEN, NIVESTYM, ZARXIO)
Adults and children. 5 mcg/kg daily for up to 2 wk or until absolute neutrophil count (ANC) has reached 10,000/mm^3 following the expected chemotherapy-induced neutrophil nadir beginning 24 hr or more after cytotoxic chemotherapy. Increased, as

needed, by 5 mcg/kg with each chemotherapy cycle.

➤ *To reduce the duration of severe neutropenia in patients with nonmyeloid malignancies after receiving myelosuppressive chemotherapy associated with a significant incidence of febril neutropenia*

SUBCUTANEOUS INJECTION

Adults and children age 1 month and older. 5 mcg/kg daily starting no earlier than 24 hr after myelosuppressive chemotherapy and continued until the neutrophil count has recovered to normal.

➤ *To reduce duration of neutropenia in patients with nonmyeloid malignancies undergoing myeloablative chemotherapy followed by bone marrow transplantation*

I.V. INFUSION (GRASTOFIL, NEUPOGEN, NIVESTYM, ZARXIO)

Adults. 10 mcg/kg daily as a continuous infusion for no longer than 24 hr beginning at least 24 hr after bone marrow infusion and cytotoxic chemotherapy. Dosage adjusted according to absolute neutrophil (ANC) count response.

➤ *To mobilize autologous hematopoietic progenitor cells into the peripheral blood for collection by leukapheresis*

SUBCUTANEOUS INJECTION (GRASTOFIL, NEUPOGEN, NIVESTYM, ZARXIO)

Adults. 10 mcg/kg daily starting at least 4 days before first leukapheresis and continuing until last day of leukapheresis.

➤ *To reduce occurrence and duration of severe neutropenia in congenital, cyclic, or idiopathic neutropenia*

SUBCUTANEOUS INJECTION (GRASTOFIL, NEUPOGEN, NIVESTYM, ZARXIO)

Adults and children. 6 mcg/kg twice daily.

➤ *To reduce the occurrence and duration of severe neutropenia in idiopathic or cyclic neutropenia*

SUBCUTANEOUS INJECTION (GRASTOFIL, NEUPOGEN, ZARXIO)

Adults and children. 5 mcg/kg daily.

➤ *To treat patients acutely exposed to myelosuppressive doses of radiation*

SUBCUTANEOUS INJECTION (NEUPOGEN)

Adults. 10 mcg/kg daily beginning as soon as possible after exposure to radiation doses greater than 2 gray and continued until ANC remains greater than 1,000/mm^3 for 3 consecutive CBCs or exceeds 10,000/mm^3 after a radiation-induced nadir.

➤ *To prevent and treat neutropenia in patients with HIV infection*

SUBCUTANEOUS INJECTION (GRASTOFIL)

Adults. 1 mcg/kg/day or 300 mcg three times weekly.

DOSAGE ADJUSTMENT Dosage adjusted according to CBC with differential and platelet count response.

Route	Onset	Peak	Duration
I.V.	In 5 min	Unknown	Unknown

Mechanism of Action

Is pharmacologically identical to human granulocyte colony-stimulating factor, an endogenous hormone synthesized by endothelial cells, fibroblasts and monocytes. Filgrastim induces formation of neutrophil progenitor cells by binding directly to receptors on the surface of granulocytes, which then divide and differentiate. It also potentiates the effects of mature neutrophils, which reduces fever and the risk of infection raised by severe neutropenia.

Incompatibilities

Don't mix filgrastim with normal saline solution because precipitate will form.

Contraindications

Hypersensitivity to filgrastim, other human granulocyte colony-stimulating factors such as pegfilgrastim, or their components

Interactions

DRUGS

None

Adverse Reactions

CNS: Fever, headache

CV: Aortitis, transient **supraventricular tachycardia**

GI: Splenic rupture, splenomegaly

GU: Glomerulonephritis

HEME: Leukocytosis, **thrombocytopenia**

MS: Arthralgia; decreased bone density (children with chronic treatment); myalgia; pain in arms, legs, lower back, or pelvis: osteoporosis (children with chronic therapy)

RESP: Acute respiratory distress syndrome (ARDS), alveolar hemorrhage, dyspnea, **hemoptysis**, wheezing

SKIN: Cutaneous vasculitis, pruritus, rash, Sweet's syndrome (acute febrile neutrophilic dermatosis)
Other: Anaphylaxis, angioedema, injection-site pain and redness, sickle cell crisis

Nursing Considerations

- Warm filgrastim to room temperature before injection. Discard drug if stored longer than 6 hours at room temperature or 24 hours in refrigerator.
- Withdraw only one dose from a vial; don't repuncture the vial.
- Don't shake the solution.
- For continuous infusion, dilute in D_5W (not normal saline solution) to produce less than 15 mcg/ml.
- For subcutaneous dose larger than 1 ml, divide and give in more than one site.
- For short I.V. infusion, give drug over 15 to 30 minutes.
- Don't give within 24 hours before or after cytotoxic chemotherapy.
- Be aware that needle cover on single-use prefilled syringe contains dry natural rubber (except for the brands Granix and Nivestym) and may cause sensitivity reaction. It shouldn't be handled by allergic people.
- Be aware that the brand Granix's prefilled syringe has a safety needle guard device for use by healthcare professionals only. To safely use the device, hold the syringe assembly by the open sides of the device and remove the needle shield. Expel any extra volume depending on dose needed. Inject Granix subcutaneously by pushing the plunger as far as it will go to inject all of the drug. Injection of the entire prefilled syringe contents is needed to activate the needle guard. With the plunger still pressed all the way down, remove the needle from the skin. Slowly let go of the plunger and allow the empty syringe to move up inside the device until the entire needle is guarded. Discard the syringe assembly in an approved container.
- Know that the Nivestym prefilled syringe with BD UltraSafe Plus Passive Needle Guard cannot be used for doses less than 0.3 ml (180 mcg), because the spring-mechanism of the needle guard apparatus affixed to the prefilled syringe interferes with the visibility of the graduation markings on the syringe barrel corresponding to 0.1 ml and 0.2 ml. For direct administration of doses less than 0.3 ml, the single-dose vial should be used instead to ensure accuracy.
- Expect to monitor CBC, hematocrit, and platelet count 2 or 3 times weekly.
- Inform prescriber and expect to stop drug if leukocytosis develops or absolute neutrophil count consistently exceeds 10,000/mm^3.
- Anticipate decreased response to drug if patient has received extensive radiation therapy or long-term chemotherapy.
- Know that aortitis has occurred in patients receiving filgrastim, occurring as early as the first week after start of therapy. Monitor patient for generalized signs and symptoms such as abdominal pain, back pain, fever, and malaise. Increased inflammatory markers (e.g., C-reactive protein and white blood cell count) help to confirm the diagnosis. Expect drug to be discontinued if aortitis is suspected.
- Monitor patient's renal function, as ordered, because drug may cause glomerulonephritis. If abnormalities occur, expect dosage to be reduced or drug discontinued.

WARNING Monitor patients with sickle cell anemia receiving filgrastim, as sickle cell crisis can occur that can be life-threatening. Notify prescriber immediately if sickle cell crisis occurs. Expect drug to be discontinued.

PATIENT TEACHING

- Review possible serious side effects (allergic reactions, capillary leak syndrome, hematological abnormalities, inflammation of blood vessels, kidney injury, respiratory distress syndrome, and sickle cell crises) with patient before drug is given and determine patient's understanding. Tell her the most common side effect is aching in the bones and muscles.
- Teach patient how to prepare, administer, and store drug. Caution her not to reuse needle, syringe, or vial.
- Alert patient that there is a difference in drug concentration between the prefilled syringe and vial of the brand Neuprogen. Tell patient to make sure she is

administering the correct volume of Neuprogen for the dose prescribed.
- Advise patient prescribed single-use prefilled syringe to notify prescriber if she has an allergy to latex, unless she is using the brands Granix or Nivestym, because needle cover may cause sensitivity reaction.
- Provide patient with puncture-resistant container for needle and syringe disposal.
- Instruct patient who is self-injecting drug to notify prescriber if a dose is missed, to obtain instructions on when to take the next dose.
- Advise patient to promptly report pain in left upper quadrant of abdomen or shoulder-tip pain. Also tell patient to report any persistent, severe, or unusual signs and symptoms to prescriber and seek emergency medical attention, if needed. For example, tell her that difficulty breathing, facial swelling, rash, or wheezing require immediate attention.
- Emphasize the importance of returning for follow-up laboratory tests.
- Advise female patient to report pregnancy to prescriber immediately and encourage her to enroll in Amgen's Pregnancy Surveillance Program by calling 1-800-77-AMGEN.
- Instruct patient to inform all prescribers of filgrastim or filgrastim-sndz use. Patient should not take any over-the-counter preparations until after speaking to prescriber.

finasteride

Propecia, Proscar

Class and Category

Pharmacologic class: 5-alpha reductase inhibitor
Therapeutic class: Benign prostatic hyperplasia agent, hair growth stimulant
Pregnancy category: X

Indications and Dosages

➤ *To treat symptomatic benign prostatic hyperplasia; to reduce the risk of symptomatic progression of benign prostatic hyperplasia when given with doxazocin*

TABLETS (PROSCAR)
Adults. 5 mg daily.

➤ *To treat male-pattern baldness*

TABLETS (PROPECIA)
Adults. 1 mg daily.

Route	Onset	Peak	Duration
P.O.*	Unknown	8 hr	24 hr†
P.O.‡	In 3 mo	Unknown	Unknown

* For benign prostatic hyperplasia.
† With single-dose therapy; 2 wk with multiple-dose therapy.
‡ For male-pattern baldness.

Mechanism of Action

Inhibits 5-alpha reductase, an intracellular enzyme that converts testosterone to its metabolite (5-alpha dihydrotestosterone) in liver, prostate, and skin. The metabolite is a potent androgen partially responsible for benign prostatic hyperplasia and hair loss.

Contraindications

Females, hypersensitivity to finasteride or its components

Interactions

DRUGS
theophylline: Decreased theophylline level

Adverse Reactions

CNS: Asthenia, depression, dizziness, headache, **progressive multifocal leukoencephalopathy** (extremely rare)
CV: **Hypotension**, peripheral edema
EENT: Lip swelling, rhinitis
ENDO: Gynecomastia, **male breast cancer**
GI: Abdominal pain, diarrhea
GU: Altered prostate-specific antigen level, decreased ejaculatory volume, decreased libido, erectile dysfunction, **high-grade prostate cancer**, impotence, male infertility, testicular pain
MS: Back pain
RESP: Dyspnea
SKIN: Pruritus, rash, urticaria
Other: **Angioedema**

Nursing Considerations

- Be aware that patient should have a urologic evaluation prior to starting finasteride therapy and periodically

throughout therapy because drug can increase the risk of prostate cancer, especially high-grade prostate cancer.
- Expect patient to have a digital rectal examination of the prostate before and periodically during finasteride therapy.
- Be aware that finasteride therapy affects PSA levels. For example, drug may decrease levels even in the presence of prostate cancer. Any increases, no matter how slight or even if increase is still within normal limits, warrant further evaluation because of finasteride's risk of high-grade prostate cancer.
- Be aware that pregnant female healthcare workers should not handle broken finasteride tablets because of potential adverse effect on male fetus.

PATIENT TEACHING

WARNING **Urge patient and female partners to use reliable contraception during therapy because semen of men who take drug can harm male fetuses. Caution women and children not to handle broken tablets.**
- Explain how to take drug, and urge patient to follow instructions that accompany it.
- Inform patient that drug may cause a variety of sexual dysfunction problems including decreased libido, erectile dysfunction, and male infertility, which may continue after drug is discontinued.
- Urge patient to have periodic follow-up to determine drug effectiveness.
- Caution patient that noncompliance with therapy may affect PSA test results.

fingolimod hydrochloride

Gilenya

Class and Category

Pharmacologic class: Sphingosine 1-phosphate receptor modulator
Therapeutic class: Antimultiple sclerotic
Pregnancy category: C

Indications and Dosages

➤ *To treat relapsing forms of multiple sclerosis (MS)*

CAPSULES

Adults and children age 10 and over weighing more than 40 kg (88 lb). 0.5 mg once daily.
Children age 10 and over weighing 40 kg (88 lb) or less. 0.25 mg once daily.

Mechanism of Action

Possibly involves reduction of lymphocyte migration into the central nervous system to produce improved physical mobility.

Contraindications

Baseline QTc interval equal to or greater than 500 msec; experience within past 6 months of class III or IV heart failure, decompensated heart failure requiring hospitalization, MI, stroke, TIA, or unstable angina; history or presence of Mobitz Type II second-degree or third-degree atrioventricular block or sick sinus syndrome unless patient has functioning pacemaker in place; hypersensitivity to fingolimod or its components; use of Class Ia or Class III antiarrhythmic drugs

Interactions

DRUGS

antineoplastics, immunosuppressives, immunomodulators: Increased immunosuppression
beta blockers such as atenolol, calcium channel blockers such as diltiazem or verapamil, digoxin: Possibly increased severity of bradycardia or slowing of atrioventricular conduction
chlorpromazine, citalopram, Class Ia and Class III antiarrhythmics, erythromycin, haloperidol, methadone: Possibly increased risk for prolonged QT interval which may lead to torsades de pointes
ketoconazole: Increased fingolimod levels
live attenuated vaccines: Increased risk of contracting disease from live virus
vaccines: Decreased effectiveness of vaccines during and up to 2 months after fingolimod therapy

Adverse Reactions

CNS: Asthenia, depression, dizziness, headache, migraine, paresthesia, **posterior reversible encephalopathy syndrome**, **progressive multifocal leukoencephalopathy**, **seizures**, **status epilepticus**, syncope

E F

CV: Atrioventricular blocks, bradycardia, elevated blood triglycerides, hypertension, **transient asystole**
EENT: Blurred vision, eye pain, macular edema, sinusitis
GI: Diarrhea, elevated liver enzymes, gastroenteritis
HEME: Leukopenia, lymphopenia
MS: Back pain, severe increase in disability with discontinuation of therapy
RESP: Bronchitis, cough, dyspnea, pulmonary dysfunction
SKIN: Alopecia, **basal cell carcinoma,** eczema, **melanoma, Merkel cell carcinoma,** pruritus, rash, tinea infections, urticaria
Other: Angioedema; flu-like symptoms; increased severity of herpes viral infections; infections such as bacterial, fungi, and viral; **lymphomas;** weight loss

Nursing Considerations

- Be aware that fingolimod therapy should not begin in a patient with an active acute or chronic infection until the infection is resolved, because drug causes a dose-dependent reduction in peripheral lymphocyte count up to 30% of baseline values.
- Immunize patient against the varicella zoster virus if he is antibody negative, as ordered. Be aware that fingolimod therapy will need to be postponed for 1 month to allow the full effect of vaccination to occur.
- Obtain an electrocardiogram on patients receiving antiarrhythmic therapy including beta-blockers and calcium channel blockers, those with cardiac risk factors, and those who have a irregular or slow heartbeat prior to beginning fingolimod therapy because drug may cause bradycardia and increased risk for atrioventricular block, especially in the first 24 hours of therapy.
- Obtain a recent complete blood count (within past 6 months) prior to starting therapy, as ordered, because drug increases risk of infection, especially bacterial, fungi, and viral, that may become serious and life-threatening. Monitor patient throughout drug therapy for signs and symptoms of infection. If present, notify prescriber, and expect drug to be discontinued if serious and infection treated according to standard of care.
- Expect patient to have an ophthalmologic evaluation prior to beginning drug therapy and then again 3 to 4 months after therapy has begun to assess for macular edema. Patients with diabetes mellitus or a history of uveitis should have ongoing evaluations because they are at increased risk for macular edema. Report any visual disturbances to prescriber during drug therapy and expect additional ophthalmologic evaluation to be performed, if present, and drug discontinued. Visual acuity loss may persist even after resolution of macular edema in some patients.
- Obtain a recent liver enzyme evaluation (within past 6 months) prior to initiating fingolimod therapy, as ordered, because drug may cause elevation of liver enzymes. Monitor periodically throughout therapy and expect drug to be discontinued if liver enzymes exceed 5 times the upper limit of normal. Also evaluate in patient who develops symptoms suggestive of hepatic dysfunction, such as unexplained abdominal pain, anorexia, dark urine, fatigue, jaundice, nausea, and vomiting. Know that patients with preexisting liver disease may be at increased risk for developing elevated liver enzymes during fingolimod therapy.
- Monitor patient for hypersensitivity reactions such as angioedema, rash, or urticaria following administration. Prepare to provide supportive care if present and expect drug to be discontinued.
- Observe patient for 24 hours after the first dose of fingolimod for signs and symptoms of bradycardia. Heart rate usually begins to decrease within an hour of the first dose. The maximal decline in heart rate usually occurs within 6 hours and recovers but not to baseline level within 10 hours after the first dose. A second decline may occur after the first within the first 24 hours after the first dose. Monitor patient closely because the second decline may be more pronounced than the first. If patient develops chest pain, dizziness, fatigue, hypotension, or palpitations, notify prescriber, initiate appropriate management, as ordered, and

continue observation until the symptoms have resolved. Know that with continued drug use, the heart rate returns to baseline within one month. Also observe patient closely for cardiac effects after drug is reinitiated if treatment is discontinued or interrupted for certain periods, as well as after dosage increases.

- Monitor patient for dyspnea throughout fingolimod therapy because drug may reduce diffusion lung capacity for carbon monoxide (DLCO) and forced expiratory volume over 1 second. Expect to perform spirometric evaluations of respiratory function and evaluation of DLCO during therapy, if clinically indicated.
- Monitor patient's blood pressure regularly to detect development of hypertension.
- Assess patient's skin for abnormalities, as drug may increase risk of basal cell carcinoma, melanoma, and Merkel cell carcinoma. Promptly report any suspicious looking lesions.
- Be aware that it takes about 2 months for drug effects to be gone after therapy is discontinued requiring patient to be monitored for adverse effects during this time. Also be aware that severe increase in disability may occur after discontinuation of drug, which may occur up to 24 weeks after drug is stopped. Assess patient's level of function during this time and expect appropriate treatment to be given, as needed.

PATIENT TEACHING

- Inform patient that he will need to be observed for at least 6 hours after the first dose. He will need to repeat this observation period again for 6 hours if treatment is interrupted for more than 1 day within the first 2 weeks of therapy, if treatment is interrupted for more than 7 days during week 3 and 4 of therapy, or if treatment is discontinued for more than 14 days and then treatment is reinitiated, as well as any time dosage is increased.
- Tell patient to report any adverse signs and symptoms of infection or any other persistent or serious abnormalities to prescriber promptly, even up to 2 months after drug has been discontinued.
- Advise patient to examine his skin regularly for skin abnormalities, because drug may increase risk of skin cancer, including melanoma. Tell patient to report any suspicious skin lesion to prescriber for evaluation. Remind patient to limit exposure to sunlight and ultraviolet light and to wear protective clothing and use a sunscreen with a high protection factor when going outdoors.
- Instruct female patients to use effective contraception to avoid pregnancy during and for 2 months after fingolimod therapy is discontinued because of potential fetal harm. Stress importance of notifying prescriber immediately if pregnancy is suspected or occurs. If confirmed, encourage patient to register with the pregnancy exposure registry by calling 877-598-7237.
- Instruct patient how to check his pulse and tell him to notify prescriber if his pulse rate drops below 60 beats per minute or becomes irregular.
- Advise patient to notify prescriber immediately if difficulty breathing or visual changes occurs.
- Tell patient to notify prescriber if he notices symptoms suggestive of liver dysfunction, such as unexplained abdominal pain, anorexia, dark urine, fatigue, jaundice, nausea, or vomiting.
- Alert patient of the need to have periodic blood work done during fingolimod therapy and urge him to be compliant with these evaluations.

flavoxate hydrochloride

Urispas

Class and Category

Pharmacologic class: Flavone derivative
Therapeutic class: Urinary tract antispasmodic
Pregnancy category: B

Indications and Dosages

➤ *To relieve dysuria; nocturia; suprapubic pain; urinary frequency, incontinence, and urgency caused by cystitis, prostatitis, urethritis, urethrocystitis, or urethrotrigonitis*

TABLETS
Adults and adolescents. 100 to 200 mg 3 times daily or 4 times daily.

Route	Onset	Peak	Duration
P.O.	55 min	112 min	Unknown

Mechanism of Action
Relaxes muscles by cholinergic blockade and counteracts smooth-muscle spasms in the urinary tract.

Contraindications
Achalasia; duodenal or pyloric obstruction; GI hemorrhage; hypersensitivity to flavoxate or its components; obstructive uropathies of the lower urinary tract

Interactions
DRUGS
bethanechol, metoclopramide: Possibly antagonized GI motility effects of these drugs

Adverse Reactions
CNS: Confusion, decreased concentration, dizziness, drowsiness, fever, headache, nervousness, vertigo
CV: Palpitations, tachycardia
EENT: Accommodation disturbances, blurred vision, dry mouth, eye pain, photophobia, worsening of glaucoma
GI: Constipation, nausea, vomiting
GU: Dysuria
HEME: Eosinophilia, **leukopenia**
SKIN: Decreased sweating, dermatoses, urticaria

Nursing Considerations
- Monitor for eye pain if patient has glaucoma because flavoxate's anticholinergic effects may worsen glaucoma.

PATIENT TEACHING
- Caution patient about possible dry mouth and photophobia. Advise her to wear sunglasses outdoors, and suggest sugarless candy or gum, ice chips, saliva substitute, or sips of water for dry mouth.
- Advise patient to avoid hazardous activities until CNS effects of flavoxate are known.
- Caution patient not to become overheated or to take hot baths or saunas during therapy because drug reduces sweating, which can lead to dizziness, fainting, or heatstroke.
- Instruct patient to notify prescriber immediately if she experiences confusion, drowsiness, dysuria, headache, high fever, hives, nausea, nervousness, palpitations, rash, tachycardia, vertigo, vision problems, vomiting, or worsening dry mouth.

flecainide acetate
Tambocor

Class and Category
Pharmacologic class: Benzamide derivative
Therapeutic class: Class IC antiarrhythmic
Pregnancy category: C

Indications and Dosages
➤ *To prevent and suppress recurrent life-threatening ventricular tachycardia*

TABLETS
Adults. *Initial:* 100 mg every 12 hr (every 8 hr for some patients). Increased by 50 mg twice daily every 4 days, as needed, until response occurs. *Maintenance:* Up to 150 mg every 12 hr. *Maximum:* 400 mg daily.

➤ *To prevent paroxysmal atrial fibrillation or flutter or paroxysmal supraventricular tachycardia*

TABLETS
Adults. *Initial:* 50 mg every 12 hr (every 8 hr for some patients). Increased by 50 mg twice daily every 4 days, as needed, until response occurs. *Maintenance:* Up to 150 mg every 12 hr. *Maximum:* 300 mg daily.

DOSAGE ADJUSTMENT Initial dose reduced to 100 mg daily or 50 mg every 12 hr for patients with creatinine clearance less than 35 ml/min.

Mechanism of Action
Achieves antiarrhythmic effect by inhibiting fast sodium channels of myocardial cell membranes, which increase myocardial recovery after repolarization, and by depressing the upstroke of the action potential. Flecainide also produces its antiarrhythmic effect by:
- slowing intracardiac conduction, which slightly increases the duration of the action potential in atrial and ventricular muscle, thus prolonging the PR interval, QRS complex, and QT interval

- shortening the action potential of Purkinje fibers without affecting surrounding myocardial tissue
- inhibiting extracellular calcium influx (at high doses)
- stopping paroxysmal reentrant supraventricular tachycardias by acting on antegrade pathways of dysfunctional AV conduction
- decreasing conduction in accessory pathways in those with Wolff–Parkinson–White syndrome.

Contraindications

Cardiogenic shock, hypersensitivity to flecainide or its components, recent MI, right bundle-branch block associated with left hemiblock or second- or third-degree AV block unless pacemaker is present

Interactions

DRUGS

amiodarone: Increased blood flecainide level
antiretrovirals: Possibly increased flecainide levels
beta blockers, disopyramide, verapamil: Possibly myocardial depression and increased blood levels of both drugs
digoxin: Possibly increased blood digoxin level

FOODS

acidic juices, foods that decrease urine pH below 5.0: Increased flecainide elimination and decreased therapeutic effects
foods that increase urine pH above 7.0, strict vegetarian diet: Decreased flecainide elimination and increased therapeutic effects

ACTIVITIES

smoking: Increased flecainide clearance

Adverse Reactions

CNS: Anxiety, depression, dizziness, drowsiness, fatigue, headache, lightheadedness, tremor, weakness
CV: **Arrhythmias**, chest pain, **heart failure**, **hypotension**
EENT: Blurred vision
GI: Abdominal pain, anorexia, constipation, **hepatic dysfunction**, nausea, vomiting
RESP: Dyspnea
SKIN: Rash

Nursing Considerations

- Monitor urine pH beginning at the start of flecainide therapy.
- Check blood pressure, fluid intake and output, and weight regularly during therapy.
- Monitor trough flecainide level, as needed; therapeutic level is 0.2 to 1 mcg/ml.
- Expect drug to cause mild to moderate negative inotropic effects, minimal cardiovascular effects, and no effect on blood pressure, heart rate, and left ventricular function.

WARNING **Know that because hypokalemia or hyperkalemia may interfere with flecainide's therapeutic effects, serum potassium level must be monitored before and during therapy as ordered, and notify prescriber immediately if potassium imbalance develops. Also monitor for and notify prescriber about prolonged PR interval, QRS complex, or QT interval; chest pain; hypotension; and signs of heart failure. Keep in mind that drug can cause fatal proarrhythmias, which is why it isn't considered a first-line antiarrhythmic.**

- Expect prolonged flecainide therapy to raise blood alkaline phosphatase level.

PATIENT TEACHING

- Instruct patient to take flecainide at regular intervals to keep a constant blood level.
- Advise patient to take a missed dose as soon as she remembers if it's within 6 hours of the scheduled time.
- Teach patient how to take her pulse, and instruct her to record it daily, along with her weight. Advise her to bring record to follow-up visits.
- Encourage family members to obtain instruction in basic cardiac life support.
- Advise patient to notify prescriber immediately about chest pain, difficulty breathing, and dizziness.
- Caution patient not to stop taking flecainide suddenly but to taper dosage gradually according to prescriber's instructions.

flibanserin

Addyi

Class and Category

Pharmacologic class: Serotonin receptor 1A agonist/serotonin receptor 2A antagonist
Therapeutic class: Sexual desire enhancer
Pregnancy category: Not classified

Indications and Dosages

➤ *To treat premenopausal women with acquired, generalized hypoactive sexual desire disorder*

TABLETS

Adults. 100 mg once daily at bedtime.

Mechanism of Action

Has high affinity for serotonin receptors with agonist activity at 5-HT1A and antagonist activity at 5-HT2A as well as antagonist activity at dopamine D4 receptors but it is unknown if this activity is the mechanism of action behind flibanserin's ability to increase sexual desire.

Contraindications

Alcohol use, concomitant use with moderate or strong CYP3A4 inhibitors, hepatic impairment, hypersensitivity to flibanserin or its components

Interactions

DRUGS

CNS depressants including benzodiazepines, hypnotics, and opioids; CYP2C19 inhibitors such as antifungals, benzodiazepines, proton pump inhibitors, selective serotonin reuptake inhibitors; CYP3A4 inhibitors (moderate or strong) such as amprenavir, atazanavir, boceprevir, ciprofloxacin, clarithromycin, conivaptan, diltiazem, erythromycin, fluconazole, fosamprenavir, indinavir, itraconazole, ketoconazole, nefazodone, nelfinavir, posaconazole, ritonavir, saquinavir, telaprevir, telithromycin, verapamil; concurrent therapy with multiple weak CYP3A4 inhibitors such as cimetidine, fluoxetine, ginkgo, oral contraceptives, ranitidine: Increased risk of CNS depression, severe hypotension and syncope

CYP3A4 inducers such as carbamazepine, phenobarbital, phenytoin, rifabutin, rifampin, rifapetine, St. John's wort: Decreased effectiveness of flibanserin

P-glycoprotein substrates such as digoxin, sirolimus: Possibly increased risk of toxicity of these drugs

FOODS

grapefruit juice: Increased risk of severe hypotension and syncope

ACTIVITIES

alcohol use: Severe hypotension with possible syncope

Adverse Reactions

CNS: Anxiety, dizziness, fatigue, insomnia, somnolence, syncope, vertigo
CV: **Hypotension (severe)**
EENT: Dry mouth
GI: Abdominal pain, constipation, nausea
GU: Metrorrhagia
SKIN: Rash

Nursing Considerations

- Know that flibanserin should not be prescribed for premenopausal women with a hypoactive sexual desire disorder that stems from a co-existing medical or psychiatric condition, effects of a medication or other drug substance, or relationship problems. It is also not indicated for treatment of hypoactive sexual desire disorders in postmenopausal women or in men and is not indicated to enhance sexual performance.
- Be aware that if patient is starting flibanserin therapy following moderate or strong CYP3A4 inhibitor use, the drug should not be started until 2 weeks after the last dose of the CYP3A4 inhibitor to avoid serious drug interactions. Know that if the patient is initiating a moderate or strong CYP3A4 inhibitor therapy following the use of flibanserin, the CYP3A4 drug therapy should not start until 2 days after the last dose of flibanserin.
- Question patient prior to flibanserin therapy being started about her alcohol intake. Know that patient must abstain from alcohol use during flibanserin therapy because hypotension and syncope resulting in accidental injury may occur. Alert prescriber if there is any concern the patient may not be able to abstain from alcohol.
- Know that flibanserin is available only through a restricted program because of the increased risk of severe hypotension and syncope due to an interaction between alcohol and flibanserin.

PATIENT TEACHING

- Instruct patient to take flibanserin at bedtime to avoid serious adverse reactions such as accidental injury from low blood pressure, sedation, sleepiness, or syncope.
- Advise patient if she has missed a dose to take the next dose at bedtime on the next day and not to double the next dose.

- Caution patient not to engage in any hazardous activities such as driving until the effects of the drug are known.

WARNING Stress importance of not taking flibanserin with alcohol or other CNS depressants because her blood pressure may fall dangerously low and she may faint. If she feels faint, tell her to lie down immediately and seek medical attention if the symptoms do not resolve.

- Tell patient to tell all prescribers she is taking flibanserin.

fluconazole

Diflucan

Class and Category

Pharmacologic class: Azole antifungal
Therapeutic class: Antifungal
Pregnancy category: C (vaginal candidiasis indication), D (all other indications)

Indications and Dosages

➤ *To treat oral and esophageal candidiasis*

ORAL SUSPENSION, TABLETS, I.V. INFUSION

Adults and adolescents. 200 mg on day 1 followed by 100 mg daily for at least 2 (oral) or 3 (esophageal) wk after symptoms resolve. I.V. dosage infused at a rate no greater than 200 mg/hr.

Children. 6 mg/kg on day 1, followed by 3 mg/kg daily for at least 2 (oral) or 3 (esophageal) wk and then for 2 wk after esophageal symptoms resolve. I.V. dosage infused at a rate no greater than 200 mg/hr.

➤ *To treat systemic candidiasis*

ORAL SUSPENSION, TABLETS, I.V. INFUSION

Adults and children. Highly individualized. *Maximum:* 400 mg daily (adults) and 12 mg/kg/day (children). I.V. dosage infused at a rate no greater than 200 mg/hr.

➤ *To treat cryptococcal meningitis*

ORAL SUSPENSION, TABLETS, I.V. INFUSION

Adults and adolescents. 400 mg on day 1, followed by 200 to 400 mg daily based on patient's response, and continued for 10 to 12 wk after CSF culture is negative. *Maintenance:* 200 mg daily to suppress relapse. I.V. dosage infused at a rate no greater than 200 mg/hr.

Children. 12 mg/kg on day 1, followed by 6 to 12 mg/kg daily and continued for 10 to 12 wk after CSF culture is negative. I.V. dosage infused at a rate no greater than 200 mg/hr.

➤ *To prevent candidiasis after bone marrow transplantation in patients who receive cytotoxic chemotherapy and/or radiation*

ORAL SUSPENSION, TABLETS, I.V. INFUSION

Adults and adolescents. 400 mg daily starting several days before procedure if severe neutropenia is expected and continued for 7 days after absolute neutrophil count exceeds 1,000/mm^3. I.V. dosage infused at a rate no greater than 200 mg/hr.

➤ *To treat vaginal candidiasis*

CAPSULES, ORAL SUSPENSION, TABLETS

Adults. 150 mg as a single dose.

DOSAGE ADJUSTMENT After initial loading dose, dosage reduced by 50% for patients with creatinine clearance of 11 to 50 ml/min.

Mechanism of Action

Damages fungal cells by interfering with a cytochrome P-450 enzyme needed to convert lanosterol to ergosterol, an essential part of the fungal cell membrane. Decreased ergosterol synthesis causes increased cell permeability, which allows cell contents to leak. Fluconazole also may inhibit endogenous respiration, interact with membrane phospholipids, inhibit transformation of yeasts to mycelial forms, inhibit purine uptake, and impair biosynthesis of triglycerides and phospholipids.

Incompatibilities

Don't add fluconazole to I.V. container that contains any other drug.

Contraindications

Coadministration of drugs known to prolong QT interval (astemizole, cisapride, erythromycin, pimozide, or quinidine) or concurrent therapy with terfenadine (when multiple dosages reach or exceed 400 mg), hypersensitivity to fluconazole or its components

Interactions

DRUGS

alfentanil, amitriptyline, celecoxib, cyclosporine, halofantrine, methadone,

E F

nortriptyline: Increased blood levels of these drugs
amiodarone, astemizole, cisapride, erythromycin, pimozide, quinidine: Increased risk of QT-interval prolongation possibly leading to torsades de pointes
benzodiazepines (short-acting): Possibly increased benzodiazepine level and psychomotor effects
calcium-channel blockers: Possibly increased systemic exposure of calcium-channel blockers causing adverse effects
carbamazepine: Possibly increased risk of carbamazepine toxicity
fentanyl: Possibly elevated fentanyl concentration that may lead to respiratory depression
glipizide, glyburide, tolbutamide: Increased risk of hypoglycemia
HMG-CoA reductase inhibitors: Increased risk of myopathy and rhabdomyolysis
hydrochlorothiazide: Increased fluconazole level from decreased excretion
losartan: Possibly decreased hypotensive effect of losartan
NSAIDs: Increased systemic exposure of NSAIDs
oral anticoagulants: Increased anticoagulant effects
phenytoin: Increased phenytoin level
prednisone: Possibly increased risk of acute adrenal cortex insufficiency
rifampin: Decreased serum fluconazole level
tacrolimus: Increased tacrolimus levels, possibly leading to nephrotoxicity
voriconazole: Increased risk of toxicity

Adverse Reactions

CNS: Chills, dizziness, drowsiness, fever, headache, **seizures**
CV: Prolonged QT interval, **torsades de pointes**
GI: Abdominal pain, anorexia, constipation, diarrhea, **hepatic failure**, nausea, vomiting
HEME: Agranulocytosis, **leukopenia**, **thrombocytopenia**
SKIN: Exfoliative dermatitis, photosensitivity, pruritus, rash
Other: Anaphylaxis, **angioedema**

Nursing Considerations

- Use fluconazole cautiously in patients with potentially proarrhythmic conditions because drug may prolong the QT interval, which can lead to life-threatening torsades de pointes.
- Expect to obtain BUN and serum creatinine levels, as well as culture, sensitivity, and liver enzymes, as ordered, before therapy starts.
- Refrigerate, but don't freeze, fluconazole oral suspension. Shake well before administering.
- Discard I.V. solution that's cloudy or contains precipitate. Don't infuse more than 200 mg/hr or add supplemental drugs to infusion.
- Monitor hepatic and renal function periodically during therapy, and notify prescriber if you detect signs of dysfunction.
- Assess for rash every 8 hours during therapy, and notify prescriber if rash occurs.
- Monitor coagulation test results and assess patient for bleeding if patient is receiving an oral anticoagulant.
- Monitor patient for symptoms of overdose, such as hallucinations and paranoia. If they occur, provide supportive treatment, gastric lavage, and, possibly, hemodialysis, which can reduce blood fluconazole level by half after about 3 hours.

PATIENT TEACHING

- Instruct patient to take fluconazole tablets or oral suspension 30 minutes before or 2 hours after meals. Inform her that tablets may be crushed for easier swallowing if needed.
- Advise patient to complete entire course of therapy, even if she feels better.
- Tell patient to inform all prescribers of fluconazole use and not to take any over-the-counter preparations without consulting prescriber first, as drug can interact with many other drugs and substances.
- Urge patient to monitor blood glucose level often if she takes an oral antidiabetic drug, because of increased risk of hypoglycemia.
- Alert patient that fluconazole may change the taste of food.
- Encourage patient to notify prescriber immediately about diarrhea, headache, nausea, rash, right-upper-quadrant abdominal pain, yellow skin or whites of eyes, or vomiting.

- Suggest that breastfeeding patient consult prescriber because breastfeeding may need to be stopped during therapy.
- Urge women of childbearing age to notify prescriber immediately if pregnancy is suspected or known, as drug may need to be discontinued.

flumazenil

Anexate (CAN), Romazicon

Class and Category

Pharmacologic class: Imidazobenzodiazepine derivative
Therapeutic class: Benzodiazepine antidote
Pregnancy category: C

Indications and Dosages

➤ *To reverse conscious sedation from benzodiazepine therapy*

I.V. INJECTION

Adults. 0.2 mg given over 15 sec, repeated after waiting 45 sec if response is inadequate and then repeated every 1 min, if needed, up to maximum dose. If sedation recurs, regimen is repeated every 20 min or more. *Maximum:* 1 mg given in 0.2 mg increments every 1 min over 5-min cycle repeated every 20 min 3 times for a total of 3 mg over 1 hr.
Children. 0.01 mg/kg over 15 sec, repeated after waiting 45 sec if response is inadequate and then repeated every 1 min, if needed, up to 4 additional doses. *Maximum:* 5 doses total, not exceeding accumulative dosage of 0.05 mg/kg or 1 mg, whichever is lower.

➤ *To reverse benzodiazepine toxicity or suspected overdose*

I.V. INJECTION

Adults. 0.2 mg given over 30 sec followed by 0.3 mg after waiting 30 sec if response is inadequate and then 0.5 mg given over 30 sec at 1-min intervals, if needed, to maximum dose. If sedation recurs, regimen is repeated every 20 min. *Maximum:* Cycle repeated every 20 min 3 times for a total of 3 mg in 1-hr period.

Route	Onset	Peak	Duration
I.V.	1–2 min	6–10 min	Variable

Mechanism of Action

Antagonizes CNS effects of benzodiazepines by competing for their binding sites.

Contraindications

Evidence of tricyclic antidepressant overdose; hypersensitivity to flumazenil, benzodiazepines, or their components; use of benzodiazepine to control intracranial pressure, status epilepticus, or a potentially life-threatening condition

Interactions

DRUGS

benzodiazepines: Benzodiazepine withdrawal symptoms, including seizures
nonbenzodiazepine agonists: Loss of effectiveness of these drugs
tetracyclic or tricyclic antidepressant overdose: High risk of seizures

Adverse Reactions

CNS: Agitation, anxiety, ataxia, confusion, dizziness, drowsiness, emotional lability, fatigue, headache, hypoesthesia, insomnia, paresthesia, resedation, **seizures**, tremor, vertigo
CV: Hot flashes, hypertension, palpitations
EENT: Blurred vision, diplopia, dry mouth
GI: Nausea, vomiting
RESP: Dyspnea, hyperventilation, **hypoventilation**
SKIN: Diaphoresis, flushing, rash
Other: Injection-site pain and thrombophlebitis

Nursing Considerations

- Use flumazenil cautiously in patients with cardiac disease. Assess for increased anxiety or stress from benzodiazepine withdrawal because patient's blood pressure may rise.
- Give flumazenil undiluted or diluted in a syringe with D_5W, lactated Ringer's solution, or normal saline solution. Administer over 15 to 30 seconds directly into tubing of a free-flowing compatible I.V. solution. Use a large vein, if possible, to minimize pain at site. Avoid extravasation because drug may irritate tissue.
- Be aware that drug may cause signs of benzodiazepine withdrawal in drug-dependent patient. Also, abrupt awakening from benzodiazepine overdose can cause agitation, dysphoria, and increased adverse reactions.

- Be aware that benzodiazepine reversal may cause an anxiety or a panic attack for patient with a history of these episodes. Expect to adjust dosage carefully.
- Monitor patient for signs of hypoventilation or resedation for at least 2 hours after giving flumazenil because drug has a short half-life. Be aware that patient shouldn't be discharged until the risk of resedation has resolved.

PATIENT TEACHING

- Caution patient to avoid alcohol and OTC drugs for 10 to 24 hours after receiving drug.
- Advise patient to avoid hazardous activities for 18 to 24 hours after discharge.
- Inform patient and family that agitation, emotional lability, fear, and panic attack (if patient has a history of them) may occur. Tell them to seek medical care if patient has depression, flushing, hyperventilation, insomnia, palpitations, tremor, or trouble breathing.
- Provide written instructions or instructions to caregiver even if patient is alert, because drug doesn't always reverse postprocedure amnesia.

fluoxetine hydrochloride

Prozac, Prozac Weekly, Sarafem

Class and Category

Pharmacologic class: Selective serotonin reuptake inhibitor (SSRI)
Therapeutic class: Antidepressant
Pregnancy category: Not classified

Indications and Dosages

➤ *To treat depression*

CAPSULES, ORAL SOLUTION, TABLETS (PROZAC)

Adults. *Initial:* 20 mg daily in the morning. Dosage increased every 4 to 8 wk as needed. Dosage greater than 20 mg daily given twice daily morning and noon. *Maximum:* 80 mg daily.

Children ages 8 and older. *Initial:* 10 mg daily. Increased after 1 wk to 20 mg daily.

DOSAGE ADJUSTMENT For lower-weight children, dosage increased to 20 mg daily only if improvement insufficient after several wk.

DELAYED-RELEASE CAPSULES (PROZAC WEEKLY)

Adults. 90 mg/wk, beginning 7 days after last 20-mg daily dose.

➤ *To treat obsessive–compulsive disorder*

CAPSULES, ORAL SOLUTION, TABLETS (PROZAC)

Adults. *Initial:* 20 mg daily in the morning. Dosage increased every 4 to 8 wk as needed. Dosage greater than 20 mg daily given twice daily morning and noon. *Maximum:* 80 mg daily.

Children ages 7 and older. *Initial:* 10 mg daily. Dosage increased after 2 wk to 20 mg daily. Subsequent dosage increased, as needed, at intervals of at least several wk. *Maintenance:* 20 to 60 mg daily.

DOSAGE ADJUSTMENT For lower-weight children, dosage should be increased above 10 mg daily only if clinical improvement remains insufficient after several wk. Maintenance dosage for such patients should not exceed 30 mg daily.

➤ *To treat moderate to severe bulimia nervosa*

CAPSULES, ORAL SOLUTION, TABLETS (PROZAC)

Adults. 60 mg daily in the morning.

➤ *To treat panic disorder with or without agoraphobia*

CAPSULES, ORAL SOLUTION, TABLETS (PROZAC)

Adults. *Initial:* 10 mg daily. Dosage increased in 1 wk to 20 mg daily, as needed. Dosage further increased after several wk, as needed. *Maximum:* 60 mg daily.

➤ *To treat premenstrual dysmorphic disorder*

CAPSULES (SARAFEM)

Adults. 20 mg daily given continuously (every day of the menstrual cycle) or intermittently (starting daily dose 14 days prior to the anticipated onset of menstruation through the first full day of menses and repeated with each new cycle). Dosage increased as needed. *Maximum:* 80 mg daily.

DOSAGE ADJUSTMENT Dose or frequency reduced for patients with concurrent illness or hepatic impairment, those who take multiple medications, and for elderly patients.

Route	Onset	Peak	Duration
P.O.*	1–6 wk†	Unknown	Unknown

* Capsules, oral solution, and tablets.
† For depression and bulimia; 5 wk for obsessive–compulsive disorder.

Mechanism of Action

Selectively inhibits reuptake of the neurotransmitter serotonin by CNS neurons and increases the amount of serotonin available in nerve synapses. An elevated serotonin level may result in elevated mood and, consequently, reduce depression, lessen obsessive–compulsive behavior, and diminish panic symptoms, as well as relieve premenstrual dysmorphic discomfort.

Contraindications

Concurrent therapy with pimozide or thioridazine; hypersensitivity to fluoxetine, other selective serotonin reuptake inhibitors or their components; use within 14 days of MAO inhibitor therapy, including reversible MAOIs such as linezolid or intravenous methylene blue

Interactions

DRUGS

alprazolam, diazepam: Possibly prolonged half-life of these drugs
anticonvulsants: Increased anticonvulsant levels
aspirin, NSAIDs, warfarin: Increased anticoagulant activity and risk of bleeding
benzodiazepines, CNS depressants: Increased risk of potentiated action and development of adverse effects
CYP2D6-metabolized drugs, such as antiarrhythmics (especially flecainide, propafenone), selected antidepressants (tricyclics), antipsychotics (phenothiazines and most atypicals), thioridazine, and vinblastine: Increased plasma levels of these drugs and increased risk of serious adverse reactions
fentanyl, intravenous methylene blue, linezolid, serotonergics (such as amphetamines and other psychostimulants, antidepressants, and dopamine agonists), St. John's wort, tramadol, tricyclic antidepressants, triptans, tryptophan: Increased risk of serotonin syndrome
highly protein-bound drugs: Possibly increased risk of elevated plasma levels of drugs increasing risk of adverse effects
lithium: Decreased or increased lithium levels; potential for serotonergic effects
MAO inhibitors: Possibly severe and life-threatening adverse effects
olanzapine: Increased blood olanzapine levels with decreased clearance resulting in possible increased risk for adverse reactions
phenytoin: Increased blood phenytoin level and risk of toxicity
pimozide, thiordazine, or other drugs that may prolong QT interval: Increased blood levels of these drugs; possibly increased risk of prolonged QT interval

Adverse Reactions

CNS: Akathisia, anxiety, ataxia, balance disorder, chills, depersonalization, dream disturbances, drowsiness, emotional lability, euphoria, fatigue, fever, headache, hypertonia, hypomania, insomnia, mania, myoclonus, nervousness, **neuroleptic malignant syndrome**, paranoid reaction, restlessness, **seizures**, **serotonin syndrome**, somnolence, **suicidal ideation**, tremor, vertigo, weakness, yawning
CV: **Arrhythmias**, **hypotension**, palpitations, **prolonged QT interval**, **torsades de pointes**, **ventricular arrhythmias**
EENT: Abnormal vision, angle-closure glaucoma, dry mouth, mydriasis, pharyngitis, sinusitis, taste perversion, teeth grinding
ENDO: Galactorrhea, gynecomastia, **hypoglycemia**, syndrome of inappropriate antidiuretic hormone secretion (SIADH)
GI: Anorexia, diarrhea, dysphagia, gastritis, gastroenteritis, indigestion, **melena**, nausea, stomach ulcer
GU: Decreased or increased libido, dysuria, ejaculation disorders, gynecological bleeding, impotence, micturition disorder
HEME: **Altered platelet function**, **unusual bleeding**
MS: Arthralgia, myalgia
RESP: Dyspnea
SKIN: Alopecia, diaphoresis, ecchymosis, pruritus, rash, urticaria
Other: Flu-like symptoms, **hyponatremia**, weight loss

Nursing Considerations

- Use fluoxetine cautiously in patients with a history of seizures and in children, because of potential for adverse effects.
- Use fluoxetine cautiously in patients with congenital long QT syndrome, previous history of QT prolongation, or family

history of long QT syndrome or sudden cardiac death. In addition, use caution in presence of other conditions that increase risk of QT prolongation and ventricular arrhythmia, such as concurrent drug therapy with drugs known to prolong the QT interval, hypokalemia, hypomagnesemia, recent MI, significant arrhythmias, uncompensated heart failure and conditions that predispose patient to increased fluoxetine exposure, such as hepatic impairment or concurrent use of drugs known to increase blood fluoxetine levels such as CYP2D6 inhibitors, CYP2D6 poor metabolizer status, or use of other highly protein-bound drugs. Obtain an ECG recording, as ordered, before fluoxetine begins in these patients and periodically throughout therapy. Expect fluoxetine to be discontinued if the QT interval becomes prolonged or patient develops a ventricular arrhythmia.

WARNING **Avoid giving fluoxetine within 14 days of an MAO inhibitor or starting MAO inhibitor therapy within 5 weeks of discontinuing fluoxetine.**

- Know that patients with depression should be screened for bipolar disorder before fluoxetine therapy is started, because treating depression alone in these patients may precipitate a manic or mixed episode.
- Monitor patient for depression (especially children, adolescents, and young adults) and watch closely for suicidal tendencies, particularly when therapy starts and dosage changes, because depression may worsen temporarily during those times.
- Monitor patient closely for evidence of GI bleeding, especially if patient takes another drug known to increase the risk, such as aspirin, an NSAID, or warfarin.
- Monitor patient—especially an elderly patient—for hypoosmolarity of serum and urine and for hyponatremia (difficulty concentrating, headache, memory impairment, unsteadiness, weakness), which may indicate fluoxetine-induced SIADH.
- Expect to taper drug when being discontinued, as ordered, to minimize adverse reactions.

WARNING **Monitor patient for possible serotonin syndrome, characterized by agitation, chills, confusion, diaphoresis, diarrhea, fever, hyperactive reflexes, poor coordination, restlessness, shaking, talking or acting with uncontrolled excitement, tremor, and twitching, especially if patient is receiving another drug that raises serotonin level (such as amphetamine, dopamine agonist, MAO inhibitor, tryptophan, or other antidepressant or psychostimulant). In its most severe form, serotonin syndrome can resemble neuroleptic malignant syndrome, which includes autonomic instability, high fever, muscle rigidity, and possible fluctuations in vital signs and mental status.**

- Monitor patient with diabetes mellitus for altered blood glucose level because drug may cause hypoglycemia during therapy and hyperglycemia when it stops. Expect to adjust dosage of antidiabetic drug, as prescribed.
- Expect patient to be reevaluated periodically to determine continued need for therapy.

PATIENT TEACHING

WARNING **Tell patient that drug increases risk of serotonin syndrome, a rare but serious complication, especially when taken with certain other drugs. Teach patient to recognize its signs and symptoms, and advise her to notify prescriber immediately if they occur.**

- Urge family or caregiver to watch patient closely for suicidal tendencies, especially when therapy starts or dosage changes, and particularly if patient is a child, teenager, or young adult.
- Caution patient to avoid hazardous activities until CNS effects of drug are known.
- Caution against stopping fluoxetine abruptly because serious adverse effects may result.
- Instruct patient to notify prescriber of any persistent, severe, or unusual signs or symptoms while taking fluoxetine.
- Inform patient that drug may cause mild pupillary dilation, which may lead to an episode of acute-angle glaucoma. Encourage patient to have an eye exam prior to starting fluoxetine therapy to see if she is at risk.
- Advise patient to consult prescriber before taking OTC or prescription drugs, if hives or a rash develop.

- Urge women of childbearing age to notify prescriber if pregnancy is suspected or occurs, because fluoxetine therapy may increase risk of serious adverse effects in the newborn. Have patient discuss alternative treatment for depression during pregnancy, explaining that coming off an antidepressant during pregnancy may cause her depression to relapse. Also tell mothers that fluoxetine is excreted in breast milk, so breastfeeding is not recommended while taking drug.
- Inform patient that drug may take several weeks to achieve full effects.

fluphenazine decanoate

Modecate (CAN),
Modecate Concentrate (CAN)

fluphenazine hydrochloride

Class and Category

Pharmacologic class: Phenothiazine
Therapeutic class: Antipsychotic
Pregnancy category: Not classified

Indications and Dosages

➤ *To control psychotic disorders*

ELIXIR, ORAL SOLUTION, TABLETS (FLUPHENAZINE HYDROCHLORIDE)

Adults and adolescents. *Initial:* 2.5 to 10 mg/day in divided doses every 6 to 8 hr. *Maintenance:* 1 to 5 mg daily. *Maximum:* 20 mg/day.

I.M. INJECTION (FLUPHENAZINE HYDROCHLORIDE)

Adults. *Initial:* 1.25 mg, increased as clinical condition tolerates up to 10 mg daily in divided doses every 6 to 8 hr. *Maximum:* 10 mg daily.

DOSAGE ADJUSTMENT For elderly or debilitated patients, initial oral dosage reduced to 1 to 2.5 mg daily in divided doses every 6 to 8 hr.

I.M. OR SUBCUTANEOUS INJECTION (FLUPHENAZINE DECANOATE)

Adults. *Initial:* 12.5 to 25 mg given every couple of weeks or longer depending on patient's needs. For doses over 50 mg, next dose increased cautiously by 12.5 mg. *Maximum:* 100 mg/dose.

Route	Onset	Peak	Duration
P.O.	In 1 hr	Variable	6–8 hr
I.M.*	In 1 hr	Variable	6–8 hr
I.M., SubQ†	In 24–72 hr	Variable	1–6 wk‡

* For hydrochloride.
† For decanoate.
‡ For decanoate.

Mechanism of Action

May block postsynaptic dopamine receptor sites in the CNS. This action may depress areas of the brain that control activity and aggression, including the cerebral cortex, hypothalamus, and limbic system.

Incompatibilities

Don't mix fluphenazine hydrochloride oral solution with beverages that contain caffeine, such as coffee and cola; pectins, such as apple juice; or tannins, such as tea. They're physically incompatible.

Contraindications

Blood dyscrasias; bone marrow depression; coma; concomitant use of large amounts of another CNS depressant; hepatic dysfunction; hypersensitivity to fluphenazine, other phenothiazines, or their components; severe CNS depression; subcortical brain damage

Interactions

DRUGS

adsorbent antidiarrheals, aluminum- or magnesium-containing antacids: Possibly inhibited absorption of fluphenazine
anticholinergics: Possibly intensified adverse effects of both drugs
antihypertensives: Possibly severe hypotension
CNS depressants: Possibly prolonged and intensified CNS depression
guanethidine: Decreased hypotensive effect of guanethidine
lithium: Possibly neurotoxicity (disorientation, extrapyramidal reactions, unconsciousness)

meperidine: Excessive sedation and hypotension

ACTIVITIES
alcohol use: Possibly increased CNS depression and increased risk of heatstroke

Adverse Reactions

CNS: Ataxia, **cerebral edema**, dizziness, drowsiness, headache, insomnia, light-headedness, nervousness, **seizures**, slurred speech, syncope, worsening psychotic symptoms
CV: AV conduction disorders, **bradycardia**, **cardiac arrest**, hypercholesterolemia, hypertension, orthostatic hypotension, **QT-interval prolongation**, **shock**, **ST-segment depression**, tachycardia
EENT: Blurred vision, dry mouth, glaucoma, increased salivation, **laryngeal edema**, **laryngospasm**, miosis, mydriasis, nasal congestion, papillary hypertrophy of the tongue, parotid gland enlargement, photophobia, pigmentary retinopathy, ptosis
ENDO: Breast engorgement (females), galactorrhea, hyperglycemia, **hypoglycemia**, mastalgia, syndrome of inappropriate ADH secretion
GI: Anorexia, constipation, diarrhea, fecal impaction, ileus, increased appetite, jaundice, nausea, vomiting
GU: Amenorrhea, bladder paralysis, decreased libido, enuresis, menstrual irregularities, polyuria, urinary frequency, urinary incontinence, urine retention
HEME: Anemia, **aplastic anemia**, eosinophilia, **leukopenia**, **nonthrombocytopenic or thrombocytopenic purpura**, **thrombocytopenia**
RESP: Bronchospasm, dyspnea, increased respiratory depth
SKIN: Contact dermatitis, dry skin, eczema, erythema, photosensitivity, pruritus, seborrhea
Other: Heatstroke, **hyponatremia**, lupus-like symptoms, weight gain

Nursing Considerations

- Be aware that fluphenazine shouldn't be used to treat dementia-related psychosis in elderly patients because of an increased mortality risk.
- Use fluphenazine cautiously in patients with a history of glaucoma or renal impairment.
- For I.M. and subcutaneous injection, use at least a 21G needle.
- Monitor temperature; a significant, unexplained rise can indicate intolerance and a need to discontinue drug. Notify prescriber immediately if this occurs.
- Watch for signs of hepatic failure, such as jaundice.
- Notify prescriber about worsening psychotic symptoms: agitation, catatonic state, confusion, depression, hallucinations, lethargy, paranoid reactions.

PATIENT TEACHING

- Instruct patient prescribed elixir form of fluphenazine to keep it in an amber or opaque bottle because drug is sensitive to light.
- Advise patient not to mix oral solution with beverages that contain caffeine (coffee, cola), pectins (apple juice), or tannins (tea).
- Caution patient about possible dizziness or light-headedness.
- Teach patient how to prevent heatstroke, orthostatic hypotension, and photosensitivity reactions.
- Warn against stopping drug abruptly.

flurazepam hydrochloride

Class, Category, and Schedule

Pharmacologic class: Benzodiazepine
Therapeutic class: Sedative-hypnotic
Pregnancy category: Not classified
Controlled substance schedule: IV

Indications and Dosages

➤ *To treat insomnia characterized by difficulty falling asleep, frequent nocturnal awakenings, or early-morning awakening*

CAPSULES
Adult women. *Initial:* 15 mg at bedtime, increased to 30 mg at bedtime, as needed.
Adult men. *Initial:* 15 or 30 mg at bedtime.

DOSAGE ADJUSTMENT Initial dose reduced to 15 mg for elderly or debilitated men until individual response is known.

Route	Onset	Peak	Duration
P.O.	15–45 min	Unknown	7–8 hr

Mechanism of Action

May potentiate the effects of gamma-aminobutyric acid (GABA) and other inhibitory neurotransmitters by binding to specific benzodiazepine receptor sites in the cortical and limbic areas of the CNS. As a result, flurazepam increases GABA's inhibitory effects and blocks cortical and limbic arousal.

Contraindications

Hypersensitivity to flurazepam, other benzodiazepines, or their components

Interactions

DRUGS

CNS depressants: Possibly potentiated CNS depression

opioids: Increased risk of profound CNS and respiratory depression and sedation

ACTIVITIES

alcohol use: Possibly potentiated CNS and respiratory depression

Adverse Reactions

CNS: Amnesia, anxiety, ataxia, bizarre behavior (such as sleep driving), confusion, delusions, depression, dizziness, drowsiness, euphoria, headache, hypokinesia, irritability, malaise, nervousness, slurred speech, tremor
CV: Chest pain, palpitations, tachycardia
EENT: Blurred vision, dry mouth, increased salivation, photophobia
GI: Abdominal pain, constipation, diarrhea, nausea, thirst, vomiting
GU: Libido changes
SKIN: Diaphoresis
Other: Anaphylaxis, angioedema, physical or psychological dependence

Nursing Considerations

- Use flurazepam cautiously in patients with severe mental depression or reduced respiratory function; drug may intensify mental depression and lead to respiratory depression.
- Expect to use lowest effective dose in debilitated or elderly patients to minimize the risk of ataxia, confusion, dizziness, and oversedation.
- Monitor liver function test results, as appropriate.

PATIENT TEACHING

- Instruct patient not to exceed prescribed dosage and not to stop drug abruptly.

WARNING Warn patient that, although rare, drug may cause swelling of the oral cavity or throat, which could cause airway obstruction. If swelling occurs, patient should seek emergency care immediately and never take flurazepam again.

- Caution patient about possible morning dizziness or drowsiness.
- Advise patient to avoid hazardous activities until drug's CNS effects are known.
- Caution patient to avoid alcohol and CNS depressants during therapy.
- Advise patient to notify prescriber if she becomes or intends to become pregnant during therapy.
- Inform patient that sleep may be disturbed for the first few nights after stopping drug.
- Warn patient and caregiver that some patients have performed bizarre activities after taking drug, such as driving a car, eating food, having sex, or making phone calls while not fully awake and often with no memory of the event. These episodes usually occur in patients who have taken the drug with alcohol or other CNS depressant or who have exceeded the recommended dose. If such an episode occurs, the prescriber should be notified and flurazepam therapy discontinued immediately.

fluticasone propionate

Armonair Respiclick, Flonase, Flonase Allergy Relief, Flovent Diskus, Flovent HFA, Xhance

fluticasone furoate

Arnuity Ellipta, Flonase Sensimist, Veramyst

Class and Category

Pharmacologic class: Corticosteroid

Therapeutic class: Antiasthmatic, anti-inflammatory
Pregnancy category: Not classified

Indications and Dosages

➤ *To prevent asthma attacks, alone or with oral corticosteroids*

INHALATION AEROSOL (FLOVENT HFA)

Adults and children age 12 and over using bronchodilator therapy. *Initial:* 88 mcg inhaled twice daily. *Maximum:* 440 mcg inhaled twice daily.
Adults and children age 12 and over switching from another inhaled corticosteroid. *Initial:* 88 to 220 mcg inhaled twice daily. *Maximum:* 440 mcg inhaled twice daily.
Adults and children age 12 and over using oral corticosteroid therapy. *Initial:* 440 mcg inhaled twice daily. *Maximum:* 880 mcg inhaled twice daily.
Children ages 4 to 11 regardless of previous therapy. 88 mcg inhaled twice daily. *Maximum:* 88 mcg twice daily.

INHALATION AEROSOL (FLOVENT DISKUS)

Adults and children age 12 and over using bronchodilator therapy. *Initial:* 100 mcg inhaled twice daily. *Maximum:* 500 mcg inhaled twice daily.
Adults and children age 12 and over switching from another inhaled corticosteroid. *Initial:* 100 to 250 mcg inhaled twice daily. *Maximum:* 500 mcg inhaled twice daily.
Adults and children age 12 and over using oral corticosteroid therapy. *Initial:* 500 to 1,000 mcg inhaled twice daily. *Maximum:* 1,000 mcg inhaled twice daily.
Children ages 4 to 11 regardless of previous therapy. *Initial:* 50 mcg inhaled twice daily. *Maximum:* 100 mcg inhaled twice daily.

INHALATION AEROSOL (ARMONAIR RESPICLICK)

Adults not on inhaled corticosteroids. 55 mcg inhaled twice daily.
Adults switching from another inhaled corticosteroid. Individualized based upon strength of previous inhaled corticosteroid and disease severity. Dosage may be low at 55 mcg inhaled twice daily, medium at 113 mcg inhaled twice daily, or high at 232 mcg inhaled twice daily, with dosage increase for lower dosages after 2 wk, if needed. *Maximum:* 232 mg inhaled twice daily.

INHALATION AEROSOL (ARNUITY ELLIPTA)

Adults and children age 12 and older not on inhaled corticosteroid therapy. 100 mcg inhaled once daily, increased after 2 wk to 200 mcg once daily, as needed.
Adults and children age 12 and older receiving other drug treatments for asthma. Highly individualized based on patient's previous asthma drug therapy and disease severity.
Children age 5 to 12. 50 mcg inhaled once daily.

➤ *To treat seasonal or perennial allergic rhinitis*

NASAL SUSPENSION (FLONASE, FLONASE ALLERGY RELIEF)

Adults. *Initial:* 50 or 100 mcg (1 to 2 sprays) in each nostril once daily. *Maximum:* 100 mcg (2 sprays) in each nostril daily.
Children ages 4 and over. 50 mcg (1 spray) in each nostril daily, increased, as needed, to 100 mcg (2 sprays) in each nostril daily. *Maximum:* 100 mcg (2 sprays) in each nostril daily.

NASAL SUSPENSION (VERAMYST)

Adults and children age 12 and over. *Initial:* 55 mcg (2 sprays) in each nostril once daily. *Maintenance:* 27.5 mcg (1 spray) in each nostril once daily.
Children ages 2 to 11. *Initial:* 27.5 mcg (1 spray) in each nostril once daily, increased to 55 mcg (2 sprays) in each nostril once daily, as needed. *Maintenance:* 27.5 mcg (1 spray) in each nostril once daily.

NASAL SUSPENSION (FLONASE SENSIMIST)

Adults and children ages 12 and over. *Initial:* 55 mcg (2 sprays) in each nostril once daily for 1 wk. Beginning wk 2 through 6 mo, 27.5 or 55 mcg (1 to 2 sprays) in each nostril once daily.
Children ages 2 to 11. 27.5 mcg (1 spray) in each nostril daily.

➤ *To treat nasal polyps*

NASAL SPRAY (XHANCE)

Adults. 1 spray (93 mcg) in each nostril twice daily, increased to 2 sprays (186 mcg) in each nostril twice daily, if needed. *Maximum:* 2 sprays (186 mcg) in each nostril twice daily for total daily dose of 744 mcg.

Route	Onset	Peak	Duration
Inhalation	In 24 hr	1–2 wk	Several days
Nasal	12 hr–3 days	4–7 days	1–2 wk

Mechanism of Action

Inhibits cells involved in the inflammatory response of asthma, such as basophils, eosinophils, lymphocytes, macrophages, mast cells, and neutrophils. Fluticasone also inhibits production or secretion of chemical mediators, such as cytokines eicosanoids, histamine, and leukotrienes.

Contraindications

Hypersensitivity to fluticasone or its components, or to milk proteins; primary treatment of status asthmaticus or other acute asthma episodes that require intensive measures; untreated nasal mucosal infection (nasal suspension)

Interactions

DRUGS

strong CYP3A4 inhibitors such as atazanavir, clarithromycin, indinavir, itraconazole, ketoconazole, nefazodone, nelfinavir, ritonavir, saquinavir, telithromycin: Possibly increased fluticasone level with increased risk of corticosteroid adverse effects

Adverse Reactions

CNS: Aggressiveness, agitation, anxiety, depression, difficulty speaking, dizziness, fatigue, fever, headache, insomnia, irritability, malaise, restlessness
EENT: Allergic rhinitis, blurred vision, cataracts, central serous chorioretinopathy, conjunctivitis, dental caries, difficulty speaking, dry mouth and throat, epistaxis, esophageal candidiasis, eye irritation, facial and **oropharyngeal edema**, glaucoma, hoarseness, impaired nasal wound healing, laryngitis, loss of voice, nasal *Candida* infection, nasal congestion or discharge, nasal discomfort (burning, dryness, irritation, soreness), nasal sinus pain, nasal septal perforation or ulceration, nasopharyngitis, oropharyngeal candidiasis, otitis media, pharyngitis, rhinitis, sinusitis, throat irritation, tonsillitis, tooth discoloration
ENDO: Adrenal insufficiency, cushingoid symptoms, hyperglycemia, slower growth in children
GI: Abdominal pain, diarrhea, indigestion, nausea, vomiting
GU: Dysmenorrhea
HEME: Churg–Strauss syndrome, easy bruising, eosinophilia
MS: Arthralgia, back pain, bone mineral density reduction (long-term use), myalgia, osteoporosis
RESP: Asthma exacerbation, bronchitis, **bronchospasm**, chest congestion and tightness, cough, dyspnea, pneumonia, upper respiratory tract infection, wheezing
SKIN: Dermatitis, ecchymosis, pruritus, rash, urticaria
Other: Anaphylaxis, angioedema, flu-like symptoms, weight gain

Nursing Considerations

- Use fluticasone cautiously in patients with ocular herpes simplex, pulmonary tuberculosis, or untreated systemic bacterial, fungal, parasitic, or viral infection. Also, use cautiously in patients with moderate or severe hepatic impairment.
- Monitor patient closely at start of therapy, especially if patient has severe allergy to milk. If hypersensitivity reaction occurs, notify prescriber, expect drug to be discontinued, and provide supportive care, as prescribed.
- Know that if patient takes a systemic corticosteroid, expect to taper dosage by no more than 2.5 mg daily at weekly intervals, starting 1 week after fluticasone therapy begins.

WARNING Be aware that if patient is switched from systemic corticosteroid to fluticasone, assess for adrenal insufficiency (fatigue, hypotension, lassitude, nausea, vomiting, weakness) early in therapy and when patient has infection, stress, surgery, trauma, or other electrolyte-depleting conditions or procedures. Notify prescriber immediately if signs or symptoms develop.

- Administer a fast-acting inhaled bronchodilator, as ordered, if bronchospasm occurs immediately after fluticasone use. Expect to stop fluticasone and start another drug therapy.
- Expect to titrate fluticasone to lowest effective dosage after asthma has stabilized.

PATIENT TEACHING

- Urge patient to use fluticasone regularly, as prescribed, and stress that drug is not for acute bronchospasm. Instruct her to have a rescue inhaler accessible if acute bronchospasm occurs.
- Teach patient how to administer drug according to the form prescribed (nasal spray or oral inhaler).
- Inform patient that Armonair Respiclick brand of fluticasone does not require priming and should not be used with a spacer or volume holding chamber. Instruct patient to shake canister for other forms of inhaled fluticasone products and use inhaler according to package instructions. On first use, advise her to spray 4 times into the air (away from her eyes and shaking inhaler between each test spray) looking for a fine mist. If inhaler hasn't been used for more than 7 days or it's dropped, it will need to be primed again by shaking well and then releasing 1 test spray into the air (away from her face).
- Tell patient prescribed 2 inhalations to wait at least 1 minute between them.
- Instruct patient to gargle and rinse her mouth after each dose of an oral inhaler to help prevent dry mouth and throat and oropharyngeal yeast infection and relieve throat irritation.
- Instruct patient prescribed more than 1 inhaler to use fluticasone last, at least 5 minutes after previous inhaler.
- Instruct patient to clean inhaler according to manufacturer guidelines at least once a week after her evening dose. Alert patient prescribed Armonair Respiclick brand never to wash or put any part of the inhaler in water, as routine mainenance is not required. Tell patient that if the mouthpiece needs cleaning, gently wipe the mouthpiece with a dry cloth or tissue.
- Inform patient that, when counter reads 020 on the inhaler, she should obtain a refill, if needed. When counter reaches 000, she should discard the inhaler.
- Instruct patient using nasal spray to shake container well before each use. If patient is using Xhance form of nasal spray, tell her to prime the container before initial use by first gently shaking and then pressing the bottle 7 times or until a fine mist appears. Tell patient if the container is not used for 7 days or more, the container will have to be reprimed by shaking and releasing 2 sprays into the air, away from the face.
- Explain that symptoms may improve within 2 days but that full improvement may not occur for 1 to 2 weeks or longer.
- Caution patient not to increase dosage but to contact prescriber after 1 week if symptoms continue or worsen.
- Urge patient to tell prescriber immediately if asthma attacks don't respond to bronchodilators during fluticasone therapy.
- Know that if patient is switching from an oral corticosteroid to fluticasone, urge her to carry medical identification indicating the need for supplemental systemic corticosteroids during stress or severe asthma attack.
- Caution patient to avoid people who have infections because fluticasone suppresses the immune system, increasing the risk of infection. Instruct patient to notify prescriber about exposure to chickenpox, measles, or other infections because additional treatment may be needed.

fluvastatin sodium

Lescol, Lescol XL

Class and Category

Pharmacologic class: HMG-CoA reductase inhibitor
Therapeutic class: Antilipemic
Pregnancy category: X

Indications and Dosages

➤ *As adjunct to lower cholesterol level in primary hypercholesterolemia and mixed dyslipidemia (Fredrickson Type IIa and II b) in patients whose response to dietary restriction and other nonpharmacologic measures has been inadequate; to decrease progression of coronary atherosclerosis; to reduce risk in patients with coronary artery disease undergoing coronary revascularization*

CAPSULES

Adults. 20 to 40 mg daily in the evening, increased up to 40 mg twice daily, as needed. *Maximum:* 40 mg twice daily.

E.R. TABLETS
Adults. 80 mg in the evening. *Maximum:* 80 mg daily.

➤ *As adjunct to lower cholesterol level in children with heterozygous familial hypercholesterolemia whose LDL-C remains 190 ml/dl or greater or whose LDL-C remains 160 mg/dl or greater combined with a positive family history of premature cardiovascular disease or two or more other cardiovascular disease risk factors are present*

CAPSULES
Boys and girls (who are at least 1 year past menarche) ages 10 to 16. *Initial:* 20 mg once daily, increased every 6 wk, as needed. *Maximum:* 40 mg twice daily.

DOSAGE ADJUSTMENT For pediatric patients, if maximum dose of 40 mg twice daily is reached with immediate-release capsules, child may be switched to extended-release tablets, 80 mg once daily. For patients taking cyclosporine or fluconazole, dosage not to exceed 20 mg twice daily.

Route	Onset	Peak	Duration
P.O.	In 1–2 wk	In 4–6 wk	Unknown
P.O. (E.R.)	In 2 wk	In 4 wk	Unknown

Mechanism of Action

Interferes with the hepatic enzyme hydroxymethylglutaryl-coenzyme A reductase, reducing formation of mevalonic acid (a cholesterol precursor) and interrupting the pathway by which cholesterol is synthesized. When cholesterol level declines in hepatic cells, LDLs are consumed, which reduces circulating total cholesterol and serum triglycerides.

Contraindications

Acute hepatic disease, breastfeeding, hypersensitivity to fluvastatin or its components, pregnancy, unexplained persistently elevated liver enzyme levels

Interactions

DRUGS
colchicine, cyclosporine, erythromycin, gemfibrozil, niacin, other fibrates: Increased risk of severe myopathy and rhabdomyolysis
cyclosporine, fluconazole: Increased fluconazole level
glyburide: Increased glyburide level
phenytoin: Increased phenytoin levels
protease inhibitors: Possible increased blood fluvastatin level; possible increased risk of myopathy and rhabdomyolysis
rifampin: Significantly decreased blood fluvastatin level, increased plasma clearance
warfarin: Possibly increased bleeding and/or increased prothrombin times

ACTIVITIES
alcohol use: Increased risk of liver dysfunction

Adverse Reactions

CNS: Dizziness, fatigue, headache, hypoesthesia, insomnia, memory loss, weakness
EENT: Pharyngitis, rhinitis, sinusitis
ENDO: Adrenal insufficiency, decreased gonadal steroid hormone production, elevated hemoglobin A1c levels, hyperglycemia
GI: Abdominal cramps and pain, anorexia, **cirrhosis**, constipation, diarrhea, elevated liver enzymes, flatulence, **fulminant hepatic necrosis**, **hepatic failure**, **hepatitis**, **hepatoma**, hyperbilirubinemia, indigestion, jaundice, nausea, **pancreatitis**, vomiting
GU: UTI
MS: Arthritis, back pain, immune-mediated necrotizing myopathy, muscle pain, myalgia, myopathy, myositis, **rhabdomyolysis**
RESP: Bronchitis, cough, **interstitial lung disease**, upper respiratory tract infection
SKIN: Pruritus, rash

Nursing Considerations

WARNING Expect to stop drug if CK level rises sharply or myopathy is suspected.

- Expect liver enzymes to be checked before fluvastatin therapy starts and then thereafter as clinically necessary.
- Assess patient for signs and symptoms of hepatic dysfunction such as dark urine or jaundice, fatigue, and/or elevation in liver enzymes to more than 3 times the upper limit of normal. Also look for hyperbilirubinemia. If present, notify prescriber and expect fluvastatin to be discontinued until cause of liver dysfunction has been identified. If no

EF

cause can be found, expect the drug to be discontinued permanently.

- Monitor patient for hyperglycemia, especially diabetic patients, and for other endocrine signs and symptoms. Notify prescriber, if present.

PATIENT TEACHING

- Urge patient to comply with monthly laboratory tests early in treatment.
- Tell patient to follow prescribed low-fat diet.
- Encourage patient to notify prescriber promptly about muscle pain or unexplained weakness.
- Instruct patient with diabetes to monitor his blood glucose level more closely.

fluvoxamine maleate

Luvox, Luvox CR

Class and Category

Pharmacologic class: Selective serotonin reuptake inhibitor (SSRI)
Therapeutic class: Antidepressant
Pregnancy category: C

Indications and Dosages

➤ *To treat obsessive–compulsive disorder*

TABLETS

Adults. *Initial:* 50 mg at bedtime, increased by 50 mg every 4 to 7 days, as needed. *Maximum:* 300 mg daily, with doses greater than 100 mg daily given as 2 divided doses and if doses are not equal, larger dose given at bedtime.

Children ages 8 to 17. *Initial:* 25 mg at bedtime, increased by 25 mg every 4 to 7 days, as needed. *Maximum:* 200 mg daily (children ages 8 to 11) and 300 mg daily (children ages 11 to 17), with doses greater than 50 mg daily divided into 2 doses, and if not divided equally, larger dose given at bedtime.

E.R. CAPSULES

Adults. *Initial:* 100 mg at bedtime, increased by 50 mg weekly, if needed. *Maximum:* 300 mg daily.

DOSAGE ADJUSTMENT For elderly patients or those with hepatic impairment, initial dosage decreased for immediate-release form and dosage increases made more slowly for both immediate-release and extended-release forms.

Route	Onset	Peak	Duration
P.O.	3–10 wk	Unknown	Unknown

Mechanism of Action

May potentiate serotonin's action by blocking its reuptake at neuronal membranes. An elevated serotonin level may elevate mood and decrease depression and anxiety, which often accompany obsessive–compulsive disorder.

Contraindications

Alosetron, pimozide, terfenadine, thioridazine, or tizanidine therapy; hypersensitivity to fluvoxamine maleate or its components; use within 14 days of MAO inhibitor, including intravenous methylene blue and linezolid

Interactions

DRUGS

alosetron: Increased plasma alosetron level
amphetamines, busipirone, fentanyl, linezolid, lithium, methylene blue (intravenous), St. John's wort, tramadol, tricyclic antidepressants, triptans, tryptophan: Increased risk of serotonin syndrome
aspirin, NSAIDs, warfarin: Risk of bleeding
astemizole, cisapride, pimozide, terfenadine, thioridazine: Possibly fatal QT prolongation
benzodiazepines such as alprazolam, diazepam, midazolam, triazolam: Decreased benzodiazepine clearance, with increased plasma levels and increased risk of adverse reactions
carbamazepine: Increased risk of carbamazepine toxicity
clozapine: Increased blood clozapine level increasing risk of orthostatic hypotension and seizures
diltiazem: Increased risk of bradycardia
lithium: Possibly increased serotonin reuptake action of fluvoxamine and increased risk of seizures
MAO inhibitors: Possibly serious or fatal reactions (such as agitation, autonomic instability, coma, delirium, fluctuating vital signs, hyperthermia, myoclonus, and rigidity)
methadone: Possibly significantly increased blood methadone level, increased risk of methadone toxicity

metoprolol, propranolol, and other beta blockers: Increased blood levels of these drugs, possibly reduced diastolic blood pressure and heart rate induced by these drugs
mexiletine: Possibly decreased clearance of mexiletine
ramelteon: Increased plasma levels of ramelteon
sympathomimetics: Possibly increased effects of sympathomimetics and increased risk of serotonin syndrome
tacrine: Increased blood level and therapeutic and adverse effects of tacrine
theophylline: Decreased theophylline clearance, increased risk of theophylline toxicity
tizanidine: Increased risk of serious adverse effects, such as hypotension and profound sedation

ACTIVITIES

smoking: Increased fluvoxamine metabolism

Adverse Reactions

CNS: Agitation, anxiety, apathy, chills, confusion, depression, dizziness, drowsiness, fatigue, headache, hypomania, insomnia, malaise, mania, nervousness, **neuroleptic malignant syndrome**, sedation, **serotonin syndrome**, **suicidal ideation**, tremor, vertigo, yawning
CV: Palpitations, tachycardia
EENT: Acute-angle glaucoma, altered taste, blurred vision, dry mouth
GI: Anorexia, constipation, diarrhea, flatulence, indigestion, nausea, **upper GI bleeding**, vomiting
GU: Decreased libido, ejaculation disorders, impotence, urinary frequency, urine retention
HEME: **Bleeding events**
MS: Muscle twitching
RESP: Dyspnea, upper respiratory tract infection
SKIN: Diaphoresis, rash
Other: Flu-like symptoms, weight gain

Nursing Considerations

- Use fluvoxamine cautiously in patients with cardiovascular disease, impaired hepatic or renal function, mania, seizures, or suicidal tendencies.

WARNING Be aware that fluvoxamine shouldn't be given within 14 days of an MAO inhibitor.

WARNING Monitor patient for possible serotonin syndrome, characterized by agitation, chills, confusion, diaphoresis, diarrhea, fever, hyperactive reflexes, poor coordination, restlessness, shaking, talking or acting with uncontrolled excitement, tremor, and twitching, especially if patient is receiving another drug that raises serotonin level (such as amphetamine, dopamine agonist, MAO inhibitor, tryptophan, or other antidepressant or psychostimulant). In its most severe form, serotonin syndrome can resemble neuroleptic malignant syndrome, which includes autonomic instability, a high fever, muscle rigidity, and possible fluctuations in vital signs and mental status.

- Watch patient closely (especially children, adolescents, and young adults), for suicidal tendencies, particularly when therapy starts and dosage changes, because depression may worsen temporarily during these times and lead to suicidal ideation.
- Monitor patient for bleeding, especially if patient also takes aspirin, an anticoagulant, or NSAID. Bleeding can range from ecchymoses, epistaxis, hematomas, and petechiae to life-threatening hemorrhage.
- Discontinue fluvoxamine therapy gradually, as ordered, to prevent unpleasant adverse reactions.

PATIENT TEACHING

- Caution patient not to drink alcohol during fluvoxamine therapy.
- Urge patient to avoid potentially hazardous activities until drug's CNS effects are known.

WARNING Inform patient that fluvoxamine increases the risk of a rare but serious problem: serotonin syndrome. Encourage her to notify prescriber immediately if symptoms develop.

- Caution patient not to stop taking drug abruptly. Explain that gradual tapering helps avoid withdrawal symptoms.
- Urge family or caregiver to watch patient closely for suicidal tendencies, especially when therapy starts or dosage changes and particularly if patient is a child, teenager, or young adult.
- Warn patient that fluvoxamine increases bleeding risk if taken with an

anticoagulant, aspirin, or an NSAID and that bleeding events could range from mild to severe. Tell patient to seek emergency care for serious or prolonged bleeding.

- Advise patient that drug may cause mild pupillary dilation, which may lead to an episode of acute-angle glaucoma. Encourage patient to have an eye exam before starting therapy to see if she is at risk.

WARNING Advise pregnant patient to consult with prescriber before her third trimester about ongoing fluvoxamine therapy because of an increased risk to her unborn child during the third trimester.

fondaparinux sodium

Arixtra

Class and Category

Pharmacologic class: Activated factor X inhibitor
Therapeutic class: Anticoagulant
Pregnancy category: B

Indications and Dosages

➤ *To provide prophylaxis against deep vein thrombosis, which may lead to pulmonary embolism in patients undergoing abdominal surgery, hip fracture surgery, hip replacement surgery, or knee replacement surgery in patients at risk for thromboembolic complications*

SUBCUTANEOUS INJECTION

Adults. *Initial:* After hemostasis has been established, 2.5 mg subcutaneously 6 to 8 hr after surgery, followed by 2.5 mg subcutaneously daily for 5 to 9 days. *Maximum:* 2.5 mg subcutaneously daily up to 10 days for abdominal surgery, up to 11 days for hip or knee replacement, and up to 24 days for hip fracture surgery.

➤ *To treat acute deep vein thrombosis (with warfarin); to treat acute pulmonary embolism (with warfarin) in a hospital setting*

SUBCUTANEOUS INJECTION

Adults weighing more than 100 kg (220 lb). 10 mg daily for at least 5 days and until INR is between 2.0 and 3.0 (usually in 5 to 9 days).
Adults weighing 50 kg (110 lb) to 100 kg (220 lb). 7.5 mg daily for at least 5 days and until INR is between 2.0 and 3.0 (usually in 5 to 9 days).
Adults weighing less than 50 kg (110 lb). 5 mg daily for at least 5 days and until INR is between 2.0 and 3.0 (usually in 5 to 9 days).

Mechanism of Action

Selectively binds to antithrombin III, which enhances the inactivation of clotting factor Xa by antithrombin III. Inactivation of factor Xa interrupts the blood coagulation pathway, which then inhibits thrombin formation. Without thrombin, fibrinogen can't convert to fibrin and clots can't form.

Incompatibilities

Don't mix fondaparinux sodium with other infusions or injections.

Contraindications

Active major bleeding; bacterial endocarditis; fondaparinux-induced thrombocytopenia associated with a positive in vitro test for antiplatelet antibodies; hypersensitivity to fondaparinux or its components; prophylactic fondaparinux therapy in patients weighing less than 50 kg (110 lb) undergoing abdominal surgery, hip repair or replacement, or knee replacement; severe renal impairment (creatinine clearance less than 30 ml/min)

Interactions

DRUGS

abciximab, thrombolytics, other drugs that increase risk of bleeding: Increased risk of hemorrhage and epidural or spinal hematoma

Adverse Reactions

CNS: Confusion, dizziness, fever, headache, insomnia
CV: Edema, elevated serum aminotransferase level, **hypotension**
GI: Constipation, diarrhea, elevated liver enzymes, indigestion, nausea, vomiting
GU: Urine retention, UTI
HEME: Anemia, **bleeding**, **elevated APTT**, hematoma, **hemorrhage**, **thrombocytopenia**, **thrombocytopenia with thrombosis**

SKIN: Bullous eruption, increased wound drainage, purpura, rash
Other: Anaphylaxis; **angioedema**; generalized pain; **hypokalemia**; injection-site bleeding, pruritus, and rash

Nursing Considerations

- Use fondaparinux cautiously in elderly patients, especially those weighing less than 50 kg (110 lb) and are receiving the drug for pulmonary embolism or deep vein thrombosis, because the risk of drug-induced bleeding increases with age.
- Don't give initial dose of fondaparinux less than 6 hours after surgery.
- Inspect fondaparinux for discoloration or particles before administration. Be aware that needle guard on prefilled syringe contains dry natural latex rubber and shouldn't be handled by those sensitive to latex.
- Alternate injection sites using left and right anterolateral or left and right posterolateral abdominal wall. Don't expel air bubble from prefilled syringe before injection to prevent expelling drug from syringe. Don't give drug by I.M. injection.

WARNING Know that if patient is receiving fondaparinux with epidural or spinal anesthesia or spinal puncture, patient must be watched closely for development of spinal hematoma, which may cause long-term or permanent paralysis. If evidence of neurologic impairment, such as changes in motor or sensory function occurs, notify prescriber immediately because urgent care is needed to minimize hematoma's effect. Risk of spinal or epidural hematoma during fondaparinux therapy is increased by concurrent use of other drugs that affect hemostasis, a history of traumatic or repeated epidural or spinal punctures, or a history of spinal deformity or spinal surgery as well as indwelling epidural catheters. Be aware that optimal timing between the administration of fondaparinux and neuraxial procedures is unknown.

- Closely monitor patient for bleeding (such as ecchymosis, epistaxis, hematemesis, hematuria, and melena), especially those at risk for decreased drug elimination (such as elderly patients and patients with mild to moderate renal impairment) and those at increased risk for bleeding (such as patients with acquired or congenital bleeding disorders; active ulcerative and angiodysplastic GI disease; diabetic retinopathy; hemorrhagic stroke; uncontrolled arterial hypertension; recent brain, spinal, or ophthalmologic surgery; history of heparin-induced thrombocytopenia; and those being treated concomitantly with platelet inhibitors). Also monitor neonates born to mothers taking fondaparinux for bleeding, because drug does cross the placenta.
- Perform periodic CBC, including platelet count, as ordered. Expect prescriber to discontinue drug if platelet count falls below 100,000/mm^3. Be aware that routine coagulation tests, such as INR and PT, are not used to monitor fondaparinux therapy; an anti-Xa assay may be used instead. Also, test stools for occult blood, as ordered.
- Monitor patient with thrombocytopenia for evidence of thrombosis that may appear similar to heparin-induced thrombocytopenia even when no exposure to heparin has taken place. If patient's platelet count falls below 100,000/mm^3, fondaparinux should be discontinued.
- Monitor renal function test results, as ordered. Expect to discontinue drug if labile renal function or severe renal impairment occurs during fondaparinux therapy because the risk of hemorrhage increases as renal function decreases.
- Store drug at a controlled room temperature.

PATIENT TEACHING

- Inform patient that fondaparinux can't be taken orally.
- Instruct patient to seek immediate help if she experiences signs of thromboembolism, such as neurologic changes and severe shortness of breath.
- Inform patient about the increased risk of bleeding. Instruct her or family member to watch for and report abdominal or lower back pain, black stools, bleeding gums, bloody urine, or severe headaches.

- Teach patient or family member how to administer fondaparinux by subcutaneous injection at home, if needed. Instruct her not to expel air bubble from a prefilled syringe to avoid expelling some of the drug. Tell her to insert the entire needle into a skinfold held between thumb and forefinger, and remind her to alternate administration sites.
- Caution patient to minimize bruising, by not rubbing the injection site after giving the drug.
- Review safe handling and disposal of syringes and needles.
- Advise patient to have follow-up appointments and prescribed laboratory tests.
- Tell patient that fondaparinux may cause serious side effects and to report any persistent, severe, or unusual signs and symptoms to prescriber.

WARNING Know that if patient is receiving fondaparinux with epidural or spinal anesthesia or spinal puncture, patient must be watched closely for development of spinal hematoma, which may cause long-term or permanent paralysis. If evidence of neurologic impairment, such as changes in sensory or motor function, occurs, notify prescriber immediately, because urgent care is needed to minimize hematoma's effect. Risk of epidural or spinal hematoma during fondaparinux therapy is increased by concurrent use of other drugs that affect hemostasis, a history of traumatic or repeated epidural or spinal punctures, or a history of spinal deformity or spinal surgery. The risk is also increased with indwelling epidural catheters.

- Advise patient to alert prescriber about any new drugs being taken, including over-the-counter drugs and especially drugs that affect clotting such as aspirin or NSAIDs.

formoterol fumarate

Oxeze Turbuhaler (CAN), Perforomist

Class and Category

Pharmacologic class: Selective $beta_2$-adrenergic agonist
Therapeutic class: Bronchodilator
Pregnancy category: Not classified

Indications and Dosages

➤ *As adjunct to inhaled corticosteroid therapy to prevent asthma-induced bronchospasm*

POWDER FOR ORAL INHALATION (OXEZE TURBUHALER)

Adults and children age 6 and over. 6 or 12 mcg every 12 hr through inhaler device. *Maximum:* 24 mcg daily (children) and 48 mcg daily (adults).

➤ *To prevent exercise-induced bronchospasm*

POWDER FOR ORAL INHALATION (OXEZE TURBUHALER)

Adults and children age 6 and over. 6 or 12 mcg at least 15 min before exercise every 12 hr as needed. *Maximum:* 24 mcg daily (children) and 48 mcg daily (adults).

➤ *To provide long-term treatment of bronchospasm in patients with chronic bronchitis and emphysema*

POWDER FOR ORAL INHALATION (OXEZE TURBUHALER)

Adults. 12 mcg every 12 hr through inhaler device. *Maximum:* 24 mcg daily.

SOLUTION FOR ORAL INHALATION (PERFOROMIST)

Adults. 20 mcg twice daily by nebulization. *Maximum:* 40 mcg daily.

Route	Onset	Peak	Duration
Oral inhalation	1–3 min	Unknown	12 hr

Mechanism of Action

Selectively attaches to $beta_2$ receptors on bronchial membranes, stimulating the intracellular enzyme adenyl cyclase to convert adenosine triphosphate to cAMP. The resulting increase in the intracellular cAMP level inhibits histamine release, relaxes bronchial smooth-muscle cells, and stabilizes mast cells.

Contraindications

Acute asthma, hypersensitivity to formoterol fumarate or its components, treatment of asthma without use of a long-term asthma control medication

Interactions

DRUGS

adrenergics: Possibly increased sympathetic effects of formoterol

beta blockers: Decreased effects of both beta blockers and formoterol
corticosteroids, non-potassium-sparing diuretics, xanthine derivatives: Possibly increased hypokalemic effect of formoterol
disopyramide, macrolides, MAO inhibitors, phenothiazines, procainamide, quinidine, tricyclic antidepressants: Possibly prolonged QT interval, increasing risk of ventricular arrhythmias

Adverse Reactions

CNS: Anxiety, dizziness, fatigue, fever, headache, insomnia, malaise, tremor
CV: Angina, **arrhythmias**, chest pain, hypertension, **hypotension**, palpitations, **prolonged QT interval**, tachycardia
EENT: Dry mouth, laryngeal irritation, **laryngeal spasm or swelling**, hoarseness, pharyngitis, rhinitis and tonsillitis (in children), sinusitis
ENDO: Hyperglycemia
GI: Abdominal pain, gastroenteritis, indigestion (in children); nausea
MS: Back pain, leg cramps, muscle spasms
RESP: Asthma exacerbation, bronchitis, **bronchospasm**, cough, dyspnea, increased sputum production, upper respiratory tract infection
SKIN: Dermatitis, pruritus, rash, urticaria
Other: Anaphylaxis, angioedema, hypokalemia, metabolic acidosis

Nursing Considerations

- Know that formoterol therapy should not be used in patients whose asthma is adequately controlled with low- or medium-dose inhaled corticosteroids. Formoterol should only be used as additional therapy for patients with asthma who are currently taking but are not adequately controlled on long-term asthma control medication, such as an inhaled corticosteroids. Once asthma is controlled and maintained, expect formoterol to be discontinued as soon as possible as long as there is no loss of asthma control.
- Use caution when administering formoterol to patients with cardiovascular disorders such as aneurysm, arrhythmias, coronary insufficiency, hypertension, or pheochromocytoma; in patients with seizure disorders or thyrotoxicosis; and in patients who are unusually responsive to sympathomimetic amines.
- Know that formoterol may interfere with uterine contractility and should be used during labor only when the benefit clearly outweighs the risk.
- Administer formoterol dry powder or solution only by oral inhalation.
- Store drug in its original packaging, and open immediately before use.
- Give inhalation solution only by standard jet nebulizer and air compressor.

WARNING Monitor patient for worsening or deteriorating asthma because asthma-related deaths have increased in patients receiving salmeterol, a drug in the same class as formoterol. Monitor patient closely, and notify prescriber immediately of any changes in patient's respiratory status.

- Watch closely for paradoxical bronchospasm; if this occurs, discontinue formoterol immediately and notify prescriber.
- Notify prescriber of any significant increases in pulse rate or blood pressure or worsening of chronic conditions because formoterol may produce cardiovascular reactions, including angina, arrhythmias, hypertension or hypotension, palpitations, and tachycardia. Drug may have to be discontinued if such reactions occur.

PATIENT TEACHING

- Advise patient, especially if she has a significant cardiac history, to inform prescriber of any other drugs she takes before beginning formoterol therapy to prevent harmful drug interactions.
- Instruct patient to use manufacturer's device for inhaling powder form of formoterol and not to use a spacer.
- Teach patient proper use of powdered formoterol delivery system. Emphasize that she should only inhale, not exhale, through device.
- For solution form, teach patient how to use, clean, and store nebulizer equipment. Tell her to leave the vial in its original foil pack until just before use.
- Instruct patient who currently uses inhaled or oral corticosteroids to continue using them, as prescribed, even if she feels better after starting formoterol.
- Caution patient not to increase formoterol dosage or frequency without consulting prescriber because she may need a rapid-acting bronchodilator.

- Urge patient to notify prescriber if her symptoms worsen, if formoterol becomes less effective, or if she needs more inhalations of short-acting beta$_2$-agonist than usual. This may indicate that her asthma is worsening.
- Instruct patient to notify prescriber immediately if she experiences chest pain, nervousness, palpitations, rapid heart rate, or tremor while taking formoterol because dosage may have to be adjusted. Also, alert patient to stop drug and seek immediate emergency care if allergic reaction occurs, such as the presence of difficulty breathing or swallowing, hives, itching, rash, or swelling.
- Ensure that patient has been informed that long-acting beta agonists, such as formoterol, increase the risk of asthma-related death and should not be used without a long-term asthma control drug prior to starting formoterol therapy.

foscarnet sodium

Foscavir

Class and Category

Pharmacologic class: Pyrophosphate analogue
Therapeutic class: Antiviral
Pregnancy category: Not classified

Indications and Dosages

➤ *To treat cytomegalovirus (CMV) retinitis in patients with acquired immunodeficiency syndrome (AIDS)*

I.V. INFUSION

Adults. *Initial:* 90 mg/kg given over 1.5 to 2 hr (not to exceed 1 mg/kg/min) every 12 hr or 60 mg/kg given over a minimum of 1 hr (not to exceed 1 mg/kg/min) every 8 hr for 2 to 3 wks, depending on clinical response. *Maintenance:* 90 mg/kg/day or 120 mg/kg/day given over 2 hr (not to exceed 1 mg/kg/min).

➤ *To treat acyclovir-resistant mucocutaneous herpes simplex virus (HSV) infections in immunocompromised patients*

I.V. INFUSION

Adults. 40 mg/kg given over a minimum of 1 hr (not to exceed 1 mg/kg/min) either every 8 or 12 hr for 2 to 3 wk or until healing has taken place.

DOSAGE ADJUSTMENT For patients with renal impairment, dosage calculated individually either by using actual 24-hr creatinine clearance (ml/min) divided by body weight (kg) or using estimated creatinine clearance in ml/min/kg from serum creatinine (mg/dl) level using the following formula:

$$\text{Males: } \frac{\text{weight in kg} \times 140 - \text{age}}{72 \times \text{serum creatinine (mg/100 ml)}}$$

Females: $0.85 \times$ above value

Mechanism of Action

Selectively inhibits the pyrophosphate binding site on virus-specific DNA polymerases, which inhibits herpes virus replication.

Contraindications

Hypersensitivity to foscarnet sodium or its components

Incompatibilities

Administer only with 5% dextrose solution or normal saline solution. Also, do not administer with any other drug or supplement concurrently via the same catheter, as a chemical or physical reaction may occur.

Interactions

DRUGS

acyclovir, aminoglycosides, amphotericin B, cyclosporine, loop diuretics, methotrexate, ritonavir, ritonavir and saquinavir, tacrolimus: Increased risk of renal dysfunction
class IA antiarrhythmics (procainamide, quinidine), class III antiarrhythmics (amiodarone, dofetilide, sotalol), phenothiazines, selected fluoroquinolones and macrolides, tricyclic antidepressants: Increased risk of QT prolongation and possible torsades de pointes
pentamidine (intravenous): Possibly hypocalcemia

Adverse Reactions

CNS: Abnormal coordination, aggressive reaction, agitation, amnesia, anxiety, aphasia, asthenia, ataxia, **coma**, confusion, dementia, depression, dizziness, EEG abnormalities, fatigue, fever, hallucination, headache, hypoesthesia, insomnia, malaise,

meningitis, nervousness, neuropathy, paresthesia, rigors, **seizures including grand mal**, sensory disturbances, somnolence, **status epilepticus**, stupor, thirst, tremors
CV: Cardiac arrest, chest pain, nonacute ECG abnormalities (first-degree AV block, nonspecific ST-T segment changes, sinus tachycardia), edema, elevated gamma GT level, hypertension, **hypotension**, palpitations, **prolonged QT interval**, **torsades de pointes**, **thrombosis**, **ventricular arrhythmia**
EENT: Conjunctivitis, dry mouth, eye abnormalities or pain, pharyngitis, rhinitis, sinusitis, **stridor**, taste perversions, vision abnormalities, ulcerative stomatitis
ENDO: Diabetes insipidus (usually nephrogenic), syndrome of inappropriate antidiuretic hormone secretion
GI: Abdominal pain, abnormal A-G ratio, anorexia, cachexia, constipation, diarrhea, dyspepsia, dysphagia, elevated liver or pancreatic enzymes, esophageal ulceration, flatulence, **GI hemorrhage**, **hepatic dysfunction**, **melena**, nausea, **pancreatitis**, **rectal hemorrhage**, vomiting
GU: Acute renal failure, **acquired Fanconi syndrome**, albuminuria, crystal-induced nephropathy, decreased creatinine clearance, dysuria, elevated BUN or serum creatinine level, glomerulonephritis, hematuria, **nephrotic syndrome**, **nephrotoxicity**, nocturia, polyuria, renal calculus or impairment, **renal tubular acidosis or necrosis**, urethral disorder, urinary retention, UTI
HEME: Anemia, **granulocytopenia**, **leukopenia**, **neutropenia**, **pancytopenia**, **thrombocytopenia**
MS: Arthralgia, back pain, generalized spasms, involuntary muscle contractions, leg cramps, muscle weakness, myalgia, myositis, **rhabdomyolysis**
RESP: Bronchospasm, coughing, dyspnea, **hemoptysis**, pneumonia, **pneumothorax**, **pulmonary infiltration**, **respiratory insufficiency**
SKIN: Diaphoresis, **erythema multiforme**, erythematous or maculopapular rash, flushing, pruritus, rash, seborrhea, skin discoloration or ulceration, **Stevens–Johnson syndrome**, **toxic epidermal necrolysis**, urticaria
Other: Acidosis, **anaphylaxis**, **angioedema**, dehydration, elevated alkaline phosphatase or LDH, flu-like symptoms, generalized pain, **hypercalcemia**, **hypernatremia**, hyperphosphatemia, **hypocalcemia**, **hypokalemia**, **hypomagnesemia**, **hypophosphatemia**, hypoproteinemia, infections (bacterial, fungal, moniliasis), injection-site inflammation or pain, localized edema, lymphadenopathy, **lymphoma-like disorder**, **sarcoma**, **sepsis**, weight loss

Nursing Considerations

- Know that foscarnet therapy should not be used in patients on a controlled sodium diet, because of the sodium content of the drug.
- Use cautiously in patients with history of prolonged QT interval, in patients taking drugs known to prolong the QT interval, in patients with electrolyte disturbances, or in patients who have other risk factors for QT prolongation, as QT prolongation and torsades de pointes have occurred with foscarnet therapy. Expect prescriber to order routine electrocardiograms and measure patient's electrolytes before foscarnet therapy is begun and periodically throughout therapy.
- Use foscarnet cautiously in patients with neurologic abnormalities (especially seizure disorders), and patients with decreased total calcium or other electrolyte abnormalities before treatment, as well as in patients receiving other drugs known to influence serum calcium levels.
- Assess patient's estimated or measured creatinine clearance before foscarnet therapy is begun, 2 to 3 times a week during initial therapy, and once weekly during maintenance therapy, as ordered, because most patients will experience some decrease in renal function as a result of foscarnet therapy. Know also that a 24-hour creatinine clearance should be determined before therapy is begun and periodically thereafter to ensure correct dosing. Expect foscarnet to be discontinued if creatinine clearance drops below 0.4 ml/min/kg.
- Determine patient's serum calcium, magnesium, phosphorus, and potassium

E F

levels before foscarnet therapy is begun, 2 to 3 times a week during initial therapy, and once weekly during maintenance therapy, as ordered, because foscarnet can chelate divalent metal ions and alter levels of serum electrolytes.

- Know that combination therapy with foscarnet and ganciclovir is indicated for patients who have relapsed after monotherapy with either drug used to treat CMV retinitis.
- Expect to calculate each dose, even in the presence of a normal serum creatinine, to reduce risk of nephrotoxicity. Know that the standard 24 mg/ml solution may be used with or without dilution when using a central venous catheter for infusion. If a peripheral vein catheter is used, the standard 24 mg/ml solution must be diluted to a 12 mg/ml concentration with 5% dextrose in water or normal saline solution prior to administration to avoid local irritation of peripheral veins. The diluted solution must be used within 24 hours.
- Maintain adequate hydration of patient to reduce the risk of nephrotoxicity. Expect to administer 750 to 1000 ml of 5% dextrose solution or normal saline prior to the first infusion of foscarnet to establish diuresis. With subsequent infusions, expect to infuse 750 to 1,000 ml of hydration fluid with a dose of 90 to 120 mg/kg of foscarnet and 500 ml of hydration fluid with a dose of 40 to 60 mg/kg. Oral hydration may be used instead if patient is able to drink the required amount of fluid.

WARNING Do not administer foscarnet by bolus or rapid intravenous injection, because toxicity increases with excessive plasma levels. An infusion pump must be used to control the rate of infusion. The rate of infusion should not exceed 1 mg/kg/min. Also know that foscarnet must be infused only in veins with adequate blood flow, because adverse reactions can occur. For example, irritation and ulcerations of penile epithelium have occurred in male patients and genital irritation and ulceration have occurred in female patients, possibly related to the presence of the drug in the urine. Ensure that patient has good personal hygiene as well as being adequately hydrated, which may minimize these effects.

- Flush eyes or skin with water if accidental contact with foscarnet occurs, because a burning sensation and local irritation may occur.
- Monitor patient for symptoms of electrolyte abnormalities (mild: perioral numbness or paresthesias; severe: seizures) regularly. If present, notify prescriber and expect serum electrolyte and mineral levels to be assessed as soon as possible and treatment initiated if abnormalities are revealed.
- Assess patient closely for hypersensitivity reactions to foscarnet. Serious acute hypersensitivity reactions have occurred in patients exposed to foscarnet. If present, notify prescriber immediately, expect foscarnet to be discontinued, and provide supportive care, as indicated and ordered.

PATIENT TEACHING

- Advise patient that foscarnet is not a cure for either CMV retinitis or mucocutaneous acyclovir-resistant HSV infection.
- Tell patient that it is important to maintain hydration during foscarnet therapy.
- Inform patient that the major adverse reactions related to foscarnet therapy are electrolyte abnormalities, kidney dysfunction, and seizures. Stress importance of reporting any abnormal, persistent, severe, or unusual signs and symptoms to prescriber, as dosage may have to be adjusted or drug discontinued.

WARNING Advise patient to get immediate emergency medical treatment if she develops any signs of an allergic reaction, such as difficulty breathing, hives, or swelling of her face, lips, tongue, or throat.

- Instruct patient to notify prescriber at once if she experiences serious adverse reactions such as confusion, feeling short of breath, increased thirst, pounding heartbeats, swelling, urinating less than usual or not at all, weakness, or weight gain.
- Caution patient to avoid performing hazardous activities such as driving until the effects of the drug on her nervous system are known and have been resolved.
- Inform mothers that breastfeeding is not recommended during foscarnet therapy, to

prevent potentially serious adverse events in the nursing infant.
- Encourage patient being treated for CMV retinitis to have regular ophthalmologic examinations.

fosfomycin tromethamine

Monurol

Class and Category

Pharmacologic class: Phosphonic acid derivative
Therapeutic class: Antibiotic
Pregnancy category: Not classified

Indications and Dosages

➤ *To treat uncomplicated UTI (acute cystitis) caused by* Enterococcus faecalis *or* Escherichia coli

GRANULES FOR ORAL SOLUTION

Women age 18 and over. 3 g as a single dose mixed with water.

Route	Onset	Peak	Duration
P.O.	2–3 days	48 hr	Unknown

Mechanism of Action

Disrupts the formation of bacterial cell walls by blocking cell wall precursors. Specifically, fosfomycin inactivates enolpyruvyl transferase, which irreversibly blocks the condensation of uridine diphosphate-*N*-acetylglucosamine with phosphoenolpyruvate, a preliminary step in bacterial cell wall synthesis. Fosfomycin also decreases adherence of bacteria to epithelial cells of the urinary tract.

Contraindications

Hypersensitivity to fosfomycin or its components

Interactions

DRUGS

metoclopramide: Decreased blood level and urinary excretion of fosfomycin

Adverse Reactions

CNS: Asthenia, dizziness, fever, headache, insomnia, nervousness, paresthesia, somnolence
EENT: Dry mouth, pharyngitis, rhinitis
GI: Abdominal pain, anorexia, constipation, diarrhea, flatulence, indigestion, nausea, **pseudomembranous colitis**, vomiting
GU: Dysmenorrhea, dysuria, hematuria, menstrual irregularities, vaginitis
MS: Back pain
SKIN: Pruritus, rash
Other: Flu-like symptoms, lymphadenopathy

Nursing Considerations

- Use fosfomycin cautiously in patients with impaired renal function because drug clearance may be decreased.
- Expect to obtain urine specimens for culture and sensitivity tests before and after fosfomycin therapy.
- To reconstitute granules, pour contents of single-dose packet into 90 to 120 ml (3 to 4 oz) of water (not hot water) and stir. Administer immediately after dissolving.

WARNING Expect adverse reactions to increase if more than one dose is used to treat a single episode of acute cystitis.

- Monitor patient for diarrhea during and for at least 2 months after drug therapy; diarrhea may signal pseudomembranous colitis caused by *Clostridium difficile.* If diarrhea occurs, notify prescriber and treat with electrolytes, fluids, and protein, as well as an antibiotic effective against *C. difficile.*

PATIENT TEACHING

- Explain how to reconstitute fosfomycin, and instruct patient to take drug immediately after it dissolves. Tell her not to take dry granules or mix them with hot water.
- Advise patient to use only a single dose, as prescribed, to avoid increasing the risk of adverse reactions.
- Urge patient to notify prescriber if symptoms don't improve in 2 to 3 days.
- Instruct patient to return to prescriber for further urine testing after taking fosfomycin.
- Urge patient to tell prescriber about diarrhea that's severe or lasts longer than 3 days. Explain that watery or bloody stools can occur 2 or more months after therapy and can be serious, requiring prompt treatment.

fosinopril sodium

Monopril

Class and Category

Pharmcologic class: Angiotensin converting enzyme (ACE) inhibitor
Therapeutic class: Antihypertensive, vasodilator
Pregnancy category: C (first trimester), D (later trimesters)

Indications and Dosages

➤ *To manage blood pressure, alone or with other antihypertensives*

TABLETS

Adults. *Initial:* 10 mg daily. *Maintenance:* 20 to 40 mg daily. *Maximum:* 80 mg daily.
Children weighing more than 50 kg (110 lb). 5 to 10 mg daily as monotherapy.

➤ *As adjunct to treat heart failure*

TABLETS

Adults. 10 mg daily. *Maintenance:* 20 to 40 mg daily. *Maximum:* 40 mg daily.
DOSAGE ADJUSTMENT Initial dosage reduced to 5 mg daily, if needed, for patients with acute heart failure, moderate to severe renal failure, or recent aggressive diuresis.

Route	Onset	Peak	Duration
P.O.	1 hr	2–6 hr	24 hr

Mechanism of Action

May reduce blood pressure by affecting renin–angiotensin–aldosterone system. By inhibiting angiotensin-converting enzyme, fosinopril:

- prevents conversion of angiotensin I to angiotensin II, a potent vasoconstrictor that also stimulates the adrenal cortex to secrete aldosterone
- may inhibit renal and vascular production of angiotensin II
- decreases serum angiotensin II level and increases serum renin activity, which decreases aldosterone secretion, slightly increasing the serum potassium level and fluid loss
- decreases vascular tone and blood pressure
- inhibits aldosterone release, which reduces sodium and water reabsorption and increases their excretion, further reducing blood pressure.

Contraindications

Hypersensitivity to fosinopril, other ACE inhibitors, or their components

Interactions

DRUGS

antacids: Impaired fosinopril absorption
diuretics, other antihypertensives: Possibly additive hypotension
lithium: Increased blood lithium level and risk of lithium toxicity
potassium-sparing diuretics, potassium supplements: Increased risk of hyperkalemia
sodium aurothiomalate: Nitritoid reactions, including facial flushing, nausea, vomiting, and hypotension

FOODS

salt substitutes: Increased risk of hyperkalemia

ACTIVITIES

alcohol use: Possibly additive hypotension

Adverse Reactions

CNS: Confusion, depression, dizziness, drowsiness, fatigue, fever, headache, insomnia, mood changes, sleep disturbance, syncope, tremor, vertigo, weakness
CV: **Angina**, **arrhythmias (including AV conduction disorders**, **bradycardia**, and tachycardia), claudication, **hypotension**, **MI**, orthostatic hypotension, palpitations
EENT: Dry mouth, epistaxis, eye irritation, hoarseness, rhinitis, sinus problems, taste perversion, tinnitus, vision changes
GI: Abdominal distention and pain, anorexia, constipation, diarrhea, flatulence, **hepatic failure**, **hepatitis**, hepatomegaly, jaundice, nausea, **pancreatitis**, vomiting
GU: Decreased libido, flank pain, **renal insufficiency**, sexual dysfunction, urinary frequency
MS: Arthralgia, gout, myalgia
RESP: **Asthma**; bronchitis; **bronchospasm**; dry, persistent, tickling cough; dyspnea; tracheobronchitis; upper respiratory tract infection
SKIN: Diaphoresis, photosensitivity, pruritus, rash, urticaria
Other: **Anaphylaxis**, **angioedema**, **hyperkalemia**, weight gain

Nursing Considerations

- Monitor serum potassium level before and during fosinopril therapy, as appropriate.
- Observe patient being treated for heart failure for at least 2 hours after giving drug to detect hypotension or orthostatic hypotension. If either develops, notify prescriber and monitor patient until blood pressure stabilizes. Keep in mind that orthostatic hypotension is unlikely to develop in patients with a systolic blood pressure over 100 mm Hg who receive a 10-mg dose.
- Separate administration times between antacids and fosinopril by at least 2 hours.
- Know that if patient also receives a diuretic or another antihypertensive, you should expect to reduce its dosage over 2 to 3 days before starting fosinopril. If blood pressure isn't controlled with fosinopril alone, other antihypertensive therapy may resume, as prescribed. If so, observe for excessive hypotension.

WARNING Know that if angioedema affects the face, glottis, larynx, limbs, lips, mucous membranes, or tongue, prescriber must be notified immediately. Expect to discontinue fosinopril and start appropriate therapy at once. If airway obstruction threatens, promptly give 0.3 to 0.5 ml of epinephrine solution 1:1,000 subcutaneously, as prescribed.

PATIENT TEACHING

- Instruct patient to take fosinopril at same time each day to improve compliance and maintain drug's therapeutic effect.
- Emphasize the importance of taking fosinopril as prescribed, even if patient feels well. Caution her not to stop taking drug without consulting prescriber.
- Explain that drug helps control—but doesn't cure—hypertension and that patient may need lifelong therapy.

WARNING Urge patient to seek immediate medical attention for difficulty breathing or swallowing, hoarseness, or swelling of the face, lips, throat, or tongue.

- Instruct patient to notify prescriber about persistent, severe diarrhea, nausea, and vomiting; resulting dehydration may lead to hypotension.
- Advise patient not to take other drugs or use salt substitutes without consulting prescriber.
- Encourage patient to keep scheduled appointments with prescriber to monitor blood pressure, blood test results, and effects of therapy.
- Caution patient about possible dizziness.
- Advise patient to rise slowly from a lying or sitting position and to dangle legs over bed for several minutes before standing to minimize effects of orthostatic hypotension.
- Reinforce prescriber's recommendations for lifestyle changes, such as alcohol avoidance, dietary improvements, smoking cessation, regular exercise, and stress reduction.
- Urge women of childbearing age to use contraception during therapy because drug may harm fetus.
- Advise patient to use caution during exercise and hot weather because of the increased risk of dehydration from excessive sweating.

fosphenytoin sodium

Cerebyx

Class and Category

Pharmacologic class: Hydantoin derivative
Therapeutic class: Anticonvulsant
Pregnancy category: Not classified

Indications and Dosages

➤ *To treat generalized tonic-clonic status epilepticus*

I.V. INFUSION, I.M. INJECTION

Adults. *Loading:* 15 to 20 mg of phenytoin equivalent (PE)/kg I.V. at 100 to 150 PE/min. *Maintenance:* 4 to 6 mg PE/kg daily I.V. at a rate no greater than 150 mg PE/min or I.M. in divided doses.

I.V. INFUSION

Neonates, infants, children, and adolescents to age 17 years. *Loading:* 15 to 20 mg PE/kg I.V. at a rate of 2 mg PE/kg/min or 150 mg PE/min for I.V. adminstration, whichever is slower. *Maintenance:* 2 to 4 mg PE/kg given 12 hr after loading dose and then continued every 12 hr at a rate of 1 to 2 mg PE/kg/min or 100 mg PE/min, whichever is slower.

➤ *To prevent or treat seizures during neurosurgery*

I.V. INFUSION, I.M. INJECTION

Adults. *Loading:* 10 to 20 mg PE/kg, not to exceed 150 mg PE/min for I.V. adminstration. *Maintenance:* 4 to 6 mg PE/kg in divided doses.

I.V. INFUSION

Neonates, infants, children, and adolescents to age 17 years. *Loading:* 10 to 15 mg PE/kg at a rate of 1 to 2 mg PE/kg/min or 150 mg PE/min, whichever is slower. *Maintenance:* 2 to 4 mg PE/kg given 12 hr after initial dose and then continued every 12 hr at a rate of 1 to 2 mg PE/kg/min or 100 mg PE/min, whichever is slower.

➤ *To substitute for oral phenytoin therapy when administration of oral phenytoin is not possible.*

I.V. INFUSION, I.M. INJECTION

Adults. Same total daily phenytoin sodium equivalents (PE) dose. I.V. infusion rate should not exceed 150 mg PE/min.

Mechanism of Action

Is converted from fosphenytoin (a prodrug) to phenytoin, which limits the spread of seizure activity and the start of new seizures. Phenytoin does so by regulating voltage-dependent sodium and calcium channels in neurons, inhibiting calcium movement across neuronal membranes, and enhancing the sodium–potassium–adenosine triphosphatase activity in neurons and glial cells. These actions may stem from phenytoin's ability to slow the recovery rate of inactivated sodium channels.

Contraindications

Concurrent delavirdine use; hypersensitivity to fosphenytoin, phenytoin, other hydantoins, or their components

Interactions

DRUGS

acyclovir: Decreased blood phenytoin level, loss of seizure control
alfentanil: Increased clearance and decreased effectiveness of alfentanil
amiodarone, calcium channel blockers, capecitabine, chloramphenicol, chlordiazepoxide, cimetidine, disulfiram, estrogen, ethosuximide, felbamate, fluconazole, fluorouracil, fluoxetine, fluvastatin, fluvoxamine, isoniazid, itraconazole, ketoconazole, methsuximide, methylphenidate, miconazole, omeprazole, oxcarbazepine, phenothiazines, salicylates, sertraline, sulfadiazine, sulfamethizole, sulfamethoxazole-trimethoprim, sulfaphenazole, ticlopidine, tolbutamide, topiramate, trimethoprim, voriconazole, warfarin: Possibly increased blood phenytoin level and risk of toxicity
antacids: Possibly decreased phenytoin effectiveness
antineoplastics, diazepam, diazoxide, fosamprenavir, nelfinavir, reserpine, rifampin, ritonavir, St. John's wort, vigabatrin: Increased phenytoin metabolism and decreased phenytoin level
beta blockers: Increased myocardial depression
bupropion, clozapine, loxapine, MAO inhibitors, maprotiline, phenothiazines, pimozide, thioxanthenes: Possibly lowered seizure threshold and decreased therapeutic effects of phenytoin, possibly intensified CNS depressant effects of these drugs
calcium: Possibly impaired phenytoin absorption
carbamazepine: Decreased blood carbamazepine level, possibly decreased blood phenytoin level
CNS depressants: Possibly increased CNS depression
corticosteroids, cyclosporine, digoxin, disopyramide, doxycycline, fosamprenavir, furosemide, levodopa, mexiletine, quinidine: Decreased therapeutic effects of these drugs
delavirdine: Possible loss of virologic response and possible resistance to delavirdine
diazoxide: Possibly decreased therapeutic effects of both drugs
dopamine: Possibly sudden hypotension or cardiac arrest after I.V. fosphenytoin administration
estrogen- and progestin-containing contraceptives: Possibly breakthrough bleeding and decreased contraceptive effectiveness
estrogens, progestins: Decreased therapeutic effects, increased blood phenytoin level
folic acid: Increased phenytoin metabolism, decreased seizure control
fosamprenavir in combination with ritonavir: Possibly increased blood fosamprenavir level

haloperidol: Possibly lowered seizure threshold and decreased therapeutic effects of phenytoin; possibly decreased blood haloperidol level
insulin, oral antidiabetic drugs: Possibly increased blood glucose level and decreased therapeutic effects of these drugs
lamotrigine: Possibly decreased therapeutic effects of lamotrigine
lidocaine: Possibly decreased blood lidocaine level, increased myocardial depression
lithium: Increased risk of lithium toxicity
methadone: Possibly increased methadone metabolism, leading to withdrawal symptoms
metronidazole, phenylbutazone, ranitidine, salicylates: Possibly impaired metabolism of these drugs, increased risk of phenytoin toxicity
molindone: Possibly lowered seizure threshold, impaired absorption, and decreased therapeutic effects of phenytoin
nondepolarizing neuromuscular blocking agents such as cisatracurium, pancuronium, rocuronium, vecuronium: Possibly more rapid recovery from neuromuscular blockade than expected
oral anticoagulants: Possibly impaired metabolism of these drugs and increased risk of phenytoin toxicity; possibly increased anticoagulant effects initially and then decreased effects with prolonged therapy
phenobarbital, valproate sodium, valproic acid: Possible decrease or increase in phenytoin serum levels
rifampin: Possibly decreased therapeutic effects of phenytoin
streptozocin: Possibly decreased therapeutic effects of streptozocin
sucralfate: Possibly decreased phenytoin absorption
tricyclic antidepressants: Possibly lowered seizure threshold and decreased therapeutic effects of phenytoin; possibly decreased blood antidepressant level
valproic acid: Increased blood valproic acid level
vitamin D analogues: Decreased vitamin D analogue activity
xanthines: Possibly inhibited phenytoin absorption and increased clearance of xanthines
zaleplon: Increased clearance and decreased effectiveness of zaleplon

ACTIVITIES
alcohol use: Possibly decreased or increased phenytoin effectiveness

Adverse Reactions

CNS: Agitation, amnesia, asthenia, ataxia, **cerebral edema**, chills, **coma**, confusion, **CVA**, decreased or increased reflexes, delusions, depression, dizziness, dyskinesia, emotional lability, **encephalitis**, **encephalopathy**, extrapyramidal reactions, fever, headache, hemiplegia, hostility, hypoesthesia, lack of coordination, malaise, **meningitis**, nervousness, neurosis, paralysis, paresthesia, personality disorder, positive Babinski's sign, **seizures**, somnolence, speech disorders, stupor, **subdural hematoma**, syncope, transient paresthesia, tremor, vertigo
CV: Atrial flutter, **bradycardia**, bundle-branch block, **cardiac arrest**, **cardiomegaly**, edema, **heart failure**, hypertension, **hypotension**, orthostatic hypotension, palpitations, **PVCs**, **serious arrhythmias**, **shock**, tachycardia, thrombophlebitis, vasodilation
EENT: Amblyopia, conjunctivitis, diplopia, dry mouth, earache, epistaxis, eye pain, gingival hyperplasia, hearing loss, hyperacusis, increased salivation, loss of taste, mydriasis, nystagmus, pharyngitis, photophobia, rhinitis, sinusitis, taste perversion, tinnitus, tongue swelling, visual field defects
ENDO: Decreased dexamethasone, metyrapone, or T4 levels; diabetes insipidus; hyperglycemia; **ketosis**
GI: Anorexia, constipation, diarrhea, dysphagia, elevated liver enzymes, flatulence, gastritis, **GI bleeding**, **hepatic necrosis**, **hepatitis**, ileus, indigestion, nausea, vomiting
GU: Albuminuria, dysuria, incontinence, oliguria, polyuria, **renal failure**, urine retention, vaginal candidiasis
HEME: Agranulocytosis, anemia, easy bruising, **granulocytopenia**, **leukopenia**, **pancytopenia**, **thrombocytopenia**
MS: Arthralgia, back or pelvic pain, dysarthria, leg cramps, muscle twitching, myalgia, myasthenia, myoclonus, myopathy
RESP: Apnea, **asthma**, **atelectasis**, bronchitis, dyspnea, **hemoptysis**, hyperventilation, **hypoxia**, increased cough,

increased sputum production, pneumonia, **pneumothorax**
SKIN: Contact dermatitis, diaphoresis, maculopapular or pustular rash, photosensitivity, pruritus, skin discoloration, skin nodule, **Stevens–Johnson syndrome**, **toxic epidermal necrolysis**, urticaria
Other: Anaphylaxis; **angioedema**; cachexia; **cryptococcosis**; dehydration; **drug reaction with eosinophilia and systemic symptoms (DRESS)**; elevated alkaline phosphatase; flu-like symptoms; **hyperkalemia**; **hypokalemia**; **hypophosphatemia**; infection; injection-site reaction such as edema, discoloration, and pain distal to the site of injection; lymphadenopathy; porphyria; **sepsis**

Nursing Considerations

- Be aware that the dosage, concentration, and infusion rate of fosphenytoin are expressed in PE units. Misreading an order or a label could result in massive overdose.
- Refrigerate unopened fosphenytoin at 2° to 8° C (36° to 46° F), but don't freeze.
- Dilute drug in D_5W or normal saline solution to 1.5 to 25 mg PE/ml.
- Inspect parenteral solution before administration. Discard solution that contains particles or is discolored.
- Be aware that drug shouldn't be given I.M. for status epilepticus because I.V. route allows faster onset and peak.
- Keep in mind that I.V. fosphenytoin administration doesn't require use of a filter, as with phenytoin administration.
- Don't give fosphenytoin solution faster than 150 mg PE/minute because of the risk of cardiac arrhythmias and severe hypotension. For a 50-kg (110-lb) patient, infusion typically takes 5 to 7 minutes. Monitor patient throughout the infusion for adverse signs and symptoms of cardiovascular toxicity. If present, notify prescriber and expect infusion rate to be slowed or drug discontinued.
- Monitor patient for signs of sensory disturbances during the infusion, such as severe burning, itching, and/or paresthesia. Know that the intensity of discomfort can be lessened by slowing or temporarily stopping the infusion.
- Follow loading dose with maintenance dosage of oral or parenteral phenytoin or parenteral fosphenytoin, as prescribed.
- Give an I.V. benzodiazepine (such as diazepam or lorazepam) as prescribed with fosphenytoin; otherwise, drug's full antiepileptic effect won't be immediate.
- Monitor blood pressure, ECG, and respiratory function for 10 to 20 minutes after infusion ends.
- Expect to obtain blood fosphenytoin (phenytoin) level 2 hours after I.V. infusion or 4 hours after I.M. injection. Therapeutic level generally ranges from 10 to 20 mcg/ml; steady-state may take several days to several weeks to reach.
- Be aware that I.V. or I.M. fosphenytoin may be substituted for oral phenytoin sodium at same total daily dose and frequency. If prescribed, give daily amount in two or more divided doses to maintain seizure control.
- Know that antiepileptic drugs such as fosphenytoin should not be discontinued abruptly, because of the possibility of increased seizure frequency, including status epilepticus.
- Remember that when switching between phenytoin and fosphenytoin, small differences in phenytoin bioavailability can lead to significant changes in blood phenytoin level and an increased risk of toxicity.
- Monitor CBC for leukopenia or thrombocytopenia—signs of hematologic toxicity. Also monitor serum albumin level and results of liver and renal function tests.
- Anticipate increased frequency and severity of adverse reactions after I.V. administration in patients with hepatic or renal impairment or hypoalbuminemia. Know that the phosphate load contained in fosphenytoin should be kept in mind when patients with severe renal impairment who require phosphate restriction are treated.
- Discontinue drug, as ordered, if signs of hypersensitivity develop: acute hepatotoxicity (hepatic necrosis and hepatitis), fever, lymphadenopathy, and skin reactions during first 2 months of therapy. Expect to rapidly substitute drug with alternative therapy not belonging to the hydantoin

chemical class because abrupt withdrawal of fosphenytoin may increase risk of seizures, including status epilepticus.

- Monitor phenytoin level to detect early signs of toxicity, such as diplopia, nausea, severe confusion, slurred speech, and vomiting. Expect to reduce or stop drug.

WARNING Monitor patient for seizures; at toxic levels, phenytoin is excitatory.

WARNING Know that if patient has bradycardia or heart block rhythm, you must notify prescriber and expect to withhold drug; severe cardiovascular reactions and death have occurred.

- Expect to provide vitamin D supplement if patient has inadequate dietary intake and is receiving long-term anticonvulsant treatment.
- Document onset, characteristics, and type of seizures and response to treatment.
- Monitor patient for injection-site reactions such as local toxicity known as Purple Glove syndrome, exhibited by discoloration, edema, and pain distal to the site of injection. Know that this may occur without extravasation being present and up to several days after injection. If present, notify prescriber and expect drug to be discontinued.

WARNING Know that patients of Asian ancestry who have the genetic allelic variant HLA-B 1502 develop serious and sometimes fatal dermatologic reactions 10 times more often than people without this variant when given carbamazepine, another antiepileptic drug. Because early data suggest a similar effect with fosphenytoin, this drug shouldn't be used as a substitute for carbamazepine in these patients.

- Monitor all patients' skin for skin reactions, because serious and sometimes fatal dermatologic reactions may occur, usually within the first 28 days of treatment. Notify prescriber at the first sign of a rash or other skin abnormalities.

PATIENT TEACHING

- Inform patient that fosphenytoin typically is used for short-term treatment.
- Inform patient that some sensory discomfort may be felt during fosphenytoin administration. Advise patient to alert the nurse, as slowing the infusion can decrease the discomfort.
- Instruct patient to notify prescriber immediately about bothersome symptoms, especially rash and swollen glands or local reaction at injection site, including discoloration, edema, and pain distal to the site, and swelling. Also notify prescriber immediately if persistent, severe, or unusual signs and symptoms occur as well as a skin rash.
- Tell patient to inform prescriber of all drugs being used, including over-the-counter preparations and alcohol products, before using.
- Emphasize need for good oral hygiene and gum massage because gingival hyperplasia may develop during long-term therapy when oral phenytoin therapy is not feasible.
- Urge patient to consume adequate amounts of vitamin D.
- Warn women of childbearing age that fosphenytoin may cause congenital malformations and developmental issues in the fetus. Advise female patient to use effective contraceptive and to notify prescriber immediately if pregnancy is suspected or occurs. Encourage her to enroll in the pregnancy exposure registry if pregnancy is confirmed by calling 888-233-2334.

fremanezumab-vfrm

Ajovy

Class and Category

Pharmacologic class: Calcitonin gene-related peptide antagonist
Therapeutic class: Antimigraine
Pregnancy category: Not classified

Indications and Dosages

➤ *To prevent migraine headaches*

SUBCUTANEOUS INJECTION

Adults. 225 mg monthly. Alternatively, 675 mg every 3 months given as 3 consecutive injections of 225 mg each.

Route	Onset	Peak	Duration
SQ	Unknown	5 to 7 days	Unknown

Mechanism of Action

Binds to the calcitonin gene-related peptide (CGRP) receptor. The CGRP receptor is thought to be responsible for transmitting signals that can cause incapacitating pain. By binding to the CGRP receptor, drug antagonizes its function, preventing pain signals from being transmitted.

Contraindications

Hypersensitivity to fremanezumab-vfrm or its components

Interactions

DRUGS

None reported

Adverse Reactions

SKIN: Pruritus, rash, urticaria
Other: Fremanezumab-vfrm antibody formation, injection-site reactions (induration, pain, redness)

Nursing Considerations

- Remove fremanezumab-vfrm from refrigerator and allow it to sit at room temperature for 30 minutes protected from direct sunlight prior to administration. Do not warm drug using a heat source such as hot water or a microwave. Discard if drug has been left at room temperature for 24 hours or longer.
- Inspect solution for discoloration or particles. Do not use if solution appears to be cloudy, discolored, or contains particles.
- Administer subcutaneously into the abdomen, thigh, or upper arm in an area that is not bruised, indurated, red, or tender. If giving 3 consecutive injections, the same body site may be used, but not the exact location of the previous injection. Do not coadminister drug with other injectable drugs at the same injection site.
- Monitor patient for an allergic reaction such as hives, itching, or a rash. Be aware that most allergic reactions occur within hours to 1 month after administration. Know that if an allergic reaction occurs, the drug may have to be discontinued and signs and symptoms treated.
- Know that when switching dosage options, the first dose of the new regimen should be administered on the next scheduled date of administration.

PATIENT TEACHING

- Tell patient that if a dose is missed, she should administer it as soon as she remembers. Thereafter, the next dose can be scheduled from the date of that dose.
- Teach patient how to prepare and administer drug subcutaneously, if self-injecting.
- Instruct patient to remove fremanezumab-vfrm from refrigerator and allow it to sit at room temperature for 30 minutes protected from direct sunlight prior to administration. Warn patient not to warm drug using a heat source such as hot water or a microwave. Tell patient to discard drug if it has been left at room temperature for 24 hours or longer.
- Tell patient to inspect solution for discoloration or particles and not to use if solution appears to be cloudy, discolored, or contains particles.
- Instruct patient to administer fremanezumab-vfrm subcutaneously into the abdomen, thigh, or upper arm in an area that is not bruised, indurated, red, or tender. If giving 3 consecutive injections, tell patient that the same body site may be used, but not the exact location of the previous injection. Warn patient not to coadminister drug with other injectable drugs at the same injection site.
- Inform patient that when switching dosage options, first dose of the new regimen should be administered on the next scheduled date of administration.
- Advise patient that drug may cause an allergic reaction within hours to up to 1 month following administration. If hives, itching, or a rash occurs, tell patient to notify prescriber immediately, because drug may have to be discontinued and the allergic reaction may require additional treatment.

frovatriptan succinate

Frova

Class and Category

Pharmacologic class: Serotonin 5-HT1 receptor agonist
Therapeutic class: Antimigraine
Pregnancy category: C

Indications and Dosages

➤ *To treat acute migraine headache*

TABLETS

Adults. 2.5 mg, as needed. If migraine returns, 2.5-mg dose repeated providing there is at least a 2-hr interval between the 2 doses. Maximum: 7.5 mg (3 2.5-mg doses) per 24 hr.

Mechanism of Action

Binds to 5-HT1 receptors on intracranial blood vessels and sensory nerves of the trigeminal system to produce cranial vessel constriction and inhibition of proinflammatory neuropeptide release, which causes pain relief.

Contraindications

Arrhythmias associated with cardiac accessory conduction pathway disorders such as Wolff–Parkinson–White syndrome; history of basilar or hemiplegic migraine, stroke, or transient ischemic attack; hypersensitivity to frovatriptan or its components; ischemic coronary artery disease or coronary artery vasospasm; ischemic bowel disease; peripheral vascular disease; uncontrolled hypertension; use within 24 hours of another 5-HT1 agonist or an ergotamine-containing or ergot-type drug such as dihydroergotamine or methysergide

Interactions

DRUGS

ergot-containing or ergot-type drugs such as dihydroergotamine, methysergide: Increased risk of prolonged vasospastic reaction

MAO inhibitors, selective serotonin reuptake inhibitors, serotonin norepinephrine reuptake inhibitors, tricyclic antidepressants: Possible development of serotonin syndrome

other 5-HT1 agonists: Potential additive effects increasing risk of serious adverse reactions

Adverse Reactions

CNS: Anxiety; **cerebral hemorrhage, CVA, and other cerebrovascular events**; dizziness; dysesthesia; exacerbation of headache; fatigue; hypoesthesia; insomnia; palpitations; paresthesia; **seizure**; **serotonin syndrome**; **subarachnoid hemorrhage**

CV: Arrhythmias, including ventricular fibrillation or tachycardia; chest, jaw, neck, or throat pain, pressure, or tightness; **MI**; **myocardial ischemia**; peripheral vascular ischemia; Prinzmetal's angina; Raynaud's syndrome

EENT: Abnormal vision, blindness (transient or permanent), dry mouth, partial vision loss, rhinitis, sinusitis, tinnitus

GI: Abdominal pain, bloody diarrhea, diarrhea, dyspepsia, **gastrointestinal vascular infarction or ischemia**, splenic infarction, vomiting

RESP: Bone pain

SKIN: Diaphoresis, flushing

Other: Anaphylaxis, angioedema, generalized pain, sensation of being cold or hot

Nursing Considerations

- Expect triptan-naïve patient with multiple cardiovascular risk factors such as diabetes, increased age, hypertension, obesity, smoking, or strong family history of coronary artery disease to have a cardiovascular evaluation prior to frovatriptan being prescribed, because drug can cause serious cardiovascular disorders such as myocardial infarction or ischemia and Prinzmetal's angina. In patients who have a negative cardiovascular evaluation, know that the first dose of frovatriptan may be administered in a medically supervised setting with an EKG performed immediately following administration to detect adverse effects. Expect periodic cardiovascular evaluations to be performed throughout frovatriptan therapy. Also expect drug to be immediately discontinued if patient develops arrhythmias, because of potential life-threatening consequences.
- Know that if patient complains of chest, jaw, neck, or throat pain, pressure, or tightness, an immediate cardiovascular evaluation should be performed even though these symptoms are usually noncardiac in nature.
- Monitor patient for signs and symptoms of cerebrovascular events, because drug use increases risk of CVAs and cerebrovascular hemorrhage.
- Monitor patient for noncardiovascular vasospasm events such as gastrointestinal vascular infarction and ischemia (abdominal pain, bloody diarrhea),

peripheral vascular ischemia, Raynaud's syndrome, or splenic infarction. If suspected, notify prescriber immediately, stop frovatriptan therapy, and be prepared to provide emergency supportive care according to institutional protocol.

WARNING Monitor patient for evidence of serotonin syndrome, such as agitation, chills, confusion, diaphoresis, diarrhea, fever, hyperactive reflexes, poor coordination, restlessness, shaking, talking or acting with uncontrolled excitement, tremor, and twitching. Be aware that risk is greater during coadministration with monoamine oxidase inhibitors, selective serotonin reuptake inhibitors, serotonin norepinephrine reuptake inhibitors, and tricyclic antidepressants. Onset of symptoms usually occurs within minutes to hours of receiving a new or a greater dose of a serotonergic medication. If serotonin syndrome is suspected, notify prescriber immediately, expect drug to be discontinued, and provide symptomatic supportive care, as prescribed.

- Monitor patient's blood pressure, because significant elevation in blood pressure, including hypertensive crisis, has been reported in patients treated with other 5-HT1 agonists.

WARNING Monitor patient for hypersensitivity reactions to frovatriptan. These reactions may be life-threatening and include anaphylaxis and angioedema. Stop drug therapy immediately and notify prescriber if a hypersensitivity reaction occurs. Provide supportive care, as prescribed.

PATIENT TEACHING

- Tell patient to take drug exactly as prescribed and not to overuse drug by using it 10 days or more in a month, because medication-overuse headache may develop. If patient begins to experience daily migraine-like headaches or a marked increase in frequency of headaches, tell him to notify prescriber. Inform him that a period of detoxification may be necessary.

WARNING Alert patient that frovatriptan therapy may cause allergic reactions that may become severe. Tell patient to notify prescriber at the first sign of an allergic reaction and to seek immediate medical attention if difficulty breathing, or swelling, especially of eyes, face, or throat, occurs.

- Advise patient to notify all prescribers of frovatriptan therapy, because serious drug interactions can occur with certain medications when taken concomitantly with frovatriptan.
- Tell women of childbearing age that drug should not be used during pregnancy. If pregnancy occurs or is suspected, tell patient to notify prescriber.

WARNING Inform patient that drug has the potential to cause a heart attack or stroke or other forms of vasospastic disorders. Instruct patient to seek immediate emergency treatment if he experiences chest pain, shortness of breath, slurring of speech, or weakness, or if he develops persistent, severe, or unusual signs and symptoms.

furosemide

Furoside (CAN), Lasix, Lasix Special (CAN), Myrosemide, Novosemide (CAN), Uritol (CAN)

Class and Category

Pharmacologic class: Loop diuretic
Therapeutic class: Antihypertensive, diuretic
Pregnancy category: C

Indications and Dosages

➤ *To reduce edema caused by cirrhosis, heart failure, and renal disease, including nephrotic syndrome*

ORAL SOLUTION, TABLETS

Adults. 20 to 80 mg as a single dose, increased by 20 to 40 mg every 6 to 8 hr until desired response occurs. *Maximum:* 600 mg daily.

Children. 2 mg/kg as a single dose, increased by 1 to 2 mg/kg every 6 to 8 hr until desired response occurs. *Maximum:* 6 mg/kg/dose.

I.V. INFUSION, I.V. OR I.M. INJECTION

Adults. 20 to 40 mg as a single dose, increased by 20 mg every 2 hr until desired response occurs. I.V. injection given slowly over 1 to 2 min. I.V. infusion given at a rate of not greater than 4 mg/min.

I.V. INJECTION

Adults with pulmonary edema. 40 mg given slowly over 1 to 2 min with dosage repeated but increased to 80 mg after 1 hr, as needed.

I.V. OR I.M INJECTION

Children. 1 mg/kg as a single dose, increased by 1 mg/kg every 2 hr until desired response occurs. *Maximum:* 6 mg/kg/dose, (children), 1 mg/kg/day (premature infants).

DOSAGE ADJUSTMENT Initial single dose limited to 20 mg for elderly patients.

➤ *To manage hypertension*

ORAL SOLUTION, TABLETS

Adults. *Initial:* 40 mg twice daily, adjusted until desired response occurs.

Route	Onset	Peak	Duration
P.O.	20–60 min	1–2 hr	6–8 hr
I.V.	5 min	In 30 min	2 hr
I.M.	30 min	Unknown	2 hr

Mechanism of Action

Inhibits sodium and water reabsorption in the loop of Henle and increases urine formation. As the body's plasma volume decreases, aldosterone production increases, which promotes sodium reabsorption and the loss of potassium and hydrogen ions. Furosemide also increases the excretion of calcium, magnesium, bicarbonate, ammonium, and phosphate. By reducing intracellular and extracellular fluid volume, the drug reduces blood pressure and decreases cardiac output. Over time, cardiac output returns to normal.

Incompatibilities

Don't mix furosemide (a milky, buffered alkaline solution) with highly acidic solutions.

Contraindications

Anuria, hypersensitivity to furosemide or its components

Interactions

DRUGS

ACE inhibitors, angiotensin II receptor blockers: Possibly first-dose hypotension, severe hypotension, deterioration in renal function
aminoglycosides, cisplatin, ethacrynic acid: Increased risk of ototoxicity
cephalosporins: Increased risk of cephalosporin-induced nephrotoxicity
chloral hydrate: Possibly diaphoresis, hot flashes, and hypertension
cyclosporine: Increased risk of gouty arthritis
digoxin: Increased risk of digitalis toxicity related to hypokalemia and exaggerated metabolic effects of hypokalemia, especially myocardial effects
ganglionic or peripheral adrenergic blocking agents: Increased furosemide effects
indomethacin: Possibly reduced natriuretic and antihypertensive effects of furosemide
insulin, oral antidiabetic drugs: Increased blood glucose level
lithium: Increased risk of lithium toxicity
methotrexate and other drugs that undergo significant renal tubular secretion: Possibly decreased therapeutic effects of furosemide
norepinephrine: Possibly decreased arterial response to norepinephrine
NSAIDs: Possibly decreased diuresis
phenytoin: Possibly decreased therapeutic effects of furosemide
propranolol: Possibly increased blood propranolol level
succinylcholine: Increased action of succinylcholine
sucralfate: Possibly reduced natriuretic and antihypertensive effects of furosemide
thiazide diuretics: Possibly profound diuresis and electrolyte imbalances
thyroid hormones: Possibly overall decrease in total thyroid hormone levels with high doses (greater than 80 mg) of furosemide
tubocurarine: Antagonized skeletal muscle relaxing effect of tubocurarine

Adverse Reactions

CNS: Dizziness, drowsiness, fever, headache, lethargy, paresthesia, restlessness, vertigo, weakness
CV: **Arrhythmias**, elevated cholesterol and triglyceride levels, orthostatic hypotension, shock, tachycardia, **thromboembolism**, thrombophlebitis vertigo
EENT: Blurred vision, deafness, dry mouth, oral irritation, ototoxicity, stomatitis, tinnitus, hearing loss (rapid I.V. injection), yellow vision
ENDO: Hyperglycemia

GI: Abdominal cramps, anorexia, constipation, diarrhea, elevated liver enzymes, gastric irritation, **hepatocellular insufficiency**, indigestion, jaundice, nausea, **pancreatitis**, vomiting
GU: Azotemia, bladder spasms, glycosuria, oliguria
HEME: Agranulocytosis (rare), anemia, **aplastic anemia (rare)**, eosinophilia, **hemolytic anemia**, **leukopenia**, **thrombocytopenia**
MS: Muscle pain or spasms
SKIN: Acute generalized exanthematous pustulosis, bullous pemphigoid, **erythema multiforme**, **exfoliative dermatitis**, photosensitivity, pruritus, purpura, rash, **Stevens–Johnson syndrome**, **toxic epidermal necrolysis**, urticaria
Other: Allergic reaction, **anaphylaxis**, dehydration, **drug reaction with eosinophilia and systemic symptoms (DRESS)**, hyperuricemia, **hypocalcemia**, hypochloremia, **hypokalemia**, **hypomagnesemia**, **hyponatremia**, hypovolemia, thirst

Nursing Considerations

WARNING Use furosemide cautiously in patients with advanced hepatic cirrhosis, especially those who also have a history of electrolyte imbalance or hepatic encephalopathy; drug may lead to lethal hepatic coma.

- Be aware that patients who are allergic to sulfonamides may also be allergic to furosemide. Monitor patient closely.
- Know that furosemide may precipitate nephrocalcinosis/nephrolithiasis in premature infants. Know that in patients with nephrotic syndrome who are hypoproteinemic, furosemide therapy may be less effective and its ototoxicity potentiated. Drug may also increase the risk of persistence of patent ductus arteriosus in premature infants.
- Obtain patient's weight before and periodically during furosemide therapy to monitor fluid loss.
- Know that for once-a-day dosing, drug should be given in the morning so patient's sleep won't be interrupted by increased need to urinate.
- Prepare drug for infusion with normal saline solution, lactated Ringer's solution, or D_5W.
- Administer drug slowly I.V. over 1 to 2 minutes to prevent ototoxicity. The risk of ototoxicity is also increased in patients who receive higher than recommended doses or who have hypoproteinemia or severe renal impairment. If high doses are prescribed, recheck with prescriber and expect to use an infusion pump so the infusion rate is no higher than 4 mg of furosemide per minute. Concomitant therapy with aminoglycoside antibiotics, ethacrynic acid, or other ototoxic drugs increases risk of ototoxicity as well.
- Expect patient to have periodic hearing tests during prolonged or high-dose I.V. therapy.
- Monitor blood pressure and hepatic and renal function as well as BUN, blood glucose, and serum creatinine, electrolyte, and uric acid levels, as appropriate.
- Be aware that elderly patients are more susceptible to hypotensive and electrolyte-altering effects and thus are at greater risk for shock and thromboembolism.
- Monitor patient for hypokalemia which may occur with brisk diuresis, inadequate oral electrolyte intake, or when cirrhosis is present. It may also occur during concomitant use of ACTH or corticosteroid therapy, intake of large amounts of licorice, or prolonged use of laxatives. Digoxin may exaggerate the metabolic effects of hypokalemia, especially cardiac effects. If patient is at high risk for hypokalemia, give potassium supplements along with furosemide, as prescribed.
- Expect to discontinue furosemide at maximum dosage if oliguria persists for more than 24 hours.
- Be aware that furosemide may worsen left ventricular hypertrophy, systemic lupus erythematosus, or renal retention and adversely affect glucose tolerance and lipid metabolism as well as increase risk of decreased renal function in patients at high risk for radiocontrast nephropathy after a procedure.
- Be aware that patients with hypoproteinemia, such as occurs with nephrotic syndrome, may weaken effect of furosemide and increase its ototoxicity potential.

- Notify prescriber if patient experiences hearing loss, vertigo, or ringing, buzzing, or sense of fullness in her ears. Drug may need to be discontinued.

PATIENT TEACHING

- Instruct patient to take furosemide at the same time each day to maintain therapeutic effects. Urge her to take it as prescribed, even if she feels well.
- Instruct patient to take the last dose of furosemide several hours before bedtime to avoid sleep interruption from diuresis. If patient receives once-daily dosing, advise her to take the dose in the morning to avoid sleep disturbance caused by nocturia.
- Advise patient to change position slowly to minimize effects of orthostatic hypotension and to take furosemide with food or milk to reduce GI distress.
- Caution patient about drinking alcoholic beverages, standing for prolonged periods, and exercising in hot weather because these actions increase the hypotensive effect of furosemide.
- Emphasize the importance of weight and diet control, especially limiting sodium intake.
- Unless contraindicated, urge patient to eat more high-potassium foods and to take a potassium supplement, if prescribed, to prevent hypokalemia.
- Instruct patient to keep follow-up appointments with prescriber to monitor progress. Urge her to notify prescriber about persistent, severe nausea, vomiting, and diarrhea because they may cause dehydration.
- Inform diabetic patient that furosemide may increase blood glucose level, and advise her to check her blood glucose level frequently.

GHI

gabapentin

Gralise, Neurontin

gabapentin enacarbil

Horizant

Class and Category

Pharmacologic class: 1-amino-methyl cyclohexaneacetic acid
Therapeutic class: Anticonvulsant
Pregnancy category: C

Indications and Dosages

➤ *To manage postherpetic neuralgia*

CAPSULES, ORAL SOLUTION, TABLETS (NEURONTIN)

Adults. *Initial:* 300 mg on day 1, increased to 300 mg twice daily on day 2, increased to 300 mg three times daily on day 3, and increased gradually thereafter according to pain response, up to 600 mg three times daily. *Maximum:* 1,800 mg daily.

TABLETS (GRALISE)

Adults. *Initial:* 300 mg once daily with evening meal on day 1, 600 mg once daily with evening meal on day 2, 900 mg once daily with evening meal on days 3 through 6, 1,200 mg once daily with evening meal on days 7 through 10, 1,500 mg once daily with evening meal on days 11 through 14, and 1,800 mg once daily with evening meal on day 15 and thereafter.

E.R. TABLETS (HORIZANT)

Adults. *Initial:* 600 mg once daily in morning for 3 days, followed by 600 mg twice daily. *Maximum*: 600 mg twice daily.

DOSAGE ADJUSTMENT For patients taking Gralise who have a reduced creatinine clearance of 30 to 60 ml/min, dosage must be individualized and may need to be reduced. Patients with a creatinine clearance of less than 30 ml/min or who are receiving hemodialysis should not receive Gralise. For patients taking Neurontin who have a reduced creatinine clearance, including patients on hemodialysis, dosage reduced but reduction is highly individualized. For patients taking Horizant with a creatinine clearance between 30 and 59 ml/min, dosage reduced to 300 mg once daily in morning for 3 days, followed by 300 mg twice daily with further increase to 600 mg twice daily, as needed. For patients taking Horizant with a creatinine clearance between 15 and 29 ml/min, dosage reduced to 300 mg once daily in morning on days 1 and 3, followed by 300 mg once daily in morning with further increase to 300 mg twice daily, if needed. For patient with a creatinine clearance less than 15 ml/min and not on dialysis, dosage reduced to 300 mg once daily in morning every other day, followed by 300 mg once daily in morning, if needed. For patient with a creatinine clearance less than 15 ml/min and on hemodialysis, 300 mg following every dialysis with further increase to 600 mg following every dialysis, if needed.

➤ *As adjunct to treat partial seizures*

CAPSULES, ORAL SOLUTION, TABLETS (NEURONTIN)

Adults and adolescents. *Initial:* 300 mg three times daily, increased gradually according to clinical response. *Maintenance:* 300 to 600 mg three times daily. *Maximum:* 3,600 mg daily with maximum time between doses not to exceed 12 hr.

Children ages 3 to 11: *Initial:* 10 to 15 mg/kg/day divided into 3 doses, increased, as needed, over a period of 3 days. *Maintenance for ages 3 to 4:* 40 mg/kg/day, given in 3 divided doses. *Maintenance for ages 5 to 11:* 25 to 35 mg/kg/day, given in 3 divided doses. *Maximum:* 50 mg/kg/day, given in 3 divided doses with maximum time between doses not to exceed 12 hr.

DOSAGE ADJUSTMENT For patients taking Neurontin who have a reduced creatinine clearance, including patients on hemodialysis, dosage reduced but reduction is highly individualized.

➤ *To treat moderate to severe primary restless legs syndrome*

E.R. TABLETS (HORIZANT)

Adults. 600 mg once daily with food at about 5 p.m.

DOSAGE ADJUSTMENT For patients taking Horizant with a creatinine clearance between 30 and 59 ml/min, dosage reduced to 300 mg daily and then increased to 600 mg, as needed. For patients taking Horizant with a creatinine clearance between 15 and 29 ml/min, dosage reduced to 300 mg daily and not increased. For patients with a creatinine clearance of less than 15 ml/min and not on hemodialysis, dosage reduced to 300 mg and given every other day. Patients taking Horizant with a creatinine clearance of less than 15 ml/min and receiving hemodialysis should not receive Horizant.

Mechanism of Action

Gabapentin is structurally like gamma-aminobutyric acid (GABA), the main inhibitory neurotransmitter in the brain. Although gabapentin's exact mechanism of action is unknown, GABA inhibits the rapid firing of neurons associated with seizures. It also may prevent exaggerated responses to painful stimuli and pain-related responses to a normally innocuous stimulus to account for its effectiveness in relieving postherpetic neuralgia and restless legs syndrome symptoms.

Contraindications

Hypersensitivity to gabapentin or its components

Interactions

DRUGS

aluminum- and magnesium-containing antacids: Decreased gabapentin bioavailability
CNS depressants: Increased CNS depression
hydrocodone: Decreased hydrocodone exposure

ACTIVITIES

alcohol use: Increased CNS depression

Adverse Reactions

CNS: Agitation, altered proprioception, amnesia, anxiety, apathy, aphasia, asthenia, ataxia, cerebellar dysfunction, chills, **CNS tumors**, delusions, depersonalization, depression, disappearance of aura, dizziness, dream disturbances, dysesthesia, dystonia, emotional lability, euphoria, facial paralysis, fatigue, fever, hallucinations, headache, hemiplegia, hostility, hyperkinesia, hyperreflexia, hypoesthesia, hypotonia, **intracranial hemorrhage**, lack of coordination, malaise, migraine headache, movement disorder, nervousness, occipital neuralgia, paranoia, paresis, paresthesia, positive Babinski's sign, psychosis, reflexes (absent or decreased), sedation, **seizures**, somnolence, stupor, **subdural hematoma**, **suicidal ideation**, syncope, tremor, vertigo
CV: Angina, hypertension, **hypotension**, murmur, palpitations, peripheral edema, peripheral vascular insufficiency, tachycardia, vasodilation
EENT: Abnormal vision, amblyopia, blepharospasm, cataracts, conjunctivitis, diplopia, dry eyes and mouth, earache, epistaxis, eye hemorrhage, eye pain, gingival bleeding, gingivitis, glossitis, hearing loss, hoarseness, increased salivation, inner ear infection, loss of taste, nystagmus, pharyngitis, photophobia, ptosis (bilateral or unilateral), rhinitis, sensation of fullness in ears, stomatitis, taste perversion, tinnitus, tooth discoloration, visual field defects
ENDO: Breast hypertrophy, hyperglycemia, **hypoglycemia**
GI: Abdominal pain, anorexia, constipation, diarrhea, elevated liver enzymes, fecal incontinence, flatulence, gastroenteritis, hemorrhoids, **hepatitis**, hepatomegaly, increased appetite, indigestion, jaundice, **melena**, nausea, thirst, vomiting
GU: Acute renal failure, anorgasmia, decreased libido, ejaculation disorders, impotence
HEME: Anemia, **coagulation defect**, **leukopenia**, **thrombocytopenia**
MS: Arthralgia, arthritis, back pain, bone fractures, dysarthria, joint stiffness or swelling, muscle twitching, myalgia, positive Romberg test, **rhabdomyolysis**, tendinitis
RESP: Apnea, cough, dyspnea, pneumonia, pseudocroup
SKIN: Acne, alopecia, cyst, diaphoresis, dry skin, eczema, **erythema multiforme**, hirsutism, pruritus, purpura, rash, seborrhea, **Stevens–Johnson syndrome**, urticaria
Other: Anaphylaxis, **angioedema**, dehydration, **drug reaction with eosinophilia and systemic symptoms (DRESS)**, elevated creatine kinase level, **hyponatremia**, increased risk of viral infection, lymphadenopathy, weight gain or loss

Nursing Considerations

- Know that gabapentin capsules may be opened and mixed with applesauce, fruit juice, pudding, or water before administration.

- Administer initial dose for Neurontin brand at bedtime to minimize adverse reactions, especially ataxia, dizziness, fatigue, and somnolence. Administer Gralise brand with evening meal and initial dose of Horizant in the morning.
- Give drug at least 2 hours after an antacid.
- Don't exceed 12 hours between doses on a three-times-a-day schedule.
- Be aware that routine monitoring of blood gabapentin level isn't needed.

WARNING **Know that to discontinue drug used to treat seizures or switch to a different anticonvulsant, expect to change gradually over at least 1 week, as prescribed, to avoid loss of seizure control. When gabapentin is discontinued after treating other indications, expect to reduce dosage, as ordered, over 1 week.**

- Monitor renal function test results, as ordered, and expect to adjust dosage, if needed.
- Monitor patient closely for evidence of suicidal thinking or behavior, especially when therapy starts or dosage changes.
- Be aware that the various brands of gabapentin are not interchangeable.
- Monitor patient for hypersensitivity, such as fever or lymphadenopathy suggestive of DRESS. Although rare, DRESS may be life-threatening. If suspected, notify prescriber immediately and expect gabapentin to be discontinued.

PATIENT TEACHING

- Tell patient who has trouble swallowing gabapentin capsules, to open them and sprinkle contents in juice or on soft food immediately before use. Tell patient taking gabapentin extended-release tablets to swallow the tablet whole and not to chew, crush, or split the tablets.

WARNING Inform patient that an allergic reaction may occur after the first dose but it may occur at any time. If he experiences difficulty breathing or swelling of his lips, throat, or tongue, he should seek immediate emergency treatment and notify prescriber as drug will need to be discontinued.

- Instruct patient not to take drug within 2 hours after taking an antacid.
- Urge patient to take a missed dose as soon as he remembers. If the next dose is in less than 2 hours, tell him to resume his regular schedule. Caution against doubling the dose.
- Caution patient not to stop drug abruptly.
- Inform patient about possible ataxia, dizziness, drowsiness, and nystagmus. Advise him to avoid hazardous activities until drug's CNS effects are known.
- Instruct patient how to prevent complications from adverse oral reactions (such as gingivitis) by encouraging patient to use good oral hygiene and to seek routine dental care.
- Explain that adverse effects usually are mild to moderate and decline with time.
- Urge patient to keep follow-up appointments with prescriber to check progress.
- Urge caregivers to watch closely for evidence of suicidal tendencies, especially when therapy starts or dosage changes, and to report concerns immediately.
- Urge woman who becomes pregnant while taking gabapentin to enroll in the North American Antiepileptic Drug Pregnancy Registry by calling 1-888-233-2334. Explain that this registry is collecting information about the safety of antiepileptic drugs during pregnancy.

galantamine hydrobromide

Razadyne, Razadyne ER

Class and Category

Pharmacologic class: Cholinesterase inhibitor
Therapeutic class: Antidementia agent
Pregnancy category: B

Indications and Dosages

➤ *To treat mild to moderate Alzheimer's-type dementia*

ORAL SOLUTION, TABLETS

Adults. *Initial:* 4 mg twice daily. Dosage increased to 8 mg twice daily after 4 wk, if tolerated and further increased to 12 mg

twice a day after an additional 4 wk, if tolerated. *Maximum:* 12 mg twice daily.
DOSAGE ADJUSTMENT For patients with moderately impaired hepatic function or a creatinine clearance between 9 and 59 ml/min, maximum dosage shouldn't exceed 16 mg daily.

E.R. CAPSULES

Adults. *Initial:* 8 mg daily. Dosage increased to 16 mg daily in 4 wk if tolerated, with further increase to 24 mg daily after another 4 wk, if tolerated. *Maximum:* 24 mg daily.

Route	Onset	Peak	Duration
P.O.	Unknown	1 hr	Unknown

Mechanism of Action

Reduces acetylcholine metabolism by competitively and reversibly inhibiting the brain enzyme acetylcholinesterase. Acetylcholine-producing neurons degenerate in the brains of patients with Alzheimer's disease. Inhibition of acetylcholinesterase increases the amount of acetylcholine, which is needed for nerve impulse transmission.

Contraindications

Hypersensitivity to galantamine hydrobromide or its components, severe hepatic or renal impairment (creatinine clearance less than 9 ml/min)

Interactions

DRUGS

amitriptyline, fluoxetine, fluvoxamine, quinidine: Possibly decreased galantamine clearance
anticholinergics: Possibly interference with cholinesterase activity
cholinergic agonists, cholinesterase inhibitors, neuromuscular blockers: Possibly exaggerated effects of these drugs and galantamine
cimetidine: Possibly increased galantamine bioavailability
ketoconazole, paroxetine: Increased galantamine bioavailability

Adverse Reactions

CNS: Aggression, asthenia, **CVA**, depression, dizziness, dysgeusia, fatigue, fever, hallucinations, headache, hypersomnia, insomnia, lethargy, malaise, **seizures**, somnolence, **suicidal ideation**, syncope, tremor
CV: AV block (including complete), **bradycardia**, chest pain, hypertension, **MI**, myocardial ischemia
EENT: Blurred vision, rhinitis, tinnitus
GI: Abdominal pain, anorexia, diarrhea, elevated liver enzymes, flatulence, **GI bleeding**, **hepatitis**, indigestion, nausea, vomiting
GU: Hematuria, incontinence, **renal failure or insufficiency**, UTI
HEME: Anemia
SKIN: Acute generalized exanthematous pustulosis, **erythema multiforme**, **Stevens–Johnson syndrome**
Other: Dehydration, hypersensitivity reactions, **hypokalemia**, weight loss

Nursing Considerations

- Give galantamine twice daily with morning and evening meals, and ensure adequate fluid intake to prevent GI symptoms.
- Know that if therapy is interrupted for several days, expect to restart drug at lowest dose because benefits are lost when it is discontinued.
- Monitor patient's cardiovascular status closely because cholinesterase inhibitors like galantamine may have a depressive effect AV and sinoatrial nodes and may lead to AV block and bradycardia.
- Monitor patient for progressive deterioration of mental status because drug is less effective as Alzheimer's disease progresses and intact cholinergic neurons decrease.

PATIENT TEACHING

- Instruct patient to take or caregiver to give regular-strength drug with morning and evening meals. Extended-release capsules should be given once in the morning, preferably with food.
- Tell patient or caregiver to stop drug immediately at the first sign of a skin rash and to notify the prescriber.
- Tell patient or caregiver to notify prescriber immediately if therapy stops for several days. Prescriber may restart at lowest dose.
- Instruct patient to maintain adequate fluid intake throughout galantamine therapy.
- Advise patient not to drive or perform activities requiring alertness, especially

during first weeks of treatment, because drug may cause dizziness and drowsiness.
- Inform patient and family members that drug isn't a cure for Alzheimer's disease.

galcanezumab-gnlm

Emgality

Class and Category

Pharmacologic class: Calcitonin gene-related peptide (CGRP) humanized monoclonal antibody
Therapeutic class: Antimigraine
Pregnancy category: Not classified

Indications and Dosages

➤ *To prevent migraine headaches*

SUBCUTANEOUS INJECTION

Adults. *Loading:* 240 mg given as 2 consecutive injections of 120 mg each, followed by 120 mg monthly.

Route	Onset	Peak	Duration
SQ	Unknown	5 days	Unknown

Mechanism of Action

Binds to calcitonin gene-related peptide ligand to block its binding to the receptor as a means of pain relief.

Contraindications

Hypersensitivity to galcanezumab-gnlm or its components

Interactions

DRUGS

None reported

Adverse Reactions

RESP: Dyspnea
SKIN: Urticaria
Other: Antibody formation to galcanezumab-gnlm, injection-site reactions (erythema, pain, pruritus)

Nursing Considerations

- Administer galcanezumab-gnlm as a subcutaneous injection using the single-dose prefilled pen or single-dose prefilled syringe. Protect drug from direct sunlight. Prior to injection, allow drug to sit at room temperature for 30 minutes. Do not warm drug by using a heat source such as hot water or a microwave. Also, do not shake the pen or syringe. Prior to injecting drug, look for discoloration and particulate matter in the solution. Do not use if solution looks cloudy or has visible particles.
- Inject drug into patient's abdomen, back of the upper arm, buttocks, or thigh subcutaneously. Do not inject into areas where the skin is bruised, hard, red or tender.
- Monitor patient for hypersensitivity reactions such as dyspnea, rash, or urticaria. If a serious or severe reaction occurs, notify prescriber, expect drug to be discontinued, and initiate supportive therapy, as prescribed. Know that a hypersensitivity reaction may occur days after administration and that reaction may be prolonged.

PATIENT TEACHING

- Instruct patient on how to administer a subcutaneous injection using the single-dose prefilled pen or single-dose prefilled syringe. Tell patient to protect drug from direct sunlight. Have patient allow drug to sit at room temperature for 30 minutes before injection. Caution patient not to warm drug by using a heat source such as hot water or a microwave. Also caution patient not to shake the pen or syringe. Tell patient to look for discoloration and particulate matter in the solution before injecting drug. Tell patient not to use if solution looks cloudy or has visible particles.
- Tell patient to administer drug into her abdomen, back of the upper arm, buttocks, or thigh subcutaneously. Reinforce that she should not inject into areas where the skin is bruised, hard, red or tender. Tell patient to dispose of pen or syringe and needle in an appropriate container.
- Advise patient that if a dose is missed, to administer drug as soon as it is remembered and then schedule the next monthly dose from the date delayed dose was given.
- Instruct patient to seek medical attention if difficulty breathing, hives, or a rash occurs. Inform patient that an allergic reaction can occur days after administration and not to delay seeking treatment, as reaction may become prolonged.

ganciclovir

Cytovene-IV

Class and Category

Pharmacologic class: Nucleoside analogue
Therapeutic class: Antiviral
Pregnancy category: Not classified

Indications and Dosages

➤ *To treat cytomegalovirus (CMV) retinitis in immunocompromised patients, including patients with acquired immunodeficiency syndrome (AIDS)*

I.V. INFUSION

Adults. *Induction:* 5 mg/kg infused over 1 hr at a constant rate every 12 hr for 14 to 21 days. *Maintenance:* 5 mg/kg infused over 1 hr at a constant rate once daily for 7 days per wk. Alternatively, 6 mg/kg infused over 1 hr at a constant rate once daily for 5 days every wk.

➤ *To prevent CMV disease in transplant recipients at risk for CMV disease*

I.V. INFUSION

Adults. *Induction:* 5 mg/kg infused over 1 hr at a constant rate every 12 hr for 14 to 21 days. *Maintenance:* 5 mg/kg infused over 1 hr at a constant rate once daily for 7 days per wk for 100 to 120 days posttransplantation. Alternatively, 6 mg/kg infused over 1 hr at a constant rate once daily for 5 days every wk for 100 to 120 days posttransplantation.

DOSAGE ADJUSTMENT For patient with a creatinine clearance between 50 and 69 ml/min, dosage for induction and maintenance reduced by 50%. For patient with a creatinine clearance between 25 and 49 ml/min, dosage for induction reduced by half and dosage interval increased to every 24 hr while maintenance dosage reduced to 1.25 mg/kg and dosage interval increased to every 24 hr. For patient with a creatinine clearance between 10 and 24 ml/min, induction dosage reduced to 1.25 mg/kg and dosage interval increased to every 24 hr while maintenance dosage reduced to 0.65 mg/kg and dosage interval increased to every 24 hr. For patient with a creatinine clearance of less than 10 ml/min, induction dosage reduced to 1.25 mg/kg with dosage interval increased to only 3 times per wk following hemodialysis while maintenance dosage decreased to 0.65 mg/kg with dosage interval increased to only 3 times per wk following hemodialysis.

Mechanism of Action

Initially, drug is phosphorylated and then slowly metabolized intracellularly into virus-infected cells. There it inhibits the viral DNA polymerase pUL54 to prevent replication of human CMV.

Incompatibilities

Do not use bacteriostatic water for injection containing parabens, because it may cause precipitation to form.

Contraindications

Hypersensitivity to ganciclovir, valganciclovir, or their components

Interactions

DRUGS

amphotericin B, cyclosporine: Increased risk of renal dysfunction
dapsone, doxorubicin, flucytosine, hydroxyurea, pentamidine, tacrolimus, trimethoprim/sulfamethoxazole, vinblastine, vincristine, zidovudine: Increased risk of myelosuppression or nephrotoxicity
didanosine: Increased risk of didanosine toxicity
imipenem-cilastatin: Increased risk of generalized seizures
mycophenolate mofetil: Increased risk for hematologic and renal toxicity
probenecid: Increased serum ganciclovir concentration with increased risk of ganciclovir toxicity

Adverse Reactions

CNS: Agitation, amnesia, anxiety, aphasia, asthenia, chills, confusion, **CVA**, depression, dizziness, dream abnormality, dysesthesia, **encephalopathy**, extrapyramidal disorder, facial paralysis, fatigue, fever, hallucinations, headache, hypoesthesia, insomnia, **intracranial hypertension**, irritability, malaise, paresthesia, peripheral neuropathy, psychotic disorder, **seizures**, somnolence, thinking abnormality, third cranial nerve paralysis, tremor
CV: **Arrhythmias**, **cardiac arrest**, chest pain, **conduction disorder**, edema, elevated

trigycerides, hypertension, **hypotension**, peripheral ischemia, phlebitis, **torsades de pointes**, vasculitis, vasodilatation, **ventricular tachycardia**
EENT: Cataracts, conjunctivitis, deafness, dry eyes or mouth, ear pain, loss of smell, macular edema, mouth ulceration, retinal detachment, taste disturbance, tinnitus, visual impairment, vitreous disorders
ENDO: Inappropriate antidiuretic hormone secretion
GI: Abdominal distention or pain, anorexia, cholelithiasis, cholestasis, constipation, diarrhea, dyspepsia, dysphagia, elevated liver enzymes, eructation, flatulence, **gastrointestinal perforation**, **hepatic dysfunction or failure**, **hepatitis**, intestinal ulcer, nausea, **pancreatitis**, vomiting
GU: Abnormal kidney function, decreased creatinine clearance, elevated serum creatinine, hematuria, **hemolytic uremic syndrome**, infertility, **kidney failure**, renal tubular disorder, testicular hypotrophy, urinary frequency
HEME: Agranulocytosis, **anemia including hemolytic**, **bone marrow failure**, **decreased platelet count**, **granulocytopenia**, **leukopenia**, **pancytopenia**, **thrombocytopenia**
MS: Arthralgia, arthritis, back pain, leg cramps, muscle spasms, myalgia, myasthenia, myelopathy, **rhabdomyolysis**
RESP: Bronchospasm, cough, dyspnea, **pulmonary fibrosis**
SKIN: Alopecia, dermatitis, diaphoresis, dry skin, **exfoliative dermatitis**, pruritus, rash, **Stevens–Johnson syndrome**, urticaria
Other: Acidosis, **anaphylaxis**, elevated blood alkaline phosphatase, generalized pain, **hypercalcemia**, **hyponatremia**, infection including *Candida,* injection-site inflammation, **multiple organ failure**, **sepsis**, weight loss

Nursing Considerations

- Be aware that ganciclovir is not recommended if the absolute neutrophil count is less than 500 cells/μL, hemoglobin is less than 8 g/dl, or the platelet count is less than 25,000 cells/μL.
- Use cautiously in patients with pre-existing cytopenias and in patients receiving myelosuppressive drugs or irradiation, because ganciclovir can cause hematologic toxicities. Also use cautiously in patients with impaired renal function, because ganciclovir levels will increase in these patients, requiring dosage adjustments.
- Expect female patients of childbearing age to have a pregnancy test done prior to receiving ganciclovir.
- Obtain a serum creatinine or creatinine clearance prior to starting ganciclovir therapy, as ordered, to establish a baseline for renal function, and then frequently throughout therapy to determine need for and degree of dosage adjustment.
- Wear disposable gloves during reconstitution and when wiping the outer surface of vial and table after reconstitution. To reconstitute ganciclovir, inject 10 ml of sterile water for injection, USP, into vial. Gently swirl vial to ensure complete wetting of contents. Continue swirling until a clear reconstituted solution is obtained. Look for particulate matter and discoloration prior to proceeding with infusion. Discard vial if present. Do not refrigerate or freeze reconstituted solution. It may be kept at room temperature for 12 hours.
- Remove the appropriate volume of reconstituted solution (based on patient's weight) and add to 100 ml of an acceptable infusion fluid such as 0.9% Sodium Chloride, 5% Dextrose, Lactate, Ringer's Injection. Know that infusion concentrations greater than 10 mg/ml are not recommended. Refrigerate diluted infusion solution and use within 24 hours.

WARNING Avoid direct contact of the skin or mucous membranes with ganciclovir. If contact occurs, wash thoroughly with soap and water; rinse eyes thoroughly with plain water. Always wear disposable gloves during preparation and handling of solution. Know that guidelines issued for antineoplastic drugs should be considered in the handling and disposal of ganciclovir because it shares some of the properties of antitumor agents.

- Administer ganciclovir as an intravenous infusion over 1 hour, preferably with a plastic cannula, into a vein with adequate blood flow. Do not administer drug by rapid or bolus injection, which may increase toxicity as a result of excessive plasma levels; do not administer drug intramuscularly or subcutaneously because it may cause severe tissue irritation due to its high pH. Do not exceed the recommended dosage and infusion rate.

- Ensure that patient has adequate hydration while receiving ganciclovir to reduce adverse effects on renal function. Monitor patient's serum creatinine levels during therapy and assess patient for signs and symptoms of renal dysfunction, especially elderly and those patients receiving concurrent therapy with nephrotoxic drugs such as amphotericin B or cyclosporine.
- Monitor patient's complete blood counts with differential and platelet counts frequently throughout therapy, especially in patients in whom ganciclovir therapy or other nucleoside analogues have previously caused cytopenias, or in whom absolute neutrophil counts are less than 1,000 cells/μL at the beginning of treatment. Granulocytopenia usually occurs during the first or second week of treatment, but may occur at any time during treatment. Notify prescriber of hematologic abnormalities and expect possibility that drug will be discontinued. Cell counts usually begin to recover within 3 to 7 days after drug is discontinued. Colony-stimulating factors may be helpful in increasing neutrophil and white blood cell counts.
- Expect patient to have frequent ophthalmologic examinations during treatment to monitor ganciclovir effectiveness.

WARNING Be aware that ganciclovir has the potential to cause cancer.

PATIENT TEACHING

- Inform patient that frequent blood tests will have to be done throughout ganciclovir therapy because drug may cause blood toxicities. Stress importance of not missing any appointments. In addition, review signs and symptoms of anemia and infections and instruct patient to notify prescriber if present.
- Instruct patient to notify prescriber of persistent, severe, or unusual adverse effects, because drug can cause many adverse reactions, some of which could be serious.
- Stress importance of maintaining adequate hydration throughout ganciclovir therapy, because of potential adverse effect of drug on the kidneys.
- Inform patient that drug may cause temporary or permanent infertility and to discuss this with prescriber if concerned.
- Instruct women of childbearing age to use effective contraception during treatment and for at least 30 days following treatment, because drug may cause fetal toxicity. Instruct men to practice barrier contraception during and for at least 90 days following treatment.
- Tell patient to inform all prescribers of ganciclovir therapy, because drug can interact with other drugs.
- Advise patient not to perform any hazardous activities, such as driving, if cognitive impairment is present.
- Remind patient that ganciclovir is not a cure for CMV retinitis and that it is important to comply with ophthalmologic follow-up examinations.
- Advise mothers not to breastfeed infant while taking ganciclovir.

gemfibrozil

Lopid, Novo-Gemfibrozil (CAN)

Class and Category

Pharmacologic class: Fibric acid derivative
Therapeutic class: Antilipemic
Pregnancy category: C

Indications and Dosages

➤ *As adjunct (with diet) to treat hyperlipidemia types IV and V; to reduce risk of coronary artery disease (CAD) in patients with type IIb hyperlipidemia who do not have a history of or symptoms of existing CAD, who have had an inadequate response to lifestyle changes or other pharmacologic agents, and have the following triad of lipid abnormalities: low HDL-cholesterol levels, elevated LDL-cholesterol levels, and elevated triglycerides*

CAPSULES, TABLETS

Adults. 600 mg 30 min before morning and evening meals.

Route	Onset	Peak	Duration
P.O.	2–5 days	4 wk	Unknown

Mechanism of Action

May decrease hepatic triglyceride production by decreasing hepatic extraction of free fatty acids, inhibiting peripheral lipolysis, and reducing VLDL synthesis. Gemfibrozil also may inhibit synthesis and increase clearance of apolipoprotein B, a carrier molecule for VLDL. In addition, it may accelerate turnover and removal of total cholesterol from the liver while increasing cholesterol excretion in the feces. As a result, total cholesterol, triglyceride, and VLDL levels decrease; the HDL level increases; and the LDL level is unaffected.

Contraindications

Concurrent therapy with dasabuvir, repaglinide, selexipag, or simvastatin; gallbladder disease; hepatic or severe renal dysfunction; hypersensitivity to gemfibrozil or its components

Interactions

DRUGS

chenodiol, ursodiol: Decreased effectiveness of gemfibrozil
colchicine: Increased toxicity of either drug; risk of myopathy, including rhabdomyolysis
CYP2C8 substrates such as dabrafenib, enzalutamide, loperamide, montelukast, paclitaxel, pioglitazone, rosiglitazone, selexipag: Increased plasma concentration of these drugs
dasabuvir: Increased dasabuvir plasma concentration increasing risk of QT prolongation
enzalutamide: Increased enzalutamide plasma concentration increasing risk of seizures
HMG-CoA reductase inhibitors: Increased risk of acute renal failure and rhabdomyolysis
OATP1B1 substrates such as atrasentan, atorvastatin, bosentan, ezetimibe, fluvastatin, glyburide, olmesartan, pitavastatin, pravastatin, rifampin, rosuvastatin, SN-38 (active metabolite of irinotecan), simvastatin, valsartan: Increased plasma concentrations of these drugs
oral anticoagulants such as warfarin: Increased anticoagulation
repaglinide: Increased serum repaglinide level and risk of severe hypoglycemia
resin-granule drugs such as colestipol: Decreased blood gemfibrozil levels

Adverse Reactions

CNS: Chills, fatigue, headache, hypoesthesia, paresthesia, **seizures**, somnolence, syncope, vertigo
CV: Vasculitis
EENT: Blurred vision, cataracts, hoarseness, retinal edema, taste perversion
GI: Abdominal or epigastric pain, cholelithiasis, colitis, diarrhea, flatulence, heartburn, **hepatoma**, jaundice, nausea, **pancreatitis**, vomiting
GU: Decreased male fertility, dysuria, impotence
HEME: Anemia, **bone marrow hypoplasia**, eosinophilia, **leukopenia**, **thrombocytopenia**
MS: Arthralgia, back pain, myalgia, myasthenia, myopathy, myositis, **rhabdomyolysis**, synovitis
RESP: Cough
SKIN: Eczema, pruritus, rash
Other: Anaphylaxis, **angioedema**, increased risk of bacterial and viral infections, lupus-like symptoms, weight loss

Nursing Considerations

- Monitor serum triglyceride and cholesterol levels, as appropriate.
- Periodically review CBC and liver enzymes, during therapy, as ordered.
- Know that if serum cholesterol and triglyceride levels don't improve within 3 months, expect to switch to a different drug, as prescribed.
- Monitor patient's prothrombin time, as ordered, if patient is also receiving warfarin therapy because gemfibrozil therapy may cause a drug interaction with warfarin. Warfarin dosage may need to be decreased to maintain prothrombin time at a level needed to prevent adverse bleeding effects.

PATIENT TEACHING

- Instruct patient to take gemfibrozil 30 minutes before breakfast and 30 minutes before dinner.

- Advise patient to take a missed dose as soon as he remembers, unless it's nearly time for the next dose. Caution against doubling the dose.
- Emphasize importance of alcohol avoidance, a low-fat diet, regular exercise, and smoking cessation, as appropriate.
- Caution patient to avoid hazardous activities until drug's CNS effects are known.
- Instruct patient to notify prescriber if he experiences chills; cough; fever; hoarseness; lower back, side, or muscle pain; painful or difficult urination; severe abdominal pain with nausea and vomiting; tiredness; or weakness.
- If patient also takes an oral anticoagulant, urge him to report unusual bleeding or bruising; anticoagulant dosage may need to be reduced.
- Advise patient to keep scheduled appointments with prescriber to check progress.

gemifloxacin mesylate

Factive

Class and Category

Pharmacologic class: Fluoroquinolone
Therapeutic class: Antibiotic
Pregnancy category: C

Indications and Dosages

➤ *To treat acute bacterial exacerbation of chronic bronchitis caused by* Haemophilus influenzae, H. parainfluenzae, Moraxella catarrhalis, *or* Streptococcus pneumoniae

TABLETS

Adults. 320 mg daily for 5 days.

➤ *To treat mild to moderate community-acquired pneumonia caused by* Chlamydia pneumoniae, H. influenzae, Klebsiella pneumoniae, M. catarrhalis, Mycoplasma pneumoniae, or S. pneumoniae *including multidrug-resistant strains*

TABLETS

Adults. 320 mg daily for 5 days (when due to *C. pneumoniae, H. influenzae, M. pneumoniae,* or *S. pneumoniae*) or 7 days (when due to *K. pneumoniae, M. catarrhalis,* or multidrug-resistant *S. pneumoniae*).

DOSAGE ADJUSTMENT Dosage should be decreased to 160 mg daily in patients with creatinine clearance of 40 ml/min or less.

Route	Onset	Peak	Duration
P.O.	0.5–2 hr	Unknown	Unknown

Mechanism of Action

Inhibits actions of the enzymes DNA gyrase and topoisomerase IV, which are required for bacterial growth, thereby causing bacterial cells to die.

Contraindications

Hypersensitivity to gemifloxacin, other fluoroquinolones, or their components; myasthenia gravis

Interactions

DRUGS

aluminum and magnesium antacids, didanosine as buffered or chewable tablets or pediatric powder for oral solution, ferrous sulfate, sucralfate, zinc or other metal cations: Reduced blood gemifloxacin level
antipsychotics; class IA antiarrhythmics, such as procainamide and quinidine; class III antiarrhythmics, such as amiodarone and sotalol; erythromycin; tricyclic antidepressants: Possibly prolonged QT interval
probenecid: Increased blood gemifloxacin level
warfarin: Possibly enhanced warfarin anticoagulant effects

Adverse Reactions

CNS: Agitation, anxiety, confusion, delirium, depression, disorientation, disturbance in attention, dizziness, fever, hallucinations, headache, **increased intracranial pressure**, insomnia, lightheadedness, memory impairment, nervousness, paranoia, peripheral neuropathy, restlessness, **seizures**, **suicidal ideation**, syncope, toxic psychosis, transient ischemic attack, tremors
CV: Aortic dissection, peripheral edema, **prolonged QT interval**, **supraventricular tachycardia**, vasculitis

EENT: Taste perversion
ENDO: Hyperglycemia, **hypoglycemia**
GI: Abdominal pain, **acute hepatic necrosis or failure**, diarrhea, elevated liver enzymes, **hepatitis**, jaundice, nausea, **pseudomembranous colitis**, vomiting
GU: Acute renal insufficiency or failure, interstitial nephritis
HEME: Agranulocytosis, **aplastic or hemolytic anemia**, **elevated international normalized ratio (INR)**, **hemorrhage**, **leukopenia**, **pancytopenia**, **thrombocytopenia**, thrombocytosis
MS: Arthralgia, muscle weakness, myalgia, tendinitis, tendon rupture
RESP: Hypersensitivity pneumonitis
SKIN: Erythema multiforme, exfoliation, photosensitivity, rash, **Stevens–Johnson syndrome**, **toxic epidermal necrolysis**, urticaria
Other: Anaphylaxis, **angioedema**, serum sickness

Nursing Considerations

- Review patient's medical history before giving gemifloxacin, which shouldn't be used in patient with a history of prolonged QT interval, patient with uncorrected electrolyte disorders, or patient receiving class IA or III antiarrhythmics because of increased risk of prolonged QT interval. Monitor elderly patients closely because they may be more susceptible to prolonged QT interval.
- Use cautiously in patients with CNS disorders, such as epilepsy, or in those prone to seizures because gemifloxacin has caused increased intracranial pressure, seizures, and toxic psychosis. Monitor patient closely; if CNS alterations occur, notify prescriber immediately and expect drug to be discontinued.
- Monitor patient closely for hypersensitivity reaction, which may occur as soon as first dose. If patient has such evidence as angioedema, bronchospasm, dyspnea, itching, rash, shortness of breath, and urticaria, notify prescriber immediately and expect drug to be discontinued.
- Monitor patients prone to tendinitis, such as athletes, the elderly, and those taking corticosteroids, for reports of tendon inflammation, pain, or rupture. If present, notify prescriber. Expect gemifloxacin to be discontinued, patient placed on bed rest with no exercise of affected limb, and diagnostic tests ordered to confirm rupture.
- Notify prescriber about severe or prolonged diarrhea; it may indicate pseudomembranous colitis caused by *Clostridium difficile*. If diarrhea occurs, notify prescriber and expect to withhold gemifloxacin and treat with electrolytes, fluids, protein, and an antibiotic effective against *C. difficile*.
- Monitor patients, especially women under age 40 and postmenopausal women receiving hormone replacement therapy, for rash. It may appear days after therapy starts and resolve in 7 days. Notify prescriber immediately if rash occurs because it can be severe in about 10% of patients.
- Assess patient for evidence of peripheral neuropathy. Notify prescriber and expect to stop drug if patient complains of burning, numbness, pain, tingling, or weakness in extremities or if physical examination reveals deficits in light touch, motor strength, pain, position sense, temperature, or vibratory sensation.
- Monitor coagulation status, as ordered, for patient who takes warfarin because adding gemifloxacin may increase risk of bleeding.
- Know that fluoroquinolones like gemifloxacin have caused disabling and potentially irreversible serious adverse reactions from different body systems that can occur together in the same patient. These reactions can occur within hours to weeks after starting the drug and usually cause central nervous system effects, peripheral neuropathy, tendinitis, and tendon rupture. All ages of patients and patients without any preexisting risk factors have experienced these reactions. Notify prescriber and expect to discontinue gemifloxacin immediately at the first sign or symptom of any serious adverse reactions.
- Monitor patient's blood glucose levels, especially in diabetic patients, and for signs and symptoms of changes in blood glucose levels. Both symptomatic hyperglycemia and hypoglycemia may occur as a result of gemifloxacin therapy. If present, alert prescriber and initiate appropriate treatment, as prescribed. Also be aware that severe hypoglycemia has

occurred with other fluoroquinolones. If a hypoglycemic reaction occurs, discontinue gemifloxacin administration immediately and initiate appropriate treatment for hypoglycemia.
- Monitor patient closely for changes in behavior or mood that may be caused by gemifloxacin-induced depression or worsening psychotic reactions potentially resulting in self-injurious behavior, such as suicide. Be aware that these reactions may occur even after just one dose. If present, notify prescriber immediately and expect to discontinue gemifloxacin therapy and institute precautions to keep patient safe until adverse effects have resolved.

PATIENT TEACHING
- Tell patient to swallow tablet whole and take with a full glass of liquid.
- Warn patient not to increase dose because doing so may cause life-threatening cardiac arrhythmias.
- Instruct patient to complete entire course of therapy, even if symptoms decrease before prescription is finished.
- Caution patient to avoid sun exposure as much as possible while taking gemifloxacin. Patient who can't avoid sun exposure should apply sunscreen and wear a hat, sunglasses, and long sleeves to cover as much skin as possible.
- Urge caregivers to monitor patient closely for suicidal tendencies; if patient develops depression or worsening of psychotic behavior during therapy, instruct them to notify prescriber.
- Instruct patient to maintain adequate hydration throughout therapy to keep urine from becoming too concentrated. Tell patient to increase fluid intake if urine darkens or amount voided decreases.
- Caution patient to avoid hazardous activities until CNS effects of drug are known.
- Instruct patient to seek medical attention and notify prescriber immediately if he has tendon pain, tenderness, or rupture; evidence of hypersensitivity reaction, such as difficulty breathing, facial swelling, rash, or urticaria; or fainting spells or palpitations. Also advise patient to stop taking gemifloxacin immediately and notify prescriber if any other persistent, serious, or worsening adverse effects occur.
- Urge patient to tell prescriber about diarrhea that's severe or lasts longer than 3 days. Explain that bloody or watery stools can occur 2 or more months after therapy and can be serious, requiring prompt treatment.
- Tell patient to consult prescriber before starting any new medications, including OTC products, because gemifloxacin may interact adversely.
- Inform patient that aluminum and/or magnesium antacids; didanosine (Videx) buffered or chewable tables and pediatric powder for oral solution (if prescribed); multivitamins containing zinc or other metal cations; and products containing iron shouldn't be taken within 3 hours before or 2 hours after gemifloxacin and that gemifloxacin should be taken at least 2 hours before sucralfate (if prescribed).
- Warn patient, especially diabetics, that gemifloxacin may alter blood glucose levels. Review signs and symptoms of hyperglycemia and hypoglycemia. Tell patient to immediately report symptomatic changes in blood glucose levels to prescriber and review how to treat hypoglycemia.

gentamicin sulfate

Cidomycin (CAN)

Class and Category

Pharmacologic class: Aminoglycoside
Therapeutic class: Antibiotic
Pregnancy category: D

Indications and Dosages

➤ *To treat serious bacterial infections caused by aerobic gram-negative organisms and some gram-positive organisms, including* Citrobacter *species,* Enterobacter *species,* Escherichia coli, Klebsiella *species,* Proteus *species,* Pseudomonas aeruginosa, Serratia *species,* Staphylococcus aureus, *and many strains of* Streptococcus *species*

I.V. INFUSION, I.M. INJECTION

Adults and adolescents. 3 mg/kg/day divided into 3 equal doses every 8 hr. *For*

life-threatening infections: Up to 5 mg/kg/day divided into 3 or 4 equal doses with dosage reduced as soon as possible to 3 mg/kg/day. Give I.V. infusion over 30 min to 2 hr.
Children. 2 to 2.5 mg/kg every 8 hr. Give I.V. infusion over 30 min to 2 hr.
Infants. 2.5 mg/kg every 8 hr. Give I.V. infusion over 30 min to 2 hr.
Premature or full-term neonates up to age 1 week. 2.5 mg/kg every 12 hr. Give I.V. infusion over 30 min to 2 hr.
DOSAGE ADJUSTMENT For adults with impaired renal function, highly individualized and dependent on degree of renal function and drug level. For patients on hemodialysis, supplemental dose of 1 to 1.7 mg/kg (2 to 2.5 mg/kg for children) after hemodialysis, based on infection severity.

Mechanism of Action

Binds to negatively charged sites on the outer cell membrane of bacteria, thereby disrupting the membrane's integrity. Gentamicin also binds to bacterial ribosomal subunits and inhibits protein synthesis. Both actions lead to cell death.

Incompatibilities

Don't administer gentamicin through same I.V. line as other drugs, especially beta-lactam antibiotics (cephalosporins and penicillins), because substantial mutual inactivation may occur. Give drugs through separate sites.

Contraindications

Hypersensitivity to gentamicin, other aminoglycosides, or their components

Interactions

DRUGS

aminoglycosides (concurrent use of two or more): Decreased bacterial uptake of each drug, increased risk of nephrotoxicity and ototoxicity
cephalosporins, enflurane, methoxyflurane, vancomycin: Increased risk of nephrotoxicity
loop diuretics: Increased risk of nephrotoxicity and ototoxicity
neuromuscular blockers: Prolonged respiratory depression, increased neuromuscular blockade
penicillins: Inactivation of gentamicin by certain penicillins, increased risk of nephrotoxicity

Adverse Reactions

CNS: Acute organic mental syndrome, confusion, depression, fever, headache, increased protein in cerebrospinal fluid, lethargy, myasthenia gravis-like syndrome, **neurotoxicity**, peripheral neuropathy or **encephalopathy**, **pseudotumor cerebri**, **seizures**
CV: Hypertension, **hypotension**, palpitations
EENT: Blurred vision, increased salivation, **laryngeal edema**, ototoxicity, stomatitis, vision changes
GI: Anorexia, nausea, splenomegaly, transient hepatomegaly, vomiting
GU: Nephrotoxicity
HEME: Anemia, eosinophilia, **granulocytopenia**, increased or decreased reticulocyte count, **leukopenia**, **thrombocytopenia**
MS: Arthralgia, leg cramps
RESP: Pulmonary fibrosis, **respiratory depression**
SKIN: Alopecia, generalized burning sensation, pruritus, purpura, rash, urticaria
Other: Anaphylaxis, injection-site pain, superinfection, weight loss

Nursing Considerations

- Expect to obtain a body fluid or tissue specimen for culture and sensitivity testing, as ordered, before gentamicin therapy begins, or check test results, if available.
- Know that drug is best absorbed when given by I.V. route. Blood level is unpredictable after I.M. administration.
- For I.V. use, dilute each dose with 50 to 200 ml normal saline solution or D_5W to yield no more than 1 mg/ml. Administer slowly over 30 minutes to 2 hours.
- Don't give gentamicin through same I.V. line as other drugs without first consulting pharmacist.
- Expect to adjust dosage based on peak and trough blood drug levels drawn after third maintenance dose, as prescribed.
- Know that drug should not be given to a pregnant patient because it can cause hearing loss in fetus.
- Know that any report of dizziness, hearing loss, or ringing in the ears should be taken very seriously. Hold drug with any report of these problems.

WARNING Be aware that when giving pediatric injectable form of drug, be alert for allergic reactions—including anaphylaxis and possibly life-threatening asthmatic episodes—because drug contains sodium bisulfite.

- Assess patient for evidence of other infections because gentamicin may cause overgrowth of nonsusceptible organisms.
- Be aware that premature infants, neonates, and elderly patients have an increased risk of nephrotoxicity.

PATIENT TEACHING

- Emphasize importance of completing full course of gentamicin therapy.
- Instruct patient to report immediately adverse reactions, such as hearing loss, to avoid permanent effects.

glimepiride

Amaryl

Class and Category

Pharmacologic class: Sulfonylurea
Therapeutic class: Antidiabetic
Pregnancy category: C

Indications and Dosages

➤ *As adjunct to control blood glucose level in type 2 diabetes mellitus*

TABLETS

Adults. *Initial*: 1 to 2 mg daily with first meal of the day. Dosage increased by 1 to 2 mg every 1 to 2 wk as needed for blood glucose control. *Maximum:* 8 mg daily.

DOSAGE ADJUSTMENT Initial dosage reduced to 1 mg daily for the elderly and patients with renal impairment.

Route	Onset	Peak	Duration
P.O.	2–3 hr	Unknown	Over 24 hr

Mechanism of Action

Stimulates insulin release from beta cells in pancreas. Glimepiride also increases peripheral tissue sensitivity to insulin, either by enhancing insulin binding to cellular receptors or by increasing the number of insulin receptors.

Contraindications

Hypersensitivity to glimepiride, sulfonamide derivatives, or their components; ketoacidosis; sole therapy for type 1 diabetes mellitus

Interactions

DRUGS

ACE inhibitors, anabolic steroids, androgens, azole antifungals, bromocriptine, chloramphenicol, clarithromycin, clonidine, cyclophosphamide, disopyramide, fibric acid derivatives, fluconazole, fluoxetine, guanethidine, H_2-receptor antagonists, insulin, magnesium salts, MAO inhibitors, methyldopa, NSAIDs, octreotide, oral anticoagulants, other oral hypoglycemic agents, oxyphenbutazone, pentoxifylline, phenylbutazone, phenyramidol, pramlintide, probenecid, propoxyphene, quinidine, quinolones, reserpine, salicylates, somatostatin analogs, sulfonamides, tetracyclines, theophylline, tricyclic antidepressants, urinary acidifiers: Increased risk of hypoglycemia
asparaginase, barbiturates, calcium channel blockers, cholestyramine, clonidine, clozapine, colesevelam, corticosteroids, danazol, diazoxide, estrogens, glucagon, hydantoins, isoniazid, laxatives, lithium, morphine, nicotinic acid, olanzapine, oral contraceptives, phenothiazines, phenytoin, protease inhibitors, reserpine, rifabutin, rifampin, somatropin, sympathomimetics, thiazide and other diuretics, thyroid hormones, urinary alkalinizers: Increased risk of hyperglycemia
beta blockers: Possibly hyperglycemia or masking of hypoglycemia signs
digoxin: Increased risk of digitalis toxicity
miconazole (oral): Increased risk of severe hypoglycemia
pentamidine: Initially hypoglycemia and then hyperglycemia if beta cell damage occurs
sympatholytic drugs such as beta blockers, clonidine, guanethidine, reserpine: Reduced or absent hypoglycemic signs and symptoms

ACTIVITIES

alcohol use: Altered blood glucose control (usually hypoglycemia)

Adverse Reactions

CNS: Abnormal gait, anxiety, asthenia, chills, depression, dizziness, fatigue, headache, hypertonia, hypoesthesia,

insomnia, malaise, migraine headache, nervousness, paresthesia, somnolence, syncope, tremor, vertigo
CV: **Arrhythmias**, edema, hypertension, vasculitis
EENT: Blurred vision, conjunctivitis, eye pain, pharyngitis, retinal hemorrhage, rhinitis, taste perversion, tinnitus
ENDO: **Hypoglycemia**, increased release of antidiuretic hormone secretion (SIADH)
GI: Anorexia, cholestasis, constipation, diarrhea, elevated liver enzymes, epigastric discomfort or fullness, flatulence, heartburn, hepatic porphyria, **hepatotoxicity**, hunger, jaundice, **liver failure**, nausea, proctocolitis, trace blood in stool, vomiting
GU: Darkened urine, decreased libido, dysuria, polyuria
HEME: **Agranulocytosis**, **aplastic anemia**, eosinophilia, **hemolytic anemia**, **leukopenia**, **pancytopenia**, **thrombocytopenia**, **thrombocytopenic purpura**
MS: Arthralgia, leg cramps, myalgia
RESP: Dyspnea
SKIN: Allergic skin reactions, alopecia, diaphoresis, eczema, **erythema multiforme**, **exfoliative dermatitis**, flushing, lichenoid reactions, maculopapular or morbilliform rash, photosensitivity, pruritus, **Stevens–Johnson syndrome**, urticaria
Other: **Anaphylaxis**, **angioedema**, disulfiram-like reaction, **hyponatremia**

Nursing Considerations

- Use cautiously in patients with glucose 6-phosphate dehydrogenase (G6PD) deficiency because glimepiride is a sulfonylurea, and sulfonylureas can cause hemolytic anemia in these patients.
- Monitor fasting blood glucose level to determine response to glimepiride. Expect to check glycosylated hemoglobin level every 3 to 6 months to evaluate long-term blood glucose control, or as ordered.
- Expect to switch patient to insulin therapy, as prescribed, during physical stress, such as infection, surgery, and trauma.

WARNING **Expect a higher risk of hypoglycemia when giving glimepiride to a debilitated or malnourished patient or one with adrenal, hepatic, pituitary, or renal insufficiency. Also be aware that hypoglycemia may be more difficult to recognize in patients with autonomic neuropathy, the elderly, and patients taking beta blockers or other sympatholytic agents. Monitor blood glucose level closely.**

- Be aware that patients taking the sulfonylurea, tolbutamide, may have an increased risk of dying from cardiovascular disease. Glimepiride has not been studied for cardiovascular mortality, but because it is also a sulfonylurea, monitor patients closely.
- Monitor patient closely for allergic reactions that could become life-threatening. If allergic reaction occurs, stop drug immediately and notify prescriber. Provide supportive care, as ordered. Give glimepiride at least 4 hours before administering colesevelam, if prescribed, to patient because colesevelam decreases exposure to glimepiride.
- Be aware that pregnant women should discontinue glimepiride at least 2 weeks before expected delivery to prevent prolonged severe hypoglycemia in the neonate and respiratory distress.

PATIENT TEACHING

- Instruct patient to take glimepiride just before first meal of the day. Caution him not to skip the meal after taking drug.
- Urge patient not to skip doses or increase dosage without consulting prescriber.
- Urge patient to seek immediate emergency care and stop taking glimepiride if an allergic reaction occurs.
- Urge patient to report signs of hypoglycemia, such as anxiety, confusion, dizziness, excessive sweating, headache, and nausea.
- Encourage patient to carry candy or other simple sugars to treat mild hypoglycemia.
- Advise patient to consult prescriber before taking any OTC drug.
- Urge patient to carry identification indicating that he has diabetes.
- Teach patient how to monitor his blood glucose level.
- Teach patient about diet, exercise, foot care, hygiene, signs of hyperglycemia and hypoglycemia, and ways to avoid infection.

- Instruct patient to notify prescriber about darkened urine, difficulty controlling his blood glucose level, easy bruising, fever, rash, sore throat, or unusual bleeding.
- Instruct patient to avoid direct sunlight and to wear sunscreen.
- Alert patient prescribed both glimepiride and colesevelam of the need to take glimepiride 4 hours before colesevelam.
- Tell women of childbearing age to notify prescriber if pregnancy is suspected or occurs. Inform pregnant women that glimepiride will have to be discontinued at least 2 weeks before expected delivery to prevent prolonged severe hypoglycemia in the newborn.
- Have mothers who are breastfeeing while taking glimepiride monitor their infant for signs of low blood sugar, which could be severe. If present, tell the mother to seek immediate emergency treatment for the infant.

glipizide

Glucotrol, Glucotrol XL

Class and Category

Pharmacologic class: Sulfonylurea
Therapeutic class: Antidiabetic
Pregnancy category: C

Indications and Dosages

➤ *As adjunct to control blood glucose level in type 2 diabetes mellitus*

E.R. TABLETS

Adults. *Initial:* 5 mg daily with breakfast. Dosage increased, as needed, based on patient's glucose response. *Maximum:* 20 mg daily.

TABLETS

Adults. *Initial:* 5 mg 30 min before first meal of day. Dosage adjusted by 2.5 to 5 mg every 2 to 3 days and given as a single dose, if dosage is 15 mg or less or given in 2 divided doses, if dosage exceeds 15 mg daily. *Maximum:* 15 mg once daily dose; or 40 mg daily for divided doses.

➤ *As adjunct to or replacement for insulin therapy in type 2 diabetes mellitus*

CAPSULES, TABLETS

Adults who need 20 units of insulin or less. Insulin discontinued and 5 mg given once a day. Dosage adjusted, as needed, every 3 to 4 days.

Adults who need more than 20 units insulin daily. *Initial:* 5 mg daily, while insulin dosage decreased by one-half. Dosage adjusted, as needed, every 3 to 4 days and further insulin reductions are made based on clinical response.

DOSAGE ADJUSTMENT Initial dosage reduced to 2.5 mg daily if needed for patients over age 65 and those with hepatic disease.

Route	Onset	Peak	Duration
P.O.	10–30 min	30 min–2 hr	12–24 hr
P.O. (E.R.)	Unknown	Unknown	18–24 hr

Mechanism of Action

Stimulates insulin release from beta cells in pancreas. Glipizide also increases peripheral tissue sensitivity to insulin, either by increasing insulin binding to cellular receptors or by increasing number of insulin receptors.

Contraindications

Hypersensitivity to glipizide, sulfonylureas, or their components; ketoacidosis; sole therapy for type 1 diabetes mellitus

Interactions

DRUGS

ACE inhibitors, anabolic steroids, androgens, angiotensin II receptor blocking agents, azole antifungals (selected), beta blockers, bromocriptine, chloramphenicol, coumarins, disopyramide, fibric acid derivatives, fluoxetine, guanethidine, H_2-receptor antagonists, insulin and other antidiabetic drugs, magnesium salts, MAO inhibitors, methyldopa, NSAIDs, octreotide, oral anticoagulants, oxyphenbutazone, pentoxifylline, phenylbutazone, pramlintide, probenecid, propoxyphene, quinidine, quinolones, salicylates, sulfonamide antibiotics, tetracycline, theophylline, tricyclic antidepressants, urinary acidifiers, voriconazole: Increased risk of hypoglycemia

asparaginase, atypical antipsychotics, calcium channel blockers, cholestyramine, clonidine, colesevelam, corticosteroids,

danazol, diazoxide, estrogen, glucagon, hydantoins, isoniazid, lithium, morphine, niacin, nicotinic acid, oral contraceptives, phenothiazines, phenytoin, protease inhibitors, rifabutin, rifampin, somatropin, sympathomimetics, thiazides and other diuretics, thyroid drugs, urinary alkalinizers: Increased risk of hyperglycemia
beta blockers, clonidine, reserpine: Possibly hyperglycemia or hypoglycemia
digitalis glycosides: Increased risk of digitalis toxicity
miconazole (oral): Possibly severe hypoglycemia
pentamidine: Initially hypoglycemia and then hyperglycemia if beta cell damage occurs
sympatholytic drugs such as beta blockers, clonidine, guanethidine, reserpine: Possible masking of hypoglycemia signs

FOODS

all foods: Possibly delayed absorption of immediate-release tablets if taken within 30 minutes of meal

ACTIVITIES

alcohol use: Altered blood glucose control (usually hypoglycemia)

Adverse Reactions

CNS: Abnormal gait, anxiety, asthenia, chills, depression, dizziness, fatigue, headache, hypertonia, hypoesthesia, insomnia, malaise, migraine headache, nervousness, paresthesia, somnolence, syncope, tremor, vertigo
CV: **Arrhythmias**, edema, hypertension, vasculitis
EENT: Blurred vision, conjunctivitis, eye pain, pharyngitis, retinal hemorrhage, rhinitis, taste perversion, tinnitus
ENDO: **Hypoglycemia**
GI: Abdominal pain, anorexia, cholestatic jaundice, constipation, diarrhea, elevated liver, enzymes, epigastric discomfort or fullness, flatulence, heartburn, hepatic porphyria, **hepatitis**, hunger, jaundice, nausea, proctocolitis, trace blood in stool, vomiting
GU: Darkened urine, decreased libido, dysuria, polyuria
HEME: **Agranulocytosis**, **aplastic anemia**, eosinophilia, **hemolytic anemia**, **leukopenia**, **pancytopenia**
MS: Arthralgia, leg cramps, myalgia
RESP: Dyspnea
SKIN: Allergic skin reactions, diaphoresis, eczema, **erythema multiforme**, **exfoliative dermatitis**, flushing, lichenoid reactions, maculopapular or morbilliform rash, photosensitivity, urticaria
Other: Disulfiram-like reaction

Nursing Considerations

- Use cautiously in patients with glucose 6-phosphate dehydrogenase deficiency because hemolytic anemia may develop. Monitor patient's CBC closely.
- Check blood glucose level at least three times daily for a patient switching from insulin to glipizide. Patients who take more than 40 units of insulin daily may need hospitalization during transition.
- Monitor fasting blood glucose level to determine response to drug. Expect to check glycosylated hemoglobin every 3 to 6 months or as ordered to evaluate long-term blood glucose control.
- Expect to switch patient to insulin therapy, as prescribed, during physical stress, such as infection, surgery, or trauma.

WARNING Be aware that the risk of hypoglycemia is higher when giving glipizide to a debilitated or malnourished patient or one with adrenal, hepatic, pituitary, or renal insufficiency.

- Expect to have glipizide discontinued 2 weeks before expected delivery in pregnant women to prevent neonatal hypoglycemia.
- Give glipizide extended release at least 4 hours before administering colesevelam, if prescribed, to patient because colesevelam decreases exposure to glipizide.

PATIENT TEACHING

- Tell patient to take immediate-release form of glipizide 30 minutes before the first meal of the day. Tell patient prescribed the extended-release form of glipizide to take it with breakfast. Caution him not to skip the meal after taking the drug.
- Advise patient not to skip doses or increase the dosage without consulting prescriber.
- Urge patient to report evidence of hypoglycemia, such as anxiety, confusion, dizziness, excessive sweating, headache, and nausea.
- Encourage patient to carry candy or other simple sugars to treat mild hypoglycemia.

- Caution patient to consult prescriber before taking any OTC drugs.
- Urge patient to carry identification indicating that he has diabetes.
- Teach patient how to monitor his blood glucose level.
- Teach patient about diet, exercise, foot care, hygiene, signs of hyperglycemia and hypoglycemia, and ways to avoid infection.
- Instruct patient to notify prescriber if he experiences darkened urine, easy bruising, fever, hypoglycemia or hyperglycemia, rash, sore throat, and unusual bleeding.
- Instruct patient to avoid direct sunlight and to wear sunscreen.
- Alert patient prescribed both extended-release form of glipizide and colesevelam of the need to take glipizide extended-release 4 hours before colesevelam.
- Advise pregnant women that glipizide will have to be temporarily withheld for about 2 weeks before expected delivery to prevent infant hypoglycemia, which could be severe. If present, tell mother to seek immediate emergency treatment for the infant.
- Tell mothers who are breastfeeding while taking glipizide to monitor their infant for hypoglycemia.

glucagon

GlucaGen, Glucagon Diagnostic Kit, Glucagon Emergency Kit

Class and Category

Pharmacologic class: Pancreatic hormone
Therapeutic class: Antihypoglycemic, diagnostic aid adjunct
Pregnancy category: B

Indications and Dosages

➤ *To provide emergency treatment of severe hypoglycemia*

I.V., I.M., OR SUBCUTANEOUS INJECTION

Adults and children weighing more than 20 kg (44 lb) or, with GlucaGen, more than 25 kg (55 lb). 1 mg, repeated in 15 min as needed. I.V. injection administered over 1 min.
Children weighing 20 kg (44 lb) or less or, with GlucaGen, 25 kg (55 lb) or less. 0.5 mg, or 0.02 to 0.03 mg/kg, repeated in 15 min, as needed. I.V. injection administered over 1 min.

➤ *To provide diagnostic assistance by inhibiting bowel peristalsis in radiologic examination of GI tract*

I.M. INJECTION

Adults. 1 to 2 mg before procedure. Dose and timing vary with segment of GI tract examined and length of procedure.

I.V. INJECTION

Adults. 0.25 to 2 mg given over 1 min before procedure. Dose and timing vary with segment of GI tract examined and length of procedure.

Route	Onset	Peak	Duration
I.V.	5–20 min*†	Unknown	90 min*‡
I.M.	15–26 min*§	Unknown	90 min*||
SubQ	30–45 min*	Unknown	90 min*

* For antihypoglycemic action.
† 45 sec to 1 min for smooth-muscle relaxation.
‡ 9 to 25 min for smooth-muscle relaxation.
§ 4 to 10 min for smooth-muscle relaxation.
|| 12 to 32 min for smooth-muscle relaxation.

Mechanism of Action

Increases production of adenylate cyclase, which catalyzes conversion of adenosine triphosphate to cAMP, a process that in turn activates phosphorylase. Phosphorylase promotes breakdown of glycogen to glucose (glycogenolysis) in the liver. As a result, blood glucose level increases and GI smooth muscles relax.

Incompatibilities

Don't mix glucagon with sodium chloride or solutions that have a pH of 3.0 to 9.5; use with dextrose solutions instead.

Contraindications

Hypersensitivity to glucagon or its components, pheochromocytoma

Interactions

DRUGS

oral anticoagulants: Possibly increased anticoagulant effects

Adverse Reactions

CV: Hypertension, **hypotension (with hypersensitivity reaction)**, tachycardia
GI: Nausea, vomiting
RESP: Bronchospasm, respiratory distress
SKIN: Necrolytic migratory erythema, urticaria
Other: Hypersensitivity reactions

Nursing Considerations

- Rouse patient as quickly as possible because prolonged hypoglycemia can cause cerebral damage.
- For I.V. use, reconstitute 1-mg vial of glucagon with 1 ml of diluent or 10-mg vial with 10 ml of diluent. Don't give more than 1 mg/ml. For large doses, dilute with sterile water for injection.
- Place unconscious patient on his side before injecting glucagon, to prevent aspiration of vomitus when he regains consciousness.
- Administer by slow I.V. injection to decrease risk of adverse reactions, such as tachycardia and vomiting.
- Expect to give I.V. dextrose if patient doesn't respond to glucagon.
- Give oral carbohydrates when patient is conscious or diagnostic procedure is completed to restore hepatic glycogen stores and prevent secondary hypoglycemia.
- Keep in mind that glucagon isn't effective in patients with depleted hepatic glycogen stores caused by such conditions as adrenal insufficiency, chronic hypoglycemia, and starvation.
- Monitor patient for necrolytic migratory erythema, a skin rash common with glucagonomas that may present with bullae, erosions, and scaly, pruritic erythematous plaques following continuous glucagon infusion. These lesions may appear on patient's face, groin, legs, or perineum or may become more widespread. Notify prescriber and expect glucagon infusion to be discontinued, if possible. Know that treatment with corticosteroids is not effective in treating necrolytic migratory erythema.

PATIENT TEACHING

- Instruct patient to monitor blood glucose level, especially with signs of hypoglycemia.
- Teach patient and family members how to recognize signs of hypoglycemia and when to notify prescriber.
- Advise patient to carry candy or other simple sugars to treat early hypoglycemia.
- Make sure unstable diabetic patients and family members know how to give glucagon subcutaneously in case of hypoglycemia. Instruct family members to keep patient on his side and give him a carbohydrate when he awakens. Advise against giving fluids by mouth until patient is fully conscious.
- Instruct patient and family members to call for emergency medical assistance after glucagon treatment, especially if patient can't ingest oral glucose or if he's taking the sulfonylurea chlorpropamide, in case secondary hypoglycemia occurs.

glyburide
(glibenclamide)

DiaBeta, Euglucon (CAN), Glynase

Class and Category

Pharmacologic class: Sulfonylurea
Therapeutic class: Antidiabetic
Pregnancy category: C (B for Glynase PresTab and Micronase)

Indications and Dosages

➤ *As adjunct to control blood glucose level in type 2 diabetes mellitus*

MICRONIZED TABLETS

Adults. *Initial:* 1.5 to 3 mg daily with first meal of day, increased by up to 1.5 mg at weekly intervals, if needed. *Maintenance:* 0.75 to 12 mg as a single dose or in divided doses with meals.

NONMICRONIZED TABLETS

Adults. *Initial:* 2.5 to 5 mg daily with first meal of the day, increased by up to 2.5 mg at weekly intervals, if needed. *Maintenance:* 1.25 to 20 mg daily as a single dose or in divided doses with meals.

DOSAGE ADJUSTMENT For conversion from insulin to glyburide for adults who use more than 40 units of insulin daily, initial dosage adjusted to 5 mg nonmicronized or 3 mg micronized glyburide as a single dose with 50% of usual insulin dose; glyburide

dosage increased gradually, as needed. For adults who use less than 40 units but more than 20 units, glyburide started at 5 mg nonmicronized or 3 mg micronized daily as a single dose and insulin stopped. If patient is taking less than 20 units of insulin daily, usual glyburide dosage is used and insulin discontinued.
For elderly patients or patients more sensitive to hypoglycemic drugs, initial dosage possibly reduced to 1.25 mg nonmicronized glyburide daily, gradually increased by 2.5 mg/wk, as needed; or 0.75 mg micronized daily, gradually increased by 1.5 mg/wk, as needed.

Route	Onset	Peak	Duration
P.O.*	1 hr	2.3–3.5 hr	12–24 hr
P.O.†	15–60 min	1–3 hr	24 hr

* Micronized.
† Nonmicronized.

Mechanism of Action
Stimulates insulin release from beta cells in the pancreas. Glyburide also increases peripheral tissue sensitivity to insulin either by enhancing insulin binding to cellular receptors or by increasing the number of insulin receptors.

Contraindications
Concurrent therapy with bosentan; diabetic ketoacidosis; hypersensitivity to glyburide, sulfonylureas, or their components; ketoacidosis; type 1 diabetes mellitus

Interactions
DRUGS
ACE inhibitors, anabolic steroids, androgens, azole antifungals, bromocriptine, chloramphenicol, clarithromycin, disopyramide, fibric acid derivatives, fluoxetine, guanethidine, H_2-receptor antagonists, insulin, magnesium salts, MAO inhibitors, methyldopa, NSAIDs, octreotide, oral anticoagulants, oxyphenbutazone, phenylbutazone, probenecid, quinidine, quinolones, salicylates, sulfonamides, tetracycline, theophylline, tricyclic antidepressants, urinary acidifiers: Increased risk of hypoglycemia
asparaginase, calcium channel blockers, cholestyramine, clonidine, colesevelam, corticosteroids, danazol, diazoxide, estrogen, glucagon, hydantoins, isoniazid, lithium, morphine, nicotinic acid, oral contraceptives, phenothiazines, rifabutin, rifampin, sympathomimetics, thiazide diuretics, thyroid drugs, urinary alkalinizers: Increased risk of hyperglycemia
beta blockers: Possibly hyperglycemia or masking of hypoglycemia signs
bosentan: Increased risk of elevated liver enzymes
cyclosporine: Increased cyclosporine plasma level and toxicity
CYP2C9 and CYP3A4 inducers or inhibitors: Possibly altered blood glucose levels
digitalis glycosides: Increased risk of digitalis toxicity
miconazole (oral): Possibly severe hypoglycemia
oral anticoagulants: Possibly potentiated or weakened anticoagulant effects
pentamidine: Initial hypoglycemia and then hyperglycemia if beta cell damage occurs
rifampin: Decreased glyburide effectiveness
topiramate: Possibly decreased effectiveness of glyburide
FOODS
high-fat foods: Reduced bioavailability of nonmicronized glyburide
ACTIVITIES
alcohol use: Altered blood glucose control (usually hypoglycemia)

Adverse Reactions
CNS: Abnormal gait, anxiety, asthenia, chills, depression, dizziness, fatigue, headache, hypertonia, hypoesthesia, insomnia, malaise, migraine headache, nervousness, paresthesia, somnolence, syncope, tremor, vertigo
CV: **Arrhythmias**, edema, hypertension, vasculitis
EENT: Blurred vision, changes in accommodation, conjunctivitis, eye pain, pharyngitis, retinal hemorrhage, rhinitis, taste perversion, tinnitus
ENDO: **Hypoglycemia**
GI: Anorexia, constipation, cholestatic jaundice, diarrhea, elevated liver enzymes, epigastric discomfort or fullness, flatulence, heartburn, **hepatic failure** or porphyria, **hepatitis**, hunger, jaundice, nausea, proctocolitis, trace blood in stool, vomiting
GU: Decreased libido, dysuria, polyuria

HEME: **Agranulocytosis**, **aplastic anemia**, eosinophilia, **hemolytic anemia**, **leukopenia**, **pancytopenia**, purpura, **thrombocytopenia**
MS: Arthralgia, leg cramps, myalgia
RESP: Dyspnea
SKIN: Allergic skin reactions, bullous reactions, diaphoresis, eczema, erythema, **erythema multiforme**, **exfoliative dermatitis**, flushing, lichenoid reactions, maculopapular or morbilliform rash, photosensitivity, porphyria cutanea tarda, pruritus, urticaria
Other: **Angioedema**, disulfiram-like reaction, **hyponatremia**, weight gain

Nursing Considerations

- Use cautiously in patients with glucose 6-phosphate dehydrogenase deficiency because hemolytic anemia may develop. Monitor patient's CBC closely.
- Give glyburide as single dose before first meal of the day. If patient takes more than 10 mg daily or if severe GI distress occurs, give in 2 divided doses before meals.
- Monitor fasting blood glucose level to determine patient's response to glyburide. Expect to check glycosylated hemoglobin every 3 to 6 months or as ordered to evaluate long-term blood glucose control.
- Know that when patient switches from insulin to glyburide, check blood glucose level three times daily before meals.
- Be aware that micronized tablets aren't equal to nonmicronized tablets; they contain smaller particles, which affects drug bioavailability.

WARNING Expect a higher risk of hypoglycemia when giving drug to a debilitated or malnourished patient or one with adrenal, hepatic, pituitary, or renal insufficiency. Also be aware that hypoglycemia may be more difficult to recognize in patients with autonomic neuropathy, the elderly, and patients who are taking beta blockers or other sympatholytic agents. Monitor blood glucose level closely.

- Monitor patient with history of allergies to other sulfonamide derivatives closely because of increased risk of allergy to glyburide. If allergic reactions persist or worsen expect drug to be discontinued.
- Administer insulin as needed and prescribed during periods of increased stress, such as infection, surgery, and trauma.
- Arrange for diabetic teaching and consultation between patient and dietitian, if appropriate.

PATIENT TEACHING

- Instruct patient to take glyburide just before first meal of the day. Caution him not to skip the meal after taking drug.
- Advise patient not to take nonmicronized glyburide with a high-fat meal because it may reduce glyburide bioavailability.
- Caution patient to avoid skipping doses, discontinuing glyburide, or taking OTC drugs without first consulting prescriber.
- Teach patient how to monitor his blood glucose level and when to notify prescriber about changes.
- Urge patient to report signs of hypoglycemia: anxiety, confusion, dizziness, excessive sweating, headache, and nausea.
- Suggest that patient carry candy or other simple sugars to treat mild hypoglycemia.
- Urge patient to avoid alcohol because it increases the risk of hypoglycemia.
- Advise patient to carry identification indicating that he has diabetes.
- Teach patient about diet, exercise, foot care, hygiene, signs of hyperglycemia and hypoglycemia, and ways to avoid infection.
- Instruct patient to notify prescriber if he experiences easy bruising, fever, hypoglycemia or hyperglycemia, rash, sore throat, and unusual bleeding.
- If photosensitivity is a problem, instruct patient to avoid direct sunlight and to wear sunscreen.

glycopyrrolate

Cuvposa, Lonhala Magnair, Seebri Neohaler

Class and Category

Pharmacologic class: Anticholinergic
Therapeutic class: Antiarrhythmic, anticholinergic, bronchodilator, cholinergic adjunct
Pregnancy category: B

Indications and Dosages

➤ *As adjunct to treat peptic ulcer disease*

TABLETS

Adults and adolescents. 1 to 2 mg twice daily or three times daily. *Maximum:* 8 mg daily.

I.V. OR I.M. INJECTION

Adults and adolescents. 0.1 to 0.2 mg every 4 hr, as needed. *Maximum:* 3 to 4 doses daily.

➤ *To reduce gastric acid and respiratory secretions before anesthesia*

I.M. INJECTION

Adults and adolescents. 0.004 mg/kg 30 to 60 min before anesthesia or when preanesthesia sedative or opioid is given.
Children over age 2. 0.004 mg/kg 30 to 60 min before anesthesia or when preanesthesia sedative or opioid is given.
Infants age 1 month to 2 years. Up to 0.009 mg/kg 30 to 60 min before anesthesia or when preanesthesia sedative or opioid is given.

➤ *To counteract intraoperative and anesthesia-induced arrhythmias*

I.V. INJECTION

Adults and adolescents. 0.1 mg, repeated every 2 to 3 min, if needed.
Children over age 2. 0.004 mg/kg. Dose repeated every 2 to 3 min, if needed. *Maximum:* 0.1 mg as a single dose.

➤ *To reverse neuromuscular blockade due to nondepolarizing muscle relaxants*

I.V. INJECTION

Adults and children over age 2. 0.2 mg glycopyrrolate for each 1 mg neostigmine or 5 mg pyridostigmine.

➤ *To reduce chronic severe drooling in patients with neurologic conditions associated with problem drooling, such as cerebral palsy*

ORAL SOLUTION

Children ages 3 to 16. *Initial:* 0.02 mg/kg three times daily 1 hr before meals or 2 hr after meals, increased in increments of 0.02 mg/kg every 5 to 7 days, as needed and based on response and adverse reactions. *Maximum:* 0.1 mg/kg three times daily not to exceed 1.5 to 3 mg per dose based on weight of child.

➤ *To provide long-term, maintenance treatment of airflow obstruction in patients with chronic obstructive pulmonary disease, including chronic bronchitis and/or emphysema*

ORAL INHALER (SEEBRI NEOHALER)

Adults. 15.6 mcg (1 capsule) inhaled using Neohaler device twice daily, once in the morning and once in the evening.

ORAL INHALATION (LONHALA MAGNAIR)

Adults. Inhalation of the contents of one vial twice daily.

Route	Onset	Peak	Duration
P.O.	60 min	Unknown	8–12 hr
Inhaled	Immediate	5 min	Unknown
I.V.	1 min	Unknown	2–3 hr*
I.M., SubQ	15–30 min	30–45 min	2–3 hr*

* For vagal blocking effect; up to 7 hr for reduction of saliva.

Mechanism of Action

Inhibits acetylcholine's action on postganglionic muscarinic receptors throughout the body. Depending on the receptors' location, glycopyrrolate produces various effects, such as:

- reducing the volume and acidity of gastric secretions
- controlling excessive bronchial, pharyngeal, and tracheal secretions and dilating the bronchi
- inhibiting vagal stimulation of the heart
- relaxing smooth muscle in the GI, GU, and respiratory tracts.

Incompatibilities

Don't mix glycopyrrolate with alkaline drugs or solutions that have a pH over 6.0 because drug stability may be affected. A pH over 6.0 may occur if glycopyrrolate is mixed with dexamethasone sodium phosphate or LR solution. Gas or precipitate may form if glycopyrrolate is mixed in same syringe as chloramphenicol, diazepam, dimenhydrinate, methohexital sodium, pentobarbital sodium, secobarbital sodium, sodium bicarbonate, or thiopental sodium.

Contraindications

Angle-closure glaucoma; asthma; concomitant use of solid oral dosage forms of potassium chloride (Cuvposa); hemorrhage with unstable cardiovascular status; hepatic disease; hypersensitivity to glycopyrrolate; its components or other anticholinergics; ileus; intestinal atony; myasthenia gravis; obstructive GI or urinary disorders; severe ulcerative colitis; toxic megacolon

Interactions

DRUGS

anticholinergics, antiparkinsonian drugs, phenothiazines, tricyclic antidepressants: Possibly increased anticholinergic effects
antidiarrheals (adsorbent): Decreased oral glycopyrrolate absorption, leading to decreased therapeutic effectiveness
antimyasthenics: Possibly reduced intestinal motility
atenolol: Possibly potentiated atenolol effects
calcium- or magnesium-containing antacids, carbonic anhydrase inhibitors, citrates, sodium bicarbonate: Possibly reduced excretion of glycopyrrolate and increased therapeutic and adverse effects
cyclopropane: Possibly ventricular arrhythmias
digoxin: Possibly potentiated digoxin effects
haloperidol, levodopa, phenothiazines: Possibly decreased effectiveness of these drugs
ketoconazole: Possibly decreased ketoconazole absorption
metformin: Possibly potentiated metformin effects
metoclopramide: Possibly antagonized effects of metoclopramide
opioids: Possibly severe constipation and urine retention, risk of ileus
potassium chloride: Possibly increased severity of potassium chloride–induced gastric lesions

Adverse Reactions

CNS: Confusion, difficulty speaking, dizziness, drowsiness, headache, insomnia, nervousness, weakness
CV: Bradycardia (low doses), **heart block**, palpitations, **prolonged QT interval**, tachycardia (high doses)
EENT: Blurred vision, cycloplegia, dilated pupils, dry mouth, increased intraocular pressure, loss of taste, mydriasis, nasal congestion, nasopharyngitis, oropharyngeal pain, photophobia, sinusitis, taste perversion
GI: Abdominal distention, constipation, dysphagia, nausea, vomiting
GU: Impotence, urinary hesitancy, urine retention UTI
RESP: Dyspnea, **paradoxical bronchospasm**
SKIN: Decreased sweating **(heat exhaustion)**, dry skin, flushing, pruritus, rash, urticaria
Other: Anaphylaxis, **angioedema**

Nursing Considerations

- Know that inhaler and inhalation forms of glycopyrrolate should not be used in patients during acutely deteriorating or potentially life-threatening episodes of COPD nor should it be used for relief of acute symptoms.
- Use glycopyrrolate cautiously in patients with autonomic neuropathy, hepatic disease, hiatal hernia, mild to moderate ulcerative colitis, narrow-angle glaucoma, or prostatic hypertrophy because drug's anticholinergic effect can worsen these conditions; gastric ulcer because drug may delay gastric emptying; and renal disease because drug excretion may be altered.
- Give tablets 30 to 60 minutes before meals.
- Give 2-mg oral dose at bedtime to ensure overnight control of symptoms, as needed and prescribed.
- For I.V. use, administer by direct injection without diluting. Or inject into tubing of flowing I.V. solution unless it contains an alkaline drug or sodium bicarbonate.
- For inhalation purpose using Seebri Neohaler, administer capsules only in the provided neohaler device and at the same time of the day (once in the morning and once in the evening). Keep capsules in the blister container and only remove immediately before use.
- For inhalation purpose using Lonhala, know that drug should only be administered with Magnair at the same time of day. Drug vials should be kept in the foil pouch and only removed immediately before use.

WARNING **Monitor patient closely after administration for an immediate hypersensitivity reaction such as patient experiencing difficulty breathing or**

swallowing; rash; swelling of the patient's face, lips, or throat; or urticaria. Notify prescriber at once, expect drug to be discontinued, and be prepared to provide emergency supportive care, as ordered.

- Be aware that closure system contains dry natural rubber that may cause hypersensitivity reaction if handled by or used to inject someone with latex sensitivity.
- Notify prescriber if patient using inhaled form of glycopyrrolate is experiencing lack of control of respiratory symptoms exhibited by increased bronchoconstriction or patient's prescribed short-acting $beta_2$-agonist becomes less effective or patient needs to use it more as these are markers of deterioration of the patient's respiratory status indicating that glycopyrrolate may no longer be effective.
- Use continuous cardiac monitoring, as ordered, to assess patient for arrhythmias during drug administration.

WARNING Check all doses carefully because even a slight overdose can lead to toxicity.

- Adjust the room temperature and make sure patient is well hydrated to prevent overheating caused by decreased sweating.

PATIENT TEACHING

- Advise patient to take glycopyrrolate tablets 30 to 60 minutes before meals or inhaler once in the morning and once in the evening.
- Instruct patient on how to load and use prescribed inhaler. Remind patient not to remove capsule from blister until immediately before use and not to push the capsule through the foil covering. Tell patient to place capsule into capsule chamber, not the mouthpiece. After closing chamber, patient should hear a click. Then tell patient to hold the inhaler upright and then press firmly both piercing buttons at the same time. Patient should hear a click signaling need to release buttons. Stress importance of not piercing capsule more than once, not swallowing capsule, using two capsules at one time or more than two capsules daily. Once drug is inhaled, instruct patient to remove the empty capsule shell as it should never be left in the device. Show patient how to clean inhaler device.
- Instruct patient how to administer inhalation form of drug using Magnair. Remind patient that device should not be used to administer any other medication. Tell patient to store the vials in the sealed foil pouch and to open the pouch only to remove a vial immediately before use. Inform patient that unopened vials should be returned to the opened foil pouch and used at his next treatment and discarded if not used within 7 days, as the drug may be ineffective. Also tell patient not to use 2 vials at one time and not to use more than 2 vials in a day. Patient should take care when discarding the plastic vials because they pose a danger of choking to young children, due to their small size.
- Inform patient that the prescribed inhaler or inhalation form of drug is not to be used to treat acute respiratory symptoms. If patient needs to use his rescue inhaler more often or his symptoms worsen, he should notify prescriber. If acute bronchospasms occur, he should stop taking drug immediately, seek emergency medical treatment, and notify prescriber as drug needs to be discontinued.
- Instruct patient to consult prescriber before taking any OTC drugs.
- Caution patient about possible dizziness and drowsiness and need to avoid hazardous activities until drug's effects are known.
- Suggest patient to use sugarless hard candy, ice, or saliva substitute to relieve dry mouth.
- Instruct patient to avoid exertion and hot environments because he's prone to heat exhaustion while taking glycopyrrolate.
- Urge patient to drink at least eight glasses of water daily, unless contraindicated.
- Tell patient to notify prescriber about abdominal distention, eye pain, irregular heartbeat, sensitivity to light, severe constipation, or trouble breathing or urinating.
- Advise patient to wear sunglasses in bright light.
- Inform male patient that reversible impotence may occur during therapy.
- Advise patient to void before taking each dose, if urinary hesitancy occurs and to notify prescriber.

golimumab

Simponi, Simponi Aria

Class and Category

Pharmacologic class: Tumor necrosis factor (TNF) blocker
Therapeutic class: Biologic disease-modifying antirheumatic drug (DMARD)
Pregnancy category: B

Indications and Dosages

➤ *To treat active psoriatic arthritis or ankylosing spondylitis with or without methotrexate or other nonbiologic Disease Modifying Antirheumatic Drugs (DMARDs)*

SUBCUTANEOUS INJECTION (SIMPONI)
Adults. 50 mg monthly.
I.V. INFUSION (SIMPONI ARIA)
Adults. 2 mg/kg infused over 30 min at weeks 0 and 4, then every 8 wk thereafter.

➤ *To treat moderate to severe active rheumatoid arthritis in combination with methotrexate*

I.V. INFUSION (SIMPONI ARIA)
Adults. 2 mg/kg infused over 30 minutes at weeks 0 and 4, then every 8 wk thereafter.
SUBCUTANEOUS INJECTION (SIMPONI)
Adults. 50 mg monthly.

➤ *To treat moderate to severe active ulcerative colitis in patients who have demonstrated corticosteroid dependence or who have had an inadequate response to or failed to tolerate 6-mercaptopurine, azathioprine, oral aminosalicylates, or oral corticosteroid*

SUBCUTANEOUS INJECTION (SIMPONI)
Adults. *Initial:* 200 mg at week 0, followed by 100 mg at week 2. *Maintenance:* 100 mg every 4 wk.

Route	Onset	Peak	Duration
SubQ	Unknown	2–6 days	Unknown

Mechanism of Action

Binds to a cytokine protein, tumor necrosis factor-alpha (TNF-alpha), to block interaction with its receptors, which prevents biological activity of TNF-alpha. Elevated TNF-alpha levels in the blood, joints, and synovium may play an important role in pathophysiology of such inflammatory diseases as ankylosing spondylitis, psoriatic arthritis, rheumatoid arthritis, and ulcerative colitis. Reduced TNF-alpha activity in these disorders improves signs and symptoms.

Incompatibilities

Don't mix golimumab solution for intravenous infusion with other drugs, as incompatibilities are unknown.

Contraindications

Hypersensitivity to golimumab or its components

Interactions

DRUGS
abatacept, anakinra, rituximab: Possibly increased risk of serious infection
cytochrome P-450 substrates such as cyclosporine, theophylline, warfarin: Effects or blood levels of these drugs may change when golimumab therapy starts or stops
live vaccines, therapeutic infectious agents such as BCG bladder instillation for treatment of cancer: Increased risk of adverse vaccine effects
methotrexate: Decreased clearance of golimumab

Adverse Reactions

CNS: Demyelinating disorders both central and peripheral, dizziness, fever, paresthesia
CV: **Congestive heart failure**, hypertension
EENT: Nasopharyngitis, oral herpes, pharyngitis, rhinitis, sinusitis
GI: Elevated liver enzymes, nausea
HEME: **Agranulocytosis**, **aplastic anemia**, **leukemia**, **leukopenia**, **neutropenia**, **thrombocytopenia**
RESP: Bronchitis, dyspnea, **interstitial lung disease**, pneumonia, tuberculosis, upper respiratory tract infection
SKIN: Bullous skin reactions, cellulitis, **melanoma**, **Merkel cell carcinoma**, new or worsening psoriasis, pruritus, rash, skin exfoliation, urticaria
Other: Abscess; **anaphylaxis**; antibody formation; bacterial (including *Legionella* and *Listeria*), fungal (including invasive), mycobacterial, parasitic, or viral infections (including **reactivation of hepatitis B infection** in chronic carriers); injection-site

erythema; lupus-like syndrome; **malignancies such as lymphomas**; sarcoidosis; **sepsis**

Nursing Considerations

- Make sure patient has a tuberculin skin test before therapy starts. If skin test is positive, treatment of latent tuberculosis must start before golimumab therapy starts, as prescribed. Also antituberculosis therapy may be started if patient has a history of active or latent tuberculosis, if adequate therapy can't be confirmed, or if patient has a negative test for latent tuberculosis but also has risk factors for tuberculosis.

WARNING **Know that if patient has evidence of an active infection when drug is prescribed, golimumab therapy shouldn't start until infection has been treated. Monitor all patients for bacterial (including *Legionella* and *Listeria*), fungal, mycobacterial, parasitic, or viral infections during therapy, especially those receiving immunosuppressants. Know that the infection could become life-threatening and affect multiple organs. If a serious infection, an opportunistic infection, or sepsis develops, expect prescriber to stop drug and start appropriate antimicrobial therapy. Monitor patient closely for tuberculosis throughout golimumab therapy because active tuberculosis has occurred in patients during and after treatment of latent tuberculosis.**

- Know that patients with a history of cancer, except those successfully treated for nonmelanoma skin cancer, should be thoroughly evaluated before golimumab therapy starts because treatment may pose more risks than benefits. Patients with rheumatoid arthritis may have a higher risk than the general population for developing leukemia while taking a TNF blocker such as golimumab.
- Use golimumab cautiously in patients with congestive heart failure, demyelinating disorders such as multiple sclerosis, and hematologic cytopenias because these disorders may develop or become worse with golimumab therapy.
- Use golimumab cautiously in patients with recurrent infection or increased risk of infection, patients who live in regions where histoplasmosis and tuberculosis are endemic, and patients with a history of hepatitis B infection because drug increases risk of infection.
- Be aware that needle cover of syringe used for subcutaneous injection contains dry rubber and should not be handled by anyone with a latex allergy.
- Take golimumab out of the refrigerator 30 minutes before giving subcutaneous injection to allow time for drug to warm up to room temperature. Never warm drug in any other way. Rotate subcutaneous injection sites. If more than one subcutaneous injection is required, administer the injections at different sites on the body.
- Know that each 4-ml vial used for intravenous infusion contains 50 mg of golimumab. Dilute the total volume of the drug solution with normal saline or half normal saline for intravenous infusion for a final volume of 100 ml. Gently mix. Discard any unused solution remaining in the vials. Use within 4 hours, keeping diluted solution at room temperature.
- Inspect diluted solution for intravenous infusion-prior to infusion for particulate matter or discoloration. Do not use if present. Use only an infusion set with an in-line, low protein-binding, nonpyrogenic, sterile filter (pore size 0.22 micrometer or less). Do not infuse concomitantly in the same intravenous line with other drugs. Infuse the diluted solution over 30 minutes.
- Monitor patient, especially young adult males, for signs and symptoms of malignancies. Although lymphomas account for about half of all malignancies associated with golimumab therapy, leukemia and rare malignancies, including melanomas and Merkel cell carcinoma, have also occurred. Report any persistent or unusual signs and symptoms to prescriber.

PATIENT TEACHING

- Explain that first injection of golimumab must be administered with a healthcare professional present.
- Teach patient or caregiver how to give golimumab as a subcutaneous injection at home, if applicable. Tell him to let prefilled syringe or autoinjector sit at room temperature outside carton for 30 minutes before injecting. Tell him not

to warm drug in any other way and not to remove needle cover or cap while letting golimumab warm up.

- Teach patient using autoinjector not to pull the device away from his skin until he hears a first "click" and then a second "click" indicating the injection is finished. It may take up to 15 seconds before second click is heard and, if device is pulled away from the skin before the second click, a full dose may not have been given.
- Emphasize need to inject full amount in prefilled syringe to obtain correct dose. Instruct patient to discard any drug left in prefilled syringe or autoinjector.
- Tell patient requiring multiple injections to administer the injections at different sites on the body.
- Alert patient that needle cover contains natural dry rubber and should not be handled by anyone with a latex allergy.
- Instruct patient or caregiver to use a puncture-resistant container to dispose of needles and syringes at home.
- Inform patient that drug must be refrigerated (not frozen).
- Urge patient to check expiration dates and not to use outdated drug.
- Teach patient to rotate injection sites and never to give injection into an area where skin bruised, hard, red or is tender.
- Explain that tuberculosis may occur during golimumab therapy. Instruct him to report low-grade fever, persistent cough, and wasting or weight loss, to prescriber.
- Teach patient how to recognize evidence of bleeding disorders and infection and to tell prescriber if they occur; drug may need to be stopped. Advise patient to avoid people with infections and to have all prescribed laboratory tests performed.
- Inform patient that golimumab therapy increases the risk of certain kinds of cancer, especially leukemias and lymphomas. Emphasize the importance of having follow-up visits and reporting unusual or sudden onset of signs or symptoms. Also, encourage patient to have regular skin examinations, as melanomas and Merkel cell carcinoma have occurred with golimumab therapy.
- Caution against receiving live-virus vaccines while taking golimumab; doing so may adversely affect the immune system.
- Tell patient to report lupus-like signs and symptoms that, although rare, may occur during therapy, such as chest pain that doesn't go away, joint pain, a rash on arms or cheeks that's sensitive to the sun or shortness of breath. Explain that drug may need to be discontinued if these occur.
- Advise patient to tell all healthcare providers about golimumab therapy and to tell prescriber about any OTC drugs, herbal remedies, and mineral and vitamin supplements being taken.
- Tell women of childbearing age to notify prescriber if pregnancy is suspected or known. This is because golimumab does cross the placenta during pregnancy and may increase the risk of infection for the neonate even up to 6 months after birth.
- Inform mothers who received golimumab therapy during pregnancy to monitor their infant for infections and not to have their infant receive live vaccines for 6 months following the mother's last golimumab dose during the pregnancy.
- Inform mothers wishing to breastfeed their infant to discuss this with prescriber before doing so.

granisetron

Sancuso, Sustol

granisetron hydrochloride

Class and Category

Pharmacologic class: Serotonin blocker (5-HT_3 receptor antagonist)
Therapeutic class: Antiemetic
Pregnancy category: B

Indications and Dosages

➤ *To prevent nausea and vomiting caused by chemotherapy*

ORAL SOLUTION, TABLETS

Adults and adolescents. 1 mg up to 1 hr before chemotherapy, repeated 12 hr later. Or, 2 mg up to 1 hr before chemotherapy.

I.V. INFUSION, I.V. INJECTION

Adults and children ages 2 and over. 10 mcg/kg diluted and infused over 5 min, starting 30 min before chemotherapy; or 10 mcg/kg undiluted and given over 30 sec, starting 30 min before chemotherapy.

TRANSDERMAL (SANCUSO)

Adults. 3.1 mg/24 hr patch applied to upper outer arm 24 to 48 hr before chemotherapy and worn up to 7 days. Patch removed no sooner than 24 hr after chemotherapy is completed.

➤ *As adjunct with other antiemetics to prevent acute and delayed nausea and vomiting associated with initial and repeat course of moderately emetogenic chemotherapy or anthracycline and cyclophosphamide combination chemotherapy regimens*

SUBCUTANEOUS INJECTION (SUSTOL)

Adults. 10 mg in combination with dexamethasone at least 30 min before chemotherapy on day 1. *Maximum:* 10 mg once every 7 days.

DOSAGE ADJUSTMENT For patients with a creatinine clearance of between 30 to 59 ml/min, Sustol brand dosage interval increased to once every 14 days.

➤ *To prevent nausea and vomiting caused by radiation therapy, including fractionated abdominal radiation and total body irradiation*

ORAL SOLUTION, TABLETS

Adults and adolescents. 2 mg daily given 1 hr before radiation therapy.

➤ *To prevent or treat postoperative nausea and vomiting*

I.V. INJECTION

Adults and adolescents. 1 mg undiluted given over 30 sec before induction of anesthesia or immediately before reversal anesthesia for prevention. 1 mg administered over 30 sec after surgery for treatment.

Mechanism of Action

Has a high affinity for serotonin receptors along vagal nerve endings in intestines. Because of this affinity, granisetron prevents nausea and vomiting that usually result when serotonin is released by damaged enterochromaffin cells.

Incompatibilities

Don't mix granisetron in same solution as other drugs.

Contraindications

Hypersensitivity to granisetron, its components, or any other 5-HT_3 receptor antagonists

Interactions

DRUGS

drugs that prolong the QT interval: Increased risk of QT-interval prolongation

Adverse Reactions

CNS: Asthenia, chills, CNS stimulation, drowsiness, fever, headache, insomnia, **serotonin syndrome**, somnolence

CV: **Bradycardia**, chest pain, hypertension, palpitations, **prolonged QT interval**, **sick sinus syndrome**

EENT: Taste perversion

GI: Abdominal pain, anorexia, constipation, diarrhea, elevated liver enzymes, gastric distention, nausea, progressive ileus, vomiting

HEME: Anemia, **leukopenia**, **thrombocytopenia**

SKIN: Alopecia, reactions at patch application site (burn, discoloration, irritation, pruritus, rash, redness, vesicles, urticaria)

Other: **Anaphylaxis**; subcutaneous injection-site reactions such as bleeding, bruising, hematomas, infections, nodules, pain, or tenderness

Nursing Considerations

- Use cautiously in patients with arrhythmias or cardiac conduction disorders because granisetron may prolong QT interval. Patients especially at risk include those with cardiac disease or electrolyte abnormalities and those receiving cardiotoxic chemotherapy or therapy with another drug that prolongs QT interval.
- For use with chemotherapy, know that drug prescribed for intravenous administration may be given diluted or undiluted. Dilute I.V. preparation of granisetron with normal saline solution or D_5W to total volume of 20 to 50 ml. Mixture may be stored up to 24 hours. Use only on days when chemotherapy is given.
- Apply transdermal patch to patient's upper outer arm 24 to 48 hours before chemotherapy, and don't remove it until at

least 24 hours after chemotherapy is completed.

- Know that the brand, Sustol, is the only granisetron that can be administered subcutaneously and comes as a refrigerated kit. Do not substitute nonkit components for any of the components from the kit. Remove kit at least 60 minutes prior to administration. Unpack the kit to allow the syringe containing the drug as well as all other contents to warm to room temperature. Activate one of the syringe warming pouches, and wrap the warming pouch around the syringe containing the drug for 5 to 6 minutes. Inspect the syringe containing the drug prior to administration for particulate matter and discoloration. Know that the syringe is amber-colored glass. Do not use if particulate matter or discoloration is seen, the tip cap is missing or has been tampered with, or if the Luer fitting is missing or dislodged.
- To administer granisetron (Sustol brand) subcutaneously, inject into abdomen at least one inch away from the umbilicus or into the back of the upper arm. Avoid injecting drug into areas that are burned, hardened, inflamed, swollen, or otherwise compromised. A topical anesthetic may be applied to the injection site prior to administration. Inject as a slow, sustained injection that may take up to 30 seconds. Know that pressing the plunger harder will not expel the drug faster.
- Be prepared to administer dexamethasone when giving granisetron subcutaneously (Sustol brand). For patients who are receiving moderately emetogenic chemotherapy, expect to administer 8 mg of dexamethasone intravenously on day 1. For patients receiving anthracycline and cyclophosphamide combination chemotherapy, expect to give 20 mg of dexamethasone intravenously on day 1, followed by 8 mg of dexamethasone twice a day on days 2, 3, and 4.
- Be aware that if Sustol brand is used with an NK_1 receptor antagonist, the dosage for dexamethasone may be different. Check the prescribing information for the NK_1 receptor antagonist for recommended dexamethasone dosage.
- Assess patient receiving subcutaneous granisetron for injection-site reactions following administration. Know that some of the reactions, such as bruising, hematoma, and infection, may develop up to 2 weeks or more after the injection. Monitor patients receiving anticogulants or antiplatelet agents closely, as bruising or hematoma formation may be more severe. When administering drug again and an injection-site reaction is still present from a previous injection, administer the drug at a site away from the affected area.

WARNING **Monitor patient for serotonin syndrome, characterized by agitation, chills, confusion, diaphoresis, diarrhea, fever, hyperactive reflexes, poor coordination, restlessness, shaking, talking tremor, twitching or uncontrolled excitement behavior.**

- Monitor patient for hypersensitivity reactions. Know that because the Sustol brand has extended-release properties, a reaction may not occur until 7 days or longer following administration and may take longer to resolve.
- Monitor patient for persistent or severe gastrointestinal effects such as constipation, gastric distention, or progressive ileus that may become severe and require hospitalization. Monitor patient closely, especially if patient is also receiving opioid medications. Consult with prescriber about using a bowel regimen, if needed. Know that the drug may mask gastric distention and/or a progressive ileus, especially in patients with recent abdominal surgery. Assess patient for decreased bowel sounds regularly.

PATIENT TEACHING

- Inform patient that granisetron is given I.V., orally, subcutaneously, or by patch before chemotherapy to help prevent nausea.
- Instruct patient to take granisetron tablet without food to avoid reducing drug bioavailability.
- Review signs and symptoms of an allergic reaction. Tell patient to seek immediate emergency care if present. Inform patient receiving drug subcutaneously to watch for allergic reactions for 7 days or longer because drug may be present in his body for up to 7 days following administration.

- Inform patient receiving drug subcutaneously about possible injection-site reactions that can occur and that these reactions may occur up to 2 weeks or more after the injection. Instruct patient to seek immediate medical care if bleeding occurs and is severe or lasts for longer than one day or the site looks infected. Tell him to notify prescriber if he experiences bruising, hematoma, persistent nodule at the injection site, or pain or tenderness severe enough to interfere with activities of daily living or for him to take pain medication.
- Advise patient to report constipation, fever, severe diarrhea, or severe headache. Also caution about possible drowsiness.
- Advise patient wearing granisetron patch to cover it with clothing if there's a risk of exposure to sunlight. Tell patient to continue covering application site with clothing for 10 days after removal of patch. Also, tell patient not to put a heating pad over or in vicinity of the patch.

WARNING **Instruct patient to seek immediate medical attention if the following symptoms occur: autonomic instability, changes in mental status, or neuromuscular symptoms, with or without gastrointestinal symptoms.**

guaifenesin

Balminil Expectorant (CAN), Benylin-E (CAN), Calmylin Expectorant (CAN), Guiatuss, Mucinex, Organidin NR, Robitussin, Scot-tussin Expectorant

Class and Category

Pharmacologic class: Glyceryl guaiacolate
Therapeutic class: Expectorant
Pregnancy category: C

Indications and Dosages

➤ *To relieve cough, especially when secretions are thick*

CAPSULES, ORAL SOLUTION, SYRUP, TABLETS

Adults and adolescents. 100 to 400 mg every 4 hr. *Maximum:* 2,400 mg daily.

CAPSULES, ORAL SOLUTION, SYRUP

Children ages 6 to 12. 100 to 200 mg every 4 hr. *Maximum:* 1,200 mg daily.
Children ages 2 to 6. 50 to 100 mg every 4 hr. *Maximum:* 600 mg daily.
Children age 6 months to 2 years. 25 to 50 mg every 4 hr. *Maximum:* 300 mg daily.

➤ *To promote productive cough*

E.R. TABLETS (MUCINEX)

Adults and adolescents. 600 to 1,200 mg every 12 hr. *Maximum:* 2,400 mg daily.

Route	Onset	Peak	Duration
P.O.	30 min	Unknown	4–6 hr

Mechanism of Action

Increases fluid and mucus removal from the upper respiratory tract by increasing the volume of secretions and reducing their adhesiveness and surface tension.

Contraindications

Hypersensitivity to guaifenesin or its components

Adverse Reactions

CNS: Dizziness, headache
GI: Nausea and vomiting (with large doses)
SKIN: Rash, urticaria

Nursing Considerations

- Give liquid forms of guaifenesin to children, as prescribed and as appropriate.
- Watch for evidence of more serious condition, such as cough that lasts longer than 1 week, fever, persistent headache, and rash.

PATIENT TEACHING

- Instruct patient to take each dose with a full glass of water.
- Advise patient not to break, chew, or crush E.R. tablets but to swallow them whole.
- Tell patient to increase fluid intake (unless contraindicated) to help thin secretions.
- Advise patient not to take drug longer than 1 week and to notify prescriber about fever, persistent headache, or rash.

guanfacine hydrochloride

Intuniv, Tenex

Class and Category

Pharmacologic class: Central $alpha_{2A}$ adrenergic receptor agonist

Therapeutic class: Antihypertensive
Pregnancy category: B

Indications and Dosages

➤ *To manage hypertension, alone or with other antihypertensives*

TABLETS (TENEX)

Adults. 1 mg daily at bedtime, increased as needed to 2 mg after 3 to 4 wk. Increased to 3 mg if needed after another 3 to 4 wk. *Maintenance:* 2 or 3 mg daily.

➤ *To treat attention deficit hyperactivity disorder (ADHD); adjunct therapy with stimulant medications*

E.R. TABLETS (INTUNIV)

Adults and children age 6 and over. *Initial:* 1 mg once daily, increased, as needed, by 1 mg/wk. *Maintenance:* 1 to 4 mg once daily. *Maximum:* 4 mg once daily.

Route	Onset	Peak	Duration
P.O.	Unknown*	8–12 hr†	24 hr

* For single dose; in 1 wk for multiple doses.
† For single dose; 1 to 3 mo for multiple doses.

Mechanism of Action

Decreases sympathetic nerve impulse outflow from the vasomotor center of the brain to the heart and blood vessels by stimulating central alpha$_2$-adrenergic receptors. This action reduces blood pressure, heart rate, peripheral vascular resistance, and renovascular resistance. Prolonged guanfacine use may reduce total peripheral vascular resistance, slightly reducing heart rate. Guanfacine also stimulates growth hormone secretion, reduces circulating plasma catecholamine levels, and reduces left ventricular hypertrophy. In addition, it enhances prefrontal cortical regulation of attention and impulse control by strengthening prefrontal cortex function.

Contraindications

Hypersensitivity to guanfacine or its components

Interactions

DRUGS

CNS depressants: Possibly increased CNS depression
ketoconazole and other strong CYP3A4/5 inhibitors: Increased plasma guanfacine level and increased risk of bradycardia, hypotension, and sedation
NSAIDs, sympathomimetics, tricyclic antidepressants: Possibly decreased antihypertensive effect of guanfacine
other antihypertensives: Possibly increased antihypertensive effect, resulting in hypotension
rifampin and other CYP3A4 inducers: Decreased plasma guanfacine level and effectiveness
valproic acid: Increased plasma valproic acid level

ACTIVITIES

alcohol use: Possibly increased CNS depression

Adverse Reactions

CNS: Anxiety, asthenia, confusion, depression, dizziness, drowsiness, fatigue, hallucinations (children), headache, irritability, lethargy, nervousness, sedation, **seizures**, somnolence, syncope, weakness
CV: Atrioventricular block, **bradycardia**, chest pain, hypertension, orthostatic hypotension, sinus arrhythmia
EENT: Conjunctivitis, dry mouth
GI: Abdominal pain, constipation, dyspepsia, elevated liver enzymes, nausea, vomiting
GU: Decreased libido, enuresis, **erectile dysfunction**, urinary frequency
RESP: Asthma
SKIN: Dermatitis, diaphoresis, pallor, pruritus, purpura, rash
Other: Increased weight

Nursing Considerations

- Use guanfacine cautiously in patients with cerebrovascular disease, chronic hepatic or renal failure, recent MI, or severe coronary insufficiency.
- Give drug at bedtime to minimize daytime sedation.
- Know that immediate-release guanfacine tablets may not be substituted on a milligram-per-milligram basis with the extended-release tablets, because of differing pharmacokinetic profiles.

WARNING **Expect to stop hypertension treatment by decreasing dosage gradually over 2 to 4 days. Typically, if patient hasn't taken drug for 2 or more days, he may have withdrawal symptoms, including abdominal cramps, anxiety, chest pain, diaphoresis, headache, increased**

salivation, insomnia, irregular heart rate and rhythm, nausea, nervousness, restlessness, tremor, and vomiting.
- Know that for patients being treated for ADHD, expect to taper dosage gradually over 3 to 7 days by no more than 1 mg every 3 to 7 days to prevent rebound hypertension and possibly hypertensive encephalopathy.
- Monitor patient for depression. If you suspect that patient has drug-related depression, notify prescriber immediately and expect to discontinue drug.

PATIENT TEACHING
- Instruct patient to take guanfacine at bedtime to reduce daytime drowsiness.
- Tell patient not to break, chew, or crush extended-release tablets before swallowing. Tell patient to swallow tablet whole with milk, water, or other beverages. Remind patient not to take drug with a high-fat meal.
- Caution patient about possible drowsiness, and advise him to avoid hazardous activities until drug's CNS effects are known.
- Urge patient to avoid consuming alcohol and other CNS depressants while taking guanfacine.
- Advise patient to report rash.
- Inform male patient that guanfacine may cause erectile dysfunction. If erectile dysfunction occurs, suggest patient discuss problem with prescriber.
- Caution patient not to stop taking drug abruptly because doing so can cause a dangerous rise in blood pressure along with anxiety and nervousness. Tell patient that if he experiences feeling very sleepy or tired, or develops seizures, severe headache, vision problems, or vomiting, to seek emergency medical care immediately.
- Advise patient to avoid becoming dehydrated or overheated.

guselkumab

Tremfya

Class and Category

Pharmacologic class: Monoclonal antibody
Therapeutic class: Antipsoriatic
Pregnancy category: Not classified

Indications and Dosages

➤ *To treat moderate to severe plaque psoriasis in patients who are candidates for systemic therapy or phototherapy*

SUBCUTANEOUS INJECTION
Adults. 100 mg at wk 0, wk 4, and every 8 wks thereafter.

Mechanism of Action

Selectively binds to the p19 subunit of interleukin 23 (IL-23) and inhibits its interaction with the IL-23 receptor, which prevents the release of proinflammatory chemokines and cytokines.

Contraindications

Hypersensitivity to guselkumab or its components

Interactions

DRUGS
CYP450 substrates: Possibly decreased effectiveness of these drugs
live vaccines: Possible decreased response to vaccine

Adverse Reactions

CNS: Headache, migraine
EENT: Nasopharyngitis, oral herpes, pharyngitis
GI: Diarrhea, elevated liver enzymes, gastroenteritis
GU: Genital herpes
MS: Arthralgia
RESP: Upper respiratory infections
SKIN: Tinea infections, urticaria
Other: Antibody formation to guselkumab; candida infections; herpes simplex infections; injection-site reactions of bruising, discoloration, edema, erythema, hematoma, hemorrhage, induration, inflammation, pain, pruritus, swelling, urticaria

Nursing Considerations

- Assess patient for tuberculosis before guselkumab therapy is begun. Expect treatment for latent tuberculosis to be given prior to starting guselkumab therapy.
- Remove prefilled syringe from refrigerator and allow to warm to room temperature before administering drug. Do not inject into any area that is bruised, hard, red, scaly, tender, thick, or affected by psoriasis.
- Know that all age-appropriate immunizations should be done before guselkumab therapy begins.

- Monitor patient for infections, as guselkumab increases risk. Institute infection precautions. Be aware that if infection occurs and is severe or does not respond to appropriate treatment, guselkumab will probably be discontinued.

PATIENT TEACHING

- Instruct patient on how to administer a subcutaneous injection. Tell patient to remove prefilled syringe from refrigerator and allow to warm to room temperature, keeping needle cap in place until ready to administer the injection. Tell him to inject the full amount of solution in the prefilled syringe. Warn patient not to inject into an area where the skin is bruised, hard, scaly, tender, thick, or affected by psoriasis.
- Review how to properly dispose of used needles and syringes.
- Tell patient to take a missed dose as soon as he remembers and then take the next dose at the scheduled time.
- Review infection prevention practices with patient. Emphasize importance of notifying prescriber if an infection should occur.

haloperidol

Apo-Haloperidol (CAN), Haldol, Novo-Peridol (CAN), Peridol (CAN)

haloperidol decanoate

Haldol Decanoate, Haldol LA (CAN)

haloperidol lactate

Haldol Concentrate

Class and Category

Pharmacologic class: Butyrophenone derivative
Therapeutic class: Antipsychotic
Pregnancy category: C (haloperidol decanoate), not classified (haloperidol, haloperidol lactate)

Indications and Dosages

➤ *To treat psychotic disorders*

ORAL SOLUTION, TABLETS

Adults and adolescents. 0.5 to 5 mg twice daily or three times daily depending on severity of disorder. *Maximum:* Usually 30 mg daily.
Children ages 3 to 12 weighing 15 kg (33 lb) to 40 kg (88 lb). 0.25 to 0.5 mg daily in divided doses twice daily or three times daily. Increased by 0.5 mg every 5 to 7 days, as needed. *Maintenance:* 0.05 to 0.15 mg/kg/day given in 2 to 3 divided doses.
DOSAGE ADJUSTMENT For debilitated or elderly patients, initial dosage reduced to 0.5 to 2 mg twice daily or three times daily, as needed.

➤ *To treat nonpsychotic behavior disorders*

Children ages 3 to 12 weighing 15 kg (33 lb) to 40 kg (88 lb). 0.5 mg daily in divided doses twice daily or three times daily. Increased by 0.5 mg every 5 to 7 days, if needed. *Maintenance:* 0.05 to 0.075 mg/kg daily divided into two or three doses.

➤ *To treat Tourette's syndrome*

ORAL SOLUTION, TABLETS

Adults and adolescents. *Initial:* 0.5 to 2 mg every 8 to 12 hr. Increased to 3 to 5 mg every 8 to 12 hr, if needed. *Maximum:* 100 mg daily in divided doses.
Children ages 3 to 12. *Initial:* 0.5 mg daily, increased by 0.5 mg every 5 to 7 days, as needed. *Maintenance:* 0.05 to 0.075 mg/kg daily divided into 2 or 3 doses.

➤ *To treat acute psychotic episodes*

PROMPT-ACTING I.M. INJECTION

Adults and adolescents. *Initial:* 2 to 5 mg, with subsequent doses up to every 60 min. Or, if symptoms are controlled, dose may be repeated every 4 to 8 hr. First oral dose may be given 12 to 24 hr after last parenteral dose. *Maximum:* 20 mg daily.

➤ *To provide long-term antipsychotic therapy for patients who require parenteral therapy*

LONG-ACTING I.M. (DECANOATE) INJECTION

Adults. *Initial:* 10 to 20 times the daily oral dose up to 100 mg. Repeated every 4 wk. *Maximum:* Initial dose should not exceed 100 mg. If conversion requires more than 100 mg as an initial dose, dose should be administered in 2 injections, the first at the maximum of 100 mg, followed by the balance in 3 to 7 days.
DOSAGE ADJUSTMENT Patients who are debilitated or elderly or who are stable on low doses of oral haloperidol (up to 10 mg/day), a range of 10 to 15 times the

previous daily dose in oral equivalents used for initial conversion.

Route	Onset	Peak	Duration
I.M.*	Unknown	3–4 days†	Unknown

* For haloperidol decanoate and lactate.
† For haloperidol decanoate only; 30 to 45 min for haloperidol lactate.

Mechanism of Action

May block postsynaptic dopamine receptors in the limbic system and increase brain turnover of dopamine, producing an antipsychotic effect.

Contraindications

Hypersensitivity to haloperidol or its components, Parkinson's disease, severe toxic CNS comatose states or depression

Interactions

DRUGS

alprazolam, buspirone, chlorpromazine, fluoxetine, fluvoxamine, itraconazole, nefazodone, promethazine, quinidine, sertraline, venlafaxine: Increased plasma haloperidol concentrations
amphetamines: Possibly decreased stimulant effects of amphetamines and decreased antipsychotic effect of haloperidol
anticholinergics, antidyskinetics, antihistamines: Increased anticholinergic effect and risk of decreased antipsychotic effect of haloperidol
anticonvulsants: Possibly decreased effectiveness of anticonvulsants and decreased blood haloperidol level
bromocriptine: Possibly decreased effectiveness of bromocriptine
bupropion: Lowered seizure threshold, increased risk of major motor seizure
carbamazepine, rifampin: Decreased plasma haloperidol levels
CNS depressants: Increased CNS depression and risk of respiratory depression and hypotension
diazoxide: Possibly hypoglycemia
dopamine (high-dose therapy): Possibly decreased vasoconstriction
ephedrine: Possibly decreased vasopressor effect of ephedrine
epinephrine: Possibly severe hypotension and tachycardia
fluoxetine: Increased risk of frequent and severe extrapyramidal effects
guanadrel, guanethidine: Decreased hypotensive effects of these drugs
ketoconazole, paroxetine: Possibly increased QT interval
levodopa, pergolide: Possibly decreased therapeutic effects of these drugs
lithium: Increased risk of neurotoxicity
MAO inhibitors, maprotiline, tricyclic antidepressants: Increased anticholinergic and sedative effects of these drugs
metaraminol: Possibly decreased vasopressor effect of metaraminol
methoxamine: Decreased vasopressor effect, shortened duration of methoxamine action
methyldopa: Possibly disorientation, difficult or slowed thought processes
phenylephrine: Decreased vasopressor response to phenylephrine

ACTIVITIES

alcohol use: Increased CNS depression and risk of hypotension and respiratory depression

Adverse Reactions

CNS: Agitation, anxiety, confusion, depression, dizziness, drowsiness, dystonia, euphoria, extrapyramidal reactions that may be irreversible, **hypothermia**, insomnia, **neuroleptic malignant syndrome**, opisthotonus, Parkinsonism, restlessness, **seizures**, slurred speech, somnolence, tremor, vertigo
CV: Cardiac arrest, edema, **extrasystoles**, hypertension, hypertensive vasculitis, orthostatic hypotension, **QT-interval prolongation**, **ventricular arrhythmias**, tachycardia, **torsades de pointes**
EENT: Blurred vision, dry mouth, increased salivation (all drug forms), **laryngeal edema**, **laryngospasm**, nystagmus, oculogyric crisis, stomatitis (oral solution)
ENDO: Breast discomfort and engorgement, galactorrhea, gynecomastia, hyperprolactinemia, inappropriate antidiuretic hormone secretion
GI: Acute hepatic failure, cholestasis, constipation, elevated liver enzymes, **hepatitis**, jaundice, nausea, vomiting

GU: Decreased or loss of libido, difficult ejaculation, impotence, menstrual irregularities, priapism, urinary retention
HEME: **Agranulocytosis**, anemia, leukocytosis, **leukopenia**, **neutropenia**, **pancytopenia**, **thrombocytopenia**
MS: Muscle rigidity or twitching, **rhabdomyolysis**, torticollis, trismus
RESP: **Bronchospasm**, dyspnea
SKIN: Acneiform skin reactions, diaphoresis, **exfoliative dermatitis**, photosensitivity, pruritis, rash, urticaria
Other: **Anaphylaxis**, **angioedema**, **heatstroke**, **hypersensitivity reactions**, weight gain or loss

Nursing Considerations

- Be aware that haloperidol shouldn't be used to treat dementia-related psychosis in the elderly because of an increased mortality risk.
- Use haloperidol cautiously in patients with a history of prolonged QT interval, patients with uncorrected electrolyte disturbances, and patients receiving Class IA or III antiarrhythmics because of an increased risk of prolonged QT interval. Monitor elderly patients closely because they may have an increased risk of prolonged QT interval.
- Dilute oral solution with a beverage, such as apple, orange, or tomato juice or cola.
- Give haloperidol decanoate (long-acting form) by deep I.M. injection into gluteal muscle using Z-track technique and 21G needle. Don't give more than 3 ml per site. Expect to reach stable plasma level after third or fourth dose.
- Know that if injection solution has a slight yellow discoloration this change doesn't affect potency.
- Assess patient for fall risks, such those who are elderly and those with conditions or diseases, or taking drugs that exacerbate central nervous system adverse effects such as motor instability, orthostatic hypotension, and somnolence. Use fall precautions in patients at risk.
- Watch for tardive dyskinesia (potentially irreversible involuntary movements) in patients receiving long-term therapy, especially elderly women who take large doses.
- Monitor CBC, especially if patient has a low WBC count or history of drug-induced leukopenia or neutropenia, often during the first few months of therapy, as ordered. If WBC count drops, especially if neutrophil count drops below 1,000/mm^3, expect haloperidol to be discontinued. If neutropenia is significant, also monitor patient for fever or other symptoms of infection and provide appropriate treatment, as prescribed.
- Know that if extrapyramidal reactions occur during the first few days of treatment, dosage should be reduced as prescribed. If symptoms persist, drug may be discontinued. Dystonia also may occur during first few days of treatment, especially in patients receiving higher doses and in males and younger age-groups. Notify prescriber.
- Avoid stopping haloperidol abruptly unless severe adverse reactions occur.
- Monitor for signs of neuroleptic malignant syndrome, a rare but possibly fatal disorder linked to antipsychotic drugs. Signs include altered mental status, arrhythmias, fever, and muscle rigidity.

WARNING Know that QT-interval prolongation, sudden death, and torsades de pointes, although uncommon, may occur in patients receiving haloperidol despite the lack of such predisposing factors.

PATIENT TEACHING

- Advise patient to take haloperidol exactly as prescribed and not to stop abruptly because withdrawal symptoms may occur.
- Instruct patient to dilute liquid form with cola or juice before taking it to prevent oral mucosal irritation.
- Caution patient to avoid skin contact with oral solution because it may cause a rash.
- Advise patient to take tablets with food or a full glass of milk or water to reduce GI distress.
- Instruct patient to consume adequate fluids and to take precautions against heatstroke.
- Urge patient not to drink alcohol during therapy.
- Caution patient to avoid driving and other hazardous activities if sedation occurs. Also warn patient to take measures to avoid falls because of adverse effects.
- Instruct patient to report repetitive movements, tremor, and vision changes.

heparin sodium

Hepalean (CAN), Heparin Leo (CAN), Heparin Lock Flush, Heparin Sodium Injection

Class and Category

Pharmacologic class: Anticoagulant
Therapeutic class: Anticoagulant
Pregnancy category: C

Indications and Dosages

➤ *To prevent and treat peripheral arterial embolism, pulmonary embolism, thromboembolic complications associated with atrial fibrillation, and venous thrombosis and its extension*

FULL-DOSE I.V. INJECTION, FULL-DOSE I.V. INFUSION

Adults receiving continuous intravenous therapy. *Loading:* 5,000 units by I.V. injection followed by 20,000 to 40,000 units infused per 24 hr.
Children. *Loading:* 50 to 100 units/kg by I.V. injection followed by infusion of 18 to 20 units/kg/hr.
Infants ages 2 months and over. *Loading:* Highly individualized followed by infusion of 25 to 30 units/kg/hr.
Infants less than 2 months. *Loading:* Highly individualized followed by individualized infusion with average of 28 units/kg/hr.
Adults receiving intermittent intravenous therapy. *Loading:* 10,000 units followed by 5,000 to 10,000 units every 4 to 6 hr.

FULL-DOSE SUBCUTANEOUS INJECTION

Adults. *Loading:* 333 units/kg followed by 250 units/kg every 12 hr.

➤ *To diagnose and treat disseminated intravascular coagulation (DIC)*

I.V. INFUSION OR INJECTION

Adults. 50 to 100 units/kg every 4 hr. Drug may be discontinued if no improvement occurs in 4 to 8 hr.
Children. 25 to 50 units/kg every 4 hr. Drug may be discontinued if no improvement occurs in 4 to 8 hr.

➤ *To prevent postoperative thromboembolism*

LOW-DOSE SUBCUTANEOUS INJECTION

Adults. 5,000 units 2 hr before surgery and then 5,000 units every 8 to 12 hr for 7 days or until patient is fully ambulatory.

➤ *To prevent clots in patients undergoing cardiovascular surgery*

I.V. INFUSION OR INJECTION

Adults. 300 units/kg for procedures that last less than 60 min; 400 units/kg for procedures that last longer than 60 min. *Minimum:* 150 units/kg.
Children. 300 units/kg for procedures that last less than 60 min. Then dosage based on coagulation test results. *Minimum:* 150 units/kg.

➤ *To provide anticoagulation with blood transfusions*

I.V. INFUSION

Adults. 400 to 600 units/100 ml of whole blood.

➤ *To provide anticoagulation with extracorporeal dialysis*

I.V. INFUSION, I.V. INJECTION

Adults. *Loading:* 25 to 30 units/kg by I.V. injection followed by infusion of 1,500 to 2,000 units/hr.

➤ *To maintain heparin lock patency*

I.V. INJECTION

Adults. 10 to 100 units/ml heparin flush solution (enough to fill device) after each use of device.

DOSAGE ADJUSTMENT Dosage possibly decreased in patients over 60 years of age, especially women, because of an increased risk of bleeding.

Route	Onset	Peak	Duration
I.V.	Immediate	Minutes	Unknown
SubQ	20–60 min	Unknown	Unknown

Mechanism of Action

Binds with antithrombin III, enhancing antithrombin III's inactivation of the coagulation enzymes thrombin (factor IIa) and factors Xa and XIa. At low doses, heparin inhibits factor Xa and prevents conversion of prothrombin to thrombin. Thrombin is needed for conversion of fibrinogen to fibrin; without fibrin, clots can't form. At high doses, heparin inactivates thrombin, preventing fibrin formation and existing clot extension.

Incompatibilities

Don't mix heparin with any other drug unless you have an order to do so and have checked with pharmacist. Heparin is incompatible with many drugs and solutions, especially ones that contain a phosphate buffer, sodium bicarbonate, or sodium oxalate.

Contraindications

Breastfeeding, infants, neonates, or pregnant woman (heparin sodium injection, USP, preserved with benzyl alcohol); history of heparin-induced thrombocytopenia or heparin-induced thrombocytopenia and thrombosis; hypersensitivity to heparin, pork, or its components; inability to monitor coagulation parameters when full-dose heparin is used; severe thrombocytopenia; uncontrolled active bleeding, except in disseminated intravascular coagulation (DIC)

Interactions

DRUGS

antihistamines, digoxin, nicotine, tetracyclines: Decreased anticoagulant effect of heparin
antithrombin III (human): Increased risk of bleeding
aspirin, dextran, dipyridamole, glycoprotein IIb/IIIa antagonists, hydroxychloroquine, NSAIDs, phenylbutazone, platelet aggregation inhibitors, sulfinpyrazone, thienopyridines: Increased platelet inhibition and risk of bleeding
cefamandole, cefoperazone, cefotetan, methimazole, plicamycin, propylthiouracil, valproic acid: Possibly hypoprothrombinemia and increased risk of bleeding
chloroquine, hydroxychloroquine: Possibly thrombocytopenia and increased risk of hemorrhage
dicumarol, warfarin: Possibly invalid prothrombin time if blood drawn sooner than 5 hours after last intravenous dose or 24 hours after last subcutaneous dose of heparin
ethacrynic acid, glucocorticoids, salicylates: Increased risk of bleeding and GI ulceration and hemorrhage
nitroglycerin (I.V.): Possibly decreased anticoagulant effect of heparin
probenecid: Possibly increased anticoagulant effect of heparin
thrombolytics: Increased risk of hemorrhage

ACTIVITIES

smoking: Decreased anticoagulant effect

Adverse Reactions

CNS: Chills, dizziness, fever, headache, peripheral neuropathy
CV: Chest pain, rebound hyperlipemia, **thrombosis**
EENT: Epistaxis, gingival bleeding, rhinitis
ENDO: Adrenal hemorrhage causing acute adrenal insufficiency
GI: Abdominal distention and pain, elevated liver enzymes, **hematemesis**, **melena**, nausea, **retroperitoneal hemorrhage**, vomiting
GU: Hematuria, hypermenorrhea, **ovarian hemorrhage**, priapism
HEME: Delayed onset of heparin-induced thrombocytopenia, easy bruising, **excessive bleeding from wounds, hemorrhage, heparin-induced thrombocytopenia, heparin-induced thrombocytopenia and thrombosis, thrombocytopenia**
MS: Back pain, myalgia, osteoporosis
RESP: Asthma, dyspnea, wheezing
SKIN: Alopecia, cutaneous necrosis following subcutaneous injection, cyanosis, petechiae, pruritus, urticaria
Other: Anaphylaxis; heparin resistance; injection-site hematoma, irritation, pain, redness, and ulceration

Nursing Considerations

- Know that heparin sodium injection, USP (porcine), preserved with benzyl alcohol, should not be given to infants, neonates, pregnant women, or women who are breastfeeding because benzyl alcohol has been associated with serious adverse events and death, especially in pediatric patients. Instead, a preservative-free heparin sodium solution should be used with these patients. Various heparin products contain the preservative benzyl alcohol, which isn't recommended for children under age 1 month because it may cause gasping syndrome, which may be fatal.
- Use heparin cautiously in alcoholics; menstruating women; patients over age 60, especially women; and patients with conditions that increase risk of hemorrhage, such as certain cardiovascular conditions (severe hypertension, subacute bacterial endocarditis), gastrointestinal conditions (continuous tube drainage of small intestine or stomach, ulcerative lesions), hematologic conditions that increase risk of bleeding (hemophilia,

thrombocytopenia, some vascular purpuras), presence of hereditary antithrombin III deficiency in patients receiving concurrent antithrombin III therapy, and during or immediately following major surgery or following spinal anesthesia or spinal tap. Also use cautiously in patients with a history of allergies or asthma.

- Read heparin label carefully. Revision has been made to state the strength of the entire container of heparin, followed by how much heparin is in 1 ml. This was done to eliminate the need to calculate the total amount of heparin in a product containing more than 1 ml, thereby reducing the risk of miscalculations that could result in medication errors.

WARNING **Give heparin only by subcutaneous or I.V. route; I.M. use causes hematoma, irritation, and pain.**

- Avoid injecting any drugs by I.M. route during heparin therapy, to decrease risk of bleeding and hematoma.

WARNING **Don't use heparin sodium injection as a catheter-lock flush because fatal errors have occurred in children when 1-ml heparin sodium injection vials were confused with 1-ml catheter-lock flush vials. Always examine vial labels closely to ensure correct product is being used.**

- Be aware that pediatric dosing is not achievable with the prefilled syringe. Another heparin product should be used when administering heparin to children to ensure an accurate dose.
- Administer subcutaneous heparin into anterior abdominal wall, above the iliac crest, and 5 cm (2 inches) or more away from the umbilicus. To minimize subcutaneous tissue trauma, lift adipose tissue away from deep tissues; don't aspirate for blood before injecting drug; don't move needle while injecting drug; and don't massage injection site before or after injection. Apply gentle pressure to the site after withdrawing needle.
- Alternate injection sites, and watch for signs of bleeding and hematoma.
- To prepare heparin for continuous infusion, invert container at least six times to prevent drug from pooling. Anticipate slight discoloration of prepared solution; this doesn't indicate a change in potency.
- During continuous I.V. therapy, expect to obtain APTT after 8 hours of therapy. Use the arm opposite the infusion site.
- For intermittent I.V. therapy, expect to adjust dose based on coagulation test results performed 30 minutes earlier. Therapeutic range is typically 1.5 to 2.5 times the control.
- Expect to periodically check patient's hematocrit and platelet count during the entire course of heparin therapy, regardless of route of administration.

WARNING **Know that bleeding is a major adverse effect of heparin therapy. Take safety precautions to prevent bleeding, such as having patient use a soft-bristled toothbrush and an electric razor. Bleeding may occur at any site and also may indicate an underlying problem, such as GI or urinary tract bleeding. Other sites of bleeding that could be fatal and require immediate attention include adrenal, ovarian, and retroperitoneal hemorrhage.**

- Be aware that heparin-induced thrombocytopenia (HIT) can occur in patients exposed to heparin and is due to the development of antibodies to a platelet factor 4-heparin complex. It may progress to the development of arterial and venous thromboses. Monitor blood test results, and observe for signs of bleeding, such as ecchymosis, epistaxis, hematemesis, hematuria, melena, and petechiae. Thrombocytopenia of any degree can occur 2 to 20 days following the onset of heparin therapy, so patient should be monitored closely. If platelet count drops below 100,000/mm^3 or recurrent thrombosis develops, notify prescriber and expect heparin to be discontinued.
- Be aware that heparin resistance may occur, especially in patients with antithrombin III deficiency, cancer, fever, infections with thrombosing tendencies, MI, thrombophlebitis, or thrombosis and postsurgery. Monitor coagulation tests closely in these patients and expect an adjustment in the heparin dose, as needed.
- Make sure all healthcare providers know that patient is receiving heparin.
- Keep protamine sulfate on hand to use as an antidote for heparin. Be aware that each milligram of protamine sulfate neutralizes 100 units of heparin.

- Be aware that prescriber may order oral anticoagulants before discontinuing heparin to avoid increased coagulation caused by heparin withdrawal. Heparin may be discontinued when full therapeutic effect of oral anticoagulant is achieved.
- Know that women over age 60 have highest risk of hemorrhage during therapy.
- Watch closely if patient is receiving heparin therapy and nitroglycerin I.V. because PTT may decrease and then rebound after nitroglycerin is discontinued. Monitor PTT closely, and be prepared to adjust heparin dose, as prescribed.

WARNING **Know that delayed-onset, heparin-induced thrombocytopenia may occur several weeks after heparin is discontinued and may progress to heparin-induced thrombocytopenia thrombosis, causing arterial and venous thromboses, including thrombus formation on a prosthetic cardiac valve.**

PATIENT TEACHING

- Explain that heparin can't be taken orally.
- Inform patient about increased risk of bleeding; urge her to avoid injuries and to use a soft-bristled toothbrush and an electric razor.
- Urge patient to report any abnormal sign or symptom to prescriber, even weeks after heparin has been discontinued, because of the potential for delayed adverse reactions.
- Advise patient to avoid drugs that interact with heparin, such as aspirin and ibuprofen.
- Instruct patient and family to watch for and report abdominal or lower back pain, black stools, bleeding gums, bloody urine, excessive menstrual bleeding, nosebleeds, and severe headaches. Also tell patient to report any persistent, severe, or unusual signs and symptoms to prescriber immediately. Alert patient receiving heparin subcutaneously that necrosis of the skin has been reported following subcutaneous administration of heparin and to alert prescriber if any abnormalities occur at injection sites.
- Explain that temporary hair loss may occur.
- Advise patient to wear or carry appropriate medical identification.

hydralazine hydrochloride

Apresoline (CAN)

Class and Category

Pharmacologic class: Vasodilator
Therapeutic class: Antihypertensive
Pregnancy category: C

Indications and Dosages

➤ *To manage essential hypertension, alone or with other antihypertensives*

TABLETS

Adults. *Initial:* 10 mg four times daily for first 2 to 4 days and then increased to 25 mg four times daily for remainder of first wk. Further increased to 50 mg four times daily beginning wk 2 and thereafter. *Maximum:* 7.5 mg/kg or 200 mg daily.
Children. 0.75 mg/kg daily in divided doses four times daily. Increased gradually over 3 to 4 wk. *Maximum:* 7.5 mg/kg daily for children older than 1 and 5 mg/kg/day for infants less than 1 year of age, not to exceed 200 mg daily for either age group.

➤ *To manage severe essential hypertension when drug can't be taken orally or when need to reduce blood pressure is urgent*

I.V. OR I.M. INJECTION

Adults. 20 to 40 mg, repeated as needed. I.V. injection given rapidly over 1 min.
Children. 1.7 to 3.5 mg/kg daily in divided doses every 4 to 6 hr, as needed. I.V. injection given rapidly over 1 min.

➤ *To treat congestive heart failure*

TABLETS

Adults. *Initial:* 10 to 25 mg 3 or 4 times daily, then gradually increased, as needed. *Maintenance:* 225 to 300 mg daily in divided doses 3 or 4 times daily. *Maximum:* 300 mg daily in divided doses.

DOSAGE ADJUSTMENT For adults with creatinine clearance of 10 to 50 ml/min, dosing interval increased to every 8 hours. For adults with creatinine clearance less than 10 ml/min who are fast acetylators, dosing interval increased to 8 to 16 hr; for slow acetylators, dosing interval increased to 12 to 24 hr.

Route	Onset	Peak	Duration
P.O.	20–30 min	1–2 hr	2–4 hr
I.V.	5–20 min	10–80 min	2–6 hr
I.M.	10–30 min	1 hr	2–6 hr

Mechanism of Action

May act in a manner that resembles organic nitrates and sodium nitroprusside, except that hydralazine is selective for arteries. It:

- exerts a direct vasodilating effect on vascular smooth muscle
- interferes with calcium movement in vascular smooth muscle by altering cellular calcium metabolism
- dilates arteries, not veins, which minimizes orthostatic hypotension and increases cardiac output and cerebral blood flow
- causes reflex autonomic response that increases, cardiac output, heart rate, and left ventricular ejection fraction
- has a positive inotropic effect on the heart.

Incompatibilities

Don't mix hydralazine in I.V. infusion solutions.

Contraindications

Coronary artery disease, hypersensitivity to hydralazine or its components, mitral valve disease

Interactions

DRUGS

beta blockers: Increased effects of both drugs
diazoxide, MAO inhibitors, other antihypertensives: Risk of severe hypotension
epinephrine: Possibly decreased vasopressor effect of epinephrine
NSAIDs: Decreased hydralazine effects
sympathomimetics: Possibly decreased antihypertensive effect of hydralazine

FOODS

all foods: Possibly increased bioavailability of hydralazine

Adverse Reactions

CNS: Chills, fever, headache, peripheral neuritis
CV: Angina, edema, orthostatic hypotension, palpitations, tachycardia
EENT: Lacrimation, nasal congestion
GI: Anorexia, constipation, diarrhea, nausea, vomiting
RESP: Dyspnea
SKIN: Blisters, flushing, pruritus, rash, urticaria
Other: Lupus-like symptoms, especially with high doses; lymphadenopathy

Nursing Considerations

- Monitor ANA titer, CBC, and lupus erythematosus cell preparation before therapy and periodically as ordered during long-term treatment.
- Anticipate that drug may change color in solution. Consult pharmacist if color changes.
- Be aware that hydralazine may change color when exposed to a metal filter.
- Give tablets with food to increase bioavailability.
- Monitor blood pressure and pulse rate regularly and weigh patient daily during therapy.
- Check blood pressure with patient in lying, sitting, and standing positions, and watch for signs of orthostatic hypotension. Expect orthostatic hypotension to be most common in the morning, during hot weather, and with exercise.

WARNING Expect to discontinue drug immediately if patient has lupus-like symptoms, such as arthralgia, fever, myalgia, pharyngitis, and splenomegaly.

- Expect prescriber to withdraw hydralazine gradually to avoid a rapid increase in blood pressure.
- Expect to treat peripheral neuritis with pyridoxine.

PATIENT TEACHING

- Instruct patient to take hydralazine tablets with food.
- Advise patient to change position slowly, especially in the morning. Caution that hot showers may increase hypotension.
- Instruct patient to immediately notify prescriber about fever, joint and muscle aches, and sore throat.
- Urge patient to report numbness and tingling in limbs, which may require treatment with another drug.
- Caution patient against stopping drug abruptly because doing so may cause severe hypertension.

hydrochlorothiazide

Microzide, Oretic, Urozide (CAN)

Class and Category

Pharmacologic class: Thiazide diuretic
Therapeutic class: Diuretic
Pregnancy category: B

Indications and Dosages

➤ *To manage hypertension*

CAPSULES

Adults. *Initial:* 12.5 to 25 mg daily increased, as needed, to 50 mg daily given as a single dose or 2 divided doses. *Maximum:* 50 mg daily.

ORAL SOLUTION, TABLETS

Adults. *Initial:* 25 mg daily, increased to 50 mg daily, as needed, and given as a single dose or in divided doses twice daily.
Children age 6 months and over. 1 to 2 mg/kg daily as a single dose or in divided doses twice daily. *Maximum:* 37.5 mg daily for children 6 months to 2 years; 100 mg daily for children age 2 to 12.
Infants under age 6 months. Up to 3 mg/kg daily in 2 divided doses.

➤ *As adjunct to treat edema caused by cirrhosis, corticosteroids, estrogen, heart failure, or renal disorders*

ORAL SOLUTION, TABLETS

Adults. 25 to 100 mg twice daily, once daily, every other day, or for 3 to 5 days/wk.

Children age 6 months and over. 1 to 2 mg/kg daily as a single dose or in divided doses twice daily. *Maximum:* 37.5 mg daily for children 6 months to 2 years; 100 mg daily for children age 2 to 12.
Infants under age 6 months. Up to 3 mg/kg daily in 2 divided doses.

Route	Onset	Peak	Duration
P.O.	2 hr	4 hr	6–12 hr

Contraindications

Anuria; hypersensitivity to hydrochlorothiazide, other thiazides, sulfonamide derivatives, or their components

Interactions

DRUGS

ACTH, amphotericin B, corticosteroids: Increased electrolyte depletion, especially potassium
amantadine: Possibly increased blood level and risk of toxicity of amantadine
amiodarone: Increased risk of arrhythmias from hypokalemia
antihypertensives: Increased antihypertensive effects
barbiturates, opioids: Possibly orthostatic hypotension
calcium: Possibly increased serum calcium level
carbamazepine: Possibly increased risk of symptomatic hyponatremia
cholestyramine, colestipol: Reduced GI absorption of hydrochlorothiazide

Mechanism of Action

A thiazide diuretic, hydrochlorothiazide promotes movement of sodium (Na^+), chloride (Cl^-), and water (H_2O) from blood in peritubular capillaries into nephron's distal convoluted tubule, as shown. Initially, it may decrease cardiac output, extracellular fluid volume, or plasma volume, which helps explain blood pressure reduction. It also may reduce blood pressure by direct arterial dilation. After several weeks, cardiac output, extracellular fluid volume, and plasma volume return to normal, and peripheral vascular resistance remains decreased.

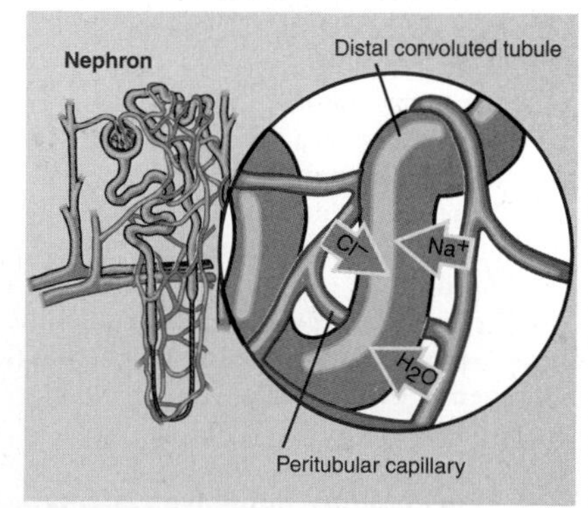

cyclosporine: Possibly increased risk of hyperuricemia and gout-type complications
diazoxide: Increased antihypertensive and hyperglycemic effects of hydrochlorothiazide
diflunisal: Possibly increased blood hydrochlorothiazide level
digoxin: Increased risk of digitalis toxicity from hypokalemia
dopamine: Possibly increased diuretic effects of both drugs
insulin, oral antidiabetic drugs: Possibly increased blood glucose level
lithium: Decreased lithium clearance, increased risk of lithium toxicity
neuromuscular blockers: Possibly enhanced neuromuscular blockade from hypokalemia
nondepolarizing skeletal muscle relaxants: Possibly increased response to muscle relaxants
NSAIDs: Decreased diuretic effect of hydrochlorothiazide, increased risk of renal failure
oral anticoagulants: Possibly decreased anticoagulant effects
sympathomimetics: Possibly decreased antihypertensive effect of hydrochlorothiazide
vitamin D: Increased risk of hypercalcemia

ACTIVITIES

alcohol use: Possibly orthostatic hypotension

Adverse Reactions

CNS: Asthenia, dizziness, fever, headache, insomnia, paresthesia, restlessness, vertigo, weakness
CV: Elevated cholesterol and triglycerides levels, **hypotension**, orthostatic hypotension, vasculitis
EENT: Acute myopia, acute angle-closure glaucoma, blurred vision, dry mouth
ENDO: Hyperglycemia
GI: Abdominal cramps, anorexia, constipation, diarrhea, indigestion, jaundice, nausea, **pancreatitis**, vomiting
GU: Decreased libido, impotence, interstitial nephritis, nocturia, polyuria, **renal failure**
HEME: Agranulocytosis, aplastic anemia, bone marrow failure, hemolytic anemia, leukopenia, neutropenia, thrombocytopenia
MS: Muscle spasms and weakness
RESP: Pneumonitis, pulmonary edema
SKIN: Alopecia, cutaneous vasculitis, **erythema multiforme, exfoliative dermatitis**, photosensitivity, purpura, rash, **Stevens–Johnson syndrome, toxic epidermal necrolysis**, urticaria
Other: Anaphylaxis, dehydration, **hypercalcemia**, hyperuricemia, hypochloremia, **hypokalemia, hypomagnesemia, hyponatremia**, hypovolemia, **metabolic alkalosis**, weight loss

Nursing Considerations

- Give hydrochlorothiazide in the morning and early evening to avoid nocturia.
- Monitor blood pressure, daily weight, fluid intake and output, and serum levels of electrolytes, especially potassium.
- Assess for evidence of hypokalemia, such as muscle spasms and weakness.
- Check blood glucose level often, as ordered, in diabetic patients, and expect to increase antidiabetic dosage, as needed and prescribed.
- Know that if patient has gouty arthritis, expect increased risk of gout attacks during therapy.
- Monitor BUN and serum creatinine levels, as ordered, especially in patients with chronic kidney disease, renal artery stenosis, severe congestive heart failure, or volume depletion, because of increased risk of acute renal failure with hydrochlorothiazide therapy. Notify prescriber if serum creatinine levels become elevated, as drug may need to be withheld or discontinued.
- Monitor patient for decreased visual acuity or ocular pain, especially within hours to weeks of beginning drug therapy and in patients with a history of penicillin or sulfonamide allergy, as acute myopia and acute angle-closure glaucoma may develop. If left untreated, permanent blindness may occur. If present, notify prescriber immediately, expect to discontinue hydrochlorothiazide, and assist with prompt medical or surgical intervention, as indicated.

WARNING Be aware that even minor alterations in fluid and electrolyte balance may precipitate hepatic coma in patients with impaired hepatic function.

PATIENT TEACHING

- Advise patient to take hydrochlorothiazide in morning and early evening to avoid awakening during the night to urinate.

- Instruct patient to take drug with food or milk if adverse GI reactions occur.
- Tell patient to weigh herself at the same time each day wearing the same amount of clothing and to notify prescriber if she gains more than 0.9 kg (2 lb) per day or 2.3 kg (5 lb) per week.
- Instruct patient to eat a diet high in potassium-rich food, including, bananas, citrus fruits, dates, and tomatoes.
- Advise patient to change position slowly to minimize effects of orthostatic hypotension.
- Urge patient to report decreased urination, muscle cramps and weakness, and unusual bleeding or bruising.

hydrocodone bitartrate

Hysingla ER, Vantrela ER, Zohydro ER

Class, Category, and Schedule

Pharmacologic class: Opioid
Therapeutic class: Opioid analgesic
Pregnancy category: C
Controlled substance schedule: II

Indications and Dosages

➤ To *manage severe pain in patients requiring continuous, around-the-clock opioid analgesia for an extended period of time and for which alternative treatment options are inadequate*

E.R. CAPSULES (ZOHYDRO ER)

Adults who are opioid naïve or opioid nontolerant. *Initial:* 10 mg every 12 hr, increased, as needed, in increments of 10 mg every 12 hr every 3 to 7 days to effective and tolerable dose. *Maximum:* 80 mg total daily dose.

Adults who are opioid tolerant and converting from another opioid. Highly individualized.

DOSAGE ADJUSTMENT For patients with renal or severe hepatic impairment, a single dose of 10 mg given, followed by close monitoring for respiratory depression and sedation. If single dose tolerated, 10 mg every 12 hr as needed and tolerated with further titration highly individualized.

E.R. TABLETS (HYSINGLA ER)

Adults who are opioid naïve or opioid nontolerant. *Initial:* 20 mg every 24 hr, increased, as needed, in increments of 10 to 20 mg daily every 3 to 5 days to effective and tolerable dose. *Maximum:* 80 mg every 24 hr.

Adults who are opioid tolerant and converting from another opioid. Highly individualized.

DOSAGE ADJUSTMENT For patients with end-stage renal disease, moderate to severe renal impairment, or severe hepatic impairment, initial dosage reduced to 10 mg every 24 hr.

E.R. TABLETS (VANTRELA ER)

Adults who are opioid naïve or opioid nontolerant. *Initial:* 15 mg every 12 hr, increased to next higher dose every 3 to 7 days as needed.

DOSAGE ADJUSTMENT For patient with end-stage renal disease, mild or moderate hepatic impairment, or moderate or severe renal impairment, initial dosage decreased by half.

Mechanism of Action

Binds to and activates opioid receptors at sites in the periaquaductal and periventricular gray matter, the ventromedial medulla, and the spinal cord to produce pain relief.

Contraindications

Acute or severe bronchial asthma or hypercarbia, children under the age of 18 for use with cold and cough medications, hypersensitivity to hydrocodone bitartrate or any of its components, known or suspected paralytic ileus, significant respiratory depression, use within 14 days of MAO inhibitor therapy

Interactions

DRUGS

anticholinergics, other drugs with anticholinergic activity: Increased risk of urinary retention or severe constipation, which may lead to paralytic ileus
antimigraine agents, cyclobenzaprine; dextromethorphan; dolasetron; granisetron; linezolid; MAO inhibitors; methylene blue; ondansetron; palonosetron; selected psychiatric drugs such as amoxapine, buspirone, lithium, maprotiline, mirtazapine, nefazodone, trazodone, vilazodone; selective

G H I

serotonin reuptake inhibitors; serotonin-norepinephrine reuptake inhibitors; St. John's wort; tricyclic antidepressants; tryptophan: Increased risk of serotonin syndrome
benzodiazepines, other opioids, sedating antihistamines, tricyclic antidepressants: Increased risk of sedation and somnolence and severe respiratory depression
CNS depressants; nonprescription or prescription drugs containing alcohol: Increased risk of coma, profound sedation, and respiratory depression that could be fatal profound sedation, coma
CYP3A4 inducers: Increased clearance of hydrocodone with decreased effectiveness
CYP3A4 inhibitors: Decreased clearance of hydrocodone resulting in increased or prolonged opioid effects
mixed agonist/antagonist analgesics such as buprenorphine, butorphanol, nalbuphine, pentazocine: Possible reduced hydrocodone effectiveness or precipitation of withdrawal symptoms

ACTIVITIES

alcohol use: Possibly increased hydrocodone plasma levels with potentially fatal overdose

Adverse Reactions

CNS: Anxiety, **CNS depression**, **coma**, depression, dizziness, fatigue, fever, headache, insomnia, lethargy, migraine, paresthesia, **seizures**, somnolence, syncope, tremor
CV: Hypercholesterolemia, **hypotension**, peripheral edema
EENT: Dry mouth
ENDO: Adrenal insufficiency (rare), hot flashes
GI: Abdominal discomfort or pain, constipation (may be severe), elevated liver enzymes, gastroesophageal reflux disease, nausea, spasm of the Sphincter of Oddi, vomiting
GU: Decreased libido, erectile dysfunction, impotence, infertility, lack of menstruation, UTI
MS: Arthralgia; back, extremity, musculoskeletal, or neck pain; muscle spasms
RESP: Cough, dyspnea, **respiratory depression**
SKIN: Pruritis, rash, sweating including night sweats
Other: Dehydration, **hypokalemia**, noncardiac chest pain, physical and psychological dependence

Nursing Considerations

- Be aware that hydrocodone increases the risk of abuse, addiction, and misuse. Know that to ensure that the benefits of hydrocodone therapy outweigh the risks, a Risk Evaluation and Mitigation Strategy (REMS) is required.
- Know that hydrocodone should not be given to a patient with impaired consciousness, nor should the drug be administered on an as-needed basis.
- Be aware that opioids like hydrocodone should not be given to women during pregnancy, while in labor, or when breastfeeding, as the newborn or infant may experience neonatal opioid withdrawal syndrome (NOWS), which could be life-threatening. This syndrome may exhibit as excessive or high-pitched crying, poor feeding, rapid breathing, or trembling. If not recognized and treated appropriately, it can become life-threatening.
- Know that hydrocodone is contraindicated in children under the age of 18 when used in cold or cough preparations.
- Use extreme caution when administering hydrocodone to patients with significant chronic obstructive pulmonary disease or cor pulmonale, and in patients having a substantially decreased respiratory reserve, hypoxia, hypercapnia, or preexisting respiratory depression, especially when initiating or titrating therapy. These patients may develop respiratory depression, even with usual therapeutic doses, because hydrocodone may decrease the patient's respiratory drive to the point of apnea.
- Use hydrocodone cautiously in cachectic, debilitated or elderly patients, especially when initiating and titrating therapy, as they are at increased risk for adverse effects, especially respiratory depression.
- Be aware that opioid therapy like hydrocodone should only be used concomitantly with benzodiazepines and other CNS depressants in patients for whom other treatment options are inadequate. If prescribed together, expect dosing and duration of hydrocodone to be limited. Monitor patient closely for signs and symptoms of decrease in consciousness, including coma, profound sedation, and significant respiratory depression. Notify prescriber immediately

and provide emergency supportive care, as death may occur.

- Be aware that patients who are considered opioid tolerant are those who have received for 1 week or longer, at least 8 mg of oral hydromorphone per day, 60 mg of oral morphine daily, 30 mg of oral oxycodone per day, 25 mg of oral oxymorphone per day, 25 micrograms transdermal fentanyl per hour, or an equianalgesic dose of another opioid.
- Do not administer hydrocodone to a patient wearing a transdermal fentanyl patch until the patch has been removed for 18 hours. Also know that close monitoring is especially important for a patient converting from methadone because methadone has a long half-life and tends to accumulate in the blood.

WARNING Be aware that hydrocodone available as an extended release formulation increases risk of overdose and death because of larger amount of drug present in this form. Also know that crushing, chewing, snorting, or injecting the contents of the Hysingla ER tablet dissolved in a liquid base will result in the uncontrolled delivery of hydrocodone and can result in overdose and death. Be aware that Zohydro ER capsules are made with a formulation that deters abuse because it forms an immediate inactive viscous gel when crushed or dissolved in liquids or solvents.

WARNING Monitor patient for respiratory depression, especially when initiating therapy or when increasing dosage, even when the drug has been used as prescribed and not abused or misused. Be aware that overestimating hydrocodone dose when converting patients from another opioid medication can result in fatal overdose with the first dose. To avoid this, know that it is recommended to underestimate a patient's 24-hour oral hydrocodone requirement and provide rescue medication, as needed, until the right dose is determined. Keep resuscitation equipment nearby.

- Monitor patients closely who may be susceptible to the intracranial effects of carbon dioxide retention from respiratory depression caused by hydrocodone therapy, such as patients with head injuries or those who have a preexisting elevation in intracranial pressure.
- Monitor patients with a seizure history or disorder because hydrocodone may cause or worsen seizures.
- Monitor effectiveness of hydrocodone in relieving pain; consult prescriber as needed.
- Assess patient for constipation and provide a high-fiber diet and adequate fluid intake, if not contraindicated, because constipation can become severe.
- Monitor patient for evidence of physical dependence or abuse. Know that addiction can occur not only in those who obtain the drug illicitly but also in patients who are appropriately prescribed the drug at recommended doses. Be aware that excessive use of hydrocodone may lead to abuse, addiction, misuse, overdose, and possibly death. Monitor patient's intake of drug closely.
- Notify prescriber if serious adverse reactions occur with hydrocodone therapy and expect dosage to be reduced.
- Expect to taper hydrocodone dosage gradually every 2 to 4 days when patient no longer requires therapy to prevent withdrawal symptoms in the physically dependent patient. Know that hydrocodone should not be discontinued abruptly.
- Monitor patient's vital signs closely, especially after initiating or titrating dose of hydrocodone. Know that in addition to respiratory depression, hydrocodone may cause severe hypotension, especially in patients whose blood pressure is already compromised by a depleted blood volume or after concurrent administration of drugs that decrease blood pressure.
- Be aware that concomitant use with CYP3A4 inhibitors or discontinuation of CYP3A inducers can result in a fatal overdose of hydrocodone.

WARNING Know that many drugs may interact with opioids like hydrocodone to cause serotonin syndrome. Monitor patient closely for signs and symptoms such as agitation, diaphoresis, diarrhea, fever, hallucinations, labile blood pressure, muscle twitching or stiffness, nausea, shakiness, shivering, tachycardia, trouble with coordination, or vomiting. Notify prescriber at once because serotonin syndrome may be life-threatening. Be prepared to discontinue drug, if possible and ordered, and provide supportive care.

- Monitor patient for adrenal insufficiency. Although rare, it can be life-threatening. Monitor patient for anorexia, dizziness, fatigue, hypotension, nausea, vomiting, or weakness. Notify prescriber if adrenal insufficiency is suspected and expect diagnostic testing to be done. If diagnosis is confirmed, expect to administer corticosteroids and wean patient off of hydrocodone, if possible.
- Monitor patient for decreased bowel motility in postoperative patients receiving hydrocodone, as the drug may obscure the development of acute abdominal conditions.

PATIENT TEACHING

- Warn parents that children under age 18 should not receive hydrocodone when mixed with cold or cough preparations.
- Instruct patient to take drug exactly as ordered and not to adjust dosage without speaking to prescriber first. Warn patient of possibility of addiction even when taken as prescribed. Inform him that excessive or prolonged use can also lead to addiction, misuse, overdose, and possibly death.
- Inform patient that capsules and tablets should be taken whole and never chewed, crushed, or dissolved. In addition, enough water should be taken with the capsule or tablet to ensure complete swallowing immediately after placing drug in mouth.
- Warn patient to keep hydrocodone away from the reach of children, as accidental consumption of even one capsule or tablet can cause significant respiratory depression and death.
- Caution patient to avoid ingesting alcohol, including medications containing alcohol, as the combination increases the risk of overdose, respiratory depression, and death, as does taking other types of depressants, including benzodiazepines, together with hydrocodone therapy. Patient should notify all prescribers of hydrocodone use.
- Advise women of childbearing age to notify prescriber if pregnancy occurs or is suspected because a fetus exposed to hydrocodone during utero may require treatment for neonatal opioid withdrawal syndrome (NOWS) when born. Also advise women not to breastfeed while taking oxycodone.
- Caution patient to avoid hazardous activities until drug's CNS effects are known.
- Instruct patient to rise slowly from a lying or sitting position and to lie or sit down if he experiences light-headedness. If effect is frequent or severe, tell him to notify prescriber.
- Urge patient to consume plenty of fluids and high-fiber foods, if not contra-indicated, to prevent constipation.
- Inform patient that long-term use of opioids like hydrocodone may decrease sex hormone levels, causing decreased libido, erectile dysfunction, impotence, infertility, or lack of menstruation. Encourage patient to report any such symptoms.
- Instruct patient to notify all prescribers of hydrocodone use.

hydrocortisone (cortisol)

Cortef, Cortenema, Hydrocortone

hydrocortisone acetate

Cortifoam, Hydrocortone Acetate

hydrocortisone cypionate

Cortef

hydrocortisone sodium phosphate

Hydrocortone Phosphate

hydrocortisone sodium succinate

A-hydroCort, Solu-Cortef

Class and Category

Pharmacologic class: Glucocorticoid
Therapeutic class: Adrenocorticoid replacement, anti-inflammatory
Pregnancy category: Not rated; C (Cortifoam)

Indications and Dosages

➤ *To treat severe inflammation or acute adrenal insufficiency*

ORAL SUSPENSION, TABLETS (HYDROCORTISONE, HYDROCORTISONE CYPIONATE)

Adults. 20 to 240 mg daily as a single dose or in divided doses.

I.V. INFUSION OR I.V., I.M., OR SUBCUTANEOUS INJECTION (HYDROCORTISONE SODIUM PHOSPHATE); I.M. INJECTION (HYDROCORTISONE)

Adults. 15 to 240 mg daily as a single dose or in divided doses. *Usual:* One-half to one-third the oral dose. For I.V. infusion, give over 20 to 30 min. For I.V. injection, give over 30 sec to 10 min depending on dose.

DOSAGE ADJUSTMENT Dosage increased to more than 240 mg daily if needed to treat acute disease.

I.V. INFUSION; I.V. OR I.M. INJECTION (HYDROCORTISONE SODIUM SUCCINATE)

Adults. 100 to 500 mg every 2, 4, or 6 hr. For I.V. infusion, give over 20 to 30 min. For I.V. injection, give over 30 sec to 10 min depending on dose.

➤ *To treat septic shock and severe sepsis*

I.V. INFUSION (HYDROCORTISONE SODIUM PHOSPHATE)

Adults. 200 mg daily given as continuous infusion.

➤ *To treat acute asthma*

I.V. INJECTION (HYDROCORTISONE SODIUM SUCCINATE)

Adults. 100 to 500 mg given over 30 sec to 10 min, depending on dose, every 6 hr.

➤ *To treat joint and tissue inflammation*

INTRA-ARTICULAR INJECTION (HYDROCORTISONE ACETATE)

Adults. 25 to 37.5 mg injected into large joints or bursae as a single dose, or 10 to 25 mg into small joints as a single dose.

INTRALESIONAL INJECTION (HYDROCORTISONE ACETATE)

Adults. 5 to 12.5 mg injected into tendon sheaths as a single dose, or 12.5 to 25 mg injected into ganglia as a single dose.

SOFT-TISSUE INJECTION (HYDROCORTISONE ACETATE)

Adults. 25 to 50 mg as a single dose. Sometimes a dose of up to 75 mg is needed.

➤ *As adjunct to treat ulcerative proctitis of the distal portion of the rectum in patients who can't retain hydrocortisone or other corticosteroid enemas*

RECTAL AEROSOL (HYDROCORTISONE ACETATE)

Adult men. Initial: 1 applicatorful once or twice daily for 2 to 3 wk; then every other day thereafter. *Maintenance:* Highly individualized.

➤ *To treat ulcerative colitis*

ENEMA (HYDROCORTISONE)

Adults. 100 mg every night for 21 days or until condition improves.

Route	Onset	Peak	Duration
P.O.†	Unknown	1 hr	1.25–1.5 days
P.O.‖	Unknown	1–2 hr	Unknown
I.V. ‡§	Rapid	Unknown	Unknown
I.M.†	Unknown	4–8 hr	Unknown
I.M.‡	Rapid	1 hr	Unknown
I.M.§	Rapid	1 hr	Variable
Other*	Unknown	24–48 hr	3 days–4 wk

* Acetate; intra-articular, intralesional, and soft-tissue injection.
† Hydrocortisone.
‡ Phosphate.
§ Succinate.
‖ Cypionate.

Mechanism of Action

Binds to intracellular glucocorticoid receptors and suppresses inflammatory and immune responses by:

- inhibiting monocyte and neutrophil accumulation at inflammation site and suppressing their bactericidal and phagocytic activity
- stabilizing lysosomal membranes
- suppressing antigen response of helper T cells and macrophages
- inhibiting synthesis of cellular mediators of inflammatory response, such as cytokines, interleukins, and prostaglandins.

Contraindications

Hypersensitivity to hydrocortisone or its components, idiopathic thrombocytopenic purpura (I.M.), intestinal conditions prohibiting intrarectal steroids (P.R.), recent live-virus vaccination, systemic fungal infection

Interactions

DRUGS

acetaminophen: Increased risk of hepatotoxicity

amphotericin B, carbonic anhydrase inhibitors: Possibly severe hypokalemia
anabolic steroids, androgens: Increased risk of edema and severe acne
anticholinergics: Possibly increased intraocular pressure
anticoagulants, thrombolytics: Increased risk of GI hemorrhage and ulceration, possibly decreased therapeutic effects of these drugs
asparaginase: Increased risk of hyperglycemia and toxicity
aspirin, NSAIDs: Increased risk of GI distress and bleeding
cholestyramine: Possibly increased hydrocortisone clearance
cyclosporine: Possibly increased action of both drugs; increased risk of seizures
digoxin: Possibly hypokalemia-induced arrhythmias and digitalis toxicity
ephedrine, phenobarbital, phenytoin, rifampin: Decreased blood hydrocortisone level
estrogens, oral contraceptives: Increased therapeutic and toxic effects of hydrocortisone
insulin, oral antidiabetic drugs: Possibly increased blood glucose level
isoniazid: Possibly decreased therapeutic effects of isoniazid
macrolide antibiotics: Possibly decreased hydrocortisone clearance
mexiletine: Decreased blood mexiletine level
neuromuscular blockers: Possibly increased neuromuscular blockade, causing apnea or respiratory depression
potassium-depleting drugs, such as thiazide diuretics: Possibly severe hypokalemia
potassium supplements: Possibly decreased effects of these supplements
somatrem, somatropin: Possibly decreased therapeutic effects of these drugs
streptozocin: Increased risk of hyperglycemia
vaccines: Decreased antibody response and increased risk of neurologic complications

ACTIVITIES

alcohol use: Increased risk of GI distress and bleeding

Adverse Reactions

CNS: Ataxia, behavioral changes, depression, dizziness, epidural lipomatosis, euphoria, fatigue, headache, **increased intracranial pressure with papilledema**, insomnia, malaise, mood changes, paresthesia, **seizures**, steroid psychosis, syncope, vertigo
CV: Arrhythmias, **fat embolism**, **heart failure**, hypertension, **hypotension**, **thromboembolism**, thrombophlebitis
EENT: Central serous chorioretinopathy, exophthalmos, glaucoma, increased intraocular pressure, nystagmus, posterior subcapsular cataracts
ENDO: Adrenal insufficiency during stress, cushingoid symptoms (buffalo hump, central obesity, moon face, supraclavicular fat pad enlargement), diabetes mellitus, growth suppression in children, hyperglycemia, negative nitrogen balance from protein catabolism
GI: Abdominal distention; hiccups; increased appetite; nausea; **pancreatitis**; peptic ulcer; rectal abnormalities, such as **bleeding**, blistering, burning, itching, or pain (rectal form); ulcerative esophagitis; vomiting
GU: Amenorrhea, glycosuria, menstrual irregularities, perineal burning or tingling
HEME: Easy bruising, leukocytosis
MS: Arthralgia; aseptic necrosis of femoral and humeral heads; compression fractures; muscle atrophy, twitching, or weakness; myalgia; osteoporosis; spontaneous fractures; steroid myopathy; tendon rupture
SKIN: Acne; altered skin pigmentation; diaphoresis; erythema; hirsutism; necrotizing vasculitis; petechiae; purpura; rash; scarring; sterile abscess; striae; subcutaneous fat atrophy; thin, fragile skin; urticaria
Other: Anaphylaxis, **hypocalcemia**, **hypokalemia**, **hypokalemic alkalosis**, impaired wound healing, masking of signs of infection, **metabolic alkalosis**, **pheochromocytoma crisis** (in presence of pheochromocytoma), suppressed skin test reaction, weight gain

Nursing Considerations

- Systemic hydrocortisone shouldn't be given to immunocompromised patients, such as those with fungal and other infections, including amebiasis, hepatitis B, tuberculosis, vaccinia, and varicella.

- Give daily dose of hydrocortisone in morning to mimic normal peak in adrenocortical secretion of corticosteroids.
- Give oral dose with food or milk to avoid GI distress.
- Don't give acetate injectable suspension by I.V. route.
- Give hydrocortisone sodium succinate as a direct I.V. injection over 30 seconds to several minutes, or as an intermittent or a continuous infusion. For infusion, dilute to 1 mg/ml or less with D_5W, normal saline solution, or dextrose 5% in normal saline solution.
- Inject I.M. form deep into gluteal muscle, and rotate injection sites to prevent muscle atrophy. Subcutaneous injection may cause atrophy and sterile abscess.
- Shake foam container vigorously for 5 to 10 seconds before each use. Gently withdraw applicator plunger past the fill line on the applicator barrel while container is upright on a level surface. Administer rectal foam only with provided applicator. After each use, wash applicator, container cap, and underlying tip with warm water.
- Be aware that high-dose therapy shouldn't be given for longer than 48 hours. Be alert for depression and psychotic episodes.
- Monitor blood pressure, electrolyte levels, and weight regularly during therapy.
- Expect hydrocortisone to worsen infections or mask signs and symptoms.
- Monitor blood glucose level in diabetic patients, and increase insulin or oral antidiabetic drug dosage, as prescribed.
- Know that elderly patients are at high risk for osteoporosis during long-term therapy.
- Anticipate the possibility of acute adrenal insufficiency with stress, such as emotional upset, fever, surgery, or trauma. Increase hydrocortisone dosage, as prescribed.

WARNING Avoid withdrawing drug suddenly after long-term therapy because adrenal crisis can result. Expect to reduce dosage gradually and monitor response.

PATIENT TEACHING

- Advise patient to take daily dose of hydrocortisone at 9 a.m.
- Instruct patient to take oral suspension or tablets with food or milk.
- Teach patient how to use enema form or foam, if prescribed.
- Caution patient not to stop drug abruptly without first consulting prescriber.
- Instruct patient to report early evidence of adrenal insufficiency: anorexia, difficulty breathing, dizziness, fainting, fatigue, joint pain, muscle weakness, and nausea.
- Inform patient that he may bruise easily.
- Advise patient on long-term therapy to have periodic eye examinations.
- If patient receives long-term therapy, urge him to carry or wear medical identification.
- Caution patient to avoid people with infections because drug can suppress immune system, increasing risk of infection. If patient comes into contact with chickenpox or measles, instruct him to call prescriber because he may need prophylactic care.

hydromorphone hydrochloride
(dihydromorphinone)

Dilaudid, Dilaudid-HP, Exalgo

Class, Category, and Schedule

Pharmacologic class: Opioid
Therapeutic class: Opioid analgesic
Pregnancy category: C
Controlled substance schedule: II

Indications and Dosages

➤ *To relieve pain severe enough to require opioid treatment and for which alternative treatment options such as nonopioid analgesics or opioid combination products are inadequate or not tolerated*

ORAL SOLUTION (DILAUDID)

Adults. 2.5 to 10 mg every 3 to 6 hr, as needed.

TABLETS (DILAUDID)

Adults. 2 to 4 mg every 4 to 6 hr, as needed.

I.V. INJECTION (DILAUDID)

Adults. 0.2 to 1 mg every 2 to 3 hr, as needed, given slowly over 2 to 3 min.

I.M. OR SUBCUTANEOUS INJECTION (DILAUDID)
Adults. 1 or 2 mg every 2 to 3 hr, as needed. Increased to 3 or 4 mg every 4 to 6 hr, as needed for severe pain.
SUPPOSITORIES (DILAUDID)
Adults. 3 mg every 6 to 8 hr, as needed.
DOSAGE ADJUSTMENT For patients with hepatic or renal impairment, initial dosage is given at 25 to 50% of normal dosage.

➤ *To treat moderate to severe pain for opioid-tolerant patients who require higher doses of opioids*

I.M., I.V. OR SUBCUTANEOUS INJECTION (DILAUDID-HP)
Adults who are not opioid-naïve. Highly individualized and dependent on patient's previous total daily 24-hour opioid use. If I.V. route is used, give slowly over 2 to 3 min. *Usual for I.M or subcutaneous injection:* 1 to 2 mg every 2 to 3 hr, as needed, with dosage adjusted according to clinical response. *Usual for I.V. injection:* 0.2 to 1 mg every 2 to 3 hr, given slowly over at least 2 to 3 min, depending on dose.
DOSAGE ADJUSTMENT For debilitated or elderly patient, I.V. injection initial dosage may be kept at 0.2 mg.

➤ *To manage moderate to severe pain in opioid-tolerant patients requiring continuous, around-the-clock opioid analgesia for an extended period of time and for which alternative treatment options are inadequate*

E.R. TABLETS (EXALGO)
Adults. Highly individualized and dependent on patient's previous total 24-hour opioid use and risk factors for abuse, addiction, and misuse. Once dosage is determined, drug is given once daily. Dosage may be increased by 4 to 8 mg every 3 to 4 days, as needed.
DOSAGE ADJUSTMENT For patients with hepatic or renal impairment, dosage started at 25% to 50% of normal dosage.

Route	Onset	Peak	Duration
P.O.	30 min	1.5–2 hr	4 hr
I.V.	10–15 min	15–30 min	2–3 hr
I.M.	15 min	30–60 min	4–5 hr
SubQ	15 min	30–90 min	4 hr
P.R.	30 min	Unknown	4 hr

Mechanism of Action
May bind with opioid receptors in the spinal cord and higher levels in the CNS. In this way, hydromorphone is believed to stimulate kappa and mu receptors, thus altering the perception of and emotional response to pain.

Contraindications
Acute asthma; history of narrowing of the GI tract or presence of blind loops in the GI tract, or GI obstruction; hypersensitivity to hydromorphone, other narcotics, or their components; increased intracranial pressure; opioid nontolerant patients (Dilaudid HP, Exalgo); paralytic ileus; severe respiratory depression; upper respiratory tract obstruction

Interactions
DRUGS
anticholinergics: Increased risk of ileus, severe constipation, or urine retention
antihypertensives, diuretics, guanadrel, guanethidine, mecamylamine: Increased risk of orthostatic hypotension
antimigraine agents; cyclobenzaprine; dextromethorphan; dolasetron; granisetron; linezolid; MAO inhibitors; methylene blue; ondansetron; palonosetron; selected psychiatric drugs such as amoxapine, buspirone, lithium, maprotiline, mirtazapine, nefazodone, trazodone, vilazodone; selective serotonin reuptake inhibitors; serotonin-norepinephrine reuptake inhibitors; St. John's wort; tricyclic antidepressants; tryptophan: Increased risk of serotonin syndrome
benzodiazepines, CNS depressants, other opioids, sedating antihistamines, tricyclic antidepressants: Increased risk of significant sedation and somnolence and severe respiratory depression
barbiturate anesthetics: Increased sedative effect of hydromorphone
belladonna alkaloids, difenoxin and atropine, diphenoxylate and atropine, kaolin pectin, loperamide, paregoric: Increased risk of CNS depression and severe constipation
buprenorphine, butorphanol, dezocine, nalbuphine, pentazocine: Possibly potentiated or suppressed symptoms of spontaneous opioid withdrawal
CNS depressants, other opioid analgesics: Additive CNS depression and hypotension,

possibly resulting in life-threatening reactions
hydroxyzine: Increased analgesia, CNS depression, and hypotension
metoclopramide: Decreased effect of metoclopramide on GI motility
naloxone: Possibly withdrawal symptoms in physically dependent patients
naltrexone: Possibly cardiac arrest or prolonged respiratory depression
neuromuscular blockers: Additive CNS depression
ACTIVITIES
alcohol use: Increased CNS and respiratory depression

Adverse Reactions

CNS: Anxiety, **CNS depression**, confusion, dizziness, drowsiness, euphoria, hallucinations, headache, nervousness, restlessness, sedation, somnolence, tremor, weakness
CV: Hypertension, orthostatic hypotension, palpitations, tachycardia
EENT: Blurred vision, diplopia, dry mouth, **laryngeal edema**, **laryngeal spasms**, nystagmus, tinnitus
ENDO: Adrenal insufficiency
GI: Abdominal cramps, anorexia, biliary tract spasm, constipation, **hepatotoxicity**, nausea, vomiting
GU: Decreased libido, dysuria, erectile dysfunction, impotence, infertility, lack of menstruation, urine retention
RESP: Dyspnea, **respiratory depression**, wheezing
SKIN: Diaphoresis, flushing
Other: Injection-site pain, redness, and swelling; physical and psychological dependence

Nursing Considerations

- Be aware that hydromorphone therapy increases risk of abuse, addiction, and misuse. A Risk Evaluation and Mitigation Strategy (REMS) is required. Monitor patient closely throughout therapy for abuse, addiction, or misuse.
- Know that chronic maternal use of hydromorphone during pregnancy can result in neonatal opioid withdrawal syndrome (NOWS), which may be life-threatening, if not recognized and treated appropriately. NOWS occurs when a newborn has been exposed to opioid drugs for a prolonged period while in utero.
- Use extreme caution when administering hydromorphone to patients with cor pulmonale or significant chronic obstructive pulmonary disease, and in patients having a substantially decreased respiratory reserve, hypercapnia, hypoxia, or preexisting respiratory depression, especially when initiating and titrating therapy. These patients may develop respiratory depression, even with usual therapeutic doses, because hydromorphone may decrease the patient's respiratory drive to the point of apnea.
- Use hydromorphone cautiously in, cachectic, debilitated, or elderly patients, especially when initiating and titrating therapy, as they are at increased risk for adverse effects, especially respiratory depression.
- Use hydromorphone cautiously in patients whose ability to maintain a normal blood pressure is already compromised by a reduced blood volume or concurrent administration of certain CNS depressant drugs; the drug may cause severe hypotension in these patients, especially when initiating or titrating the dose of hydromorphone.
- Be aware that hydromorphone should only be used concomitantly with benzodiazepines and other CNS depressants in patients for whom other treatment options are inadequate. If prescribed together, expect dosing and duration of hydromorphone to be limited. Monitor patient closely for signs and symptoms of decrease in consciousness, including coma, profound sedation, and significant respiratory depression. Notify prescriber immediately, expect drug to be discontinued, and provide emergency supportive care, as death may occur.
- Be aware that to improve analgesic action, give hydromorphone before pain becomes intense.
- Give I.V. form by direct injection over at least 2 minutes. For infusion, mix drug with D_5W, normal saline solution, or Ringer's solution.
- Rotate I.M. and subcutaneous injection sites.

WARNING Monitor patient for respiratory depression, especially within the first 72 hours of initiating therapy or when increasing dosage, even when the drug has been used as prescribed and not abused or misused. Patients who are especially vulnerable include the elderly and those who are cachectic or debilitated. Be aware that overestimating hydromorphone dose when converting patients from another opioid medication can result in fatal overdose with the first dose. To avoid this, know that it is recommended to underestimate a patient's 24-hour oral hydromorphone requirement and provide rescue medication, as needed, until the right dose is determined. Keep resuscitation equipment and naloxone nearby.

- Monitor patient for coma, hypotension, profound sedation, or respiratory depression when administering hydromorphone around-the-clock; these reactions can occur if alcohol or illicit drugs are being used without the prescriber's knowledge.

WARNING Know that many drugs may interact with opioids like hydromorphone to cause serotonin syndrome. Monitor patient closely for signs and symptoms such as agitation, diaphoresis, diarrhea, fever, hallucinations, labile blood pressure, muscle twitching or stiffness, nausea, shakiness, shivering, tachycardia, trouble with coordination, or vomiting. Notify prescriber at once because serotonin syndrome may be life-threatening. Be prepared to discontinue drug, if possible and ordered, and provide supportive care.

- Monitor patient for adrenal insufficiency. Although rare, it can be life-threatening. Monitor patient for anorexia, dizziness, fatigue, hypotension, nausea, vomiting, or weakness. Notify prescriber if adrenal insufficiency is suspected and expect to do diagnostic testing. If diagnosis is confirmed, expect to administer corticosteroids and wean patient off hydromorphone, if possible.
- Monitor patients with seizure disorders because hydromorphone therapy may aggravate or induce convulsions.
- Monitor effectiveness of hydromorphone in relieving pain; consult prescriber as needed.
- Assess patient for constipation.
- Monitor patient for evidence of physical abuse or dependence. Be aware that excessive use of opioids such as hydromorphone may lead to abuse, addiction, misuse, overdose, and possibly death. Monitor patient's intake of drug closely.
- Anticipate that drug may mask or worsen gallbladder pain.
- Be aware that all other around-the-clock opioid analgesics should be stopped when E.R. tablets are prescribed. Expect to give immediate-release nonopioid analgesics for exacerbation of pain and for preventing pain during certain activities.
- Know that E.R. tablets may be visible on abdominal X-rays under certain circumstances, especially when digital enhancing techniques are utilized, because the tablet is nondeformable and does not change much in shape in the GI tract.
- Expect to taper dosages of hydromorphone that have been administered for an extended period of time to the opioid-tolerant patient gradually by 25 to 50% every 2 to 3 days, down to a dose of 8 mg before the drug is discontinued. This will help prevent signs and symptoms of withdrawal.

PATIENT TEACHING

- Instruct patient to take drug exactly as prescribed and before pain is severe. Also, tell her not to take more drug than prescribed and not to take it longer than absolutely needed, because excessive or prolonged use can lead to abuse, addiction, misuse, overdose, and possibly death.
- Alert patient that drug is a controlled substance. She should take steps to protect drug from theft.
- Advise patient to take drug with food to avoid GI distress.
- Tell patient not to break, chew, crush, or dissolve E.R. tablets, but to swallow them whole.
- Instruct patient to refrigerate suppositories.
- Inform patient about potentially fatal additive effects of combining hydromorphone with a benzodiazepine. In addition, other serious drug reactions can

occur. Instruct patient to inform all prescribers of hydromorphone use.
- Caution patient to avoid alcohol and OTC drugs during therapy, unless prescriber approves.
- Instruct patient to report constipation, difficulty breathing, severe nausea, or vomiting.
- Inform patient that drug may cause drowsiness and sedation. Advise her to avoid hazardous activities until drug's CNS effects are known.
- Tell patient to change position slowly to minimize orthostatic hypotension.
- Instruct physically dependent patient not to stop taking hydromorphone abruptly to avoid withdrawal.
- Warn patient to keep drug out of reach of children, as accidental ingestion may cause death.
- Advise women of childbearing age to notify prescriber immediately if they suspect they are pregnant or become pregnant because hydromorphone may cause fetal harm or neonatal withdrawal that could be life-threatening.
- Advise patients when hydromorphone tablets or solution are no longer needed to remit to authorities at a certified drug take-back program.
- Inform patient that long-term use of opioids like hydromorphone may decrease sex hormone levels, causing decreased libido, erectile dysfunction, impotence, infertility, or lack of menstruation. Encourage patient to report any such symptoms.

hydroxychloroquine sulfate

Plaquenil

Class and Category

Pharmacologic class: Aminoquinoline
Therapeutic class: Antimalarial, antirheumatic, lupus erythematosus suppressant
Pregnancy category: C

Indications and Dosages

➤ *To prevent malaria*

TABLETS

Adults. 400 mg the same day of each week starting 2 wk before entering endemic area and continuing until departure from endemic area.

Children age 6 and over. 6.5 mg/kg the same day of each week, starting 2 wk before entering endemic area and continuing until departure from endemic area. *Maximum:* 400 mg once weekly.

➤ *To treat acute attacks of malaria caused by* Plasmodium falciparum, P. malariae, P. ovale, or P. vivax

TABLETS

Adults. *Initial:* 800 mg, followed by 400 mg in 6 hr, 24 hr, and 49 hr after initial dose.

Children age 6 and over. *Initial:* 13 mg/kg (up to 800 mg), then 6.5 mg/kg (up to 400 mg) at 6 hr, 24 hr, and 48 hr after initial dose.

➤ *To treat chronic discoid and systemic lupus erythematosus*

TABLETS

Adults. 200 to 400 mg once or in 2 divided doses for several weeks or months. *Maximum:* 400 mg daily.

➤ *To treat acute or chronic rheumatoid arthritis*

TABLETS

Adults. *Initial:* 400 to 600 mg daily as a single dose or in 2 divided doses. Following a good response, dosage reduced by 50%. *Maintenance:* 200 mg to 400 mg daily as a single dose or in 2 divided doses. *Maximum:* 600 mg daily or 6.5 mg/kg daily, whichever is lower.

DOSAGE ADJUSTMENT For patients with rheumatoid arthritis who develop troublesome adverse reactions, initial dosage decreased for 5 to 10 days and then gradually increased to optimum response level.

Mechanism of Action

May mildly suppress the immune system, inhibiting production of rheumatoid factor and acute phase reactants.

Hydroxychloroquine also accumulates in WBCs, stabilizing lysosomal membranes and inhibiting enzymes such as collagenase and proteases that cause cartilage breakdown. These actions may decrease symptoms of rheumatoid arthritis and lupus erythematosus.

Hydroxychloroquine also binds to and alters DNA of malaria parasite to prevent it from reproducing. It also may increase the pH of acid vesicles, which interferes with vesicle function and may inhibit parasitic phospholipid metabolism in erythrocytes, thereby halting plasmodial activity.

Contraindications

Hypersensitivity to hydroxychloroquine, other 4-aminoquinoline compounds, or their components; long-term therapy in children, retinal or visual changes related to 4-aminoquinoline compounds

Interactions

DRUGS

ampicillin: Possibly significant decrease in bioavailability of ampicillin, decreasing its effectiveness
antacids, kaolin: Possible reduced absorption of hydroxychloroquine
antidiabetic drugs, insulin: Possible increased risk of hypoglycemia
antiepileptics, mefloquine, other drugs that lower seizure threshold: Increased risk of seizures
aurothioglucose: Increased risk of blood dyscrasias
cimetidine: Possibly increased plasma hydroxychloroquine levels
cyclosporin: Increased plasma cyclosporin levels
digoxin: Increased digoxin concentrations
drugs that prolong QT interval, including other arrhythmogenic drugs: Increased risk of arrhythmias
hepatotoxic or nephrotoxic drugs: Possibly increased risk of kidney or liver toxicity
methotrexate: Possible increased risk of adverse reactions
praziquantel: Possible reduced bioavailability of praziquantel affecting its effectiveness
tamoxifen: Increased risk of irreversible retinal damage

Adverse Reactions

CNS: Abnormal nerve conduction, ataxia, dizziness, emotional lability, fatigue, extrapyramidal disorders, headache, irritability, lassitude, nervousness, neuromuscular sensory abnormalities, nightmares, psychosis, **seizures**, **suicidal ideation**, vertigo
CV: Atrioventricular blocks, bundle branch block, **cardiomyopathy** (prolonged high doses), **prolonged QT interval**, **torsades de pointes**, **ventricular arrhythmias**
EENT: Abnormal pigmentation (bullseye appearance) or colored vision, blurred vision, central scotoma with decreased visual acuity, corneal deposits, decreased corneal sensitivity, diplopia, irreversible retinal damage, halo vision, lassitude, macular atrophy or edema, nerve-related hearing loss, nystagmus, paracentral or pericentral scotoma, photophobia, retinal fundus changes, tinnitus, visual abnormalities including visual fields
ENDO: Hypoglycemia
GI: Abdominal cramps, **acute or fulminant hepatic failure**, anorexia, diarrhea, elevated liver enzymes, nausea, vomiting
HEME: Agranulocytosis, anemia, **aplastic anemia**, **bone marrow failure**, **hemolysis** (in patients with glucose-6 phosphate dehydrogenase [G6PD] deficiency), **leukopenia**, **thrombocytopenia**
MS: Atrophy of proximal skeletal muscle groups, depressed tendon reflexes, muscle weakness, myopathy
RESP: Bronchospasm
SKIN: Acute generalized exanthematous pustulosis, alopecia, altered mucosal and skin pigmentation, bleaching of hair, dermatitis (including bullous and **exfoliative dermatitis**), **erythema multiforme**, non-light-sensitive psoriasis, photosensitivity, pruritus, psoriasis exacerbation, rash, **Stevens–Johnson syndrome**, **toxic epidermal necrolysis**, urticaria
Other: Angioedema, **drug reaction with eosinophilia and systemic symptoms (DRESS)**, porphyria including worsening, weight loss

Nursing Considerations

- Use hydroxychloroquine cautiously in patients with G6PD deficiency, patients with alcoholism or hepatic or renal disease, and patients taking hepatotoxic drugs. Also use cautiously in patients with blood, gastrointestinal, or neurological disorders and in patients who are sensitive to quinine.
- Monitor children closely for adverse reactions because they're especially

sensitive to 4-aminoquinoline compounds.
- Observe patients with psoriasis closely because hydroxychloroquine may lead to severe psoriasis attack. Also monitor patients with porphyria closely because hydroxychloroquine may worsen it. Expect to use hydroxychloroquine in patients with porphyria or psoriasis only after risks and benefits have been considered.
- Obtain periodic blood cell counts, as ordered, during prolonged therapy to detect adverse hematologic effects. Expect to stop drug if severe adverse effects occur.
- Monitor patient's vision when giving hydroxychloroquine, because irreversible retinal damage may occur in some patients during high-dose or long-term therapy. Ask regularly about vision abnormalities, such as light flashes or streaks that may indicate retinopathy. Expect patient to have an initial ophthalmologic examination, followed by examinations every 3 months. Be aware that in patients of Asian descent, retinal toxicity may first be noticed outside the macula. Report changes to prescriber immediately, and expect drug to be stopped. Retinal changes may progress even after therapy stops.
- Monitor patient on long-term therapy for muscle weakness and abnormal ankle and knee reflexes. If present, notify prescriber and expect drug to be stopped.
- Expect drug to be stopped if patient with rheumatoid arthritis shows no improvement, such as reduced joint swelling or increased mobility, in 6 months.
- Notify prescriber immediately if serious adverse reactions occur. Expect drug to be stopped. Also expect to give ammonium chloride (8 g daily in divided doses for adults) 3 or 4 days weekly for several months because acidification of urine increases renal excretion of drug.

PATIENT TEACHING

- Instruct patient to take drug with meals or milk to minimize stomach upset.
- Tell patient to take hydroxychloroquine exactly as prescribed because taking too much may cause serious adverse reactions and taking too little or skipping doses decreases effectiveness.
- Caution patient to notify prescriber about troublesome adverse reactions. Hydroxychloroquine dosage may need to be adjusted or drug stopped.
- Caution patient about possible visual reactions and the need for periodic eye examinations. Tell patient to notify prescriber about abnormal visual changes, including blurred vision, halos around lights, and light flashes or streaks; explain that drug will need to be stopped.
- Tell patient receiving prolonged therapy about the need for periodic blood tests to detect adverse effects.
- Advise patient to notify prescriber if muscle weakness develops.
- Review early signs and symptoms of toxicity. Tell patient to notify prescriber immediately, if present.
- Inform mothers wishing to breastfeed that drug is excreted in breast milk and that infants are extremely sensitive to the toxic effects of drug. Advise them to discuss breastfeeding with prescriber before doing so.
- Warn patient to keep drug out of reach of children, as fatalities have occurred when drug has been accidentally ingested, even in small amounts.

hydroxyzine hydrochloride

Atarax (CAN)

hydroxyzine pamoate

Vistaril

Class and Category

Pharmacologic class: Piperazine derivative
Therapeutic class: Anxiolytic, Antiemetic, antihistamine, sedative-hypnotic
Pregnancy category: C

Indications and Dosages

➤ *To relieve anxiety*

CAPSULES, ORAL SUSPENSION, SYRUP, TABLETS

Adults and adolescents. 50 to 100 mg four times daily.

Children age 6 and over. 50 to 100 mg daily in divided doses.
Children under 6 years of age. 50 mg daily in divided doses.

I.M. INJECTION

Adults and adolescents. 50 to 100 mg every 4 to 6 hr, as needed (antianxiety).

➤ *To treat pruritus*

CAPSULES, ORAL SUSPENSION, SYRUP, TABLETS

Adults and adolescents. 25 mg three times daily or four times daily, as needed.
Children age 6 and over. 50 to 100 mg daily in divided doses.
Children under 6 years of age. 50 mg daily in divided doses.

➤ *As adjunct to permit reduction in preoperative and postoperative opioid dosage*

I.M. INJECTION

Adults and adolescents. 50 to 100 mg given with prescribed opioid.
Children. 0.6 mg/kg given with prescribed opioid.

DOSAGE ADJUSTMENT For elderly patients, treatment is started at lowest possible dosage.

Route	Onset	Peak	Duration
P.O.	15–60 min	Unknown	4–6 hr
I.M.	20–30 min	Unknown	4–6 hr

Mechanism of Action

Competes with histamine for histamine$_1$ receptor sites on surfaces of effector cells. This suppresses results of histaminic activity, including edema, flare, and pruritus. Sedative actions occur at subcortical level of CNS and are dose related.

Contraindications

Breastfeeding; early pregnancy; hypersensitivity to cetirizine, hydroxyzine, or their components; prolonged QT interval

Interactions

DRUGS

antibiotics such as azithromycin, erythromycin, clarithromycin, gatifloxacin, or moxifloxacin; antidepressants such as citalopram or fluoxetine; antipsychotics such as chlorpromazine, clozapine, iloperidone, quetiapine, or ziprasidone; class IA antiarrhythmics such as procainamide or quinidine; class III antiarrhythmics such as amiodarone or sotalol; droperidol; methadone; ondansetron; pentamidine: Increased risk of QT prolongation
CNS depressants: Increased CNS depression

ACTIVITIES

alcohol use: Increased CNS depression

Adverse Reactions

CNS: Drowsiness, hallucinations, headache, involuntary motor activity, **seizures**, tremor
CV: Prolonged QT interval, torsades de pointes
EENT: Dry mouth
SKIN: Fixed drug eruptions, pruritus, rash, urticaria
Other: Hypersensitivity reactions, injection-site pain

Nursing Considerations

- Use hydroxyzine cautiously in patients with risk factors for QT prolongation such as concomitant arrhythmogenic drug use, electrolyte imbalance, or preexisting heart disease. Also use cautiously in patients with bradyarrhythmias, congenital or family history of long QT syndrome, other conditions that predispose patient to QT prolongation and ventricular arrhythmia, recent MI, or uncompensated heart failure.
- Don't give hydroxyzine by subcutaneous or I.V. route because tissue necrosis may occur.
- Inject I.M. form deep into large muscle, using Z-track method.
- Observe for oversedation if patient takes another CNS depressant.

PATIENT TEACHING

- Urge patient to avoid alcohol.
- Caution patient about drowsiness; tell her to avoid hazardous activities until drug's CNS effects are known.
- Instruct woman to tell prescriber if she is or could be pregnant because drug is contraindicated in early pregnancy.

ibalizumab-uiyk

Trogarzo

Class and Category

Pharmacologic class: CD4-directed post-attachment HIV-1 inhibitor
Therapeutic class: Antiretroviral
Pregnancy category: Not classified

Indications and Dosages

➤ *As adjunct to treat human immunodeficiency virus (HIV) type 1 infection in heavily treatment-experienced patients with multidrug-resistant HIV-1 infection who are failing their current antiretroviral regimen*

I.V. INFUSION

Adults. *Loading:* 2,000 mg infused over at least 30 min. *Maintenance:* 800 mg infused 2 wk later and every 2 wk thereafter. Infused over 15 min providing no infusion reaction occurred with loading dose; otherwise infused over at least 30 min.

Mechanism of Action

Blocks HIV-1 from infecting CD4 T cells by binding to domain 2 of CD4 and interfering with post-attachment steps required for entry of HIV-1 virus particles into host cells. Also prevents the viral transmission that occurs via cell–cell infusion.

Contraindications

Hypersensitivity to ibalizumab-uiyk or its components

Interactions

DRUGS

None reported

Adverse Reactions

CNS: Dizziness
ENDO: Hyperglycemia
GI: Diarrhea, elevated bilirubin and lipase levels, nausea
GU: Elevated creatinine level
HEME: Anemia, **decreased platelet count, leukopenia, neutropenia**
SKIN: Rash
Other: Antibody formation to ibalizumab-uiyk, elevated uric acid level, immune reconstitution inflammatory syndrome

Nursing Considerations

- Use 10 vials to prepare the loading dose of 2,000 mg and 4 vials to prepare each maintenance dose of 800 mg. To prepare, insert sterile syringe needle into each vial through center of stopper, withdraw 1.33 ml of drug, and transfer into a 240-ml intravenous bag of 0.9% sodium chloride injection, USP. Do not use any other diluent solutions. Once diluted, administer immediately or store at room temperature for up to 4 hours or refrigerated for up to 24 hours. If refrigerated, allow diluted drug solution to stand at room temperature for at least 30 minutes but no more than 4 hours prior to administration.
- Administer infusion in the cephalic vein of patient's left or right arm. If this vein is not accessible, know that an appropriate vein located elsewhere can be used. Never administer drug as an IV bolus or IV push.
- Infuse loading dose over at least 30 minutes or more. If no infusion-associated adverse reactions occur, maintenance infusion time can be decreased to no less than 15 minutes. After infusion is complete, flush intravenous line with 30 ml of 0.9% sodium chloride injection, USP.
- Observe patient for 1 hour after loading-dose infusion is complete. If no infusion-associated adverse reactions occur, time of observation can be decreased to 15 minutes for subsequent maintenance infusions.
- Know that if a maintenance dose is missed by 3 days or longer beyond the scheduled dosing day, a loading dose of 2,000 mg should be administered as early as possible and the maintenance dosing of 800 mg resumed 2 weeks later.
- Monitor patient for signs and symptoms of infection, which could be caused by immune reconstitution inflammatory syndrome. Although rare, this syndrome may occur in combination with other antiretroviral therapy in patients whose immune systems respond during the initial phase causing an inflammatory reaction to indolent or residual opportunistic infections. If present, further evaluation and treatment will be needed.

PATIENT TEACHING

- Stress importance of compliance with dosage schedule of every 2 weeks. Remind patient that if dose is missed for 3 days or longer, a loading dosage will have to be repeated before maintenance dosing can be reestablished.
- Instruct patient to immediately report any signs and symptoms of an infection to prescriber.

- Inform women of childbearing age to notify prescriber if pregnancy occurs, and encourage patient to enroll in the pregnancy exposure registry.
- Advise mothers not to breastfeed their infant while receiving ibalizumab-uiyk.

ibandronate sodium

Boniva

Class and Category

Pharmacologic class: Bisphosphonate
Therapeutic class: Antiosteoporotic
Pregnancy category: C

Indications and Dosages

➤ *To prevent osteoporosis in postmenopausal women*

TABLETS

Adult women. 150 mg once monthly taken same day of each month.

➤ *To treat osteoporosis in postmenopausal women*

TABLETS

Adult women. 150 mg once monthly taken same day of each month.

I.V. INJECTION

Adults. 3 mg injected over 15 to 30 sec every 3 mo.

Mechanism of Action

Based on its affinity for hydroxyapatite, which is part of the mineral matrix of bone, osteoclast activity is inhibited and bone resorption and turnover is reduced. In postmenopausal women, the elevated rate of bone turnover is reduced leading to, on average, a net gain in bone mass.

Incompatibilities

Do not mix with calcium-containing solutions or other intravenously administered drugs.

Contraindications

Esophageal abnormalities that delay esophageal emptying, such as achalasia or stricture (oral form); hypersensitivity to ibandronate or its components; uncorrected hypocalcemia

Interactions

DRUGS

aspirin, NSAIDs: Increased risk of GI irritation
calcium-containing preparations, including antacids: Impaired absorption of ibandronate

FOODS

all foods: Decreased ibandronate bioavailability

Adverse Reactions

CNS: Asthenia, depression, dizziness, fatigue, headache, insomnia, nerve root lesion, vertigo
CV: Hypercholesterolemia, hypertension
EENT: Nasopharyngitis, pharyngitis, tooth disorder
GI: Abdominal pain, constipation, diarrhea, dyspepsia, gastritis, gastroenteritis, nausea, vomiting
GU: Cystitis, UTI
MS: Arthralgia; arthritis; atypical subtrochanteric and diaphyseal femoral fractures; back, bone, extremity, joint, or muscle pain; joint disorder; localized osteoarthritis; myalgia; osteonecrosis of jaw and other orofacial sites
RESP: **Asthma exacerbations**, bronchitis, **bronchospasm**, pneumonia, upper respiratory infection
SKIN: Dermatitis bullous, **erythema multiforme**, rash, **Stevens–Johnson syndrome**
Other: **Anaphylaxis**, **angioedema**, **hypersensitivity reactions**, infection, flu-like symptoms, **hypocalcemia**, injection-site reactions such as redness or swelling

Nursing Considerations

- Be aware that hypocalcemia, hypovitaminosis D, and other disturbances of bone and mineral metabolism must be effectively treated before starting ibandronate therapy.
- Know that ibandronate should not be administered to patients with severe renal impairment or to women who are not postmenopausal.
- Use cautiously in patients with active upper gastrointestinal problems (such as known Barrett's esophagus, dysphagia, other esophageal diseases, duodenitis, gastritis, ulcers because drug may cause

local irritation of the upper gastrointestinal mucosa).
- Make sure patient has had a dental checkup before having invasive dental procedures during ibandronate therapy, especially if patient has cancer; is receiving chemotherapy, head or neck radiation, or a corticosteroid; or has poor oral hygiene, because the risk of jaw osteonecrosis has increased in these patients taking other bisphosphonates, a class of drugs of which ibandronate is a member.
- Obtain serum creatinine level in patients receiving injection form of ibandronate prior to administering each dose because other bisphosphonates have been associated with serious renal toxicity. If renal deterioration occurs, expect drug to be withheld.
- Administer parenteral ibandronate intravenously over 15 to 30 seconds using the needle provided. Prefilled syringes are for single use only. Be careful not to inject drug intra-arterially or paravenously, as this could lead to tissue damage.
- Administer drug as soon as possible after a missed appointment for parenteral ibandronate therapy. Schedule next injection from the date of the last injection, as drug must not be administered more frequently than once every 3 months.

PATIENT TEACHING
- Instruct patient prescribed oral ibandronate to take the tablet at least 1 hour before first food or drink of day (except water) while in an upright position and with 6 to 8 oz of water. Caution against lying down for at least 60 minutes after taking drug to keep it from lodging in esophagus and causing irritation. Also instruct patient not to chew or suck on tablet because doing so may irritate mouth or throat.
- Inform patient of need and importance of taking supplemental calcium and vitamin D on daily basis.
- Instruct patient to take calcium supplements at least 2 hours before or after oral ibandronate.
- Advise patient to stop taking drug and to notify prescriber if GI symptoms appear or become worse.
- Alert patient that drugs in the same class as ibandronate have caused severe bone, joint, or muscle pain. If such symptoms appear while taking ibandronate, advise patient to contact prescriber. Also, tell him to report new or worsening groin or thigh pain.
- Tell patient to stop taking drug and notify prescriber if he develops dysphagia, pain while swallowing, retrosternal pain, or new or worsening heartburn.
- Inform women of childbearing age that drug is not used in their age group because of risk to fetal skeleton if pregnancy were to occur.
- Instruct patient on proper oral hygiene and on the need to notify prescriber about invasive dental procedures because risk of developing osteonecrosis of the jaw decreases in the absence of bisphosphonate therapy.

ibuprofen

Actiprofen Caplets (CAN), Advil, Apo-Ibuprofen (CAN), Bayer Select Ibuprofen Pain Relief Formula Caplets, Caldolor, Children's Advil, Children's Motrin, Dolgesic, Excedrin IB, Genpril, Haltran, Ibifon 600 Caplets, Ibuprin, Ibuprohm Caplets, Ibu-Tab, Medipren, Midol IB, Motrin, Motrin-IB, Novo-Profen (CAN), Nu-Ibuprofen (CAN), Nuprin, Pamprin-IB, Q-Profen, Rufen, Trendar

Class and Category

Pharmacologic class: NSAID
Therapeutic class: Analgesic, anti-inflammatory, antipyretic
Pregnancy category: C (before 30 weeks gestation); D (starting at 30 weeks gestation)

Indications and Dosages

➤ *To relieve pain in rheumatoid arthritis and osteoarthritis*

CAPSULES, CHEWABLE TABLETS, ORAL SUSPENSION, TABLETS

Adults. 300 mg four times daily; or 400, 600, or 800 mg three times daily; or four times daily. Range: 1.2 to 3.2 g daily.

➤ *To relieve pain in juvenile arthritis*
CAPSULES, CHEWABLE TABLETS, ORAL SUSPENSION, TABLETS
Children ages 6 months and over. 20 to 40 mg/kg daily in 3 or 4 divided doses. *Maximum:* 40 mg/kg daily.
➤ *To relieve mild to moderate pain*
CAPSULES, CHEWABLE TABLETS, ORAL SUSPENSION, TABLETS
Adults. 400 mg every 4 to 6 hr, as needed.
I.V. INFUSION
Adults. 400 to 800 mg infused over at least 30 min, every 6 hr, as needed. *Maximum:* 3,200 mg daily.
Adolescents. 400 mg infused over at least 10 min, every 4 to 6 hr, as needed. *Maximum:* 2,400 mg daily.
Children ages 6 months to 12 years. 10 mg/kg up to 400 mg maximum for single dose infused over at least 10 min, every 4 to 6 hr, as needed. *Maximum:* 40 mg/kg or 2,400 mg daily, whichever is less.
➤ *To relieve pain in primary dysmenorrhea*
CAPSULES, CHEWABLE TABLETS, ORAL SUSPENSION, TABLETS
Adults. 400 mg every 4 hr, as needed.
➤ *To relieve moderate to severe pain as an adjunct to opioid analgesics*
I.V. INFUSION
Adults. 400 to 800 mg infused over at least 30 min, every 6 hr, as needed.
➤ *To reduce fever*
CAPSULES, CHEWABLE TABLETS, ORAL SUSPENSION, TABLETS
Adults and adolescents. 200 to 400 mg every 4 to 6 hr, as needed.
Children age 11 weighing 33 to 43 kg (72 to 95 lb). 300 mg every 6 to 8 hr, as needed.
Children ages 9 and 10 weighing 28 to 32 kg (60 to 71 lb). 250 mg every 6 to 8 hr, as needed.
Children ages 6 to 8 weighing 22 to 27 kg (48 to 59 lb). 200 mg every 6 to 8 hr, as needed.
Children ages 4 and 5 weighing 16 to 21 kg (36 to 47 lb). 150 mg every 6 to 8 hr, as needed.
Children ages 2 and 3 weighing 11 to 16 kg (24 to 35 lb). 100 mg every 6 to 8 hr, as needed.
I.V. INFUSION
Adults. 400 mg infused over at least 30 min, followed by 400 mg infused over at least 30 min, every 4 to 6 hr. Or, 100 to 200 mg infused over at least 30 min, every 4 hr, as needed. *Maximum:* 3,200 mg daily.
Adolescents. 400 mg infused over at least 10 min, every 4 to 6 hr, as needed. *Maximum:* 2,400 mg daily.
Children ages 6 months to 12 years. 10 mg/kg up to 400 mg maximum for single dose infused over at least 10 min, every 4 to 6 hr, as needed. *Maximum:* 40 mg/kg or 2,400 mg daily, whichever is less.
➤ *To treat patent ductus arteriosus (ibuprofen lysine).*
I.V. INFUSION
Gestational age 32 weeks or less and weighing between 500 and 1,500 g
Initial: 10 mg/kg infused over at least 15 min, followed by 5 mg/kg 24 hr later and 5 mg/kg 24 hr after second dose.

Route	Onset	Peak	Duration
P.O.*	30 min	Unknown	4–6 hr
P.O.†	Up to 7 days	1–2 wk	Unknown
P.O.†	In 1 hr	2–4 hr	6–8 hr
I.V.	10–30 min	Unknown	Unknown

* For analgesic effects.
† For anti-inflammatory effects.
‡ For antipyretic effects.

Mechanism of Action

Blocks activity of cyclooxygenase, the enzyme needed to synthesize prostaglandins, which mediate inflammatory response and cause local pain, swelling, and vasodilation. By inhibiting prostaglandins, this NSAID reduces inflammatory symptoms and relieves pain. Ibuprofen's antipyretic action probably stems from its effect on the hypothalamus, which increases peripheral blood flow, causing vasodilation and encouraging heat dissipation.

Contraindications

Angioedema, asthma, bronchospasm, nasal polyps, rhinitis, or urticaria caused by hypersensitivity to aspirin, iodides, or other NSAIDs; hypersensitivity to ibuprofen, its components, or other fever reducers or pain relievers; pain with coronary artery bypass graft (CABG) surgery; pediatric heart surgery (before and after)

Interactions

DRUGS

acetaminophen: Possibly increased renal effects with long-term use of both drugs
antihypertensives: Decreased effectiveness of these drugs
aspirin: Possibly decreased cardioprotective and stroke-preventive effects of aspirin
aspirin, other NSAIDs: Increased risk of bleeding and adverse GI effects
bone marrow depressants: Possibly increased leukopenic and thrombocytopenic effects of bone marrow depressants
cefamandole, cefoperazone, cefotetan: Increased risk of hypoprothrombinemia and bleeding
colchicine, platelet aggregation inhibitors: Increased risk of GI bleeding, hemorrhage, and ulcers
corticosteroids, potassium supplements: Increased risk of adverse GI effects
cyclosporine: Increased risk of nephrotoxicity from both drugs, increased blood cyclosporine level
digoxin: Increased blood digoxin level and risk of digitalis toxicity
diuretics (loop, potassium-sparing, and thiazide): Decreased diuretic and antihypertensive effects
gold compounds, nephrotoxic drugs: Increased risk of adverse renal effects
heparin, oral anticoagulants, thrombolytics: Increased anticoagulant effects, increased risk of hemorrhage
insulin, oral antidiabetics: Possibly increased hypoglycemic effects of these drugs
lithium: Increased blood lithium level
methotrexate: Decreased methotrexate clearance and increased risk of toxicity
plicamycin, valproic acid: Increased risk of hypoprothrombinemia and GI bleeding, hemorrhage, and ulcers
probenecid: Possibly increased blood level, effectiveness, and risk of toxicity of ibuprofen

ACTIVITIES

alcohol use: Increased risk of adverse GI effects

Adverse Reactions

CNS: Aseptic meningitis, **CVA**, dizziness, headache, nervousness, **seizures**
CV: Fluid retention, **heart failure**, hypertension, **MI**, peripheral edema, tachycardia
EENT: Amblyopia, epistaxis, stomatitis, tinnitus
GI: Abdominal cramps, distention, or pain; anorexia; constipation; diarrhea; diverticulitis; dyspepsia; dysphagia; elevated liver enzymes; epigastric discomfort; esophagitis; flatulence; gastritis; gastroenteritis; gastroesophageal reflux disease; **GI bleeding**, **hemorrhage**, **perforation**, or ulceration; heartburn; hemorrhoids; **hepatic failure**; **hepatitis**; hiatal hernia; indigestion; **melena**; nausea; stomatitis; vomiting
GU: Cystitis, hematuria, **renal failure (acute)**
HEME: Agranulocytosis, anemia, **aplastic anemia**, eosinophilia, **hemolytic anemia**, **leukopenia**, **neutropenia**, **pancytopenia**, **prolonged bleeding time**, **thrombocytopenia**
RESP: Bronchospasm, dyspnea, wheezing
SKIN: Blisters, **erythema multiforme**, photosensitivity, pruritus, rash, **Stevens–Johnson syndrome**, **toxic epidermal necrolysis**, urticaria
Other: Anaphylaxis, **angioedema**, flu-like symptoms, **hypokalemia**, weight gain

Nursing Considerations

- Be aware that ibuprofen should not be used in pregnant women starting at 30 weeks gestation because premature closure of the ductus arteriosus may occur in the fetus.
- Be aware that NSAIDs like ibuprofen should be avoided in patients with a recent MI because risk of reinfarction increases with NSAID therapy. If therapy is unavoidable, monitor patient closely for signs of cardiac ischemia.
- Know that the risk of heart failure increases with use of NSAIDs such as

ibuprofen. Ibuprofen should not be used in patients with severe heart failure but, if unavoidable, monitor patient for worsening of heart failure.

- Use ibuprofen with extreme caution in patients with a history of GI bleeding or ulcer disease because NSAIDs, such as ibuprofen, increase risk of GI bleeding and ulceration. Expect to use ibuprofen for shortest time possible in these patients.

WARNING **Be aware that the risk of serious cardiovascular thrombotic events such as a MI or stroke increases the longer ibuprofen is used. Expect to give drug for shortest time possible. These events may occur early in treatment and happen even in patients who do not have a history or risk factors for cardiovascular disease. Monitor patient for warning signs such as chest pain, slurring of speech, shortness of breath, or weakness. If any signs and symptoms develop, withhold ibuprofen, alert prescriber immediately, and provide supportive care as prescribed.**

- For I.V. use, dilute Caldolor brand of ibuprofen to final concentration of 4 mg/ml or less using 0.9% sodium chloride injection, 5% dextrose injection, or lactated Ringer's solution. For an 800-mg dose, dilute 8 ml Caldolor in at least 200 ml diluent; for a 400-mg dose, dilute 4 ml Caldolor in at least 100 ml diluent. Diluted solutions may be kept at room temperature up to 24 hours. When infusing ibuprofen intravenously, infusion time must be at least 30 minutes for adults and 10 minutes for children.
- Keep in mind that serious GI tract bleeding, perforation, and ulceration may occur without warning symptoms. Elderly patients are at greater risk. To minimize risk, give oral drug with food. If GI distress occurs, withhold drug and notify prescriber immediately.
- Use ibuprofen cautiously in patients with hypertension, and monitor blood pressure closely throughout therapy. Drug may cause hypertension or worsen it.

WARNING Monitor patient closely for thrombotic events, including MI and stroke, because NSAIDs increase the risk.

- Monitor patient—especially if he's elderly or receiving long-term oral ibuprofen therapy—for less common but serious adverse GI reactions, including anorexia, constipation, diverticulitis, dysphagia, esophagitis, gastritis, gastroenteritis, gastroesophageal reflux disease, hemorrhoids, hiatal hernia, melena, stomatitis, and vomiting.
- Monitor liver enzymes, as ordered, because, in rare cases, elevations may progress to severe hepatic reactions, including fatal hepatitis, hepatic failure, or liver necrosis.
- Monitor BUN and serum creatinine levels in elderly patients, patients taking ACE inhibitors or diuretics, and patients with heart failure, hepatic dysfunction or impaired renal function; drug may cause renal failure.
- Monitor CBC for decreased hemoglobin and hematocrit. Drug may worsen anemia.

WARNING **Be aware that if patient has bone marrow suppression or is receiving an antineoplastic drug, monitor laboratory results (including WBC count), and watch for evidence of infection. Ibuprofen's anti-inflammatory and antipyretic actions may mask signs and symptoms, such as fever and pain.**

- Assess patient's skin regularly for signs of rash or other hypersensitivity reaction because ibuprofen is an NSAID and may cause serious skin reactions without warning, even in patients with no history of NSAID sensitivity. At first sign of reaction, stop drug and notify prescriber.
- Expect higher doses for rheumatoid arthritis than for osteoarthritis.
- Be aware that ibuprofen oral suspension may contain sucrose, which may affect blood glucose level in diabetic patients.

PATIENT TEACHING

- Instruct patient to take tablets with a full glass of water, and caution him not to lie down for 15 to 30 minutes to prevent esophageal irritation.
- Advise patient to take drug with food or after meals to reduce GI distress.
- Urge patient not to take higher doses of drug or for a longer time than prescribed because stomach bleeding may occur and risk of MI or stroke may increase.
- Instruct patient to consult prescriber if he needs to take drug for more than 3 days for fever or 10 days for pain; if stomach problems (heartburn, pain, or upset)

recur; if he has a history of bleeding problems, heart or renal disease, hypertension, or ulcers; if he takes a diuretic; or if he's over age 65.

- Inform patient with phenylketonuria that Motrin chewable tablets contain aspartame.
- Inform patient that full therapeutic effect for arthritis may take 2 weeks or longer.
- Urge patient to avoid taking two different NSAIDs at the same time, unless directed, and to alert prescriber before taking ibuprofen if he has ever had an allergic reaction to any other analgesic or fever-reducing drug or has a history of asthma.
- Urge patient to avoid alcohol, aspirin, and corticosteroids while taking ibuprofen, unless prescribed. If patient takes aspirin as prevention of MI or stroke, explain that ibuprofen may interfere with this effect.
- Suggest that patient wear sunscreen and protective clothing when outdoors.
- Advise patient to report flu-like symptoms, rash, signs of GI bleeding, swelling, vision changes, and weight gain.
- Urge parents to tell prescriber promptly if child receiving drug develops headache, high fever, nausea, persistent diarrhea, severe persistent sore throat, or vomiting or hasn't been drinking fluids.
- Advise parents to consult prescriber before giving OTC ibuprofen to a child if the child has asthma, bleeding problems, heart or kidney disease, high blood pressure, or ulcers; a need for diuretic therapy; serious adverse effects from previous use of fever reducers or pain relievers; or persistent stomach problems, such as heartburn, stomach pain or upset stomach.
- Caution pregnant patient not to take NSAIDs such as ibuprofen during last trimester because they may cause premature closure of the ductus arteriosus.
- Explain that ibuprofen may increase risk of serious adverse cardiovascular reactions; urge patient to seek immediate medical attention if signs or symptoms arise, such as chest pain, edema, shortness of breath, slurring of speech, swelling in legs, unexplained weight gain, or weakness.
- Explain that ibuprofen may increase risk of serious adverse GI reactions; stress importance of seeking immediate medical attention for such signs and symptoms as abdominal or epigastric pain, black or tarry stools, indigestion, or vomiting blood or material that looks like coffee grounds.
- Alert patient to rare but serious skin reactions. Urge him to seek immediate medical attention for blisters, fever, itching, rash, or other indications of hypersensitivity.

ibutilide fumarate

Corvert

Class and Category

Pharmacologic class: Methanesulfonanilide derivative
Therapeutic class: Class III antiarrhythmic
Pregnancy category: C

Indications and Dosages

➤ *To rapidly convert recent-onset atrial flutter or fibrillation to sinus rhythm*

I.V. INFUSION

Adults weighing 60 kg (132 lb) or more. 1 mg over 10 min. Dose repeated 10 min after first dose is finished if arrhythmia persists.

Adults weighing less than 60 kg (132 lb). 0.01 mg/kg over 10 min. Dose is repeated 10 min after first dose is completed if arrhythmia persists.

DOSAGE ADJUSTMENT Infusion stopped if arrhythmia is terminated or if nonsustained or sustained ventricular tachycardia or prolonged QT or QTc interval develops.

Mechanism of Action

May promote sodium movement through slow inward sodium channels in myocardial cell membranes. Ibutilide also may inhibit potassium channels in myocardial cell membranes involved in cardiac repolarization. These actions prolong cardiac action potential by delaying repolarization and increasing atrial and ventricular refractoriness. As a result, sinus rate slows and AV conduction is delayed.

Contraindications
Hypersensitivity to ibutilide or components

Interactions
DRUGS
amiodarone, astemizole, disopyramide, maprotiline, phenothiazines, procainamide, quinidine, sotalol, tricyclic antidepressants: Possibly prolonged QT interval, leading to increased risk of proarrhythmias

Adverse Reactions
CNS: Headache, syncope
CV: **AV block, bradycardia**, bundle-branch block, **heart failure**, hypertension, **hypotension, idioventricular rhythm**, orthostatic hypotension, palpitations, **prolonged QT interval**, sinus tachycardia, **supraventricular arrhythmias, ventricular arrhythmias**
GI: Nausea
GU: **Renal failure**

Nursing Considerations
- Know that before giving ibutilide, check serum electrolyte levels and expect to correct abnormalities, as prescribed. Be especially alert for hypokalemia and hypomagnesemia, which can lead to arrhythmias.
- Give drug undiluted or dilute in 50 ml normal saline solution or D_5W. Add contents of 10-ml vial (0.1 mg/ml) to 50 ml solution to obtain 0.017 mg/ml. Use polyvinyl chloride plastic bags or polyolefin bags for admixtures. Give drug within 24 hours (48 hours if refrigerated).
- Infuse drug slowly over 10 minutes.
- As ordered, monitor patient's cardiac rhythm continuously during infusion and for at least 4 hours afterward—longer if arrhythmias appear or if patient has abnormal hepatic function. Observe patient for ventricular ectopy.
- Make sure defibrillator and drugs to treat sustained ventricular tachycardia are available during therapy and when monitoring patient after therapy.

PATIENT TEACHING
- Inform patient that ibutilide will be given by I.V. infusion and that his heart rhythm will be monitored continuously.
- Ask patient to report chest pain, faintness, numbness, palpitations, shortness of breath, and tingling.
- Advise patient to keep follow-up appointments to monitor heart rhythm.

icosapent ethyl
Vascepa

Class and Category
Pharmacologic class: Lipid-regulating agent
Therapeutic class: Antilipemic
Pregnancy category: C

Indications and Dosages
➤ *Adjunct to diet to reduce triglyceride levels in patients with severe (equal to or greater than 500 mg/dl) hypertriglyceridemia*

CAPSULES
Adults. 2 g twice daily with food.

Mechanism of Action
Reduces very low-density lipoprotein triglycerides (VLDL-TG) synthesis and/or secretion in the liver and enhances triglyceride clearance from circulating VLDL particles. Mechanisms used to accomplish this may include decreased lipogenesis in the liver, increased beta oxidation, increased lipoprotein lipase activity, and inhibition of acyl-CoA:1,2-diacylglycerol acyltransferase. These mechanisms work together to lower triglyceride levels.

Contraindications
Hypersensitivity to icosapent ethyl or its components

Interactions
DRUGS
antiplatelet drugs: Possibly increased bleeding time

Adverse Reactions
EENT: Oropharyngeal pain
MS: Arthralgia

Nursing Considerations
- Use icosapent ethyl cautiously in patients with a known hypersensitivity to fish and/or shellfish because the drug contains

ethyl esters of the omega-3 fatty acid obtained from the oil of fish.

- Be aware that patient should have been placed on a lipid-lowering diet and exercise regimen before starting icosapent ethyl therapy.
- Know that efforts should be made to control conditions that may increase lipid abnormalities, such as alcohol intake, diabetes mellitus, and hypothyroidism.
- Expect medications known to exacerbate hypertriglyceridemia, such as beta blockers, estrogen therapy, and immunosuppressants to be changed or discontinued prior to icosapent ethyl therapy.
- Obtain lipid levels prior to initiating icosapent ethyl therapy, as ordered, to determine a baseline. Monitor lipid levels periodically throughout icosapent ethyl therapy to determine effectiveness.
- Monitor alanine aminotransferase and aspartate aminotransferase levels periodically, as ordered, in patients with hepatic impairment.

PATIENT TEACHING

- Tell patient that icosapent ethyl therapy is not a substitution for diet and exercise but that these lifestyle changes need to continue during icosapent ethyl therapy.
- Instruct patient to take capsules whole and not to break, chew, crush, or dissolve open the capsules.
- Inform patient that periodic blood tests will be needed to monitor effectiveness of icosapent ethyl therapy.

idarucizumab

Praxbind

Class and Category

Pharmacologic class: Humanized monoclonal antibody fragment
Therapeutic class: Antidote
Pregnancy category: Not classified

Indications and Dosages

➤ *To reverse anticoagulant effects of dabigatran*

I.V. INFUSION, I.V. INJECTION

Adults. 5 g given in 2.5 g doses consecutively, and repeated one time, as needed.

Mechanism of Action

Binds to dabigatran and its acyl-glucuronide metabolites with higher affinity than the binding of dabigatran to thrombin, thereby neutralizing their anticoagulant effect and reversing the effects of dabigatran.

Contraindications

Hypersensitivity to idarucizumab or its components

Adverse Reactions

CNS: Delirium, fever
CV: Thrombotic events
GI: Constipation
RESP: Bronchospasm, hyperventilation, pneumonia
SKIN: Pruritus, rash
Other: Anaphylaxis, formation of idarucizumab antibodies, **hypokalemia**

Nursing Considerations

- Use extreme caution when administering idarucizumab to a patient with hereditary fructose intolerance because idarucizumab contains 4 g of sorbitol. The amount of sorbitol that may cause serious or even fatal adverse reactions is not known.
- Administer idarucizumab solution within 1 hour after it is removed from the vial. Expect to use two 2.5 g/50 ml vials and administer drug as 2.5 g doses back to back either as an intravenous infusion or injection. Flush intravenous line with 0.9% sodium chloride solution prior to administering drug. Do not coadminister any other drug in the same intravenous line.
- Provide standard supportive measures to control dabigatran induced bleeding, as needed, in conjunction with idarucizumab treatment.
- Monitor the patient's coagulation parameters such as activated partial thromboplastin time (aPTT) or ecarin clotting time (ECT), as ordered.
- Be prepared to administer an additional 5 g of idarucizumab, as ordered, if patient redevelops significant bleeding together with elevated coagulation parameters or if patient requires a second emergency surgery or urgent procedure and has elevated coagulation parameters.

WARNING Monitor patient closely for thrombotic events because reversing dabigatran with idarucizumab increases the risk of such events. Know that resumption of anticoagulant therapy should be done as soon as possible. For example, dabigatran may be resumed 24 hours after the administration of idarucizumab.

- Monitor patient for an allergic reaction to idarucizumab. If present, stop administration immediately, notify prescriber, and provide emergency supportive care, as indicated.

PATIENT TEACHING

- Instruct patient to alert medical personnel immediately if she experiences difficulty breathing or develops skin reactions such as itchiness or a rash during or after idarucizumab has been administered.
- Alert patient that she will continue to need anticoagulant therapy once the bleeding episode has been resolved to prevent future blood clots. She may be able to resume dabigatran therapy 24 hours after idarucizumab therapy is given, if ordered.
- Tell her she will need blood tests to monitor effectiveness of idarucizumab therapy and that a second dose of idarucizumab may be required if bleeding reoccurs or an emergency procedure or surgery is required.

iloperidone

Fanapt

Class and Category

Pharmacologic class: Atypical antipsychotic
Therapeutic class: Second-generation antipsychotic
Pregnancy category: C

Indications and Dosages

➤ *To treat schizophrenia*

TABLETS

Adults. *Initial:* 1 mg twice daily, adjusted to target dosage range as follows: 2 mg twice daily on day 2, 4 mg twice daily on day 3, and 6 mg twice daily on day 4. Dosage may be further increased, as needed, as follows: 8 mg twice daily on day 5, 10 mg twice daily on day 6, and 12 mg twice daily on day 7. *Maximum:* 12 mg twice daily.

DOSAGE ADJUSTMENT For patients taking strong CYP2D6 inhibitors, such as fluoxetine and paroxetine, or CYP3A4 inhibitors, such as clarithromycin and ketoconazole, dosage reduced by half.

Route	Onset	Peak	Duration
P.O.	1–2 wk	2–4 hr	Unknown

Mechanism of Action

Selectively blocks dopamine type 2 (D_2) and serotonin type 2 (5-HT_2) receptors in CNS, thereby suppressing psychotic symptoms.

Contraindications

Hypersensitivity to iloperidone or its components

Interactions

DRUGS

antibiotics such as fluoroquinolones or macrolides, class IA antiarrhythmics such as procainamide or quinidine, class III antiarrhythmics such as amiodarone or sotalol, other antipsychotic drugs such as chlorpromiazine or thioridazine, or any other drug that affects the QT interval, such as methadone or pentamidine: Possibly prolonged QT interval
antihypertensive drugs: Increased antihypertensive effects
CYP2D6 inhibitors such as fluoxetine or paroxetine, CYP3A4 inhibitors such as ketoconazole: Increased plasma iloperidone level
dextromethorphan: Increased blood dextromethorphan level

Adverse Reactions

CNS: Aggression, delusion, dizziness, extrapyramidal effects, fatigue, lethargy, **neuroleptic malignant syndrome**, restlessness, **seizures**, somnolence, **suicidal ideation**, tremor
CV: Congestive heart failure, dyslipidemia, orthostatic hypotension, palpitations, **QT-interval prolongation**, tachycardia
EENT: Blurred vision, conjunctivitis, dry mouth, nasal congestion, nasopharyngitis, **oropharyngeal swelling**, **throat tightness**, upper respiratory tract infection
ENDO: Diabetic ketoacidosis, elevated prolactin levels, hyperglycemia, **hyperosmolar coma**

GI: Abdominal discomfort, diarrhea, nausea
GU: Ejaculation failure, erectile dysfunction, priapism, urinary incontinence
HEME: Leukopenia
MS: Arthralgia, musculoskeletal stiffness, spasms, myalgia
RESP: Dyspnea
SKIN: Pruritus, rash, urticaria
Other: Anaphylaxis, angioedema, weight gain

Nursing Considerations

- Know that iloperidone shouldn't be used in patients with a history of cardiovascular disease such as cardiac arrhythmias, QT-interval prolongation, recent MI, or uncompensated heart failure. It also shouldn't be used in patients taking other drugs known to prolong the QT interval and in patients with hepatic impairment.

WARNING Be aware that iloperidone shouldn't be used to treat patients with dementia-related psychosis, especially elderly patients, because of an increased risk of death.

- Use cautiously in patients who have a history of seizures or who have conditions that lower the seizure threshold, such as Alzheimer's dementia. Also use cautiously in patients who are at risk for aspiration pneumonia or who have moderate hepatic impairment (not recommended for use in patients with severe hepatic impairment).
- Expect to restart dosage adjustment schedule in patients who have been off iloperidone therapy for more than 3 days.
- Obtain baseline serum magnesium and potassium levels in patients at risk for electrolyte imbalances, and then monitor periodically throughout therapy, as ordered, because electrolyte imbalances increase risk of prolonged QT interval or arrhythmia. If patient reports dizziness, palpitations, or syncope, notify prescriber and expect further evaluation to be done.

WARNING Know that neuroleptic malignant syndrome has occurred in patients taking other antipsychotic drugs. Monitor patient for altered mental status, autonomic instability, hyperpyrexia, and muscle rigidity. If present, notify prescriber immediately, expect drug to be discontinued, and start intensive treatment, as prescribed. Watch for recurrence if patient resumes antipsychotic therapy.

- Monitor patient for tardive dyskinesia, which has occurred with other antipsychotic drugs. If patient develops involuntary, dyskinetic movements, notify prescriber and expect to discontinue drug.
- Monitor blood glucose level, especially in patients with diabetes mellitus, because iloperidone may alter blood glucose enough to induce life-threatening hyperosmolar coma or ketoacidosis.
- Monitor patient's CBC periodically, as ordered, especially during first few months of therapy, because iloperidone may cause neutropenia. Also, be aware that other antipyschotic drugs have caused sometimes fatal agranulocytosis and leukopenia. If patient's WBC count decreases, expect drug to be discontinued.
- Monitor patient closely for abnormal tendencies that may suggest suicidal thinking, especially when iloperidone therapy starts or dosage is changed.

PATIENT TEACHING

- Inform patient that when iloperidone therapy starts, dosage must be adjusted for up to a week to reach target level. Also explain that adjustment process will need to be repeated if she skips drug for more than 3 days.
- Advise patient or caregiver to notify prescriber about persistent severe, or unusual adverse reactions because drug may need to be discontinued.
- Urge patient or caregiver to report evidence of abnormal thinking, especially when therapy starts or dosage changes.
- Tell diabetic patient to monitor blood glucose levels closely and to report persistent elevations immediately to prescriber.
- Caution patient to avoid hazardous activities until CNS effects of drug are known. Patient should also avoid alcohol.
- Instruct patient to avoid activities that might raise body temperature, such as being exposed to extreme heat, being subjected to dehydration, doing strenuous exercise or taking other drugs with anticholinergic activity.
- Emphasize the need to comply with follow-up appointments and laboratory tests.
- Tell patient to rise slowly from lying to sitting position and from sitting position to standing to avoid dizziness or lightheadedness during therapy.

- Advise female patient of childbearing age to notify prescriber if she intends to become or suspects that she is pregnant during therapy.

imipramine hydrochloride

Novo-pramine (CAN), Tipramine, Tofranil

imipramine pamoate

Tofranil-PM

Class and Category

Pharmacologic class: Tricyclic antidepressant (TCA)
Therapeutic class: Antidepressant
Pregnancy category: Not classified

Indications and Dosages

➤ *To treat depression*

CAPSULES

Adults. *Initial:* 75 mg (outpatient) or 100 to 150 mg (hospitalized) daily at bedtime or in divided doses, gradually increased as needed and tolerated. *Maximum:* 300 mg daily (hospitalized patients), 200 mg/day (outpatients).

TABLETS

Adults. *Initial:* 25 mg three times daily (outpatient) or four times daily (hospitalized) gradually increased as needed and tolerated. *Maximum:* 300 mg daily (hospitalized patients), 200 mg daily (outpatients).
Adolescents and elderly. *Initial:* 30 to 40 mg daily at bedtime or in divided doses, adjusted as needed and tolerated. *Maximum:* 100 mg daily.

➤ *As adjunct to treat childhood enuresis*

TABLETS

Children age 6 and over. 25 mg 1 hr before bedtime. Increased to 50 mg if no response occurs within 1 wk and child is under age 12; increased to 75 mg if child is age 12 or over. *Maximum:* 2.5 mg/kg daily.

Route	Onset	Peak	Duration
P.O.	2–3 wk*	Unknown	Unknown

* For antidepressant effect.

Mechanism of Action

May interfere with reuptake of serotonin (and possibly other neurotransmitters) at presynaptic neurons, thus enhancing serotonin's effects at postsynaptic receptors. Mood elevation may result from restoration of normal levels of neurotransmitters at nerve synapses. This tricyclic antidepressant also blocks acetylcholine receptors, which may explain how it relieves enuresis.

Contraindications

Acute recovery period after MI; hypersensitivity to imipramine, other tricyclic antidepressants, or their components; use within 14 days of MAO inhibitor therapy, including intravenous methylene blue and linezolid

Interactions

DRUGS

amantadine, anticholinergics, antidyskinetics, antihistamines: Risk of increased anticholinergic effects, including confusion, hallucinations, and nightmares
anticonvulsants: Decreased effectiveness of imipramine, increased risk of CNS depression, increased risk of seizures
antithyroid drugs: Possibly agranulocytosis
barbiturates, carbamazepine: Possibly decreased imipramine level and effects
cimetidine, fluoxetine: Possibly increased blood imipramine level
clonidine, guanadrel, guanethidine: Possibly decreased antihypertensive effects of these drugs, increased CNS depression (clonidine)
CNS depressants: Increased CNS depression, hypotension, and respiratory depression
disulfiram, ethchlorvynol: Risk of delirium, increased CNS depression (ethchlorvynol)
estramustine, estrogen-containing oral contraceptives, estrogens: Risk of increased bioavailability of imipramine, increased depression
MAO inhibitors: Increased risk of hypertensive crisis, severe seizures, and death
oral anticoagulants: Possibly increased anticoagulant activity
pimozide, probucol: Risk of arrhythmias
sympathomimetics (including ophthalmic epinephrine and vasoconstrictive local anesthetics): Increased risk of arrhythmias, hyperpyrexia, hypertension, tachycardia

thyroid hormones: Risk of increased therapeutic and adverse effects of both drugs

ACTIVITIES

alcohol use: Increased alcohol effects and CNS depression

sun exposure: Increased risk of photosensitivity

Adverse Reactions

CNS: Anxiety, ataxia, chills, confusion, **CVA**, delirium, dizziness, drowsiness, excitation, extrapyramidal reactions, fever, hallucinations, headache, insomnia, nervousness, nightmares, Parkinsonism, **seizures**, **serotonin syndrome**, **suicidal ideation**, tremor

CV: Arrhythmias, orthostatic hypotension, palpitations

EENT: Blurred vision, dry mouth, increased intraocular pressure, pharyngitis, taste perversion, tinnitus, tongue swelling

ENDO: Gynecomastia, syndrome of inappropriate ADH secretion

GI: Constipation, diarrhea, heartburn, ileus, increased appetite, jaundice, nausea, vomiting

GU: Impotence, libido changes, testicular swelling, urine retention

HEME: Agranulocytosis, **bone marrow depression**

RESP: Wheezing

SKIN: Alopecia, diaphoresis, photosensitivity, pruritus, rash, urticaria

Other: Angioedema, **hypersensitivity reactions**, weight gain

Nursing Considerations

- Use imipramine cautiously in patients with a history of angle-closure glaucoma or urine retention because drug's anticholinergic effects may cause increased intraocular pressure and urine retention.

WARNING Know that MAO inhibitors should not be given within 2 weeks of imipramine, including intravenous methylene blue and linezolid. Patient may experience hypertensive crisis, seizures, and death.

WARNING Monitor patient for possible serotonin syndrome, characterized by agitation, chills, confusion, diaphoresis, diarrhea, fever, hyperactive reflexes, poor coordination, restlessness, shaking, talking or acting with uncontrolled excitement, tremor, and twitching. Notify prescriber immediately if serotonin syndrome is suspected because it can become life-threatening. Expect to discontinue imipramine therapy if serotonin syndrome is confirmed.

- Frequently assess for adverse reactions during first 2 hours of therapy.
- Check standing and supine blood pressure for orthostatic hypotension before and during imipramine therapy and before dosage increases.
- Anticipate increased risk of arrhythmias in patients with a history of cardiac disease.
- Know that when drug is used for depression, expect mood elevation to take 2 to 3 weeks. Watch patient closely for suicidal tendencies, especially children and adolescents and especially when therapy starts or dosage changes, because depression may worsen temporarily at these times.
- Avoid abrupt withdrawal of drug in patients on long-term therapy. Such withdrawal may cause headache, malaise, nausea, sleep disturbance, and vomiting.
- Taper drug gradually, as ordered, a few days before surgery to avoid risk of hypertension during surgery.
- Obtain CBC, as ordered, if patient experiences signs and symptoms of infection, such as fever or pharyngitis.
- Limit amount of drug given to potentially suicidal patient.

PATIENT TEACHING

- Advise patient to take imipramine exactly as prescribed. Warn that stopping drug abruptly may cause headache, malaise, nausea, trouble sleeping, and vomiting.
- Caution parents to monitor child or adolescent closely for suicidal tendencies, especially when therapy starts or dosage changes.
- Urge patient to report chills, dizziness, excess sedation, fever, palpitations, signs of allergic reaction, sore throat, and trouble urinating.
- Caution patient to avoid hazardous activities until drug's CNS effects are known.
- Urge patient to avoid alcohol during imipramine therapy because it increases alcohol effects and CNS depression.
- Suggest that patient eat frequent, small meals to help relieve nausea.

- Instruct patient to avoid prolonged exposure to sunlight because of the risk of photosensitivity.
- Inform male patient about possible impotence and decreased or increased libido.
- If patient reports dry mouth, suggest sugarless candy or gum to relieve it. Tell him to check with prescriber if dry mouth persists after 2 weeks.

immune globulin intramuscular (human)

(gamma globulin, IG)

BayGam, GamaSTAN S/D, WinRho SDF

immune globulin intravenous (human)

Bivigam 10% Liquid; Carimune NF, Nanofiltered; Gammaplex 5% Liquid, Octagam 10%

(IGIV, immune serum globulin, ISG, IVIG)

Flebogamma 5% DIF, Flebogamma 10% DIF, Gamimune N 5% S/D, Gamimune N 10% S/D, Gammagard Liquid, Gammagard S/D, Gammagard S/D 0.5 g, Gammar-P IV, Gamunex-C 10%, Iveegam EN, Octagam 5%, Privigen, Rhophylac, WinRho SDF

immune globulin subcutaneous (human)

Cuvitru 20%, Gammagard Liquid, Gamunex-C 10%, Hizentra 20%, Vivaglobin

Class and Category

Pharmacologic class: Immune serum
Therapeutic class: Antibody production stimulator
Pregnancy category: C

Indications and Dosages

➤ *To treat primary immunodeficiency*

I.M. INJECTION (BAYGAM)

Adults. 0.66 ml/kg (at least 100 mg/kg) every 3 to 4 wk; initial dose may be doubled.

I.V. INFUSION (GAMIMUNE N 5% S/D OR 10% S/D)

Adults. 300 to 600 mg/kg every 3 to 4 wk.

I.V. INFUSION (GAMMAGARD S/D)

Adults. 300 to 600 mg/kg every 3 to 4 wk. If response is inadequate, dose or frequency may be adjusted.

I.V. INFUSION (GAMMAR-P IV)

Adults. 200 to 400 mg/kg every 3 to 4 wk.
Adolescents and children. 200 mg/kg every 3 to 4 wk.

I.V. INFUSION (GAMUNEX-C 10%)

Adults and children ages 2 and over. 300 to 600 mg/kg every 3 or 4 wk.

I.V. INFUSION (IVEEGAM EN)

Adults. 200 mg/kg every mo.

I.V. INFUSION (OCTAGAM 5%)

Adults. *Initial:* 30 mg/kg/hr for first 30 min; increased, if tolerated, to 60 mg/kg/hr for second 30 min and, if tolerated, to 120 mg/kg/hr for another 30 min; followed by maintenance infusion of up to 200 mg/kg/hr.

I.V. INFUSION (CARIMUNE NF, NANOFILTERED)

Adults and children. 0.4 to 0.8 g/kg once every 3 to 4 wk initially infused at 0.5 mg/kg/min. If tolerated, after 30 min, infusion rate increased to 1 mg/kg/min for 30 min. If tolerated, infusion rate gradually increased to maximum rate of 3 mg/kg/min. For patients at risk for renal dysfunction or thrombosis development, rate of infusion should be less than 2 mg/kg/min.

I.V. INFUSION (GAMMAPLEX 5% LIQUID)

Adults. 300 to 800 mg/kg once every 3 to 4 wk, initially infused at 0.5 mg/kg/min and then gradually rate increased every 15 min, if tolerated, to final infusion rate of 4 mg/kg/min.

SUBCUTANEOUS INJECTION (GAMUNEX-C 10%, VIVAGLOBIN)

Adults. Highly individualized and begun 1 wk after patient's last immune globulin intravenous (IGIV) infusion with initial weekly dosage obtained by multiplying the previous IGIV dose by 1.37; this number is then divided by the number of weeks between doses during the patient's previous IGIV treatment. Average weekly dose falls in the range of 100 to 200 mg/kg.

SUBCUTANEOUS INJECTION (GAMUNEX-C 10%)
Adults and children ages 2 and over. Highly individualized and begun 1 wk after patient's last immune globulin intravenous (IGIV) infusion, with initial weekly dosage obtained by multiplying the previous IGIV dose in grams by 1.37; this number is then divided by the number of weeks between dosages during the patient's previous IGIV treatment.
SUBCUTANEOUS INJECTION (CUVITRU 20%)
Adults and children ages 2 and over. Highly individualized and begun 1 wk after patient's last immune globulin intravenous (IGIV) infusion or adult's last immune globulin infusion 10% (human) with recombinant human hyaluronidase (HYQVIA), with initial weekly dosage obtained by dividing the previous IGIV or HYQVIA dose in grams by the number of weeks between intravenous doses, then multiplying this dose by 1.30.

➤ *To treat primary immunodeficiency disorders associated with defects in humoral immunity*

I.V. INFUSION (FLEBOGAMMA 5% DIF, FLEBOGAMMA 10% DIF, GAMMAGARD LIQUID)
Adults and children ages 2 and over. 300 to 600 mg/kg every 3 to 4 wk.
I.V. INFUSION (PRIVIGEN)
Adults and children ages 3 and over. 200 to 800 mg/kg every 3 to 4 wk.
I.V. INFUSION (BIVIGAM 10% LIQUID)
Adults. 300 to 800 mg/kg every 3 to 4 wk. Infuse 0.5 mg/kg/min for the first 10 min, then increase infusion rate every 20 min, if tolerated, by 0.8 up to 6 mg/kg/min.
SUBCUTANEOUS INFUSION (HIZENTRA 20%)
Adults and children age 2 and over. Highly individualized and begun 1 wk after patient's last IGIV infusion with initial weekly dosage, obtained by multiplying the previous IGIV dose in grams by the dose adjustment factor of 1.37; this number is then divided by the number of weeks between doses during the patient's previous IGIV treatment, followed by multiplying the calculated dose by 5 to convert the dose calculated in grams to milliliters.
SUBCUTANEOUS INFUSION (GAMMAGARD LIQUID)
Adults and children age 2 and over. Highly individualized and begun 1 wk after patient's last immune globulin intravenous (IGIV) infusion with initial weekly dosage obtained by multiplying the previous IGIV dose in grams by the dose adjustment factor of 1.37; this number is then divided by the number of weeks between doses during the patient's previous IGIV treatment, followed by multiplying the calculated dose by 10 to convert the dose calculated in grams to milliliters.

➤ *To treat idiopathic thrombocytopenic purpura (ITP)*

I.V. INFUSION (GAMIMUNE N 5% S/D)
Adults and children. 400 mg/kg daily for 5 days. Or, 1,000 mg/kg for 1 or 2 days for patients not at risk for increased fluid volume.
I.V. INFUSION (PRIVIGEN)
Adults and adolescents age 15 and over. 1 g/kg daily for 2 consecutive days for patients not at risk for increased fluid volume.
I.V. INFUSION (FLEBOGAMMA 10% DIF)
Adults and children ages 2 and over. 1 g/kg daily for 2 consecutive days.
I.V. INFUSION (GAMIMUNE N 10% S/D)
Adults and children. 1,000 mg/kg for 1 or 2 days for patients not at risk for increased fluid volume.
I.V. INFUSION (OCTAGAM 10%)
Adults. 1 g/kg (10 ml/kg) daily for 2 consecutive days. Initially infuse at 0.01 ml/kg/min for 30 min. If tolerated, increase infusion rate to 0.02 ml/kg/min for next 30 min. If tolerated, further increase infusion rate to 0.04 ml/kg/min for 30 min. If tolerated, further increase infusion rate to 0.08 ml/kg/min for 30 min. If tolerated, infusion rate may be increased up to 0.12 mg/kg/min for remainder of infusion.
I.V. INFUSION (GAMUNEX-C 10%)
Adults. 2 g/kg/dose.
I.V. INFUSION (CARIMUNE NF, NANOFILTERED)
Adults and children. 0.4 g/kg on 2 to 5 consecutive days, initially infused at 0.5 mg/kg/min. If tolerated, after 30 min, infusion rate increased to 1 mg/kg/min for 30 min. If tolerated, infusion rate gradually increased to maximum rate of 3 mg/kg/min.
I.V. INFUSION (GAMMAPLEX 5% LIQUID)
Adults. 1 g/kg on 2 consecutive days, initially infused at 0.5 mg/kg/min and then gradually rate increased every 15 min, if tolerated, to final infusion rate of 4 mg/kg/min.

DOSAGE ADJUSTMENT In acute ITP of childhood, I.V. Carimune NF therapy may be discontinued after second day of 5-day course if initial platelet count response is adequate (30,000 to 50,000/mm^3). In chronic ITP, an additional I.V. infusion of 400 mg/kg (Carimune NF, or Gamimune) may be prescribed if platelet count falls below 30,000/mm^3 or if patient develops significant bleeding. If response remains inadequate, an additional I.V. infusion of 800 to 1,000 mg/kg may be given. In chronic ITP, dosage of Gammaplex 5% liquid may need to be reduced in patients at risk for thrombosis, hemolysis, acute kidney injury, or volume overload.

I.V. INFUSION (GAMMAGARD S/D)

Adults. 1 g/kg. If response is inadequate, up to 3 separate doses may be administered on alternate days.

I.V. INFUSION (RHOPHYLAC)

Adults. 50 mcg/kg at 2 ml/15 to 60 sec.

➤ *To treat acute or chronic pediatric ITP; to treat chronic adult-onset ITP; to treat pediatric- and adult-onset ITP secondary to HIV infection*

I.V. INJECTION (WINRHO SDF)

Adults and children. *Initial:* 250 international units/kg given as a single injection over 3 to 5 min. Or, 125 international units/kg given as a single injection over 3 to 5 min and repeated once on a separate day. *Maintenance:* Frequency and dosage highly individualized based on patient's hemoglobin and platelet levels.

DOSAGE ADJUSTMENT For patients with hemoglobin level less than 10 g/dl, dose reduced to 125 to 200 international units.

➤ *As adjunct to treat Kawasaki disease*

I.V. INFUSION (GAMMAGARD S/D)

Adults and adolescents. 1 g/kg as a single dose; or, 400 mg/kg daily for 4 consecutive days.

➤ *To treat chronic inflammatory demyelinating polyneuropathy (CIDP)*

INTRAVENOUS INFUSION (GAMUNEX-C 10%)

Adults. *Loading dose:* 2 g/kg. *Maintenance dose:* 1 g/kg.

INTRAVENOUS INFUSION (PRIVIGEN 10%)

Adults. *Initial:* 2 g/kg given in divided doses over 2 to 5 consecutive days with each dose infused at a rate of 0.5mg/kg/min and, if tolerated, infusion rate gradually increased up to a maximum of 8 mg/kg/min. *Maintenance:* 1 g/kg as a single infusion or divided into 2 doses given on 2 consecutive days, every 3 wk for up to 6 months. Minimum infusion rate is 0.5 mg/kg/min and maximum infusion rate is 8 mg/kg/min.

SUBCUTANEOUS INFUSION (HIZENTRA 20%)

Adults. 0.2 g/kg/wk administered in 1 or 2 sessions over 1 or 2 consecutive days.

DOSAGE ADJUSTMENT For patient receiving Hizentra in whom CIDP symptoms worsen, an IGIV-approved drug initiated while Hizentra is being discontinued. If patient improves and stablizes during IGIV teatment, Hizentra may be reinitiated at a dose of 0.4 g/kg/wk administered in 2 sessions per wk over 1 or 2 days while IGIV therapy is being discontinued. If symptoms worsen on the 0.4 g/kg/wk dosage, drug discontinued.

➤ *To decrease the risk of graft-versus-host disease, interstitial pneumonia, septicemia, and other infections during first 100 days after bone marrow transplantation*

I.V. INFUSION (GAMIMUNE N 5% S/D OR 10% S/D)

Adults over age 20. 500 mg/kg on 7th and 2nd days before transplant (or at time when conditioning therapy for transplantation begins), and then weekly through 90th day after transplant.

➤ *As adjunct to treat bacterial infections secondary to B-cell chronic lymphocytic leukemia*

I.V. INFUSION (GAMMAGARD S/D)

Adults and adolescents. 400 mg/kg every 3 to 4 wk.

➤ *To prevent bacterial infection in children with HIV who are immunosuppressed*

I.V. INFUSION (GAMIMUNE N 5% S/D OR 10% S/D)

Children. 400 mg/kg daily every 28 days.

➤ *To prevent hepatitis A*

I.M. INJECTION (BAYGAM)

Adults with household or institutional contacts. 0.02 ml/kg (0.01 ml/lb).

Adults traveling to areas where hepatitis A is common. 0.02 ml/kg if staying less than 3 mo, 0.06 ml/kg (repeated every 4 to 6 mo) if staying 3 mo or longer.

I.M. INJECTION (GAMASTAN S/D)

Adults and children with household or institutional contacts. 0.02 ml/kg.

Adults traveling for less than 3 months to areas where hepatitis A is common. 0.02 ml/kg.
Adults traveling for 3 months or longer to areas where hepatitis A is common. 0.06 ml/kg, repeated every 4 to 6 mo, as needed.

➤ *To prevent or lessen severity of measles (rubeola) in susceptible persons*

I.M. INJECTION (BAYGAM)
Adults exposed fewer than 6 days previously. 0.25 ml/kg (0.11 ml/lb).

I.M. INJECTION (GAMASTAN S/D)
Adults and children exposed fewer than 6 days previously. 0.25 ml/kg (0.11 ml/lb).
Children exposed to rubeola and are immunocompromised. 0.5 ml/kg immediately. *Maximum:* 15 ml dose.

➤ *To provide passive immunization against varicella in immunosuppressed patients*

I.M. INJECTION (BAYGAM, GAMASTAN S/D)
Adults. 0.6 to 1.2 ml/kg if varicella-zoster immune globulin (human) is unavailable.

➤ *To improve muscle strength and disability as maintenance therapy in patients with multifocal motor neuropathy*

I.V. INFUSION (GAMMAGARD LIQUID)
Adults. *Maintenance:* 0.5 to 2.4 g/kg/mo. Initially infused at 0.5 ml/kg/hr (0.8 mg/kg/min) with rate increased, as needed, up to 5.4 ml/kg/hr (9 mg/kg/min).

➤ *To reduce the risk of infection and fetal damage in women who have been exposed to rubella in early pregnancy*

I.M. INJECTION (BAYGAM, GAMASTAN S/D)
Adults. 0.55 ml/kg.

➤ *To suppress Rh isoimmunization*

I.M. INJECTION, I.V. INFUSION (RHOPHYLAC)
Adult pregnant women. 1,500 international units as a single dose at 28- to 30-wk gestation, followed by 1,500 international units within 72 hr after delivery of an Rh-positive newborn.

I.M. INJECTION (WINRHO SDF)
Adult pregnant women. 1,500 international units as a single dose at 28-wk gestation, followed by 600 international units within 72 hr after delivery of an Rh-positive newborn.

I.V. INJECTION (WINRHO SDF)
Adult pregnant women. 1,500 international units as a single dose infused at a rate of 2 ml/5 to 15 sec at 28-wk gestation, followed by 600 international units infused at a rate of 2 ml/5 to 15 sec within 72 hr after delivery of an Rh-positive newborn.
DOSAGE ADJUSTMENT For patients with more than 34-wk gestation and having an abortion, amniocentesis, or other manipulative procedure, 600 international units given within 72 hr but preferably immediately after procedure. For patients with 34-wk gestation or less and having amniocentesis or chorionic villus sampling, 1,500 international units given immediately after procedure and repeated every 12 wk for duration of pregnancy. For patients with threatened abortion at any stage of pregnancy, 1,500 international units given immediately.

➤ *To treat incompatible blood transfusions*

I.M. INJECTION, I.V. INFUSION (RHOPHYLAC)
Adults exposed to Rh-positive RBCs. 100 international units/2 ml transfused blood or per 1 ml erythrocyte concentrate within 72 hr of exposure.

I.M. INJECTION (WINRHO SDF)
Adults exposed to Rh-positive whole blood. 6,000 international units every 12 hr until total dose (60 international units/ml of blood) is given.
Adults exposed to Rh-positive RBCs. 6,000 international units every 12 hr until total dose (120 international units/ml of cells) is given.

I.V. INJECTION (WINRHO SDF)
Adults exposed to Rh-positive whole blood. 3,000 international units infused at a rate of 2 ml/5 to 15 sec every 8 hr until total dose (45 international units/ml of blood) is given.
Adults exposed to Rh-positive RBCs. 3,000 international units infused at a rate of 2 ml/5 to 15 sec every 8 hr until total dose (90 international units/ml of cells) is given.

➤ *To treat massive fetomaternal hemorrhage*

I.M. INJECTION, I.V. INFUSION (RHOPHYLAC)
Adults exposed to Rh-positive RBCs. 1,500 international units plus 100 international units for every 1 ml of fetal RBCs exceeding 15 ml if transplacental bleeding is quantified, or an additional 1,500 international units if transplacental bleeding can't be quantified within 72 hr of hemorrhage.

I.M. INJECTION (WINRHO SDF)
Adults exposed to Rh-positive whole blood. 6,000 international units every 12 hr

until total dose (60 international units/ml of blood) is given.
Adults exposed to Rh-positive RBCs. 6,000 international units every 12 hr until total dose (120 international units/ml of cells) is given.

I.V. INJECTION (WINRHO SDF)

Adults exposed to Rh-positive whole blood. 3,000 international units infused at a rate of 2 ml/5 to 15 sec every 8 hr until total dose (45 international units/ml of blood) is given.
Adults exposed to Rh-positive RBCs. 3,000 international units infused at a rate of 2 ml/5 to 15 sec every 8 hr until total dose (90 international units/ml of cells) is given.

Route	Onset	Peak	Duration
I.M.	Unknown	Unknown	Unknown
I.V.	Unknown	Unknown	21–28 days
SubQ	Unknown	Unknown	Unknown

Mechanism of Action

Releases antibody-specific globulins to produce an antibody–antigen reaction that results in bacterial lysis and facilitates bacterial phagocytosis. In treatment of ITP, immune globulin blocks iron receptors on macrophages to increase immunoglobulin action. Immune globulin also increases cytokine production and improves B-cell immune function by regulating macrophage and T-cell activity. Newly formed antigen–antibody complexes produce split complement components that cause bacterial lysis.

In Kawasaki disease and bacterial infections with B-cell chronic lymphocytic leukemia, immune globulin neutralizes bacterial and viral toxins that harm immune and inflammatory responses.

Incompatibilities

Don't mix immune globulin with any other drugs, including other immune globulins, or with any I.V. solutions other than D_5W or manufacturer's supplied diluent because effects of doing so are unknown.

Contraindications

Hypersensitivity to immune globulin (human) or its components; IgA deficiency in patients with known antibody to IgA

Interactions

DRUGS

live-virus vaccines: Possibly decreased response to vaccine

Adverse Reactions

CNS: Aseptic meningitis (rare), headache, malaise
CV: Chest discomfort, hypertension, tachycardia, **thrombotic events, volume overload**
EENT: Blurred vision, oropharyngeal pain
GI: Nausea, vomiting
GU: Acute renal dysfunction or failure, osmotic nephrosis
HEME: Acute hemolysis, delayed hemolytic anemia, disseminated intravascular coagulation (DIC), positive Coombs' test
MS: Arthralgia, back or extremity pain, muscle spasms or weakness, myalgia
RESP: Dyspnea, **pulmonary edema or embolism**
Other: Hyperproteinemia, **hyponatremia**, increased serum viscosity

Nursing Considerations

- Know that before giving immune globulin, monitor patient's fluid volume and BUN and serum creatinine levels, as ordered, to determine risk for acute renal failure. Those at increased risk include patients with diabetes mellitus, paraproteinemia, renal insufficiency, sepsis, or volume depletion; those taking nephrotoxic drugs; and those over age 65. Expect drug to be discontinued if renal function deteriorates.
- Use caution when administering immune globulin, regardless of the route of administration, because of risk for thrombosis. Monitor closely patients with increased risk of thrombosis such as advanced age, coagulation disorders, a history of atherosclerosis, impaired cardiac output, multiple cardiovascular risk factors, or prolonged periods of immobilization, and/or hyperviscosity. In such patients, obtain a baseline assessment of blood viscosity, as ordered. Ensure patient is adequately hydrated prior to administration. When administering drug intravenously, expect to infuse at the lowest rate possible. Report any signs and symptoms suggestive of a thrombotic event

immediately to prescriber and be prepared to administer treatment, as ordered.

- Keep in mind when preparing immune globulin, verify that appropriate form is being used—either immune globulin intramuscular for I.M. injection, immune globulin intravenous for I.V. infusion or immune globulin subcutaneous for subcutaneous infusion.
- To reconstitute drug if required, follow manufacturer's guidelines and use only diluent recommended by manufacturer. Don't shake solution; excessive shaking causes foaming. If drug or diluent is cold, drug may take up to 20 minutes to dissolve.
- Know that if drug reconstituted outside of sterile laminar airflow conditions, administer it immediately and discard unused portions.
- Be aware that an in-line filter may be required for intravenous infusion of drug. Check manufacturer's guidelines for specific product being used.
- Consult manufacturer's guidelines to determine appropriate flow rate for starting infusion. Expect to increase flow rate after 15 to 30 minutes, as specified, except for Hizentra 20%, which has a flow adjustment rate done after the first infusion is completed and Privigen, which may adjust flow rate, as needed.
- Be aware that when giving drug by I.M. injection, inject it only into deltoid muscle of upper arm or anterolateral aspect of upper thigh. If giving a dose larger than 5 ml, divide it and administer at separate sites.
- Know that when giving Hizentra by subcutaneous infusion, infuse in the abdomen, lateral hip, thigh, or upper arm with no more than 4 sites used simultaneously. Infusion sites should be at least 2 inches apart and sites changed with each weekly administration. For first infusion, do not infuse more than 15 ml/hr/site. The volume may be increased to 20 ml/hr/site after the fourth infusion and to a maximum of 25 ml/hr/site as tolerated. However, do not exceed a maximum flow rate of more than a total of 50 ml/hr for all sites combined at any time. Use an infusion pump to administer the drug.
- Keep in mind when giving Gamunex-C by subcutaneous infusion, infuse in the abdomen, lateral hip, thigh, or upper arm with no more than 8 sites used simultaneously. Infusion sites should be at least 2 inches apart and sites changed with each weekly administration. Be aware that the average infusion rate for Gamunex-C as a subcutaneous infusion is 20 ml/hr/site. Know that if dilution is required, Gamunex-C is not compatible with saline. It may be diluted with 5% dextrose in water. Content of Gamunex-C vials may be pooled under aseptic conditions into sterile infusion bags and infused within 8 hours after pooling. Use an infusion pump to administer the drug.
- Administer Vivaglobin by subcutaneous injection into patient's abdomen, lateral hip, thighs, or upper arms. Rotate injection sites weekly. Never inject intravenously.
- Watch for an acute inflammatory reaction in patients who have never received immune globulin therapy before, in those whose last treatment was more than 8 weeks before, and in those whose initial infusion rate exceeded 1 ml/min. Within 30 minutes to 1 hour after beginning infusion, assess for chills, diaphoresis, dizziness, facial flushing, feeling of tightness in chest, fever, hypotension, nausea, and vomiting. Notify prescriber immediately if such symptoms occur, and be prepared to stop infusion until symptoms have subsided.
- Monitor patient closely for signs and symptoms of hemolysis, especially patients with risk factors. For patients at increased risk, expect to obtain a baseline measurement of hematocrit or hemoglobin prior to infusion and within 36 to 96 hours post infusion. Notify prescriber of any abnormalities.

WARNING Be aware that after immune globulin administration, monitor patient closely for aseptic meningitis. Notify prescriber if patient develops drowsiness, fever, nausea, nuchal rigidity, painful eye movements, photophobia, severe headache, or vomiting.

- Be aware that immune globulin intravenous is made from human plasma and therefore may contain infectious agents, such as viruses. Risk of transmitting a virus by infusion has been reduced by inactivating or removing certain viruses from the product, screening blood donors, or testing donated blood.

- Monitor patient with preexisting renal insufficiency who is receiving Bivigam to be sure the patient is not volume-depleted. If renal function deteriorates, notify prescriber and expect drug to be discontinued. For the patient at risk for renal dysfunction or thrombotic events, administer Bivigam at the minimum infusion rate practicable.
- Be aware that for patient receiving WinRho SDF to treat ITP, assess clinical response by monitoring patient's hemoglobin level, platelet count, RBC count, and reticulocyte level.
- Be aware that for patient receiving WinRho SDF for exposure to incompatible blood transfusions or massive fetal hemorrhage, give drug within 72 hours of incident, as ordered.

PATIENT TEACHING

- Instruct patient to report immediately any symptoms he experiences after receiving immune globulin.
- Inform patient to postpone live-virus vaccinations for up to 11 months after receiving immune globulin because drug may delay or inhibit response to vaccine.

indacaterol maleate

Arcapta Neohaler

Class and Category

Pharmacologic class: Long-acting $beta_2$-adrenergic agonist
Therapeutic class: Bronchodilator
Pregnancy category: C

Indications and Dosages

➤ *To alleviate airflow obstruction in patients with chronic obstructive pulmonary disease (COPD), including chronic bronchitis and/or emphysema*

INHALATION AEROSOL

Adults. 75 mcg once daily.

Mechanism of Action

Selectively attaches to $beta_2$ receptors on bronchial membranes, stimulating the intracellular enzyme adenyl cyclase to convert adenosine triphosphate to cAMP. The resulting increase in the intracellular cAMP level relaxes bronchial smooth-muscle cells, which allows greater airflow through the airways.

Contraindications

Asthma, hypersensitivity to indacaterol or its components

Interactions

DRUGS

adrenergic drugs: potentiated sympathetic effects
beta blockers: Possible interference with the effect of beta blockers and indacaterol, cytochrome P-450 3A4, P-gp efflux transporter such as erythromycin
diuretics, steroids, xanthine derivatives: Possible increased risk of hypokalemic effect
MAO inhibitors, tricyclic antidepressants: Potentiated adrenergic action on the cardiovascular system
nonpotassium-sparing diuretics: Increased risk of ECG changes or hypokalemia
QT prolonging drugs: Increased risk of ventricular arrhythmias

Adverse Reactions

CNS: Dizziness, headache, nervousness, tremor
CV: Angina, **atrial fibrillation**, peripheral edema, palpitations, tachycardia
EENT: Nasopharyngitis, oropharyngeal pain, sinusitis
ENDO: Hyperglycemia
GI: Nausea
MS: Muscle spasm, musculoskeletal pain
RESP: COPD exacerbation, cough, dyspnea, **paradoxical bronchospasm**, pneumonia, upper respiratory tract infection
SKIN: Pruritus, rash, urticaria
Other: Angioedema, hypokalemia, immediate hypersensitivity reactions

Nursing Considerations

- Be aware that indacaterol should not be given to patients with acutely deteriorating COPD nor should it be used for relief of acute symptoms. Instead acute symptoms should be treated with an inhaled short-acting $beta_2$-agonist.
- Use cautiously in patients with cardiovascular disorders, especially cardiac arrhythmias, coronary insufficiency, and hypertension because drug can increase blood pressure, pulse rate, and cause ECG

changes, such as flattening of the T wave, prolongation of the QT interval, and ST segment depression.

- Use cautiously in patients with convulsive disorders or thyrotoxicosis, or in patients who are unusually responsive to sympathomimetic amines as drug may aggravate these conditions.
- Monitor the patient's vital signs for an increase in blood pressure or pulse rate. If such effects occur, notify prescriber as indacaterol may need to be discontinued.

WARNING Monitor patient for immediate hypersensitivity reactions after administering indacaterol that may include difficulties in breathing or swallowing; rash; swelling of face, lips, and tongue; or urticaria. If present, discontinue drug immediately, notify prescriber, and provide supportive care, as indicated.

PATIENT TEACHING

- Instruct patient who has been taking inhaled, short-acting beta$_2$-agonists on a regular basis to discontinue the regular use of these drugs, as directed by prescriber, and use them only for symptomatic relief of acute respiratory symptoms, as ordered.
- Tell patient indacaterol capsules are only for use in inhaler device and should never be swallowed.
- Instruct patient to store capsules in their original packaging and to open immediately before use.
- Teach patient how to use delivery system. Tell them to place capsule in well of inhaler device and then to press and release buttons on side of device only once to pierce capsule. A click-type of sound will occur. Have patient place the inhaler into his mouth with the buttons to the left and right (not up and down). Then have him inhale rapidly and deeply through mouthpiece; drug is dispersed into airways as patient inhales. A whirring noise should be heard when inhaling. If not, the capsule may be stuck in the capsule cavity. If this occurs, have the patient open the inhaler and carefully loosen the capsule by tapping the base of the device. Tell him not to press the piercing buttons to loosen the capsule. Have him repeat these steps, if needed.
- Remind patient that indacaterol is not to be used to relieve acute symptoms. Instead, he should use his short-acting beta$_2$-agonist.
- Inform patient to notify prescriber if any of the following situations occur: if indacterol no longer seems to control his symptoms, if he needs to use his short-acting beta$_2$-agonist more often than usual; or if the short-acting beta$_2$-agonist becomes less effective.

indapamide

Apo-Indapamide (CAN), Gen-Indapamide (CAN), Lozide (CAN), Novo-Indapamide (CAN), Nu-Indapamide (CAN)

Class and Category

Pharmacologic class: Thiazide-like diuretic
Therapeutic class: Diuretic
Pregnancy category: B

Indications and Dosages

➤ *To treat edema caused by heart failure*

TABLETS

Adults. 2.5 mg daily in the morning, increased to 5 mg daily after 1 wk, if indicated.

➤ *To manage hypertension*

TABLETS

Adults. *Initial:* 1.25 mg daily, increased to 2.5 mg daily after 4 wk, if needed. Increased to 5 mg daily after additional 4 wk, if needed.

Route	Onset	Peak	Duration
P.O.*	1–2 hr	Unknown	36 hr
P.O.†	1–2 wk	8–12 wk	Up to 8 wk

* For edema.
† For hypertension (with multiple doses).

Mechanism of Action

Acts mainly on distal convoluted tubules, where it enhances excretion of chloride, sodium, and water by inhibiting sodium ion movement across renal tubules. The resulting decrease in extracellular fluid volume and plasma decreases peripheral vascular resistance and reduces blood pressure. This thiazide diuretic also may cause arterial vasodilation by blocking calcium channels in smooth-muscle cells.

Contraindications

Anuria; hypersensitivity to indapamide, other thiazide or related diuretics, sulfonamide-derived drugs, or their components

Interactions

DRUGS

amiodarone: Increased risk of arrhythmias if hypokalemia develops
cholestyramine, colestipol: Decreased indapamide absorption
diazoxide: Increased risk of hyperglycemia
digoxin: Increased risk of digitalis toxicity if hypokalemia develops
hypotension-producing drugs: Increased antihypertensive or diuretic effects
lithium: Increased risk of lithium toxicity
neuromuscular blockers: Possibly increased neuromuscular blockade, risk of respiratory depression
oral anticoagulants: Possibly decreased anticoagulant effects

Adverse Reactions

CNS: Anxiety, dizziness, drowsiness, fatigue, fever, headache, mood changes, nervousness, sleep disturbance, vertigo, weakness
CV: **Arrhythmias**, hypercholesterolemia, orthostatic hypotension, palpitations
EENT: Dry mouth
ENDO: Hyperglycemia, **hypoglycemia**
GI: Anorexia, constipation, diarrhea, **hepatitis**, jaundice, nausea, **pancreatitis**, thirst, vomiting
GU: Impotence, nocturia
MS: Gout, muscle spasms
SKIN: Necrotizing vasculitis, photosensitivity, pruritus, rash, urticaria
Other: Dilutional hypochloremia and hyponatremia, **hypokalemia**, **metabolic alkalosis**, weight loss

Nursing Considerations

- Administer indapamide with food or milk to reduce adverse GI reactions.
- Give drug early in the day to avoid nocturia.
- Weigh patient daily, and monitor blood pressure, fluid intake and output, and serum electrolyte levels, especially in elderly women, because severe hypokalemia and hyponatremia may occur. Report electrolyte abnormalities, and expect to provide corrective measures, as prescribed.
- Monitor BUN and serum creatinine levels regularly, as ordered.
- Know that if muscle cramps and weakness develop from hypokalemia, expect prescriber to order potassium-sparing diuretic or potassium supplement.
- Be aware that when managing hypertension, expect therapeutic response to indapamide to take several weeks.

PATIENT TEACHING

- Advise patient to take indapamide early in the day to avoid nighttime urination and to take it with food or milk to minimize GI distress.
- Encourage patient to eat high-potassium foods, such as bananas and oranges.
- Caution patient to change position slowly to minimize effects of orthostatic hypotension.
- Instruct patient to weigh himself daily at the same time and wearing similar clothing. Direct him to report a weight gain of more than 0.9 kg (2 lb) per day or 2.3 kg (5 lb) per week.
- Inform patient about possible photosensitivity.
- Suggest sugarless gum or hard candy if patient has a dry mouth.

indinavir

Crixivan

Class and Category

Pharmacologic class: Protease inhibitor
Therapeutic class: Antiretroviral
Pregnancy category: C

Indications and Dosages

➤ *As adjunct to treat human immunodeficiency virus (HIV) infection*

CAPSULES

Adults. 800 mg every 8 hr given 1 hr before or 2 hr after a meal.

DOSAGE ADJUSTMENT For patient who has mild to moderate hepatic insufficiency due to cirrhosis and for patients who are taking delavirdine at a dosage of 400 mg three times daily, itraconazole at a dosage of 200 mg twice daily, or ketoconazole, dosage reduced to 600 mg every 8 hr. For patients taking rifabutin concomitantly, dosage increased to 1000 mg every 8 hr with rifabutin dosage reduced by half.

Mechanism of Action

Binds to the protease active site to inhibit the activity of the HIV-1 protease enzyme. This inhibition prevents cleavage of the viral polyproteins, resulting in the formation of immature noninfectious viral particles.

Contraindications

Concurrent therapy with alfuzosin, alprazolam, amiodarone, cisapride, dihydroergotamine, ergonovine, ergotamine, lovastatin, lurasidone, methylergonovine, midazolam (oral), pimozide, sildenafil (when used to treat pulmonary arterial hypertension), simvastatin, or triazolam; hypersensitivity to indinavir or its components

Interactions

DRUGS

alfuzosin: Possibly increased alfuzosin concentrations leading to hypotension
alprazolam, midazolam (oral), triazolam: Possible risk of increased or prolonged respiratory depression or sedation
amiodarone, cisapride: Increased risk for serious or life-threatening adverse reactions such as cardiac arrhythmias
atazanavir: Increased risk of unconjugated hyperbilirubinemia
atorvastatin, bepridil, bosentan, calcium channel blockers, colchicine, fluticasone, lidocaine (systemic), midazolam (parenteral), quetiapine, quinidine, rosuvastatin, trazodone: Increased concentration of these drugs
carbamazepine, efavirenz, nevirapine, phenobarbital, phenytoin, venlafaxine: Decreased indinavir concentration, lowering effectiveness
clarithromycin: Increased concentrations of both clarithromycin and indinavir
cyclosporine, sirolimus, tacrolimus: Increased immunosuppressant effects
delavirdine, itraconazole, ketoconazole, nelfinavir, ritonavir, saquinavir: Increased indinavir concentration, increasing risk of adverse reactions
didanosine: Possibly interference with absorption of indinavir
dihydroergotamine, ergonovine, ergotamine, methylergonovine: Possible acute ergot toxicity
lovastatin, simvastatin: Increased risk of myopathy and rhabdomyolysis
lurasidone, pimozide: Possibly increased risk of serious or life-threatening adverse reactions
rifabutin: Decreased indinavir concentration and effectiveness; increased rifabutin concentration and possibly adverse reactions
rifampin, St. John's wort: Possible loss of virologic response and resistance to indinavir
salmeterol: Possibly increased risk of cardiovascular adverse effects such as palpitations, prolonged QT, and sinus tachycardia
sildenafil (used to treat of pulmonary arterial hypertension), tadalafil, vardenafil: Possible increased risk of PDE5-inhibitor-induced adverse reactions such as hypotension, prolonged erection, syncope, and visual disturbances

Adverse Reactions

CNS: Asthenia, **cerebrovascular disorders**, depression, dizziness, fatigue, fever, headache, malaise, somnolence
CV: Angina pectoris, elevated cholesterol and triglyceride levels, **MI**, vasculitis
EENT: Oral paresthesia, pharyngitis, taste perversion
ENDO: Cushingoid appearance, exacerbation of preexisting diabetes mellitus, fat redistribution, hyperglycemia, new-onset diabetes mellitus
GI: Abdominal distention or pain, acid regurgitation, anorexia, diarrhea, dyspepsia, elevated amylase or liver enzymes, **hepatic dysfunction or failure**, **hepatitis**, hyperbilirubinemia, increased appetite, jaundice, nausea, **pancreatitis**, vomiting
GU: **Acute renal failure**, dysuria, elevated creatinine level, flank pain, hematuria, interstitial nephritis, leukocyturia,

nephrolithiasis, pyelonephritis, **renal insufficiency**, urolithiasis
HEME: Acute hemolytic anemia, anemia, decreased hemoglobin, **neutropenia**, **spontaneous bleeding in patients with hemophilia**, **thrombocytopenia**
MS: Arthralgia, back pain, periarthritis
RESP: Cough, dyspnea, shortness of breath, upper respiratory infection
SKIN: Alopecia, dry skin, **erythema multiforme**, hyperpigmentation, paronychia, pruritus, rash, **Stevens–Johnson syndrome**, urticaria
Other: Anaphylaxis

Nursing Considerations

- Review patient's drug history before starting indinavir therapy, because drug interacts with many other drugs, some of which are contraindicated during indinavir use.
- Administer indinavir 1 hour before or 2 hours after a meal. Know that drug can be administered with other liquids such as coffee, juice, skim milk, or tea or with a light meal (such as dry toast with jelly or corn flakes with skim milk and sugar). Know that a meal high in calories, fat, and protein reduces the absorption of indinavir.
- Monitor patient for signs and symptoms of nephrolithiasis or urolithiasis, such as flank pain with or without hematuria. Notify prescriber if patient complains of flank pain or exhibits hematuria. Expect drug to be temporarily stopped for up to 3 days or discontinued. Ensure that patient receives adequate hydration throughout therapy.
- Monitor patient's complete blood count, because acute hemolytic anemia has occurred with indinavir therapy, ending in death for some patients. Report any change in complete blood count and signs and symptoms of anemia to prescriber. Be prepared to provide supportive care as ordered. Expect indinavir to be discontinued.
- Monitor patient's liver enzymes and assess patient for signs and symptoms of liver dysfunction, because hepatitis including hepatic failure has occurred with indinavir therapy.
- Check patient's blood glucose levels routinely, because indinavir therapy may cause hyperglycemia and exacerbate glucose control in patients with diabetes or even induce diabetes mellitus in patients not diagnosed with diabetes mellitus before therapy was begun.
- Be aware that immune reconstitution syndrome has occurred in patients treated with combination antiretroviral therapy, including indinavir. The inflammatory response predisposes susceptible patients to opportunistic infections such as cytomegalovirus, *Mycobacterium avium* infection, *Pneumocystis jiroveci* pneumonia, or tuberculosis. Autoimmune disorders such as Graves' disease, Guillain–Barré syndrome, or polymyositis have also occurred. Report sudden or unusual adverse reactions to prescriber.
- Perform a urinalysis periodically, as ordered. Notify prescriber if leukocyturia occurs, as further evaluation and possible discontinuation of indinavir may be needed.

PATIENT TEACHING

- Instruct patient to take indinavir 1 hour before or 2 hours after a meal. Tell patient that alternatively, she may take the drug with other liquids such as coffee, juice, skim milk, or tea, or with a light meal such as dry toast with jelly or corn flakes with skim milk and sugar.
- Tell patient to store drug in original container and that the desiccant should remain in the bottle because the capsules are sensitive to moisture.
- Inform patient that she must maintain adequate hydration throughout therapy. She should drink at least 48 ounces of liquids daily.
- Instruct patient who is also taking didanosine to take the two drugs 1 hour apart on an empty stomach.
- Advise patient to notify all prescribers of indinavir therapy, because of potential drug interactions, and advise patient not to take over-the-counter preparations (including herbal drugs and preparations) without consulting prescriber first.
- Warn male patient of the danger of taking drugs used to treat erectile dysfunction,

because very serious adverse reactions can occur if taken with indinavir.
- Inform patient that indinavir therapy may cause changes in her body appearance because of fat redistribution. Prepare her for the possibility of developing breast enlargement, central obesity, dorsocervical fat enlargement (buffalo hump), facial wasting, and peripheral wasting.
- Instruct patient to report any persistent, severe, or unusual signs and symptoms.
- Encourage women of childbearing age to report known or suspected pregnancy.
- Alert mothers that breastfeeding is not recommended during indinavir therapy, because drug is present in human breast milk.
- Inform patients with hemophilia that indinavir may cause spontaneous bleeding and to seek immediate medical attention if bleeding occurs.

indomethacin

Apo-Indomethacin (CAN), Indocid (CAN), Indocin, Indocin SR, Indo-Lemmon, Novo-Methacin (CAN), Nu-Indo (CAN), Tivorbex

indomethacin sodium trihydrate

Indocin I.V.

Class and Category

Pharmacologic class: NSAID
Therapeutic class: Analgesic
Pregnancy category: Not classified

Indications and Dosages

➤ *To relieve symptoms of ankylosing spondylitis, osteoarthritis, and rheumatoid arthritis*

CAPSULES, ORAL SUSPENSION

Adults and adolescents over age 14. 25 to 50 mg twice daily to four times daily, increased by 25 or 50 mg daily every wk, as needed. *Maximum:* 200 mg daily. After adequate response, dosage reduced as low as possible.

E.R. CAPSULES (ANTIRHEUMATIC)

Adults and adolescents over age 14. 75 mg daily, increased to 75 mg twice daily, if needed.

SUPPOSITORIES

Adults and adolescents over age 14. 50 mg up to four times daily.

➤ *To relieve symptoms of acute gouty arthritis*

CAPSULES, ORAL SUSPENSION, SUPPOSITORIES

Adults. 50 mg three times daily until gout attack relieved and then drug discontinued.

➤ *To treat inflammation and relieve acute shoulder pain from bursitis or tendinitis*

CAPSULES, ORAL SUSPENSION

Adults and adolescents over age 14. 75 to 150 mg daily in divided doses three times daily or four times daily for 7 to 14 days.

E.R. CAPSULES

Adults and adolescents over age 14. 75 mg twice daily for 7 to 14 days.

SUPPOSITORIES

Adults and adolescents over age 14. 50 mg up to three times daily for 7 to 14 days. *Maximum:* 200 mg daily.

➤ *To treat mild to moderate acute pain*

CAPSULES (TIVORBEX)

Adults. 20 mg three times daily or 40 mg two or three times daily.

DOSAGE ADJUSTMENT Dosage reduced for elderly patients.

➤ *To treat hemodynamically significant patent ductus arteriosus in premature infants weighing 500 to 1,750 g (1 to 3.9 lb)*

I.V. INFUSION

Infants over age 7 days. *Initial:* 200 mcg/kg (0.2 mg/kg) over 20 to 30 min; 1 or 2 additional doses of 250 mcg/kg (0.25 mg/kg) given at 12- to 24-hr intervals, if needed.

Neonates ages 2 to 7 days. *Initial:* 200 mcg/kg (0.2 mg/kg) over 20 to 30 min; 1 or 2 additional doses of 200 mcg/kg (0.2 mg/kg) given at 12- to 24-hr intervals, if needed.

Neonates under age 48 hours. *Initial:* 200 mcg/kg (0.2 mg/kg) over 20 to 30 min; 1 or 2 additional doses of 100 mcg/kg (0.1 mg/kg) given at 12- to 24-hr intervals, if needed.

Route	Onset	Peak	Duration
P.O.*	2–4 hr	2–5 days	Unknown
P.O.†	30 min	Unknown	4–6 hr
P.O.‡	In 7 days	1–2 wk	Unknown

* For antigout effects.
† For anti-inflammatory effects.
‡ For antirheumatic effects.

Mechanism of Action

Blocks activity of cyclooxygenase, the enzyme needed to synthesize prostaglandins, which mediate inflammatory response and cause local vasodilation, pain, and swelling. By blocking cyclooxygenase and inhibiting prostaglandins, this NSAID reduces inflammatory symptoms and helps relieve pain.

Incompatibilities

Don't give indomethacin suspension with alkaline antacids or liquids. Don't mix reconstituted indomethacin sodium with other I.V. infusion solutions.

Contraindications

Allergy or hypersensitivity to aspirin, indomethacin, iodides, other NSAIDs, or their components; history of proctitis or recent rectal bleeding (suppositories); postoperative pain with coronary artery bypass graft (CABG) surgery

Interactions

DRUGS

Note: All effects listed are for oral forms and suppositories unless indicated.
acetaminophen: Increased risk of adverse renal effects (long-term use of both drugs)
aluminum- and magnesium-containing antacids: Possibly decreased blood indomethacin level
aminoglycosides: Increased risk of aminoglycoside toxicity
antihypertensives: Decreased effectiveness of these drugs
aspirin, other NSAIDs: Increased risk of adverse GI effects and non-GI bleeding
bone marrow depressants: Possibly increased leukopenic or thrombocytopenic effects of these drugs
cefamandole, cefoperazone, cefotetan: Increased risk of hypoprothrombinemia and bleeding
colchicine, platelet aggregation inhibitors: Increased risk of GI bleeding, hemorrhage, and ulcers
corticosteroids, potassium supplements: Increased risk of adverse GI effects
cyclosporine: Increased risk of nephrotoxicity from both drugs, increased blood cyclosporine level
diflunisal: Increased blood indomethacin level and risk of GI bleeding
digoxin: Increased blood digoxin level and risk of digitalis toxicity (all forms)
diuretics (loop, potassium-sparing, and thiazide): Decreased antihypertensive and diuretic effects
gold compounds, nephrotoxic drugs: Increased risk of adverse renal effects
heparin, oral anticoagulants, thrombolytics: Possibly increased anticoagulant effects and risk of hemorrhage
lithium: Increased blood lithium level and risk of toxicity
methotrexate: Increased risk of methotrexate toxicity
plicamycin, valproic acid: Increased risk of hypoprothrombinemia and GI bleeding, hemorrhage, and ulcers
probenecid: Increased blood level and effectiveness of indomethacin, increased risk of indomethacin toxicity
zidovudine: Increased blood zidovudine level and risk of toxicity, increased risk of indomethacin toxicity

ACTIVITIES

alcohol use: Increased risk of adverse GI effects

Adverse Reactions

Note: All reactions are for oral forms and suppositories unless indicated.
CNS: Confusion, **CVA**, depression, dizziness, drowsiness, fatigue, hallucinations, headache, **intraventricular hemorrhage (I.V.)**, peripheral neuropathy, **seizures**, syncope, vertigo
CV: **Arrhythmias**, chest pain, edema, fluid retention (all forms), **heart failure**, hypertension, **MI**, **pulmonary hypertension (I.V.)**, tachycardia
EENT: Blurred vision, corneal and retinal damage, epistaxis, hearing loss, stomatitis, tinnitus

ENDO: Hypoglycemia (I.V.)
GI: Abdominal cramps or pain, abdominal distention (I.V.), anorexia, constipation, diarrhea, diverticulitis, dyspepsia, dysphagia, elevated liver enzymes, epigastric discomfort, esophagitis, gastritis, gastroenteritis, gastroesophageal reflux disease, **GI bleeding** and ulceration (all forms), hemorrhoids, **hepatic dysfunction (I.V.)**, **hepatic failure**, hiatal hernia, ileus (I.V.), indigestion, **melena**, nausea, **necrotizing enterocolitis (I.V.)**, **pancreatitis**, peptic ulcer, **perforation of intestine or stomach**, vomiting (all forms)
GU: Acute renal failure, hematuria, interstitial nephritis, **nephrotic syndrome**, oliguria (I.V.), proteinuria, renal dysfunction (I.V.), vaginal bleeding
HEME: Agranulocytosis, anemia, **aplastic anemia**, **bone marrow depression**, **decreased platelet aggregation (I.V.)**, **disseminated intravascular coagulation (DIC)**, **hemolytic anemia**, iron deficiency anemia, **leukopenia**, **neutropenia**, **pancytopenia**, **thrombocytopenia**, **unusual bleeding** or bruising (all forms)
RESP: Asthma, **respiratory depression**
SKIN: Ecchymosis, **erythema multiforme**, erythema nodosum, photosensitivity, pruritus, rash, **Stevens–Johnson syndrome**, **toxic epidermal necrolysis**, urticaria
Other: Anaphylaxis, **angioedema**, **hyperkalemia (I.V.)**, **hyponatremia (I.V.)**, injection-site irritation

Nursing Considerations

- Be aware that NSAIDs like indomethacin should be avoided in patients with a recent MI because risk of reinfarction increases with NSAID therapy. If therapy is unavoidable, monitor patient closely for signs of cardiac ischemia.
- Know that the risk of heart failure increases with indomethacin use because it is a NSAID. This class of drugs should not be used in patients with severe heart failure but, if unavoidable, monitor patient for worsening of heart failure.
- Use indomethacin with extreme caution in patients with history of GI bleeding or ulcer disease because NSAIDs, such as indomethacin, increase risk of GI bleeding and ulceration. Expect to use drug for shortest time possible in these patients.
- Be aware that serious GI tract, bleeding, perforation, and ulceration may occur without warning symptoms. Elderly patients are at greater risk. To minimize risk, give oral indomethacin with an antacid, food, or a full glass of water (not suspension), to reduce GI distress.
- Know that if GI distress occurs, withhold drug and notify prescriber immediately.
- Use indomethacin cautiously in patients with hypertension, and monitor blood pressure closely throughout therapy. Drug may cause hypertension or worsen it.
- Shake suspension well before giving it.
- Make sure suppository stays in rectum at least 1 hour to improve absorption.
- To reconstitute I.V. form, add 1 to 2 ml of preservative-free sodium chloride for injection or preservative-free sterile water to vial. Solution made with 1 ml diluent contains 100 mcg (0.1 mg) indomethacin/0.1 ml. Solution made with 2 ml diluent contains 50 mcg (0.05 mg) indomethacin/0.1 ml. Use solution immediately because it contains no preservatives. Discard unused portion.
- Be aware that scheduled I.V. doses may be withheld if infant or neonate has anuria or a significant decrease in urine output (less than 0.6 ml/kg/hr).
- Be aware that when using I.V. form, avoid extravasation to protect surrounding tissue.
- Anticipate a second course (3 more doses) of I.V. indomethacin if patent ductus arteriosus fails to close or reopens. After 2 courses, surgery may be performed.

WARNING Monitor patient closely for thrombotic events, including MI and stroke, because NSAIDs increase the risk. These events may occur early in treatment and risk increases with duration of use. Be aware that these events have occurred even in patients who do not have a history or risk factors for cardiovascular disease. Monitor patient for warning signs such as chest pain, slurring of speech, shortness of breath, or weakness. If any signs and symptoms develop, withhold indomethacin, alert prescriber immediately, and provide supportive care as prescribed.

- Monitor patient—especially if he's elderly or receiving long-term indomethacin therapy—for less common but serious adverse GI reactions, including anorexia, constipation, diverticulitis, dysphagia, esophagitis, gastritis, gastroenteritis, gastroesophageal reflux disease, hemorrhoids, hiatal hernia, melena, stomatitis, and vomiting.
- Monitor liver enzymes because, rarely, elevations may progress to severe hepatic reactions, including fatal hepatitis, hepatic failure, and liver necrosis.
- Monitor BUN and serum creatinine levels in elderly patients, those taking ACE inhibitors or diuretics, and those with heart failure, hepatic dysfunction, or impaired renal function; drug may cause renal failure.
- Monitor CBC for decreased hemoglobin and hematocrit. Drug may worsen anemia.

WARNING Know that if patient has bone marrow suppression or is receiving an antineoplastic drug, monitor laboratory results (including WBC count), and watch for evidence of infection because anti-inflammatory and antipyretic actions of indomethacin may mask signs and symptoms, such as fever and pain.

- Assess patient's skin regularly for signs of rash or other hypersensitivity reaction because indomethacin is an NSAID and may cause serious skin reactions without warning, even in patients with no history of NSAID sensitivity. At first sign of reaction, stop drug and notify prescriber.
- Monitor weight and blood pressure, especially if patient has hypertension, because indomethacin causes sodium retention.
- Keep in mind when drug is used to treat gouty arthritis, expect its action to peak in 24 to 36 hours and significant swelling to gradually disappear over 3 to 5 days.
- Be aware that E.R. form shouldn't be used to treat gouty arthritis.
- Expect to use suppositories for patients who can't swallow oral form.
- Assess for improved joint mobility and reduced pain and inflammation to evaluate drug effectiveness.
- Expect patient to have intermittent checkups during long-term therapy and an ophthalmologic examination if vision changes.

PATIENT TEACHING

- Urge patient to take indomethacin capsules with full glass of water and to avoid lying down for 15 to 30 minutes afterward. This helps prevent drug from lodging in esophagus and causing irritation. Caution patient not to crush or open capsules.
- Instruct patient to take drug with food or an antacid to reduce GI distress.
- Instruct patient to make sure suppository stays in rectum at least 1 hour.
- Urge patient to avoid alcohol during indomethacin therapy.
- Remind patient that improvement may not occur for 2 to 4 weeks after starting indomethacin to treat arthritis or ankylosing spondylitis and that he should continue taking drug, as prescribed.
- Inform breastfeeding patient that indomethacin appears in breast milk and may cause seizures in infants. Urge her to use another feeding method during therapy.
- Caution against prolonged sun exposure during therapy.
- Urge patient to notify prescriber immediately about changes in hearing or vision, fever, itching, rash, sore throat, or swelling in arms or legs.
- Emphasize importance of having ordered laboratory tests and eye examinations during long-term therapy.
- Caution pregnant patient not to take NSAIDs such as indomethacin during last trimester because they may cause premature closure of the ductus arteriosus.
- Explain that indomethacin may increase risk of serious adverse cardiovascular reactions; urge patient to seek immediate medical attention if signs or symptoms arise, such as chest pain, edema, shortness of breath, slurring of speech, unexplained weight gain, or weakness.
- Explain that indomethacin may increase risk of serious adverse GI reactions; emphasize need to seek immediate medical attention for such signs and symptoms as abdominal or epigastric pain, indigestion, black or tarry stools, or vomiting blood or material that looks like coffee grounds.

- Alert patient to rare but serious skin reactions. Urge him to seek immediate medical attention for blisters, fever, itching, rash, or other indications of hypersensitivity.

infliximab
Remicade
infliximab abda
Renflexis
infliximab dyyb
Inflectra

Class and Category
Pharmacologic class: Monoclonal antibody (tumor necrosis factor [TNF] blocker)
Therapeutic class: Anti-inflammatory
Pregnancy category: C

Indications and Dosages
➤ *To control moderate to severe Crohn's disease long-term*

I.V. INFUSION

Adults and children ages 6 and over. *Initial:* 5 mg/kg infused over 2 hr, repeated 2 and 6 wk after first infusion. *Maintenance:* 5 mg/kg infused over 2 hr every 8 wk.

DOSAGE ADJUSTMENT For adults who respond and then lose response, dosage may be increased to 10 mg/kg.

➤ *To reduce signs and symptoms, to induce and maintain remission and mucosal healing, and to eliminate corticosteroid use in patients with moderate to severe active ulcerative colitis who have had an inadequate response to conventional therapy; to treat chronic severe plaque psoriasis in patients who are candidates for systemic therapy and when other systemic therapies are medically less appropriate*

I.V. INFUSION

Adults. *Initial:* 5 mg/kg infused over 2 hr, repeated 2 and 6 wk after first infusion. *Maintenance:* 5 mg/kg infused over 2 hr every 8 wk.

➤ *As adjunct to reduce signs and symptoms, inhibit progression of structural damage, and improve physical function in patients with moderate to severe active rheumatoid arthritis*

I.V. INFUSION

Adults. *Initial:* 3 mg/kg infused over 2 hr, with methotrexate, repeated 2 and 6 wk after first infusion. *Maintenance:* 3 mg/kg infused over 2 hr every 8 wk.

DOSAGE ADJUSTMENT For adults who have an incomplete response, dosage increased up to 10 mg/kg per infusion or treatment frequency increased to every 4 wk.

➤ *To treat active ankylosing spondylitis*

I.V. INFUSION

Adults. *Initial:* 5 mg/kg infused over 2 hr, repeated 2 and 6 wk after first infusion. *Maintenance:* 5 mg/kg infused over 2 hr every 6 wk.

➤ *To reduce signs and symptoms, inhibit progression of structural damage, and improve physical function in patients with psoriatic arthritis*

I.V. INFUSION

Adults. *Initial:* 5 mg/kg infused over 2 hr, with or without methotrexate, repeated 2 and 6 wk after first infusion. *Maintenance:* 5 mg/kg infused over 2 hr every 8 wk.

Mechanism of Action
Binds with cytokine tumor necrosis factor-alpha (TNF-alpha), preventing it from binding with its receptors. As a result, TNF-alpha can't produce proinflammatory cytokines and endothelial permeability. Infiltration of inflammatory cells into inflamed intestine and joints declines.

Incompatibilities
Don't infuse infliximab in same I.V. line with other drugs or through plasticized polyvinyl chloride infusion equipment or devices.

Contraindications
Breastfeeding; doses greater than 5 mg/kg in patients with moderate to severe heart failure; hypersensitivity to infliximab, murine proteins, or their components

Interactions
DRUGS

abatacept, anakinra, etanercept, tocilizumab: Increased risk of neutropenia and serious infections *live vaccines, therapeutic infectious agents such as BCG in bladder instillation:* Increased risk of adverse vaccine effects

Adverse Reactions

CNS: Chills, **CVA**, dizziness, fatigue, fever, headache, **meningitis**, neuritis, neuropathies, numbness, paresthesia, peripheral demyelinating disorders, **seizures**, syncope, tingling
CV: Arrhythmias, **bradycardia**, chest pain, edema, hypertension, **hypotension**, **MI**, myocardial ischemia, myelitis, neuropathies, **pericardial effusion**, systemic and cutaneous vasculitis, thrombophlebitis
EENT: Laryngeal/pharyngeal edema, oral candidiasis, pharyngitis, rhinitis, sinusitis, transient vision loss, visual changes
GI: Abdominal hernia; abdominal pain; **acute hepatic failure**; cholecystitis; cholestasis; constipation; diarrhea; dyspepsia; elevated aminotranferases; **GI hemorrhage**; **hepatitis**, **hepatotoxicity**; ileus; **intestinal obstruction**, **perforation**, or stenosis; jaundice; **melena**; nausea; **pancreatitis**; splenic infarction; splenomegaly; vomiting
GU: Cervical cancer, kidney infection, **renal failure**, ureteral obstruction, UTI, vaginal candidiasis, vaginitis
HEME: Agranulocytosis, anemia, **aplastic anemia**, **hemolytic anemia**, **leukemia**, **leukopenia**, **neutropenia**, **pancytopenia**, **thrombocytopenia**, **thrombocytopenic purpura**
MS: Ankylosing spondylitis, arthralgia, back pain, limb weakness, myalgia, psoriatic arthritis, transverse myelitis
RESP: Adult respiratory distress syndrome, bronchitis, cough, dyspnea, **interstitial lung disease**, pleurisy, pneumonia, **pulmonary edema**, tuberculosis, respiratory tract infection, **severe bronchospasm**, wheezing
SKIN: Cellulitis, diaphoresis, **erythema multiforme**, facial flushing, **melanoma**, **Merkel cell cancer**, pruritus, psoriasis (new or worsening), rash, **Stevens–Johnson syndrome**, **toxic epidermal necrolysis**, urticaria
Other: Anaphylaxis; antibody formation to infliximab; bacterial (including *Legionella* and *Listeria*), fungal, mycobacterial, parasitic, or viral infections; dehydration; infusion reaction; lupus-like symptoms; lymphadenopathy; **malignancies**, **such as lymphomas**, **including hepatosplenic T-cell lymphoma**; sarcoidosis; **sepsis**; serum sickness

Nursing Considerations

- Know that infliximab therapy shouldn't be started in a patient with an active infection, including serious localized infection.
- Know that because drug increases risk of developing tuberculosis or reactivating latent tuberculosis, expect prescriber to evaluate patient's risk and start tuberculosis treatment, as needed, before starting infliximab.
- Use with extreme caution if patient has a history of chronic or recurrent infection, known exposure to tuberculosis, an underlying condition that predisposes to infection, or residence or travel to areas of endemic tuberculosis or mycoses, such as blastomycosis, coccidioidomycosis, or histoplasmosis.
- Use cautiously in elderly patients because they have a higher risk of infection.
- Use cautiously in patients with previous or ongoing hematologic abnormalities because infliximab may cause serious or even life-threatening adverse hematologic effects. Monitor patient's CBC regularly, as ordered. If adverse effects occur, expect drug to be discontinued.
- Be aware that use of TNF-blocking therapy, including infliximab, may reactivate hepatitis B virus in patients who are chronic carriers of this virus. Ensure that patient has been tested for hepatitis B infection before infliximab therapy is begun. For patients who develop reactivation of hepatitis B, know that therapy should be stopped and antiviral therapy with appropriate supportive treatment begun.

WARNING Be aware that infliximab increases risk of serious or fatal opportunistic infections, including invasive fungal infections, as well as bacterial (including *Legionella* and *Listeria*), mycobacterial, parasitic, and viral infections. The most common ones include aspergillosis, blastomycosis, candidiasis, coccidioidomycosis, cryptococcosis, histoplasmosis, legionellosis, listeriosis, pneumocytosis, salmonellosis, and tuberculosis.

WARNING Watch for infection, especially if patient receives immunosuppressant therapy or has a chronic infection. Upper respiratory tract infections and UTI are most common, but sepsis and fatal infections have occurred. If infection is suspected, notify prescriber, and if a serious infection is confirmed, expect drug to be discontinued.

- Reconstitute infliximab, by using a 21G (or smaller) needle to add 10 ml sterile water for injection to each vial of drug. Swirl to mix; don't shake. Solution may foam and be clear or light yellow.
- Withdraw volume equal to amount of reconstituted drug from a 250-ml glass bottle or polypropylene or polyolefin infusion bag of normal saline solution. Then add reconstituted infliximab to bottle to dilute to 250 ml. Use within 3 hours.
- Know that the infusion should be given over at least 2 hours using polyethylene-lined infusion set and in-line, sterile, nonpyrogenic, low–protein-binding filter with pores 1.2 microns or less. Don't reuse.
- Expect to premedicate patient, as prescribed, with acetaminophen, antihistamines, and/or corticosteroids to decrease an infusion reaction. If a mild to moderate infusion reaction occurs, notify prescriber and expect to slow or suspend infusion. If infusion was suspended, know that once the reaction has been resolved, the infusion may be restarted at a lower infusion rate and patient premedicated if not done before. If a severe infusion reaction occurs, know that infusion should be stopped and drug permanently discontinued. Be prepared to provide supportive emergency care according to protocol.
- Be aware that a reaction may occur 2 hours to 12 days after infusion.
- Monitor patient closely for the first 24 hours after the initial drug infusion because serious cardiovascular and cerebrovascular reactions may occur during and after infusion. Also, monitor patient for transient visual loss during or within 2 hours of infusion. If serious reactions occur, stop infusion, notify prescriber, and expect to provide supportive emergency care, as ordered.
- Monitor liver function because severe hepatic reactions may occur. Expect to stop drug if jaundice develops or liver enzymes are five times or more the upper limit of normal.
- Be aware that infliximab is a tumor necrosis factor (TNF) blocker. Malignancies, especially leukemia and such rare lymphomas as hepatosplenic T-cell lymphoma, have been reported in patients, particularly children and adolescents, receiving TNF blockers. Patients at increased risk of leukemia are those with rheumatoid arthritis. Patients at increased risk of lymphomas are those with ankylosing spondylitis, Crohn's disease, plaque psoriasis, psoriatic arthritis, and rheumatoid arthritis, especially those with long-term or very active disease. Other malignancies, such as cervical cancer and skin cancer, have also occurred. Monitor them closely.

PATIENT TEACHING

- Inform patient that infliximab should take effect within 1 to 2 weeks.
- Urge patient to report evidence of infection, such as cough, painful urination, and sore throat. Infusion reaction (chest pain, chills, dyspnea, facial flushing, fever, itching, headache, rash) may occur for up to 12 days.
- Explain that infliximab increases the risk of lymphoma; urge prompt medical attention for suspicious signs or symptoms. Also, advise patient to have regular skin examinations because drug increases risk of skin cancer and for female patients to have periodic screening for cervical cancer.
- Advise patient not to receive vaccinations using live vaccines. Also advise parents not to have their infant exposed to live vaccines for up to 6 months after birth if the mother was taking infliximab during the pregnancy.

insulin, inhaled (rapid-acting)

Afrezza

Class and Category

Pharmacologic class: Human insulin
Therapeutic class: Antidiabetic
Pregnancy category: C

Indications and Dosages

➤ *To improve glycemic control in patients with diabetes mellitus*

ORAL INHALATION

Adults who are not currently taking insulin. *Initial:* 4 units at beginning of each meal with dosage increased, as needed.
Adults converting from subcutaneous mealtime (prandial) insulin. Dosage dependent upon subcutaneous insulin dosage as follows: 4 units at beginning of each meal if up to 4 units of subcutaneous mealtime insulin was being used; 8 units at beginning of each meal if 5 to 8 units of subcutaneous mealtime insulin was used; 12 units at beginning of each meal if 9 to 12 units of subcutaneous mealtime insulin was used; 16 units if 13 to 16 units of subcutaneous mealtime insulin was used; 20 units at beginning of each meal if 17 to 20 units of subcutaneous mealtime insulin was used; and 24 units at beginning of each meal if 21 to 24 units of subcutaneous mealtime insulin was used. *Maintenance*: Dosage based on blood glucose monitoring results, glycemic control goal, and metabolic needs.
Adults converting from subcutaneous premixed insulin. Both basal and mealtime dosages required for conversion. *Mealtime dosage:* Beginning-of-mealtime injected dose estimated by dividing half of the total daily injected premixed insulin dose equally among the three meals of the day. Then each estimated injected mealtime dose converted as follows: 4 units if up to 4 units of subcutaneous premixed insulin was used; 8 units if 5 to 8 units of subcutaneous premixed insulin was used; 12 units if 9 to 12 units of subcutaneous premixed insulin was used; 16 units if 13 to 16 units of subcutaneous premixed insulin was used; 20 units if 17 to 20 units of subcutaneous premixed insulin was used; and 24 units if 21 to 24 units of subcutaneous premixed insulin was used. *Basal dosage:* The remaining half of the total daily injected premixed dose injected as a basal insulin dose. *Maintenance:* Mealtime and basal dosages based on, blood glucose monitoring results, glycemic control goal, and metabolic needs.

DOSAGE ADJUSTMENT Dosage may need to be decreased if patient is taking any of the following drugs concurrently: ACE inhibitors, angiotensin II receptor blocking agents, disopyramide, fibrates, fluoxetine, monoamine oxidase inhibitors, other antidiabetic agents, pentoxifylline, pramlintide, propoxyphene, salicylates, somatostatin analogues, or sulfonamide antibiotics. Dosage may have to be increased if patient is taking any of the following drugs concurrently: atypical antipsychotics, corticosteroids, danazol, diuretics, estrogens, glucagon, isoniazid, niacin, oral contraceptives, phenothiazines, progestogens, protease inhibitors, somatropin, sympathomimetic agents, or thyroid hormones. Dosage may have to be increased or decreased if patient is taking any of the following concurrently: alcohol, beta blockers, clonidine, lithium, or pentamidine

Mechanism of Action

Lowers blood glucose levels by stimulating peripheral glucose uptake by fat and skeletal muscle, and by inhibiting hepatic glucose production. Also enhances protein synthesis, inhibits lipolysis in adipocytes, and inhibits proteolysis.

Contraindications

Chronic lung disease (asthma, chronic obstructive pulmonary disease), during episodes of hypoglycemia, hypersensitivity to regular human insulin or any of its components

Interactions

DRUGS

ACE inhibitors, angiotensin II receptor blocking agents, disopyramide, fibrates, fluoxetine, monoamine oxidase inhibitors, other antidiabetic agents, pentoxifylline,

pramlintide, propoxyphene, salicylates, somatostatin analogues, sulfonamide antibiotics: Increased risk of hypoglycemia
atypical antipsychotics, corticosteroids, danazol, diuretics, estrogens, glucagon, isoniazid, niacin, oral contraceptives, phenothiazines, progestogens, protease inhibitors, somatropin, sympathomimetic agents, thyroid hormones: Decreased effectiveness of inhaled insulin
beta blockers, clonidine, lithium, or pentamidine: Possibly decreased or increased blood glucose levels
beta blockers, clonidine, guanethidine, reserpine: Blunted hypoglycemic signs and symptoms
thiazolidinediones: Increased risk of fluid retention and heart failure

ACTIVITIES
alcohol use: Possibly decreased or increased blood glucose levels

Adverse Reactions

CNS: Confusion, dizziness, drowsiness, fatigue, headache
CV: Tachycardia
EENT: Throat irritation or pain
ENDO: Diabetic ketoacidosis, hypoglycemia
GI: Diarrhea, nausea
GU: UTI
RESP: Acute bronchospasm, bronchitis, cough, decline in pulmonary function, dyspnea, **lung cancer** (rare), shortness of breath
SKIN: Diaphoresis, rash
Other: Anaphylaxis, **angioedema**, anti-insulin antibodies, **hypokalemia**, weight gain

Nursing Considerations

- Be aware that inhaled insulin is not a substitute for long-acting insulin and must be used in combination with long-acting insulin in patients with type 1 diabetes mellitus.
- Know that inhaled insulin should not be used to treat diabetic ketoacidosis, nor should it be used in patients who smoke or who have recently stopped smoking. Also know that drug is not recommended in patients with active lung cancer or who have a prior history of lung cancer or risk factors for lung cancer because, although rare, lung cancer has occurred in nonsmokers prescribed inhaled insulin.
- Ensure that patient has had a complete medical history, physical examination, and spirometry before inhaled insulin therapy is begun to identify potential lung disease, as the drug is contraindicated in patients with chronic lung disease. Spirometry should be repeated after the first 6 months of therapy and annually thereafter. Expect drug to be discontinued if patient experiences a 20% or more decline in pulmonary function.
- Administer inhaled insulin using only the Afrezza inhaler. Each cartridge provides a single inhalation.

WARNING Monitor patient closely for signs and symptoms of hypoglycemia, which could become severe, causing seizures or even death. If present, withhold inhaled insulin, treat according to standard of care, and notify prescriber.

- Monitor patient's blood glucose level closely to detect need for dosage adjustment, as ordered. Expect dosage adjustments with changes in patient's hepatic or renal function, meal patterns, and physical activity, or during acute illness.
- Monitor patient for hypersensitivity reactions. If present, withhold drug, treat according to standard of care, and monitor patient closely until signs and symptoms resolve. Notify prescriber and expect drug to be discontinued and replaced with subcutaneous forms of insulin therapy.
- Monitor patient's serum potassium levels throughout inhaled insulin therapy in patients at risk for hypokalemia, such as those using, drugs sensitive to serum potassium concentrations, intravenously administered insulin or potassium lowering drugs.

PATIENT TEACHING

- Teach patient how to use the inhaler device.
- Tell patient that doses that exceed 8 units per mealtime will require more than one cartridge.
- Instruct patient to keep the inhaler level, the white mouthpiece on the top, and the purple base on the bottom after a cartridge has been inserted into the

inhaler. Remind patient that loss of drug effect can occur if the inhaler is turned upside down, held with the mouthpiece pointing down, or shaken (or dropped) after the cartridge has been inserted but before the dose has been administered. If any of these events occur, tell patient to replace the cartridge before use.

WARNING Review signs and symptoms of hypoglycemia and how to treat them. If frequent or severe, tell patient to notify prescriber, as dosage may need to be adjusted. Stress importance of monitoring blood glucose levels.

- Stress importance of not ingesting alcoholic beverages or smoking while using inhaled insulin.
- Tell patient to avoid performing hazardous activities such as driving until the effects of inhaled insulin on her nervous system is known.

ipratropium bromide

Apo-Ipravent (CAN), Atrovent, Atrovent HFA, Kendral-Ipratropium (CAN)

Class and Category

Pharmacologic class: Anticholinergic
Therapeutic class: Bronchodilator
Pregnancy category: B

Indications and Dosages

➤ *To treat bronchitis and COPD*

INHALATION AEROSOL

Adults. 2 to 4 inhalations (36 to 72 mcg) three times daily or four times daily. *Maximum:* Up to 12 inhalations (216 mcg)/24 hr.

INHALATION SOLUTION FOR NEBULIZER

Adults. 250 to 500 mcg dissolved in preservative-free sterile normal saline solution every 6 to 8 hr. For severe COPD exacerbations, 500 mcg every 4 to 8 hr.

➤ *To treat perennial and allergic rhinitis*

NASAL SPRAY

Adults and children age 6 and over. 2 sprays of 0.03% (21 mcg/spray) per nostril twice daily or three times daily *Maximum:* 12 sprays (252 mcg)/24 hr.

➤ *To treat rhinorrhea caused by seasonal allergic rhinitis*

NASAL SPRAY

Adults and children age 5 and over. 2 sprays of 0.06% (42 mcg/spray) per nostril four times daily for up to 3 wk. *Maximum:* 16 sprays (672 mcg)/24 hr.

➤ *To treat rhinorrhea associated with the common cold*

NASAL SPRAY

Adults and adolescents. 2 sprays of 0.06% (42 mcg/spray) per nostril three or four times daily for up to 4 days.

Children ages 5 to 11. 2 sprays of 0.06% (42 mcg/spray) per nostril three times daily for up to 4 days.

Route	Onset	Peak	Duration
Inhalation	5–15 min	1–2 hr	3–8 hr
Nasal	5 min	1–4 hr	4–8 hr

Contraindications

Hypersensitivity to atropine, ipratropium bromide, or their components; hypersensitivity to peanuts, soya lecithin, soybeans, or related products (with aerosol inhaler)

Interactions

DRUGS

anticholinergics: Increased anticholinergic effects
tacrine: Decreased effects of both drugs

Adverse Reactions

CNS: Dizziness, insomnia
CV: **Atrial fibrillation** (oral inhalation), **bradycardia** (nasal spray), edema, hypertension, palpitations, **supraventricular tachycardia** (oral inhalation), tachycardia
EENT: Acute eye pain, dry mouth or pharyngeal area, increased intraocular pressure, **laryngospasm**, taste perversion, **oropharyngeal edema** (all drug forms); blurred vision, conjunctival and corneal congestion, eye irritation and pain, mydriasis, visual halos (if nasal spray comes in contact with eyes); epistaxis, mydriasis,

Mechanism of Action

After acetylcholine is released from cholinergic fibers, ipratropium prevents it from attaching to muscarinic receptors on membranes of smooth-muscle cells, as shown at right. By blocking acetylcholine's effects in bronchi and bronchioles, ipratropium relaxes smooth muscles and causes bronchodilation.

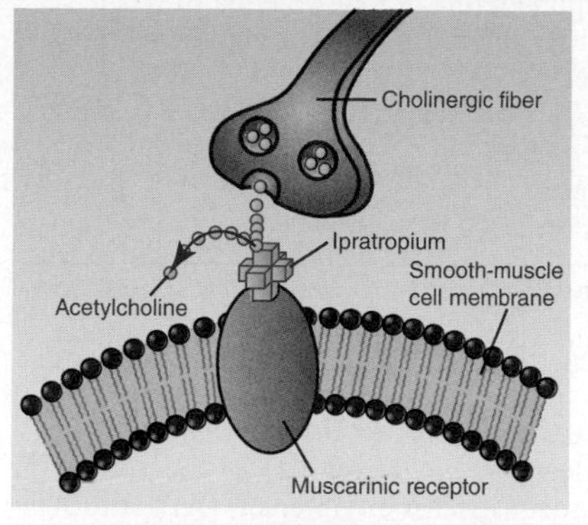

nasal dryness and irritation, pharyngitis, rhinitis, sinusitis, tinnitus (with nasal spray)
GI: Bowel obstruction, constipation, diarrhea, ileus, nausea, vomiting
GU: Prostatitis, urine retention
MS: Arthritis
RESP: Bronchitis, **bronchospasm**, cough, dyspnea, increased sputum production, wheezing
SKIN: Dermatitis, pruritus, rash, urticaria
Other: Anaphylaxis, **angioedema**, flu-like symptoms

Nursing Considerations

- Use ipratropium cautiously in patients with angle-closure glaucoma, benign prostatic hyperplasia, or bladder neck obstruction and in patients with hepatic or renal dysfunction.
- When using a nebulizer, apply a mouthpiece to prevent drug from leaking out around mask and causing blurred vision or eye pain.

WARNING Monitor patient for hypersensitivity reactions that could be life-threatening. If present, stop drug use immediately, notify prescriber, and provide supportive care, as needed.

PATIENT TEACHING

- Caution patient not to use ipratropium to treat acute bronchospasm.
- Inform patient that although some people feel relief within 24 hours of drug use, maximum effect may take up to 2 weeks.
- Teach patient to use inhaler or nasal spray. Tell him to shake inhaler well at each use.
- Advise patient to keep spray out of his eyes because it may irritate them or blur his vision. If spray comes in contact with eyes, instruct patient to flush them with cool tap water for several minutes and to contact prescriber.
- Instruct patient to rinse mouth after each nebulizer or inhaler treatment to help minimize throat dryness and irritation.
- Teach patient to track canister contents by counting and recording number of doses.
- Advise patient to report decreased response to ipratropium as well as difficulty voiding, eye pain, nasal dryness, nose bleeds, palpitations, and vision changes.

irbesartan

Avapro

Class and Category

Pharmacologic class: Angiotensin II receptor antagonist
Therapeutic class: Antihypertensive
Pregnancy category: D

Indications and Dosages

➤ *To manage hypertension, alone or with other antihypertensives*

TABLETS

Adults and adolescents. *Initial:* 150 mg daily. *Maximum:* 300 mg daily.

DOSAGE ADJUSTMENT Initial dosage reduced to 75 mg daily for patients with hyponatremia or hypovolemia from such causes as hemodialysis or vigorous diuretic therapy.

➤ *To treat nephropathy in type 2 diabetes mellitus*

TABLETS

Adults. 300 mg daily.

Route	Onset	Peak	Duration
P.O.	Unknown	In 4–6 wk	Unknown

Mechanism of Action

Selectively blocks binding of the potent vasoconstrictor angiotensin (AT) II to AT_1 receptor sites in many tissues, including adrenal glands and vascular smooth-muscle. This inhibits the aldosterone-secreting and vasoconstrictive effects of AT II, which reduces blood pressure.

Contraindications

Concurrent aliskiren use in patients with diabetes or patients with renal impairment (GFR less than 60 ml/min), hypersensitivity to irbesartan or its components

Interactions

DRUGS

ACE inhibitors, aliskiren (patients with diabetes or renal impairment), other angiotensin receptor blockers: Increased risk of hyperkalemia, hypotension, and renal dysfunction

diuretics: Possibly additive hypotensive effects

lithium: Possibly increased serum lithium level

NSAIDs: Possible decreased renal function in patients who are elderly, volume-depleted, or have a compromised renal function

potassium-sparing diuretics, potassium supplements, or salt substitutes containing potassium: Possible hyperkalemia

Adverse Reactions

CNS: Anxiety, dizziness, fatigue, headache, nervousness

CV: Chest pain, **hypotension**, peripheral edema, tachycardia

EENT: Pharyngitis, rhinitis, tinnitus

GI: Abdominal pain, diarrhea, elevated liver enzymes, heartburn, **hepatitis**, indigestion, jaundice, nausea, vomiting

GU: Impaired renal function, **renal failure**, UTI

MS: Musculoskeletal pain

HEME: Thrombocytopenia

MS: Increased CPK level, **rhabdomyolysis**

RESP: Upper respiratory tract infection

SKIN: Rash, urticaria

Other: Anaphylaxis including shock, **angioedema**, **hyperkalemia**

Nursing Considerations

- Know that if patient has known or suspected hypovolemia, provide treatment, such as I.V. normal saline solution, as prescribed, to correct this condition before beginning irbesartan therapy. Or expect to begin therapy with a lower dosage.
- Check blood pressure often to evaluate drug's effectiveness.
- Be aware that if blood pressure isn't controlled with irbesartan alone, expect to also give a diuretic, such as hydrochlorothiazide, as prescribed.

WARNING Be alert for hypotension in a patient who receives a diuretic or another antihypertensive during irbesartan therapy. Frequently monitor blood pressure. If patient experiences symptomatic hypotension, expect to stop drug temporarily. Immediately place him in supine position and prepare to give I.V. normal saline solution, as prescribed. Expect to resume drug therapy after blood pressure stabilizes.

- Be aware that if patient receives a diuretic, provide adequate hydration, as appropriate, to help prevent hypovolemia. Also monitor patient for signs and symptoms of hypovolemia, such as dizziness, fainting, and hypotension.

WARNING Monitor patient for increased BUN and serum creatinine levels if he has heart failure or impaired renal function because drug may cause acute renal failure. If increases are significant or persistent, notify prescriber immediately.

PATIENT TEACHING

- Advise patient to take drug at the same time each day to maintain its therapeutic effect.
- Explain importance of regular exercise, proper diet, and other lifestyle changes in controlling hypertension.

- Caution patient to avoid hazardous activities until drug's CNS effects are known.
- Instruct patient to consult prescriber before taking any new drug.
- To reduce risk of dehydration and hypotension, advise patient to drink adequate fluids during hot weather and exercise.
- Instruct patient to contact prescriber if diarrhea, severe nausea, or vomiting, occurs and continues, because of the risk of dehydration and hypotension.

WARNING Advise female patient to notify prescriber immediately about known or suspected pregnancy. Explain that if she becomes pregnant, prescriber may replace irbesartan with another antihypertensive that's safe to use during pregnancy.

- Urge patient to keep follow-up appointments with prescriber to monitor progress.

iron dextran

(contains 50 mg of elemental iron per milliliter)

DexFerrum, DexIron (CAN), InFeD

Class and Category

Pharmacologic class: Iron mineral
Therapeutic class: Hematinic
Pregnancy category: C

Indications and Dosages

➤ *To treat iron deficiency anemia*

I.M. INJECTION (INFED)

Adults and children weighing more than 15 kg (33 lb). Calculated using following formula: Dose (ml) = 0.0442 (desired hemoglobin – observed hemoglobin) × lean body weight (LBW) in kg (Males = 50 kg + 2.3 kg for each inch of patient's height over 5 feet. Females = 45.5 kg + 2.3 kg for each inch of patient's height over 5 feet.) + (0.26 × LBW). Or, consult dosage table in package insert. *Test dose on day 1:* 0.5 ml by Z-track technique followed in 1 hr or more with remainder of dose, if no reaction occurs. Total dosage repeated once daily thereafter.
Children over age 4 months weighing 5 to 15 kg (11 to 33 lb). Calculated using following formula: Dose (ml) = 0.0442 (desired hemoglobin – observed hemoglobin) × weight in kg + (0.26 × weight in kg). Or, consult dosage table in package insert. *Test dose on day 1:* 0.5 ml by Z-tack technique followed in 1 hr or more with remainder of dose, if no reaction occurs. Total dosage repeated once daily thereafter.

I.V. INFUSION

Adults and children weighing more than 15 kg (33 lb). Calculated using following formula: Dose (ml) = 0.0442 (desired hemoglobin – observed hemoglobin) × lean body weight (LBW) in kg (Males = 50 kg + 2.3 kg for each inch of patient's height over 5 feet. Females = 45.5 kg + 2.3 kg for each inch of patient's height over 5 feet.) + (0.26 × LBW). Or, consult dosage table in package insert. *Test dose on day 1:* 0.5 ml over at least 5 min followed in 1 hr or more with remainder of dose, if no reaction occurs. Total dosage repeated once daily thereafter. *Maximum:* 2 ml (100 mg) daily.
Children over age 4 months weighing 5 to 15 kg (11 to 33 lb). Calculated using following formula: Dose (ml) = 0.0442 (desired hemoglobin – observed hemoglobin) × weight in kg + (0.26 × weight in kg)
Test dose on day 1: 0.5 ml over at least 5 min followed in 1 hr or more with remainder of dose, if no reaction occurs. Total dosage repeated once daily thereafter. *Maximum:* 1 ml (50 mg) daily.

➤ *To replace iron lost in blood loss*

I.V. INFUSION

Adults. Replacement iron (mg) = Blood loss (ml) × hematocrit. Infuse at a slow gradual rate that does not exceed 50 mg (1 ml)/min.

Mechanism of Action

Restores hemoglobin and replenishes iron stores. Iron, an essential component of hemoglobin, myoglobin, and several enzymes (including catalase, cytochromes, and peroxidase), is needed for catecholamine metabolism and normal neutrophil function.

In iron dextran therapy, iron binds to available protein parts after the drug has been split into dextran and iron by cells of the reticuloendothelial system. The bound iron forms hemosiderin or ferritin, physiologic forms of iron, and transferrin, which replenish hemoglobin and deplete iron stores. Dextran is metabolized or excreted.

Incompatibilities

Don't mix iron dextran with blood for transfusion, other drugs, or parenteral nutrition solutions for I.V. infusion.

Contraindications

Anemia other than iron deficiency, hypersensitivity to iron dextran or its components

Adverse Reactions

CNS: Chills, disorientation, dizziness, fever, headache, malaise, paresthesia, **seizures**, syncope, unconsciousness, weakness
CV: Arrhythmias, **bradycardia**, chest pain, hypertension, **hypotension**, **shock**, tachycardia
EENT: Altered taste
GI: Abdominal pain, diarrhea, nausea, vomiting
GU: Hematuria
HEME: Leukocytosis
MS: Arthralgia, arthritis, backache, myalgia, **rhabdomyolysis**
RESP: Bronchospasm, **cyanosis**, dyspnea, **respiratory arrest**, wheezing
SKIN: Diaphoresis, rash, pruritus, purpura, urticaria
Other: Anaphylaxis, infusion-site phlebitis

Nursing Considerations

- Be aware that iron dextran is given only when oral therapy isn't feasible.
- Expect to monitor hematocrit, hemoglobin level, serum ferritin level, and transferrin saturation, as ordered, before, during, and after iron dextran therapy.

WARNING Expect with first dose to administer a test dose as prescribed, and monitor patient closely for anaphylactic reaction. Expect to wait 1 or more hours before giving remainder of dose if no reaction occurs.

- Infuse undiluted iron dextran slowly, at no more than 1 ml/minute (50 mg/minute).
- Change needle after drawing up iron dextron into syringe if giving by intramuscular injection. Administer intramuscular injection using Z-track method. Inject deep into the upper outer quadrant of the patient's buttock. Do not inject drug into any other site. Use a 2- to 3-inch, 19G or 20G needle.

WARNING Monitor patient closely for signs and symptoms of anaphylaxis (such as collapse, dyspnea, loss of consciousness, seizures, and severe hypotension) during and after drug administration. Patients with a history of allergies or asthma are at increased risk for anaphylaxis, possibly death. Institute emergency resuscitation measures as needed, including epinephrine administration, as prescribed.

WARNING Assess blood pressure often after iron dextran administration, especially if given intravenously, because hypotension is a common adverse effect that may be related to infusion rate; avoid rapid infusion.

- Be aware that patient may have adverse reactions, including arthralgia, backache, chills, and vomiting, 1 to 2 days after drug therapy. Symptoms should resolve within 3 to 4 days.
- Assess patients with a history of rheumatoid arthritis for exacerbation of joint pain and swelling.
- Know that if patient has cardiovascular disease, watch for worsening from drug's adverse effects.
- Assess patient for iron overload, characterized by bleeding in GI tract and lungs, decreased activity, pale eyes, and sedation.
- Store iron dextran at 15° to 30° C (59° to 86° F).

PATIENT TEACHING

- Instruct patient to report immediately signs of adverse reaction, such as rash, shortness of breath, or wheezing, during iron dextran therapy.
- Advise patient not to take any oral iron without first consulting prescriber.
- Urge patient to plan periods of activity and rest to avoid excessive fatigue.
- Emphasize need to follow dosage regimen and keep follow-up medical and laboratory appointments.

iron sucrose

(contains 100 mg of elemental iron per 5 ml)
Venofer

Class and Category

Pharmacologic class: Iron mineral
Therapeutic class: Hematinic
Pregnancy category: B

Indications and Dosages

➤ *To treat iron deficiency anemia in patients with hemodialysis dependent-chronic kidney disease*

I.V. INJECTION

Adults. *Initial:* 100 mg elemental iron injected undiluted over 2 to 5 min during dialysis. *Usual:* 100 mg elemental iron every wk to 3 times/wk to total dose of 1,000 mg. Dosage repeated as needed to maintain target levels of hemoglobin and hematocrit and acceptable blood iron level. *Maximum:* 100 mg/dose.

I.V. INFUSION

Adults. *Initial:* 100 mg elemental iron infused diluted over 15 min during dialysis. *Usual:* 100 mg elemental iron every wk to 3 times/wk to a total dose of 1,000 mg. Dosage repeated as needed to maintain target levels of hemoglobin and hematocrit and acceptable blood iron level. *Maximum:* 100 mg/dose.

➤ *To treat iron-deficiency anemia patients with peritoneal dialysis dependent-chronic kidney disease*

I.V. INFUSION

Adults. *Initial:* 300 mg elemental iron infused diluted over 1.5 hr on days 1 and 14, followed by 400 mg elemental iron infused over 2.5 hr on day 28. Dosage repeated as needed to maintain target levels of hemoglobin and hematocrit and acceptable blood iron level. *Maximum:* 1,000 mg/28 days.

➤ *To maintain iron therapy in children with chronic kidney disease who are nondialysis-dependent receiving erythropoietin or who are peritoneal–dialysis-dependent receiving erythropoietin; to maintain iron therapy in children with hemodialysis dependent-chronic kidney disease (HDD-CKD)*

I.V. INJECTION

Children age 2 years and over. 0.5 mg/kg, not to exceed 100 mg/dose, every 2 wk (HDD-CKD) or 4 wk (other indications) for 12 wk given undiluted over 5 min. Treatment repeated, as needed.

I.V. INFUSION

Children age 2 years and over. 0.5 mg/kg, not to exceed 100 mg/dose, every 2 wk (HDD-CKD) or 4 wk (other indications) for 12 wk diluted in 25 ml of 0.9% NaCl and given over 5 to 60 min. Treatment repeated, as needed.

➤ *To treat iron deficiency anemia in nondialysis patients with chronic renal disease.*

I.V. INJECTION

Adults. *Initial:* 200 mg elemental iron injected undiluted over 2 to 5 min and repeated 4 more times over a 14-day period for a total dose of 1,000 mg. Dosage repeated as needed to maintain target levels of hemoglobin and hematocrit and acceptable blood iron level. *Maximum:* 1,000 mg/14 days.

I.V. INFUSION

Adults. 500 mg elemental iron infused diluted over 3.5 to 5 hr on days 1 and 14. Dosage repeated as needed to maintain target levels of hemoglobin and hematocrit and acceptable blood iron level. *Maximum:* 1,000 mg/14 days.

Mechanism of Action

Acts to replenish iron stores lost during dialysis because of increased erythropoiesis and insufficient absorption of iron from GI tract. Iron is an essential component of hemoglobin, myoglobin, and several enzymes, including catalase, cytochromes, and peroxidase, and is needed for catecholamine metabolism and normal neutrophil function. Iron sucrose injection also normalizes RBC production by binding with hemoglobin or being stored as ferritin in reticuloendothelial cells of the bone marrow, liver, or spleen.

Incompatibilities
Don't mix with other drugs or parenteral nutrition solutions for I.V. infusion.

Contraindications
Anemia other than iron deficiency, hypersensitivity to iron salts or their components, iron overload

Interactions
DRUGS

chloramphenicol: Possibly decreased effectiveness of iron sucrose
oral iron preparations: Possibly reduced absorption of oral iron supplements

Adverse Reactions
CNS: Asthenia, **collapse**, confusion, dizziness, fatigue, fever, headache, hypoesthesia, light-headedness, loss of consciousness, malaise, **seizures**
CV: Bradycardia, chest pain, edema, **heart failure**, hypertension, **hypotension**, peripheral edema, **shock**
EENT: Conjunctivitis, ear pain, nasal congestion, nasopharyngitis, rhinitis, sinusitis, taste perversion
ENDO: Hyperglycemia, **hypoglycemia**
GI: Abdominal pain, constipation, diarrhea, elevated liver enzymes, nausea, occult-positive feces, peritoneal infection, vomiting
GU: Chromaturia, UTI
MS: Arthralgia, arthritis, back pain, joint swelling, leg cramps, muscle pain or weakness, myalgia
RESP: Bronchospasm, cough, dyspnea, pneumonia, upper respiratory tract infection
SKIN: Hyperhidrosis, pruritus, rash
Other: Anaphylaxis; **angioedema**; **iron overload**; gout; infusion or injection-site burning, pain, redness, or skin discoloration (with extravasation); **sepsis**

Nursing Considerations
- Reconstitute iron sucrose injection for infusion, by diluting 100 mg elemental iron in maximum of 100 ml normal saline solution (for hemodialysis patients) or 250 ml (for nondialysis and peritoneal dialysis patients) immediately before infusion. Discard any unused diluted solution.
- Give drug directly into dialysis line by slow I.V. injection or by infusion.

WARNING Monitor patient closely for evidence of anaphylaxis, such as collapse, dyspnea, loss of consciousness, seizures, or severe hypotension during and for at least 30 minutes after therapy. Institute emergency resuscitation measures as needed.

WARNING Assess blood pressure often after drug administration because hypotension is a common adverse reaction that may be related to infusion rate (avoid rapid infusion) or total cumulative dose.

- Expect to monitor hematocrit, hemoglobin, serum ferritin, and transferrin saturation, as ordered, before, during, and after iron sucrose therapy. Test serum iron level 48 hours after last dose, as ordered. Notify prescriber and expect to stop therapy if blood iron levels are normal or elevated, to prevent iron toxicity.
- Watch for evidence of iron overload, such as bleeding in GI tract and lungs, decreased activity, pale eyes, and sedation.

PATIENT TEACHING

- Tell patient to inform prescriber if she has a prior history of reactions to parenteral iron products before drug is given.
- Inform patient that symptoms of iron deficiency may include decreased stamina, fatigue, learning problems, and shortness of breath.
- Instruct patient to report any of the following signs and symptoms of an allergic reaction that may develop during and following the infusion of iron sucrose: breathing problems, dizziness, itching, light-headedness, rash, and swelling.
- Tell mothers who are breastfeeding while receiving iron sucrose to monitor their infant for constipation or diarrhea. If present, pediatrician should be notified, as this may indicate gastrointestinal toxicity.

isocarboxazid
Marplan

Class and Category
Pharmacologic class: Monoamine oxidase inhibitor (MAOI)

Therapeutic class: Antidepressant
Pregnancy category: C

Indications and Dosages

➤ *To treat major depression*

TABLETS

Adults and adolescents over age 16. *Initial:* 10 mg twice daily, increased by 10 mg daily every 2 to 4 days, as needed and tolerated to achieve a daily dose of 40 mg by end of first week with further increases in increments up to 20 mg weekly, as needed. *Maximum:* 60 mg daily.

Route	Onset	Peak	Duration
P.O.	7–10 days	Unknown	10 days

Mechanism of Action

Irreversibly binds to MAO, reducing its activity and increasing levels of neurotransmitters, including serotonin and the catecholamine neurotransmitters dopamine, epinephrine, and norepinephrine. This regulation of CNS neurotransmitters helps to ease depression. With long-term use, drug results in down-regulation (desensitization) of $alpha_2$- or beta-adrenergic and serotonin receptors after 2 to 4 weeks, which also produces an antidepressant effect.

Contraindications

Cardiovascular disease; cerebrovascular disease; heart failure; hepatic disease; history of headaches; hypersensitivity to isocarboxazid or its components; hypertension; pheochromocytoma; severe renal impairment; use of anesthetics, antihypertensives, bupropion, buspirone, carbamazepine, CNS depressants, cyclobenzaprine, dextromethorphan, meperidine, selective serotonin reuptake inhibitors, sympathomimetics, or tricyclic antidepressants; use within 14 days of another MAO inhibitor

Interactions

DRUGS

anticholinergics, antidyskinetics, antihistamines: Increased anticholinergic effect, prolonged CNS depression (with antihistamines)
anticonvulsants: Increased CNS depression, possibly altered seizure pattern
antihypertensives, diuretics: Increased hypotensive effect
bromocriptine: Possibly interference with bromocriptine effects
bupropion: Increased risk of bupropion toxicity
buspirone, guanadrel, guanethidine: Increased risk of hypertension
caffeine-containing drugs: Increased risk of dangerous arrhythmias and severe hypertension
carbamazepine, cyclobenzaprine, maprotiline, other MAO inhibitors: Increased risk of hyperpyretic crisis, hypertensive crisis, severe seizures, and death; altered pattern of seizures (with carbamazepine)
CNS depressants: Increased CNS depression
dextromethorphan: Increased risk of excitation, hyperpyrexia, and hypertension
doxapram: Increased vasopressor effects of either drug
fluoxetine, paroxetine, sertraline, trazodone, tricyclic antidepressants: Increased risk of life-threatening serotonin syndrome
haloperidol, loxapine, molindone, phenothiazines, pimozide, thioxanthenes: Prolonged and intensified anticholinergic, hypotensive, and sedative effects
insulin, oral antidiabetic drugs: Increased hypoglycemic effects
levodopa: Increased risk of sudden, moderate to severe hypertension
local anesthetics (with epinephrine or levonordefrin): Possibly severe hypertension
meperidine, other opioid analgesics: Increased risk of coma, hyperpyrexia, hypotension, immediate excitation, rigidity, seizures, severe hypertension, severe respiratory depression, shock, sweating, and death
methyldopa: Increased risk of hallucinations, headache, hyperexcitability, and severe hypertension
methylphenidate: Increased CNS stimulation
metrizamide: Decreased seizure threshold and increased risk of seizures
oral anticoagulants: Increased anticoagulant activity
phenylephrine (nasal or ophthalmic): Potentiated vasopressor effect of phenylephrine

Rauwolfia alkaloids: Increased risk of moderate to severe hypertension, CNS depression (when isocarboxazid is added to Rauwolfia alkaloid therapy), CNS excitation and hypertension (when Rauwolfia alkaloid is added to isocarboxazid therapy)
spinal anesthetics: Increased risk of hypotension
sympathomimetics: Prolonged and intensified cardiac stimulant and vasopressor effects
tryptophan: Increased risk of confusion, disorientation, hyperreflexia, hyperthermia, hyperventilation, mania or hypomania, and shivering

FOODS

aged cheese; avocados; bananas; fava or broad beans; cured meat or sausage; overripe fruit; pickled or smoked fish, meats or poultry; protein extract; soy sauce; yeast extract; and other foods high in tyramine or other pressor amines: Increased risk of dangerous arrhythmias and severe hypertensive crisis

ACTIVITIES

alcohol-containing products that also may contain tyramine, such as beer (including reduced-alcohol and alcohol-free beer), hard liquor, liqueurs, sherry, and wines (red and white): Increased risk of developing hypertensive crisis

Adverse Reactions

CNS: Agitation, dizziness, drowsiness, fever, headache, insomnia, **intracranial bleeding**, overstimulation, restlessness, sedation, **suicidal ideation**, tremor, weakness
CV: Bradycardia, chest pain, edema, **hypertensive crisis**, orthostatic hypotension, palpitations, tachycardia
EENT: Blurred vision, dry mouth, mydriasis, photophobia, yellowing of sclera
GI: Abdominal pain, anorexia, constipation, diarrhea, elevated liver enzymes, increased appetite, jaundice, nausea
GU: Dark urine, oliguria, sexual dysfunction
HEME: Leukopenia
MS: Muscle spasms, myoclonus, neck stiffness
SKIN: Clammy skin, diaphoresis, rash
Other: Unusual weight gain

Nursing Considerations

- Monitor patient's blood pressure during isocarboxazid therapy to detect hypertensive crisis and decrease risk of orthostatic hypotension.

WARNING Notify prescriber immediately if patient has evidence of hypertensive crisis (drug's most serious adverse effect), such as chest pain, headache, neck stiffness, and palpitations. Expect to stop drug immediately if these occur.

- Keep phentolamine readily available to treat hypertensive crisis. Give 5 mg by slow I.V. infusion, as prescribed, to reduce blood pressure without causing excessive hypotension. Use external cooling measures, as prescribed, to manage fever.
- Know that to avoid hypertensive crisis, expect to wait 10 to 14 days when switching patient from one MAO inhibitor to another or when switching from a dibenzazepine-related drug, such as amitriptyline or perphenazine.
- Monitor patient with a history of epilepsy for seizures because isocarboxazid may alter seizure threshold. Institute seizure precautions according to facility protocol.
- Monitor liver enzymes, and assess patient for abdominal pain, dark urine, and jaundice because isocarboxazid may cause hepatic dysfunction.
- Expect to observe some therapeutic effect in 7 to 10 days, but keep in mind that full effect may not occur for 4 to 8 weeks.
- Be aware that, for maintenance therapy, the smallest possible dose should be used. Once clinical effect has been achieved, expect to decrease the dosage slowly over several weeks.
- Keep dietary restrictions in place for at least 2 weeks after stopping isocarboxazid because of slow recovery from drug's enzyme-inhibiting effects.
- Ideally, expect to stop drug 10 days before elective surgery, as prescribed, to avoid hypotension.
- Anticipate that coadministration with a selective serotonin reuptake inhibitor may cause confusion, diaphoresis, diarrhea, seizures, and other less severe symptoms.
- Monitor depressed patient for suicidal tendencies, especially when therapy starts or dosage changes, because depression

may worsen temporarily. If suicidal tendencies arise, institute suicide precautions, as appropriate and according to facility policy, and notify prescriber immediately.
- Monitor patient for sudden insomnia. If it develops, notify prescriber and be prepared to give drug early in the day.

PATIENT TEACHING
- Inform patient and family members that therapeutic effects of isocarboxazid may take several weeks to appear and that he should continue taking drug as prescribed.
- Caution caregivers to monitor patients, closely for suicidal tendencies, especially when therapy starts or dosage changes.
- Caution patient to rise slowly from a lying or sitting position to minimize effects of orthostatic hypotension.

WARNING Instruct patient to avoid the following foods, beverages, and drugs during isocarboxazid therapy and for 2 weeks afterward: alcohol-free and reduced-alcohol beer and wine; appetite suppressants; beer; broad beans; cheese (except cottage and cream cheese); chocolate and caffeine in large quantities; dry sausage (including Genoa salami, hard salami, Lebanon bologna, and pepperoni); hay fever drugs; inhaled asthma drugs; liver; meat extract; OTC cold and cough medicines (including those containing dextromethorphan); nasal decongestants (drops, tablets, or spray); pickled herring; products that contain tyramine; protein-rich foods that may have undergone protein changes by aging, fermenting, pickling, or smoking; sauerkraut; sinus drugs; weight-loss products; yeast extracts (including brewer's yeast in large quantities); yogurt; and wine.
- Advise patient to notify prescriber immediately about chest pain, dizziness, headache, nausea, neck stiffness, palpitations, rapid heart rate, sweating, and vomiting.
- Advise patient to inform all healthcare providers (including dentists) that he takes an MAO inhibitor because certain drugs are contraindicated within 2 weeks of it.
- Urge patient to avoid hazardous activities until drug's adverse effects are known.
- Urge patient with diabetes mellitus who's taking insulin or an oral antidiabetic to check blood glucose level often during therapy because isocarboxazid may affect glucose control.
- Caution patient not to stop taking drug abruptly to avoid recurrence of original symptoms.

isoniazid
(isonicotinic acid hydrazide, INH)

Isotamine (CAN)

Class and Category
Pharmacologic class: Isonicotinic acid derivatives
Therapeutic class: **Antitubercular agent**
Pregnancy category: C

Indications and Dosages
➤ *To prevent tuberculosis*

SYRUP, TABLETS

Adults. 300 mg daily for 6 to 12 mo.
Children. 10 mg/kg daily (up to 300 mg) for up to 1 yr.

➤ *As adjunct to treat active tuberculosis*

SYRUP, TABLETS I.M. INJECTION

Adults. 5 mg/kg up to 300 mg daily or 15 mg/kg (up to 900 mg) 2 or 3 times/wk, based on treatment regimen.
Children. 10 to 20 mg/kg (up to 300 mg) daily or 20 to 40 mg/kg (up to 900 mg) 2 or 3 times/wk, based on treatment regimen.

Mechanism of Action
Interferes with lipid and nucleic acid synthesis in actively growing tubercule bacilli cells. Isoniazid also disrupts bacterial cell wall synthesis and may interfere with mycolic acid synthesis in mycobacterial cells.

Contraindications
History of severe adverse reactions (acute liver disease of any etiology, including drug-induced hepatitis, arthritis, chills, drug fever); hypersensitivity to isoniazid or its components

Interactions
DRUGS

acetaminophen: Increased risk of hepatotoxicity and possibly nephrotoxicity

alfentanil: Decreased alfentanil clearance and increased duration of effects
aluminum-containing antacids: Decreased isoniazid absorption
benzodiazepines: Decreased benzodiazepine clearance
carbamazepine: Increased blood carbamazepine level and toxicity, increased risk of isoniazid toxicity
corticosteroids: Decreased isoniazid effects
cycloserine: Increased risk of adverse CNS effects and CNS toxicity
disulfiram: Changes in behavior and coordination
enflurane: Increased risk of high-output renal failure
halothane: Increased risk of hepatotoxicity and hepatic encephalopathy
hepatotoxic drugs, rifampin: Increased risk of hepatotoxicity
ketoconazole: Possibly decreased blood ketoconazole level and resistance to antifungal treatment
meperidine: Risk of hypotensive episodes or CNS depression
nephrotoxic drugs: Increased risk of nephrotoxicity
oral anticoagulants: Increased anticoagulation
phenytoin: Increased blood phenytoin level, increased risk of phenytoin toxicity
theophylline: Increased theophylline level

FOODS

histamine-containing foods, such as tuna, skipjack, and other tropical fish: Inhibited action of the enzyme diamine oxidase in foods, possibly resulting in flushing, headache, hypotension, palpitations and sweating.
tyramine-containing foods, such as cheese and fish: Increased response to tyramine in foods, possibly resulting in chills; diaphoresis; headache; light-headedness; and red, itchy, clammy skin

ACTIVITIES

alcohol use: Increased risk of hepatotoxicity and increased isoniazid metabolism

Adverse Reactions

CNS: Clumsiness, confusion, dizziness, **encephalopathy**, fatigue, fever, hallucinations, **neurotoxicity**, paresthesia, peripheral neuritis, psychosis, **seizures**, weakness
CV: Vasculitis
EENT: Optic neuritis
ENDO: Gynecomastia, hyperglycemia
GI: Abdominal pain, anorexia, elevated liver enzymes, epigastric distress, **hepatitis**, jaundice, nausea, **pancreatitis**, vomiting
GU: Glycosuria
HEME: Agranulocytosis, **aplastic anemia**, eosinophilia, **hemolytic anemia**, sideroblastic anemia, **thrombocytopenia**
MS: Arthralgia, joint stiffness
SKIN: Pruritus, rash, **Stevens–Johnson syndrome**, **toxic epidermal necrolysis**
Other: Anaphylaxis, **hypocalcemia**, **drug reaction with eosinophilia and systemic symptoms (DRESS)**, hypophosphatemia, injection-site irritation, lupus-like symptoms, lymphadenopathy

Nursing Considerations

- Administer isoniazid cautiously to alcoholic, diabetic, or malnourished patients and those at risk for peripheral neuritis.
- Give oral drug 1 hour before or 2 hours after meals to promote absorption. If GI distress occurs, give drug with a small amount of food or an antacid that doesn't contain aluminum 1 hour before or 2 hours after meal.
- Monitor liver enzyme studies, which may be ordered monthly, because isoniazid can cause severe (possibly fatal) hepatitis.
- Know that about 50% of patients metabolize isoniazid slowly, which may lead to increased toxic effects. Watch for adverse reactions, such as peripheral neuritis; if they occur, expect to decrease dosage.
- Give isoniazid with other antituberculotic drugs, as prescribed, to prevent development of resistant organisms.
- Be aware that patients with advanced HIV infection may experience more severe adverse reactions in greater numbers.

PATIENT TEACHING

- Instruct patient to take isoniazid exactly as prescribed and not to stop without first consulting prescriber. Explain that treatment may take months or years.
- Direct patient to take drug on an empty stomach 1 hour before or 2 hours after meals. If GI distress occurs, instruct him to take drug with food or an antacid that doesn't contain aluminum.

- Advise patient to report signs of hepatic dysfunction, including dark urine, decreased appetite, fatigue, and jaundice.
- Caution patient not to drink alcohol while taking isoniazid because alcohol increases the risk of hepatotoxicity.
- Give patient a list of tyramine-containing foods to avoid when taking isoniazid, such as cheese, fish, red wine, salami, and yeast extracts. Explain that consuming these foods during isoniazid therapy may cause unpleasant adverse reactions, such as chills, pounding heartbeat, and sweating.
- Tell patient to avoid histamine-containing foods such as tuna, skipjack, and other tropical fish during therapy to avoid such adverse reactions as flushing, headache, low blood pressure, rapid heartbeat and sweating.
- Tell patient that he'll need periodic laboratory tests and physical examinations.
- Urge patient to report fever, nausea, numbness and tingling in arms and legs, rash, vision changes, vomiting, and yellowing skin.

isoproterenol hydrochloride

Isuprel

Class and Category

Pharmacologic class: Sympathomimetic
Therapeutic class: Antiarrhythmic, bronchodilator
Pregnancy category: B (inhalation), C (I.V. infusion)

Indications and Dosages

➤ *To manage bronchospasm during anesthesia*

I.V. INJECTION

Adults. 0.01 to 0.02 mg, repeated as needed.

➤ *To treat hypoperfusion states and shock*

I.V. INFUSION

Adults. 0.5 mcg to 5 mcg/min.

➤ *To treat Adams–Stokes attacks, cardiac arrest, or heart block*

I.V. INFUSION

Adults. *Initial:* 5 mcg/min.

Route	Onset	Peak	Duration
I.V.*	Unknown	Unknown	1–2 hr
I.V.†	In 5 min	Unknown	10 min

* For treatment of bronchospasm.
† For treatment of bradycardia.

Mechanism of Action

Stimulates $beta_1$ receptors in the cardiac and myocardium conduction system, resulting in positive chronotropic and inotropic effects. Isoproterenol also shortens AV conduction time and refractory period in patients with AV block. This action increases ventricular rate and halts bradycardia and associated syncope.

In addition, isoproterenol attaches to $beta_2$ receptors on bronchial cell membranes. This action stimulates the intracellular enzyme adenylate cyclase to convert adenosine triphosphate to cyclic adenosine monophosphate (cAMP). An increased intracellular cAMP level inhibits histamine release, relaxes bronchial smooth-muscle cells, and stabilizes mast cells.

Contraindications

Angina pectoris, heart block or tachycardia from digitalis toxicity; hypersensitivity to isoproterenol or its components, tachyarrhythmias, including ventricular arrhythmias that require inotropic therapy

Interactions

DRUGS

alpha blockers, other drugs with this action: Possibly decreased peripheral vasoconstricting and hypertensive effects of isoproterenol
anesthetics (hydrocarbon inhalation): Increased risk of atrial and ventricular arrhythmias
astemizole, cisapride, drugs that prolong QTc interval, terfenadine: Possibly prolonged QTc interval
beta blockers (ophthalmic): Decreased effects of isoproterenol, increased risk of bronchospasm, decreased pulmonary function, respiratory failure, and wheezing
beta blockers (systemic): Increased risk of bronchospasm, decreased effects of both drugs

G H I

digoxin: Increased risk of arrhythmias, digitalis toxicity, and hypokalemia
diuretics, other antihypertensives: Possibly decreased antihypertensive effects
ergot alkaloids: Increased vasoconstriction and vasopressor effects
MAO inhibitors: Intensified and extended cardiac stimulation and vasopressor effects
quinidine, other drugs that affect myocardial reaction to sympathomimetics: Increased risk of arrhythmias
theophylline: Increased risk of cardiotoxicity, decreased blood theophylline level
thyroid hormones: Increased effects of both drugs, increased risk of coronary insufficiency in patients with coronary artery disease
tricyclic antidepressants: Increased vasopressor response, increased risk of arrhythmias and prolonged QTc interval

Adverse Reactions

CNS: Dizziness, headache, insomnia, nervousness, syncope, tremor, weakness
CV: Angina, **arrhythmias**, **bradycardia**, hypertension, **hypotension**, palpitations, tachycardia, **ventricular arrhythmias**
EENT: Dry mouth, **oropharyngeal edema**, taste perversion
ENDO: Hyperglycemia
GI: Heartburn, nausea, vomiting
MS: Muscle spasms and twitching
RESP: Bronchitis, **bronchospasm**, cough, dyspnea, increased sputum production, **pulmonary edema**, wheezing
SKIN: Dermatitis, diaphoresis, **erythema multiforme**, flushing, pallor, pruritus, rash, **Stevens–Johnson syndrome**, urticaria
Other: **Angioedema**, **hypokalemia**

Nursing Considerations

- Expect to give lowest possible dose of isoproterenol for shortest possible time to minimize tolerance.
- Don't administer I.V. isoproterenol if solution is pink or brown or contains precipitate.
- Administer isoproterenol infusion through a large vein, and monitor patient for signs of extravasation.
- Monitor blood pressure, cardiac rhythm, central venous pressure, and urine output when giving I.V. drug. Adjust infusion rate to response, as ordered.
- Notify prescriber immediately if heart rate increases significantly or exceeds 110 beats/minute during I.V. infusion.
- Know that drug may increase pulse pressure and cause hypotension. Expect to reduce I.V. infusion slowly to decrease risk of hypotension.

WARNING Be aware that drug markedly increases risk of arrhythmias. If an arrhythmia develops, expect to give a cardioselective beta blocker, such as atenolol.

WARNING Know that if drug aggravates a ventilation-perfusion problem, expect blood oxygen level to fall even as breathing seems to improve.

PATIENT TEACHING

- Instruct patient to notify medical staff immediately about chest pain, dizziness, hyperglycemic symptoms (such as abdominal cramps, lethargy, nausea, and vomiting), insomnia, irregular heartbeat, palpitations, tremor, and weakness.

isosorbide dinitrate

Dilatrate-SR, ISDM (CAN), Isordil

isosorbide mononitrate

Apo-ISMN (CAN), Monoket

Class and Category

Pharmacologic class: Nitrate
Therapeutic class: Antianginal
Pregnancy category: C

Indications and Dosages

➤ *To prevent angina*

E.R. CAPSULES

Adults. *Initial:* 40 mg (dinitrate), increased as needed with nitrate free 14 hr interval daily. *Maximum:* 160 mg daily.

E.R. TABLETS

Adults. *Initial:* 5 to 20 mg two to three times daily with nitrate free 14 hr interval daily (dinitrate); 30 to 60 mg daily, increased gradually no less than every 3 days as tolerated to 240 mg daily (mononitrate).

Mechanism of Action

Isosorbide may interact with nitrate receptors in vascular smooth-muscle cell membranes. By interacting with receptors' sulfhydryl groups, drug is reduced to nitric oxide. Nitric oxide activates the enzyme guanylate cyclase, increasing intracellular formation of cyclic guanosine monophosphate (cGMP). An increased cGMP level may relax vascular smooth muscle by forcing calcium out of muscle cells, causing vasodilation. This improves cardiac output by reducing mainly preload but also afterload.

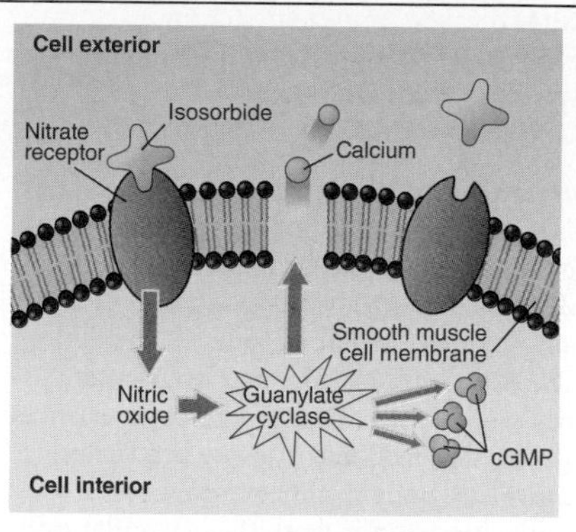

S.L. TABLETS

Adults. 2.5 to 5 mg as needed about 15 min before any activity that could cause an anginal attack (dinitrate).

TABLETS

Adults. 5 to 40 mg two or three times daily with nitrate free 14 hr interval daily. (dinitrate); 20 mg in 2 doses given 7 hr apart (mononitrate).

➤ *To treat acute angina attack*

S.L. TABLETS

Adults. 2.5 to 5 mg, repeated every 5 to 10 min, as needed, for no more than 3 doses in a 15 to 30 min period.

Route	Onset	Peak	Duration
P.O.*	1 hr†	Unknown	5–6 hr
P.O. (E.R.)*	30 min	Unknown	6–8 hr
P.O. (S.L.)*	In 3 min	Unknown	2 hr

* For dinitrate.

† For mononitrate, onset also is 1 hr; peak and duration are unknown.

Contraindications

Angle-closure glaucoma; cerebral hemorrhage; concurrent use of phosphodiesterase inhibitors (sildenafil, tadalafil, vardenafil) or riociguat; head trauma; hypersensitivity to isosorbide, other nitrates, or their components; orthostatic hypotension; severe anemia

Interactions

DRUGS

acetylcholine, norepinephrine: Possibly decreased effectiveness of these drugs
antihypertensives, calcium channel blockers, opioid analgesics, other vasodilators: Increased risk of orthostatic hypotension
aspirin: Increased blood level and pharmacologic action of isosorbide
other vasodilators: Additive effects
phosphodiesterase inhibitors such as sildenafil, tadalafil, vardenafil: Increased risk of hypotension, myocardial ischemia, syncope, and possibly death
riociguat: Increased risk of hypotension
sympathomimetics: Increased risk of hypotension, possibly decreased therapeutic effects of isosorbide

ACTIVITIES

alcohol use: Increased risk of orthostatic hypotension

Adverse Reactions

CNS: Agitation, confusion, dizziness, headache, insomnia, restlessness, syncope, vertigo, weakness
CV: Arrhythmias, orthostatic hypotension, palpitations, peripheral edema, tachycardia
EENT: Blurred vision, diplopia (all forms); sublingual burning (S.L. form)
GI: Abdominal pain, diarrhea, indigestion, nausea, vomiting
GU: Dysuria, impotence, urinary frequency
HEME: Hemolytic anemia

MS: Arthralgia, muscle twitching
RESP: Bronchitis, pneumonia, upper respiratory tract infection
SKIN: Diaphoresis, flushing, rash

Nursing Considerations

- Use isosorbide cautiously in patients with hypovolemia or mild hypotension. Monitor patient for increased hypotension and reduced cardiac output.
- Give drug 1 hour before or 2 hours after meals. Give with meals if patient experiences adverse GI reactions or severe headaches.
- Know that patient may experience daily headaches from isosorbide's vasodilating effects. Give acetaminophen, as prescribed, to relieve pain.

WARNING Be aware that stopping drug abruptly may cause angina and increase the risk of MI.

- Monitor blood pressure often during isosorbide therapy, especially in elderly patients; drug may cause severe hypotension.
- Keep isosorbide protected from heat and light.

PATIENT TEACHING

- Teach patient and family to recognize signs and symptoms of angina, including chest pain, fullness, or pressure, which commonly is accompanied by nausea and sweating. Pain may radiate down the left arm or into the neck or jaw. Inform female patients and those with diabetes mellitus or hypertension that they may experience only fatigue and shortness of breath.
- Caution patient not to crush or chew isosorbide E.R. capsules or tablets or S.L. tablets unless specifically ordered to do so by prescriber.
- Instruct patient to place S.L. tablet under tongue and not to swallow it, but to let it dissolve. Explain that moisture in mouth promotes drug absorption and that burning or tingling in the mouth indicates drug effectiveness.
- Advise patient to carry S.L. isosorbide with him at all times, if prescribed.
- Caution patient that abrupt drug discontinuation may cause angina and increase the risk of MI.
- Instruct patient to notify prescriber about blurred vision, fainting, increased angina attacks, rash, and severe or persistent headaches.
- Teach patient to reduce the effects of orthostatic hypotension by changing position slowly. Advise him to lie down if he becomes dizzy.
- Inform patient that drug commonly causes headache, which typically resolves after a few days of continuous therapy. Suggest that patient take acetaminophen as needed and as prescribed.
- Advise patient to avoid potentially hazardous activities until drug's CNS effects are known.
- Urge patient to avoid alcohol consumption.
- Instruct patient to store drug in a tightly closed container and protect from heat and light.
- Advise male patient with erectile dysfunction to alert prescriber that he is taking isosorbide because sildenafil, tadalafil, and vardenafil can cause fatal reactions when taken with isosorbide.

isotretinoin

Absorica, Amnesteem, Claravis, Myorisan, Zenatane

Class and Category

Pharmacologic class: Retinoid
Therapeutic class: Acne inhibitor
Pregnancy category: X

Indications and Dosages

➤ *To treat severe recalcitrant nodular acne unresponsive to conventional therapy*

CAPSULES

Adults. *Initial:* 0.5 mg to 1 mg/kg daily in 2 divided doses, increased as needed up to 2 mg/kg daily given in 2 divided doses. *Maximum:* 2 mg/kg daily. Course of therapy given for 15 to 20 wk with second course given, as needed, after a period of 2 mo or more off therapy.

Mechanism of Action

Inhibits sebaceous gland function and keratinization, which results in diminished nodular formation associated with recalcitrant nodular acne.

Contraindications

Hypersensitivity to isotretinoin or any of its components, hypersensitivity to parabens, pregnancy

Interactions

DRUGS

corticosteroids (systemic): Possibly increased risk of osteoporosis
hormonal contraceptives including levonorgestrel implants medroxyprogesterone injection, microdosed progesterone preparations: Possibly decreased effectiveness of contraceptive
phenytoin: Possibly increased risk of osteomalacia
tetracyclines: Increased risk of benign intracranial hypertension
vitamin A supplements: Increased risk of additive toxic effects

Adverse Reactions

CNS: Aggressive or violent behavior, **violent behavior**, **CVA**, depression, dizziness, drowsiness, emotional instability, fatigue, headache, insomnia, lethargy, malaise, nervousness, paresthesias, **pseudotumor cerebri**, psychosis, **seizures**, **suicidal ideation**, syncope, weakness
CV: Chest pain, decreased high-density lipoprotein level, edema, elevated creatinine phosphokinase level, hypercholesteremia, hypertriglyceridemia, palpitation, tachycardia, **vascular thrombotic disease**, vasculitis
ENDO: Abnormal menses, hyperglycemia, **hypoglycemia**
EENT: Bleeding and inflammation of gums, cataracts, color vision disorder, conjunctivitis, corneal opacities, decreased night vision, dry eyes, dry mouth or nose, epistaxis, eyelid inflammation, hearing impairment, keratitis, optic neuritis, photophobia, tinnitus, visual disturbances, voice alteration
GI: Colitis, **hepatitis**, ileitis, inflammatory bowel disease, elevated liver enzymes, nausea, **pancreatitis**
GU: Glomerulonephritis, hematuria, proteinuria, WBCs in urine
HEME: Anemia, **agranulocytosis**, **neutropenia**, sedimentation rate elevation, **thrombocytopenia**, thrombocytosis
MS: Arthralgia, arthritis, bone abnormalities, calcification of ligaments and tendons, premature epiphyseal closure, tendonitis
RESP: **Bronchospasms**, respiratory infection
SKIN: Alopecia, bruising, diaphoresis, disseminated herpes simplex, dry lips or skin, eczema, eruptive xanthomas, **erythema multiforme**, facial erythema, flushing, fulminant acne, hair abnormalities, hirsutism, hyperpigmentation, hypopigmentation, increased sunburn susceptibility, infections, nail dystrophy, paronychia, peeling of palms and soles, photoallergic or photosensitizing reactions, pruritus, pyogenic granuloma, rash, seborrhea, skin fragility, **Stevens–Johnson syndrome**, **toxic epidermal necrolysis**, urticaria
Other: Abnormal wound healing, alkaline phosphatase increase, **hypersensitivity reactions**, hyperuricemia, lymphadenopathy, weight loss

Nursing Considerations

- Be aware that drug is only available through a restricted program called iPLEDGE.
- Ensure that women of childbearing age have had two negative serum or urine pregnancy tests with a sensitivity of at least 50 mIU/ml, joined the Accutane Survey, signed the consent form, and watched the videotape provided by manufacturer prior to beginning isotretinoin therapy.

WARNING Notify prescriber if elevated serum triglyceride levels can't be controlled or if symptoms of pancreatitis occur (abdominal pain, nausea, vomiting). Drug may need to be discontinued because fatal hemorrhagic pancreatitis has occurred with drug use.

- Obtain serum lipid level before therapy and periodically thereafter, as ordered, to detect elevated lipid levels that result from isotretinoin therapy.
- Monitor liver enzyme levels periodically, as ordered, because drug can cause hepatitis.
- Assess patient frequently for adverse reactions and report to prescriber any that occur; drug may have serious adverse effects that require discontinuation.

PATIENT TEACHING

- Alert patient that Absorica brand of isotretinoin contains the color additive FD&C Yellow No. 5 (tartrazine), which may cause allergic reactions, especially in patients with an allergy to aspirin or who have asthma.
- Instruct patient to take isotretinoin with food or milk.
- Advise women of childbearing age that two forms of contraceptives must be used simultaneously (unless absolute abstinence is the chosen method) 1 month before therapy and for 1 month after therapy has stopped because of potential for fetal harm. Inform women who use oral contraceptives that drug may lessen effectiveness of oral contraceptives. Urge patient to notify prescriber immediately if pregnancy occurs.
- Emphasize importance of picking up isotretinoin prescription within 7 days of a pregnancy test or, for male patients or women not of childbearing potential, within 30 days of prescription.
- Urge patient to report headache, nausea, vomiting and visual disturbances immediately to prescriber because drug will need to be discontinued immediately and patient referred to a neurologist.
- Caution patient and family that isotretinoin may cause aggressive or violent behavior, depression, psychosis, and suicidal ideation. Instruct patient to notify prescriber immediately if changes in mood occur.
- Tell patient to report, hearing changes or tinnitus; painful or trouble swallowing; rectal bleeding; severe abdominal, bowel, or chest pain; severe diarrhea or skin reactions to prescriber because drug may have to be discontinued.
- Advise patient to avoid hazardous activities until drug's CNS effects are known. Caution that changes in night vision may occur suddenly.
- Caution patient not to donate blood during therapy and for 1 month after therapy has stopped because blood might be given to a pregnant woman.
- Warn patient that transient exacerbation of acne may occur, especially during initial therapy and to notify prescriber if this occurs.
- Instruct patient to avoid wax epilation and skin resurfacing procedures during therapy and for at least 6 months thereafter because of scarring potential.
- Caution patient to avoid exposure to direct sunlight or UV light and to wear sunscreen when outdoors.
- Inform patient that contact lens tolerance may decrease during and after isotretinoin therapy.
- Alert patient to the potential for mild musculoskeletal adverse reactions, which usually clear rapidly after drug is discontinued. Urge patient to notify prescriber if symptoms become bothersome or serious because drug may need to be discontinued.
- Advise patient not to take vitamin A supplements while on isotretinoin therapy because of potentially additive toxic effects.
- Instruct patient to notify all prescribers of isotretinoin use because of the risk of interactions.
- Inform patient of need for frequent laboratory tests and importance of complying with scheduled appointments.

isradipine

DynaCirc

Class and Category

Pharmacologic class: Calcium channel blocker
Therapeutic class: Antihypertensive
Pregnancy category: C

Indications and Dosages

➤ *To manage essential hypertension*

CAPSULES

Adults. *Initial:* 2.5 mg twice daily, increased by 5 mg every 2 to 4 wk, as needed. *Maximum:* 20 mg daily.

Route	Onset	Peak	Duration
P.O.	2–3 hr	2–4 wk	Unknown

Mechanism of Action

Inhibits calcium movement into coronary vascular smooth-muscle cells by blocking the slow calcium channels in their membranes. By decreasing intracellular calcium level, isradipine inhibits smooth-muscle cell contractions. The result is decreased peripheral vascular resistance, reduced diastolic and systolic blood pressure, and relaxation of coronary and vascular smooth muscle, all of which decrease myocardial oxygen demand.

Contraindications

Hypersensitivity to isradipine or its components

Interactions

DRUGS

anesthetics (hydrocarbon inhalation), antihypertensives, hydrochlorothiazide, prazocin: Increased risk of hypotension
beta blockers: Increased adverse effects of beta blockers
cimetidine: Increased blood level and bioavailability of isradipine
digoxin: Transiently increased blood digoxin level and risk of digitalis toxicity
estrogens: Possibly decreased isradipine effectiveness and increased fluid retention
lithium: Increased risk of neurotoxicity
NSAIDs, sympathomimetics: Possibly decreased therapeutic effects of isradipine
procainamide, quinidine: Increased risk of prolonged QT interval

FOODS

grapefruit juice: Doubled isradipine bioavailability
other foods: Prolonged time to achieve peak blood level

Adverse Reactions

CNS: Asthenia, **CVA**, dizziness, fatigue, headache, paresthesia, somnolence, syncope, transient ischemic attack, weakness
CV: Angina, **atrial fibrillation**, **heart failure**, **hypotension**, **MI**, orthostatic hypotension, palpitations, peripheral edema, tachycardia, **ventricular fibrillation**
EENT: Gingival hyperplasia, pharyngitis, rhinitis
GI: Abdominal cramps, constipation, diarrhea, elevated liver enzymes, indigestion, nausea, vomiting
HEME: **Leukopenia**
MS: Back pain
RESP: Cough
SKIN: Flushing, photosensitivity, rash, urticaria
Other: **Angioedema**

Nursing Considerations

- Monitor blood pressure and heart rate often during isradipine therapy.
- Monitor patient with impaired hepatic or renal function for an increased blood isradipine level.
- Avoid giving isradipine with food because doing so increases time to peak effect by about 1 hour.
- Observe for mild peripheral edema caused by vasodilation of small blood vessels. Know that this type of edema doesn't result from fluid retention or heart failure.

PATIENT TEACHING

- Inform patient that isradipine therapy will be long-term and will require laboratory tests and follow-up visits to monitor drug effects.
- Instruct patient to take drug exactly as prescribed and to swallow capsules whole, not chewing or crushing them.
- Advise patient to take drug on an empty stomach 1 hour before or 2 hours after meals.
- Instruct patient to take a missed dose as soon as he remembers it unless it's nearly time for the next dose. In that case, advise him to wait and take next scheduled dose, but not to double the dose. If more than one dose is missed, tell him to contact prescriber.

WARNING Urge patient not to stop taking drug suddenly. Doing so may lead to life-threatening problems.

- Inform patient that fragments of capsules may be visible in stool.
- Caution patient not to drink grapefruit juice during isradipine therapy.
- Urge patient to avoid potentially hazardous activities until isradipine's CNS effects are known.
- Caution patient to change position slowly to minimize orthostatic hypotension.
- Urge patient to contact prescriber if he experiences chest pain, fainting, irregular heartbeat, rash, or swollen ankles while taking isradipine.

- Instruct patient to maintain good oral hygiene, perform gum massage, and see a dentist every 6 months to prevent gum bleeding and gum disorders.
- Caution patient to avoid direct sunlight and to wear protective clothing and apply sunscreen when outdoors.
- Instruct patient to store drug at room temperature in a dry place.

itraconazole

Onmel, Sporanox

Class and Category

Pharmacologic class: Triazole derivative
Therapeutic class: Antifungal
Pregnancy category: Not classified

Indications and Dosages

➤ *To treat blastomycosis caused by* Blastomyces dermatitidis *and histoplasmosis caused by* Histoplasma capsulatum

CAPSULES

Adults and adolescents. *Initial:* 200 mg daily, increased, in 100 mg increments, as needed. *Maximum:* 400 mg daily, with dosage greater than 200 mg given in divided doses twice daily.

➤ *To treat aspergillosis unresponsive to amphotericin B*

CAPSULES

Adults and adolescents. 200 to 400 mg daily, with dosage greater than 200 mg daily given in divided doses twice daily.

➤ *To prevent fungal infections in neutropenic patients*

ORAL SOLUTION

Adults. 5 mg/kg daily divided into 2 doses until recovery of neutrophils for up to 8 wk.

➤ *To treat oropharyngeal candidiasis in HIV-positive or other immunocompromised patients*

ORAL SOLUTION

Adults and adolescents. 200 mg once a day or 100 mg twice daily for 7 to 14 days.

➤ *To treat fluconazole resistant oropharyngeal candidiasis in HIV-positive or other immunocompromised patients*

ORAL SOLUTION

Adults and adolescents. 200 mg daily or 100 mg twice daily for 14 days, increased, if no response, to 400 mg daily for 2 wk.

➤ *To treat onychomycosis of toenails only or of toenails and fingernails in non-immunocompromised patients*

CAPSULES

Adults and adolescents. 200 mg daily for 12 wk.

➤ *To treat onychomycosis of fingernails only in non-immunocompromised patients*

CAPSULES

Adults and adolescents. 200 mg twice daily for 7 days; then repeated after 3 wk.

➤ *To treat onychomycosis of toenails only*

TABLETS (ONMEL)

Adults. 200 mg once daily for 12 wk.

DOSAGE ADJUSTMENT For some immunocompromised patients taking capsule form of drug, dosage may have to be increased because oral bioavailability of capsule form may be decreased.

Mechanism of Action

Inhibits the synthesis of ergosterol, an essential component of fungal cell membranes, by binding with a cytochrome P-450 enzyme needed to convert lanosterol to ergosterol. Lack of ergosterol results in increased cellular permeability and leakage of cell contents. Itraconazole also may lead to fungal cell death by inhibiting fungal respiration under aerobic conditions.

Contraindications

Concurrent therapy with avanafil, cisapride, disopyramide, dofetilide, dronedarone, eplerenone, ergot alkaloids, felodipine, HMG-CoA inhibitors (lovastatin and simvastatin), irinotecan, isavuconazole, ivabradine, levomethadyl, lomitapide, lurasidone, methadone, naloxegol, nisoldipine, oral midazolam, pimozide, quinidine, ranolazine, ticagrelor, or triazolam; concurrent therapy with colchicine, fesoterodine, or solifenacin in patients with hepatic or renal impairment; concurrent therapy with eliglustat in patients who are poor or intermediate metabolizers of CYP2D6 or are taking moderate or strong CYP2D6 inhibitors; evidence of ventricular dysfunction, as in congestive heart failure (CHF) or a history of it (onychomycosis treatment); hepatic or renal impairment; hypersensitivity to itraconazole or its components; pregnancy or contemplating pregnancy during onychomycosis treatment

Interactions

DRUGS

alfentanil, budesonide, buspirone, busulfan, carbamazepine, cyclosporine, dexamethasone, digoxin, docetaxel, felodipine, fluticasone, indinavir, methylprednisolone, phenytoin, pimozide, rifabutin, ritonavir, saquinavir, sirolimus, tacrolimus, trimetrexate, vinca alkaloids: Possibly increased blood levels of these drugs and serious adverse effects

alprazolam, diazepam, oral midazolam, triazolam: Elevated blood levels and possibly prolonged sedative effects of these drugs

antacids, anticholinergics, H_2-receptor antagonists, proton pump inhibitors, sucralfate: Possibly decreased itraconazole absorption

atorvastatin, lovastatin, simvastatin: Increased blood levels of these drugs; possibly rhabdomyolysis

avanafil, cisapride, colchicine, dofetilide, dronedarone, eplerenone, ergot alkaloids, felodipine, fesoterodine, halofantrine, irinotecan, isavuconazole, ivabradine, levomethadyl, lovastatin, lurasidone, methadone, midazolam (oral), naloxegol, nisoldipine, pimozide, quinidine, ranolazine, simvastatin, solifenacin, ticagrelor, triazolam: Possibly increased plasma levels of these drugs leading to potentially life-threatening cardiovascular complications such as cardiac arrest, prolonged QT interval, torsades de pointes, ventricular tachycardia, and sudden death

calcium channel blockers: Possibly edema and increased risk of CHF; increased blood levels of these drugs

carbamazepine, isoniazid, nevirapine, phenobarbital, phenytoin, rifabutin, rifampin: Possibly decreased blood itraconazole level

cilostazol; eletriptan; glucocorticosteroids such as budesonide, dexamethasone, fluticasone, and methylprednisolone; trimetrexate: Possibly inhibited metabolism of these drugs

clarithromycin, erythromycin, indinavir, ritonavir: Possibly increased blood itraconazole level

didanosine: Possibly decreased therapeutic effects of itraconazole

ergot alkaloids: Possibly increased plasma ergot alkaloid elevation, leading to cerebral ischemia and ischemia of the extremities

fentanyl: Possibly increased plasma fentanyl level, causing potentially fatal respiratory depression

nisoldipine: Increased plasma nisoldipine levels that do not decrease after drug dosage is reduced

oral antidiabetic drugs: Possibly increased blood levels of these drugs and risk of hypoglycemia

warfarin: Increased anticoagulant effect of warfarin

Adverse Reactions

CNS: Chills, confusion, dizziness, drowsiness, fatigue, fever, headache, hypoesthesia, paresthesia, peripheral neuropathy, tremor, vertigo

CV: **Cardiac failure**, chest pain, **congestive heart failure**, hypertension, hypertriglyceridemia, **hypotension**, **left ventricular failure**, peripheral edema, tachycardia

EENT: Altered sense of taste, blurred vision, diplopia, dysphonia, transient or permanent hearing loss, tinnitis

ENDO: Hyperglycemia

GI: Abdominal pain, anorexia, constipation, diarrhea, elevated liver enzymes, flatulence, **hepatic failure**, **hepatitis**, **hepatotoxicity**, hyperbilirubinemia, indigestion, jaundice, nausea, **pancreatitis**, vomiting

GU: Erectile dysfunction, menstrual irregularities, pollakiuria, renal impairment, urinary incontinence

HEME: Leukopenia, **neutropenia**, **thrombocytopenia**

MS: Arthralgia, myalgia

RESP: Cough, dyspnea, **pulmonary edema**

SKIN: Acute generalized exanthematous pustulosis, alopecia, diaphoresis, **erythema multiforme**, **exfoliative dermatitis**, leukocytoclastic vasculitis, photosensitivity, pruritus, rash, **Stevens–Johnson syndrome**, **toxic epidermal necrolysis**, urticaria

Other: Anaphylaxis, **angioedema**, **hyperkalemia**, **hypokalemia**, **hypomagnesemia**, serum sickness

Nursing Considerations

- Know that itraconazole should not be used for the treatment of onychomycosis in patients with evidence of ventricular dysfunction such as congestive heart failure (CHF) or a history of CHF. If signs and symptoms of CHF develops during therapy, notify prescriber immediately and expect drug to be discontinued.
- Use itraconazole with extreme caution in patients with risk factors for CHF, such as ischemic or valvular heart disease, renal failure and other edematous disorders, or significant pulmonary disease such as chronic obstructive pulmonary disease because of increased risk of developing CHF during itraconazole treatment.
- Use itraconazole cautiously in patients with hypersensitivity to other azole antifungals (because cross-hypersensitivity is unknown) and in patients with hepatic or renal impairment.
- Know that because itraconazole has been linked to serious adverse cardiac and hepatic effects, expect to send appropriate nail specimens for laboratory testing to confirm onychomycosis before beginning therapy.

WARNING **Keep in mind that itraconazole is a potent inhibitor of the cytochrome P-450 3A4 (CYP3A4) isoenzyme system, which may increase blood levels of drugs metabolized by this system. Patients taking such drugs as cisapride with itraconazole or other CYP3A4 inhibitors have experienced life-threatening cardiovascular complications, such as prolonged QT interval, torsades de pointes, and ventricular tachycardia, as well as sudden death.**

- Administer itraconazole capsules (not oral solution) and tablets with a meal to ensure maximal absorption.
- Know that capsules and oral solution forms are not interchangeable because drug exposure is greater with oral solution. Tablet form is used only for the treatment of onychomycosis of the toenail.
- Keep in mind that a patient with AIDS may have hypochlorhydria, which reduces drug absorption. For such a patient, expect to administer higher doses of itraconazole.
- Monitor liver enzymes in patients with impaired hepatic function and those who have experienced hepatotoxicity with other drugs.
- Be aware that if patient develops signs and symptoms of peripheral neuropathy or CHF, such as dyspnea, fatigue and peripheral edema, expect to discontinue drug.
- Assess patient for rash every 8 hours during therapy; notify prescriber if rash occurs.
- Know that if patient also receives warfarin, monitor PT and assess patient for signs and symptoms of bleeding.
- Keep in mind that if patient also receives digoxin, monitor blood digoxin level as appropriate to detect toxic level, and assess patient for signs and symptoms of digitalis toxicity, such as nausea and yellow vision.
- Know that if a patient with cystic fibrosis does not respond to itraconazole therapy, alternative therapy should be considered.

PATIENT TEACHING

- Instruct patient to take itraconazole capsules or tablets with a meal and to swallow capsules whole, but oral solution without food.
- Tell patient with diabetes who takes an oral antidiabetic drug to check his blood glucose level often because of the increased risk of hypoglycemia.
- Advise patient to avoid taking antacids with oral itraconazole.
- Advise patient to notify prescriber immediately of changes in other drugs, such as new drugs and dosage changes.
- Advise patient to notify prescriber immediately about abdominal pain, diarrhea, headache, hearing loss, nausea, peripheral neuropathy, or vomiting.
- Instruct patient to stop itraconazole and notify prescriber immediately if he experiences an allergic reaction.
- Tell him to stop itraconazole and notify prescriber immediately if he notices fluid retention.
- Instruct patient to notify prescriber if he experiences signs of liver problems, such as abdominal pain, dark urine, fatigue, loss of appetite, pale stools, weakness, or yellow eyes or skin.
- Caution patient to avoid performing hazardous activities such as driving until

CNS effects such as dizziness or change in vision are not present.
- Tell women of childbearing age to begin therapy on the second or third day following the onset of menses. Also, advise patient to use effective contraception to prevent pregnancy during itraconazole therapy and for 2 months following the end of treatment. Tell patient to notify prescriber immediately if pregnancy is suspected or occurs.
- Caution breastfeeding patient to consult prescriber about continuation of breast-feeding during itraconazole therapy.

ivabradine

Corlanor

Class and Category

Pharmacologic class: Nucleotide-gated channel blocker
Therapeutic class: Cardiac pacemaker regulator
Pregnancy category: Not classified

Indications and Dosages

➤ *To reduce risk of hospitalization for worsening heart failure in patients with stable, symptomatic chronic heart failure who have a left ventricular ejection fraction of 35% or less, who are in sinus rhythm with a resting heart rate of 70 beats/minute or more and either are on maximally tolerated doses of beta-blockers or have a contraindication to beta-blocker use*

TABLETS

Adults. *Initial:* 5 mg twice daily with meals followed by a dosage adjustment in 2 weeks to achieve a resting heart rate between 50 and 60 beats/minute.

DOSAGE ADJUSTMENT For a patient with a resting heart rate greater than 60 beats/minute, dosage increased by 2.5 mg given twice daily up to a maximum dose of 7.5 mg twice daily, as needed. For a patient with a resting heart rate below 50 beats/minute or who experience signs and symptoms of bradycardia, dosage decreased by 2.5 mg given twice daily; if current dose is already 2.5 mg twice daily, drug discontinued.

Mechanism of Action

Blocks the hyperpolarization-activated cyclic nucleotide-gated (HCN) channel responsible for the cardiac pacemaker, which regulates heart rate. This results in a reduction in heart rate

Contraindications

Acute decompensated heart failure; blood pressure less than 90/50 mm Hg; concomitant use of strong cytochrome P-4503A4 (CYP3A4) inhibitors such as azole antifungals, HIV protease inhibitors, macrolide antibiotics, and nefazodone or concurrent use of diltiazem or verapamil; hypersensitivity to ivabradine or its components; pacemaker dependence; severe hepatic impairment; sick sinus syndrome, sinoatrial block, or third degree AV block, unless a functioning demand pacemaker is present

Interactions

DRUGS

CYP3A4 inducers such as barbiturates, phenytoin, rifampicin, St. John's wort: Decreased ivabradine plasma concentrations decreasing effectiveness
CYP3A4 inhibitors such as azole antifungals, diltiazem, HIV protease inhibitors, macrolide antibiotics, nefazodone, verapamil: Increased ivabradine plasma concentrations, which may exacerbate bradycardia and conduction disturbances
negative chronotropes such as amiodarone, beta-blockers, digoxin, diltiazem, verapamil: Increased risk of bradycardia

FOODS

grapefruit juice: Increased ivabradine plasma concentrations, which may exacerbate bradycardia and conduction disturbances

Adverse Reactions

CNS: Syncope, vertigo
CV: Atrial fibrillation, **bradycardia**, **heart block**, hypertension, **hypotension**, **sinus arrest**, **torsades de pointes**, **ventricular fibrillation and tachycardia**
EENT: Diplopia, colored bright lights, halos, image decomposition such as

GHI

kaleidoscopic or stroboscopic effects, multiple images, transiently enhanced brightness in a limited area of the visual field, visual impairment
SKIN: Erythema, pruritus, rash, urticaria
Other: Angioedema, fetal toxicity

Nursing Considerations

- Be aware that ivabradine should not be given to patients with demand pacemakers set to a rate of 60 beats/minute or greater because these patients will not be able to achieve a target heart rate of less than 60 beats/minute.
- Know that although drug is not contraindicated, it is not recommended for use in patients with a second degree heart block unless a functioning demand pacemaker is in place.
- Monitor patient's cardiac rhythm regularly because ivabradine increases the risk of atrial fibrillation and conduction disturbances. Also monitor patient's heart rate, because drug may cause bradycardia. Risk factors for bradycardia include conduction defects, sinus node dysfunction, ventricular dysfunction, and use of other negative chronotropic drugs such as amiodarone, digoxin, diltiazem, or verapamil. Be aware that bradycardia may increase risk of prolonged QT interval, which may lead to life-threatening ventricular arrhythmias. Notify prescriber if arrhythmias such as atrial fibrillation or conduction disturbances occurs or the patient's heart rate drops below 50 beats/minute. Expect drug to be discontinued in these situations.

PATIENT TEACHING

- Instruct patient to take ivabradine with meals.

WARNING Advise female patients of childbearing age that ivabradine may cause fetal toxicity and an effective contraceptive must be used during therapy. Tell patient to notify prescriber immediately if pregnancy is suspected or occurs.

- Instruct patient to notify all prescribers of ivabradine therapy.
- Tell patient to notify prescriber if pulse becomes irregular or less than 50 beats/minute or visual disturbances occurs.

ixekizumab

Taltz

Class and Category

Pharmacologic class: Interleukin-17 A antagonist
Therapeutic class: Immunomodulator
Pregnancy category: Not classified

Indications and Dosages

➤ *To treat moderate-to-severe plaque psoriasis in patients who are candidates for phototherapy or systemic therapy*

SUBCUTANEOUS INJECTION

Adults. *Initial:* 160 mg (two 80-mg injections) at wk 0, followed by 80 mg at wks 2, 4, 6, 8, 10, and 12; then 80 mg every 4 wk.

➤ *To treat active psoriatic arthritis*

SUBCUTANEOUS INJECTION

Adults. *Initial:* 160 mg (two 80-mg injections), followed by 80 mg every 4 wk.

Mechanism of Action

Selectively binds with the interleukin 17A cytokine and inhibits its interaction with the IL-17 receptor. This inhibits the release of proinflammatory cytokines and chemokines involved in normal inflammatory and immune responses. Binding of IL-17 receptors prevents inflammation-related signals from being relayed, which reduces the inflammatory response and relieves signs and symptoms of plaque psoriasis

Incompatibilities

Don't mix ixekizumab with other drugs.

Contraindications

Hypersensitivity to ixekizumab or its components

Interactions

DRUGS

CYP450 substrates with a narrow therapeutic index such as cyclosporine, warfarin: Possibly decreased plasma levels of these drugs with decreased effectiveness
live vaccines: Increased risk of adverse vaccine effects

Adverse Reactions

EENT: Conjunctivitis, oral candidiasis, rhinitis
GI: Crohn's disease (new onset or exacerbation), nausea, ulcerative colitis (new onset or exacerbation)
HEME: Neutropenia, thrombocytopenia
RESP: Upper respiratory infections
SKIN: Tinea infections, urticaria
Other: Anaphylaxis, angioedema, anti-ixekizumab antibodies, flu-like symptoms, infection including activation of latent infections such as tuberculosis, injection-site reactions such as erythema and pain

Nursing Considerations

- Check patient's immunization history and make sure all age-appropriate immunizations according to current guidelines have been administered prior to initiating ixekizumab therapy. Live vaccines should be avoided during ixekizumab therapy.
- Make sure patient has a tuberculin skin test before therapy starts. If skin test is positive, tuberculosis treatment will need to be started before ixekizumab can begin. Even patients who have tested negative for tuberculosis may develop tuberculosis during therapy. Monitor patient for low-grade fever, persistent cough, and wasting or weight loss; report such findings to prescriber.
- Know that if patient has evidence of an active infection when drug is prescribed, therapy shouldn't start until infection has been treated. Monitor patients for the development of infections such as conjunctivitis, oral candidiasis, tinea infections, and upper respiratory tract infections during therapy; report such findings to prescriber. Know that if a patient develops a serious infection or does not respond to treatment prescribed for the infection, ixekizumab may have to be temporarily withheld until the infection is resolved.
- Remove autoinjector or prefilled syringe from the refrigerator and allow about 30 minutes for drug to reach room temperature. Don't remove the needle cap during this time. Inspect solution for particulate matter or discoloration. Solution should appear clear and colorless to slightly yellow. Because the solution does not contain a preservative, discard any unused solution.
- Administer ixekizumab as a subcutaneous injection using either the autoinjector or prefilled syringe. Inject the full amount (1 ml), which provides 80 mg of ixekizumab into any quadrant of the abdomen, thighs, or upper arms. Rotate injection sites and do not inject into areas where the skin is affected by psoriasis or is bruised, erythematous, or indurated.

WARNING **Monitor patient closely for hypersensitivity. If a serious reaction occurs, such as angioedema or urticaria, discontinue drug immediately, notify prescriber, and provide supportive care, as prescribed.**

- Monitor patient closely for evidence of inflammatory bowel disease. Know that Crohn's disease and ulcerative colitis may occur. During treatment, monitor patient for onset or exacerbation of inflammatory bowel disease.

PATIENT TEACHING

- Instruct patient or caregiver on how to administer drug subcutaneously, if self-administration is prescribed. Provide instructions on how to use the autoinjector or prefilled syringe correctly. Tell patient how to dispose of syringe or autoinjector properly and to keep out of reach of children and pets, including those already used.
- Tell patient to keep drug refrigerated in between doses but to allow the drug to warm to room temperature for about 30 minutes before administering. Tell patient to inject the full amount of the drug into any quadrant of the abdomen, thighs, or upper arms. Stress importance of avoiding areas where the skin is affected by psoriasis or is bruised, indurated, or red and to rotate sites. Alert him to the possibility of experiencing redness or pain at injection site, but advise him that these are not usually severe.
- Review the signs and symptoms of an allergic reaction (difficulty breathing, hives, swollen face) and tell patient to seek emergency care immediately if these occur.

- Inform patient that infections, including activation of latent infections such as tuberculosis, may occur during ixekizumab therapy. Instruct him to report persistent, severe, or unusual signs and symptoms to prescriber. Advise patient to avoid people with infections.
- Alert patient that irritable bowel syndrome may occur or be aggravated by ixekizumab therapy. Tell him to notify prescriber of adverse reactions such as abdominal distention or pain or diarrhea that is persistent or severe.
- Warn patient not to receive immunizations that contain live vaccines while taking ixekizumab.

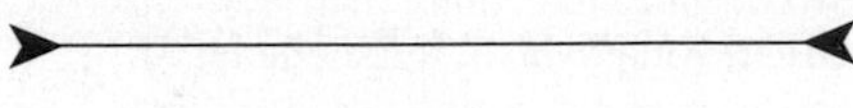

JKL

ketoprofen

Apo-Keto (CAN), Nexcede

Class and Category

Pharmacologic class: NSAID
Therapeutic class: Analgesic
Pregnancy category: B

Indications and Dosages

➤ *To treat symptoms of osteoarthritis or rheumatoid arthritis*

CAPSULES, TABLETS

Adults. *Initial:* 75 mg three times daily or 50 mg four times daily. *Maximum:* 300 mg daily.

E.R. CAPSULES

Adults. *Maintenance:* 200 mg daily.

➤ *To relieve mild to moderate pain; pain associated with dysmenorrhea*

TABLETS

Adults. *Initial:* 25 to 50 mg every 6 to 8 hr as needed. May be increased to 75 mg every 6 to 8 hr, as needed. *Maximum:* 300 mg daily.

DOSAGE ADJUSTMENT For debilitated, elderly, and small patients, dosage reduced. For patients with mild renal dysfunction, maximum daily dose reduced to 150 mg daily; for patients with more severe renal impairment (glomerular filtration rate less than 25 ml/min), end-stage renal disease, or liver dysfunction, maximum daily dose reduced to 100 mg.

Mechanism of Action

Blocks activity of cyclooxygenase, the enzyme needed for prostaglandin synthesis. Prostaglandins, important mediators of inflammatory response, cause local vasodilation with pain and swelling. By blocking cyclooxygenase and inhibiting prostaglandins, this NSAID reduces inflammatory symptoms and relieves pain.

Contraindications

Angioedema; aspirin-, iodide-, or NSAID-induced asthma, bronchospasm, nasal polyps, rhinitis, or urticaria; hypersensitivity to ketoprofen or its components

Interactions

DRUGS

ACE inhibitors: Possibly decreased hypotensive effect of ACE inhibitors
acetaminophen: Possibly increased adverse renal effects with long-term acetaminophen use
aspirin, other NSAIDs: Increased risk of bleeding and adverse GI effects, increased and prolonged blood ketoprofen levels
cefamandole, cefoperazone, cefotetan: Increased risk of hypoprothrombinemia and bleeding
colchicine, platelet aggregation inhibitors: Increased risk of GI bleeding, hemorrhage, and ulcers
corticosteroids, potassium supplements: Increased risk of adverse GI effects
cyclosporine: Increased risk of nephrotoxicity from both drugs, increased blood cyclosporine level
diuretics (loop, potassium-sparing, and thiazide): Decreased diuretic and antihypertensive effects
gold compounds, nephrotoxic drugs: Increased risk of adverse renal effects
heparin, oral anticoagulants, thrombolytics: Increased anticoagulant effects, increased risk of hemorrhage
insulin, oral antidiabetic drugs: Possibly increased hypoglycemic effects of these drugs
lithium: Increased blood lithium level and possibly toxicity
methotrexate: Decreased methotrexate clearance, increased risk of methotrexate toxicity
plicamycin, valproic acid: Increased risk of hypoprothrombinemia and GI bleeding, hemorrhage, and ulcers
probenecid: Possibly increased blood level, effectiveness, and risk of toxicity of ketoprofen

ACTIVITIES

alcohol use: Increased risk of adverse GI effects

Adverse Reactions

CNS: CVA, headache, irritability, nervousness, **seizures**
CV: Edema, hypertension, **MI**, tachycardia
EENT: Tinnitus, vision changes

GI: Abdominal pain, anorexia, constipation, diarrhea, diverticulitis, dyspepsia, dysphagia, elevated liver enzymes, flatulence, gastritis, gastroenteritis, gastroesophageal reflux disease, **GI bleeding** and ulceration, **hepatic failure**, hiatal hernia, indigestion, **melena**, nausea, **perforation of intestine or stomach**, stomatitis, vomiting
GU: Acute renal failure, decreased urine output
HEME: Agranulocytosis, anemia, easy bruising, **hemolytic anemia**, **leukopenia**, **neutropenia**, **pancytopenia**, **thrombocytopenia**
RESP: Asthma, **respiratory depression**
SKIN: Erythema multiforme, **Stevens–Johnson syndrome**, **toxic epidermal necrolysis**, rash
Other: Anaphylaxis, **angioedema**, rapid weight gain

Nursing Considerations

- Use ketoprofen with extreme caution in patients with history of GI bleeding or ulcer disease because NSAIDs, such as ketoprofen, increase risk of GI bleeding and ulceration. Expect to use ketoprofen for shortest time possible in these patients.
- Be aware that serious GI tract bleeding, perforation, and ulceration may occur without warning symptoms. Elderly patients are at greater risk. To minimize risk, give drug with food. If GI distress occurs, withhold drug and notify prescriber immediately.
- Use ketoprofen cautiously in patients with hypertension, and monitor blood pressure closely throughout therapy. Drug may cause hypertension or worsen it.

WARNING Monitor patient closely for thrombotic events, including MI and stroke, because NSAIDs increase the risk.

- Monitor patient—especially if he's elderly or receiving long-term ketoprofen therapy—for less common but serious adverse GI reactions, including anorexia, constipation, diverticulitis, dysphagia, esophagitis, gastritis, gastroenteritis, gastroesophageal reflux disease, hemorrhoids, hiatal hernia, melena, stomatitis, and vomiting.
- Monitor liver enzymes, as ordered, because, rarely, elevations may progress to severe hepatic reactions, including fatal hepatitis, liver necrosis, and hepatic failure. Monitor BUN and serum creatinine levels in elderly patients, patients taking ACE inhibitors or diuretics, and patients with heart failure or impaired renal function; drug may cause renal failure in these patients.
- Monitor CBC for decreased hematocrit and hemoglobin level because drug may worsen anemia.

WARNING If patient has bone marrow suppression or is receiving an antineoplastic drug, monitor laboratory results (including WBC count), and watch for evidence of infection because anti-inflammatory and antipyretic actions of ketoprofen may mask signs and symptoms, such as fever and pain.

- Assess patient's skin regularly for signs of rash or other hypersensitivity reaction because ketoprofen is an NSAID and may cause serious skin reactions without warning, even in patients with no history of NSAID sensitivity. At first sign of reaction, stop drug and notify prescriber.
- Be aware that if patient takes acetaminophen, BUN level, fluid intake and output, and serum creatinine level should be monitored for evidence of adverse renal effects.

PATIENT TEACHING

- Instruct patient to take ketoprofen with food or after meals to prevent GI upset. Advise him to take drug with a full glass of water and to avoid lying down for 15 to 30 minutes afterward to prevent drug from lodging in esophagus and causing irritation.
- Advise patient to swallow drug whole and not to break, chew, crush, or open capsules.
- Instruct patient to avoid alcohol, aspirin, and aspirin-containing products while taking ketoprofen to decrease risk of adverse GI effects.
- Tell patient not to take more drug than prescribed because stomach bleeding may occur.
- Warn patient taking an anticoagulant to watch for and immediately report bleeding problems, such as bloody or tarry stools and bloody vomitus.
- Advise patient taking insulin or an oral antidiabetic agent to monitor blood glucose level closely. Urge him to carry candy or other simple sugars to treat mild

hypoglycemia. If he has frequent or severe episodes, instruct him to consult prescriber.
- Inform patient that he may be nervous and irritable while taking ketoprofen.
- Instruct patient to notify prescriber immediately if he develops decreased urine output, dark brown or yellow urine, rash, or signs of fluid retention, including swelling of extremities and unexplained rapid weight gain.
- Caution pregnant patient not to take NSAIDs such as ketoprofen during last trimester because drug may cause premature closure of the ductus arteriosus.
- Explain that ketoprofen may increase risk of serious adverse cardiovascular reactions; urge patient to seek immediate medical attention if signs or symptoms arise, such as chest pain, shortness of breath, slurring of speech, or weakness.
- Explain that ketoprofen may increase risk of serious adverse GI reactions; emphasize importance of seeking immediate medical attention for such signs and symptoms as abdominal or epigastric pain, black or tarry stools, indigestion, or vomiting blood or material that looks like coffee grounds.
- Alert patient to rare but serious skin reactions. Urge him to seek immediate medical attention for blisters, fever, itching, rash, or other indications of hypersensitivity.

ketorolac tromethamine

Sprix, Toradol

Class and Category

Pharmacologic class: NSAID
Therapeutic class: Analgesic
Pregnancy category: C

Indications and Dosages

➤ *To treat moderate to severe pain*

TABLETS

Adults ages 17 to 64. *Initial:* 20 mg as single dose, followed by 10 mg every 4 to 6 hr as needed, up to four times a day. *Maximum:* 40 mg daily for no more than 5 days.
DOSAGE ADJUSTMENT For elderly patients, patients with impaired renal function, or patients weighing less than 50 kg (110 lb), initial dose reduced to 10 mg.

I.M. INJECTION

Adults ages 17 to 64. *Initial:* 60 mg as single dose, followed by oral ketorolac if needed; or 30 mg every 6 hr as needed. *Maximum:* 120 mg daily for no more than 5 days.
DOSAGE ADJUSTMENT For elderly patients, patients with impaired renal function, or patients weighing less than 50 kg (110 lb), initial dose reduced to 30 mg, followed by oral ketorolac if needed; or 15 mg every 6 hr as needed, up to maximum of 60 mg daily for no more than 5 days.

I.V. INJECTION

Adults ages 17 to 64. *Initial:* 30 mg given over no less than 15 sec as single dose, followed by oral ketorolac if needed; or 30 mg every 6 hr as needed. *Maximum:* 120 mg daily for no more than 5 days.
DOSAGE ADJUSTMENT For elderly patients, patients with impaired renal function, or patients weighing less than 50 kg (110 lb), initial dose reduced to 15 mg, followed by oral ketorolac if needed; or 15 mg every 6 hr as needed, up to maximum of 60 mg daily for no more than 5 days.

NASAL SPRAY (SPRIX)

Adults less than 65 years of age. 15.75 mg (1 spray) in each nostril every 6 to 8 hr. *Maximum:* 126 mg (four doses) daily for no more than 5 days.
DOSAGE ADJUSTMENT For elderly patients, patients with impaired renal function, or patients weighing less than 50 kg (110 lb), 15.75 mg in only one nostril every 6 to 8 hr with maximum dose of 63 mg (four doses) daily for no more than 5 days.

Route	Onset	Peak	Duration
P.O.	30–60 min	2–3 hr	5–6 hr
I.M., I.V.	30–60 min	1–2 hr	4–6 hr
Nasal	30–60 min	Unknown	6–8 hr

Mechanism of Action

Blocks cyclooxygenase, an enzyme needed to synthesize prostaglandins. Prostaglandins mediate inflammatory response and cause local vasodilation, pain, and swelling. They also promote pain transmission from periphery to spinal cord. By blocking cyclooxygenase and inhibiting prostaglandins, this NSAID reduces inflammation and relieves pain.

Contraindications

Advanced renal impairment or risk of renal impairment due to volume depletion; before or during surgery if hemostasis is critical; breastfeeding; cerebrovascular bleeding; concurrent use of aspirin or other salicylates, other NSAIDs, or probenecid; hemorrhagic diathesis; history of GI bleeding, GI perforation, or peptic ulcer disease; hemophilia or other bleeding problems, including coagulation or platelet function disorders; hypersensitivity to ketorolac tromethamine, aspirin, other NSAIDs, or their components; incomplete hemostasis; labor and delivery; postoperative pain after coronary artery bypass graft (CABG) surgery

Interactions

DRUGS

ACE inhibitors, angiotensin II receptor antagonists: Increased risk of renal impairment; decreased effectiveness of these drugs
acetaminophen, gold compounds: Increased risk of adverse renal effects
amphotericin, penicillamine, and other nephrotoxic drugs: Increased risk or severity of adverse renal reactions
antihypertensives, diuretics: Possibly reduced effects of these drugs
aspirin and other salicylates, other NSAIDs: Additive toxicity
cefamandole, cefoperazone, cefotetan: Possibly hypoprothrombinemia
corticosteroids, potassium supplements: Increased risk of gastric ulcers or hemorrhage
furosemide: Decreased effects of furosemide
heparin, oral anticoagulants, platelet aggregation inhibitors, thrombolytics: Increased risk of GI bleeding and I.M. hematoma formation
lithium: Possibly increased blood lithium level and increased risk of lithium toxicity
methotrexate: Possibly methotrexate toxicity
nondepolarizing muscle relaxants: Increased risk of apnea
pentoxifylline, selective serotonin reuptake inhibitors: Increased risk of bleeding
plicamycin, valproic acid: Possibly hypoprothrombinemia and increased risk of bleeding
probenecid: Decreased elimination of ketorolac, increased risk of adverse effects

ACTIVITIES

alcohol use: Increased risk of adverse GI effects

Adverse Reactions

CNS: **Aseptic meningitis**, **cerebral hemorrhage**, **coma**, **CVA**, dizziness, drowsiness, headache, psychosis, **seizures**
CV: Edema, hypertension
EENT: **Laryngeal edema**, stomatitis
ENDO: Hyperglycemia
GI: Abdominal pain; **acute pancreatitis**; bloating; constipation; diarrhea; diverticulitis; elevated liver enzymes; flatulence; **GI bleeding**, **perforation**, or ulceration; **hepatitis**; **hepatic failure**; jaundice; indigestion; nausea; vomiting; worsening of inflammatory bowel disease
GU: Interstitial nephritis, **renal failure**, urine retention
HEME: **Agranulocytosis**, anemia, **aplastic or hemolytic anemia**, eosinophilia, **leukopenia**, lymphadenopathy, **pancytopenia**, **thrombocytopenia**
RESP: **Bronchospasm**, pneumonia, **respiratory depression**
SKIN: Diaphoresis, **erythema multiforme**, **exfoliative dermatitis**, photosensitivity, pruritus, rash, **Stevens–Johnson syndrome**, **toxic epidermal necrolysis**, urticaria
Other: **Anaphylaxis**, **angioedema**, **hyperkalemia**, **hyponatremia**, injection-site pain, **sepsis**, unusual weight gain

Nursing Considerations

- Be aware that NSAIDs like ketorolac should be avoided in patients with a recent MI because risk of reinfarction increases with NSAID therapy. If therapy is unavoidable, monitor patient closely for signs of cardiac ischemia.
- Know that the risk of heart failure increases with ketorolac use because drug is a NSAID. This class of drugs should not be used in patients with severe heart

failure but, if unavoidable, monitor patient for worsening of heart failure.

- Read ketorolac label carefully. Don't use I.M. form for I.V. route. Know that ketorolac isn't for epidural or intrathecal use.
- Inject I.M. ketorolac slowly, deep into a large muscle mass. Monitor site for bleeding, bruising, or hematoma.
- Give I.V. injection over at least 15 seconds.
- Notify prescriber if pain relief is inadequate or if breakthrough pain occurs between doses because supplemental doses of an opioid analgesic may be required.

WARNING Monitor liver enzymes, as ordered. If elevated levels persist or worsen, notify prescriber and expect to stop drug, as ordered, to prevent hepatic impairment.

WARNING Monitor patients with a history of peripheral edema, heart failure, or hypertension for adequate fluid balance because drug can promote fluid retention and worsen these conditions. Assess patient for decreased activity tolerance, dyspnea, edema, and unexplained rapid weight gain. Notify prescriber if such symptoms develop.

- Use ketorolac with extreme caution in patients with history of GI bleeding or ulcer disease because NSAIDs like ketorolac increase risk of GI bleeding and ulceration. Use ketorolac in these patients for shortest length of time possible.
- Know that serious GI tract bleeding and ulceration and perforation of intestine or stomach can occur without warning or symptoms. Elderly patients are at greater risk. To minimize risk, give drug with food. If GI distress occurs, withhold drug and notify prescriber immediately.
- Monitor patient with history of inflammatory bowel disease, such as Crohn's disease or ulcerative colitis, because ketorolac may worsen these conditions.
- Use ketorolac cautiously in patients with hypertension, and monitor blood pressure closely throughout therapy because drug can lead to onset of hypertension or worsen existing hypertension.

WARNING Monitor patient closely for thrombotic events including MI and stroke because NSAIDs such as ketorolac increase risk. These events may occur early in treatment and risk increases with duration of use. Be aware that these events have occurred even in patients who do not have a history of or risk factors for cardiovascular disease. Monitor patient for warning signs such as chest pain, slurring of speech, shortness of breath, or weakness. If any signs and symptoms develop, withhold ketorolac, alert prescriber immediately, and provide supportive care, as prescribed.

- Monitor patient—especially if elderly—for less common but serious adverse GI reactions, including anorexia, constipation, diverticulitis, dysphagia, esophagitis, gastritis, gastroenteritis, gastroesophageal reflux disease, hemorrhoids, hiatal hernia, melena, stomatitis, and vomiting.
- Monitor BUN and serum creatinine levels in the elderly; patients with heart failure, hepatic impairment, or impaired renal function; and those who are taking ACE inhibitors or diuretics because drug may cause renal failure.
- Monitor CBC for decreased hemoglobin and hematocrit because drug may worsen anemia.

WARNING In patient who has bone marrow suppression or is receiving antineoplastic drug therapy, monitor laboratory results (including WBC) and assess for evidence of infection because ketorolac has anti-inflammatory and antipyretic actions that may mask signs and symptoms, such as fever and pain.

- Assess patient's skin routinely for rash or other evidence of hypersensitivity reactions because ketorolac is an NSAID and may cause serious skin reactions without warning, even in patients with no history of NSAID hypersensitivity. Stop drug at first sign of reaction, and notify prescriber.

PATIENT TEACHING

- Instruct patient to take ketorolac tablets with an antacid, a meal, or a snack to prevent stomach upset. Advise him to take drug with a full glass of water and to stay upright for at least 15 minutes afterward.
- Teach patient how to prime bottle and administer nasal spray form, if prescribed. Remind patient that nasal spray form is not to be inhaled. Tell patient not to use

any single nasal spray bottle for more than 1 day, as it will not deliver the intended dose after 24 hours.

- Advise patient not to take aspirin, other NSAIDs, or other salicylates while taking ketorolac without consulting prescriber. Urge patient to limit use of acetaminophen to only a few days during ketorolac therapy and to notify prescriber of use.
- Caution patient not to use ketorolac for more than 5 days, as serious adverse effects may occur.
- Instruct him to immediately report blood in urine, easy bruising, itching, rash, swelling, or yellow eyes or skin.
- Caution pregnant patient that NSAIDs like ketorolac shouldn't be taken during last trimester because drug may cause premature closure of the ductus arteriosus.
- Explain that ketorolac may increase risk of serious adverse cardiovascular reactions; urge patient to seek immediate medical attention if signs or symptoms arise, such as chest pain, edema, shortness of breath, slurring of speech, unexplained weight gain, or weakness.
- Tell patient that ketorolac also may increase risk of serious adverse GI reactions; stress importance of seeking immediate medical attention if signs or symptoms occur, such as abdominal or epigastric pain, black tarry stools, indigestion, and vomiting blood or coffee ground material.
- Alert patient to the possibility of serious skin reactions, although rare, occurring with ketorolac therapy. Urge patient to seek immediate medical attention if signs or symptoms occur, such as blisters, fever, a rash, or other signs of hypersensitivity, such as itching.
- Caution patient to avoid hazardous activities until drug's CNS effects are known.
- Urge patient to avoid alcohol while taking ketorolac.
- Encourage patient to have dental procedures performed before starting drug therapy because of increased risk of bleeding.
- Teach patient proper oral hygiene measures, and encourage him to use a soft-bristled toothbrush while taking ketorolac.

labetalol hydrochloride

Normodyne, Trandate

Class and Category

Pharmacologic class: Noncardioselective beta-blocker/alpha$_1$ blocker
Therapeutic class: Antihypertensive
Pregnancy category: C

Indications and Dosages

➤ *To manage hypertension*

TABLETS

Adults. *Initial:* 100 mg twice daily, increased by 100 mg twice daily as needed and tolerated every 2 to 3 days. *Maintenance:* 200 to 400 mg twice daily. For severe hypertension, 1.2 to 2.4 g daily in divided doses twice daily or three times daily.

➤ *To manage severe hypertension and treat hypertensive emergencies*

I.V. INFUSION

Adults. 2 mg/min until desired response occurs.

I.V. INJECTION

Adults. 20 mg given over 2 min; additional doses given in increments of 40 to 80 mg every 10 min as indicated until desired response occurs. *Maximum:* 300 mg.

Route	Onset	Peak	Duration
P.O.	20 min–2 hr	1–4 hr	8–24 hr
I.V.	2–5 min	5–15 min	2–4 hr

Mechanism of Action

Selectively blocks alpha$_1$ and beta$_2$ receptors in vascular smooth muscle and beta$_1$ receptors in heart to reduce blood pressure and peripheral vascular resistance. Potent beta blockade prevents reflex tachycardia, which commonly occurs when alpha blockers reduce cardiac output, resting heart rate, or stroke volume.

Incompatibilities

Don't dilute labetalol in sodium bicarbonate solution or give through same I.V. line as alkaline drugs, such as furosemide; doing so may cause white precipitate to form.

Contraindications

Asthma, cardiogenic shock, heart failure, hypersensitivity to labetalol or its components, second- or third-degree heart block, severe bradycardia

Interactions

DRUGS

allergen immunotherapy, allergenic extracts for skin testing: Increased risk of serious systemic reaction or anaphylaxis
beta blockers, digoxin: Increased risk of bradycardia
calcium channel blockers, clonidine, diazoxide, guanabenz, reserpine: Possibly hypotension
cimetidine: Possibly increased labetalol effects
estrogens, NSAIDs: Possibly reduced antihypertensive effect of labetalol
general anesthetics: Increased risk of hypotension and myocardial depression
insulin, oral antidiabetic drugs: Increased risk of hyperglycemia
nitroglycerin: Possibly hypertension
phenoxybenzamine, phentolamine: Possibly additive $alpha_1$-blocking effects
sympathomimetics with alpha- and beta-adrenergic effects (such as pseudoephedrine): Possibly hypertension, excessive bradycardia, or heart block
xanthines (aminophylline and theophylline): Possibly decreased therapeutic effects of both drugs

FOODS

all food: Increased blood labetalol level

ACTIVITIES

alcohol use: Increased labetalol effects

Adverse Reactions

CNS: Anxiety, confusion, depression, dizziness, drowsiness, fatigue, paresthesia, syncope, vertigo, weakness, yawning
CV: **Bradycardia**, chest pain, edema, **heart block**, **heart failure**, **hypotension**, orthostatic hypotension, **ventricular arrhythmias**
EENT: Nasal congestion, taste perversion
GI: Elevated liver enzymes, **hepatic necrosis**, **hepatitis**, indigestion, jaundice, nausea, vomiting
GU: Ejaculation failure, impotence
RESP: Dyspnea, wheezing
SKIN: Pruritus, rash, scalp tingling

Nursing Considerations

- During I.V. labetalol use, expect to monitor blood pressure according to facility policy, usually every 5 minutes for 30 minutes, then every 30 minutes for 2 hours, and then every hour for 6 hours.
- Keep patient in supine position for 3 hours after I.V. administration.

WARNING Be aware that labetalol masks common signs of shock.

- Monitor blood glucose level in diabetic patient because labetalol may conceal symptoms of hypoglycemia.
- Be aware that stopping labetalol tablets abruptly after long-term therapy could result in angina, MI, or ventricular arrhythmias. Expect to taper dosage over 2 weeks while monitoring response.

PATIENT TEACHING

- Advise patient to report confusion, difficulty breathing, rash, slow pulse, and swelling in arms or legs.
- Caution patient not to stop drug abruptly because doing so could cause angina and rebound hypertension.
- Suggest that patient minimize effects of orthostatic hypotension by avoiding sudden position changes, rising to a sitting or standing position slowly, and taking labetalol at bedtime, if approved by prescriber.
- Instruct diabetic patient to check blood glucose level often and to be alert for signs and symptoms of hypoglycemia.
- Inform patient that scalp tingling may occur early in treatment but is transient.
- Urge patient to avoid alcohol during labetalol therapy.
- Advise patient to inform eye healthcare provider if he needs cataract surgery because intraoperative floppy iris syndrome has occurred during cataract surgery in some patients treated with the class of drugs of which labetalol is a member.

lacosamide

Vimpat

Class and Category

Pharmacologic class: Functionalized amino acid
Therapeutic class: Anticonvulsant
Pregnancy category: C

Indications and Dosages

➤ *To treat partial-onset seizures*

ORAL SOLUTION, TABLETS

Adults and adolescents age 17 and over. 100 mg twice daily, increased by 50 mg twice daily every week to recommended maintenance dose. Alternatively, 200 mg given as single loading dose, followed 12 hr later by 100 mg twice daily for 1 wk. Dosage increased at weekly intervals by 50 mg twice daily, as needed, up to recommended maintenance dose. *Maintenance:* 300 to 400 mg daily.

Children ages 4 to 17 weighing 50 kg (110 lb) or more. 50 mg twice daily, increased by 50 mg twice daily every week to recommended maintenance dose. *Maintenance:* 150 mg to 200 mg twice daily.

Children ages 4 to 17 weighing 30 kg (66 lb) to less than 50 kg (110 lb). 1 mg/kg twice daily, increased by 1 mg/kg twice daily every week to recommended maintenance dose. *Maintenance:* 2 mg/kg to 4 mg/kg twice daily.

Children ages 4 to 17 weighing 11 kg (24.2 lb) to less than 30 kg (66 lb). 1 mg/kg twice daily, increased by 1 mg/kg twice daily every week to recommended maintenance dose. *Maintenance:* 3 mg/kg to 6 mg/kg twice daily.

I.V. INFUSION

Adults and adolescents age 17 and over. *Initial:* 100 mg infused over 30 to 60 min twice daily for 1 wk. Dosage increased by 50 mg/day at weekly intervals. Alternatively, 200 mg given as single loading dose infused over 30 to 60 min, followed 12 hr later by 100 mg infused over 30 to 60 min twice daily for 1 wk. Dosage increased at weekly intervals by 50 mg twice daily, as needed, up to recommended maintenance dose. *Maintenance:* 300 to 400 mg daily.

➤ *As adjunct to treat partial-onset seizures*

ORAL SOLUTION, TABLETS

Adults and adolescents age 17 and over. *Initial:* 50 mg twice daily, increased by 50 mg twice daily at weekly intervals based on response and tolerance. Alternatively, 200 mg given as single loading dose, followed 12 hr later by 100 mg twice daily for 1 wk. Dosage increased at weekly intervals by 50 mg twice daily, as needed, up to recommended maintenance dose. *Maintenance:* 200 to 400 mg daily.

Children ages 4 to 17 weighing 50 kg (110 lb) or more. 50 mg twice daily, increased by 50 mg twice daily every week to recommended maintenance dose. *Maintenance:* 100 mg to 200 mg twice daily.

Children ages 4 to 17 weighing 30 kg (66 lb) to less than 50 kg (110 lb). 1 mg/kg twice daily, increased by 1 mg/kg twice daily every week to recommended maintenance dose. *Maintenance:* 2 mg/kg to 4 mg/kg twice daily.

Children ages 4 to 17 weighing 11 kg (24.2 lb) to less than 30 kg (66 lb). 1 mg/kg twice daily, increased by 1 mg/kg twice daily every week to recommended maintenance dose. *Maintenance:* 3 mg/kg to 6 mg/kg twice daily.

I.V. INFUSION

Adults and adolescents age 17 and over. *Initial:* 50 mg infused over 30 to 60 min twice daily, increased by 50 mg twice daily, at weekly intervals based on response and tolerance. Alternatively, 200 mg given as a single loading dose infused over 30 to 60 min, followed 12 hr later by 100 mg twice daily infused over 30 to 60 min for 1 wk. Dosage increased at weekly intervals by 50 mg twice daily, as needed, up to recommended maintenance dose. *Maintenance:* 200 to 400 mg daily.

DOSAGE ADJUSTMENT For patients with mild to moderate hepatic impairment or severe renal impairment (creatinine clearance of 30 ml/min or less) including end-stage renal disease, dosage reduced by 25% of maximum dosage recommended. Following a 4-hr hemodialysis treatment, dosage supplementation of up to 50% may be required. For patients with hepatic impairment taking strong CYP2C9 or CYP3A4 inhibitors concurrently, dosage may need to be reduced.

Mechanism of Action

May selectively inactivate voltage-gated sodium channels, which prevents seizure activity by inhibiting repetitive neuronal firing in the brain and stabilizing hyperexcitable neuronal membranes.

Contraindications

Hypersensitivity to lacosamide and its components

Interactions

DRUGS

CYP2C9 inhibitors or CYP3A4 inhibitors (in presence of hepatic or renal impairment): Possibly significant increase in lacosamide exposure and adverse effects

drugs that may prolong the QT interval: Possibly further QT-interval prolongation

Adverse Reactions

CNS: Aggression, agitation, asthenia, ataxia, attention deficit, cerebellar syndrome, confusion, depression, dizziness, feeling drunk, fever, hallucinations, headache, hypoesthesia, impaired balance, insomnia, irritability, memory impairment, mood alteration, paresthesia, psychotic disorder, somnolence, **suicidal ideation**, tremor, vertigo

CV: Atrial fibrillation or flutter, **AV block**, **bradycardia**, **conduction disturbances**, palpitations, prolonged PR interval, **prolonged QT interval**

EENT: Blurred vision, diplopia, dry mouth, nystagmus, oral hypoesthesia, tinnitus

GI: Constipation, diarrhea, dyspepsia, nausea, vomiting

HEME: Agranuloctyosis, anemia, **neutropenia**

MS: Dysarthria, muscle spasms

SKIN: Pruritus, rash, **Stevens–Johnson syndrome**, **toxic epidermal necrolysis**, urticaria

Other: Angioedema; **delayed multiorgan hypersensitivity reaction**; injection-site erythema, irritation, and pain

Nursing Considerations

- Use cautiously in patients with concomitant drug therapy with drugs that prolong the PR interval, conduction problems (such as AV block, sick sinus syndrome and no pacemaker in place), severe cardiac disease (such as heart failure, myocardial ischemia), or sodium channel disorders such as Brugada syndrome, because lacosamide may affect conduction. For these patients, ensure an ECG has been done, as ordered, prior to starting therapy and after dosage titration.
- Use cautiously in patients with cardiovascular disease or diabetic neuropathy because drug may predispose them to atrial fibrillation or flutter.
- Know that in patients who are already taking a single antiepileptic and being converted to lacosamide monotherapy, the maintenance dose of lacosamide should be maintained for at least 3 days before beginning the withdrawal of the concomitant antiepileptic drug, as ordered. A gradual withdrawal of the concomitant antiepileptic drug over at least 6 weeks is recommended.
- Administer drug intravenously without further dilution or know that it may be mixed with diluents such as 0.9% sodium chloride injection, 5% dextrose injection, or lactated Ringer's injection. If diluted, do not store diluted solution for more than 4 hours at room temperature.
- Watch patient closely for suicidal tendencies, particularly when therapy starts and dosage changes, because depression may worsen temporarily during these times and lead to suicidal ideation.
- Be aware that lacosamide therapy should be discontinued gradually over at least 1 week to minimize seizure frequency.
- Monitor patient closely for hypersensitivity reactions to lacosamide, such as pruritus, rash, and more than one organ abnormality, such as elevated liver enzymes and myocarditis or pancreatitis. Be aware that drug reaction with eosinophilia and systemic symptoms (DRESS) has occurred with use of other antiepileptics and therefore may possibly occur with lacosamide use. Monitor patient closely and if signs and symptoms are present to suggest DRESS, notify prescriber immediately and expect that drug may be discontinued.

PATIENT TEACHING

- Tell patient that lacosamide tablet or oral solution may be taken with or without food. If using oral solution, remind patient to measure and administer the dose using a calibrated measuring device because a household teaspoon or tablespoon may not deliver correct dose.
- Alert patient that the oral solution of lacosamide contains aspartame, a source of phenylalanine that could be harmful to patients with phenylketonuria (PKU).
- Urge family or caregiver to watch patient closely for suicidal tendencies, especially when therapy starts or dosage changes.

- Instruct patient to report any persistent, severe, or unusual signs and symptoms to prescriber immediately. If allergic reaction occurs, counsel patient to seek immediate emergency medical care.
- Caution patient to avoid hazardous activities until drug's CNS effects are known.
- Encourage patient to carry medical identification that indicates her diagnosis and drug therapy.
- Tell women of childbearing age to notify prescriber if pregnancy is suspected or occurs. If pregnancy is confirmed, encourage patient to enroll in the North American Antiepileptic Drug pregnancy registry.

lactulose

Cholac, Constilac, Constulose, Enulose

Class and Category

Pharmacologic class: Disaccharide
Therapeutic: Colonic acidifier
Pregnancy category: B

Indications and Dosages

➤ *To treat constipation*

POWDER, SYRUP

Adults. *Initial:* 10 to 20 g daily, increased as needed. *Maximum:* 40 g daily.

➤ *To prevent and treat hepatic encephalopathy*

POWDER, SYRUP

Adults. *Initial:* 20 to 30 g three times daily or four times daily until two or three soft stools occur daily. *Usual:* 60 to 100 g daily in divided doses. For acute episodes, 20 to 30 g every 2 hr initially to achieve rapid laxative effect and then reduced to usual dosage.

RETENTION ENEMA

Adults. 200 g (300 ml) diluted in 700 ml water or normal saline solution and given every 4 to 6 hr, as needed.

Route	Onset	Peak	Duration
P.O.	24–48 hr	Unknown	Unknown
P.R.	Unknown	Unknown	Unknown

Mechanism of Action

Arrives unchanged in the colon, where it breaks down into lactic acid and small amounts of acetic and formic acids, acidifying fecal contents. Acidification leads to increased osmotic pressure in the colon, which, in turn, increases stool water content and softens stool.

Also, lactulose makes intestinal contents more acidic than blood. This prevents ammonia diffusion from intestine into blood, as occurs in hepatic encephalopathy. The trapped ammonia is converted into ammonia ions and, by lactulose's cathartic effect, is expelled in feces with other nitrogenous wastes.

Contraindications

Hypersensitivity to lactulose or its components, low-galactose diet

Interactions

DRUGS

antacids, antibiotics (especially oral neomycin), other laxatives: Decreased effectiveness of lactulose

Adverse Reactions

ENDO: Hyperglycemia
GI: Abdominal cramps and distention, diarrhea, flatulence
Other: Hypernatremia, hypokalemia hypovolemia

Nursing Considerations

- When giving lactulose by retention enema, use a rectal tube with a balloon to help patient retain enema for 30 to 60 minutes. If not retained for at least 30 minutes, repeat dose. Be sure to deflate balloon and remove rectal tube after completing administration.
- Expect to periodically check serum electrolyte levels of debilitated or elderly patient who uses oral drug longer than 6 months.
- Monitor blood ammonia level in patient with hepatic encephalopathy. Also watch for dehydration, hypernatremia, and hypokalemia when giving higher lactulose doses to treat this condition.
- Monitor diabetic patient for hyperglycemia because lactulose contains galactose and lactose.
- Plan to replace fluids if frequent bowel movements cause hypovolemia.

PATIENT TEACHING

- Advise patient to take lactulose with food or dilute with juice to reduce sweet taste.

- Direct patient not to use other laxatives while taking lactulose.
- Instruct patient to report abdominal distention or severe diarrhea.
- Advise diabetic patient to check blood glucose level often and to report hyperglycemia.
- Instruct patient to increase fluid intake if frequent bowel movements occur.
- Teach patient with chronic constipation the importance of exercising, increasing fiber in diet, and increasing fluid intake.
- Inform patient that because oral lactulose must reach the colon to work, bowel movement may not occur for 24 to 48 hours after taking drug.

lamivudine

3TC (CAN), Epivir, Epivir-HBV

Class and Category

Pharmacologic class: Synthetic nucleoside analogue
Therapeutic class: Antiviral
Pregnancy category: Not classified

Indications and Dosages

➤ *To treat chronic hepatitis B virus (HBV) infection associated with active liver inflammation and evidence of hepatitis B viral replication*

ORAL SOLUTON, TABLETS (EPIVIR-HBV)

Adults. 100 mg once daily.
Children ages 2 to 17. 3 mg/kg once daily. *Maximum:* 100 mg once daily.

➤ *As adjunct to treat human immunodeficiency virus type 1 (HIV-1) infection*

ORAL SOLUTON, TABLETS (EPIVIR)

Adults. 300 mg once daily or 150 mg twice daily.
Children ages 3 months and over. 4 mg/kg

DOSAGE ADJUSTMENT For adults receiving Epivir-HBV, dosage adjustment is as follows: Adults with creatinine clearance between 30 and 49 ml/min, 100 mg first dose, then reduced to 50 mg once daily thereafter. For adults with creatinine clearance between 15 and 29 ml/min, 100 mg first dose, then reduced to 25 mg once daily thereafter. For adults with creatinine clearance between 5 and 14 ml/min, first dose reduced to 35 mg, then reduced to 10 mg once daily thereafter. There is no recommendation for pediatric patients with renal impairment for Epivir-HBV.
For adults receiving Epivir, dosage adjustment is as follows: Adults with creatinine clearance between 30 and 49 ml/min, dosage reduced to 150 mg once daily. For adults with creatinine clearance between 15 and 29 ml/min, 150 mg first dose, then reduced to 100 mg once daily thereafter. For adults with creatinine clearance between 5 and 14 ml/min, 150 mg first dose, then reduced to 50 mg once daily thereafter. For adults with creatinine clearance less than 5 ml/min, 50 mg first dose, then reduced to 25 mg once daily. For pediatric patients with renal impairment taking Epivir, dosage may be reduced or dosing interval increased.

Mechanism of Action

After being phosphorylated to its active metabolite, lamivudine inhibits the DNA- and RNA-dependent polymerase activities of HBV and HIV-1 reverse transcriptases via DNA chain termination after incorporation of the nucleotide analogue into viral DNA. This destroys the activity of the hepatitis B and HIV-1 viruses.

Contraindications

Hypersensitivity to lamivudine or its components

Interactions

DRUGS

None

Adverse Reactions

CNS: Chills, depression, dizziness, fatigue, fever, headache, insomnia, malaise, neuropathy, paresthesia, peripheral neuropathy, sleep disorders, weakness
EENT: Ear, nose, throat infections; nasal congestion or discharge; sore throat; stomatitis
ENDO: Cushingoid appearance, fat redistribution, hyperglycemia
GI: Abdominal pain, anorexia, bilirubin increase, diarrhea, dyspepsia, elevated lipase and liver enzyme levels, **exacerbation of hepatitis posttreatment**, **hepatic decompensation in patient co-infected with HIV-1 and hepatitis C**, **hepatomegaly**

with steatosis, nausea, **pancreatitis**, vomiting
HEME: Anemia, **severe anemias including pure red cell aplasia and neutropenia**, splenomegaly, **thrombocytopenia**
MS: Abdominal cramps, arthralgia, elevated CPK level, musculoskeletal pain, myalgia, **rhabdomyolysis**
RESP: Abnormal breath sounds, cough, wheezing
SKIN: Alopecia, pruritus, rash, urticaria
Other: Anaphylaxis, emergence of resistant HBV infection or HIV-1 infection, immune reconstitution syndrome, **lactic acidosis**, lymphadenopathy

Nursing Considerations

- Be aware that Epivir-HBV oral solution and tablets contain a lower dose of lamivudine than used to treat HIV-1 infection and should not be used to treat patients co-infected with HBV and HIV-1 infections. Patients with unrecognized or untreated HIV infection exposed to Epivir-HBV may develop a rapid emergence of HIV-1 resistance. Make sure appropriate HIV counseling and testing have been done before treatment and periodically during treatment with lamivudine to ensure this does not happen.
- Use extreme caution when administering lamivudine to patient with known risk factors for liver disease.
- Monitor patient throughout treatment for evidence of loss of therapeutic response. Indicators include increasing levels of HBV DNA over time after an initial decline below assay limit, progression of clinical signs or symptoms of hepatic disease and/or worsening of hepatic necroinflammatory findings, or return of persistently elevated ALT levels. These findings may require drug to be discontinued.
- Be aware that a switch to an alternative regimen may be needed for patients in whom serum HBV DNA remains detectable after 24 weeks of treatment to reduce the risk of resistance in patients receiving monotherapy with Epivir-HBV.

WARNING Know that lactic acidosis and severe hepatomegaly with steatosis have occurred with lamivudine therapy, and death has occurred in some patients. Risk factors include presence of obesity, prolonged nucleoside exposure, and being a woman. However, know that lactic acidosis and severe hepatomegaly with steatosis have also occurred in patients with no known risk factors. Expect lamivudine to be discontinued in any patient who develops clinical or laboratory findings suggestive of lactic acidosis or pronounced hepatotoxicity, even in the absence of marked transaminase elevations.

- Monitor patient's ALT and HBV DNA levels during treatment to determine treatment options if viral mutants emerge.
- Monitor patients co-infected with HIV-1 and hepatitis C closely for signs and symptoms of liver dysfunction, because hepatic decompensations, some of which resulted in death, have occurred in patients receiving combination antiretroviral therapy for HIV-1 that included interferon alfa.
- Be aware that immune reconstitution syndrome has occurred in patients treated with combination antiretroviral therapy, including lamivudine. The inflammatory response predisposes susceptible patients to opportunistic infections such as cytomegalovirus, *Mycobacterium avium* infection, *Pneumocystis jiroveci* pneumonia, or tuberculosis. Autoimmune disorders such as Graves' disease, Guillain–Barré syndrome, or polymyositis have also occurred. Report sudden or unusual adverse reactions to prescriber.
- Observe patient for redistribution of body fat, including breast enlargement, central obesity, development of buffalo hump, facial wasting, and peripheral wasting, which may produce a cushingoid-type appearance.
- Expect patient to be closely monitored for at least several months after lamivudine has been discontinued, because exacerbation of hepatitis may occur.

PATIENT TEACHING

- Instruct patient to take lamivudine once daily. If he misses a dose, tell him to take it as soon as he remembers but not to double the next dose or take more than the prescribed dose.
- Advise patient that treatment with lamivudine does not reduce the risk of

transmission of HBV or HIV to others through blood contamination or sexual contact.

- Inform diabetic patient using oral solution that each 2-ml dose contains 4 g of sucrose.
- Tell patient being treated for hepatitis B to report immediately any new or worsening symptoms to prescriber, because emergence of resistant hepatitis B virus may occur or disease may worsen during treatment.
- Instruct patient with hepatitis B on the importance of testing for HIV before therapy begins and then periodically throughout therapy to avoid development of resistance to HIV treatment.
- Warn patient with hepatitis B that acute severe exacerbations of hepatitis B may occur following discontinuation of lamivudine. He should not discontinue drug without prescriber knowledge. Tell patient to report any reappearance of signs and symptoms of hepatitis B.
- Instruct mothers not to breastfeed while receiving lamivudine therapy, as drug is present in human breast milk.
- Warn patient that fat distribution may occur with lamivudine therapy and may alter his appearance.
- Tell women of childbearing age to report a known or suspected pregnancy.

WARNING Alert patient that severe conditions may develop while taking lamivudine. Encourage him to stop taking drug and seek medical attention immediately if he experiences any persistent, severe, or unusual symptoms.

lamotrigine

Lamictal, Lamictal ODT, Lamictal XR

Class and Category

Pharmacologic class: Phenyltriazine
Therapeutic class: Anticonvulsant
Pregnancy category: C

Indications and Dosages

➤ *As adjunct to treat partial seizures; to treat generalized seizures of Lennox–Gastaut syndrome; to treat primary generalized tonic–clonic seizures*

CHEWABLE TABLETS, ORALLY DISINTEGRATING TABLETS, TABLETS

Adults and children age 13 and over taking valproate. 25 mg every other day for 2 wk, followed by 25 mg once daily for 2 wk. Increased by 25 to 50 mg every 1 to 2 wk, if needed. *Maintenance:* 100 to 200 mg daily.

Children ages 2 to 12 taking valproate. 0.15 mg/kg daily as a single dose or in divided doses twice daily for 2 wk and then 0.3 mg/kg daily as single dose or in divided doses twice daily for next 2 wk. Increased by 0.3 mg/kg every 1 to 2 wk, if needed, to reach maintenance dosage. *Maintenance:* 1 to 3 mg/kg daily as single dose or in divided doses twice daily. *Maximum:* 200 mg daily.

Adults and children age 13 and over taking an antiepileptic drug other than carbamazepine, phenobarbital, phenytoin, primidone, or valproate. 25 mg once daily for 2 wk, followed by 50 mg once daily for 2 wk. Increased by 50 mg every 1 to 2 wk, if needed. *Maintenance:* 225 to 375 mg daily in 2 divided doses.

Children ages 2 to 12 taking an antiepileptic drug other than carbamazepine, phenobarbital, phenytoin, primidone, or valproate. 0.3 mg/kg daily in 1 or 2 divided doses for 2 wk; followed by 0.6 mg/kg daily in 2 divided doses for 2 wk. Increased by 0.6 mg/kg daily every 1 to 2 wk, if needed. *Maintenance:* 4.5 to 7.5 mg/kg daily in 2 divided doses. *Maximum:* 300 mg daily.

Adults and children age 13 and over taking carbamazepine, phenobarbital, phenytoin, or primidone but NOT valproate. 50 mg once daily for 2 wk and then 100 mg daily in 2 divided doses for 2 wk. Increased by 100 mg every 1 to 2 wk, if needed. *Maintenance:* 300 to 500 mg daily in 2 divided doses

Children ages 2 to 12 taking carbamazepine, phenobarbital, phenytoin, or primidone but NOT valproate. 0.6 mg/kg daily in 2 divided doses for 2 wk and then 1.2 mg/kg daily in 2 divided doses for 2 wk. Increased by 1.2 mg/kg every 1 to 2 wk, if needed to reach maintenance dosage. *Maintenance:* 5 to 15 mg/kg daily in 2 divided doses. *Maximum:* 400 mg daily in 2 divided doses.

➤ *To treat partial seizures with conversion from carbamazepine, phenobarbital, phenytoin, primidone, or valproate*

CHEWABLE TABLETS, ORALLY DISINTEGRATING TABLETS, TABLETS

Adults and adolescents age 16 and over converting from carbamazepine, phenytoin, phenobarbital, or primidone. 50 mg once daily for 2 wk, followed by 50 mg twice daily for next 2 wk. Increased by 100 mg daily every 1 to 2 wk (while continuing to take carbamazepine, phenobarbital, or primidone), until usual maintenance dosage—500 mg daily in 2 divided doses is achieved. Then carbamazepine, phenobarbital, phenytoin, or primidone dosage tapered in 20% decrements weekly over 4 wk and then discontinued.

Adults and adolescents age 16 and over converting from valproate. 25 mg every other day for 2 wk followed by 25 mg once daily for 2 wk. Then increased by 25 to 50 mg daily every 1 to 2 wk until maintenance dosage of 200 mg daily is achieved. (At this time valproate dosage decreased to 500 mg daily by decrements no greater than 500 mg daily every wk and then maintained at 500 mg daily for 1 wk.) After valproate dosage has been at 500 mg for 1 wk, lamotrigine dosage increased to 300 mg daily while valproate dosage decreased to 250 mg daily for 1 wk. Then lamotrigine dosage increased by 100 mg daily every wk until maintenance dose of 500 mg daily is reached (given in 2 divided doses). Valproate therapy is then discontinued.

E.R. TABLETS

Adults and adolescents age 13 and over converting from carbamazepine, phenobarbital, phenytoin, or primidone. 50 mg once daily for first 2 wk, then increased as follows: 100 mg once daily for wk 3 and 4, then 200 mg once daily for wk 5, then 300 mg once daily for wk 6, then 400 mg once daily for wk 7, and 500 mg for wk 8. Once maintenance dosage of 500 mg daily has been reached, carbamazepine, phenobarbital, phenytoin, or primidone dosage tapered in 20% decrements weekly over 4 wk and then discontinued. Two weeks after carbamazepine, phenobarbital, phenytoin, or primidone has been discontinued, lamotrigine dosage decreased no faster than 100 mg/day each week until monotherapy maintenance dosage of 250 to 300 mg daily has been reached.

Adults and adolescents age 13 and over converting from valproate. 25 mg every other day for 2 wk, then increased as follows: 25 mg once daily for wk 3 and 4, then 50 mg once daily for wk 5, then 100 mg once daily for wk 6, then 150 mg once daily for wk 7, and 200 mg once daily for wk 8, with dosage increased to 250 mg once daily, if needed, for wk 9. Once lamotrigine dosage has reached 150 mg once daily, valproate dosage decreased by decrements no greater than 500 mg/day/wk to 500 mg/day and then maintained for 1 wk, followed by dosage decrease to 250 mg/day for 1 wk and then discontinued.

➤ *To treat partial seizures with conversion from a single antiepileptic drug other than carbamazepine, phenobarbital, phenytoin, primidone, or valproate*

E.R. TABLETS

Adults and adolescents age 13 and over converting from an antiepileptic drug other than carbamazepine, phenobarbital, phenytoin, primidone, or valproate. 25 mg once daily for 2 wk, followed by 50 mg once daily for next 2 wk. Increased to 100 mg once daily for wk 5, followed by 150 mg once daily for wk 6 and 200 mg once daily for wk 7. Further increased by 100 mg once daily at weekly intervals beginning at week 8 and onward until usual maintenance dosage—300 to 400 mg daily—is reached. Once dosage has reached 250 to 300 mg once daily, antiepileptic drug tapered in 20% decrements weekly over 4 wk and then discontinued.

➤ *As adjunct to treat primary generalized tonic-clonic seizures and partial-onset seizures*

E.R. TABLETS

Adults and children age 13 and over taking valproate. 25 mg every other day for 2 wk, followed by 25 mg once daily for 2 wk, followed by 50 mg once daily for 1 wk. Then 100 mg once daily for 1 wk, then 150 mg once daily. Dosage increased further, as needed, but increase not greater than 100 mg weekly. *Maintenance:* 200 to 250 mg once daily.

Adults and children age 13 and over NOT taking carbamazepine,

phenobarbital, phenytoin, primidone, or valproate. 25 mg once daily for 2 wk, followed by 50 mg once daily for 2 wk, followed by 100 mg once daily for 1 wk. Then 150 mg once daily for 1 wk, followed by 200 mg once daily. Dosage increased further, as needed, but increase not greater than 100 mg weekly. *Maintenance:* 300 to 400 mg once daily.
Adults and children age 13 and over taking carbamazepine, phenobarbital, phenytoin, or primidone and NOT taking valproate. 50 mg once daily for 2 wk, followed by 100 mg once daily for 2 wk, followed by 200 mg once daily for 1 wk. Then, 300 mg once daily for 1 wk, followed by 400 mg once daily. Dosage increased further, as needed, but increase not greater than 100 mg weekly. *Maintenance:* 400 to 600 mg once daily.
DOSAGE ADJUSTMENT For women taking estrogen-containing oral contraceptives, maintenance dose may need to be increased gradually by as much as twofold over recommended target maintenance dose. For women discontinuing estrogen-containing oral contraceptives who have been stabilized on lamotrigine prior to discontinuation, maintenance dose may need to be decreased gradually by as much as half. For patient with moderate to severe hepatic impairment without ascites, all dosages decreased by 25%, and for patient with severe hepatic impairment with ascites, all dosages decreased by 50%. For patient with significant renal impairment, maintenance dosage may need to be reduced on individual basis.

➤ *As maintenance therapy for bipolar 1 disorder to delay occurrence of mood episodes (depression, mania, hypomania, mixed episodes)*

CHEWABLE TABLETS, ORALLY DISINTEGRATING TABLETS, TABLETS

Adults not taking carbamazepine, phenobarbital, phenytoin, primidone, rifampin, or valproate. 25 mg once daily for 2 wk, followed by 50 mg once daily for 2 wk, followed by 100 mg once daily for 1 wk, and then increased to 200 mg once daily as maintenance dose. *Maximum:* 200 mg daily.
Adults taking valproate. 25 mg every other day for 2 wk, followed by 25 mg once daily for 2 wk, followed by 50 mg once daily for 1 wk, and then increased to 100 mg once daily as maintenance dose.
Adults taking carbamazepine, phenobarbital, phenytoin, primidone, or rifampin, but not valproate. 50 mg once daily for 2 wk, followed by 100 mg once daily in divided doses for 2 wk, followed by 200 mg once daily in divided doses for 1 wk, then increased to 300 mg daily in divided doses for 1 wk, and then increased to 400 mg daily in divided doses as maintenance dose.
DOSAGE ADJUSTMENT For patient starting or stopping estrogen-containing oral contraceptives, lamotrigine dosage may need to be adjusted on individual basis. For patient with moderate to severe liver impairment without ascites, dosage reduced by 25%. For patient with severe liver impairment with ascites, dosage reduced by 50%.

Route	Onset	Peak	Duration
P.O.	Days to weeks	Unknown	Unknown

Mechanism of Action

May stabilize neuron membranes by blocking their sodium channels and inhibiting release of excitatory neurotransmitters, such as aspartate and glutamate through these channels. By blocking the release of neurotransmitters, lamotrigine inhibits the spread of seizure activity in the brain, reduces seizure frequency and diminishes mood swings.

Contraindications

Hypersensitivity to lamotrigine or its components

Interactions

DRUGS

acetaminophen (long-term use): Possibly decreased blood lamotrigine level
atazanavir/ritonavir, lopinavir/ritonavir, rifampin: Decreased blood lamotrigine level
carbamazepine: Decreased blood lamotrigine level; possibly increased risk of ataxia, blurred vision, diplopia, and dizziness

folate inhibitors such as cotrimoxazole and methotrexate: Increased blood lamotrigine level
oral contraceptives: Decreased blood lamotrigine level during 3 weeks of active hormonal therapy and increased blood lamotrigine level during 1 week of inactive hormonal therapy; possibly reduced effectiveness of oral contraceptives
oxcarbazepine: Possibly increased risk of dizziness, headache, nausea, and somnolence
phenobarbital, phenytoin, primidone: Decreased blood lamotrigine level, possibly increased CNS depression
topiramate: Increased topiramate level
valproic acid: Increased lamotrigine level

ACTIVITIES

alcohol use: Possibly increased CNS depression

Adverse Reactions

CNS: Amnesia, anxiety, **aseptic meningitis**, ataxia, confusion, depression, dizziness, drowsiness, emotional lability, exacerbation of parkinsonian symptoms, fever, headache, **increased seizure activity**, lack of coordination, **suicidal ideation**
CV: Chest pain, vasculitis
EENT: Blurred vision, diplopia, dry mouth, nystagmus
GI: Abdominal pain, anorexia, constipation, diarrhea, esophagitis, **hepatic failure**, **pancreatitis**, vomiting
HEME: Agranulocytosis, anemia, **aplastic or hemolytic anemia**, **disseminated intravascular coagulation (DIC)**, eosinophilia, **hemophagocytic lymphohistiocytosis**, **leukopenia**, **neutropenia**, **pancytopenia**, **severe anemia such as pure red cell aplasia**, **thrombocytopenia**
MS: Rhabdomyolysis
RESP: Apnea
SKIN: Petechiae, photosensitivity, pruritus, rash, **Stevens–Johnson syndrome**, **toxic epidermal necrolysis**
Other: Angioedema, **drug reaction with eosinophilia and systemic symptoms (DRESS)**, flu-like symptoms, lupus-like reaction, lymphadenopathy, progressive immunosuppression

Nursing Considerations

- Use cautiously in patients with illnesses that could affect elimination or metabolism of lamotrigine, such as cardiac hepatic, or renal functional impairment.
- Be aware that the patient may be converted directly from immediate-release lamotrigine to extended-release lamotrigine with the initial dose of extended-release matching the total daily dose of immediate-release lamotrigine. However, monitor effects closely, especially for patient who is receiving an enzyme-inducing agent that may lower plasma levels of lamotrigine on conversion. If drug effectiveness appears to be altered, notify prescriber and expect a dosage adjustment.

WARNING Be aware that lamotrigine may cause potentially life-threatening rash. Notify prescriber at first sign, and expect to discontinue drug. Lamotrigine therapy shouldn't be restarted after rash subsides.

- Monitor patient for adverse reactions, especially suicidal thoughts, at start of therapy and with each dosage increase.

WARNING Monitor patient for hypersensitivity, such as fever, rash, or lymphadenopathy in association with other organ system dysfunction that may be suggestive of DRESS. Although rare, DRESS may be life-threatening. If suspected, notify prescriber immediately and expect lamotrigine to be discontinued.

WARNING Monitor patient closely for signs and symptoms of aseptic meningitis such as fever, headache, nausea, nuchal rigidity, or vomiting. Additional signs and symptoms may include altered consciousness, chills, myalgia, photophobia, rash, and somnolence. These symptoms may occur within 1 day to 1.5 months following the initiation of lamotrigine therapy. Notify prescriber immediately, if suspected, and expect drug to be discontinued.

- Monitor patient for seizure activity during lamotrigine therapy.

WARNING Monitor patient closely for signs and symptoms of hemophagocytic lymphohistiocytosis such as coagulation abnormalities, cytopenias, fever, hepatosplenomegaly, liver dysfunction, lymphadenopathy, neurologic symptoms, and rash that may occur within 8 to 24 days from start of lamotrigine therapy. Be aware that this is a life-threatening condition of extreme systemic inflammation.

- Expect to taper dosage over at least 2 weeks, even for treatment of bipolar disorder to avoid stopping lamotrigine abruptly, which may increase seizure activity.

PATIENT TEACHING

- Advise patient to take lamotrigine exactly as prescribed and not to stop abruptly because seizure activity may increase.
- Instruct patient to seek immediate emergency help or call local poison control center if too much lamotrigine is taken.
- Advise patient to notify prescriber immediately if rash or other symptoms of hypersensitivity, such as a fever or swollen glands, occur.
- Instruct patient to report increased seizure activity, vision changes, and vomiting.

WARNING Inform patient that excessive immune activation may occur with lamotrigine therapy and to immediately report fever, rash, or swollen lymph nodes.

- Caution patient to avoid hazardous activities until drug's CNS effects are known.
- Advise patient to avoid direct sunlight and to wear protective clothing to minimize risk of photosensitivity.
- Instruct patient to wear or carry medical identification stating that she takes lamotrigine.
- Caution patient or caregiver about possibility of suicidal thoughts, especially when therapy begins or dosage changes.

WARNING Advise patient to notify prescriber immediately if she develops any combination of an abnormal sensitivity to light, chills, confusion, drowsiness fever, headache, myalgia, nausea, rash, stiff neck, or vomiting while taking lamotrigine.

- Tell female patient to notify prescriber if she becomes pregnant, is considering pregnancy, or starts or stops an oral hormonal contraceptive or other female hormonal preparation.
- Urge woman who becomes pregnant while taking lamotrigine to enroll in the North American Antiepileptic Drug Pregnancy Registry by calling 1-888-233-2334. Explain that registry is collecting information about safety of antiepileptic drugs during pregnancy.

lansoprazole

Prevacid, Prevacid I.V., Prevacid SoluTab

dexlansoprazole

Dexilant

Class and Category

Pharmacologic class: Proton pump inhibitor
Therapeutic class: Antiulcer
Pregnancy category: B

Indications and Dosages

➤ *To treat duodenal ulcers and maintain healed duodenal ulcers*

DELAYED-RELEASE CAPSULES, DELAYED-RELEASE SUSPENSION, DELAYED-RELEASE ORALLY DISINTEGRATING TABLETS

Adults. 15 mg daily before morning meal for 4 wk. *Maintenance:* 15 mg daily.

➤ *To treat benign gastric ulcers*

DELAYED-RELEASE CAPSULES, DELAYED-RELEASE SUSPENSION, DELAYED-RELEASE ORALLY DISINTEGRATING TABLETS

Adults. 30 mg daily before morning meal for up to 8 wk.

➤ *To treat symptomatic gastroesophageal reflux disease (GERD)*

DELAYED-RELEASE CAPSULES, DELAYED-RELEASE SUSPENSION, DELAYED-RELEASE ORALLY DISINTEGRATING TABLETS

Adults. 15 mg daily before morning meal for up to 8 wk.

➤ *To treat symptomatic nonerosive gastroesophageal reflux disease*

CAPSULES (DEXLANSOPRAZOLE)

Adults. 30 mg once daily for 4 wk.

➤ *To heal all grades of erosive esophagitis*

CAPSULES (DEXLANSOPRAZOLE)

Adults. 60 mg once daily for up to 8 wk.

➤ *To maintain healed erosive esophagitis*

CAPSULES (DEXLANSOPRAZOLE)

Adults. 30 mg once daily.

➤ *To treat erosive esophagitis*

DELAYED-RELEASE CAPSULES, DELAYED-RELEASE SUSPENSION, DELAYED-RELEASE ORALLY DISINTEGRATING TABLETS
Adults. *Initial:* 30 mg daily before morning meal for up to 8 wk. Continued another 8 wk if indicated. *Maintenance:* 15 mg daily.

➤ *To treat erosive esophagitis short-term (up to 7 days) in patients unable to take oral medication*

I.V. INFUSION
Adults. 30 mg daily infused over 30 min for up to 7 days.

➤ *To treat pathological hypersecretory conditions, such as Zollinger–Ellison syndrome*

DELAYED-RELEASE CAPSULES, DELAYED-RELEASE SUSPENSION, DELAYED-RELEASE ORALLY DISINTEGRATING TABLETS
Adults. *Initial:* 60 mg daily before morning meal, increased as needed according to patient's condition. Doses exceeding 120 mg/day administered in divided doses.

➤ *To eradicate* Helicobacter pylori *and reduce risk of duodenal ulcer recurrence*

DELAYED-RELEASE CAPSULES, DELAYED-RELEASE SUSPENSION, DELAYED-RELEASE ORALLY DISINTEGRATING TABLETS
Adults. 30 mg plus 1 g amoxicillin and 500 mg clarithromycin every 12 hr before meals for 10 to 14 days. Or, 30 mg plus 1 g amoxicillin t.i.d. before meals for 14 days.

➤ *To treat symptomatic pediatric gastroesophageal reflux disease*

DELAYED-RELEASE CAPSULES, DELAYED-RELEASE SUSPENSION, DELAYED-RELEASE ORALLY DISINTEGRATING TABLETS
Children ages 12 to 17. 15 mg daily for up to 8 wk.
Children ages 1 to 11 weighing 30 kg (66 lb) or less. 15 mg daily for up to 12 wk.
Children ages 1 to 11 weighing more than 30 kg. 30 mg daily for up to 12 wk.

➤ *To treat symptomatic pediatric erosive esophagitis*

DELAYED-RELEASE CAPSULES, DELAYED-RELEASE SUSPENSION, DELAYED-RELEASE ORALLY DISINTEGRATING TABLETS
Children ages 12 to 17. 30 mg daily for up to 8 wk.
Children ages 1 to 11 weighing 30 kg (66 lb) or less. 15 mg daily for up to 12 wk.
Children ages 1 to 11 weighing more than 30 kg. 30 mg daily for up to 12 wk.

➤ *To treat frequent heartburn*

E.R. CAPSULES (PREVACID 24-HR)
Adults. 15 mg daily for 14 days. May repeat course every 4 months.

DOSAGE ADJUSTMENT For patients with moderate hepatic impairment, dosage reduced.

Route	Onset	Peak	Duration
P.O.	1–3 hr	Unknown	Over 24 hr

Mechanism of Action
Binds to and inactivates the hydrogen-potassium adenosine triphosphate enzyme system (also called the proton pump) in gastric parietal cells. This action blocks the final step of gastric acid production.

Incompatibilities
Don't give any other drugs with parenteral lansoprazole, and dilute only with solutions recommended by manufacturer (sterile water for initial reconstitution and D_5W, lactated Ringer's solution, or normal saline solution for further dilution).

Contraindications
Concurrent therapy with rilpivirine-containing products, hypersensitivity to lansoprazole or its components

Interactions
DRUGS
ampicillin, dasatinib, erlotinib, iron salts, itraconazole, ketoconazole, mycophenolate mofetil, nilotinib, other drugs that depend on low gastric pH for bioavailability: Inhibited absorption of these drugs
antiretrovirals such as atazanavir, nelfinavir, rilpivirine: Possible decreased antiviral effect and increased risk of drug resistance to antiretroviral
digoxin: Increased digoxin absorption with possible toxicity
methotrexate: Possibly elevated methotrexate levels, which may cause toxicity
ritonavir, St. John's wort: Decreased plasma levels of dexlansoprazole
saquinavir: Possibly increased toxicity of saquinavir
sucralfate: Delayed lansoprazole absorption
tacrolimus: Possibly increased blood tacrolimus levels
theophylline: Slightly decreased blood theophylline level

voriconazole: Increased exposure of dexlansoprazole possibly causing toxicity
warfarin: Increased INR and PT with possibly increased risk of serious bleeding

ACTIVITIES

alcohol: Possibly decreased effectiveness of delayed-release form of drug

Adverse Reactions

CNS: CVA, dizziness, headache, transient ischemic attack
EENT: Blurred vision, deafness, oral edema oropharyngeal pain, **pharyngeal edema, throat tightness**
GI: Abdominal pain, anorexia, ***Clostridium difficile*-associated diarrhea**, diarrhea, elevated liver enzymes, flatulence, fundic gland polyps, **hepatitis, hepatotoxicity**, increased appetite, nausea, **pancreatitis**, vomiting
GU: Acute renal failure, interstitial nephritis, urine retention
HEME: Agranulocytosis, aplastic anemia, decreased hemoglobin, **hemolytic anemia, idiopathic thrombocytopenic purpura, leukopenia, neutropenia, pancytopenia, thrombocytopenia, thrombotic thrombocytopenic purpura**
MS: Arthralgia, bone fracture, bursitis, myositis
RESP: Upper respiratory tract infection
SKIN: Cutaneous lupus erythematosus, **erythema multiforme, exfoliative dermatitis**, leucocytoclastic vasculitis, pruritus, rash, **Stevens–Johnson syndrome, toxic epidermal necrolysis**
Other: Anaphylaxis, angioedema, hyperkalemia, hypomagnesemia, hyponatremia, injection-site reaction, systemic lupus erythematosus, vitamin B_{12} deficiency

Nursing Considerations

- Give lansoprazole before meals. Dexlansoprazole may be taken with or without food. Antacids may be given as well, if needed.
- Keep in mind that if patient is prescribed capsules and has trouble swallowing them, open and sprinkle granules on applesauce, cottage cheese, Ensure pudding, strained pears, or yogurt. Don't crush granules. Have patient swallow mixture immediately. Or, empty granules into 2 ounces apple, orange, or tomato juice; mix quickly, and have patient swallow immediately. Then add 2 or more ounces of juice to glass and have patient drink immediately to ensure full dose.
- For delayed-release orally disintegrating tablets, place tablet on patient's tongue and let it dissolve, with or without water, until patient can swallow particles.
- For patient with nasogastric tube, don't use oral suspension. Instead use capsules or orally disintegrating tablets. For capsule form, open capsule, mix granules in 40 ml apple juice only, and inject through tube. Then flush tube with apple juice only. For disintegrating tablets, place tablet in syringe and draw up 4 ml (for 15-mg tablet) or 8 ml (for 30-mg tablet) of water. Shake gently, and inject through tube within 15 minutes. Then refill syringe with 5 ml of water, shake gently, and inject through tube.
- For delayed-release oral suspension, empty packet contents into a container with 2 tablespoons water (no other liquids or foods), stir well, and have patient drink immediately. If any particles remain in container, add more water, stir, and have patient drink again immediately.
- Reconstitute parenteral form by injecting 5 ml sterile water into 30-mg drug vial. Mix gently until powder dissolves. Use within 1 hour. After reconstitution, dilute with 50 ml D_5W lactated Ringer's solution, or normal saline solution. Give within 12 hours if mixed with D_5W or 24 hours if mixed with lactated Ringer's solution or normal saline solution.
- Give parenteral drug with a filter following manufacturer's guidelines. Change filter every 24 hours. Give as I.V. infusion over 30 minutes. Flush line with D_5W lactated Ringer's solution, or normal saline solution before and after giving lansoprazole.
- Expect to give lansoprazole with antibiotics when used to eradicate *H. pylori* because decreased gastric acid secretion helps antibiotics eradicate *H. pylori.*
- Be aware that diarrhea from *C. difficile* infection can occur with or without concurrent antibiotics when lansoprazole is used. If *C. difficile*-associated diarrhea occurs, notify prescriber and expect to withhold drug and treat with an antibiotic

effective against *C. difficile,* electrolytes, fluids, and protein.

- Monitor patient for bone fracture, especially in patients receiving multiple daily doses for more than a year, because proton pump inhibitors, such as lansoprazole, increase risk for osteoporosis-related fractures of the hip, spine, or wrist.
- Monitor the patient, especially the patient on long-term therapy for hypomagnesemia. If patient is to remain on lansoprazole long term, expect to monitor the patient's serum magnesium level, as ordered, and if level becomes low, anticipate that magnesium replacement therapy and lansoprazole will be discontinued.
- Monitor patient for renal dysfunction because drug may cause acute interstitial nephritis at any point during lansoprazole therapy. Expect drug to be discontinued if it occurs.
- Be aware that drug may cause false-positive results in diagnostic investigations for neuroendocrine tumors. Expect drug to be temporarily discontinued for at least 14 days before testing is done. Also know that drug can cause a hyper-response in gastrin secretion in response to secretin stimulation test. Expect lansoprazole to be temporarily withheld at least 30 days before assessment is done. Be aware that false-positive urine screening tests for tetrahydrocannabinol may occur during lansoprazole therapy.
- Monitor patient for cutaneous and systemic lupus erythematosus either as new onset or exacerbation of existing disorder. Know that cutaneous lupus erythematosus occurs more commonly. Expect lansoprazole to be discontinued if present.
- Be aware that long-term use (especially more than one year) of lansoprazole increases risk for the development of fundic gland polyps. Be aware that the drug should be given for the shortest duration possible for the condition being treated.

PATIENT TEACHING

- Urge patient to take lansoprazole exactly as prescribed, usually before a meal (preferably breakfast) to decrease gastric acid output. Tell patient taking dexlansoprazole that drug may be taken with or without food.
- Tell patient who is having trouble swallowing dexlansoprazole capsules to open them and sprinkle granules on 1 tablespoon of applesauce and swallow immediately. If patient has trouble swallowing lansoprazole capsules, tell her to open them and sprinkle granules on applesauce, cottage cheese, Ensure pudding, strained pears, or yogurt and to swallow immediately without chewing. Or, she may empty lansoprazole granules into 2 ounces of apple, orange, or tomato juice, mix quickly, and swallow immediately. Tell her to refill glass with 2 or more ounces of juice and drink immediately to ensure a full dose.
- Tell patient prescribed delayed-release orally disintegrating tablets to place tablet on tongue, let it dissolve, and then swallow particles with or without water. Also tell her not to break, cut, or chew the tablets.
- Tell patient prescribed delayed-release oral suspension to empty contents of packet into a container with 2 tablespoons of water (no other liquids or foods), stir well, and drink immediately. If particles remain in container, she should add water, stir, and drink immediately.
- Warn patient to avoid alcoholic beverages when taking dexlansoprazole form of drug.
- Inform patient that she may take antacids with lansoprazole.
- Tell patient to stop taking drug and report to prescriber blood in urine or decrease in urination, joint pain that is new or worsening, or a rash on arms or cheeks that gets worse in the sun.
- Advise patient to report severe headache, or worsening of symptoms immediately to prescriber.
- Urge patient to tell prescriber about diarrhea that's severe or lasts longer than 3 days. Remind patient that bloody or watery stools can occur 2 or more months after antibiotic therapy and can be serious, requiring prompt treatment.
- Alert women of childbearing age that lansoprazole may pose a potential risk for fetal harm and to notify prescriber if pregnancy is suspected or known.
- Advise mothers wishing to breastfeed while taking lansoprazole to check with prescriber first.

lanthanum carbonate

Fosrenol

Class and Category

Pharmacologic class: Rare earth element
Therapeutic class: Phosphate binder
Pregnancy category: C

Indications and Dosages

➤ *To reduce serum phosphate levels in patients with end-stage renal disease*

ORAL POWDER, TABLETS (CHEWABLE)

Adults. *Initial:* 500 mg three times daily with meals or immediately after meals; increased, as needed, by 750 mg daily every 2 to 3 wk until acceptable serum phosphate level is reached.

Contraindications

Bowel obstruction, fecal impaction, hypersensitivity to lanthanum carbonate or any of its components, hypophosphatemia, ileus

Interactions

DRUGS

ACE inhibitors; antibiotics such as ampicillin, fluoroquinolones or tetracyclines; antimalarials; drugs with narrow therapeutic range; statins; thyroid hormones: Possibly reduced bioavailability with these drugs
calcium channel blockers: Increased risk of adverse gastrointestinal effects

Adverse Reactions

CNS: Headache
CV: Hypotension
EENT: Rhinitis, tooth injury while chewing tablet
GI: Abdominal pain, constipation, diarrhea, dyspepsia, fecal impaction, **GI obstruction or perforation**, ileus, nausea, subileus, vomiting
GU: Dialysis graft occlusion
RESP: Bronchitis
SKIN: Pruritus, rash, urticaria
Other: Hypercalcemia, **hypocalcemia**, **hypophosphatemia**

Mechanism of Action

During digestion, phosphate is released into the upper GI tract (below left) and absorbed into the bloodstream, increasing serum phosphate levels. In patients with end-stage renal disease, however, inefficient phosphate clearance from the blood leads to abnormally elevated levels.

Lanthanum dissociates in the upper GI tract, releasing ions that attach to unbound phosphate to form an insoluble complex (below right). Unabsorbed into the bloodstream, these altered phosphate molecules can't elevate the patient's serum phosphate level.

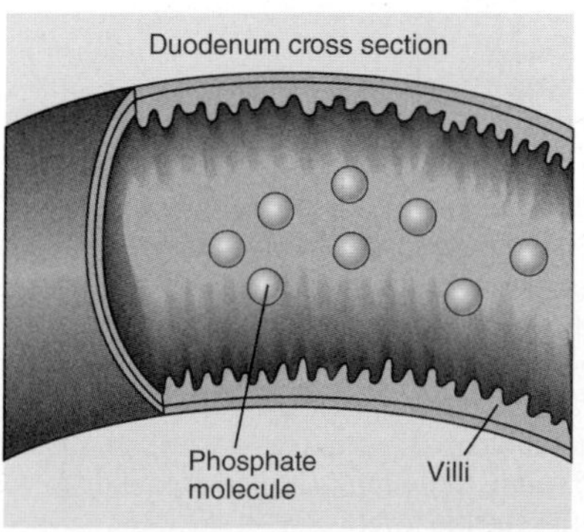

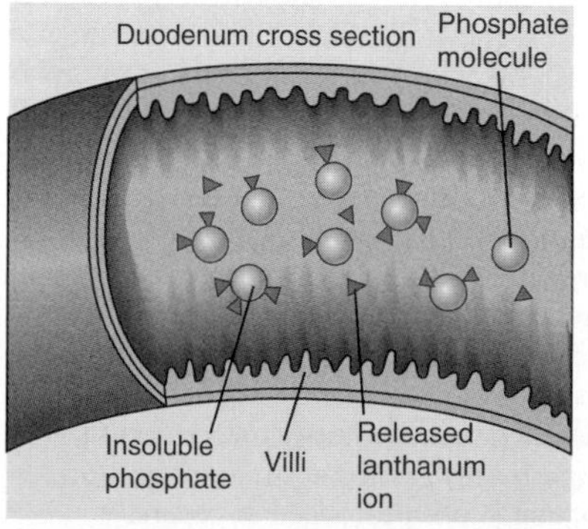

Nursing Considerations

- Use lanthanum carbonate cautiously in patients with acute peptic ulcer, bowel obstruction, Crohn's disease, or ulcerative colitis because drug effects are unknown in these patients.
- Monitor the patient's serum phosphate levels, as ordered, especially during dosage adjustment, to determine effectiveness of lanthanum carbonate therapy. Serum phosphate levels should fall below 6 mg/dl.
- Monitor patient closely for signs and symptoms of bowel obstruction, fecal impaction, or ileus, especially the patient with a history of colon cancer, gastrointestinal surgery, or hypomotility disorders, as well as the patient receiving calcium channel blockers. Notify prescriber, if present, because these gastrointestinal adverse effects may become serious enough to require hospitalization or surgery.
- Administer tetracyclines and drugs with a narrow therapeutic range at least 1 hour before or 3 hours after lanthanum administration; quinolone antibiotics at least 1 hour before or 4 hours after lanthanum administration; and levothyroxine at least 2 hours before or 2 hours after lanthanum administration to prevent a reduction in bioavailability.

PATIENT TEACHING

- Instruct patient to take lanthanum carbonate with or immediately after meals.
- Advise patient to chew each tablet thoroughly before swallowing. If patient has trouble chewing tablets, tell her she may crush them.
- Tell patient to sprinkle the prescribed oral powder form on a small quantity of applesauce or other similar foods and consume immediately.
- Urge patient to take drug exactly as prescribed, and explain that it may take weeks to reach a desired serum phosphate level.
- Advise patient to notify prescriber if she experiences gastrointestinal discomfort that becomes prolonged or severe.

leflunomide

Arava

Class and Category

Pharmacologic class: Pyrimidine synthesis inhibitor
Therapeutic class: Antirheumatic
Pregnancy category: X

Indications and Dosages

➤ *To relieve symptoms of active rheumatoid arthritis, improve physical function and slow disease progression*

TABLETS

Adults who are at low risk for hepatotoxicity and myelosuppression. *Loading:* 100 mg daily for 3 days, followed by 20 mg daily. *Maximum:* 20 mg/day.
Adults at high risk for hepatotoxicity or myelosuppression. 20 mg daily without a loading dose. *Maximum:* 20 mg/day.
DOSAGE ADJUSTMENT Dosage reduced to 10 mg daily if poorly tolerated.

Mechanism of Action

Inhibits dihydroorotate dehydrogenase, the enzyme in autoimmune process that leads to rheumatoid arthritis. With this action, leflunomide relieves inflammation and prevents alteration of the autoimmune process.

Contraindications

Hypersensitivity to leflunomide, teriflunomide, or their components; pregnancy

Interactions

DRUGS

activated charcoal, cholestyramine: Decreased blood leflunomide level
live-virus vaccines: Possibly adverse reactions to vaccines caused by leflunomide-induced immunosuppression
methotrexate: Risk of hepatotoxicity
NSAIDs: Possibly impaired NSAID metabolism
rifampin, tolbutamide: Increased blood leflunomide level

Adverse Reactions

CNS: Anxiety, dizziness, drowsiness, fatigue, fever, headache, paresthesia, peripheral neuropathy
CV: Chest pain, hypertension, palpitations, tachycardia, vasculitis
EENT: Blurred vision, conjunctivitis, dry mouth, epistaxis, mouth ulcers, pharyngitis, rhinitis, sinusitis
GI: Abdominal pain, **acute hepatic necrosis**, cholestasis, colitis, constipation, diarrhea, elevated liver enzymes, flatulence, gastritis, gastroenteritis, **hepatic injury or failure**, **hepatitis**, jaundice, nausea, **pancreatitis**, vomiting
GU: Hypophosphaturia, UTI
HEME: Agranulocytosis, anemia, **leukopenia**, **neutropenia**, **pancytopenia**, **thrombocytopenia**
MS: Back pain, synovitis, tendinitis
RESP: Asthma, bronchitis, dyspnea, **interstitial lung disease**, **pulmonary fibrosis or hypertension**, respiratory tract infection
SKIN: Alopecia (transient), cutaneous lupus erythematosus, cutaneous necrotizing vasculitis, **erythema multiforme**, erythematous rash, pruritus, pustular psoriasis, **Stevens–Johnson syndrome**, **toxic epidermal necrolysis**, urticaria, worsening psoriasis
Other: Angioedema, **drug reaction with eosinophilia and systemic symptoms (DRESS)**, opportunistic infections, **sepsis**, weight loss

Nursing Considerations

- Know that leflunomide isn't recommended for patients with severe immunodeficiency, or severe, uncontrolled infections because of its immunosuppressant effect. It is also not recommended for patients with liver disease or those with a serum alanine aminotransferase level greater than two times the upper level normal prior to initiation of therapy because drug may worsen liver dysfunction.
- Use cautiously in patients who are over 60 years of age, in patients taking concomitant neurotoxic drugs, or in patients with diabetes because of an increased risk of developing peripheral neuropathy. If peripheral neuropathy occurs during leflunomide therapy, notify prescriber and expect drug to be discontinued and possibly cholestyramine washout to be ordered.
- Test patient for latent tuberculosis before starting leflunomide, as ordered. If positive, expect standard medical treatment to be given before leflunomide therapy starts.
- Ensure that women of childbearing age have a negative pregnancy test result prior to starting leflunomide therapy.
- Obtain baseline blood pressure before starting leflunomide, and monitor periodically thereafter because drug may cause hypertension.
- Know that patients at high risk for drug-associated hepatotoxicity are those who are taking concomitant methotrexate. Patients at high risk for drug-associated myelosuppression are those who are taking concomitant immunosuppressants.
- Assess liver enzyme (ALT and AST) levels at start of therapy, monthly during first 6 months, and if stable, every 6 to 8 weeks thereafter, as ordered. If levels become elevated greater than threefold upper level normal, notify prescriber and expect leflunomide therapy to be withheld until underlying cause is determined. If the elevation is thought to be leflunomide induced, expect to start cholestyramine washout, as ordered, and monitor liver test weekly until normalized. If another cause is found for the elevation, expect to resume leflunomide therapy.
- Obtain platelet count, hemoglobin or hematocrit, and WBC count at start of therapy and every 4 to 8 weeks thereafter, as ordered.
- Notify prescriber if patient develops serious infection because drug may need to be interrupted and charcoal or cholestyramine given to eliminate drug rapidly.

WARNING Monitor patient's respiratory function closely because drug may cause interstitial lung disease that could become life-threatening. If patient develops a cough and dyspnea, notify prescriber; drug will need to be stopped, and patient may need charcoal or cholestyramine to eliminate drug rapidly.

WARNING Assess patient's skin regularly for evidence of serious skin reactions. If present, notify prescriber, as drug will need to be discontinued, and patient may need charcoal or cholestyramine to eliminate drug rapidly.

PATIENT TEACHING

- Advise patient that leflunomide doesn't cure arthritis but may relieve its symptoms and improve physical function.
- Inform patient that reversible hair loss may occur.
- Caution woman of childbearing potential not to become pregnant while taking drug because of the high risk of birth defects.
- Instruct patient to report signs of hepatotoxicity, such as mouth ulcers, unusual bleeding or bruising, and yellow skin or eyes.
- Tell patient to report signs of respiratory dysfunction, such as cough and dyspnea, and signs of persistent or serious skin reactions.
- Advise patient to avoid live vaccines during leflunomide therapy.
- Instruct patient to notify prescriber if she develops an infection.

lesinurad

Zurampic

Class and Category

Pharmacologic class: Uric acid transporter 1 inhibitor
Therapeutic class: Antigout
Pregnancy category: Not classified

Indications and Dosages

➤ *Adjunct to treat hyperuricemia associated with gout in patients who have not achieved target serum uric acid levels with a xanthine oxidase inhibitor alone*

TABLETS

Adults. 200 mg once daily in the morning with a meal and coadministered with a xanthine oxidase inhibitor such as allopurinol or febuxostat.

Mechanism of Action

Reduces serum uric acid levels by inhibiting the function of transporter proteins involved in uric acid reabsorption in the kidney. This increases renal clearance and excretion of uric acid, which lowers serum uric acid level in the body.

Contraindications

Dialysis, end-stage renal disease, hypersensitivity to lesinurad or its components, kidney transplant recipients, Lesch–Nyhan syndrome, severe renal impairment (creatinine clearance less than 30 ml/min), tumor lysis syndrome

Interactions

DRUGS

amlodipine, antihypertensives which are CYP3A substrates, HMG-CoA reductase inhibitors, sildenafil: Possibly reduced plasma concentrations of these drugs.
aspirin above 325 mg daily: Possibly decreased effectiveness of lesinurad
CYP2C9 inducers such as carbamazepine, rifampin: Decreased effectiveness of lesinurad
CYP2C9 inhibitors such as amiodarone, fluconazole: Increased lesinurad exposure with increased risk of adverse reactions
hormonal contraceptives: Possibly decreased effectiveness of the contraceptive regardless of the form used to administer it
valproic acid: Possibly interference with lesinurad metabolism

Adverse Reactions

CNS: CVA, headache
CV: MI
GI: GI reflux disease
GU: Acute or chronic renal failure, elevated serum creatinine level, nephrolithiasis
Other: Flu-like symptoms, gout flare

Nursing Considerations

- Be aware that lesinurad should not be given to a patient who is taking less than 300 mg of allopurinol daily or less than 200 mg of allopurinol daily who has an estimated creatinine clearance less than 60 ml/min.

- Know that lesinurad should not be given to patients who have a creatinine clearance less than 45 ml/min.
- Use cautiously in patients who are CYP2C9 poor metabolizers because lesinurad exposure is increased possibly increasing risk of adverse reactions.
- Assess patient's renal function, as ordered, prior to starting lesinurad therapy and periodically thereafter by monitoring serum creatinine levels, as ordered. Know that frequency of monitoring should be increased in patients with a serum creatinine elevation 1.5 to 2 times the pretreatment value or in patients who have a decline in creatinine clearance below 60 ml/min. Expect drug therapy to be interrupted if serum creatinine level becomes elevated above two times the pretreatment value or the patient experiences symptoms that may indicate acute uric acid nephropathy such as flank pain, nausea, or vomiting. Expect drug to be discontinued if creatinine clearance persistently falls below 45 ml/min during treatment or no other explanation is found for serum creatinine abnormalities.
- Expect to withhold lesinurad therapy, as ordered, if the treatment with the prescribed xanthine oxidase inhibitor is interrupted because of an increased risk of serious renal dysfunction.
- Monitor patient for gout flares after lesinurad therapy is begun because of changing serum uric acid levels resulting in the mobilization of urate from tissue deposits. Institute flare prophylaxis, as ordered, when lesinurad therapy begins. If a gout flare occurs during therapy, know that lesinurad is not usually discontinued but the gout flare is managed concurrently.
- Monitor patient closely for adverse cardiovascular reactions because lesinurad therapy has caused serious effects such as myocardial infarctions or strokes.

PATIENT TEACHING

- Instruct patient to take lesinurad with food and water at the same time as his morning dose of prescribed xanthine oxidase inhibitor.
- Stress importance of staying well hydrated by drinking at least 2 liters of fluid daily.
- Tell patient that if for any reason his prescribed xanthine oxidase inhibitor therapy is discontinued, he should consult his prescriber and expect to discontinue taking lesinurad also.
- Teach patient that if he should miss a dose of lesinurad, he should not take it later in the day but wait to take his normal dose the next day. The dose should never be doubled.
- Alert patient that he will need periodic blood tests to monitor his kidney function while taking lesinurad.
- Warn patient that a gout flare up may occur during lesinurad so he should be compliant with taking gout flare prophylaxis medication. If a gout flare should occur, tell him to notify his prescriber but not to stop taking lesinurad.

letermovir

Prevymis

Class and Category

Pharmacologic class: CMV DNA terminase complex inhibitor
Therapeutic class: Antiviral
Pregnancy category: Not classified

Indications and Dosages

➤ *To prevent cytomegalovirus (CMV) infection and disease in CMV-seropositive recipients of an allogenic hematopoietic stem cell transplant*

I.V. INFUSION, TABLETS

Adults. 480 mg once daily initiated between day 0 and day 28 post transplantation and continued through day 100 post-transplantation. Infusion should be administered at a constant rate over 1 hr.

DOSAGE ADJUSTMENT For patients taking concurrent therapy with cyclosporine, dosage deceased to 240 mg once daily. If cyclosporine is discontinued, dosage resumed at 450 mg once daily. If cyclosporine dosing is interrupted due to high cyclosporine levels, no dose adjustment is needed.

Mechanism of Action

Inhibits the CMV DNA terminase complex, which is required for viral DNA processing and packaging. This affects the production of proper unit length genomes and interferes with virion maturation to produce the antiviral effects.

Incompatibilities

Don't administer through the same cannula or intravenous line or with any of the following drugs: amiodarone, amphotericin B (liposomal), aztreonam, cefepime, ciprofloxacin, cyclosporine, diltiazem, filgrastim, gentamicin, levofloxacin, linezolid, lorazepam, midazolam, mycophenolate mofetil, ondansetron, or palonosetron. Don't administer letermovir using a polyurethane-containing IV administration set tubing. Use only manufacturer-recommended catheters, infusion sets, IV bags, or plasticizers.

Contraindications

Concurrent therapy with ergot alkaloids, pimozide, or with pitavastatin or simvastatin if cyclosporine is also given; hypersensitivity to letermovir or its components

Interactions

DRUGS

alfentanil, amiodarone, atorvastatin, fentanyl, fluvastatin, glyburide, lovastatin, midazolam, OATP1B1/3 transporters, pravastatin, quinidine, repaglinide, rosiglitazone, rosuvastatin, sirolimus, tacrolimus: Increased plasma concentration of these drugs with possible increase in adverse reactions

cyclosporine: Increased plasma levels of both cyclosporine and letermovir with increased risk of adverse reactions

ergot alkaloids such as dihydroergotamine, ergotamine: Increased risk of ergotism

OATP1B1/3 transporters inhibitors: Possibly increased plasma letermovir level

omeprazole, pantoprazole, phenytoin, voriconazole, warfarin: Decreased plasma concentrations of these drugs with possible decrease in effectiveness

pimozide: Increased plasma concentration of pimozide with increased risk of QT prolongation and torsades de pointes

pitavastatin, simvastatin: Increased plasma concentrations of these drugs and increased risk of myopathy or rhabdomyolysis

rifampin: Decreased letermovir concentration with possible decreased effectiveness

Adverse Reactions

CNS: Fatigue, headache

CV: **Atrial fibrillation**, peripheral edema, tachycardia

GI: Abdominal pain, diarrhea, nausea, vomiting

GU: Decreased serum creatinine level

HEME: Anemia, **neutropenia, thrombocytopenia**

RESP: Cough, dyspnea

Other: **Hypersensitivity reactions**

Nursing Considerations

- Know that tablet and parenteral formulations may be used interchangeably and no dosage adjustment is necessary when switching formulations. However, expect to administer letermovir intravenously only in patients unable to take drug orally, and be aware that route should be switched as soon as patient is able to take oral medication.
- Dilute parenteral formulation of letermovir by adding one single-dose vial to a 250-ml prefilled IV bag containing either 0.9% sodium chloride injection, USP, or 5% Dextrose Injection, USP, and mix bag gently. Do not shake. Once diluted, solution should be clear and colorless to yellow. Diluted solution is stable for up to 24 hours at room temperature or up to 48 hours under refrigeration. These times include storage of the diluted solution in the intravenous bag through the duration of infusion, which is 1 hour.
- Know that only compatible IV bags and infusion sets should be used. See manufacturer list of approved materials in package insert. Be aware that letermovir should not be administered via a polyurethane-containing IV administration set tubing.
- Administer the entire contents of the intravenous bag by intravenous infusion

via a central venous line or peripheral catheter at a constant rate over 1 hour.

- Monitor patient for drug interactions, as letermovir interacts with many drugs that may increase risk of adverse reactions or reduce therapeutic effect of letermovir or the concomitant drug.

PATIENT TEACHING

- Instruct patient that it is important not to miss or skip doses and to take letermovir for the duration that it is prescribed. If a dose is missed, tell patient to take it as soon as it is remembered. If she does not remember until it is time for the next dose, tell patient to skip the missed dose and go back to the regular schedule. Tell her never to double the dose or take more than prescribed.
- Advise patient to store the tablets in the original package until use.
- Inform patient that letermovir interacts with many drugs. Advise patient to tell prescriber of any drug taken—even over-the-counter drugs and herbal preparations—before using them.
- Tell patient that if an allergic reaction occurs, she should seek immediate emergency attention.

leuprolide acetate

Eligard, Lupron, Lupron Depot, Lupron Depot-3 Month 11.25 mg, Lupron Depot-3 Month 22.5 mg, Lupron Depot-4 Month 30 mg, Lupron Depot-6 Month 45 mg, Lupron Depot-Ped-1 Month, Lupron Depot-Ped-3 Month

Class and Category

Pharmacologic class: Gonadoptropin-releasing hormone analogue
Therapeutic class: Antineoplastic, gonadotropin inhibitor
Pregnancy category: X

Indications and Dosages

➤ *To provide palliative treatment of advanced prostate cancer*

SUBCUTANEOUS INJECTION (ELIGARD)
Adults. 7.5 mg/mo, 22.5 mg every 3 mo, 30 mg every 4 mo, or 45 mg every 6 mo.

SUBCUTANEOUS INJECTION (LUPRON)
Adults. 1 mg daily.

I.M. INJECTION (LUPRON, LUPRON DEPOT-3 MONTH, LUPRON DEPOT-4 MONTH, LUPRON DEPOT-6 MONTH)
Adults. 7.5 mg/mo, 22.5 mg every 3 mo, 30 mg every 4 mo, or 45 mg every 6 mo.

➤ *To treat central precocious puberty*

I.M. INJECTION (LUPRON DEPOT-PED-1 MONTH)
Children weighing more than 37.5 kg (83 lb). 15 mg every 4 wk. *Maximum:* 15 mg every 4 wk.
Children weighing 26 to 37.5 kg (57 to 83 lb). *Initial:* 11.25 mg every 4 wk. Dosage increased as needed to next available dose at next monthly injection. *Maximum:* 15 mg every 4 wk.
Children weighing 25 kg (55 lb) or less. *Initial:* 7.5 mg every 4 wk. Dosage increased as needed to next available dose at next monthly injection. *Maximum:* 15 mg every 4 wk.

I.M. INJECTION (LUPRON DEPOT-PED-3 MONTH)
Children age 2 and over. 11.25 or 30 mg once every 3 mo (dose not based on weight).

SUBCUTANEOUS INJECTION (LEUPROLIDE ACETATE INJECTION)
Children. 50 mcg/kg daily. Dosage increased in increments of 10 mcg/kg daily, as needed.

➤ *To treat endometriosis*

I.M. INJECTION (LUPRON DEPOT, LUPRON DEPOT-3 MONTH)
Adults. 3.75 mg every mo or 11.25 mg every 3 mo for up to 6 mo. *Maximum:* 22.5 mg total dose.

➤ *As adjunct to treat anemia due to uterine leiomyomas*

I.M. INJECTION (LUPRON DEPOT, LUPRON DEPOT-3 MONTH)
Adults. 3.75 mg every mo up to 3 mo or 11.25 mg single dose. *Maximum:* 11.25 mg total dose.

Route	Onset	Peak	Duration
I.M., SubQ*	1 wk	Unknown	4–12 wk after therapy
I.M., SubQ†	2–4 wk	After 1–2 mo	60–90 days after therapy

* Gonadotropin inhibitor.
†Antiendometrionic, antineoplastic.

Mechanism of Action

After stimulating follicle-stimulating hormone (FSH) and luteinizing hormone (LH), continuous leuprolide therapy suppresses secretion of gonadotropin-releasing hormone, decreasing estradiol and testosterone levels. In children with central precocious puberty, this stops menses and reproductive organ development.

In adult men, continuous suppression decreases testosterone levels and causes pharmacologic castration, which slows the activity of prostatic neoplastic cells. In women with endometriosis or uterine leiomyomas, leuprolide suppresses ovarian function, inactivating endometrial tissues and resulting in amenorrhea.

Contraindications

Women and children (leuprolide acetate injectable suspension); hypersensitivity to benzyl alcohol, gonadorelin, and gonadotropin-releasing hormone analogues, including leuprolide, and their components; pregnancy; undiagnosed abnormal vaginal bleeding

Adverse Reactions

CNS: Aggression, anger, anxiety, **CVA**, depression, dizziness, emotional lability, fatigue, fever, headache, hyperkinesia, insomnia, lethargy, malaise, memory loss, mood changes, nervousness (adult women), paresthesia, paralysis (from spinal fracture), peripheral neuropathy, rigors, **seizures**, somnolence, **suicidal ideation**, syncope, transient ischemic attacks, weakness
CV: Arrhythmias, **bradycardia**, **deep vein thrombosis**, edema, hypertension, **hypotension**, palpitations, peripheral vascular disorder, **prolonged QT interval**, vasodilation; angina, **MI**, thrombophlebitis (adult men)
EENT: Blurred vision, decreased vision, epistaxis, gingivitis, hearing disorder, pharyngitis, rhinitis, sinusitis
ENDO: Amenorrhea, androgenic effects in women, breast tenderness or swelling, decreased testicle size, goiter, growth retardation, gynecomastia, hot flashes, hyperglycemia, **pituitary apoplexy**
GI: Colitis, constipation in adult men, dyspepsia, dysphagia, gastroenteritis, **hepatic dysfunction**, increased appetite, nausea, vomiting
GU: Bladder spasm, cervix disorder, **cervical neoplasm**, decreased libido, decreased penis size, dysmenorrhea and other menstrual disorders, dysuria, endometriosis flare-up, impotence, incontinence, nocturia, **prostate cancer flare-up**, prostate pain, urinary incontinence, uterine bleeding, vaginal discharge in girls, vaginitis
HEME: Leukopenia, purpura
MS: Arthralgia, body pain in children, bone density loss, bone or limb pain, fibromyalgia, joint disorder, myalgia, myopathy, spinal fracture, tenosynovitis
RESP: Asthmatic attack, dyspnea, **interstitial lung disease**, **pulmonary embolism**
SKIN: Alopecia, clamminess, hirsutism, leukoderma, nail disorder, night sweats, photosensitivity, rash, skin hypertrophy, urticaria
Other: Aggravation of preexisting tumor; **anaphylaxis**; elevated uric acid; flu-like symptoms; infection; injection-site abscess, burning, edema, induration, itching, pain, or redness; **tumor flare**; weight gain

Nursing Considerations

- Use cautiously in patients at risk for prolonged QT interval, such as in the presence of congenital long QT syndrome, congestive heart failure, or frequent electrolyte abnormalities, and in patients taking drugs that may prolong the QT interval. Know that electrolyte abnormalities should be corrected, as ordered, prior to therapy beginning. Monitor patient's electrocardiogram and electrolytes regularly throughout therapy, as ordered. Notify prescriber of any abnormalities.
- Let drug come to room temperature before using. Reconstitute leuprolide acetate depot suspension with diluent provided by manufacturer. Add diluent to powder for suspension and thoroughly shake vials to

disperse particles into a uniform milky suspension. Use within 30 minutes after mixing, and discard any unused portion. If using a prefilled dual-chamber syringe, follow manufacturer's instructions to release diluent into chamber containing powder. Shake gently after diluted to disperse particles evenly in solution. No dilution or reconstitution is needed for leuprolide acetate injection for subcutaneous administration. Rotate injection sites.

WARNING **Know that leuprolide acetate for injectable suspension (Eligard) is approved only for use in men for palliative treatment of prostate cancer. Use provided syringes and delivery system, and read and follow instructions carefully to ensure proper mixing of product; shaking alone is inadequate to mix it.**

WARNING **Be aware that life-threatening hypersensitivity reactions such as anaphylaxis and asthmatic attacks have occurred with leuprolide therapy. Patients at higher risk for an asthma attack include those with a preexisting history of asthma, drug and environmental allergies, and sinusitis. If present, alert prescriber and provide supportive emergency care, as prescribed. Also monitor patient for possible allergic reaction (erythema and induration) at injection site because leuprolide injections contain benzyl alcohol. Manufacturer recommends that injection be given by physician.**

- Be aware that during first weeks of leuprolide therapy, patient being treated for prostate cancer should be monitored for initial worsening of symptoms, such as difficulty urinating, increased bone pain, and paralysis or paresthesia (in patients with vertebral metastasis). Also be aware that, following the first dose of leuprolide depot form used to treat endometriosis, an increase in symptoms may occur during the initial days of therapy because of a temporary rise in the hormone levels. These symptoms usually abate with time.
- During treatment for prostate cancer, monitor patient's PSA and serum testosterone levels periodically, as ordered, to determine response to leuprolide therapy.
- Monitor patient's blood glucose level, as ordered, because leuprolide therapy may elevate blood glucose levels, leading to a diagnosis of diabetes mellitus, or may adversely affect glycemic control in patients with diabetes.
- Watch patient closely for signs and symptoms of cardiovascular disease because leuprolide therapy increases risk of myocardial infarction, stroke, and sudden cardiac death.
- Expect to stop drug before age 11 in female patients and age 12 in male patients treated for precocious central puberty.
- Monitor bone density test results, as ordered, of women at risk for osteoporosis who are receiving leuprolide because of possible drug-induced estrogen loss, which may result in decreased bone density.
- Be aware that therapeutic doses of leuprolide suppress the pituitary–gonadal system and that normal function doesn't return for 4 to 12 weeks after drug is stopped.

WARNING **Monitor patient for evidence of pituitary apoplexy, such as altered mental status, and possibly cardiovascular collapse, ophthalmoplegia, sudden headache, visual changes, and vomiting. Although rare, it may occur within 2 weeks of first dose, sometimes within the first hour. Notify prescriber immediately and provide supportive care.**

- Institute seizure precautions, especially in patients with a history of central nervous system dysfunction or tumors, cerebrovascular disorders, epilepsy, or history of seizures or in patients who are taking medications that may cause seizures.

PATIENT TEACHING

- Instruct patient who is self-administering leuprolide injection to use syringe provided by manufacturer. If manufacturer's syringe is unavailable, advise her to use only a 0.5-ml disposable, low-dose, U-100 insulin syringe to ensure accurate dosage. Substitution of syringes is not recommended for leuprolide acetate for injectable suspension.

J
K
L

- Advise women to report monthly menses or breakthrough bleeding to prescriber immediately.
- Instruct female patient of childbearing age to use a nonhormonal form of contraception during leuprolide therapy. Advise her to stop taking drug and notify prescriber at once if she becomes pregnant. Be aware that patient should not breastfeed while receiving leuprolide.
- Inform patient with osteoporosis or at risk for developing it that drug may increase bone density loss.
- Inform parents of child being treated for central precocious puberty that they should expect normal gonadal-pituitary function to return 4 to 12 weeks after therapy ends.
- Advise patient to report symptoms of depression or memory problems.
- Caution patient being treated for prostate cancer that drug may initially worsen such symptoms as bone pain and that it may cause new signs or symptoms to occur during first few weeks of treatment. Also inform women receiving drug for treatment of endometriosis that an increase in symptoms may occur during the initial days of therapy. Reassure these patients that these reactions are transient.
- Instruct patient to report to prescriber any symptoms that are new, prolonged, or worsen.
- Advise patient with diabetes to monitor his blood glucose level closely.
- Emphasize importance of seeking immediate emergency care if patient develops symptoms suggestive of a heart attack or stroke, or symptoms of an allergic reaction.
- Inform caregivers to watch for emotional lability such as aggression, anger, crying, depression, impatience, or irritability. Also warn caregivers that although rare, suicidal behaviors and thoughts have occurred during leuprolide therapy. If present, tell caregiver to notify prescriber.
- Review seizure precautions with patient and family or caregiver.

levalbuterol hydrochloride

Xopenex,

levalbuterol tartrate

Xopenex HFA

Class and Category

Pharmacologic class: $Beta_2$ agonist
Therapeutic class: Bronchodilator
Pregnancy category: C

Indications and Dosages

➤ *To prevent or treat bronchospasm in reversible obstructive airway disease*

INHALATION AEROSOL (XOPENEX HFA)

Adults and children age 4 and over. 45 or 90 mcg (1 or 2 inhalations) every 4 to 6 hr.

INHALATION SOLUTION (XOPENEX)

Adults and children age 12 and over. 0.63 to 1.25 mg three times daily every 6 to 8 hr. *Maximum:* 1.25 mg three times daily.
Children ages 6 to 11. 0.31 to 0.63 mg three times daily. *Maximum:* 0.63 mg three times daily.

DOSAGE ADJUSTMENT For elderly patients, dosage limited to 0.63 mg three times daily every 6 to 8 hr.

Route	Onset	Peak	Duration
Inhalation	10–17 min	1.5 hr	5–6 hr

Mechanism of Action

Attaches to $beta_2$ receptors on bronchial cell membranes, which stimulates the intracellular enzyme adenyl cyclase to convert adenosine triphosphate to cAMP. Increased intracellular cAMP level relaxes bronchial smooth muscle and inhibits histamine release from mast cells.

Contraindications

Hypersensitivity to levalbuterol, other sympathomimetic amines, or their components

Interactions

DRUGS

beta blockers: Blocked effects of both drugs
digoxin: Decreased blood digoxin level

loop or thiazide diuretics: Increased risk of hypokalemia
MAO inhibitors, sympathomimetics, tricyclic antidepressants: Increased risk of adverse cardiovascular effects

Adverse Reactions

CNS: Anxiety, chills, dizziness, dysphonia, hypertonia, insomnia, migraine headache, nervousness, paresthesia, syncope, tremor
CV: Arrhythmias, chest pain, hypertension, **hypotension**, tachycardia
EENT: Dry mouth and throat, rhinitis, sinusitis
GI: Diarrhea, gastroesophageal reflux disease (GERD), indigestion, nausea, vomiting
MS: Leg cramps, myalgia
RESP: Asthma exacerbation, cough, dyspnea, **paradoxical bronchospasm**
SKIN: Rash, urticaria
Other: Anaphylaxis, **angioedema**, flu-like symptoms, lymphadenopathy, **metabolic acidosis**

Nursing Considerations

- Use levalbuterol cautiously in patients with arrhythmias, diabetes mellitus, hypertension, hyperthyroidism, or a history of seizures.
- Give oral solution form only by nebulizer.
- Monitor blood pressure and pulse rate before and after nebulizer treatment.
- Observe for dyspnea, increased coughing and wheezing, because drug may provoke paradoxical bronchospasm.

PATIENT TEACHING

- Teach patient how to use levalbuterol nebulizer and to measure correct dose.
- Instruct patient to prime inhaler before using it for the first time or when it hasn't been used for more than 3 days by releasing 4 test sprays into the air, aiming it away from her face. Tell patient that inhaler canister must be shaken well before each use, including when priming.
- Show patient how to clean nebulizer or inhaler, and explain the need to do so at least once weekly.
- Instruct patient to notify prescriber if drug fails to work or if she needs more treatments because asthma is worsening.
- Inform patient that common side effects with levalbuterol use include chest pain, nervousness, palpitations, rapid heart rate, and tremor.
- Instruct patient not to increase dosage or frequency unless told by prescriber.
- Urge patient to stop drug and call prescriber if she has paradoxical bronchospasm.
- Instruct patient to use inhalation solution within 2 weeks of opening the foil pouch and to protect drug from heat and light.
- Inform patient that inhaler canister has a dose indicator display, which will change after every tenth actuation. When nearing the end of usable inhalations, the color behind the number in the dose indicator window will change to red. Tell patient to discard the inhaler when the display window shows zero.
- Urge patient to consult prescriber before using OTC or other drugs.
- Tell women of childbearing age to notify prescriber if pregnancy is suspected or known. Also tell mothers wishing to breastfeed to discuss this with prescriber before doing so.

levetiracetam

Keppra, Keppra XR, Spritam

Class and Category

Pharmacologic class: Pyrrolidine derivative
Therapeutic class: Anticonvulsant
Pregnancy category: C

Indications and Dosages

➤ *As adjunct to treat partial seizures*

I.V. INFUSION, ORAL SOLUTION

Adults and adolescents age 16 and over. *Initial:* 500 mg (I.V.: infused over 15 min) twice daily, increased by 1,000 mg daily every 2 wk if needed, and given in 2 divided doses. *Maximum:* 3,000 mg daily.
Children ages 4 to 16. *Initial:* 10 mg/kg (I.V.: infused over 15 min) twice daily, increased by 20 mg/kg daily every 2 wk until recommended daily dose of 60 mg/kg

given in 2 divided doses is reached. *Maximum:* 3,000 mg daily.
Children 6 months to 4 years. *Initial:* 10 mg/kg (I.V.: infused over 15 min) twice daily, increased by 20 mg/kg daily every 2 wk until the recommended daily dose of 50 mg/kg given in 2 divided doses is reached.
Infants 1 to 6 months of age. *Initial:* 7 mg/kg (I.V.: infused over 15 min) twice daily, increased by 14 mg/kg every 2 wk until recommended daily dose of 42 mg/kg given in 2 divided doses is reached.

TABLETS (KEPPRA)

Adults and adolescents ages 16 and over. *Initial:* 500 mg twice daily, increased by 1,000 mg daily every 2 wk if needed, and given in 2 divided doses. *Maximum:* 3,000 mg daily.
Children ages 4 to 16 weighing more than 40 kg (88 lb). *Initial:* 10 mg/kg twice daily, increased by 20 mg/kg daily every 2 wk until recommended daily dose of 60 mg/kg given in 2 divided doses is reached.
Children ages 4 to 16 weighing 20 to 40 kg (44 to 88 lb): *Initial:* 250 mg twice daily, increased by 500 mg daily every 2 wk. *Maximum:* 750 mg twice daily.

TABLETS (SPRITAM)

Adults and children age 4 and over weighing over 40 kg (88 lb). *Initial:* 500 mg twice daily, increased by 1,000 mg daily every 2 wk. *Maximum:* 3,000 mg daily given in 2 divided doses.
Children age 4 and over weighing 20 to 40 kg (44 to 88 lb). *Initial:* 250 mg twice daily, increased by 500 mg every 2 wk until recommended daily dose of 1,500 mg given in 2 divided doses is reached.

XR TABLETS

Adults and children age 12 and over. 1,000 mg once daily, increased by 1,000 mg daily every 2 wk until recommended daily dose of 3,000 mg is reached.

➤ *As adjunct to treat myoclonic seizures in patients with juvenile myoclonic epilepsy*

I.V. INFUSION, ORAL SOLUTION, TABLETS

Adults and children age 12 and over. *Initial:* 500 mg (I.V.: infused over 15 min) twice daily, increased by 1,000 mg daily every 2 wk. *Maximum:* 3,000 mg daily.

➤ *As adjunct to treat primary generalized tonic–clonic seizures in patients with idiopathic generalized epilepsy*

I.V. INFUSION, ORAL SOLUTION, TABLETS (KEPPRA)

Adults and children age 16 and over. *Initial:* 500 mg (I.V.: infused over 15 min) twice daily, increased by 1,000 mg daily every 2 wk, as needed. *Maximum:* 3,000 mg daily.
Children ages 6 to 16. *Initial:* 10 mg/kg (I.V.: infused over 15 min) twice daily, increased by 20 mg/kg daily every 2 wk, if needed, and given in 2 divided doses. *Maximum:* 60 mg/kg daily in 2 divided doses.

TABLETS (SPRITAM)

Adults and children age 6 and over weighing over 40 kg (88 lb). *Initial:* 500 mg twice daily, increased by 1,000 mg daily every 2 wk to recommended daily dose of 3,000 mg given in 2 divided doses.
Children age 6 and over weighing 20 to 40 kg (44 to 88 lb): *Initial:* 250 mg twice daily, increased by 500 mg every 2 wk to the recommended daily dose of 1,500 mg given in 2 divided doses.

DOSAGE ADJUSTMENT Maximum dosage reduced to 2,000 mg daily for patients with creatinine clearance of 50 to 80 ml/min; to 1,500 mg daily for clearance of 30 to 49 ml/min; and to 1,000 mg daily for clearance less than 30 ml/min. For patients with end-stage renal disease who are having dialysis, expect to give another 250 to 500 mg, as prescribed, after each dialysis session. For children who can't tolerate maximum daily dose, dosage reduced to point of tolerance.

Mechanism of Action

May protect against secondary generalized seizure activity by preventing coordination of epileptiform burst firing. Levetiracetam doesn't seem to involve inhibitory and excitatory neurotransmission.

Contraindications

Hypersensitivity to levetiracetam or its components

Adverse Reactions

CNS: Abnormal gait, aggression, agitation, anger, anxiety, apathy, asthenia, ataxia, behavioral difficulties (children), choreoathetosis, confusion, coordination

difficulties, depersonalization, depression, dizziness, dyskinesia, emotional lability, fatigue, hallucinations, headache, hostility, increased reflexes, insomnia, involuntary movements, irritability, mental or mood changes, nervousness, neurosis, panic attacks, paranoia, paresthesia, personality disorder, psychosis, **seizures**, somnolence, **suicidal ideation**, vertigo
CV: Elevated diastolic blood pressure (children up to 4 years of age), **hypotension**
EENT: Amblyopia, conjunctivitis, diplopia, ear pain, nasopharyngitis, pharyngitis, rhinitis, sinusitis
GI: Anorexia, constipation, diarrhea, elevated liver enzymes, gastroenteritis, **hepatic failure**, **hepatitis**, **pancreatitis**, vomiting
GU: Acute kidney injury, albuminuria
HEME: Agranulocytosis; decreased hematocrit, hemoglobin, and red blood cell counts; elevated eosinophil count; **leukopenia**; **neutropenia**; **pancytopenia**; **thrombocytopenia**
MS: Muscle weakness, neck pain
RESP: Asthma, cough, dyspnea
SKIN: Alopecia, ecchymosis, **erythema multiforme**, pruritus, rash, skin discoloration, **Stevens–Johnson syndrome**, **toxic epidermal necrolysis**, vesiculobullous rash, urticaria
Other: Anaphylaxis, **angioedema**, dehydration, **drug reaction with eosinophilia and systemic symptoms (DRESS)**, **hyponatremia**, infection, influenza, weight loss

Nursing Considerations

- Know that children weighing 20 kg or less should be given only the oral solution form.
- Know that the intravenous form of levetiracetam should be used only as an alternative for patients when oral administration is temporarily not possible.
- Keep in mind that when switching patient from oral dosing to intravenous dosing and from intravenous dosing to oral dosing, no dosage or frequency changes are needed.
- For I.V. use, dilute parenteral levetiracetam in 100 ml of compatible diluent, such as normal saline injection, lactated Ringer's injection, or dextrose 5% injection. Use within 24 hours. Infuse each dose over 15 minutes.

WARNING **Monitor patient for hypersensitivity reactions. Know that anaphylaxis or angioedema have occurred with levetiracetam therapy as early as after the first dose, but also at other times during treatment. Monitor patient for difficulty breathing, hives, hypotension, rash, and swelling. If present, withhold drug, notify prescriber immediately, and provide emergency supportive care, as ordered. Expect drug to be discontinued.**

- Monitor patient for seizure activity during therapy. As appropriate, implement seizure precautions according to facility policy.
- Avoid stopping drug abruptly because doing so may increase seizure activity. Expect to taper dosage gradually.
- Monitor patient for bleeding, fever, recurrent infections, or significant weakness. If present, notify prescriber and expect to obtain a complete blood count to assess patient's hematological status.
- Assess compliance, especially during the first 4 weeks of therapy, when certain adverse effects, including abnormal behaviors, coordination problems, fatigue, and somnolence may be more likely to occur.
- Monitor blood pressure in children because increased diastolic blood pressure may occur in patients up to 4 years old.
- Monitor patient closely for evidence of suicidal thinking or behavior, especially when therapy starts or dosage changes.
- Monitor patient for a rash and other adverse skin reactions because serious dermatological reactions have occurred with levetiracetam therapy. Although these adverse reactions usually appear within 14 to 17 days after therapy has begun, some have occurred as late as 4 months later. Notify prescriber at the first sign of a rash and expect drug to be discontinued.
- Monitor pregnant patient closely, especially during third trimester, because

physiological changes associated with pregnancy may gradually decrease plama levetiracetam levels. Monitoring should continue through the postpartum period.

PATIENT TEACHING

- Instruct patient prescribed Spritam form of levetiracetam to place tablet on tongue with a dry hand and immediately follow with a sip of water as it is intended to disintegrate in the mouth when taken with a sip of water.
- Tell patient to seek immediate emergency care if an allergic reaction occurs, especially if he experiences difficulty breathing, hives, low blood pressure, rash, or swelling.
- Caution patient that levetiracetam may cause dizziness and drowsiness, especially during first 4 weeks of therapy.
- Advise patient to avoid hazardous activities until drug's CNS effects are known.
- Caution patient not to stop taking levetiracetam abruptly; inform her that drug dosage should be tapered under prescriber's direction to reduce the risk of breakthrough seizures.
- Explain to patient and family that levetiracetam may cause mental and behavioral changes, such as aggression, depression, irritability, and rarely psychotic symptoms. The prescriber should be contacted about any bothersome changes.
- Advise patient to keep taking other anticonvulsants, as ordered, while taking levetiracetam.
- Encourage patient to avoid alcohol during therapy because alcohol can increase incidence of dizziness and drowsiness.
- Instruct patient to see prescriber regularly so that her progress can be monitored.
- Urge caregivers to watch patient closely for evidence of suicidal tendencies, especially when therapy starts or dosage changes, and to report concerns immediately.
- Urge woman who becomes pregnant while taking levetiracetam to enroll in the North American Antiepileptic Drug Pregnancy Registry by calling 1-888-233-2334. Explain that registry is collecting information about safety of antiepileptic drugs during pregnancy.
- Emphasize importance of notifying prescriber at the first sign of a rash.

levocetirizine

Xyzal

Class and Category

Pharmacologic class: H_1-receptor antagonist
Therapeutic class: Antihistamine
Pregnancy category: B

Indications and Dosages

➤ *To treat chronic idiopathic urticaria; to treat perennial allergic rhinitis*

TABLETS, ORAL SOLUTION

Adults under the age of 65 and children age 12 and over. 5 mg once daily in evening. *Maximum:* 5 mg daily.
Children ages 6 to 11. 2.5 mg once daily in evening. *Maximum:* 2.5 mg daily.
Children 6 months to age 5. 1.25 mg once daily in evening. *Maximum:* 1.25 mg daily.

DOSAGE ADJUSTMENT For adult patient with mild renal impairment (creatinine clearance 50 to 80 ml/min), dosage shouldn't exceed 2.5 mg daily. For adult patient with moderate renal impairment (creatinine clearance 30 to 50 ml/min), dosage shouldn't exceed 2.5 mg once every other day. For adult patient with severe renal impairment (creatinine clearance 10 to 30 ml/min), dosage shouldn't exceed 2.5 mg once every 3 to 4 days. Dosages for children should not exceed maximum dose because systemic exposure is about twice that of adults.

Mechanism of Action

Binds to central and peripheral H_1 receptors, competing with histamine for these sites and preventing it from reaching its site of action. By blocking histamine, levocetirizine produces antihistamine effects, inhibiting respiratory, vascular, and GI smooth-muscle contraction; decreasing capillary permeability, which reduces wheals, flares, and itching; and decreasing salivary and lacrimal gland secretions to relieve chronic urticaria and signs and symptoms of allergic rhinitis.

Contraindications

Children ages 6 to 11 with impaired renal function; creatinine clearance less than 10 ml/min; end-stage renal disease in adults and children age 12 and over; hypersensitivity to levocetirizine, cetirizine or their components; renal failure

Interactions

DRUGS

CNS depressants: Possibly increased CNS depression
MAO inhibitors: Possibly intensified and prolonged anticholinergic effects
ritonavir: Possibly increased risk of adverse effects of levocetirizine
theophylline: Possibly decreased clearance of levocetirizine

ACTIVITIES

alcohol use: Possibly increased CNS depression

Adverse Reactions

CNS: Aggression, agitation, asthenia, depression, dizziness, fatigue, fever, hallucinations, insomnia, movement disorders, myoclonus and extrapyramidal symptoms, paraesthesia, **seizures**, somnolence, **suicidal ideation**, syncope, tic, tremor, vertigo
CV: Edema, palpitations, tachycardia
EENT: Blurred vision, dry mouth, epistaxis, nasopharyngitis, pharyngitis, visual disturbances
GI: Hepatitis, increased appetite, nausea, vomiting
GU: Dysuria, urinary retention
MS: Arthralgia, myalgia
RESP: Cough, dyspnea
SKIN: Acute generalized exanthematous pustulosis, fixed drug eruption, pruritus, rash, urticaria
Other: Anaphylaxis, **angioedema**, weight gain

Nursing Considerations

- Use levocetirizine cautiously in patients with predisposing risk factors for urinary retention, such as prostatic hyperplasia or spinal cord lesion. Monitor patient's intake and output closely. If urinary retention is suspected, notify prescriber and expect drug to be discontinued if confirmed.
- Monitor patient for abnormal thinking, such as desire to harm oneself. Notify prescriber immediately if present.
- Expect to stop drug at least 72 hours before skin tests for allergies because drug may inhibit cutaneous histamine response, thus producing false-negative results.

PATIENT TEACHING

- Instruct patient to take drug exactly as prescribed. For oral solution, patient should use appropriate measuring device.
- Urge patient to avoid alcohol while taking levocetirizine
- Advise patient to avoid hazardous activities until drug's CNS effects are known.
- Tell patient to notify prescriber if he is feeling bladder fullness or notices that his urine output is significantly less than his intake.
- Warn patient that if he develops abnormal thoughts, especially thoughts of harming himself, he should notify prescriber immediately.
- Alert patient taking levocetirizine long-term that rebound itching may occur within days after drug is discontinued.

levofloxacin

Levaquin

Class and Category

Pharmacologic class: Fluoroquinolone
Therapeutic class: Antibiotic
Pregnancy category: C

Indications and Dosages

➤ *To reduce incidence or progression of inhalation anthrax after exposure to aerosolized* Bacillus anthracis; *to treat plague, including pneumonic and septicemic plague, caused by* Yersinia pestis; *to provide prophylaxis for plague*

TABLETS, I.V. INFUSION, ORAL SOLUTION

Adults and children weighing more than 50 kg (110 lb). 500 mg (over 60 min for I.V. infusion) daily for 60 days for treatment of inhalation anthrax and 10 to 14 days for treatment of plague.
Children weighing less than 50 kg (110 lb) (but no less than 30 kg for tablet form) and 6 months of age or older. 8 mg/kg (over 60 min for I.V. infusion) every 12 hr for 60 days for treatment of inhalation anthrax and 10 to 14 days for treatment of plague.
Maximum: 250 mg/dose.

➤ *To treat acute bacterial sinusitis caused by* Haemophilus influenzae, Moraxella catarrhalis, *or* Streptococcus pneumoniae

TABLETS, I.V. INFUSION, ORAL SOLUTION

Adults. 500 mg daily (over 60 min for I.V. infusion) for 10 to 14 days. Or 750 mg daily for 5 days.

➤ *To treat acute exacerbation of chronic bacterial bronchitis caused by* H. influenzae, H. parainfluenzae, M. catarrhalis, S. pneumoniae, *or* Staphylococcus aureus

TABLETS, I.V. INFUSION, ORAL SOLUTION

Adults. 500 mg daily (over 60 min for I.V. infusion) for 7 days.

➤ *To treat community-acquired pneumonia caused by* Chlamydia pneumoniae, H. influenzae, H. parainfluenzae, Klebsiella pneumoniae, Legionella pneumophila, M. catarrhalis, Mycoplasma pneumoniae, S. aureus, *or* S. pneumoniae

TABLETS, I.V. INFUSION, ORAL SOLUTION

Adults. 500 mg daily (over 60 min for I.V. infusion) for 7 to 14 days. Alternatively, for infection caused by *C. pneumoniae, H. influenzae, H. parainfluenzae, M. pneumoniae,* or *S. pneumoniae,* 750 mg daily (over 90 min for I.V. infusion) for 5 days.

➤ *To treat uncomplicated UTI caused by* Escherichia coli, K. pneumoniae, *or* Staphylococcus saprophyticus

TABLETS, I.V. INFUSION, ORAL SOLUTION

Adults. 250 mg daily (over 60 min for I.V. infusion) for 3 days.

➤ *To treat complicated UTI caused by* Enterococcus faecalis, E. cloacae, E. coli, K. pneumoniae, Proteus mirabilis, *or* Pseudomonas aeruginosa; *acute pyelonephritis caused by* E. coli

TABLETS, I.V. INFUSION, ORAL SOLUTION

Adults. 250 mg daily (over 60 to 90 min for I.V. infusion) for 10 days.

➤ *To treat complicated UTI caused by* E. coli, K. pneumoniae, *or* P. mirabilis *or acute pyelonephritis caused by* E. coli

TABLETS, I.V. INFUSION, ORAL SOLUTION

Adults. 750 mg daily (over 90 min for I.V. infusion) for 5 days.

➤ *To treat mild to moderate skin and soft-tissue infections caused by* S. aureus *or* Streptococcus pyogenes

TABLETS, I.V. INFUSION, ORAL SOLUTION

Adults. 500 mg daily (over 60 min for I.V. infusion) for 7 to 10 days.

➤ *To treat complicated skin and soft-tissue infections caused by methicillin-sensitive* Enterococcus faecalis, Proteus mirabilis, S. aureus, *or* S. pyogenes; *to treat nosocomial pneumonia caused by* E. coli, H. influenzae, K. pneumoniae, Pseudomonas aeruginosa, S. aureus, *or* Serratia marcescens

TABLETS, I.V. INFUSION, ORAL SOLUTION

Adults. 750 mg daily (over 60 min for I.V. infusion) for 7 to 14 days.

➤ *To treat chronic bacterial prostatitis caused by* E. coli, E. faecalis, *or* S. epidermidis

TABLETS, I.V. INFUSION, ORAL SOLUTION

Adults. 500 mg daily (over 60 to 90 min for I.V. infusion) for 28 days.

DOSAGE ADJUSTMENT For patients with creatinine clearance of 20 to 49 ml/min and normal dosage is 750 mg, dosage interval increased to every 48 hr; for normal dosage of 500 mg, one dose of 500 mg given, followed by 250 mg every 24 hr. For patients with creatinine clearance of 10 to 19 ml/min or who are receiving dialysis, and normal dosage is 750 mg, one dose of 750 mg given, followed by 500 mg every 48 hr; for normal dosage of 500 mg, one dose of 500 mg given, followed by 250 mg every 48 hr; and for normal dosage of 250 mg (no information on dosing adjustment available for patient on dialysis at this dosage), dosage interval increased to every 48 hr unless the 250 mg dosage is used to treat uncomplicated UTI, then no dosage adjustment is required. Supplemental doses of levofloxacin are not required following continuous ambulatory peritoneal dialysis or hemodialysis because dialysis is not effective in removing levofloxacin from the body.

Mechanism of Action

Interferes with bacterial cell replication by inhibiting the bacterial enzyme DNA gyrase, which is essential for repair and replication of bacterial DNA.

Contraindications

Hypersensitivity to levofloxacin, other fluoroquinolones, or their components; myasthenia gravis

Interactions

DRUGS

aluminum-, calcium-, or magnesium-containing antacids; didanosine; iron; sucralfate; zinc: Reduced GI absorption of levofloxacin
antineoplastics: Decreased blood levofloxacin level
cimetidine: Increased blood levofloxacin level
cyclosporine: Increased risk of nephrotoxicity
NSAIDs: Possibly increased CNS stimulation and risk of seizures
oral anticoagulants: Increased anticoagulant effect and risk of bleeding
oral antidiabetic drugs: Possibly hyperglycemia or hypoglycemia
theophylline: Increased blood theophylline level and risk of toxicity

ACTIVITIES

sun exposure: Increased risk of photosensitivity

Adverse Reactions

CNS: Agitation, anxiety, CNS stimulation, confusion, delirium, depression, disorientation, disturbance in attention, dizziness, electroencephalogram abnormalities, **encephalopathy** (rare), fever, hallucinations, headache, hoarse voice, **increased intracranial pressure**, insomnia, light-headedness, memory impairment, nervousness, nightmares, paranoia, peripheral neuropathy, **pseudotumor cerebri**, psychosis, restlessness, **seizures**, sleep disturbance, **suicidal ideation**, toxic psychoses, tremors
CV: Aortic dissection, **arrhythmias**, leukocytoclastic vasculitis, **prolonged QT interval**, **rupture of aortic aneurysm**, tachycardia, **torsades de pointes**, vasculitis, vasodilation
EENT: Blurred vision, decreased visual acuity, diplopia, dysphonia, scotoma, smell or taste perversion, tinnitus, uveitis
ENDO: Hyperglycemia, **hypoglycemia**
GI: Abdominal pain, **acute hepatic failure or necrosis**, anorexia, constipation, diarrhea, flatulence, **hepatitis**, **hepatotoxicity**, indigestion, jaundice, nausea, **pseudomembranous colitis**, vomiting
GU: Acute renal failure or insufficiency, crystalluria, interstitial nephritis, vaginal candidiasis
HEME: Agranulocytosis, **aplastic anemia**, eosinophilia, **hemolytic anemia**, **leukopenia**, **pancytopenia**, **prolonged International Normalized Ratio (INR) and prothrombin time**, **thrombocytopenia**
MS: Arthralgia, arthritis, back pain, elevated muscle enzymes, gait abnormality, myalgia, **rhabdomyolysis**, tendon or muscle rupture, tendinopathy
RESP: Hypersensitivity pneumonitis
SKIN: Erythema multiforme, photosensitivity, pruritus, rash, **Stevens–Johnson syndrome**, **toxic epidermal necrolysis**, urticaria
Other: Anaphylaxis, **angioedema**, exacerbation of myasthenia gravis, **multiorgan failure**, serum sickness

Nursing Considerations

- Use levofloxacin cautiously in patients with renal insufficiency. Monitor renal function as appropriate during treatment.
- Use drug cautiously in patients with CNS disorders, such as epilepsy or renal dysfunction, as well as certain drug therapies, that may lower the seizure threshold. Also use cautiously in patients taking corticosteroids, especially elderly patients, because of increased risk of tendon rupture.
- Expect to obtain culture and sensitivity tests before levofloxacin treatment begins.
- Know that levofloxacin therapy should begin as soon as possible after suspected or confirmed exposure to *Y. pestis*.
- Avoid giving drug within 2 hours of antacids.
- Give parenteral form over 60 to 90 minutes, depending on dosage, because bolus or rapid I.V. delivery may cause hypotension.

WARNING Stop levofloxacin at first sign of hypersensitivity, including jaundice and rash, because drug may lead to anaphylaxis. Reaction may occur after first dose. Expect to give epinephrine and provide supportive care.

- Monitor blood glucose level, especially in diabetic patient who takes an oral antidiabetic or uses insulin, because levofloxacin may alter blood glucose level. If so, notify prescriber, stop drug immediately if patient has hypoglycemia, and provide prescribed treatment.
- Monitor QT interval if needed. If it lengthens, notify prescriber at once and stop drug. Patients with cardiomyopathy, hypokalemia, or significant bradycardia and those receiving a class IA or III antiarrhythmic shouldn't receive levofloxacin.
- Notify prescriber if patient has symptoms of peripheral neuropathy (altered sensations of light touch, pain, temperature, position sense, or vibration sense), which could be permanent; or CNS or psychiatric abnormalities (i.e., CNS stimulation, increased ICP, psychosis, or seizures), which may lead to more serious adverse reactions, such as suicidal ideation. In each case, expect to discontinue levofloxacin.
- Watch for evidence of tendon rupture (inflammation, pain, swelling) during and up to several months after therapy, especially in children, elderly patients, patients receiving corticosteroids, and patients with heart, kidney, and lung transplants. Notify prescriber about suspected tendon rupture, and have patient rest and refrain from exercise until tendon rupture has been ruled out. If present, expect to provide supportive care, as ordered.
- Be aware that children have a higher incidence of musculoskeletal adverse reactions, especially arthralgia, arthritis, gait abnormality, and tendinopathy. Report any complaint involving the musculoskeletal system promptly to prescriber.
- Monitor patient's bowel elimination. If diarrhea develops, obtain stool culture to check for pseudomembranous colitis. If confirmed, expect to stop drug and give antibiotics effective against *Clostridium difficile*, electrolytes, and fluids.
- Know that fluoroquinolones like levofloxacin have caused disabling and potentially irreversible serious adverse reactions from different body systems that can occur together in the same patient. These reactions can occur within hours to weeks after starting the drug and usually cause central nervous system effects, peripheral neuropathy, tendinitis, and tendon rupture. All ages of patients and patients without any preexisting risk factors have experienced these reactions. Notify prescriber and expect to discontinue levofloxacin immediately at the first signs or symptoms of any serious adverse reactions.

PATIENT TEACHING

- Tell patient prescribed oral solution to take it 1 hour before or 2 hours after eating.
- Advise patient to increase fluid intake during therapy to prevent crystalluria.
- Direct patient to take an antacid, didanosine, iron, sucralfate, or zinc at least 2 hours before or after levofloxacin.
- Tell patient to complete the drug as prescribed, even if symptoms subside.
- Urge patient to avoid excessive sun exposure and to wear sunscreen because of increased risk of photosensitivity. Tell patient to notify prescriber at first sign of photosensitivity.
- Caution patient to avoid hazardous activities until drug's CNS effects are known.
- Tell patient to stop drug and notify prescriber if he develops abnormal changes in motor or sensory function, or tendon inflammation or pain.
- Urge patient experiencing a rash or other allergic reactions to stop drug and tell prescriber.
- Advise diabetic patient to monitor blood glucose level and report changes.
- Urge patient to tell prescriber about severe diarrhea, even if it's more than 2 months after drug therapy ends. Additional treatment may be needed.
- Advise patient to notify prescriber about heart palpitations or loss of consciousness.
- Advise patient to stop taking levofloxacin immediately and notify prescriber if any persistent, serious, or worsening adverse effects occur.

levomilnacipran

Fetzima

levomilnacipran hydrochloride

Savella

Class and Category

Pharmacologic class: Selective norepinephrine and serotonin reuptake inhibitor (SSNRI)
Therapeutic class: Antidepressant
Pregnancy category: C

Indications and Dosages

➤ *To treat major depressive disorder*

E.R. CAPSULES

Adults. *Initial:* 20 mg once daily for 2 days then increased to 40 mg once daily. Dosage further increased in 40-mg increments at intervals of 2 or more days, as needed. *Maximum:* 120 mg once daily.

DOSAGE ADJUSTMENT For patients with moderate renal impairment (creatinine clearance of 30 to 59 ml/min), maintenance dosage should not exceed 80 mg once daily. For patients with severe renal impairment (creatinine clearance of 15 to 29 ml/min), maintenance dosage should not exceed 40 mg once daily.

➤ *To manage fibromyalgia*

TABLETS (SAVELLA)

Adults. *Initial:* 12.5 mg once daily on day 1, 12.5 mg twice daily on days 2 and 3, 25 mg twice daily on days 4 through 7, and then 50 mg twice daily. Further increased to 100 mg twice daily, if needed. *Maintenance:* 50 mg twice daily. *Maximum:* 200 mg daily.

DOSAGE ADJUSTMENT For patient with severe renal impairment (creatinine clearance of 5 to 29 ml/min), maintenance dose reduced by 50% to 25 mg twice daily.

Mechanism of Action

Inhibits reuptake of norepinephrine and serotonin by CNS neurons without affecting uptake of dopamine or other neurotransmitters, thereby increasing amount of norepinephrine and serotonin available in nerve synapses in the central nervous system. Elevated norepinephrine and serotonin levels may relieve symptoms of depression and may improve symptoms of fibromyalgia, including central analgesic effect.

Contraindications

Hypersensitivity to levomilnacipran, milnacipran, or its components; uncontrolled narrow-angle glaucoma; use within 14 days of MAO inhibitor therapy, including reversible agents such as intravenous methylene blue or linezolid

Interactions

DRUGS

antipsychotics or other dopamine antagonists, MAO inhibitors, other serotonergic drugs (buspirone, fentanyl, lithium, St. John's wort, tramadol, tricyclic antidepressants, triptans, tryptophan), selective serotonin reuptake inhibitors, serotonin-norepinephrine reuptake inhibitors: Possibly development of neuroleptic malignant syndrome-like reactions or serotonin syndrome
aspirin, NSAIDs, warfarin: Increased risk of bleeding
CNS-active drugs: Possibly increased CNS effects
ketoconazole: Increased exposure of levomilnacipran resulting in increased risk of adverse reactions

ACTIVITIES

alcohol use: Increased risk of adverse reactions

Adverse Reactions

CNS: Activation of hypomania or mania, aggression, agitation, anger, anxiety, delirium, depression, dizziness, extrapyramidal disorder, fatigue, fever, hallucinations, headache, hypoesthesia, insomnia, irritability, loss of consciousness, migraine, panic attack, paresthesia, **seizures**, **serotonin syndrome**, **suicidal ideation**, syncope, thirst, tremor
CV: Chest pain, elevated cholesterol levels, **extrasystoles**, hypertension, **hypertensive crisis**, **hypotension**, increased heart rate, palpitations, peripheral edema, **supraventricular tachycardia**, tachycardia, **Takotsubo cardiomyopathy**

EENT: Angle-closure glaucoma, blurred vision, conjunctival hemorrhage, dry eye, epistaxis, mydriasis
ENDO: Hot flashes
GI: Abdominal distention or pain, anorexia, constipation, diarrhea, elevated liver enzymes, flatulence, nausea, vomiting
GU: Decreased libido, dysuria, ejaculation disorder, erectile dysfunction, hematuria, prostatitis, proteinuria, scrotal or testicular pain, testicular swelling, urinary hesitation or retention
HEME: Ecchymosis, hematoma, **hemorrhage**, petechiae
RESP: Dyspnea,
SKIN: Dry skin, **erythema multiforme**, excessive sweating including night sweats, flushing, pruritus, rash, urticaria

Nursing Considerations

- Use levomilnacipran cautiously in patients with cardiac disease or significant hypertension and in patients with renal impairment. Also use cautiously in patients with a history of dysuria, especially men with prostatic hypertrophy, prostatitis, and other lower urinary tract obstructive disorders.
- Know that at least 14 days should elapse between stopping an MAO inhibitor and starting levomilnacipran. At least 7 days should elapse between stopping levomilnacipran and starting an MAO inhibitor antidepressant.
- Measure patient's blood pressure and heart rate before starting and periodically during levomilnacipran therapy because drug can raise blood pressure and heart rate. If hypertension or tachycardia occurs and persists, notify prescriber and expect to reduce dosage or discontinue drug.
- Watch closely for suicidal tendencies, especially when therapy starts and after dosage changes.

WARNING Monitor patient closely for serotonin syndrome, a rare but serious adverse effect of selective serotonin reuptake inhibitors such as levomilnacipran. Signs and symptoms include agitation, confusion, diaphoresis, diarrhea, fever, hyperactive reflexes, poor coordination, restlessness, shaking, talking or acting with uncontrolled excitement, tremor, and twitching. In its most severe form, it can resemble neuroleptic malignant syndrome with autonomic instability with possible rapid fluctuation of vital signs, mental status changes, and muscle rigidity. If symptoms occur, notify prescriber immediately, expect to discontinue drug, and provide supportive care.

- Assess effectiveness of levomilnacipran periodically being aware that therapy may be required for several months or longer. Expect to taper drug when no longer needed, as ordered, to minimize adverse reactions.

PATIENT TEACHING

- Instruct patient to take levomilnacipran capsules whole and not to chew, crush, or open capsules.
- Advise patient that drug may cause mild pupillary dilation, which may lead to an episode of acute-closure glaucoma. Encourage patient to have an eye exam before starting therapy to see if he is at risk.
- Urge family or caregiver to watch patient closely for suicidal tendencies, especially when therapy starts or dosage changes.
- Caution patient against stopping drug abruptly because serious adverse effects may result.
- Instruct patient to alert all prescribers of levomilnacipran therapy.
- Tell patient to have his blood pressure monitored regularly throughout levomilnacipran therapy.
- Advise patient to avoid activities, such as driving, that require alertness until the CNS effects of levomilnacipran are known.
- Monitor patient to avoid aspirin and NSAIDs, if possible, while taking levomilnacipran.
- Instruct patient to report any persistent, severe, or unusual adverse effects to prescriber immediately.
- Tell mothers wishing to breastfeed to discuss this with prescriber first, as there is a potential for serious adverse reactions in nursing infants.

levothyroxine sodium
(L-thyroxine sodium, T_4, thyroxine sodium)

Eltroxin (CAN), Euthyrox, Levo-T, Levoxyl, Synthroid, Tirosint, Unithroid

Class and Category

Pharmacologic class: Synthetic thyroxine (T_4)
Therapeutic class: Thyroid hormone replacement
Pregnancy category: A

Indications and Dosages

➤ *To treat mild hypothyroidism*

CAPSULES, TABLETS

Adults younger than 50 or those older than 50 who have been recently treated for hyperthyroidism or have been hypothyroid for a short time. 1.7 mcg/kg once daily. *Usual maintenance dose:* 100 to 125 mcg daily.
Adults younger than 50 with underlying cardiac disease or adults older than 50. *Initial:* 25 to 50 mcg daily, increased by 12.5 to 25 mcg daily every 6 to 8 wk, as needed.
Elderly patients with cardiac disease. *Initial:* 12.5 to 25 mcg daily, increased gradually every 4 to 6 wk, as needed.
Children in whom growth and puberty are complete. 1.7 mcg/kg daily.
Children age 12 and over in whom growth and puberty are incomplete. 2 to 3 mcg/kg daily.
Children ages 6 to 12. 4 to 5 mcg/kg daily.
Children ages 1 to 5. 5 to 6 mcg/kg daily.
Infants ages 6 to 12 months. 6 to 8 mcg/kg daily.
Infants ages 3 to 6 months. 8 to 10 mcg daily.
Infants and neonates birth to age 3 months. 10 to 15 mcg/kg daily. *Usual:* 75 to 100 mcg daily.

➤ *To treat severe hypothyroidism*

CAPSULES, TABLETS

Adults. *Initial:* 12.5 to 25 mcg daily. Increased by 25 mcg every 2 to 4 wk until desired response occurs or therapeutic blood level is reached. *Maintenance:* 75 to 125 mcg daily. *Maximum:* 200 mcg daily.
Children. *Initial:* 25 mcg daily, increased by 25 mcg daily every 2 to 4 wk, as needed.
Infants. *Initial:* 50 mcg daily and adjusted, as needed.

➤ *To treat myxedema coma*

I.V. INJECTION

Adults. *Initial as loading dose:* 300 to 500 mcg, followed by 50 to 100 mcg once daily until patient able to tolerate drug orally.

DOSAGE ADJUSTMENT Dosage adjustment highly individualized according to patient's response and tolerance as well as age, degree of hypothyroidism present, general physical condition, and severity of cardiac risk factors. Dosage possibly increased during pregnancy.

Route	Onset	Peak	Duration
P.O.	3–5 days	3–4 wk	1–3 wk
I.V.	6–8 hr	24 hr	Unknown

Mechanism of Action

Replaces endogenous thyroid hormone, which may exert its physiologic effects by controlling DNA transcription and protein synthesis. Levothyroxine has all the following actions of endogenous thyroid hormone. The drug:

- increases energy expenditure
- accelerates the rate of cellular oxidation, which stimulates body tissue growth, maturation, and metabolism
- regulates differentiation and proliferation of stem cells
- aids in myelination of nerves and development of synaptic processes in the nervous system
- regulates growth
- decreases blood and hepatic cholesterol concentrations
- enhances carbohydrate and protein metabolism, increasing gluconeogenesis and protein synthesis.

Contraindications

Acute MI, hypersensitivity to levothyroxine or its components, uncorrected adrenal insufficiency, untreated thyrotoxicosis

Interactions

DRUGS

5-fluorouracil, clofibrate, estrogens (oral), estrogen-containing oral contraceptives, heroin, methadone, mitotane, tamoxifen:

Possibly increased serum thyroxine-binding globulin (TBG) concentration
adrenocorticoids: Possibly altered blood adrenocorticoid level
aluminum- and magnesium-containing antacids, calcium carbonate, cation exchange resins, ferrous sulfate, orlistat, phenobarbital, rifampin: Possibly decreased absorption and reduced effects of levothyroxine
amiodarone, glucocorticoids, iodide: Possibly hyperthyroidism from decreased peripheral conversion of T_4 to T_3, leading to decreased T_3 levels
anabolic steroids, androgens, asparaginase, glucocorticoids, slow-release nicotinic acid: Possibly decreased serum TBG concentration
beta blockers: Possibly impaired action of beta blockers and decreased conversion of T_4 to triiodothyronine (T_3)
carbamazepine, fenamates, furosemide (greater than 80 mg IV), heparin, hydantoins, NSAIDs, salicylates (greater than 2 g/day): Transient increase in FT4 followed by decreased serum T_4 and normal FT4 and TSH concentrations with continued administration
cholestyramine, colestipol, colesevelam, kayexalate, proton pump inhibitors, sevelamer, simethicone, sucralfate: Delayed or inhibited levothyroxine absorption
digoxin: Reduced digoxin effects
estrogen, phenylbutazone, phenytoin: Possibly decreased levothyroxine effectiveness.
insulin, oral antidiabetic drugs: Decreased effectiveness of these drugs
ketamine: Possibly hypertension and tachycardia
oral anticoagulants: Altered anticoagulant activity
selective serotonin reuptake inhibitors, tricyclic and tetracyclic antidepressants: Increased therapeutic and toxic effects of both drugs
sympathomimetics: Increased risk of coronary insufficiency in patients with coronary artery disease
theophylline: Decreased theophylline clearance
tyrosine-kinase inhibitors: Possible decreased effectiveness of levothyroxine leading to hypothyroidism

FOODS

cottonseed meal, dietary fiber, soybean flour (infant formula), walnuts: Possibly decreased absorption of levothyroxine from GI tract
grapefruit juice: Possible delayed absorption of levothyroxine and reduced bioavailability

Adverse Reactions

CNS: Anxiety, craniosynostosis (infants with overtreatment), emotional lability, fatigue, fever, headache, heat intolerance, hyperactivity, insomnia, irritability, nervousness, **pseudotumor cerebri** (children), **seizures** (rare), somnolence, tremors
CV: Angina, **arrhythmias**, **cardiac arrest**, **heart failure**, increased blood pressure and pulse, **MI**, palpitations, tachycardia
ENDO: Hyperthyroidism (with over-replacement), **myxedema coma (with undertreatment)**, worsening of diabetic control
GI: Abdominal cramps or pain, diarrhea, dysphagia, elevated liver enzymes, increased appetite, nausea, vomiting
GU: Impaired fertility, menstrual irregularities
MS: Arthralgia, decreased bone mineral density (with over-replacement), premature closure of the epiphysis (children), muscle spasm or weakness, myalgia, slipped capital femoral epiphysis (children)
RESP: Dyspnea, wheezing
SKIN: Alopecia (transient), diaphoresis, flushing, pruritus, rash, urticaria
Other: Angioedema, serum sickness, weight gain or loss

Nursing Considerations

- Be aware that levothyroxin therapy is not to be used for treatment of obesity or for weight loss.
- Use levothyroxine cautiously in the elderly and patients with underlying cardiovascular disease. Know that levothyroxine should be started at a lower dose in these patients because overtreatment can increase cardiac contractility, cardiac wall thickness, and heart rate, which can precipitate angina or arrhythmias. Also use caution in patients with coronary artery disease undergoing surgery while receiving suppressive levothyroxin therapy and in patients receiving sympathomimetic drugs concurrently. Monitor for signs and symptoms of coronary insufficiency.
- Use caution when administering levothyroxine to children to avoid overtreatment or undertreatment. Be aware that overtreatment may cause craniosynostosis in infants, may adversely

affect brain maturation, and may accelerate the bone age and result in premature epiphyseal closure, which will compromise stature for life. Undertreatment may cause adverse effects on intellectual development and linear growth of the child.
- Administer levothyroxine capsules or tablets as a single daily dose 30 to 60 minutes before breakfast. Capsules must be swallowed whole. If patient has difficulty swallowing or patient is an infant or small child, crush tablet and suspend in a small amount of water or food avoiding liquids that decrease absorption of levothyroxine, such as soybean infant formula. Once mixed, do not store the suspension.
- Give oral levothyroxine at least 4 hours before or after aluminum- or magnesium-containing antacids, bile acid sequestrants, calcium carbonate, cation exchange resins, cholestyramine, colestipol, ferrous sulfate, kayexalate, or sucralfate to prevent decreased drug absorption.
- Expect to give drug I.V. if patient can't take tablets.
- For I.V. use, reconstitute drug by adding 5 ml of normal saline solution.
- Monitor PT of patient who is receiving anticoagulants; she may require a dosage adjustment.
- Monitor blood glucose level of diabetic patient because drug may worsen glycemic control and result in increased antidiabetic agent or insulin requirement. Carefully monitor patient after starting, changing, or discontinuing levothyroxine.
- Expect patient to undergo thyroid function tests regularly during levothyroxine therapy. Monitor patient for signs and symptoms of over- or undertreatment with levothyroxine because drug has a narrow therapeutic index. Be aware that atrial fibrillation is the most common arrhythmia with levothyroxine overtreatment in the elderly.
- Keep in mind when interpreting TBG levels that many disorders and medications can decrease TBG concentration, causing a TBG deficiency.

PATIENT TEACHING
- Inform patient that levothyroxine replaces a hormone that is normally produced by the thyroid gland and that she'll probably need to take drug for life.
- Instruct patient to take drug at least 30 minutes before breakfast because drug absorption is increased on an empty stomach and evening doses may cause insomnia.
- Emphasize the need to take levothyroxine with a full glass of water to avoid choking, gagging, having tablet stick in throat, and developing heartburn afterward.
- Instruct patient to separate antacids and calcium or iron supplements by at least 4 hours from levothyroxine doses.
- Inform patient that drug may require a few weeks to take effect.
- Advise patient not to stop drug or change dosage unless instructed by prescriber.
- Instruct patient to report signs of hyperthyroidism, such as chest pain, diarrhea, excessive sweating, fever, headache, heat intolerance, insomnia, irritability, leg cramps, nervousness, palpitations, weight loss, shortness of breath, tremors, and vomiting.
- Tell patient to notify prescriber if hives or rash develop during drug use.
- Inform patient that transient hair loss may occur during first few months of levothyroxine therapy.
- Instruct female patient of childbearing age to notify prescriber immediately if she becomes pregnant because levothyroxine dosage may have to be increased.

lidocaine hydrochloride
(lignocaine hydrochloride)

Alphacaine (CAN), Anestacon, DermaFlex, Dilocaine, L-Caine, Lidoderm, Xylocaine, Xylocard (CAN), Zingo

Class and Category
Pharmacologic class: Amide derivative
Therapeutic class: Class IB antiarrhythmic, local anesthetic
Pregnancy category: B

Indications and Dosages

➤ *To treat ventricular fibrillation or ventricular tachycardia*

I.V. INFUSION AND INJECTION

Adults. *Loading:* 50 to 100 mg (or 1 to 1.5 mg/kg), given at 25 to 50 mg/min. If desired response isn't achieved after 5 to 10 min, second dose of 25 to 50 mg (or 0.5 to 0.75 mg/kg) given every 5 to 10 min until maximum loading dose (300 mg in 1 hr) has been given. *Maintenance:* 20 to 50 mcg/kg/min (1 to 4 mg/min) by continuous infusion. Smaller bolus dose repeated 15 to 20 min after start of infusion if needed to maintain therapeutic blood level. *Maximum:* 300 mg (or 3 mg/kg) over 1 hr.

Children. *Loading:* 1 mg/kg. *Maintenance:* 30 mcg/kg/min by continuous infusion. *Maximum:* 3 mg/kg.

DOSAGE ADJUSTMENT For elderly patients and for patients with acute hepatitis or decompensated cirrhosis, loading dose and continuous infusion rate reduced by 50%. For patients with severe renal impairment (creatinine clearance estimated glomerular filtration rate less than 30 ml/min), maintenance infusion rate reduced. For children, if infusion is not initiated within 15 min of the initial bolus dose, bolus dose repeated.

➤ *To provide topical anesthesia for mucous membranes or skin*

FILM-FORMING GEL, JELLY, OR OINTMENT

Adults. Thin layer applied to skin or mucous membranes as needed before procedure.

➤ *To provide pain relief postherpetic neuralgia*

TRANSDERMAL PATCH

Adults. 1 to 3 patches applied over most painful area only once for up to 12 hr within a 24-hr period.

➤ *To provide topical anesthesia before venous access procedures*

POWDER

Children ages 3 to 18. Compressed gas application of powder to selected skin site 1 to 3 min before procedure.

Route	Onset	Peak	Duration
I.V.	45–90 sec	Immediate	10–20 min
Topical	2–5 min	Unknown	0.5–1 hr

Mechanism of Action

Combines with fast sodium channels in myocardial cell membranes, which inhibits sodium influx into cells and decreases ventricular depolarization, as well as automaticity and excitability during diastole. Lidocaine also blocks nerve impulses by decreasing the permeability of neuronal membranes to sodium, which produces local anesthesia.

Incompatibilities

Do not mix lidocaine with blood transfusions because of the possibility of hemolysis or pseudoagglutination. Also do not administer with solutions containing amphotericin, cephazolin, or phenytoin because of precipitate formation.

Contraindications

Adams–Stokes syndrome; hypersensitivity to lidocaine, amide anesthetics, or their components; severe heart block (without artificial pacemaker); Wolff–Parkinson–White syndrome

Interactions

DRUGS

amiodarone, phenytoin, procainamide, propranolol, quinidine: Additive cardiac effects possibly resulting in toxicity; antagonistic cardiac effects

beta blockers, CYP1A2 inhibitors such as fluvoxamine, CYP3A4 inhibitors such as propofol, cimetidine: Increased blood lidocaine level and risk of toxicity

CYP1A2 inducers, CYP3A4 inducers: Decreased blood lidocaine level with decreased effectiveness

MAO inhibitors, tricyclic antidepressants: Risk of severe, prolonged hypertension

mexiletine, tocainide: Additive cardiac effects

neuromuscular blockers: Possibly increased neuromuscular blockade

phenytoin, procainamide: Increased cardiac depression

Adverse Reactions

CNS: Agitation; anxiety; apprehension; confusion; difficulty speaking; disorientation; dizziness; drowsiness; euphoria; hallucinations; lethargy; light-headedness; **malignant hyperthermia**; paresthesia; **seizures**; sensation of cold, heat, or numbness; tremors; twitching; unconsciousness

CV: **Bradycardia**, **cardiac arrest**, **hypotension**, **new or worsening arrhythmias**, tachycardia
EENT: Blurred vision, diplopia, oral hypoesthesia, tinnitus
GI: Nausea, vomiting
HEME: **Methemoglobinemia**
MS: Dysarthria, muscle weakness, myalgia
RESP: **Respiratory arrest or depression**
Other: **Anaphylaxis**; other less severe hypersensitivity reactions; injection-site burning, irritation, petechiae, redness, stinging, swelling, and tenderness; worsened pain

Nursing Considerations

- Use caution in patients with severe hepatic or renal disease because accumulation of lidocaine may occur and lead to toxicity. Also, use caution in patients with any form of AV block, including AV block caused by digitalis toxicity, as well as in patients with hypovolemia and shock.
- Use caution when administering lidocaine to patients with compromised myocardial function because of risk of electrolyte disturbances or fluid overload.
- Observe for respiratory depression after bolus injection and during I.V. infusion of lidocaine.
- Keep life-support equipment and vasopressors nearby during I.V. use in case of respiratory depression or other reactions. Hypersensitivity reactions, including anaphylaxis, have occurred with lidocaine-containing solutions.
- Carefully check prefilled syringes before using. Use only syringes labeled "for cardiac arrhythmias" for I.V. administration.
- As ordered, titrate I.V. dose to minimum amount needed to prevent arrhythmias. If administration is controlled by a pumping device, stop pump before container runs dry because an air embolism may result. Change intravenous administration apparatus at least once every 24 hours.
- During I.V. administration, place patient on cardiac monitor, as ordered, and closely observe her at all times. Monitor for prolonged PR interval, widening QRS complex, or worsening arrhythmias—possible signs of drug toxicity. If present, notify prescriber and expect to discontinue lidocaine therapy immediately. Although infrequent, also monitor her for hypersensitivity reactions that can be as severe as anaphylaxis following lidocaine administration. If anaphylaxis occurs, discontinue drug, notify prescriber, and provide supportive care.
- Check blood drug level, as ordered. Therapeutic level is 2 to 5 mcg/ml.
- If signs of toxicity, such as dizziness, occur, notify prescriber and expect to discontinue or slow infusion.
- Monitor for malignant hyperthermia. If present, stop lidocaine administration immediately, notify prescriber, and provide therapeutic countermeasures, as indicated and ordered.
- Apply lidocaine jelly or ointment to gauze or bandage before applying to skin.
- Monitor vital signs as well as BUN and serum creatinine and electrolyte levels during and after therapy.

PATIENT TEACHING

- Inform patient who receives lidocaine as an anesthetic that she'll feel numbness.
- Advise patient to report difficulty speaking, dizziness, injection-site pain, nausea, numbness or tingling, and vision changes.
- Caution patient to keep lidocaine topical preparations and patches out of reach of children and pets.
- Tell patient to wash hands thoroughly after handling lidocaine topical forms or patch and to avoid getting drug in eyes.
- Remind patient using patches to store them in their sealed envelopes until needed and to apply immediately after removing from the envelope. Tell patient to remove patch if burning or irritation occurs at the site and not to reapply until irritation is gone.
- Tell patient to fold used patches so that the adhesive side sticks to itself and discard where children or pets cannot get to them.
- Warn patient prescribed a lidocaine patch not to place external heat sources, such as electric blanket or heating pad, on it while wearing it, because heat may cause the drug to be absorbed faster, increasing the risk of adverse effects.
- Instruct women of childbearing age to alert prescriber if pregnancy is suspected or known, because lidocaine may cross the

placental barrier. Inform mothers wishing to breastfeed that lidocaine is present in breast milk and to discuss wisdom of breastfeeding with prescriber before doing so.

linaclotide

Linzess

Class and Category

Pharmacologic class: Guanylate cyclase-C agonist
Therapeutic class: Bowel stimulator
Pregnancy category: C

Indications and Dosages

➤ *To treat irritable bowel syndrome with constipation*

CAPSULES

Adults. 290 mcg once daily on an empty stomach, at least 30 min prior to the first meal of the day.

➤ *To treat chronic, idiopathic constipation*

CAPSULES

Adults. 145 mcg once daily on an empty stomach, at least 30 min prior to the first meal of the day.

Mechanism of Action

Acts locally on the luminal surface of the intestinal epithelium through activation of guanylate cyclase-C, which increases both extracellular and intracellular concentrations of cyclic guanosine monophosphate (cGMP). Elevation in intracellular cGMP stimulates secretion of bicarbonate and chloride into the intestinal lumen, which increases intestinal fluid and accelerates GI transit to relieve constipation. Increased extracellular cGMP decreases the activity of pain-sensing nerves, resulting in a reduction of intestinal pain present with constipation and irritable bowel syndrome.

Contraindications

Hypersensitivity to linaclotide or its components, known or suspected mechanical gastrointestinal obstruction, pediatric patients under 6 years of age

Adverse Reactions

CNS: Fatigue, headache
EENT: Sinusitis
GI: Abdominal distention or pain, defecation urgency, diarrhea (may become severe), dyspepsia, fecal incontinence, flatulence, gastroesophageal reflux, hematochezia, **melena**, **rectal hemorrhage**, viral gastroenteritis, vomiting
RESP: Upper respiratory infection
SKIN: Urticaria
Other: **Hypersensitivity reactions**

Nursing Considerations

- Be aware that although linaclotide is contraindicated in children under 6 years of age, it also is not recommended to be given to children between the ages of 6 and 17 years.
- Monitor patient for diarrhea that may become severe. If severe diarrhea occurs, assess patient for dizziness, electrolyte abnormalities (hypokalemia and hyponatremia), hypotension, and syncope. Notify prescriber if diarrhea occurs. Expect to withhold drug. Also know that if severe, patient may require hospitalization and intravenous fluid administration.
- Open capsules for patients having difficulty swallowing capsules and sprinkle contents on 1 teaspoon of applesauce or mix with 1 ounce of room-temperature bottled water (swirl beads and water for at least 20 seconds) just prior to administration. Linaclotide can also be administered through a gastrostomy or nasogastric tube by mixing first with 1 ounce room-temperature bottled water (swirling beads and water for at least 20 seconds) immediately before administration.

PATIENT TEACHING

- Instruct patient to swallow the capsules whole and to avoid breaking the capsule apart or chewing it. However, if patient has difficulty swallowing capsules, tell patient to open capsule and mix with either 1 teaspoon of applesauce or 1 ounce of room-temperature bottled water (swirl beads in the for at least 20 seconds) immediately before ingesting.
- Tell patient that linaclotide is to be taken on an empty stomach 30 minutes before the first meal of the day.
- Advise patient to stop taking linaclotide if severe diarrhea occurs and to contact prescriber immediately because

hospitalization and intravenous fluid replacement may be necessary.

- Instruct patient to store linaclotide out of the reach of children.

linagliptin

Tradjenta

Class and Category

Pharmacologic class: Dipeptidyl peptidase-4 (DDP-4) enzyme inhibitor
Therapeutic class: Antidiabetic
Pregnancy category: B

Indications and Dosages

➤ *As adjunct to improve glycemic control in type 2 diabetes mellitus*

TABLETS

Adults. 5 mg once daily.

DOSAGE ADJUSTMENT For patients taking a supplemental oral hypoglycemic agent or insulin, dosage may need to be reduced.

Mechanism of Action

Inhibits the enzyme, dipeptidyl peptidase-4, that degrades incretin hormones responsible for glucose elevation. This allows levels of incretin hormones to rise, stimulating the release of insulin in a glucose-dependent manner while decreasing the glucagon level in the blood. In addition, glucagon secretion from pancreatic alpha cells is reduced, resulting in a reduction in the amount of glucose released by the liver. These combined actions reduce blood glucose levels, thereby improving glycemic control in type 2 diabetes.

Contraindications

Hypersensitivity to linagliptin or its components, ketoacidosis, type 1 diabetes mellitus

Interactions

DRUGS

CYP3A4 or P-gp inducers (strong) such as rifampin: Decreased linagliptin effectiveness
insulin, sulfonylureas: Increased risk of hypoglycemia

Adverse Reactions

CNS: Headache
CV: Hyperlipidemia, hypertriglyceridemia
EENT: Mouth ulceration, nasopharyngitis, stomatitis
ENDO: Hypoglycemia
GI: Acute pancreatitis, constipation, diarrhea, elevated lipase level
GU: UTI
MS: Arthralgia (may be disabling and severe); back, extremity, or joint pain; myalgia
RESP: Bronchial hyperreactivity, cough
SKIN: Localized skin exfoliation, rash, urticaria
Other: Anaphylaxis, **angioedema**, elevated uric acid, weight gain

Nursing Considerations

WARNING Know that linagliptin's hypersensitivity may be exhibited through serious adverse reactions such as anaphylaxis, angioedema, bronchial hyperreactivity, exfoliative skin conditions, or urticaria. Monitor patient closely for hypersensitivity reactions. If present, withhold drug immediately, notify prescriber, and be prepared to administer emergency care, as ordered.

- Be aware that heart failure has been linked to two other drugs in the same class as linagliptin. Use caution when administering linagliptin, especially to patients with a prior history of heart failure or renal impairment. Monitor patient for signs and symptoms of heart failure and report any to prescriber immediately.
- Monitor patient closely for hypoglycemia, especially if another antidiabetic drug, such as insulin or a sulfonylurea is used concomitantly. If signs and symptoms of hypoglycemia occur, check patient's blood glucose level. If confirmed, administer 15 g of an oral rapid-acting carbohydrate. After 15 minutes, repeat blood glucose and, if needed, administer 15 g of an oral rapid-acting carbohydrate again. (Administer glucagon 1 mg parenterally, as ordered; if patient is unresponsive, and repeat dose in 15 minutes, if needed.) Notify prescriber of incident, as dosage of the other antidiabetic drug may need to be reduced.
- Monitor the patient's blood glucose level routinely to determine response to drug. Expect to check the patient's glycosylated hemoglobin every 3 to 6 months or as ordered to evaluate long-term blood glucose control.

- Monitor patient for signs and symptoms of pancreatitis such as abdominal pain, fever, nausea, sweating, and vomiting. Notify prescriber if present, and expect drug to be discontinued, as acute pancreatitis may become life-threatening.

PATIENT TEACHING

- Urge patient to report evidence of hypoglycemia, such as anxiety, confusion, dizziness, excessive sweating, headache, and nausea.
- Encourage patient to carry hard candy or other simple sugars to treat mild hypoglycemia.
- Urge patient to carry identification indicating that he has diabetes.
- Teach patient how to monitor his blood glucose level.
- Instruct patient about diet, exercise, foot care, hygiene, signs of hyperglycemia and hypoglycemia, and ways to avoid infection.
- Tell patient to stop drug if he experiences signs and symptoms of an allergic reaction such as difficulty breathing, hives, rash, or swelling of face or skin or signs and symptoms of acute pancreatitis such as persistent severe abdominal pain radiating to the back, which may or may not be accompanied by vomiting, and to seek medical attention immediately.
- Review signs and symptoms of heart failure with patient such as difficulty breathing; swelling or fluid retention, especially in ankles, feet, or legs; unusual tiredness; or fast weight gain. Tell patient to report any such symptoms immediately.
- Inform mother wishing to breastfeed that linagliptin is present in breast milk, so she should discuss breastfeeding with prescriber before doing so.

lincomycin hydrochloride

Lincocin

Class and Category

Pharmacologic class: Lincosamide
Therapeutic class: Antibiotic
Pregnancy category: C

Indications and Dosages

➤ *To treat serious respiratory, skin, and soft-tissue infections caused by susceptible strains of pneumococci, staphylococci, and streptococci*

CAPSULES

Adults and adolescents. 500 mg every 6 to 8 hr.
Children over age 1 month. 7.5 to 15 mg/kg every 6 hr or 10 to 20 mg/kg every 8 hr.

I.V. INFUSION

Adults. 600 mg to 1 g infused over at least 1 hr for each gram given every 8 to 12 hr. *Maximum:* 8 g daily in divided doses for life-threatening infection.
Children over age 1 month. 10 to 20 mg/kg/day infused over at least 1 hr for each gram given in divided doses every 8 to 12 hr, depending on severity of infection.

I.M. INJECTION

Adults and adolescents. 600 mg every 12 to 24 hr.
Children over age 1 month. 10 mg/kg every 12 to 24 hr.

DOSAGE ADJUSTMENT Dosage reduced by 25% to 30% for patients with severely impaired renal function.

Mechanism of Action

Inhibits protein synthesis in susceptible bacteria by binding to 50S subunit of bacterial ribosomes and preventing peptide bond formation, causing bacterial cells to die.

Incompatibilities

Don't give lincomycin with kanamycin or novobiocin.

Contraindications

Hypersensitivity to lincomycin, clindamycin, or their components

Interactions

DRUGS

antimyasthenic drugs: Possibly antagonized effects of these drugs
chloramphenicol, clindamycin, erythromycin: Possibly blocked access of lincomycin to its site of action
hydrocarbon inhalation anesthetics, neuromuscular blockers: Increased neuromuscular blockade, possibly severe respiratory depression
opioid analgesics: Increased risk of increased or prolonged respiratory depression

Adverse Reactions

CNS: Dizziness, fever, headache, somnolence, tinnitus, vertigo
CV: **Cardio-respiratory arrest**, **hypotension**, thrombophlebitis (intravenous administration)
EENT: Glossitis, stomatitis, tinnitus
GI: Abdominal cramps or pain, anal pruritus, colitis, ***Clostridium difficile*-associated diarrhea**, diarrhea, elevated liver enzymes, jaundice, nausea, **pseudomembranous colitis**, rectal candidiasis, vomiting
GU: **Azotemia**, oliguria, proteinuria, renal impairment, vaginal candidiasis
HEME: **Agranulocytosis**, **aplastic anemia**, eosinophilia, **leukopenia**, **neutropenia**, **pancytopenia**, **thrombocytopenia**
SKIN: Acute generalized exanthematous pustulosis, bullous dermatitis, **erythema multiforme**, **exfoliative dermatitis**, pruritus, rash, **Stevens–Johnson syndrome**, **toxic epidermal necrolysis**, urticaria
Other: **Anaphylaxis**; **angioedema**; injection-site abscess, induration, irritation, or pain; serum sickness

Nursing Considerations

- Expect to obtain a specimen for culture and sensitivity testing before giving first dose of lincomycin.

WARNING Be aware that some lincomycin preparations contain benzyl alcohol, which can cause a fatal toxic syndrome in neonates or premature infants characterized by circulatory, CNS, renal, and respiratory impairment and metabolic acidosis. Because drug enters breast milk, breastfeeding patient may need to stop drug or stop breastfeeding.

- Dilute 600-mg dose in at least 100 ml D_5W, $D_{10}W$, normal saline solution, dextrose 5% in normal saline solution, or other compatible diluent recommended by manufacturer. Dilute higher doses in 100 ml of a compatible diluent for each gram being given—for example, dilute a 3-g dose in at least 300 ml of diluent. Use diluted solution within 24 hours if stored at room temperature.

WARNING Give lincomycin over at least 1 hour for each gram being administered. For example, infuse 1 g over 1 hour and 3 g over 3 hours. Too-rapid infusion may result in cardiac arrest or hypotension.

WARNING Monitor patient for hypersensitivity reaction, such as pruritus, rash, wheezing, and dysphagia from laryngeal edema. Also monitor patient for severe cutaneous adverse reactions. If a reaction occurs, stop infusion and notify prescriber immediately. If anaphylaxis occurs, provide care according to medical protocol. Be aware that patients with a history of asthma or significant allergies are at increased risk of hypersensitivity.

- Observe patient for evidence of superinfection, such as vaginal itching and sore mouth.
- Monitor patient for signs of pseudomembranous colitis, such as loose, watery stools. Patients with a history of GI disease, particularly colitis or regional enteritis, are at increased risk for colitis. In elderly patients, antibiotic-related diarrhea may be less well-tolerated or more severe. Notify prescriber if prolonged or severe diarrhea develops; it may indicate pseudomembranous colitis caused by *C. difficile.* Expect to withhold lincomycin and treat with an antibiotic effective against *C. difficile,* as well as electrolytes, fluids, and protein.
- Monitor results of CBC, platelet counts, and liver and renal function tests periodically during lincomycin therapy.
- Before diluting drug, store it at a controlled room temperature of 20° to 25°C (68° to 77°F).

PATIENT TEACHING

- Advise patient to take lincomycin capsules with a full glass of water on an empty stomach 1 hour before or 2 hours after meals to maximize drug's effectiveness.
- Review with patient possibly serious adverse reactions, such as chest tightness, difficulty breathing, and rash, and tell the patient to report any that occur.
- Inform patient that buttermilk or yogurt can help maintain intestinal flora and may decrease the risk of diarrhea.
- Urge patient to tell prescriber about diarrhea that's severe or lasts longer than 3 days. Remind patient that bloody or watery stools can occur 2 or more months

after antibiotic therapy and can be serious, requiring prompt treatment.
- Emphasize the importance of following dosage regimen and keeping follow-up laboratory and medical appointments.

linezolid

Zyvox

Class and Category

Pharmacologic class: Oxazolidinone
Therapeutic class: Antibiotic
Pregnancy category: C

Indications and Dosages

➤ *To treat vancomycin-resistant* Enterococcus faecium *infections, including bacteremia*

ORAL SUSPENSION, TABLETS, I.V. INFUSION

Adults and adolescents. 600 mg every 12 hr for 14 to 28 days.
Neonates age 7 days and over, infants, and children. 10 mg/kg every 8 hr for 14 to 28 days.
Neonates younger than 7 days. 10 mg/kg every 12 hr, increased to every 8 hr when neonate is 7 days old. Given for 14 to 28 days.

➤ *To treat nosocomial pneumonia caused by* Staphylococcus aureus *(methicillin-susceptible and resistant strains) or* Streptococcus pneumoniae *(penicillin-susceptible strains only) and community-acquired pneumonia, including accompanying bacteremia, caused by* S. aureus *(methicillin-susceptible strains only) or* S. pneumoniae *(penicillin-susceptible strains only); to treat complicated skin and soft-tissue infections, including diabetic foot infections without concomitant osteomyelitis, caused by* S. aureus *(methicillin-susceptible and resistant strains),* Streptococcus *agalactiae, or* Streptococcus pyogenes

ORAL SUSPENSION, TABLETS, I.V. INFUSION

Adults and adolescents. 600 mg every 12 hr for 10 to 14 days. I.V. infused over 30 min to 2 hr.
Neonates age 7 days or older, infants, and children. 10 mg/kg every 8 hr for 10 to 14 days. I.V. infused over 30 min to 2 hr.
Neonates younger than 7 days. 10 mg/kg every 12 hr, increased to every 8 hr when neonate is 7 days old. Given for 10 to 14 days. I.V. infused over 30 min to 2 hr.

➤ *To treat uncomplicated skin and soft-tissue infections caused by* S. aureus *(methicillin-susceptible strains only) or* S. pyogenes

ORAL SUSPENSION, TABLETS

Adults. 400 mg every 12 hr for 10 to 14 days.
Adolescents. 600 mg every 12 hr for 10 to 14 days.
Children age 5 to 11. 10 mg/kg every 12 hr for 10 to 14 days.
Neonates age 7 days and over, infants, and children to age 5. 10 mg/kg every 8 hr.
Neonates younger than 7 days. 10 mg/kg every 12 hr, increased to every 8 hr when neonate is 7 days old. Given for 10 to 14 days.

Incompatibilities

Don't add other drugs to linezolid solution. Don't infuse linezolid in same I.V. line as amphotericin B, chlorpromazine hydrochloride, cotrimoxazole, diazepam, erythromycin lactobionate, pentamidine isethionate, or phenytoin sodium because these drugs are physically incompatible. Don't infuse linezolid with ceftriaxone sodium because these drugs are chemically incompatible.

Contraindications

Carcinoid syndrome; concurrent therapy with buspirone, dopaminergic agents, meperidine, serotonin 5-HT_1 receptor agonists, serotonin reuptake inhibitors, sympathomimetic agents, tricyclic antidepressants, or vasopressive agents without careful monitoring; hypersensitivity to linezolid or its components; phenylketonuria; thyrotoxicosis; uncontrolled hypertension; use within 14 days of an MAO inhibitor

Interactions

DRUGS

adrenergics, including phenylpropanolamine and pseudoephedrine, dopaminergic agents, serotonergic agents, vasopressive agents such as epinephrine or norepinephrine: Possibly increased blood pressure

buspirone, meperidine, serotonergics, tricyclic antidepressants: Possibly serotonin syndrome
carbamazepine, phenytoin, phenobarbital, rifampin: Possibly decreased plasma linezolid level
MAO inhibitors: Increased risk of life-threatening adverse effects
FOODS
tyramine-containing beverages and foods: Possibly hypertension

Adverse Reactions

CNS: Dizziness, fever, headache, insomnia, peripheral neuropathy, **seizures**, **serotonin syndrome**, vertigo
CV: Hypertension
EENT: Optic neuropathy with possible loss of vision, oral candidiasis, taste alteration, tooth or tongue discoloration
GI: Abdominal pain, constipation, diarrhea, elevated liver enzymes, indigestion, nausea, **pseudomembranous colitis**, vomiting
GU: Vaginal candidiasis
HEME: Anemia, eosinophilia, **leukopenia**, **pancytopenia**, **siberoblastic anemia**, **thrombocytopenia**
SKIN: Bullous dermatitis, pruritus, rash, **Stevens–Johnson syndrome**, **toxic epidermal necrolysis**
Other: **Anaphylaxis**, **angioedema**, fungal infections, **lactic acidosis**

Mechanism of Action

Linezolid inhibits bacterial protein synthesis by interfering with translation of ribonucleic acid (RNA) to protein. In bacteria, protein synthesis begins with binding of a 30S ribosomal subunit and a 50S ribosomal subunit to a messenger RNA (mRNA) molecule to form a 70S initiation complex. The 50S ribosomal subunit consists of 23S ribosomal RNA (rRNA) and other ribosomal subunits. Then translation begins. Transfer RNA (tRNA) attaches to the 50S subunit and brings specific amino acids into place. As the tRNA and amino acids fall into place, they are joined together by peptide bonds and elongate to form a polypeptide chain, as shown below left. This chain eventually combines with other polypeptide chains to form a complete protein molecule. After translation is complete, the ribosomal subunits fall away and are ready to combine with more mRNA to start the translation process over again.

Linezolid binds to a site on the bacterial 23S rRNA of the 50S subunit. This action prevents formation of a functional 70S initiation complex, an essential component of the bacterial translation. Without proper protein production, as shown below right, susceptible bacteria are unable to multiply. Linezolid is bactericidal against most streptococci and bacteriostatic against staphylococci and enterococci.

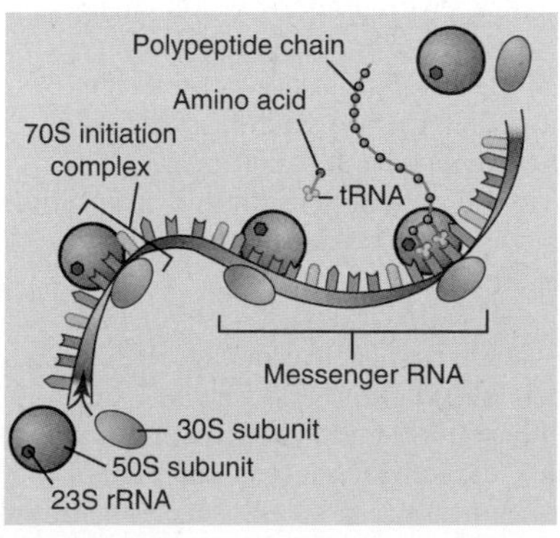

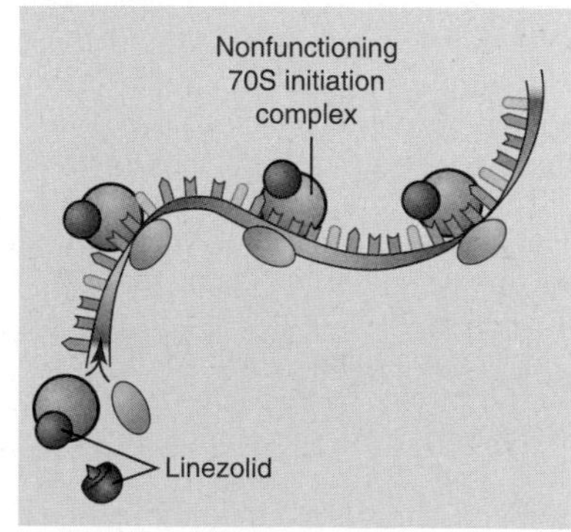

J K L

Nursing Considerations

- Obtain body tissue and fluid specimens for culture and sensitivity tests, as ordered, before giving first dose of linezolid. Expect to start drug before test results are known.
- Be aware that linezolid shouldn't be used to treat catheter-related bloodstream infections, catheter-site infections, or infections caused by gram-negative bacteria because the risk of death is higher in these infections.
- Infuse I.V. solution over 30 to 120 minutes with D_5W, normal saline solution, or lactated Ringer's solution.

WARNING Monitor CBC weekly, as ordered, to detect or track worsening myelosuppression in patients who need more than 2 weeks of therapy, who have preexisting myelosuppression and are receiving drugs that produce bone marrow suppression, or who have chronic infection and are receiving or have received antibiotic therapy.

- Notify prescriber if patient develops visual impairment that suggests optic neuropathy, such as blurred vision, changes in color vision or visual acuity, lost vision, or visual field defect. If optic or peripheral neuropathy develops, the drug may need to be stopped.
- Know that if patient takes a dopaminergic agent, sympathomimetic agent, or vasopressive agent, monitor blood pressure closely; if monitoring isn't possible, know that linezolid shouldn't be prescribed.
- Be aware that while linezolid should not be given to patients receiving serotonergic drugs, there are some conditions that may be life-threatening and require the use of linezolid, such as the presence of vancomycin-resistent *Enterococcus faecium* (VRE) or infections such as nosocomial pneumonia and complicated skin and skin structure infections, including those caused by *methicillin-resistant Staphylococcus aureus* (MRSA). If patient takes buspirone, meperidine, or a serotonergic or tricyclic antidepressant, watch closely for signs and symptoms of serotonin syndrome; if monitoring isn't possible, know that linezolid shouldn't be prescribed.
- Assess bowel pattern daily. Also watch for secondary infection, including oral candidiasis and profuse, watery diarrhea.
- Monitor patient with diabetes who is also taking antidiabetic medication because hypoglycemia has been linked to linezolid use in these patients. If hypoglycemia occurs, treat appropriately and notify prescriber, as the dosage of the antidiabetic medication may have to be decreased.

PATIENT TEACHING

- Caution patient with phenylketonuria that oral suspension contains phenylalanine and that he should receive tablets instead.
- Tell patient to store oral suspension at room temperature and to discard any unused portion after 21 days.
- Advise patient not to take OTC cold remedies without consulting prescriber because medications that contain propanolamine or pseudoephedrine may cause or worsen hypertension.
- Instruct patient to avoid beverages and foods that contain large amounts of tyramine, including aged cheese, air-dried or fermented meats, protein-rich foods that have been stored for long periods or poorly refrigerated, red wines, soy sauce, and tap beers.
- Instruct patient to notify prescriber at once about severe diarrhea, even up to 2 months after linezolid therapy has ended, because additional treatment may be needed.
- Tell patient to report changes in limb sensation (such as numbness, pins and needles, or tingling) or vision changes because drug may have to be stopped. Also, tell patient to notify prescriber immediately if persistent, severe, or unusual signs and symptoms develop.
- Reassure patient with tooth discoloration that professional dental cleaning can restore tooth color.
- Advise diabetic patients prescribed antidiabetic medications to monitor their blood glucose closely and be prepared to treat hypoglycemia if it should occur. If present, tell patient to notify prescriber as a dosage adjustment may be required in his antidiabetic medication.

liothyronine sodium

(L-triiodothyronine, sodium L-triiodothyronine, T_3, thyronine sodium)

Cytomel, Triostat

Class and Category

Pharmacologic class: Synthetic triiodothyronine (T_3)
Therapeutic class: Thyroid hormone replacement
Pregnancy category: A

Indications and Dosages

➤ *To treat mild hypothyroidism*

TABLETS (CYTOMEL)

Adults. *Initial:* 25 mcg daily. Increased by 12.5 to 25 mcg every 1 to 2 wk until response occurs. *Maintenance:* 25 to 75 mcg daily.

➤ *To treat congenital hypothyroidism*

TABLETS (CYTOMEL)

Adults and children. *Initial:* 5 mcg daily. Increased by 5 mcg every 3 to 4 days until desired response occurs. *Maintenance:* Highly individualized.

➤ *To treat simple nontoxic goiter*

TABLETS (CYTOMEL)

Adults. *Initial:* 5 mcg daily. Increased by 5 to 10 mcg every 1 to 2 wk up to 25 mcg daily. Then increased by 12.5 to 25 mcg/wk, as indicated. *Maintenance:* 75 mcg daily.

➤ *To treat myxedema*

TABLETS (CYTOMEL)

Adults. *Initial:* 5 mcg daily. Increased 5 to 10 mcg every 1 to 2 wk up to 25 mcg daily. Then increased by 5 to 25 mcg every 1 to 2 wk, as indicated. *Maintenance:* 50 to 100 mcg daily.

DOSAGE ADJUSTMENT For elderly and pediatric patients and those with cardiovascular disease, initial dose reduced to 5 mcg daily and then increased by 5 mcg at recommended intervals.

➤ *To treat myxedema coma or premyxedema coma (severe hypothyroidism)*

I.V. INJECTION (TRIOSTAT)

Adults. *Initial:* 25 to 50 mcg. Repeated every 4 to 12 hr according to patient's response. Then P.O. therapy is resumed as soon as possible.

DOSAGE ADJUSTMENT When treating myxedema coma in patients with known or suspected cardiovascular disease, initial dose decreased to 10 to 20 mcg.

➤ *To differentiate hyperthyroidism from euthyroidism (T_3 suppression test)*

TABLETS (CYTOMEL)

Adults. 75 to 100 mcg daily for 7 days.

Route	Onset	Peak	Duration
P.O.	24–72 hr	48–72 hr	Up to 72 hr
I.V.	2–4 hr	2 days	Unknown

Mechanism of Action

Replaces endogenous thyroid hormone, which may exert its physiologic effects by controlling DNA transcription and protein synthesis. Like endogenous thyroid hormone, liothyronine:

- accelerates the rate of cellular oxidation, which stimulates body tissue growth, maturation, and metabolism
- aids in myelination of nerves and development of synaptic processes in the nervous system
- decreases blood and hepatic cholesterol concentrations
- enhances carbohydrate and protein metabolism, increasing gluconeogenesis and protein synthesis
- increases energy expenditure
- regulates differentiation and proliferation of stem cells
- regulates growth.

Contraindications

Acute MI (unless caused or complicated by hypothyroidism), hypersensitivity to liothyronine or its components, uncorrected adrenal insufficiency, untreated thyrotoxicosis

Interactions

DRUGS

adrenocorticoids: Possibly need for adrenocorticoid dosage adjustments as thyroid status changes

beta blockers: Possibly impaired action of beta blockers
cholestyramine, colestipol: Decreased liothyronine absorption
digoxin: Reduced therapeutic effects of digoxin
estrogen, phenylbutazone, phenytoin: Reduced binding of liothyronine to protein, possibly requiring increased liothyronine dosage
insulin, oral antidiabetic: Possibly uncontrolled diabetes mellitus, requiring increased dosage of insulin or oral antidiabetic
ketamine: Possibly hypertension and tachycardia
maprotiline: Increased risk of arrhythmias
oral anticoagulants: Altered anticoagulant activity, possibly need for anticoagulant dosage adjustment
sympathomimetics: Increased risk of coronary insufficiency in patients with coronary artery disease
theophylline: Decreased theophylline clearance
tricyclic antidepressants: Increased therapeutic and toxic effects of both drugs

Adverse Reactions

CNS: Insomnia
ENDO: Hyperthyroidism (with overdose)
SKIN: Alopecia (transient), rash, urticaria

Nursing Considerations

- Be aware that liothyronine is used most often for rapid onset or rapidly reversible thyroid hormone replacement.
- Administer tablet as a single daily dose before breakfast.
- Give I.V. injections more than 4 hours but less than 12 hours apart.
- Evaluate response to therapy by monitoring blood pressure and pulse rate.
- Expect patient to undergo regular tests of thyroid function during therapy.
- Monitor PT of patient receiving anticoagulants because patient may require a dosage adjustment.
- Frequently monitor blood glucose level of diabetic patient. Prescriber may reduce antidiabetic drug dosage as thyroid hormone level enters therapeutic range.
- Be aware that liothyronine is used in T_3 suppression test to differentiate hyperthyroidism from euthyroidism (normal thyroid function). For this test, ^{131}I uptake test is performed before and after liothyronine administration. Suppression of ^{131}I uptake by 50% indicates normal thyroid function.

PATIENT TEACHING

- Inform patient that liothyronine usually is taken for life. Caution her not to change dosage or discontinue drug unless instructed by prescriber.
- Instruct patient to take drug before breakfast; evening doses may cause insomnia.
- Advise patient to report signs of hyperthyroidism, such as chest pain, excessive sweating, heat intolerance, increased pulse rate, nervousness, and palpitations.
- Inform patient that transient hair loss may occur during first few months of therapy.
- Instruct diabetic patient to monitor blood glucose level frequently because antidiabetic drug dosage may need to be reduced.
- Inform patient of need for periodic blood tests to monitor drug effectiveness.

liraglutide

Saxenda, Victoza

Class and Category

Pharmacologic class: Glucagon-like peptide-1 receptor agonist
Therapeutic class: Antidiabetic
Pregnancy category: C (Victoza), X (Saxenda)

Indications and Dosages

➤ *To improve glycemic control as an adjunct to diet and exercise in patients with type 2 diabetes mellitus; to reduce risk of major adverse cardiovascular events such as CVA or MI in patients with type 2 diabetes mellitus and established cardiovascular disease*

SUBCUTANEOUS INJECTION (VICTOZA)
Adults. *Initial:* 0.6 mg daily for 1 wk, then increased to 1.2 mg daily. *Maximum:* 1.8 mg daily.

➤ *Adjunct for chronic weight management in patients with an initial body mass index of 30 kg/m² or greater, or 27 kg/m² or greater in the presence of at least one weight-related comorbid condition such as dyslipidemia, hypertension, or type 2 diabetes mellitus*

SUBCUTANEOUS INJECTION (SAXENDA)

Adults. *Initial:* 0.6 mg daily for wk 1, increased to 1.2 mg daily for wk 2, increased to 1.8 mg daily for wk 3, increased to 2.4 mg daily for wk 4, and increased to 3 mg daily for wk 5 and onward. *Maintenance:* 3 mg daily.

Route	Onset	Peak	Duration
SubQ	Unknown	8–12 hr	Unknown

Mechanism of Action

Activates the glucagon-like peptide-1 site on pancreatic beta cells, which increases intracellular cyclic AMP, which increases insulin release when blood glucose level is elevated. In addition, because glucagon and insulin levels occur in an inverse relationship to plasma glucose level, increased insulin level will decrease glucagon level, which inhibits glucagon stimulation of the liver that increases plasma glucose level. Although its exact mechanism is unclear, liraglutide also delays gastric emptying, which helps prevent a sudden rise in plasma glucose level after eating. Together these actions work to lower plasma glucose level.

Binds to the glucagon-like peptide-1 receptor and activates it to regulate appetite and calorie intake, resulting in weight loss.

Contraindications

Family or personal history of medullary thyroid cancer, hypersensitivity to liraglutide or its components, ketoacidosis, pregnancy (Saxenda), presence of multiple endocrine neoplasia syndrome type 2, pregnancy, type 1 diabetes mellitus

Interactions

DRUGS

oral hypoglycemic agents such as sulfonylureas: Increased risk of hypoglycemia

orally administered drugs: Possibly decreased absorption of these drugs

Adverse Reactions

CNS: Anxiety, asthenia, dizziness, fatigue, headache, insomnia, malaise, **suicidal ideation**

CV: Edema, hypertension, **hypotension**, palpitations

EENT: Dry mouth, nasopharyngitis, sinusitis, taste distortion

ENDO: Elevated calcitonin levels, **hypoglycemia**, **thyroid C-cell hyperplasia**, **thyroid cancer**

GI: Abdominal distention or pain, **acute pancreatitis**, anorexia, cholecystitis, cholelithiasis, constipation, diarrhea, dyspepsia, elevated liver or pancreatic enzymes, eructation, flatulence, gastroenteritis, **hemorrhagic and necrotizing pancreatitis**, **hepatitis**, hyperbilirubinemia, jaundice, nausea, slowed gastric emptying, vomiting

GU: Acute renal failure, elevated serum creatinine level, UTI, **worsening of chronic renal failure**

MS: Back pain

RESP: Dyspnea, upper respiratory tract infection

SKIN: Pruritus, rash, urticaria

Other: Anaphylaxis; **angioedema**; antiliraglutide antibodies; dehydration; influenza-like symptoms; injection-site reaction including erythema, pruritus, rash

Nursing Considerations

- Be aware that liraglutide isn't recommended as first-line therapy for patients with type 2 diabetes mellitus not well controlled with diet and exercise. It also isn't a substitute for insulin therapy. Saxenda brand shouldn't be given with insulin, nor should it be combined with other products intended for weight loss, including herbal preparations, over-the-counter products, or prescription drugs.
- Know that liraglutide shouldn't be given to a patient with a history of thyroid C-cell tumors, including medullary thyroid carcinoma, or to patients with multiple endocrine neoplasia syndrome type 2 because drug may stimulate tumor growth.
- Use liraglutide cautiously in patients with a history of pancreatitis because drug can cause pancreatitis, in patients with impaired hepatic function because drug

effects in these patients are unknown, and in patients with renal dysfunction because liraglutide may adversely affect renal function.

- Be aware that dosage of liraglutide given during first week of therapy to lower blood glucose level isn't enough to provide glycemic control, but is given to minimize adverse effects when dosage is increased.
- Monitor patient closely for signs and symptoms of a hypersensitivity reaction that may become serious, especially in patients with a history of angioedema to other medications. If any hypersensitivity reaction occurs, discontinue liraglutide and notify the prescriber.
- Monitor patient's fluid intake, especially if gastrointestinal dysfunction occurs, because dehydration can lead to renal dysfunction that can become severe enough to require dialysis.
- Monitor patient's serum calcitonin levels, as indicated. Be aware that elevations occur more often when liraglutide dosage is 1.8 mg daily.
- Monitor patient for pancreatitis, especially when therapy starts or dosage increases. Report persistent severe abdominal pain; it may radiate to the back and may be accompanied by vomiting. If pancreatitis is confirmed, expect to stop drug and know that it should not be restarted after episode has been resolved.
- Also monitor patient for acute gallbladder disease. Risk is increased in patients who experience a rapid or substantial weight loss, although it may also occur in patients who have lost weight more slowly or less significantly. Notify prescriber if signs and symptoms occur and expect diagnostic testing to be performed.
- Monitor patient for hypoglycemia, especially if he takes another antidiabetic, such as a sulfonylurea. Report any episode of hypoglycemia because dosage of other antidiabetic may need adjustment. Treat hypoglycemia with a glucose-containing beverage or food, or give glucagon, as ordered, to raise blood glucose level.
- Monitor patient's blood glucose level and hemoglobin A_{1C} regularly, as ordered, to assess effectiveness of drug when used to treat diabetes mellitus.
- Monitor effectiveness of all other oral drugs because liraglutide slows gastric emptying and may impair their absorption. Alert prescriber to any concerns.
- Be aware that if more than 3 days has elapsed since the last liraglutide dose, the drug should be reinitiated at the initial dose of 0.6 mg.
- Monitor patient closely for suicidal ideation such as depression, or unusual changes in behavior or mood. If patient becomes suicidal, take safety precautions immediately, discontinue liraglutide therapy, as ordered, and notify prescriber.

PATIENT TEACHING

- Teach patient how to use prefilled multi-dose pen and how to give a subcutaneous injection. Explain that he'll need to inject drug daily but that he can do it at any time of day, independent of meals. Tell patient to inject drug into his abdomen, thigh, or upper arm and to rotate sites to minimize injection-site reactions. Warn patient not to share his pen with anyone.
- Instruct patient to maintain an adequate fluid intake, as dehydration may cause kidney dysfunction.
- Advise patient of possible risk of medullary thyroid cancer or multiple endocrine neoplasia syndrome type 2 and the need to report any symptoms, such as dysphagia, dyspnea, a neck mass, or persistent hoarseness.
- Tell caregivers to monitor patient closely for depression or changes in behavior or mood. If suicidal, have them take safety precautions, stop the drug, and seek emergency medical help for patient.
- Emphasize that liraglutide therapy (Victoza brand) isn't a substitute for diet and exercise when used to treat diabetes mellitus but is used to enhance the effectiveness of these measures. However, alert patient that hypoglycemia can occur with drug use. Review signs and symptoms of low blood sugar with patient and appropriate treatment.
- Instruct patient to discontinue drug immediately and seek emergency care if he experiences a serious hypersensitivity reaction, such as difficulty breathing, feeling acutely ill, or swelling of the face or throat area.

- Inform patient that drug may increase risk for gallbladder disease. If abdominal pain, nausea, and vomiting occur, instruct patient to notify prescriber. Also, tell patient to report yellowing of skin or white of the eye along with gastrointestinal signs and symptoms to prescriber.
- Inform patient that drug may increase risk for acute pancreatitis. Tell patient to report persistent severe abdominal pain that may radiate to the back and may be accompanied by vomiting and to stop taking drug.
- Instruct female patients prescribed Saxenda to notify prescriber immediately if pregnancy is suspected or occurs, as drug will have to be discontinued.
- Have patient monitor her weight to assess effectiveness of drug (Saxenda) when prescribed for weight management. Tell patient that Saxenda used for weight loss must be discontinued if she has not achieved a 4% weight loss by 16 weeks.
- Tell patient prescribed Saxenda brand of drug that it should not be given with insulin, nor should it be combined with other products intended for weight loss, including herbal preparations, over-the-counter products, and prescription drugs.
- Alert women that liraglutide does have an effect on preexisting breast neoplasia that may increase risk of breast cancer. In addition, inform all patients that there may be an increase in the development of colorectal neoplasms. Encourage all patients to have cancer screenings done as recommended by their doctor.
- Advise patient not to share her pen with another person, even if the needle is changed, because of an increased risk of transmitting an infection.

lisdexamfetamine dimesylate

Vyvanse

Class, Category, and Schedule

Pharmacologic class: Amphetamine
Therapeutic class: CNS stimulant
Pregnancy category: C
Controlled substance schedule: II

Indications and Dosages

➤ *To treat attention deficit hyperactivity disorder (ADHD)*

CAPSULES

Adults, adolescents, and children age 6 and over. *Initial:* 30 mg once daily in the morning, increased as needed in increments of 10 or 20 mg daily every wk. *Maximum:* 70 mg daily.

➤ *To treat moderate to severe binge eating disorder*

CAPSULES

Adults. *Initial:* 30 mg once daily, increased as needed in increments of 20 mg weekly to reach target dosage of 50 to 70 mg/day. *Maximum:* 70 mg daily.

DOSAGE ADJUSTMENT For patients with severe renal impairment (GFR from 15 ml/min to less than 30 ml/min), maximum dose is limited to 50 mg daily. For patients with end-stage renal disease (GFR less than 15 ml/min), maximum dose is limited to 30 mg daily. For patients taking agents that alter urinary pH, dosage adjustments are individualized.

Route	Onset	Peak	Duration
P.O.	Unknown	1 hr	Unknown

Mechanism of Action

Produces CNS stimulant effects, probably by facilitating release and blocking reuptake of norepinephrine at adrenergic nerve terminals and by stimulating alpha and beta receptors in peripheral nervous system. The drug also releases and blocks reuptake of dopamine in limbic regions of brain. These actions cause decreased motor restlessness and increased alertness. Lisdexamfetamine's action in the treatment of binge eating is unknown.

Contraindications

Advanced arteriosclerosis; agitation; glaucoma; history of drug abuse, hypersensitivity, or idiosyncratic reaction to lisdexamfetamine, other sympathomimetic amines, or their components; history of seizures; hyperthyroidism; MAO inhibitor therapy including intravenous methylene blue and linzolid within 14 days; moderate to severe hypertension; symptomatic cardiovascular disease

Interactions

DRUGS

acetazolamide, alkalinizers (such as sodium bicarbonate), some thiazides: Increased blood level and effects of lisdexamfetamine
adrenergic blockers: Inhibited adrenergic blockade
antihistamines: Possibly reduced sedation from antihistamine
antihypertensives: Possibly decreased antihypertensive effects
buspirone, fentanyl, lithium, MAO inhibitors, selective serotonin reuptake inhibitors, serotonin-norepinephrine reuptake inhibitors, St. John's wort, tricyclic antidepressants, triptans, tryptophan: Increased risk of serotonin syndrome
chlorpromazine: Inhibited CNS stimulant effects of lisdexamfetamine
ethosuximide: Possibly delayed ethosuximide absorption
GI acidifiers (such as ascorbic acid), reserpine: Decreased amphetamine absorption
guanethine: Decreased antihypertensive effect and decreased lisdexamfetamine absorption
guanfacine: Possibly increased blood guanfacine level
haloperidol: Decreased CNS stimulation
lithium carbonate: Possibly decreased anorectic and stimulant effects of lisdexamfetamine
MAO inhibitors: Potentiated effects of lisdexamfetamine, possibly hypertensive crisis
meperidine: Increased analgesia
methenamine: Increased urine excretion and decreased effects of lisdexamfetamine
norepinephrine: Possibly increased adrenergic effect of norepinephrine
phenobarbital: Synergistic anticonvulsant action
phenytoin: Possible delayed absorption of phenytoin; increased synergistic anticonvulsant action
propoxyphene: Increased CNS stimulation, potentially fatal seizures
sympathomimetic drugs: Increased stimulant effect
tricyclic antidepressants: Possibly increased antidepressant effects and decreased lisdexamfetamine effects
urinary acidifiers (such as ammonium chloride and sodium acid phosphate): Increased amphetamine excretion and decreased amphetamine blood level and effects
veratrum alkaloids: Decreased hypotensive effect

Adverse Reactions

CNS: Affect lability, aggression, agitation, anxiety, depression, dizziness, dyskinesia, dysphoria, energy increase, euphoria, fever, hallucinations, headache, insomnia, irritability, jittery feeling, mania, mood swings, nightmare, paranoia, psychomotor hyperactivity, psychotic episodes, restlessness, **seizures**, **serotonin syndrome**, somnolence, tics, tremor
CV: Cardiomyopathy, chest pain, hypertension, palpitations, peripheral vasculopathy, including Raynaud's phenomenon, tachycardia, ventricular hypertrophy
EENT: Blurred vision, diplopia, dry mouth, mydriasis, oropharyngeal pain, taste alterations, teeth grinding, visual accommodation difficulties
ENDO: Long-term growth suppression
GI: Anorexia, constipation, diarrhea, **hepatitis**, nausea, upper abdominal pain, vomiting
GU: Decreased libido, erectile dysfunction, frequent or prolonged erections, priapism, UTI
MS: Rhabdomyolysis
RESP: Dyspnea
SKIN: Alopecia, diaphoresis, rash, **Stevens–Johnson syndrom**e, **toxic epidermal necrolysis**, uncontrolled picking at skin, urticaria
Other: Anaphylaxis, **angioedema**, physical or psychological dependence, weight loss

Nursing Considerations

WARNING Keep in mind lisdexamfetamine shouldn't be given to patients with cardiac abnormalities (structural), cardiomyopathy, or other serious heart problems or rhythm abnormalities because even usual CNS-stimulant dosages increase risk of sudden death in patients with these conditions.

- Use lisdexamfetamine cautiously in patients with heart failure, hypertension, recent MI, or ventricular arrhythmia because drug may increase blood pressure and worsen these conditions.

- Know that patient should be screened for psychiatric risk factors such as a family or personal history of bipolar disorder, depression, or suicidal ideation because lisdexamfetamine may cause psychiatric adverse reactions. Monitor patients with bipolar disorder for mania.
- Monitor patient's blood pressure closely; stimulant drugs such as lisdexamfetamine may increase it.

WARNING Monitor patient closely for serotonin syndrome, a rare but serious adverse effect of lisdexamfetamine. Signs and symptoms include agitation, confusion, diaphoresis, diarrhea, fever, hyperactive reflexes, poor coordination, restlessness, shaking, talking or acting with uncontrolled excitement, tremor, and twitching. If symptoms occur, notify prescriber immediately, expect drug to be discontinued, and provide supportive care.

- Know that chest pain or fainting should be reported to prescriber immediately.
- Monitor patients with bipolar illness, a history of aggression or hostility or psychosis; CNS stimulation may worsen symptoms.
- Assess growth pattern in pediatric patients because stimulants such as lisdexamfetamine may suppress growth. If so, notify prescriber and expect therapy to be halted.
- Know that if patient has a history of seizures or EEG abnormality, watch for seizure activity because stimulants may lower seizure threshold. Rarely, lisdexamfetamine may cause seizures in a patient with no history of them. Take seizure precautions in all patients, and notify prescriber if a seizure occurs. Expect to discontinue lisdexamfetamine, as prescribed.
- Take safety precautions because stimulants may alter accommodation and cause blurred vision. Although these effects haven't been reported with lisdexamfetamine, the drug is a known stimulant.
- Be aware that therapy may be stopped temporarily to assess continued need for it, as evidenced by a return of attention deficit and hyperactivity.
- Know that lisdexamfetamine can cause a significant elevation in plasma corticosteroid levels, especially in the evening, which may interfere with urinary steroid determinations.

PATIENT TEACHING

- Warn patient or caregiver that drug must be taken exactly as prescribed and dosage increased only at prescriber's instruction because drug can be abused or lead to dependence.
- Instruct patient or caregiver that capsule may be opened and contents dissolved in a glass of orange juice or water and drunk immediately. Alternatively, the contents of the capsule may be mixed with yogurt until completely dispersed; the entire mixture must be consumed immediately.
- Tell patient or caregiver that drug should only be taken in the morning because taking it later in the day may cause insomnia.
- Tell patient with symptoms such as chest pain or fainting to contact prescriber immediately.

WARNING Instruct patient to tell all prescribers about lisdexamfetamine therapy, as serious drug interactions can occur. Stress importance of seeking immediate medical care if persistent, severe, or unusual adverse reactions occur.

- Advise patient or caregiver to report any symptoms that suggest heart disease, such as exertional chest pain or unexplained syncope.
- Urge patient to avoid hazardous activities until drug effects are known.
- Warn male patients and parents of male children that painful or prolonged penile erections may occur while taking the drug, especially after a dose increase or during a period of drug withdrawal. In the event this happens, immediate medical attention should be sought.
- Instruct patient or parents to monitor fingers and toes for soft tissue breakdown and/or ulceration. If noticed, prescriber should be notified. Reassure patient that signs and symptoms generally improve after the dose is reduced or drug is discontinued.

- Tell female patient of childbearing age to notify prescriber if pregnancy is suspected or occurs. Also inform women wanting to breastfeed that breastfeeding is not recommended during lisdexamfetamine therapy.

lisinopril

Prinivil, Qbrelis, Zestril

Class and Category

Pharmacologic class: Angiotensin-converting enzyme (ACE) inhibitor
Therapeutic class: Antihypertensive
Pregnancy category: D

Indications and Dosages

➤ *To treat hypertension*

ORAL SOLUTION, TABLETS

Adults. *Initial:* 10 mg daily. *Maintenance:* 20 to 40 mg daily. *Maximum:* 80 mg daily.
Children age 6 and over with a GFR of at least 30 ml/min. *Initial:* 0.07 mg/kg daily, adjusted according to blood pressure response up to 5 mg daily. *Maximum:* 0.61 mg/kg or 40 mg daily.

➤ *As adjunct with digitalis and diuretics to treat heart failure*

ORAL SOLUTION, TABLETS

Adults. *Initial:* 5 mg daily. *Maintenance:* 5 to 20 mg daily. *Maximum:* 80 mg daily.
DOSAGE ADJUSTMENT For patients with hyponatremia or creatinine clearance of 30 ml/min or less, initial dosage reduced to 2.5 mg daily.

➤ *To improve survival in hemodynamically stable patient within 24 hours of an acute MI*

ORAL SOLUTION, TABLETS

Adults. 5 mg within 24 hr after onset of symptoms, followed by 5 mg after 24 hr and 10 mg after 48 hr. *Maintenance:* 10 mg daily for 6 wk.
DOSAGE ADJUSTMENT For patients with baseline systolic blood pressure of 120 mm Hg or less, initial dosage decreased to 2.5 mg daily for first 3 days after MI. If systolic blood pressure falls to 100 mm Hg or less during therapy, maintenance dosage decreased to 2.5 or 5 mg as tolerated; if systolic blood pressure is 90 mm Hg or less for more than 1 hr, drug discontinued. For adult patients, regardless of indication, with impaired renal function (creatinine clearance of 10 to 30 ml/min), initial dosage reduced by half; for patients on hemodialysis or with a creatinine clearance of less than 10 ml/min, initial dose reduced to 2.5 mg once daily.

Route	Onset	Peak	Duration
P.O.	1 hr	6–8 hr	24 hr

Mechanism of Action

May reduce blood pressure by inhibiting conversion of angiotensin I to angiotensin II. Angiotensin II is a potent vasoconstrictor that also stimulates adrenal cortex to secrete aldosterone. Lisinopril may also inhibit renal and vascular production of angiotensin II. Decreased release of aldosterone reduces sodium and water reabsorption and increases their excretion, thereby reducing blood pressure.

Contraindications

Concurrent aliskiren use in patients with diabetes or patients with renal impairment (GFR less than 60 ml/min); hereditary or idiopathic angioedema or history of angioedema related to previous treatment with an ACE inhibitor; hypersensitivity to lisinopril, other ACE inhibitors, or their components; use of a neprilysin inhibitor such as sacubitril within 36 hours

Interactions

DRUGS

aliskiren (in presence of diabetes or renal impairment), other ACE inhibitors, angiotension receptor blockers: Increased risk of hypotension, hyperkalemia, and renal impairment
allopurinol, bone marrow depressants (such as methotrexate), procainamide, systemic corticosteroids: Increased risk of potentially fatal agranulocytosis or neutropenia
cyclosporine, potassium-sparing diuretics, potassium supplements: Increased risk of hyperkalemia
diuretics, other antihypertensives: Increased hypotensive effect
gold: Possibly nitritoid reaction (facial flushing, hypotension, nausea, vomiting)
insulin, oral antidiabetics: Increased risk of hypoglycemia
lithium: Increased blood lithium level and risk of lithium toxicity

neprilysin inhibitors such as sacubitril: Increased risk for angioedema
NSAIDs: Possibly reduced antihypertensive effect; possibly reduced renal function in patients with preexisting renal dysfunction, the elderly and patients who are volume-depleted
sympathomimetics: Possibly reduced antihypertensive effect
thiazide diuretics: Increased risk of hypokalemia
FOODS
high-potassium diet, potassium-containing salt substitutes: Increased risk of hyperkalemia
ACTIVITIES
alcohol use: Possibly increased hypotensive effect

Adverse Reactions

CNS: Ataxia, confusion, **CVA**, depression, dizziness, fatigue, hallucinations, headache, insomnia, irritability, memory impairment, mood alterations, nervousness, paresthesia, peripheral neuropathy, somnolence, syncope, transient ischemic attack, tremor, vertigo
CV: Arrhythmias, chest pain, fluid overload, **hypotension**, **MI**, orthostatic hypotension, palpitations, peripheral edema, vasculitis
ENDO: Hyperglycemia, syndrome of inappropriate ADH secretion
EENT: Blurred vision, diplopia, dry mouth, olfactory or taste disturbance, photophobia, tinnitus, visual loss
GI: Abdominal pain, anorexia, cholestatic jaundice, constipation, diarrhea, elevated liver enzymes, flatulence, **fulminant hepatic necrosis**, gastritis, **hepatitis**, indigestion, nausea, **pancreatitis**, vomiting
GU: Acute renal failure, decreased libido, impotence, pyelonephritis
HEME: Agranulocytosis, anemia, **hemolytic anemia**, **neutropenia**, **thrombocytopenia**
MS: Arthralgia, arthritis, bone or joint pain, muscle spasms, myalgia
RESP: Bronchospasm, cough, dyspnea, paroxysmal nocturnal dyspnea, **pulmonary embolism and infarction**, upper respiratory tract infection
SKIN: Alopecia, cutaneous pseudolymphoma, diaphoresis, erythema, flushing, herpes zoster, infections, pemphigus, photosensitivity, pruritus, psoriasis, rash, **Stevens–Johnson syndrome**, **toxic epidermal necrolysis**, urticaria
Other: Anaphylaxis, **angioedema**, dehydration, gout, **hyperkalemia**, **hyponatremia**, weight gain or loss

Nursing Considerations

- Be aware that lisinopril should not be given to a patient who is hemodynamically unstable after an acute MI.
- Use lisinopril cautiously in patients with fluid volume deficit, heart failure, impaired renal function, or sodium depletion.
- Also use cautiously in patients with severe aortic stenosis or hypertrophic cardiomyopathy because symptomatic hypotension may occur.
- Prepare pediatric suspension by adding 10 ml purified water to a polyethylene terephthalate (PET) bottle containing 10 20-mg tablets and shake for at least 1 minute. Add 30 ml of Bicitra diluent and 160 ml of Ora-Sweet SF to concentrate in PET bottle and shake gently for several seconds. Refrigerate up to 4 weeks. Shake suspension before each use.
- Monitor blood pressure often, especially during the first 2 weeks of therapy and whenever the dose of lisinopril and/or prescribed diuretic is increased. If excessive hypotension develops, expect to withhold drug for several days.

WARNING Keep in mind if angioedema, affects face, glottis, larynx, limbs, lips, mucous membranes, or tongue, notify prescriber immediately and expect to stop lisinopril and start appropriate therapy at once. If airway obstruction threatens, promptly give 0.3 to 0.5 ml of epinephrine 1:1000 solution subcutaneously, as prescribed.

- Monitor patient for anaphylaxis, especially patient being dialyzed with high-flux membranes. If anaphylaxis occurs, stop dialysis immediately and treat aggressively (antihistamines are ineffective in this situation), as ordered. Anaphylaxis has also occurred with some patients undergoing low-density lipoprotein apheresis with dextran sulfate absorption.

- Notify prescriber if patient has persistent, nonproductive cough, a common adverse effect of ACE inhibitors such as lisinopril.
- Monitor for dehydration, which can lead to hypotension especially if patient experiences diarrhea or vomiting.
- Monitor patient for hepatic dysfunction because lisinopril, an ACE inhibitor, may rarely cause a syndrome that starts with cholestatic jaundice or hepatitis and progresses to fulminant hepatic necrosis. If patient develops jaundice or a marked elevation in liver enzymes, withhold drug and notify prescriber.
- Monitor patient's serum creatinine, as ordered because changes in renal function can occur with lisinopril use. If renal function decreases, alert prescriber and expect drug to be withheld or discontinued.
- If patient takes insulin or an oral antidiabetic, monitor blood glucose level closely because risk of hypoglycemia increases, especially during first month of therapy.
- Monitor patient's serum potassium level, as ordered because drugs that inhibit the renin–angiotensin system such as lisinopril can cause hyperkalemia. Patients at increased risk for developing hyperkalemia include patients with diabetes or renal insufficiency or who are also taking potassium-sparing diuretics, potassium containing salt substitutes, or potassium supplements.

PATIENT TEACHING

- Explain that lisinopril helps to control, but doesn't cure, hypertension and that patient may need lifelong therapy.

WARNING Warn patient to seek immediate emergency treatment if she experiences difficulty breathing or swallowing or notices swelling of her eyes, extremities, face, lips, or tongue.

- Advise patient to take lisinopril at the same time every day.
- Emphasize need to take drug as ordered, even if patient feels well; caution her not to stop drug without consulting prescriber.
- Instruct patient to report dizziness, especially during first few days of therapy.
- Caution her to avoid hazardous activities such as driving until dizziness or other nervous system symptoms abates.
- Inform patient that persistent, nonproductive cough may develop during lisinopril therapy. Urge her to notify prescriber immediately if cough becomes difficult to tolerate.
- Advise patient to drink adequate fluids and avoid excessive sweating, which can lead to dehydration and hypotension. Make sure she understands that diarrhea excessive perspiration, and vomiting can also cause hypotension.
- Caution patient not to use salt substitutes that contain potassium.
- Instruct patient to report signs of infection, such as fever and sore throat, which may indicate neutropenia.
- Advise patient to change position slowly to minimize orthostatic hypotension.
- If patient has diabetes and takes insulin or an oral antidiabetic, urge her to monitor her blood glucose level closely and watch for symptoms of hypoglycemia.
- Caution female patient to notify prescriber immediately if she is or could be pregnant because lisinopril must be discontinued. Also inform her that breastfeeding is not recommended during lisinopril therapy because severe adverse reactions may develop in the infant.
- Advise patient to inform all prescribers of lisinopril therapy.

lithium carbonate

Carbolith (CAN), Duralith (CAN), Lithane (CAN), Lithobid

lithium citrate

Class and Category

Pharmacologic class: Alkali metal
Therapeutic class: Antimanic
Pregnancy category: D

Indications and Dosages

➤ *To treat acute mania episodes of bipolar disorder; to maintain patients with bipolar disorder*

CAPSULES, TABLETS

Adults and children age 7 and over weighing 30 kg (66 lb) or more. *Initial:* 300 mg three times daily, increased in 3 days by 300 mg, as needed. *Acute goal:* 600 mg two to three times daily. *Maintenance:* 300 to 600 mg two to three times daily.

Children ages 7 and over weighing 20 (44 lb) to 30 kg (66 lb). *Initial:* 300 mg twice daily, increased in 1 wk by 300 mg. *Acute goal:* 600 mg to 1,500 mg in divided doses daily. *Maintenance:* 600 mg to 1,200 mg in divided doses daily.

E.R. TABLETS

Adults and children age 12 and over. *Initial:* 900 mg twice daily. Alternatively, 600 mg three times daily. *Maintenance:* 600 mg twice daily. Alternatively, 400 mg three times daily.

ORAL SOLUTION

Adults and children age 7 and over weighing 30 kg (66 lb) or more. *Initial:* 8 mEq (5 ml) three times daily, increased by 8 mEq (5 ml) in 3 days, as needed. *Acute goal:* 16 mEq (10 ml) two to three times daily. *Maintenance:* 8 to 16 mEq (5 to 10 ml) two to three times daily.

Children age 7 and over weighing 20 kg (44 lb) to 30 kg (66 lb). *Initial:* 8 mEq (5 ml) twice daily, increased by 8 mEq (5 ml) weekly, as needed. *Acute goal:* 16 to 40 mEq (10 to 25 ml) in divided doses daily. *Maintenance:* 16 to 32 mEq (10 to 20 ml) in divided doses daily.

SYRUP (LITHIUM CITRATE)

Adults and children age 12 and over. *Initial:* 16 mEq (10 ml) three times daily. *Maintenance:* 8 mEq (5 ml) three or four times daily.

DOSAGE ADJUSTMENT For elderly patient and patient at risk for lithium toxicity, such as in the presence of severe debilitation or dehydration, or significant cardiovascular or renal disease or who is taking drugs that may affect kidney function such as angiotensin-converting enzyme inhibitors, angiotensin receptor blockers, diuretics, or NSAIDS, initial dosage may have to be reduced and titration done slowly.

Route	Onset	Peak	Duration
P.O.	1–3 wk	Unknown	Unknown

Mechanism of Action

May increase presynaptic degradation of the catecholamine neurotransmitters dopamine, norepinephrine, and serotonin; inhibit their release at neuronal synapses; and decrease postsynaptic receptor sensitivity. These actions may correct overactive catecholamine systems in patients with mania.

Contraindications

Concurrent use of diuretics, hypersensitivity to lithium or its components, hyponatremia, significant cardiovascular or renal disease, severe debilitation or dehydration

Interactions

DRUGS

ACE inhibitors, ARBs, diuretics, metronidazole, NSAIDs, piroxicam: Possibly increased blood lithium level and increased risk of toxicity

acetazolamide, sodium bicarbonate, urea, xanthines: Decreased blood lithium level

buspirone, fentanyl, MAO inhibitors, norepinephrine reuptake inhibitors, selective serotonin reuptake inhibitors, St. John's wort, tramadol, tricyclic antidepressants, triptans, tryptophan: Increased risk of serotonin syndrome

calcium channel blockers, molindone: Increased risk of neurotoxicity from lithium

calcium iodide, iodinated glycerol, potassium iodide: Possibly increased hypothyroid effects of both drugs

carbamazepine, methyldopa, phenytoin: Possibly increased risk of adverse reactions with these drugs

chlorpromazine, other phenothiazines: Possibly impaired GI absorption and decreased blood levels of these drugs; possibly masking of early signs of lithium toxicity

desmopressin, lypressin, vasopressin: Possibly impaired antidiuretic effects of these drugs

diuretics (loop and osmotic): Increased lithium reabsorption by kidneys, possibly leading to lithium toxicity

fluoxetine: Decreased or increased serum lithium concentrations

haloperidol and other antipyschotics: Increased risk of brain damage and irreversible neurotoxicity

neuromuscular blockers: Risk of prolonged paralysis or weakness
norepinephrine: Possibly decreased therapeutic effects of norepinephrine and severe respiratory depression
thyroid hormones: Possibly hypothyroidism
FOODS
high-sodium foods: Increased excretion and possibly decreased therapeutic effects of lithium

Adverse Reactions

CNS: Ataxia, coma, confusion, depression, disorientation, dizziness, drowsiness, fatigue, headache, lethargy, **seizures**, **serotonin syndrome**, syncope, tremor (in hands), vertigo
CV: Arrhythmias, **bradycardia**, **ECG changes**, edema, **hypotension**, palpitations, **peripheral circulatory collapse**, tachycardia, unmasking of **Brugada syndrome**
EENT: Blurred vision, dental caries, dry mouth, exophthalmos
ENDO: Diabetes insipidus, euthyroid goiter, hypothyroidism, **myxedema**, polydipsia
GI: Abdominal distention and pain, anorexia, diarrhea, nausea, vomiting
GU: Nephrotic syndrome, polyuria, stress incontinence, urinary frequency
HEME: Leukocytosis
MS: Muscle twitching and weakness
RESP: Dyspnea
SKIN: Acne; alopecia; dermatitis; dry, thin hair; pruritus; rash
Other: Cold sensitivity, weight gain or loss

Nursing Considerations

- Administer lithium after meals to slow absorption from GI tract and reduce adverse reactions. Dilute syrup with juice or other flavored drink before giving.
- Note that 5 ml of lithium citrate equals 8 mEq of lithium ion or 300 mg of lithium carbonate.
- Expect to monitor blood lithium level two or three times weekly during first month, and then weekly to monthly during maintenance therapy and when starting or stopping NSAID therapy. In uncomplicated cases, plan to monitor lithium level every 2 to 3 months.
- Be aware that lithium has a narrow therapeutic range. Even a slightly high blood level is dangerous, and some patients show signs of toxicity at normal levels. Be aware that risk of toxicity is increased in patients with electrolyte changes (especially potassium and sodium), recent onset of a concurrent febrile illness, severe debilitation or dehydration, or significant cardiovascular or renal disease, and in patients taking other drugs that affect kidney function, such as angiotensin-converting enzyme inhibitors, angiotensin receptor blockers, diuretics, and NSAIDs. Lithium toxicity signs and symptoms affect many areas of the body and can range from mild to severe and life-threatening symptoms. No antidote for lithium toxicity is available.
- Expect prescriber to decrease dosage after acute manic episode is controlled.

WARNING Be aware that lithium affects extracellular and intracellular potassium ion shift, which can cause ECG changes, such as flattened or inverted T waves; it also can increase the risk of cardiac arrest.

- Monitor ECGs, renal and thyroid function test results, and serum electrolyte levels, as appropriate, during lithium treatment. Know that nephrotic syndrome has occurred with lithium use but has resulted in remission after lithium was discontinued.

WARNING Be aware that lithium can cause reversible leukocytosis, which usually peaks within 7 to 10 days of starting therapy; WBC count typically returns to baseline within 10 days after therapy stops.

- Weigh patient daily to detect sudden weight changes.
- Monitor blood glucose level often in diabetic patient because lithium alters glucose tolerance.
- Palpate thyroid gland to detect enlargement because drug may cause goiter.
- Ensure that patient's fluid and sodium intake is adequate during treatment.
- Monitor patient closely for unexplained palpitations or syncope after starting lithium therapy as these symptoms may be caused by the unmasking of Brugada syndrome by lithium. Know that Brugada syndrome is a disorder in which electrocardiographic abnormalities occur and can result in sudden death. Patients at risk include those

with a family history of Brugada syndrome or a family history of sudden death before the age of 45 years. Notify prescriber if palpitations or syncope occur and expect to discontinue lithium therapy.

WARNING Monitor patient closely for serotonin syndrome, a rare but serious adverse effect of lithium. Signs and symptoms include agitation, confusion, diaphoresis, diarrhea, fever, hyperactive reflexes, poor coordination, restlessness, shaking, talking or acting with uncontrolled excitement, tremor, and twitching. If symptoms occur, notify prescriber immediately, expect drug to be discontinued, and provide supportive care.

PATIENT TEACHING

- Advise patient to take lithium with or after meals to minimize adverse reactions.
- Instruct patient to swallow E.R. form whole.
- Direct patient to mix syrup form with juice or other flavored drink before taking.
- Inform patient that frequent urination, nausea, and thirst may occur during the first few days of treatment.
- Caution patient not to stop taking lithium or adjust dosage without first consulting prescriber.
- Instruct patient to report signs of toxicity, such as diarrhea, drowsiness, muscle weakness, tremor, uncoordinated body movements, and vomiting.
- Urge patient to avoid hazardous activities until drug's CNS effects are known.
- Advise patient to maintain normal fluid and sodium intake.
- Emphasize importance of complying with scheduled checkups and laboratory tests.
- Instruct patient to seek immediate emergency care if he experiences abnormal heart beats, fainting, lightheadedness, or shortness of breath.

lixisenatide

Adlyxin

Class and Category

Pharmacologic class: Glucagon-like peptide receptor agonist
Therapeutic class: Antidiabetic
Pregnancy category: Not classified

Indications and Dosages

➤ *Adjunct to diet and exercise to improve glycemic control in patients with type 2 diabetes mellitus*

SUBCUTANEOUS INJECTION

Adults. *Initial:* 10 mcg within 1 hr before first meal of day once daily for 14 days. Increased to 20 mcg once daily on day 15 and thereafter. *Maintenance:* 20 mcg once daily.

Mechanism of Action

As a glucagon-like peptide receptor agonist, lixisenatide decreases glucagon secretion, increases glucose-dependent insulin release, and slows gastric emptying. All of these actions work together to reduce blood glucose levels.

Contraindications

Hypersensitivity to lixisenatide or its components

Interactions

DRUGS

basal insulin, sulfonylureas: Increased risk of hypoglycemia
orally administered drugs: Possibly delayed absorption of orally administered drugs resulting in decreased effectiveness

Adverse Reactions

CNS: Dizziness, headache
EENT: Laryngeal edema
GI: Abdominal distention or pain, **acute pancreatitis**, constipation, diarrhea, dyspepsia, nausea, vomiting
GU: Acute kidney injury, **worsening of chronic renal failure**
RESP: Bronchospasms
SKIN: Urticaria
Other: Anaphylaxis; **angioedema**; injection-site reactions such as erythema, pain, and pruritus; lixisenatide-induced antibodies

Nursing Considerations

- Administer lixisenatide subcutaneously 1 hour before the patient's first meal of the day into the patient's abdomen, thighs, or upper arm. Rotate sites.
- Protect the pen device containing the drug from light by keeping it in its original packaging. Write date that pen was first used on packaging and discard 14 days later.

WARNING Monitor patient closely for hypersensitivity reactions that could become serious, especially if patient has a history of hypersensitivity to other drugs in the same class.

- Monitor patient for signs and symptoms of pancreatitis including persistent severe abdominal pain, sometimes radiating to the back, that may or may not be accompanied with vomiting. Know that risk increases in patients who have a history of alcohol abuse or cholelithiasis. If pancreatitis is suspected, notify prescriber, discontinue drug, and provide supportive care, as ordered.
- Monitor patient for hypoglycemia, especially in patients who also take basal insulin and/or a sulfonylurea. Be prepared to treat hypoglycemia should it occur. Notify prescriber of persistent or severe hypoglycemic episodes as a dosage reduction in the insulin or sulfonylurea may be needed.
- Monitor patient's renal function before lixisenatide is initiated and during therapy, as ordered. Know that acute kidney injury can occur quickly even in patients who have no history of kidney disease. Patients are at increased risk when they experience dehydration, diarrhea, nausea, or vomiting. Notify prescriber immediately if patient's fluid balance is compromised.

PATIENT TEACHING

- Instruct patient or caregiver on how to administer drug subcutaneously, if self-administration is prescribed. Provide instructions on how to use the pen device correctly. Tell patient how to dispose of pen properly and to keep out of reach of children and pets.
- Tell patient to inspect solution in pen before administering. It should appear clear and colorless.
- Instruct patient to administer lixisenatide 1 hour before the first meal of the day by injecting into her abdomen, thigh, or upper arm. Stress importance of rotating sites. Tell her it is best to administer the drug before the same meal each day.
- Inform patient that if she forgets a dose, she should administer the drug within 1 hour prior to the next meal but never double the dose to make up for a missed dose.
- Tell patient to protect the pen from light by keeping it in the original packaging. She should also write down the date the pen was first used, as pen must be discarded 14 days later.
- Inform women who are taking oral contraceptives that lixisenatide may interfere with absorption and effectiveness of oral contraceptive. To avoid this, tell patient to take oral contraceptive 1 hour before or 11 hours after administering lixisenatide each day.
- Tell all patients taking oral medication to take them at least 1 hour before administering lixisenatide; if a prescribed drug requires food intake, take it with a meal or snack that does not coincide with lixisenatide administration.
- Warn patient never to share the pen used to inject lixisenatide even if the needle is changed, because of an increased risk for transmission of blood-borne diseases.
- Remind patient that lixisenatide does not take the place of dietary measures and exercise also used to control blood sugar.
- Advise patient to maintain adequate hydration. Emphasize importance of alerting prescriber immediately if she does become dehydrated or develops diarrhea, nausea, or vomiting.

WARNING Instruct patient to seek immediate medical attention if she develops an allergic reaction to drug.

- Review signs and symptoms of pancreatitis with patient and urge her to stop taking drug and notify the prescriber, if present.
- Encourage patient to be on the alert for hypoglycemia, especially if she is taking basal insulin or sulfonylurea. Review the signs and symptoms and how to treat it. If episodes occur frequently or become severe, tell her to notify prescriber, as a dosage reduction may be needed for her basal insulin or sulfonylurea.

lofexidine

Lucemyra

Class and Category

Pharmacologic class: Central alpha$_2$-agonist
Therapeutic class: Opioid withdrawal
Pregnancy category: Not classified

Indications and Dosages

➤ *To mitigate opioid withdrawal symptoms in order to facilitate abrupt opioid discontinuation*

TABLETS

Adults. 3 tablets (0.18 mg each) four times daily with 5 to 6 hr between each dose and continued during the period of peak withdrawal (usually first 5 to 7 days following last use of an opioid, although peak withdrawal may last up to 14 days). Then, dosage gradually reduced over 2 to 4 days by reducing 1 tablet per dose every 1 to 2 days. *Maximum:* 4 tablets (total 0.72 mg) for a single dose, 16 tablets (total 2.88 mg) daily.

DOSAGE ADJUSTMENT For patients experiencing drug-related adverse reactions, dosage reduced, held, or drug discontinued depending on severity of reactions. Dosage may be reduced as opioid withdrawal symptoms wane. For patient with moderate hepatic or renal impairment, dosage reduced to 2 tablets four times daily; for patient with severe hepatic or renal impairment, dosage reduced to 1 tablet four times daily.

Mechanism of Action

Binds to receptors on adrenergic neurons to reduce the release of norepinephrine and decrease sympathetic tone, thereby reducing opioid withdrawal symptoms.

Contraindications

Hypersensitivity to lofexidine or its components

Interactions

DRUGS

benzodiazepines: Potentiates the CNS effects of benzodiazepines

CNS depressants such as barbiturates and other sedating drugs: Possibly potentiates effects of CNS depressants

CYP2D6 inhibitors such as paroxetine: Increased absorption of lofexidine, increasing risk for bradycardia and orthostatic hypotension

methadone: Increased risk of QT prolongation leading to life-threatening arrythmias

naltrexone (oral): Possibly reduced effectiveness of oral naltrexone if administered within 2 hours of lofexidine

ACTIVITIES

alcohol use: Possibly potentiates CNS depressant effect of alcohol

Adverse Reactions

CNS: Dizziness, insomnia, sedation, somnolence, syncope

CV: Bradycardia, hypotension, orthostatic hypotension, **QT prolongation, torsades de pointes**

EENT: Dry mouth, tinnitus

Other: Discontinuation effects (anxiety, chills, diarrhea, elevation of blood pressure, extremity pain, hyperhidrosis, insomnia)

Nursing Considerations

- Be aware that lofexidine should not be used in patients with cerebrovascular disease, congenital long QT syndrome, marked bradycardia, recent myocardial infarction, or severe coronary insufficiency.
- Monitor vital signs before administering each dose of lofexidine, because drug may cause a decrease in blood pressure or pulse and cause syncope.

WARNING Know that lofexidine prolongs the QT interval. Expect to monitor patient's ECG if he has a history of bradyarrhythmias, congestive heart failure, or hepatic or renal impairment; ECG should also be monitored in patients with electrolyte abnormalities such as hypokalemia or hypomagnesemia. Know that electrolyte imbalances should be corrected before lofexidine therapy begins.

- Be aware that lofexidine therapy should not be stopped abruptly but gradually withdrawn to reduce the risk of discontinuation symptoms such as a sudden rise in blood pressure along with anxiety, chills, diarrhea, excessive sweating, extremity pain, and insomnia. If patient stops drug use abruptly, symptoms can be managed by administering the previous lofexidine dose and then subsequently gradually tapering drug dosage downward.

PATIENT TEACHING

- Instruct patient to take lofexidine exactly as prescribed. Warn patient that stopping drug abruptly can result in a sudden rise in blood pressure along with anxiety, chills, diarrhea, excessive sweating, extremity pain, and insomnia. Caution him that drug must be gradually withdrawn.

- Tell patient that lofexidifne therapy will help with opioid withdrawal symptoms but will not completely prevent them.
- Inform patient that lofexidine may cause a sudden drop in blood pressure or pulse. Instruct patient to rise slowly from a lying or sitting position and to maintain adequate hydration, as well as avoid becoming overheated, to help minimize these effects. Tell patient that if he experiences low blood pressure or decreased pulse rate to withhold the drug and notify the prescriber for guidance on how to adjust his dose.
- Tell patient to inform all prescribers of lofexidine therapy and not to take any over-the-counter preparations, including herbal products, without consulting prescriber, as the combination may cause an excessive drop in blood pressure or pulse rate.
- Instruct patient to avoid performing hazardous activities such as driving until the drug's effects on his nervous system are known.

WARNING Alert patient that lofexidine is not a treatment for opioid use. Tell patient that upon complete opioid discontinuation, he is more likely to have a reduced tolerance to opioids and is at increased risk for a fatal overdose should he resume opioid use. Make sure both patient and caregivers are aware of the increased risk of overdose.

- Warn patient to avoid taking any CNS depressant drugs such as barbiturates, benzodiazepines, or other sedating drugs while taking lofexidine, because severe respiratory depression and sedation may occur. Also warn patient not to drink alcohol while taking drug, for the same reason.

lomitapide mesylate

Juxtapid

Class and Category

Pharmacologic class: Microsomal triglyceride transfer protein (MTP) inhibitor
Therapeutic class: Antilipemic
Pregnancy category: X

Indications and Dosages

➤ *To control lipid levels as adjunct to diet and other lipid-lowering treatments in homozygous familial hypercholesterolemia*

CAPSULES

Adults. *Initial:* 5 mg once daily with full glass of water 2 hr after evening meal with dosage increased to 10 mg once daily after 2 wk, as needed. Dosage further increased in 4 wk increments to 20 mg once daily, then to 40 mg once daily to 60 mg once daily, as needed. *Maximum*: 60 mg once daily.

DOSAGE ADJUSTMENT For patients with mild hepatic impairment or with end-stage renal impairment requiring dialysis, dosage not to exceed 40 mg once daily. For patients receiving weak CYP3A4 inhibitors such as alprazolam, amiodarone, amlodipine, atorvastatin, bicalutamide, cilostazol, cimetidine, cyclosporine, fluoxetine, fluvoxamine, ginkgo, goldenseal, isoniazid, lapatinib, nilotinib, pazopanib, ranitidine, ranolazine, ticagrelor, or zileuton, initial dosage of 10 mg or more reduced by half and maximum dosage not to exceed 30 mg once daily. However, for patient taking oral contraceptives which are also weak CYP3A4 inhibitors, maximum daily dosage reduced to 40 mg daily. For patients who develop elevated transaminases three times or greater but less than five times upper normal limits during therapy, daily dosage reduced with degree of reduction individualized.

Mechanism of Action

Binds and inhibits microsomal triglyceride transfer protein, located in the lumen of the endoplasmic reticulum of cells which in turn prevents the assembly of apo B-containing lipoproteins in enterocytes and hepatocytes. This then prevents the synthesis of chylomicrons and very low-density lipoproteins (VLDL). Lower VLDL levels leads to reduced levels of plasma low-density lipoprotein-cholesterol.

Contraindications

Active liver disease, concurrent therapy with moderate or strong CYP3A4 inhibitors, hypersensitivity to lomitapide or its components, moderate or severe hepatic impairment, pregnancy, unexplained persistent elevations of serum transaminases

Interactions

DRUGS

bile acid sequestrants: Possibly decreased absorption of lomitapide
CYP3A inhibitors: Increased lomitapide exposure with possible increased risk of adverse reactions
lovastatin, simvastatin: Increased risk of myopathy, including rhabdomyolysis
P-glycoprotein substrates such as aliskiren, colchicine, dabigatran etexilate, digoxin, everolimus, fexofenadine, imatinib, lapatinib, maraviroc, nilotinib, posaconazole, ranolazine, saxagliptin, sirolimus, sitagliptin, talinolol, tolvaptan, topotecan: Increased absorption of these drugs resulting in higher drug levels
warfarin: Increased plasma warfarin levels with possible increased risk of bleeding events

FOODS

grapefruit juice: Increased lomitapide exposure and adverse reactions

ACTIVITIES

alcohol use: Possibly increased risk of hepatic steatosis

Adverse Reactions

CNS: Dizziness, fatigue, fever, headache
CV: Chest pain, palpitations
EENT: Nasal congestion, nasopharnygitis, pharyngolaryngeal pain
GI: Abdominal distention or pain, constipation, defecation urgency, diarrhea (may become severe), dyspepsia, elevated liver enzymes, flatulence, gastroenteritis, gastroesophageal reflux disease, hepatic steatosis, **hepatotoxicity**, nausea, rectal tenesmus, transaminase elevations, vomiting
MS: Back pain, myalgia
SKIN: Alopecia
Other: Fat-soluble vitamin deficiency, flu-like symptoms, serum fatty acid deficiency, weight loss

Nursing Considerations

- Be aware that lomitapide should not be given to patients with rare, hereditary problems of galactose intolerance, glucose–galactose malabsorption, or Lapp lactase deficiency because drug may cause diarrhea and malabsorption in these patients.
- Know that because lomitapide increases risk of hepatotoxicity, the drug can only be administered through the Juxtapid REMS program.
- Determine patient has had ALT, AST, alkaline phosphatase and total bilirubin measured, has had a negative pregnancy test if patient is female, and has initiated a low-fat diet supplying less than 20% of energy from fat prior to initiating lomitapide therapy.
- Be aware that ALT and AST levels should be measured prior to potential dosage increase or monthly, whichever comes first, for first year of therapy and then before each actual dosage increase and every 3 months thereafter. If transaminase values are equal to or greater than three times upper limit normal but less than five times upper limit normal, expect to confirm elevation with a repeat measurement within 1 week. If confirmed, expect dosage to be decreased and additional liver-related tests done, such as measurement of alkaline phosphatase, total bilirubin, and patient's INR. Repeat tests weekly, as ordered, and expect to withhold drug if there are signs of abnormal liver function such as an elevation in patient's bilirubin or an increase in patient's INR. If transaminase levels are above five times upper limit normal, or if transaminase levels do not fall below three times upper limit normal within about 4 weeks, expect drug to be withheld or discontinued. Know that if drug therapy is resumed, dosage should be reduced and more frequent liver-related tests ordered.
- Monitor patient closely for signs and symptoms of liver impairment, such as presence of abdominal pain, fever, flu-like symptoms, jaundice, or lethargy; a bilirubin result that is equal to or greater than two times upper limit normal, or active liver disease is suspected because risk of hepatotoxicity increases with lomitapide therapy.
- Monitor patient for fat-soluble vitamin and fatty acids deficiencies, especially patients with chronic bowel or pancreatic

diseases that predispose to malabsorption, because lomitapide reduces the absorption of fat-soluble vitamins.
- Monitor patient for adverse reactions, especially gastrointestinal reactions, which are the most common reactions associated with lomitapide therapy. Give drug with a full glass of water 2 hours after evening meals. Ensure patient is adhering to a low-fat diet that supplies less than 20% of energy needs from fat to reduce the risk of adverse gastrointestinal reactions.
- Know that lomitapide may cause severe diarrhea in some patients, requiring hospitalization because of diarrhea-induced volume depletion. Monitor patients closely, especially the elderly and those who are taking drugs that can lead to hypotension or volume depletion.

PATIENT TEACHING
- Advise patient to take lomitapide with a full glass of water 2 hours after the evening meal because taking drug with food may increase the risk of gastrointestinal adverse reactions.
- Caution patient to swallow capsule whole and not to chew, crush, dissolve, or open capsule.
- Instruct patient to take daily supplements of 400 international units of vitamin E and at least 210 mg alpha-linolenic acid, 110 mg eicosapentaenoic acid, and 80 mg of docosahexaenoic acid to prevent deficiencies.
- Remind patient of importance of adhering to the low-fat diet prescribed as lomitapide therapy is not a replacement for dietary control of fat in her diet.
- Tell patient to inform all prescribers about lomitapide therapy because of potential drug interactions.
- Review signs and symptoms of liver impairment, and emphasize importance of reporting such to prescriber. Inform patient of need for blood tests to monitor her liver function and importance of compliance with test schedule.
- Instruct patient to stop taking drug and notify prescriber if severe diarrhea occurs or if he experiences symptoms such as decreased urine output, lightheadedness, or unexplainable tiredness that accompanies diarrhea.

WARNING Instruct patient not to consume more than one alcoholic beverage daily.

WARNING Caution women of childbearing age to notify prescriber immediately if pregnancy occurs or is suspected because drug will have to be discontinued. Also, encourage them to enroll in the pregnancy exposure registry that monitors pregnancy outcomes in women exposed to the drug during pregnancy.

lorazepam

Apo-Lorazepam (CAN), Ativan, Lorazepam Intensol, Novo-Lorazem (CAN), Nu-Loraz (CAN)

Class, Category, and Schedule

Pharmacologic class: Benzodiazepine
Therapeutic class: Anxiolytic
Pregnancy category: D (parenteral), Not rated (oral)
Controlled substance schedule: IV

Indications and Dosages

➤ *To treat anxiety*

ORAL CONCENTRATE, TABLETS

Adults. 1 to 3 mg twice daily or three times daily. *Maximum:* 10 mg daily.

DOSAGE ADJUSTMENT For elderly or debilitated patients, initial dosage may be reduced to 0.5 to 2 mg daily in divided doses.

➤ *To treat insomnia caused by anxiety*

ORAL CONCENTRATE, TABLETS

Adults. 2 to 4 mg at bedtime.

DOSAGE ADJUSTMENT Dosage possibly reduced for elderly or debilitated patients.

➤ *To provide preoperative sedation*

I.V. INJECTION

Adults. 0.044 mg/kg or 2 mg, whichever is less, given at 2 mg/min 2 hr before procedure. *Maximum:* 0.05 mg/kg or total of 4 mg.

I.M. INJECTION

Adults. 0.05 mg/kg 2 hr before procedure. *Maximum:* 4 mg.

➤ *To treat status epilepticus*

I.V. INJECTION

Adults. *Initial:* 4 mg at a rate of 2 mg/min. Repeated in 10 to 15 min if seizures don't subside. *Maximum:* 8 mg/24 hr.

Route	Onset	Peak	Duration
I.V.	5 min	Unknown	12–24 hr
I.M.	15–30 min	Unknown	12–24 hr

Mechanism of Action

May potentiate the effects of gamma-aminobutyric acid (GABA) and other inhibitory neurotransmitters by binding to specific benzodiazepine receptors in cortical and limbic areas of CNS. GABA inhibits excitatory stimulation, which helps control emotional behavior. Limbic system contains a highly dense area of benzodiazepine receptors, which may explain drug's antianxiety effects. Also, lorazepam hyperpolarizes neuronal cells, thereby interfering with their ability to generate seizures.

Incompatibilities

Don't mix I.V. lorazepam in same syringe as buprenorphine.

Contraindications

Acute angle-closure glaucoma; hypersensitivity to lorazepam, its components, or benzodiazepines; intra-arterial delivery; premature infants; psychosis

Interactions

DRUGS

aminophylline, theophylline: Possibly reduced sedative effects of lorazepam
clozapine: Increased risk of ataxia, delirium, excessive salivation, hypotension, marked sedation, and respiratory arrest
CNS depressants: Additive CNS depression, potentially fatal respiratory depression
digoxin: Possibly increased blood digoxin level and risk of digitalis toxicity
fentanyl: Possibly decreased therapeutic effects of fentanyl
probenecid: Possibly increased therapeutic and adverse effects of lorazepam
other benzodiazepines, sedating antihistamines, opioids, tricyclic antidepressants: Increased risk of profound respiratory depression, sedation, and somnolence

ACTIVITIES

alcohol use: Increased CNS depression and severe respiratory depression

Adverse Reactions

CNS: Amnesia, anxiety, ataxia, **coma**, confusion, delusions, depression, dizziness, drowsiness, euphoria, extrapyramidal symptoms, fatigue, headache, hypokinesia, irritability, malaise, nervousness, **seizures**, slurred speech, **suicidal ideation**, tremor, unsteadiness, vertigo
CV: Chest pain, palpitations, tachycardia
EENT: Blurred vision, diplopia, dry mouth, increased salivation, photophobia
ENDO: Syndrome of inappropriate ADH
GI: Abdominal pain, constipation, diarrhea, elevated liver enzymes, jaundice, nausea, thirst, vomiting
GU: Libido changes
HEME: Agranulocytosis, **pancytopenia**, **thrombocytopenia**
RESP: Apnea, **respiratory depression**, worsening of obstructive pulmonary disease or sleep apnea
SKIN: Diaphoresis
Other: Anaphylaxis, injection-site pain (I.M.) or phlebitis (I.V.), physical and psychological dependence, withdrawal symptoms

Nursing Considerations

- Be aware that parenteral form of lorazepam is contraindicated in premature infants because the formulation contains benzyl alcohol, increasing risk of gasping syndrome, kernicterus, and toxicity. Lorazepam should be used with extreme caution in neonates because although the amount of benzyl alcohol is well below that associated with toxicity, a total daily metabolic load of benzyl alcohol from combined sources may increase the risk of toxicity.
- Before starting lorazepam therapy in a patient with depression, make sure he already takes an antidepressant, because of the increased risk of suicide in patients with untreated depression.
- Be aware that the combination of general anesthesia and sedation drugs like lorazepam used during procedures or surgeries in pregnant women in their third trimester is not recommended because it may affect brain development in the fetus.
- Use extreme caution when giving lorazepam to elderly patients, especially

those with compromised respiratory function, because drug can cause hypoventilation, respiratory depression, sedation, and unsteadiness. Also, use extreme caution when administering lorazepam to children under the age of 3 because of the risk of neurotoxicity, especially if exposed to drug longer than 3 hours or with repeated exposure.

- Use drug cautiously in patients with a history of alcohol or drug abuse or a personality disorder because of an increased risk of physical and psychological dependence. Also use cautiously in patients with encephalopathy or severe hepatic insufficiency because drug may worsen hepatic encephalopathy.
- Be aware that benzodiazepine therapy such as lorazepam should only be used concomitantly with opioids in patients for whom other treatment options are inadequate because adverse effects could be profound and possibly result in death. If prescribed together, expect dosing and duration of the opioid to be limited. Monitor patient closely for signs and symptoms of profound decrease in consciousness, including coma, sedation, and respiratory depression. Notify prescriber immediately and provide emergency supportive care.
- For I.M. use, inject lorazepam deep into large muscle mass, such as gluteus maximus.
- For I.V. use, dilute lorazepam with equal amount of D_5W, sterile water for injection, or sodium chloride for injection. Give diluted lorazepam slowly, at no more than 2 mg/min.
- Monitor patient's respirations every 5 to 15 minutes and keep emergency resuscitation equipment readily available.

WARNING Monitor patient's respiratory status closely because drug may cause life-threatening respiratory depression.

- Know that because stopping drug abruptly increases risk of withdrawal symptoms, dosage should be tapered gradually, especially in epileptic patients.

PATIENT TEACHING

- Instruct patient to take lorazepam exactly as prescribed and not to stop without consulting prescriber because of the risk of withdrawal symptoms.
- Advise patient to avoid hazardous activities until drug's CNS effects are known.
- Urge patient to avoid alcohol while taking lorazepam because it increases drug's CNS depressant effects and can cause severe respiratory depression which may lead to death.
- Instruct patient to report excessive drowsiness and nausea.
- Inform pregnant patient that lorazepam therapy will need to be discontinued early in third trimester to avoid possible withdrawal symptoms in newborn.
- Warn patient about potentially fatal additive effects of combining lorazepam with an opioid. Instruct him to inform all prescribers of lorazepam use, especially when pain medication may be prescribed.

lorcaserin hydrochloride

Belviq, Belviq XR

Class, Category, and Schedule

Pharmacologic class: Serotonin 2C receptor agonist
Therapeutic class: Appetite suppressant
Pregnancy category: X
Controlled substance schedule: IV

Indications and Dosages

➤ *Adjunct to reduced-calorie diet and increased physical activity for chronic weight management in patients with an initial body mass index of 30 kg/m² or greater (obese), or 27 kg/m² or greater (overweight) in the presence of at least one weight-related comorbid condition such as dyslipidemia, hypertension, or type 2 diabetes*

TABLETS

Adults. 10 mg twice daily.

E.R. TABLETS

Adults. 20 mg once daily.

Mechanism of Action

Selectively activates 5-HT_{2C} receptors on anorexigenic pro-opiomelanocortin neurons located in the hypothalamus to decrease food consumption and promote satiety.

Contraindications

Hypersensitivity to lorcaserin or its components, pregnancy

Interactions

DRUGS

antidiabetic agents, insulin: Possible risk of hypoglycemia that could be severe
bupropion, dextromethorphan, linezolid, lithium, MAOIs, selective serotonin norepinephrine reuptake inhibitors (SSNRIs), selective serotonin reuptake inhibitors (SSRIs), St. John's wort, tramadol, tricyclic antidepressants (TCAs), triptans, tryptophan: Increased risk for serotonin syndrome
cytochrome P450 (2D6) substrates: Increased exposure of these drugs
dopaminergic and serotonergic drugs (e.g., cabergoline): Increased risk for cardiac valvulopathy
phosphodiesterase type 5 inhibitors: Possibly increased risk of priapism

Adverse Reactions

CNS: Anxiety, cognitive impairment, depression, dizziness, euphoria, fatigue, headache, insomnia, **neuroleptic malignant syndrome-like reaction, serotonin syndrome, suicidal ideation**
CV: Bradycardia, hypertension, peripheral edema, valvulopathy
EENT: Abnormal ocular sensations; blurred vision; cataracts; conjunctival infections, inflammation, or irritation; dry eyes or mouth; nasopharyngitis; ocular sensation disorders; oropharyngeal pain; sinus congestion; toothache; visual impairment
ENDO: Elevated prolactin level, **hypoglycemia**, worsening of diabetes mellitus
GI: Constipation, decreased appetite, diarrhea, gastroenteritis, nausea, vomiting
GU: UTI
HEME: Anemia; **leukopenia, lymphopenia, neutropenia**
MS: Back or musculoskeletal pain
RESP: Cough, upper respiratory infection
SKIN: Rash
Other: Hypersensitivity reactions, seasonal allergy

Nursing Considerations

- Use extreme caution when administering lorcaserin with any drug that affects the serotonergic neurotransmitter system, especially when drug is initiated and during dosage changes, because of the risk of serotonin syndrome.
- Use caution when administering lorcaserin to patients with congestive heart failure or hemodynamically significant valvular heart disease because lorcaserin has been linked to regurgitant cardiac valvular disease, primarily affecting the aortic and/or mitral valves. Monitor patient closely for congestive heart failure, dependent edema, dyspnea, or a new cardiac murmur. If present, notify prescriber and expect drug to be discontinued.
- Use caution when administering lorcaserin to men who have conditions that might predispose them to priapism (e.g., leukemia, multiple myeloma, or sickle cell anemia), or in men with anatomical deformation of the penis (e.g., angulation, cavernosal fibrosis, or Peyronie's disease) because priapism is a potential effect of 5-HT_{2C} receptor agonism.
- Use lorcaserin cautiously in patients with bradycardia or a history of heart block greater than first degree because a decrease in heart rate may occur with lorcaserin therapy.
- Use lorcaserin cautiously in patients with moderate renal impairment or severe hepatic impairment because the effects of lorcaserin in these patients are unknown. The drug is not recommended for patients with severe renal impairment or end-stage renal disease.
- Be aware that daily dosage should not exceed 10 mg twice a day for immediate-release formulation and 20 mg once daily for extended-release formulation, because of increased risk of psychiatric disorders such as dissociation, euphoria, or hallucinations.
- Assess patient's weight loss at the end of 12 weeks. If patient has not lost at least 5% of his baseline body weight, notify prescriber and expect lorcaserin to be discontinued, as no further benefits are likely.

WARNING Monitor patient for signs and symptoms of serotonin syndrome, which may include autonomic instability (e.g., hyperthermia, labile blood pressure, tachycardia), gastrointestinal symptoms (e.g., diarrhea, nausea, vomiting), mental status changes (e.g., agitation, coma, hallucinations), and/or neuromuscular aberrations (e.g., hyperreflexia, incoordination). Know that serotonin syndrome, in its most severe form, can resemble neuroleptic malignant syndrome, which includes autonomic instability with possible rapid fluctuation of vital signs, hyperthermia, mental status changes, and muscle rigidity. If present, discontinue lorcaserin immediately, notify prescriber, and provide supportive care.

- Monitor patient's blood glucose level, especially patient with type 2 diabetes mellitus who is also being treated with insulin and/or oral hypoglycemic agents. As weight is lost, the risk of hypoglycemia increases. If hypoglycemia develops, treat appropriately and notify prescriber, as a dosage reduction may be needed with the patient's antidiabetic drug regimen.
- Monitor patient's complete blood count (CBC) periodically, as ordered, as hematological changes may occur during lorcaserin therapy.
- Monitor patient for signs and symptoms of prolactin excess (e.g., galactorrhea, gynecomastia) because lorcaserin moderately elevates prolactin levels. If present, notify prescriber and expect to obtain a prolactin level to confirm.
- Monitor patient for emergence or worsening of depression, suicidal behavior or thoughts, and/or any unusual changes in behavior or mood, because some drugs such as lorcaserin that target the central nervous system may be associated with depression or suicidal ideation. Monitor patient closely and expect drug to be discontinued if patient experiences suicidal behavior or thoughts.

PATIENT TEACHING

- Warn patient not to exceed prescribed dosage because serious adverse effects may occur.
- Instruct patient prescribed extended-release form that tablet must be swallowed whole and must not be chewed, crushed, or divided.
- Tell patient using drug for weight loss that drug is not a replacement for a diet and exercise regimen. Instruct patient to stop drug after 12 weeks if patient has not achieved a 5% weight loss.
- Advise patient to avoid hazardous activities until drug's CNS effects on cognition are known.
- Instruct patient with type 2 diabetes mellitus who is also taking insulin or an oral hypoglycemic agent to monitor his blood glucose level closely. If hypoglycemia develops, tell him to notify prescriber, as a dosage adjustment of his antidiabetic agent(s) may be needed.
- Inform a male patient to seek emergency care if he develops a painful erection that lasts longer than 4 hours and to discontinue lorcaserin therapy immediately.
- Instruct patient to tell prescriber of all medications being taken, including over-the-counter drugs and any weight loss products.
- Advise patient to inform prescriber of any persistent, severe, or unusual signs and symptoms.
- Tell women of childbearing age to notify prescriber immediately if pregnancy is suspected or has occurred.
- Inform mothers that breastfeeding is not recommended, because of the risk for serious adverse reactions in a breastfed infant.
- Caution family and caregivers to monitor patient for emergence or worsening of depression, suicidal behavior or thoughts, and/or any unusual changes in behavior or mood. If present, urge them to contact prescriber immediately.

losartan potassium

Cozaar

Class and Category

Pharmacologic class: Angiotensin II receptor blocker (ARB)
Therapeutic class: Antihypertensive
Pregnancy category: D

Indications and Dosages

➤ *To manage hypertension*

SUSPENSION, TABLETS

Adults. *Initial:* 50 mg daily. *Maintenance:* 25 to 100 mg as a single dose or in 2 divided doses.

Children age 6 and over with an estimated glomerular filtration rate 30 ml/min or greater. *Initial:* 0.7 mg/kg (up to 50 mg total) once daily, with dosage adjusted, as needed. *Maximum:* 1.4 mg/kg or 100 mg daily.

➤ *To treat nephropathy in patients with type 2 diabetes and hypertension*

TABLETS

Adults. *Initial:* 50 mg daily, increased to 100 mg daily, as needed.

➤ *To reduce stroke risk in patients with hypertension and left ventricular hypertrophy*

TABLETS

Adults. *Initial:* 50 mg daily, followed by 12.5 mg hydrochlorothiazide daily. Dosage increased to 100 mg daily, as needed, followed by 25 mg hydrochlorothiazide daily, as needed.

DOSAGE ADJUSTMENT Initial losartan dosage reduced to 25 mg daily for patients with impaired hepatic function or volume depletion.

Route	Onset	Peak	Duration
P.O.	Unknown	6 hr	Over 24 hr

Mechanism of Action

Blocks binding of angiotensin II to receptor sites in many tissues, including adrenal glands and vascular smooth muscle. Angiotensin II is a potent vasoconstrictor that also stimulates the adrenal cortex to secrete aldosterone. The inhibiting effects of angiotensin II reduce blood pressure.

Decreases left ventricular mass index in patients with left ventricular hypertrophy who also have hypertension. By targeting the renin–angiotensin system, a renoprotective action occurs through the lowering of the albumin excretion rate in patients with type 2 diabetes.

Contraindications

Concurrent aliskiren therapy (in patients with diabetes or renal impairment [GFR less than 60 ml/min]), hypersensitivity to losartan or its components

Interactions

DRUGS

ACE inhibitors, aliskiren (in patients with diabetes or renal impairment), other angiotensin receptor blockers: Increased risk of hyperkalemia, hypotension, and renal dysfunction

antihypertensives, diuretics: Possibly hypotension

cyclosporine, potassium-sparing diuretics, potassium supplements: Increased risk of hyperkalemia

indomethacin, sympathomimetics: Possibly decreased antihypertensive effect of losartan

lithium: Increased serum lithium levels and risk of lithium toxicity

NSAIDs: Possibly decreased renal function in elderly patients or those with renal dysfunction or volume depletion; possibly decreased effectiveness of losartan

FOODS

high-potassium diet, potassium-containing salt substitutes: Increased risk of hyperkalemia

Adverse Reactions

CNS: Dizziness, fatigue, headache, insomnia, malaise

CV: Hypotension

EENT: Nasal congestion

GI: Diarrhea, indigestion, nausea, vomiting

HEME: Thrombocytopenia

MS: Back pain, leg pain, muscle spasms

RESP: Cough, upper respiratory tract infection

SKIN: Erythroderma

Other: Angioedema, hyperkalemia, hyponatremia

Nursing Considerations

- Know that in some patients, losartan is more effective when given in 2 divided doses daily; it may be used with other antihypertensives.
- Know that patients of African descent with hypertension and left ventricular hypertrophy may not benefit from losartan to reduce stroke risk.

WARNING Be aware that patients who have renal artery stenosis or severe heart failure may experience acute renal failure from losartan therapy because losartan inhibits the angiotensin–aldosterone system, on which renal function depends.

- Monitor blood pressure and renal function studies, as ordered, to evaluate drug effectiveness.
- Periodically monitor patient's serum potassium level, as ordered, to detect hyperkalemia.

- Monitor patient for muscle pain; rarely, rhabdomyolysis has developed in patients taking other angiotensin II receptor blockers.

PATIENT TEACHING

- Instruct patient to avoid potassium-containing salt substitutes because they may increase risk of hyperkalemia.
- Advise patient to avoid exercising in hot weather and drinking excessive amounts of alcohol; instruct her to notify prescriber if she has prolonged diarrhea, nausea, or vomiting.
- Warn patient to tell all prescribers of losartan therapy.
- Instruct women to notify prescriber immediately if pregnancy occurs or is suspected as drug may cause fetal harm and will need to be discontinued.

lovastatin
(mevinolin)

Altoprev, Mevacor

Class and Category

Pharmacologic class: HMG-CoA reductase inhibitor (statin)
Therapeutic class: Antilipemic
Pregnancy category: X

Indications and Dosages

➤ *To reduce LDL and total cholesterol levels in patients with primary hypercholesterolemia; to reduce risk of coronary revascularization procedures, myocardial infarction, or unstable angina in patients without symptomatic cardiovascular disease and who have average to moderately elevated total-C and LDL-C, and below average HDL-C as primary prevention of coronary heart disease; to slow progression of coronary atherosclerosis in patients with coronary heart disease*

TABLETS (MEVACOR)

Adults. *Initial:* 20 mg as a single dose with evening meal for LDL-C reduction of 20% or more, 10 mg daily for LDL-C reduction of less than 20%; dosage adjusted after at least 4 wk. *Maintenance:* 10 to 80 mg daily as a single dose or in 2 divided doses with meals. *Maximum:* 80 mg daily.

E.R. TABLETS (ALTOPREV)

Adults. *Initial:* 10, 20, 40, or 60 mg as single dose at bedtime, increased, as needed, every 4 wk, up to maximum dose. *Maintenance:* 10 to 60 mg daily as single dose. *Maximum:* 60 mg daily.

➤ *To reduce apolipoprotein B, LDL, and total cholesterol levels in adolescents with heterozygous familial hypercholesterolemia*

TABLETS

Adolescents 1 yr postmenarche (ages 10 to 17). *Initial:* 20 mg daily for LDL-C reduction of 20% or more, 10 mg daily for LDL-C reduction of less than 20%; dosage adjusted after at least 4 wk. *Maintenance:* 10 to 40 mg daily. *Maximum:* 40 mg daily.

DOSAGE ADJUSTMENT For patients who also take amiodarone, maximum dosage limited to 40 mg daily. For patients who also take danazol, diltiazem, dronedarone, or verapamil, initial therapy begun at 10 mg daily and maximum dosage limited to 20 mg daily. For patients with creatinine clearance less than 30 ml/min, maximum dosage limited to 20 mg daily or increased, if needed, very carefully.

Route	Onset	Peak	Duration
P.O.	In 2 wk	Unknown	4–6 wk

Mechanism of Action

Interferes with the hepatic enzyme hydroxymethylglutaryl-coenzyme A reductase. By doing so, lovastatin reduces formation of mevalonic acid (a cholesterol precursor), thus interrupting the pathway by which cholesterol is synthesized. When cholesterol level declines in hepatic cells, LDLs are consumed, which also reduces amount of circulating total cholesterol and serum triglycerides. The decrease in LDLs may result in decreased level of apolipoprotein B, which is found in each LDL particle.

Contraindications

Acute hepatic disease; breastfeeding; concomitant therapy with cobicistat-containing products, cyclosporine, gemfibrozil, or strong CYP3A4 inhibitors (such as boceprevir, clarithromycin, erythromycin, HIV protease inhibitors, itraconazole, ketoconazole, nefazodone, posaconazole, telaprevir, telithromycin, voriconazole); hypersensitivity to lovastatin or its components; pregnancy; unexplained elevated liver enzymes

Interactions

DRUGS

amiodarone, boceprevir, cobicistat-containing products, clarithromycin, colchicine, cyclosporine, danazol, erythromycin, fibric acid derivatives, gemfibrozil and other fibrates, HIV protease inhibitors, immunosuppressants, itraconazole, ketoconazole, nefazodone, niacin (1 g daily or more), posaconazole, ranolazine, telaprevir, telithromycin, verapamil, voriconazole: Increased risk of severe myopathy or rhabdomyolysis
bile acid sequestrants, cholestyramine, colestipol: Decreased bioavailability of lovastatin
cimetidine, spironolactone: Possibly decreased activity or level of endogenous steroid hormones
isradipine: Increased hepatic clearance of lovastatin
itraconazole, ketoconazole: Increased lovastatin blood level
oral anticoagulants: Increased anticoagulant effect and risk of bleeding
voriconazole: Possibly increased blood lovastatin levels

FOODS

all foods: Increased lovastatin absorption
grapefruit juice (more than 1 qt daily): Increased risk of myopathy or rhabdomyolysis

ACTIVITIES

alcohol use: Increased lovastatin blood level

Adverse Reactions

CNS: Anxiety, asthenia, cognitive impairment, chills, confusion, cranial nerve dysfunction, depression, dizziness, fatigue, fever, headache, insomnia, malaise, memory loss, paresthesia, peripheral nerve palsy, peripheral neuropathy, psychic disturbances, tremor, vertigo
CV: Vasculitis
EENT: Blurred vision, cataracts, ophthalmoplegia, pharyngitis, rhinitis, sinusitis
ENDO: Elevated glycosylated hemoglobin levels, gynecomastia, hyperglycemia, thyroid function abnormalities
GI: Abdominal cramps and pain, anorexia, cholestatic jaundice, **cirrhosis**, constipation, diarrhea, elevated liver enzymes, flatulence, **fulminant hepatic necrosis**, **hepatic failure** (rare), **hepatitis**, hyperbilirubinemia, indigestion, nausea, hepatoma, **pancreatitis**, vomiting
GU: Erectile dysfunction, loss of libido
HEME: Elevated ESR, eosinophilia, **hemolytic anemia**, **leukopenia**, positive ANA, purpura, **thrombocytopenia**
MS: Arthralgias, arthritis, back pain, immune-mediated necrotizing myopathy, muscle pain, myalgia, myopathy, myositis, polymyalgia rheumatica, **rhabdomyolysis**
RESP: Cough, dyspnea, **interstitial lung disease**, upper respiratory tract infection
SKIN: Alopecia, changes to hair and nails, dermatomyositis, discolored or dry skin, **erythema multiforme**, flushing, photosensitivity, pruritus, rash, **Stevens–Johnson syndrome**, **toxic epidermal necrolysis**, urticaria
Other: **Anaphylaxis**, **angioedema**, elevated alkaline phosphatase, lupus erythematosus-like syndrome

Nursing Considerations

- Give lovastatin cautiously in patients who have a history of liver disease and patients who consume large amounts of alcohol.
- Give drug 1 hour before or 4 hours after bile acid sequestrant, cholestyramine, or colestipol.
- Expect patient to be prescribed a standard low-cholesterol diet during therapy.
- Be aware that drug affects mainly total cholesterol and LDL levels; it has only slight effects on HDL and triglyceride levels.
- Monitor liver enzymes before therapy begins, as ordered. If indicated, expect to measure them during therapy, as ordered. If ALT or AST level reaches or exceeds three times upper limit of normal and persists at that level, expect to discontinue lovastatin.

- Monitor patient closely for muscle pain, tenderness, or weakness suggestive of myopathy. Also monitor creatinine kinase, as ordered. If patient becomes symptomatic or creatine kinase becomes highly elevated, withhold drug, notify prescriber and expect drug to be discontinued. Be especially alert for myopathy that could become its more severe form, rhabdomyolysis, in patients with other disorders such as diabetes complicated with renal dysfunction.
- Expect to withhold drug temporarily in patients who develop an acute or serious condition predisposing the patient to the development of renal failure secondary to rhabdomyolysis. Conditions to be watchful for include hypotension; major surgery or trauma; sepsis; or severe electrolyte, endocrine, or metabolic disorders; or uncontrolled epilepsy. Be mindful that the drug interactions may not be the same for the extended-release formulation of lovastatin as for those encountered with the immediate-release formulation.

PATIENT TEACHING

- Tell patient who takes drug once daily to do so with evening meal to enhance absorption.
- Advise patient to report muscle aches, pains, tenderness, or weakness, being especially watchful of these symptoms when dosage is increased. If present, tell him to stop taking lovastatin immediately and notify prescriber.
- Instruct patient to report severe GI distress or vision changes, as well as the development of dark urine, fatigue, loss of appetite, right upper abdominal pain or yellowing of skin.
- Advise patient to avoid performing any hazardous activity, such as driving, if cognitive impairment develops and to notify prescriber.
- Tell patient to alert prescriber of any over-the-counter or prescription drugs being taken because serious drug interactions could occur.
- Urge patient to avoid consuming alcohol or more than 1 quart of grapefruit juice daily while taking drug.
- Direct patient to follow a low-cholesterol diet during therapy. Recommend exercise and weight loss programs as appropriate.
- Emphasize the importance of periodic eye examinations during therapy.
- Teach female patients appropriate contraceptive methods and the need to report suspected pregnancy immediately.
- Tell mothers that breastfeeding is contraindicated while taking lovastatin.

lubiprostone

Amitiza

Class and Category

Pharmacologic class: Chloride channel activator
Therapeutic class: GI motility
Pregnancy category: Not classified

Indications and Dosages

➤ *To treat chronic idiopathic constipation; to treat opioid-induced constipation in patients with chronic noncancer pain*

CAPSULES

Adults. 24 mcg twice daily.

➤ *To treat irritable bowel syndrome with constipation*

CAPSULES

Women at least 18 years of age. 8 mcg twice daily.

DOSAGE ADJUSTMENT For patients with chronic idiopathic constipation or opioid-induced constipation who have moderate liver impairment, dosage reduced to 16 mcg twice daily. For patients being treated for any listed indication who have severe liver impairment, dosage reduced to 8 mcg once daily.

Mechanism of Action

Enhances a chloride-rich intestinal fluid secretion specifically by activating CIC-2, which is a normal constituent of the apical membrane of the human intestine. By increasing intestinal fluid secretion, motility in the intestine is increased, which facilitates the passage of stool to alleviate the symptoms associated with chronic idiopathic constipation. In addition, activation of the apical CIC-2 channels in intestinal epithelial cells bypasses the antisecretory action of opiates through suppression of secretomotor neuron excitability.

Contraindications

Hypersensitivity to lubiprostone or its components, mechanical gastrointestinal obstruction

Interactions

DRUGS

diphenylheptaine opioids such as methadone: Decreased effectiveness of lubiprostone

Adverse Reactions

CNS: Anxiety, asthenia, depression, dizziness, fatigue, headache, lethargy, malaise, syncope, tremor
CV: Chest discomfort or pain, **hypotension**, palpitations, peripheral edema, tachycardia
EENT: Distortion of sense of smell, dry mouth, pharyngolaryngeal pain, **throat tightness**
GI: Abdominal distention or pain, anorexia, constipation, defecation urgency, diarrhea, dyspepsia, elevated liver enzymes, eructation, fecal incontinence, flatulence, frequent bowel movements, gastritis, gastroesophageal reflux disease, intestinal functional disorder, **ischemic colitis**, nausea, **rectal hemorrhage**, vomiting
GU: Pollakiuria, UTI
MS: Fibromyalgia, joint swelling, muscle cramps or spasms, myalgia
RESP: Cough, dyspnea
SKIN: Cold sweat, erythema, excessive diaphoresis, rash
Other: Flu-like symptoms, generalized pain, **hypokalemia**, swelling, weight gain

Nursing Considerations

- Be aware that lubiprostone should not be given to patients with severe diarrhea. If severe diarrhea occurs while patient is taking drug, notify prescriber and expect drug to be discontinued.
- Administer lubiprostone with food and water to reduce nausea.
- Monitor patient's blood pressure for hypotension. Syncope and hypotension have occurred with lubiprostone therapy and sometimes within 1 hour after drug administration, including the first dose. Risk factors include the presence of diarrhea or vomiting or taking drugs known to lower blood pressure.
- Assess patient for dyspnea, which generally has occurred as an acute onset within 30 to 60 minutes after being given the first dose of lubiprostone. Although dysnpea usually resolves within 3 hours after taking drug, it may reoccur with subsequent doses. If it becomes severe or reoccurs, notify prescriber.

PATIENT TEACHING

- Instruct patient to swallow capsules whole and not to break apart or chew the capsules.
- Tell patient to take lubiprostone with food and water.
- Inform patient of the possibility of diarrhea occurring with lubiprostone therapy. If diarrhea becomes severe, tell patient to stop taking drug and notify prescriber.
- Tell patient that drug may lower his blood pressure to the point of fainting. Caution patient to avoid performing hazardous activities until the effects of drug are known.
- Instruct patient to inform all prescribers of lubiprostone therapy, because drugs known to lower blood pressure increase patient's risk of low blood pressure and possibly fainting.
- Alert patient that difficulty breathing may occur after the first dose of lubiprostone but generally resolves within 3 hours. Tell patient to notify prescriber if dyspnea occurs.
- Tell mothers who are breastfeeding while taking lubiprostone to monitor the infant for diarrhea.

lurasidone hydrochloride

Latuda

Class and Category

Pharmacologic class: Atypical antipsychotic
Therapeutic class: Antipsychotic
Pregnancy category: B

Indications and Dosages

➤ *To treat schizophrenia*

TABLETS

Adults. *Initial:* 40 mg once daily (with a meal consisting of at least 350 calories), increased as needed. *Maximum:* 160 mg once daily.

Adolescents ages 13 to 17. *Initial:* 40 mg once daily (with a meal consisting of at least 350 calories), increased as needed. *Maximum:* 80 mg daily.

➤ *To treat depressive episodes associated with bipolar I disorder as monotherapy or adjunctive therapy with either lithium or valproate*

TABLETS

Adults. *Initial:* 20 mg once daily (with a meal consisting of at least 350 calories), increased as needed. *Maximum:* 120 mg once daily (with a meal consisting of at least 350 calories).

➤ *To treat depressive episodes associated with bipolar I disorder as monotherapy*

TABLETS

Children age 10 to 17 years. *Initial:* 20 mg once daily (with a meal consisting of at least 350 calories), increased weekly, after one week, as needed. *Maximum:* 80 mg daily.

DOSAGE ADJUSTMENT For patients already taking a moderate CYP3A4 drug or who have moderate hepatic impairment or moderate (creatinine clearance 30 to less than 50 ml/min) or severe (creatinine clearance less than 30 ml/min) renal impairment, maximum dose should not exceed 80 mg once daily. For patient with severe hepatic impairment, maximum dose should not exceed 40 mg once daily. For patient newly prescribed a moderate CYP3A4 inhibitor, dosage reduced to half of the original dose of lurasidone prescribed. For patient receiving a moderate CYP3A4 inducer, dosage may have to be increased after CYP3A4 inducer therapy has been in place for at least 7 days.

Mechanism of Action

Possibly mediated through a combination of central dopamine type 2 and serotonin type 2 receptor antagonism to suppress psychotic symptoms.

Contraindications

Concurrent therapy with strong CYP3A4 inducers such as rifampin, and strong CYP3A4 inhibitors such as ketoconazole; hypersensitivity to lurasidone or its components

Interactions

DRUGS

CNS depressants: Additive CNS depression
CYP3A4 inducers: Possibly decreased effect of lurasidone
CYP3A4 inhibitors: Possibly increased effect of lurasidone
digoxin, midazolam: Possibly increased blood levels of these drugs

ACTIVITIES

alcohol use: Additive CNS depression

Adverse Reactions

CNS: Agitation, akathisia, anxiety, **CVA**, dizziness, dystonia, extrapyramidal symptoms, fatigue, hypomania or mania activation, impaired cognitive and motor function, insomnia, **neuroleptic malignant syndrome**, parkinsonism, psychomotor hyperactivity, restlessness, **seizures**, somnolence, **suicidal ideation**, syncope, tardive dyskinesia, transient ischemic attacks
CV: Hypertension, orthostatic hypotension, tachycardia
EENT: Blurred vision, dry mouth, increased salivation, oropharyngeal pain, rhinitis, **throat swelling**, tongue swelling
ENDO: Hyperglycemia, hyperprolactinemia
GI: Abdominal pain, anorexia, diarrhea, dyspepsia, dysphagia, nausea, vomiting
GU: Elevated creatinine level
HEME: Agranulocytosis, **leukopenia**, **neutropenia**
MS: Back pain, **rhabdomyolysis**
RESP: Dyspnea
SKIN: Pruritus, rash, urticaria
Other: Elevated CPK level, **hyponatremia**, weight gain

Nursing Considerations

WARNING Be aware that lurasidone should not be used to treat dementia-related psychosis in the elderly because of an increased risk of death nor in patients at risk for aspiration pneumonia because drug may cause esophageal dysmotility, resulting in dysphagia.

- Use lurasidone cautiously in patients with cardiovascular disease, cerebrovascular disease, or conditions that would predispose them to hypotension. Also, use cautiously in those with a history of seizures or with conditions that lower the seizure threshold, such as Alzheimer's disease.

- Also, use cautiously in elderly patients because of increased risk of serious adverse cerebrovascular effects, such as stroke and transient ischemic attack.

WARNING Monitor patient closely for neuroleptic malignant syndrome, seizures, and tardive dyskinesia throughout therapy, and take safety precautions, as needed. Notify prescriber immediately of any occurrence.

- Monitor patient's blood glucose level routinely; risk of hyperglycemia may increase.
- Watch patients closely for suicidal tendencies, especially in children and young adults, and particularly when therapy starts and dosage changes, because depression may worsen temporarily during these times.
- Monitor patient's CBC, as ordered, because serious adverse hematologic reactions may occur, such as agranulocytosis, leukopenia, and neutropenia. Assess more often during first few months of therapy if patient has a history of drug-induced leukopenia or neutropenia or a significantly low WBC count. If abnormalities occur during therapy, watch for fever or other signs of infection, notify prescriber, and, if severe, expect drug to be discontinued.
- Know that extrapyramidal symptoms and withdrawal symptoms may occur in newborns following delivery to mothers taking lurasidone during the third trimester.
- Be aware that the occurrence of tardive dyskinesia and the chances of the dyskinesia being irreversible increase the longer therapy continues, as well as with the total cumulative dose. Although less common, tardive dyskinesia may also occur after relatively short periods of therapy at low doses and may even occur after therapy has been discontinued. Monitor patient closely and notify prescriber at once if present.
- Assess patient for fall risk and institute fall precautions.

PATIENT TEACHING

- Instruct patient or caregiver that lurasidone must be taken with a meal consisting of at least 350 calories.
- Urge patient to avoid alcohol during lurasidone therapy.
- Instruct patient to avoid hazardous activities until drug's effects are known. Warn patient that falls can also occur due to the effects of drug on the nervous system. Review fall precautions with patient.
- Alert women of childbearing age to report known or suspected pregnancy to prescriber. If pregnancy is confirmed, encourage patient to enroll in the pregnancy exposure registry by calling 866-961-2388.
- Caution patient to avoid dehydration, exercising strenuously, exposure to extreme heat or taking medication with anticholinergic activity because lurasidone therapy may interfere with being able to reduce the body's core body temperature.

M

magnesium chloride

(contains 64 mg of elemental magnesium per tablet, 100 mg of elemental magnesium per enteric-coated tablet, 64 mg of elemental magnesium per E.R. tablet, and 200 mg of elemental magnesium per 1 ml of injection)
Chloromag, Mag-L-100, Slow-Mag

magnesium citrate (citrate of magnesia)

(contains 40.5 to 47 mg elemental magnesium per 5 ml oral solution)
Citroma, Citro-Mag (CAN)

magnesium gluconate

(contains 54 mg elemental magnesium per 5 ml oral solution and 27 to 29.3 mg elemental magnesium per tablet)
Almora, Maglucate (CAN), Magonate, Magtrate

magnesium hydroxide (milk of magnesia)

(contains 135 mg elemental magnesium per tablet, 129 to 130 mg elemental magnesium per chewable tablet, and 164 to 328 mg elemental magnesium per 5 ml liquid, liquid concentrate, or oral solution)
Phillips' Chewable Tablets, Phillips' Magnesia Tablets (CAN), Phillips' Milk of Magnesia, Phillips' Milk of Magnesia Concentrate

magnesium lactate

(contains 84 mg elemental magnesium per E.R. tablet)
Mag-Tab SR Caplets

magnesium oxide

(contains 84.5 mg elemental magnesium per capsule and 50 to 302 mg elemental magnesium per tablet)
Mag-200, Mag-Ox 400, Maox, Uro-Mag

magnesium sulfate

(contains 100 to 500 mg elemental magnesium per 1 ml of injection, 1 to 5 g elemental magnesium per 10 ml of injection, and 40 mEq per 5 mg of crystals)

Class and Category

Pharmacologic class: Mineral
Therapeutic class: Electrolyte replacement
Pregnancy category: D (parenteral magnesium sulfate), Not classified (others)

Indications and Dosages

➤ *To correct magnesium deficiency caused by alcoholism, magnesium-depleting drugs, malnutrition, or restricted diet; to prevent magnesium deficiency based on U.S. and Canadian recommended daily allowances*

CAPSULES, CHEWABLE TABLETS, CRYSTALS, ENTERIC-COATED TABLETS, E.R. TABLETS, LIQUID, LIQUID CONCENTRATE, ORAL SOLUTION, TABLETS (MAGNESIUM CHLORIDE, CITRATE, GLUCONATE, HYDROXIDE, LACTATE [EXCEPT IN CHILDREN], OXIDE, SULFATE)

Dosage individualized based on severity of deficiency and normal recommended daily allowances listed below.

Adult men and children over age 10. 270 to 400 mg daily (*Canada:* 130 to 250 mg daily).
Adult women and children over age 10. 280 to 300 mg daily (*Canada:* 135 to 210 mg daily).
Pregnant women. 320 mg daily (*Canada:* 195 to 245 mg daily).
Breastfeeding women. 340 to 355 mg daily (*Canada:* 245 to 265 mg daily).
Children ages 7 to 10. 170 mg daily (*Canada:* 100 to 135 mg daily).
Children ages 4 to 6. 120 mg daily (*Canada:* 65 mg daily).
Children from birth to age 3. 40 to 80 mg/day (*Canada:* 20 to 50 mg daily).

➤ *To treat mild magnesium deficiency*
I.M. INJECTION (MAGNESIUM SULFATE)
Adults and adolescents. 1 g every 6 hr for 4 doses.
➤ *To treat severe hypomagnesemia*
I.V. INFUSION (MAGNESIUM CHLORIDE)
Adults. 4 g diluted in 250 ml D_5W and infused at no more than 3 ml/min. *Maximum:* 40 g daily.
I.V. INFUSION (MAGNESIUM SULFATE)
Adults and adolescents. 5 g diluted in 1 L I.V. solution and infused over 3 hr.
➤ *To prevent and control seizures in preeclampsia or eclampsia*
I.V. INFUSION OR INJECTION (MAGNESIUM SULFATE)
Adults. *Loading:* 4 g of a 10% to 20% solution and given very slowly following manufacturer's guidelines for type of solution used. *Maintenance:* 1 to 2 g/hr by continuous infusion. *Maximum*: 40 g/day and for no longer than 5 to 7 days.
I.M. INJECTION (MAGNESIUM SULFATE)
Adults. 4 to 5 g of a 50% solution every 4 hr, as needed.
➤ *To treat acute nephritis in children*
I.M. INJECTION (MAGNESIUM SULFATE)
Children. 20 to 40 mg/kg of a 20% solution, repeated as needed.
➤ *To treat torsades de pointes*
I.V. INFUSION
Adults. *For patient with pulse:* 1 to 2 g diluted in 50 to 100 ml D_5W and infused over 5 to 60 min, followed by 0.5 to 1 g/hr. *For patient in cardiac arrest:* 1 to 2 g diluted in 10 ml D_5W and infused over 5 to 20 min.
➤ *To relieve indigestion with hyperacidity*
CHEWABLE TABLETS, LIQUID, LIQUID CONCENTRATE, ORAL SOLUTION TABLETS (MAGNESIUM HYDROXIDE)
Adults and adolescents. 400 to 1,200 mg (5 to 15 ml liquid or 2.5 to 7.5 ml liquid concentrate) up to four times daily with water, or 622 to 1,244 mg (tablets or chewable tablets) up to four times daily.
CAPSULES, TABLETS (MAGNESIUM OXIDE)
Adults and adolescents. 140 mg (capsules) three times daily or four times daily with water or milk, or 400 to 800 mg daily (tablets).
➤ *To relieve constipation, to evacuate colon for rectal or bowel examination*
LIQUID, LIQUID CONCENTRATE (MAGNESIUM HYDROXIDE)
Adults and children age 12 and over. 2.4 to 4.8 g (30 to 60 ml) daily as single dose or divided doses.
Children ages 6 to 11. 1.2 to 2.4 g (15 to 30 ml)/day as a single dose or in divided doses.
Children ages 2 to 5. 0.4 to 1.2 g (5 to 15 ml) daily as single dose or divided doses.
ORAL SOLUTION (MAGNESIUM CITRATE)
Adults and children age 12 and over. Up to 10 ounces with 8 ounces of water.
Children ages 6 to 11. Up to 5 ounces with 8 ounces of water.
Children ages 2 to 5. Highly individualized.
CRYSTALS (MAGNESIUM SULFATE)
Adults and children age 12 and over. 10 to 30 g daily as single dose or divided doses. *Maximum:* two times daily.
DOSAGE ADJUSTMENT Dosage limited to 20 g of magnesium sulfate every 48 hr for patients with severe renal impairment.
CAPSULES, TABLETS (MAGNESIUM OXIDE)
Adults. 1 to 2 g with a full glass of water or milk, usually at bedtime.

Route	Onset	Peak	Duration
P.O.*	0.5–3 hr	Unknown	Unknown
P.O.†	20 min	Unknown	20–180 min
I.M.‡	1 hr	Unknown	3–4 hr
I.V.‡	Immediate	Unknown	About 30 min

* For laxative effect.
† For antacid effect.
‡ For anticonvulsant effect.

Mechanism of Action
Assists all enzymes involved in phosphate transfer reactions that use adenosine triphosphate (ATP). Magnesium is required for normal function of the ATP-dependent sodium–potassium pump in muscle membranes. It may effectively treat digitalis glycoside–induced arrhythmias because correction of hypomagnesemia improves the sodium–potassium pump's ability to distribute potassium into intracellular spaces and because magnesium decreases calcium uptake and potassium outflow through myocardial cell membranes.

As a laxative, magnesium exerts a hyperosmotic effect in the small intestine. It causes water retention that distends the bowel and causes the duodenum to secrete cholecystokinin. This substance stimulates fluid secretion and intestinal motility.

As an antacid, magnesium reacts with water, converting magnesium oxide to magnesium hydroxide. Magnesium hydroxide rapidly reacts with gastric acid to form water and magnesium chloride, which increases gastric pH.

As an anticonvulsant, magnesium depresses the CNS and blocks peripheral neuromuscular impulse transmission by decreasing available acetylcholine.

Incompatibilities

Don't combine magnesium sulfate with alkali carbonates and bicarbonates, alkali hydroxides, arsenates, calcium, clindamycin phosphate, dobutamine, fat emulsions, heavy metals, hydrocortisone sodium succinate, phosphates, polymyxin B, procaine hydrochloride, salicylates, sodium bicarbonate, strontium, and tartrates.

Contraindications

Hypersensitivity to magnesium salts or any component of magnesium-containing preparations
For magnesium chloride: Coma, heart disease, renal impairment
For magnesium sulfate: Heart block, MI, preeclampsia 2 hours or less before delivery (I.V. form)
For use as laxative: Acute abdominal problem (as indicated by abdominal pain, nausea, or vomiting), diverticulitis, fecal impaction, intestinal obstruction or perforation, colostomy or ileostomy, severe renal impairment, ulcerative colitis

Interactions

DRUGS

amphotericin B, cisplatin, cyclosporine, gentamicin: Possibly magnesium wasting and need for magnesium dosage adjustment
anticholinergics: Possibly decreased absorption and therapeutic effects of these drugs
calcium salts (I.V.): Possibly neutralization of magnesium sulfate's effects
cellulose sodium phosphate: Possibly binding with magnesium, possibly decreased therapeutic effectiveness of cellulose
CNS depressants: Increased CNS depression
digoxin (I.V.): Possibly heart block and conduction changes, especially when calcium salts are also administered
digoxin, fluoroquinolones, folic acid, H_2-receptor blockers, iron preparations, isoniazid, ketoconazole, penicillamine, phenothiazines, phenytoin, phosphates (oral), tetracyclines: Possibly decreased absorption and blood levels of these drugs
diuretics (loop or thiazide): Possibly hypomagnesemia
edetate sodium, sodium polystyrene sulfonate: Possibly binding with magnesium
enteric-coated drugs: Possibly quicker dissolution of these drugs and increased risk of adverse GI reactions
etidronate (oral): Decreased etidronate absorption
mecamylamine: Possibly prolonged effects of mecamylamine
methenamine, streptomycin, sucralfate, tetracyclines, tobramycin (oral), urinary acidifiers: Possibly decreased therapeutic effects of these drugs
misoprostol: Increased misoprostol-induced diarrhea
neuromuscular blockers: Possibly increased neuromuscular blockade
nifedipine: Possibly increased hypotensive effects when taken with magnesium sulfate
potassium-sparing diuretics: Increased risk of hypermagnesemia
salicylates: Possibly increased excretion and lower blood levels of salicylates
sodium polystyrene sulfonate resin: Possibly metabolic alkalosis

FOODS

high glucose intake: Increased urinary excretion of magnesium

ACTIVITIES

alcohol use: Increased urinary excretion of magnesium

Adverse Reactions

CNS: Confusion, decreased reflexes, dizziness, syncope
CV: Arrhythmias, hypotension
GI: Flatulence, vomiting

M

MS: Muscle cramps
RESP: Dyspnea, **respiratory depression or paralysis**
SKIN: Diaphoresis
Other: Hypermagnesemia, hypersensitivity reactions, injection-site pain or irritation (I.M. form), laxative dependence, **magnesium toxicity**

Nursing Considerations

- Be aware that magnesium sulfate is the elemental form of magnesium. Oral preparations aren't all equivalent.
- Be aware that drug isn't metabolized. Drug remaining in the GI tract produces watery stool within 30 minutes to 3 hours.
- Make sure patient chews chewable tablets thoroughly before swallowing.
- Avoid giving other oral drugs within 2 hours of magnesium-containing antacid.
- Before giving drug as laxative, shake oral solution, liquid, or liquid concentrate well and give with a large amount of water.

WARNING Observe for and report early evidence of hypermagnesemia: bradycardia, depressed deep tendon reflexes, diplopia, dyspnea, flushing, hypotension, nausea, slurred speech, vomiting, and weakness.

WARNING Be aware that magnesium may precipitate myasthenic crisis by decreasing patient's sensitivity to acetylcholine.

- Frequently assess cardiac status of patient taking drugs that lower heart rate, such as beta blockers because magnesium may aggravate symptoms of heart block.

WARNING Be aware that magnesium chloride for injection contains the preservative benzyl alcohol, which may cause fatal toxic syndrome in neonates and premature infants.

- Provide adequate diet, exercise, and fluids for patient being treated for constipation.
- Monitor serum electrolyte levels in patients with renal insufficiency because they're at risk for magnesium toxicity.
- Be aware that magnesium salts aren't intended for long-term use. For example, magnesium sulfate may cause fetal abnormalities if administered for more than 5 to 7 days to pregnant women. When magnesium sulfate is administered by continuous I.V. infusion (especially for more than 24 hours preceding delivery) to control convulsions in a toxemic woman, monitor newborn for signs of magnesium toxicity, such as neuromuscular or respiratory depression.

PATIENT TEACHING

- Advise patient to chew magnesium chewable tablets thoroughly before swallowing, and then drink a full glass of water. Mention that tablets have a chalky taste.
- Instruct patient to take magnesium-containing antacid between meals and at bedtime. Urge him not to take other drugs within 2 hours of the antacid.
- Tell patient to notify prescriber and avoid using magnesium-containing laxative if he has abdominal pain, nausea, or vomiting.
- Instruct patient to refrigerate magnesium citrate solution.
- Caution patient about risk of dependence with long-term laxative use.
- Teach patient to prevent constipation by increasing dietary fiber and fluid intake and exercising regularly.
- Inform patient that magnesium supplements used to replace electrolytes can cause diarrhea.

mannitol

Osmitrol, Resectisol

Class and Category

Pharmacologic class: Osmotic diuretic
Therapeutic class: Diuretic
Pregnancy category: B

Indications and Dosages

➤ *To reduce intracranial or intraocular pressure*

I.V. INFUSION

Adults and adolescents. 0.25 to 2 g/kg as 15% to 25% solution given over 30 to 60 min. If used before eye surgery, 1.5 to 2 g/kg 60 to 90 min before procedure.

DOSAGE ADJUSTMENT For small or debilitated patients, dosage reduced to 0.5 g/kg.

➤ *To diagnose oliguria or inadequate renal function*

I.V. INFUSION

Adults and adolescents. 200 mg/kg or 12.5 gas 15% to 20% solution given over 3 to 5 min. Second dose given only if patient fails to excrete 30 to 50 ml of urine in 2 to 3 hr. Drug discontinued if no response after second dose.

➤ *To prevent oliguria or acute renal failure*

I.V. INFUSION

Adults and adolescents. 50 to 100 g as 5% to 25% solution.

➤ *To treat oliguria*

I.V. INFUSION

Adults and adolescents. 50 to 100 g as 15% to 25% solution given over 90 min to several hr.

➤ *To promote diuresis in drug toxicity*

I.V. INFUSION

Adults and adolescents. *Loading:* 25 g. *Maintenance:* Up to 200 g as 5% to 25% solution given continuously to maintain urine output of 100 to 500 ml/hr with positive fluid balance of 1 to 2 L.

➤ *To provide irrigation during transurethral resection of prostate gland*

IRRIGATION SOLUTION

Adults. 2.5% or 5% solution, as needed.

Route	Onset	Peak	Duration
I.V.*	1–3 hr	Unknown	Up to 8 hr
I.V.†	30–60 min	Unknown	4–8 hr
I.V.‡	In 15 min	Unknown	3–8 hr

* To produce diuresis.
† To decrease intraocular pressure.
‡ To decrease intracranial pressure.

Mechanism of Action

Elevates plasma osmolality, causing water to flow from tissues, such as brain and eyes, and from CSF, into extracellular fluid, thereby decreasing intracranial and intraocular pressure.

As an osmotic diuretic, mannitol increases the osmolarity of glomerular filtrate, which decreases water reabsorption. This leads to increased excretion of chloride, sodium, water, and toxic substances.

As an irrigant, mannitol minimizes the hemolytic effects of water used as an irrigant and reduces the movement of hemolyzed blood from the urethra to the systemic circulation, which prevents hemoglobinemia and serious renal complications.

Incompatibilities

Don't administer mannitol through same I.V. line as blood or blood products.

Contraindications

Active intracranial bleeding (except during craniotomy), anuria due to severe renal insufficiency, hypersensitivity to mannitol or its components, severe congestion or pulmonary edema, severe hypovolemia

Interactions

DRUGS

digoxin, drugs that prolong the QT interval, neuromuscular blocking agents: Increased risk of electrolyte imbalances resulting in serious cardiac adverse reactions; increased risk of digitalis toxicity from hypokalemia
diuretics; nephrotoxic drugs such as aminoglycosides, cyclosporine: Increased risk of renal failure and toxicity
lithium: Initial increased elimination of lithium followed by increased risk of lithium toxicity in patients with hypovolemia or renal impairment
neurotoxic drugs such as aminoglycosides: Increased risk of CNS toxicity

Adverse Reactions

CNS: Asthenia, chills, **coma**, confusion, dizziness, fever, headache, lethargy, malaise, **rebound increased intracranial pressure**, **seizures**
CV: Chest pain, **heart failure**, hypertension, **hypotension**, palpitations, peripheral edema, tachycardia, thrombophlebitis
EENT: Blurred vision, dry mouth, rhinitis
GI: Diarrhea, nausea, vomiting
GU: **Acute kidney injury**, **anuria**, **azotemia**, hematuria, oliguria, osmotic nephrosis, polyuria, urine retention
MS: Musculoskeletal stiffness, myalgia
RESP: Cough, dyspnea, **pulmonary edema**
SKIN: Diaphoresis, pruritus, rash, urticaria
Other: **Anaphylaxis**, dehydration, extravasation (with compartment syndrome, swelling, and tissue necrosis), generalized discomfort or pain, **hyperkalemia**, **hypernatremia**,

hyperosmolarity, hypervolemia, **hypokalemia**, hyponatremia (dilutional), infusion-site reactions (erythema, inflammation, pain, phlebitis, pruritus, or extravasation complications of compartment syndrome, tissue necrosis), **metabolic acidosis**, thirst

Nursing Considerations

- Know that if crystals form in mannitol solution exposed to low temperature, solution should be placed in hot-water bath to redissolve crystals.
- Know that elderly patients and patients with preexisting renal disease are at greater risk for developing adverse reactions. Expect to evaluate patient's cardiac, pulmonary, and renal status and correct any preexisting fluid and electrolyte imbalances before therapy begins, as ordered.
- Use a 5-micron in-line filter when administering drug solution of 15% or greater. Know that infusion of hypertonic solutions of mannitol should be administered through a large central vein, if possible, because administration through a peripheral vein can cause severe infusion-site reactions, such as compartment syndrome and swelling associated with extravasation.
- Be aware that depending on dosage and duration of mannitol administration, acid–base and electrolyte imbalances may occur, which can be severe and potentially fatal. Monitor central venous pressure, fluid intake and output, and vital signs every hour during I.V. infusion of mannitol. Measure urine output with indwelling urinary catheter, as appropriate. Notify prescriber if renal function worsens and expect mannitol to be discontinued.

WARNING Assess patient for hypersensitivity reactions, including anaphylaxis, dyspnea, and hypotension; cardiac arrest and death have occurred. If hypersensitivity reactions present, stop infusion immediately, notify prescriber, and expect to provide supportive emergency care. Be aware that concomitant administration of nephrotoxic drugs or other diuretics should be avoided during mannitol therapy.

- Check weight and monitor BUN and serum creatinine electrolyte levels daily, as ordered.
- Expect to monitor patient's cardiac, pulmonary, and renal function as well as signs and symptoms of hyper- or hypovolemia for patient receiving mannitol therapy for reduction in intracranial pressure. Also expect to monitor this patient's acid–base balance, intracranial pressure, osmol gap, and serum electrolytes and osmolarity.

WARNING Monitor patient, especially patient with impaired renal function, for CNS toxicity such as coma, confusion, or lethargy. This may occur as a result of high serum mannitol concentrations or disturbances of electrolyte and acid–base balance caused by mannitol administration. Patients with preexisting compromise of the blood–brain barrier are at increased risk for increasing cerebral edema with mannitol use. Monitor patient closely for a rebound increase in intracranial pressure for at least several hours after mannitol has been discontinued. Know that use of neurotoxic drugs should be avoided, if possible, during mannitol administration.

- Provide frequent mouth care to relieve dry mouth and thirst.
- Know that high concentrations of mannitol may produce false low results for inorganic phosphorus blood concentrations. Mannitol therapy may also produce false positive results in tests for blood ethylene glycol concentrations.

PATIENT TEACHING

- Inform patient that he may experience dry mouth and thirst during mannitol therapy.
- Instruct patient to report chest pain, difficulty breathing, or pain at I.V. site, along with any other new, persistent, or severe adverse reactions.

maprotiline hydrochloride

Ludiomil

Class and Category

Pharmacologic class: Tetracyclic antidepressant
Therapeutic class: Antidepressant
Pregnancy category: B

Indications and Dosages

➤ *To treat mild to moderate depression*

TABLETS

Adults and adolescents. *Initial:* 75 mg once daily or given in divided doses for 2 wk. Increased in 25-mg increments as needed and tolerated. *Maintenance:* 75 to 150 mg once daily or given in divided doses.

➤ *To treat hospitalized patients with severe depression*

TABLETS

Adults and adolescents. *Initial:* 100 to 150 mg once daily or given in divided doses, increased as needed and tolerated. *Maintenance:* 150 to 225 mg once daily or given in divided doses.

DOSAGE ADJUSTMENT For patients over age 60, initial dosage reduced to 25 mg daily and then increased by 25 mg/wk up to maintenance dosage of 50 to 75 mg once daily or given in divided doses.

Route	Onset	Peak	Duration
P.O.	1–3 wk	3–6 wk	Unknown

Mechanism of Action

Blocks norepinephrine's reuptake at adrenergic nerve fibers. Normally, when a nerve impulse reaches an adrenergic nerve fiber, norepinephrine is released from storage sites and metabolized in the nerve or at the synapse. Some norepinephrine reaches receptor sites on target organs and tissues, but most is taken back into the nerve and stored by way of reuptake mechanism. By blocking norepinephrine reuptake, maprotiline increases its level at nerve synapses. Elevated norepinephrine level may decrease depression by improving mood.

Contraindications

Hypersensitivity to maprotiline, mirtazapine, or their components; use within 14 days of MAO inhibitor therapy

Interactions

DRUGS

anticholinergics, antihistamines: Increased atropine-like adverse effects, such as blurred vision, constipation, dizziness, and dry mouth
anticonvulsants: Increased risk of CNS depression, possibly lower seizure threshold and increased risk of seizures
bupropion, clozapine, haloperidol, loxapine, molindone, other tricyclic antidepressants, phenothiazines, pimozide, thioxanthenes, trazodone: Possibly increased anticholinergic effects, possibly lowered seizure threshold and increased risk of seizures
cimetidine: Possibly increased blood maprotiline level
clonidine, guanadrel, guanethidine: Possibly decreased antihypertensive effects of these drugs, possibly increased CNS depression (with clonidine)
CNS depressants: Increased risk of CNS depression
estrogens, oral contraceptives containing estrogen: Possibly decreased therapeutic effects and increased adverse effects of maprotiline
MAO inhibitors: Increased risk of hyperpyrexia, hypertensive crisis, severe seizures, or death
sympathomimetics: Increased risk of arrhythmias, hyperpyrexia, hypertension, or tachycardia
thyroid hormones: Increased risk of arrhythmias

ACTIVITIES

alcohol use: Increased risk of CNS depression

Adverse Reactions

CNS: Agitation, dizziness, drowsiness, fatigue, headache, insomnia, **seizures**, **suicidal ideation**, tremor, weakness
EENT: Blurred vision, dry mouth, increased intraocular pressure
ENDO: Gynecomastia
GI: Constipation, diarrhea, epigastric distress, increased appetite, nausea, vomiting
GU: Impotence, libido changes, testicular swelling, urinary hesitancy, urine retention
HEME: Agranulocytosis
SKIN: Diaphoresis, photosensitivity, pruritus, rash
Other: Weight loss

Nursing Considerations

- Give maprotiline at bedtime if daytime drowsiness occurs.
- Check CBC, as ordered, if fever, sore throat, or other evidence of agranulocytosis develops.
- Take seizure precautions according to facility policy.

- Watch patient (especially adolescents and young adults) closely for suicidal tendencies, particularly when therapy starts and dosage changes because depression may worsen temporarily during these times, possibly leading to suicidal ideation.
- Expect to taper drug gradually because stopping abruptly may produce withdrawal symptoms.

PATIENT TEACHING

- Advise patient to take maprotiline exactly as prescribed. Caution him not to stop drug abruptly because of risk of withdrawal symptoms, including headache, nausea, nightmares, and vertigo.
- Inform patient that he may not feel drug's effects for several weeks.
- Suggest that patient take drug with food if adverse GI reactions develop.
- Urge patient to report difficulty urinating, excessive drowsiness, fever, or sore throat.
- Advise patient to avoid hazardous activities until drug's CNS effects are known.
- Caution patient to avoid alcohol and other CNS depressants while taking drug.
- Urge family or caregiver to watch patient closely for suicidal tendencies, especially when therapy starts or dosage changes and particularly if patient is a teenager or young adult.

maraviroc

Selzentry

Class and Category

Pharmacologic class: CCR5 co-receptor antagonist
Therapeutic class: Antiretroviral
Pregnancy category: Not classified

Indications and Dosages

➤ *As adjunct to treat CCR5-tropic human immunodeficiency virus type 1 (HIV-1) infection*

ORAL SOLUTION, TABLETS

Adults taking potent CYP3A inhibitors such as boceprevir, delavirdine, clarithromycin, elvitegravir/ritonavir, itraconazole, ketoconazole, nefazodone, protease inhibitors except tipranavir/ritonavir, or telithromycin; children age 2 and over weighing 40 kg (88 lb) or more. 150 mg twice daily.
Children age 2 and over weighing at least 30 kg (66 kg) to less than 40 kg (88 lb) taking potent CYP3A inhibitors such as boceprevir, delavirdine, clarithromycin, elvitegravir/ritonavir, itraconazole, ketoconazole, nefazodone, protease inhibitors except tipranavir/ritonavir, or telithromycin. 100 mg twice daily.
Children age 2 and over weighing at least 20 kg (44 lb) to less than 30 kg (66 lb) taking potent CYP3A inhibitors such as boceprevir, delavirdine, clarithromycin, elvitegravir/ritonavir, itraconazole, ketoconazole, nefazodone, protease inhibitors except tipranavir/ritonavir, or telithromycin. 75 mg (tablet) or 80 mg (oral solution) twice daily.
Children age 2 and over weighing at least 10 kg (22 lb) to less than 20 kg (44 lb) taking potent CYP3A inhibitors such as boceprevir, delavirdine, clarithromycin, elvitegravir/ritonavir, itraconazole, ketoconazole, nefazodone, protease inhibitors except tipranavir/ritonavir, or telithromycin. 50 mg twice daily.
Adults taking potent CYP3A inducers (without a potent CYP3A inhibitor) such as carbamazepine, efavirenz, etravirine, phenobarbital, phenytoin, or rifampin. 600 mg twice daily.
Adults and children age 2 and over weighing at least 30 kg (66 lb) taking drugs that are not potent CYP3A inducers or inhibitors. 300 mg twice daily.
DOSAGE ADJUSTMENT For adult patients experiencing orthostatic hypotension and taking 300 mg twice daily, dosage reduced to 150 mg twice daily.

Mechanism of Action

Selectively binds to the human chemokine receptor CCR5 present on the cell membrane, preventing an interaction that would allow CCR5-tropic HIV-1 to enter the cell. This prevents replication of the CCR5-tropic human immunodeficiency virus type I.

Contraindications

End-stage renal disease treated with hemodialysis or severe renal impairment in patients receiving potent CYP3A inducers or inhibitors, hypersensitivity to maraviroc or its components

Interactions

DRUGS

CYP3A and P-gp inducers: Decreased effectiveness of maraviroc
CYP3A and P-gp inhibitors: Increased plasma concentration of maraviroc with increased risk of adverse reactions
St. John's wort: Decreased plasma concentration of maraviroc with substantially decreased effectiveness; increased risk of development of resistance to maraviroc

Adverse Reactions

CNS: Anxiety, changes in levels of consciousness including loss of consciousness, **CVA**, depression, dizziness, dysesthesias, facial palsy, fever, malaise, memory loss excluding dementia, paresthesias, peripheral neuropathies, sensory abnormalities, sleep disturbances, **seizures**, syncope, tremor
CV: Acute heart failure, coronary artery disease, **coronary artery occlusion**, **endocarditis**, hypertension, **MI**, myocardial ischemia, orthostatic hypotension, **unstable angina**
EENT: Conjunctivitis, ear disorders, hemianopia, nasal or ocular infections or inflammations, oral lesions, paranasal sinus disorders, visual field defects
GI: Abdominal distention, appetite disorders, bilirubin increase, bloating, cholestatic jaundice, constipation, elevated pancreatic and liver enzymes, flatulence, gastrointestinal atonic and hypomotility disorders, **hepatic cirrhosis or failure**, **hepatitis**, **hepatotoxicity**, jaundice, **portal vein thrombosis**
GU: Ejaculation and erection disorders, urinary tract signs and symptoms
HEME: Anemias, eosinophilia, **hypoplastic anemia**, **marrow depression**, **neutropenia**
MS: Elevated creatine kinase, joint or muscle aches or pains, myositis, osteonecrosis, **rhabdomyolysis**
RESP: Breathing difficulties, cough, respiratory infections
SKIN: Acne, alopecia, apocrine and eccrine gland disorders, benign skin neoplasms, blisters, erythemas, lipodystrophies, nail and nail bed disorders, pruritus, rash (could be severe), **Stevens–Johnson syndrome**, **toxic epidermal necrolysis**
Other: Angioedema; drug reaction with eosinophilia and systemic symptoms (DRESS); elevated IgE; generalized discomfort or pain; immune reconstitution syndrome; infections such as bacterial, herpes, *Neisseria*, respiratory, tinea, and viral

Nursing Considerations

- Know that maraviroc is not recommended in patients with dual/mixed- or CXCR4-tropic HIV-1 infections.
- Be sure patient has been checked for CCR5 tropism before treatment with maraviroc is started, because it is only effective against this type of infection.

WARNING Check patient's bilirubin and liver enzyme levels before maraviroc treatment is started and periodically throughout treatment, as ordered, because drug increases risk of hepatotoxicity. Know that patients with a history of liver dysfunction or patients with co-infection with hepatitis B and/or C virus may require additional monitoring. Severe rash or evidence of systemic allergic reactions (including DRESS, eosinophilia, elevated IgE, and other systemic symptoms) has occurred with hepatotoxicity about 1 month after maraviroc therapy was started in some patients. Know that cases of hepatitis have occurred in some patients in the absence of allergic manifestations or who have had no history of hepatic disease.

WARNING Monitor patient closely for severe skin reactions. Notify prescriber and expect maraviroc to be discontinued immediately if patient develops a rash that is accompanied by blisters, conjunctivitis, eosinophilia, facial edema, fever, joint or muscle aches, lip swelling, malaise, or oral lesions. Be aware that a delay in discontinuing the drug may result in a life-threatening situation.

- Monitor patient's cardiovascular status throughout maraviroc therapy because, although uncommon, major events such as acute heart failure, endocarditis, hypertension, myocardial infarction or ischemia and unstable angina have been reported with maraviroc therapy. Pay close attention to the patient's blood pressure if renal impairment is present, because of risk of orthostatic hypotension. Patients with severe renal impairment or end-stage renal disease experiencing orthostatic hypotension should be evaluated for a dosage reduction.

- Be aware that immune reconstitution syndrome has occurred in patients treated with combination antiretroviral therapy, including maraviroc. The inflammatory response predisposes susceptible patients to opportunistic infections such as cytomegalovirus, *Mycobacterium avium* infection, *Pneumocystis jiroveci* pneumonia, or tuberculosis. Autoimmune disorders such as Graves' disease, Guillain–Barré syndrome, or polymyositis have also occurred. Report sudden or unusual adverse reactions to prescriber.
- Assess patient frequently for signs and symptoms of infection, because maraviroc affects some immune cells placing patient at increased risk.
- Be aware that maraviroc may put patient at increased risk for malignant tumors because of its effect on the immune system.

PATIENT TEACHING

- Advise patient to avoid missing doses of maraviroc, as it can result in the development of resistance to drug. If she misses a dose, she should take it as soon as she remembers, but should not double the next dose or take more than prescribed.

WARNING Inform patient to seek immediate medical attention if signs and symptoms of hepatitis or an allergic reaction occurs.

- Advise patients with a history of cardiovascular disease or postural hypotension to notify prescriber if signs and symptoms develop or increase, as such patients are at increased risk for cardiovascular events.
- Tell patient to avoid hazardous activities, such as driving, until drug's CNS effects are known. Urge her to take safety precautions to prevent falling if she has adverse reactions, such as dizziness.
- Instruct patient to alert all prescribers of maraviroc therapy and not to take any over-the-counter medication, including herbal products, without the consent of the prescriber. Inform her that St. John's wort should not be taken while on maraviroc therapy.
- Advise female patient to alert prescriber if pregnancy is suspected or has occurred, and encourage her to register with the Antiretroviral Pregnancy Registry by calling 1-800-258-4263.
- Inform mothers that breastfeeding is not recommended during maraviroc therapy.
- Instruct patient prescribed oral solution to throw away any unused solution 60 days after first opening the bottle.

meclizine hydrochloride
(meclozine hydrochloride)

Antivert, Bonamine (CAN), Bonine, Dramamine Less Drowsy, Meclicot, Meni-D

Class and Category

Pharmacologic class: Antihistamine
Therapeutic class: Antiemetic, antivertigo
Pregnancy category: B

Indications and Dosages

➤ *To prevent and treat vertigo*

CAPSULES, CHEWABLE TABLETS, TABLETS

Adults and adolescents. 25 to 100 mg daily, as needed, in divided doses.

➤ *To treat motion sickness*

CAPSULES, TABLETS

Adults. 25 to 50 mg 1 hr before travel and then every 24 hr, as needed, for duration of trip.

Route	Onset	Peak	Duration
P.O.	1 hr	Unknown	8–24 hr

Mechanism of Action

May inhibit nausea and vomiting by blocking cholinergic synapses in the brain's vomiting center and reducing sensitivity of labyrinthine apparatus.

Contraindications

Hypersensitivity to meclizine or its components

Interactions

DRUGS

anticholinergics: Possibly potentiated anticholinergic effects
apomorphine: Possibly decreased emetic response to apomorphine
CNS depressants: Possibly potentiated CNS depression

CYP2D6 inhibitors: Possibly decreased effectiveness of meclizine

ACTIVITIES

alcohol use: Possibly potentiated CNS depression

Adverse Reactions

CNS: Dizziness, drowsiness, euphoria, excitement, fatigue, hallucinations, headache, insomnia, nervousness, restlessness, vertigo
CV: **Hypotension**, palpitations, tachycardia
EENT: Blurred vision; diplopia; dry mouth, nose, and throat; tinnitus
GI: Abdominal pain, anorexia, constipation, diarrhea, jaundice, nausea, vomiting
GU: Urinary frequency and hesitancy, urine retention
RESP: **Bronchospasm**, thickening of respiratory secretions
SKIN: Rash, urticaria

Nursing Considerations

- Use meclizine cautiously in patients with asthma, glaucoma, or prostate gland enlargement.
- Also, use cautiously in the elderly and in patients with hepatic or renal impairment because of potential increase of drug blood levels under these conditions.
- Be aware that drug may mask signs of brain tumor, intestinal obstruction, or ototoxicity.

PATIENT TEACHING

- Explain that meclizine works best for motion sickness when taken before travel.
- Instruct patient to chew meclizine chewable tablets thoroughly before swallowing.
- Instruct patient to report blurred vision or other adverse effects that are prolonged or severe.
- Urge patient to avoid alcohol while taking drug.
- Caution patient to avoid hazardous activities until drug's CNS effects are known.
- Advise patient to have regular eye examinations during long-term therapy.
- Tell mothers who are breastfeeding not to take large doses of drug for a prolonged period of time, because drug may have adverse effects on the nursing infant or may decrease milk supply.

meclofenamate sodium

Meclomen

Class and Category

Pharmacologic class: NSAID
Therapeutic class: Analgesic
Pregnancy category: C

Indications and Dosages

➤ *To relieve pain and inflammation in rheumatoid arthritis and osteoarthritis*

CAPSULES

Adults and adolescents over age 14. 50 to 100 mg every 6 to 8 hr, as needed. *Maximum:* 400 mg/day.

➤ *To relieve mild to moderate pain*

CAPSULES

Adults and adolescents over age 14. 50 mg every 4 to 6 hr, as needed. Increased to 100 mg every 4 to 6 hr, as needed. *Maximum:* 400 mg daily.

➤ *To treat hypermenorrhea and primary dysmenorrhea*

CAPSULES

Adults and adolescents over age 14. 100 mg three times daily for up to 6 days starting with the onset of menstrual flow.

Route	Onset	Peak	Duration
P.O.*	1 hr	0.5–2 hr	4–6 hr
P.O.†	Few days	2–3 wk	Unknown

* For analgesic effect.
† For antirheumatic effect.

Mechanism of Action

Blocks cyclooxygenase, the enzyme needed to synthesize prostaglandins, which mediate the inflammatory response and cause local pain, swelling, and vasodilation. By inhibiting prostaglandins, this NSAID reduces inflammatory symptoms. It also relieves pain because prostaglandins promote pain transmission from periphery to spinal cord.

Contraindications

Hypersensitivity to aspirin, iodides, meclofenamate, other NSAIDs, or their components

M

Interactions

DRUGS

acetaminophen: Increased risk of adverse renal effects with long-term use of both drugs
anticoagulants, thrombolytics: Prolonged PT and increased risk of bleeding
antihypertensives: Decreased effectiveness of antihypertensives
beta blockers: Impaired antihypertensive effect of beta blockers
cefamandole, cefoperazone, cefotetan, plicamycin, valproic acid: Possibly hypoprothrombinemia and increased risk of bleeding
cimetidine: Altered meclofenamate level
colchicine, glucocorticoids, potassium supplements: Increased risk of GI bleeding and irritability
cyclosporine, gold compounds, nephrotoxic drugs: Increased risk of nephrotoxicity
digoxin: Increased blood digoxin level
insulin, oral antidiabetic drugs: Decreased effectiveness of these drugs
lithium: Increased risk of lithium toxicity
loop diuretics: Decreased effects of these drugs
methotrexate: Increased risk of methotrexate toxicity
NSAIDs, salicylates: Increased risk of GI bleeding and irritability, decreased meclofenamate effectiveness
phenytoin: Increased blood phenytoin level
probenecid: Increased risk of meclofenamate toxicity

ACTIVITIES

alcohol use: Increased risk of GI bleeding and irritability

Adverse Reactions

CNS: **CVA**, dizziness, drowsiness, fatigue, headache, insomnia, **seizures**
CV: Hypertension, **MI**, peripheral edema, tachycardia
EENT: Stomatitis, tinnitus
GI: Abdominal pain; anorexia; constipation; diarrhea; diverticulitis; dyspepsia; dysphagia; elevated liver enzymes; esophagitis; flatulence; gastritis; gastroenteritis; gastroesophageal reflux disease; **GI bleeding**, **perforation**, and ulceration; **hepatic failure**; indigestion; jaundice; **melena**; nausea; stomatitis; vomiting
GU: **Acute renal failure**, dysuria, elevated BUN and serum creatinine levels
HEME: **Agranulocytosis**, anemia, easy bruising, **hemolytic anemia**, **leukopenia**, **neutropenia**, **pancytopenia**, **thrombocytopenia**
RESP: **Asthma**, **respiratory depression**
SKIN: **Erythema multiforme**, pruritus, rash, **Stevens–Johnson syndrome**, **toxic epidermal necrolysis**, urticaria
Other: **Anaphylaxis**, **angioedema**

Nursing Considerations

- Use meclofenamate with extreme caution in patients with a history of GI bleeding or ulcer disease because NSAIDs, such as meclofenamate, increase risk of GI bleeding, and ulceration. Expect to use drug for shortest time possible in these patients.
- Be aware that serious GI tract bleeding, perforation, and ulceration may occur without warning symptoms. Elderly patients are at greater risk. To minimize risk, give drug with food and a full glass of water. If GI distress occurs, withhold drug and notify prescriber immediately.
- Use meclofenamate cautiously in patients with hypertension, and monitor blood pressure closely throughout therapy. Drug may cause hypertension or worsen it.

WARNING Monitor patient closely for thrombotic events, including MI and stroke, because NSAIDs increase the risk.

- Monitor patient—especially if he's elderly or taking meclofenamate long-term—for less common but serious adverse GI reactions, including anorexia, constipation, diverticulitis, dysphagia, esophagitis, gastritis, gastroenteritis, gastroesophageal reflux disease, hemorrhoids, hiatal hernia, melena, stomatitis, and vomiting.
- Monitor liver enzymes, as ordered, because, rarely, elevations may progress to severe hepatic reactions, including fatal hepatitis, hepatic failure, or liver necrosis.
- Monitor BUN and serum creatinine levels in elderly patients, patients taking ACE inhibitors or diuretics, and patients with heart failure, hepatic dysfunction, or impaired renal function; drug may cause renal failure in these patients.

- Monitor CBC for decreased hemoglobin and hematocrit because drug may worsen anemia.

WARNING If patient has bone marrow suppression or is receiving an antineoplastic drug, monitor laboratory results (including WBC count), and watch for evidence of infection because anti-inflammatory and antipyretic actions of meclofenamate may mask signs and symptoms, such as fever and pain.

- Assess patient's skin regularly for rash or other hypersensitivity reaction because meclofenamate is an NSAID and may cause serious skin reactions without warning, even in patients with no history of NSAID sensitivity. At first sign of reaction, stop drug and notify prescriber.
- Expect lower doses of meclofenamate to be used for long-term therapy.

PATIENT TEACHING

- Tell patient to take drug with a full glass of water to keep it from lodging in esophagus and causing irritation. Suggest taking drug with food or milk to avoid GI distress.
- Instruct patient to report itching, rash, severe diarrhea, and swelling in ankles or fingers.
- Caution patient to avoid hazardous activities until drug's CNS effects are known.
- Caution pregnant patient not to take NSAIDs, such as meclofenamate, during last trimester because drug may cause premature closure of fetal ductus arteriosus.
- Explain that meclofenamate may increase risk of serious adverse cardiovascular reactions; urge patient to seek immediate medical attention if signs or symptoms arise, such as chest pain, shortness of breath, slurring of speech, or weakness.
- Explain that meclofenamate may increase risk of serious adverse GI reactions; stress importance of seeking immediate medical attention for such signs and symptoms as abdominal or epigastric pain, black or tarry stools, indigestion, or vomiting blood or material that looks like coffee grounds.
- Alert patient to rare but serious skin reactions to meclofenamate. Urge him to seek immediate medical attention for blisters, fever, itching, rash, or other indications of hypersensitivity.

meloxicam

Mobic, Vivlodex

Class and Category

Pharmacologic class: NSAID
Therapeutic class: Analgesic
Pregnancy category: C

Indications and Dosages

➤ *To relieve signs and symptoms of osteoarthritis*

ORAL SUSPENSION, TABLETS (MOBIC)

Adults. 7.5 mg daily. *Maximum:* 15 mg daily.

CAPSULES (VIVLODEX)

Adults. 5 mg once daily. *Maximum:* 10 mg once daily (5 mg once daily for patient on hemodialysis).

➤ *To relieve signs and symptoms of rheumatoid arthritis*

ORAL SUSPENSION, TABLETS (MOBIC)

Adults. 7.5 mg daily. *Maximum:* 15 mg daily.

➤ *To relieve pauciarticular or polyarticular signs and symptoms of juvenile rheumatoid arthritis*

ORAL SUSPENSION, TABLETS (MOBIC)

Children age 2 and over. 0.125 mg/kg daily. *Maximum:* 7.5 mg daily.

Mechanism of Action

Blocks cyclooxygenase, the enzyme needed to synthesize prostaglandins, which mediate the inflammatory response and cause local pain, swelling, and vasodilation. By inhibiting prostaglandins, the NSAID meloxicam reduces inflammatory symptoms. It also relieves pain because prostaglandins promote pain transmission from the periphery to the spinal cord.

Contraindications

History of angioedema, asthma, bronchospasm, nasal polyps, rhinitis, or urticaria induced by hypersensitivity to aspirin or other NSAIDs; hypersensitivity to meloxicam or its components; setting of coronary artery bypass graft (CABG) surgery

Interactions

DRUGS

ACE inhibitors: Decreased antihypertensive effect, increased risk of renal failure
aspirin: Increased risk of GI ulceration

furosemide: Decreased diuretic effect of furosemide, possibly renal impairment
kayexalate: Increased risk of intestinal necrosis
lithium: Elevated blood lithium level, possibly lithium toxicity
oral anticoagulants, warfarin: Increased risk of bleeding

ACTIVITIES

alcohol use, smoking: Increased risk of GI bleeding

Adverse Reactions

CNS: Confusion, **CVA**, dizziness, fever, headache, insomnia, mood alteration, **seizures**
CV: Chest pain, edema, **heart failure**, hypertension, **MI**, tachycardia, vasculitis
EENT: Laryngitis, pharyngitis, sinusitis
GI: Abdominal pain, anorexia, colitis, constipation, diarrhea, diverticulitis, dyspepsia, dysphagia, elevated liver enzymes, esophagitis, flatulence, gastritis, gastroenteritis, gastroesophageal reflux disease, **GI bleeding** and ulceration, **hepatic failure**, **hepatitis**, indigestion, **melena**, nausea, **pancreatitis**, **perforation of intestines or stomach**, stomatitis, vomiting
GU: Acute renal failure, acute urine retention (children), urinary frequency, UTI
HEME: Agranulocytosis, anemia, easy bruising, **hemolytic anemia**, **leukopenia**, **neutropenia**, **pancytopenia**, **thrombocytopenia**
MS: Arthralgia; back pain; joint crepitation, effusion, or swelling; muscle spasms; myalgia
RESP: Asthma, **bronchospasm**, cough, dyspnea, **respiratory depression**, upper respiratory tract infection
SKIN: Erythema multiforme, **exfoliative dermatitis**, photosensitivity, pruritus, rash, **Stevens–Johnson syndrome**, **toxic epidermal necrolysis**
Other: Anaphylaxis, **angioedema**, flu-like symptoms

Nursing Considerations

- Be aware that NSAIDs like meloxicam should be avoided in patients with a recent MI because risk of reinfarction increases with NSAID therapy. If therapy is unavoidable, monitor patient closely for signs of cardiac ischemia.
- Know that the risk of heart failure increases with NSAID use. Meloxicam should not be used in patients with severe heart failure but, if unavoidable, monitor patient for worsening of heart failure.
- Use meloxicam with extreme caution in patients with history of GI bleeding or ulcer disease because NSAIDs, such as meloxicam, increase risk of GI bleeding and ulceration. Expect to use drug for shortest time possible in these patients.
- Be aware that capsules are not interchangeable with other formulations of oral meloxicam even if the total milligram strength is the same. Do not substitute similar dose strengths of other meloxicam products for capsule form.
- Be aware that serious GI tract bleeding, perforation, and ulceration may occur without warning symptoms. Elderly patients are at greater risk. To minimize risk, give drug with food and a full glass of water. If GI distress occurs, withhold drug and notify prescriber immediately.
- Use meloxicam cautiously in patients with hypertension, and monitor blood pressure closely throughout therapy. Drug may cause hypertension or worsen it.

WARNING Monitor patient closely for thrombotic events, including MI and stroke, because NSAIDs increase the risk. These events may occur early in treatment and risk increases with duration of use. Be aware that these events have occurred even in patients who do not have a history or risk factors for cardiovascular disease. Monitor patient for warning signs such as chest pain, slurring of speech, shortness of breath, or weakness. If any signs and symptoms develop, withhold meloxicam, alert prescriber immediately, and provide supportive care, as prescribed.

- Monitor patient—especially if elderly or taking meloxicam long-term—for less common but serious adverse GI reactions, including anorexia, constipation, diverticulitis, dysphagia, esophagitis, gastritis, gastroenteritis, gastroesophageal reflux disease, hemorrhoids, hiatal hernia, melena, stomatitis, and vomiting.
- Monitor liver enzymes because, rarely, elevations may progress to severe hepatic

reactions, including fatal hepatitis, hepatic failure, or liver necrosis.

- Monitor BUN and serum creatinine levels in elderly patients; patients taking ACE inhibitors, angiotensin II receptor antagonists, or diuretics; and patients with heart failure, hepatic dysfunction, or impaired renal function. Drug may cause renal failure.
- Monitor CBC for decreased hemoglobin and hematocrit. Drug may worsen anemia.

WARNING Keep in mind if patient has bone marrow suppression or is receiving an antineoplastic drug, monitor laboratory results (including WBC count), and watch for evidence of infection because anti-inflammatory and antipyretic actions of meloxicam may mask signs and symptoms, such as fever and pain.

- Assess patient's skin regularly for rash or other hypersensitivity reaction because meloxicam is an NSAID and may cause serious skin reactions without warning, even in patients with no history of NSAID sensitivity. At first sign of reaction, stop drug and notify prescriber.
- Monitor patient for adequate hydration before beginning meloxicam therapy to decrease risk of renal dysfunction.

PATIENT TEACHING

- Instruct patient to take meloxicam with food or after meals if she has stomach upset.
- For oral suspension, tell patient to shake container gently before use.
- Caution patient to avoid using other NSAIDs, aspirin, or products containing aspirin while taking meloxicam.
- Advise patient to refrain from alcohol use or smoking because these activities may increase risk of adverse GI reactions.
- Instruct patient to notify prescriber if she develops signs or symptoms of hepatic dysfunction, such as dark yellow or brown urine, fatigue, fever, itching, lethargy, nausea, or yellowing of eyes or skin.
- Advise patient, especially if she's taking an oral anticoagulant such as warfarin, to report immediately signs of bleeding, such as black or tarry stools, blood in urine, easy bruising, or stomach pain.
- Alert women of childbearing age that meloxicam may cause a reversible delay in ovulation that may make conception more difficult. If pregnancy is desired, she should consult with prescriber about discontinuing meloxicam therapy and using an alternative drug to treat her condition.
- Caution pregnant patient not to take NSAIDs, such as meloxicam, during the last trimester because they may cause premature closure of ductus arteriosus.
- Explain that meloxicam may increase risk of serious adverse cardiovascular reactions including heart failure; urge patient to seek immediate medical attention if signs or symptoms arise, such as chest pain, edema, shortness of breath, slurring of speech, unexplained weight gain, or weakness.
- Explain that meloxicam may increase risk of serious adverse GI reactions; emphasize importance of seeking immediate medical attention for such signs and symptoms as abdominal or epigastric pain, black or tarry stools, indigestion, or vomiting blood or material that looks like coffee grounds.
- Alert patient to rare but serious skin reactions. Urge her to seek immediate medical attention for blisters, fever, itching, rash, or other indications of hypersensitivity.

memantine hydrochloride

Namenda, Namenda XR

Class and Category

Pharmacologic class: N-methyl-D-aspartate (NMDA) receptor antagonist
Therapeutic class: Antidementia agent
Pregnancy category: B

Indications and Dosages

➤ *To treat moderate-to-severe dementia of the Alzheimer's type*

ORAL SOLUTION, TABLETS

Adults. *Initial:* 5 mg daily, increased by 5 mg/wk, as needed, to 10 mg daily in two

Mechanism of Action

Memantine blocks the excitatory amino acid glutamate on N-methyl-D-aspartate (NMDA) receptor cells in the CNS. In Alzheimer's disease, glutamate levels are abnormally high when brain cells are both active and at rest. Normally, when certain brain cells are resting, magnesium ions block NMDA receptors and prevent influx of calcium and sodium ions and outflow of potassium ions. When learning and memory cells in the brain are active, glutamate engages with NMDA receptors, magnesium ions are removed from NMDA receptors, and cells are depolarized. During depolarization, calcium and sodium ions enter brain cells, and potassium ions leave. In Alzheimer's disease, excessive circulating glutamate permanently removes magnesium ions and opens ion channels. Excessive influx of calcium may damage brain cells and play a major role in Alzheimer's disease. What's more, dying brain cells release additional glutamate, worsening the cycle of brain cell destruction.

Memantine replaces magnesium on NMDA receptors of brain cells, closing ion channels and preventing calcium influx and the resulting damage to brain cells. By preventing excessive brain cell death, memantine slows progression of Alzheimer's disease.

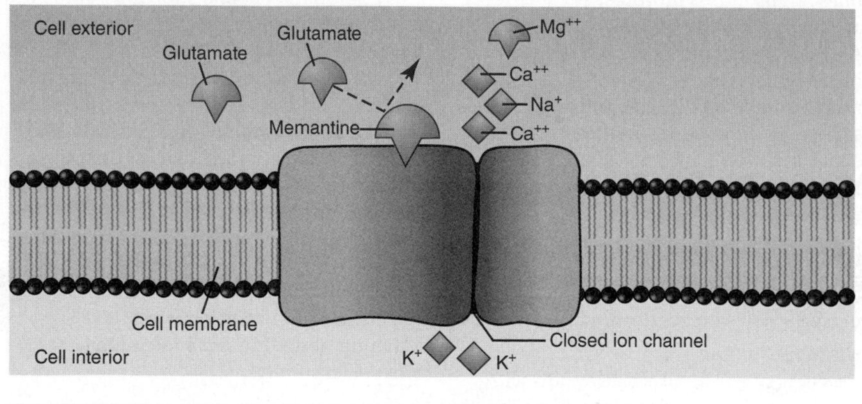

divided doses; then 15 mg daily with one 5-mg and one 10-mg dose daily; then 20 mg daily in two divided doses. *Maintenance:* 20 mg daily.

E.R. CAPSULES

Adults. *Initial:* 7 mg once daily, increased by 7 mg/wk, as needed, to 28 mg once daily. *Maximum:* 28 mg once daily.

DOSAGE ADJUSTMENT For patients with severe renal impairment, maintenance dosage reduced to 5 mg twice daily for oral solution and tablet form and 14 mg once daily for extended-release capsules.

Contraindications

Hypersensitivity to memantine, amantadine, or their components

Interactions

DRUGS

amantadine, dextromethorphan, ketamine: Possibly additive effects

carbonic anhydrase inhibitors, sodium bicarbonate: Decreased memantine clearance, leading to increased blood drug levels and risk of adverse effects

cimetidine, hydrochlorothiazide, metformin, nicotinic acid, quinidine, ranitidine, triamterene: Possibly increased blood levels of both agents

Adverse Reactions

CNS: Abnormal gait, agitation, akathisia, anxiety, confusion, **CVA**, delirium, delusions, depression, dizziness, drowsiness, dyskinesia, fatigue,

hallucinations, headache, hyperexcitability, insomnia, **neuroleptic malignant syndrome**, psychosis, restlessness, **seizures**, somnolence, **suicidal ideation**, tardive dyskinesia
CV: AV block, chest pain, **congestive heart failure**, hypertension, peripheral edema, **prolonged QT interval**, **supraventricular tachycardia**, tachycardia
ENDO: Hypoglycemia
GI: Acute pancreatitis, anorexia, colitis, constipation, diarrhea, **hepatic failure**, **hepatitis**, ileus, nausea, **pancreatitis**, vomiting
GU: Acute renal failure, elevated creatinine levels, impotence, **renal insufficiency**, urinary incontinence, UTI
HEME: Agranulocytosis, **leukopenia**, **neutropenia**, **pancytopenia**, **thrombocytopenia**, **thrombotic thrombocytopenic purpura**
MS: Arthralgia, back pain
RESP: Bronchitis, cough, dyspnea, upper respiratory tract infection
SKIN: Stevens–Johnson syndrome
Other: Generalized pain, flu-like symptoms

Nursing Considerations

- Use memantine cautiously in patients with renal tubular acidosis or severe UTI because these conditions make urine alkaline, reducing memantine excretion and increasing the risk of adverse reactions.
- Use cautiously in patients with severe hepatic impairment because drug undergoes partial hepatic metabolism, which may increase risk of adverse reactions.
- Monitor patient's response to memantine, and notify prescriber if bothersome or serious adverse reactions occur.
- Monitor patient closely for suicidal thoughts.

PATIENT TEACHING

- Instruct patient to take memantine exactly as prescribed. Inform him to notify the prescriber if he fails to take the drug for several days, as dosage adjustments may be necessary. Caution him not to double dose if he misses a single dose. Instead, tell him to take the next dose as scheduled.
- Advise patient to avoid a diet excessively high in fruits and vegetables because these foods contribute to alkaline urine, which can alter memantine clearance and increase adverse reactions.
- Tell patient that capsule should be swallowed whole and not chewed, crushed, or opened. If patient has difficulty swallowing the capsule, instruct him to open capsule, sprinkle contents on applesauce, and immediately consume entire amount of applesauce.
- Caution patient to avoid hazardous activities until drug's CNS effects are known.
- Alert patient or caregiver that memantine has the potential to cause suicidal thoughts. If present, prescriber should be notified immediately.

meperidine hydrochloride (pethidine hydrochloride)

Demerol

M

Class, Category, and Schedule

Pharmacologic class: Opioid
Therapeutic class: Opioid analgesic
Pregnancy category: C
Controlled substance schedule: II

Indications and Dosages

➤ *To relieve pain severe enough to require opioid treatment and for which alternative treatment options such as nonopioid analgesics or opioid combination products are inadequate or not tolerated*

SYRUP, TABLETS, I.M. OR SUBCUTANEOUS INJECTION

Adults. 50 to 150 mg every 3 to 4 hr, as needed.
Children. 1.1 to 1.8 mg/kg (0.5 to 0.8 mg/lb) every 3 to 4 hr, as needed.

➤ *To provide preoperative sedation*

I.V. INFUSION, I.V. INJECTION

Adults. 15 to 35 mg/hr, as needed. Alternatively, dosage highly individualized using patient-controlled analgesia device.

I.M. OR SUBCUTANEOUS INJECTION
Adults. 50 to 100 mg (0.5 to 1 mg/lb) 30 to 90 min before surgery.
Children. 1 to 2 mg/kg 30 to 90 min before surgery. *Maximum:* 100 mg every 3 to 4 hr.

➤ *As adjunct to anesthesia*

I.V. INFUSION OR INJECTION
Adults. Individualized. Repeated slow injections of 10 mg/ml solution or continuous infusion of dilute solution (1 mg/ml) titrated as needed.

➤ *To provide obstetric analgesia*

I.M. OR SUBCUTANEOUS INJECTION
Adults. 50 to 100 mg given with regular, painful contractions; repeated every 1 to 3 hr.

DOSAGE ADJUSTMENT For patients with creatinine clearance of 10 to 50 ml/min, 75% of usual dose is used; with creatinine clearance of less than 10 ml/min, 50% of usual dose is used. For elderly patients, total daily dosage decreased. For patients receiving CNS depressants, phenothiazines, and tranquilizers concurrently, dosage proportionately reduced by 25% to 50%.

Route	Onset	Peak	Duration
P.O.	15 min	1–1.5 hr	2–4 hr
I.V.	1 min	5–7 min	2–4 hr
I.M., SubQ	10–15 min	30–50 min	2–4 hr

Mechanism of Action

Binds with opiate receptors in the spinal cord and higher levels of the CNS. In this way, meperidine stimulates kappa and mu receptors, which alters the perception of and emotional response to pain.

Incompatibilities

Don't mix meperidine in same syringe with aminophylline, barbiturates, heparin, iodides, methicillin, morphine sulfate, phenytoin, sodium bicarbonate, sulfadiazine, or sulfisoxazole.

Contraindications

Acute asthma; hypersensitivity to meperidine, opioids, or their components; increased intracranial pressure; severe respiratory depression; upper respiratory tract obstruction; use within 14 days of MAO inhibitor therapy

Interactions

DRUGS

acyclovir, ritonavir: Possibly increased blood meperidine level
agonist or antagonist analgesics such as buprenorphine, butorphanol, nalbuphine, pentazocine: Possibly decreased therapeutic effects of meperidine and increased risk of precipitating withdrawal symptoms
alfentanil, CNS depressants, fentanyl, sufentanil: Increased risk of CNS and respiratory depression and hypotension
amphetamines, MAO inhibitors: Risk of increased CNS depression or excitation with possibly fatal reactions
anticholinergics: Increased risk of severe constipation
antidiarrheals (such as loperamide and difenoxin and atropine): Increased risk of increased CNS depression and severe constipation
antihypertensives: Increased risk of hypotension
antimigraine agents, cyclobenzaprine; dextromethorphan; dolasetron; granisetron; linezolid; MAO inhibitors; methylene blue; ondansetron; palonosetron; selected psychiatric drugs such as amoxapine, buspirone, lithium, maprotiline, mirtazapine, nefazodone, trazodone, vilazodone; selective serotonin reuptake inhibitors; serontonin-norepinephrine reuptake inhibitors; St. John's wort; tricyclic antidepressants; tryptophan: Increased risk of serotonin syndrome
benzodiazepines, CNS depressants, other opioids, sedating antihistamines, tricyclic antidepressants: Increased risk of significant respiratory depression and other life-threatening adverse effects
buprenorphine: Increased risk of respiratory depression
cimetidine: Reduced clearance and volume of distribution of meperidine
CYP3A4 inducers: Increased clearance of meperidine with decreased effectiveness
CYP3A4 inhibitors: Decreased clearance of meperidine resulting in increased or prolonged opioid effects
hydroxyzine: Increased risk of CNS depression and hypotension
metoclopramide: Possibly decreased effects of metoclopramide

MAO inhibitors: Increased risk of coma, hypotension, or severe respiratory depression
naloxone, naltrexone: Decreased pharmacologic effects of meperidine
neuromuscular blockers: Increased risk of prolonged CNS and respiratory depression
oral anticoagulants: Possibly increased anticoagulant effect and risk of bleeding
phenytoin: Possibly enhanced hepatic metabolism of meperidine

ACTIVITIES

alcohol use: Possibly increased CNS and respiratory depression and hypotension

Adverse Reactions

CNS: Agitation, confusion, delirium, depression, dizziness, drowsiness, headache, **increased intracranial pressure**, lack of coordination, malaise, mood changes, nervousness, nightmares, restlessness, **seizures**, syncope, transient hallucinations or disorientation, tremor, weakness
CV: Hypotension, orthostatic hypotension, tachycardia
EENT: Blurred vision, diplopia, dry mouth
ENDO: Adrenal insufficiency
GI: Abdominal cramps or pain, anorexia, constipation, ileus, nausea, vomiting
GU: Decreased libido, dysuria, erectile dysfunction, impotence, infertility, lack of menstruation, urinary frequency, urine retention
MS: Involuntary muscle movements
RESP: Dyspnea, **respiratory arrest or depression**, wheezing
SKIN: Diaphoresis, flushing, pruritus, rash, urticaria
Other: Anaphylaxis; injection-site pain, redness, or swelling; physical and psychological dependence

Nursing Considerations

- Be aware that excessive use of opioids like meperidine may lead to abuse, addiction, misuse, overdose, and possibly death. Because of this, a Risk Evaluation and Mitigation Strategy (REMS) is required. Monitor patient's intake of drug closely and for evidence of physical dependence.
- Know that chronic maternal use of meperidine during pregnancy can result in neonatal opioid withdrawal syndrome (NOWS), which may be life-threatening if not recognized and treated appropriately. NOWS occurs when a newborn has been exposed to opioid drugs like meperidine for a prolonged period while in utero.
- Use meperidine with extreme caution in patients with acute abdominal conditions, hepatic or renal disorders, hypothyroidism, prostatic hyperplasia, seizures, or supraventricular tachycardia.
- Use cautiously in debilitated patients or patients with adrenocortical insufficiency, pheochromocytoma, sickle cell anemia, toxic psychosis, and any other condition that might worsen with CNS depression, such as acute alcoholism.
- Be aware that meperidine should only be used concomitantly with benzodiazepine and other CNS depressants therapy in patients for whom other treatment options are inadequate. If prescribed together, expect dosing and duration of meperidine to be limited. Monitor patient closely for signs and symptoms of a decrease in consciousness, including coma, profound sedation, and significant respiratory depression. Notify prescriber immediately and provide emergency supportive care, as death may occur.
- Be aware that dosing errors related to confusion between milligrams (mg) and milliliters (ml) and different concentrations of oral solutions can result in accidental overdose and death. Check dosage and concentration of oral solution very carefully before administering.
- Dilute meperidine syrup with water before use to minimize local anesthetic effect.
- Give I.V. dose slowly by direct injection or as a slow continuous infusion. Mix with D_5W, normal saline solution, or Ringer's or lactated Ringer's solution.
- Keep naloxone available when giving I.V. meperidine.
- Be aware that subcutaneous injection is painful and isn't recommended unless no other route can be used.
- Be aware that oral form of meperidine is less than half as effective as parenteral meperidine. Give I.M. form when possible, and expect to increase dosage when switching patient to oral form.

WARNING Monitor patient's respiratory and cardiovascular status during treatment.

M

Notify prescriber immediately and expect to discontinue drug if respiratory rate falls to less than 12 breaths/minute or if respiratory depth decreases because serious, life-threatening, or fatal respiratory depression may occur. Monitor patient especially during initiation or following a dose increase.
- Monitor patient's bowel function to detect constipation, and assess the need for stool softeners.
- Know that prolonged use may increase risk of toxicity exhibited by seizures from the accumulation of the meperidine metabolite, normeperidine.
- Expect withdrawal symptoms to occur if drug is abruptly withdrawn after long-term use.
- Be aware that concomitant use with CYP3A4 inhibitors or discontinuation of CYP3A4 inducers can result in fatal overdose of meperidine.

WARNING Know that many drugs may interact with opioids like meperidine to cause serotonin syndrome. Monitor patient closely for signs and symptoms such as agitation, diaphoresis, diarrhea, fever, hallucinations, labile blood pressure, muscle twitching or stiffness, nausea, shakiness, shivering, tachycardia, trouble with coordination, or vomiting. Notify prescriber at once because serotonin syndrome may be life-threatening. Be prepared to discontinue drug, if possible and ordered, and provide supportive care.
- Monitor patient for adrenal insufficiency. Although rare, it can be life-threatening. Monitor patient for anorexia, dizziness, fatigue, hypotension, nausea, vomiting, or weakness. Notify prescriber if adrenal insufficiency is suspected and expect diagnostic testing to be done. If confirmed, expect to administer corticosteroids and wean patient off meperidine, if possible.

PATIENT TEACHING
- Inform patient that meperidine is a controlled substance.
- Instruct patient to use only a calibrated measuring device when measuring a dose of oral solution and never use a teaspoon or tablespoon, because a spoon is inexact and it is easy to use the wrong size spoon when measuring. Advise patient to dilute oral solution in half a glass of water before taking, because the undiluted solution may exert a slight topical anesthetic effect on mucous membranes.
- Advise patient to take drug exactly as prescribed. Warn patient that excessive or prolonged use can lead to abuse, addiction, misuse, overdose, and possibly death. If patient has been receiving meperidine for more than a few weeks and the drug is to be discontinued, advise patient to taper dosage off, as abrupt discontinuation could precipitate withdrawal symptoms.
- Instruct patient to report constipation, severe nausea, and shortness of breath.
- Advise patient to avoid hazardous activities until drug's CNS effects are known.
- Instruct patient to prevent postoperative atelectasis by turning, coughing, and deep breathing.
- Warn patient not to consume alcohol or take a benzodiazepine without prescriber knowledge, as severe respiratory depression can occur and may lead to death.
- Urge patient to avoid alcohol, sedatives, and tranquilizers during therapy.
- Inform patient that long-term use of opioids like meperidine may decrease sex hormone levels, causing decreased libido, erectile dysfunction, impotence, infertility, or lack of menstruation. Encourage patient to report any symptoms to prescriber.
- Caution pregnant patient not to increase dosage or take drug for a prolonged period, as adverse effects can cause infant to experience life-threatening withdrawal when born.
- Instruct patient to notify all prescribers of opioid use.
- Stress importance of keeping meperidine out of the reach of children, as ingestion may lead to a fatal overdose.

mepolizumab

Nucala

Class and Category

Pharmacologic class: Monoclonal antibody (interleukin-5 antagonist)

Therapeutic class: Antiasthmatic
Pregnancy category: Not classified

Indications and Dosages

➤ *Adjunct to maintenance treatment of patients with severe asthma who have an eosinophilic phenotype*

SUBCUTANEOUS INJECTION

Adults and children age 12 and over. 100 mg once every 4 wk.

➤ *To treat eosinophilic granulomatosis with polyangiitis (EGPA)*

SUBCUTANEOUS INJECTION

Adults. 300 mg once every 4 wk given as 3 separate 100-mg injections.

Mechanism of Action

Binds to IL-5 to inhibit the bioactivity of IL-5 by blocking its ability to bind to the alpha chain of the IL-5 receptor complex on the eosinophil cell surface. This action inhibits IL-5 signaling, which reduces the production and survival of eosinophils that play a role in inflammation.

Contraindications

Hypersensitivity to mepolizumab or its components

Adverse Reactions

CNS: Asthenia, dizziness, fatigue, fever, headache
CV: Hypertension, **hypotension**
EENT: Nasal congestion, nasopharyngitis, rhinitis, **stridor**
GI: Abdominal pain (upper), gastroenteritis, nausea, vomiting
GU: Cystitis, UTI
MS: Back or other musculoskeletal pain, muscle spasms, myalgia
RESP: Bronchitis, **bronchospasm**, dyspnea
SKIN: Eczema, feeling of cold in extremities, flushing, pruritus, rash, urticaria, warm sensation in neck and trunk
Other: Anaphylaxis; **angioedema**; antimepolizumab antibody formation; flu-like symptoms; herpes zoster; injection-site reactions such as burning sensation, erythema, pain, and swelling

Nursing Considerations

WARNING Know that mepolizumab should not be used to treat acute asthma exacerbations or symptoms, bronchospasms, or status asthmaticus.

- Anticipate the patient receiving a varicella vaccination, if needed, prior to mepolizumab therapy being started because herpes zoster has occurred during treatment. Also expect patients with a preexisting helminth infection to be treated before mepolizumab therapy is begun.
- Reconstitute a mepolizumab vial with 1.2 ml sterile water for injection, USP, preferably using a 2- or 3-ml syringe and a 21-gauge needle. Direct the stream of sterile water vertically onto the center of the lyophilized cake. Gently swirl the vial for 10 seconds with a circular motion at 15-second intervals until the powder is dissolved, which may take up to 5 minutes or more. Do not shake the reconstituted solution as foaming or precipitation may occur. If using a mechanical reconstitution device such as a swirler, swirl at 450 rpm for no longer than 10 minutes or 1,000 rpm for no longer than 5 minutes. The resulting solution will contain a concentration of 100 mg of mepolizumab per ml. Use reconstituted solution immediately or store at a temperature below 30°C (86°F) for up to 8 hours. Discard if not used within 8 hours.
- Prepare to administer by removing 1 ml of the reconstituted solution using a 1-ml polypropylene syringe fitted with a disposable 21- to 27-gauge, one-half inch needle. Do not shake the reconstituted solution during the procedure. Administer drug by subcutaneous injection into the patient's abdomen, thigh or upper arm.
- Administer 300-mg dose as three separate 100-mg injections into the abdomen, thigh, or upper arm. If using the same site for more than one injection, administer the injections at least 5 cm (2 inches) apart.

WARNING Monitor patient for hypersensitivity reactions such as anaphylaxis, angioedema, bronchospasm, hypotension, rash, or urticaria. Be aware these reactions can occur within hours to days after administration. If present, notify prescriber, expect mepolizumab to be discontinued, and provide supportive care.

- Know that if the patient has been taking systemic or inhaled corticosteroid therapy, a gradual reduction, may be warranted but an abrupt discontinuation of the corticosteroid should be avoided.
- Expect mepolizumab therapy to be temporarily discontinued in a patient who develops a parasitic infection during mepolizumab therapy and does not respond to antihelminth treatment. Mepolizumab therapy may be resumed once the infection has resolved.

PATIENT TEACHING

- Advise patient to notify prescriber immediately if an allergic reaction occurs even days after receiving mepolizumab and to seek emergency care, if serious.
- Caution patient taking a corticosteroid not to change his corticosteroid dosage without prescriber knowledge.
- Encourage patient to receive a varicella vaccination before therapy starts, if needed.
- Urge patient to seek medical care if his asthma remains uncontrolled or worsens after mepolizumab therapy is initiated.
- Alert female patients of childbearing age to notify prescriber if pregnancy occur or is suspected during mepolizumab therapy. Encourage them to enroll in the pregnancy exposure registry by calling 1-877-311-8972.

meropenem

Merrem I.V.

Class and Category

Pharmacologic class: Carbapenem
Therapeutic class: Antibiotic
Pregnancy category: B

Indications and Dosages

➤ *To treat complicated appendicitis and peritonitis caused by susceptible strains of alpha-hemolytic streptococci,* Bacteroides fragilis, B. thetaiotaomicron, Escherichia coli, Klebsiella pneumoniae, Peptostreptococcus species, *or* Pseudomonas aeruginosa

I.V. INFUSION OR INJECTION

Adults and children weighing more than 50 kg (110 lb). 1 g every 8 hr infused over 15 to 30 min or given as a bolus over 3 to 5 min.

Children over age 3 months weighing less than 50 kg (110 lb). 20 mg/kg every 8 hr infused over 15 to 30 min or given as bolus over 3 to 5 min. *Maximum:* 1 g every 8 hr.

I.V. INFUSION

Infants with gestational age of 32 weeks and over and postnatal age of 2 weeks and over. 30 mg/kg every 8 hr given over 30 min.

Infants with gestational age of 32 weeks and over but postnatal age less than 2 weeks or infants with gestational age less than 32 weeks but postnatal age of 2 weeks or over. 20 mg/kg every 8 hr given over 30 min.

Infants with gestational age less than 32 weeks and postnatal age less than 2 weeks. 20 mg/kg every 12 hr given over 30 min.

➤ *To treat complicated skin and skin structure infections caused by* Bacteroides fragilis, Enterococcus faecalis *(excluding vancomycin-resistant isolates),* E. coli, Peptostreptococcus species, Proteus mirabilis, P. aeruginosa, Staphylococcus aureus, Streptococcus agalactiae, S. pyogenes, *and viridans group streptococci*

I.V. INFUSION

Adults and children weighing more than 50 kg (110 lb). 500 mg (1 g if caused by *Pseudomonas aeruginosa* every 8 hr infused over 15 to 30 min.

Children over age 3 months weighing 50 kg (110 lb) or less. 10 mg/kg (20 mg/kg if caused by *Pseudomonas aeruginosa* every 8 hr infused over 15 to 30 min. *Maximum:* 500 mg every 8 hr.

➤ *To treat bacterial meningitis caused by* Haemophilus influenzae, Neisseria meningitidis, *or* Streptococcus pneumoniae *in children*

I.V. INFUSION OR INJECTION

Children weighing more than 50 kg (110 lb). 2 g every 8 hr infused over 15 to 30 min or given as a bolus over 3 to 5 min.

Children over age 3 months weighing less than 50 kg (110 lb). 40 mg/kg every 8 hr

infused over 15 to 30 min or given as bolus over 3 to 5 min. *Maximum:* 2 g every 8 hr.
DOSAGE ADJUSTMENT For adult patients with a creatinine clearance of 10 to 25 ml/min, dosage reduced by half and given every 12 hr. For those with creatinine clearance less than 10 ml/min, dosage reduced by half and given every 24 hr.

Mechanism of Action
Penetrates cell walls of most gram-negative and gram-positive bacteria, inactivating penicillin-binding proteins. This action inhibits bacterial cell wall synthesis and causes cell death.

Incompatibilities
Don't mix meropenem in same solution with other drugs.

Contraindications
Hypersensitivity to meropenem, other carbapenem drugs, beta-lactams, or their components

Interactions
DRUGS
probenecid: Inhibited renal excretion of meropenem
valproic acid: Possibly reduced blood level of valproic acid to subtherapeutic level

Adverse Reactions
CNS: Headache, paresthesias, **seizures**
CV: Shock
EENT: Epistaxis, glossitis, oral candidiasis
GI: Anorexia, constipation, diarrhea, elevated liver enzymes, nausea, **pseudomembranous colitis**, vomiting
GU: Elevated BUN and serum creatinine levels, hematuria, **renal failure**
HEME: Agranulocytosis, hemolytic anemia, leukopenia, neutropenia, positive Coombs' test
RESP: Apnea, dyspnea
SKIN: Acute generalized exanthematous pustulosis, diaper rash from candidiasis (children), **erythema multiforme**, pruritus, rash, **Stevens–Johnson syndrome**, **toxic epidermal necrolysis**
Other: Anaphylaxis; angioedema; drug reaction with eosinophilia and systemic symptoms (DRESS); injection-site inflammation, pain, phlebitis, or thrombophlebitis; **sepsis**

Nursing Considerations
- Obtain body fluid and tissue samples, as ordered, for culture and sensitivity testing. Expect to review test results, if possible, before giving first dose of meropenem.
- For I.V. bolus, add 10 ml sterile water for injection to 500 mg/20-ml vial, or 20 ml diluent to 1 g/30-ml vial of drug. Shake to dissolve.

WARNING Be aware that fatal hypersensitivity reactions have occurred with meropenem use. Determine whether patient has had previous reactions to antibiotics or other allergens. Monitor patient closely and stop drug immediately if signs and symptoms of anaphylaxis occur. Notify prescriber, and expect to provide supportive emergency care that may include airway management, epinephrine and I.V. steroid administration, and oxygen.

- Monitor patient closely for diarrhea, which may indicate pseudomembranous colitis caused by *Clostridium difficile.* If diarrhea occurs, notify prescriber and expect to withhold meropenem and treat with an antibiotic effective against *C. difficile*, and electrolytes, fluids, and protein.
- Monitor patient for blister formation, rash, and other cutaneous abnormalities, because drug may cause severe cutaneous adverse reactions that may become life-threatening. At first sign of skin abnormality, stop drug therapy immediately and notify prescriber.
- Take seizure precautions according to facility policy, especially for patients with bacterial meningitis or CNS or renal disorders because of an increased risk of seizures with meropenem.
- Monitor patient with creatinine clearance of 10 to 26 ml/min for signs and symptoms of heart failure, renal failure, seizures, or shock.

PATIENT TEACHING
- Tell patient to report immediately difficulty breathing, injection-site pain, skin changes (blister formation, rash), and sore mouth.
- Urge patient to tell prescriber about diarrhea that's severe or lasts longer than 3 days. Remind patient that bloody or

watery stools can occur 2 or more months after antibiotic therapy and can be serious, requiring prompt treatment.

- Instruct patient to avoid hazardous activities until drug's CNS effects are known.

mesalamine

Apriso, Asacol, Asacol HD, Canasa, Delzicol, Lialda, Mesasal (CAN), Pentasa, Rowasa, Salofalk (CAN), sfRowasa

Class and Category

Pharmacologic class: Aminosalicylate
Therapeutic class: Anti-inflammatory
Pregnancy category: C

Indications and Dosages

➤ *To treat and maintain remission of mildly to moderately active ulcerative colitis*

DELAYED-RELEASE TABLETS (ASACOL), DELAYED-RELEASE CAPSULES (DELZICOL)

Adults. *Initial:* 0.8 g three times daily for 6 wk. *Maintenance:* 1.6 g daily in divided doses.

DELAYED-RELEASE TABLETS (MESASAL)

Adults. 1.5 to 3 g daily in divided doses for 6 wk.

DELAYED-RELEASE TABLETS (SALOFALK)

Adults. 1 g three times daily or four times daily for 6 wk.

➤ *To induce remission in patients with active mild to moderate ulcerative colitis.*

TABLETS (LIALDA)

Adults. 2.4 or 4.8 g once daily with a meal for up to 8 wk.

➤ *To treat mildly to moderately active ulcerative colitis*

DELAYED-RELEASE TABLETS (ASACOL HD)

Adults. 1,600 mg three times daily for 6 wk. *Maximum:* 4.8 g daily.

DELAYED-RELEASE TABLETS (ASACOL), DELAYED-RELEASE CAPSULES (DELZICOL)

Children age 5 and over weighing 54 to 90 kg (119 to 198 lb): 27 to 44 mg/kg/day in two divided doses morning and afternoon for 6 wk. *Maximum:* 2.4 g daily.
Children age 5 and over weighing 33 to 54 kg (72.5 to 119 lb): 37 to 61 mg/kg daily in two divided doses morning and afternoon for 6 wk. *Maximum:* 2 g daily.
Children age 5 and over weighing 17 to 33 kg (37.5 to 72.5 lb): 36 to 71 mg/kg daily in two divided doses morning and afternoon. *Maximum:* 1.2 g daily.

➤ *To maintain remission of ulcerative colitis*

E.R. CAPSULES (APRISO)

Adults. 1.5 g once daily in morning.

TABLETS (LIALDA)

Adults. 2.4 g once daily with a meal.

➤ *To treat mild to moderate distal ulcerative colitis, proctitis, and proctosigmoiditis*

RECTAL SUSPENSION (ROWASA, SFROWASA)

Adults. 4 g (60 ml) daily at bedtime for 3 to 6 wk.

➤ *To treat active ulcerative proctitis*

SUPPOSITORIES (CANASA)

Adults. 1 g at bedtime for 3 to 6 wk.

Mechanism of Action

May reduce inflammation by inhibiting the enzyme cyclooxygenase and decreasing production of arachidonic acid metabolites, which may be increased in patients with inflammatory bowel disease. Cyclooxygenase is needed to form prostaglandins from arachidonic acid. Prostaglandins mediate inflammatory activity and produce signs and symptoms of inflammation. Mesalamine also may reduce inflammation by interfering with leukotriene synthesis and inhibiting the enzyme lipoxygenase, both of which take part in inflammatory response.

Contraindications

Hypersensitivity to mesalamine, other salicylates including aminosalicylates, or their components

Interactions

DRUGS

azathioprine, 6-mercaptopurine: Possibly increased risk for blood disorders
digoxin: Possibly decreased absorption and bioavailability of digoxin
lactulose: Possibly interference with delayed-release tablets or E.R. capsules
nephrotoxic agents including NSAIDs: Possibly increased risk of nephrotoxicity
omeprazole: Increased mesalamine absorption

Adverse Reactions

CNS: Chills, confusion, depression, dizziness, emotional lability, fatigue, fever, **Guillain–Barré syndrome**, headache (severe), **intracranial hypertension**, peripheral neuropathy, somnolence, transverse myelitis, tremor, vertigo, weakness
CV: Myocarditis, pericardial effusion, pericarditis
EENT: Blurred vision, dry mouth, rhinitis, swelling of eye, taste perversion, tinnitus
GI: Abdominal cramps or pain (severe), anal pruritus, anorexia, bloody diarrhea, cholecystitis, colitis, constipation, diarrhea, discoloration of feces, distention (abdomen), elevated liver enzymes, feeling of incomplete defecation, flatulence, gastritis, **GI bleeding**, **hepatitis**, **hepatotoxicity**, indigestion, jaundice, Kawasaki-like syndrome, **liver failure or necrosis**, mucous stools, nausea, **pancreatitis**, **perforated peptic ulcer**, rectal discharge or pain, vomiting
GU: Acute or chronic renal failure, interstitial nephritis, nephrogenic diabetes insipidus, **nephrotoxicity**, reversible oligospermia
HEME: Agranulocytosis, anemia, **aplastic anemia**, eosinophilia, **granulocytopenia**, **leukopenia**, lymphadenopathy, **neutropenia**, **pancytopenia**, **thrombocytopenia**
MS: Back pain, dysarthria, myalgia
RESP: Allergic alveolitis, **Allergic alveolitis**, **asthma exacerbation**, **eosinophilic or interstitial pneumonitis**, **fibrosing alveolitis**, pleuritis, pneumonitis
SKIN: Acne, alopecia, dryness, erythema including erythema nodosum, photosensitivity, psoriasis, pruritus, pyoderma gangrenosum, rash, **Stevens–Johnson syndrome**, urticaria
Other: Acute intolerance syndrome, **anaphylaxis**, **angioedema**, **drug reaction with eosinophilia and systemic symptoms (DRESS)**, gout, systemic lupus erythematosus or lupus-like syndrome

Nursing Considerations

WARNING Use mesalamine cautiously in patients with sulfite sensitivity. Some drug formulations contain sulfites, which may cause hypersensitivity reactions in these patients. Know that hypersensitivity reactions may affect internal organs such as the heart (myocarditis, pericarditis), kidneys (nephritis), liver (hepatitis), and lungs (pneumonitis), as well as cause hematologic adverse effects. If hypersensitivity is suspected, notify prescriber immediately, expect mesalamine to be discontinued, and provide supportive care, as ordered.

- Use mesalamine cautiously in patients with liver disease because hepatic dysfunction may occur. Monitor patient's liver enzymes, as ordered, for elevations.
- Expect to assess patient's renal function prior to the initiation of mesalamine therapy and then periodically throughout therapy, as ordered, because drug may cause renal impairment.
- Ensure that suppository is firm before inserting it. If it's too soft, chill in refrigerator for 30 minutes or run under cold water before removing wrapper. Moisten with water-soluble lubricant or tap water before insertion. Have patient retain suppository for 1 to 3 hours, as directed.
- Give rectal suspension at bedtime, and have patient retain for prescribed time—about 8 hours, if possible. Retention time ranges from 3.5 to 12 hours.
- Be aware that rectal suspension may darken slightly over time but that this change doesn't affect potency. Discard rectal suspension that turns dark brown.
- Assess patient for evidence of acute intolerance similar to flare-up of inflammatory bowel disease: acute abdominal cramps and pain, bloody diarrhea, and, possibly, fever, headache, and rash. If present, notify prescriber.
- Monitor patient's CBC with differential for eosinophilia, which may indicate an allergic reaction, and other hematological adverse reactions. Know that patients age 65 and over are at increased risk for blood dyscrasias such as agranulocytosis, neutropenia, and pancytopenia.
- Be aware that mesalamine may interfere with the measurement of urinary normetanephrine producing falsely elevated test results if the test is done by

liquid chromatography with electrochemical detection.
- Monitor patient for signs and symptoms of acute intolerance syndrome, such as acute abdominal pain, bloody diarrhea, fever, headache, and rash. If suspected, expect to discontinue mesalamine therapy and provide supportive care, as ordered.
- Be aware that patients with preexisting skin conditions such as atopic dermatitis and atopic eczema are at higher risk for more severe photosensitivity reactions.

PATIENT TEACHING
- Instruct patient taking oral drug to swallow tablets or capsules whole and not to break outer coating by cutting or chewing.
- Tell patient taking extended-release product to take it with a meal unless prescribed otherwise.
- Teach patient how to use rectal suspension or suppositories correctly. Emphasize shaking suspension bottle well before using. Tell patient not to break or cut suppository. Remind him to retain the suppository for 1 to 3 hours or longer, if possible. Caution patient not to use two suppositories at the same time to make up for a missed dose. Make patient aware that suppository will cause staining if drug comes into direct contact with surfaces, such as clothing, floors, enamel, granite, marble, painted surfaces, and vinyl.
- Advise patient to notify prescriber immediately about abdominal cramps or pain, bloody diarrhea, fever, headache, or rash or any other adverse effects that are persistent, severe, or worsen during mesalamine therapy.
- Inform woman who is breastfeeding to monitor her infant for diarrhea and report if diarrhea occurs.
- Advise patient to take sun precautions such as using sunscreen and protective clothing while outdoors, as drug may cause photosensitivity reactions that could be severe, especially in patient with preexisting skin conditions.
- Tell patient to alert all prescribers of mesalamine therapy because of potential drug interactions, especially those drugs that increase sensitivity to sun and UV light.

metaxalone

Skelaxin

Class and Category

Pharmacologic class: Oxazolidinone derivative
Therapeutic class: Skeletal muscle relaxant
Pregnancy category: Not classified

Indications and Dosages

➤ *To relieve discomfort caused by acute, painful musculoskeletal conditions*

TABLETS

Adults and children over age 12. 800 mg three times daily or four times daily.

Route	Onset	Peak	Duration
P.O.	Usually in 1 hr	Unknown	4–6 hr

Mechanism of Action

May depress CNS, causing sedation, which in turn may reduce skeletal muscle spasms to provide pain relief. Metaxalone doesn't directly relax tense skeletal muscles.

Contraindications

Hypersensitivity to metaxalone or its components, significant hepatic or renal disease, tendency to develop drug-induced, hemolytic, or other anemias

Interactions

DRUGS

CNS depressants: Increased CNS depression

ACTIVITIES

alcohol use: Increased CNS depression

Adverse Reactions

CNS: Dizziness, drowsiness, excitement, **CNS depression**, headache, insomnia, irritability, nervousness, restlessness
GI: Abdominal cramps or pain, GI upset, jaundice, **hepatotoxicity**, nausea, vomiting
HEME: Hemolytic anemia, leukopenia
SKIN: Pruritus, rash

Nursing Considerations

- Know that metaxalone may not be prescribed for women who are or may become pregnant unless potential

benefits outweigh risks, because drug's effect on fetus is unknown.
- Expect to avoid giving metaxalone with food because food may increase CNS depression, especially in elderly patients.
- Monitor patient for excessive drowsiness, which may lead to respiratory depression.
- Monitor liver enzymes for elevations, especially in patients with preexisting hepatic disease.
- Monitor renal function test results, as prescribed, for signs of impaired renal function because drug is excreted by kidneys.
- Provide rest and other pain-relief measures.
- Store drug at 15° to 30°C (59° to 86°F).

PATIENT TEACHING
- Advise patient to take metaxalone tablets exactly as prescribed and not to increase dosage or frequency.
- Instruct patient to take metaxalone tablets on an empty stomach.
- Caution patient to avoid hazardous activities, such as driving or operating machinery, until drug's CNS effects are known.
- Instruct patient to avoid alcohol and other CNS depressants during therapy.
- Caution patient to consult prescriber before taking other drugs, such as allergy or cold preparations, antidepressants, opioid analgesics, or sleeping pills.
- Urge patient to notify prescriber if he notices itching or a rash, which may signify a hypersensitivity reaction, or if he develops signs of hepatotoxicity, such as flu-like symptoms, tiredness, nausea, or yellow skin.

metformin hydrochloride

Fortamet, Gen-Metformin (CAN), Glucophage, Glucophage XR, Glumetza, Glycon (CAN), Novo-Metformin (CAN), Riomet

Class and Category

Pharmacologic class: Biguanide
Therapeutic class: Antidiabetic
Pregnancy category: B

Indications and Dosages

➤ *To reduce blood glucose level in type 2 diabetes mellitus*

ORAL SOLUTION (RIOMET), TABLETS (GLUCOPHAGE)

Adults. *Initial:* 500 mg twice daily or 850 mg daily, increased as prescribed by 500 mg/wk or by 850 mg every 2 wk until desired response occurs. *Usual:* 500 to 850 mg twice daily or three times daily. *Maximum:* 2,550 mg daily.
Children ages 10 to 17. 500 mg twice daily, increased as prescribed by 500 mg/wk until desired response occurs. *Maximum:* 2,000 mg daily in divided doses.
DOSAGE ADJUSTMENT If patient uses insulin, initial dosage reduced to 500 mg daily and then increased as prescribed by 500 mg weekly until blood glucose level is controlled.

E.R. TABLETS (GLUCOPHAGE XR, GLUMETZA)

Adults and adolescents age 17 and over. *Initial:* 500 mg daily with evening meal. Increased as prescribed by 500 mg/wk. *Maximum:* 2,000 mg daily.

E.R. TABLETS (FORTAMET)

Adults and adolescents age 17 and over. *Initial:* 500 to 1,000 mg once daily in evening. Increased in increments of 500 mg weekly, as needed. *Maximum:* 2,500 mg daily. If control isn't achieved after 4 wk at maximum dosage, an oral sulfonylurea may be prescribed.

Route	Onset	Peak	Duration
P.O.	Unknown	Up to 2 wk	2 wk after drug discontinued

Mechanism of Action

May promote storage of excess glucose as glycogen in the liver, which reduces glucose production. Metformin also may improve glucose use by adipose tissue and skeletal muscle by increasing glucose transport across cell membranes. This drug also may increase the number of insulin receptors on cell membranes and make them more sensitive to insulin. In addition, metformin modestly decreases blood total cholesterol and triglyceride levels.

Contraindications

Advanced renal disease (estimated glomerular filtration rate below 30 ml/min), hypersensitivity to metformin or its components, metabolic acidosis, use of iodinated contrast media within preceding 48 hours.

Interactions

DRUGS

calcium channel blockers, corticosteroids, estrogens, isoniazid, nicotinic acid, oral contraceptives, phenothiazines, phenytoin, sympathomimetics, thiazide and other diuretics, thyroid drugs: Possibly hyperglycemia

carbonic anhydrase inhibitors such as acetazolamide, dichlorphenamide, topiramate, zonisamide: Possibly increased risk of lactic acidosis

cationic drugs (such as amiloride, cimetidine, digoxin, dolutegravir, morphine, procainamide, quinidine, quinine, ranitidine, ranolazine, triamterene, trimethoprim, vancomycin), nifedipine, vandetanib: Increased blood metformin level and possibly increased risk of lactic acidosis

insulin, sulfonylureas: Increased risk of hypoglycemia

FOODS

all foods: Possibly delayed metformin absorption

ACTIVITIES

alcohol use: Increased risk of hypoglycemia and lactate formation

Adverse Reactions

CNS: Headache

EENT: Metallic taste

ENDO: Hypoglycemia

GI: Abdominal distention, anorexia, constipation, diarrhea, flatulence, **hepatic injury**, indigestion, nausea, vomiting

HEME: Aplastic anemia, megaloblastic anemia, **thrombocytopenia**

SKIN: Photosensitivity, rash

Other: Lactic acidosis, vitamin B_{12} deficiency (with immediate-release formulation), weight loss

Nursing Considerations

- Know that metformin should never be given to a patient with severe renal impairment (eGFR below 30 ml/min). Also be aware that metformin is not recommended for use in patients with hepatic impairment because of risk of lactic acidosis.
- Give metformin tablets with food, which decreases and slightly delays absorption, thus reducing risk of adverse GI reactions. Give E.R. tablets with evening meal; don't break or crush them.
- Expect prescriber to alter dosage if patient has a condition that decreases or delays gastric emptying, such as diarrhea, gastroparesis, GI obstruction, ileus, or vomiting.
- Expect to assess patient's estimated glomerular filtration rate (eGFR) at least annually. Anticipate that the elderly and those at increased risk for renal impairment may be tested more frequently. Be aware that initiation of metformin is not recommended in patients who have an eGFR between 45 and 60 ml/min.

WARNING Monitor patient closely for signs and symptoms of lactic acidosis that often are subtle and nonspecific, such as abdominal pain, increased somnolence, malaise, myalgias, and respiratory distress. Know that hypotension and resistant bradyarrhythmias have occurred with severe acidosis. Be aware that most cases of lactic acidosis have occurred in patients with significant renal impairment because metformin is substantially excreted by the kidneys. Other risk factors include being age 65 or older; certain drug interactions, such as carbonic anhydrase inhibitors; excessive alcohol intake; hepatic impairment; hypoxic states; radiologic studies with contrast; and withholding of fluids and food, which increases risk of volume depletion. If lactic acidosis is suspected, notify prescriber, expect metformin to be immediately discontinued, and provide appropriate supportive care. Know that prompt hemodialysis may be needed to correct the acidosis and remove the accumulated metformin.

- Monitor patient's blood glucose level to evaluate drug effectiveness. Assess for hyperglycemia and the need for insulin during times of increased stress, such as infection and surgery.
- Withhold drug, as ordered, if patient becomes dehydrated or develops hypoxemia or sepsis because these conditions increase the risk of lactic acidosis.

- Know that iodinated contrast media used in radiographic studies increase risk of renal failure and lactic acidosis during metformin therapy. Expect to withhold drug for 48 hours before and after testing.
- Expect yearly measurements of patient's hematologic status as well as vitamin B_{12} level. Be aware that vitamin B_{12} deficiency has occurred with use of the immediate-release formulation of metformin.

PATIENT TEACHING

- Instruct patient to take immediate-release metformin tablet at breakfast if taking drug once a day, or at breakfast and dinner if taking drug twice a day. Instruct him to take E.R. tablets once daily with evening meal and to swallow them whole without chewing or crushing.
- Direct patient to take drug exactly as prescribed and not to change the dosage or frequency unless instructed.
- Emphasize importance of checking blood glucose level regularly, controlling weight, exercising regularly, and following prescribed diet.
- Teach patient how to measure blood glucose level and recognize hyperglycemia and hypoglycemia. Urge him to notify prescriber of abnormal blood glucose level.
- Caution patient to avoid alcohol, which can increase the risk of hypoglycemia and lactic acidosis.
- Instruct patient to report early signs of lactic acidosis, including drowsiness, hyperventilation, malaise, and muscle pain.
- Advise patient to expect laboratory testing of glycosylated hemoglobin every 3 months until blood glucose is controlled.
- Alert women of childbearing age that metformin may cause ovulation in some premenopausal anovulatory women, which may lead to unintended pregnancy.

methadone hydrochloride

Dolophine, Methadose

Class, Category, and Schedule

Pharmacologic class: Opioid
Therapeutic class: Opioid agonist
Pregnancy category: C
Controlled substance schedule: II

Indications and Dosages

➤ *To manage opioid detoxification and then maintenance of opioid abstinence*

DISPERSIBLE TABLETS, ORAL CONCENTRATE, ORAL SOLUTION, TABLETS

Adults. *Initial on day 1:* 20 to 30 mg as a single dose, followed by 5 to 10 mg 2 to 4 hr later, if needed. *Maximum for day 1:* 40 mg. *Maintenance*: Highly individualized with dosage adjustments made until opioid withdrawal symptoms have ceased for 24 hr. *Maximum:* 120 mg daily.

I.V., I.M., OR SUBCUTANEOUS INJECTION

Hospitalized adults unable to take drug orally. Highly individualized. If oral methodone had been used prior to hospitalization, dosage initially decreased by 50%.

➤ *To manage moderate to severe pain when a continuous, around-the-clock opioid analgesic is needed for an extended period of time*

ORAL SOLUTION, TABLETS

Adults. *Initial:* 2.5 to 10 mg every 8 to 12 hr. *Maintenance:* Dosage adjustments made every 1 to 2 days, as needed. *Maximum:* 120 mg/day.

I.V., I.M., OR SUBCUTANEOUS INJECTION

Hospitalized adults unable to take drug orally. Highly individualized. If oral methodone dosage had been used prior to hospitalization, dosage initially decreased by 50%.

➤ *To treat pain severe enough to require opioid treatment not responsive to non-narcotic analgesics*

I.V., I.M., OR SUBCUTANEOUS INJECTION, ORAL SOLUTION, TABLETS

Hospitalized opioid nontolerant adults. *Initial:* 2.5 to 10 mg every 8 to 12 hr, slowly titrated to effect with dosage interval decreased, as needed.

Hospitalized opioid tolerant adults. Highly individualized.

DOSAGE ADJUSTMENT Addison's disease, debilitated patients, elderly patients, hypothyroidism, patients with severe hepatic or renal dysfunction, prostatic hyperplasia, or urethral stricture; and patients who are taking CNS depressants such as anxiolytics, hypnotics, neuroleptics, other opioids, or sedatives or who are suspected of alcohol or illicit drug use need individualized reduced dosages.

Route	Onset	Peak	Duration
P.O.	30–60 min	1.5–2 hr	4–6 hr
I.M., SubQ	10–20 min	1–2 hr	4–5 hr
I.V.	Unknown	15–30 min	Unknown

Mechanism of Action

Binds with and activates opioid receptors (primarily mu receptors) in spinal cord and higher levels of CNS to produce analgesia and euphoric effects.

Contraindications

Acute or severe bronchial asthma in unmonitored setting or in absence of resuscitative equipment, hypersensitivity to methadone or its components, paralytic ileus, significant respiratory depression

Interactions

DRUGS

amitriptyline, chloripramine, nortriptyline: Increased CNS and respiratory *depression*
ammonium chloride, ascorbic acid, potassium, sodium phosphate: May precipitate methadone withdrawal symptoms
anticholinergics: Possibly severe constipation leading to ileus; urine retention
antiemetics, general anesthetics, hypnotics, phenothiazines, sedatives, tranquilizers: Possibly coma, hypotension, respiratory depression, and severe sedation
antihistamines, choral hydrate, glutethimide, MAO inhibitors, methocarbamol: Increased CNS and respiratory depressant effects of methadone
antihypertensives, hypotension-producing drugs: Increased hypotension, risk of orthostatic hypotension
antimigraine agents, cyclobenzaprine; dextromethorphan; dolasetron; granisetron; linezolid; MAO inhibitors; methylene blue; ondansetron; palonosetron; selected psychiatric drugs such as amoxapine, buspirone, lithium, maprotiline, mirtazapine, nefazodone, trazodone, vilazodone; selective serotonin reuptake inhibitors; serontonin-norepinephrine reuptake inhibitors; St. John's wort; tricyclic antidepressants; triptans, tryptophan: Increased risk of serotonin syndrome
benzodiazepines, CNS depressants, other opioids, sedating antihistamines, tricyclic antidepressants: Increased risk of significant respiratory depression and other life-threatening adverse effects
buprenorphine, butorphanol, nalbuphine, pentazocine: Decreased therapeutic effect of methadone, increased respiratory depression, possibly withdrawal symptoms
calcium channel blockers, class IA and class III antiarrhythmics, diuretics, laxatives, mineralocorticoid hormones, neuroleptics, tricyclic antidepressants: Increased risk of electrolyte disturbances and prolonged QT interval
cimetidine: Increased analgesic and CNS and respiratory depressant effects of methadone
CYP3A4, CYP2B6, CYP2C19, CYP2C9 inducers such as carbamazepine, phenobarbital, phenytoin, rifampin, St. John's wort: Decreased methadone concentration, resulting in decreased efficacy or onset of withdrawal symptoms in patients dependent on methadone
CYP3A4, CYP2B6, CYP2C19, CYP2C9, CYP2D6 inhibitors such as azole-antifungal agents, macrolide antibiotics, protease inhibitors, some selective serotonin reuptake inhibitors (fluvoxamine, sertraline): Increased methadone concentration, resulting in increased or prolonged opioid effects that may result in a fatal overdose
desipramine: Increased plasma desipramine level
didanosine, stavudine: Decreased plasma levels of these drugs
diuretics: Decreased diuresis
efavirenz, nevirapine, ritonavir, ritonavir, lopinavir, and other antiretroviral agents, alone or in combination: Decreased or increased blood methadone level
hydroxyzine: Increased analgesic, CNS depressant, and hypotensive effects of methadone
loperamide, paregoric: Increased CNS depression, possibly severe constipation
MAO inhibitors: Possibly increased risk of severe adverse reactions
metoclopramide: Possibly antagonized metoclopramide effects on GI motility

mixed agonist-antagonist analgesics: Possibly withdrawal symptoms
naloxone: Antagonized analgesic and CNS and respiratory depressant effects of methadone, and possibly withdrawal symptoms
naltrexone: Possibly induction or worsening of withdrawal symptoms if methadone given within 7 days before naltrexone
neuromuscular blockers: Increased or prolonged respiratory depression
opioid analgesics (such as alfentanil and sufentanil): Increased CNS and respiratory depression, increased hypotension
selective serotonin reuptake inhibitors: Possibly increased blood methadone levels and increased risk of methadone toxicity
zidovudine: Increased blood zidovudine level and risk of toxicity

ACTIVITIES

alcohol use: Increased CNS and respiratory depression, possibly hypotension

Adverse Reactions

CNS: Agitation, amnesia, anxiety, asthenia, **coma**, confusion, decreased concentration, delirium, delusions, depression, dizziness, drowsiness, euphoria, fever, hallucinations, headache, insomnia, lethargy, light-headedness, malaise, psychosis, restlessness, sedation, **seizures**, syncope, tremor
CV: Bradycardia, **cardiac arrest**, **cardiomyopathy**, edema, **heart failure**, **hypotension**, orthostatic hypotension, palpitations, phlebitis, **prolonged QT interval**, **shock**, tachycardia, **torsades de pointes**, T-wave inversion on ECG, **ventricular fibrillation or tachycardia**
EENT: Blurred vision, diplopia, dry mouth, glossitis, **laryngeal edema or laryngospasm**, miosis, nystagmus, rhinitis
ENDO: Adrenal insufficiency
GI: Abdominal cramps or pain, anorexia, biliary tract spasm, constipation, diarrhea, dysphagia, elevated liver enzymes, gastroesophageal reflux, hiccups, ileus and **toxic megacolon** (in patients with inflammatory bowel disease), indigestion, nausea, vomiting
GU: Amenorrhea, decreased ejaculate potency, decreased libido, difficult ejaculation, impotence, infertility, lack of menstruation, prolonged labor, urinary hesitancy, urine retention
HEME: Anemia, **leukopenia**, **thrombocytopenia**
MS: Arthralgia
RESP: Apnea, **asthma exacerbation**, **atelectasis**, **bronchospasm**, depressed cough reflex, **hypoventilation**, **pulmonary edema**, **respiratory arrest or depression**, wheezing
SKIN: Diaphoresis, flushing
Other: Allergic reaction; **angioedema**; **hypokalemia**; **hypomagnesemia**; injection-site edema, pain, rash, or redness; physical and psychological dependence; weight gain; withdrawal symptoms

Nursing Considerations

- Make sure opioid antagonist and equipment for administering oxygen and controlling respiration are nearby before giving methadone.
- Assess patient's current drug use, including all prescription and OTC drugs before therapy begins. Be aware that excessive use of methadone may lead to abuse, addiction, misuse, overdose, and possibly death. Monitor patient's intake of drug closely.
- Be aware that use of methadone requires a Risk Evaluation and Mitigation Strategy (REMS) before drug can be dispensed, to ensure that the benefits outweigh the risks of abuse, addiction, and misuse.
- Know that benzodiazepine and other CNS depressant therapy should only be used concomitantly in patients for whom other treatment options are inadequate. If prescribed together, expect dosing and duration of methadone to be limited. Monitor patient closely for signs and symptoms of a decrease in consciousness, including coma, profound sedation, and significant respiratory depression. Notify prescriber immediately and provide emergency supportive care, as death may occur.
- Use extreme caution when administering methadone to patients with conditions accompanied by hypercapnia or hypoxia or decreased respiratory reserve such as asthma, chronic obstructive pulmonary disease or cor pulmonale, CNS depression

or coma, kyphoscoliosis, myxedema, severe obesity, or sleep apnea syndrome. This is because methadone, even with usual therapeutic doses, may decrease respiratory drive while simultaneously increasing airway resistance to the point of apnea. Know that the peak respiratory depressant effect of methadone occurs later and persists longer than the peak analgesic effect. Monitor patient's respiratory status closely, especially when initiating drug or following a dosage increase.

WARNING Give drug cautiously to patients at risk for a prolonged QT interval, such as those with cardiac hypertrophy, hypokalemia, or hypomagnesemia; those with a history of cardiac conduction abnormalities; and those taking diuretics or medications that affect cardiac conduction.

- Dilute oral concentrate with water or another liquid to volume of at least 30 ml, but preferably to 90 ml or more, before administration. Dissolve dispersible tablets in 120 ml of water or another liquid before giving. Know that the dispersible tablet may not completely dissolve in water. If a residue remains in the cup after initial administration with water, add a small amount of liquid to the cup and give to patient to drink to ensure all of the drug has been ingested.
- Monitor patient for expected excessive confusion, drowsiness, or unsteadiness during first 3 to 5 days of therapy, and notify prescriber if effects continue to worsen or persist beyond this time.

WARNING Monitor circulatory and respiratory status carefully and often during methadone therapy, especially when drug therapy is initiated and when patient is being converted to methadone, because cardiac arrest, circulatory or respiratory depression, hypotension, respiratory arrest, and shock, can develop. Life-threatening respiratory depression can occur even when drug is being used as prescribed and is not abused or misused. Be especially vigilant with cachectic, debilitated, and elderly patients, who are at higher risk for developing respiratory depression. Assess patient for excessive or persistent sedation; dosage may need to be adjusted.

- Be aware that patients tolerant to other opioids may be incompletely tolerant to methadone. A high degree of "opioid tolerance" does not eliminate the possibility of methadone toxicity. Some patients have died during conversion from chronic high-dose therapy with other opioid agonists. Monitor patient closely during the conversion process.
- Watch for drug tolerance, especially in patients with a history of chronic drug abuse, because methadone can cause physical and psychological dependence.
- Monitor patient for pain because maintenance dosage doesn't provide pain relief; patients with tolerance to opiate agonists, including those with chronic cancer pain, may require a higher dosage.
- Know that chronic maternal use of methadone during pregnancy can result in NOWS, which may be life-threatening, if not recognized and treated appropriately. Monitor patients who are pregnant or who have liver or renal impairment for increased adverse effects from methadone because drug may have a prolonged duration and cumulative effect in these patients. Methadone may prolong labor by reducing duration, frequency, strength of uterine contractions, so expect dosage to be tapered before third trimester of pregnancy. Breast-feeding mothers on maintenance therapy put their infants at risk of withdrawal symptoms if they abruptly stop breastfeeding or discontinue methadone therapy. Methadone also accumulates in CNS tissue, increasing the risk of seizures in infants.
- Check plasma amylase and lipase levels in patients who develop biliary tract spasms because levels may increase up to 15 times normal. Notify prescriber immediately of any significant or sustained increase.
- Monitor patients who have head injuries or other conditions that may increase intracranial pressure (ICP) because methadone may further increase ICP.
- Assess patient for withdrawal symptoms and tolerance to therapy because physiologic dependence can occur with long-term methadone use. Avoid abrupt discontinuation because withdrawal

symptoms will occur within 3 to 4 days after last dose.

- Monitor patients, especially the elderly, for cardiac arrhythmias, hypotension, hypovolemia, orthostatic hypotension, and vasovagal syncope because methadone may produce cholinergic effects in patients with cardiac disease, resulting in bradycardia and peripheral vasodilation; dosage decrease may be indicated.
- Monitor patients with prostatic hypertrophy, renal disease, or urethral stricture for urine retention and oliguria because methadone can increase tension of detrusor muscle.
- Be prepared to treat patient's symptoms of anxiety; be aware that anxiety may be confused with symptoms of opioid abstinence and that methadone doesn't have antianxiety effects.
- Monitor patients with seizure disorders because methadone may induce or aggravate seizure activity.

WARNING Know that many drugs may interact with opioids like methadone to cause serotonin syndrome. Monitor patient closely for signs and symptoms such as agitation, diaphoresis, diarrhea, fever, hallucinations, labile blood pressure, muscle twitching or stiffness, nausea, shakiness, shivering, tachycardia, trouble with coordination, or vomiting. Notify prescriber at once because serotonin syndrome may be life-threatening. Be prepared to discontinue drug, if possible and ordered, and provide supportive care. Also be aware that concomitant use of methadone with CYP3A4, CYP2B6, CYP2C19, or CYP2D6 inhibitors or discontinuation of concomitantly used CYP3A4, CYP2B6, CYP2C19, or CYP2C9 inducers can result in a fatal overdose.

- Monitor patient for adrenal insufficiency. Although rare, it can be life-threatening. Monitor patient for anorexia, dizziness, fatigue, hypotension, nausea, vomiting, or weakness. Notify prescriber if adrenal insufficiency is suspected and expect diagnostic testing to be done. If confirmed, expect to administer corticosteroids and wean patient off methadone, if possible.

PATIENT TEACHING

- Inform patient that misuse of drug either by taking excessive amounts or by taking drug for prolonged periods of time can lead to addiction, overdose, or even death. Therefore, tell patient to take drug exactly as prescribed and for the shortest time possible.
- Instruct patient taking oral concentrate form of methadone to dilute it with water or another liquid to a volume of at least 30 ml, and preferably to 90 ml or more, before administration.
- Instruct patient to dissolve dispersible tablets in 120 ml of water or other liquid immediately before administration. Alert patient that if water is used and residue is left in the cup after ingesting, he should add a little more liquid to the cup and drink to ensure all the drug was consumed.
- Advise patient to notify prescriber of all other drugs he's currently taking, including benzodiazepines, and to avoid alcohol and other depressants, such as sleeping pills and tranquilizers, because they may increase drug's CNS depressant effects and cause severe respiratory depression that could result in death.
- Inform patient that abrupt cessation of methadone therapy can precipitate withdrawal symptoms. Urge him to notify prescriber if he develops any concerns over therapy.
- Urge patient to notify prescriber if he experiences dizziness, light-headedness, palpitations, or syncope, which may be caused by methadone-induced arrhythmias.
- Instruct patient to avoid potentially hazardous activities or those that require mental alertness because methadone therapy may cause drowsiness or sleepiness.
- Teach patient to change positions slowly to minimize the effects of orthostatic hypotension.
- Instruct patient to notify prescriber of worsening or breakthrough pain because dosage may need to be adjusted.
- Instruct female patient to notify prescriber immediately if she becomes pregnant during methadone therapy

because drug may cause physical dependence in fetus and withdrawal symptoms in neonate.

- Caution mother who is breastfeeding not to stop doing so abruptly and not to stop taking methadone without prescriber's approval, because infant may experience withdrawal symptoms. Caution mother to monitor infant for signs of methadone toxicity, which may include breathing difficulties, difficulty breastfeeding, increased sleepiness, or limpness. If present, instruct patient to seek immediate medical attention for her infant.
- Instruct patient or parents to keep methadone out of the reach of children because accidental ingestion can be fatal.
- Inform patient that long-term use of opioids like methadone may decrease sex hormone levels, causing decreased libido, erectile dysfunction, impotence, infertility, or lack of menstruation. Encourage patient to report any symptoms.
- Advise patient that drug may cause severe constipation and to take measures to avoid constipation. If unresolved or severe, tell patient to seek medical attention.

methenamine hippurate

Hiprex, Urex

methenamine mandelate

Mandelamine

Class and Category

Pharmacologic class: Urinary tract antiseptic
Therapeutic class: Antibiotic
Pregnancy category: C

Indications and Dosages

➤ *To prevent or suppress frequently recurring UTI caused by a wide variety of gram-negative and gram-positive bacteria (including enterococci,* E. coli, Micrococcus pyogenes, *and staphylococci) when long-term therapy is necessary, such as in intermittently catheterized patients with neurogenic bladder*

ENTERIC-COATED TABLETS, ORAL SUSPENSION (METHENAMINE MANDELATE)

Adults and adolescents. 1 g four times daily before meals and at bedtime.
Children ages 6 to 12. 500 mg four times daily.

TABLETS (METHENAMINE HIPPURATE)

Adults and adolescents. 1 g twice daily.
Children ages 6 to 12. 0.5 to 1 g every 12 hr.

Mechanism of Action

Hydrolyzes to ammonia and formaldehyde in an acidic environment, such as urine, producing greater amounts of formaldehyde as pH decreases. Formaldehyde has bactericidal action, possibly by denaturing proteins. To facilitate hydrolysis, methenamine is formulated with weak organic acid, such as hippuric acid or mandelic acid.

Contraindications

Concurrent therapy with sulfonamides, hypersensitivity to methenamine or its components, renal insufficiency, severe dehydration, severe hepatic disease

Interactions

DRUGS

bicarbonate-containing antacids, urinary alkalinizers: Decreased methenamine effect
sulfonamides, such as sulfamethizole: Possibly formation of insoluble precipitate in urine

FOODS

milk, milk products, most fruits: Possibly decreased effectiveness of methenamine

Adverse Reactions

CNS: Headache
CV: Edema
EENT: Stomatitis
GI: Abdominal cramps, anorexia, diarrhea, nausea, upset stomach, vomiting
GU: Bladder irritation, crystalluria, dysuria, hematuria, proteinuria, urinary frequency
RESP: Pulmonary hypersensitivity
SKIN: Pruritus, rash, urticaria

Nursing Considerations

- Be aware that methenamine is used for prophylaxis; it isn't recommended as primary treatment for UTI.

- Know that drug shouldn't be given to patients with creatinine clearance less than 50 ml/min.
- Expect to obtain urine specimen for culture and sensitivity tests and to review test results if available before giving first dose.
- Make sure patient receives adequate fluids.
- Expect to repeat culture and sensitivity tests if patient fails to improve.

PATIENT TEACHING

- Instruct patient to take methenamine with food to avoid GI distress.
- Direct patient to drink extra fluids; avoid alkaline foods, such as milk, milk products, and most fruits; and avoid antacids that contain sodium bicarbonate or carbonate during methenamine therapy.
- Instruct patient to report painful urination, rash, or severe GI distress.
- Urge patient to comply with urine testing before and during long-term therapy.

methimazole

Tapazole

Class and Category

Pharmacologic class: Thyroid hormone antagonist
Therapeutic class: Antithyroid
Pregnancy category: D

Indications and Dosages

➤ *To treat mild hyperthyroidism*

TABLETS

Adults and adolescents. *Initial:* 15 mg daily in divided doses three times daily 8 hr apart for 6 to 8 wk or until euthyroid level is reached. *Maintenance:* 5 to 15 mg daily.
Children. *Initial:* 0.4 mg/kg daily in divided doses three times daily 8 hr apart. *Maintenance:* 0.2 mg/kg daily.

➤ *To treat moderate hyperthyroidism*

TABLETS

Adults and adolescents. *Initial:* 30 to 40 mg/day three times daily 8 hr apart for 6 to 8 wk or until euthyroid level is reached. *Maintenance:* 5 to 15 mg daily.
Children. *Initial:* 0.4 mg/kg daily in divided doses three times daily 8 hr apart. *Maintenance:* 0.2 mg/kg daily.

➤ *To treat severe hyperthyroidism*

TABLETS

Adults and adolescents. *Initial:* 60 mg daily in divided doses three times daily 8 hr apart for 6 to 8 wk or until euthyroid level is reached. *Maintenance:* 5 to 15 mg daily.
Children. *Initial:* 0.4 mg/kg daily in divided doses three times daily 8 hr apart. *Maintenance:* 0.2 mg/kg daily.

Route	Onset	Peak	Duration
P.O.	5 days	7 wk	Unknown

Mechanism of Action

Directly interferes with thyroid hormone synthesis in the thyroid gland by inhibiting iodide incorporation into thyroglobulin. Iodination of thyroglobulin is an important step in synthesizing the thyroid hormones thyroxine and triiodothyronine. Eventually, thyroglobulin is depleted and the circulating thyroid hormone level drops.

Contraindications

Breastfeeding; hypersensitivity to methimazole, other antithyroid drugs, or their components

Interactions

DRUGS

amiodarone, iodine, potassium iodide: Decreased response to methimazole
digoxin: Possibly increased blood digoxin level
oral anticoagulants: Possibly a need for altered anticoagulant dosage

Adverse Reactions

CNS: Drowsiness, headache, paresthesia, vertigo
CV: Edema
EENT: Loss of taste
ENDO: Hypothyroidism
GI: Diarrhea, indigestion, jaundice, nausea, vomiting
HEME: Agranulocytosis, aplastic anemia, leukopenia, thrombocytopenia
MS: Arthralgia, myalgia
SKIN: Alopecia, pruritus, rash, skin discoloration, urticaria
Other: Lupus-like symptoms, lymphadenopathy

Nursing Considerations

- Closely monitor thyroid function test results during methimazole therapy.

M

- Check CBC results to detect abnormalities caused by inhibition of myelopoiesis.
- Watch for signs and symptoms of hypothyroidism, such as cold intolerance, depression, and edema.
- Be aware that hyperthyroidism may increase metabolic clearance of beta blockers and theophylline and that dosages of these drugs may need to be reduced as the patient's thyroid condition becomes corrected.

PATIENT TEACHING

- Instruct patient to take drug with meals to avoid adverse GI reactions.
- Explain about possible hair loss or thinning during and for months after therapy.
- Instruct patient to notify prescriber immediately about cold intolerance, fever, sore throat, tiredness, and unusual bleeding or bruising.

methocarbamol

Robaxin, Robaxin 750

Class and Category

Pharmacologic class: Carbamate derivative
Therapeutic class: Skeletal muscle relaxant
Pregnancy category: C

Indications and Dosages

➤ *To relieve discomfort caused by acute, painful musculoskeletal conditions*

TABLETS

Adults and adolescents. *Initial:* 1,500 mg four times daily for 2 to 3 days; for severe discomfort 8,000 mg daily. *Maintenance:* 1,000 mg four times daily, or 1,500 mg three times daily.

I.M. INJECTION, I.V. INJECTION

Adults and adolescents. Up to 3,000 mg daily administered at 8-hr intervals for no more than three consecutive days. Regimen repeated as prescribed after patient is drug-free for 48 hr. I.V. injection administered at a maximum rate of 300 mg/min.

➤ *To provide supportive therapy for tetanus*

TABLETS

Adults and adolescents. Up to 24,000 mg daily given by NG tube.

I.V. INFUSION OR INJECTION

Adults and adolescents. *Initial:* 1 to 2 g directly into I.V. tubing slowly, at a maximum rate of 3 ml/min, followed by an additional 1 to 2 g by I.V. infusion at a maximum rate of 300 mg/min for a total dose of up to 3 g. Dosing procedure repeated every 6 hr, as needed, until nasogastric tube can be inserted and oral therapy begun. *Maximum:* 300 mg (3 ml)/min.

Children. 15 mg/kg at a rate of 180 mg/m^2 every 6 hr, as needed. *Maximum*: 1.8 g/m^2/day for 3 days only.

Route	Onset	Peak	Duration
P.O.	30 min	Unknown	Unknown
I.V.	Immediate	Unknown	Unknown

Mechanism of Action

May depress CNS, which leads to sedation and reduced skeletal muscle spasms. Methocarbamol also alters perception of pain.

Contraindications

Hypersensitivity to methocarbamol or its components, renal disease (injectable form)

Interactions

DRUGS

CNS depressants: Increased CNS depression

ACTIVITIES

alcohol use: Increased CNS depression

Adverse Reactions

CNS: Dizziness, drowsiness, fever, headache, light-headedness, **seizures (I.V.)**, syncope, vertigo, weakness
CV: Bradycardia, hypotension, and thrombophlebitis (parenteral)
EENT: Blurred vision, conjunctivitis, diplopia, metallic taste, nasal congestion, nystagmus
GI: Nausea
GU: Black, brown, or green urine
SKIN: Flushing, pruritus, rash, urticaria
Other: Anaphylaxis (parenteral), **angioedema**, injection-site irritation or pain (I.M.), injection-site sloughing (I.V.)

Nursing Considerations

- Crush methocarbamol tablets and mix with water or saline solution for administration by NG tube.
- Give I.V. form directly through infusion line at 3 ml/min. To prepare solution, add 10 ml to no more than 250 ml D_5W or

normal saline solution. Infuse at no more than 300 mg (3 ml)/min to avoid hypotension and seizures.

- Keep patient recumbent during I.V. administration and for at least 15 minutes afterward. Then have him rise slowly.
- Monitor I.V. site regularly for signs of phlebitis.
- Inject I.M. form deep into large muscle, such as the gluteus. Give no more than 5 ml/dose every 8 hours. One dose is usually adequate.
- Don't give methocarbamol by subcutaneous route.
- Keep antihistamines, corticosteroids, and epinephrine available in case patient experiences anaphylactic reaction.
- Be aware that the parenteral dosage form shouldn't be used in patients with renal dysfunction because the polyethylene glycol 300 vehicle is nephrotoxic.

PATIENT TEACHING

- Tell patient to take drug exactly as prescribed.
- Advise patient to take drug with food or milk to avoid nausea.
- Inform patient that urine may turn black, brown, or green until methocarbamol is discontinued.
- Advise patient to avoid hazardous activities until drug's CNS effects are known.
- Instruct patient to avoid alcohol and other CNS depressants during therapy.

methotrexate (amethopterin)

Rasuvo, Rheumatrex, Xatmep

methotrexate sodium

Otrexup, Trexall

Class and Category

Pharmacologic class: Folate antagonist (antimetabolite)
Therapeutic class: Antineoplastic
Pregnancy category: X

Indications and Dosages

➤ *To treat severe psoriasis unresponsive to other therapy*

TABLETS (RHEUMATREX, TREXALL)
Adults. 2.5 mg every 12 hr for 3 doses/wk, increased as ordered by 2.5 mg/wk. *Maximum:* 30 mg/wk. Alternatively, 10 to 25 mg as a single dose weekly.

I.V. OR I.M INJECTION (METHOTREXATE SODIUM), SUBCUTANEOUS INJECTION (OTREXUP, RASUVO)
Adults. 10 to 25 mg as a single dose weekly. *Maximum:* 30 mg weekly. I.V. injection rate dependent upon dose. Follow manufacturer instructions.

➤ *To treat severe rheumatoid arthritis unresponsive to other therapy*

TABLETS (RHEUMATREX, TREXALL)
Adults. 2.5 to 5 mg every 12 hr for 3 doses/wk, increased as ordered by 2.5 mg/wk. *Maximum:* 20 mg/wk. Alternatively, 7.5 mg as a single dose weekly.

SUBCUTANEOUS INJECTION (RASUVO, TREXALL)
Adults. 7.5 mg once weekly, then gradually increased to achieve an optimal response. *Maximum:* 20 mg/wk.

➤ *To treat active polyarticular juvenile idiopathic arthritis unresponsive to other therapy*

ORAL SOLUTION (XATMEP), SUBCUTANEOUS INJECTION (OTREXUP, RASUVO), TABLETS (RHEUMATREX, TREXALL)
Children. 10 mg/m^2 once weekly.

Route	Onset	Peak	Duration
P.O., I.V., I.M.	3–6 wk	Unknown	Unknown
SubQ	Unknown	Unknown	Unknown

Mechanism of Action

May exert immunosuppressive effects by inhibiting replication and function of T and possibly B lymphocytes. Methotrexate also slows rapidly growing cells, such as epithelial skin cells in psoriasis. This action may result from the drug's inhibition of dihydrofolate reductase, the enzyme that reduces folic acid to tetrahydrofolic acid. Inhibition of tetrahydrofolic acid interferes with DNA synthesis and cell reproduction in rapidly proliferating cells.

Contraindications

Breastfeeding, hypersensitivity to methotrexate or its components, pregnancy

Interactions

DRUGS

bone marrow depressants: Possibly increased bone marrow depression
chloramphenicol, neomycin, tetracycline: Possibly decreased methotrexate absorption
co-trimoxazole: Possibly increased bone marrow suppression
folic acid: Possibly decreased effectiveness of methotrexate
hepatotoxic drugs: Increased risk of hepatotoxicity
nitrous oxide anesthesia: Increased risk of methotrexate toxicity
NSAIDs, penicillins, phenylbutazone, phenytoin, probenecid, salicylates, sulfonamides: Increased risk of methotrexate toxicity
oral anticoagulants: Increased bleeding risk
proton pump inhibitors such as esomeprazole, omeprazole, pantoprazole: Increased risk of methotrexate toxicities
sulfonamides: Increased risk of hepato-toxicity
theophylline: Possibly increased risk of theophylline toxicity
vaccines: Risk of disseminated infection with live-virus vaccines, risk of suppressed response to killed-virus vaccines

ACTIVITIES

alcohol use: Increased risk of hepatotoxicity

Adverse Reactions

CNS: Aphasia, **cerebral thrombosis**, chills, dizziness, drowsiness, fatigue, fever, headache, hemiparesis, **leukoencephalopathy**, malaise, paresis, **seizures**
CV: Chest pain, **deep vein thrombosis**, **hypotension**, **pericardial effusion**, **pericarditis**, **thromboembolism**
ENDO: Gynecomastia
EENT: Blurred vision, conjunctivitis, gingivitis, glossitis, pharyngitis, stomatitis, transient blindness, tinnitus
GI: Abdominal pain, anorexia, **cirrhosis**, diarrhea, elevated liver enzymes, enteritis, **GI bleeding** and ulceration, **hepatitis**, **hepatotoxicity**, nausea, **pancreatitis**, vomiting
GU: Cystitis, hematuria, infertility, menstrual dysfunction, nephropathy, **renal failure**, **tubular necrosis**, vaginal discharge
HEME: Anemia, **aplastic anemia**, **leukopenia**, **neutropenia**, **pancytopenia**, **thrombocytopenia**
MS: Arthralgia, dysarthria, myalgia, stress fracture
RESP: Dry nonproductive cough, dyspnea, **interstitial pneumonitis**, pneumonia, **pulmonary fibrosis or failure**, **pulmonary infiltrates**
SKIN: Acne, alopecia, altered skin pigmentation, ecchymosis, **erythema multiforme**, **exfoliative dermatitis**, furunculosis, necrosis, photosensitivity, pruritus, psoriatic lesions, rash, **Stevens–Johnson syndrome**, telangiectasia, **toxic epidermal necrolysis**, ulceration, urticaria
Other: **Anaphylaxis**, increased risk of infection, lymphadenopathy, **lymphoproliferative disease**

Nursing Considerations

- Know that nitrous oxide anesthesia increases the risk for methotrexate toxicity and should not be used in patients receiving methotrexate. Use methotrexate cautiously in patients who have a recent history of nitrous oxide administration.
- Follow facility policy for preparing and handling drug; parenteral form poses a risk of carcinogenicity, mutagenicity, and teratogenicity. Avoid skin contact.
- Use only preservative-free formulation of methotrexate when administering high-dose therapy.
- Monitor results of CBC, chest x-ray, liver and renal function tests, and urinalysis before and during treatment.
- Administer subcutenaous injection into patient's abdomen or thigh.
- Increase patient's fluid intake to 2 to 3 L daily, unless contraindicated, to reduce the risk of adverse GU reactions.
- Assess patient for bleeding and infection.

WARNING Expect renal impairment to severely alter drug elimination.

- Be aware that high doses of methotrexate can impair renal elimination by forming crystals that obstruct urine flow. To prevent drug precipitation, alkalinize patient's urine with sodium bicarbonate tablets, as ordered.

- Follow standard precautions because drug can cause immunosuppression.
- Be aware that if patient becomes dehydrated from vomiting, prescriber should be notified, and expect to withhold drug until patient recovers.
- Be aware that if patient receives high doses of drug, leucovorin should be kept readily available as antidote.
- Be aware that methotrexate resistance may develop with prolonged use.

PATIENT TEACHING

- Prepare a calendar of treatment days for patient, and emphasize importance of following instructions exactly.
- Advise parents or caregivers administering oral solution form of methotrexate to use a calibrated measuring device and never to use a household measuring teaspoon because it is not an accurate measuring device.
- Teach patient prescribed weekly subcutaneous injections, how to administer the injection using the single-dose auto-injector. Tell him to give the injection into his abdomen or thigh and to rotate injection sites.
- Instruct patient to avoid alcohol during methotrexate therapy.
- Encourage frequent mouth care to reduce the risk of mouth sores.
- Instruct patient to use sunblock when exposed to sunlight.
- Advise patient to notify prescriber about bruising, chills, cough, dark or bloody urine, fever, mouth sores, shortness of breath, sore throat, and yellow skin or eyes.
- Urge women of childbearing age to use reliable contraception during methotrexate therapy.

methoxypolyethylene glycol-epoetin beta

Mircera

Class and Category

Pharmacological class: Erythropoietin stimulating protein
Therapeutic class: Antianemic
Pregnancy category: C

Indications and Dosages

➤ *To treat anemia associated with chronic renal failure in dialysis-dependent and dialysis-independent patients*

I.V. INJECTION, SUBCUTANEOUS INJECTION

Adults not currently being treated with an erythropoiesis-stimulating agent. *Initial:* 0.6 mcg/kg every 2 wk, increased or decreased by 25% monthly as needed. *Maintenance:* 1.2 mcg/kg every 4 wk.

Adults stabilized on less than 8,000 units/wk of epoetin alfa or 40 mcg/wk of darbepoetin alfa. 60 mcg every 2 wk or 120 mcg every 4 wk.

Adults stabilized on 8,000 to 16,000 units/wk of epoetin alfa or 40 to 80 mcg/wk of darbepoetin alfa. 100 mcg every 2 wk or 200 mcg every 4 wk.

Adults stabilized on more than 16,000 units/wk of epoetin alfa or more than 80 mcg/wk of darbepoetin alfa. 180 mcg every 2 wk or 360 mcg every 4 wk.

DOSAGE ADJUSTMENT If hemoglobin increase is greater than 1 g/dl during any 2-wk period or hemoglobin is increasing and approaching 11 g/dl, dosage reduced by 25% or more. If hemoglobin continues to increase despite this reduction, drug discontinued until hemoglobin begins to decrease; then drug restarted at a dose 25% less than previously given. If hemoglobin doesn't increase by 1 g/dl after 4 wk of therapy, dosage increased by 25%.

Route	Onset	Peak	Duration
I.V., SubQ	7–15 days	72 hr	72 hr

Mechanism of Action

Stimulates release of reticulocytes from bone marrow into the bloodstream, where they develop into mature RBCs.

Incompatibilities

Don't mix methoxypolyethylene glycol-epoetin beta with any other drug.

Contraindications

Hemoglobin greater than 11 g/dl, hypersensitivity to methoxypolyethylene glycolepoetin beta or its components, red cell aplasia, uncontrolled hypertension

Adverse Reactions

CNS: CVA, headache, **seizures**
CV: Chest pain, **congestive heart failure, deep vein thrombosis**, hypertension, **hypotension, MI**, tachycardia, vascular access thrombosis
EENT: Nasopharyngitis
GI: Constipation, diarrhea, **GI bleeding**, vomiting
GU: UTI
HEME: Severe anemia including pure red cell aplasia
MS: Back or limb pain, muscle spasms
RESP: Bronchospasms, cough, upper respiratory tract infection
SKIN: Erythema, pruritus, rash, **Stevens–Johnson syndrome, toxic epidermal necrolysis**, urticaria
Other: Anaphylaxis, angioedema, antibody formation to drug

Nursing Considerations

- Use drug cautiously in patients who have conditions that could decrease or delay response to drug, such as aluminum intoxication, folic acid deficiency, hemolysis, infection, inflammation, iron deficiency, malignant neoplasm, osteitis (birrosa cystica), or vitamin B_{12} deficiency.
- Also use drug cautiously in patients with a cardiovascular disorder caused by a history of seizures, hypertension, vascular disease. Also use cautiously in patients with a hematologic disorder, such as hypercoagulation, myelodysplastic syndrome, or sickle cell disease.
- Be aware that if patient's blood pressure is difficult to control even with dietary measures or drug therapy, dose of methoxypolyethylene glycol-epoetin beta should be reduced or drug withheld until blood pressure is controlled.
- Don't shake vial during preparation to avoid denaturing glycoprotein, inactivating drug. Protect prefilled syringes and vials from light by storing in original cartons.
- Discard unused portion of single-dose vial because it contains no preservatives.

WARNING Know that target hemoglobin shouldn't exceed 11 g/dl because it increases risk of life-threatening adverse cardiovascular effects.

- Monitor drug effectiveness by checking hemoglobin every 2 weeks until stabilized and maintenance dose has been established. Then expect hemoglobin to be monitored at least monthly unless dosage adjustment is needed.
- Expect to give an iron supplement because iron requirements rise when erythropoiesis consumes existing iron stores.
- Notify prescriber if patient has sudden loss of response to drug, evidenced by low reticulocyte count or severe anemia. Anti-erythropoietin antibody-related anemia may be present, which requires stopping drug and any other erythropoietic proteins.
- Take seizure precautions, especially during the first couple months of therapy.
- Keep in mind the risk of hypertensive or thrombotic complications increases if hemoglobin rises more than 1 g/dl over 2 weeks.

PATIENT TEACHING

- Teach patient how to administer drug and how to dispose of needles properly. Caution against reusing needles.
- Stress importance of complying with dosage regimen and keeping follow-up laboratory and medical appointments.
- Review possible adverse reactions, and urge patient to notify prescriber about chest pain, headache, hives, rapid heartbeat, rash, seizures, shortness of breath, or swelling.

WARNING Warn patient to stop taking drug immediately if an allergic reaction occurs and notify prescriber. If serious, tell patient to seek emergency treatment.

- Advise patient that the risk of seizures is highest during the first couple of months of methoxypolyethylene glycol-epoetin beta therapy. Urge him to avoid hazardous activities during this time.
- Encourage patient to eat iron-rich foods.

methsuximide

Celontin

Class and Category

Pharmacologic class: Succinimide
Therapeutic class: Anticonvulsant
Pregnancy category: Not classified

Indications and Dosages

➤ *To treat absence seizures unresponsive to other drugs*

CAPSULES

Adults and children. *Initial:* 300 mg daily. Increased by 300 mg daily every wk for 3 additional weeks until maximum dosage of 1.2 g daily is reached until control is achieved with minimal adverse reactions. *Maximum:* 1.2 g daily.

Mechanism of Action

Elevates seizure threshold and reduces frequency of seizures by depressing motor cortex and elevating threshold of CNS response to convulsive stimuli. Methsuximide is metabolized to active metabolite N-demethylmethsuximide, which may add to the anticonvulsant effects of the drug.

Contraindications

Hypersensitivity to methsuximide, succinimides, or their components

Interactions

DRUGS

carbamazepine, phenobarbital, phenytoin, primidone: Possibly decreased blood methsuximide level
CNS depressants: Possibly increased CNS depression
haloperidol: Altered seizure pattern; possibly decreased blood haloperidol level
loxapine, MAO inhibitors, maprotiline, molindone, phenothiazines, pimozide, thioxanthenes, tricyclic antidepressants: Possibly lowered seizure threshold and reduced therapeutic effect of methsuximide

ACTIVITIES

alcohol use: Possibly increased CNS depression

Adverse Reactions

CNS: Aggressiveness, ataxia, decreased concentration, dizziness, drowsiness, fatigue, fever, headache, insomnia, irritability, mental depression, nightmares, **seizures**, **suicidal ideation**
EENT: Periorbital edema, pharyngitis
GI: Abdominal cramps, abdominal and epigastric pain, abnormal liver enzymes, diarrhea, hiccups, nausea, vomiting
GU: Microscopic hematuria, proteinuria
HEME: Agranulocytosis, aplastic anemia, eosinophilia, **leukopenia**, **pancytopenia**
MS: Muscle pain
SKIN: Erythematous and pruritic rash, **Stevens–Johnson syndrome**, systemic lupus erythematosus, urticaria
Other: Lymphadenopathy

Nursing Considerations

- Monitor CBC and platelet count and assess patient for signs of infection, such as cough, fever, and pharyngitis, because methsuximide may cause blood dyscrasias.
- Monitor liver enzymes and urinalysis results in patients with a history of hepatic or renal disease; methsuximide may cause functional changes in kidneys and liver.
- When giving drug to patient with a history of mixed-type epilepsy, institute seizure precautions because drug may increase risk of generalized tonic–clonic seizures.
- Expect the dosage to be carefully and slowly adjusted according to patient's response and needs and withdrawn slowly to avoid precipitating seizures.
- Notify prescriber if patient develops aggressiveness or depression.
- Monitor patient closely for evidence of suicidal thinking or behavior, especially when therapy starts or dosage changes.

PATIENT TEACHING

- Advise patient to take a missed dose as soon as he remembers unless it's nearly time for the next dose. Warn him not to double the dose.
- Instruct patient to take drug with food or milk to reduce gastric irritation.
- Advise patient to notify prescriber if he develops cough, fever, or pharyngitis.
- Urge patient to avoid alcohol because of increased risk of CNS depression.
- Instruct patient to avoid hazardous activities until drug's adverse effects are known.
- Caution patient not to stop taking drug abruptly to avoid risk of absence seizures reoccurring.
- Urge caregivers to watch patient closely for evidence of suicidal tendencies, especially when therapy starts or dosage changes, and to report concerns immediately.

- Urge woman who becomes pregnant while taking methsuximide to enroll in the North American antiepileptic drug pregnancy registry by calling 1-888-233-2334. Explain that this registry is collecting information about the safety of antiepileptic drugs during pregnancy.

methyldopa

methyldopate hydrochloride

Class and Category

Pharmacologic class: Central alpha agonist
Therapeutic class: Antihypertensive
Pregnancy category: B (oral form), C (parenteral form)

Indications and Dosages

➤ *To manage hypertension*

ORAL SUSPENSION, TABLETS (METHYLDOPA)

Adults. *Initial:* 250 mg twice daily or three times daily for first 48 hr, decreased or increased as needed after 2 days with adjustments made no less than every 2 days. *Maintenance:* 500 to 2,000 mg daily in divided doses twice daily to four times daily. *Maximum:* 3,000 mg daily.
Children. *Initial:* 10 mg/kg daily in divided doses twice daily to four times daily for first 48 hr, decreased or increased as needed after 2 days with adjustments made no less than every 2 days. *Maximum:* 65 mg/kg or 3,000 mg daily, whichever is less.

I.V. INFUSION (METHYLDOPATE HYDROCHLORIDE)

Adults. 250 to 500 mg diluted in D_5W and infused over 30 to 60 min every 6 hr. *Maximum:* 1,000 mg every 6 hr.
Children. 20 to 40 mg/kg/day in divided doses every 6 hr and infused over 30 to 60 min. *Maximum:* 65 mg/kg or 3,000 mg daily.

Route	Onset	Peak	Duration
P.O.	Unknown	4–6 hr*	12–24 hr†
I.V.	Unknown	4–6 hr	10–16 hr

* For single dose; 2 to 3 days for multiple doses.

† For single dose; 24 to 48 hr for multiple doses.

Mechanism of Action

Is decarboxylated in the body to produce alpha-methylnorepinephrine, a metabolite that stimulates central inhibitory alpha-adrenergic receptors. This action may reduce blood pressure by decreasing sympathetic stimulation of heart and peripheral vascular system.

Incompatibilities

Don't administer methyldopate through same I.V. line as barbiturates or sulfonamides.

Contraindications

Active hepatic disease, hypersensitivity to methyldopa or its components, impaired hepatic function from previous methyldopa therapy, use within 14 days of MAO inhibitor

Interactions

DRUGS

antihypertensives: Increased hypotension
appetite suppressants, NSAIDs, tricyclic antidepressants: Possibly decreased therapeutic effects of methyldopa or methyldopate
central anesthetics: Possibly need for reduced anesthetic dosage
CNS depressants: Possibly increased CNS depression
haloperidol: Increased risk of adverse CNS effects
levodopa: Possibly decreased therapeutic effects of levodopa and increased risk of adverse CNS effects
lithium: Increased risk of lithium toxicity
MAO inhibitors: Possibly hallucinations, headaches, hyperexcitability, and severe hypertension
oral anticoagulants: Possibly increased therapeutic effects of anticoagulants
sympathomimetics: Possibly decreased therapeutic effects of methyldopa and methyldopate and increased vasopressor effects of sympathomimetics

ACTIVITIES

alcohol use: Possibly increased CNS depression

Adverse Reactions

CNS: Decreased concentration, depression, dizziness, drowsiness, fever, headache, involuntary motor activity,

memory loss (transient), nightmares, paresthesia, Parkinsonism, sedation, vertigo, weakness
CV: Angina, **bradycardia**, edema, **heart failure**, **myocarditis**, orthostatic hypotension
EENT: Black or sore tongue, dry mouth, nasal congestion
ENDO: Gynecomastia
GI: Constipation, diarrhea, flatulence, **hepatic necrosis**, **hepatitis**, jaundice, nausea, **pancreatitis**, vomiting
GU: Decreased libido, impotence
HEME: **Agranulocytosis**, **hemolytic anemia**, **leukopenia**, positive Coombs' test, positive tests for ANA and rheumatoid factor, **thrombocytopenia**
SKIN: Eczema, rash, urticaria
Other: Weight gain

Nursing Considerations

- For I.V. infusion, add methyldopate to 100 ml of D_5W and administer over 30 to 60 minutes.
- Expect to monitor CBC and differential results before and periodically during methyldopa therapy.
- Monitor blood pressure regularly during therapy.
- Monitor results of Coombs' test; a positive result after several months of treatment indicates that patient has hemolytic anemia. Expect to discontinue drug.
- Assess for edema and weight gain. If they develop, give a diuretic, as prescribed.
- Notify prescriber if patient has signs of heart failure (dyspnea, edema, hypertension) or involuntary, rapid, jerky movements.
- Be aware that hypertension may return within 48 hours after stopping drug.

PATIENT TEACHING

- Instruct patient to take methyldopa exactly as prescribed and not to skip a dose. Explain that hypertension can return within 48 hours after stopping drug.
- Suggest that patient take drug at bedtime to minimize daytime drowsiness.
- Instruct patient to weigh himself daily and to report a gain of more than 5 lb (2.3 kg) in 2 days.
- Advise patient to change position slowly to minimize orthostatic hypotension.
- Direct patient to notify prescriber about bruising, chest pain, fever, involuntary jerky movements, prolonged dizziness, rash, and yellow eyes or skin.
- Caution patient not to stop drug abruptly; doing so may cause withdrawal symptoms, such as headache, hypertension, increased sweating, nausea, and tremor.

methylnaltrexone bromide

Relistor

Class and Category

Pharmacologic class: Peripheral mu-opioid receptor antagonist
Therapeutic class: GI effector
Pregnancy category: B

Indications and Dosages

➤ *To treat opioid-induced constipation in patients receiving palliative care and not responsive to laxative therapy.*

SUBCUTANEOUS INJECTION

Adults weighing more than 114 kg (251 lb). 0.15 mg/kg every other day, as needed. *Maximum:* 0.15 mg/kg daily.
Adults weighing 62 to 114 kg (136 to 251 lb). 12 mg every other day, as needed. *Maximum:* 12 mg daily.
Adults weighing 38 to less than 62 kg (84 to less than 136 lb). 8 mg every other day, as needed. *Maximum:* 8 mg daily.
Adults weighing less than 38 kg (84 lb). 0.15 mg/kg every other day, as needed. *Maximum:* 0.15 mg/kg daily.
DOSAGE ADJUSTMENT For patient with moderate to severe renal impairment, dosage reduced by half and given one dose every other day.

➤ *To treat opioid-induced constipation in patients with chronic noncancer pain*

SUBCUTANEOUS INJECTION

Adults. 12 mg once daily.

TABLETS

Adults. 450 mg once daily in the morning.
DOSAGE ADJUSTMENT For patients with moderate to severe renal failure (creatinine clearance less than 60 ml/min), dosage reduced by half for subcutaneous injection. For patients with moderate to severe

hepatic or renal impairment taking tablet form, daily dosage reduced to 150 mg daily.

Route	Onset	Peak	Duration
SubQ	Unknown	0.5 hr	Unknown

Mechanism of Action

Binds to peripherally acting mu-opioid receptors in the GI tract, preventing opioid-induced slowing of GI motility and transit time. When motility and transit time are restored to normal, constipation is relieved.

Contraindications

Hypersensitivity to methylnaltrexone bromide or its components, GI obstruction, I.V. administration

Adverse Reactions

CNS: Anxiety, chills, dizziness, headache, malaise, tremor
EENT: Rhinorrhea
ENDO: Hot flashes
GI: Abdominal distention, pain, or tenderness; diarrhea; flatulence; GI cramping, **GI perforation**; nausea; vomiting
MS: Muscle spasms
SKIN: Excessive diaphoresis, piloerection

Nursing Considerations

- Use methylnaltrexone cautiously in patients with known or suspected lesions of the gastrointestinal (GI) tract as well as conditions that may affect the structural integrity of the GI tract wall, such as diverticular disease, infiltrative GI tract malignancies, Ogilvie's syndrome, peptic ulcer disease, and peritoneal metastases, because of increased risk of GI perforation.
- Know that food affects absorption of tablet form of drug. Give on an empty stomach only with water 30 minutes before the first meal of the day.
- To determine volume of drug to give subcutaneously to patients who weigh more than 114 kg (251 lb) or less than 38 kg (84 lb), multiply patient's weight in pounds by 0.0034 and round up to the nearest 0.1 ml. Or, multiply patient's weight in kilograms by 0.0075 and round up to the nearest 0.1 ml. For patients who weigh 62 to 114 kg (136 to 251 lb), injection volume administered should be 0.6 ml. For patients who weigh 38 to less than 62 kg (84 to less than 136 lb), injection volume administered should be 0.4 ml.
- Inspect vial before giving drug subcutaneously to make sure solution is clear and colorless to pale yellow.
- Give parenteral form of drug only as subcutaneous injection into patient's abdomen, thigh, or upper arm and no more than once in 24 hours. Make sure to rotate injection sites.
- Once parenteral form of drug is drawn into syringe, it should be given immediately. However, if needed, it may be stored at room temperature for up to 24 hours.
- Notify prescriber about persistent or severe diarrhea, and expect drug to be discontinued. Be aware that elderly patients experience a higher incidence of diarrhea.
- Monitor patient for development of persistent, severe, or worsening abdominal pain because gastrointestinal perforation may occur with severe constipation that has not responded to methylnaltrexone therapy. Notify prescriber immediately and expect drug to be discontinued.
- Monitor patient for symptoms of opioid withdrawal such as abdominal pain, anxiety, chills, diaphoresis, diarrhea, or yawning that has occurred with methylnaltrexone therapy. Patients at greatest risk for opioid withdrawal are those who have disruptions to the blood–brain barrier with opioid administration.

PATIENT TEACHING

- Instruct patient prescribed tablet form to take it on an empty stomach with water 30 minutes before the first meal of the day.
- Teach patient or caregiver how to prepare and give methylnaltrexone subcutaneously. Stress need to rotate injection sites.
- Inform patient that a bowel movement may occur within 30 minutes after drug has been administered.
- Advise patient that if abdominal pain, nausea, persistent or severe diarrhea, or vomiting that is new or worsens occurs, prescriber should be notified and drug discontinued.

- Reassure patient that drug is not a controlled substance.
- Tell women of childbearing age to alert prescriber if pregnancy occurs, as the use of methylnaltrexone during pregnancy may precipitate opioid withdrawal in a fetus.
- Tell patient to stop taking methylnaltrexone if she stops taking opioid pain medication.

methylphenidate hydrochloride

Aptensio XR, Concerta, Cotempla XR-ODT, Daytrana, Jornay PM, Metadate CD, Metadate ER, Methylin, Methylin ER, PMS-Methylphenidate (CAN), Quillivant XR, Riphenidate (CAN), Ritalin, Ritalin-LA, Ritalin SR (CAN), Ritalin-SR

Class, Category, and Schedule

Pharmacologic class: Piperidine
Therapeutic class: CNS stimulant
Pregnancy category: C
Controlled substance schedule: II

Indications and Dosages

➤ *To treat attention-deficit hyperactivity disorder (ADHD)*

CAPSULES, E.R. TABLETS, ORAL SOLUTION, S.R. TABLETS, TABLETS (METHYLIN, RITALIN)
Adults *Initial:* 10 mg twice daily or three times daily 30 to 45 min before breakfast and lunch, and a third dose between 2 and 4 pm, if needed. Increased by 5 to 10 mg weekly, as needed. *Maximum:* 60 mg daily in two or three divided doses.
Children age 6 and over. *Initial:* 2.5 to 5 mg twice daily 30 to 45 min before breakfast and lunch; increased by 5 to 10 mg daily at 1-wk intervals. *Maximum:* 60 mg daily in two to three divided doses.

E.R. CAPSULES (RITALIN LA)
Adults. *Initial:* 20 mg once daily in morning before breakfast
Adults who have been taking immediate release form. Initial: For patient switching from 10 mg twice daily, 20 mg once daily before breakfast; for patient switching from 15 mg twice daily, 30 mg once daily before breakfast; for patient switching from 20 mg twice daily, 40 mg once daily before breakfast; for patient switching from 30 mg twice daily, 60 mg once daily before breakfast. Dosage increased by 10 mg daily once a wk, as needed. Maximum: 60 mg once daily.

E.R. ORAL SUSPENSION (QUILLIVANT XR)
Adults and children age 6 and over. *Initially:* 20 mg once daily in morning; increased weekly in increments of 10 to 20 mg, as needed. *Maximum:* 60 mg daily.

SUSTAINED RELEASE TABLETS (METADATE ER, RITALIN SR)
Adults and children age 6 and over who are switching from immediate release to sustained release form. *Initial:* If dosage same as immediate release and not taken more frequently than every 8 hr, sustained release dosage same taken once daily before breakfast, increased by 10 mg weekly, as needed. *Maximum:* 60 mg once daily before breakfast.

E.R. ONCE-DAILY TABLETS (CONCERTA)
Adults and children age 6 and over who are methylphenidate-naive. 18 mg daily before breakfast; increased in 18-mg increments at 1-wk intervals. *Maximum:* 72 mg daily (adults and children over age 12), 54 mg/day (children ages 6 to 12), not to exceed 2 mg/kg daily.
Adults and children age 6 and over who are currently taking immediate-release methylphenidate tablets. Switch to E.R. tablets dependent on immediate release tablet dose. *Maximum:* 72 mg (adults and children over age 12) and 54 mg (children ages 6 to 12) once daily in the morning before breakfast.

E.R. ONCE-DAILY CAPSULES (METADATE CD)
Adults and children age 6 and over. *Initial:* 20 mg daily in the morning before breakfast, increased by 20 mg daily every wk, as needed. *Maximum:* 60 mg daily.

E.R. CAPSULES (APTENSIO XR)
Adults and children age 6 and over. *Initial:* 10 mg once daily in morning, increased by 10 mg once daily weekly, as needed. *Maximum:* 60 mg once a day in the morning.

ORALLY DISINTEGRATING TABLET (COTEMPLA XR-ODT)
Children ages 6 to 17. *Initial:* 17.3 mg once daily in the morning, then titrated weekly

in increments of 8.6 mg to 17.3 mg. *Maximum:* 51.8 mg daily.

E.R. CAPSULES (JORNAY PM)

Adults and children age 6 and over. 20 mg once daily in evening, increased weekly in increments of 20 mg, as needed. *Maximum:* 100 mg once daily.

TRANSDERMAL PATCH (DAYTRANA)

Adults and children age 6 and over. *Initial:* 10-mg (12.5-cm^2) patch worn 9 hr daily for wk 1; 15-mg (18.75-cm^2) patch worn 9 hr daily for wk 2; 20-mg (25-cm^2) patch worn 9 hr daily for wk 3; 30-mg (37.5-cm^2) patch worn 9 hr daily for wk 4 and thereafter. *Maximum:* 30-mg (37.5-cm^2) patch worn 9 hr daily.

➤ *To treat narcolepsy*

ORAL SOLUTION, TABLETS (METHYLIN, RITALIN)

Adults. *Initial:* 10 mg twice daily or three times daily 30 to 45 min before meals, increased by 5 to 10 mg daily every wk, as needed. *Maximum:* 60 mg daily in two or three divided doses.

SUSTAINED RELEASE TABLETS (METADATE ER, RITALIN SR)

Adults who are switching from immediate release to sustained release form. *Initial:* If dosage same as immediate release and not taken more frequently than every 8 hr, dosage same for sustained release taken once daily before breakfast, increased by 10 mg weekly, as needed. *Maximum:* 60 mg once daily before breakfast.

E.R. CAPSULES (METADATE CD)

Adults. *Initial:* 20 mg once daily in morning before breakfast, increased by 20 mg daily each wk, as needed. *Maximum:* 60 mg once daily in morning before breakfast.

E.R. TABLETS (CONCERTA)

Adults who are methylphenidate naive. *Initial:* 18 mg once daily in morning before breakfast, increased by 18 mg daily at weekly intervals, as needed. *Maximum:* 72 mg once daily in morning before breakfast.

Adults who are currently receiving methylphenidate as immediate release tablets. Switch to E.R. tablets dependent on current dose of immediate release tablets.

Mechanism of Action

Blocks the reuptake mechanism of dopaminergic neurons in the cerebral cortex and subcortical structures of the brain, including the thalamus, decreasing motor restlessness, and improving concentration.

Methylphenidate also may trigger sympathomimetic activity. This action produces decreased fatigue and increased alertness and motor activity in patients with narcolepsy.

Contraindications

Angina pectoris, anxiety, cardiac arrhythmias, depression, fructose intolerance, glaucoma, glucose-galactose malabsorption, heart failure, hypersensitivity to methylphenidate or its components, hyperthyroidism, motor tics, recent MI, severe agitation, severe hypertension, sucrase-isomaltase insufficiency, tension, thyrotoxicosis, Tourette's syndrome or family history of it, use of halogenated anesthetics, use within 14 days of an MAO inhibitor

Interactions

DRUGS

anticholinergics: Possibly increased anticholinergic effects of both drugs

anticonvulsants, oral anticoagulants, phenylbutazone, tricyclic antidepressants: Inhibited metabolism and increased blood levels of these drugs

buspirone, fentanyl, lithium, MAO inhibitors, selective serotonin reuptake inhibitors, serotonin-norepinephrine reuptake inhibitors, St. John's wort, tricyclic antidepressants, triptans, tryptophan: Increased risk of serotonin syndrome

dopamine agonists and antagonists: Possibly altered effectiveness of these drugs

diuretics, antihypertensives: Decreased therapeutic effects of these drugs

halogenated anesthetics: Possibly sudden decrease in blood pressure during surgery

MAO inhibitors: Possibly increased adverse effects of methylphenidate, possibly severe hypertension

Route	Onset	Peak	Duration
P.O. (tablets)	Unknown	Unknown	3–6 hr
P.O. (E.R., S.R.)	Unknown	Unknown	About 8 hr
P.O. (E.R. once daily)	Unknown	Unknown	About 12 hr

FOODS
caffeine: Increased methylphenidate effects
ACTIVITIES
alcohol use: Possibly increased CNS effects; with long-acting forms, possible increased adverse effects

Adverse Reactions

CNS: Aggressiveness, agitation, anxiety, cerebral arteritis, **cerebral occlusion**, confusion, **CVA**, depression, disorientation, dizziness, drowsiness, dyskinesia, emotional lability, fatigue, fever, hallucinations, headache, hyperactivity, insomnia, irritability, ischemic neurologic defects (reversible), lethargy, mania, migraine, motor tics, nervousness, **neuroleptic malignant syndrome**, obsessive–compulsive disorder (rare), paresthesia, psychosis, sedation, **seizures**, somnolence, stroke, **suicidal ideation**, transient mood depression, tension, tremor, Tourette's syndrome (rare), toxic psychosis, vertigo
CV: Angina, **arrhythmias**, **bradycardia**, **cardiac arrest**, chest discomfort or pain, **extrasystoles**, hypertension, **hypotension**, **MI**, necrotizing vasculitis, palpitations, peripheral vasculopathy including Raynaud's phenomenon, **sudden death**, tachycardia
EENT: Accommodation abnormality, blurred vision, diplopia, dry mouth or throat, mydriasis, pharyngitis, rhinitis, sinusitis, vision changes
ENDO: Dysmenorrhea, growth suppression in children with long-term use
GI: Abdominal pain, anorexia, constipation, diarrhea, dyspepsia, elevated bilirubin and liver enzymes, **hepatotoxicity**, nausea, **severe hepatic injury**, vomiting
GU: Decreased libido, priapism
HEME: Anemia, **leukopenia**, **pancytopenia**, **thrombocytopenia**, **thrombocytopenic purpura**
MS: Arthralgia, myalgia, muscle tightness or twitching, **rhabdomyolysis**
RESP: Increased cough, upper respiratory tract infection
SKIN: Allergic contact dermatitis, alopecia, application-site reactions (transdermal patch), bullous skin conditions, chemical leukoderma (persistent loss of skin pigmentation with transdermal patch) diaphoresis, erythema, **erythema multiforme**, exanthemas, **exfoliative dermatitis**, pruritus, rash, urticaria
Other: **Anaphylaxis**, **angioedema**, elevated alkaline phosphatase, physical and psychological dependence, weight loss (prolonged use)

Nursing Considerations

WARNING Be aware that methylphenidate may induce CNS stimulation and psychosis and may worsen behavior disturbances and thought disorders in patients who already have psychosis. Use drug cautiously in patients with psychosis.

- Keep in mind that, when signs and symptoms of ADHD occur with acute stress reactions or with preexisting structural cardiac abnormalities or other serious heart problems, methylphenidate usually isn't indicated because of possible worsened reaction or sudden death.
- Reconstitute oral suspension form by first tapping bottle until powder flows freely. Remove bottle cap and add specified amount of water to the drug bottle (53 ml of water to 300-mg drug bottle, 105 ml of water to 600-mg drug bottle, 131 ml of water to 750-mg drug bottle, or 158 ml of water to 900-mg drug bottle). Insert bottle adapter into neck of bottle and replace cap. Shake vigorously using a back and forth motion for at least 10 seconds. Know that reconstituted oral suspension is stable up to 4 months.
- Monitor children and adolescents for first-time psychotic or manic symptoms. If present, notify prescriber and expect drug to be discontinued.

WARNING Know that the E.R. tablet form (Concerta) shouldn't be given to patients with esophageal motility disorders; drug may cause GI obstruction because tablet doesn't change shape in GI tract.

- Monitor blood pressure and pulse rate to detect hypertension and excessive stimulation. Notify prescriber if present. For patient with hypertension, expect to increase antihypertensive dosage or add another antihypertensive to regimen.

WARNING Watch for signs of physical or psychological dependence. Methylphenidate's abuse potential is similar to that of amphetamines; use cautiously in patients with a history of drug abuse.

- Stopping drug abruptly after long-term use may unmask dysphoria, paranoia, severe depression, or suicidal thoughts.
- Monitor growth in children. Report failure to grow or gain weight, and expect to stop drug.
- Watch closely (especially children, adolescents, and young adults), for suicidal tendencies, particularly when therapy starts and dosage changes, because depression may worsen temporarily during these times, possibly leading to suicidal ideation.
- Monitor transdermal patch application site for erythema. If more intense reactions occur with erythema, such as local edema or papule or vesicle formation that doesn't improve within 48 hours after patch is removed from irritated site or that spreads beyond the patch site, further diagnostic testing is required to determine presence of allergic contact dermatitis.
- Know that patients with allergic contact dermatitis from transdermal patch may develop systemic allergy reaction if methylphenidate is taken by another route, such as by mouth. Monitor patient closely if route of administration changes, and report any evidence of flare-up of previous dermatitis or positive patch-test sites, generalized skin eruptions in previously unaffected skin, or other symptoms such as arthralgia, diarrhea, fever, headache, malaise, or vomiting because drug may need to be discontinued.
- Observe patient for paradoxical aggravation of symptoms or other serious adverse reactions. If present, notify prescriber and expect dosage to be reduced or drug discontinued.

WARNING Monitor patient closely for serotonin syndrome, a rare but serious adverse effect of methylphenidate when taken in combination with serotonergic drugs. Signs and symptoms include agitation, confusion, diaphoresis, diarrhea, fever, hyperactive reflexes, poor coordination, restlessness, shaking, talking or acting with uncontrolled excitement, tremor, and twitching. If symptoms occur, notify prescriber immediately, expect drug to be discontinued, and provide supportive care.

- Inspect patient's fingers and toes for signs of peripheral vasculopathy, such as digital ulceration and/or soft tissue breakdown. Although usually mild and intermittent, more severe manifestation may occur. Notify prescriber if present, and expect dose to be reduced or drug discontinued.

PATIENT TEACHING

- Emphasize need to take drug exactly as prescribed because misuse may cause serious adverse cardiovascular reactions, including sudden death.
- For transdermal form, teach patient to apply patch to a clean, dry location in his hip area 2 hours before effect is needed and to remove it 9 hours after application.
- Caution patient to avoid applying patch to skin that's damaged, irritated, or oily and to avoid the waistline, where clothing may dislodge the patch. Tell patient to rotate application sites between hips.
- Instruct patient to apply patch immediately after opening pouch and removing protective liner. Tell him to press patch firmly in place with palm of his hand for about 30 seconds. Reassure patient that exposing site to water shouldn't cause patch to fall off. If a patch does fall off, explain that a new patch may be applied but that the total exposure time for the day shouldn't exceed 9 hours.
- Urge patient not to chew or crush E.R. tablets.
- Tell patient to take tablets at least 6 hours before bedtime to avoid insomnia and to take E.R. once-daily tablets in the morning.
- Advise patient taking E.R. once-daily tablets (Concerta) that he may see intact tablet in stool. Explain that drug is slowly released from nonabsorbable tablet shell.
- Tell patient taking capsule form to swallow it whole or sprinkle contents onto a tablespoon of applesauce and take immediately, followed by a liquid such as water.
- Instruct patient taking E.R. capsules (Jornay PM brand) to take drug only in the evening, starting at 8:00 pm, with timing adjustment of between 6:30 pm and 9:30 pm, as needed. Stress importance of not taking this form of drug in the morning.
- Instruct patient taking E.R. oral suspension form to vigorously shake the

bottle for at least 10 seconds before measuring dose to ensure that the proper dose is being taken. If using the oral dosing dispenser, tell patient to remove the bottle cap and confirm that the bottle adapter has been inserted into the top of the bottle. Tell him to insert the tip of the oral dosing dispenser provided into the bottle adapter, turn bottle upside down, and withdraw prescribed amount of liquid into the oral dosing dispenser. Then have patient remove the filled oral dosing dispenser from bottle and dispense drug directly into his mouth. Tell him to then replace the bottle cap and wash the oral dosing dispenser after each use (components are dishwasher-safe). Also alert patient taking drug long term that prescriber may take patient off of drug periodically to determine continued need.

- Tell patient taking ODT tablet not to remove the tablet from the blister pack until just prior to dosing and to take the tablet immediately after opening the blister pack. Tell him to use dry hands when opening the blister pack and remove tablet by peeling back the foil on the blister pack. Caution him not to push the tablet through the foil. Tell patient to place the whole tablet on his tongue and allow it to disintegrate without chewing or crushing it. Inform patient that no liquid is needed to take the tablet.
- Direct patient to notify prescriber about excessive nervousness, fever, insomnia, palpitations, rash, or vomiting.

WARNING Instruct patient to tell all prescribers about methylphenidate therapy, as serious drug interactions can occur. Stress importance of seeking immediate medical care if persistent, severe, or unusual adverse reactions occur.

- Warn patient with seizure disorder that drug may cause seizures.
- Inform parents of children on long-term therapy that drug may delay growth.
- Warn male patients and parents of male children that painful or prolonged penile erections may occur while taking the drug, especially after a dosage increase or during period of drug withdrawal. In the event that this happens, immediate medical attention should be sought.
- Instruct patient or parents to monitor fingers and toes for ulceration and/or soft tissue breakdown. If noticed, prescriber should be called. Reassure patient that signs and symptoms generally improve after the dose is reduced or drug is discontinued.
- Urge family or caregiver to watch patient closely for suicidal tendencies, especially when therapy starts or dosage changes and particularly if patient is a child, teenager, or young adult. Alert patient prescribed transdermal patch that a persistent loss of skin pigmentation, most commonly at and around the application site, may occur. Tell patient to notify prescriber if this occurs and expect this form of methylphenidate to be discontinued.

methylprednisolone

Medrol

methylprednisolone acetate

Depo-Medrol

methylprednisolone sodium succinate

A-methaPred, Solu-Medrol

Class and Category

Pharmacologic class: Glucocorticoid
Therapeutic class: Corticosteroid
Pregnancy category: C

Indications and Dosages

➤ *To treat immune and inflammatory disorders*

TABLETS (METHYLPREDNISOLONE)

Adults. 4 to 48 mg daily as a single dose or in divided doses. Alternatively, twice the daily dose every other day.
Children. 0.42 to 1.67 mg/kg daily in divided doses three times daily or four times daily.

I.V. INFUSION, I.M. INJECTION (METHYLPREDNISOLONE SODIUM SUCCINATE)

Adults. *Initial:* 10 to 40 mg infused over several min. Later doses given I.V. or I.M., based on patient's condition and response.

I.M. INJECTION (METHYLPREDNISOLONE ACETATE)
Adults. *Initial:* 4 to 120 mg daily according to clinical response.
Children: 0.14 to 0.84 mg/kg every 12 to 24 hr.
INTRA-ARTICULAR, INTRALESIONAL, OR SOFT-TISSUE INJECTION (METHYLPREDNISOLONE ACETATE)
Adults. 4 to 80 mg every 1 to 5 wk, according to clinical response.

➤ *To treat acute exacerbations of multiple sclerosis*

TABLETS (METHYLPREDNISOLONE)
Adults. 160 mg daily for 7 days followed by 64 mg every other day for 1 mo.
I.V. OR I.M. INJECTION (METHYLPREDNISOLONE ACETATE, METHYLPREDNISOLONE SODIUM SUCCINATE)
Adults. 160 mg daily for 1 wk followed by 64 mg every other day for 1 mo. I.V. injection given over at least 1 min.

Route	Onset	Peak	Duration
P.O.	In 60 min	1–2 hr	1.25–1.5 days
I.V.	Rapid	30 min	Unknown
I.M.	6–48 hr	4–8 days	1–4 wk

Mechanism of Action

Binds to intracellular glucocorticoid receptors and suppresses inflammatory and immune responses by inhibiting accumulation of monocytes and neutrophils at inflammation sites, stabilizing lysosomal membranes, suppressing the antigen response of macrophages and helper T cells, and inhibiting the synthesis of inflammatory response mediators, such as cytokines, interleukins, and prostaglandins.

Incompatibilities

Don't mix methylprednisolone with any drug without first consulting pharmacist. Don't dilute methylprednisolone acetate with any other drug.

Contraindications

Fungal infection, hypersensitivity to cow's milk for Solu-Medrol 40-mg formulation, hypersensitivity to methylprednisolone or its components, idiopathic thrombocytopenic purpura (I.M.), intrathecal administration, premature infants (preparations containing benzyl alcohol)

Interactions

DRUGS
acetaminophen: Increased risk of hepatotoxicity
aminoglutethimide: Possibly loss of methylprednisolone-induced adrenal suppression
amphotericin B, carbonic anhydrase inhibitors: Possibly severe hypokalemia
anabolic steroids, androgens: Increased risk of edema and worsening of acne
anticholinergics: Possibly increased intraocular pressure
asparaginase: Increased risk of hyperglycemia and toxicity
aspirin, NSAIDs: Increased risk of adverse GI effects and bleeding
barbiturates, carbamazepine, phenytoin, rifampin: Decreased blood methylprednisolone level
cholestyramine: Possibly increased methylprednisolone clearance
cyclosporine: Increased risk of seizures
digoxin: Possibly hypokalemia-induced arrhythmias and digitalis toxicity
estrogens, oral contraceptives: Possibly increased therapeutic and toxic effects of methylprednisolone
insulin, oral antidiabetic drugs: Possibly increased blood glucose level
isoniazid: Possibly decreased therapeutic effects of isoniazid
ketoconazole, macrolide antibiotics such as erythromycin and troleandomycin: Decreased methylprednisolone clearance and increased risk of adverse effects
mexiletine: Possibly decreased blood mexiletine level
neuromuscular blockers: Possibly increased neuromuscular blockade, causing respiratory depression or apnea
oral anticoagulants, thrombolytics: Increased risk of GI hemorrhage and ulceration, possibly decreased therapeutic effects of these drugs
potassium supplements: Possibly decreased effects of these supplements
somatrem, somatropin: Possibly decreased therapeutic effects of these drugs
streptozocin: Increased risk of hyperglycemia

troleandomycin: Increased blood methylprednisolone level
vaccines: Decreased antibody response and increased risk of neurologic complications
ACTIVITIES
alcohol use: Increased risk of adverse GI effects including bleeding

Adverse Reactions

CNS: Ataxia, behavioral changes, depression, dizziness, euphoria, fatigue, headache, **increased intracranial pressure with papilledema**, insomnia, malaise, mood changes, neuropathy, paresthesia, restlessness, **seizures**, steroid psychosis, syncope, vertigo
CV: **Arrhythmias**, **cardiac arrest**, edema, **fat embolism**, **heart failure**, hypertension, **hypertrophic cardiomyopathy** (premature infants), **hypotension**, **myocardial rupture following recent MI**, tachycardia, **thromboembolism**, thrombophlebitis
EENT: Exophthalmos, glaucoma, increased intraocular pressure, nystagmus, posterior subcapsular cataracts
ENDO: **Adrenal insufficiency**, cushingoid symptoms (buffalo hump, central obesity, moon face, supraclavicular fat pad enlargement), diabetes mellitus, growth suppression in children, hyperglycemia
GI: Abdominal distention, **acute hepatitis**, elevated liver enzymes, hepatomegaly, hiccups, increased appetite, **melena**, nausea, **pancreatitis**, peptic ulcer, ulcerative esophagitis, vomiting
GU: Amenorrhea, glycosuria, menstrual irregularities, perineal burning or tingling
HEME: Easy bruising, leukocytosis
MS: Arthralgia; aseptic necrosis of femoral and humeral heads; Charcot-like arthropathy; compression fractures; muscle atrophy, twitching, or weakness; myalgia; osteoporosis; spontaneous fractures; steroid myopathy; tendon rupture
RESP: **Pulmonary edema**
SKIN: Acne; allergic dermatitis; altered skin pigmentation; diaphoresis; dry, scaly skin; erythema; hirsutism; necrotizing vasculitis; petechiae; purpura; rash; scarring; sterile abscess; striae; subcutaneous fat atrophy; thin, fragile skin; urticaria
Other: Activation of latent infections, **anaphylaxis**, **angioedema**, exacerbation of systemic fungal infections, **hypernatremia**, **hypocalcemia**, **hypokalemia**, **hypokalemic alkalosis**, impaired wound healing, masking of signs of infection, **metabolic alkalosis**, negative nitrogen balance from protein catabolism, suppressed skin test reaction, weight gain

Nursing Considerations

- Know that high doses of systemic corticosteroids, including methylprednisolone, should not be used for the treatment of traumatic brain injury because of increased risk of death or in patients with active ocular herpes simplex because of risk of corneal perforation. Preparations containing benzyl alcohol should not be used to treat pediatric patients because of risk of "gasping syndrome."
- Administer methylprednisolone with extreme caution in patients with a recent myocardial infarction because corticosteroid use may increase risk of left ventricular free wall rupture.
- Use cautiously in patients with congestive heart failure or renal insufficiency because sodium retention and edema can occur in patients taking a corticosteroid. Also use cautiously in patients with diverticulitis, fresh intestinal anastomoses, nonspecific ulcerative colitis, or peptic ulcer; these conditions increase risk of perforation during corticosteroid therapy. In addition, use caution in patients with systemic sclerosis, because drug may increase risk of scleroderma renal crisis.
- Give methylprednisolone tablets with food to minimize GI irritation and indigestion. For once-daily dosing, give in the morning to coincide with normal cortisol secretion. Expect prescriber to add an antacid or H_2-receptor antagonist to regimen.
- Discard parenteral products that are discolored or contain particles. Discard any remaining Depo-Medrol suspension after prescribed dose is drawn from vial.
- Inject I.M. form deep into gluteal muscle. Avoid injecting into deltoid muscle because of risk of subcutaneous atrophy.
- Arrange for low-sodium diet with added potassium, as prescribed.
- Protect patient from falling, especially elderly patient at risk for fractures from osteoporosis.

- Closely monitor patient for signs of infection because drug may mask them or may worsen systemic fungal infections or active latent disease. Be aware that chickenpox and measles can become life-threatening in patients taking a corticosteroid.
- Assess for possible depression or psychotic episodes during therapy.
- Monitor blood glucose level; dosage of insulin or oral antidiabetic drug may need to be adjusted in diabetic patient.

WARNING To avoid possibly fatal acute adrenocortical insufficiency, expect to taper long-term therapy when discontinuing it, but expect dosage to be increased during times of stress.

- Be aware that changes in thyroid function, such as development of hyperthyroidism or hypothyroidism, may require dosage adjustment in chronic therapy because metabolic clearance of methylprednisolone is affected by thyroid activity.
- Know that skin testing should be avoided during methylprednisolone therapy because drug may suppress reaction.
- Monitor patient's liver enzymes, as ordered, especially in patients receiving high doses such as 1 g/day intravenously (usually for treatment of exacerbations of multiple sclerosis). This is important because, although rare, this can develop into a toxic form of acute hepatitis. The onset of liver dysfunction can occur several weeks or even longer after administration of methylprednisolone. Notify prescriber if liver dysfunction is suspected and expect drug to be discontinued, as condition can develop into acute liver failure and death.

PATIENT TEACHING

- Caution patient not to stop taking methylprednisolone abruptly or to change dosage without consulting prescriber.
- Tell patient to take a missed dose as soon as he remembers unless it's nearly time for the next dose. Caution against double-dosing.
- Urge patient to notify prescriber immediately about dark or tarry stools; signs of impending adrenocortical insufficiency, such as anorexia, dizziness, fainting, fatigue, fever, joint pain, muscle weakness, or nausea; and swelling or sudden weight gain.
- Instruct patient not to obtain vaccinations unless approved by prescriber.
- Urge patient to take calcium supplements, vitamin D, or both if recommended by prescriber.
- Inform patient that insomnia and restlessness usually resolve after 1 to 3 weeks.
- Caution patient to avoid people with contagious diseases.
- Explain the need for regular exercise or physical therapy to maintain muscle mass.
- Advise patient to carry medical identification that documents his need for long-term corticosteroid therapy.

metoclopramide hydrochloride

Metozolv, Reglan

Class and Category

Pharmacologic class: Dopamine-2 receptor antagonist
Therapeutic class: Antiemetic, upper GI stimulant
Pregnancy category: B

Indications and Dosages

➤ *To treat diabetic gastroparesis*

ORAL SOLUTION, ORAL SOLUTION CONCENTRATE, TABLETS

Adults experiencing mild symptoms. 10 mg 30 min before meals and at bedtime up to four times daily for 2 to 8 wk.

I.V. OR I.M. INJECTION

Adults experiencing severe symptoms. 10 mg 30 min before meals and at bedtime. I.V. injection given slowly over 1 to 2 min for up to 10 days before being switched to oral formulation and continued for another 2 to 8 wk.

➤ *To treat gastroesophageal reflux disease*

ORAL SOLUTION, ORAL SOLUTION CONCENTRATE, TABLETS

Adults. 10 to 15 mg 30 min before meals and at bedtime.

➤ *To prevent or reduce nausea and vomiting from emetogenic cancer chemotherapy*

I.V. INFUSION

Adults receiving less emetogenic regimens. 1mg/kg infused over at least 15 min 30 min before chemotherapy and repeated every 2 hr for 2 doses, then every 3 hr for 3 doses.

Adults receiving highly emetogenic regimens with drugs such as cisplatin or dacarbaxine. 2 mg/kg infused over at least 15 min 30 min before chemotherapy and repeated in 2 hr. Dosage decreased to 1 mg/kg and given 2 hr after second dose, followed by 1 mg/kg every 3 hr for 3 doses.

➤ *To prevent postoperative nausea and vomiting*

I. M. INJECTION

Adults. 10 to 20 mg given near end of surgery.

➤ *To facilitate small bowel intubation; to aid in radiological examinations*

I.V. INJECTION

Adults and adolescents over age 14. 10 mg undiluted given slowly over 1 to 2 min.

Children ages 6 to 14 years. 2.5 to 5 mg undiluted given slowly over 1 to 2 min.

Children under 6 years. 0.1 mg/kg undiluted given slowly over 1 to 2 min.

DOSAGE ADJUSTMENT Reduced by half if creatinine clearance is less than 40 ml/min.

Route	Onset	Peak	Duration
P.O.	30–60 min	Unknown	1–2 hr
I.V.	1–3 min	Unknown	1–2 hr
I.M.	10–15 min	Unknown	1–2 hr

Mechanism of Action

Antagonizes the inhibitory effect of dopamine on GI smooth muscle. This causes gastric contraction, which promotes gastric emptying and peristalsis, thus reducing gastroesophageal reflux. Metoclopramide also blocks dopaminergic receptors in the chemoreceptor trigger zone, preventing nausea and vomiting.

Incompatibilities

Don't administer metoclopramide through same I.V. line as calcium gluconate, cephalothin sodium, chloramphenicol sodium, cisplatin, erythromycin lactobionate, furosemide, methotrexate, penicillin G potassium, or sodium bicarbonate.

Contraindications

Concurrent use of butyrophenones, phenothiazines, or other drugs that may cause extrapyramidal reactions; GI hemorrhage, mechanical obstruction, or perforation; history of a dystonic reaction to metoclopramide; history of tardive dyskinesia; hypersensitivity to metoclopramide or its components; pheochromocytoma; seizure disorders

Interactions

DRUGS

anticholinergics, antidiarrheals, antiperistaltics, opioid analgesics: Decreased absorption of metoclopramide, thus decreasing effectiveness

antipsychotic drugs: Potential for additive effects, including increased frequency and severity of neuroleptic malignant syndrome, other extrapyramidal symptoms, and tardive dyskinesia

apomorphine, bromocriptine, cabergoline, levodopa, pramipexole, ropinirole, rotigotine: Decreased effectiveness of metoclopramide; potential for exacerbation of symptoms such as Parkinsonian symptoms

atovaquone, cimetidine, digoxin, fosfomycin, posaconazole (oral suspension): Decreased absorption and reduced effectiveness of these drugs

CNS depressants: Possibly increased CNS depression

cyclosporine, sirolimus, tacrolimus: Increased absorption and risk of adverse effects

CYP2D6 inhibitors (strong) such as bupropion, fluoxetaine, paroxetine, quinidine: Increased plasma concentrations of metoclopramide; risk of exacerbation of extrapyramidal symptoms

hepatotoxic drugs: Increased risk of hepatotoxicity characterized by elevated liver enzymes and jaundice

levodopa: Possibly decreased levodopa effects

MAO inhibitors: Increased risk of severe hypertension if patient has essential hypertension

mexiletine: Possibly faster mexiletine absorption

mivacurium, succinylcholine: Enhanced neuromuscular blockade

serotonergic drugs: Possible development of serotonin syndrome

ACTIVITIES
alcohol use: Risk of increased CNS depression

Adverse Reactions

CNS: Agitation, anxiety, confusion, depression, dizziness, drowsiness, extrapyramidal reactions (motor restlessness, Parkinsonism, tardive dyskinesia), fatigue, hallucinations, headache, insomnia, irritability, lassitude, nervousness, **neuroleptic malignant syndrome**, panic reaction, restlessness, **seizures**, **suicidal ideation**
CV: **AV block**, **bradycardia**, fluid retention, **heart failure**, hypertension, **hypotension**, **supraventricular tachycardia**
EENT: Dry mouth, glossal edema, **laryngeal edema**, visual disturbances
ENDO: Galactorrhea, gynecomastia, hyperprolactinemia
GI: Constipation, diarrhea, nausea
GU: Impotence, menstrual irregularities, urinary frequency or incontinence
HEME: **Agranulocytosis**, **leukopenia**, **methemoglobinemia**, **neutropenia**, **sulfhemoglobinemia**
RESP: **Bronchospasm**
SKIN: Rash, urticaria
Other: **Angioedema**, porphyria, restless leg syndrome

Nursing Considerations

- Be aware that metoclopramide therapy should not be used in patients with depression because of increased risk of suicidal ideation. Also know that drug should not be given to patients with a history of hypertension or patients taking monoamine oxidase inhibitors, because of increased risk of hypertension that could lead to a hypertensive crisis.
- Use metoclopramide cautiously in patients with hypertension because it may increase catecholamine levels.

WARNING Watch closely for tardive dyskinesia, especially in the elderly, women, and patients with diabetes, because this serious adverse effect is often irreversible even after therapy stops. Therapy lasting longer than 12 weeks isn't recommended because risk of tardive dyskinesia increases the longer the patient takes metoclopramide. Risk also has been linked to total cumulative dose so prescriber must take this into account when setting dosage. Also be aware that drug can cause other extrapyramidal symptoms besides tardive dyskinesia. For example, though rare, drug may cause dystonic reactions such as dyspnea and stridor, possibly caused by laryngospasm. At first sign of involuntary movements of face, tongue, or limbs, or any other abnormal sign or symptom, notify prescriber and expect to discontinue drug.

- Monitor patient with NADH-cytochrome b5 reductase deficiency because metoclopramide increases risk of methemoglobinemia and sulfhemoglobinemia, and patient can't receive methylene blue.
- Assess patient for signs of intestinal obstruction, such as abnormal bowel sounds, diarrhea, nausea, and vomiting, before administering metoclopramide. Notify prescriber if you detect them.
- For I.V. use, do not dilute doses of 10 mg or less. Give drug over 1 to 2 minutes. For doses larger than 10 mg, dilute in 50 ml normal saline solution, half-normal (0.45) saline solution, D_5W, or lactated Ringer's solution and infuse over at least 15 minutes.
- Avoid rapid I.V. delivery because it may cause anxiety, restlessness, and drowsiness.

WARNING Notify prescriber if patient shows signs of toxicity, such as disorientation, drowsiness, and extrapyramidal reactions.

- Monitor patient, especially one with heart failure or cirrhosis, for possible fluid retention or volume overload due to transient increase in plasma aldosterone level.

WARNING Monitor patient closely for neuroleptic malignant syndrome, a rare but potentially fatal disorder characterized by hyperthermia, muscle rigidity, altered level of consciousness, irregular pulse or blood pressure, tachycardia, diaphoresis, and arrhythmias. Know that risk increases in patients experiencing a toxic reaction to metoclopramide as a result of overdosage or receiving concomitant treatment with another drug associated with neuroleptic malignant syndrome.

- Store drug in a light-resistant container; discard if discolored or contains particulate.

- Monitor patient for abnormal behaviors or thoughts suggestive of suicidal ideation because depression may occur while taking metoclopramide even in patients without a history of depression.

PATIENT TEACHING

- Advise against activities that require alertness for about 2 hours after each dose.
- Urge patient to avoid alcohol and CNS depressants while taking metoclopramide. They may increase CNS depression.
- Tell patient to immediately report involuntary movements of face, eyes, tongue, or hands, including lip smacking, chewing, puckering of mouth, frowning, scowling, sticking out tongue, blinking, moving eyes, or shaking arms and legs.
- Explain that stopping metoclopramide may cause withdrawal symptoms that include dizziness, nervousness, and headache.
- Warn patient's family or caregiver to monitor patient for abnormal behavior or thoughts that may be suggestive of suicidal ideation. If concerns are raised, urge them to contact prescriber.
- Tell women of childbearing age to alert prescriber if pregnancy occurs, as metoclopramide crosses the placental barrier and may cause adverse effects in the neonate if mother is taking drug at time of delivery.
- Inform women wishing to breastfeed that doing so is not recommended while taking metoclopramide because drug may cause adverse effects in the nursing infant.
- Urge patient to tell all prescribers about metoclopramide therapy.

metolazone

Zaroxolyn

Class and Category

Pharmacologic class: Thiazide-like diuretic
Therapeutic class: Diuretic
Pregnancy category: B

Indications and Dosages

➤ *To manage mild to moderate hypertension*

TABLETS

Adults. 2.5 to 5 mg daily.

➤ *To manage edema from heart failure or renal disease*

TABLETS

Adults. 5 to 20 mg daily.

Route	Onset	Peak	Duration
P.O.	1 hr	2 hr	12–24 hr

Mechanism of Action

Promotes renal excretion of sodium and water by inhibiting their reabsorption in distal convoluted tubules. The resulting reduction in extracellular fluid volume and plasma reduces blood pressure. Metolazone also helps reduce blood pressure by decreasing peripheral vascular resistance.

Contraindications

Anuria; hepatic coma; hypersensitivity to metolazone, other sulfonamide derivatives, quinethazones, thiazides, or their components; renal failure

Interactions

DRUGS

allopurinol: Increased risk of hypersensitivity to allopurinol
amiodarone: Increased risk of arrhythmias from hypokalemia
amphotericin B: Increased risk of electrolyte imbalances
anesthetics: Increased effects of anesthetics
antigout drugs: Increased blood uric acid level and risk of gout attack
antihypertensives: Increased hypotension
antineoplastics: Prolonged antineoplastic-induced leukopenia
calcium salts: Increased risk of hypercalcemia
cholestyramine, colestipol: Decreased metolazone absorption
diazoxide: Increased risk of hyperglycemia
digoxin: Increased risk of electrolyte imbalances and digoxin-induced arrhythmias
diuretics: Additive effects of both drugs, possibly leading to electrolyte imbalances and severe hypovolemia
dopamine: Increased diuretic effect
insulin, oral antidiabetic drugs: Decreased effectiveness of these drugs, increased risk of hyperglycemia
lithium: Increased risk of lithium toxicity
methenamine: Decreased metolazone effectiveness from urinary alkalinization

methyldopa: Possibly hemolytic anemia
neuromuscular blockers: Increased risk of hypokalemia and neuromuscular blockade, increased risk of respiratory depression
NSAIDs, sympathomimetics: Possibly decreased metolazone effectiveness
oral anticoagulants: Decreased anticoagulation
vitamin D: Increased vitamin D action, increased risk of hypercalcemia

Adverse Reactions

CNS: Anxiety, chills, depression, dizziness, drowsiness, headache, insomnia, neuropathy, paresthesia, restlessness, syncope, weakness
CV: Chest pain, cold extremities, orthostatic hypotension, palpitations, peripheral edema, vasculitis, **venous thrombosis**
EENT: Bitter taste, blurred vision, dry mouth, epistaxis, pharyngitis, sinus congestion, tinnitus
ENDO: Hyperglycemia
GI: Abdominal pain, anorexia, cholecystitis, constipation, diarrhea, **hepatic dysfunction**, **hepatitis**, indigestion, nausea, **pancreatitis**, vomiting
GU: Decreased libido, glycosuria, impotence
HEME: Agranulocytosis, **aplastic anemia**, **leukopenia**, **thrombocytopenia**
MS: Arthralgia, gout, myalgia
RESP: Cough
SKIN: Dry skin, necrosis, petechiae, photosensitivity, pruritus, rash, urticaria
Other: Hypochloremia, **hypokalemia**, **hyponatremia**, hypovolemia, **metabolic alkalosis**

Nursing Considerations

- Anticipate giving metolazone with a loop diuretic if patient responds poorly to loop diuretic alone.
- Measure patient's fluid intake and output and daily weight to monitor drug's diuretic effect.
- Monitor blood chemistry test results and assess for evidence of hypochloremia, hypokalemia, and, possibly, mild metabolic alkalosis.
- Monitor serum calcium and uric acid levels, especially if patient has a history of gout or renal calculi. Metolazone may slightly increase calcium reabsorption and decrease uric acid excretion.

PATIENT TEACHING

- Inform patient that metolazone controls but doesn't cure hypertension. Discuss possible need for lifelong therapy and consequences of uncontrolled hypertension.
- Instruct patient to take drug at the same time each day.
- Direct patient to take drug with food or milk to minimize adverse GI reactions.
- Advise patient to change position slowly to minimize orthostatic hypotension.
- Urge patient to notify prescriber about persistent, severe diarrhea, nausea, or vomiting, which can cause dehydration and orthostatic hypotension.
- Emphasize the importance of diet control, especially limiting sodium intake, and maintaining a normal weight.
- Inform diabetic patient that metolazone may increase blood glucose level and that he should check his level often.

metoprolol succinate

Toprol-XL

metoprolol tartrate

Apo-Metoprolol (CAN), Betaloc (CAN), Betaloc Durules (CAN), Lopresor (CAN), Lopresor SR (CAN), Lopressor, Novometoprol (CAN)

Class and Category

Pharmacologic class: Beta$_1$-adrenergic blocker
Therapeutic class: Antianginal, antihypertensive
Pregnancy category: C

Indications and Dosages

➤ *To manage hypertension, alone or with other antihypertensives*

E.R. TABLETS (METOPROLOL SUCCINATE)

Adults. *Initial:* 25 to 100 mg daily, adjusted weekly as prescribed. *Maximum:* 400 mg daily.
Children 6 years and over. *Initial:* 1 mg/kg daily, not to exceed 50 mg daily with initial dose, adjusted weekly as prescribed. *Maximum:* 2 mg/kg daily, not to exceed 200 mg daily.

TABLETS (METOPROLOL TARTRATE)
Adults. *Initial:* 100 mg daily as a single dose or in divided doses, adjusted weekly as prescribed. *Maximum:* 450 mg daily as a single dose or in divided doses.

➤ *To treat acute MI or evolving acute MI*

TABLETS (METOPROLOL TARTRATE), I.V. INJECTION (METOPROLOL TARTRATE)
Adults. *Initial:* 5 mg by I.V. bolus every 2 min for three doses followed by 50 mg P.O. for patients who tolerate total I.V. dose (25 to 50 mg P.O. for patients who can't tolerate total I.V. dose) every 6 hr for 48 hr, starting 15 min after final I.V. dose; after 48 hr, 100 mg twice daily. *Maintenance:* 100 mg P.O. twice daily for at least 3 mo.

➤ *To treat angina pectoris and chronic stable angina*

E.R. TABLETS (METOPROLOL SUCCINATE)
Adults. 100 mg daily, increased weekly as prescribed. *Maximum:* 400 mg daily.

TABLETS (METOPROLOL TARTRATE)
Adults. *Initial:* 50 mg twice daily, adjusted weekly as prescribed. *Maximum:* 400 mg daily.

➤ *To treat stable, symptomatic (New York Heart Association [NYHA] class II or III), ischemic, hypertensive, or cardiomyopathic heart failure*

E.R. TABLETS (METOPROLOL SUCCINATE)
Adults. *Initial:* 25 mg daily (NYHA Class II) or 12.5 mg daily (NYHA Class III or more severe heart failure) for 2 wk. Then dosage doubled every 2 wk as tolerated. *Maximum:* 200 mg daily.

DOSAGE ADJUSTMENT For elderly patients or patients with hepatic impairment, initial dosage reduced with gradual dose titration.

Route	Onset	Peak	Duration
P.O.	60 min	1–2 hr	Unknown
P.O. (E.R.)	Unknown	6–12 hr	Unknown
I.V.	Unknown	20 min	Unknown

Mechanism of Action

Inhibits stimulation of $beta_1$-receptor sites, located mainly in the heart, resulting in decreased cardiac excitability, cardiac output, and myocardial oxygen demand. These effects help relieve angina, minimize cardiac tissue damage from a myocardial infarction, and help relieve symptoms of heart failure. Metoprolol also helps reduce blood pressure by decreasing renal release of renin.

Contraindications

Acute heart failure; cardiogenic shock; hypersensitivity to metoprolol, its components, or other beta blockers; pheochromocytoma; pulse less than 45 beats/minute; second- or third-degree AV block; severe peripheral arterial disorders; sick sinus syndrome

Interactions

DRUGS

alpha-adrenergic agents such as alpha-methyldopa, betanidine, guanethidine: Possibly increased antihypertensive effects
aluminum salts, barbiturates, calcium salts, cholestyramine, colestipol, NSAIDs, rifampin, salicylates, sulfinpyrazone: Decreased therapeutic effects of metoprolol
amiodarone, digoxin, diltiazem, verapamil: Increased risk of complete AV block
calcium channel blockers: Increased risk of heart failure and increased effects of both drugs
catecholamine-depleting drugs such as reserpine, monoamine oxidase (MAO) inhibitors: Possibly additive effect resulting in hypotension or marked bradycardia
cimetidine; CYP2D6 inhibitors such as antiarrhythmics, antidepressants, antifungals, antihistamines, antimalarials, antipsychotics, antiretrovirals; hydralazine: Increased plasma metoprolol level causing decrease in the cardioselectivity of metoprolol
clonidine: Increased risk of bradycardia and hypotension; increased risk of rebound hypertension when clonidine is discontinued
digoxin, diltiazem, other beta-blockers, verapamil: Decreased heart rate and slowed atrioventricular conduction
dipyridamole: Possibly altered heart rate
estrogens: Possibly decreased anti-hypertensive effect of metoprolol
ergot alkaloids: Possibly enhanced vasoconstrictive action of ergot alkaloids
general anesthetics: Increased risk of heart failure and hypotension
insulin, oral antidiabetic drugs: Decreased blood glucose control, possibly masking of signs and symptoms of hypoglycemia (by metoprolol)
lidocaine: Increased risk of lidocaine toxicity
neuromuscular blockers: Possibly enhanced and prolonged neuromuscular blockade

other antihypertensives: Additive hypotensive effect
phenothiazines: Possibly increased blood levels of both drugs
prazosin: Possibly increased postural hypotensive effect of first dose of prazosin
propafenone: Increased blood level and half-life of metoprolol
sympathomimetics, xanthines: Possibly decreased therapeutic effects of both drugs
FOODS
all foods: Increased bioavailability of metoprolol

Adverse Reactions

CNS: Anxiety, confusion, **CVA**, depression, dizziness, drowsiness, fatigue, hallucinations, headache, insomnia, nightmares, paresthesia, short-term memory loss, somnolence, syncope, tiredness, vertigo, weakness
CV: Angina, **arrhythmias (including AV block and bradycardia)**, **arterial insufficiency**, **cardiac arrest**, **cardiogenic shock**, chest pain, decreased HDL level, increased triglyceride levels, gangrene of extremity, **heart failure**, hypertension, orthostatic hypotension, palpitations, peripheral edema
EENT: Blurred vision, dry eyes or mouth, nasal congestion, rhinitis, taste disturbance, tinnitus
GI: Constipation, diarrhea, flatulence, heartburn, **hepatitis**, nausea, vomiting
GU: Decreased libido, impotence
HEME: Agranulocytosis, **leukopenia**, **thrombocytopenia**
MS: Arthralgia, back pain, myalgia
RESP: Bronchospasm, dyspnea, shortness of breath
SKIN: Alopecia, diaphoresis, photosensitivity, pruritus, rash, urticaria, worsening of psoriasis

Nursing Considerations

- Know that patients undergoing noncardiac major surgery should not begin a high-dose regimen using extended-release metoprolol because such use in patients with cardiovascular risk factors has been associated with bradycardia, hypotension, stroke, and death. However, also be aware that beta-blocker therapy such as metoprolol that is already in place should not be routinely discontinued prior to major surgery.
- Use metoprolol with extreme caution in patients with bronchospastic disease who don't respond to or can't tolerate other antihypertensives. Expect to give smaller doses more often to avoid the higher plasma levels in longer dosage intervals.
- Use cautiously in patients with angina or hypertension who have congestive heart failure because beta blockers such as metoprolol can further depress myocardial contractility, worsening heart failure.
- Expect patients with acute MI who can't tolerate initial dosage or who delay treatment to start with maintenance dosage, as prescribed and tolerated.
- Before starting therapy for heart failure, expect to give an ACE inhibitor, digoxin, and a diuretic to stabilize patient.
- Be aware that if patient has pheochromocytoma, alpha blocker therapy should start first, followed by metoprolol to prevent paradoxical increase in blood pressure from attenuation of beta-mediated vasodilation in skeletal muscle.
- Be aware that metoprolol dosage for heart failure is highly individualized. Monitor patient for evidence of worsening heart failure during dosage increases. If heart failure worsens, expect to increase diuretic dosage and possibly decrease metoprolol dosage or temporarily discontinue drug, as prescribed. Metoprolol dosage shouldn't be increased until worsening heart failure has been stabilized.
- If patient with heart failure develops symptomatic bradycardia, expect to decrease the metoprolol dosage.

WARNING Know that if dosage exceeds 400 mg daily, patient should be monitored for bronchospasm and dyspnea because metoprolol competitively blocks $beta_2$-adrenergic receptors in bronchial and vascular smooth muscles.

WARNING When substituting metoprolol for clonidine, expect to gradually reduce clonidine and increase metoprolol dosage over several days. Given together, these drugs have additive hypotensive effects.

- Assess ECG of patients who take metoprolol because they may be at risk for AV block. If AV block results from depressed AV node conduction, prepare to give appropriate drug, as ordered, or assist with insertion of temporary pacemaker.

- Check for signs of poor glucose control in patient with diabetes mellitus. Metoprolol may interfere with therapeutic effects of insulin and oral antidiabetic drugs. It also may mask evidence of hypoglycemia, such as palpitations, tachycardia, and tremor.
- Monitor patient with hyperthyroidism closely because beta-adrenergic blockers such as metoprolol may mask signs of hyperthyroidism, such as tachycardia. Also know that abrupt discontinuation of metoprolol should be avoided because thyroid storm could be precipitated.
- Monitor patient with peripheral vascular disease for evidence of arterial insufficiency (coldness, pain, and pallor in affected extremity). Metoprolol can precipitate or aggravate peripheral vascular disease.
- Be aware that patients with a history of severe anaphylactic reactions may be more reactive to repeated challenges of the allergen while taking beta-blocker therapy, such as metoprolol, and may be unresponsive to the usual doses of epinephrine used to treat an allergic reaction.

WARNING Expect to taper dosage over 1 to 2 weeks when drug is discontinued; stopping abruptly can cause myocardial ischemia, MI, severe hypertension, or ventricular arrhythmias, especially in patients with cardiac disease.

PATIENT TEACHING

- Instruct patient to take metoprolol with food at the same time each day—once daily for E.R. tablets. Explain that he may halve tablets but not chew or crush them.
- Advise patient to notify prescriber if pulse rate falls below 60 beats/minute or is significantly lower than usual.
- Urge diabetic patient to check blood glucose level often during therapy.
- Caution patient not to stop drug abruptly.

metronidazole

Flagyl, Flagyl ER, Protostat, Trikacide (CAN)

metronidazole hydrochloride

Flagyl I.V. RTU

Class and Category

Pharmacologic class: Nitroimidazole
Therapeutic class: Antiprotozoal
Pregnancy category: B

Indications and Dosages

➤ *To treat systemic anaerobic infections caused by* Bacteroides fragilis, Clostridium difficile, Clostridium perfringens, Eubacterium, Fusobacterium, Peptococcus, Peptostreptococcus, *and* Veillonella *species*

CAPSULES, TABLETS

Adults. 7.5 mg/kg up to 1,000 mg every 6 hr for 7 days or longer. *Maximum:* 4,000 mg daily.

I.V. INFUSION

Adults. *Initial:* 15 mg/kg infused over 1 hr and then 7.5 mg/kg up to 1,000 mg infused over 1 hr every 6 hr for 7 days or longer. *Maximum:* 4,000 mg daily.

➤ *To treat amebiasis (*Entamoeba histolytica*)*

CAPSULES, TABLETS

Adults. 750 mg three times daily for 5 to 10 days.

Children. 11.6 to 16.7 mg/kg three times daily for 10 days.

➤ *To treat trichomoniasis (*Trichomonas vaginalis*)*

CAPSULES, TABLETS

Adults. 2,000 mg as a single dose, 1,000 mg twice daily for 1 day, or 250 mg three times daily for 7 days.

➤ *To prevent perioperative bowel infection*

I.V. INFUSION

Adults. 15 mg/kg infused 30 to 60 min 1 hr before surgery and then 7.5 mg/kg infused over 30 to 60 min 6 and 12 hr after initial dose.

➤ *To treat bacterial vaginosis*

M

E.R. TABLETS

Adult nonpregnant women. 750 mg once daily for 7 days.

DOSAGE ADJUSTMENT For patients with severe hepatic impairment, dosage reduced by 50%.

*Topical and vaginal forms presented in appendix.

Mechanism of Action

Undergoes intracellular chemical reduction during anaerobic metabolism. After metronidazole is reduced, it damages DNA's helical structure and breaks its strands, which inhibits bacterial nucleic acid synthesis and causes cell death.

Incompatibilities

Don't administer I.V. metronidazole with aluminum needles or hubs or through same I.V. line as other drugs.

Contraindications

Breastfeeding, disulfiram use within past 2 weeks, hypersensitivity to metronidazole or its components, trichomoniasis during first trimester of pregnancy

Interactions

DRUGS

5-fluorouracil: Decreased clearance of 5-fluorouracil and potential for 5-fluorouracil toxicity

amiodarone, carbamazepine, cyclosporine, phenytoin, quinidine, tacrolimus: Increased plasma levels of these drugs

busulfan: Increased risk of serious busulfan toxicity

cimetidine: Possibly delayed elimination and increased blood level of metronidazole

disulfiram: Possibly combined toxicity, with confusion and psychotic reactions

lithium: Possible development of elevated lithium levels with potential for toxicity in patients on high doses

neurotoxic drugs: Increased risk of neurotoxicity

oral anticoagulants: Possibly increased anticoagulant effect

phenobarbital, phenytoin: Possibly accelerated elimination of metronidazole and decreased effectiveness

vecuronium: Possibly increased effects of vecuronium

ACTIVITIES

alcohol use: Possibly disulfiram-like effects

Adverse Reactions

CNS: Aseptic meningitis (parenteral form), ataxia, asthenia, chills, confusion, depression, dizziness, dysarthria, **encephalopathy**, fever, headache, hypoesthesia, incoordination, insomnia, irritability, jumpy eye movements, lightheadedness, malaise, numbness, paresthesia, peripheral neuropathy, psychosis, **seizures** (high doses), somnolence, syncope, weakness, vertigo

CV: Chest pain, palpitations, peripheral edema, tachycardia

EENT: Dry mouth, lacrimation (topical form), metallic taste, nasal congestion, nystagmus, optic neuropathy, pharyngitis

GI: Abdominal cramps or pain, anorexia, diarrhea, elevated liver enzymes, **hepatic failure or hepatotoxicity** (patients with Cockayne syndrome), nausea, **pancreatitis**, vomiting

GU: Burning or irritation of sexual partner's penis, candidal cervicitis or vaginitis, chromaturia, dark urine, decreased libido, dryness of vagina or vulva, dyspareunia, dysuria, proctitis, urinary frequency

HEME: Agranulocytosis, eosinophilia, **leukopenia, neutropenia, thrombocytopenia**

MS: Arthralgia, back pain, dysarthria, muscle spasms, myalgia

RESP: Dyspnea

SKIN: Burning or stinging sensation, erythema, flushing, hyperhidrosis, pruritus, rash, **Stevens–Johnson syndrome, toxic epidermal necrolysis**, urticaria

Other: Anaphylaxis; angioedema; drug reaction with eosinophilia and systemic symptoms (DRESS); infusion-site edema, pain, or tenderness

Nursing Considerations

- Use parenteral metronidazole with extreme caution in patients with Cockayne syndrome, because acute hepatic failure and severe hepatotoxicity have occurred, with some fatalities. If no other treatment is available, expect to obtain liver function studies before metronidazole is given parenterally, again

within the first 2 to 3 days after treatment is initiated, frequently during therapy, and at the end of therapy. If liver enzymes become elevated, expect metronidazole to be discontinued and liver enzymes monitored until they have returned to baseline values.
- Use cautiously in patients with CNS diseases.
- Use cautiously in patients with blood dyscrasias or a history of such because metronidazole therapy has caused agranulocytosis, leukopenia, and neutropenia in some patients.
- Don't give I.V. administration by direct I.V. injection.
- Discontinue primary I.V. infusion during metronidazole infusion.

WARNING Know that if patient has adverse CNS reactions, such as peripheral neuropathy or seizures, prescriber must be told and drug stopped immediately.

- Monitor patient with severe liver disease because slowed metronidazole metabolism may cause drug to accumulate in body and increase the risk of adverse effects.
- Monitor patients with end-stage renal disease who are not on hemodialysis or patients with severe renal impairment for adverse reactions, because reduced urinary excretion may cause metronidazole and its metabolites to accumulate in the body.
- Monitor CBC and culture and sensitivity tests if therapy lasts longer than 10 days or if second course of treatment is needed.
- Monitor patient's neurologic status throughout metronidazole therapy. If abnormal neurologic signs and symptoms occur, notify prescriber and expect to discontinue drug.
- Be aware that parenteral form of metronidazole contains 790 mg of sodium per 100 ml. Monitor patients predisposed to edema or who are receiving corticosteroids or a reduced-sodium diet.
- Assess patient for fungal superinfections. Candidiasis may occur and present with more serious symptoms during therapy with metronidazole and requires treatment with a candidacidal agent.
- Be aware that metronidazole may interfere with certain chemistry values, such as alanine aminotransferase (AST, SGOT), aspartate aminotransferase, glucose hexokinase, lactate dehydrogenase (LDH), and triglycerides.
- Monitor patient with Crohn's disease exposed to metronidazole at high doses for extended periods of time because these patients have an increased risk of extraintestinal and gastrointestinal cancers such as breast and colon cancers.

PATIENT TEACHING

- Instruct female patient to notify prescriber if she is pregnant, intends to get pregnant, or is breastfeeding, because breastfeeding is contraindicated during metronidazole therapy.
- Urge patient to take metronidazole at evenly spaced intervals during the day and with food to minimize adverse GI reactions. except for E.R. tablets, which should be taken 1 hour before or 2 hours after a meal.
- Urge patient to complete the entire course of therapy.
- Caution patient to avoid alcohol during therapy and for at least 3 days afterward.
- Advise patient to avoid hazardous activities until drug's CNS effects are known and to report any abnormal neurologic signs or symptoms, such as numbness, seizures, weakness, or vision changes.
- If patient reports dry mouth, suggest ice chips or sugarless hard candy or gum; suggest a dental visit if dryness lasts longer than 2 weeks.
- Instruct patient to notify prescriber if no improvement occurs within a few days of taking tablets or capsules.
- Inform patient with trichomoniasis that her male sexual partners should wear condoms during her treatment and that they may need treatment themselves to prevent reinfection.
- Urge patient to follow up with prescriber to make sure infection is gone.
- Tell patient with Cockayne syndrome who is receiving metronidazole to stop drug immediately if signs and symptoms of liver dysfunction occur, such as abdominal pain, change in skin or stool color, or nausea, and to notify prescriber.

metyrosine

Demser

Class and Category

Pharmacologic class: Tyrosine hydroxylase inhibitor
Therapeutic class: Antipheochromocytoma agent
Pregnancy category: C

Indications and Dosages

➤ *To control hypertension and related symptoms until pheochromocytomectomy is performed, to treat chronic malignant pheochromocytoma*

CAPSULES

Adults and adolescents. *Initial:* 250 mg four times daily, increased as ordered by 250 to 500 mg daily. *Maintenance:* 2,000 to 3,000 mg daily in divided doses four times daily. Preoperative dosage given for at least 7 days. *Maximum:* 4,000 mg daily in divided doses.

Mechanism of Action

Blocks activity of tyrosine hydroxylase, the enzyme that controls rate of catecholamine synthesis. This action decreases production of the catecholamines epinephrine and norepinephrine, which, in patients with pheochromocytoma, are produced in excessive amounts.

Contraindications

Hypersensitivity to metyrosine or its components

Interactions

DRUGS

CNS depressants: Increased sedation
haloperidol, phenothiazines: Increased extrapyramidal effects

ACTIVITIES

alcohol use: Increased sedation

Adverse Reactions

CNS: Anxiety, confusion, depression, disorientation, extrapyramidal reactions (difficulty speaking, drooling, Parkinsonism, tremor, trismus), hallucinations, headache, sedation
CV: Peripheral edema
EENT: Dry mouth, nasal congestion, pharyngeal edema
ENDO: Galactorrhea, gynecomastia
GI: Abdominal pain, diarrhea, elevated serum AST level, nausea, vomiting
GU: Crystalluria, dysuria (transient), ejaculation failure, hematuria, impotence, urolithiasis
HEME: Anemia, eosinophilia, **thrombocytopenia**, thrombocytosis
SKIN: Urticaria

Nursing Considerations

- Expect patient taking metyrosine to experience moderate to severe sedation at low and high dosages. Sedation begins during first 24 hours, peaks after 2 to 3 days, and tends to wane during next few days. It usually subsides after 1 week unless dosage is increased or exceeds 2 g daily.
- Obtain urine specimens as ordered to check for crystalluria and urolithiasis. If crystalluria develops, increase fluid intake to achieve daily urine output of 2,000 ml or more with doses above 2 g daily. If crystalluria persists, reduce dosage or stop drug, as ordered.
- Expect to adjust dosage, as prescribed, based on clinical response and urine catecholamine level.
- If signs and symptoms aren't adequately controlled by metyrosine, expect to add an alpha-adrenergic blocker, such as phenoxybenzamine, as prescribed.

PATIENT TEACHING

- Inform patient about metyrosine's sedative effects. Advise him to avoid alcohol and CNS depressants, which may increase sedation.
- Instruct patient to increase fluid intake, as appropriate.
- Urge patient to report drooling, severe diarrhea, shaking and trembling of hands and fingers, or trouble speaking.
- Inform patient that he may experience changes in sleep pattern for 2 to 3 days after stopping drug.
- Advise patient to keep regular visits with prescriber to monitor progress.

micafungin sodium

Mycamine

Class and Category

Pharmacologic class: Echinocandin
Therapeutic class: Antifungal
Pregnancy category: C

Indications and Dosages

➤ *To treat esophageal candidiasis*

I.V. INFUSION

Adults. 150 mg infused over 1 hr once daily.

Children age 4 months and over weighing more than 30 kg. 2.5 mg/kg infused over 1 hr once daily. *Maximum:* 150 mg once daily.

Children age 4 months and over weighing 30 kg or less. 3 mg/kg infused over 1 hr once daily.

➤ *To prevent* Candida *infection in patients undergoing hematopoietic stem cell transplantation*

I.V. INFUSION

Adults. 50 mg infused over 1 hr once daily.

Children age 4 months and over. 1 mg/kg infused over 1 hr once daily. *Maximum:* 50 mg once daily.

➤ *To treat candidemia, acute disseminated candidiasis, and* Candida *peritonitis and abscesses*

I.V. INFUSION

Adults. 100 mg infused over 1 hr once daily.

Children age 4 months and over. 2 mg/kg infused over 1 hr once daily. *Maximum*: 100 mg once daily.

Mechanism of Action

Inhibits synthesis of 1,3-beta-D-glucan, which is an essential component of the *Candida* fungal cell wall. Without 1,3-beta-D-glucan, the fungal cell dies.

Contraindications

Hypersensitivity to micafungin, its components, or other echinocandins

Incompatibilities

Mixing or infusing with other drugs may cause micafungin to precipitate.

Interactions

DRUGS

immunosuppressants: Possibly additive adverse hematologic effects
itraconazole, nifedipine, sirolimus: Increased plasma levels of these drugs

Adverse Reactions

CNS: Anxiety, delirium, dizziness, dysgeusia, fatigue, fever, headache, insomnia, **intracranial hemorrhage**, rigors, **seizures**, somnolence
CV: Arrhythmia, **atrial fibrillation**, **bradycardia**, **cardiac arrest**, **deep vein thrombosis**, hypertension, **hypotension**, **MI**, peripheral edema, phlebitis, tachycardia, **shock**, vasodilation
EENT: Epistaxis, mucosal inflammation
ENDO: Hyperglycemia, **hypoglycemia**
GI: Abdominal pain, anorexia, constipation, diarrhea, dyspepsia, elevated liver enzymes, **hepatic dysfunction**, hiccups, hyperbilirubinemia, jaundice, nausea, vomiting
GU: Acute renal failure, **anuria**, elevated blood urea and serum creatinine levels, oliguria, **renal tubular necrosis**
HEME: Anemia, **coagulopathy**, **disseminated intravascular coagulation (DIC)**, eosinophilia, **hemolytic anemia**, **leukopenia**, **lymphopenia**, **neutropenia**, **pancytopenia**, **thrombocytopenia**
RESP: Apnea, cough, **cyanosis**, dyspnea, **hypoxia**, pneumonia, **pulmonary embolism**
SKIN: Erythema, **erythema multiforme**, flushing, necrosis, pruritus, rash, **Stevens–Johnson syndrome**, **toxic epidermal necrolysis**, urticaria
Other: Acidosis, **anaphylaxis**, **angioedema**, bacteremia, **hyperkalemia**, **hypernatremia**, **hypocalcemia**, **hypokalemia**, **hypomagnesemia**, **hyponatremia**, **hypophosphatemia**, injection-site reactions including phlebitis and thrombophlebitis, **sepsis**

Nursing Considerations

- Use cautiously in patients with hepatic insufficiency.
- Reconstitute micafungin by adding 5 ml 0.9% sodium chloride injection, USP or 5% dextrose injection, USP solution to each 50-mg vial being used (to yield 10 mg

micafungin/ml) and to each 100-mg vial being used (to yield 20 mg micafungin/ml). Swirl vial gently to minimize excessive foaming. For adult patients, add reconstituted solution to 100 ml 0.9% sodium chloride injection, USP or 5% dextrose injection, USP. For pediatric patients, follow manufacturer guidelines for calculating volume to use for dilution. Give solution for both adults and children over 1 hour after flushing an existing I.V. line with 0.9% sodium chloride injection, USP. Protect diluted solution from light, although the infusion drip chamber or tubing does not need to be covered.
- Administer concentrations greater than 1.5 mg/ml through a central catheter to minimize risk of infusion reactions.
- Monitor infusion rate carefully because infusions that took less than 1 hour to infuse have been associated with more frequent hypersensitivity reactions.

WARNING Monitor patient closely for hypersensitivity reactions, including anaphylaxis and angioedema. Stop infusion immediately if present, notify prescriber, and provide supportive care, as prescribed.
- Monitor patient's liver and renal function closely throughout therapy because liver and renal abnormalities may occur in patients receiving micafungin.
- Monitor hematologic status closely because hematologic abnormalities may occur. If they do, monitor patient closely. If patient's condition worsens, expect micafungin to be discontinued.

PATIENT TEACHING
- Instruct patient to report any infusion-site discomfort immediately.
- Tell patient to report any unusual or persistent signs and symptoms to prescriber.

midazolam hydrochloride

Versed

Class, Category, and Schedule

Pharmacologic class: Benzodiazepine
Therapeutic class: Sedative-hypnotic
Pregnancy category: D
Controlled substance schedule: IV

Indications and Dosages

➤ *To induce preoperative sedation or amnesia, to control preoperative anxiety*

SYRUP

Children ages 6 months to 16 years. 0.25 to 0.5 mg/kg as a single dose 30 to 45 min before surgery. *Usual:* 0.5 mg/kg. *Maximum:* 20 mg.

I.V. INJECTION

Adults age 60 and over and adults who are debilitated or chronically ill. *Initial:* 1.5 mg over 2 min immediately before procedure. *Maintenance:* After 2-min waiting period, dosage adjusted to desired level in 25% increments, as ordered. *Maximum:* 1 mg in 2 min.

Adults under age 60 and adolescents. *Initial:* Up to 2.5 mg over 2 min immediately before procedure. After 2-min waiting period, dosage adjusted to desired level in 25% increments, as ordered. *Maximum:* 5 mg.

Children ages 6 to 12. *Initial:* 0.025 to 0.05 mg/kg, over 2 min up to 0.4 mg/kg, if needed immediately before procedure. *Maintenance:* After a 2- to 3-min waiting period, dosage adjusted as needed. *Maximum:* 10 mg.

Children ages 6 months to 5 years. *Initial:* 0.05 to 0.1 mg/kg, over 2 min up to 0.6 mg/kg, if needed immediately before procedure. *Maintenance:* After waiting 2 to 3 min, dosage adjusted, as needed. *Maximum:* 6 mg.

I.M. INJECTION

Adults age 60 and over. 0.02 to 0.05 mg/kg as a single dose 30 to 60 min before surgery.

Adults under age 60 and adolescents. 0.07 to 0.08 mg/kg as a single dose 30 to 60 min before surgery.

Children ages 6 months to 12 years. 0.1 to 0.15 mg/kg, up to 0.5 mg/kg for more anxious patients as a single dose 30 to 60 min before surgery. *Maximum:* 10 mg.

DOSAGE ADJUSTMENT For elderly patients and patients who are chronically ill, maintenance dosage reduced by 50%. For adults who have been premedicated with an opiate, maintenance dosage reduced by 25%.

➤ *To relieve agitation and anxiety in mechanically ventilated patients*

I.V. INFUSION
Adults. *Initial:* 0.01 to 0.05 mg/kg infused over several min, repeated at 10- to 15-min intervals until adequate sedation occurs. *Maintenance:* 0.02 to 0.1 mg/kg/hr initially, adjusted to desired level in 25% to 50% increments, as ordered. After achieving desired level of sedation, infusion rate decreased by 10% to 25% every few hr, as ordered, until minimum effective infusion rate is determined.
Children. *Initial:* 0.05 to 0.2 mcg/kg over 2 to 3 min. *Maintenance:* 0.06 to 0.12 mg/kg/hr by continuous infusion with dosage adjusted, as needed, to maintain effect.
Infants over age 32 weeks. 0.06 mg/kg/hr by continuous infusion with rate adjusted, as needed.
Infants under age 32 weeks. *Initial:* 0.03 mg/kg/hr by continuous infusion with rate adjusted, as needed.

Route	Onset	Peak	Duration
I.V.*	1.5–5 min	Rapid	2–6 hr
I.M.*	5–15 min	15–60 min	2–6 hr
I.M.†	30–60 min	Unknown	Unknown

* For sedation.
† For amnesia.

Mechanism of Action
May exert sedating effect by increasing activity of gamma-aminobutyric acid, a major inhibitory neurotransmitter in the brain. As a result, midazolam produces a calming effect, relaxes skeletal muscles, and—at high doses—induces sleep.

Contraindications
Acute angle-closure glaucoma; alcohol intoxication; coma; hypersensitivity to midazolam, other benzodiazepines, or their components; shock

Interactions
DRUGS
antihypertensives: Increased risk of hypotension
cimetidine, diltiazem, erythromycin, fluconazole, indinavir, itraconazole, ketoconazole, ranitidine, ritonavir, saquinavir, verapamil: Intense and prolonged sedation caused by reduced midazolam metabolism
CNS depressants: Possibly increased CNS and respiratory depression and hypotension
rifampin: Decreased blood midazolam level
FOODS
grapefruit, grapefruit juice: Possibly increased blood midazolam level and risk of toxicity
ACTIVITIES
alcohol use: Possibly intense, prolonged sedative effect and increased respiratory depression and hypotension

Adverse Reactions
CNS: Agitation, delirium, or dreaming during emergence from anesthesia; anxiety; ataxia; chills; combativeness; confusion; dizziness; drowsiness; euphoria; excessive sedation; headache; insomnia; lethargy; nervousness; nightmares; paresthesia; prolonged emergence from anesthesia; restlessness; retrograde amnesia; sleep disturbance; slurred speech; weakness; yawning
CV: Cardiac arrest, hypotension, nodal rhythm, PVCs, tachycardia, **vasovagal episodes**
EENT: Blurred vision, diplopia, or other vision changes; increased salivation; **laryngospasm**; miosis; nystagmus; toothache
GI: Hiccups, nausea, retching, vomiting
RESP: Airway obstruction, bradypnea, bronchospasm, coughing, decreased tidal volume, dyspnea, hyperventilation, **respiratory arrest, shallow breathing,** tachypnea, wheezing
SKIN: Pruritus, rash, urticaria
Other: Injection-site burning, edema, induration, pain, redness, and tenderness

Nursing Considerations
- Determine whether patient consumes alcohol or takes antibiotics, antihypertensives, or protease inhibitors because these substances can produce an intense and prolonged sedative effect when taken with midazolam.

WARNING Know that I.V. midazolam is given only in hospital or ambulatory care settings that allow continuous monitoring of cardiac and respiratory function. Keep resuscitative drugs and equipment at hand.

- Know that repeated or lengthy use of sedation drugs such as midazolam and general anesthetics during procedures or surgeries should be avoided in children younger than 3 years of age or in pregnant women during their third trimester, because the combined use may affect the development of children's brains.
- Know that midazolam injection may be combined with D_5W, normal saline solution or lactated Ringer's solution. With D_5W and normal saline, solution is stable for 24 hours. With lactated Ringer's, solution is stable for 4 hours.
- Mix injection in same syringe with atropine sulfate, meperidine hydrochloride, morphine sulfate, or scopolamine hydrobromide, if needed. The resulting solution is stable for 30 minutes.
- Assess level of consciousness frequently because the range between sedation and unconsciousness or disorientation is narrow with midazolam.
- Be aware that recovery time is usually 2 hours but may be up to 6 hours.

PATIENT TEACHING

- Inform patient that he may not remember procedure because midazolam produces amnesia.
- Advise patient to avoid hazardous activities until drug's adverse CNS effects, such as dizziness and drowsiness, have worn off.
- Instruct patient to avoid alcohol and other CNS depressants for 24 hours after receiving drug, as directed by prescriber.

miglitol

Glyset

Class and Category

Pharmacologic class: Alpha glucosidase inhibitor
Therapeutic class: Antidiabetic
Pregnancy category: B

Indications and Dosages

➤ *To manage type 2 diabetes mellitus*

TABLETS

Adults. *Initial:* 25 mg three times daily with first bite of each meal. Or, 25 mg daily, increased gradually to 25 mg three times daily. *Maximum:* 100 mg three times daily.

DOSAGE ADJUSTMENT After 4 to 8 wk, dosage increased, if ordered, to 50 mg three times daily. for about 3 mo; then dosage adjusted based on glycosylated hemoglobin (HbA_{1C}) level.

Route	Onset	Peak	Duration
P.O.	Rapid	2–3 hr	Unknown

Mechanism of Action

Inhibits intestinal glucoside hydrolase enzymes, which normally hydrolyze disaccharides and oligosaccharides to glucose and other monosaccharides. This action delays carbohydrate absorption and digestion and reduces postprandial blood glucose level.

Contraindications

Acute or chronic bowel disorder, diabetic ketoacidosis, hypersensitivity to miglitol or its components

Interactions

DRUGS

digestive enzyme preparations, intestinal adsorbents (activated charcoal): Decreased miglitol effects
digoxin: Decreased blood digoxin level
insulin, sulfonylureas: Increased risk and severity of hypoglycemia
propranolol, ranitidine: Decreased bioavailability of these drugs

Adverse Reactions

GI: Abdominal distention or pain, diarrhea, flatulence, **hepatotoxicity**, ileus including paralytic ileus, nausea, pneumatosis cystoides intestinalis (rare), subileus
HEME: Low serum iron level
SKIN: Rash (transient)

Nursing Considerations

- Use miglitol cautiously in patient with serum creatinine level above 2 mg/dl.
- Be aware that some patients with type 2 diabetes also may receive insulin or a sulfonylurea as an adjunct to miglitol

therapy. Monitor these patients closely for hypoglycemia because insulin and sulfonylureas may cause hypoglycemia, and miglitol therapy may make it more severe. If hypoglycemia occurs, use an oral glucose product such as dextrose to treat mild-to-moderate hypoglycemia rather than sucrose, whose hydrolysis to fructose and glucose is inhibited by miglitol.
- Give miglitol with first bite of each meal. Drug must have arrived at site of enzymatic action when carbohydrates reach small intestine.
- Review patient's HbA_{1C} level, as appropriate, to monitor long-term glucose control.
- Monitor patient for evidence of overdose, such as transient increases in abdominal discomfort, diarrhea, and flatulence (but not hypoglycemia).
- Monitor patient for constipation, diarrhea, mucus discharge, or rectal bleeding suggestive of pneumatosis cystoides intestinalis. If suspected, notify prescriber and prepare patient for diagnostic imaging, as ordered. If confirmed, expect drug to be discontinued.

PATIENT TEACHING

- Explain that miglitol is an adjunct to diet, which is the primary treatment for type 2 diabetes mellitus.
- Instruct patient to take drug with first bite of each meal.
- Describe signs and symptoms of hypoglycemia and pathophysiology of diabetes to patient and family members.
- Alert patient that if miglitol is the only drug patient takes to control blood glucose level, it won't cause hypoglycemia.
- Instruct patient who takes insulin or a sulfonylurea with miglitol to keep a source of glucose readily available to reverse hypoglycemia.
- Explain importance of monitoring blood glucose levels.
- Explain that adverse GI reactions usually decrease in frequency and intensity over time.
- Teach obese patient about calorie restriction, diet, regular exercise, and weight loss, as indicated.
- Instruct patient to report to prescriber persistent or severe constipation, diarrhea, mucus discharge, or rectal bleeding.

milnacipran hydrochloride

Savella

Class and Category

Pharmacologic class: Selective norepinephrine and serotonin reuptake inhibitor (SSNRI)
Therapeutic class: Antifibromyalgia
Pregnancy category: C

Indications and Dosages

➤ *To manage fibromyalgia*

TABLETS

Adults. *Initial:* 12.5 mg on day 1; 12.5 mg twice daily on days 2 and 3; 25 mg twice daily on days 4 through 7; and then 50 mg twice daily, increased if needed to 100 mg twice daily. *Maximum:* 100 mg twice daily.
DOSAGE ADJUSTMENT For patients with severe renal impairment (creatinine clearance of 5 to 29 ml/min), maintenance dosage reduced by half.

Route	Onset	Peak	Duration
P.O.	Unknown	2–4 hr	Unknown

Mechanism of Action

Inhibits reuptake of norepinephrine and serotonin by CNS neurons without affecting uptake of dopamine or other neurotransmitters, thereby increasing amount of norepinephrine and serotonin available in nerve synapses. Elevated norepinephrine and serotonin levels may improve symptoms of fibromyalgia, including central analgesic effect.

Contraindications

Hypersensitivity to milnacipran or its components, uncontrolled narrow-angle glaucoma, use within 14 days of MAO inhibitor, including I.V. methylene blue and linezolid

Interactions

DRUGS

antipsychotics or other dopamine antagonists, MAO inhibitors, selective serotonin reuptake inhibitors, serotonin-norepinephrine reuptake inhibitors: Possibly development of

neuroleptic malignant syndrome-like reactions or serotonin syndrome
aspirin, NSAIDs, warfarin: Increased risk of bleeding
clomipramine: Increased risk of euphoria and postural hypotension
clonidine: Possibly inhibited antihypertensive effect
CNS-active drugs: Possibly increased CNS effects
digoxin (I.V.): Possibly increased risk of postural hypotension and tachycardia
epinephrine, norepinephrine: Increased risk of arrhythmias and paroxysmal hypertension
lithium: Increased risk of serotonin syndrome
MAO inhibitors: Possibly hyperpyretic episodes, hypertensive crisis, serotonin syndrome, and severe seizures
serotonergic drugs such as SSRIs, tramadol, and *triptans:* Increased risk of coronary artery vasoconstriction and hypertension

ACTIVITIES

alcohol use: Increased risk of liver impairment

Adverse Reactions

CNS: Aggression, anger, anxiety, chills, delirium, depression, dizziness, fatigue, fever, hallucinations, headache, **homicidal ideation**, hypoesthesia, insomnia, irritability, loss of consciousness, migraine, **neuroleptic malignant syndrome**, Parkinsonism, paresthesia, **seizures**, **serotonin syndrome**, **suicidal ideation**, tremor
CV: Chest pain, hypercholesterolemia, hypertension, **hypertensive crisis**, increased heart rate, palpitations, peripheral edema, **supraventricular tachycardia**, tachycardia, **Takotsubo cardiomyopathy**
EENT: Accommodation abnormality, angle closure glaucoma, blurred vision, dry mouth, mydriasis
ENDO: Galactorrhea, hot flashes, hyperprolactinemia
GI: Abdominal distention or pain, **acute pancreatitis**, anorexia, constipation, diarrhea, dyspepsia, elevated liver enzymes, gastroesophageal reflux, flatulence, **hepatitis**, jaundice, liver dysfunction, nausea, vomiting
GU: **Acute renal failure**, cystitis, decreased libido, dysuria, ejaculation disorder, erectile dysfunction, prostatitis, scrotal or testicular pain, testicular swelling, urinary hesitation, urine retention, urethral pain, UTI
HEME: **Leukopenia**, **neutropenia**, **thrombocytopenia**
MS: **Rhabdomyolysis**
RESP: Dyspnea, upper respiratory infection
SKIN: **Erythema multiforme**, flushing, hyperhidrosis, night sweats, pruritus, rash, **Stevens–Johnson syndrome**
Other: **Hyponatremia**, weight gain or loss

Nursing Considerations

- Keep in mind that because milnacipran may aggravate liver disease, it shouldn't be given to patients with alcohol addiction or chronic liver disease.
- Ensure patient has had an opthalmic examination before milnacipran therapy is begun because pupillary dilation that occurs with drug use may trigger an angle closure attack in a patient with anatomically narrow angles who does not have a patent iridectomy.
- Use cautiously in patients with cardiac disease, mild to moderate renal impairment and patients with significant hypertension. Also use cautiously in patients with a history of dysuria, especially men with prostatic hypertrophy, prostatitis, and other lower urinary tract obstructive disorders.
- Know that at least 14 days should elapse between stopping an MAO inhibitor and starting milnacipran. At least 5 days should elapse between stopping milnacipran and starting an MAO inhibitor.
- Measure patient's blood pressure and heart rate before starting and periodically during milnacipran therapy because drug can raise blood pressure and heart rate. If hypertension or tachycardia occurs and persists, notify prescriber and expect to reduce dosage or discontinue drug.
- Watch closely for suicidal tendencies, especially when therapy starts and dosage changes.

WARNING Monitor patient closely for serotonin syndrome, a rare but serious

adverse effect of selective serotonin reuptake inhibitors such as milnacipran. Signs and symptoms include agitation, confusion, diaphoresis, diarrhea, fever, hyperactive reflexes, poor coordination, restlessness, shaking, talking or acting with uncontrolled excitement, tremor, and twitching. In its most severe form, it can resemble neuroleptic malignant syndrome with autonomic instability with possible rapid fluctuation of vital signs, mental status changes, and muscle rigidity. If symptoms occur, notify prescriber immediately, expect to discontinue drug, and provide supportive care.
- Monitor patient's liver function. If jaundice or signs and symptoms of liver dysfunction occur, notify prescriber and expect drug to be discontinued.
- Watch for hypersensitivity reactions, especially in patients with aspirin sensitivity, because drug contains the yellow dye tartrazine.
- Check patient's serum sodium level, as ordered, because drug may cause hyponatremia, especially in elderly patients, patients taking diuretics, and patients who are volume-depleted.
- Expect to taper drug when no longer needed, as ordered, to minimize adverse reactions.

PATIENT TEACHING
- Urge family or caregiver to watch patient closely for suicidal tendencies, especially when therapy starts or dosage changes.
- Caution patient against stopping drug abruptly because serious adverse effects may result.
- Instruct patient to alert all prescribers that he takes milnacipran.
- Tell patient to have his blood pressure monitored regularly throughout milnacipran therapy.
- Advise patient to avoid activities, such as driving, that require alertness until the CNS effects of milnacipran are known.
- Caution patient to avoid aspirin and NSAIDs, if possible, while taking milnacipran.
- Instruct patient to notify prescriber if any persistent, severe, or unusual signs or symptoms occur.

milrinone lactate

Primacor

Class and Category
Pharmacologic class: Phosphodiesterase 3 inhibitor
Therapeutic class: Inotropic
Pregnancy category: C

Indications and Dosages
➤ *To provide short-term treatment of acute heart failure*

I.V. INFUSION

Adults. *Loading:* 50 mcg/kg over 10 min (at least 0.375 mcg/kg/min). *Usual:* 0.375 to 0.75 mcg/kg/min. *Maximum:* 1.13 mg/kg daily.

DOSAGE ADJUSTMENT Dosage adjusted according to cardiac output, pulmonary artery wedge pressure (PAWP), and clinical response. If creatinine clearance is 30 to 39 ml/min, infusion rate reduced to 0.33 mcg/kg/min; if 20 to 29 ml/min, to 0.28 mcg/kg/min; if 10 to 19 ml/min, to 0.23 mcg/kg/min; and if less than 9 ml/min, to 0.2 mcg/kg/min.

Route	Onset	Peak	Duration
I.V.	5–15 min	Unknown	3–6 hr

Incompatibilities
Don't administer milrinone through same I.V. line as furosemide because precipitate will form. Don't add other drugs to premixed milrinone flexible containers.

Contraindications
Hypersensitivity to milrinone or its components

Interactions
DRUGS

antihypertensives: Possibly hypotension

Adverse Reactions
CNS: Headache, tremor
CV: Angina, **hypotension, supraventricular arrhythmias, torsades de pointes, ventricular ectopic activity ventricular fibrillation and tachycardia, torsades de pointes**
GI: Liver function test abnormalities
HEME: Thrombocytopenia

M

Mechanism of Action

An inotropic drug, milrinone increases the force of myocardial contraction—and cardiac output—by blocking the enzyme phosphodiesterase. Normally, this enzyme is activated by hormones binding to cell membrane receptors. As shown below left, phosphodiesterase normally degrades intracellular cAMP, which restricts calcium movement into myocardial cells.

By inhibiting phosphodiesterase, as shown below right, milrinone slows the rate of cAMP degradation, increasing the intracellular cAMP level and the amount of calcium that enters myocardial cells. In blood vessels, increased cAMP causes smooth-muscle relaxation, which improves cardiac output by reducing preload and afterload.

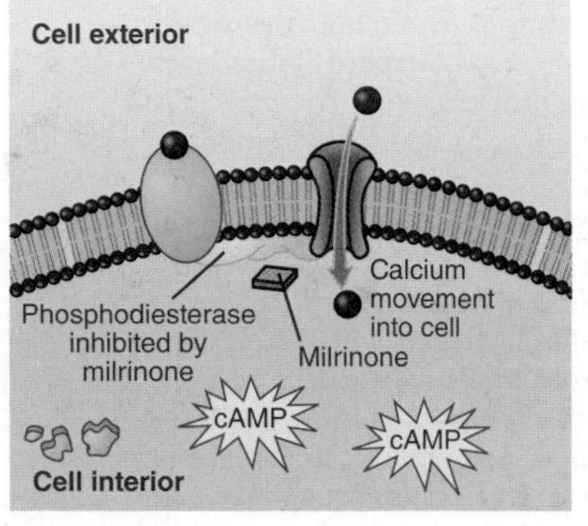

RESP: Bronchospasm
SKIN: Rash
Other: Anaphylactic shock, hypokalemia, infusion-site reactions (pain, redness, swelling)

Nursing Considerations

- Make sure ECG equipment is available for continuous monitoring during milrinone therapy.
- Discard drug if it's discolored or contains particles.
- For loading dose, infuse undiluted drug directly into I.V. line with compatible infusing solution. For continuous infusion, dilute drug with half-normal (0.45) saline solution, normal saline solution, or D_5W. Dilution isn't needed when using premixed milrinone flexible containers.
- Give loading dose using a controlled-rate infusion device. For continuous infusion, use a calibrated electronic infusion device.
- Check platelet count before and periodically during infusion, as ordered. Expect to discontinue drug if platelet count falls below 150,000/mm^3.
- Monitor blood pressure, cardiac output, fluid status, heart rate, pulmonary artery wedge pressure, and weight during therapy to determine drug effectiveness.
- Monitor liver and renal function test results and serum electrolyte levels. Notify prescriber of abnormalities.
- If severe hypotension develops, notify prescriber at once and expect to stop drug.
- Expect patient to receive digoxin before starting milrinone, which can increase ventricular response rate.

PATIENT TEACHING

- Reassure patient that he will be monitored constantly during therapy.

minocycline

Minocin

minocycline hydrochloride

Dynacin, Minocin, Novo-Minocycline (CAN), Solodyn

Class and Category

Pharmacologic class: Tetracycline
Therapeutic class: Antibiotic
Pregnancy category: D

Indications and Dosages

➤ *To treat bartonellosis, brucellosis, chancroid, granuloma inguinale, inclusion conjunctivitis, lymphogranuloma venereum, nongonococcal urethritis, plague, psittacosis, Q fever, relapsing fever, respiratory tract infections (including pneumonia), rickettsial pox, Rocky Mountain spotted fever, tularemia, typhus, and UTI caused by gram-negative organisms (including* Bartonella bacilliformis, Brucella *species,* Haemophilus ducreyi, Haemophilus influenzae, Vibriocholerae, *and* Yersinia pestis), *susceptible gram-positive organisms (including certain strains of* Streptococcus pneumoniae), *and other organisms (including* Actinomyces *species,* Bacillus anthracis, Borrelia recurrentis, Chlamydia *species,* Mycoplasma pneumoniae, *and* Rickettsiae); *as adjunct to treat intestinal amebiasis and as alternative to treat listeriosis caused by* Listeria monocytogenes, *and yaws caused by* Treponema pertenue *for nonpregnant patients allergic to penicillin*

CAPSULES, ORAL SUSPENSION, TABLETS

Adults and adolescents. *Initial:* 200 mg. *Maintenance:* 100 mg every 12 hr. Or 100 to 200 mg initially, followed by 50 mg every 6 hr.

Children over age 8. *Initial:* 4 mg/kg. *Maintenance:* 2 mg/kg every 12 hr.

I.V. INFUSION

Adults and adolescents. *Initial:* 200 mg infused over 60 min. *Maintenance:* 100 mg every 12 hr.

Children over age 8. *Initial:* 4 mg/kg. *Maintenance:* 2 mg/kg every 12 hr.

DOSAGE ADJUSTMENT For patient with renal impairment, dosage decreased or dosage interval increased; dosage not to exceed 200 mg daily.

E.R. TABLETS

Adults and adolescents age 12 and over. 1 mg/kg once daily for 12 weeks.

DOSAGE ADJUSTMENT For patient with renal impairment, dosage reduced or time interval between doses extended.

➤ *To treat uncomplicated gonorrhea from* Neisseria gonorrhoeae *in nonpregnant patients allergic to penicillin*

CAPSULES, ORAL SUSPENSION, TABLETS

Adults and adolescents. *Initial:* 200 mg. *Maintenance:* 100 mg every 12 hr for at least 4 days.

➤ *To treat uncomplicated gonococcal urethritis in men allergic to penicillin*

CAPSULES, ORAL SUSPENSION, TABLETS

Adults. 100 mg every 12 hr for 5 days.

➤ *To treat asymptomatic meningococcal carriers with* Neisseria meningitidis *in nasopharynx*

CAPSULES, ORAL SUSPENSION, TABLETS

Adults and adolescents. 100 mg every 12 hr for 5 days.

Children over age 8. *Initial:* 4 mg/kg. *Maintenance:* 2 mg/kg every 12 hr for 5 days.

➤ *To treat infections caused by* Mycobacterium marinum

CAPSULES, ORAL SUSPENSION, TABLETS

Adults. 100 mg every 12 hr for 6 to 8 wk.

➤ *To treat uncomplicated nongonococcal endocervical, rectal, or urethral infection caused by* Chlamydia trachomatis or Ureaplasma urealyticum

CAPSULES, ORAL SUSPENSION, TABLETS

Adults. 100 mg every 12 hr for at least 7 days.

➤ *To treat syphilis caused by* Treponema pallidum *in patients allergic to penicillin*

CAPSULES, ORAL SUSPENSION, TABLETS

Adults. *Initial:* 200 mg, followed by 100 mg every 12 hr for 10 to 15 days.

Route	Onset	Peak	Duration
P.O.	Unknown	2–4 hr	6–12 hr
I.V.	Unknown	Unknown	6–12 hr

Mechanism of Action
Inhibits bacterial protein synthesis by competitively binding to the 30S ribosomal subunit of the mRNA–ribosome complex of certain organisms.

Incompatibilities
Don't mix minocycline in same syringe with solution that contains calcium because precipitate will form.

Contraindications
Hypersensitivity to minocycline, other tetracyclines, or their components

Interactions
DRUGS
aluminum-, calcium-, or magnesium-containing antacids; calcium supplements; choline and magnesium salicylates; iron-containing preparations; magnesium-containing laxatives; sodium bicarbonate: Possibly formation of nonabsorbable complex, impaired minocycline absorption
cholestyramine, colestipol: Possibly impaired cholestyramine or colestipol absorption
cimetidine: Possibly decreased GI absorption and effectiveness of minocycline
digoxin: Possibly increased blood digoxin level and risk of digitalis toxicity
insulin: Possibly decreased need for insulin
iron salts: Possibly decreased GI absorption and antimicrobial effect of minocycline
isotretinoin: Possibly increased risk of pseudotumor cerebri
lithium: Possibly increased or decreased blood lithium level
methoxyflurane: Increased risk of nephrotoxicity
oral anticoagulants: Possibly potentiated anticoagulant effects
oral contraceptives containing estrogen: Decreased contraceptive effectiveness, increased risk of breakthrough bleeding
penicillin: Interference with bactericidal action of penicillin
vitamin A: Possibly benign intracranial hypertension

Adverse Reactions
CNS: Dizziness, fever, headache, **intracranial hypertension**, light-headedness, unsteadiness, vertigo
CV: **Myocarditis, pericarditis**
EENT: Blurred vision, darkened or discolored tongue, glossitis, papilledema, tooth discoloration, vision changes
ENDO: Thyroid function abnormality, **thyroid cancer**
GI: Abdominal cramps or pain, anorexia, diarrhea, dysphagia, enterocolitis, esophageal irritation and ulceration, **hepatitis, hepatotoxicity, jaundice**, indigestion, nausea, **pancreatitis, pseudomembranous colitis**, vomiting
GU: Genital candidiasis, **nephritis, nephrotoxicity**
HEME: Eosinophilia, **hemolytic anemia, neutropenia, thrombocytopenia, thrombocytopenic purpura**
MS: Arthralgia, myopathy (transient)
RESP: **Pneumonitis, pulmonary infiltrates**
SKIN: **Erythema multiforme, exfoliative dermatitis**, Brown pigmentation of skin and mucous membranes, **erythema multiforme, exfoliative dermatitis**, erythematous and maculopapular rash, onycholysis, photosensitivity, pruritus, purpura (anaphylactoid), rash, **Stevens–Johnson syndrome**, urticaria
Other: **Anaphylaxis, angioedema**, serum sickness-like reaction, systemic lupus erythematosus exacerbation

Nursing Considerations
- Use minocycline cautiously in patients with hepatic or renal dysfunction and in those taking other hepatotoxic drugs because drug may cause nephrotoxicity or hepatotoxicity.
- Use minocycline cautiously in patients with a history of predisposition to oral candidiasis, because safety and effectiveness of drug have not been established for treatment of periodontitis in patients with coexistent oral candidiasis.

WARNING Notify prescriber if patient is breastfeeding because drug appears in breast milk and may have toxic effects.

- Monitor blood, hepatic, and renal tests before and during long-term therapy.
- Shake oral suspension well before use.

- Prepare drug for I.V. use by reconstituting each 100-mg vial with 5 to 10 ml sterile water for injection. Further dilute in 500 to 1,000 ml normal saline solution, D_5W, dextrose 5% in normal saline solution, or Ringer's or lactated Ringer's solution. Administer final dilution immediately, but avoid rapid administration.
- Store reconstituted drug for I.V. administration at room temperature and use within 24 hours.
- Assess patient for signs of superinfection; if signs appear, notify prescriber, discontinue minocycline, and start appropriate therapy, as ordered.
- Monitor patient for development of foul-smelling diarrhea, which suggests *Clostridium difficile.* If present, notify prescriber, obtain stool culture, and expect to withhold minocycline and provide supportive care, as indicated and ordered.
- Monitor PT in patient who also takes an anticoagulant during minocycline therapy.
- Monitor patient for signs and symptoms of thyroid cancer such as alteration in thyroid function or presence of nodule in patients receiving minocycline therapy over prolonged periods.

WARNING Monitor patient for blurred vision or headache because benign intracranial hypertension has occurred with the use of minocycline. If present, notify prescriber and expect drug to be discontinued. Know that although intracranial hypertension usually resolves after drug is discontinued, permanent visual loss can occur. Expect patient with suspected intracranial hypertension to undergo a prompt ophthalmologic evaluation and be monitored until vision is stabilized as intracranial pressure can remain elevated for weeks after drug is discontinued.

PATIENT TEACHING

- Instruct patient to shake oral suspension well and to use calibrated measuring device.
- Advise patient to take minocycline with a full glass of water, with food or milk, and in an upright position to minimize esophageal and GI irritation.
- Direct patient to take a missed dose as soon as he remembers unless it's nearly time for the next dose. Caution against double-dosing.
- Instruct patient not to take minocycline within 2 hours of an antacid or 3 hours of an iron preparation.
- Urge patient to complete full course of treatment even if he feels better before finishing.
- Instruct patient to notify prescriber if no improvement occurs in a few days.
- Advise patient to avoid prolonged exposure to sun or sunlamps during therapy.
- Counsel female patient to avoid becoming pregnant because minocycline should be avoided, if possible, during tooth development (last half of gestation up to age 8). Drug may permanently turn teeth brown, gray, or yellow and cause enamel hypoplasia. It also may slow skeletal growth and cause congenital anomalies, including limb reduction.
- Encourage patient who uses an oral contraceptive to use additional contraceptive method during minocycline therapy.
- Instruct patient to notify prescriber immediately about blurred vision, dizziness, headache, known or suspected pregnancy, and unsteadiness.
- Explain that diarrhea may occur up to 2 months after completing therapy; urge patient to notify prescriber if it occurs.

minoxidil (oral)

Loniten

Class and Category

Pharmacologic class: Vasodilator
Therapeutic class: Antihypertensive
Pregnancy category: C

Indications and Dosages

➤ *To treat hypertension*

TABLETS

Adults and adolescents. *Initial:* 5 mg as a single dose daily. Increased, as directed, after at least 3 days with dosage above 10 mg given once daily or divided in two equal

doses daily. *Maintenance:* 10 to 40 mg daily. *Maximum:* 100 mg daily.
Children. *Initial:* 0.2 mg/kg daily. Increased, after at least 3 days. *Maintenance:* 0.25 to 1 mg/kg daily as a single dose or in divided doses twice daily. *Maximum:* 50-mg starting dose, 50 mg daily.
DOSAGE ADJUSTMENT For patient with a decrease in supine diastolic pressure more than 30 mm Hg, dosage divided into two equal doses daily. For elderly patients and those who have renal failure or are having dialysis, dosage possibly reduced.
*Topical use found in Appendix.

Route	Onset	Peak	Duration
P.O.	30 min	2–3 hr	24–48 hr

Mechanism of Action
Reduces blood pressure by inhibiting intracellular phosphodiesterase, an enzyme that facilitates hydrolysis of cAMP and cGMP. This action decreases the intracellular cAMP level, relaxes arterial smooth muscles, and lowers blood pressure. Oral minoxidil produces greater dilation in arteries than in veins. It also reduces peripheral resistance and increases cardiac output, heart rate, and stroke volume.

Contraindications
Acute MI; dissecting aortic aneurysm; hypersensitivity to minoxidil or its components, including propylene glycol; pheochromocytoma

Interactions
DRUGS
guanethidine: Possibly severe hypotension, increased risk of orthostatic hypotension
nitrates, other hypotension-producing drugs, potent parenteral antihypertensives: Possibly severe hypotension
NSAIDs, sympathomimetics: Decreased antihypertensive effects

Adverse Reactions
CNS: Fatigue, light-headedness, headache, lightheadedness, paresthesia
CV: Angina, **ECG changes**, edema, **fast or irregular heartbeat**, **heart failure**, **pericardial tamponade**, **pericarditis**, peripheral effusion rebound hypertension
ENDO: Breast tenderness
GI: Abdominal distention, ascites, nausea, vomiting
GU: Elevated BUN and serum creatinine levels
HEME: **Leukopenia**; **thrombocytopenia**; transient decrease in erythrocyte counts, and in hematocrit and hemoglobin
RESP: Dyspnea, **pulmonary hypertension**
SKIN: Bullous eruptions, flushing, hyperpigmentation, hypertrichosis, rash, **Stevens–Johnson syndrome**, **toxic epidermal necrolysis**
Other: **Hypernatremia**, weight gain

Nursing Considerations
WARNING Be aware that patient who receives guanethidine should be hospitalized before starting oral minoxidil therapy so that his blood pressure can be monitored.
- Be aware that drug isn't usually prescribed for mild hypertension.
- For rapid management of hypertension, expect to adjust dosage up to every 6 hours and to monitor patient as prescribed. Also expect to give a beta blocker and diuretic.
- Monitor progress by measuring blood pressure often and weight daily. Evaluate for signs of fluid and sodium retention and for other systemic adverse reactions.
- Watch for signs of pericardial effusion. Be prepared to stop minoxidil, if ordered.
- Expect to discontinue minoxidil gradually because abrupt discontinuation may lead to rebound hypertension.

PATIENT TEACHING
- Inform patient that minoxidil controls but doesn't cure hypertension.
- Advise him to take tablets at the same time every day.
- Teach patient to take his radial pulse, and advise him to take it daily. Instruct him to notify prescriber if it exceeds normal rate by 20 beats/minute or more.
- Emphasize the importance of daily blood pressure and weight measurements.
- Instruct patient to notify prescriber immediately about bloating, breathing problems, a fast or irregular heartbeat, flushed or red skin, swelling of feet or lower legs, or weight gain of more than 5 lb (2.3 kg) in 1 day.
- Advise patient to have regular checkups with prescriber to monitor progress.

- Urge patient to consult prescriber before taking other prescription or OTC drugs.
- Tell females of childbearing age to report known or suspected pregnancy to prescriber as neonatal hypertrichosis may occur following exposure to the drug during pregnancy.

mipomersen sodium

Kynamro

Class and Category

Pharmacologic class: Oligonucleotide
Therapeutic class: Antilipemic
Pregnancy category: B

Indications and Dosages

➤ *As adjunct to diet and lipid-lowering medications to reduce apolipoprotein B (apo B), low density lipoprotein-cholesterol (LDL-C), non-high density lipoprotein-cholesterol (non-HDL-C), and total cholesterol (TC) in patients with homozygous familial hypercholesterolemia*

SUBCUTANEOUS INJECTION
Adults. 200 mg once weekly.

Mechanism of Action

Targets human messenger ribonucleic acid (mRNA) for apo B-100, the principal apolipoprotein of low density lipoproteins (LDL) and its metabolic precursor, very low density lipoprotein (VLDL). Once targeted, translation of the apo B-100 protein is inhibited, resulting in lower lipid levels.

Contraindications

Active liver disease, hypersensitivity to mipomersen or its components, moderate or severe hepatic impairment, unexplained persistent elevations of serum transaminases

Interactions

DRUGS
other hepatotoxic drugs such as acetaminophen, amiodarone, isotretinoin, methotrexate, tamoxifen, tetracyclines: Increased risk of hepatotoxicity and hepatic steatosis

ACTIVITIES
alcohol use: Possibly increased risk of hepatic steatosis

Adverse Reactions

CNS: Chills, fatigue, fever, headache, insomnia
CV: Angina pectoris, hypertension, palpitations, peripheral edema
GI: Abdominal pain, elevated liver enzymes, hepatic steatosis, **hepatotoxicity**, nausea, transaminase elevations, vomiting
HEME: Alterations in platelet count, idiopathic thrombocytopenic purpura
MS: Extremity or musculoskeletal pain
SKIN: Rash, urticaria
Other: Angioedema, flu-like symptoms; injection-site reactions such as discoloration, erythema, hematoma, local swelling, pain, pruritus, tenderness

Nursing Considerations

- Know that because mipomersen increases risk of hepatotoxicity, the drug can only be administered through the Kynamro REMS program.
- Determine that patient has had alkaline phosphatase, transaminase levels, and total bilirubin measured prior to initiating mipomersen therapy to rule out liver impairment.
- Administer mipomersen only by subcutaneous route. Never administer drug intramuscularly or intravenously.
- Know that each vial or prefilled syringe contains 200 mg of mipomersen in 1 ml of solution and is intended for single dose only.
- Remove vial or prefilled syringe from refrigerated storage and allow to reach room temperature for at least 30 minutes prior to administration.
- Give injection on the same day every week. If a dose is missed, give injection at least 3 days from the next weekly dose. Administer injection into the patient's abdomen, outer region of the upper arm, or thigh region. Never inject drug in areas of active skin disease or injury such as inflammation, skin infections or rashes, sunburns, or psoriasis areas that are active. Also, do not inject drug into scar areas or tattooed skin.

- Be aware that transaminase levels should be measured monthly for first year of therapy and then every 3 months thereafter. If transaminase values are equal to or greater than three times upper limit normal but less than five times upper limit normal, expect to confirm elevation with a repeat measurement within 1 week. If confirmed, expect dosage to be withheld and additional liver-related tests done, such as measurement of alkaline phosphatase, total bilirubin, and INR. If transaminase elevations are five times or greater, expect drug to be withheld immediately and additional liver-related tests performed. Once transaminases level are less than three times upper limit normal, know that drug may be resumed and liver function assessed more frequently. If transaminase elevations are accompanied by signs of abnormal liver function such as abdominal pain, doubling or greater bilirubin values of upper limit normal, fever, flu-like symptoms, jaundice, lethargy, nausea, or vomiting, expect drug to be discontinued.

PATIENT TEACHING

- Remind patient of importance of adhering to the low-fat diet prescribed, as mipomersen therapy is not a replacement for dietary control of fat in her diet.
- Teach patient how to administer a subcutaneous injection and where on body to administer drug. Remind patient to rotate sites and to discard syringe and needle appropriately.
- Warn patient that flu-like symptoms may occur within 2 days of injection but does not occur with all injections. If significant, tell patient to notify prescriber.
- Tell patient to inform all prescribers about mipomersen therapy because of potential drug interactions.
- Review signs and symptoms of liver impairment and emphasize importance of reporting such to prescriber, especially stomach pain that gets worse, does not go away, or changes. Inform patient of need for blood tests to monitor her liver function and importance of compliance with test schedule.

WARNING Instruct patient not to consume more than one alcoholic beverage daily.

mirabegron

Myrbetriq

Class and Category

Pharmacologic class: Beta-3 adrenergic agonist
Therapeutic class: Bladder antispasmodic
Pregnancy category: Not classified

Indications and Dosages

➤ *To treat overactive bladder with symptoms of urge urinary incontinence, urgency, and urinary frequency as monotherapy or in combination with solifenacin succinate*

E.R. TABLETS

Adults. *Initially*: 25 mg once daily, increased as needed to 50 mg once daily (after 4 to 8 wk if used with solifenacin succinate).

DOSAGE ADJUSTMENT For patients with severe hepatic or renal impairment, dosage should not exceed 25 mg once daily.

Mechanism of Action

Relaxes the detrusor smooth muscle during the storage phase of the urinary bladder fill-void cycle by activating the beta-3 adrenergic receptor, which increases bladder capacity. With increased bladder capacity, urge sensation is decreased, which in turn decreases urinary frequency.

Contraindications

Hypersensitivity to mirabegron or its components

Interactions

DRUGS

CYP2D6 substrates such as desipramine, flecainide, metoprolol, propafenone, thioridazine: Increased blood levels of these drugs
digoxin: Increased risk of digoxin toxicity

Adverse Reactions

CNS: Anxiety, confusion, dizziness, fatigue, hallucinations, headache, insomnia
CV: Atrial fibrillation, hypertension, elevated LDH levels, palpitations, tachycardia

EENT: Dry mouth, glaucoma, nasopharyngitis, rhinitis, sinusitis
GI: Abdominal distention or pain, constipation, diarrhea, dyspepsia, elevated liver enzymes, gastritis, nausea
GU: Bladder pain, cystitis, nephrolithiasis, **prostate cancer**, urinary retention, UTI, vaginal infections, vulvovaginal pruritis
MS: Arthralgia, back pain
SKIN: Pruritis, rash, **Stevens–Johnson syndrome**
Other: **Angioedema**, influenza-like infection

Nursing Considerations

- Know that mirabegron should not be given to patients with severe uncontrolled hypertension (defined as systolic blood pressure 180 mm Hg or higher and/or diastolic blood pressure 110 mm Hg or higher) because drug can increase blood pressure. Monitor patient's blood pressure regularly and report persistent or significant increases to prescriber.
- Be aware that mirabegron should not be given to patients with end stage renal disease or in patients with severe hepatic impairment because drug has not been studied in these conditions, and adverse effects are unknown.
- Use mirabegron cautiously in patients with bladder outlet obstruction and in patients taking antimuscarinic drugs for the treatment of this condition because the drug may cause urinary retention.

WARNING Monitor patient closely for angioedema of the face, larynx, lips, and tongue, which may occur as soon as the first dose or hours after the first dose or after multiple doses. Be prepared to administer emergency treatment for life-threatening upper airway swelling, as ordered, and maintain a patent airway. Notify prescriber and expect drug to be discontinued.

- Keep in mind that it may take up to 8 weeks to observe efficacy with 25 mg strength

PATIENT TEACHING

- Instruct patient to take mirabegron with water and to swallow tablet whole. Caution patient not to chew, crush, or divide tablets prior to ingesting.
- Warn patient that drug may increase blood pressure. Encourage patient to have his blood pressure checked regularly, especially if he has hypertension.
- Review common adverse effects of drug with patient. Tell patient to notify prescriber if he experiences a decrease in urinary output despite a normal intake. Also remind patient that drug may cause itching, rapid heartbeat, rash, or urinary tract infections and to alert prescriber if present.

mirtazapine

Remeron, Remeron SolTab

Class and Category

Pharmacologic class: Tetracyclic antidepressant
Therapeutic class: Antidepressant
Pregnancy category: C

Indications and Dosages

➤ *To treat major depression*

DISINTEGRATING TABLETS, TABLETS

Adults. *Initial:* 15 mg daily, preferably at bedtime. Increased as needed and tolerated at 1- to 2-wk intervals. *Maximum:* 45 mg daily.

Route	Onset	Peak	Duration
P.O.	1–2 wk	6 wk or longer	Unknown

Mechanism of Action

May inhibit neuronal reuptake of norepinephrine and serotonin. By doing so, this tetracyclic antidepressant increases the action of these neurotransmitters in nerve cells. Increased neuronal serotonin and norepinephrine levels may elevate mood.

Contraindications

Hypersensitivity to mirtazapine or its components; use within 14 days of an MAO inhibitor, including I.V. methylene blue and linezolid

Interactions

DRUGS

antihypertensives: Increased hypotensive effects of these drugs or enhanced mirtazapine effects
anxiolytics, hypnotics, other CNS depressants (including sedatives): Increased CNS depression

MAO inhibitors, I.V. methylene blue and linezolid, other serotonergic drugs: Possibly hyperpyrexia, hypertension, seizures, and serotonin syndrome

ACTIVITIES

alcohol use: Increased CNS depression

Adverse Reactions

CNS: Agitation, akathisia, amnesia, anxiety, apathy, asthenia, ataxia, **cerebral ischemia**, chills, confusion, delirium, delusions, depersonalization, depression, dizziness, dream disturbances, drowsiness, dyskinesia, dystonia, emotional lability, euphoria, extrapyramidal reactions, fever, hallucinations, hostility, hyperkinesia, hyperreflexia, hypoesthesia, hypokinesia, lack of coordination, malaise, mania, migraine headache, **neuroleptic malignant syndrome-like reactions**, neurosis, paranoia, paresthesia, psychomotor restlessness, **seizures**, **serotonin syndrome**, somnolence, syncope, tremor, vertigo
CV: Angina, **bradycardia**, edema, hypercholesterolemia, hypertension, hypertriglyceridemia, **hypotension**, **MI**, orthostatic hypotension, peripheral edema, **PVCs**, **torsades de pointes**, vasodilation, **ventricular arrhythmia**
EENT: Accommodation disturbances, conjunctivitis, dry mouth, earache, epistaxis, eye pain, gingival bleeding, glaucoma, glossitis, hearing loss, hyperacusis, keratoconjunctivitis, lacrimation, pharyngitis, sinusitis, stomatitis
ENDO: Breast pain
GI: Abdominal distention and pain, anorexia, cholecystitis, colitis, constipation, elevated ALT level, eructation, increased appetite, nausea, thirst, vomiting
GU: Amenorrhea, cystitis, dysmenorrhea, dysuria, hematuria, impotence, increased libido, leukorrhea, renal calculi, urinary frequency and incontinence, urine retention, UTI, vaginitis
HEME: Agranulocytosis, **neutropenia**
MS: Arthralgia, back pain, dysarthria, elevated creatine kinase blood level, muscle twitching, myalgia, myasthenia, neck pain and rigidity, **rhabdomyolysis**
RESP: Asthma, bronchitis, cough, dyspnea, pneumonia
SKIN: Acne, alopecia, bullous dermatitis, dry skin, **erythema multiforme**, **exfoliative dermatitis**, photosensitivity, pruritus, rash, **Stevens–Johnson syndrome**, **toxic epidermal necrolysis**
Other: Angioedema, dehydration, flu-like symptoms, herpes simplex, **hyponatremia**, weight change

Nursing Considerations

- Use mirtazapine cautiously in elderly patients and in those receiving concurrent medication known to cause hyponatremia because drug may lower the serum sodium level in these patients.
- Administer mirtazapine before bedtime.
- Expect disintegrating tablet to dissolve on patient's tongue within 30 seconds.

WARNING Don't give drug within 14 days of an MAO inhibitor or concurrent therapy with serotonin-precursors such as L-tryptophan and oxitriptan to avoid serious, possibly fatal, serotonin syndrome reaction. Use drug cautiously in patients receiving other serotonergic drugs such as lithium, St. John's wort, tramadol, triptans, and most tricyclic antidepressants because of increased risk for serotonin syndrome. Know that both disorders can occur as an adverse drug reaction to mirtazapine therapy without the concomitant use of other drugs. Monitor patient closely for signs and symptoms of serotonin syndrome such as alteration in vital signs, gastrointestinal symptoms, mental status changes, or neuromuscular abnormalities. Its most severe form resembles neuroleptic malignant syndrome and presents with autonomic instability with possible rapid changes in vital signs, hyperthermia, mental status changes, and muscle rigidity. If any of these symptoms occur, notify prescriber immediately, provide supportive care, as ordered, and expect mirtazapine to be discontinued.

- Monitor patient closely, especially during the first few weeks of therapy, for the development of akathisia, an unpleasant or distressing restlessness and need to move, often accompanied by an inability to sit or stand still. Notify prescriber, if present, and know that increasing the dose may worsen patient's condition.
- Watch closely for suicidal tendencies, especially when therapy starts or dosage changes, because depression may briefly worsen.

- Monitor patient closely for infection (fever, pharyngitis, stomatitis), which may be linked to a low WBC count. If these signs occur, notify prescriber and expect to stop drug.
- Expect mirtazapine therapy to last 6 months or longer for acute depression.
- Be aware that mirtazapine therapy should not be discontinued abruptly because adverse reactions may occur.

PATIENT TEACHING

- Instruct patient not to swallow disintegrating tablet. Tell him to hold tablet on tongue and let it dissolve. Inform him that tablet will dissolve within 30 seconds.
- Inform phenylketonuric patient that mirtazapine disintegrating tablets contain phenlyalanine 2.6 mg per 15-mg tablet, 5.2 mg per 30-mg tablet, and 7.8 mg per 45-mg tablet.
- Advise patient that drug may cause mild pupillary dilation, which may lead to an episode of acute closure glaucoma. Encourage patient to have an eye exam before starting therapy to see if he is at risk.
- Instruct patient to avoid alcohol and other CNS depressants during therapy and for up to 7 days after drug is discontinued.
- Advise patient to avoid hazardous activities until drug's CNS effects are known.
- Direct patient to change position slowly to minimize the effects of orthostatic hypotension.
- Instruct patient to notify prescriber at once about chills, fever, mouth irritation, sore throat, and other signs of infection.
- Encourage patient to visit prescriber regularly during therapy to monitor progress.
- Caution patient not to discontinue mirtazapine therapy abruptly.

misoprostol

Cytotec

Class and Category

Pharmacologic class: Prostaglandin E_1 analogue
Therapeutic class: Antiulcer
Pregnancy category: X

Indications and Dosages

➤ *To prevent NSAID-induced gastric ulcers*

TABLETS

Adults. 200 mcg four times daily with last dose at bedtime every day.

DOSAGE ADJUSTMENT Dosage reduced to 100 mcg four times daily if patient can't tolerate 200-mcg dose.

Route	Onset	Peak	Duration
P.O.	30 min	60–90 min	3–6 hr

Mechanism of Action

May protect the stomach from NSAID-induced mucosal damage by increasing gastric mucus production and mucosal bicarbonate secretion. Misoprostol also inhibits gastric acid secretion caused by such stimuli as coffee, food, and histamine.

Contraindications

Hypersensitivity to misoprostol, other prostaglandins or their analogues; pregnancy

Interactions

DRUGS

magnesium-containing antacids: Increased misoprostol-induced diarrhea

Adverse Reactions

CNS: Anxiety, asthenia, chills, confusion, **CVA**, depression, drowsiness, dizziness, fatigue, fever, headache, neuropathy, neurosis, rigors, syncope, thirst
CV: **Arrhythmias**, chest pain, edema, hypertension, **hypotension**, **increased cardiac enzyme levels**, **MI**, phlebitis, **thromboembolism**
EENT: Abnormal taste or vision, conjunctivitis, deafness, earache, epistaxis, gingivitis, tinnitus
ENDO: Hyperglycemia
GI: Abdominal pain, constipation, diarrhea, dysphagia, flatulence, **GI bleeding** or inflammation, **hepatobiliary dysfunction**, indigestion, nausea, reflux, vomiting
GU: Dysmenorrhea, dysuria, hematuria, hypermenorrhea, impotence, loss of libido, menstrual irregularities, polyuria, urinary tract infection, vaginal bleeding

M

HEME: Anemia, **abnormal differential thrombocytopenia purpura**, increased erythrocyte sedimentation rate
MS: Arthralgia, back pain, myalgia, muscle cramps or stiffness
RESP: Bronchitis, **bronchospasm**, dyspnea, pneumonia, **pulmonary embolism**, upper respiratory tract infection
SKIN: Alopecia, diaphoresis, dermatitis, pallor, rash
Other: **Anaphylaxis**, gout, weight changes

Nursing Considerations

WARNING Anticipate female patients having a pregnancy test done before misoprostol therapy is begun, because it can cause teratogenic effects in the fetus. In addition, it may cause contractions, spontaneous abortion, and uterine bleeding or rupture if patient is pregnant. Drug is contraindicated in pregnancy for these reasons.

- Use drug cautiously in patients with cerebrovascular disease, coronary artery disease, or uncontrolled epilepsy because of the risk of severe complications.
- Also use misoprostol cautiously in patients with inflammatory bowel disease because drug may worsen intestinal inflammation and cause diarrhea. If diarrhea causes severe dehydration, misoprostol may need to be discontinued.

PATIENT TEACHING

- Caution female patient about risk of taking misoprostol during pregnancy, and urge her to use reliable contraception during therapy. Urge her to notify prescriber at once if she is or might be pregnant.
- Instruct patient to take misoprostol with meals and at bedtime.
- Advise patient that he may take NSAIDs, if prescribed, during misoprostol therapy.
- Explain that diarrhea is dose related and usually resolves after 8 days. Tell patient to avoid magnesium-containing antacids because they may worsen diarrhea and to call prescriber if diarrhea lasts more than 8 days.
- Urge female patient to notify prescriber immediately about postmenopausal bleeding; she may need diagnostic tests.

mitoxantrone hydrochloride

Novantrone

Class and Category

Pharmacologic class: Anthracenedione
Therapeutic class: Antineoplastic
Pregnancy category: D

Indications and Dosages

➤ *To reduce neurologic disability and frequency of relapses in patients with secondary (chronic) progressive, progressive relapsing, or worsening relapsing-remitting multiple sclerosis (patients whose neurologic status is significantly abnormal between relapses)*

I.V. INFUSION

Adults. 12 mg/m^2 over 5 to 15 min every 3 mo. *Maximum:* Cumulative dose of 140 mg/m^2.

➤ *As adjunct to treat pain related to advanced hormone-refractory prostate cancer*

I.V. INFUSION

Adults. 12 to 14 mg/m^2 over 5 to 15 min every 21 days.

➤ *As adjunct to treat acute nonlymphocytic leukemia (ANLL)*

I.V. INFUSION

Adults. *Initial:* 12 mg/m^2 over 5 to 15 min on days 1 to 3 with 100 mg/m^2 of cytarabine as a continuous 24-hr infusion on days 1 to 7. If patient's antileukemic response is inadequate or incomplete, second induction course is given at same dosage but only for 2 days with mitoxantrone and 5 days for cytarabine.

Mechanism of Action

Binds to DNA, causing cross-linkage and strand breakage, interfering with RNA synthesis, and inhibiting topoisomerase II, an enzyme that uncoils and repairs damaged DNA. Mitoxantrone produces a cytocidal effect on proliferating and nonproliferating cells and doesn't appear to be cell-cycle specific. It's known to inhibit B-cell, T-cell, and macrophage proliferation and impair antigen function.

Incompatibilities

Don't mix mitoxantrone in the same infusion as heparin (because a precipitate may form); don't mix with any other drugs.

Contraindications

Hypersensitivity to mitoxantrone or its components

Interactions

DRUGS

allopurinol, colchicine, probenecid, sulfinpyrazone: Possibly interference with antihyperuricemic action of these drugs
blood-dyscrasia-causing drugs (such as cephalosporins and sulfasalazine): Increased risk of leukopenia and thrombocytopenia
bone marrow depressants, such as carboplatin and lomustine: Possibly additive bone marrow depression
daunorubicin, doxorubicin: Increased risk of cardiotoxicity
methotrexate and other antineoplastics: Risk of developing leukemia
vaccines, killed virus: Decreased antibody response to vaccine
vaccines, live virus: Increased risk of replication of and adverse effects of vaccine virus, decreased antibody response to vaccine

Adverse Reactions

CNS: Headache, **seizures**
CV: **Arrhythmias**, **cardiotoxicity**, chest pain, **congestive heart failure**, decreased left ventricular ejection fraction, **ECG changes**
EENT: Blue-colored cornea, conjunctivitis, mucositis, stomatitis
GI: Abdominal pain, diarrhea, elevated liver enzymes, **GI bleeding**, jaundice, nausea, vomiting
GU: Blue-green urine, **renal failure**
HEME: **Acute myelogenous leukemia**, **leukopenia**, **other leukemias**, **thrombocytopenia**
MS: Myelodysplasia
RESP: Cough, dyspnea
SKIN: Alopecia, extravasation
Other: **Anaphylaxis**, **hypersensitivity reactions**, hyperuricemia, infection, infusion-site pain or redness

Nursing Considerations

- Before mitoxantrone therapy and before each dose, expect patient to have an ECG and evaluation of left ventricular ejection fraction. Expect to obtain CBC with platelet count, and hematocrit and hemoglobin level(s). If patient's left ventricular ejection fraction drops below normal, expect drug to be discontinued.
- Be aware that drug shouldn't be given to patient with multiple sclerosis whose neutrophil count is less than $1,500/mm^3$ or who has a below-normal left ventricular ejection fraction.
- Check liver enzymes, as ordered, before each course of therapy. Expect that drug won't be given to multiple sclerosis patient with abnormal liver function.
- Assess patient for cardiac dysfunction throughout therapy. Watch for evidence of cardiotoxicity, such as arrhythmias and chest pain, in patient with heart disease. Risk increases when cumulative dose reaches 140 mg/m^2 in cancer or 100 mg/m^2 in multiple sclerosis. Notify prescriber of any significant changes, and expect drug to be discontinued. Be aware that congestive heart failure may occur months or years after drug has been discontinued.
- Anticipate obtaining pregnancy test before each course of therapy for women of childbearing age with multiple sclerosis.
- Follow facility policy for handling antineoplastics. Be aware that manufacturer recommends goggles, gloves, and a gown during drug preparation and delivery.
- Before infusing drug, dilute it in at least 50 ml of normal saline solution or D_5W.

WARNING **Know that drug shouldn't be given intrathecally because paralysis may occur.**

- Know that if mitoxantrone solution contacts skin or mucosa, the area should be washed thoroughly with warm water. If it contacts eyes, irrigate them thoroughly with water or normal saline solution.
- Discard unused diluted solution because it contains no preservatives. After penetration of stopper, store undiluted drug for up to 7 days at room temperature or 14 days refrigerated. Avoid freezing drug.

M

- If extravasation occurs, stop infusion immediately and notify prescriber. Reinsert I.V. line in another vein and resume infusion. Although mitoxantrone is a nonvesicant, observe the extravasation site for signs of necrosis or phlebitis.
- Monitor patients with chickenpox or recent exposure and patients with herpes zoster for severe, generalized disease.
- Monitor blood uric acid level for hyperuricemia in patients with a history of gout or renal calculi. Expect to give allopurinol, as prescribed, to patients with leukemia or lymphoma and elevated blood uric acid level to prevent uric acid nephropathy.

WARNING **Be aware that if severe or life-threatening nonhematologic or hematologic toxicity occurs during first induction course, the second course will probably be withheld until it resolves.**

- Know that if patient develops thrombocytopenia, precautions should be taken per facility policy.
- Assess patient for evidence of infection, such as fever, if leukopenia occurs. Expect to obtain appropriate specimens for culture and sensitivity testing.
- Be aware that patients receiving mitoxantrone in combination with other antineoplastics or radiation therapy or who have multiple sclerosis are at risk for developing secondary leukemia, including acute myelogenous leukemia.

PATIENT TEACHING

- Advise patient to complete dental work, if possible, before treatment begins or defer it until blood counts return to normal; drug may delay healing and cause gingival bleeding. Teach patient proper oral hygiene, and advise use of a toothbrush with soft bristles.
- Urge patient to drink plenty of fluid to increase urine output and uric acid excretion.
- Advise patient to contact prescriber immediately if GI upset occurs, but to continue taking drug unless otherwise directed.
- Emphasize the importance of complying with the dosage regimen and keeping follow-up medical and laboratory appointments.
- Explain that urine may appear blue-green for 24 hours after treatment and that the whites of the eyes may appear blue. Emphasize that these effects are temporary and harmless. Explain that hair loss is possible, but that hair should return after therapy ends.
- Caution patient not to receive immunizations unless approved by prescriber. Also, advise persons who live in same household as patient to avoid receiving immunization with oral polio vaccine. Tell patient to avoid persons who recently received the oral polio vaccine or to wear a mask over his nose and mouth.
- Instruct patient to avoid persons with infections if bone marrow depression occurs. Advise patient to contact prescriber if chills, cough, fever, hoarseness, lower back or side pain, or difficult or painful urination occurs; these changes may signal an infection.
- Tell patient to contact prescriber immediately if he has black or tarry stools, unusual bleeding or bruising, blood in urine or stool, or pinpoint red spots on his skin.
- Urge patient not to touch his eyes or the inside of his nose unless he has just washed his hands.
- Emphasize the need to avoid accidental cuts, as from fingernail clippers or a razor, because of possible excessive bleeding or infection.
- Caution patient to avoid contact sports or activities that may cause bruising or injury.
- Urge patient to comply with yearly examinations after therapy ends to check for late-occurring drug-induced heart problems. Tell patient to report trouble breathing, swelling in ankles or legs, or a fast or uneven heartbeat even after drug has been discontinued.

modafinil

Provigil

Class, Category, and Schedule

Pharmacologic class: Analeptic
Therapeutic class: CNS stimulant
Pregnancy category: C
Controlled substance schedule: IV

Indications and Dosages

➤ *To improve daytime wakefulness in patients with narcolepsy, obstructive sleep apnea hypopnea syndrome, and shift work sleep disorder*

TABLETS

Adults. 200 mg daily in the morning or 1 hr before starting work shift. *Maximum:* 400 mg daily.

DOSAGE ADJUSTMENT For patients with severe hepatic impairment, dosage should be reduced by 50%.

Mechanism of Action

May inhibit the release of gamma-aminobutyric acid (GABA), the most common inhibitory neurotransmitter, or CNS depressant, in the brain. Modafinil also increases the release of glutamate, an excitatory neurotransmitter, or CNS stimulant, in the hippocampus and thalamus. These two actions may improve wakefulness.

Contraindications

Hypersensitivity to modafinil or its components

Interactions

DRUGS

amitriptyline, citalopram, clomipramine, diazepam, imipramine, propranolol, tolbutamide, topiramate: Possibly prolonged elimination time and increased blood levels of these drugs

carbamazepine: Possibly decreased modafinil effectiveness and decreased blood carbamazepine level

cimetidine, clarithromycin, erythromycin, fluconazole, fluoxetine, fluvoxamine, itraconazole, ketoconazole, nefazodone, sertraline: Possibly inhibited metabolism, decreased clearance, and increased blood level of modafinil

contraceptive-containing implants or devices, oral contraceptives: Possibly contraceptive failure

cyclosporine: Possibly decreased blood cyclosporine level and increased risk of organ transplant rejection

dexamethasone, phenobarbital and other barbiturates, primidone, rifabutin, rifampin: Possibly decreased blood level and effectiveness of modafinil

dextroamphetamine, methylphenidate: Possibly 1-hour delay in modafinil absorption when these drugs are given together

fosphenytoin, mephenytoin, phenytoin: Possibly decreased effectiveness of modafinil, increased blood phenytoin level, and increased risk of phenytoin toxicity

theophylline: Possibly decreased blood level and effectiveness of theophylline

triazolam: Possibly decreased effectiveness of triazolam

warfarin: Possibly decreased warfarin metabolism and increased risk of bleeding

FOODS

all foods: 1-hour delay in modafinil absorption and possibly delayed onset of action

caffeine: Increased CNS stimulation

grapefruit juice: Possibly decreased modafinil metabolism

Adverse Reactions

CNS: Aggressiveness, agitation, anxiety, confusion, delusions, depression, hallucinations, headache, insomnia, mania, nervousness, psychomotor hyperactivity, psychosis, **suicidal ideation**

GI: Nausea

HEME: Agranulocytosis

SKIN: Rash, **Stevens–Johnson syndrome**, **toxic epidermal necrolysis**

Other: Anaphylaxis, **angioedema**, **drug reaction with eosinophilia and systemic symptoms (DRESS)**, infection, **multiorgan hypersensitivity**

Nursing Considerations

- Keep in mind that modafinil shouldn't be given to patients with mitral valve prolapse syndrome or a history of left ventricular hypertrophy because drug may cause ischemic changes.
- Use cautiously in patients with recent MI or unstable angina because effect of drug is unknown in these disorders.
- Use cautiously in patients with a history of depression, mania, or psychosis because these conditions may worsen during therapy and may require modafinil to be stopped.

WARNING Monitor patient with a history of alcoholism, stimulant abuse, or other substance abuse for compliance with

M

modafinil therapy. Observe for signs of abuse or misuse, including drug seeking behavior, frequent prescription refill requests, or increased frequency of dosing. Also watch for evidence of excessive modafinil dosage, including aggressiveness, anxiety, confusion, decreased prothrombin time, diarrhea, irritability, nausea, nervousness, palpitations, sleep disturbances, and tremor.

- Be aware that modafinil, like other CNS stimulants, may alter feelings, judgment mood, motor skills, perception, thinking, and signs that patient needs sleep.
- Know that if giving drug to patient with emotional instability, a history of psychosis, or psychological illness with psychotic features, be prepared to perform baseline behavioral assessments or frequent clinical observation.
- Stop drug at first sign of rash, and notify prescriber. Although rare, rash may indicate a potentially life-threatening event.
- Monitor patient for signs and symptoms of multisystem organ hypersensitivity, such as asthenia, fever, hematologic abnormalities, hepatitis, myocarditis, pruritus, rash, or any other serious abnormality, because multiorgan hypersensitivity may vary in its presentation. Notify prescriber if suspected, and expect to discontinue drug and provide supportive care, as ordered.
- Watch closely for suicidal tendencies, especially in patients with a psychiatric history.

PATIENT TEACHING

- Inform patient that modafinil can help, but not cure, narcolepsy and that drug's full effects may not be seen right away.
- Advise patient to avoid taking modafinil within 1 hour of eating because food may delay drug's absorption and onset of action. If he drinks grapefruit juice, encourage him to drink a consistent amount daily.
- Instruct patient to stop taking modafinil and to notify prescriber if he develops a fever, rash, or other serious effect.
- Urge patient to report anxiety, chest pain, depression, or evidence of mania or psychosis to prescriber.
- Inform patient that drug can affect concentration and function and can hide signs of fatigue. Urge him not to drive or perform activities that require mental alertness until full CNS effects are known.
- Advise patient to avoid alcohol while taking modafinil.
- Encourage a regular sleeping pattern.
- Caution patient to avoid excessive intake of beverages, foods, and OTC drugs that contain caffeine because caffeine may lead to increased CNS stimulation.
- Inform female patient that modafinil can decrease the effectiveness of certain contraceptives, including birth control pills and implantable hormonal contraceptives. If she uses such contraceptives, urge her to use an alternate birth control method during modafinil therapy and for up to 1 month after she stops taking the drug.
- Advise patient to keep follow-up appointments with prescriber so that her progress can be monitored.
- Urge family or caregiver to watch patient closely for abnormal behaviors, including suicidal tendencies, especially if patient has a psychiatric history.

moexipril hydrochloride

Univasc

Class and Category

Pharmacologic class: Angiotensin converting enzyme (ACE) inhibitor
Therapeutic class: Antihypertensive
Pregnancy category: D

Indications and Dosages

➤ *To manage hypertension without diuretic therapy*

TABLETS

Adults. *Initial:* 7.5 mg daily 1 hr before a meal. *Maintenance:* 7.5 to 30 mg as a single dose or in divided doses twice daily. 1 hr before meals. *Maximum:* 30 mg/day.

DOSAGE ADJUSTMENT For patients with creatinine clearance of 40 ml/min or less, initial dosage reduced to 3.75 mg daily and increased, as ordered, to maximum of 15 mg daily.

➤ *To manage hypertension with diuretic therapy*

TABLETS

Adults. *Initial:* 3.75 mg daily 1 hr before a meal. Increased gradually, as ordered, until blood pressure is controlled.

Route	Onset	Peak	Duration
P.O.	1 hr	3–6 hr	24 hr

Mechanism of Action

Is converted to the active metabolite moexiprilat, which reduces blood pressure by inhibiting ACE activity. ACE normally catalyzes conversion of angiotensin I to angiotensin II—a vasoconstrictor that stimulates aldosterone secretion by adrenal cortex and directly suppresses renin release. Inhibited ACE activity results in decreased aldosterone secretion, decreased peripheral arterial resistance, and increased plasma renin activity. Decreased aldosterone secretion causes water and sodium excretion.

Contraindications

Concurrent aliskiren (in patients with diabetes), history of angioedema with previous ACE inhibitor use, hypersensitivity to moexipril or its components

Interactions

DRUGS

aliskiren (in patients with diabetes), angiotensin receptor blockers, other ACE inhibitors: Increased risk of hyperkalemia, hypotension, and renal dysfunction
allopurinol, bone marrow depressants, corticosteroids (systemic), cytostatic drugs, procainamide: Increased risk of possibly fatal neutropenia or agranulocytosis
antacids: Possibly decreased moexipril bioavailability
cyclosporine, heparin, potassium-containing drugs, potassium-sparing diuretics, potassium supplements: Increased risk of hyperkalemia
digoxin: Possibly increased digoxin level
diuretics, other hypotension-producing drugs: Hypotension, risk of renal failure (from sodium or volume depletion), possibly decreased secondary aldosteronism and hypokalemia caused by diuretics
lithium: Increased blood lithium level and risk of lithium toxicity
NSAIDs: Decreased antihypertensive effect of moexipril; possible decreased renal function in patients who are elderly or have volume-depletion or preexisting renal dysfunction
phenothiazines: Increased pharmacologic effects of moexipril
sympathomimetics: Decreased antihypertensive effect of moexipril
sodium aurothiomalate: Possibly nitritoid reaction with facial flushing, hypotension, nausea, and vomiting

FOODS

all foods: Decreased moexipril absorption
low-salt milk, salt substitutes: Possibly hyperkalemia

ACTIVITIES

alcohol use: Possibly hypotension

Adverse Reactions

CNS: Anxiety, chills, confusion, **CVA**, dizziness, drowsiness, fatigue, fever, headache, malaise, mood changes, nervousness, sleep disturbance, syncope
CV: Angina, **arrhythmias**, chest pain, **hypotension**, **MI**, orthostatic hypotension, palpitations, peripheral edema
EENT: Dry mouth, hoarseness, **laryngeal edema**, mouth or tongue swelling, pharyngitis, rhinitis, sinusitis, taste perversion, tinnitus
GI: Abdominal distention or pain, anorexia, constipation, diarrhea, dysphagia, elevated liver enzymes, **hepatitis**, increased appetite, nausea, **pancreatitis**, vomiting
GU: **Azotemia**, elevated BUN and serum creatinine and uric acid levels, interstitial nephritis, oliguria, proteinuria, **renal insufficiency**, urinary frequency
HEME: **Agranulocytosis**, **bone marrow depression**, elevated erythrocyte sedimentation rate, **hemolytic anemia**, leukocytosis, **leukopenia**, **neutropenia**, **thrombocytopenia**
MS: Arthralgia, leg heaviness or weakness, myalgia, myositis
RESP: **Bronchospasm**, cough, dyspnea, upper respiratory tract infection

SKIN: Alopecia, diaphoresis, flushing, onycholysis, pallor, pemphigus, photosensitivity, pruritus, rash, **Stevens–Johnson syndrome**, urticaria
Other: **Anaphylaxis**, **angioedema**, flu-like symptoms, **hyperkalemia**, **hyponatremia**, positive ANA titer

Nursing Considerations

WARNING Contact prescriber if patient is or may be pregnant. Moexipril may cause fetal or neonatal harm or death if used during second or third trimester.

- Be aware that patient who already takes a diuretic should be medically supervised for several hours after first moexipril dose.
- Administer drug 1 hour before meals.
- Monitor blood pressure, leukocyte count, and liver and renal function test results during moexipril therapy.
- Be aware that black patients may be less responsive to antihypertensive effect if moexipril is used alone to control blood pressure.

PATIENT TEACHING

- Urge female patient to notify prescriber immediately if she is or may be pregnant.
- Instruct patient to take moexipril at the same time each day, 1 hour before meals.
- Direct patient to take a missed dose as soon as he remembers unless it's nearly time for the next dose. Caution against doubling the dose.

WARNING Instruct patient to stop drug and seek immediate medical attention for hoarseness; swelling of face, feet, glottis, hands, larynx, or tongue; or sudden difficulty breathing or swallowing.

- Caution patient not to stop drug without consulting prescriber, even if he feels better.
- Inform patient about possible dizziness, especially after first dose and if he takes a diuretic.
- Advise patient to change position slowly to minimize orthostatic hypotension.
- Caution patient to avoid hazardous activities until drug's CNS effects are known.
- Instruct patient to notify prescriber if he faints or experiences persistent dizziness.
- Instruct patient to report evidence of infection (such as chills, fever, and sore throat), diarrhea, nausea, or vomiting, which may lead to dehydration-induced hypotension.
- Advise patient to avoid alcohol during moexipril therapy because it may cause hypotension.
- Instruct patient to check with prescriber before taking OTC drugs.
- Urge patient to avoid potassium supplements and potassium-containing salt substitutes unless prescriber allows them.
- Advise patient to visit prescriber regularly to monitor progress.
- Discuss importance of weight control and low-salt diet in managing hypertension.

mometasone furoate

Asmanex Twisthaler

mometasone furoate monohydrate

Nasonex

Class and Category

Pharmacologic class: Glucocorticoid
Therapeutic class: Anti-inflammatory
Pregnancy category: C

Indications and Dosages

➤ *To manage symptoms of seasonal or perennial allergic rhinitis*

NASAL SPRAY

Adults and children 12 years and over. 100 mcg (2 sprays) in each nostril daily.
Children ages 2 to 12. 50 mcg (1 spray) in each nostril daily.

➤ *To prevent seasonal allergic rhinitis*

NASAL SPRAY (NASONEX)

Adults and adolescents 12 years and over. 100 mcg (2 sprays) in each nostril daily, started 2 to 4 wk prior to anticipated start of pollen season, if known.

➤ *To treat nasal polyps*

NASAL SPRAY (NASONEX)
Adults. 100 mcg (2 sprays) in each nostril once or twice daily.
➤ *To maintain asthma control*
ORAL INHALATION (ASMANEX TWISTHALER)
Adults and children age 12 and over who have been taking bronchodilators alone or inhaled corticosteroids. *Initial:* 220 mcg (1 inhalation) once daily in evening. *Maximum:* 440 mcg (2 inhalations) daily given as 220 mcg (1 inhalation) twice daily or 440 mcg (1 inhalation) once daily.
Adults and children age 12 and over who have taken oral corticosteroids. 440 mcg (2 inhalations) twice daily.
Children ages 4 to 11. 110 mcg (1 inhalation) once daily in evening.

Mechanism of Action

Inhibits the activity of cells and mediators active in the inflammatory response, possibly by decreasing influx of inflammatory cells into nasal passages and thereby decreasing nasal inflammation.

Inflammation is a key component in asthma pathophysiology. Decreasing the inflammatory response in lung tissue helps to relieve asthma symptoms.

Contraindications

Hypersensitivity to mometasone or its components or to milk proteins; recent nasal surgery, nasal trauma, or septal ulcers; status asthmaticus or other asthma episodes that require emergency care

Interactions

DRUGS
strong CYP4503A4 inhibitors such as atazanavir, clarithromycin, cobicistat-containing products, indinavir, itraconazole, ketoconazole, nefazodone, nelfinavir, ritonavir, saquinavir, telithromycin: Increased plasma mometasone levels leading to possible increased adverse reactions

Adverse Reactions

CNS: Headache
CV: Chest pain
EENT: Blurred vision, cataracts, conjunctivitis, dry mouth, earache, epistaxis, glaucoma, nasal irritation, oral and pharyngeal candidiasis, otitis media, pharyngitis, rhinitis, sinusitis, throat tightness, unpleasant taste
ENDO: **Adrenal insufficiency**, growth suppression
GI: Diarrhea, dyspepsia, nausea, vomiting
GU: Dysmenorrhea
MS: Arthralgia, decreased bone mineral density, myalgia, pain
RESP: **Asthma**, bronchitis, **bronchospasm**, increased cough, upper respiratory tract infection, wheezing
SKIN: Pruritus, rash, urticaria
Other: **Anaphylaxis**, **angioedema**, flu-like symptoms, viral infection

Nursing Considerations

WARNING Be aware that Asmanex brand of mometasone contains small amounts of lactose, which contains trace levels of milk proteins. Do not administer to patients with a milk protein allergy because anaphylactic reactions have occurred.

- Use mometasone cautiously if patient has ocular herpes simplex; tubercular infection; or untreated bacterial, fungal, or systemic viral infection.
- If patient takes an oral corticosteroid, expect to taper it slowly 1 week after changing to mometasone. If patient takes prednisone, expect to reduce it by no more than 2.5 mg daily at weekly intervals, beginning at least 1 week after mometasone therapy starts. Monitor patient for symptoms of systemically active corticosteroid withdrawal such as depression, joint and muscle pain, and lassitude, despite maintenance or even improvement of respiratory symptoms.

WARNING Assess patient switched from systemic corticosteroid to mometasone for adrenal insufficiency (fatigue, hypotension, lassitude, nausea, vomiting, weakness) during initial treatment and during infection, stress, surgery, trauma, or an electrolyte-depleting condition. Notify prescriber immediately if signs or symptoms arise because adrenal insufficiency may be life-threatening. Hypothalamic-pituitary-adrenal axis function may take several months to recover after systemic corticosteroids are discontinued. Abrupt withdrawal of mometasone also may precipitate adrenal insufficiency.

- Notify prescriber immediately if patient has bronchospasm after mometasone oral inhalation, and expect to give a fast-acting inhaled bronchodilator, discontinue mometasone, and use an alternate drug.
- Closely monitor a child's growth pattern; drug may stunt growth.
- Report oropharyngeal candidiasis, and expect patient to receive appropriate antifungal therapy while remaining on mometasone therapy. If candidiasis is severe, however, mometasone therapy may need to be temporarily halted.

PATIENT TEACHING

- For nasal spray, instruct patient to shake container before each use. Instruct her to blow her nose, tilt her head slightly forward, and insert tube into a nostril, pointing toward inner corner of eye, away from nasal septum. Tell her to hold the other nostril closed and spray while inhaling gently. Then have her repeat the procedure in the other nostril.
- For oral inhalation, give patient these instructions for using inhaler: Remove cap only after placing inhaler in an upright position. Twist cap in counterclockwise while holding colored base, making sure indented arrow (on white portion of the inhaler directly above the colored base) is pointing to the dose counter. Removing the cap loads inhaler with drug, and the dose counter on the base will count down by one. Tell her to take a full breath in and out, and then place mouthpiece in her mouth. Firmly close her lips around mouthpiece, taking care not to cover ventilation holes on the inhaler. Then take a fast, deep breath. Remind her she may not taste, smell, or feel anything with the inhalation. After taking the breath, she should remove inhaler from her mouth and hold her breath for about 10 seconds. She should not exhale into the inhaler. Then, she should wipe the mouthpiece dry, if needed, and replace the cap right away, turning it clockwise as she presses down. She should hear a click when the cap is fully closed. Tell her to write down the date inhaler is opened, and discard it 45 days from that date or when dose counter reads 00, whichever comes first.
- Instruct patient to gargle or rinse after each use of oral inhaler to help prevent mouth and throat dryness, relieve throat irritation, and prevent oropharyngeal infection.

WARNING Caution patient not to use mometasone oral inhalation to relieve acute bronchospasm and to notify prescriber if rescue inhaler is required more often or doesn't seem to be as effective.

- Keep in mind that if patient switches from an oral corticosteroid to mometasone, she should be advised to carry or wear medical identification indicating the need for supplemental systemic corticosteroids during stress or severe asthma attack. Tell her to seek emergency care if either occurs.
- Instruct patient to contact prescriber if symptoms persist or worsen after 3 weeks.
- Caution patient to avoid exposure to chickenpox and measles and, if exposed, to contact prescriber immediately.

montelukast sodium

Singulair

Class and Category

Pharmacologic class: Leukotriene receptor antagonist
Therapeutic class: Antiallergen, antiasthmatic
Pregnancy category: B

Indications and Dosages

➤ *To prevent or treat asthma*

ORAL GRANULES

Children ages 1 to 5. 4 mg daily in the evening. *Maximum:* 4 mg daily.

CHEWABLE TABLETS

Children ages 6 to 14. 5 mg daily in the evening. *Maximum:* 5 mg daily.
Children ages 2 to 5. 4 mg daily in the evening. *Maximum:* 4 mg daily.

TABLETS

Adults and adolescents age 15 and over. 10 mg daily in the evening. *Maximum:* 10 mg daily.

➤ *To treat seasonal allergic rhinitis*

ORAL GRANULES

Children ages 2 to 5. 4 mg daily.

CHEWABLE TABLETS
Children ages 6 to 14. 5 mg daily.
Children ages 2 to 5. 4 mg daily.
TABLETS
Adults and adolescents age 15 and over. 10 mg daily.

➤ *To treat perennial allergic rhinitis*
ORAL GRANULES
Children ages 6 months to 5 years. 4 mg daily.
CHEWABLE TABLETS
Children ages 6 to 14. 5 mg daily.
Children ages 2 to 5. 4 mg daily.
TABLETS
Adults and adolescents age 15 and over. 10 mg daily.

➤ *To prevent exercise-induced bronchoconstriction*
TABLETS
Adults and adolescents age 15 and over. 10 mg at least 2 hr before exercise. *Maximum:* 10 mg in 24 hr.
CHEWABLE TABLETS
Children ages 6 to 14. 5 mg at least 2 hr before exercise. *Maximum:* 5 mg in 24 hr.

Route	Onset	Peak	Duration
P.O.	Unknown	Unknown	24 hr

Mechanism of Action
Antagonizes receptors for cysteinyl leukotrienes, produced by arachidonic acid metabolism and released from eosinophils, mast cells, and other cells. When cysteinyl leukotrienes bind to receptors in bronchial airways, they increase endothelial membrane permeability, which leads to airway edema, smooth-muscle contraction, and altered activity of cells in asthma's inflammatory process. Also, antagonizes receptors for cysteinyl leukotrienes in nasal tissue that are responsible for producing rhinitis caused by allergens. Montelukast blocks these effects.

Interactions
DRUGS
phenobarbital: Decreased amount of circulating montelukast

Adverse Reactions
CNS: Aggression, agitation, anxiousness, asthenia, attention disturbance, depression, disorientation, dizziness, dream abnormalities, drowsiness, fatigue, fever, hallucinations, headache, hostility, hypoesthesia, insomnia, irritability, memory impairment, obsessive–compulsive symptoms, paresthesia, restlessness, **seizures**, sleep walking, somnolence, **suicidal ideation**, tic, tremor
CV: Palpitations, edema
EENT: Dental pain, epistaxis, laryngitis, nasal congestion, otitis media, pharyngitis, sinusitis
GI: Abdominal pain, **cholestatic hepatitis**, diarrhea, dyspepsia, elevated liver enzymes, **hepatic eosinophilic infiltration**, **hepatotoxicity**, indigestion, infectious gastroenteritis; diarrhea, nausea, **pancreatitis**, vomiting
GU: Enuresis (children), pyuria
HEME: Increased bleeding tendency, systemic eosinophilia, **thrombocytopenia**
MS: Arthralgia, muscle cramps, myalgia
RESP: Cough, upper respiratory tract infection, **pulmonary eosinophilia**
SKIN: Erythema multiforme, erythema nodosum, pruritus, rash, **Stevens–Johnson syndrome**, **toxic epidermal necrolysis**, urticaria
Other: Anaphylaxis, **angioedema** (in all patients); flu-like syndrome, viral infection (in children)

Nursing Considerations
WARNING Know that montelukast isn't for acute asthma attack or status asthmaticus.

- Keep in mind that montelukast shouldn't be abruptly substituted for inhaled or oral corticosteroids; expect to taper corticosteroid dosage gradually, as directed.
- Monitor patient for adverse reactions, such as eosinophilia, cardiac and pulmonary symptoms, and vasculitis, in patient undergoing corticosteroid withdrawal. Notify prescriber if such reactions occur.
- Watch patient closely for suicidal tendencies during montelukast therapy, especially when therapy starts or dosage changes.
- Monitor patient for adverse neuropsychiatric effects and notify prescriber if present. Drug may need to be discontinued.

M

PATIENT TEACHING

- Advise patient to take montelukast daily as prescribed, even when he feels well. Urge him not to decrease dosage or stop taking other prescribed allergy or asthma drugs unless instructed by prescriber.
- Caution patient prescribed drug for asthma not to use drug for acute asthma attack or status asthmaticus; make sure he has appropriate short-acting rescue drug available.
- Tell parents administering oral granules to pour contents directly into the child's mouth or mix with ice cream or cold or room temperature applesauce, carrots, or rice—but not liquids or other foods—just before administration. Liquids may be given after drug has been administered. Once packet is opened, the full dose must be administered within 15 minutes. Drug must not be stored for future use if mixed with food.
- Instruct patient prescribed drug for asthma to notify prescriber if he needs a short-acting inhaled bronchodilator more often than usual, or more often than prescribed, to control symptoms.
- Teach patient prescribed drug for asthma to use a peak flowmeter to determine his personal best expiratory volume.
- Caution patient with aspirin sensitivity to avoid aspirin and NSAIDs during montelukast therapy. Montelukast may not effectively reduce bronchospasm in such a patient.
- Inform patient (or parents of child) with phenylketonuria that chewable tablet contains phenylalanine.
- Instruct patient to notify prescriber if she is or could be pregnant.
- Urge family or caregiver to watch patient closely for abnormal behaviors, including suicidal tendencies, during therapy, and urge them to notify prescriber if present.
- Instruct patient to report increased bleeding tendency or severe skin reaction that occurs without warning immediately to prescriber.
- Inform mothers wishing to breastfeed that montelukast is present in breast milk. Advise patient to discuss breastfeeding with prescriber before doing so to avoid adverse reactions in the breastfed infant.

morphine sulfate

Arymo ER, Astramorph PF, Duramorph, Kadian, M-Eslon (CAN), MorphaBond ER, MS Contin, MSIR, Oramorph SR, Roxanol, Statex (CAN)

Class, Category, and Schedule

Pharmacologic class: Opioid
Therapeutic class: Opioid analgesic
Pregnancy category: C
Controlled substance schedule: II

Indications and Dosages

➤ *To relieve pain severe enough to require opioid treatment and for which alternative treatment options such as nonopioid analgesics or opioid combination products are inadequate or not tolerated*

CAPSULES, ORAL SOLUTION, SYRUP, TABLETS
Adults. 5 to 30 mg every 3 to 4 hr, as needed.
Children. Individualized dosage based on patient's age, size, and need.

I.V. INFUSION
Adults. *Initial:* 0.8 to 10 mg/hr, increased, as needed. *Maintenance:* 0.8 to 80 mg/hr.
Children. 0.01 to 0.04 mg/kg/hr postoperatively, 0.025 to 0.206 mg/kg/hr for severe chronic cancer pain or sickle cell crisis.

I.V. INJECTION
Adults. 4 to 15 mg injected slowly every 3 to 4 hr, as needed.
Children. 0.5 to 0.1 0.05 to 0.2 mg/kg given slowly every 4 hr, as needed.

I.M. OR SUBCUTANEOUS INJECTION
Adults. 2.5 to 20 mg every 3 to 4 hr, as needed.
Children. *Initial:* 0.05 to 0.2 mg/kg every 4 hr, as needed. *Maximum:* 15 mg/dose.

EPIDURAL INJECTION (PRESERVATIVE-FREE)
Adults. *Initial:* 5 mg as a single dose. If pain isn't relieved after 1 hr, 1- to 2-mg doses given at appropriate intervals to relieve pain. *Maximum:* 10 mg/24 hr.

INTRATHECAL INJECTION (PRESERVATIVE-FREE)
Adults. 0.2 to 1 mg as a single dose.

SUPPOSITORIES
Adults. 10 to 30 mg every 4 hr, as needed.
Children. Individualized dosage based on patient's age, size, and need.

➤ *To manage moderate to severe pain when a continuous, around-the-clock opioid analgesic is needed for an extended period of time*

E.R. CAPSULES (KADIAN)

Adults who are not opioid tolerant. *Initial:* 30 mg every 24 hr, as needed.

Adults converting from other oral morphine formulations: Total previous daily dose every 24 hr. Alternatively, one-half total previous daily dose every 12 hr.

Adults converting from parenteral morphine. Highly individualized. *Usual:* Three times the previous daily parenteral morphine dosage.

Adults converting from other nonmorphine opioids (oral or parenteral). Highly individualized. *Usual:* Half of the estimated daily morphine requirements every 24 hr, and then increased as needed.

E.R. TABLETS (MORPHABOND, MS CONTIN)

Adults who are not opioid tolerant. 15 mg every 8 or 12 hr, as needed.

Adults converting from other oral morphine formulations. One-half of patient's previous 24-hr requirements every 12 hr. Alternatively for MS Contin, one-third of patient's previous 24-hr requirements every 8 hr.

Adults converting from parenteral morphine. Highly individualized. *Usual:* Three times the previous daily parenteral morphine dosage.

Adults converting from other parenteral or oral nonmorphine opioids. Highly individualized. *Usual:* Half of the estimated daily morphine requirements, and then increased as needed.

E.R. TABLETS (ARYMO ER)

Adults who are not opioid tolerant. 15 mg every 8 or 12 hr.

Adults converting from other oral morphine formulations. One-half of patient's previous 24-hr requirements every 12 hr. Alternatively, one-third of patient's previous 24-hr requirements every 8 hr.

Adults converting from parenteral morphine. Highly individualized. *Usual:* Three times the previous daily parenteral morphine dosage.

Adults converting from other opioids. 15 mg every 8 to 12 hr.

Route	Onset	Peak	Duration
P.O.	Unknown	1–2 hr	4–5 hr
P.O. (E.R.)	Unknown	Unknown	8–12 hr
I.V.	Unknown	20 min	4–5 hr
I.M.	10–30 min	30–60 min	4–5 hr
SubQ	10–30 min	50–90 min	4–5 hr
Epidural	15–60 min	Unknown	Up to 24 hr
Intrathecal	15–60 min	Unknown	Up to 24 hr
P.R.	20–60 min	Unknown	Unknown

Mechanism of Action

Binds with and activates opioid receptors (mainly mu receptors) in brain and spinal cord to produce analgesia and euphoria.

Contraindications

For all drug forms: Acute or severe bronchial asthma in an unmonitored setting or in the absence of resuscitative equipment, Hypersensitivity to montelukast sodium or any of its components, labor (premature delivery), prematurity (in infants), respiratory depression, upper airway obstruction

For E.R. formulations: Paralytic ileus

For oral solution: Acute abdominal disorders, acute alcoholism, alcohol withdrawal syndrome, arrhythmias, brain tumor, head injuries, heart failure caused by chronic lung disease, increased cerebrospinal or intracranial pressure, recent biliary tract surgery, respiratory insufficiency, seizure disorders, severe CNS depression, surgical anastomosis, use within 14 days of an MAO inhibitor

For I.M., I.V., or subcutaneous injection: Acute alcoholism, alcohol withdrawal syndrome, arrhythmias, brain tumor, heart failure caused by chronic lung disease, seizure disorders

For epidural or intrathecal injection: Anticoagulant therapy, bleeding tendency, injection-site infection, parenteral corticosteroid treatment (or other treatment or condition that prohibits drug delivery by intrathecal or epidural route) within 2 weeks

Interactions

DRUGS

amitriptyline, clomipramine, nortriptyline: Increased CNS and respiratory depression
anticholinergics: Possibly severe constipation leading to ileus, urine retention
antidiarrheals (such as loperamide and paregoric): CNS depression, possibly severe constipation
antihistamines, chloral hydrate, glutethimide, MAO inhibitors, methocarbamol: Increased CNS and respiratory depressant effects
antihypertensives, hypotension-producing drugs: Increased hypotension, risk of orthostatic hypotension
antimigraine agents, cyclobenzaprine; dextromethorphan; dolasetron; granisetron; linezolid; MAO inhibitors; methylene blue; ondansetron; palonosetron; selected psychiatric drugs such as amoxapine, buspirone, lithium, maprotiline, mirtazapine, nefazodone, trazodone, vilazodone; selective serotonin reuptake inhibitors; serontonin-norepinephrine reuptake inhibitors; St. John's wort; tricyclic antidepressants; tryptophan: Increased risk of serotonin syndrome
benzodiazepines, CNS depressants, other opioids, sedating antihistamines, tricyclic antidepressants: Increased risk of significant sedation and somnolence and severe respiratory depression
bupivacaine: Increased serum morphine level and possibly significant adverse effects
buprenorphine: Decreased therapeutic effects of morphine, increased respiratory depression, possibly withdrawal symptoms
cimetidine: Increased analgesic and CNS and respiratory depressant effects
CNS depressants (antiemetics, general anesthetics, hypnotics, opioids, phenothiazines, sedatives, tranquilizers): Possibly coma, hypotension, respiratory depression, severe sedation
diuretics: Decreased diuretic efficacy
hydroxyzine: Increased analgesic, CNS depressant, and hypotensive effects of morphine
metoclopramide: Possibly antagonized metoclopramide effect on GI motility
mixed agonist-antagonist analgesics: Possibly withdrawal symptoms
naloxone: Antagonized analgesic and CNS and respiratory depressant effects of morphine, possibly withdrawal symptoms
naltrexone: Possibly induction or worsening of withdrawal symptoms if morphine given within 7 to 10 days before naltrexone
neuromuscular blockers: Increased or prolonged respiratory depression
opioid analgesics (such as alfentanil and sufentanil): Increased CNS and respiratory depression, increased hypotension
zidovudine: Decreased zidovudine clearance

ACTIVITIES

alcohol use: Increased CNS and respiratory depression, increased hypotension

Adverse Reactions

CNS: Agitation, amnesia, anxiety, ataxia, chills, **coma**, confusion, decreased concentration, delirium, delusions, depression, dizziness, dream abnormalities, drowsiness, edema, euphoria, fever, gait disturbance, hallucinations, headache, **increased intracranial pressure**, insomnia, lethargy, light-headedness, malaise, mood alterations, psychosis, restlessness, rigidity, sedation, **seizures**, syncope, thinking disturbances, tremor, uncoordinated muscle movements, unresponsiveness, vertigo, weakness
CV: Bradycardia, **cardiac arrest**, edema, hypertension, **hypotension**, orthostatic hypotension, palpitations, **shock**, tachycardia, vasodilation
EENT: Amblyopia, blurred vision, diplopia, dry mouth, eye pain, hiccup, **laryngeal edema or laryngospasm** (allergic), miosis, nystagmus, rhinitis, taste or voice alteration
ENDO: Adrenal insufficiency (rare), hypogonadism
GI: Abdominal cramps or pain, anorexia, biliary tract spasm, constipation, diarrhea, dysphagia, elevated liver enzymes, gastroenteritis, gastroesophageal reflux, hiccups, ileus (in patients with inflammatory bowel disease), **toxic megacolon** (in patients with inflammatory bowel disease), indigestion, **intestinal obstruction**, nausea, vomiting
GU: Decreased ejaculate potency, decreased libido, difficult ejaculation, dysuria, impotence, infertility, menstrual irregularities, oliguria, prolonged labor, urinary hesitancy, urine retention
HEME: Anemia, **leukopenia**, **thrombocytopenia**

MS: Arthralgia, decreased bone mineral density, skeletal muscle rigidity
RESP: Apnea, **asthma exacerbation**, **atelectasis**, **bronchospasm**, depressed cough reflex, **hypoventilation**, **pulmonary edema**, **respiratory arrest and depression**, wheezing
SKIN: Diaphoresis, dryness, flushing, pallor, pruritus, rash, urticaria
Other: Allergic reaction; **anaphylaxis**; **angioedema**; injection-site edema, pain, rash, or redness; physical and psychological dependence; weight loss; withdrawal symptoms

Nursing Considerations

- Be aware that morphine can lead to abuse, addiction, and misuse. To ensure that benefits of morphine therapy outweigh risks, a Risk Evaluation and Mitigation Strategy (REMS) is required.
- Know that chronic maternal use of morphine during pregnancy can result in NOWS, which may be life-threatening if not recognized and treated appropriately. NOWS occurs when a newborn has been exposed to opioid drugs like morphine for a prolonged period while in utero.
- Use extreme caution when administering morphine to patients with conditions accompanied by hypercapnia, hypoxia, or decreased respiratory reserve such as asthma, chronic obstructive pulmonary disease (COPD), or cor pulmonale. This is because, even with usual therapeutic doses, morphine may decrease respiratory drive while simultaneously increasing airway resistance to the point of apnea. Monitor patient's respiratory status closely, especially during the initiation of therapy or following a dose increase.
- Use morphine with extreme caution in patients who may be at risk for carbon dioxide retention (e.g., those with brain tumors or increased intracranial pressure). Monitor for signs of sedation and respiratory depression, especially when initiating therapy. Morphine may reduce respiratory drive, and the resultant carbon dioxide retention can further increase intracranial pressure. Also know that opioids like morphine may obscure signs and symptoms in a patient with a head injury.
- Know that morphine should only be used concomitantly with benzodiazepine and other CNS depressant therapy in patients for whom other treatment options are inadequate. If prescribed together, expect dosing and duration of morphine to be limited. Monitor patient closely for signs and symptoms of a decrease in consciousness, including coma, profound sedation, and significant respiratory depression. Notify prescriber immediately and provide emergency supportive care, as death may occur.
- Use cautiously in patients about to undergo surgery of the biliary tract and patients with acute pancreatitis secondary to biliary tract disease because morphine may cause spasm of the sphincter of Oddi.
- Be aware that MorphaBond ER formulation has an added abuse deterrent property that makes it difficult to break, crush, or cut the tablet. It also resists extraction and forms a viscous liquid when physically compromised and placed in a liquid. This abuse deterrent helps prevent abuse when attempts are made to administer it intranasally or by injection.
- Store morphine at room temperature.
- Ensure that before giving morphine, opioid antagonist and equipment for oxygen delivery and respiration are available.
- Assess patient's drug use, including all prescription and OTC drugs before therapy begins.
- Expect prescriber to usually start patient who has never received opioids on immediate-release form and then switch to E.R. form if therapy must last longer than a few days.
- Keep in mind that when morphine is given by epidural route, dosage must be individualized according to patient's age, body mass, physical status, previous experience with opioids, risk factors for respiratory depression, and drugs to be coadministered before or during surgery.
- Give oral form with food or milk to minimize adverse GI reactions, if needed. Solution can be mixed with fruit juice to improve taste.
- Open E.R. capsules and sprinkle contents on applesauce (at room temperature or

cooler) just before giving to patient, if needed. Make sure patient doesn't chew or crush capsules or dissolve capsule's pellets in his mouth.

- Be aware that E.R. forms of morphine aren't interchangeable.
- Discard injection solution that is discolored or darker than pale yellow or that contains precipitates that don't dissolve with shaking.

WARNING **Don't use highly concentrated solutions (such as 10 to 25 mg/ml) for single-dose I.V., I.M., or subcutaneous administration. These solutions are intended for use in continuous, controlled microinfusion devices.**

- For direct I.V. injection, dilute appropriate dose with 4 to 5 ml of sterile water for injection. Inject 2.5 to 15 mg directly into tubing of free-flowing I.V. solution over 4 to 5 minutes. Rapid I.V. injection may increase adverse reactions.
- For continuous I.V. infusion, dilute drug in D_5W and administer with infusion-control device. Adjust dose and rate based on patient response, as prescribed.
- Avoid I.M. route for long-term therapy because of injection-site irritation.
- During subcutaneous injection, take care to avoid injecting drug intradermally.
- For intrathecal injection, expect prescriber to give no more than 2 ml of 0.5-mg/ml solution or 1 ml of 1-mg/ml solution. Expect intrathecal dosage to be about one-tenth of epidural dosage.
- Keep in mind if rectal suppository is too soft to insert, refrigerate for 30 minutes or run wrapped suppository under cold tap water.

WARNING **Monitor circulatory and respiratory status carefully and frequently during morphine therapy, especially when drug therapy is initiated and when patient is being converted to morphine because respiratory depression and severe hypotension can develop. Be especially vigilant with cachectic, debilitated, and elderly patients who are at higher risk. Know that life-threatening depression can occur even when morphine is taken as prescribed and is not misused or abused.**

- Monitor patient with seizure disorder for increased seizure activity because morphine may worsen the disorder.
- Monitor patient for excessive or persistent sedation; dosage may need to be adjusted.
- Know that if patient is receiving a continuous morphine infusion, watch for and notify prescriber about new neurologic signs or symptoms. Inflammatory masses (such as granulomas) have caused serious neurologic reactions, including paralysis.
- Expect morphine to cause physical and psychological dependence; watch for drug tolerance and withdrawal, such as body aches, diaphoresis, diarrhea, fever, piloerection, rhinorrhea, sneezing, and yawning.
- Keep in mind if tolerance to morphine develops, expect prescriber to increase dosage.
- Know that morphine may have a prolonged duration and cumulative effect in patients with impaired hepatic or renal function. It also may prolong labor.

WARNING **Know that many drugs may interact with opioids like morphine to cause serotonin syndrome. Monitor patient closely for signs and symptoms such as agitation, diaphoresis, diarrhea, fever, hallucinations, labile blood pressure, muscle twitching or stiffness, nausea, shakiness, shivering, tachycardia, trouble with coordination, or vomiting. Notify prescriber at once because serotonin syndrome may be life-threatening. Be prepared to discontinue drug, if possible and ordered, and provide supportive care.**

- Monitor patient for adrenal insufficiency. Although rare, it can be life-threatening. Monitor patient for anorexia, dizziness, fatigue, hypotension, nausea, vomiting, and weakness. Notify prescriber if adrenal insufficiency is suspected and expect diagnostic testing to be done. If confirmed, expect to administer corticosteroids and wean patient off morphine, if possible.
- Keep in mind when discontinuing morphine in patients receiving more than 30 mg daily, expect prescriber to reduce

daily dose by about one-half for 2 days and then by 25% every 2 days thereafter until total dose reaches initial amount recommended for patients who haven't received opioids (15 to 30 mg daily). This regimen minimizes the risk of withdrawal symptoms.

PATIENT TEACHING

- Instruct patient to take morphine exactly as prescribed and not to change dosage without consulting prescriber. Tell patient this is because excessive or prolonged use can lead to abuse, addiction, misuse, overdose, and possibly death.
- Explain that patient may take tablets or capsules with food or milk to relieve GI distress and may mix oral solution with juice to improve taste.
- Urge patient not to break, chew, or crush E.R. capsules and tablets to avoid rapid release and, possibly, toxicity.
- Tell patient who has difficulty swallowing, suggest that he can open E.R. capsules and sprinkle contents on food or liquids. Urge him to take drug immediately and not let capsule contents dissolve in his mouth.
- Instruct patient to moisten rectal suppository before inserting it.
- Urge patient to avoid alcohol and other CNS depressants, including benzodiazepines, during therapy without prescriber knowledge, as severe respiratory depression can occur and may lead to death.
- Advise patient to avoid potentially hazardous activities during morphine therapy.
- Tell patient to change positions slowly to minimize the orthostatic hypotension.
- Instruct patient to notify prescriber about worsening or breakthrough pain.
- Explain that morphine may be habit-forming. Urge him to notify prescriber if he experiences anxiety, decreased appetite, excessive tearing, irritability, muscle aches or twitching, rapid heart rate, or yawning.
- Advise female patient to notify prescriber if she becomes pregnant. Regular morphine use during pregnancy may cause physical dependence in fetus and withdrawal in neonate.
- Tell patient to alert all prescribers of morphine use. This is important because a potentially fatal effect can occur when an opioid like morphine is combined with a benzodiazepine.
- Warn patient not to discontinue morphine use abruptly if more than a few weeks of use has occurred, as withdrawal symptoms may develop.
- Caution patient to keep drug out of reach of children because accidental consumption by a child may be fatal.
- Inform patient that long-term use of opioids like morphine may decrease sex hormone levels, causing decreased libido, erectile dysfunction, impotence, infertility, or lack of menstruation. Encourage patient to report any symptoms.

moxifloxacin hydrochloride

Avelox, Avelox IV

Class and Category

Pharmacologic class: Fluoroquinolone
Therapeutic class: Antibiotic
Pregnancy category: C

Indications and Dosages

➤ *To treat acute sinusitis caused by* Haemophilus influenzae, Moraxella catarrhalis, *or* Streptococcus pneumoniae; *to treat mild to moderate community-acquired pneumonia caused by* Chlamydia pneumoniae, H. influenzae, M. catarrhalis, Mycoplasma pneumoniae, *or* S. pneumoniae *(including penicillin- or multi-drug-resistant strains)*

TABLETS, I.V. INFUSION

Adults. 400 mg every 24 hr for 10 days for acute sinusitis and 7 to 14 days for community-acquired pneumonia. I.V. infusion given over 1 hr.

➤ *To treat acute exacerbation of chronic bronchitis caused by* H. influenzae, H. parainfluenzae, Klebsiella pneumoniae, M. catarrhalis, S. pneumoniae, *or* Staphylococcus aureus

TABLETS, I.V. INFUSION
Adults. 400 mg every 24 hr for 5 days. I.V. infusion given over 1 hr.

➤ *To treat uncomplicated skin and soft-tissue infections caused by* S. aureus *or* Streptococcus pyogenes

TABLETS, I.V. INFUSION
Adults. 400 mg every 24 hr for 7 days. I.V. infusion given over 1 hr.

➤ *To treat complicated skin and skin structure infections caused by* S. aureus, E. coli, K. pneumoniae, *or* Enterobacter cloacae

TABLETS, I.V. INFUSION
Adults. 400 mg every 24 hr for 7 to 21 days. I.V. infusion given over 1 hr.

➤ *To treat complicated intra-abdominal infections, including polymicrobial infections such as abscesses caused by* E. coli, Bacteroides fragilis, Streptococcus anginosus, Streptococcus constellatus, Enterococcus faecalis, Proteus mirabilis, Clostridium perfringens, Bacteroides thetaiotaomicron, *or* Peptostreptococcus *species*

TABLETS, I.V. INFUSION
Adults. 400 mg every 24 hr for 5 to 14 days with initial dosage given as I.V. infusion over 1 hr.

➤ *To prevent or treat plague, including pneumonic and septicemic plague, caused by* Yersinia pestis

I.V. INFUSION, TABLETS
Adults. 400 mg every 24 hr for 10 to 14 days after exposure confirmed or suspected. I.V. infusion given over 1 hr.

Mechanism of Action

Inhibits synthesis of bacterial enzyme DNA gyrase by counteracting excessive supercoiling of DNA during replication or transcription. Inhibiting DNA gyrase causes rapid- and slow-growing bacterial cells to die.

Incompatibilities

Don't infuse I.V. moxifloxacin simultaneously through the same I.V. line with other I.V. additives, drugs, or substances.

Contraindications

Hypersensitivity to moxifloxacin, other fluoroquinolones, or their components; myasthenia gravis

Interactions

DRUGS
aluminum- or magnesium-containing antacids; drug formulations with divalent or trivalent cations, such as didanosine chewable buffered tablets or powder for oral solution; metal cations, such as iron; multivitamins containing iron or zinc; sucralfate: Possibly substantial interference with moxifloxacin absorption, causing low blood moxifloxacin level
class IA antiarrhythmics, such as quinidine; class III antiarrhythmics, such as sotalol; other drugs known to prolong QTc interval, such as disopyramide and pentamidine: Possibly prolonged QTc interval
corticosteroids: Increased risk of Achilles and other tendon ruptures
NSAIDs: Increased risk of CNS stimulation and seizures
warfarin: Possibly increased anticoagulation

Adverse Reactions

CNS: Abnormal gait, agitation, altered coordination, anxiety, confusion, delirium, depression, disorientation, disturbance in attention, dizziness, fever, hallucinations, headache, **increased intracranial pressure (including pseudotumor cerebri)**, insomnia, memory impairment, paranoia, peripheral neuropathy, nervousness, psychosis, psychotic reaction, **seizures**, **suicidal ideation**, syncope, **toxic psychosis**, tremors
CV: Aortic dissection, hypertension, **hypotension** palpitations, peripheral edema, **prolonged QT interval**, **rupture of aortic aneurysm**, tachycardia, vasculitis, vasodilation, **ventricular tachyarrhythmias**
EENT: Altered taste, deafness or other hearing impairments, **laryngeal edema**, vision loss
ENDO: Hyperglycemia, **hypoglycemia**
GI: Abdominal pain, abnormal liver enzymes, **acute hepatic necrosis**, **cholestatic hepatitis**, diarrhea, dyspepsia, **hepatic failure**, **hepatitis**, jaundice, nausea, **pseudomembranous colitis**, vomiting
GU: Acute renal insufficiency or failure, interstitial nephritis
HEME: Agranulocytosis, **aplastic anemia**, eosinophilia, **hemolytic anemia**, **leukopenia**, **pancytopenia**, **prolonged prothrombin time**, **thrombocytopenia**

MS: Arthralgia; muscle weakness; myalgia; tendon inflammation, pain, or rupture
RESP: Allergic pneumonitis
SKIN: Photosensitivity, rash, **Stevens–Johnson syndrome, toxic epidermal necrolysis**
Other: Anaphylaxis, anaphylactic shock, angioedema, serum sickness, worsening of myasthenia gravis

Nursing Considerations

- Be aware that if patient has hypokalemia, expect to correct it before beginning moxifloxacin therapy to prevent arrhythmias.
- Determine if patient has a history of CNS disorder, such as cerebral arteriosclerosis or epilepsy, because drug may lower seizure threshold. Notify prescriber before starting drug, and take seizure precautions.
- Use cautiously in patients with liver dysfunction, including cirrhosis, because drug may adversely affect liver function.
- Obtain a fluid or tissue specimen for culture and sensitivity, as ordered. Expect to begin therapy before results are available.

WARNING Keep in mind before starting moxifloxacin therapy, determine if patient takes a class IA antiarrhythmic, such as quinidine; a class III antiarrhythmic, such as sotalol; or other drugs that prolong the QTc interval, such as antipsychotics, cisapride, erythromycin, or tricyclic antidepressants. These drugs should be avoided in patients taking moxifloxacin because they may prolong the QTc interval and lead to life-threatening ventricular tachycardia or torsades de pointes. Monitor patient closely throughout therapy, especially if he has significant acute myocardial ischemia or bradycardia because these conditions increase risk of prolonging the QTc interval.

- Infuse drug over 60 minutes with ready-to-use flexible bags with 400 mg of moxifloxacin in 250 ml of 0.8% saline. Don't dilute further.
- Know that if giving through Y-type tubing or piggyback, stop other solutions during moxifloxacin infusion, and flush the line before and after infusion with a compatible solution, such as 1M sodium chloride, 5% dextrose, sterile water for injection, 10% dextrose, lactated Ringer's or normal saline solution. Also flush line before and after giving other drugs in same I.V. line.
- Don't refrigerate I.V. moxifloxacin ready-to-use bags because precipitation will occur. Discard any unused portion; premixed bags are for single-use only.
- Expect to obtain a 12-lead ECG to assess patient for prolonged QTc interval. Ask patient if he or a blood relative has a history of prolonged QTc interval. Monitor elderly patients closely; they may have increased risk of prolonged QT interval.
- Monitor patient for central nervous system (including psychiatric) adverse reactions such as confusion, depression, dizziness, hallucinations, peripheral neuropathy, psychosis, suicidal ideation, and tremors. If any occurs, notify prescriber and expect moxifloxacin to be discontinued.
- Monitor patient for diarrhea. If profuse, watery diarrhea develops, contact prescriber and expect to obtain a stool specimen to rule out pseudomembranous colitis caused by *Clostridium difficile*. If diarrhea occurs, notify prescriber and expect to withhold moxifloxacin and treat with fluids, an antibiotic effective against *C. difficile*, electrolytes, fluids, and protein, as ordered.
- Monitor serum potassium level, as ordered, during therapy to assess for hypokalemia.
- Keep emergency resuscitation equipment readily available, and observe for evidence of hypersensitivity, such as angioedema, dyspnea, and urticaria. If you suspect anaphylaxis, prepare to give epinephrine, corticosteroids, diphenhydramine, and epinephrine, as prescribed.
- Monitor patients who are prone to tendinitis, such as athletes, the elderly, and those taking corticosteroids, for complaints of tendon inflammation, pain, or rupture. If present, notify prescriber and expect to discontinue moxifloxacin, place patient on bedrest with no exercise of affected limb, and obtain diagnostic tests to confirm rupture.

- Monitor patient's blood glucose, especially in diabetic patients receiving concomitant treatment with insulin or an oral hypoglycemic agent, for changes in blood glucose levels that could become decreased or increased. If dysglycemia occurs, treat according to standard of care and expect that drug may need to be discontinued.
- Know that fluoroquinolones like moxifloxacin have caused disabling and potentially irreversible serious adverse reactions from different body systems that can occur together in the same patient. These reactions can occur within hours to weeks after starting the drug and usually cause central nervous system effects, peripheral neuropathy, tendinitis and tendon rupture. All ages of patients and patients without any preexisting risk factors have experienced these reactions. Notify prescriber and expect to discontinue moxifloxacin immediately at the first signs or symptoms of any serious adverse reactions.

PATIENT TEACHING

- Urge patient to notify prescriber at once about fainting or palpitations because they may indicate a serious arrhythmia.
- Teach patient to take drug at least 4 hours before and 8 hours after aluminum- or magnesium-containing antacids, didanosine chewable buffered tablets or oral solution prepared from powder, multivitamins containing iron or zinc, or sucralfate.
- Urge patient to drink plenty of fluids while taking moxifloxacin.
- Caution patient to stop drug and notify prescriber if he has a rash, trouble breathing, or other signs of an allergic reaction. Also advise patient to stop taking moxifloxacin immediately and notify prescriber if any persistent, serious, or worsening adverse effects occur.
- Urge patient to stop any exercise and contact prescriber immediately if he develops tendon inflammation, pain, or rupture.
- Tell patient to notify prescriber if motor or sensory changes occur.
- Caution patient to avoid hazardous activities until adverse CNS effects are known.
- Urge patient to tell prescriber if diarrhea develops, even more than 2 months after moxifloxacin therapy ends.
- Caution patient to complete the prescribed course of therapy even if he feels better before it's completed.
- Tell patient to avoid excessive exposure to sunlight or artificial ultraviolet light because severe sunburn may result. Instruct patient to notify prescriber if sunburn develops because moxifloxacin may have to be discontinued.
- Warn patient, especially diabetics, that moxifloxacin may alter blood glucose levels. Review signs and symptoms of hyperglycemia and hypoglycemia. Tell patient to report symptomatic changes in blood glucose levels to prescriber and review how to treat hypoglycemia.

mycophenolate mofetil

CellCept, CellCept Oral Suspension

mycophenolate mofetil hydrochloride

CellCept Intravenous

mycophenolic acid

Myfortic

Class and Category

Pharmacologic class: Mycophenolic acid
Therapeutic class: Immunosuppressant
Pregnancy category: D

Indications and Dosages

➤ *To prevent organ rejection in patients receiving allogenic kidney transplants*

CAPSULES, ORAL SUSPENSION, TABLETS, I.V. INFUSION

Adults. 1 g (over 2 hr for I.V. infusion) twice daily

E.R. TABLETS

Adults. 720 mg twice daily.
Children age 5 to 16. 400 mg/m^2 twice daily. *Maximum:* 540 mg twice daily if body

surface area is between 1.19 to 1.58 m^2 or 720 mg twice daily if body surface area is greater than 1.58 m^2.

ORAL SUSPENSION

Children age 3 months to 18 years. 600 mg/m^2 twice daily. *Maximum:* 2 g (10 ml) daily.

CAPSULES

Children with body surface area of 1.25 m^2 to 1.5 m^2. 750 mg twice daily.

CAPSULES, TABLETS

Children with body surface area greater than 1.5 m^2. 1 g twice daily.

➤ *To prevent organ rejection in patients receiving allogenic heart transplants*

CAPSULES, ORAL SUSPENSION, TABLETS, I.V. INFUSION

Adults. 1.5 g (over 2 hr for I.V. infusion) twice daily.

➤ *To prevent organ rejection in patients receiving allogenic liver transplants*

I.V. INFUSION

Adults. 1 g infused over 2 hr twice daily.

CAPSULES, ORAL SUSPENSION, TABLETS

Adults. 1.5 g twice daily.

Mechanism of Action

Hydrolyzes to form mycophenolic acid (MPA), which inhibits guanosine nucleotide synthesis and proliferation of T and B lymphocytes. MPA also suppresses antibody formation by B lymphocytes and prevents glycosylation of lymphocyte and monocyte glycoproteins involved in adhesion to endothelial cells. MPA also may inhibit leukocytes from sites of inflammation and graft rejection, which may explain how mycophenolate mofetil prolongs allogeneic transplant survival.

Incompatibilities

Don't mix or give mycophenolate mofetil hydrochloride in same infusion catheter with other I.V. admixtures or drugs.

Contraindications

Hypersensitivity to mycophenolate mofetil, mycophenolic acid, or any of its components; hypersensitivity to polysorbate 80 (I.V. form)

Interactions

DRUGS

acyclovir, ganciclovir, probenecid: Increased plasma levels of both drugs
aminoglycosides, bile acid sequestrants, cephalosporins, fluoroquinolones, penicillins, rifampin, sevelamer, sulfamethoxazole/trimethoprim, telmisartan: Decreased effectiveness of mycophenolate mofetil
amoxicillin plus clavulanic acid, cholestyramine, cyclosporine, metronidazole, norfloxacin, rifampin: Decreased plasma level of mycophenolate mofetil
antacids with aluminum and magnesium hydroxides, sevelamer: Decreased absorption of oral mycophenolate mofetil
azathioprine: Increased bone marrow suppression
cyclosporine, telmisartan: Decreased effectiveness of mycophenolate mofetil
isavuconazole: Increased risk of adverse reactions caused by mycophenolate mofetil
live vaccines: Decreased effectiveness of live vaccines
oral contraceptives: Possibly decreased effectiveness of oral contraceptives
proton pump inhibitors: Possibly decreased effectiveness of mycophenolate mofetil

Adverse Reactions

CNS: Agitation, anxiety, chills, confusion, delirium, depression, dizziness, emotional lability, fever, hallucinations, headache, hypertonia, hypesthesia, insomnia, malaise, meningitis, nervousness, neuropathy, paresthesia, **progressive multifocal leukoencephalopathy**, psychosis, **seizures**, somnolence, syncope, thinking abnormality, tremor, vertigo
CV: Angina pectoris, **arrhythmias**, **arterial thrombosis**, **atrial fibrillation or flutter**, **bradycardia**, **cardiac arrest**, CV disorder, **congestive heart failure**, **extrasystoles**, generalized edema, **hemorrhage**, hypercholesterolemia, hyperlipemia, hypertension, **hypotension**, increased lactic dehydrogenase, increased SGOT and SGPT, increased venous pressure, **infectious endocarditis**, orthostatic hypotension, palpitations, **pericardial effusion**, peripheral edema, peripheral vascular disorder, **supraventricular tachycardia**, **thrombosis**, vasodilation, vasospasm, **ventricular extrasystole**, **ventricular tachycardia**
EENT: Amblyopia, cataract, conjunctivitis, deafness, dry mouth, ear disorder or pain, epistaxis, eye hemorrhage, gingivitis, gum

M

hyperplasia, lacrimation disorder, mouth ulceration, oral candidiasis, pharyngitis, rhinitis, sinusitis, stomatitis, tinnitus, vision abnormality, voice alteration
ENDO: Cushing's syndrome, diabetes mellitus, hypercalcemia, **hypoglycemia**, hypothyroidism, parathyroid disorder
GI: Abdomen enlargement or pain, anorexia, ascites, cholangitis, cholestatic jaundice, colitis, constipation, diarrhea, dyspepsia, dysphagia, elevated liver enzymes, esophagitis, flatulence, gastritis, gastroenteritis, **GI hemorrhage or perforation**, GI infection, GI candidiasis, **hepatitis**, hernia, ileus, jaundice, **liver damage**, **melena**, nausea, **pancreatitis**, **peritonitis**, rectal disorder, stomach ulcer, vomiting
GU: Albuminuria; bilirubinemia; BK virus-related nephropathy; dysuria; hematuria; hydronephrosis; impotence; increased BUN or creatinine levels; **kidney tubular necrosis**; nocturia; oliguria; pain; polyomavirus-associated nephropathy; prostatic disorder; pyelonephritis; **renal failure**; scrotal edema, urinary tract disorder or infection; urine abnormality, frequency, incontinence, or retention
HEME: Anemia, **coagulation disorder**, hypochromic anemia, hypogammaglobulinemia, **increased prothrombin time or thromboplastin time**, leukocytosis, **leukopenia**, polyhemia, pure red cell aplasia, **thrombocytopenia**
MS: Arthralgia; back, neck or pelvic pain; joint disorder; leg cramps; myalgia; myasthenia; osteoporosis
RESP: Apnea; **asthma**; **atelectasis**; bronchitis; candidiasis; cough; dyspnea; **hemoptysis**; hyperventilation; **hypoxia**; **neoplasm**; pleural effusion; pneumonia; **pneumothorax**; **pulmonary edema, fibrosis, or hypertension**; **respiratory acidosis**; sputum increase
SKIN: Abscess; acne; alopecia, cellulite; ecchymosis; fungal dermatitis; hirsutism; pallor; petechia; pruritus; rash; benign neoplasm, **carcinoma**, hypertrophy, or ulcer; sweating; vesiculobullous rash
Other: Abnormal healing; **acidosis**; activation of latent infections (such as tuberculosis) or **reactivation of hepatitis B or hepatitis C**; **alkalosis**; **angioedema**; bacterial, fungal, protozoal, and viral infections, including opportunistic infections; congenital defects; cyst; dehydration; flu-like syndrome; gout; hiccup; **hyperkalemia**; hyperuricemia; hypervolemia; hypochloremia; **hypocalcemia**; **hypokalemia**; **hypomagnesemia**; **hyponatremia**; hypophosphatemia; hypoproteinemia; increased alkaline phosphatase; increased gamma glutamyl transpeptidase; loss of pregnancy during first trimester; **lymphoma**; **malignancies**; **sepsis**; thirst; weight gain or loss

Nursing Considerations

- Keep in mind, before starting mycophenolate therapy in a woman of childbearing potential, to make sure she has a negative pregnancy test within 1 week of starting therapy, using a test with a sensitivity of at least 25 mIU/ml. Therapy shouldn't start until results are confirmed.
- Know that mycophenolate mofetil therapy should be avoided in patients with hypoxanthine-guanine phosphoribosyl-transferase deficiency, because drug may exacerbation of disease symptoms.
- Expect to give I.V. form within 24 hours of transplantation and for no longer than 14 days. Expect to switch patient to oral form as soon as possible, as ordered.
- Keep in mind when preparing I.V. form or oral suspension, avoid inhalation, or direct contact with skin or mucous membranes. If contact occurs, wash area thoroughly with soap and water and rinse eyes with water.
- Prepare oral suspension tapping closed bottle several times to loosen powder and then measure 94 ml of water in a graduated cylinder. Add half of the water to the bottle and shake for about 1 minute. Then add remainder of water and shake again for 1 minute. Remove child-resistant cap and push bottle adapter into neck of bottle. Close bottle tightly with child-resistant cap. Be aware that the suspension bottle may become cold immediately after reconstitution.
- Know that oral suspension can be administered by 8F or larger nasogastric tube.
- Be aware that when giving oral suspension, don't mix with any other drugs. Ask patient about history of

phenylketonuria before initial administration because oral suspension contains aspartame.

- Don't open or crush capsules. If necessary, use the oral suspension.
- Handle I.V. form similarly to a chemotherapeutic drug because mycophenolate mofetil is embryotoxic and genotoxic and may have mutagenic properties.
- Know that I.V. form must be reconstituted and diluted to 6 mg/ml using 5% dextrose injection USP. Inject 14 ml 5% dextrose injection USP into each vial (2 vials will be needed for each 1-g dose; 3 vials for each 1.5-g dose), then shake gently. Further dilute a 1-g dose by adding 2 reconstituted vials to 140 ml of 5% dextrose injection USP; dilute a 1.5-g dose by adding 3 reconstituted vials to 210 ml of 5% dextrose injection USP.
- Be aware that I.V. form should be administered within 4 hours of once reconstituted, as an infusion and over no less than 2 hours. Never administer by rapid or bolus I.V. injection because of increased risk of local reactions such as phlebitis and thrombosis.
- Know that extended release form of mycophenolate mofetil should not be given to children who have a body surface area of less than 1.19 m^2. Also be aware that extended release form is not interchangeable with other forms of the drug.
- Know that corticosteroids and cyclosporine should be used with mycophenolate mofetil therapy.
- Obtain CBC weekly during first month of therapy, twice monthly for the second and third months of therapy, and then monthly through the first year, as ordered. Notify prescriber of any abnormalities. If significant, anticipate dosage reduction if absolutely necessary because reduced immunosuppression increases the risk of organ rejection. Also provide supportive care.
- Monitor patient's serum creatinine levels, as ordered, to detect changes in kidney function because drug may cause polyomavirus-associated nephropathy. Notify prescriber if changes occur and expect dosage to be reduced, if needed.
- Monitor patient closely for adverse reactions because drug has many adverse effects, some of which can be serious or severe, such as the development of lymphoma and other malignancies, especially of the skin. Also know that patient may be at increased risk for bacterial, fungal, protozoal, and viral infections, including opportunistic infections and viral reactivation of hepatitis B and C, which may lead to hospitalization and possibly fatal outcome.
- Expect to stop drug or reduce the dose and provide supportive care, as ordered, if neutropenia develops.

WARNING Know that mycophenolate mofetil therapy has been associated with progressive multifocal leukoencephalopathy that can be life-threatening. Monitor patient for apathy, ataxia, cognitive deficiencies, and confusion. Report suspicions of disorder immediately to prescriber.

PATIENT TEACHING

- Advise women of childbearing age that two forms of contraceptives should be used simultaneously before beginning mycophenolate mofetil therapy and for 6 weeks following discontinuation of therapy because of potential for fetal harm. Inform women who use oral contraceptives that drug may decrease effectiveness of oral contraceptives. Urge patient to notify prescriber immediately if pregnancy occurs because drug increases risk of first-trimester pregnancy loss and congenital malformations. If pregnancy occurs, encourage patient to enroll in the pregnancy exposure registry by calling 800-617-8191.
- Tell patient about increased risk of lymphomas or other malignancies, especially of the skin, before therapy starts. Tell patient to report any unusual signs or symptoms to prescriber.
- Tell patient to take oral form of drug on an empty stomach.
- Inform patient prescribed oral suspension that it contains aspartame, which is a source of phenylalanine.
- Instruct patient not to crush tablets or capsules or open capsules.
- Inform patient not to receive live vaccines during therapy. Urge him to avoid people who have received such vaccines or to wear a protective mask when he's around them.

- Tell patient to report any serious or ongoing adverse reactions, especially neurologic abnormalities, to prescriber immediately.
- Caution patient to avoid contact with people who have infections because drug causes immunosuppression, placing patient at increased risk for developing an infection.
- Urge patient to report any signs of infection, unexpected bleeding or bruising, or any other sign of bone marrow depression immediately.
- Tell patient that frequent laboratory tests may be needed during therapy. Emphasize that having these tests done is essential to continuing therapy.
- Advise patient to avoid exposure to direct sunlight and UV light and to wear sunscreen when outdoors because of increased risk for skin cancer.
- Advise patient not to take antacids at the same time as oral mycophenolate mofetil because some antacids can decrease drug's absorption.
- Tell patient to report dizziness, fainting, lack of energy, paleness, or unusual tiredness because dosage may have to be reduced or drug discontinued.
- Emphasize importance of follow-up care to monitor the drug's effectiveness and possible adverse effects because of the increased risk for cancer and infections as a result of immunosuppression. Inform patient of the need for periodic laboratory tests.
- Caution patient not to donate blood during therapy and for at least 6 weeks following discontinuation of drug. Tell male patients not to donate semen during therapy and for 90 days following discontinuation of drug.

NO

nabumetone

Class and Category
Pharmacologic class: NSAID
Therapeutic class: Anti-inflammatory
Pregnancy category: C (first trimester), Not classified (later trimesters)

Indications and Dosages
➤ *To relieve symptoms of acute and chronic osteoarthritis and rheumatoid arthritis*

TABLETS

Adults. *Initial:* 1 g daily as a single dose or in divided doses twice daily, increased to 1.5 to 2 g daily, as needed. *Maintenance:* Adjusted according to clinical response. *Maximum:* 2 g daily.

Mechanism of Action
Blocks activity of cyclooxygenase, the enzyme needed to synthesize prostaglandins, which mediate the inflammatory response and cause local vasodilation, which can lead to pain and swelling. Prostaglandins also promote pain transmission from periphery to spinal cord. By blocking cyclooxygenase and inhibiting prostaglandins, the NSAID nabumetone reduces inflammatory symptoms and relieves pain.

Contraindications
Angioedema, asthma, bronchospasm, nasal polyps, rhinitis, or urticaria induced by aspirin, iodides, or other NSAIDs

Interactions
DRUGS

acetaminophen (long-term use): Increased risk of adverse renal effects
anticoagulants, thrombolytics: Increased risk of GI bleeding
antihypertensives: Decreased antihypertensive effectiveness
beta blockers: Decreased antihypertensive effects of beta blockers
bone marrow depressants, such as aldesleukin and cisplatin: Increased risk of leukopenia and thrombocytopenia
cefamandole, cefoperazone, cefotetan, plicamycin, valproic acid: Increased risk of hypoprothrombinemia and bleeding
colchicine, other NSAIDs, salicylates: Increased GI irritability and bleeding
cyclosporine, gold compounds, nephrotoxic drugs: Increased risk of nephrotoxicity
digoxin: Increased blood digoxin level and risk of digitalis toxicity
diuretics: Decreased diuretic effectiveness
glucocorticoids, potassium supplements: Increased GI bleeding and irritability
insulin, oral antidiabetic drugs: Increased effects of these drugs; risk of hypoglycemia
lithium: Increased risk of lithium toxicity
methotrexate: Increased risk of methotrexate toxicity
probenecid: Increased risk of nabumetone toxicity

ACTIVITIES

alcohol use: Increased GI bleeding and irritability

Adverse Reactions
CNS: CVA, drowsiness, fatigue, fever, headache, nervousness, **seizures**, vertigo
CV: Edema, hypertension, **MI**, tachycardia
EENT: Dry mouth, pharyngitis, stomatitis, tinnitus
GI: Abdominal pain, anorexia, constipation, diarrhea, diverticulitis, dyspepsia, dysphagia, esophagitis, flatulence, gastritis, gastroenteritis, gastroesophageal reflux disease, **GI bleeding** and ulceration, **hepatic dysfunction**, indigestion, jaundice, **melena**, nausea, **perforation of intestines or stomach**, stomatitis, vomiting
GU: Albuminuria, **azotemia**, interstitial nephritis, **nephrotic syndrome**
HEME: Agranulocytosis, anemia, eosinophilia, **granulocytopenia**, **hemolytic anemia**, **leukopenia**, **neutropenia**, **pancytopenia**, **thrombocytopenia**
MS: Muscle spasms, myalgia
RESP: Asthma, **pneumonitis**, **respiratory depression**
SKIN: Alopecia, **erythema multiforme**, photosensitivity, pruritus, rash, **Stevens–Johnson syndrome**, **toxic epidermal necrolysis**
Other: Anaphylaxis, **angioedema**

Nursing Considerations

- Use nabumetone with extreme caution in patients with a history of GI bleeding or ulcer disease because NSAIDs, such as nabumetone, increase risk of GI bleeding and ulceration. Expect to use nabumetone for shortest time possible in these patients.
- Be aware that serious GI tract bleeding, perforation, and ulceration may occur without warning symptoms. Elderly patients are at greater risk. To minimize risk, give drug with food. If GI distress occurs, withhold drug and notify prescriber immediately.
- Use nabumetone cautiously in patients with hypertension, and monitor blood pressure closely throughout therapy. Drug may cause hypertension or worsen it.

WARNING Monitor patient closely for thrombotic events, including MI and stroke because NSAIDs increase the risk.

- Monitor patient—especially if elderly or receiving long-term nabumetone therapy—for less common but serious adverse GI reactions, including anorexia, constipation, diverticulitis, dysphagia, esophagitis, gastritis, gastroenteritis, gastroesophageal reflux disease, hemorrhoids, hiatal hernia, melena, stomatitis, and vomiting.
- Monitor liver enzymes, as ordered, because, rarely, elevations may progress to severe hepatic reactions, including fatal hepatitis, hepatic failure, and liver necrosis.
- Monitor BUN and serum creatinine levels in elderly patients, patients taking ACE inhibitors or diuretics, and patients with heart failure, hepatic dysfunction, or impaired renal function; nabumetone may cause renal failure.
- Monitor CBC for decreased hemoglobin and hematocrit; drug may worsen anemia.

WARNING Be aware that if patient has bone marrow suppression or is receiving treatment with an antineoplastic, laboratory results (including WBC count) should be monitored; also watch for evidence of infection because anti-inflammatory and antipyretic actions of nabumetone may mask signs and symptoms, such as fever and pain.

- Assess patient's skin regularly for signs of rash or other hypersensitivity reaction because nabumetone is an NSAID and may cause serious skin reactions without warning, even in patients with no history of NSAID sensitivity. At first sign of reaction, stop drug and notify prescriber.
- Assess patient for severe hepatic reactions, including jaundice. Stop drug, as prescribed, if symptoms persist.

PATIENT TEACHING

- Instruct patient to take nabumetone with food to reduce GI distress.
- Advise patient to take drug with a full glass of water and to remain upright for 15 to 30 minutes afterward to prevent drug from lodging in esophagus and causing irritation.
- Tell patient not to increase dose or frequency without consulting prescriber.
- Urge patient to avoid alcohol to reduce risk of GI bleeding.
- Inform patient that regular laboratory tests are needed to check for drug toxicity during long-term therapy.
- Caution pregnant patient not to take NSAIDs such as nabumetone during the last trimester because they may cause premature closure of the ductus arteriosus.
- Explain that nabumetone may increase the risk of serious adverse cardiovascular reactions; urge patient to seek immediate medical attention if signs or symptoms arise, such as chest pain, shortness of breath, slurring of speech, and weakness.
- Explain that nabumetone may increase the risk of serious adverse GI reactions; emphasize the importance of seeking immediate medical attention for such signs and symptoms as abdominal or epigastric pain, black or tarry stools, indigestion, or vomiting blood or material that looks like coffee grounds.
- Alert patient to rare, but serious, skin reactions. Urge her to seek immediate medical attention for blisters, fever, itching, rash, or other indications of hypersensitivity.

nadolol

Corgard, Syn-Nadolol (CAN)

Class and Category

Pharmacologic class: Nonselective beta blocker
Therapeutic class: Antianginal, antihypertensive
Pregnancy category: C

Indications and Dosages

➤ *To manage hypertension, alone or with other antihypertensives*

TABLETS

Adults. *Initial:* 40 mg daily, increased by 40 to 80 mg daily every 7 days, as needed. *Maintenance:* 40 to 80 mg daily. *Maximum:* 320 mg daily.

➤ *To manage angina pectoris as long-term therapy*

TABLETS

Adults. *Initial:* 40 mg daily, increased by 40 to 80 mg daily every 3 to 7 days, as needed. *Maintenance:* 40 to 80 mg daily. *Maximum:* 240 mg daily.

DOSAGE ADJUSTMENT Interval possibly increased to every 24 to 36 hr if creatinine clearance is 31 to 50 ml/min; to every 24 to 48 hr if it's 10 to 30 ml/min; or to every 40 to 60 hr if it's less than 10 ml/min.

Route	Onset	Peak	Duration
P.O.	Up to 5 days	4 hr	24 hr

Mechanism of Action

Selectively blocks $alpha_1$ and $beta_2$ receptors in vascular smooth muscle and $beta_1$ receptors in the heart, thereby reducing peripheral vascular resistance and blood pressure. Potent beta blockade decreases cardiac excitability, cardiac output, and myocardial oxygen demand, thus reducing angina. It also prevents reflex tachycardia, which typically occurs with most alpha blockers.

Contraindications

Asthma; bronchospasm; cardiogenic shock; heart failure; hypersensitivity to nadolol, other beta blockers, or their components; second- or third-degree AV block; severe COPD; sinus bradycardia

Interactions

DRUGS

allergen immunotherapy, allergenic extracts for skin testing: Increased risk of serious systemic reactions, including anaphylaxis
amiodarone: Increased risk of conduction abnormalities and negative inotropic effects
beta blockers, calcium channel blockers, digoxin: Increased risk of bradycardia
calcium channel blockers: Increased risk of bradycardia
cimetidine: Possibly increased effects of nadolol
clonidine, guanabenz: Impaired blood pressure control
diazoxide, nitroglycerin: Increased risk of hypotension
estrogens, NSAIDs: Possibly reduced antihypertensive effect of nadolol
general anesthetics: Increased risk of hypotension and myocardial depression
insulin, oral antidiabetic drugs: Possibly increased risk of hyperglycemia and impaired recovery from hypoglycemia, masking of signs of hypoglycemia
lidocaine: Increased risk of lidocaine toxicity
neuromuscular blockers: Possibly prolonged action of these drugs
phenothiazines: Possibly increased blood levels of both drugs
reserpine: Increased risk of bradycardia and hypotension
sympathomimetics with alpha- and beta-adrenergic effects, such as pseudoephedrine: Possibly excessive bradycardia, heart block, and hypertension
xanthines, such as theophyllines: Possibly decreased therapeutic effects of both drugs

Adverse Reactions

CNS: Anxiety, depression, dizziness, drowsiness, fatigue, headache, paresthesia, syncope, vertigo, weakness, yawning
CV: **Bradycardia**, chest pain, edema, **heart block**, **heart failure**, **hypotension**, orthostatic hypotension, **ventricular arrhythmias**
EENT: Nasal congestion, taste perversion
GI: Dyspepsia, elevated liver enzymes, **hepatic necrosis**, **hepatitis**, jaundice, nausea, vomiting
GU: Ejaculation failure, impotence
RESP: Cough, dyspnea, wheezing
SKIN: Pruritus, scalp tingling

Nursing Considerations

- Use nadolol cautiously in patients with diabetes mellitus because it may prolong or worsen hypoglycemia by interfering with glycogenolysis.
- Anticipate that drug may worsen psoriasis; in patients with myasthenia gravis, it may worsen muscle weakness and diplopia.
- Be aware that chronic beta blocker therapy such as nadolol is not routinely withheld prior to major surgery because the benefits outweigh the risks associated with

its use with general anesthesia and surgical procedures.

WARNING Withdraw drug gradually over 2 weeks, or as ordered, to avoid MI caused by unopposed beta stimulation or thyroid storm caused by underlying hyperthyroidism. Expect drug to mask tachycardia caused by hyperthyroidism.

PATIENT TEACHING

- Teach patient how to take her radial pulse, and direct her to do so before each dose of nadolol.
- Instruct patient to notify prescriber if pulse rate falls below 60 beats/minute.
- Caution patient not to stop taking nadolol abruptly or change dosage. Tell her to take a missed dose as soon as possible unless it's within 8 hours of the next scheduled dose.
- Advise patient with diabetes to check blood glucose level often because nadolol may mask signs of hypoglycemia, such as tachycardia.
- Review signs of impending heart failure, and urge patient to notify prescriber immediately if they occur.

nafcillin sodium

Class and Category

Pharmacologic class: Penicillin
Therapeutic class: Antibiotic
Pregnancy category: B

Indications and Dosages

➤ *To treat infections caused by penicillinase-producing* Staphylococcus aureus

I.V. INFUSION

Adults. 500 to 1,000 mg given over 30 to 60 min every 4 hr. Duration of therapy varies depending on type and severity of infection, but is continued for at least 48 hr after patient is afebrile, asymptomatic, and cultures are negative. Severe infections require at least 14 days of therapy.

Mechanism of Action

Binds to certain penicillin-binding proteins in bacterial cell walls, thereby inhibiting the final stage of bacterial cell wall synthesis. The result is cell lysis. Nafcillin's action is bolstered by its chemical composition; its unique side chain resists destruction by beta-lactamases.

Incompatibilities

Don't mix nafcillin in same I.V. bag as aminoglycosides; they're chemically incompatible.

Contraindications

Hypersensitivity to nafcillin, other penicillins, or their components

Interactions

DRUGS

aminoglycosides: Substantial mutual inactivation
chloramphenicol, erythromycins, sulfonamides, tetracyclines: Possibly decreased therapeutic effects of nafcillin
hepatotoxic drugs: Increased risk of hepatotoxicity
methotrexate: Increased risk of methotrexate toxicity
probenecid: Increased blood nafcillin level

Adverse Reactions

CNS: Depression, fever, headache, **seizures**
CV: Hypotension, vascular collapse
EENT: Black or hairy tongue, **laryngospasm**, oral candidiasis, stomatitis
GI: Abdominal pain, cholestasis, diarrhea, elevated liver enzymes, nausea, **pseudomembranous colitis**, vomiting
GU: Acute kidney injury, hematuria, interstitial nephritis, proteinuria, **renal tubular damage**, vaginitis
HEME: Agranulocytosis, bone marrow depression, leukopenia, neutropenia
RESP: Bronchospasm
SKIN: Exfoliative dermatitis, pruritus, rash, urticaria
Other: Anaphylaxis; **angioedema**; **hypokalemia**; injection-site pain, redness, and swelling; phlebitis; serum sickness-like reaction; skin sloughing; thrombophlebitis; tissue necrosis (severe)

Nursing Considerations

- Obtain body fluid or tissue samples for culture and sensitivity testing, as prescribed, and obtain test results, if possible, before giving nafcillin, as ordered.
- Expect to have the following laboratory tests ordered before and then periodically

during nafcillin therapy: alkaline phosphatase, bilirubin, blood urea nitrogen, creatinine, liver enzymes, and urinalysis; this provides a baseline and then allows monitoring for adverse effects stemming from nafcillin therapy.
- For intermittent I.V. infusion, infuse over 30 to 60 minutes.
- Give nafcillin at least 1 hour before or after aminoglycosides, especially if patient has renal disease.
- When giving nafcillin to patient at risk for fluid overload or hypertension, be aware that each gram contains 2.5 mEq sodium.
- Watch for evidence of superinfection, such as oral candidiasis and pseudomembranous colitis, especially in elderly, immunocompromised, or debilitated patients who receive large doses of nafcillin. If profuse, watery diarrhea develops, contact prescriber and expect to obtain a stool specimen to rule out pseudomembranous colitis caused by *Clostridium difficile.* If diarrhea occurs, notify prescriber and expect to withhold nafcillin and treat with electrolytes, fluids, protein, and an antibiotic effective against *C. difficile.*

PATIENT TEACHING
- Advise patient to notify prescriber if she experiences chills, fever, GI distress, or rash.
- Urge patient to tell prescriber if diarrhea develops, even 2 or more months after nafcillin therapy ends.

nalbuphine hydrochloride

Nubain (CAN)

Class and Category

Pharmacologic class: Opioid
Therapeutic class: Opioid analgesic
Pregnancy category: B

Indications and Dosages

➤ *To relieve pain severe enough to require opioid-like treatment and for which alternative treatment options such as nonopioid analgesics or opioid combination products are inadequate or not tolerated*

I.M., I.V., OR SUBCUTANEOUS INJECTION
Adults weighing 70 kg (154 lb). 10 mg every 3 to 6 hr, as needed. Dosage adjusted for patients weighing more or less.

➤ *As adjunct to anesthesia*

I.V. INJECTION
Adults. 0.3 to 3 mg/kg over 10 to 15 min followed by 0.25 to 0.5 mg/kg, as needed.
DOSAGE ADJUSTMENT For patients who have repeatedly received an opioid agonist, initial dose possibly reduced to 25% of usual. For patients in whom tolerance to drug's effects hasn't developed, maximum usually is 20 mg/dose or 160 mg daily.

Route	Onset	Peak	Duration
I.M.	In 15 min	1 hr	3–6 hr
I.V.	2–3 min	30 min	3–4 hr
SubQ	In 15 min	Unknown	3–6 hr

Mechanism of Action

Binds with and stimulates kappa and mu opiate receptors in the spinal cord and higher levels in the CNS. In this way, nalbuphine alters the perception of and emotional response to pain.

Incompatibilities

Don't give nalbuphine with diazepam or pentobarbital. Use separate I.V. line or flush line well before and after administration.

Contraindications

Hypersensitivity to nalbuphine or its components

Interactions

DRUGS
alfentanil, benzodiazepines, CNS depressants, fentanyl, sedating antihistamines, sufentanil tricyclic antidepressants: Increased risk of significant CNS and respiratory depression and hypotension
anticholinergics: Increased risk of severe constipation and urine retention
antidiarrheals, such as difenoxin and atropine, loperamide, and paregoric: Increased risk of severe constipation and increased CNS depression
antihypertensives: Increased risk of hypotension
antimigraine agents, cyclobenzaprine; dextromethorphan; dolasetron; granisetron; linezolid; MAO inhibitors; methylene blue;

ondansetron; palonosetron; selected psychiatric drugs such as amoxapine, buspirone, lithium, maprotiline, mirtazapine, nefazodone, trazodone, vilazodone; selective serotonin reuptake inhibitors; serotonin-norepinephrine reuptake inhibitors; St. John's wort; tricyclic antidepressants; tryptophan: Increased risk of serotonin syndrome
benzodiazepines, CNS depressants, other opioids, sedating antihistamines, tricyclic antidepressants: Increased risk of severe respiratory depression and significant sedation and somnolence
buprenorphine: Possibly decreased therapeutic effects of nalbuphine and increased risk of respiratory depression
hydroxyzine: Increased risk of CNS depression and hypotension
MAO inhibitors: Risk of possibly fatal increased CNS depression or excitation
metoclopramide: Possibly antagonized effects of metoclopramide
naloxone, naltrexone: Decreased pharmacologic effects of nalbuphine
neuromuscular blockers: Increased risk of prolonged CNS and respiratory depression

ACTIVITIES

alcohol use: Increased risk of coma, hypotension, profound sedation, and respiratory depression

Adverse Reactions

CNS: Confusion, depression, dizziness, euphoria, fatigue, hallucinations, headache, nervousness, restlessness, **seizures**, syncope, tiredness, weakness
CV: Hypertension, **hypotension**, tachycardia
EENT: Blurred vision, diplopia, dry mouth
ENDO: Adrenal insufficiency
GI: Abdominal cramps, anorexia, constipation, nausea, vomiting
GU: Decreased libido, decreased urine output, impotency, infertility, lack of menstruation, ureteral spasm
RESP: Dyspnea, **pulmonary edema**, **respiratory depression**, wheezing
SKIN: Diaphoresis, flushing, pruritus, rash, sensation of warmth, urticaria
Other: Injection-site burning, pain, redness, swelling, and warmth

Nursing Considerations

- Be aware that excessive use of opioids like nalbuphine may lead to abuse, addiction, misuse, overdose, and possibly death. Monitor patient's intake of drug closely and for evidence of physical dependence.
- Know that chronic maternal use of nalbuphine during pregnancy can result in neonatal opioid withdrawal syndrome (NOWS), which may be life-threatening if not recognized and treated appropriately. NOWS occurs when a newborn has been exposed to opioid drugs like nalbuphine for a prolonged period while in utero.
- Use nalbuphine cautiously in patients taking other drugs that can cause respiratory depression.

WARNING Be aware that nalbuphine should only be used concomitantly with benzodiazepine therapy in patients for whom other treatment options are inadequate. If prescribed together, expect dosing and duration of nalbuphine to be limited. Monitor patient closely for signs and symptoms of a decrease in consciousness, including coma, profound sedation, and significant respiratory depression. Notify prescriber immediately and provide emergency supportive care, as death may occur.

- Keep resuscitation equipment and naloxone readily available to reverse nalbuphine's effects, if needed.
- For direct I.V. injection through an I.V. line with a compatible infusing solution, give drug slowly—no more than 10 mg over 3 to 5 minutes. Inject into free-flowing D_5W, lactated Ringer's solution, or normal saline solution.
- Be aware that during prolonged use, a stool softener may be given to minimize constipation.
- Know that if patient is opioid-dependent, drug will usually not be discontinued abruptly. Monitor patient for withdrawal symptoms, such as abdominal cramps, anorexia, anxiety, backache, bone or joint pain, confusion, depression, diaphoresis, dysphoria, erythema, fear, fever, irritability, labile blood pressure and pulse, lacrimation, muscle spasms, myalgia, mydriasis, nasal congestion, nausea, opioid craving, piloerection, restlessness,

rhinorrhea, sensation of crawling skin, sleep disturbances, tremor, uneasiness, vomiting, and yawning.

WARNING Know that many drugs may interact with opioids like nalbuphine to cause serotonin syndrome. Monitor patient closely for signs and symptoms such as agitation, diaphoresis, diarrhea, fever, hallucinations, labile blood pressure, muscle twitching or stiffness, nausea, shakiness, shivering, tachycardia, trouble with coordination, or vomiting. Notify prescriber at once because serotonin syndrome may be life-threatening. Be prepared to discontinue drug, if possible and ordered, and provide supportive care.

- Monitor patient for adrenal insufficiency. Although rare, it can be life-threatening. Monitor patient for anorexia, dizziness, fatigue, hypotension, nausea, vomiting, or weakness. Notify prescriber if adrenal insufficiency is suspected and expect to do diagnostic testing. If confirmed, expect to administer corticosteroids and wean patient off nalbuphine, if possible.

WARNING Be aware that drug may obscure neurologic assessment findings if patient has a cerebral aneurysm, head injury, or increased intracranial pressure.

PATIENT TEACHING

- Warn patient not to take drug longer than absolutely needed because excessive or prolonged use can lead to abuse, addiction, misuse, overdose, and possibly death.
- Advise patient to avoid hazardous activities until nalbuphine's CNS effects are known.

WARNING Warn patient not to consume alcohol or take a benzodiazepine without prescriber knowledge while taking nalbuphine, as severe respiratory depression can occur and may lead to death. Inform patient about potentially fatal additive effects of combining a benzodiazepine with an opioid. Instruct patient to inform all prescribers of nalbuphine use.

- Counsel patient against making important decisions while receiving drug because it may cloud her judgment.
- Inform patient that long-term use of opioids like nalbuphine may decrease sex hormone levels, causing decreased libido, erectile dysfunction, impotence, infertility, or lack of menstruation. Encourage patient to report any symptoms to prescriber.
- Instruct patient to notify all prescribers of opioid use.

naldemedine

Symproic

Class and Category

Pharmacologic class: Opioid receptor antagonist
Therapeutic class: Opioid antagonist of GI tract
Pregnancy category: Not classified

Indications and Dosages

➤ *To treat opioid-induced constipation in patients with chronic noncancer pain*

TABLETS

Adults. 0.2 mg once daily.

Route	Onset	Peak	Duration
P.O.	Unknown	0.75 hr	Unknown

Mechanism of Action

Functions as a peripherally acting mu-opioid receptor antagonist in the gastrointestinal tract to decrease the constipating effects of opioids.

Contraindications

Gastrointestinal obstruction or increased risk of recurrent obstruction due to the potential for gastrointestinal perforation, hypersensitivity to naldemedine or its components

Interactions

DRUGS

moderate CYP3A inhibitors such as aprepitant, atazanavir, diltiazem, erythromycin, fluconazole; P-glycoprotein inhibitors such as amiodarone, captopril, cyclosporine, quercetin, quinidine, verapamil; strong CYP3A inhibitors such as itraconazole: Increased plasma naldemedine concentrations increasing risk of adverse reactions
other opioid antagonists: Possible additive effect of opioid receptor antagonism and increased risk of opioid withdrawal

strong CYP3A inducers such as carbamazepine, phenytoin, rifampin, St. John's wort: Significant decrease in plasma naldemedine concentrations, which may decrease effectiveness

Adverse Reactions

GI: Abdominal pain, diarrhea, gastroenteritis, **GI perforation**, nausea, vomiting
RESP: Bronchospasm
SKIN: Rash
Other: Opioid withdrawal

Nursing Considerations

- Know that patients receiving opioids for less than a month may be less responsive to naldemedine therapy.
- Expect naldemedine to be discontinued if treatment with an opioid pain medication is discontinued.
- Monitor patient closely for abdominal pain. Know that gastrointestinal perforation has occurred with use of another peripherally acting opioid antagonist in patients with conditions that affect the gastrointestinal tract wall integrity, such as diverticular disease, infiltrative gastrointestinal tract malignancies, Ogilvie's syndrome, peptic ulcer disease, or peritoneal metastases. Patients with Crohn's disease may be at increased risk for gastrointestinal perforation. Notify prescriber immediately if abdominal pain becomes persistent, severe, or worsens. Expect drug to be discontinued.
- Monitor patient for signs and symptoms of opioid withdrawal such as abdominal pain, chills, diarrhea, feeling cold, fever, flushing, hyperhidrosis, increased lacrimation, nausea, and vomiting. Patients who develop disruptions to the bloodbrain barrier may be at increased risk for opioid withdrawal or reduced analgesia.

PATIENT TEACHING

- Inform patient that naldemedine should be discontinued if treatment with the opioid pain medication is discontinued.
- Tell patient that the most common side effects of naldemedine include abdominal pain, diarrhea, nausea, and vomiting.
- Advise patient to seek immediate emergency care if persistent, severe, or worsening abdominal pain occurs.
- Review the signs and symptoms of withdrawal with patient and tell her to notify prescriber if these symptoms occur.
- Inform women of childbearing age to notify prescriber if pregnancy occurs, as naldemedine does cross the placenta and may precipitate opioid withdrawal in the fetus.
- Inform mothers wishing to breastfeed that drug does appear in breast milk, increasing risk of adverse reactions for the nursing infant. Therefore, breastfeeding is not recommended.

naloxegol

Movantik

Class and Category

Pharmacologic class: Opioid receptor antagonist
Therapeutic class: Opioid antagonist of gastrointestinal tract
Pregnancy category: C

Indications and Dosages

➤ *To treat opioid-induced constipation in patients with chronic noncancer pain*

TABLETS

Adults. 25 mg once daily in the morning.
DOSAGE ADJUSTMENT For patients unable to tolerate naloxegol at the normal dose, patients with renal impairment (creatinine clearance less than 60 ml/min), and patients taking moderate CYP3A4 inhibitor drugs such as diltiazem, erythromycin, or verapamil, dosage reduced to 12.5 mg once daily in the morning. If dose is well tolerated in patients with renal impairment, dosage increased to 25 mg once daily in the morning.

Mechanism of Action

Functions as a peripherally acting mu-opioid receptor antagonist in tissues such as the gastrointestinal tract, thereby decreasing the constipating effects of opioids.

Contraindications

Concomitant therapy with strong CYP3A4 inhibitors such as clarithromycin and ketoconazole, gastrointestinal obstruction or risk of recurrent obstruction, hypersensitivity to naloxegol or its components

Interactions

DRUGS

CYP3A4 inducers such as carbamazepine, rifampin, St. John's wort: Decreased plasma naloxegol levels and effectiveness
CYP3A4 inhibitors such as clarithromycin, diltiazem, erythromycin, itraconazole, ketoconazole, verapamil: Increased plasma naloxegol levels, possibly increasing risk of adverse reactions including opioid withdrawal
other opioid antagonists: Potential for additive effects and increased risk of opioid withdrawal

FOOD

grapefruit, grapefruit juice: Increased plasma naloxegol levels

Adverse Reactions

CNS: Headache
GI: Abdominal pain (may become severe), diarrhea, flatulence, nausea, vomiting
SKIN: Diaphoresis
Other: Opioid withdrawal

Nursing Considerations

- Expect all maintenance laxative therapy to be discontinued prior to patient starting naloxegol therapy but know that laxatives may be given, as ordered and if needed, after 3 days of naloxegol therapy.
- Know that tablet can be crushed to a powder and mixed with 4 ounces of water for patient who is unable to swallow tablet whole. Once mixed, patient must drink mixture immediately. To ensure that all of the dosage was ingested, refill same glass with 4 ounces of water, stir, and have patient drink contents again.
- Know that naloxegol may be administered through a nasogastric tube. Begin by flushing tube with 30 ml of water using a 60 ml syringe. Crush tablet to a powder in a container and mix with 60 ml of water. Draw up mixture using the 60 ml syringe and administer contents through the nasogastric tube. Add about 60 ml of water to same container used to prepare the dose. Draw up the water using the same 60 ml syringe and use all the water to flush the nasogastric tube and any remaining drug from the nasogastric tube into the stomach.
- Monitor patient for the development of persistent, severe, or worsening abdominal pain and/or diarrhea because gastrointestinal perforation has occurred with use of naloxegol. Symptoms generally occur within a few days of starting naloxegol therapy. If this type of abdominal pain occurs, withhold drug and notify prescriber. Know that drug may be restarted at a lower dose (12.5 mg daily), once symptoms have resolved and if drug is still needed.
- Monitor patient's reaction to naloxegol therapy, especially in patients who have taken opioids for at least 4 weeks prior to starting naloxegol, because sustained exposure to opioids may cause an increased response to naloxegol.
- Monitor patient for opioid withdrawal symptoms such as abdominal pain, anxiety, chills, diaphoresis, diarrhea, irritability, and yawning. Clusters of these symptoms may occur with naloxegol therapy, especially if patient is receiving methadone or has a disruption in opioid therapy.
- Know that if opioid therapy is discontinued, naloxegol therapy should be discontinued.

PATIENT TEACHING

- Tell patient to stop all maintenance laxative therapy prior to starting naloxegol therapy. Reassure him that laxatives may be used, if needed, after the first 3 days of therapy.
- Instruct patient to take naloxegol at least 1 hour prior to the first meal of the day or 2 hours after the meal.
- Tell patient who is unable to swallow tablet whole to crush it to a fine powder, mix it with 4 ounces of water and drink the mixture immediately. To ensure that all the drug has been ingested, have patient refill the same glass with 4 ounces of water again, stir, and drink entire content.
- Teach caregiver how to administer drug via a nasogastric tube, if necessary.
- Remind patient not to consume grapefruit or grapefruit juice while taking naloxegol.
- Tell patient to notify prescriber if opioid therapy is discontinued.
- Advise patient to inform prescriber of all medications being taken, including over-the-counter drugs and any new drug therapy begun once naloxegol therapy begins.
- Instruct patient to stop drug and seek medical attention promptly if he develops persistent, severe, or worsening abdominal pain and/or diarrhea. Tell

patient symptoms may occur a few days after starting treatment.
- Warn patient that opioid withdrawal symptoms may occur while taking naloxegol and to notify prescriber.
- Caution female patients of childbearing age to notify prescriber immediately if pregnancy is suspected or has occurred, as the drug may precipitate opioid withdrawal in a fetus, due to the undeveloped blood–brain barrier, as well as in the pregnant woman.
- Advise females who might wish to breastfeed their infants not to do so, as the infant may experience opioid withdrawal symptoms because of the drug's presence in breast milk.

naloxone hydrochloride

Evzio, Narcan

Class and Category

Pharmacologic class: Opioid antagonist
Therapeutic class: Antidote
Pregnancy category: B

Indications and Dosages

➤ *To treat known or suspected opioid overdose*

I.V., I.M., OR SUBCUTANEOUS INJECTION (NARCAN)
Adults. 0.4 to 2 mg repeated every 2 to 3 min, as needed (in divided doses for children). If no response after 10 mg, patient may not have opioid-induced respiratory depression.
Infants 1 month and over and children. 0.01 mg/kg as a single dose; if no improvement, 0.1 mg/kg given in divided doses.

I.V., I.M., OR SUBCUTANEOUS INJECTION (NARCAN)
Neonates. 0.01 mg/kg repeated every 2 to 3 min, as needed, until desired response occurs.

I.M. OR SUBCUTANEOUS INJECTION (EVZIO)
Adults and children. 0.4 mg, repeated every 2 to 3 min, as needed, until desired response occurs.

NASAL SPRAY (NARCAN)
Adults and children. 2 mg (1 spray) to 4 mg (1 spray) repeated every 2 to 3 min, as needed, alternating nostrils with each dose.

➤ *To treat postoperative opioid-induced respiratory depression*

I.V. INJECTION
Adults. *Initial:* 0.1 to 0.2 mg every 2 to 3 min until desired response occurs. Additional doses given every 1 to 2 hr, if needed, based on patient response.
Children. *Initial:* 0.005 to 0.01 mg every 2 to 3 min until desired response occurs. Additional doses given every 1 to 2 hr, as needed, based on patient response.

➤ *To reverse opioid-induced asphyxia*

I.V., I.M., OR SUBCUTANEOUS INJECTION
Neonates. *Initial:* 0.01 mg/kg every 2 to 3 min until desired response occurs. Additional doses given every 1 to 2 hr, if needed, based on patient response.

➤ *As adjunct to treat hypotension caused by septic shock*

I.V. INFUSION OR INJECTION
Adults. Highly individualized.

Route	Onset	Peak	Duration
I.V.	1–2 min	5–15 min	45 min or longer
I.M., SubQ	2–5 min	5–15 min	45 min or longer
Nasal spray	1–3 min	Unknown	Unknown

Mechanism of Action

Briefly and competitively antagonizes mu, kappa, and sigma receptors in the CNS, thus reversing analgesia, hypotension, respiratory depression, and sedation caused by most opioids. Mu receptors are responsible for analgesia, euphoria, miosis, and respiratory depression. Kappa receptors are responsible for analgesia and sedation. Sigma receptors control dysphoria and other delusional states.

Incompatibilities

Don't mix naloxone with any other solution unless you verify that the drugs are compatible; drug is incompatible with alkaline, bisulfite, and metabisulfite solutions.

Contraindications

Hypersensitivity to naloxone or its components

Interactions

DRUGS

butorphanol, nalbuphine, pentazocine: Reversal of these drugs' analgesic and adverse effects

opioid analgesics: Reversal of these drugs' analgesic and adverse effects, possibly withdrawal symptoms in opioid-dependent patients

Adverse Reactions

CNS: Excitement, headache, irritability, nervousness, restlessness, **seizures**, tremor, violent behavior

CV: **Cardiac arrest**, hypertension (severe), **hypotension**, **ventricular fibrillation**, **ventricular tachycardia**

EENT: Nasal congestion, dryness, edema, inflammation, or pain (spray form); toothache

GI: Constipation, nausea, vomiting

MS: Muscle spasms, musculoskeletal pain

RESP: Dyspnea, **pulmonary edema**

SKIN: Diaphoresis, xeroderma

Other: Withdrawal symptoms

Nursing Considerations

- Keep resuscitation equipment readily available during naloxone administration.
- Administer parenteral Narcan brand by I.V. route whenever possible.
- Be aware that each Narcan nasal spray contains a single dose of naloxone and cannot be reused. Place patient in supine position to administer making sure device nozzle is inserted in either nostril of the patient. Provide support to the back of the patient's neck to allow the head to tilt back. Do not prime or test the device prior to administration. Press firmly on the device plunger to administer the dose. Remove the device nozzle from the patient's nostril after use and turn patient on side.
- Administer Evzio brand only by I.M. or subcutaneous route following printed instructions on the device label. Be aware that an electronic voice will guide user through each step but if it does not operate properly, the device will still deliver the intended dose. Once the red safety guard is removed, drug must be used immediately or disposed of properly. Do not attempt to replace the red safety guard once it is removed.
- Know that upon actuation, Evzio brand will automatically insert the needle I.M. or subcutaneously, deliver 0.4 mg naloxone, and retract needle fully into its housing. Post injection, the black base locks in place, a red indicator appears in the viewing window, and the electronic visual and audible instructions signal that Evzio has delivered the intended dose.
- Give repeat doses as prescribed, depending on patient's response.
- Anticipate that rapid reversal of opioid effects can cause diaphoresis, nausea, and vomiting in addition to serious adverse effects such as hypotension, pulmonary edema, seizures, and ventricular arrhythmias. Monitor patient closely, especially patients at risk because of the presence of preexisting cardiovascular disorders or who are receiving drugs that cause similar adverse cardiovascular effects.

WARNING Watch for opioid withdrawal symptoms, especially when giving naloxone to opioid-dependent patient. Symptoms may include abdominal cramps, anorexia, anxiety, backache, bone or joint pain, confusion, depression, diaphoresis, dysphoria, erythema, fear, fever, irritability, labile blood pressure and pulse, lacrimation, muscle spasms, myalgia, mydriasis, nasal congestion, nausea, opioid craving, piloerection, restlessness, rhinorrhea, sensation of crawling skin, sleep disturbances, tremor, uneasiness, vomiting, and yawning.

- Monitor patients in postoperative setting who have received naloxone because abrupt postoperative reversal of opioid depression after using naloxone may cause serious adverse effects. Excessive doses of naloxone in the postoperative setting have also caused significant reversal of analgesia and have caused patient to become agitated.
- Expect patient with hepatic or renal dysfunction to have increased circulating blood naloxone level.

PATIENT TEACHING

- Inform patient or family that naloxone will reverse opioid-induced adverse reactions.
- Urge opioid-dependent patient to seek drug rehabilitation.

- Instruct family on how to administer naloxone by nasal spray, if prescribed for emergency use at home. Tell family to administer drug as quickly as possible if patient is unresponsive and an opioid overdose is suspected. Instruct family to lay patient on his back and administer the nasal spray into one nostril while providing support to the back of the neck to allow the head to tilt back. Tell them to use each nasal spray only one time. They should then turn the patient on his side and call for help by calling 911. Tell family to monitor patient while help is coming and to readminister nasal spray using a new NARCAN Nasal Spray every 2 to 3 minutes, if patient is not responding or responds and then relapses back into respiratory depression. Tell them to administer the nasal spray in alternate nostrils with each dose.

naltrexone

Vivitrol

naltrexone hydrochloride

ReVia

Class and Category

Pharmacologic class: Opioid antagonist
Therapeutic class: Opioid and alcohol blocker
Pregnancy category: C

Indications and Dosages

➤ *To treat opioid dependence*

TABLETS (REVIA)

Adults. *Initial:* 25 mg, and if no withdrawal symptoms occur, dosage increased following day to 50 mg and then 50 mg given once daily thereafter. *Maintenance:* 50 mg every weekday with 100 mg dose on Saturday. Alternatively, 100 mg every other day or 150 mg every third day.

➤ *To prevent relapse to opioid dependence following opioid detoxification*

I.M. INJECTION (VIVITROL)

Adults. 380 mg every 4 wk or once monthly.

➤ *As adjunct to treat alcoholism*

TABLETS (REVIA)

Adults. 50 mg daily (up to 100 mg daily for some patients) for 12 wk.

I.M. INJECTION (VIVITROL)

Adults. 380 mg every 4 wk or once monthly.

Route	Onset	Peak	Duration
P.O.	15–30 min	In 12 hr	24 hr*
I.M.	Unknown	2 hr	Unknown

* For 50 mg; 48 hr for 100 mg; 72 hr for 150 mg.

Mechanism of Action

Displaces opioid agonists from—or blocks them from binding with—delta, kappa, and mu receptors. Opioid receptor blockade reverses the euphoric effect of opioids. Naltrexone also inhibits the effects of endogenous opioids, thus reducing alcohol craving.

Contraindications

Acute hepatitis, acute opioid withdrawal, concurrent use of opioid analgesics (including opioid agonists, such as levo-alpha-acetyl-methadol [LAAM] or methadone, or partial agonists such as buprenorphine), failure of naloxone challenge test, hepatic failure, hypersensitivity to naltrexone or its components, opioid dependence, positive urine screen for opioids

Interactions

DRUGS

opioid analgesics: Reversal of analgesic and adverse effects of these drugs, possibly withdrawal symptoms in opioid-dependent patients
thioridazine: Increased lethargy and somnolence

Adverse Reactions

CNS: Abnormal thinking, agitation, anxiety, asthenia, chills, confusion, depression, dizziness, euphoria, fatigue, fever, hallucinations, headache, hyperkinesia, insomnia, irritability, malaise, nervousness, restlessness, somnolence, **suicidal ideation**, syncope, tremor
CV: Chest pain, edema, hypertension, palpitations, tachycardia
EENT: Blurred vision, burning eyes, conjunctivitis, dry mouth, eyelid swelling,

hoarseness, pharyngitis, rhinitis, sneezing, tinnitus, vision abnormalities
ENDO: Hot flashes
GI: Abdominal cramps, anorexia, constipation, diarrhea, elevated liver enzymes, GI ulceration, **hepatotoxicity** (excessive doses), nausea, vomiting
GU: Difficult ejaculation, urinary frequency
HEME: Idiopathic thrombocytopenic purpura
MS: Arthralgia, back pain or stiffness, joint stiffness, muscle cramps, myalgia
RESP: Cough, dyspnea, **eosinophilic pneumonia**, upper respiratory tract infection
SKIN: Increased sweating, pruritus, rash
Other: Injection-site reactions, such as bruising, erythema, induration, pain, tenderness; thirst

Nursing Considerations

- Use naltrexone cautiously in patients with hemophilia, severe hepatic failure, severe renal impairment, or thrombocytopenia.
- To avoid withdrawal symptoms, wait 7 to 10 days after last opioid dose, as prescribed, before starting naltrexone. Because urine testing isn't always conclusive, prepare patient for naloxone challenge test if there are any doubts about patient's abstinence.
- Give oral drug with antacids or food to decrease adverse GI reactions.
- Dilute parenteral form using only diluent supplied in carton. Inject intramuscularly in gluteal muscle using only needle supplied in carton. Don't substitute any components for components in carton. Store entire dose pack in refrigerator; unrefrigerated drug can be stored at room temperature for no more than 7 days. Avoid administering as a subcutaneous injection because of increased risk of severe injection-site reactions.
- Inspect injection site for reactions, such as induration, redness, swelling, or tenderness. Ask if patient feels itching or pain at the site. Report any such findings to prescriber because abscesses and site necrosis may occur and require surgical intervention.

WARNING Never give parenteral form intravenously.

- Be aware that patients who receive naltrexone and need pain management are more likely to have longer, deeper respiratory depression and histamine-release reactions (such as bronchoconstriction, facial swelling, generalized erythema, and itching) if given an opioid analgesic. Expect alternative analgesics to be used, such as conscious sedation with a benzodiazepine, general anesthesia, nonopioid analgesics, or regional anesthesia. If an opioid analgesic must be used, monitor patient closely.
- Watch patient closely for suicidal tendencies throughout naltrexone therapy.
- Anticipate that some patients may need treatment for up to 1 year.
- Be aware that after opioid detoxification, patients may have lowered tolerance to opioids that could result in life-threatening circulatory collapse or respiratory compromise if patient uses previously tolerated doses of opioids.

PATIENT TEACHING

WARNING Caution patient against taking opioids during naltrexone therapy or in the future because she'll be more sensitive to them. In fact, strongly warn patient that taking large doses of heroin or any other opioid (including LAAM or methadone) while taking naltrexone could lead to coma, serious injury, or death.

- Explain that patient may have nausea after first injection but that it is usually mild and subsides within a few days. Most patients don't have nausea with repeat doses.
- Tell patient to report adverse reactions promptly, especially abdominal pain, coughing, dyspnea, jaundice, and wheezing. Also, tell patient to report any injection-site reactions to prescriber, especially if reaction does not improve in 1 month following the injection or worsens as further treatment may be necessary.
- Caution patient to avoid performing hazardous activities, such as driving, until CNS effects of drug are known.
- Urge family or caregiver to watch patient closely for abnormal behaviors, including suicidal tendencies, even after patient stops taking naltrexone.
- Inform patient that naltrexone doesn't eliminate or diminish alcohol withdrawal symptoms.

- Urge patient to have comprehensive rehabilitation in addition to receiving naltrexone.
- Inform patient about nonopioid treatments for cough, diarrhea, and pain.
- Warn patient that drug may cause liver damage. Tell her to report any signs of liver dysfunction, such as anorexia, digestive problems, or yellowing of skin or whites of her eyes.
- Instruct patient to carry medical identification that lists naltrexone therapy.
- Instruct women of childbearing age to notify prescriber if pregnancy is suspected.

naproxen

Apo-Naproxen (CAN), EC-Naprosyn, Naprosyn, Novo-Naprox (CAN), Nu-Naprox (CAN)

naproxen sodium

Aleve, Anaprox, Anaprox DS, Apo-Napro-Na (CAN), Naprelan, Naprosyn-SR (CAN), Novo-Naprox Sodium (CAN)

Class and Category

Pharmacologic class: NSAID
Therapeutic class: Analgesic
Pregnancy category: C

Indications and Dosages

➤ *To relieve mild to moderate musculoskeletal inflammation, including ankylosing spondylitis, osteoarthritis, and rheumatoid arthritis*

DELAYED-RELEASE TABLETS, ORAL SUSPENSION, TABLETS (NAPROXEN)

Adults. 250 to 500 mg twice daily. *Maximum:* 1,500 mg daily for limited periods, as prescribed.

E.R. TABLETS (NAPROXEN SODIUM)

Adults. 750 to 1,000 mg daily. *Maximum:* 1,500 mg daily.

TABLETS (NAPROXEN SODIUM)

Adults. 275 to 550 mg twice daily. *Maximum:* 1,650 mg daily for limited periods, as prescribed.

SUPPOSITORIES (NAPROXEN SODIUM)

Adults. 500 mg at bedtime in addition to daytime P.O. administration. *Maximum:* 1,500 mg daily (P.O. and suppository combined).

➤ *To relieve symptoms of juvenile rheumatoid arthritis and other inflammatory conditions in children*

ORAL SUSPENSION, TABLETS (NAPROXEN)

Children. 10 mg/kg daily in divided doses twice daily.

➤ *To relieve symptoms of acute gouty arthritis*

DELAYED-RELEASE TABLETS, ORAL SUSPENSION, TABLETS (NAPROXEN)

Adults. *Initial:* 750 mg, then 250 mg every 8 hr until symptoms subside.

E.R. TABLETS (NAPROXEN SODIUM)

Adults. *Initial:* 1,000 to 1,500 mg on day 1; then 1,000 mg daily until symptoms subside. *Maximum:* 1,500 mg daily.

TABLETS (NAPROXEN SODIUM)

Adults. *Initial:* 825 mg, then 275 mg every 8 hr until symptoms subside.

➤ *To relieve mild to moderate pain, including acute tendinitis and bursitis, arthralgia, dysmenorrhea, and myalgia*

DELAYED-RELEASE TABLETS (NAPROXEN)

Adults. *Initial:* 1,000 mg daily. *Maximum:* 1,500 mg daily.

E.R. TABLETS (NAPROXEN SODIUM)

Adults. *Initial:* 1,100 mg daily, increased as prescribed. *Maximum:* 1,500 mg daily.

ORAL SUSPENSION, TABLETS (NAPROXEN)

Adults. *Initial:* 500 mg, then 250 mg every 6 to 8 hr, as needed. *Maximum:* 1,250 mg daily.

TABLETS (NAPROXEN SODIUM)

Adults. *Initial:* 550 mg, then 275 mg every 6 to 8 hr, as needed. *Maximum:* 1,375 mg daily.

➤ *To relieve fever and mild to moderate musculoskeletal inflammation or pain*

TABLETS (OTC NAPROXEN SODIUM)

Adults. 220 mg every 8 to 12 hr; or 440 and 220 mg 12 hr later. *Maximum:* 660 mg daily for 10 days unless directed otherwise.

DOSAGE ADJUSTMENT For patients over age 65, 220 mg every 12 hr. *Maximum:* 440 mg for 10 days unless directed otherwise.

Route	Onset	Peak	Duration
P.O. (naproxen)*	1 hr†	2–4 hr†‡	7–12 hr†
P.O. (naproxen sodium)*	30 min†	1 hr†‡	7–12 hr†

* For antirheumatism, onset is in 14 days, peak is unknown, and duration is 2 to 4 wk.

† For analgesia.

‡ For gout, 1 to 2 days.

Mechanism of Action

Blocks cyclooxygenase, the enzyme needed to synthesize prostaglandins, which mediate the inflammatory response and cause local pain, swelling, and vasodilation. Thus, naproxen, an NSAID, reduces symptoms of inflammation and relieves pain. Antipyretic action probably stems from effects on the hypothalamus, which increases peripheral blood flow, causing vasodilation and heat dissipation.

Contraindications

Angioedema, asthma, bronchospasm, nasal polyps, rhinitis, or urticaria induced by aspirin, iodides, or other NSAIDs; hypersensitivity to naproxen or its components; postoperatively after coronary artery bypass graft (CABG) surgery

Interactions

DRUGS

angiotensin converting enzyme (ACE) inhibitors, angiotensin receptor blockers (ARBs): Decreased antihypertensive effects; increased risk of renal dysfunction, especially in the elderly and those with impaired renal function or volume depletion
acetaminophen: Increased risk of adverse renal effects with combined long-term use
aluminum hydroxide or magnesium oxide antacids, cholestyramine, sucralfate: Possibly delayed absorption of naproxen
anticoagulants, thrombolytics: Prolonged PT, increased risk of bleeding
antihypertensives: Decreased effectiveness of antihypertensive
aspirin: Decreased aspirin effectiveness
beta blockers: Decreased antihypertensive effects of these drugs
bone marrow depressants, such as aldesleukin and cisplatin: Increased risk of leukopenia and thrombocytopenia
cefamandole, cefoperazone, cefotetan, plicamycin, valproic acid: Increased risk of hypoprothrombinemia and bleeding
cimetidine: Altered blood naproxen level
colchicine, glucocorticoids, other NSAIDs, potassium supplements, salicylates: Increased GI bleeding and irritability
cyclosporine, gold compounds, nephrotoxic drugs: Increased risk of nephrotoxicity
digoxin: Increased blood digoxin level and risk of digitalis toxicity
diuretics: Decreased diuretic effectiveness
furosemide: Decreased natriuretic effect
insulin, oral antidiabetic drugs: Increased effectiveness of these drugs; risk of hypoglycemia
lithium: Increased risk of lithium toxicity
methotrexate: Increased risk of methotrexate toxicity
naproxen-containing products: Increased risk of toxicity
phenytoin: Increased blood phenytoin level
probenecid: Increased risk of naproxen toxicity

ACTIVITIES

alcohol use, smoking: Increased risk of naproxen-induced GI ulceration

Adverse Reactions

CNS: Aseptic meningitis, chills, cognitive impairment, **CVA**, decreased concentration, depression, dizziness, dream disturbances, drowsiness, fever, headache, insomnia, light-headedness, malaise, **seizures**, vertigo
CV: Edema, **heart failure**, hypertension, **MI**, palpitations, tachycardia, vasculitis
EENT: Papilledema, papillitis, retrobulbar optic neuritis, stomatitis, tinnitus, vision or hearing changes
ENDO: Hyperglycemia, **hypoglycemia**
GI: Abdominal pain, anorexia, colitis, constipation, diarrhea, diverticulitis, dyspepsia, dysphagia, elevated liver enzymes, esophagitis, flatulence, gastritis, gastroenteritis, gastroesophageal reflux disease, **GI bleeding** and ulceration, heartburn, hematemesis, **hepatitis**, indigestion, **melena**, nausea, **pancreatitis**, **perforation of intestines or stomach**, stomatitis, vomiting
GU: Elevated serum creatinine level, glomerulonephritis, hematuria, infertility (in women), interstitial nephritis, menstrual

irregularities, **nephrotic syndrome**, **renal failure**, **renal papillary necrosis**
HEME: **Agranulocytosis**, anemia, **aplastic anemia**, eosinophilia, **granulocytopenia**, **hemolytic anemia**, **leukopenia**, **neutropenia**, **pancytopenia**, **thrombocytopenia**
MS: Muscle weakness, myalgia
RESP: **Asthma**, dyspnea, **eosinophilic pneumonitis**, **respiratory depression**
SKIN: Alopecia, diaphoresis, ecchymosis, **erythema multiforme**, photosensitivity, pruritus, pseudoporphyria, purpura, rash, **Stevens–Johnson syndrome** systemic lupus erythematosus, **toxic epidermal necrolysis**, urticaria
Other: Anaphylaxis, **angioedema**, **hyperkalemia**

Nursing Considerations

- Be aware that NSAIDs like naproxen should be avoided in patients with a recent MI because risk of reinfarction increases with NSAID therapy. If therapy is unavoidable, monitor patient closely for signs of cardiac ischemia.
- Know that the risk of heart failure increases with use of NSAIDs such as naproxen. NSAIDs should not be used in patients with severe heart failure but, if unavoidable, monitor patient for worsening of heart failure.
- Use naproxen with extreme caution in patients with a history of GI bleeding or ulcer disease because NSAIDs, such as naproxen, increase risk of GI bleeding and ulceration. Expect to use naproxen for the shortest time possible in these patients.
- Use naproxen cautiously in patients with hypertension, and monitor blood pressure closely. Drug may cause hypertension or worsen it. Because of naproxen's sodium content, watch for fluid retention.
- Use naproxen cautiously in patients with heart failure, hypovolemia, liver dysfunction, renal dysfunction, salt depletion, or patients taking ACE inhibitors or ARBs and diuretics, and the elderly because of increased risk of renal decompensation. Be aware that naproxen is not recommended for patients with advanced renal disease.
- Monitor patient for serious GI tract bleeding, perforation, and ulceration, which may occur without warning symptoms. Elderly patients are at greater risk. To minimize risk, give drug with food. If GI distress occurs, withhold drug and notify prescriber immediately.
- Rehydrate a dehydrated patient before giving drug. If patient has renal disease, monitor renal function closely during therapy.

WARNING Monitor patient closely for thrombotic events, including MI and stroke, because NSAIDs increase the risk, especially if used in higher doses than recommended or for extended periods of time. These events have occurred even in patients who do not have a history or risk factors for cardiovascular disease. Monitor patient for warning signs such as chest pain, slurring of speech, shortness of breath, or weakness. If present, withhold naproxen, alert prescriber immediately, and provide supportive care as prescribed.

- Monitor patient—especially if elderly or receiving long-term naproxen therapy—for less common but serious adverse GI reactions, including anorexia, constipation, diverticulitis, dysphagia, esophagitis, gastritis, gastroenteritis, gastroesophageal reflux disease, hemorrhoids, hiatal hernia, melena, stomatitis, and vomiting.
- Monitor liver enzymes because, in rare cases, elevations may progress to severe hepatic reactions, including fatal hepatitis, hepatic failure, or liver necrosis
- Monitor BUN and serum creatinine levels in elderly patients, patients taking diuretics or ACE inhibitors, and patients with heart failure, hepatic dysfunction, or impaired renal function; naproxen may cause renal failure.
- Monitor CBC for decreased hemoglobin and hematocrit because drug may worsen anemia.

WARNING Know that if patient has bone marrow suppression or is receiving treatment with an antineoplastic drug, laboratory results (including WBC count) must be monitored; watch for evidence of infection because anti-inflammatory and antipyretic actions of naproxen may mask signs and symptoms, such as fever and pain.

- Assess patient's skin regularly for signs of rash or other hypersensitivity reaction

because naproxen is an NSAID and may cause serious skin reactions without warning, even in patients with no history of NSAID sensitivity. At first sign of reaction, stop drug and notify prescriber.
- Assess drug effectiveness in ankylosing spondylitis, as evidenced by decreased morning stiffness, night pain, and pain at rest; in osteoarthritis: decreased joint pain or tenderness and increased ability to perform daily activities, mobility, and range of motion; in rheumatoid arthritis: decreased joint swelling and morning stiffness and increased mobility; in acute gouty arthritis: decreased heat, pain, swelling, and tenderness in affected joints.
- Tell prescriber if patient complains of vision changes; patient may need ophthalmic exam.

PATIENT TEACHING

- Caution patient not to exceed recommended dosage, take for longer than directed, or take for more than 10 days without consulting prescriber because serious adverse reactions may occur.
- Tell patient to swallow delayed-release tablets whole and not to break, chew, or crush them.
- Advise patient to take drug with food to reduce GI distress.
- Tell patient to take drug with a full glass of water and to remain upright for 15 to 30 minutes after taking it to prevent drug from lodging in esophagus and causing irritation.
- Caution patient to avoid hazardous activities until drug's CNS effects are known.
- Urge patient to keep scheduled appointments with prescriber to monitor progress.
- Tell pregnant patient to avoid taking naproxen-containing products late in pregnancy.
- Explain that naproxen may increase risk of serious adverse cardiovascular reactions; urge patient to seek immediate medical attention if signs or symptoms arise, such as chest pain, edema, shortness of breath, slurring of speech, unexplained weight gain, and weakness.
- Inform patient that naproxen may increase risk of serious adverse GI reactions; stress the importance of seeking immediate medical attention for such signs and symptoms as abdominal or epigastric pain, black or tarry stools, indigestion, or vomiting blood or material that looks like coffee grounds.
- Alert patient to rare but serious skin reactions. Urge her to seek immediate medical attention for blisters, fever, itching, rash, or other indications of hypersensitivity.
- Advise patient to consult prescriber before taking naproxen-containing OTC products if he has asthma, bleeding problems, heart or kidney disease, high blood pressure, or ulcers; a need for diuretic therapy; persistent stomach problems, such as heartburn, stomach pain, or upset stomach; or serious adverse effects from previous use of fever reducers or pain relievers.

naratriptan hydrochloride

Amerge

Class and Category

Pharmacologic class: Selective serotonin 5-HT receptor agonist
Therapeutic class: Antimigraine
Pregnancy category: C

Indications and Dosages

➤ *To relieve acute migraine with or without aura*

TABLETS

Adults. 1 or 2.5 mg as a single dose, repeated once in 4 hr as needed if headache returns or only partial relief obtained. *Maximum:* 5 mg daily.

DOSAGE ADJUSTMENT For patients with mild to moderate hepatic or renal impairment, initial dose not to exceed 1 mg and maximum dosage reduced to 2.5 mg daily.

Mechanism of Action

Binds to receptors on intracranial blood vessels and sensory nerves in trigeminal-vascular system to stimulate negative feedback, which halts serotonin release. Thus, naratriptan selectively constricts dilated and inflamed cranial vessels in the carotid circulation and inhibits production of proinflammatory neuropeptides.

Contraindications

Basilar or hemiplegic migraine; cerebrovascular, coronary artery, or peripheral vascular disease (ischemic or vasospastic); hypersensitivity to naratriptan or its components; hypertension (uncontrolled); severe hepatic or renal dysfunction; use within 24 hours of another 5-HT agonist or an ergotamine-containing or ergot-type drug, such as dihydroergotamine or methysergide

Interactions

DRUGS

ergot-containing drugs: Possibly additive or prolonged vasospastic reactions
fluoxetine, fluvoxamine, paroxetine, sertraline: Possibly weakness, hyperreflexia, and incoordination
oral contraceptives: Possibly reduced clearance and increased blood level of naratriptan
other selective serotonin 5-HT receptor agonists (including rizatriptan, sumatriptan, and zolmitriptan): Possibly additive effects
selective serotonin reuptake inhibitors, serotonin norepinephrine reuptake inhibitors, other triptans: Increased risk of serotonin syndrome

Adverse Reactions

CNS: Dizziness, drowsiness, fatigue, malaise, paresthesia
CV: **Chest heaviness**, **pain**, **or pressure**; hypertension; **hypertensive crisis**
EENT: Decreased salivation, otitis media, pharyngitis, photophobia, rhinitis, **throat tightness**
GI: Nausea, vomiting
Other: **Anaphylaxis**, **angioedema**

Nursing Considerations

WARNING Know that because naratriptan therapy can cause coronary artery vasospasm, monitor patient with coronary artery disease for signs or symptoms of angina while taking drug. Because naratriptan may also cause peripheral vasospastic reactions, such as ischemic bowel disease, monitor patient for abdominal pain and bloody diarrhea.

- Monitor patient for hypertension during naratriptan therapy even in patients with no history of hypertension because drug can cause significant elevation in blood pressure.
- Be prepared to perform complete neurovascular assessment in any patient who reports an unusual headache or who fails to respond to first dose of naratriptan.

WARNING Monitor patient closely for serotonin syndrome if she is taking naratriptan along with a selective serotonin reuptake inhibitor or serotonin norepinephrine reuptake inhibitor. Notify prescriber immediately if the patient exhibits agitation, coma, diarrhea, hallucinations, hyperreflexia, hyperthermia, incoordination, labile blood pressure, nausea, tachycardia, or vomiting because serotonin syndrome can be life-threatening. Provide supportive care.

PATIENT TEACHING

- Inform patient that naratriptan is used to treat acute migraine attacks and that it won't prevent or reduce the number of migraines.
- Tell patient if she has no relief from initial dose of naratriptan, instruct her to notify prescriber rather than taking another dose in 4 hours; she may need a different drug.
- Advise patient not to take more than maximum prescribed amount of naratriptan during any 24-hour period or to exceed 10 times or more instances of drug use each month. Overuse can cause headaches to become worse or increase frequency of migraine attacks. Tell patient that if she is using naratriptan 10 times or more in a 30-day period she should notify prescriber, as drug may need to be discontinued. Also tell patient that she may need to be treated for withdrawal symptoms upon discontinuation.
- Advise patient to seek reevaluation by prescriber if she has more than four headaches during any 30-day period while taking naratriptan.
- Urge patient to inform all prescribers that she is receiving naratriptan therapy because serious drug interactions may occur.

natalizumab

Tysabri

Class and Category

Pharmacologic class: Monoclonal antibody
Therapeutic class: Immunomodulator
Pregnancy category: C

Indications and Dosages

➤ *To delay physical disability and reduce frequency of clinical exacerbations in relapsing forms of multiple sclerosis; to induce and maintain remission in moderately to severely active Crohn's disease with evidence of inflammation in patients who had inadequate response to or are unable to tolerate conventional therapy and inhibitors of tumor necrosis factor alpha*

I.V. INFUSION

Adults. 300 mg infused over 1 hr every 4 wk.

Route	Onset	Peak	Duration
I.V.	Unknown	24 wk	Unknown

Mechanism of Action

Inhibits migration of leukocytes from vascular space, increasing the number of circulating leukocytes. It does this by binding to integrins on the surface of leukocytes (except neutrophils) and inhibiting adhesion of leukocytes to their counter receptors. In multiple sclerosis, lesions probably occur when activated inflammatory cells, including T-lymphocytes, cross the blood–brain barrier.

Contraindications

History of or presence of progressive multifocal leukoencephalopathy, hypersensitivity to natalizumab or its components

Interactions

DRUGS

antineoplastics, immunomodulating agents, immunosuppressants: Increased risk of life-threatening infection

Adverse Reactions

CNS: Depression, dizziness, **encephalitis**, fatigue, headache, **herpes encephalitis**, **meningitis**, **progressive multifocal leukoencephalopathy (PML)**, rigors, somnolence, **suicidal ideation**, vertigo
CV: Chest discomfort, peripheral edema
EENT: Acute retinal necrosis, sinusitis, tonsillitis, tooth infection
GI: Abdominal discomfort, cholelithiasis, diarrhea, elevated liver enzymes, gastroenteritis, **hepatotoxicity**, jaundice, nausea
GU: Amenorrhea; dysmenorrhea; irregular menstruation; ovarian cysts; UTI; urinary frequency, incontinence, or urgency; vaginitis
HEME: Hemolytic anemia
MS: Arthralgia, back or limb pain, joint swelling, muscle cramp
RESP: Cough, pneumonia, or other respiratory tract infection
SKIN: Dermatitis, night sweats, pruritus, rash, urticaria
Other: Acute hypersensitivity reaction, anaphylaxis, antibody formation, flu-like illness, herpes, immune reconstitution inflammatory syndrome, opportunistic infections, weight gain or loss

Nursing Considerations

- Make sure patient has enrolled in the TOUCH prescribing program before giving natalizumab. Once patient has signed and initialed the TOUCH program enrollment form, place original signed form in the patient's medical record, send a copy to Biogen Idec, and give a copy to patient.
- Be aware that all atypical and serious opportunistic infections must be reported to Biogen Idec at 1-800-456-2255 and the FDA's MedWatch Program at 1-800-FDA-1088.
- Make sure patient with multiple sclerosis has had an MRI of the brain before starting natalizumab therapy. It will help distinguish evidence of multiple sclerosis from PML symptoms if they occur after therapy starts. Also know that the following three factors increase the risk of PML in patients treated with natalizumab: longer treatment duration, especially beyond 2 years; prior treatment with an immunosuppressant; and the presence of anti-JCV antibodies.

- Dilute natalizumab concentrate 300 mg/15 ml in 100 ml of normal saline injection. Gently invert solution to mix completely. Do not shake.
- Infuse drug immediately after dilution over 1 hour. After infusion, flush line with normal saline injection.
- Do not give natalizumab by I.V. push or bolus injection.
- Refrigerate drug and use within 8 hours if not used immediately.
- Observe patient during and for 1 hour after infusion for hypersensitivity reaction, evidenced by chest pain, dizziness, dyspnea, fever, flushing, hypotension, nausea, pruritis, rash, rigors, and urticaria. Reaction is more likely to occur if natalizumab therapy was interrupted. If hypersensitivity reaction occurs, notify prescriber; expect to withhold drug and provide supportive care.

WARNING Monitor patient closely for evidence of PML, a viral brain infection that may be disabling or fatal, because natalizumab increases the risk. Patients at increased risk include those who have received natalizumab for longer than 2 years, have had prior treatment with an immunosuppressant, and who have anti-JCV antibodies. If patient has unexplained neurologic changes, notify prescriber, withhold natalizumab, and prepare patient for a gadolinium-enhanced brain MRI and possible cerebrospinal fluid analysis, as ordered. Be aware that immune reconstitution inflammatory syndrome may occur in patients who develop PML, even when drug has been discontinued. Monitor such patients for evidence of an overwhelming inflammatory response either to an opportunistic infection or the paradoxical symptomatic relapse of a prior infection despite it having been treated successfully in the past.

- Expect that patient will be reevaluated 3 months after first infusion, 6 months after first infusion, and every 6 months thereafter.
- Assess patient for evidence of infection because natalizumab may adversely affect immune system, increasing risk of infection. For example, the drug increases the risk for encephalitis and meningitis as well as acute retinal necrosis caused by herpes simplex and varicella zoster viruses that could become life-threatening or result in blindness. Other infections that may occur but are uncommon may include aspergilloma, Candida pneumonia, cryptococcal fungemia, or pulmonary mycobacterium avium intracellulare. If infection occurs, expect to obtain appropriate specimens for culture and sensitivity and to treat accordingly. If infection is serious, expect drug to be discontinued.
- Be aware that if patient with Crohn's disease has no therapeutic response after 12 weeks, natalizumab should be discontinued. If patient is on chronic oral corticosteroid therapy, expect tapering of oral corticosteroid dose to begin. If patient can't be tapered off oral corticosteroids within 6 months of starting natalizumab therapy, expect natalizumab to be discontinued. Likewise, if patient needs additional steroid use that extends beyond 3 months in a calendar year to control signs and symptoms of Crohn's disease, expect natalizumab to be discontinued.
- Assess patient's liver function regularly, as ordered, because natalizumab may cause significant liver damage. Expect drug to be discontinued if patient becomes jaundiced or liver enzymes become elevated.
- Ensure that when natalizumab is discontinued, patient completes the "Initial Discontinuation Questionnaire" and then has an appointment in 6 months to complete the "6-Month Discontinuation Questionnaire."

PATIENT TEACHING

- Instruct patient on benefits and risks of natalizumab therapy, and provide medication guide for patient to read before therapy begins.
- Encourage patient to ask questions before signing the enrollment form.
- Emphasize need to report any worsening symptoms that persist over several days.
- Tell patient to inform all healthcare providers that he is receiving natalizumab therapy.
- Stress the need to have follow-up visits 3 months after first infusion, 6 months after first infusion, and at least every 6 months thereafter.

- Instruct patient to report evidence of allergic reaction.
- Instruct patient to avoid people who have infections. Advise him or family members to report confusion, cough, fever, headache, lower-back or side pain, or other unexplained signs and symptoms because they may indicate infection. Also tell patient to report decreased visual acuity or eye pain or redness, as these may be early signs of acute retinal necrosis caused by a herpes virus.
- Alert patient that signs and symptoms suggestive of PML can occur up to 6 months after drug is discontinued and should be reported immediately.

nateglinide

Starlix

Class and Category

Pharmacologic class: Meglitinide
Therapeutic class: Antidiabetic
Pregnancy category: C

Indications and Dosages

➤ *To control blood glucose level in type 2 diabetes mellitus, either as monotherapy or with metformin or a thiazolidinedione*

TABLETS

Adults. 120 mg three times daily within 30 min before meals.

DOSAGE ADJUSTMENT Dosage reduced to 60 mg three times daily in patients with near-goal glycosylated hemoglobin (HbA_{1c}) level.

Route	Onset	Peak	Duration
P.O.	20 min	1 hr	4 hr

Contraindications

Hypersensitivity to nateglinide or its components

DRUGS

corticosteroids, phenytoin, rifampin, somatropin, St. John's wort, sympathomimetics, thiazide diuretics, thyroid products: Possibly reduced hypoglycemic effects of nateglinide

Mechanism of Action

Nateglinide stimulates the release of insulin from functioning beta cells of the pancreas. In patients with type 2 diabetes mellitus, a lack of functioning beta cells diminishes blood levels of insulin and causes glucose intolerance. By interacting with the adenosine triphosphatase (ATP)-potassium channel on the beta cell membrane, nateglinide prevents potassium (K^+) from leaving the cell. This causes the beta cell to depolarize and the cell membrane's calcium channel to open. Consequently, calcium (Ca^{++}) moves into the cell and insulin moves out of it. The extent of insulin release is glucose dependent; the lower the glucose level, the less insulin is secreted from the cell.

By promoting insulin secretion in patients with type 2 diabetes mellitus, nateglinide improves glucose tolerance.

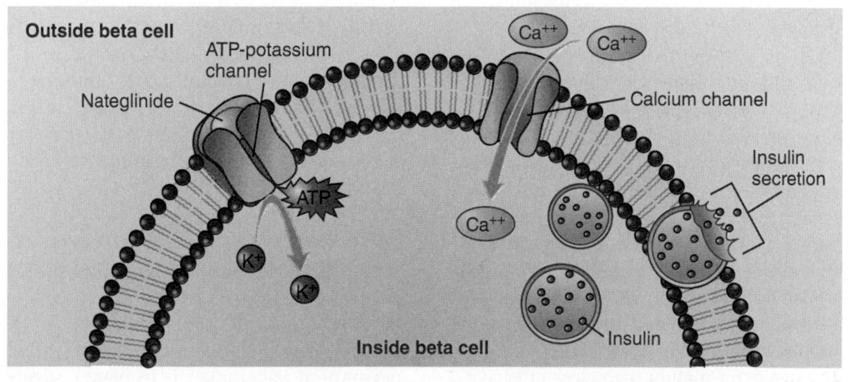

N O

MAO inhibitors, nonselective beta-adrenergic blockers, NSAIDs, salicylates, somatostatin analogues: Possibly additive hypoglycemic effects of nateglinide

Adverse Reactions

CNS: Dizziness
ENDO: **Hypoglycemia**
GI: **Cholestatic hepatitis**, diarrhea, elevated liver enzymes, jaundice
MS: Accidental trauma, arthropathy, back pain
RESP: Bronchitis, cough, upper respiratory tract infection
SKIN: Pruritus, rash, urticaria
Other: Flu-like symptoms

Nursing Considerations

- Give nateglinide within 30 minutes before meals to reduce the risk of hypoglycemia.
- Monitor fasting glucose and HbA_{1c} levels periodically, as ordered, to evaluate treatment effectiveness.
- Monitor patient often in event of fever, infection, surgery, or trauma because transient loss of glucose control may occur, requiring an alteration in therapy.
- Know that patients who are poor metabolizers of CYP2CP substrates are at increased risk of developing hypoglycemia because they may experience an additive hypoglycemic effect from nateglinide therapy.

PATIENT TEACHING

- Instruct patient to take nateglinide within 30 minutes before meals. Advise her to skip scheduled dose if she skips a meal to reduce the risk of hypoglycemia.
- Teach patient to measure blood glucose level and recognize hyperglycemia and hypoglycemia. Advise her to notify prescriber if blood glucose level is persistently abnormal.
- Inform patient that persistent consumption of alcohol, insufficient calorie intake, and strenuous exercise increase risk of hypoglycemia.
- Advise patient to monitor blood glucose level as prescribed and to keep follow-up appointments to monitor HbA_{1c} level because drug may become less effective over time.
- Tell patient to inform all prescribers of nateglinide therapy and not to take any over-the-counter drugs, including herbal preparations, without prescriber's knowledge.

nebivolol hydrochloride

Bystolic

Class and Category

Pharmacologic class: Beta-adrenergic blocker
Therapeutic class: Antihypertensive
Pregnancy category: C

Indications and Dosages

➤ *To treat hypertension*

TABLETS

Adults. *Initial:* 5 mg once daily, increased at 2-wk intervals, as needed. *Maximum:* 40 mg once daily.

DOSAGE ADJUSTMENT For patients with moderate hepatic impairment (Child-Pugh Class B) or moderate renal impairment (creatinine clearance less than 30 ml/min, initial dose reduced to 2.5 mg.

Route	Onset	Peak	Duration
P.O.	Unknown	1.5–4 hr	Unknown

Mechanism of Action

May prevent arterial dilation and inhibit renin secretion, although precise mechanism of action isn't known. Negative chronotropic effects may slow resting heart rate, and negative inotropic effects may reduce cardiac output, myocardial contractility, and myocardial oxygen consumption during exercise or stress. All of these actions may work together to lower systolic and diastolic blood pressure.

Contraindications

Advanced AV block, cardiogenic shock, decompensated cardiac failure, hypersensitivity to nebivolol or its components, sick sinus syndrome (unless permanent pacemaker is in place), severe bradycardia, severe hepatic impairment

Interactions

DRUGS

antiarrhythmias such as disopyramide, beta blockers, digoxin, selected calcium antagonists such as diltiazem and verapamil: Increased effect on AV conduction and myocardial depression; increased risk of bradycardia

fluoxetine, paroxetine, propafenone, quinidine: Increased hypertensive effect of nebivolol

guanethidine, reserpine: Possibly excessive reduction of sympathetic activity

Adverse Reactions

CNS: Asthenia, dizziness, fatigue, headache, insomnia, paresthesia, somnolence, syncope, vertigo
CV: Allergic vasculitis, **AV block**, **bradycardia**, chest pain, hypercholesterolemia, hyperuricemia, **hypotension**, **MI**, peripheral edema, peripheral ischemia, Raynaud's phenomenon
ENDO: Hyperglycemia, mask symptoms of **hypoglycemia**
GI: Abdominal pain, diarrhea, elevated bilirubin and liver enzymes, nausea, vomiting
GU: **Acute renal failure**, elevated BUN level, erectile dysfunction
HEME: **Leukopenia**, **thrombocytopenia**
RESP: **Acute pulmonary edema**, **bronchospasms**, dyspnea
SKIN: Pruritus, psoriasis, rash, urticaria
Other: **Angioedema** (rare)

Nursing Considerations

- Know that patients with bronchospastic disease usually shouldn't be treated with beta blocker therapy such as nebivolol.
- Use nebivolol cautiously in patients with impaired hepatic or renal function.
- Expect to administer an alpha blocker, as ordered, before starting nebivolol therapy in patients with pheochromocytoma.
- Monitor blood pressure and pulse rate often, especially at start of nebivolol therapy and during dosage adjustments. Also monitor fluid intake and output and daily weight, and watch for evidence of heart failure, such as dyspnea, edema, fatigue, and jugular vein distention. If heart failure occurs or worsens, expect drug to be discontinued.
- Be aware that nebivolol shouldn't be stopped abruptly because MI, myocardial ischemia, severe hypertension, or ventricular arrhythmias may result.
- Expect nebivolol therapy to continue throughout the perioperative period of major surgery. However, monitor patient closely for protracted severe hypotension and difficulty restarting and keeping a heartbeat. Be prepared to administer a beta agonist such as dobutamine or isoproterenol, as ordered, to reverse the effects of nebivolol, if needed.
- Assess distal circulation and peripheral pulses in patient with peripheral vascular disease because drug can worsen it.
- Be aware that nebivolol may mask tachycardia from hyperthyroidism and that abrupt withdrawal can cause thyroid storm. Drug also can decrease blood glucose level, prolong or mask symptoms of hypoglycemia, promote hyperglycemia in patient with diabetes mellitus, or worsen psoriasis.
- Monitor patient closely for hypersensitivity reactions that may occur with beta blockers, especially patients with a history of severe anaphylactic reactions who may not be responsive to usual doses of epinephrine used to treat allergic reactions.
- Monitor neonates born to mothers treated with beta blockers such as nebivolol during the third trimester of pregnancy. Watch for bradycardia, hypoglycemia, hypotension, and respiratory depression.

PATIENT TEACHING

- Instruct patient to take nebivolol exactly as prescribed and not to stop using it abruptly.
- Tell patient to weigh herself daily during nebivolol therapy and to notify prescriber if she gains more than 2 lb (0.9 kg) in 1 day or 5 lb (2.3 kg) in 1 week.
- Advise patient to rise slowly from a lying or seated position to minimize effects of orthostatic hypotension.
- Advise patient to avoid hazardous activities until drug's CNS effects are known.
- Instruct patient to contact prescriber about bleeding or bruising, cough at night, dizziness, edema, rash, shortness of breath, or slow pulse rate.
- Advise diabetic patient to monitor her blood glucose level more often during

nebivolol therapy because drug may mask symptoms of hypoglycemia.
- Inform patient with psoriasis that drug may aggravate this condition.

nelfinavir mesylate

Viracept

Class and Category

Pharmacologic class: Protease inhibitor
Therapeutic class: Antiretroviral
Pregnancy category: B

Indications and Dosages

➤ *As adjunct to treat human immunodeficiency virus-1 (HIV-1) infection*

ORAL POWDER, TABLETS

Adults and adolescents. 1,250 mg twice daily or 750 mg three times daily with food.
Children ages 2 years and over. 45 to 55 mg/kg twice daily or 25 to 35 mg/kg three times daily with food.
Maximum: 2,500 mg daily.

Mechanism of Action

Selectively inhibits the virus-specific processing of specific polyproteins in HIV-1-infected cells to prevent formation of mature virions.

Contraindications

Concomitant therapy with alfuzosin, amiodarone, cisapride, dihydroergotamine, ergotamine, lovastatin, methylergonovine, midazolam (oral), pimozide, quinidine, rifampin, St. John's wort, sildenafil (for treatment of pulmonary arterial hypertension), simvastatin, or triazolam; hypersensitivity to nelfinavir or its components; moderate to severe hepatic impairment

Interactions

DRUGS

atorvastatin, azithromycin, bosentan, colchicine, fluticasone, PDE5 inhibitors (sildenafil, tadalafil, vardenafil), quetiapine, rosuvastatin: Increased concentration of these drugs, with possible increased effect and risk of adverse reactions
carbamazepine, ethinyl estradiol, norethindrone, phenobarbital, phenytoin: Decreased concentration of these drugs and nelfinavir, interfering with their effectiveness
cyclosporine, sirolimus, tacrolimus: Increased concentrations of these drugs and nelfinavir when nelfinavir is given with atorvastatin and rosuvastatin along with any of these immunosuppressants, with possible increased effect of the immunosuppressants and nelfinavir and risk of adverse reactions
delavirdine: Decreased concentrations of delavirdine and its effectiveness and increased concentration of nelfinavir, with possible increased effect and risk of adverse reactions
indinavir, salmeterol, saquinavir: Increased concentration of these drugs and nelfinavir, with possible increased effects and risk of adverse reactions
methadone: Decreased concentration of methadone and possible reduced effectiveness
omeprazole, ritonavir: Increased concentration of nelfinavir, with possible increased effect and risk of adverse reactions
rifabutin: Decreased concentration of nelfinavir and effectiveness and increased concentration of rifabutin, with possible increased effects and risk of adverse reactions
trazodone: Increased concentration of trazodone, with possible increased effect and risk of dizziness, hypotension, nausea, and syncope
vevirapine: Decreased concentration of nelfinavir and effectiveness
warfarin: Possible changes in international normalized ratio (INR) requiring dosage change of warfarin

Adverse Reactions

CNS: Anxiety, asthenia, depression, dizziness, emotional lability, fever, headache, hyperkinesia, insomnia, malaise, migraine, paresthesia, **seizures**, sleep disorder, somnolence, **suicidal ideation**
CV: Edema, hyperlipidemia, **prolonged QT interval**, **torsades de pointes**
EENT: Acute iritis, eye disorders, mouth ulcers, pharyngitis, rhinitis, sinusitis
ENDO: Fat redistribution, hyperglycemia, **hypoglycemia**
GI: Abdominal pain, anorexia, bilirubinemia, diarrhea, dyspepsia, elevated liver and pancreatic enzymes, epigastric pain, flatulence, **GI bleeding**, **hepatitis**, jaundice, nausea, **pancreatitis**, vomiting

GU: Kidney calculus, sexual dysfunction, urine abnormality
HEME: Anemia, **leukopenia**, **neutropenia**, **thrombocytopenia**
MS: Arthralgia, arthritis, back pain, cramps, elevated creatine kinase, myalgia, myasthenia, myopathy
RESP: Bronchospasms, dyspnea
SKIN: Dermatitis including fungal, diaphoresis, folliculitis, maculopapular rash, pruritus, rash, urticaria
Other: Dehydration, generalized pain, **hypersensitivity reactions**, hyperuricemia, immune reconstitution syndrome, **metabolic acidosis**

Nursing Considerations

- Administer nelfinavir with food.
- Know that for patients who cannot swallow tablets, the tablets may be placed in a small amount of water. Once dissolved, the mixture should be stirred well and consumed immediately. Add water to the container the tablets were mixed in and then have the patient swallow the rinse to ensure that the entire dose has been consumed.
- Prepare oral powder for consumption by mixing with a small amount of a dietary supplement, formula, milk, soy formula, or water. Have patient consume the mixture immediately, but know that it can be refrigerated up to 6 hours. Know that acidic foods or juices are not recommended for mixing the oral powder because it may result in a bitter taste. Do not reconstitute oral powder in its original container.
- Monitor patient's blood glucose level, because nelfinavir may cause changes in blood glucose levels. Other drugs in the same class as nelfinavir have caused exacerbation of preexisting diabetes mellitus and new-onset diabetes mellitus, including diabetic ketoacidosis.
- Assess patients who have hemophilia type A or B closely for bleeding, because spontaneous skin hematomas and hemarthrosis have occurred with other protease inhibitors. In some cases, treatment with factor VIII was required.
- Be aware that immune reconstitution syndrome has occurred in patients treated with combination antiretroviral therapy, including nelfinavir. The inflammatory response predisposes susceptible patients to opportunistic infections such as cytomegalovirus, *Mycobacterium avium* infection, *Pneumocystis jiroveci* pneumonia, or tuberculosis. Autoimmune disorders such as Graves' disease, Guillain–Barré syndrome, or polymyositis have also occurred. Report sudden or unusual adverse reactions to prescriber.

PATIENT TEACHING

- Advise patient to avoid missing doses of nelfinavir. If she misses a dose, she should take it as soon as she remembers but should not double the next dose or take more than prescribed.
- Instruct patient or caregiver that drug must be taken with food.
- Inform patients who cannot swallow tablets that the tablets may be placed in a small amount of water. Once dissolved, the mixture should be stirred well and consumed immediately. Tell patient to then add water to the container the tablets were mixed in and swallow the rinse to ensure that the entire dose has been consumed.
- Instruct patient or caregiver on how to prepare oral powder for consumption by mixing with a small amount of a dietary supplement, formula, milk, soy formula, or water. Consumption of the mixture should occur immediately, but tell patient/caregiver that it can be refrigerated for up to 6 hours. Warn that acidic foods or juices are not recommended for mixing the oral powder because it may result in a bitter taste. The oral powder should not be reconstituted in its original container.
- Alert patient or caregiver that oral powder form contains phenylalanine and could be harmful to patients with phenylketonuria.
- Review signs and symptoms of hyperglycemia and hypoglycemia even if patient is not a diabetic. Urge patient to report any such findings to prescriber.
- Warn patients with hemophilia that nelfinavir may increase the risk of bleeding and to seek immediate medical attention if bleeding occurs.
- Inform patient that nelfinavir therapy may cause changes in his body appearance because of fat redistribution. Prepare him for the possibility of developing breast enlargement, central

obesity, dorsocervical fat enlargement (buffalo hump), facial wasting, and peripheral wasting.

- Instruct patient to report any persistent, severe, or unusual signs and symptoms.
- Inform women using oral contraceptives that an alternative or additional contraceptive should be used during nelfinavir therapy, because drug may make the oral contraceptive unreliable. Encourage women of childbearing age to report known or suspected pregnancy.
- Alert mothers that breastfeeding is not recommended during nelfinavir therapy.
- Tell patient to report all drugs being taken, including over-the-counter medications and herbals, as serious drug interactions may occur. Advise patient not to begin any new drug therapy without first checking with prescriber.
- Warn male patients who are taking a PDE5 inhibitor to discuss use with prescriber before continuing and, if used, to seek immediate medical attention for prolonged penile erection.
- Inform patient that the most common side effect of nelfinavir is diarrhea, which can be controlled with over-the-counter drugs such as loperamide if prescriber so advises.

neomycin sulfate

Neo-Fradin

Class and Category

Pharmacologic class: Aminoglycoside
Therapeutic class: Antibiotic
Pregnancy category: D

Indications and Dosages

➤ *To suppress intestinal bacterial growth in preoperative bowel preparation*

TABLETS (24-HR REGIMEN)

Adults. 1 g every hr for four doses and then 1 g every 4 hr for remainder of 24 hr before surgery. Or, for 8 a.m. surgery, 1 g of neomycin with erythromycin at 1, 2, and 11 p.m. the day before surgery.
Children. 25 mg/kg at 1, 2, and 11 p.m. the day before surgery.

TABLETS (2- TO 3-DAY REGIMEN)

Adults and children. 88 mg/kg every 4 hr in six equally divided doses for 2 to 3 days before surgery.

➤ *As adjunct in hepatic encephalopathy*

TABLETS

Adults. 4 to 12 g daily in divided doses every 6 hr for 5 to 6 days.
Children. 50 to 100 mg/kg daily in divided doses every 6 hr for 5 to 6 days.

➤ *To treat infectious diarrhea caused by enteropathic* Escherichia coli

TABLETS

Adults. 3 g daily in divided doses four times daily for 2 to 3 days.
Children. 50 mg/kg daily in divided doses four times daily for 2 to 3 days.

Mechanism of Action

Is transported into bacterial cells, where it competes with messenger RNA to bind with a specific receptor protein on the 30S ribosomal subunit of DNA. This action causes abnormal, nonfunctioning proteins to form. A lack of functional proteins causes bacterial cell death.

Contraindications

Hypersensitivity or serious reaction to neomycin, other aminoglycosides, or their components; inflammatory or ulcerative GI disease; intestinal obstruction

Interactions

DRUGS

digoxin, spironolactone: Possibly reduced absorption rate of these drugs
dimenhydrinate: Possibly masked symptoms of neomycin-induced ototoxicity
methotrexate: Possibly decreased absorption and bioavailability of methotrexate
neuromuscular blockers: Potentiated neuromuscular blockade, increased risk of prolonged respiratory depression
oral anticoagulants: Possibly potentiated anticoagulant effects

Adverse Reactions

EENT: Ototoxicity
GI: Diarrhea, malabsorption syndrome nausea, **pseudomembranous colitis**, vomiting
GU: Nephrotoxicity

Nursing Considerations

- Monitor patient's BUN and serum creatinine levels to assess renal function before and during neomycin therapy. Expect to decrease dosage or stop drug if nephrotoxicity develops.
- Monitor blood neomycin level, as directed, to assess for therapeutic range of 5 to 10 mcg/ml.

WARNING Know that neomycin is highly ototoxic and may cause hearing loss and tinnitus.

- Watch for evidence of pseudomembranous colitis, such as severe abdominal cramps and severe, watery diarrhea.
- Anticipate that neomycin's curare-like effect may worsen muscle weakness in patients with neuromuscular disorders, such as myasthenia gravis and Parkinsonism.

PATIENT TEACHING

- Urge patient to complete full course of neomycin therapy.
- Unless contraindicated, urge patient to drink plenty of fluids to prevent nephrotoxicity.
- Urge patient undergoing bowel preparation to comply with recommended regimen, including, bisacodyl enema administration, low-residue diet, and neomycin use.
- Advise patient to notify prescriber about hearing loss or ringing in ears.

neostigmine methylsulfate

Bloxiverz, Neostigmine Methylsulfate

Class and Category

Pharmacologic class: Cholinesterase inhibitor
Therapeutic class: Curare antidote (muscle stimulant)
Pregnancy category: C

Indications and Dosages

➤ *To reverse nondepolarizing neuromuscular blockade after surgery*

I.V. INJECTION

Adults and children. 0.03 mg/kg (drugs with shorter half-lives) or 0.07 mg/kg (drugs with longer half-lives or need for more rapid recovery) given over at least 1 min with atropine or glycopyrrolate administered prior to or concomitantly. *Maximum:* 0.07 mg/kg or 5 mg, whichever is less.

Route	Onset	Peak	Duration
I.V.	4–8 min	30 min	2–4 hr

Mechanism of Action

Inhibits action of cholinesterase, an enzyme that destroys acetylcholine at myoneuronal junctions, thereby increasing acetylcholine accumulation at myoneuronal junctions. This action competes for the same binding sites as nondepolarizing neuromuscular blocking agents thereby reversing the neuromuscular blockade.

Contraindications

Hypersensitivity to neostigmine, other anticholinesterases, bromides, or their components; mechanical obstruction of intestinal or urinary tract; peritonitis

Interactions

DRUGS

aminoglycosides, anesthetics, capreomycin, colistimethate, colistin, lidocaine, lincomycins, polymyxin B, quinine: Increased risk of neuromuscular blockade
anticholinergics: Possibly masked signs of cholinergic crisis
guanadrel, guanethidine, mecamylamine, trimethaphan: Possibly antagonized effects of neostigmine, possibly decreased antihypertensive effects
neuromuscular blockers: Possibly prolonged action of depolarizing—and antagonized action of nondepolarizing—neuromuscular blockers
procainamide, quinidine: Possibly antagonized effects of neostigmine
quinine: Decreased neostigmine effectiveness

Adverse Reactions

CNS: Dizziness, drowsiness, headache, **seizures**, syncope, weakness
CV: Arrhythmias (**AV block**, **bradycardia**, **nodal rhythm**, tachycardia), **cardiac arrest**, **ECG changes**, **hypotension**
EENT: Increased salivation, lacrimation, miosis, vision changes

GI: Abdominal cramps, diarrhea, flatulence, increased peristalsis, nausea, vomiting
GU: Urinary frequency
MS: Arthralgia, dysarthria, muscle spasms
RESP: **Bronchospasm**, dyspnea, increased bronchial secretions, **respiratory arrest or depression**
SKIN: Flushing, diaphoresis, rash, urticaria

Nursing Considerations

- Keep in mind when giving neostigmine I.V., make sure patient is well ventilated and airway remains patent until normal respiration is assured.
- When administering neostigmine methylsulfate know that a peripheral nerve stimulation device should be used to time the initial dose and any further doses, if needed.

WARNING Monitor patient for evidence of neostigmine overdose, which can cause possibly fatal cholinergic crisis (increased muscle weakness, including respiratory muscles). Expect to stop neostigmine as ordered.

PATIENT TEACHING

- Reassure patient prior to surgery that drug therapy like neostigmine is available to help her recover from anesthesia.

nesiritide

Natrecor

Class and Category

Pharmacologic class: Human B-type natriuretic peptide
Therapeutic class: Vasodilator
Pregnancy category: C

Indications and Dosages

➤ *To reduce dyspnea at rest or with minimal activity in patients with acute decompensated congestive heart failure*

I.V. INFUSION, I.V. INJECTION

Adults. 2 mcg/kg bolus given over 1 min and then continuous infusion of 0.01 mcg/kg/min with dosage adjustment upward, as needed, no more frequently than every 3 hr. *Maximum:* 0.03 mcg/kg/min.

DOSAGE ADJUSTMENT For patients starting therapy with a systolic blood pressure below 110 mm Hg or for patients recently treated with afterload reducers, bolus dosage may need to be eliminated. For patients developing hypotension during treatment, dosage reduced or drug discontinued. If drug restarted after patient has stabilized, dose reduced by 30% with no initial bolus given.

Route	Onset	Peak	Duration
I.V.	In 15 min	1 hr	3 hr

Mechanism of Action

Binds to guanylate cyclase receptor of vascular smooth muscle. This action increases intracellular levels of cyclic guanosine monophosphate, which leads to arterial and venous smooth muscle cell relaxation. Ultimately, nesiritide reduces pulmonary capillary wedge pressure and systemic arterial pressure in patients with congestive heart failure, which decreases the heart's workload and subsequently relieves dyspnea.

Incompatibilities

Don't infuse nesiritide through same I.V. line as bumetanide, enalaprilat, ethacrynate sodium, furosemide, heparin, hydralazine, or insulin because these drugs are chemically and physically incompatible with nesiritide. Don't infuse drugs that contain the preservative sodium metabisulfite through same I.V. line as nesiritide.

Contraindications

Cardiogenic shock, hypersensitivity to nesiritide or its components, persistent systolic blood pressure less than 100 mm Hg

Interactions

DRUGS

ACE inhibitors: Increased risk of symptomatic hypotension

Adverse Reactions

CNS: Anxiety, dizziness, headache, insomnia
CV: Angina, **bradycardia**, **hypotension**, **PVCs**, **ventricular tachycardia**
GI: Abdominal pain, nausea, vomiting
GU: Elevated serum creatinine level, worsening of renal function
MS: Back pain
Other: **Anaphylaxis and other hypersensitivity reactions**

Nursing Considerations

WARNING Be aware that nesiritide isn't recommended for patients suspected to have low cardiac filling pressures or patients for whom vasodilating drugs aren't appropriate, such as those with constrictive pericarditis, pericardial tamponade, obstructive or restrictive cardiomyopathy, significant valvular stenosis, or other conditions in which cardiac output depends on venous return.

- Reconstitute 1.5-mg vial by adding 5 ml diluent removed from a 250-ml plastic I.V. bag containing preservative-free D_5W, normal saline solution, dextrose 5% in half-normal (0.45) saline solution, or dextrose 5% in quarter-normal (0.2) saline solution.
- Don't shake vial. Rock it gently so all surfaces, including the stopper, are in contact with diluent to ensure complete reconstitution. Inspect drug for discoloration and particulate matter; if present, discard drug.
- Withdraw entire contents of reconstituted solution and add it to 250-ml plastic I.V. bag used to withdraw diluent to yield a solution of about 6 mcg/ml. Invert I.V. bag several times to ensure complete mixing.
- After preparing infusion bag, withdraw bolus volume from infusion bag and give it over about 60 seconds. Immediately after bolus, infuse drug at 0.1 ml/kg/hr, which will deliver 0.01 mcg/kg/min.
- Prime I.V. tubing with 25 ml of solution before connecting to the I.V. line and before administering the bolus dose or starting the infusion.
- Flush the I.V. line between doses of nesiritide and incompatible drugs.
- Know that because nesiritide binds to heparin and therefore could bind to the heparin lining of a heparin-coated catheter, it should not be given through a central heparin-coated catheter.
- Store reconstituted vials at room temperature (20° to 25°C [68° to 77°F]) or refrigerate (2° to 8°C [36° to 46°F]) for up to 24 hours.
- Discard the reconstituted solution after 24 hours because nesiritide contains no antimicrobial preservatives.
- Monitor blood pressure and heart rate and rhythm frequently during therapy. If hypotension occurs, notify prescriber and expect to reduce dosage or discontinue the drug. Implement measures to support blood pressure as prescribed.
- Assess patient's breath sounds and respiratory depth, quality, rate, and rhythm frequently during drug therapy.
- Monitor serum creatinine level during and after therapy has been completed. Notify prescriber of abnormal results because nesiritide may decrease renal function.

WARNING Monitor patient for serious hypersensitivity reactions following nesiritide administration. Reactions can become serious, requiring emergency supportive care.

- Store unopened drug at controlled room temperature or refrigerate. Keep in carton until time of use.

PATIENT TEACHING

- Instruct patient to notify you or another nurse if she becomes dizzy because this may indicate hypotension.
- Reassure patient that her blood pressure, breathing, and heart rate will be monitored frequently.
- Emphasize importance of reporting an allergic reaction immediately.

nevirapine

Viramune, Viramune XR

Class and Category

Pharmacologic class: Non-nucleoside reverse transcriptase inhibitor (NNRTI)
Therapeutic class: Antiretroviral
Pregnancy category: Not classified

Indications and Dosages

➤ *As adjunct to treat human immunodeficiency virus (HIV-1) infection*

ORAL SUSPENSION, TABLETS

Adults. 200 mg (immediate-release tablets) once a day for 14 days. *Maintenance:* 200 mg (immediate-release tablets or oral suspension) twice daily.
Infants 15 days and over and children. 150 mg/m^2 once a day for 14 days.

Maximum during first 14 days: 200 mg/day. *Maintenance:* 150 mg/m^2 twice daily.

E.R. TABLETS

Adults. 400 mg once daily after an initial dose of 200 mg (immediate-release tablets) given for 14 days.

Children age 6 and over with a body surface area (BSA) 1.17 m^2 or greater. 400 mg once a day after an initial dose of 150 mg/m^2 (immediate-release tablets) given once a day for 14 days.

Children age 6 and over with a BSA 0.84 to 1.16 m^2. 300 mg once a day after an initial dose of 150 mg/m^2 (immediate-release tablets) given once a day for 14 days.

Children age 6 and over with a BSA 0.58 to 0.83 m^2. 200 mg once a day after an initial dose of 150 mg/m^2 (immediate-release tablets) given once a day for 14 days.

DOSAGE ADJUSTMENT For patient experiencing a mild to moderate rash without constitutional symptoms during the 14-day lead-in period of 200 mg/day for adults and 150 mg/m^2 for infants and children using immediate-release formulation, maintenance dosage not increased to twice daily until rash is resolved. If rash not resolved after 28 days of taking nevirapine once daily, drug discontinued. For adult patient with end-stage renal disease receiving dialysis, an additional dose of 200 mg given following each dialysis session.

Mechanism of Action

Binds directly to reverse transcriptase and blocks the RNA-dependent and DNA-dependent DNA polymerase activities by causing a disruption of the enzymes' catalytic site.

Contraindications

Hypersensitivity to nevirapine or its components, moderate to severe hepatic impairment, use as part of nonoccupational and occupational postexposure prophylaxis regimens

Interactions

DRUGS

amiodarone, boceprevir, cisapride, clarithromycin, cyclophosphamide, cyclosporine, diltiazem, disopyramide, efavirenz, ergotamine, ethinyl estradiol, fentanyl, ketoconazole, indinavir, itraconazole, lidocaine, lopinavir/ritonavir, nelfinavir, nifedipine, norethindrone, saquinavir/ritonavir, sirolimus, tacrolimus, telaprevir, verapamil: Possible decreased concentration of these drugs with possible decreased effectiveness

atazanavir/ritonavir, fosamprenavir, fosamprenavir/ritonavir: Decreased amprenavir concentration with these drugs with possible decreased effectiveness and increased nevirapine concentration with possible risk of prolonged action and adverse reactions

carbamazepine, clonazepam, ethosuximide: Decreased concentrations of these drugs and nevirapine with possible decreased effectiveness

fluconazole: Increased nevirapine concentration with possible increased risk of prolonged action and adverse reactions

methadone: Decreased concentration of methadone, increasing risk of opiate withdrawal

other NNRTI agents such as delavirdine, etravirine, rilpivirine: Possible plasma concentration alteration

rifabutin: Increased concentration of rifabutin with possible risk of prolonged action and adverse reactions

rifampin: Decreased concentration of nevirapine with possible decreased effectiveness

St. John's wort: Substantially decreased concentration of nevirapine with decreased effectiveness

warfarin: Possible increased concentration of warfarin with possible alteration in anticoagulation

Adverse Reactions

CNS: Fatigue, fever, headache, **hepatic encephalopathy**, malaise, paresthesia, somnolence

EENT: Conjunctivitis, oral lesions, ulcerative stomatitis

ENDO: Cushingoid appearance, fat redistribution

GI: Abdominal pain, anorexia, **cholestatic and fulminant hepatitis**, diarrhea, elevated liver enzymes, **hepatic failure or necrosis, hepatotoxicity**, hyperbilirubinemia, jaundice, liver tenderness, nausea, vomiting

GU: Renal dysfunction

HEME: Anemia, **granulocytopenia, leukopenia, neutropenia, prolonged partial thromboplastin time, thrombocytopenia**
MS: Arthralgia, joint and muscle aches, myalgia, **rhabdomyolysis**
SKIN: Blisters, bullous eruptions, pruritus, rash, **Stevens–Johnson syndrome, toxic epidermal necrolysis**, urticaria
Other: Anaphylaxis, angioedema, drug reaction with eosinophilia and systemic symptoms (DRESS), drug withdrawal symptoms, flu-like symptoms, **hypophosphatemia**, immune reconstitution syndrome, lymphadenopathy, organ dysfunction

Nursing Considerations

- Know that nevirapine should never be used as monotherapy, because a resistant virus emerges rapidly.
- Check patient's liver enzymes before initiating nevirapine therapy, as ordered and regularly thereafter.
- Shake oral suspension container gently prior to measuring dose. Use an oral syringe or dosing cup to measure dosage, especially if volume to be administered is 5 ml or less. If a dosing cup is used, thoroughly rinse the cup with water and have patient drink the rinse.
- Expect to strictly follow the initial 14-day period of once-daily dosing to decrease the incidence of a rash. If a mild to moderate rash develops, know that the 14-day once-daily dosing period should be extended to as long as 28 days total. However, if rash continues to persist after 28 days of therapy, expect drug to be discontinued. Report a severe rash or any rash that is accompanied by other signs and symptoms to prescriber immediately and expect drug to be discontinued.
- Be aware that the oral suspension formulation is not recommended for use initially in adult female patients with a CD4+ cell count greater than 250 cells/mm^3 or adult male patients with a CD4+ cell count greater than 400 cells/mm^3, because of risk for serious or life-threatening hepatotoxicity.
- Know that if nevirapine therapy is interrupted for more than 7 days, the initial dosage regimen using the immediate-release formulation can be expected to be repeated for the first 14 days.

WARNING Monitor patient closely during the first 18 weeks of therapy to detect potentially life-threatening hepatotoxicity or skin reactions. Know that the greatest risk occurs during the first 6 weeks of therapy; patients at greatest risk include females and those having higher CD4+ cell counts at the initiation of therapy. Women with CD4+ cell count greater than 250 cells/mm^3 are at greatest risk. Patients coinfected with hepatitis B or C and/or who have increased transaminase levels at the start of therapy are at a greater risk of symptomatic events that may appear 6 weeks or more after starting nevirapine therapy. However, monitor all patients at all times, as these adverse reactions have also occurred in patients not considered at risk. Monitor patient closely for rash that may be combined with signs and symptoms of hepatitis that may progress to hepatic failure. If patient develops signs and symptoms of hepatitis or presents with increased transaminases accompanied with a rash or systemic symptoms such as blisters, conjunctivitis, facial edema, fatigue, fever, joint or muscle aches, malaise, oral lesions, or renal dysfunction, notify prescriber immediately; check transaminases levels, as ordered; and expect nevirapine to be discontinued.

- Be aware that immune reconstitution syndrome has occurred in patients treated with combination antiretroviral therapy, including nevirapine. The inflammatory response predisposes susceptible patients to opportunistic infections such as cytomegalovirus, *Mycobacterium avium* infection, *Pneumocystis jiroveci* pneumonia, or tuberculosis. Autoimmune disorders such as Graves' disease, Guillain–Barré syndrome, or polymyositis have also occurred. Report sudden or unusual adverse reactions to prescriber.

PATIENT TEACHING

- Advise patient to avoid missing doses of nevirapine. If she misses a dose, she should take it as soon as she remembers, but should not double the next dose or take more than prescribed.

- Tell patient prescribed oral suspension to shake oral suspension container gently prior to measuring dose. Use an oral syringe or dosing cup to measure dosage, especially if volume to be administered is 5 ml or less. If a dosing cup is used, tell patient to thoroughly rinse the cup with water and drink the rinse.

WARNING Inform patient about severe liver disease that may occur with nevirapine. Tell her to report signs and symptoms of liver disease such as acholic stools, anorexia, fatigue, malaise, nausea, tenderness over liver area, or yellowing of skin or whites of the eyes, and to seek immediate medical attention.

- Stress importance of being compliant with tests ordered to screen for adverse effects of nevirapine therapy.

WARNING Advise patient that nevirapine therapy may cause severe hypersensitivity or skin reactions. Tell her to report a rash, especially if it is accompanied by blisters, conjunctivitis, facial edema, fatigue, fever, joint or muscle aches, liver problems, or oral lesions, and to seek immediate medical attention.

- Inform patient that nevirapine therapy may cause changes in her body appearance because of fat redistribution. Prepare her for the possibility of developing breast enlargement, central obesity, dorsocervical fat enlargement (buffalo hump), facial wasting, and peripheral wasting.
- Instruct patient to report any persistent, severe, or unusual signs and symptoms.
- Inform women using oral contraceptives that an alternative or additional contraceptive should be used during nevirapine therapy, because drug may make the oral contraceptive unreliable. Encourage women of childbearing age to report known or suspected pregnancy. Also inform female patients of childbearing age that nevirapine may impair fertility.
- Alert mothers that breastfeeding is not recommended during nevirapine therapy.
- Tell patient to report all drugs being taken, including over-the-counter medications and herbals, as serious drug interactions may occur. Advise patient not to begin any new drug therapy without first checking with prescriber.

nicardipine hydrochloride

Cardene, Cardene IV, Cardene SR

Class and Category

Pharmacologic class: Calcium channel blocker
Therapeutic class: Antianginal, antihypertensive
Pregnancy category: C

Indications and Dosages

➤ *To manage angina pectoris and Prinzmetal's angina*

CAPSULES

Adults. 20 to 40 mg three times daily, increased every 3 days, as prescribed.

➤ *To manage hypertension*

CAPSULES

Adults. 20 mg three times daily, increased every 3 days, as needed. *Maintenance:* 20 to 40 mg three times daily.

E.R. CAPSULES

Adults. 30 mg twice daily.

➤ *To control acute hypertension*

I.V. INFUSION

Adults. *Initial:* 5 mg/hr by continuous infusion; increased by 2.5 mg/hr every 5 to 15 min, as prescribed. *Maximum:* 15 mg/hr.

DOSAGE ADJUSTMENT For patients with impaired liver function or reduced hepatic blood flow, dosage may be decreased. For patients with impaired renal function, titration should be done gradually when drug is given intravenously.

Route	Onset	Peak	Duration
P.O.	20 min	1–2 hr	Unknown
P.O. (E.R.)	20 min	1–2 hr	12 hr
I.V.	Immediate	Unknown	Unknown

Mechanism of Action

May slow extracellular calcium movement into myocardial and vascular smooth-muscle cells by deforming calcium channels in cell membranes, inhibiting ion-controlled gating mechanisms, and interfering with calcium release from the sarcoplasmic reticulum. By decreasing the intracellular calcium level, nicardipine inhibits smooth-muscle cell contraction and dilates coronary and systemic arteries. As with other calcium channel blockers, these actions lead to decreased myocardial oxygen requirements and reduced afterload, blood pressure, and peripheral resistance.

Incompatibilities
Don't mix nicardipine with sodium bicarbonate or lactated Ringer's solution, and don't administer through same I.V. line.

Contraindications
Advanced aortic stenosis, hypersensitivity to any calcium channel blocker including nicardipine and its components, second- or third-degree AV block in patient without artificial pacemaker

Interactions
DRUGS
anesthetics (hydrocarbon inhalation): Possibly hypotension
beta blockers, other antihypertensives, prazosin: Increased risk of hypotension
calcium supplements: Possibly impaired action of nicardipine
cimetidine: Increased nicardipine bioavailability
cyclosporine: Increased plasma cyclosporine levels
digoxin: Transiently increased blood digoxin level, increased risk of digitalis toxicity
disopyramide, flecainide: Increased risk of bradycardia, conduction defects, and heart failure
estrogens: Possibly increased fluid retention and decreased therapeutic effects of nicardipine
lithium: Increased risk of neurotoxicity
NSAIDs, sympathomimetics: Possibly decreased therapeutic effects of nicardipine
procainamide, quinidine: Possibly prolonged QT interval
tacrolimus: Increased plasma tacrolimus levels

FOODS
grapefruit, grapefruit juice: Possibly increased bioavailability of nicardipine
high-fat meals: Decreased blood nicardipine level

ACTIVITIES
alcohol use: Increased hypotensive effect

Adverse Reactions
CNS: Anxiety, asthenia, ataxia, confusion, dizziness, drowsiness, headache, nervousness, paresthesia, psychiatric disturbance, syncope, tremor, weakness
CV: **Bradycardia**, chest pain, exacerbation of angina (chronic therapy), **heart failure**, **hypotension**, orthostatic hypotension, palpitations, peripheral edema, tachycardia
EENT: Altered taste, blurred vision, dry mouth, epistaxis, gingival hyperplasia, pharyngitis, rhinitis, tinnitus
ENDO: Gynecomastia, hyperglycemia
GI: Anorexia, constipation, diarrhea, elevated liver enzymes, indigestion, nausea, thirst, vomiting
GU: Dysuria, nocturia, polyuria, sexual dysfunction, urinary frequency
HEME: Anemia, **leukopenia**, **thrombocytopenia**
MS: Joint stiffness, muscle spasms
RESP: Bronchitis, cough, **decreased oxygen saturation**, upper respiratory tract infection
SKIN: Dermatitis, diaphoresis, **erythema multiforme**, flushing, photosensitivity, pruritus, rash, **Stevens-Johnson syndrome**, urticaria
Other: **Hypokalemia**, injection-site irritation, weight gain

Nursing Considerations
- Check blood pressure and pulse rate before nicardipine therapy begins, during dosage changes, and periodically throughout therapy. During prolonged therapy, periodically assess ECG tracings for arrhythmias and other changes.
- Dilute each 25-mg ampule of nicardipine with 240 ml of solution to yield 0.1 mg/ml. Mixture is stable at room temperature for 24 hours.
- Know that if using premixed nicardipine for intravenous infusion, strength must

be checked carefully because drug comes as single strength (20 mg nicardipine in 200 ml of solution, providing 0.1 mg/ml) or double strength (40 mg nicardipine in 200 ml of solution, providing 0.2 mg/ml).

- Administer continuous infusion by I.V. pump or controller, and adjust according to patient's blood pressure, as prescribed. Be aware that the I.V. dosage should be titrated slowly in patients receiving a beta blocker and in patients with heart failure or significant left ventricular dysfunction because of possible negative inotropic effects. Also, patients with renal impairment require a more gradual titration when given drug intravenously.
- Administer drug through large peripheral veins or central veins to reduce the possibility of extravasation, local irritation, phlebitis, swelling, vascular impairment, or venous thrombosis. Change peripheral I.V. site every 12 hours, if feasible, to minimize these effects.
- Give first dose of oral nicardipine 1 hour before stopping I.V. infusion, as ordered.
- Monitor fluid intake and output and daily weight for signs of fluid retention, which may precipitate heart failure. Also assess for signs of heart failure, such as crackles, dyspnea, jugular vein distention, peripheral edema, and weight gain.
- During prolonged therapy, expect to periodically monitor liver and renal function test results. Anticipate drug dosage to be titrated slowly in these patients. Expect elevated liver enzymes to return to normal after drug is discontinued.
- Monitor patient with angina for increases in duration, frequency, or severity of symptoms because with chronic use of oral nicardipine (rarely with I.V. administration), exacerbation of angina may occur.
- Monitor serum potassium level during prolonged therapy. Hypokalemia increases the risk of arrhythmias.
- Monitor patients who take a beta blocker or have heart failure or significant left ventricular dysfunction because of drug's negative inotropic effect on some patients.

WARNING Expect to taper dosage gradually before discontinuing drug. Otherwise, angina or dangerously high blood pressure could result.

PATIENT TEACHING

- Urge patient to take nicardipine as prescribed, even if she feels well.
- Instruct patient to swallow E.R. capsules whole, not to chew, crush, cut, or open them.
- Advise patient not to take drug within 1 hour of eating a high-fat meal or grapefruit product. Urge her not to alter the amount of grapefruit products in her diet without consulting prescriber.

WARNING Caution patient against stopping nicardipine abruptly because angina or dangerously high blood pressure could result.

- Teach patient how to take her pulse, and urge her to notify prescriber immediately if it falls below 50 beats/minute.
- Teach patient how to measure blood pressure, and urge her to do so weekly if drug was prescribed for hypertension. Suggest that she keep a log of blood pressure readings and take it to follow-up visits.
- Advise patient to change position slowly to minimize orthostatic hypotension.
- Urge patient to avoid potentially hazardous activities until drug's CNS effects are known.
- Advise patient to notify prescriber immediately about chest pain that's not relieved by rest or nitroglycerin, constipation, irregular heartbeats, nausea, pronounced dizziness, severe or persistent headache, and swelling of hands or feet.
- Encourage patient to comply with suggested lifestyle changes, such as alcohol moderation, low-fat or low-sodium diet, regular exercise, smoking cessation, stress management, and weight reduction.
- Inform patient that hot tubs, prolonged hot showers, or saunas may cause dizziness or fainting.
- Instruct patient to avoid prolonged sun exposure and to use sunscreen when going outdoors.

nicotine for inhalation

Nicotrol Inhaler

nicotine nasal solution

Nicotrol NS

nicotine polacrilex

Nicorette, Nicorette Plus (CAN), Thrive

nicotine transdermal system

Habitrol, Nicoderm, NicoDerm CQ, Nicotrol, Nicrotrol CQ, ProStep

Class and Category

Pharmacologic class: Nicotinic agonist
Therapeutic class: Smoking cessation adjunct
Pregnancy category: C (nicotine polacrilex), D (other forms of nicotine)

Indications and Dosages

➤ *To relieve nicotine withdrawal symptoms, including craving*

CHEWING GUM

Adults. *Initial:* For patient who smokes less than 25 cigarettes a day, 2 mg (1 piece) or for patient who smokes more than 25 cigarettes a day, 4 mg (1 piece) every 1 to 2 hr, for 1 to 6 wk; then 2 or 4 mg every 2 to 4 hr for 7 to 9 wk; and then 2 or 4 mg every 4 to 8 hr for 10 to 12 wk. *Maximum:* 24 pieces daily for no longer than 12 wk.

THIN FILM STRIPS

Adults who smoke first cigarette 30 minutes or more after waking. 1 strip (2.5 mg) every 1 to 2 hr for 1 to 6 wk followed by 1 strip every 2 to 4 hr for 7 to 9 wk followed by 1 strip every 4 to 8 hr for 10 to 12 wk.

NASAL SOLUTION

Adults. 1 to 2 sprays (1 to 2 mg) in each nostril/hr. *Maximum:* 5 mg/hr or 40 mg daily for up to 3 mo.

LOZENGES

Adults who smoke first cigarette more than 30 min after waking up. 2 mg (1 lozenge) when needed using at least 9 lozenges daily for 6 wk, then daily amount decreased for remaining 6 wk.

Adults who smoke first cigarette within 30 min after waking up. 4 mg (1 lozenge), when needed using at least 9 lozenges daily for 6 wk, then daily amount decreased for remaining 6 wk. *Maximum:* No more than 1 lozenge at a time, no use of lozenges continuously one after another, no more than 5 lozenges in 6 hr; no more than 20 lozenges daily. Not to be used longer than 12 wk.

ORAL INHALATION

Adults and adolescents. 6 to 16 cartridges (24 to 64 mg) daily for up to 12 wk; then dosage gradually reduced over 12 wk or less. *Maximum:* 16 cartridges (64 mg) daily for 6 mo.

TRANSDERMAL PATCH (NICOTROL)

Adults. 15 mg patch worn for 16 hr daily for 6 wk.

TRANSDERMAL SYSTEM HABITROL, NICODERM, NICODERM CQ, NICOTROL CQ, PROSTEP)

Adults. *Initial:* 11 to 22 mg daily, adjusted to lower-dose systems over 6 to 12 wk.

DOSAGE ADJUSTMENT For adolescents and for adults weighing less than 45 kg (100 lb) and who smoke less than 10 cigarettes daily or have heart disease, initial dosage reduced to 11 to 14 mg daily and adjusted to lower-dose systems.

Mechanism of Action

Binds selectively to nicotinic-cholinergic receptors at autonomic ganglia, in the adrenal medulla, at neuromuscular junctions, and in the brain. By providing a lower dose of nicotine than cigarettes, this drug reduces nicotine craving and withdrawal symptoms.

Contraindications

Hypersensitivity to nicotine, its components, components of transdermal system or soy (mint flavor lozenges); life-threatening arrhythmias; nonsmokers; recovery from acute MI; severe angina pectoris; skin disorders (transdermal); temporomandibular joint disease (chewing gum)

Interactions

DRUGS

acetaminophen, beta blockers, imipramine, insulin, oxazepam, pentazocine, theophylline: Possibly increased therapeutic effects of these drugs (chewing gum, nasal spray, transdermal system)
alpha blockers, bronchodilators: Possibly increased therapeutic effects of these drugs (chewing gum, transdermal system)
bupropion: Potentiated therapeutic effects of nicotine, possibly increased risk of hypertension
sympathomimetics: Possibly decreased therapeutic effects of these drugs (chewing gum, transdermal system)
theophylline, tricyclic antidepressants: Possibly altered pharmacologic actions of these drugs (oral inhalation)

FOODS

acidic beverages (citrus juices, coffee, soft drinks, tea, wine): Decreased nicotine absorption from gum if beverages consumed within 15 minutes before or while chewing gum
caffeine: Increased effects of caffeine (chewing gum, nasal spray, transdermal system)

Adverse Reactions

CNS: Dizziness, dream disturbances, drowsiness, headache, irritability, lightheadedness, nervousness (chewing gum, transdermal system); amnesia, confusion, difficulty speaking, headache, migraine headache, paresthesia (nasal spray); chills, fever, headache, paresthesia (oral inhalation)
CV: **Arrhythmias** (all forms); hypertension (chewing gum, transdermal system); peripheral edema (nasal spray)
EENT: Increased salivation, injury to teeth or dental work, mouth injury, oral blistering, pharyngitis, stomatitis (chewing gum); altered taste, dry mouth (chewing gum, transdermal system); altered smell and taste, burning eyes, dry mouth, earache, epistaxis, gum disorders, hoarseness, lacrimation, mouth and tongue swelling, nasal blisters, nasal irritation or ulceration, pharyngitis, rhinitis, sinus problems, sneezing, vision changes (nasal spray); altered taste, lacrimation, pharyngitis, rhinitis, sinusitis, stomatitis (oral inhalation)
GI: Eructation (chewing gum); abdominal pain, constipation, diarrhea, flatulence, increased appetite, indigestion, nausea, vomiting (chewing gum, transdermal system); abdominal pain, constipation, diarrhea, flatulence, hiccups, indigestion, nausea (nasal spray); diarrhea, flatulence, hiccups, indigestion, nausea, peptic ulcer (transdermal), vomiting (oral inhalation)
GU: Dysmenorrhea (chewing gum, transdermal system); menstrual irregularities (nasal spray)
MS: Jaw and neck pain (chewing gum); arthralgia, myalgia (chewing gum, transdermal system); arthralgia, back pain, myalgia (nasal spray); back pain (oral inhalation)
RESP: Cough (chewing gum, transdermal system); bronchitis, **bronchospasm**, chest tightness, cough, dyspnea, increased sputum production (nasal spray); chest tightness, cough, dyspnea, wheezing (oral inhalation)
SKIN: Diaphoresis, erythema, pruritus, rash, urticaria (chewing gum, transdermal system); acne, flushing of face, pruritus, purpura, rash (nasal spray); pruritus, rash, urticaria (oral inhalation)
Other: Delayed wound healing (transdermal); flu-like symptoms, generalized pain, physical dependence (nasal spray); **hypersensitivity reactions** (chewing gum, transdermal system); withdrawal symptoms (oral inhalation)

Nursing Considerations

- Know that transdermal system (Habitrol brand) should not be used in patients who have a history of diabetes, peptic ulcer, or seizures.
- Know that when administering nicotine by oral inhalation, expect optimal effect to result from continuous puffing for 20 minutes.
- Keep in mind to avoid possible burns, remove patch before patient has an MRI.

PATIENT TEACHING

- Instruct patient to read and follow package instructions to obtain best results with nicotine product.
- Advise patient to notify prescriber about other conditions or drugs she takes. For example, the transdermal system (Habitrol

brand) should not be used in patients who have a history of diabetes, peptic ulcer, or seizures.

- Emphasize that patient must stop smoking as soon as nicotine treatment starts to avoid toxicity.
- Tell patient to stop taking drug and notify prescriber or seek emergency medical care if she develops an allergic reaction such as difficulty breathing or a rash or experiences an irregular heartbeat or palpitations, or signs of nicotine overdose.
- For chewing gum therapy, instruct patient to wait at least 15 minutes after drinking coffee, juice, soft drink, tea, or wine. Advise her to chew gum until she detects a tingling sensation or peppery taste and then to place gum between her cheek and gum until tingling or peppery taste subsides. Then direct her to move gum to a different site until tingling or taste subsides, repeating until she no longer feels the sensation—usually about 30 minutes. Caution against swallowing the gum. Advise her to stop use and contact prescriber if she experiences oral blistering.
- For nasal spray, tell patient to tilt her head back and spray into a nostril. Caution against inhaling, sniffing, or swallowing spray because nicotine is absorbed through nasal and oral mucosa.
- Warn patient that prolonged use of nasal form may cause dependence.
- For oral inhalation, tell patient to use 6 to 16 cartridges daily to prevent or relieve withdrawal symptoms and craving. Starting with 1 or 2 cartridges daily yields poor success. Direct patient to inhale through device like a cigarette, puffing often for 20 minutes.
- For transdermal system, tell patient not to open package until just before use because nicotine is lost in the air. Advise her to apply system to clean, dry, hairless site on upper outer arm or upper body. Instruct her to change systems and rotate sites every 24 hours and not to use the same site for 7 days. To avoid possible burns, advise patient to remove patch before undergoing any MRI procedure.

WARNING Urge patient to keep all unused nicotine forms safely away from children and pets and to discard used forms carefully. (Enough nicotine may remain in used systems to poison children and pets.) Instruct her to contact a poison control center immediately if she suspects that a child has ingested nicotine.

- Explain to patient with asthma or COPD that nicotine may cause bronchospasm.
- Inform patient that it may take several attempts to stop smoking. Urge her to join a smoking cessation program.

nifedipine

Adalat CC, Adalat XL (CAN), Afeditab CR, Apo-Nifed (CAN), Procardia, Procardia XL

Class and Category

Pharmacologic class: Calcium channel blocker
Therapeutic class: Antianginal, antihypertensive
Pregnancy category: C

Indications and Dosages

➤ *To manage angina*

CAPSULES (APO-NIFED, PROCARDIA)

Adults. *Initial:* 10 mg three times daily, increased over 1 to 2 wk as needed. *Maintenance:* 10 to 20 mg three times daily *Maximum:* 180 mg daily, 30 mg/dose.

E.R. TABLETS (ADALAT XL, PROCARDIA XL)

Adults. *Initial:* 30 to 60 mg daily, increased or decreased over 7 to 14 days based on patient response. *Maximum:* 90 mg daily.

➤ *To manage hypertension*

E.R. TABLETS (ADALAT CC, AFEDITAB CR)

Adults. *Initial:* 30 mg daily. *Maintenance:* 30 to 60 mg daily, increased or decreased over 7 to 14 days based on patient response. *Maximum:* 90 mg daily.

E.R. TABLETS (ADALAT XL)

Adults. *Initial:* 30 to 60 mg daily, increased or decreased over 7 to 14 days based on patient response. *Maintenance:* 60 to 90 mg daily. *Maximum:* 120 mg daily.

E.R. TABLETS (PROCARDIA XL)

Adults. 30 to 60 mg daily, increased or decreased over 7 to 14 days based on patient response. *Maximum:* 120 mg daily.

DOSAGE ADJUSTMENT Dosage may be reduced for elderly patients and those with heart failure or impaired hepatic or renal function.

Route	Onset	Peak	Duration
P.O. (caps)	20 min	Unknown	Unknown

Mechanism of Action

May slow movement of calcium into myocardial and vascular smooth-muscle cells by deforming calcium channels in cell membranes, inhibiting ion-controlled gating mechanisms, and disrupting calcium release from sarcoplasmic reticulum. Decreasing intracellular calcium level inhibits smooth-muscle cell contraction and dilates arteries, which decreases myocardial oxygen demand, peripheral resistance, blood pressure, and afterload.

Contraindications

Hypersensitivity to nifedipine or its components, second- or third-degree AV block without artificial pacemaker, sick sinus syndrome

Interactions

DRUGS

anesthetics (hydrocarbon inhalation): Possibly hypotension
antiviral drugs, cimetidine, cisapride, clarithromycin, dalfopristin, diltiazem, erythromycin, fluconazole, fluoxetine, indinavir, itraconazole, ketoconazole, nefazodone, nelfinavir, other antihypertensives, prazosin, quinupristin, saquinavir, timolol, valproic acid, verapamil: Increased risk of hypotension
benazepril: Possibly increased heart rate and hypotensive effect
beta blockers: Increased risk of profound hypotension, heart failure, and worsening of angina
calcium supplements: Possibly interference with action of nifedipine
carbamazepine, NSAIDs, phenobarbital, phenytoin, rifabutin, rifampin, rifapentine, St. John's wort, sympathomimetics: Possibly decreased therapeutic effects of nifedipine
digoxin: Transiently increased blood digoxin level, increased risk of digitalis toxicity
disopyramide, flecainide: Increased risk of bradycardia, conduction defects, and heart failure
doxazosin: Decreased doxazosin effectiveness; increased nifedipine effectiveness
estrogens: Possibly increased fluid retention and decreased nifedipine effects
lithium: Increased risk of neurotoxicity
metformin: Increased metformin absorption and plasma level
tacrolimus: Decreased tacrolimus metabolism

FOODS

grapefruit, grapefruit juice: Possibly increased bioavailability of nifedipine
high-fat meals: Possibly delayed nifedipine absorption

ACTIVITIES

alcohol use: Additive hypotensive effect

Adverse Reactions

CNS: Anxiety, ataxia, confusion, dizziness, drowsiness, headache, nervousness (possibly extreme), nightmares, paresthesia, psychiatric disturbance, syncope, tremor, weakness
CV: **Bradycardia**, chest pain, **heart failure**, **hypotension**, palpitations, peripheral edema, tachycardia
EENT: Altered taste, blurred vision, dry mouth, epistaxis, gingival hyperplasia, nasal congestion, pharyngitis, sinusitis, tinnitus
ENDO: Gynecomastia, hyperglycemia
GI: Anorexia; constipation; diarrhea; dyspepsia; elevated liver enzymes; **GI bleeding**, irritation, or **obstruction**; **hepatitis**; nausea; vomiting
GU: Dysuria, nocturia, polyuria, sexual dysfunction, urinary frequency
HEME: Anemia, **leukopenia**, positive Coombs' test, **thrombocytopenia**
MS: Joint stiffness, muscle cramps
RESP: Chest congestion, cough, dyspnea, respiratory tract infection, wheezing
SKIN: Acute generalized exanthematous pustulosis, diaphoresis, **erythema multiforme**, **exfoliative dermatitis**, flushing, photosensitivity, pruritus, rash, **Stevens–Johnson syndrome**, **toxic epidermal necrolysis**, urticaria

Nursing Considerations

- Be aware that patients with galactose intolerance should not take nifedipine because the drug contains lactose. The capsule form of nifedipine should not be used to treat hypertension because its effects on blood pressure are not known.

- Use cautiously in patients with cirrhosis because it is unknown how nifedipine exposure may be altered in these patients.
- Know that when starting and stopping nifedipine therapy, taper it, as prescribed, over 7 to 14 days.
- Keep in mind that because of drug's negative inotropic effect on some patients, frequently monitor heart rate and rhythm, as well as blood pressure, especially in patients who take a beta blocker or have heart failure, significant left ventricular dysfunction, or tight aortic stenosis.
- Monitor fluid intake/output and daily weight; fluid retention may lead to heart failure. Also assess for signs of heart failure, such as crackles, dyspnea, jugular vein distention, peripheral edema, and weight gain.

PATIENT TEACHING

- Instruct patient to swallow E.R. tablets whole, not to break, chew, or crush them. Inform her that their empty shells may appear in stool.
- Urge patient to take nifedipine exactly as prescribed, even when she's feeling well. Advise her to notify prescriber if she misses two or more doses.
- Urge patient not to take drug within 1 hour of a high-fat meal or grapefruit. Urge her not to alter the amount of grapefruit in her diet without consulting prescriber.

WARNING Caution patient against stopping nifedipine abruptly because angina or dangerously high blood pressure could result.

- Teach patient to measure blood pressure and pulse rate, and advise her to call prescriber if they drop below accepted levels. Suggest keeping a log of weekly measurements and taking it to follow-up visits.
- Instruct patient to notify prescriber immediately about chest pain, difficulty breathing, ringing in ears, and swollen gums.
- Advise patient to avoid hazardous activities until drug's CNS effects are known.
- Urge patient to avoid alcoholic beverages because they may worsen dizziness, drowsiness, and hypotension.
- Teach patient to minimize constipation by increasing her intake of fluids, if allowed, and dietary fiber.
- Emphasize the need to comply with prescribed lifestyle changes, such as alcohol moderation, low-fat or low-sodium diet, regular exercise, smoking cessation, stress reduction, and weight reduction.
- Emphasize the need for good oral hygiene and regular dental visits.
- Caution patient that hot tubs, prolonged hot showers, and saunas may cause dizziness and fainting.
- Advise patient to avoid prolonged sun exposure and to wear sunscreen outdoors.

nisoldipine

Sular

Class and Category

Pharmacologic class: Calcium channel blocker
Therapeutic class: Antihypertensive
Pregnancy category: C

Indications and Dosages

➤ *To manage hypertension*

E.R. TABLETS

Adults. *Initial:* 17 mg once daily, then increased by 8.5 mg weekly or longer, as needed. *Maintenance:* 17 to 34 mg once daily. *Maximum:* 34 mg daily.

DOSAGE ADJUSTMENT For patients over age 65 and patients with hepatic impairment, initial dosage reduced to 8.5 mg daily.

Mechanism of Action

May slow extracellular calcium movement into myocardial and vascular smooth-muscle cells by deforming calcium channels in cell membranes, inhibiting ion-controlled gating mechanisms, and interfering with calcium release from the sarcoplasmic reticulum. By decreasing the intracellular calcium level, nisoldipine inhibits smooth-muscle cell contraction and dilates coronary and systemic arteries. As with other calcium channel blockers, these actions lead to decreased myocardial oxygen requirements and reduced afterload, blood pressure, and peripheral resistance.

Contraindications

Hypersensitivity to calcium channel blockers, including nisoldipine and its components, second- or third-degree AV block with no artificial pacemaker, sick sinus syndrome

Interactions

DRUGS

beta blockers: Possibly increased risk of hypotension
CYP3A4 inducers such as phenytoin: Decreased nisoldipine levels and effectiveness
CYP3A4 inhibitors such as cimetidine: Increased blood nisoldipine level; increased risk of adverse reactions
NSAIDs: Decreased antihypertensive effect of nisoldipine
quinidine: Increased plasma quinidine concentration

FOODS

grapefruit, grapefruit juice: Possibly increased bioavailability of nisoldipine
high-fat meals: Possibly delayed nisoldipine absorption

ACTIVITIES

alcohol use: Additive hypotensive effect

Adverse Reactions

CNS: Dizziness, headache
CV: Angina, **hypotension**, palpitations, peripheral edema, vasodilation
EENT: Pharyngitis, sinusitis
GI: Constipation, nausea
GU: Impotence
RESP: **Bronchospasm**, dyspnea
SKIN: Rash
Other: **Hypersensitivity reactions**

Nursing Considerations

- Monitor blood pressure and pulse rate and rhythm before starting nisoldipine therapy, during dosage adjustments, and periodically throughout therapy.
- Don't break or crush E.R. tablets.
- Know that for optimal absorption, give drug should be given 1 hour before or 2 hours after meals.
- Monitor fluid intake and output and daily weight to assess for signs of fluid retention, which may lead to heart failure. Also assess for signs of heart failure, such as crackles, dyspnea, jugular vein distention, peripheral edema, and weight gain.
- Monitor patient for allergic-type reaction that may include bronchospasm, especially if patient has aspirin sensitivity, because drug contains FD&C yellow no. 5 dye.

PATIENT TEACHING

- Instruct patient to swallow E.R. nisoldipine tablets whole, not to break, chew, or crush them.
- Advise patient to take drug 1 hour before or 2 hours after meals. Urge her not to alter amount of grapefruit products in her diet without consulting prescriber.
- Urge patient to continue taking drug as prescribed, even if she feels well.

WARNING Caution patient against stopping drug abruptly because blood pressure could rise dangerously high.

- Instruct patient to notify prescriber about constipation, difficulty breathing, dizziness, irregular heartbeat, nausea, severe headache, and swelling of hands or feet.
- Teach patient and family how to measure blood pressure, and instruct them to notify prescriber if systolic blood pressure falls below 90 mm Hg. Suggest that patient keep a log of weekly measurements and take it to follow-up visits.
- Advise patient to change positions slowly to minimize the effects of orthostatic hypotension. Inform her that hot tubs, prolonged hot showers, and saunas may worsen this adverse reaction.
- Caution patient to avoid hazardous activities until drug's CNS effects are known.
- Urge patient to avoid alcohol and OTC alcohol-containing drugs without consulting prescriber. Many OTC preparations can raise blood pressure.
- Emphasize the need to adhere to prescribed lifestyle changes, such as alcohol moderation, low-fat and low-sodium diet, regular exercise, smoking cessation, stress reduction, and weight reduction.

nitrofurantoin

Apo-Nitrofurantoin (CAN), Furadantin, Macrobid, Macrodantin, Novo-Furantoin (CAN)

Class and Category

Pharmacologic class: Nitrofuran
Therapeutic class: Antibiotic
Pregnancy category: B (except near term)

Indications and Dosages

➤ *To treat acute cystitis*

CAPSULES, ORAL SUSPENSION

Adults and children age 12 and over. 50 to 100 mg four times daily and continued for 1 wk or at least 3 days after urine is negative for bacteria.

Children over age 1 month. 5 to 7 mg/kg/day in four divided doses, continued for 1 wk or at least 3 days after urine is negative for bacteria. *Maximum:* 400 mg daily.

MACROCRYSTAL CAPSULES

Adults and children age 12 and over. 100 mg every 12 hr for 7 days.

➤ *To suppress chronic cystitis*

CAPSULES, ORAL SUSPENSION

Adults. 50 to 100 mg at bedtime.

Children over age 1 month. 1 to 2 mg/kg daily at bedtime or divided into two doses and given q 12 hr. *Maximum*: 100 mg daily.

Mechanism of Action

Alters or inactivates bacterial ribosomal proteins and other macromolecules. This action of nitrofurantoin inhibits aerobic energy metabolism, bacterial protein synthesis, cell wall synthesis, DNA synthesis, and RNA synthesis. Nitrofurantoin is bacteriostatic at low doses and bactericidal at higher doses.

Contraindications

Age under 1 month, anuria, creatinine clearance less than 60 ml/min; history of cholestatic jaundice or hepatic dysfunction with previous nitrofurantoin therapy; hypersensitivity to nitrofurantoin, parabens or their components; oliguria; pregnancy near term

Interactions

DRUGS

hepatotoxic drugs: Increased risk of hepatotoxicity

magnesium trisilicate: Decreased nitrofurantoin absorption

methyldopa, procainamide, hemolytics: Increased risk of toxic effects from nitrofurantoin

nalidixic acid: Possibly impaired therapeutic effects of this drug

neurotoxic drugs: Increased risk of neurotoxicity

probenecid, sulfinpyrazone: Increased blood nitrofurantoin level and increased risk of toxicity

Adverse Reactions

CNS: Chills, confusion, depression, headache, **neurotoxicity**, peripheral neuropathy

CV: Vasculitis

EENT: Optic neuritis, parotitis, tooth discoloration

GI: Abdominal pain, anorexia, cholestatic jaundice, diarrhea, **hepatic necrosis, hepatitis**, jaundice, nausea, **pancreatitis, pseudomembranous colitis**, vomiting

GU: Rust-colored to brown urine

HEME: Aplastic anemia, granulocytopenia, hemolytic anemia, leukopenia, megaloblastic anemia, **methemoglobinemia, thrombocytopenia**

MS: Arthralgia, myalgia

RESP: Asthma (in asthmatic patients), **cyanosis, interstitial pneumonitis, pulmonary fibrosis**

SKIN: Alopecia; eczematous, erythematous, or maculopapular eruptions; **erythema multiforme; exfoliative dermatitis;** pruritus; rash; **Stevens–Johnson syndrome**

Other: Anaphylaxis, angioedema, drug-induced fever, lupus-like syndrome

Nursing Considerations

- Obtain a specimen of patient's urine for culture and sensitivity tests, as ordered; review test results if possible before giving nitrofurantoin.
- Give drug with food or milk to avoid staining teeth.
- Don't break or crush capsules.
- Shake oral nitrofurantoin suspension before pouring dose, and mix with food or milk, as needed.
- Monitor patient for evidence of superinfection, such as abdominal pain, diarrhea, and fever. If patient develops diarrhea, it may indicate pseudomembranous colitis caused by *Clostridium difficile.* Notify prescriber and expect to withhold nitrofurantoin and treat with electrolytes, fluids, protein, and an antibiotic effective against *C. difficile.*
- Monitor patient for hepatic and pulmonary abnormalities because rare but

severe reactions have occurred with nitrofurantoin use, especially in the elderly.
- Observe patient for changes in nervous function because peripheral neuropathy, although uncommon, may become severe or irreversible. Patients with anemia, debilitating disease, diabetes mellitus, electrolyte imbalance, renal impairment, or vitamin B deficiency are at higher risk for peripheral neuropathy.

PATIENT TEACHING
- Instruct patient to shake nitrofurantoin oral suspension before measuring dose and to take drug with food or milk.
- Caution patient against taking any preparations that contain magnesium trisilicate during therapy.
- Explain that urine may turn brown, orange, or rust-colored during therapy.
- Instruct patient to complete prescribed course of therapy even if symptoms subside before course is completed.
- Urge patient to tell prescriber about diarrhea that's severe or lasts longer than 3 days. Explain that bloody or watery stools can occur 2 or more months after nitrofurantoin therapy and can be serious, requiring prompt treatment.

nitroglycerin
(glyceryl trinitrate)

Gen-Nitro (CAN), GoNitro, Minitran, Nitro-Bid, Nitrocot, Nitro-Dur, Nitrolingual Pumpspray, NitroMist, NitroQuick, Nitrostat, Nitro-Time, Rectiv, Transderm-Nitro, Trinipatch (CAN)

Class and Category
Pharmacologic class: Nitrate
Therapeutic class: Antianginal, vasodilator
Pregnancy category: B (Nitrostat), C

Indications and Dosages
➤ *To prevent acute anginal attacks*

E.R. CAPSULES

Adults. 2.5, 6.5, or 9 mg two to four times daily.

TRANSDERMAL OINTMENT

Adults. *Initial:* 1/2 inch of 2% ointment twice daily, increasing in 1/2 inch increments and/or dosing frequency to three or four times daily, as needed. *Usual maintenance:* 1/2 to 2 inches every 6 to 8 hr.

TRANSDERMAL PATCH

Adults. *Initial:* 0.2 to 0.4 mg/hr worn 12 to 14 hr, with dosage increased or decreased, as needed. *Maintenance:* 0.1 to 0.8 mg/hr, worn 12 to 14 hr.

S.L. POWDER

Adults. 400 mcg (1 packet) sprinkled under tongue 5 to 10 min before exertion.

➤ *To treat acute angina pectoris; to reduce or limit anginal attacks before exercise*

S.L. TABLETS

Adults. 0.3 to 0.6 mg, repeated every 5 min. *Maximum:* 3 tabs in 15 min or 10 mg daily.

S.L. POWDER

Adults. 400 or 800 mcg (1 or 2 packets) sprinkled under tongue, repeated every 5 min, as needed. *Maximum*: 1,200 mcg (3 packets) in 15 min.

TRANSLINGUAL SPRAY

Adults. 1 or 2 metered doses (400 or 800 mcg) onto or under tongue, repeated every 5 min, as needed, for an acute attack or taken 5 to 10 min before exercise. *Maximum:* 3 sprays within 15 min.

➤ *To treat acute angina when oral therapy has been ineffective; to manage hypertension related to surgery or heart failure following an acute myocardial infarction*

I.V. INFUSION

Adults. 5 mcg/min, increased by 5 mcg/min every 3 to 5 min to 20 mcg/min, as needed, and then by 10 to 20 mcg/min every 3 to 5 min, if higher dosage is needed.

➤ *To treat moderate to severe pain associated with chronic anal fissure*

OINTMENT

Adults. 1 inch (375 mg of ointment equivalent to 1.5 mg of nitroglycerin) to intra-anal area every 12 hr for up to 3 wk.

Route	Onset	Peak	Duration
P.O.*	20–45 min	Unknown	8–12 hr
I.V.	1–2 min	Unknown	3–5 min
S.L.	1–3 min	Unknown	30–60 min

Route	Onset	Peak	Duration
Trans-dermal†	In 30 min	Unknown	4–8 hr
Trans-dermal‡	In 30 min	Unknown	8–24 hr
Trans-lingual	2 to 4 min	Unknown	30–60 min

* E.R.

† Ointment.

‡ Patch.

Mechanism of Action

May interact with nitrate receptors in vascular smooth-muscle cell membranes. This interaction reduces nitroglycerin to nitric oxide, which activates the enzyme guanylate cyclase, increasing intracellular formation of cGMP. Increased cGMP level may relax vascular smooth muscle by forcing calcium out of muscle cells, causing vasodilation. Venous dilation decreases venous return to the heart, reducing left ventricular end-diastolic pressure and pulmonary artery wedge pressure. Arterial dilation decreases systemic arterial pressure, systemic vascular resistance, and mean arterial pressure. Thus, nitroglycerin reduces preload and afterload, decreasing myocardial workload and oxygen demand. It also dilates coronary arteries, increasing blood flow to ischemic myocardial tissue and provides analgesic effects in anal tissue.

Incompatibilities

Don't administer I.V. nitroglycerin through I.V. bags or tubing made of polyvinyl chloride. Don't mix drug with other solutions.

Contraindications

Acute MI (S.L.), angle-closure glaucoma, cerebral hemorrhage, circulatory failure and shock, concurrent use of phosphodiesterase inhibitors (avanafil, sildenafil, tadalafil, vardenafil) or riociguat, constrictive pericarditis (I.V.), head trauma, hypersensitivity to adhesive in transdermal form, hypersensitivity to nitrates, or their components, hypotension (I.V.), hypovolemia (I.V.), inadequate cerebral circulation (I.V.), increased intracranial pressure, orthostatic hypotension, pericardial tamponade, severe anemia

Interactions

DRUGS

acetylcholine, norepinephrine: Possibly decreased therapeutic effects of these drugs
ergotamine and related drugs: Possibly precipitate angina (oral nitroglycerin)
heparin: Possibly decreased anticoagulant effect of heparin (I.V. nitroglycerin)
opioid analgesics, other antihypertensives, including beta blockers, vasodilators: Possibly increased orthostatic hypotension
phosphodiesterase inhibitors (such as avanafil, sildenafil, tadalafil, vardenafil), riociguat: Possibly severe hypotensive effect of nitroglycerin
sympathomimetics: Possibly decreased antianginal effect of nitroglycerin and increased risk of hypotension

ACTIVITIES

alcohol use: Possibly increased orthostatic hypotension

Adverse Reactions

CNS: Agitation, anxiety, dizziness, drowsiness, headache, insomnia, restlessness, syncope, weakness
CV: **Arrhythmias**, edema, **hypotension**, orthostatic hypotension, palpitations, tachycardia
EENT: Blurred vision, burning or tingling in mouth (S.L. forms), dry mouth
GI: Abdominal pain, diarrhea, indigestion, nausea, vomiting
GU: Dysuria, impotence, urinary frequency
HEME: **Methemoglobinemia**
MS: Arthralgia
RESP: Bronchitis, pneumonia, transient hypoxemia
SKIN: Contact dermatitis (transdermal forms), **exfoliative dermatitis**, flushing of face and neck, rash
OTHER: **Hypersensitivity reactions**

Nursing Considerations

- Know that patients receiving oral nitroglycerin should not receive ergotamine and related drugs, if possible, because oral administration of nitroglycerin significantly increases effects of ergotamine and related drugs.

- Use nitroglycerin cautiously in elderly patients, especially those who are volume-depleted or taking several medications, because of the increased risk of falls and hypotension. Hypotension may be accompanied by angina and paradoxical slowing of the heart rate. Hypotension may become severe, especially in patients in an upright position, even with small doses, particularly in patients with aortic or mitral stenosis, constrictive pericarditis, or who are already experiencing hypotension. Symptoms of severe hypotension include collapse, nausea, pallor, perspiration, syncope, vomiting, and weakness. Notify prescriber immediately if these occur, and provide appropriate treatment, as ordered.
- Use nitroglycerin cautiously in patients with hypertrophic obstructive cardiomyopathy because nitrate therapy may aggravate angina in this condition.
- Plan a nitroglycerin-free period of about 10 hours each day, as prescribed, to maintain therapeutic effects and avoid tolerance.
- Don't break or crush E.R. capsules. Have patient swallow them whole with a full glass of water.
- Place S.L. tablet under patient's tongue and make sure it dissolves completely.
- Place patient in sitting position, if possible, when administering S.L. powder. Have patient open mouth, sprinkle powder under tongue. Have patient close mouth and breath normally. Allow powder to dissolve without patient swallowing. Do not allow patient to rinse mouth or spit for five minutes after administration.
- When applying transdermal ointment, apply correct amount on dose-measuring paper. Then place paper on hairless area of body and spread in a thin, even layer over an area at least 2 inches by 3 inches. Don't place on cuts or irritated areas. Wash hands after application. Rotate sites. Store at room temperature.
- Open transdermal patch package immediately before use. Apply patch to hairless area, and press edges to seal. Rotate sites. Store at room temperature. If patient needs cardioversion or defibrillation, remove transdermal patch before procedure.
- Don't shake translingual spray container before administering. Have patient inhale and hold her breath, and then spray drug under or on her tongue.
- Be aware that I.V. nitroglycerin should be diluted only in D_5W or normal saline solution and shouldn't be mixed with other infusions. The pharmacist should add drug to a glass bottle, not a container made of polyvinyl chloride. Don't use a filter because plastic absorbs drug. Administer with infusion pump.
- Check vital signs before every dosage adjustment and often during therapy.
- Monitor frequently heart and breath sounds, level of consciousness, fluid intake and output, and pulmonary artery wedge pressure, if possible.
- Store premixed containers in the dark; don't freeze them.

WARNING Assess patient for evidence of overdose, such as confusion, diaphoresis, dyspnea, flushing, headache, hypotension, nausea, palpitations, tachycardia, vertigo, vision changes, and vomiting. Treat as prescribed by removing nitroglycerin source, if possible; elevating legs above heart level; and administering an alpha-adrenergic agonist, such as phenylephrine, as prescribed, to treat severe hypotension.

PATIENT TEACHING

- Teach patient to recognize signs and symptoms of angina pectoris, including chest fullness, pain, and pressure, possibly with sweating and nausea. Pain may radiate down left arm or into neck or jaw. Inform women and those with diabetes mellitus or hypertension that they may feel only fatigue and shortness of breath.
- Instruct patient to read and follow package instructions to obtain full benefits of drug.
- Inform patient that prescriber may order a 10- to 12-hour drug-free period at night (or at another time if she has chest pain at night or in the morning) to prevent drug tolerance. Also inform patient that drug should be taken as prescribed as excessive use may lead to tolerance as well.
- Instruct patient to swallow E.R. capsules whole—not to break, chew, or crush them—with a full glass of water.
- For sublingual use, advise patient to place 1 or 2 packets of powder or 1 tablet under her tongue or in buccal pouch (tablet

form only) when angina starts and then to sit or lie down. Instruct her not to swallow drug, but to let it dissolve. Explain that moisture in her mouth helps drug absorption. Remind patient not to rinse mouth or spit for 5 minutes after using drug. If angina doesn't subside, instruct patient to place another packet of powder or tablet under her tongue or in buccal pouch (tablet form only) after 5 minutes and to repeat, if needed, for three doses total. If pain doesn't subside after 15 minutes, urge patient to call 911 or another emergency service.

- Advise patient to carry S.L. packets of powder or tablets in their original brown bottle in a purse or jacket pocket, but not one that will be affected by body heat. Instruct her to store drug in a dry place at room temperature and to discard cotton from container. Advise her to discard and replace S.L. tablets after 6 months. Tell her to note date on packets of powder and not to use beyond the expiration date printed.
- Advise patient using transdermal ointment or patch to rotate sites to avoid skin sensitization.
- Inform patient that swimming or bathing doesn't affect transdermal forms but that electric blankets, hot tubs, magnetic therapy, prolonged hot showers, and saunas over the site may increase drug absorption and cause dizziness and hypotension.
- Caution against inhaling translingual spray. Before first use, tell patient to press actuator button 10 times to prime container and then hold container upright with forefinger on top of actuator button. Tell her to open her mouth, bring container as close as possible, press actuator button firmly to release spray onto or under tongue, and release button and immediately close her mouth. Remind her to replace plastic cover on container and to not spit out the drug or rinse her mouth for 5 to 10 minutes. Tell her to reprime container by pressing actuator button twice if container hasn't been used for more than 6 weeks. Remind patient to periodically check level of fluid in container. If it reaches the top or middle hole on side of container, more should be obtained. Caution patient not to let level of liquid get to bottom of hole.
- Inform patient that nitroglycerin commonly causes headache, which typically resolves after a few days of continuous therapy. Suggest taking acetaminophen, as needed, and not contraindicated.
- Advise patient to notify prescriber immediately about blurred vision, dizziness, and severe headache.
- Suggest that patient change positions slowly to minimize orthostatic hypotension.
- Advise patient to avoid hazardous activities until drug's CNS effects are known.
- Urge patient to avoid alcohol and erectile dysfunction drugs during therapy.
- Advise patient to alert all prescribers of nitroglycerin use because of potential drug interactions.
- Advise patient to alert all prescribers of nitroglycerin use because of potential drug interactions.

nitroprusside sodium

Nipride (CAN), Nitropress

Class and Category

Pharmacologic class: Vasodilator
Therapeutic class: Antihypertensive, vasodilator
Pregnancy category: C

Indications and Dosages

➤ *To treat hypertensive crisis and acute heart; to produce controlled hypotension in order to reduce bleeding during surgery*

I.V. INFUSION

Adults and children. *Initial:* 0.3 mcg/kg/min, increased gradually every few minutes until blood pressure reaches desired level. *Maximum:* 10 mcg/kg/min.

DOSAGE ADJUSTMENT For children weighing less than 10 kg, infusion rate may be reduced.

Route	Onset	Peak	Duration
I.V.	1–2 min	Immediate	1–10 min

Mechanism of Action

May interact with nitrate receptors in vascular smooth-muscle cell membranes. This action reduces nitroprusside to nitric oxide and then activates intracellular guanylate cyclase, which increases the cGMP level. Increased cGMP level may relax vascular smooth muscle by forcing calcium out of muscle cells. Smooth-muscle relaxation causes arteries and veins to dilate, which reduces peripheral vascular resistance and blood pressure.

Incompatibilities

Don't mix nitroprusside with any other drug.

Contraindications

Acute heart failure with decreased peripheral vascular resistance, congenital optic atrophy, decreased cerebral perfusion, hypersensitivity to nitroprusside or its components, hypertension from aortic coarctation or AV shunting, tobacco-induced amblyopia

Interactions

DRUGS

dobutamine: Increased cardiac output, decreased pulmonary artery wedge pressure
ganglionic blockers, general anesthetics, hypotension-producing drugs: Increased hypotensive effect
sympathomimetics: Decreased antihypertensive effect of nitroprusside

Adverse Reactions

CNS: Anxiety, dizziness, headache, **increased intracranial pressure,** nervousness, restlessness
CV: Hypotension, tachycardia
ENDO: Hypothyroidism
GI: Abdominal pain, ileus, nausea, vomiting
HEME: Methemoglobinemia
MS: Muscle twitching
SKIN: Diaphoresis, flushing, rash
Other: Infusion-site phlebitis

Nursing Considerations

- Obtain baseline vital signs before administering nitroprusside.

WARNING Don't give drug undiluted. Reconstitute with 2 ml D_5W, and add solution to 250 to 500 ml D_5W to produce 200 or 100 mcg/ml, respectively.

- Be aware that solution is stable at room temperature for 24 hours when protected from light. Don't use reconstituted solution if it contains particles or is blue, green, red, or darker than faint brown.
- Use an infusion pump. Place opaque cover over infusion container because drug is metabolized by light. I.V. tubing doesn't need to be covered.
- Keep patient supine when starting drug or titrating dose up or down.
- Monitor blood pressure continuously with intra-arterial pressure monitor. Record blood pressure every 5 minutes at start of infusion and every 15 minutes thereafter.
- Be aware that if patient has severe heart failure, expect to administer an inotropic drug, such as dopamine or dobutamine, as prescribed.

WARNING Know that patient who receives prolonged nitroprusside therapy or short-term high-dose therapy should be watched for evidence of thiocyanate toxicity (ataxia, blurred vision, delirium, dizziness, dyspnea, headache, hyperreflexia, loss of consciousness, nausea, tinnitus, and vomiting). Toxicity can cause arrhythmias, metabolic acidosis, severe hypotension, and death.

- Monitor serum thiocyanate level at least every 72 hours; levels above 100 mcg/ml are associated with toxicity.

WARNING Assess patient for evidence of cyanide toxicity (absence of reflexes, coma, distant heart sounds, hypotension, metabolic acidosis, mydriasis, pink skin, shallow respirations, and weak pulse). If detected, discontinue nitroprusside, as ordered, and give 4 to 6 mg/kg sodium nitrite over 2 to 4 minutes to convert hemoglobin to methemoglobin. Follow with 150 to 200 mg/kg sodium thiosulfate. Repeat this regimen at half the original doses after 2 hours, as ordered.

PATIENT TEACHING

- Advise patient to change position slowly to minimize dizziness from sudden, severe hypotension.

nizatidine

Axid, Axid AR

Class and Category

Pharmacologic class: $Histamine_2$ (H_2) receptor antagonist
Therapeutic class: Antiulcer
Pregnancy category: B

Indications and Dosages

➤ *To manage active duodenal ulcer; to manage acute benign gastric ulcer*

CAPSULES

Adults and adolescents. 300 mg at bedtime or 150 mg twice daily for up to 8 wk.

➤ *To prevent recurrence of duodenal ulcer*

CAPSULES

Adults and adolescents. 150 mg at bedtime.

➤ *To manage gastroesophageal reflux disease*

CAPSULES

Adults and adolescents. 150 mg twice daily.

➤ *To prevent or relieve acid indigestion or heartburn*

TABLETS

Adults and adolescents. 75 mg 30 min to 1 hr before meals.

Route	Onset	Peak	Duration
P.O.	Unknown	Unknown	10–12 hr*

* For nocturnal acid secretion; up to 4 hr for food-stimulated acid secretion.

Mechanism of Action

Inhibits basal and nocturnal secretion of gastric acid by competitively and reversibly blocking H_2 receptors, especially those in gastric parietal cells. Nizatidine also inhibits gastric acid secretion in response to stimuli, including caffeine and food.

Contraindications

Hypersensitivity to nizatidine or other H_2-receptor antagonists

Interactions

DRUGS

antacids: Decreased nizatidine bioavailability

itraconazole, ketoconazole: Decreased absorption of these drugs

salicylates: Increased blood level of these drugs

sucralfate: Possibly decreased nizatidine absorption

Adverse Reactions

CNS: Agitation, anxiety, confusion, depression, dizziness, fatigue, fever, hallucinations, headache, insomnia, somnolence

CV: **Arrhythmias**, chest pain, vasculitis

EENT: Amblyopia, dry mouth, **laryngeal edema**, pharyngitis, rhinitis, sinusitis

ENDO: Gynecomastia

GI: Abdominal pain, constipation, diarrhea, **hepatitis**, jaundice, nausea, vomiting

GU: Decreased libido, hyperuricemia not associated with gout or nephrolithiasis, impotence

HEME: Anemia, **aplastic anemia**, eosinophilia, **hemolytic anemia**, **leukopenia**, **neutropenia**, **thrombocytopenia**

MS: Back pain, myalgia

RESP: **Bronchospasm**, cough

SKIN: Alopecia, diaphoresis, **erythema multiforme**, **exfoliative dermatitis**, pruritus, rash, **Stevens–Johnson syndrome**, **toxic epidermal necrolysis**, urticaria

Other: **Anaphylaxis**, **angioedema**, serum sickness-like reaction

Nursing Considerations

- Monitor BUN, CBC, and serum creatinine levels, and liver enzymes, as ordered, before and periodically during nizatidine therapy.
- Don't give within 1 hour of an antacid.

PATIENT TEACHING

- Instruct patient not to take nizatidine within 1 hour of an antacid.
- Urge patient to take nizatidine exactly as prescribed, even if she feels better before prescription is finished. Inform her that ulcer may take up to 8 weeks to heal.
- Urge smoking patient to stop because smoking increases gastric acid production.
- Teach patient to minimize constipation by drinking plenty of fluids (if allowed), eating high-fiber foods, and exercising regularly.
- Instruct patient to notify prescriber immediately about abdominal pain, bloody vomitus, bloody or tarry stools, easy bruising, extreme fatigue, yellow skin or sclera, or trouble swallowing food.
- Urge patient not to take nizatidine with other acid reducers.

norepinephrine bitartrate (levarterenol bitartrate)

Levophed

Class and Category

Pharmacologic class: Sympathomimetic
Therapeutic class: Vasopressor
Pregnancy category: C

Indications and Dosages

➤ *To manage blood pressure in acute hypotensive states such as blood transfusion, drug adverse effect, myocardial infarction, pheochromocytomectomy, poliomyelitis, spinal anesthesia, and sympathectomy reactions; adjunct in treatment of cardiac arrest and profound hypotension*

I.V. INFUSION

Adults. *Initial:* 8 to 12 mcg/min of base. Then titrated to maintain systolic blood pressure between 80 to 100 mm Hg in patients previously not hypertensive and 40 mm Hg below preexisting systolic blood pressure in patients previously hypertensive. *Maintenance:* 2 to 4 mcg/min.

Route	Onset	Peak	Duration
I.V.	Rapid	Unknown	1–2 min

Mechanism of Action

At more than 4 mcg/min, inhibits adenyl cyclase and directly stimulates alpha-adrenergic receptors, which inhibits cAMP production. Inhibition of cAMP constricts arteries and veins and increases peripheral vascular resistance and systolic blood pressure.

Contraindications

Concurrent use of hydrocarbon inhalation anesthetics, hypersensitivity to norepinephrine or its components, hypovolemia, mesenteric or peripheral vascular thrombosis

Interactions

DRUGS

alpha blockers: Decreased vasopressor effects of norepinephrine
beta blockers: Decreased cardiac-stimulating effect of norepinephrine, possibly decreased therapeutic effects of both drugs
digoxin: Increased risk of arrhythmias, possibly potentiated inotropic effect
doxapram: Possibly increased vasopressor effects of both drugs
ergonovine, ergotamine, methylergonovine, methysergide, oxytocin: Possibly increased vasoconstriction
general anesthetics: Risk of arrhythmias
guanadrel, guanethidine: Increased vasopressor response to norepinephrine, possibly severe hypertension
MAO inhibitors: Possibly life-threatening arrhythmias, hyperpyrexia, severe headache, severe hypertension, and vomiting
maprotiline, tricyclic antidepressants: Possibly potentiated cardiovascular and pressor effects of norepinephrine, including arrhythmias, hyperpyrexia, and severe hypertension
methylphenidate: Possibly potentiated vasopressor effect of norepinephrine
nitrates: Possibly decreased therapeutic effects of both drugs
phenoxybenzamine: Possibly arrhythmias or hypotension
sympathomimetics: Increased risk of adverse cardiovascular effects
thyroid hormones: Increased risk of coronary insufficiency

Adverse Reactions

CNS: Anxiety, dizziness, headache, insomnia, nervousness, tremor, weakness
CV: Angina, **bradycardia**, **ECG changes**, edema, hypertension, **hypotension**, palpitations, peripheral vascular insufficiency (including gangrene), **PVCs**, sinus tachycardia
GI: Nausea, vomiting
GU: Decreased renal perfusion
RESP: Apnea, dyspnea
SKIN: Pallor
Other: Infusion-site sloughing and tissue necrosis, **metabolic acidosis**

Nursing Considerations

- Dilute norepinephrine concentrate for infusion by adding a 4 ml ampule (contains 4 mg) of drug to 1,000 ml of a 5% dextrose-containing solution. Each ml of this dilution contains 4 mcg of the base of the drug.
- Make sure solution contains no particles and isn't discolored before administering.
- Give drug with a flow-control device.
- Check blood pressure every 2 to 3 minutes, preferably by direct intra-arterial monitoring, until stabilized and then every 5 minutes.

WARNING Because extravasation can cause severe tissue damage and necrosis, expect prescriber to give multiple subcutaneous injections of phentolamine

(5 to 10 mg diluted in 10 to 15 ml normal saline solution) around extravasated infusion site.
- If blanching occurs along vein, change infusion site and notify prescriber at once.
- Monitor continuous ECG during therapy.

PATIENT TEACHING
- Urge patient to immediately report burning, leaking, or tingling around I.V. site.

nortriptyline hydrochloride

Aventyl (CAN), Pamelor

Class and Category

Pharmacologic class: Tricyclic antidepressant (TCA)
Therapeutic class: Antidepressant
Pregnancy category: D

Indications and Dosages

➤ *To treat depression*

CAPSULES, ORAL SOLUTION

Adults. *Initial:* 25 mg three times a day or four times a day. Alternatively, total daily dose once daily. *Maximum:* 150 mg daily.
Adolescents. 30 to 50 mg daily in divided doses. Alternatively, total daily dose once daily.

DOSAGE ADJUSTMENT Dosage reduced to 30 to 50 mg daily (in divided doses or total dose at bedtime) for elderly patients.

Route	Onset	Peak	Duration
P.O.	2–3 wk	Unknown	Unknown

Mechanism of Action

May interfere with reuptake of serotonin (and possibly other neurotransmitters) at presynaptic neurons, thus enhancing serotonin's effects at postsynaptic receptors. By restoring normal neurotransmitter levels at nerve synapses, this tricyclic antidepressant may elevate mood.

Contraindications

Acute recovery phase of MI or stroke; hypersensitivity to nortriptyline, other tricyclic antidepressants, or their components; use within 14 days of MAO inhibitor therapy including intravenous methylene blue or linezolid

Interactions

DRUGS

amantadine, anticholinergics, antidyskinetics, antihistamines: Possibly increased anticholinergic effects, confusion, hallucinations, nightmares; increased CNS depression
anticonvulsants: Possibly increased CNS depression and risk of seizures, possibly decreased anticonvulsant effectiveness
antithyroid drugs: Possibly agranulocytosis
barbiturates, carbamazepine: Possibly decreased level and effects of nortriptyline
bupropion, clozapine, cyclobenzaprine, haloperidol, loxapine, maprotiline, molindone, phenothiazines, thioxanthenes: Possibly increased anticholinergic and sedative effects, possibly increased risk of seizures
cimetidine, fluoxetine: Possibly increased blood nortriptyline level and risk of toxicity
clonidine: Possibly decreased antihypertensive effect and increased CNS depression
disulfiram: Possibly delirium
ethchlorvynol: Possibly delirium, increased CNS depression
guanadrel, guanethidine: Possibly decreased antihypertensive effect of these drugs
MAO inhibitors: Increased risk of hypertensive crisis, severe seizures, and death
oral anticoagulants: Possibly increased anticoagulant activity
pimozide, probucol: Possibly arrhythmias
sympathomimetics, including ophthalmic epinephrine and vasoconstrictive local anesthetics: Increased risk of arrhythmias, hyperpyrexia, hypertension, tachycardia
thyroid hormones: Possibly increased therapeutic and toxic effects of both drugs

ACTIVITIES

alcohol use: Increased alcohol effects, CNS and respiratory depression, hypertension

Adverse Reactions

CNS: Ataxia, confusion, **CVA**, delirium, dizziness, drowsiness, excitation, hallucinations, headache, insomnia, nervousness, nightmares, Parkinsonism, **serotonin syndrome**, **suicidal ideation**, tremor
CV: Arrhythmias, orthostatic hypotension

EENT: Angle-closure glaucoma, blurred vision, dry mouth, increased intraocular pressure, taste perversion
GI: Constipation, diarrhea, heartburn, ileus, increased appetite, nausea, vomiting
GU: Sexual dysfunction, urine retention
HEME: Bone marrow depression
RESP: Wheezing
SKIN: Diaphoresis, urticaria
Other: Weight gain

Nursing Considerations

- Expect to stop MAO inhibitor therapy, including intravenous methylene blue and linezolid, 10 to 14 days before starting nortriptyline.
- Watch patient closely (especially adolescents and young adults), for suicidal tendencies, particularly when therapy starts and dosage changes because depression may worsen temporarily during these times, possibly leading to suicidal ideation.
- Be aware that oral solution (10 mg/5 ml) is 4% alcohol.

WARNING Monitor patient for possible serotonin syndrome, characterized by agitation, chills, confusion, diaphoresis, diarrhea, fever, hyperactive reflexes, poor coordination, restlessness, shaking, talking or acting with uncontrolled excitement, tremor, and twitching. Notify prescriber immediately if serotonin syndrome is suspected because it can become life-threatening and expect to discontinue nortriptyline therapy.

- Give nortriptyline with food to reduce GI reactions.
- Monitor blood nortriptyline level; therapeutic range is 50 to 150 ng/ml.
- Monitor ECG tracing to detect arrhythmias.

PATIENT TEACHING

- Explain that oral solution contains alcohol.
- Discourage alcohol consumption during therapy.
- Explain that improvement may take weeks.
- Advise patient that drug may cause mild pupillary dilation, which may lead to an episode of acute closure glaucoma. Encourage patient to have an eye exam before starting therapy to see if he is at risk.
- Advise patient to avoid hazardous activities until drug's CNS effects are known.
- Urge family or caregiver to watch patient closely for suicidal tendencies, especially when therapy starts or dosage changes and particularly if patient is a teenager or young adult.
- Instruct patient to change position slowly to minimize orthostatic hypotension.
- Suggest that patient minimize constipation by drinking plenty of fluids (if allowed), exercising regularly, and eating high-fiber foods.

nystatin

Nystop, Pedi-Dri

Class and Category

Pharmacologic class: Polyene macrolide
Therapeutic class: Antifungal
Pregnancy category: Not classified

Indications and Dosages

➤ *To treat oropharyngeal candidiasis (thrush)*

LOZENGES (PASTILLES)

Adults and children over age 5. 200,000 to 400,000 units (1 or 2 lozenges) dissolved in mouth three to five times daily for up to 14 days.

ORAL SUSPENSION

Adults and children. 400,000 to 600,000 units (4 to 6 ml) swished and swallowed four times a day until at least 48 hr after symptoms subside.
Infants. 100,000 units (1 ml) applied to each side of mouth four times a day until at least 48 hr after symptoms subside.

TABLETS

Adults and adolescents. 500,000 to 1,000,000 units (1 to 2 tablets) three times a day until at least 48 hr after symptoms subside.
Children age 5 and over. 500,000 units (1 tablet) four times a day until at least 48 hr after symptoms subside.

➤ *To treat cutaneous and mucocutaneous candidiasis*

CREAM, OINTMENT, POWDER

Adults and children. 100,000 units (1 g) on affected area twice daily or three times a day for at least 2 wk.

Mechanism of Action
Binds to sterols in fungal cell membranes, impairing membrane integrity. Cells lose intracellular potassium and other cellular contents and, eventually, die.

Contraindications
Hypersensitivity to nystatin or its components

Adverse Reactions
ENDO: Hyperglycemia (lozenge, oral suspension)
GI: Abdominal pain, diarrhea, nausea, vomiting (oral forms)
SKIN: Irritation (topical forms)

Nursing Considerations
- Prepare nystatin powder for oral suspension for each dose; it has no preservatives.
- Gently rub nystatin cream or ointment into skin at affected area. Keep area dry and avoid occlusive dressings.
- Don't get topical form in patient's eyes.
- Dust patient's shoes, socks, and feet when treating candidal infection of feet.

PATIENT TEACHING
- Instruct patient to let nystatin lozenges dissolve slowly in her mouth, not to chew or swallow them.
- Tell patient to swish oral suspension in her mouth as long as possible before swallowing.
- Advise patient to gently rub ointment or cream into skin at affected area, to keep area dry, and to avoid occlusive dressings.
- Caution patient to keep topical away from her eyes.
- Advise patient with candidal infection of feet to dust her shoes, socks, and feet with nystatin.

obiltoxaximab
Anthim

Class and Category
Pharmacologic class: Monoclonal antibody
Therapeutic class: Antianthrax agent
Pregnancy category: B

Indications and Dosages
➤ *To prevent inhalational anthrax due to* Bacillus anthracis *when alternative therapies are not appropriate or available; to treat inhalational anthrax due to* B. anthracis *in combination with appropriate antibacterial drugs*

I.V. INFUSION
Adults and children weighing more than 40 kg (88 lb). 16 mg/kg over 90 min as a single dose.
Adults and children weighing more than 15 kg (33 lb) to 40 kg (88 lb): 24 mg/kg over 90 min as a single dose.
Children weighing 15 kg (33 lb) or less. 32 mg/kg over 90 min as a single dose.

Mechanism of Action
Binds to the PA component of the *B. anthracis* toxin to inactivate it.

Contraindications
Hypersensitivity to obiltoxaximab or its components

Interactions
DRUGS
None reported

Adverse Reactions
CNS: Dizziness, dysphonia, fatigue, fever, headache
CV: Chest discomfort or pain, palpitations
EENT: Dry mouth, nasal congestion, oropharyngeal pain, rhinorrhea, sinus congestion
GI: Vomiting
HEME: leukopenia, **lymphopenia**, **neutropenia**
MS: Extremity pain, myalgia, musculoskeletal pain
RESP: Cough, **cyanosis**, dyspnea, upper respiratory infections
SKIN: Pruritus, urticaria
Other: Anaphylaxis; antibody formation against obiltoxaximab; increased creatine phosphokinase; infusion-site reactions of bruising, discoloration, pain, swelling, or urticaria

Nursing Considerations
- Know that obiltoxaximab should only be used for prophylaxis when its benefit for

prevention of inhalational anthrax outweighs the risk of anaphylaxis and other hypersensitivity reactions.

- Be aware that because obiltoxaximab does not have antibacterial activity, it must be used in combination with appropriate antibacterial drugs.
- Expect to premedicate patient with diphenhydramine because drug can cause serious hypersensitivity reactions including anaphylaxis.
- Do not shake drug vial. Know that there are two ways to prepare and dilute the drug for infusion. To prepare and dilute drug in infusion bag, first calculate the required dosage and volume according to manufacturer guidelines. Know that each single vial allows delivery of 6 ml of obiltoxaximab. Select an appropriate size bag of 0.9% sodium chloride injection, USP. Withdraw a volume of solution from the bag equal to the calculated volume in milliliters of the drug to be administered and discard. Then withdraw the required volume of the drug from the drug vial(s) and discard any unused portion remaining in the vial(s). Transfer the required volume of the drug into the selected infusion bag. Gently invert the bag to mix the solution. Do not shake. Know that the prepared solution is stable for 8 hours stored in the refrigerator or at room temperature. To prepare and dilute the drug using the syringe for infusion method, first calculate the required dosage and volume of the drug according to manufacturer guidelines. Select an appropriate size syringe for the total volume of infusion to be administered. Using the selected syringe, withdraw the required volume of drug. Discard any unused portion remaining in the vial(s). Withdraw an appropriate amount of 0.9% sodium chloride injection, USP, using the syringe containing the drug to prepare the total infusion volume specified in manufacturer guidelines. Gently mix the solution. Do not shake. Once diluted in the syringe, administer immediately. Do not store solution in syringe.
- Administer drug intravenously as an infusion using either of the stated methods of dilution. Use a 0.22-micron inline filter and infuse at the rate specified in the manufacturer guidelines in order for the drug to be administered over 90 minutes. Flush the intravenous line with 0.9% sodium chloride injection, USP, at the end of the intravenous infusion.

WARNING Be aware that because of the risk for serious hypersensitivity reactions, including anaphylaxis, the drug should be administered in an environment conducive to treating anaphylaxis. Monitor patient closely for signs and symptoms of hypersensitivity that may progress rapidly to anaphylaxis. Know that hypersensitivity reactions were the most common adverse reactions that occurred in the safety trials for obiltoxaximab. Observe the patient throughout the infusion and for a period of time after administration. Stop infusion immediately if hypersensitivity or anaphylaxis occurs, notify prescribe and provide supportive care, as ordered.

PATIENT TEACHING

- Inform patient of the possibility of an allergic reaction that could become severe with obiltoxaximab administration. Reassure him that he will be given a drug to help prevent this before obiltoxaximab is given. Review the signs and symptoms of an allergic reaction with the patient and stress importance of alerting the healthcare staff administering the drug if any should occur. Tell him that if he experiences any reactions after going home, he should seek immediate medical attention.
- Tell patient that he will only need to receive the drug one time.

ocrelizumab

Ocrevus

Class and Category

Pharmacologic class: Monoclonal antibody
Therapeutic class: Antimultiple sclerotic
Pregnancy category: Not classified

Indications and Dosages

➤ *To treat primary progressive or relapsing forms of multiple sclerosis*

I.V. INFUSION

Adults. *Initial:* 300 mg, followed 2 wk later by a second 300-mg infusion. Initial dose infused starting at 30 ml per hour, then increased by 30 ml per hour every 30 min to maximum infusion rate of 180 ml per hour with an infusion duration of 2.5 hours or longer. *Maintenance:* Single infusion of 600 mg every 6 months. Maintenance dose infused starting at 40 ml per hour, increased by 40 ml per hour every 30 min with maximum infusion of 200 ml per hour and duration of infusion 3.5 hours or longer.

Route	Onset	Peak	Duration
I.V.	Unknown	14 days	Unknown

Mechanism of Action

Although precise mechanism is unknown, ocrelizumab binds to CD20, a cell surface antigen on pre-B and mature B lymphocytes, which results in antibody-dependent cellular cytolysis and complement-mediated lysis to help relieve symptoms of multiple sclerosis.

Incompatibilities

Don't dilute ocrelizumab in any solution other than 0.9% sodium chloride injection, and use a dedicated line to infuse ocrelizumab because potential reactions are unknown if other drugs are infused through the same line.

Contraindications

Active hepatitis B virus infection, hypersensitivity to ocrelizumab or its components

Interactions

DRUGS

other immune-modulating or immunosuppressants: Increased risk of immunosuppression

Adverse Reactions

CNS: Depression, dizziness, fatigue, fever, headache
CV: Hypotension, peripheral edema, tachycardia
EENT: Laryngeal or pharyngeal edema, oropharyngeal pain, throat irritation
GI: Diarrhea, nausea
HEME: Neutropenia
MS: Back or extremity pain
RESP: Bronchospasms, cough, dyspnea, respiratory infections
SKIN: Erythema, flushing, pruritus, rash, skin infections, urticaria
Other: Antiocrelizumab antibody formation, decreased immunoglobulins, herpes virus-associated infections, infusion reactions

Nursing Considerations

- Expect to perform hepatitis B virus (HBV) screening, as ordered, prior to initiating ocrelizumab therapy because drug is contraindicated in patients with active HBV that has been confirmed by positive test results.
- Administer all necessary immunizations, as ordered, according to guidelines at least 6 weeks prior to initiation of ocrelizumab therapy because vaccination with live-attenuated or live vaccines is not recommended during treatment and after discontinuation of drug until B-cell repletion.
- Assess patient for evidence of an active infection prior to every infusion of ocrelizumab. If present, know that the infusion must be delayed until the infection is resolved.
- Expect to premedicate the patient with 100 mg of methylprednisolone (or an equivalent corticosteroid) intravenously about 30 minutes before each ocrelizumab infusion to reduce the frequency and severity of infusion reactions. Also expect to premedicate the patient with an antihistamine such as diphenhydramine about 30 to 60 minutes prior to each ocrelizumab infusion to further reduce infusion reactions. Know that the administration of an antipyretic such as acetaminophen may also be ordered.
- Do not shake drug vial. Withdraw prescribed dose and further dilute into an infusion bag containing 0.9% sodium chloride injection to a final drug concentration of approximately 1.2 mg/ml. For example, withdraw 10 mg (300 mg) from vial and inject into a 250-ml infusion bag containing 0.9% sodium chloride injection solution or withdraw 20 ml (600 mg) from vial and inject into a 500-ml infusion bag containing 0.9% sodium chloride injection solution. Do not use any other diluents to dilute ocrelizumab.
- Know that prepared infusion solution should be at room temperature prior to starting the intravenous infusion.

Administer the prepared infusion immediately. However, know that the prepared solution can be stored for up to 24 hours in the refrigerator or 8 hours at room temperature, which includes the infusion time.
- Administer the diluted ocrelizumab solution through a dedicated line using an infusion set with a 0.2 or 0.22 micron in-line filter.
- Monitor patient for infusion reactions for at least 1 hour after completion of the infusion.
- Expect to administer a planned infusion that is missed as soon as possible. Know that it should not be withheld until the next scheduled dose. Reset the dose schedule to administer the next sequential dose 6 months after the missed dose is administered, because doses must be separated by at least 5 months.

WARNING Monitor patient for life-threatening infusion reactions. If present, stop infusion immediately, provide supportive care, as ordered, and know that drug will be permanently discontinued. If infusion reaction is not life-threatening but severe, expect to immediately interrupt the infusion and provide supportive treatment, as ordered and needed. Expect to restart the infusion only after all symptoms have resolved. When restarting, expect to restart at half the infusion rate at the time of onset of the infusion reaction. If this rate is tolerated, increase the rate per the standard protocol. If patient is experiencing a mild to moderate infusion reaction, expect to reduce the infusion rate to half the rate at the onset of the infusion reaction and maintain the reduced rate for at least 30 minutes. If this rate is tolerated, expect to increase the rate per the standard protocol.

WARNING Know that progressive multifocal leukoencephalopathy (PML) has occurred in patients treated with other anti-CD20 antibodies and other multiple sclerosis therapies. Patients at risk included patients who were immunocompromised or received polytherapy with immunosuppressants. Monitor patient for PML, which may include changes in memory, orientation, or thinking that could lead to confusion and personality changes. Other symptoms include clumsiness of limbs, disturbance of vision, and progressive weakness on one side of the body. If present, notify prescriber immediately, because PML usually leads to death or severe disability.

PATIENT TEACHING
- Explain the importance of as well as the risks associated with ocrelizumab therapy.
- Tell patient she will receive medication before the infusion to lessen or prevent infusion reactions. However, inform patient that infusion reactions may occur up to 24 hours after the infusion and include allergic types of signs and symptoms. If adverse reactions occur in this time frame, patient should notify prescriber and if reactions are severe, seek immediate emergency medical care.
- Instruct patient to report changes in memory, orientation, or thinking that could lead to confusion and personality changes. Other symptoms to report include clumsiness of limbs, disturbance of vision, and progressive weakness on one side of the body. If present, urge patient to notify prescriber immediately.
- Inform patient that ocrelizumab may increase risk of breast cancer. Stress importance of following standard breast cancer screening guidelines.

octreotide acetate

Sandostatin, Sandostatin LAR Depot

Class and Category

Pharmacologic class: Octapeptide
Therapeutic class: Somatotropic hormone
Pregnancy category: B

Indications and Dosages

➤ *To control symptoms associated with vasoactive intestinal peptide tumors (watery diarrhea) and metastatic carcinoid tumors (diarrhea and flushing)*

I.M. INJECTION (SANDOSTATIN LAR DEPOT)
Adults currently receiving Sandostatin. 20 mg every 4 wk for 2 mo, with subcutaneous doses continued for 2 to 4 wk after I.M. injections start. If

patient has positive response to initial 2-mo regimen, dosage reduced to 10 mg every 4 wk. If symptoms persist or increase after initial 2-mo regimen, dosage increased to 30 mg every 4 wk, as prescribed.

I.V. INFUSION, I.V. OR SUBCUTANEOUS INJECTION (SANDOSTATIN)

Adults with vasoactive intestinal peptide tumors. *Initial:* 200 to 300 mcg daily in divided doses twice daily to four times a day, for first 2 wk. *Maintenance:* Individualized. *Maximum:* 450 mcg daily. I.V. infusion given over 15 to 30 min and I.V. injection given over 3 min.

Adults with carcinoid tumors. *Initial*: 100 to 600 mcg daily in divided doses twice daily to four times a day, for first 2 wk. *Maintenance*: Individualized. I.V. infusion given over 15 to 30 min and I.V. injection given over 3 min.

➤ *To treat symptoms of acromegaly, to suppress the release of growth hormone from pituitary tumors*

I.V. INFUSION, I.V. OR SUBCUTANEOUS INJECTION (SANDOSTATIN)

Adults. *Initial:* 50 mcg three times a day. *Usual*: 100 mcg three times a day. *Maximum:* 1,500 mcg daily. I.V. infusion given over 15 to 30 min and I.V. injection given over 3 min.

I.M. INJECTION (SANDOSTATIN LAR DEPOT)

Adults currently receiving Sandostatin. 20 mg every 4 wk for 3 mo; then adjusted as prescribed in response to serum growth hormone level. *Maximum:* 40 mg every 4 wk.

DOSAGE ADJUSTMENT For patients with hepatic impairment or renal failure requiring dialysis, starting dose of Sandostatin LAR Depot decreased to 10 mg every 4 weeks.

Route	Onset	Peak	Duration
SubQ	Unknown	Unknown	Up to 12 hr

Mechanism of Action

Controls many types of secretory diarrhea by inhibiting secretion of GI, pituitary, and serotonin hormones (including insulin, glucagon, growth hormone, thyrotropin, and, possibly, thyroid-stimulating hormone) as well as pancreatic polypeptides and vasoactive intestinal peptides (including gastrin, motilin, and secretin). Inhibiting peptides and serotonin increases intestinal absorption of electrolytes and water, decreases gastric acid and pancreatic secretions, and increases intestinal transit time by slowing gastric motility.

By inhibiting hormones involved in vasodilation, octreotide increases splanchnic arterial resistance and decreases GI and hepatic blood flow, hepatic vein wedge pressure, intravariceal pressure, and portal vein pressure, thus raising seated and standing blood pressures. By inhibiting serotonin secretion, octreotide eases symptoms of acromegaly, including diarrhea, flushing, urinary excretion of 5-hydroxyindoleacetic acid, and wheezing.

Incompatibilities

Don't mix octreotide in same syringe with fat emulsions or total parenteral nutrition solutions.

Contraindications

Hypersensitivity to octreotide or its components

Interactions

DRUGS

beta blockers, calcium channel blockers: Additive cardiovascular effects of these drugs
bromocriptine: Increased blood bromocriptine level
cisapride: Decreased effectiveness of both drugs
cyclosporine: Decreased cyclosporine level
diuretics: Increased risk of fluid and electrolyte imbalances
insulin, oral antidiabetic drugs: Increased risk of hypoglycemia
quinidine, terfenadine: Decreased clearance and increased blood levels of these drugs
vitamin B_{12}: Decreased vitamin B_{12} level

Adverse Reactions

CNS: Dizziness, drowsiness, fatigue, headache, **intracranial hemorrhage**, migraine, paranoia, **seizures**, **suicidal ideation**
CV: Arrhythmias (including conduction abnormalities), edema, hypertension, **hypotension**, **MI**, orthostatic hypotension, Raynaud's syndrome

EENT: Deafness, epistaxis, glaucoma, retinal vein thrombosis, sinusitis, vision changes
ENDO: Hyperglycemia, **hypoglycemia**, hypothyroidism, **pituitary apoplexy**
GI: Abdominal pain, acute cholecystitis, ascending cholangitis, biliary obstruction, cholelithiasis, **cholestatic hepatitis**, constipation, diarrhea, elevated liver enzymes, flatulence, gastric or peptic ulcer, **GI hemorrhage**, **intestinal obstruction**, nausea, **pancreatitis**, vomiting
GU: Decreased libido, hematuria, increased urine output, **renal failure**
HEME: Anemia, **pancytopenia**, **thrombocytopenia**
MS: Arthropathy, back pain, myalgia
RESP: Status asthmaticus, **pulmonary hypertension**, upper respiratory tract infection
SKIN: Alopecia, petechiae, pruritus, rash, urticaria
Other: Anaphylaxis, **angioedema**, dehydration, **electrolyte imbalances**, flu-like symptoms, injection-site irritation or pain

Nursing Considerations

- Prepare depot injection (long-acting suspension form) by letting powder and diluent warm to room temperature and then reconstitute according to manufacturer's instructions. Gently inject 2 ml of supplied diluent down side of vial without disturbing depot powder. Let diluent saturate powder. After 2 to 5 minutes, check sides and bottom of vial without inverting it. Once powder is completely saturated, swirl—don't shake—vial for 30 to 60 seconds to form suspension. Use immediately after reconstituting.
- Don't give depot injection by subcutaneous route; give only by I.M. route and only to patients who respond to and tolerate subcutaneous drug, as prescribed.
- For I.V. administration, dilute in 50 to 200 ml using 5% Dextrose in Water or 0.9% Normal Saline Solution and infuse over 15 to 30 minutes, or give by I.V. push over 3 min.
- Use smallest injection volume to deliver dose, and rotate injection sites to minimize pain.
- Avoid deltoid site for I.M. use because injection-site reaction and pain may result. Intragluteal injection is recommended.
- Be aware that octreotide increases risk of acute cholecystitis, ascending cholangitis, biliary obstruction, cholestatic hepatitis, and pancreatitis.
- Monitor bowel sounds, stool consistency, and vital signs. Assess for abdominal pain and signs of gallbladder disease.
- Monitor serum liver enzyme levels, as ordered.
- Monitor patient for signs of dehydration and electrolyte imbalances.
- Carefully monitor diabetic patient for altered glucose control.
- Monitor patient's thyroid function, as ordered, because octreotide suppresses secretion of thyroid-stimulating hormone, which may cause hypothyroidism.
- Be aware that if patient has periodic symptom flare-ups, expect to give additional subcutaneous octreotide temporarily, as prescribed.

PATIENT TEACHING

- Emphasis importance of complying with scheduled return visits in order to minimize exacerbation of symptoms.
- Advise patient to change position slowly to minimize orthostatic hypotension.
- Instruct patient to notify prescriber about adverse reactions, especially abdominal pain, which may indicate pancreatitis.
- Urge diabetic patient to check blood glucose level often.
- Caution female patient of childbearing age that drug may restore fertility and, if pregnancy isn't desired, that contraception should be used during octreotide therapy.

ofloxacin

Class and Category

Pharmacologic class: Fluoroquinolone
Therapeutic class: Antibiotic
Pregnancy category: C

Indications and Dosages

➤ *To treat acute, uncomplicated cystitis caused by* Escherichia coli *or* Klebsiella pneumoniae

TABLETS

Adults. 200 mg every 12 hr for 3 days.

➤ *To treat uncomplicated cystitis caused by* Citrobacter diversus, Enterobacter aerogenes, Proteus mirabilis, *or* Pseudomonas aeruginosa

TABLETS

Adults. 200 mg every 12 hr for 7 days.

➤ *To treat complicated UTI caused by* C. diversus, E. coli, K. pneumoniae, P. mirabilis, *or* P. aeruginosa

Adults. 200 mg every 12 hr for 10 days.

➤ *To treat uncomplicated gonorrhea*

TABLETS

Adults and adolescents. 400 mg as single dose.

➤ *To treat urethritis or cervicitis caused by* Chlamydia trachomatis *or* Neisseria gonorrhoeae

TABLETS

Adults and adolescents. 300 mg twice daily for 7 days as an alternative to doxycycline or azithromycin.

➤ *To treat pelvic inflammatory disease caused by susceptible organisms*

TABLETS

Adults and adolescents. 400 mg twice daily with metronidazole P.O. for 10 to 14 days.

➤ *To treat prostatitis caused by* E. coli

TABLETS

Adults. 300 mg every 12 hr for 6 wk.

➤ *To treat lower respiratory tract infections caused by* Haemophilus influenzae *or* Streptococcus pneumoniae *and skin and soft-tissue infections caused by* Staphylococcus aureus *or* Streptococcus pyogenes

TABLETS

Adults. 400 mg every 12 hr for 10 days.

DOSAGE ADJUSTMENT If creatinine clearance is 20 to 50 ml/min, dosing interval possibly reduced to every 24 hr; if clearance is less than 10 ml/min, dosage possibly reduced by 50% and given every 24 hr. For patients with severe liver dysfunction, maximum dose limited to 400 mg daily.

Mechanism of Action

Inhibits synthesis of the bacterial enzyme DNA gyrase by counteracting excessive supercoiling of DNA during replication or transcription. Inhibition of DNA gyrase causes rapid- and slow-growing bacterial cells to die.

Contraindications

Hypersensitivity to ofloxacin, other fluoroquinolones, or their components; myasthenia gravis

Interactions

DRUGS

aluminum-, calcium-, or magnesium-containing antacids; didanosine; ferrous sulfate; magnesium-containing laxatives; multivitamins; sevelamer; sucralfate; zinc: Decreased absorption of ofloxacin

probenecid: Decreased ofloxacin excretion, increased risk of toxicity

procainamide: Decreased renal clearance of procainamide

warfarin: Possibly increased anticoagulant activity and risk of bleeding

Adverse Reactions

CNS: Aggressiveness, agitation, ataxia, **CVA**, delirium, disorientation, disturbance in attention, dizziness, drowsiness, emotional lability, exacerbation of extrapyramidal disorders and myasthenia gravis, fever, headache, incoordination, insomnia, light-headedness, mania, memory impairment, nervousness, peripheral neuropathy, psychotic reactions, restlessness, **suicidal ideation**, syncope

CV: Arrhythmias, **prolonged QT interval**, **severe hypotension**, **torsades de pointes**, vasculitis

EENT: Blurred vision; diplopia; disturbances in equilibrium, hearing, smell, and taste

ENDO: Hyperglycemia, **hypoglycemia**

GI: Abdominal cramps or pain, **acute hepatic necrosis or failure**, diarrhea, **hepatitis**, jaundice, nausea, **pseudomembranous colitis**, vomiting

GU: Acute renal insufficiency or failure, interstitial nephritis, renal calculi, vaginal candidiasis

HEME: **Agranulocytosis, aplastic or hemolytic anemia, leukopenia, pancytopenia, thrombocytopenia**
MS: Arthralgia; myalgia; **rhabdomyolysis**; tendinitis; tendon inflammation, pain, or rupture
RESP: **Hypersensitivity pneumonitis, pulmonary edema**
SKIN: Blisters, diaphoresis, erythema, **erythema multiforme, exfoliative dermatitis**, photosensitivity, pruritus, rash, **Stevens–Johnson syndrome, toxic epidermal necrolysis**, urticaria
Other: **Acidosis, anaphylaxis**, infusion-site phlebitis, serum sickness

Nursing Considerations

- Know that because of increased risk of prolonged QT interval, ofloxacin shouldn't be used if patient has had a prolonged QT interval, has an uncorrected electrolyte disorder, or takes a Class IA or III antiarrhythmic. Monitor elderly patients closely because risk of prolonged QT interval may be increased in this group.
- Monitor patient closely for hypersensitivity, which may occur as early as first dose. Reaction may include angioedema, bronchospasm, dyspnea, itching, jaundice, rash, shortness of breath, and urticaria. If these signs or symptoms appear, notify prescriber immediately and expect to discontinue drug.
- Know that fluoroquinolones like ofloxacin have caused disabling and potentially irreversible serious adverse reactions from different body systems that can occur together in the same patient. These reactions can occur within hours to weeks after starting the drug and usually cause central nervous system effects, peripheral neuropathy, tendinitis and tendon rupture. All ages of patients and patients without any preexisting risk factors have experienced these reactions. Notify prescriber and expect to discontinue ofloxacin immediately at the first signs or symptoms of any serious adverse reactions.
- Notify prescriber if patient has symptoms of peripheral neuropathy (burning, numbness, pain, tingling, weakness, or altered sensations of light touch, pain, position sense, temperature, or vibration sense), which could be permanent; tendon rupture (inflammation and pain), which may occur more often in patients (especially elderly ones) taking corticosteroids and requires immediate rest; or a severe photosensitivity reaction. In each case, expect to stop ofloxacin.
- Maintain adequate hydration to prevent development of highly concentrated urine and crystalluria.
- Expect an increased risk of toxicity in severe hepatic disease, including cirrhosis.
- Be aware that ofloxacin may stimulate the CNS and aggravate seizure disorders. Also know that the drug may cause many psychiatric adverse reactions. Monitor patient closely.
- If diarrhea develops, notify prescriber because it may indicate pseudomembranous colitis. Ofloxacin may have to be discontinued and additional therapy started.
- Be alert for secondary fungal infection.
- Monitor patient closely for hypoglycemia, especially if patient is elderly, has diabetes or renal insufficiency, or is taking hypoglycemic drugs such as sulfonylureas. Hypoglycemia can become severe and result in coma. Treat hypoglycemia quickly and effectively. Notify prescriber of incident and expect that drug may be replaced with a different antibiotic for this patient.

PATIENT TEACHING

- Encourage patient to take each dose with a full glass of water.
- Tell patient to complete full course of ofloxacin therapy exactly as prescribed, even if he feels better before it's complete.
- Urge patient not to take antacids, iron or zinc preparations, or other drugs (such as didanosine and sucralfate), within 2 hours of ofloxacin to prevent decreased or delayed drug absorption.
- Advise patient to avoid hazardous activities until CNS effects of drug are known.
- Tell patient to limit exposure to sun and ultraviolet light to prevent phototoxicity.

- Advise patient to notify prescriber immediately about abnormal motor or sensory function, burning skin, hives, itching, rapid heart rate, rash, and tendon pain. Also advise patient to stop taking ofloxacin immediately and notify prescriber if any other persistent, serious, or worsening adverse effects occur.
- Urge patient to seek medical care immediately for trouble breathing or swallowing, which may signal an allergic reaction.
- Instruct diabetic patient who takes an antidiabetic agent or insulin to notify prescriber immediately if he develops a hypoglycemic reaction.
- Advise patient to notify prescriber if diarrhea develops, even up to 2 months after ofloxacin therapy ends. Additional therapy may be needed.

olanzapine

Zydis, Zyprexa

olanzapine pamoate monohydrate

Zyprexa Relprevv

Class and Category

Pharmacologic class: Thienobenzodiazepine derivative
Therapeutic class: Antipsychotic
Pregnancy category: C

Indications and Dosages

➤ *To treat schizophrenia*

ORALLY DISINTEGRATING TABLETS, TABLETS

Adults. *Initial:* 5 to 10 mg daily. Once 10 mg daily dosage reached, additional dosage adjustment made in 5 mg increments every wk, as needed. *Maintenance:* 10 mg daily. *Maximum:* 20 mg daily.
Adolescents age 13 and over. *Initial:* 2.5 to 5 mg daily. *Maintenance*: 10 mg daily. *Maximum:* 20 mg daily.

I.M. INJECTION-ER (ZYPREXA RELPREVV)

Adults who have been taking 10 mg daily orally. *Initial:* 210 mg every 2 wk for first 8 wk, then decreased to 150 mg every 2 wk. Alternatively, 405 mg every 4 wk for first 8 wk, then decreased to 300 mg every 4 wk.
Adults who have been taking 15 mg daily orally. *Initial:* 300 mg every 2 wk for 8 wk, then decreased to 210 mg every 2 wk or 405 mg every 4 wk.
Adults who have been taking 20 mg daily orally. *Initial:* 300 mg every 2 wk.

➤ *To treat manic phase of bipolar I disorder (manic or mixed episodes)*

ORALLY DISINTEGRATING TABLETS, TABLETS

Adults. *Initial:* 10 to 15 mg daily decreased or increased in 5 mg increments every 24 hr, as needed. *Maintenance*: 5 to 20 mg daily. *Maximum:* 20 mg daily.
Adolescents age 13 and over. *Initial:* 2.5 to 5 mg daily, increased, as needed, in 2.5 or 5 mg increments weekly. *Maintenance:* 10 mg daily. *Maximum:* 20 mg daily.

➤ *As adjunct to treat bipolar I disorder*

ORALLY DISINTEGRATING TABLETS, TABLETS

Adults. *Initial:* 10 mg daily with lithium or valproate sodium, increased or decreased by 5 mg every 24 hr, as needed. *Maintenance*: 5 to 20 mg/day. *Maximum:* 20 mg daily.
DOSAGE ADJUSTMENT Initial dosage possibly reduced to 5 mg for debilitated patients, those prone to hypotension, and female nonsmokers over age 65.

➤ *To treat agitation associated with schizophrenia and bipolar I mania*

I.M. INJECTION

Adults. 5 to 10 mg, as needed. Repeat as needed every 2 to 4 hr. *Maximum:* Three doses of 10 mg administered 2 to 4 hr apart providing patient is not exhibiting orthostatic hypotension.
DOSAGE ADJUSTMENT Dosage decreased to 5 mg for elderly patients and 2.5 mg for debilitated patients, those prone to hypotension, and female nonsmokers over age 65.

Route	Onset	Peak	Duration
P.O., I.M.–E.R.	1 wk	Unknown	Unknown
I.M.	Unknown	Unknown	Unknown

Mechanism of Action

May achieve antipsychotic effects by antagonizing dopamine and serotonin

N O

receptors. Anticholinergic effects may result from competitive binding to and antagonism of the muscarinic receptors M_1 through M_5.

Contraindications

Blood dyscrasias, bone marrow depression, cerebral arteriosclerosis, coma, coronary artery disease, hepatic dysfunction, high-dose CNS depressants, hypersensitivity to olanzapine or its components, hypertension, hypotension, myeloproliferative disorders, severe CNS depression, subcortical brain damage

Interactions

DRUGS

anticholinergics: Increased anticholinergic effects, altered thermoregulation
antihypertensives: Increased effects of both drugs, increased risk of hypotension
benzodiazepines (parenteral): Increased risk of cardiorespiratory depression and excessive sedation
carbamazepine, omeprazole, rifampin: Increased olanzapine clearance
CNS depressants: Additive CNS depression, potentiated orthostatic hypotension
diazepam: Increased CNS depressant effects
fluvoxamine: Decreased olanzapine clearance
levodopa: Decreased levodopa efficacy
lorazepam (parenteral): Possibly increased somnolence with I.M. olanzapine injection

ACTIVITIES

alcohol use: Additive CNS depression, potentiated orthostatic hypotension
smoking: Decreased blood olanzapine level

Adverse Reactions

CNS: Abnormal gait, agitation, akathisia, altered thermoregulation, amnesia, anxiety, asthenia, dizziness, euphoria, fatigue, fever, headache, hypertonia, insomnia, motor and sensory instability, nervousness, **neuroleptic malignant syndrome**, restless leg syndrome, restlessness, somnolence, stuttering, **suicidal ideation**, syncope, tardive dyskinesia, thirst, tremor
CV: Bradycardia, chest pain, hyperlipidemia, hypertension, **hypotension**, orthostatic hypotension, peripheral edema, tachycardia, **venous thromboembolic events**
EENT: Amblyopia, dry mouth, increased salivation, pharyngitis, rhinitis
ENDO: Diabetic coma, **diabetic ketoacidosis**, hyperglycemia, **hyperprolactinemia**
GI: Abdominal pain, constipation, dysphagia, elevated liver enzymes, **hepatitis**, increased appetite, jaundice, liver injury, nausea, **pancreatitis**, vomiting
GU: Priapism, urinary incontinence, UTI
HEME: Agranulocytosis, **leukopenia**, **neutropenia**
MS: Arthralgia; back, joint, or limb pain; muscle spasms and twitching; **rhabdomyolysis**
RESP: Cough, **pulmonary embolism**
SKIN: Ecchymosis, photosensitivity, pruritus, rash, urticaria
Other: Anaphylaxis, **angioedema**, **drug reaction with eosinophilia and systemic symptoms (DRESS)**, flu-like symptoms, weight gain

Nursing Considerations

WARNING Olanzapine shouldn't be used for elderly patients with dementia-related psychosis because drug increases risk of death in these patients.

- Use cautiously in patients with hepatic impairment or conditions associated with limited hepatic functional reserve and in patients who are being treated with potentially hepatotoxic drugs. Also use cautiously in patients with known cardiovascular or cerebrovascular disease and conditions that would predispose patient to hypotension, such as presence of dehydration, hypovolemia, or treatment with antihypertensive medications because of the increased risk for bradycardia, hypotension, and syncope.

WARNING Keep in mind that there are two formulations for I.M. injection. One is an immediate release formulation and one is an extended release. They are not interchangeable. When administering drug intramuscularly, make sure the right formulation is being administered.

- Reconstitute parenteral immediate-release olanzapine by dissolving contents of vial in 2.1 ml sterile water to yield 5 mg/ml. Solution should be clear yellow. Use within 1 hour.

- Inject I.M. immediate-release olanzapine slowly, deep into muscle mass.
- Reconstitute parenteral extended-release olanzapine using only the diluent provided as follows: for 150 or 210 mg dose, use 1.3 ml of diluent; for 300 mg dose, use 1.8 ml of diluent; and for 405 mg dose, use 2.3 ml diluent. Withdraw predetermined diluent into syringe. Inject into powder vial and withdraw air to equalize pressure. Remove needle and hold vial upright. Pad a hard surface, then tap vial firmly and repeatedly on the surface until no powder is visible. Shake vial vigorously until suspension appears smooth and consistent in color and texture (yellow and opaque). If foam has formed, let vial stand until it has dissipated. Administer immediately or if stored for up to 24 hr, remember drug vial must be vigorously shaken to resuspend solution prior to administration. Attach new needle to syringe and slowly withdraw desired amount into the syringe. Remove needle from syringe.
- Administer parenteral extended-release olanzapine by first attaching a 19 gauge needle or larger to syringe to prevent clogging. Inject intramuscularly deeply into the gluteal muscle. Withdraw needle. Do not massage injection site.
- Keep patient recumbent after I.M. injection of olanzapine if drowsiness, dizziness, bradycardia, or hypoventilation occurs. Don't let patient sit or stand up until blood pressure and heart rate have returned to baseline.
- Be aware that following the injection of extended-release olanzapine, patient may experience a syndrome similar to an olanzapine overdose, with delirium and sedation being the primary symptoms. Know that patient must be observed for 3 hours following each injection for this syndrome. Notify prescriber immediately if it should occur.
- Monitor patient's blood pressure routinely during therapy because olanzapine may cause orthostatic hypotension.
- Be aware that olanzapine may worsen such conditions as angle-closure glaucoma, benign prostatic hyperplasia, and seizures. Monitor patient closely.
- Assess daily weight to detect fluid retention or metabolic changes.
- Notify prescriber if patient develops tardive dyskinesia or urinary incontinence.
- Be alert for and immediately report signs of neuroleptic malignant syndrome.
- Watch patient closely (especially adolescent and young adults), for suicidal tendencies, particularly when therapy starts and dosage changes, because depression may worsen temporarily during these times, possibly leading to suicidal ideation.
- Monitor patient's lipid levels throughout therapy, as ordered, because olanzapine may cause significant elevations.
- Monitor patient's blood glucose level routinely because olanzapine may increase risk of hyperglycemia.
- Monitor CBC often during first few months of therapy, especially if patient has low WBC count or history of drug-induced leukopenia or neutropenia. If WBC count declines, and especially if neutrophil count drops below 1,000/mm^3, expect olanzapine to be discontinued. If neutropenia is significant, also monitor patient for fever or other evidence of infection and provide appropriate treatment, as prescribed.
- Be aware that drug may cause hyperprolactinemia, which, in turn, may reduce pituitary gonadotropin secretion. This then inhibits reproductive function by impairing gonadal steroidogenesis in both female and male patients. In addition, longstanding hyperprolactinemia may decrease bone density in patient when it is associated with hypogonadism.
- Know that olanzapine may cause a drug reaction with eosinophilia and systemic symptoms called DRESS. Although uncommon, it can become fatal. Assess patient regularly for a cutaneous reaction exhibited by eosinophilia, exfoliative dermatitis, fever, lymphadenopathy, or rash. Know that systemic complications such as hepatitis, myocarditis and/or pericarditis, nephritis, or pneumonitis also may occur. If suspected, stop olanzapine

and notify presriber immediately. Expect to provide supportive care, as ordered.
- Institute fall precautions, especially in patients with conditions, diseases, or concurrent drug therapy that could exacerbate effects of motor and sensory instability, postural hypotension, and somnolence.

PATIENT TEACHING
- Advise patient to avoid alcohol and smoking during olanzapine therapy.
- Teach patient to open orally disintegrating tablet sachet by peeling back foil on the blister, not by pushing tablet through the foil. Immediately after opening blister, tell him to use dry hands to remove tablet and place it in his mouth. Explain that tablet will disintegrate rapidly in saliva so he can easily swallow it without liquid.
- Caution patient with phenylketonuria that disintegrating olanzapine tablets contain phenylalanine.
- Tell patient receiving the extended-release parenteral form of olanzapine, that she will need to be monitored for at least 3 hours following the injection. Stress importance of reporting any unusual symptoms including altered thoughts and lethargy immediately to healthcare professional.
- Urge patient to avoid hazardous activities until drug's CNS effects are known. Also inform patient of increased risk for falls because of potential CNS effects. Review fall precautions with patient.
- Instruct patient to change position slowly to minimize effects of orthostatic hypotension.
- Encourage patient to weigh self frequently to detect weight gain. If diabetes is present, also instruct patient to monitor blood glucose level closely.
- Urge family or caregiver to watch patient closely for suicidal tendencies, especially when therapy starts or dosage changes and particularly if patient is a teenager or young adult.
- Warn patient that chronic olanzapine therapy may alter reproductive function through olanzapine-induced hyperprolactinemia causing amenorrhea and impotence. If reproductive adverse effects occur, patient should notify prescriber.
- Advise female patient of childbearing age to notify prescriber if she intends to become or suspects that she is pregnant during therapy.
- Instruct patient to notify prescriber of any persistent, severe, or worsening adverse reactions, including fever, rash, or swollen glands or change in body function.

olmesartan medoxomil

Benicar

Class and Category

Pharmacologic class: Angiotensin II receptor blocker (ARB)
Therapeutic class: Antihypertensive
Pregnancy category: D

Indications and Dosages

➤ *To manage or as adjunct to manage hypertension*

SUSPENSION, TABLETS

Adults, adolescents, and children age 6 and over who weigh 35 kg (77 lb) or more. *Initial:* 20 mg daily, increased in 2 wk to 40 mg daily, as needed. *Maximum:* 40 mg daily.
Adolescents and children age 6 and over who weigh 20 kg to less than 35 kg (44 to 77 lb). *Initial:* 10 mg daily, increased in 2 wk to 20 mg daily, as needed. *Maximum:* 20 mg daily.

DOSAGE ADJUSTMENT Lower starting dosage is recommended for patients with possible depletion of intravascular volume, such as those treated with diuretics, especially if impaired renal function is present.

Contraindications

Aliskiren therapy in patients with diabetes or renal impairment (GFR less than 60 ml/min), children under age 1, hypersensitivity to olmesartan medoxomil or its components

Interactions

DRUGS

ACE inhibitors, aliskiren (in patients with diabetes or renal impairment), other angiotensin receptor blockers: Increased risk of hyperkalemia, hypotension, and renal dysfunction

Mechanism of Action

Olmesartan medoxomil blocks angiotensin II from binding to receptor sites in many tissues, including adrenal glands and vascular smooth muscle. Angiotensin II, a potent vasoconstrictor, is then free to stimulate the adrenal cortex to secrete aldosterone, and the inhibiting effects of angiotensin II reduce blood pressure.

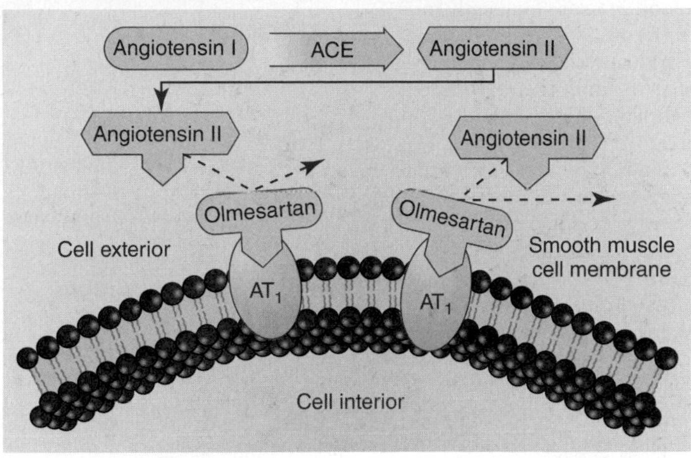

colesevelam: Reduced effectiveness of olmesartan
lithium: Increased serum lithium level with possible toxicity
NSAIDs: Increased risk of renal dysfunction in elderly patients and patients who are volume-depleted or have preexisting renal dysfunction; increased antihypertensive effect of olmesartan

Adverse Reactions

CNS: Asthenia, dizziness, fatigue, headache, insomnia, vertigo
CV: Chest pain, hypercholesterolemia, hyperlipidemia, hypertriglyceridemia, peripheral edema, tachycardia
EENT: Pharyngitis, rhinitis, sinusitis
ENDO: Hyperglycemia
GI: Abdominal pain, diarrhea, gastroenteritis, indigestion, nausea, sprue-like enteropathy, vomiting
GU: Acute renal failure, elevated BUN and serum creatinine levels, hematuria, UTI
MS: Arthralgia, arthritis, back pain, myalgia, **rhabdomyolysis**, skeletal pain
RESP: Bronchitis, cough, upper respiratory tract infection
SKIN: Alopecia, pruritus, rash, urticaria
Other: Anaphylaxis, angioedema, hyperkalemia, hyperuricemia, increased CK level, flu-like symptoms, pain

Nursing Considerations

- Expect to provide treatment such as normal saline solution I.V., as prescribed, to correct known or suspected hypovolemia before beginning olmesartan therapy.
- Make 200 ml of a 2-mg/ml suspension for children or adults who cannot swallow tablets by adding 50 ml of purified water to an amber polyethylene terephthalate (PET) bottle containing twenty 20-mg tablets and allow to stand for a minimum of 5 minutes. Shake the container for at least 1 minute and allow the suspension to stand for at least 1 minute. Repeat 1-minute shaking and 1-minute standing for four additional times. Add 100 ml of Ora-Sweet and 50 ml of Ora-Plus to the suspension and shake well for at least 1 minute. Refrigerate the suspension for up to 4 weeks. Shake the suspension well before each use and return promptly to the refrigerator.

- Monitor patient for increased BUN and serum creatinine levels, especially in a patient with impaired renal function, because drug may cause acute renal failure. If increased levels are significant or persist, notify prescriber immediately.
- Monitor blood pressure frequently to assess effectiveness of therapy. If blood pressure isn't controlled with olmesartan alone, expect to administer a diuretic, such as hydrochlorothiazide, as prescribed.

WARNING Monitor patient's blood pressure frequently if he receives a diuretic or other antihypertensive during olmesartan therapy because of an increased risk of hypotension.

- Expect to discontinue drug temporarily if patient experiences hypotension. Place patient in supine position immediately and prepare to administer normal saline solution I.V., as prescribed. Expect to resume drug therapy after blood pressure stabilizes.
- Know that if patient also receives a diuretic, adequate hydration should be provided, as appropriate, to help prevent hypovolemia. Watch for evidence of hypovolemia, such as hypotension with dizziness and fainting.
- Monitor patient's electrolytes regularly, as ordered, and observe patient for signs and symptoms of electrolyte imbalances, especially hyperkalemia, because drug inhibits the renin–angiotensin system and may cause hyperkalemia.

PATIENT TEACHING

- Teach patient, parent, or caregiver how to mix olmesartan suspension if patient is unable to swallow tablets.
- Advise patient to avoid exercise in hot weather and excessive alcohol use to reduce the risk of dehydration and hypotension. Also instruct him to notify prescriber if he has prolonged diarrhea, nausea, or vomiting.
- Caution patient to avoid hazardous activities until drug's CNS effects are known.
- Explain the importance of proper diet, regular exercise, and other lifestyle changes in controlling hypertension.
- Advise female patient to notify prescriber immediately about known or suspected pregnancy. Explain that if she becomes pregnant, prescriber may replace olmesartan with another antihypertensive that's safe to use during pregnancy.

olodaterol

Striverdi Respimat

Class and Category

Pharmacologic class: Long-acting beta$_2$-adrenergic agonist
Therapeutic class: Bronchodilator
Pregnancy category: C

Indications and Dosages

➤ *To treat long-term airflow obstruction in patients with chronic obstructive pulmonary disease (COPD)*

ORAL INHALATION

Adults. 5 mcg (2 inhalations) once daily at same time each day.

Mechanism of Action

By binding and activating beta$_2$-adrenoceptors in the airways, intracellular adenyl cyclase (an enzyme that mediates the synthesis of cyclic-3′ 5′-adenosine monophosphate [cAMP]) is stimulated. Elevated levels of cAMP cause bronchodilation by relaxing airway smooth muscle cells.

Contraindications

Asthma without use of a long-term asthma control drug, hypersensitivity to olodaterol or its components

Interactions

DRUGS

adrenergic agents: Potentiated effects
beta blockers: Decreased effectiveness of olodaterol; possibly severe bronchospasm
diuretics, steroids, xanthine derivatives: Increased risk of hypokalemia
drugs known to prolong QT interval, MAO inhibitors, tricyclic antidepressants: Possibly adverse cardiovascular effects
ketoconazole: Possibly increased serum olodaterol level
non-potassium-sparing diuretics: Possibly increased risk of ECG changes and hypokalemia

Adverse Reactions

CNS: Dizziness, fever
CV: **Atrial fibrillation**, chest pain, **ECG changes**, palpitations, tachycardia
EENT: Nasopharyngitis
ENDO: Hyperglycemia
GI: Constipation, diarrhea
GU: UTI
MS: Arthralgia, back pain
RESP: Bronchitis, COPD exacerbation, cough, **paradoxical bronchospasms**, pneumonia, upper respiratory infection
SKIN: Rash
Other: Anaphylaxis, angioedema, hypokalemia, immediate hypersensitivity reactions

Nursing Considerations

- Know that olodaterol therapy should not be used in patients with acutely deteriorating COPD, which may be a life-threatening condition. It should also not be used for relief of acute episodes of bronchospasm.
- Use caution when administering olodaterol to patients with cardiovascular disorders, such as arrhythmias, coronary insufficiency, hypertension, or hypertrophic obstructive cardiomyopathy; to patients with seizure disorders or thyrotoxicosis; and to patients who are unusually responsive to sympathomimetic amines or are at risk for developing prolonged QT interval.
- Administer olodaterol only by oral inhalation. Remember to prime inhaler before using for the first time.
- Watch patient closely for paradoxical bronchospasm. If present, discontinue olodaterol therapy immediately, notify prescriber, and implement treatment according to standard of care.

WARNING Monitor patient for worsening or deteriorating asthma because asthma-related deaths have increased in patients receiving salmeterol, a drug in the same class as olodaterol. Be aware that use of long-acting beta$_2$-adrenergic agonists such as olodaterol is contraindicated in patients with asthma without the use of a long-term asthma control medication, such as an inhaled corticosteroid. Monitor patient closely and notify prescriber immediately of any changes in patient's respiratory status.

- Monitor patients with a history of cardiovascular disorders. Notify prescriber of any significant increases in blood pressure or pulse rate or worsening of chronic conditions. Olodaterol may also cause ECG changes such as flattening of the T wave, prolonged QT interval, and ST-segment depression. Drug may need to be discontinued if such reactions occur.

WARNING Watch patient closely for hypersensitivity reactions. If present, stop olodaterol therapy immediately, notify prescriber, and provide emergency treatment according to standard of care.

- Monitor patient's serum potassium level and assess for signs and symptoms of hypokalemia, especially if patient has severe COPD, because hypokalemia may be made worse by hypoxia and concomitant treatment.

PATIENT TEACHING

- Advise patient, especially if she has a significant cardiac history, to inform prescriber of any other drugs she is taking before beginning olodaterol therapy and to keep prescriber informed of any new drug therapies while taking olodaterol.
- Caution patient not to increase olodaterol dosage or frequency without consulting prescriber because serious adverse reactions may occur.
- Instruct patient on how to load the cartridge into the inhaler. Remind patient that after insertion, the unit must be primed before first use by actuating the inhaler toward the ground until an aerosol cloud is visible and then repeating the process three more times. If not used for more than 3 days, remind patient to actuate the inhaler once before use; if not used for more than 21 days, tell patient to prime inhaler as if using for the first time.
- Teach patient how to use inhaler. Stress importance of using inhalation spray only with the Striverdi Respimat inhaler and that the inhaler should not be used for administering other drugs.

WARNING Caution patient that immediate hypersensitivity reactions, including swelling of face or throat, may occur after administration of olodaterol. If present, patient should stop taking drug, seek immediate medical treatment, and notify prescriber.

- Urge patient to notify prescriber if her symptoms worsen, if olodaterol becomes less effective, or if she needs more inhalations of her prescribed short-acting beta$_2$-agonist than usual. This may indicate that her condition is worsening.
- Instruct patient to notify prescriber immediately if she experiences chest pain, palpitations, rapid heart rate, or other troublesome effects while taking olodaterol because dosage may have to be adjusted.
- Tell patient that olodaterol may cause paradoxical bronchospasms. If present, tell patient to discontinue drug and notify prescriber. If severe or unrelieved, stress importance of seeking emergency treatment to relieve bronchospasms.

olsalazine sodium

Dipentum

Class and Category

Pharmacologic class: Salicylate
Therapeutic class: Anti-inflammatory
Pregnancy category: C

Indications and Dosages

➤ *To maintain remission of ulcerative colitis in patients who are intolerant of sulfasalazine*

CAPSULES, TABLETS

Adults and adolescents. 500 mg twice daily.

Mechanism of Action

Exerts anti-inflammatory action in GI tract after being converted by colonic bacteria to mesalamine (5-aminosalicylic acid), which inhibits cyclooxygenase. Inhibition of cyclooxygenase reduces prostaglandin production in intestinal mucosa. This in turn reduces production of arachidonic acid metabolites, which may be increased in patients with inflammatory bowel disease. Olsalazine also exerts an anti-inflammatory effect by indirectly inhibiting leukotriene synthesis, which normally catalyzes production of arachidonic acid.

Contraindications

Hypersensitivity to olsalazine, salicylates, or their components

Interactions

DRUGS

6-mercaptopurine, thioguanine: Increased risk of myelosuppression
low-molecular-weight heparins or heparinoids: Increased risk of bleeding after neuraxial anesthesia
oral anticoagulants: Possibly prolonged PT
varicella vaccine: Increased risk of Reye's syndrome

Adverse Reactions

CNS: Anxiety, depression, dizziness, drowsiness, fatigue, fever, headache, insomnia, lethargy, paresthesia, peripheral neuropathy, vertigo
CV: Cardiac arrest, hypotension, myocarditis, pericarditis, prolonged QT interval, second-degree AV block
ENDO: Hot flashes
EENT: Dry eyes and mouth, lacrimation, **laryngeal edema**, **stridor**, stomatitis, tinnitus
GI: Abdominal pain, anorexia, cholestatic jaundice, **cirrhosis**, diarrhea, dyspepsia, elevated liver enzymes, **hepatic failure or necrosis**, **hepatitis**, **hepatotoxicity**, nausea, vomiting
GU: Dysuria, hematuria, interstitial nephritis, **nephrotic syndrome**, urinary frequency
HEME: Aplastic or hemolytic anemia, lymphopenia, neutropenia, pancytopenia
MS: Arthralgia, joint pain, muscle spasms, myalgia
RESP: Bronchospasms, dyspnea, **interstitial lung disease**, shortness of breath
SKIN: Acne, alopecia, erythema nodosum, flushing, photosensitivity, pruritus, rash
Other: Anaphylaxis, **angioedema**, dehydration

Nursing Considerations

- Assess patient for aspirin allergy before giving olsalazine.
- Know that if patient has severe allergies or asthma, he should be watched closely for worsening symptoms during olsalazine therapy; notify prescriber immediately if they occur.

- Assess consistency and quantity of stools and frequency of bowel movements before, during, and after therapy.
- Give drug with food to decrease adverse GI reactions.
- Monitor skin for adequate hydration.
- Assess patient for abdominal pain and hyperactive bowel sounds.
- Monitor hepatic and renal status in patient with underlying hepatic or renal dysfunction because drug may further impair these functions.

PATIENT TEACHING

- Instruct patient to take olsalazine with food.
- Urge patient to continue taking drug as prescribed, even if symptoms improve.
- Advise patient to watch for signs of dehydration.
- Tell patient to report unusual, persistent, or severe adverse effects to prescriber.

omadacycline

Nuzyra

Class and Category

Pharmacologic class: Aminomethylcycline of the tetracycline class
Therapeutic class: Antibacterial
Pregnancy category: Not classified

Indications and Dosages

➤ *To treat community-acquired bacterial pneumonia caused by* Chlamydophila pneumoniae, Haemophilus influenzae, H. parainfluenzae, Klebsiella pneumoniae, Legionella pneumophilia, Mycoplasma pneumoniae, Staphylococcus aureus *(methicillin-susceptible isolates), or* Streptococcus pneumoniae

I.V. INFUSION, TABLETS

Adults. *Loading:* 200 mg I.V. infused over 60 min on day 1. Alternatively, 100 mg I.V. infused over 30 min twice on day 1. *Maintenance:* 100 mg I.V. infused over 30 min once daily for 7 to 14 days. Alternatively, 300 mg P.O. once daily for 7 to 14 days.

➤ *To treat acute bacterial skin structure and skin infections caused by* Enterobacter cloacae, Enterococcus faecalis, K. pneumoniae, S. aureus *(methicillin-susceptible and-resistant isolates),* S. lugdunensis, S. anginosus *group, or* S. pyogenes

I.V. INFUSION, TABLETS

Adults. *Loading:* 200 mg I.V. infused over 60 min on day 1. Alternatively, 100 mg I.V. infused over 30 min twice on day 1 or 450 mg P.O. once daily on day 1 and day 2. *Maintenance:* 100 mg I.V. infused over 30 min once daily for 7 to 14 days if loading dose was 200 mg administered I.V. once on day 1. Alternatively, 300 mg P.O. once daily for 7 to 14 days if loading dose was 100 mg administered I.V. twice on day 1 or 450 mg P.O. once on day 1 and day 2.

Mechanism of Action

Binds to the 30S ribosomal subunit and blocks protein synthesis, exerting a bacteriostatic effect as well as a bactericidal effect against some isolates of *S. pneumoniae* and *H. influenzae.*

Incompatibilities

Do not administer omadacycline intravenously with any solution containing multivalent cations such as calcium and magnesium through the same intravenous line.

Contraindications

Hypersensitivity to omadacycline, other tetracycline-class antibacterial drugs or their components

Interactions

DRUGS

antacids containing aluminum, calcium, or magnesium; bismuth subsalicylate; iron preparations: Decreased absorption of oral omadacycline
anticoagulant drugs: Depressed plasma prothrombin activity

FOODS

all foods, especially dairy products: Decreased absorption of oral omadacycline

Adverse Reactions

CNS: Fatigue, headache, insomnia, lethargy, vertigo
CV: **Atrial fibrillation**, hypertension, tachycardia
EENT: Oral candidiasis, oropharyngeal pain, taste distortion
GI: Abdominal pain, **Clostridium difficile-associated diarrhea (CDAD)**, constipation,

diarrhea, dyspepsia, elevated bilirubin and liver enzymes, elevated lipase levels, nausea, vomiting
GU: Vulvovaginal mycotic infection
HEME: Anemia, thrombocytosis
MS: Elevated creatinine phosphokinase
SKIN: Excessive diaphoresis, erythema, pruritus, urticaria
Other: Elevated alkaline phosphatase, **hypersensitivity reactions**, infusion-site reactions (erythema, induration, inflammation, irritation, pain, swelling)

Nursing Considerations

- Know that omadacycline must be reconstituted and then further diluted prior to administration. Reconstitute each 100-mg vial with 5 ml of sterile water for injection. Gently swirl contents and let vial stand until the cake has completely dissolved and any foam disperses. Do not shake vial. If needed, invert vial to dissolve any remaining powder and swirl gently, to prevent foaming. Reconstituted solution should be yellow to dark orange in color; if not, discard solution.
- Dilute further immediately (within 1 hour) by withdrawing reconstituted solution from vial and adding it to a 100 ml or more of 0.9% sodium chloride injection, USP, or 5% Dextrose Injection USP intravenous bag. Concentration of the final diluted infusion solution will be either 1 mg/ml or 2 mg/ml depending on number of vials reconstituted. Use within 24 hours if diluted drug is left at room temperature or within 48 hours if refrigerated. If refrigerated, remove infusion bag from refrigerator and place in a vertical position at room temperature 60 minutes before use.
- Administer total infusion over 60 minutes for a 200-mg dose or a total infusion time of 30 minutes for a 100-mg dose. Infuse through a dedicated line or through a Y-site. If the same intravenous line is used for sequential infusion of several drugs, flush with 0.9% sodium chloride injection, USP, or 5% Dextrose Injection, USP, before and after infusion of omadacycline.
- Administer oral tablets of omadacycline with water after patient has fasted for at least 4 hours. After administration, patient should not drink (except water) or eat for 2 hours and not ingest any antacids, dairy products, iron preparations, or multivitamins for 4 hours after administration.

WARNING Be aware that patients treated for community-acquired bacterial pneumonia with omadacycline may have a higher risk of death, especially patients over the age of 65 and patients with multiple disorders. Monitor patients with pneumonia closely for worsening and/or complications of infection and underlying conditions.

- Know that omadacycline, as a tetracycline, may cause permanent discoloration of the teeth, enamel hypoplasia, and inhibition of bone growth in the neonate if administered during the last half of pregnancy.

WARNING Monitor patient for hypersensitivity reactions, because other tetracyclines have caused reactions, including anaphylaxis. If patient develops a reaction, notify prescriber and expect drug to be discontinued. Provide supportive care, as ordered and required.

- Assess patient for signs of secondary infection, such as profuse, watery diarrhea. If such diarrhea develops, contact prescriber and expect to obtain a stool specimen to rule out pseudomembranous colitis caused by *Clostridium difficile*. If diarrhea occurs, notify prescriber and expect to withhold omadacycline and treat with electrolytes, fluids, protein, and an antibiotic effective against *C. difficile*.
- Monitor patient for tetracycline-class effects such as abnormal liver function tests, acidosis, azotemia, hyperphosphatemia, increased BUN, pancreatitis, photosensitivity, and pseudotumor cerebri. Expect omadacycline to be discontinued if any of these adverse reactions occurs.

PATIENT TEACHING

- Instruct patient taking oral tablets of omadacycline to take drug with water after patient has fasted for at least 4 hours. After administration, patient should not drink (except water) or eat for 2 hours. Also tell patient not to ingest any antacids, dairy products, iron preparations, or multivitamins for 4 hours after administration.

- Inform patient that nausea and vomiting may occur with omadacycline use, especially if patient received the oral loading dose for treatment of acute bacterial skin and skin structure infections.
- Alert women who are pregnant that omadacycline may cause tooth discoloration and enamel hypoplasia later in life and inhibition of bone growth in the unborn child if the mother is exposed to omadacycline during the second or third trimester of her pregnancy.
- Alert patient that diarrhea is a common problem with antibacterial drugs. Tell patient that bloody or watery stools can occur even after omadacycline therapy has been discontinued. Stress importance of reporting diarrhea to prescriber.

WARNING Instruct patient to stop taking drug and seek medical attention if an allergic reaction occurs.

- Advise mothers not to breastfeed their infant during omadacycline therapy and for 4 days after the last dose of drug.

omalizumab

Xolair

Class and Category

Pharmacologic class: Monoclonal antibody
Therapeutic class: Antiallergenic, antiasthmatic
Pregnancy category: B

Indications and Dosages

➤ *To treat moderate to severe persistent asthma in patients with positive skin test or in vitro reactivity to a perennial aeroallergen whose symptoms have been inadequately controlled with inhaled corticosteroids*

SUBCUTANEOUS INJECTION

Adults and adolescents age 6 and over. 75 to 375 mg every 2 or 4 wk. Dose and frequency determined by body weight and blood IgE levels.

DOSAGE ADJUSTMENT Dosage adjusted for significant changes in body weight.

➤ *To treat chronic idiopathic urticaria in patients who remain symptomatic despite H_1 antihistamine treatment*

SUBCUTANEOUS INJECTION

Adults and adolescents age 12 and over. 150 or 300 mg every 4 wk.

Mechanism of Action

Helps reduce inflammation by binding to circulating IgE and keeping it from binding to mast cells. This action inhibits degranulation and blocks release of histamine and other chemical mediators. In asthma, inflammation results when antigen reexposure causes mast cells to degranulate and release histamine and chemical mediators. By blocking these responses, asthma symptoms and urticaria are less likely to develop.

Contraindications

Hypersensitivity to omalizumab or its components

Adverse Reactions

CNS: Dizziness, fatigue, fever, headache, vertigo
EENT: Earache, epistaxis, nasopharyngitis, otitis media, pharyngitis, sinusitis
GI: Gastroenteritis, nausea, upper abdominal pain
HEME: Eosinophilic conditions, **thrombocytopenia (severe)**
MS: Arm or leg pain, arthralgia, fractures
RESP: Bronchitis, cough, upper respiratory tract infection
SKIN: Alopecia, dermatitis, pruritus, rash, urticaria
Other: Anaphylaxis; antibodies to omalizumab; generalized pain; injection-site bruising, burning, hive or mass formation, induration, inflammation, itching, pain, redness, stinging, and warmth; lymphadenopathy; **malignancies**

Nursing Considerations

- Record patient's weight, and obtain blood IgE levels, as ordered, before starting omalizumab prescribed to treat asthma; dosage and dosing frequency are based on these factors.
- Reconstitute using sterile water for injection, and allow 15 to 20 minutes (on average) for lyophilized product to dissolve. Draw 1.4 ml sterile water for injection into a 3-ml syringe with a 1-in 18G needle.

Place omalizumab vial upright, and inject sterile water into vial using aseptic technique. Gently swirl upright vial for about 1 minute to evenly wet powder. Don't shake. Every 5 minutes, gently swirl for 5 to 10 seconds until solution contains no gel-like particles. Discard if powder takes longer than 40 minutes to dissolve, and start with a new vial. Once reconstituted, solution should be clear or slightly opalescent and may have a few small bubbles or foam around edge of vial. Use omalizumab within 8 hours if refrigerated or 4 hours if stored at room temperature.

- Remove reconstituted omalizumab from vial by inverting vial for 15 seconds to let solution drain toward stopper. Using a new 3-ml syringe with a 1-in 18G needle, insert needle into inverted vial and position needle tip at the very bottom of solution in the vial stopper. Then pull plunger all the way back to end of syringe barrel to remove all solution from inverted vial. To obtain full 150-mg dose (1 vial containing 1.2 ml of reconstituted omalizumab), all product must be withdrawn from vial before expelling any air or excess solution from syringe.
- Be aware that omalizumab is also available as a prefilled syringe. However, know that the needle cover on the prefilled syringe contains dry natural rubber, which is a derivative of latex and may cause allergic reactions in individuals sensitive to latex.
- Don't give more than 150 mg of omalizumab per injection site.
- Be prepared to inject omalizumab over 5 to 10 seconds because solution is slightly viscous.

WARNING Monitor patient closely for hypersensitivity reactions, particularly for first 2 hours after administration. Although rare, anaphylaxis has occurred as early as first dose and more than 1 year after starting regular treatment. Keep emergency medication and equipment readily available.

WARNING Monitor patient closely for signs of cancer. Report any abnormal findings to prescriber.

PATIENT TEACHING

- Instruct patient to notify prescriber immediately about possible hypersensitivity, such as difficulty breathing, hives, or rash.
- Caution patient that any improvement in his condition may take time.
- Encourage patient to comply with regularly scheduled prescriber visits.
- Inform patient of risk of malignancy and suggest routine cancer screening.
- Explain that omalizumab prescribed for the treatment of asthma isn't used to treat acute bronchospasm or status asthmaticus.
- Tell patient not to abruptly stop any prescribed systemic or inhaled corticosteroid when starting omalizumab therapy for asthma treatment because steroid dosage must be tapered gradually under prescriber's supervision.
- If female patient becomes pregnant within 8 weeks before or during omalizumab therapy, urge her to enroll in the Xolair Pregnancy Exposure Registry at 1-866-496-5247. Also, tell her to notify prescriber because drug may need to be changed.

omega-3-acid ethyl esters

Lovaza

Class and Category

Pharmacologic class: Ethyl esters
Therapeutic class: Antilipemic
Pregnancy category: C

Indications and Dosages

➤ *As adjunct to diet to reduce triglyceride level that is equal to or exceeds 500 mg/dl*

CAPSULES

Adults. 4 g once daily or 2 g twice daily.

Mechanism of Action

Omega-3-acid ethyl esters are essential fatty acids that may inhibit very-low-density lipoprotein and triglyceride synthesis in the liver. With less triglyceride synthesis, plasma triglyceride levels decrease.

Contraindications

Hypersensitivity to omega-3-acid ethyl esters or their components

Interactions

DRUGS

anticogulants: Possibly increased bleeding time

Adverse Reactions
CV: Angina pectoris
EENT: Halitosis, nosebleeds, taste perversion
GI: Diarrhea, dyspepsia, eructation, nausea, vomiting
HEME: Prolonged bleeding time
MS: Back pain
SKIN: Bruising, rash
Other: Anaphylaxis, flu-like symptoms

Nursing Considerations
- Be aware that drugs known to increase triglyceride levels—such as beta blockers, thiazide diuretics, and estrogens—should be discontinued or changed, if possible, before omega-3 ethyl ester therapy starts.
- Expect to check patient's triglyceride level before starting and periodically throughout omega-3-acid ethyl ester therapy to determine effectiveness.
- Administer drug with meals.
- Expect to stop omega-3-acid ethyl ester therapy after 2 months if patient's trigylceride level doesn't decrease as expected.
- Monitor patient with history of paroxysmal or persistent atrial fibrillation for recurrences of symptomatic atrial fibrillation or flutter, especially within the first 2 to 3 months of initiating omega-3 ethyl ester therapy.

PATIENT TEACHING
- Explain to patient the importance of dietary measures, an exercise program, and controlling other factors—such as blood glucose level—that may contribute to elevated triglyceride levels.
- Advise patient to take drug with meals.
- Explain that patient will need periodic laboratory tests to evaluate therapy.
- Instruct patient to seek immediate medical attention if an allergic reaction or chest pain occurs.

omega 3-carboxylic acids
Epanova

Class and Category
Pharmacologic class: Fish oil derivative
Therapeutic class: Antilipemic
Pregnancy category: Not classified

Indications and Dosages
➤ *To reduce triglyceride levels in patients with severe (equal to or greater than 500 mg/dl) hypertriglyceridemia*

CAPSULES
Adults. 2 or 4 g once daily.

Mechanism of Action
Possibly reduces synthesis of triglycerides in the liver by inhibiting acyl-CoA-1,2 diacylglycerol acyltransferase, increasing mitochondrial and peroxisomal beta oxidation in the liver, decreasing lipogenesis in the liver, and increasing plasma lipoprotein lipase activity.

Contraindications
Hypersensitivity to omega 3-carboxylic acids or its components

Interactions
DRUGS
anticoagulants, antiplatelet agents: Possibly increased risk of bleeding

Adverse Reactions
CNS: Fatigue
CV: Elevated LDL-C levels
EENT: Difficulty swallowing, nasopharyngitis
GI: Abdominal discomfort, distention, or pain; constipation; diarrhea; eructation; flatulence; nausea; vomiting
MS: Arthralgia

Nursing Considerations
- Use cautiously in patients with fish and/or shellfish allergy because omega 3-carboxylic acids contain polyunsaturated free fatty acids derived from fish oils and it is not known if cross-sensitivity exists.
- Monitor LDL-C levels, as ordered, periodically during therapy with omega 3-carboxylic acids because drug may increase these levels in some patients.

PATIENT TEACHING
- Instruct patient to swallow capsules whole and not to break open, chew, crush, or dissolve the capsules.
- Advise patient that if a dose is missed, take it as soon as it is remembered, but never to double the next dose to make up for the missed dose.

- Inform patient that drug therapy is not a substitution for dietary measures. Adherence to dietary restrictions must be continued.
- Tell patient to notify prescriber if any signs or symptoms of an allergic reaction occur and to seek immediate emergency care, if severe.

omeprazole

Losec (CAN), Prilosec

Class and Category

Pharmacologic class: Proton pump inhibitor
Therapeutic class: Antiulcer
Pregnancy category: Not classified

Indications and Dosages

➤ *To treat symptomatic gastroesophageal reflux disease (GERD)*

DELAYED-RELEASE CAPSULES, DELAYED-RELEASE TABLETS, DELAYED-RELEASE ORAL SUSPENSION

Adults and adolescents 16 years and over. 20 mg daily for 4 wk.
Children age 1 to 16 years of age weighing 20 kg (44 lb) or more. 20 mg once daily for up to 4 wk.
Children age 1 to 16 weighing 10 kg (22 lb) to less than 20 kg (44 lb). 10 mg once daily for up to 4 wk.
Children age 1 to 16 weighing 5 kg (11 lb) to less than 10 kg (22 lb). 5 mg once daily for up to 4 wk.

➤ *To treat erosive esophagitis due to acid-mediated GERD*

DELAYED-RELEASE CAPSULES, DELAYED-RELEASE TABLETS, DELAYED-RELEASE ORAL SUSPENSION

Adults and adolescents age 16 and over. 20 mg daily for 4 to 8 wk.

➤ *To treat pediatric erosive esophagitis due to acid-mediated GERD*

DELAYED-RELEASE CAPSULES, DELAYED-RELEASE ORAL SUSPENSION

Children age 1 to 16 years of age weighing 20 kg (44 lb) or more. 20 mg daily for 4 to 8 wk.
Children age 1 to 16 weighing 10 kg (22 lb) to less than 20 kg (44 lb). 10 mg daily for 4 to 8 wk.
Children age 1 to 16 weighing 5 kg (11 lb) to less than 10 kg (22 lb). 5 mg daily for 4 to 8 wk.
Children ages 1 month to less than 1 year weighing 10 kg (22 lb) or more. 10 mg once daily up to 6 wk.
Children ages 1 month to less than 1 year weighing 5 kg (11 b) to less than 10 kg (22 lb). 5 mg once daily up to 6 wk.
Children ages 1 month to less than 1 year weighing 3 kg (6.6 lb) to less than 5 kg (11 lb). 2.5 mg once daily up to 6 wk.

➤ *To provide maintenance of healing of erosive esophagitis due to acid-mediated GERD*

DELAYED-RELEASE CAPSULES, DELAYED-RELEASE ORAL SUSPENSION, DELAYED-RELEASE TABLETS

Adults and adolescents age 16 and over. 20 mg once daily up to 12 mo.
Children age 1 to 16 years of age weighing 20 kg (44 lb) or more. 20 mg once daily up to 12 mo.
Children age 1 to 16 weighing 10 kg (22 lb) to less than 20 kg (44 lb). 10 mg once daily up to 12 mo.
Children age 1 to 16 weighing 5 kg (11 lb) to less than 10 kg (22 lb). 5 mg once daily for up to 12 mo.

DOSAGE ADJUSTMENT For adult patients with hepatic impairment and Asian patients, dosage reduced to 10 mg once daily.

➤ *To provide short-term treatment of active benign gastric ulcer*

DELAYED-RELEASE CAPSULES, DELAYED-RELEASE ORAL SUSPENSION

Adults. 40 mg daily for 4 to 8 wk.

DELAYED-RELEASE TABLETS

Adults. 20 mg daily for 4 to 8 wk, increased to 40 mg daily, as needed.

➤ *To treat active duodenal ulcer short-term*

DELAYED-RELEASE CAPSULES, DELAYED-RELEASE ORAL SUSPENSION

Adults. 20 mg once daily for 4 wk, with an additional 4 wk of therapy, as needed.

➤ *To eradicate* Helicobacter pylori *in order to reduce risk of duodenal ulcer recurrence*

DELAYED-RELEASE CAPSULES, DELAYED-RELEASE ORAL SUSPENSION

Adults. 40 mg daily with clarithromycin 500 mg three times daily for 14 days. If ulcer present at start of therapy, 20 mg daily for an additional 14 days. Alternatively, 20 mg twice daily with amoxicillin 1,000 mg twice daily, and clarithromycin 500 mg twice daily for 10 days. If ulcer present at start of therapy, 20 mg once daily for an additional 18 days.

DELAYED-RELEASE TABLETS

Adults. 20 mg twice daily with amoxicillin 1,000 mg twice daily and clarithromycin

Mechanism of Action

Omeprazole interferes with gastric acid secretion by inhibiting the hydrogen potassium adenosine triphosphatase (H+ K+ -ATPase) enzyme system, or proton pump, in gastric parietal cells. Normally, the proton pump uses energy from hydrolysis of adenosine triphosphate to drive hydrogen (H^+) and chloride (Cl^-) out of parietal cells and into the stomach lumen in exchange for potassium (K^+), which leaves the stomach lumen and enters parietal cells. After this exchange, H^+ and Cl^- combine in the stomach to form hydrochloric acid (HCl), as shown below left. Omeprazole irreversibly blocks the exchange of intracellular H^+ and extracellular K^+, as shown below right. By preventing H^+ from entering the stomach lumen, omeprazole keeps additional HCl from forming.

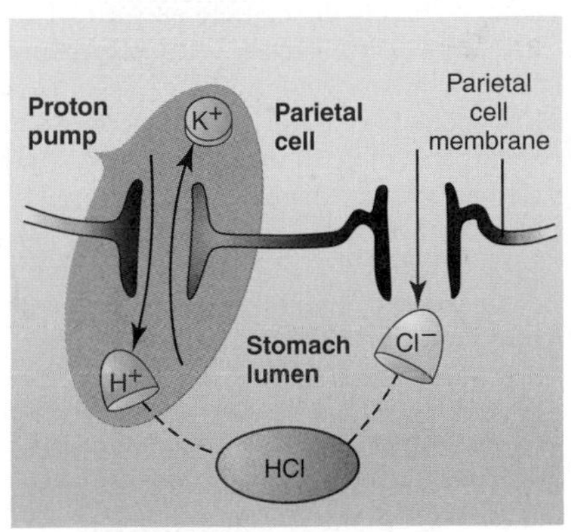

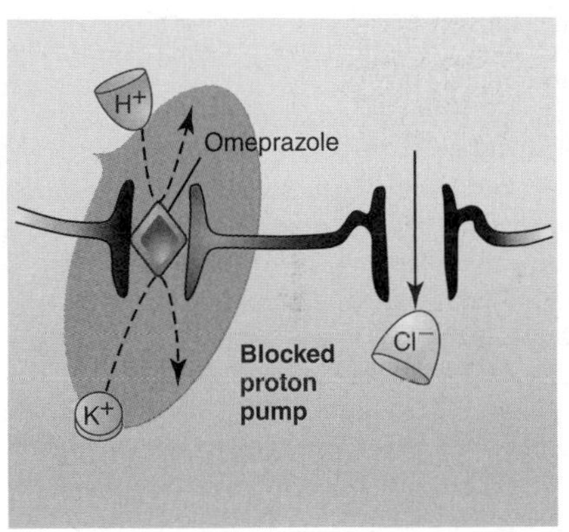

500 mg twice daily for 7 days. Alternatively, 20 mg twice daily with clarithromycin 250 mg twice daily and metronidazole 500 mg twice daily for 7 days. Then 20 mg daily for up to 3 wk (for duodenal ulcer) or 20 to 40 mg daily for up to 12 wk (for gastric ulcer).

➤ *To provide long-term treatment of gastric hypersecretory conditions, such as multiple endocrine adenoma syndrome, systemic mastocytosis, and Zollinger–Ellison syndrome*

DELAYED-RELEASE CAPSULES, DELAYED-RELEASE TABLETS, DELAYED-RELEASE ORAL SUSPENSION

Adults. 60 mg daily or in divided doses for doses greater than 80 mg. *Maximum:* 120 mg three times daily.

Route	Onset	Peak	Duration
P.O.	1 hr	In 2 hr	72–96 hr

Contraindications

Concurrent therapy with rilpivirine-containing products; hypersensitivity to omeprazole, other proton pump inhibitors, substituted benzimidazoles, or their components

Interactions

DRUGS

alprazolam, astemizole, carbamazepine, cisapride, cyclosporine, diazepam, diltiazem, disulfiram, erythromycin, felodipine, lidocaine, lovastatin, midazolam, quinidine, simvastatin, terfenadine, triazolam, verapamil, voriconazole: Decreased clearance and increased blood levels of these drugs

ampicillin, atazanavir, etlontinib, iron salts, itraconazole, ketoconazole, mycophenolate mofetil, vitamin B_{12}: Impaired absorption of these drugs

atazanavir, nelfinavir: Decreased plasma levels of these agents

cilostazol: Increased blood cilostazol

clopidogrel: Reduced effectiveness of clopidogrel

clarithromycin: Increased blood levels of omeprazole and clarithromycin

N O

digoxin: Increased digoxin bioavailability, possibly digitalis toxicity
levobupivacaine: Increased risk of levobupivacaine toxicity
methotrexate: Possibly delayed methotrexate elimination and increased risk of toxicity
nifedipine: Decreased nifedipine clearance, increased risk of hypotension
phenytoin: Decreased phenytoin clearance, increased risk of phenytoin toxicity
saquinavir: Increased plasma saquinavir level
St. John's wort, rifampin: Decreased plasma omeprazole level
sucralfate: Decreased omeprazole absorption
tacrolimus: Possibly increased tacrolimus level
warfarin: Possibly increased risk of abnormal bleeding

Adverse Reactions

CNS: Agitation, asthenia, dizziness, drowsiness, fatigue, fever, headache, malaise, psychic disturbance, somnolence
CV: Chest pain, hypertension, peripheral edema
EENT: Anterior ischemic optic neuropathy, optic atrophy or neuritis, otitis media, stomatitis
ENDO: Hypoglycemia
GI: Abdominal pain, acid regurgitation, constipation, diarrhea, ***Clostridium difficile*-associated diarrhea**, dyspepsia, elevated liver enzymes, flatulence, fundic gland polyps (long-term use), **hepatic dysfunction or failure**, indigestion, nausea, **pancreatitis**, vomiting
GU: Interstitial nephritis
HEME: Agranulocytosis, anemia, **hemolytic anemia**, **leukopenia**, leukocytosis, **neutropenia**, **pancytopenia**, **thrombocytopenia**
MS: Back pain, bone fracture, joint pain
RESP: Bronchospasms, cough, upper respiratory infection
SKIN: Cutaneous lupus erythematosis, **erythema multiforme**, photosensitivity, pruritus, rash, **Stevens–Johnson syndrome**, **toxic epidermal necrolysis**, urticaria
Other: Anaphylaxis, **angioedema**, **hypomagnesemia**, **hyponatremia**, systemic lupus erythematosus, vitamin B_{12} deficiency (long-term use)

Nursing Considerations

- Give omeprazole before meals, preferably in the morning for once-daily dosing. If needed, also give an antacid, as prescribed.
- If needed, open capsule and sprinkle enteric-coated granules on applesauce or yogurt or mix with water or acidic fruit juice, such as apple or cranberry juice. Give immediately.
- Give drug via NG tube, when needed by mixing granules in acidic juice, because enteric coating dissolves in alkaline pH, or using the delayed-release oral suspension form by mixing with water.
- Know that because drug can interfere with absorption of vitamin B_{12}, monitor patient for macrocytic anemia.
- Monitor patient for bone fracture, especially in patients receiving multiple daily doses for more than a year because proton pump inhibitors, such as omeprazole, increase risk for osteoporosis-related fractures of the hip, spine, or wrist.
- Be aware that long-term use of omeprazole may increase the risk of gastric carcinoma and symptomatic response to omeprazole therapy does not rule out the presence of gastric tumors.
- Know that omeprazole therapy may produce false elevations of serum chromogranin levels, used to help diagnosis presence of neuroendocrine tumors. If test results are high, withhold omeprazole therapy temporarily and repeat test, as ordered.
- Keep in mind that if omeprazole is given with antibiotics, watch for diarrhea from *C. difficile*. If diarrhea occurs, notify prescriber and expect to withhold drug and treat with electrolytes, fluids, protein, and an antibiotic effective against *C. difficile*.
- Monitor patient's urine output because omeprazole may cause acute interstitial nephritis. Notify prescriber if urine output decreases or there is blood in patient's urine.
- Monitor the patient, especially the patient on long-term therapy, for hypomagnesemia. If patient is to remain on omeprazole long term, expect to monitor the patient's serum magnesium level, as ordered, and if level becomes low,

anticipate magnesium replacement therapy and omeprazole to be discontinued.
- Know that both cutaneous and systemic lupus erythematosus have occurred within days to years after proton pump therapy such as omeprazole was initiated. The most common symptoms presented were arthralgia, cytopenia, and rash. Report such findings to prescriber.
- Know that proton pump inhibitors such as omeprazole should not be prescribed longer than medically necessary.

PATIENT TEACHING
- Tell patient to take drug before eating—usually before breakfast—and to swallow delayed-release capsules or tablets whole. If needed, patient may sprinkle contents of capsule onto 1 tablespoon of applesauce and swallow immediately without chewing pellets. Tell him to follow with a glass of cool water and not to keep any leftover mixture.
- Tell patient prescribed the oral suspension form to empty package into a small cup containing 2 tablespoons of water (no other beverage should be used), stir the mixture well, drink it immediately, refill the cup with water, and drink again.
- Encourage patient to avoid alcohol, aspirin products, ibuprofen, and foods that may increase gastric secretions during therapy. Tell him to notify all prescribers about prescription drug use.
- Advise patient to notify prescriber immediately about abdominal pain or diarrhea. Also, tell patient to stop taking omeprazole and notify prescriber if a rash or joint pain occurs.
- Urge female patient of childbearing age to use effective contraception during therapy and to inform prescriber immediately if she is or suspects she may be pregnant.
- Instruct patient to inform all prescribers of omeprazole therapy.
- Advise patient to notify prescriber if patient notices he is experiencing a decrease in the amount of urine voided or there is blood in his urine. Also tell him to notify prescriber if he experiences new or worsening joint pain or a rash on his arms or cheeks that gets worse in the sun.

ondansetron hydrochloride

Zofran, Zofran ODT, Zuplenz

Class and Category

Pharmacologic class: Selective serotonin ($5\text{-}HT_3$) receptor antagonist
Therapeutic class: Antiemetic
Pregnancy category: B

Indications and Dosages

➤ *To prevent nausea and vomiting associated with highly emetogenic cancer chemotherapy*

DISINTEGRATING TABLETS, ORAL SOLUTION, ORAL SOLUBLE FILM, TABLETS

Adults. 24 mg 30 min before chemotherapy. Films and tablets given as three 8-mg doses (allowing each 8-mg film or disintegrating tablet to dissolve completely before another given).

I.V. INFUSION

Adults and children ages 6 months to 18 years. Three 0.15-mg/kg doses, each infused over 15 min, starting with first dose given 30 min before chemotherapy and second and third doses given 4 and 8 hr after first dose.

➤ *To prevent nausea and vomiting associated with moderately emetogenic cancer chemotherapy*

DISINTEGRATING TABLETS, ORAL SOLUTION, ORAL SOLUBLE FILM, TABLETS

Adults and adolescents age 12 and over. *Initial:* One 8-mg dose given 30 min before chemotherapy and one 8-mg dose given 8 hr after the first dose. Then, one 8-mg dose given every 12 hr for 1 to 2 days after completion of chemotherapy.
Children ages 4 to 11. *Initial:* One 4-mg dose given 30 min before chemotherapy with one 4-mg dose given 4 and 8 hr after the first dose. Then, one 4-mg dose given every 8 hr for 1 to 2 days after completion of chemotherapy.

➤ *To prevent nausea and vomiting associated with initial and repeat courses of emetogenic chemotherapy*

I.V. INFUSION

Adults and children ages 6 months to 18 years. Three 0.15-mg/kg doses, each infused over 15 min, starting with first dose given 30 min before chemotherapy and second and third doses given 4 and 8 hr after first dose. *Maximum*: 16 mg per dose.

➤ *To prevent nausea and vomiting associated with radiotherapy in patients receiving either total body irradiation, single high-dose fraction to the abdomen, or daily fractions to the abdomen*

DISINTEGRATING TABLETS, ORAL SOLUTION, ORAL SOLUBLE FILM, TABLETS

Adults. One 8-mg dose given three times a day.

DOSAGE ADJUSTMENT For patient receiving total body irradiation, one 8-mg dose given 1 to 2 hr before each fraction of radiotherapy administered each day; for patient receiving single high-dose fraction radiotherapy to the abdomen, one 8-mg dose given 1 to 2 hr before radiotherapy, with subsequent doses given every 8 hr after the first dose for 1 to 2 days after completion of radiotherapy; for patient receiving daily fractionated radiotherapy to the abdomen, one 8-mg dose given 1 to 2 hr before radiotherapy with subsequent doses given every 8 hr after the first dose for each day radiotherapy is given.

➤ *To prevent postoperative nausea and vomiting*

DISINTEGRATING TABLETS, ORAL SOLUTION, TABLETS

Adults. 16 mg as a single dose 1 hr before anesthesia induction.

ORAL SOLUBLE FILM

Adults. 16 mg given as two 8-mg films (first 8-mg film allowed to dissolve completely before second 8-mg film given) 1 hr before induction of anesthesia.

I.V. INJECTION

Adults and children age 12 and over. 4 mg undiluted as a single dose over 2 to 5 min just before anesthesia induction or if nausea or vomiting develops after surgery, providing no prophylactic antiemetics had been given preoperatively.

Children ages 2 to 12 weighing more than 40 kg (88 lb). 4 mg as a single dose over 2 to 5 min just before anesthesia induction or if nausea or vomiting develops shortly after surgery, providing no prophylactic antiemetics had been given preoperatively.

Children ages 1 month to 12 years weighing less than 40 kg (88 lb). 0.1 mg/kg as a single dose over 2 to 5 min just before or immediately after anesthesia induction or if nausea or vomiting develops shortly after surgery.

I.M. INJECTION

Adults and children age 12 and over. 4 mg undiluted as a single dose just before anesthesia induction or if nausea or vomiting develops shortly after surgery.

DOSAGE ADJUSTMENT For patients with hepatic impairment, maximum dosage limited to 8 mg daily I.V. or P.O.

Mechanism of Action

Blocks serotonin receptors centrally in the chemoreceptor trigger zone and peripherally at vagal nerve terminals in the intestine. This action reduces nausea and vomiting by preventing serotonin release in the small intestine (probable cause of chemotherapy- and radiation-induced nausea and vomiting) and by blocking signals to the CNS. Ondansetron may also bind to other serotonin receptors and to mu-opioid receptors.

Incompatibilities

Don't give ondansetron in same I.V. line as acyclovir, allopurinol, aminophylline, amphotericin B, ampicillin, ampicillin and sulbactam, amsacrine, cefepime, cefoperazone, furosemide, ganciclovir, lorazepam, methylprednisolone, mezlocillin, piperacillin, or sargramostim. Alkaline solutions and highly concentrated fluorouracil solutions are physically incompatible.

Contraindications

Concomitant use of apomorphine, congenital long QT syndrome, hypersensitivity to ondansetron or its components

Interactions

DRUGS

cisplatin, cyclophosphamide: Possibly altered blood levels of these drugs

drugs that increase QT interval: Augmented effect on QT interval increasing risk of torsades de pointes

ACTIVITIES
alcohol use: Increased stimulant and sedative effects, including mood and physical sensations

Adverse Reactions

CNS: Agitation, akathisia, anxiety, ataxia, dizziness, drowsiness, dystonia, fever, headache, **hypotension**, restlessness, seizures, **serotonin syndrome**, syncope, somnolence, thirst, weakness
CV: Arrhythmias, cardiopulmonary arrest (parenteral form), chest pain, **hypotension**, palpitations, **prolonged QT interval, shock**, tachycardia, **torsades de pointes**,
EENT: Accommodation disturbances, altered taste, blurred vision, dry mouth, **laryngeal edema, laryngospasm, stridor**, transient blindness
GI: Abdominal pain, anorexia, constipation, diarrhea, elevated liver enzymes, flatulence, indigestion, **intestinal obstruction**, masking of progressive gastric and ileus distention
RESP: Bronchospasms, pulmonary embolism, shortness of breath
SKIN: Flushing, hyperpigmentation, maculopapular rash, pruritus, **Stevens–Johnson syndrome, toxic epidermal necrolysis**, urticaria
Other: Anaphyolaxis; angioedema; hiccups; injection-site burning, pain, and redness

Nursing Considerations

WARNING Be aware that oral disintegrating tablets may contain aspartame, which is metabolized to phenylalanine and must be avoided in patients with phenylketonuria.

- Know that if hypokalemia or hypomagnesemia is present, these electrolyte imbalances should be corrected before ondansetron is administered because of increased risk for QT-interval prolongation, which could predispose the patient to develop torsades de pointes.
- Place disintegrating tablet or oral soluble film on patient's tongue immediately after opening package. It dissolves in seconds.
- Use calibrated container or oral syringe to measure dose of oral solution.
- Dilute drug in 50 ml of D_5W or normal saline solution when indicated. However, know that when used to treat postoperative nausea and vomiting in adults, drug is administered undiluted intramuscularly or intravenously.
- Monitor patient closely for signs and symptoms of hypersensitivity to ondansetron because hypersensitivity reactions, including anaphylaxis and bronchospasm, may occur. If present, discontinue drug, notify prescriber, and provide supportive care.

WARNING Monitor patient closely for serotonin syndrome, which may include agitation, chills, confusion, diaphoresis, diarrhea, fever, hyperactive reflexes, poor coordination, restlessness, shaking, talking or acting with uncontrolled excitement, tremor, and twitching.

- Monitor patient's electrocardiogram, as ordered, and especially in patients with bradyarrhythmias, congestive heart failure, hypokalemia, or hypomagnesemia or in patients taking other medications known to prolong the QT interval because ondansetron therapy can prolong the QT interval resulting in life-threatening arrhythmias such as torsades de pointes. Be aware that no dosage greater than 16 mg should be given intravenously at any one time due to increased risk of prolonged QT interval.

WARNING Be aware that ondansetron may mask symptoms of adynamic progressive ileus or gastric distention after abdominal surgery. Monitor patient for decreased bowel activity, especially if patient has risk factors for gastrointestinal obstruction.

PATIENT TEACHING

- Advise patient to use calibrated container or oral syringe to measure oral solution.

WARNING Tell patient that oral disintegrating tablets may contain aspartame, which is metabolized to phenylalanine and must be used cautiously in patients with phenylketonuria. Tell patient each 4- and 8-mg orally disintegrating tablet contains less than 0.03 mg phenylalanine.

- Instruct patient to place ondansetron disintegrating tablet or oral soluble film on his tongue immediately after opening package and to let it dissolve on his tongue before swallowing.

- Advise patient to immediately report signs of hypersensitivity, such as rash.

WARNING Advise patients to seek immediate medical attention if patient experiences persistent, severe, unusual, or worsening symptoms.

- Reassure patient with transient blindness that it will resolve within a few minutes to 48 hours.

oritavancin

Orbactiv

Class and Category

Pharmacologic class: **Lipoglycopeptide**
Therapeutic class: Antibiotic
Pregnancy category: C

Indications and Dosages

➤ *To treat acute bacterial skin and skin structure infections caused by gram-positive microorganisms such as* Enterococcus faecalis *(vancomycin-susceptible isolates only),* Staphylococcus aureus *(including methicillin-susceptible and methicillin-resistant isolates),* Streptococcus agalactiae, S. anginosus *group (*S. anginosus, S. constellatus, S. intermedius*), and* S. pyogenes

I.V. INFUSION

Adults. 1,200 mg given over 3 hr as a one-time dose.

Mechanism of Action

Kills bacteria by inhibiting cell wall synthesis.

Incompatibilities

Do not mix or administer oritavancin in normal saline solution, as a precipitation of the drug may occur. Also, do not administer with other drugs, including those formulated at a basic or neutral pH, as they may be incompatible with oritavancin.

Contraindications

Hypersensitivity to oritavancin and its components, intravenous unfractionated heparin sodium administration used within 5 days following oritavancin administration

Interactions

DRUGS

drugs with a narrow therapeutic window that are predominantly metabolized by CYP450 enzymes: Possibly decreased or increased concentration of these drugs
warfarin: Increased risk of bleeding

Adverse Reactions

CNS: Dizziness, headache
CV: Peripheral edema, tachycardia
ENDO: **Hypoglycemia**
GI: ***Clostridium difficile*-associated diarrhea**, diarrhea, elevated liver enzymes, nausea, vomiting
HEME: Anemia, eosinophilia
MS: Myalgia, osteomyelitis, tenosynovitis
RESP: **Bronchospasm**, wheezing
SKIN: **Erythema multiforme**, leucocytoclastic vasculitis, pruritus, rash, urticaria
Other: **Angioedema**; hyperuricemia; infusion reactions such as erythema, flushing of the upper body, pruritus, or urticaria; infusion-site extravasation, induration, or phlebitis

Nursing Considerations

- Use oritavancin cautiously in patients with a history of hypersensitivity to glycopeptides because of the possibility of cross-sensitivity.
- Reconstitute drug by adding 40 ml of sterile water for injection to each vial (three vials are needed to provide a dose of 1,200 mg), to provide a 10 mg/ml solution per vial. Gently swirl to avoid foaming and to completely dissolve the powder. Solution should appear clear, colorless to pale yellow.
- Withdraw and discard 120 ml from a 1,000-ml intravenous bag of D_5W (never use normal saline). Then, withdraw 40 ml from each of the three reconstituted vials and add to D_5W intravenous bag to bring bag volume back to 1,000 ml. This will yield a concentration of 1.2 mg/ml. Once mixed in infusion bag, use within 3 hours when stored at room temperature or within 9 hours when refrigerated to allow the additional 3 hours needed for administration.

- Monitor patient for infusion reactions such as red man syndrome, including flushing of the upper body, pruritus, rash, and/or urticaria. Notify prescriber immediately, because slowing or stopping the infusion may resolve these symptoms.
- Flush intravenous line with D_5W solution before and after administering drug.
- Monitor patient closely for signs of bleeding, especially if patient is taking warfarin therapy, because drug may artificially prolong prothrombin time (PT) and INR for up to 12 hours, making monitoring of the effectiveness of warfarin unreliable for at least 12 hours after the administration of oritavancin. Drug may also artificially prolong activated partial thromboplastin time (aPTT) for up to 120 hours and activated clotting time (ACT) for up to 24 hours after a single 1,200-mg dose of oritavancin.
- Infuse oritavancin over 3 hours. If patient develops an infusion-related reaction such as flushing, pruritus, or urticaria, slow or stop the infusion and notify prescriber.

WARNING Monitor patient closely for signs of hypersensitivity reactions because some reactions may be serious. If present, discontinue infusion immediately, notify prescriber, and implement appropriate standard of care.

- Assess patient for signs of secondary infection, such as profuse, watery diarrhea. If such diarrhea develops, contact prescriber and expect to obtain a stool specimen to rule out pseudomembranous colitis caused by *C. difficile*. If confirmed, expect to withhold drug and treat with electrolytes, fluids, protein, and an antibiotic effective against C. *difficile*.
- Monitor patient for osteomyelitis, as drug has been shown to produce more cases of osteomyelitis than vancomycin used to treat similar infections. If present, be prepared to institute appropriate alternative antibacterial therapy.

PATIENT TEACHING

- Alert patient that an allergic reaction can occur up to a day after oritavancin has been administered. Instruct him to notify prescriber of any signs of an allergic reaction and seek immediate medical attention if signs are severe or prolonged.
- Urge patient to tell prescriber if diarrhea develops, even 2 months or more after oritavancin ends.

orlistat

Alli, Xenical

Class and Category

Pharmacologic class: Lipase inhibitor
Therapeutic class: Antiobesity
Pregnancy category: X

Indications and Dosages

➤ *To promote weight loss in patients with body mass index 30 kg (66 lb)/m² (27 kg [59.4 lb]/m² or above in those with diabetes mellitus, hyperlipidemia, or hypertension) and to reduce the risk of weight regain*

GELCAPS

Adults and adolescents. 120 mg three times a day with fat-containing meals.

Contraindications

Cholestasis, chronic malabsorption syndrome, hypersensitivity to orlistat or its components, pregnancy

Interactions

DRUGS

amiodarone: Decreased effectiveness of amiodarone
anticoagulants: Altered therapeutic coagulation
antiepileptics: Possibly increased risk of seizures
cyclosporine: Altered cyclosporine absorption
fat-soluble vitamins: Decreased vitamin absorption, especially vitamin E and beta-carotene
insulin, oral antidiabetic agents: Possibly increased risk of hypoglycemia as weight loss occurs, necessitating lower insulin or oral antidiabetic dosage
levothyroxine: Possibly decreased levothyroxine effectiveness, resulting in hypothyroidism
pravastatin: Potentiated lipid-lowering effect

Mechanism of Action

In the GI tract, orlistat binds with and inactivates gastric and pancreatic enzymes known as lipases, as shown. Normally, lipase enzymes convert ingested triglycerides into absorbable free fatty acids and monoglycerides. By inactivating lipase, orlistat allows undigested triglycerides to pass through the GI tract and exit the body in feces. Blocking the absorption of some of these fats lowers the number of calories received from food, which promotes weight loss.

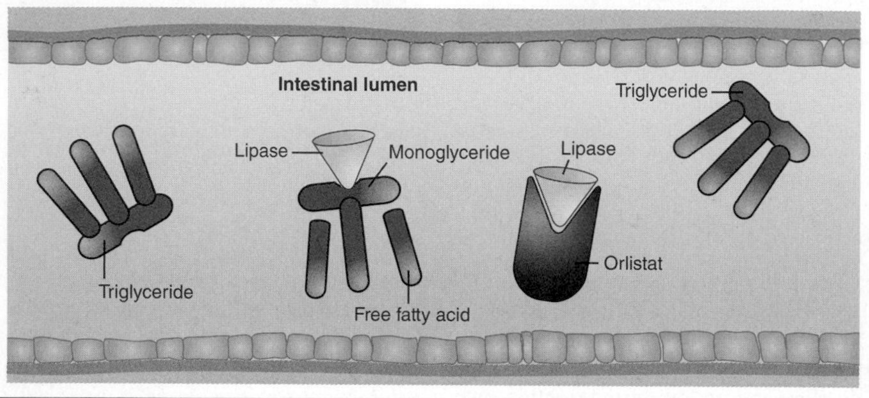

Adverse Reactions

CNS: Anxiety, depression, dizziness, fatigue, headache, **seizures**, sleep disturbance
CV: Leukocytoclastic vasculitis (rare), pedal edema
EENT: Gingival or tooth disorder, otitis
GI: Abdominal discomfort or pain, **acute hepatic failure**, cholelithiasis, diarrhea (infectious), elevated liver enzymes, fatty or oily stool, fecal incontinence or urgency, flatulence with discharge, **hepatitis**, **hepatocellular necrosis**, increased frequency of bowel movements, **lower GI bleeding**, nausea, **pancreatitis**, rectal pain, vomiting
GU: Elevated urinary oxalate levels, menstrual irregularities, nephrolithiasis, **renal failure**, UTI, vaginitis
MS: Arthralgia, arthritis, back pain, leg pain, myalgia, tendinitis
RESP: **Bronchospasm**, respiratory tract infection
SKIN: Dry skin, pruritus, rash, urticaria
Other: Anaphylaxis, **angioedema**, flu-like symptoms

Nursing Considerations

- Use cautiously in patients with a history of calcium oxalate nephrolithiasis or hyperoxaluria, as orlistat may increase levels of urinary oxalate and cause nephrolithiasis and oxalate nephropathy, which may lead to renal failure. Monitor serum creatinine levels closely, as ordered.
- Give orlistat with or up to 1 hour after meals that contain fat.
- Give levothyroxine and orlistat at least 4 hours apart because orlistat may decrease levothyroxine effectiveness, resulting in hypothyroidism.
- Also, give cyclosporine 3 hours after administering orlistat because orlistat can decrease plasma cyclosporine levels.
- Consult prescriber if you think patient has an eating disorder, such as anorexia nervosa or bulimia.

WARNING Monitor patient's liver enzymes, as ordered. Notify prescriber if abnormalities occur and expect to discontinue orlistat immediately. Be aware that severe liver injury has occurred in some patients, resulting in the need for a liver transplant or death.

PATIENT TEACHING

- Instruct patient to take orlistat with or shortly after meals that contain fat.
- Advise patient to take a multivitamin that contains fat-soluble vitamins and beta-

carotene at least 2 hours before or after orlistat, if indicated.

- Stress importance of notifying prescriber if patient takes a heart medicine called amiodarone.
- Advise patient taking levothyroxine to separate it from orlistat by at least 4 hours.
- Explain orlistat's adverse GI effects and that reducing dietary fat may decrease them. Instruct him to notify prescriber if they become too unpleasant.
- Help patient plan a reduced-fat diet (less than 30% of daily calories) and an exercise program to promote weight loss.
- Advise patient to weigh himself daily, at the same time and wearing similar clothes, to check his progress in losing weight.
- Urge patient to report anorexia, dark urine, jaundice, light-colored stools, pruritus, or right upper quadrant pain immediately to prescriber and to stop taking orlistat.
- Tell patient to notify prescriber if he is receiving drug treatment for seizures. Also, notify prescriber if seizures happen more often or get worse.

oseltamivir phosphate

Tamiflu

Class and Category

Pharmacologic class: Selective neuraminidase inhibitor
Therapeutic class: Antiviral
Pregnancy category: C

Indications and Dosages

➤ *To treat acute uncomplicated illness due to influenza A and B infection in patients who have been symptomatic for no more than 48 hours*

CAPSULES, ORAL SUSPENSION

Adults and adolescents. 75 mg twice daily for 5 days.
Children ages 1 to 12 years weighing more than 40 kg (88 lb). 75 mg twice daily.
Children ages 1 to 12 years weighing 23.1 kg (50.82 lb) to 40 kg (88 lb). 60 mg twice daily.
Children ages 1 to 12 years weighing 15.1 kg (33.22 lb) to 23 kg (50.6 lb). 45 mg twice daily.
Children ages 1 to 12 years weighing 15 kg (33 lb) or less. 30 mg twice daily.
Infants 2 weeks to less than 1 year at any weight. 3 mg/kg twice daily.

➤ *To prevent influenza A and B infection*

CAPSULES, ORAL SUSPENSION

Adults and adolescents. 75 mg once daily for at least 10 days following close contact with an infected individual, up to 6 wk during a community outbreak, and up to 12 wk for immunocompromised patients.
Children ages 1 to 12 years weighing more than 40 kg (88 lb). 75 mg twice daily for at least 10 days following close contact with an infected individual, up to 6 wk during a community outbreak, and up to 12 wk for immunocompromised patients.
Children ages 1 to 12 years weighing 23.1 kg (50.82 lb) to 40 kg (88 lb). 60 mg twice daily for at least 10 days following close contact with an infected individual, up to 6 wk during a community outbreak, and up to 12 wk for immunocompromised patients.
Children ages 1 to 12 years weighing 15.1 (33.22 lb) to 23 kg (50.6 lb). 45 mg twice daily for at least 10 days following close contact with an infected individual, up to 6 wk during a community outbreak, and up to 12 wk for immunocompromised patients.
Children ages 1 to 12 years weighing 15 kg (33 lb) or less. 30 mg twice daily for at least 10 days following close contact with an infected individual, up to 6 wk during a community outbreak, and up to 12 wk for immunocompromised patients.

DOSAGE ADJUSTMENT For adult patients with a creatinine clearance between 30 and 60 ml/min, dosage reduced to 30 mg twice daily for 5 days to treat influenza A and B infection and 30 mg once daily to prevent influenza A and B infection. For adult patients with a creatinine clearance of between 10 to 30 ml/min, dosage reduced to 30 mg once daily for 5 days to treat influenza A and B infection and 30 mg every other day to prevent influenza A and B infection. For adult patients with end-stage renal disease on hemodialysis, dosage reduced to 30 mg given immediately and then 30 mg after each hemodialysis cycle (treatment duration not to exceed 5 days) to treat influenza A and B infection and 30 mg given immediately and then 30 mg after alternate hemodialysis cycles to prevent influenza A and B infection. For patients with end-stage renal disease on continuous ambulatory peritoneal dialysis, dosage reduced to a single 30-mg dose administered immediately to treat influenza A and B infection and 30 mg given immediately and then 30 mg once weekly to prevent influenza A and B infection.

Mechanism of Action

After conversion to its active form, oseltamivir inhibits influenza virus neuraminidase, affecting release of viral particles.

Contraindications

Hypersensitivity to oseltamivir phosphate or its components

Interactions

DRUGS

live attenuated influenza vaccine: Possibly decreased effectiveness

Adverse Reactions

CNS: Abnormal behavior, agitation, altered level of consciousness, anxiety, delirium, delusions, headache, **hypothermia**, nightmares, **seizures**
CV: **Arrhythmia**
ENDO: Aggravation of diabetes mellitus
GI: Diaper rash, diarrhea, elevated liver enzymes, **GI bleeding**, **hemorrhagic colitis**, **hepatitis**, nausea, vomiting
SKIN: Dermatitis, eczema, **erythema multiforme**, rash, **Stevens–Johnson syndrome**, **toxic epidermal necrolysis**, urticaria
Other: **Anaphylaxis**, **angioedema**, generalized pain

Nursing Considerations

WARNING Monitor patient for serious hypersensitivity and skin reactions when administering oseltamivir. Know that anaphylaxis and skin reactions such as erythema multiforme, Stevens–Johnson syndrome, and toxic epidermal necrolysis have occurred. If present, discontinue oseltamivir therapy immediately, notify prescriber, and be prepared to provide emergency supportive care as ordered.

- Be aware that although uncommon, abnormal behavior and delirium have occurred after administration of oseltamivir, especially in children. While the onset is abrupt, rapid resolution usually occurs once oseltamivir is discontinued.

PATIENT TEACHING

- Instruct patient that for oseltamivir to be most effective, therapy should begin as soon as possible with the first appearance of flu symptoms: no later than 48 hours of onset of symptoms and as soon as possible after exposure.
- Tell patient to take a missed dose as soon as he remembers it, except if it is within 2 hours of the next scheduled dose.
- Warn patient that oral suspension contains above-normal maximum daily limits of sorbitol and may cause dyspepsia and diarrhea, especially in patients with hereditary fructose intolerance.
- Inform patient who cannot swallow capsules, when oral suspension is not available, that capsules may be opened and mixed with sweetened liquids such as caramel topping, corn syrup, light brown sugar dissolved in water, or regular or sugar-free chocolate syrup.
- Instruct patient, parent, or caregiver to use the oral dispenser device that comes with the product.

WARNING Advise patient to seek immediate medical attention if he experiences an allergic reaction or unusual or severe skin reactions.

- Alert patient and parents that, although uncommon, abnormal behavior and delirium have occurred, especially in children. Notify prescriber if present and expect drug to be discontinued.
- Inform patient that oseltamivir is not a substitute for receiving an annual flu vaccination.

oxacillin sodium

Class and Category

Pharmacologic class: Penicillin
Therapeutic class: Antibiotic
Pregnancy category: B

Indications and Dosages

➤ *To treat mild to moderate infections caused by penicillinase-producing strains of* Staphylococcus *or other susceptible organisms*

I.V. INFUSION, I.M. OR I.V. INJECTION

Adults and children weighing 40 kg (88 lb) or more. 250 to 500 mg every 4 to 6 hr. I.V. infusion given over 60 min. I.V. injection given over 10 min.
Infants and children weighing less than 40 kg (88 lb). 50 mg/kg daily in equally divided doses every 6 hr. I.V. infusion given over 60 min. I.V. injection given over 10 min.

➤ *To treat severe infections caused by penicillinase-producing strains of* Staphylococcus *or other susceptible organisms*

I.V. INFUSION, I.M. OR I.V. INJECTION

Adults and children weighing 40 kg (88 lb) or more. 1,000 mg every 4 to 6 hr.
Infants and children weighing less than 40 kg (88 lb). 100 mg/kg daily in divided doses every 4 to 6 hr. I.V. infusion given over 30 min. I.V. injection given over 10 min.
Neonates and premature infants. 25 kg/day.

Mechanism of Action

Inhibits bacterial cell wall synthesis. In susceptible bacteria, the rigid, cross-linked cell wall is assembled in several steps. Oxacillin affects final stage of cross-linking process by binding with and inactivating penicillin-binding proteins (enzymes responsible for linking the cell wall strands). This action causes bacterial cell lysis and death.

Incompatibilities

Don't give oxacillin at same time or in same admixture as aminoglycosides because they are chemically and physically incompatible and will inactivate each other.

Contraindications

Hypersensitivity to oxacillin, penicillins, or their components

Interactions

DRUGS

aminoglycosides: Inactivation of both drugs
chloramphenicol, erythromycins, sulfonamides, tetracyclines: Decreased therapeutic effects of oxacillin
oral contraceptives: Decreased contraceptive efficacy
probenecid: Increased blood oxacillin level

FOODS

all foods: Altered absorption of oxacillin

Adverse Reactions

CNS: Anxiety, depression, fatigue, hallucinations, headache, **seizures**
EENT: Oral candidiasis
GI: Diarrhea, nausea, **peudomembranous colitis**, vomiting
GU: Interstitial nephritis, vaginal candidiasis
HEME: Agranulocytosis, anemia, **granulocytopenia**, **neutropenia**
SKIN: Exfoliative dermatitis, pruritus, rash, urticaria
Other: Anaphylaxis

Nursing Considerations

- Know that before reconstitution, bottle should be tapped several times to loosen powder. For I.M. injection, reconstitute with sterile water for injection, half-normal (0.45) saline solution, or normal saline solution. Shake until solution is clear.
- For I.V. infusion, reconstitute only with normal saline solution or D_5W.
- When giving drug to patient at risk for hypertension or fluid overload, be aware that each gram of oxacillin contains 4.02 mEq of sodium.
- Monitor patient closely for diarrhea, which may indicate pseudomembranous colitis caused by *Clostridium difficile.* If diarrhea occurs, notify prescriber and expect to withhold oxacillin and treat with electrolytes, fluids, protein, and an antibiotic effective against *C. difficile.*

PATIENT TEACHING

- Instruct patient to notify prescriber immediately should a rash develop.
- Advise female patient who uses an oral contraceptive to use an additional contraceptive method during oxacillin therapy.
- Urge patient to tell prescriber about diarrhea that's severe or lasts longer than 3 days. Remind patient that watery or bloody stools can occur 2 or more months after antibiotic therapy and can be serious, requiring prompt treatment.

oxandrolone

Oxandrin

Class, Category, and Schedule

Pharmacologic class: Androgen
Therapeutic class: Appetite stimulant
Pregnancy category: X
Controlled substance schedule: III

Indications and Dosages

➤ *To promote weight gain after chronic infection, extensive surgery, failure to maintain weight despite no evidence of pathology, or severe trauma; to offset protein catabolism from prolonged use of corticosteroids*

TABLETS

Adults. 2.5 to 20 mg in divided doses given twice daily to four times a day for 2 to 4 wk; intermittent therapy repeated as prescribed. *Maximum:* 20 mg daily.
Children. 0.1 mg/kg or less daily; intermittent therapy repeated as prescribed.
DOSAGE ADJUSTMENT Dosage shouldn't exceed 5 mg twice daily for elderly patients.

Mechanism of Action

Promotes tissue-building processes and reverses catabolic or tissue-depleting processes by promoting protein anabolism.

Contraindications

Breast cancer (males); breast cancer with hypercalcemia (females); hypersensitivity to oxandrolone, anabolic steroids, or their components; nephrosis; pregnancy; prostate cancer

Interactions

DRUGS

corticosteroids: Increased risk of edema and severe acne
hepatotoxic drugs: Increased risk of hepatotoxicity
insulin, oral antidiabetic drugs: Possibly hypoglycemia
NSAIDs, oral anticoagulants, salicylates: Increased anticoagulant effects
sodium-containing drugs: Increased risk of edema
somatrem, somatropin: Possibly accelerated epiphyseal closure
warfarin: Increased warfarin half-life and risk of bleeding

FOODS

high-sodium foods: Increased risk of edema

Adverse Reactions

CNS: Depression, excitement, insomnia
CV: Decreased serum HDL level, edema, hyperlipidemia, hypertension
ENDO: Feminization in postpubertal males (epididymitis, gynecomastia, impotence, oligospermia, priapism, testicular atrophy); glucose intolerance; virilism in females (acne, clitoral enlargement, decreased breast size, deepened voice, diaphoresis, emotional lability, flushing, hirsutism, hoarseness, libido changes, male-pattern baldness, menstrual irregularities, nervousness, oily skin or hair, vaginal bleeding, vaginitis, weight gain), virilism in prepubertal males (acne, decreased ejaculatory volume, penis enlargement, prepubertal closure of epiphyseal plates, unnatural growth of body and facial hair)
GI: Diarrhea, elevated liver enzymes, **hepatocellular carcinoma**, jaundice, nausea, vomiting
GU: Benign prostatic hyperplasia, **prostate cancer**, urinary frequency, urine retention (elderly men)
HEME: Iron deficiency anemia, **leukemia, prolonged bleeding time**
Other: Fluid retention, **hypercalcemia** (females), physical and psychological dependence, sodium retention

Nursing Considerations

- Use oxandrolone cautiously in patients with heart disease because drug has hypercholesterolemic effects.
- Provide adequate calories and protein, as ordered, to maintain a positive nitrogen balance during oxandrolone therapy.
- Anticipate an increased risk of fluid and sodium retention in patients with cardiac, hepatic, or renal dysfunction.
- Weigh patient daily to detect fluid retention. If patient has fluid retention, expect a sodium-restricted diet or diuretics.

WARNING Be aware that oxandrolone may suppress spermatogenesis in males and cause permanent virilization in females.

- Monitor blood glucose level frequently in patient with diabetes mellitus.
- Know that if patient takes an oral anticoagulant, check INR or PT should be checked as ordered.

PATIENT TEACHING

- Advise patient to consume a diet high in calories and protein to achieve maximum therapeutic effect of oxandrolone.
- Urge patient to weigh himself daily during therapy and to report swelling or unexplained weight gain at once.
- Explain that drug may alter libido.
- Inform woman that drug may cause permanent physical changes, such as clitoral enlargement, deepened voice, and hair growth.
- Advise female patient of childbearing age that she must use contraception during oxandrolone therapy and should notify prescriber immediately about suspected or known pregnancy.
- Instruct diabetic patient to monitor blood glucose level frequently.
- Advise bleeding precautions (such as an electric shaver and soft toothbrush) if patient takes warfarin. Tell patient to notify prescriber immediately if bleeding occurs.

oxaprozin

Daypro

oxaprozin potassium

Daypro Alta

Class and Category

Pharmacologic class: NSAID
Therapeutic class: Anti-inflammatory, antirheumatic
Pregnancy category: C (first trimester), Not classified (later trimesters)

Indications and Dosages

➤ *To treat osteoarthritis and rheumatoid arthritis*

TABLETS

Adults. *Initial:* 1,200 mg once daily. Dosage adjusted based on response. *Maximum:* 1,800 mg daily or 26 mg/kg daily (whichever is less) in divided doses twice daily or three times a day.

DOSAGE ADJUSTMENT Initial dose limited to 600 mg daily for patients with low body weight or severe renal impairment.

➤ *To treat juvenile rheumatoid arthritis*

TABLETS

Children ages 6 to 16 years weighing 55 kg (121 lb) or more. 1,200 mg once daily.
Children ages 6 to 16 weighing 32 to 54 kg (70.4 to 118.8 lb). 900 mg once daily.
Children ages 6 to 16 weighing 22 to 31 kg (48.4 to 68.2). 600 mg once daily.

Route	Onset	Peak	Duration
P.O.	In 7 days	Unknown	Unknown

Mechanism of Action

Blocks cyclooxygenase, the enzyme needed to synthesize prostaglandins, which mediate the inflammatory response and cause local vasodilation, pain, and swelling. By blocking cyclooxygenase and prostaglandins, the NSAID oxaprozin relieves pain.

Contraindications

Angioedema, asthma, bronchospasm, nasal polyps, rhinitis, or urticaria induced by aspirin, iodides, or other NSAIDs; hypersensitivity to oxaprozin or its components; postoperatively after coronary artery bypass graft (CABG) surgery

Interactions

DRUGS

ACE inhibitors, antihypertensives: Decreased antihypertensive response, possibly impaired renal function
acetaminophen: Increased risk of adverse renal effects with long-term use of both drugs
anticoagulants, thrombolytics: Prolonged PT, increased risk of bleeding
beta blockers: Decreased antihypertensive effect
bone marrow depressants: Increased risk of leukopenia and thrombocytopenia
cefamandole, cefoperazone, cefotetan, plicamycin, valproic acid: Increased risk of hypoprothrombinemia and bleeding
cimetidine: Decreased oxaprozin clearance
corticosteroids, potassium supplements: Increased risk of adverse GI effects
digoxin: Increased blood digoxin level and risk of digitalis toxicity
diuretics: Possibly decreased diuretic effect

insulin, oral antidiabetic drugs: Increased effects of these drugs; risk of hypoglycemia
lithium: Increased blood lithium level
methotrexate: Increased blood methotrexate level and risk of methotrexate toxicity
other NSAIDs, salicylates: Increased GI irritability and bleeding
probenecid: Increased risk of oxaprozin toxicity

ACTIVITIES
alcohol use, smoking: Increased risk of adverse GI effects

Adverse Reactions

CNS: **Aseptic meningitis**, confusion, **CVA**, dizziness, drowsiness, fatigue, headache, insomnia, nervousness, sedation, transient ischemic attacks, vertigo, weakness
CV: **Deep vein thrombosis**, hypertension, **hypotension**, **MI**, peripheral edema
EENT: Tinnitus
ENDO: **Hypoglycemia**
GI: Abdominal pain, constipation, diarrhea, dyspepsia, elevated liver enzymes, **GI bleeding** or ulceration, **hepatitis**, jaundice, **liver failure**, nausea, **perforation of intestine or stomach**, vomiting
GU: **Acute renal failure**, dysuria, interstitial nephritis, urinary frequency
HEME: **Agranulocytosis**, anemia, **aplastic anemia**, **leukopenia**, **pancytopenia**, **thrombocytopenia**
SKIN: Alopecia, **erythema multiforme**, **exfoliative dermatitis**, maculopapular rash, photosensitivity, **Stevens-Johnson syndrome**, **toxic epidermal necrolysis**
Other: Anaphylaxis, angioedema

Nursing Considerations

- Be aware that NSAIDs like oxaprozin should be avoided in patients with a recent MI because risk of reinfarction increases with NSAID therapy. If therapy is unavoidable, monitor patient closely for signs of cardiac ischemia.
- Know that the risk of heart failure increases with use of NSAIDs such as oxaprozin. NSAIDs should not be used in patients with severe heart failure, but if unavoidable, monitor patient for worsening of heart failure.
- Use oxaprozin with extreme caution in patients with a history of GI bleeding or ulcer disease because NSAIDs, such as oxaprozin, increase risk of GI bleeding and ulceration. Expect to use oxaprozin for the shortest time possible in these patients.
- Be aware that serious GI tract bleeding, perforation, and ulceration may occur without warning symptoms. Elderly patients are at greater risk. To minimize risk, give drug with food. If GI distress occurs, withhold drug and notify prescriber at once.
- Use oxaprozin cautiously in patients with hypertension, and monitor blood pressure closely throughout therapy. Drug may cause hypertension or worsen it.

WARNING Monitor patient closely for thrombotic events, including MI and stroke, because NSAIDs increase the risk. These events have occurred even in patients who do not have a history or risk factors for cardiovascular disease. Monitor patient for warning signs such as chest pain, slurring of speech, shortness of breath, or weakness. If present, withhold oxaprozin, alert prescriber immediately, and provide supportive care as prescribed.

WARNING If patient has bone marrow suppression or is receiving antineoplastic drug therapy, monitor laboratory results (including WBC count), and watch for evidence of infection because anti-inflammatory and antipyretic actions of oxaprozin may mask signs and symptoms, such as fever and pain.

- Watch for less common but serious adverse GI reactions, including anorexia, constipation, diverticulitis, dysphagia, esophagitis, gastritis, gastroenteritis, gastroesophageal reflux disease, hemorrhoids, hiatal hernia, melena, stomatitis, and vomiting. The risk is higher if patient is elderly or taking oxaprozin long term.
- Monitor liver enzymes because, in rare cases, elevated levels may progress to severe hepatic reactions, including fatal hepatitis, hepatic failure, and liver necrosis.
- Monitor BUN and serum creatinine levels in patients with heart failure, hepatic

dysfunction, or impaired; those taking ACE inhibitors or diuretics; and elderly patients because drug may cause renal failure.

- Monitor CBC for decreased hemoglobin level and hematocrit because drug may worsen anemia.
- Assess patient's skin routinely for rash or other signs of hypersensitivity reaction because oxaprozin and other NSAIDs may cause serious skin reactions without warning, even in patients with no history of NSAID hypersensitivity. Stop drug at first sign of reaction, and notify prescriber.

PATIENT TEACHING

- Instruct patient to take oxaprozin exactly as prescribed.
- Advise patient to take drug with a full glass of water and to stay upright for 15 to 30 minutes afterward to keep drug from lodging in esophagus and causing irritation.
- Urge patient to avoid alcohol as well as aspirin and other NSAIDs during oxaprozin therapy to avoid bleeding complications.
- Advise patient to avoid excessive sun exposure to reduce the risk of photosensitivity.
- Caution patient to avoid hazardous activities until drug's CNS effects are known.
- Inform patient that risk of bleeding may continue up to 2 weeks after stopping drug.
- Explain that oxaprozin may increase the risk of serious adverse cardiovascular reactions; urge patient to seek immediate medical attention if signs or symptoms arise, such as chest pain, edema, shortness of breath, slurring of speech, unexplained weight gain, or weakness.
- Inform patient that oxaprozin also may increase the risk of serious adverse GI reactions; stress need to seek immediate medical attention for such signs and symptoms as abdominal or epigastric pain, black or tarry stools, indigestion or vomiting blood, or material that looks like coffee grounds.
- Alert patient to rare but serious skin reactions. Urge him to seek immediate medical attention for blisters, fever, itching, rash, or other indications of hypersensitivity.

oxazepam

Apo-Oxazepam (CAN), Novoxapam (CAN), Serax

Class, Category, and Schedule

Pharmacologic class: Benzodiazepine
Therapeutic class: Anxiolytic
Pregnancy category: Not classified
Controlled substance schedule: IV

Indications and Dosages

➤ *To treat anxiety*

CAPSULES, TABLETS

Adults. 10 to 15 mg three times a day or four times a day for mild to moderate anxiety; up to 30 mg three times a day or four times a day for severe anxiety.

➤ *To help manage acute alcohol withdrawal symptoms*

CAPSULES, TABLETS

Adults. 15 to 30 mg three times a day or four times a day.

DOSAGE ADJUSTMENT For elderly or debilitated patients, initial dose of 10 mg three times a day increased cautiously to 15 mg three times a day or four times a day.

Mechanism of Action

May potentiate the effects of gamma-aminobutyric acid (GABA) and other inhibitory neurotransmitters by binding to specific benzodiazepine receptors in limbic and cortical areas of the CNS. GABA inhibits excitatory stimulation, which helps control emotional behavior. The limbic system contains highly dense areas of benzodiazepine receptors, which may explain oxazepam's antianxiety effects.

Contraindications

Acute angle-closure glaucoma; concurrent use of itraconazole or ketoconazole; hypersensitivity to oxazepam, benzodiazepines, or their components; psychoses

Interactions

DRUGS

cimetidine, oral contraceptives: Impaired metabolism and elimination of oxazepam

clozapine: Increased risk of respiratory depression and arrest
CNS depressants: Increased risk of apnea and CNS depression
levodopa: Decreased therapeutic effects of levodopa
probenecid: Increased therapeutic effects of oxazepam and risk of oversedation
ACTIVITIES
alcohol use: Increased risk of apnea and CNS depression

Adverse Reactions

CNS: Anxiety (in daytime), ataxia, confusion, depression, dizziness, drowsiness, fatigue, headache, insomnia, nightmares, sleep disturbance, slurred speech, syncope, talkativeness, tremor, vertigo
GI: Nausea
Other: Drug tolerance, physical and psychological dependence, withdrawal symptoms

Nursing Considerations

WARNING Oxazepam may cause physical and psychological dependence.

- Be aware that drug shouldn't be stopped abruptly after prolonged use; doing so may cause seizures or withdrawal symptoms, such as insomnia, irritability, and nervousness.
- Be aware that withdrawal symptoms can occur when therapy lasts only 1 or 2 weeks.

WARNING Monitor respiratory status in patients with pulmonary disease (such as severe COPD), respiratory depression, or sleep apnea; drug may worsen ventilatory failure.

- Expect an increased risk of falls among elderly patients from impaired cognition and motor function. Take safety precautions.
- Be aware that drug may worsen acute intermittent porphyria, myasthenia gravis, and severe renal impairment.
- Expect patient with late-stage Parkinson's disease to experience decreased cognition or coordination and, possibly, increased psychosis.

PATIENT TEACHING

- Instruct patient to take oxazepam exactly as prescribed and not to stop taking it without consulting prescriber.
- Caution patient about possible drowsiness and reduced coordination.
- Urge patient to avoid alcohol, which increases oxazepam's sedative effects.

oxcarbazepine

Oxtellar XR, Trileptal

Class and Category

Pharmacologic class: Carboxamide derivative
Therapeutic class: Anticonvulsant
Pregnancy category: C

Indications and Dosages

➤ *As adjunct to treat partial seizures*
ORAL SUSPENSION, TABLETS
Adults and adolescents over age 16. *Initial:* 300 mg twice daily. Dosage increased by 600 mg/day every wk. *Usual:* 1,200 mg daily. *Maximum:* 2,400 mg daily.
Children ages 2 to 16. *Initial:* 4 to 5 mg/kg twice daily to maximum initial dose of 600 mg daily. *Usual:* 900 mg daily for children weighing 20 to 29 kg (44 to 64 lb); 1,200 mg daily for those weighing 29.1 to 39 kg (65 to 86 lb); 1,800 mg daily for those weighing more than 39 kg. *Maximum:* 1,800 mg daily.
XR TABLETS
Adults and adolescents over age 16. *Initial:* 600 mg once daily for 1 wk, increased in 600 mg a day increments weekly to reach target dose. *Maintenance:* 1,200 to 2,400 mg once daily. *Maximum:* 2,400 mg once daily.
Children ages 6 to 17. *Initial:* 8 to 10 mg/kg once daily, not to exceed initial dose of 600 mg in first wk, then increased in 8 to 10 mg/kg in once daily increments weekly. *Usual:* 900 mg daily for children weighing 20 to 29 kg (44 to 64 lb); 1,200 mg daily for those weighing 29.1 to 39 kg (65 to 86 lb); 1,800 mg daily for those weighing more than 39 kg (more than 86 lb). *Maximum:* 1,800 mg daily.
➤ *As monotherapy to treat partial seizures*
ORAL SUSPENSION, TABLETS
Adults and adolescents over age 16. *Initial:* 300 mg twice daily. Dosage increased

by 300 mg/day every 3 days, as needed. *Usual:* 1,200 mg daily. *Maximum:* 2,400 mg daily.
Children ages 4 to 16. *Initial:* 4 to 5 mg/kg twice daily, increased by 5 mg/kg daily every third day to maximum maintenance dosage, as needed. *Maximum:* 900 mg daily for children weighing 20 to 24.9 kg (44 to 55 lb); 1,200 mg daily for those weighing 25 to 34.9 kg (55 to 77 lb); 1,500 mg daily for those weighing 35 to 49.9 kg (77 to 110 lb); 1,800 mg daily for those weighing 50 to 59.9 kg (110 to 132 lb); 2,100 mg daily for those weighing 60 to 70 kg (132 to 154 lb).

➤ *To convert to monotherapy in treating partial seizures*

ORAL SUSPENSION, TABLETS

Adults and adolescents over age 16. *Initial:* 300 mg twice daily. Dosage increased by 600 mg daily every wk over 2 to 4 wk, as needed, while dosage of other anticonvulsant is reduced. *Usual:* 1,200 mg daily. *Maximum:* 2,400 mg daily.
Children ages 4 to 16. *Initial:* 4 to 5 mg/kg twice daily, increased by 10 mg/kg daily weekly as needed to maximum maintenance dosage while dosage of other anticonvulsant is reduced over 3 to 6 wk. *Maximum:* 900 mg daily for children weighing 20 to 24.9 kg (44 to 55 lb); 1,200 mg daily for those weighing 25 to 34.9 kg (55 to 77 lb); 1,500 mg daily for those weighing 35 to 49.9 kg (77 to 110 lb); 1,800 mg daily for those weighing 50 to 59.9 kg (110 to 132 lb); 2,100 mg daily for those weighing 60 to 70 kg (132 to 154 lb).

DOSAGE ADJUSTMENT For all patients with creatinine clearance less than 30 ml/min and elderly patients prescribed XR tablets, usual initial dosage reduced by 50%.

Mechanism of Action

May prevent or halt seizures by blocking or closing sodium channels in neuronal cell membrane. By preventing sodium from entering the cell, oxcarbazepine may slow nerve impulse transmission, thus decreasing the rate at which neurons fire.

Contraindications

Hypersensitivity to oxcarbazepine, eslicarbazepine acetate, or their components

Interactions

DRUGS

carbamazepine, phenobarbital, phenytoin, rifampin, valproic acid: Decreased blood oxcarbazepine level, possibly increased blood levels of phenobarbital and phenytoin
cyclosporine, dihydropyridine calcium antagonists, oral contraceptives: Decreased effectiveness of these drugs
felodipine, verapamil: Decreased blood levels of these drugs

FOODS

all food (XR tablets): Increased risk of adverse effects

ACTIVITIES

alcohol use: Possibly additive CNS depressant effects

Adverse Reactions

CNS: Abnormal coordination or gait, agitation, amnesia, asthenia, ataxia, confusion, difficulty concentrating, dizziness, EEG abnormalities, emotional lability, fatigue, fever, headache, hypoesthesia, insomnia, language or speech problems, nervousness, psychomotor slowing, **seizures**, somnolence, **status epilepticus**, **suicidal ideation**, tremor, vertigo
CV: **AV block**, chest pain, **hypotension**, peripheral edema
EENT: Abnormal vision, diplopia, earache, ear infection, epistaxis, nystagmus, pharyngitis, rhinitis, sinusitis, taste perversion
ENDO: Hot flashes, hypothyroidism, syndrome of inappropriate antidiuretic hormone secretion
GI: Abdominal pain, anorexia, constipation, diarrhea, elevated liver or pancreatic enzymes, gastritis, indigestion, nausea, **pancreatitis**, vomiting
GU: Frequent urination, UTI, vaginitis
HEME: Agranulocytosis, **aplastic anemia**, eosinophilia, **leukopenia**, **pancytopenia**, purpura
MS: Arthralgia, back pain, decreased bone mineral density, dysarthria, fractures, muscle weakness, osteoporosis (long-term therapy with immediate-release form)
RESP: Bronchitis, cough, respiratory tract infection

SKIN: Acne, acute generalized exanthematous pustulosis, diaphoresis, **erythema multiforme**, maculopapular rash, rash, **Stevens–Johnson syndrome**, **toxic epidermal necrolysis**
Other: **Anaphylaxis**, **drug reaction with eosinophilia and systemic symptoms (DRESS)**, **hyponatremia**, lymphadenopathy, **multiorgan hypersensitivity**

Nursing Considerations

- Know that patient with allergic reaction to carbamazepine may have hypersensitivity to oxcarbazepine.
- Administer XR tablets to patients 1 hour before or 2 hours after a meal because adverse reactions are more likely to occur when taken with food.
- Monitor serum sodium level for signs of hyponatremia, especially during first 3 months. Know that elderly patients may be at higher risk for hyponatremia because of age-related reductions in creatinine clearance.
- Monitor therapeutic oxcarbazepine levels during initiation and titration, and expect to adjust dosage accordingly.
- Implement seizure precautions as needed, especially in patients who are pregnant, because physiological changes during pregnancy may cause oxcarbazepine levels to decrease gradually throughout pregnancy, increasing the risk of seizures. Patient should also be monitored closely throughout the postpartum period for adverse reactions, as the level of oxcarbazepine may return to normal after delivery. Aggravation of seizures can also occur in other patients, especially children. If seizures occur, expect oxcarbazepine to be discontinued.

WARNING Monitor patient's skin closely. If a reaction develops, notify prescriber at once because skin reactions caused by oxcarbazepine may be serious or life-threatening. Be aware that patients carrying the HLA-B*1502 allele may be at increased risk for Stevens–Johnson syndrome or toxic epidermal necrolysis.

WARNING Watch closely for evidence of multiorgan hypersensitivity, such as arthralgia, asthenia, fever, hematologic abnormalities, hepatitis, hepatorenal syndrome, liver function abnormalities, lymphadenopathy, nephritis, oliguria, organ dysfunction, pruritus, and rash. If suspected, notify prescriber and expect to stop drug. Provide supportive care, as prescribed.

- Monitor patient closely for evidence of suicidal thinking or behavior, especially when therapy starts or dosage changes.
- Monitor patient for CNS adverse reactions that may involve cognitive symptoms, coordination abnormalities, fatigue, and somnolence.
- Expect to discontinue oxcarbazepine gradually, as abrupt withdrawal may increase risk of seizure frequency and development of status epilepticus.

PATIENT TEACHING

- Teach patient to shake suspension well and measure dose immediately afterward. Tell him to then withdraw prescribed amount using supplied oral dosing syringe. Instruct him to mix dose in a small glass of water just before taking it, or tell him that he can swallow drug directly from syringe. Instruct him to close bottle and rinse syringe with warm water and let it dry thoroughly. Instruct patient to discard any unused oral suspension after 7 weeks of first opening the bottle.
- Instruct patient prescribed XR tablets not to break, chew, or crush tablets but to swallow whole.
- Inform patient that he may experience dizziness, double vision, and unsteady gait as well as other adverse CNS signs and symptoms. Caution him not to drive or perform any other hazardous activity if these effects occur.
- Instruct patient not to drink alcohol during oxcarbazepine therapy.
- Alert patient to possibility of hypersensitivity or serious skin reactions and importance of reporting them to prescriber.
- Review signs and symptoms of low sodium level with patient. Tell him to report signs and symptoms such as confusion, increase in severity of seizures, lack of energy, nausea, or tiredness to prescriber.
- Warn patient to notify prescriber immediately if he develops difficulty breathing or swallowing; fever; rash;

swelling of face, eyes, lips, tongue; or other evidence of hypersensitivity because drug may have to be stopped and emergency medical care given.
- Alert woman of childbearing age that oxcarbazepine may render hormonal contraceptives ineffective. Urge patient to use an additional or a different contraceptive during oxcarbazepine therapy.
- Urge caregivers to watch patient closely for evidence of suicidal tendencies, especially when therapy starts or dosage changes, and to report concerns to prescriber at once.
- Urge female patient who becomes pregnant while taking oxcarbazepine to enroll in the North American antiepileptic drug pregnancy registry by calling 1-888-233-2334. Explain that the registry is collecting information about the safety of antiepileptic drugs during pregnancy.
- Warn patient not to stop taking oxcarbazepine abruptly, as an increase in seizure activity may occur and possibly lead to status epilepticus.

oxybutynin chloride

Ditropan XL, Gelnique 3%, Gelnique 10%, Oxytrol

Class and Category

Pharmacologic class: Anticholinergic
Therapeutic class: Antispasmodic (urinary)
Pregnancy category: B

Indications and Dosages

➤ *To treat overactive bladder with urge urinary frequency, incontinence or urgency*

E.R. TABLETS (DITROPAN XL)

Adults. *Initial:* 5 or 10 mg daily, adjusted by 5 mg/wk, as prescribed. *Maximum:* 30 mg daily.

TRANSDERMAL SYSTEM (OXYTROL)

Adults. System supplying 3.9 mg daily, applied twice weekly.

TOPICAL GEL (GELNIQUE)

Adults. 1 sachet (10%) or 3 pumps (3%) applied once daily to dry, intact skin on the abdomen, upper arms, shoulders, or thighs.

➤ *To treat symptoms of detrusor muscle overactivity of bladder associated with a neurological condition such as spina bifida*

E.R. TABLETS (DITROPAN XL)

Children age 6 and over. *Initial:* 5 mg once daily, increased in 5 mg increments weekly, as needed. *Maximum:* 20 mg once daily.

Route	Onset	Peak	Duration
Gel	Unknown	Unknown	72 hr
P.O.	30–60 min	3–6 hr	6–10 hr
Transdermal	Unknown	24–48 hr	96 hr

Mechanism of Action

Exerts antimuscarinic (atropine-like) and potent direct antispasmodic (papaverine-like) actions on smooth muscle in the bladder and decreases detrusor muscle contractions. The result is increased bladder capacity and a decreased urge to void.

Contraindications

Acute hemorrhage, angle-closure glaucoma, gastric retention (gel form), GI obstruction, hypersensitivity to oxybutynin or its components, ileus, intestinal atony in debilitated or elderly patients, myasthenia gravis, obstructive uropathy, toxic megacolon with ulcerative colitis, urine retention (gel form)

Interactions

DRUGS

amantadine, amitriptyline, amoxapine, antimuscarinics, brompheniramine, bupropion, carbinoxamine, chlorpheniramine, chlorpromazine, clemastine, clomipramine, clozapine, cyclobenzaprine, dimenhydrinate, diphenhydramine, disopyramide, doxepin, doxylamine, imipramine, maprotiline, mesoridazine, methdilazine, nortriptyline, procainamide, promazine, promethazine, protriptyline, thioridazine, triflupromazine, trimeprazine, trimipramine: Increased anticholinergic effects
CNS depressants: Increased sedation
ketoconazole: Possibly altered total absorption rate and blood level of ketoconazole
opioid agonists: Increased depressive effects on GI motility and bladder function

N O

other anticholinergics: Possibly decreased absorption of other drugs leading to decreased effectiveness; increased risk of frequency and severity of certain adverse reactions such as constipation, dry mouth and somnolence
parasympathomimetics: Decreased antimuscarinic action of oxybutynin
prokinetic agents such as metoclopramide: Possibly antagonized effects of prokinetic agents
ACTIVITIES
alcohol use: Increased sedation

Adverse Reactions

CNS: Abnormal behaviors, agitation, asthenia, confusion, delirium, depression, dizziness, drowsiness, fatigue, hallucinations, headache, insomnia, memory impairment, nervousness, psychosis, restlessness, **seizures**, somnolence, thirst
CV: Arrhythmias, chest discomfort, edema, hypertension, **hypotension**, palpitations, peripheral edema, **QT-interval prolongation**, tachycardia, vasodilation
EENT: Abnormal or blurred vision; cycloplegia; dry eyes, mouth, nose, and throat; eye irritation; glaucoma; keratoconjunctivitis sicca; mydriasis; nasal congestion; nasopharyngitis; rhinitis; sinusitis
ENDO: Hot flashes, hyperglycemia, suppression of lactation
GI: Abdominal pain, anorexia, constipation, decreased GI motility, diarrhea, dysphagia, esophagitis, flatulence, gastroesophageal reflux, indigestion, nausea, vomiting
GU: Cystitis, dysuria, impotence, urinary hesitancy, urine retention, UTI
MS: Arthralgia, arthritis, back pain
RESP: Asthma, bronchitis, cough, dysphonia, upper respiratory tract infection
SKIN: Decreased sweating, dry skin, flushing, pruritus, rash, urticaria
Other: Anaphylaxis, angioedema, application-site reactions (anesthesia, dermatitis, erythema, irritation, papules, pruritus), flu-like symptoms, fungal infections, **heatstroke**

Nursing Considerations

- Use oxybutynin cautiously in patients with diarrhea because it may signal incomplete GI obstruction, especially in patients with colostomy or ileostomy. Also use cautiously in patients with dementia treated with cholinesterase inhibitors because drug may aggravate symptoms.
- Use cautiously in patients with GI disorders such as autonomic neuropathy, myasthenia gravis, or Parkinson's disease because drug may adversely affect these conditions. If exacerbation of symptoms occurs, notify prescriber and expect drug to be discontinued.
- Assess urinary symptoms before and after treatment.
- Make sure patient swallows E.R. tablets whole and doesn't chew, crush, or divide them. Expect to see portions of drug in stool.
- Apply transdermal system to dry, intact skin of abdomen, buttock, or hip; avoid using same site for at least 7 days by rotating sites.
- Apply gel form to dry, intact skin on patient's abdomen, shoulders, thighs, or upper arms. Rotate application sites.

WARNING Monitor patient for angioedema of the face, lips, tongue, and/or larynx, even after just the first dose. If present, notify prescriber, stop oxybutynin therapy, as ordered, and provide emergency supportive care.

WARNING Watch for adverse cardiovascular reactions in patients with arrhythmias, coronary artery disease, heart failure, or hypertension because drug's anti-muscarinic effects may increase their risk.

- Keep in mind that decreased GI motility can cause adynamic ileus; assess for abdominal pain and ileus. Also use with caution in patients who have intestinal atony or ulcerative colitis, because of decreased gastrointestinal motility.
- Be aware that drug may aggravate benign prostatic hyperplasia, gastroesophageal reflux disease, and hyperthyroidism.
- Monitor patient for anticholinergic CNS effects, such as agitation, confusion, hallucinations, and somnolence, especially in the first few months of therapy or when dosage is increased. If such effects occur, notify prescriber and expect dosage to be reduced or drug discontinued.

PATIENT TEACHING

- Instruct patient to take oxybutynin on an empty stomach. If adverse GI reactions develop, suggest taking drug with food or milk.
- Advise patient to swallow E.R. tablets whole and not to break, chew, or crush them.
- Instruct patient how to apply gel transdermal system. Tell her to apply to clean, dry skin, avoiding areas that have been recently shaved or have open sores or rashes. Remind patient to wash hands after handling product.
- Warn patient that gel is flammable and that she should avoid open fire or smoking until gel has dried. Also tell patient to avoid bathing, exercising, showering, swimming, or immersing application site in water for 1 hour after application and to cover site with clothing once gel has dried.
- Warn of possible decreased alertness, and advise patient against performing hazardous activities until drug's CNS effects are known.
- Caution patient to avoid excessive sun exposure and strenuous exercise because of increased risk of heatstroke.
- Urge patient to avoid alcohol during therapy.
- Instruct patient to seek immediate emergency care if he experiences swelling of his face, lips, throat, or tongue, or if he has difficulty breathing.

oxycodone hydrochloride

Oxecta, OxyContin, Roxicodone, Supeudol (CAN), Xtampza ER

Class, Category, and Schedule

Pharmacologic class: Opioid
Therapeutic class: Opioid analgesic
Pregnancy category: Not classified
Controlled substance schedule: II

Indications and Dosages

➤ *To relieve pain severe enough to require opioid treatment and for which alternative treatment options such as nonopioid analgesics or opioid combination products are inadequate or not tolerated*

ORAL SOLUTION (ROXICODONE), TABLETS (OXECTA, ROXICODONE)
Adults. 5 to 15 mg every 4 to 6 hr, as needed.

SUPPOSITORY (SUPEUDOL)
Adults. 1 suppository three to four times daily, as needed.

TABLETS (SUPEUDOL)
Adults. 5 to 10 mg every 6 hr, as needed.

➤ *To manage moderate to severe pain when a continuous around-the-clock opioid analgesic is needed for an extended period of time*

CONTROLLED-RELEASE TABLETS, E.R. TABLETS (OXYCONTIN)
Adults who haven't received opioids before; adults converting from other opioids. *Initial:* 10 mg every 12 hr, increased by 25% to 50% of current total daily dosage every 1 to 2 days, as needed.
Adults converting from other oral oxycodone formulations. Highly individualized. *Usual:* Half the 24-hr oxycodone dose every 12 hr.
Adults converting from methadone. Highly individualized.
Adults and children age 11 and over converting from fentanyl transdermal patch. Highly individualized. *Usual:* 10 mg oxycodone for each 25 mcg/hr of fentanyl patch dosage every 12 hr, beginning 18 hr after removing patch.
Children age 11 and over who are already receiving opioids for at least 5 consecutive days and requiring at least 20 mg of oxycodone daily. *Initial:* 20 mg every 12 hr, increased by 25% of total daily dosage every 1 to 2 days, as needed.

E.R. CAPSULES (XTAMPZA ER)
Adults who are opioid-naive, not opioid tolerant, or converting from other opioids. 9 mg every 12 hr with food, increased as needed with dose adjusted to obtain balance between management of pain and opioid-related adverse reactions. *Maximum:* 288 mg daily in split doses.
Adults converting from other oral oxycodone formulations. Highly individualized. *Usual:* Half the 24-hr oxycodone dose every 12 hr.
Adults converting from methadone. Highly individualized.

DOSAGE ADJUSTMENT For elderly patients, patients with hepatic impairment, or patients currently taking a CNS depressant, one-third to one-half the usual starting dose and then adjusted, as needed.

Route	Onset	Peak	Duration
P.O.	10–15 min	1 hr	3–4 hr
P.R.	15–30 min	Unknown	Unknown

Mechanism of Action

Alters perception of and emotional response to pain at spinal cord and higher levels of CNS by blocking release of inhibitory neurotransmitters, such as acetylcholine and gamma-aminobutyric acid.

Contraindications

Acute or severe bronchial asthma or hypercarbia in an unmonitored setting or in the absence of resuscitative equipment, gastrointestinal obstruction, hypersensitivity to oxycodone or its components, paralytic ileus, significant respiratory depression

Interactions

DRUGS

anticholinergics: Possibly severe constipation and ileus
antidiarrheals: Possibly severe constipation and additive CNS depression
antihypertensives: Possibly exaggerated antihypertensive effects and risk of orthostatic hypotension
antimigraine agents, cyclobenzaprine; dextromethorphan; dolasetron; granisetron; linezolid; MAO inhibitors; methylene blue; ondansetron; palonosetron; selected psychiatric drugs such as amoxapine, buspirone, lithium, maprotiline, mirtazapine, nefazodone, trazodone, vilazodone; selective serotonin reuptake inhibitors; serotonin-norepinephrine reuptake inhibitors; St. John's wort; tricyclic antidepressants; tryptophan: Increased risk of serotonin syndrome
benzodiazepines, CNS depressants, other opioids, sedating antihistamines, tricyclic antidepressants: Increased risk of severe respiratory depression and significant sedation and somnolence
butorphanol, pentazocine: Possibly acute withdrawal symptoms in opioid-dependent patients, decreased analgesic effects
carbamazepine, phenytoin, primidone, rifampin: Possibly need for increased oxycodone dosage to achieve analgesia and prevent withdrawal symptoms in opioid-dependent patients
cimetidine: Possibly apnea, confusion, disorientation, and seizures from respiratory depression and impaired CNS function
CNS depressants: Possibly increased CNS and respiratory depression and orthostatic hypotension that could result in life-threatening reactions
CYP3A4 inhibitors such as azole-antifungal drugs, macrolide antibiotics, and protease inhibitors: Possibly increased plasma oxycodone levels and prolonged opioid effects with possible overdose effects
MAO inhibitors: Possibly fatal reactions, including cardiac arrest, coma, respiratory depression, seizures, and severe hypertension
nalbuphine, nalmefene, naloxone, naltrexone: Blocked oxycodone effects, withdrawal symptoms in opioid-dependent patients

ACTIVITIES

alcohol use: Additive CNS and respiratory depressive effects that may become severe

Adverse Reactions

CNS: Abnormal dreams, anxiety, asthenia, chills, dizziness, drowsiness, euphoria, excitation, headache, insomnia, nervousness, sedation, **seizures**, somnolence, syncope, twitching
CV: Bradycardia, chest pain, **hypotension**, orthostatic hypotension, palpitations
EENT: Blurred vision, **choking** or difficulty swallowing tablets (OxyContin), dry eyes or mouth, lens opacities, miosis
ENDO: Adrenal insufficiency (rare), syndrome of inappropriate antidiuretic hormone secretion
GI: Abdominal pain, anorexia, constipation, diarrhea, dyspepsia, dysphagia, elevated liver enzymes, gastritis, hiccups, ileus, nausea, vomiting
GU: Amenorrhea, decreased libido, erectile dysfunction, impotence, infertility, lack of menstruation, oliguria, urinary hesitancy, urine retention

RESP: Dyspnea, **respiratory depression**
SKIN: Diaphoresis, pruritus, rash
Other: Anaphylaxis, drug tolerance, **hyponatremia**, physical and psychological dependence, withdrawal symptoms

Nursing Considerations

- Be aware that excessive use of opioids like oxycodone may lead to abuse, addiction, misuse, overdose, and possibly death. For this reason, a Risk Evaluation and Mitigation Strategy (REMS) is required for oxycodone to be prescribed. Monitor patient's intake of drug closely and for evidence of physical dependence.
- Know that chronic maternal use of oxycodone during pregnancy can result in NOWS, which may be life-threatening if not recognized and treated appropriately. NOWS occurs when a newborn has been exposed to opioid drugs like oxycodone for a prolonged period while in utero.
- Use extreme caution when administering oxycodone to patients with conditions accompanied by hypoxia or decreased respiratory reserve such as asthma, COPD, or cor pulmonale. This is because even with usual therapeutic dosages, oxycodone may decrease respiratory drive while simultaneously increasing airway resistance to the point of apnea. Monitor patient's respiratory status closely, especially in cachectic, debilitated, and elderly patients and in patients with chronic pulmonary disease. Respiratory depression may occur at any time, but it is most likely to occur during the initiation of therapy or following a dose increase. Have resuscitative equipment nearby.
- Use oxycodone with extreme caution in patients who may be at risk for carbon dioxide retention (e.g., those with increased intracranial pressure or brain tumors). Monitor for signs of sedation and respiratory depression, especially when initiating therapy. Oxycodone may reduce respiratory drive, and the resultant carbon dioxide retention can further increase intracranial pressure. Also know that opioids like oxycodone may obscure signs and symptoms in a patient with a head injury.

WARNING Be aware that oxycodone should only be used concomitantly with benzodiazepine therapy in patients for whom other treatment options are inadequate. If prescribed together, expect dosing and duration of oxycodone to be limited. Monitor patient closely for signs and symptoms of a decrease in consciousness, including coma, profound sedation, and significant respiratory depression. Notify prescriber immediately and provide emergency supportive care, as death may occur.

- Assess patient's pain level regularly, and give drug as prescribed before pain becomes severe.
- Be careful to have patient swallow one controlled-release tablet (OxyContin) at a time, with enough water to ensure complete swallowing immediately after the patient places the tablet in his mouth; otherwise, choking on tablets or difficulty swallowing the tablets may occur due to the swelling and hydrogelling property of the tablet if left in the mouth too long.
- Be prepared to adjust dosage for patient who hasn't previously received opioids, as prescribed, until he can tolerate drug effects.
- Expect to give controlled-release tablets only to opioid-tolerant adult patients who need at least 160 mg daily.
- Monitor patient's blood pressure closely, especially when initiating oxycodone therapy and when titrating the dose, because oxycodone may cause severe hypotension and syncope in ambulatory patients due to its vasodilatory effects. Risk of hypotension is greater in patients who already have been compromised by a reduced blood volume or concurrent administration of certain CNS depressant drugs, such as general anesthetics and phenothiazines.
- Assess patient for possible paradoxical excitation during dosage titration.
- Assess patient for abdominal pain because oxycodone may mask underlying GI disorders.

WARNING Know that many drugs may interact with opioids like oxycodone to cause serotonin syndrome. Monitor patient closely for signs and symptoms such as agitation, diaphoresis, diarrhea, fever, hallucinations, labile blood pressure, muscle twitching or stiffness, nausea, shakiness, shivering, tachycardia, trouble with coordination, or vomiting. Notify prescriber at once because serotonin syndrome may be life-threatening. Be prepared to discontinue drug, if possible and ordered, and provide supportive care.

- Monitor patient for adrenal insufficiency. Although rare, it can be life-threatening. Monitor patient for anorexia, dizziness, fatigue, hypotension, nausea, vomiting, or weakness. Notify prescriber if adrenal insufficiency is suspected and expect diagnostic testing to be done. If confirmed, expect to administer corticosteroids and wean patient off oxycodone, if possible.
- Monitor patients with seizure disorders closely because oxycodone may induce or aggravate seizures.

WARNING Be aware that oxycodone given concomitantly with CYP3A4 inhibitors (or if CYP3A4 inducers are discontinued) can result in a fatal overdose of oxycodone.

WARNING Be aware that abuse of crushed controlled-release tablets poses a hazard of overdose and death. If you suspect abuse and determine that patient also is abusing alcohol or illicit substances, notify prescriber immediately because risk of overdose and death is increased. If you suspect parenteral abuse, be aware that tablet excipients, especially talc, may result in endocarditis, infection, local tissue necrosis, pulmonary granulomas, and valvular heart injury.

- Know that oxycodone therapy should not be stopped abruptly in a physically dependent patient.

PATIENT TEACHING

WARNING Strongly warn patient to swallow oxycodone tablets whole and not to break, chew, or crush them because taking broken, chewed, or crushed tablets leads to rapid release and absorption of a potentially fatal dose.

- Remind patient that Xtampza ER capsules must be taken with food. Tell patient to consume about the same amount of food for every dose in order to maintain consistent blood levels of the drug.
- Instruct patient not to take oxycodone more often than prescribed and not to take it longer than absolutely needed because excessive or prolonged use can lead to abuse, addiction, misuse, overdose, and possibly death. Also warn patient not to stop abruptly after long-term use.
- Caution patient prescribed controlled-release tablets to take one tablet at a time; not to presoak, lick, or otherwise wet the tablet prior to placing in his mouth; and to take each tablet with enough water to ensure complete swallowing of tablet.
- Advise patient prescribed suppository form to store drug in refrigerator for 30 minutes or run under cold water if it is too soft to administer.

WARNING Warn patient not to consume alcohol or take a benzodiazepine without prescriber knowledge, as severe respiratory depression can occur and may lead to death.

- Caution patient to avoid hazardous activities such as driving during oxycodone therapy.
- Tell patient to notify prescriber about signs of possible toxicity or hypersensitivity, such as excessive light-headedness, extreme dizziness, itching, swelling, and trouble breathing.
- Warn patient to keep drug out of reach of children because ingestion of the drug by a child can be fatal.
- Inform patient that long-term use of opioids like oxycodone may decrease sex hormone levels, causing decreased libido, erectile dysfunction, impotence, infertility, or lack of menstruation. Encourage patient to report any symptoms to prescriber.
- Caution pregnant patient not to increase dosage or take drug for a prolonged period, as adverse effects can cause infant to experience life-threatening withdrawal when born.
- Instruct patient to notify all prescribers of opioid use.

oxymorphone hydrochloride

Numorphan, Opana

Class, Category, and Schedule

Pharmacologic class: Opioid

Therapeutic class: Opioid analgesic
Pregnancy category: Not classified
Controlled substance schedule: II

Indications and Dosages

➤ *To relieve pain severe enough to require opioid treatment and for which alternative treatment options such as nonopioid analgesics or opioid combination products are inadequate or not tolerated.*

TABLETS (OPANA)

Adults receiving an opioid for first time. *Initial:* 5 to 20 mg every 4 to 6 hr, as needed.

Adults converting from parenteral oxymorphone. *Initial:* 10 times the patient's total daily parenteral oxymorphone dose divided by 4 or 6 to provide four or six equally divided doses every 4 to 6 hr.

Adults converting from other oral opioids. Highly individualized.

DOSAGE ADJUSTMENT For opioid-naive patients with mild hepatic impairment or who have a creatinine clearance less than 50 ml/min or for opioid-naive patients over the age of 65, initial dosage started at 5 mg. For patients on prior opioid therapy with creatinine clearance less than 50 ml/min or who are over the age of 65, initial dosage decreased by 50%. For patients receiving other CNS depressants, dosage started at one-third to one-half the usual starting dose.

➤ *To provide support for anesthesia and use as preoperative medication; to relieve anxiety in patients with dyspnea from pulmonary edema caused by acute left ventricular dysfunction; to relieve obstetrical pain*

I.V. INJECTION (NUMORPHAN)

Adults. *Initial:* 0.5 mg, repeated every 3 to 6 hr, as needed.

I.M. OR SUBCUTANEOUS INJECTION (NUMORPHAN)

Adults. *Initial:* 1 to 1.5 mg, repeated every 4 to 6 hr, as needed.

SUPPOSITORIES (NUMORPHAN)

Adults. 5 mg every 4 to 6 hr, as needed.

➤ *To relieve obstetric pain during labor*

I.M. INJECTION (NUMORPHAN)

Adults. 0.5 to 1 mg as a single dose.

DOSAGE ADJUSTMENT For patients with renal impairment with a creatinine clearance rate less than 50 ml/min, dosage reduced. For patients receiving concomitant CNS depressants, dosage for injection form reduced by one-third to one-half.

Route	Onset	Peak	Duration
I.V.	5–10 min	15–30 min	3–4 hr
I.M.	10–15 min	30–90 min	3–6 hr
SubQ	10–20 min	30–90 min	3–6 hr
P.R.	15–30 min	2 hr	3–6 hr

Mechanism of Action

Alters perception of and emotional response to pain at spinal cord and higher levels of CNS by blocking release of inhibitory neurotransmitters, such as acetylcholine and gamma-aminobutyric acid.

Contraindications

Acute or severe asthma; gastrointestinal obstruction including paralytic ileus; hypercarbia; hypersensitivity to oxymorphone, other morphine analogues, or their components; moderate to severe hepatic impairment; pulmonary edema from a chemical respiratory irritant; severe respiratory depression; upper airway obstruction

Interactions

DRUGS

anticholingerics: Increased risk of urine retention, severe constipation

antidiarrheals, antiperistaltics: Increased risk of severe CNS depression, constipation

antihypertensives, diuretics, hypotension-producing drugs: Increased hypotensive effects

antimigraine agents, cyclobenzaprine; dextromethorphan; dolasetron; granisetron; linezolid; MAO inhibitors; methylene blue; ondansetron; palonosetron; selected psychiatric drugs such as amoxapine, buspirone, lithium, maprotiline, mirtazapine, nefazodone, trazodone, vilazodone; selective serotonin reuptake inhibitors; serotonin-norepinephrine reuptake inhibitors; St. John's wort; tricyclic antidepressants; tryptophan: Increased risk of serotonin syndrome

benzodiazepines, CNS depressants, other opioids, sedating antihistamines, tricyclic

antidepressants: Increased risk of severe respiratory depression and significant sedation and somnolence
buprenorphine: Reduced oxymorphone effectiveness if buprenorphine is given first, possibly withdrawal symptoms in oxymorphone-dependent patients
hydroxyzine, other opioid analgesics: Increased analgesia, CNS depression, and hypotensive effects
MAO inhibitors: Increased risk of unpredictable, severe, sometimes fatal adverse reactions
metoclopramide: Antagonized effects of metoclopramide on GI motility
naloxone: Antagonized analgesic, CNS, and respiratory depressant effects of oxymorphone
naltrexone: Withdrawal symptoms in oxymorphone-dependent patients
neuromuscular blockers: Additive respiratory depression

ACTIVITIES

alcohol use: Additive CNS and respiratory depressant effects which could be severe, increased risk of habituation

Adverse Reactions

CNS: Agitation, asthenia, CNS depression, confusion, delusions, depersonalization, dizziness, drowsiness, euphoria, fatigue, hallucinations, headache, insomnia, light-headedness, nervousness, nightmares, restlessness, **seizures**, somnolence, tiredness, tremor, weakness
CV: **Bradycardia**, hypertension, **hypotension**, palpitations, tachycardia
EENT: Blurred vision, diplopia, dry mouth, **laryngeal edema**, **laryngospasm**, miosis, tinnitus
ENDO: **Adrenal insufficiency**
GI: Abdominal cramps or pain, anorexia, bilary colic, constipation, elevated serum amylase level, **hepatotoxcity**, ileus, nausea, spasm of the sphincter of Oddi (E.R. tablets), vomiting
GU: Decreased urine output, decreased libido, dysuria, erectile dysfunction, impotence, infertility, lack of menstruation, urinary frequency and hesitancy, urine retention
MS: Muscle rigidity (with large doses), uncontrolled muscle movements
RESP: **Apnea**, **atelectasis**, **bradypnea**, **bronchospasm**, dyspnea, irregular breathing, **irregular breathing**, **respiratory depression**, wheezing
SKIN: Dermatitis, diaphoresis, erythema, flushing of face, pruritus, urticaria
Other: **Angioedema**; injection-site burning, pain, redness, and swelling; psychological and physical dependence

Nursing Considerations

- Be aware that excessive use of opioids like oxymorphone may lead to abuse, addiction, misuse, overdose, and possibly death. Monitor patient's intake of drug closely and watch for evidence of physical dependence. Know that drug use now requires a Risk Evaluation and Mitigation Strategy (REMS) for a prescription.
- Know that chronic maternal use of oxymorphone during pregnancy can result in NOWS, which may be life-threatening if not recognized and treated appropriately. NOWS occurs when a newborn has been exposed to opioid drugs like oxymorphone for a prolonged period while in utero.
- Use extreme caution when administering oxymorphone to patients with conditions accompanied by decreased respiratory reserve or hypoxia, such as asthma, COPD, or cor pulmonale. This is because oxymorphone, even with usual therapeutic dosages, may decrease respiratory drive while simultaneously increasing airway resistance to the point of apnea.
- Use oxymorphone with extreme caution in patients who may be at risk for carbon dioxide retention (e.g., those with brain tumors or increased intracranial pressure). Monitor for signs of respiratory depression and sedation, especially when initiating therapy. Oxymorphone may reduce respiratory drive, and the resultant carbon dioxide retention can further increase intracranial pressure. Also know that opioids like oxymorphone may obscure signs and symptoms in a patient with a head injury.
- Use cautiously in patients with biliary tract disease because drug may cause spasm of sphincter of Oddi; mild

hepatic impairment because drug is metabolized in liver; and impaired renal function because drug is excreted by kidneys.

- Use cautiously in patients receiving mixed agonist-antagonist opioid analgesics because these drugs may reduce analgesic effect of oxymorphone or may cause withdrawal symptoms.
- Use cautiously in elderly patients because plasma oxymorphone levels in the elderly are higher than in younger patients.
- Know that oral hydromorphone shouldn't be used "as needed" or for first 24 hours after surgery in patients not already taking opioids because of the risk of oversedation and respiratory depression.
- Taper dosage, as ordered, before stopping therapy to prevent withdrawal in physically dependent patients.

WARNING Monitor patient's respiratory status closely for respiratory depression, especially in cachectic, debilitated, or elderly patients; when initiating or titrating dosages; or when other drugs that depress respiration are given together. Have resuscitative equipment nearby. Report respiratory depression immediately, because severe respiratory depression may occur. Be prepared to provide supportive care.

- Monitor patient's blood pressure closely, especially when initiating oxymorphone therapy and when titrating the dose because oxymorphone may cause severe hypotension and syncope in ambulatory patients due to its vasodilatory effects. Risk of hypotension is greatest in patients who already have been compromised by a reduced blood volume or concurrent administration of certain CNS depressant drugs, such as general anesthetics and phenothiazines.

WARNING Know that many drugs may interact with opioids like oxymorphone to cause serotonin syndrome. Monitor patient closely for signs and symptoms such as agitation, diaphoresis, diarrhea, fever, hallucinations, labile blood pressure, muscle twitching or stiffness, nausea, shakiness, shivering, tachycardia, trouble with coordination, or vomiting. Notify prescriber at once because serotonin syndrome may be life-threatening. Be prepared to discontinue drug, if possible and ordered, and provide supportive care.

- Monitor patient for adrenal insufficiency. Although rare, it can be life-threatening. Monitor patient for anorexia, dizziness, fatigue, hypotension, nausea, vomiting, or weakness. Notify prescriber if adrenal insufficiency is suspected and expect diagnostic testing to be done. If confirmed, expect to administer corticosteroids and wean patient off oxymorphone, if possible.
- Monitor patient for signs of excessive opioid-related adverse reactions. If present, notify prescriber and expect next dose to be reduced.
- Monitor bowel and urinary status; constipation may be so severe it causes ileus.
- Offer fluids to relieve dry mouth.

WARNING Be aware that oxymorphone should only be used concomitantly with benzodiazepine therapy in patients for whom other treatment options are inadequate. If prescribed together, expect dosing and duration of oxymorphone to be limited. Monitor patient closely for signs and symptoms of a decrease in consciousness, including coma, profound sedation, and significant respiratory depression. Notify prescriber immediately and provide emergency supportive care, as death may occur.

PATIENT TEACHING

- Instruct patient to take oxymorphone exactly as prescribed and not to stop abruptly; warn that drug can cause abuse, misuse, overdose, physical dependence, and possibly death.
- Emphasize importance of taking drug before pain becomes severe.
- Instruct patient prescribed oxymorphone in tablet form to take it on an empty stomach.
- Instruct patient to store suppositories in refrigerator.
- Encourage patient to increase fluid and fiber intake during therapy to prevent constipation.
- Emphasize need to avoid alcohol, benzodiazepine therapy, and CNS depressants during therapy because of risk of severe life-threatening adverse reactions.

- Caution patient to avoid potentially hazardous activities until drug's CNS effects are known.
- Advise female patient to notify prescriber about known or suspected pregnancy because if fetus is exposed to opioids for a prolonged period, the baby may experience withdrawal when born.
- Warn patient to keep drug out of the reach of children, as accidental ingestion may be fatal.
- Inform patient that long-term use of opioids like oxymorphone may decrease sex hormone levels, causing decreased libido, erectile dysfunction, impotence, infertility, or lack of menstruation. Encourage patient to report any symptoms to prescriber.
- Instruct patient to notify all prescribers of opioid use.

P

paliperidone
Invega
paliperidone palmitate
Invega Sustenna, Invega Trinza

Class and Category
Pharmacologic class: Benzisoxazole derivative
Therapeutic class: Antipsychotic (atypical)
Pregnancy category: C

Indications and Dosages
➤ *To treat schizophrenia*
E.R. TABLETS (INVEGA)
Adults. *Initial:* 6 mg once daily in the morning; then increased or decreased in increments of 3 mg daily every 6 or more days, as needed. *Maximum:* 12 mg daily.
Adolescents 12 to 17. *Initial:* 3 mg once daily; then increased in increments of 3 mg daily every 6 or more days, as needed.
I.M. INJECTION (INVEGA SUSTENNA)
Adults. *Initial:* 234 mg on day 1 and 156 mg 1 wk later. *Maintenance:* 39 to 234 mg monthly. Maintenance dosage decreased or increased monthly according to patient's response and tolerance. *Maximum:* 234 mg monthly.
I.M. INJECTION (INVEGA TRINZA)
Adults who have been adequately treated with Invega Sustenna for at least 4 mo. *Initial:* 273 mg if last monthly Sustenna dose was 78 mg; 410 mg if last monthly Sustenna dose was 117 mg; 546 mg if last monthly Sustenna dose was 156 mg; or 819 mg if last monthly Sustenna dose was 234 mg, administered within 7 days before or after next monthly Sustenna dose would have been given with dosage adjustment made thereafter every 3 mo, as needed. *Maintenance:* 273 to 819 mg every 3 mo. *Maximum:* 819 mg every 3 mo.
➤ *To treat schizoaffective disorder*
E.R. TABLETS (INVEGA)
Adults. *Initial:* 6 mg once daily; then increased or decreased in increments of 3 mg daily every 4 or more days, as needed. *Maximum:* 12 mg daily.
I.M. INJECTION (INVEGA SUSTENNA)
Adults. *Initial:* 234 mg on day 1 and 156 mg 1 wk later. *Maintenance:* 78 to 234 mg monthly. Maintenance dosage decreased or increased monthly according to patient's response and tolerance. *Maximum:* 234 mg monthly.
DOSAGE ADJUSTMENT For patients taking E.R. tablets with mild renal impairment (creatinine clearance 50 to 79 ml/min), initial dosage decreased to 3 mg daily then increased to maximum dosage 6 mg daily; moderate to severe renal impairment (creatinine clearance less than 50 ml/min), initial dose decreased to 1.5 mg daily, then increased to maximum dosage of 3 mg daily. For patient receiving Invega Sustenna with mild renal impairment (creatinine clearance equal to or greater than 50 ml/min but less than 80 ml/min), initial dosage decreased to 156 mg on day 1 and second dose given 1 wk later decreased to 117 mg, followed by 78 mg monthly. For patient receiving Invega Sustenna and a strong CYP3A4 inducer such as carbamazepine, rifampin, or St. John's wort, dosage may have to be increased, and when the strong CYP3A4 inducer is discontinued, dosage may have to be decreased. For patient receiving Invega Trinza with mild renal impairment, dosage adjustment follows Invega sustenna guidelines.

Route	Onset	Peak	Duration
P.O.	Unknown	24 hr	Unknown
I.M.	1 day	13 days	126 days

Mechanism of Action
The main active metabolite of risperidone, paliperidone selectively blocks serotonin and dopamine receptors in mesocortical tract of CNS to suppress psychotic symptoms.

Contraindications
AV block, cardiac arrhythmias, congenital heart disease, history of congenital long-QT syndrome; hypersensitivity to paliperidone, risperidone, or its components

Interactions
DRUGS
alpha agonists, alpha blockers, angiotensin-converting enzyme (ACE) inhibitors,

angiotensin II receptor blockers (ARBs), beta blockers, calcium channel blockers, diuretics including thiazide, nitrates, vasodilators: Increased risk of hypotension, including orthostatic
antiarrhythmics of class IA (such as quinidine, procainamide) and class III (such as amiodarone, sotalol), antibiotics (such as gatifloxacin, moxifloxacin), antipsychotics (such as chlorpromazine, thioridazine): Increased risk of QT-interval prolongation
bromocriptine, levodopa, pergolide: Possibly antagonized effects of these drugs
CNS depressants: Additive CNS depression
CYP3A4 and P-gp strong inducers (carbamazepine, rifampin, St. John's wort): Decreased plasma paliperidone level and effectiveness
paroxetine: Possible increased blood paliperidone level

ACTIVITIES

alcohol use: CNS depression

Adverse Reactions

CNS: Agitation, akathisia, anxiety, asthenia, bradykinesia, cogwheel rigidity, **CVA**, dizziness, drooling, dyskinesia, dystonia, extrapyramidal disorder, fatigue, fever, headache, hyperkinesia, hypertonia, insomnia, lethargy, **neuroleptic malignant syndrome**, nightmares, nuchal rigidity, Parkinsonism, psychomotor hyperactivity, restlessness, **seizures**, somnolence, **suicidal ideation**, syncope, tardive dyskinesia, transient ischemic attack, tremor, vertigo
CV: Bradycardia, bundle branch block, elevated cholesterol and triglyceride level, first-degree heart block, hypertension, ischemia, orthostatic hypotension, palpitations, peripheral edema, **prolonged QT interval**, tachycardia, **venous thrombosis**
EENT: Blurred vision, dry mouth, eye movement disorder, nasal congestion, nasopharyngitis, oromandibular dystonia, pharyngolaryngeal pain, rhinitis, salivary hypersecretion, swollen tongue, toothache
ENDO: Breast engorgement, pain, or tenderness; gynecomastia; hyperglycemia; hyperprolactinemia
GI: Abdominal discomfort, constipation, diarrhea, dyspepsia, flatulence, ileus, nausea, **small intestinal obstruction**, upper abdominal pain, vomiting
GU: Erectile dysfunction, menstrual abnormalities, priapism, urinary incontinence or retention, UTI
HEME: Agranulocytosis, **leukopenia**, **neutropenia**, **thrombocytopenia**, **thrombotic thrombocytopenic purpura**
MS: Arthralgia; back or limb pain; dysarthria; joint stiffness; muscle rigidity, spasms, tightness, or twitching; myalgia; torticollis, trismus
RESP: Cough, dyspnea, upper respiratory tract infection
SKIN: Drug eruption, pruritus, rash, urticaria
Other: Anaphylaxis, **angioedema**, injection-site reactions, weight gain

Nursing Considerations

- Keep in mind paliperidone shouldn't be used to treat dementia-related psychosis in the elderly because of an increased mortality risk. Parenteral paliperidone is not recommended for patients with moderate to severe renal impairment.
- Know that drug shouldn't be given if patient has a condition that severely narrows GI tract because tablet doesn't change shape as it passes and could cause blockage.
- Use paliperidone cautiously in patients with cardiovascular disease, because drug may cause orthostatic hypotension. Also use cautiously in patients with Lewy bodies, because these patients are more sensitive to antipsychotic drugs. Monitor patient for increased sensitivity manifested as confusion, extrapyramidal symptoms, neuroleptic malignant syndrome clinical features, postural instability with frequent falls, and obtundation.
- Be aware that the long-acting preparation (Invega Sustenna) should be initiated only after patient has been established with oral paliperidone or oral risperidone therapy. Also know that Invega Trinza should not be given until patient has received Invega Sustenna for at least 4 months.
- Administer parenteral paliperidone slowly as a deep intramuscular injection. The first two injections should be administered in the deltoid muscle; thereafter, the injection may be administered in the deltoid or gluteal muscle. Use a 1.5-inch 22G needle for gluteal administration or, if

the patient weighs more than 200 pounds, for injecting drug into the deltoid muscle. If patient weighs less than 200 pounds, use a 1-inch 23G needle when administering drug in the deltoid muscle.

- Know that if the due date for the parenteral dose is missed, the recommended reinitiation depends on the length of time that has elapsed since the patient's last injection. To avoid missing a dose, the prescriber may order the parenteral dose to be given up to 7 days before or after the due date.
- Be aware that when a patient who has been taking a long-acting injectable antipsychotic consistently is now switching to the long-lasting 1 month preparation of paliperidone, the first dose of paliperidone is given in place of the next scheduled injection of the other medication. Parenteral long-acting 1 month preparation of paliperidone therapy is then continued at monthly intervals. The 1-week initiation dosing is not required.
- Know that the patient may switch from the 3-month long-acting paliperidone preparation to the 1 month preparation or to E.R. tablets. When doing so the new preparation is begun 3 months after the last dose of the long-acting 3-month preparation and dosage adjustment made according to the new preparation guidelines.

WARNING Notify prescriber immediately and expect to stop drug if patient shows signs of neuroleptic malignant syndrome (altered mental status, autonomic instability, hyperpyrexia, muscle rigidity). Patients at risk for developing neuroleptic malignant syndrome are patients with dementia with Lewy bodies or Parkinson's disease because these patients can experience increased sensitivity to paliperidone.

- Monitor patient for involuntary, dyskinetic movements. Notify prescriber if present, and expect to stop therapy. In some cases, therapy may have to continue despite tardive dyskinesia.
- Monitor blood glucose level because drug increases risk of hyperglycemia and possible hyperosmolar coma or ketoacidosis.
- Keep in mind dosage adjustments of paliperidone may be needed when carbamazepine therapy is started or discontinued because of carbamazepine's interaction with paliperidone.
- Check CBC often during first few months of therapy, especially if patient has low WBC count or history of drug-induced leukopenia or neutropenia. If WBC count declines, and especially if neutrophil count goes below 1,000/mm^3, expect to stop drug. If neutropenia is significant, also watch for evidence of infection and provide appropriate treatment, as prescribed.
- Watch patient closely for suicidal tendencies, especially when therapy starts or dosage changes.
- Institute fall measures because of potential for adverse CNS effects.

PATIENT TEACHING

- Instruct patient to take tablet whole with liquid beverage. Caution against chewing, crushing, or splitting it because it's designed to release drug at a controlled rate.
- Explain that shell of tablet will be eliminated in stool and that patient need not worry if he sees tablet in stool.
- Urge patient to rise slowly from sitting or lying position to minimize orthostatic hypotension.
- Caution patient to avoid hazardous activities until CNS effects of drug are known. Review fall precautions with patient as well.
- Advise patient to avoid activities that may cause overheating, such as becoming dehydrated, being exposed to extreme heat, or exercising strenuously.
- Urge family or caregiver to watch patient closely for suicidal tendencies, especially when therapy starts or dosage changes.
- Advise female patient of childbearing age to notify prescriber if she intends to become or suspects that she is pregnant during therapy because neonates exposed to paliperidone during the third trimester of pregnancy are at risk for extrapyramidal and/or withdrawal symptoms following delivery. If pregnancy occurs, encourage patient to enroll in the pregnancy registry.
- Inform mothers who wish to breastfeed to discuss breastfeeding with prescriber before doing so, because paliperidone is present in breast milk and may cause

adverse effects in infant. If breastfeeding occurs, instruct mother to monitor her infant for abnormal muscle movements, excess sedation, failure to thrive, jitteriness, or tremors.

- Alert the patient who experiences hyperprolactinemia as a result of paliperidone therapy that reproductive function may become impaired. If this is a concern for the patient, she should consult prescriber.
- Instruct patient to alert prescriber immediately if he experiences any persistent, severe, or unusual signs and symptoms.
- Tell patient to contact prescriber if abnormal movements occur.
- Instruct patient with diabetes to monitor her blood glucose level closely, as drug can affect glycemic control. Also review signs and symptoms of hyperglycemia with all patients and tell them to notify prescriber if present.
- Tell male patients that painful or prolonged penile erections can occur while taking paliperidone. Instruct him to seek immediate emergency medical attention if this occurs.
- Advise patient to notify all prescribers of paliperidone therapy and not to take over-the-counter preparations, including herbal products, without consulting prescriber.

palonosetron hydrochloride

Aloxi

Class and Category

Pharmacologic class: Selective serotonin subtype 3 (5-HT_3) receptor antagonist
Therapeutic class: Antiemetic
Pregnancy category: B

Indications and Dosages

➤ *To prevent acute and delayed nausea and vomiting from chemotherapy*

CAPSULES

Adults. 0.5 mg 1 hr before chemotherapy.

I.V. INJECTION

Adults. 0.25 mg over 30 sec about 30 min before start of chemotherapy.
Infants 1 month of age and over, children, and adolescents ages 12 to 17. 20 mcg/kg over 15 sec about 30 min before start of chemotherapy. *Maximum:* 1.5 mg.

➤ *To prevent postoperative nausea and vomiting for up to 24 hr after surgery*

I.V. INJECTION

Adults. 0.075 mg over 10 sec immediately before induction of anesthesia.

Incompatibilities

Palonosetron shouldn't be mixed with any other drug.

Contraindications

Hypersensitivity to palonosetron or its components

Adverse Reactions

CNS: Anxiety, dizziness, drowsiness, dyskinesia, fatigue, headache, insomnia, **serotonin syndrome**, weakness
CV: Bradycardia, hypotension, prolonged QT interval, tachycardia
GI: Abdominal pain, constipation, diarrhea
SKIN: Dermatitis, pruritus, rash
Other: Hyperkalemia, hypersensitivity reactions, injection-site reaction (burning, discomfort, induration, pain)

Nursing Considerations

- Use palonosetron cautiously in patients who have or may develop prolonged cardiac conduction intervals—especially QT interval—such as those with congenital QT syndrome, hypokalemia, or hypomagnesemia; those taking an antiarrhythmic, a diuretic known to induce electrolyte abnormalities, or another drug that may prolong QT interval; and those who have received cumulative high-dose anthracycline therapy. With these patients, obtain a baseline ECG before giving palonosetron; repeat the ECG 15 minutes or 24 hours after giving drug, as ordered. Notify prescriber of any delayed conduction.
- Flush I.V. line with normal saline solution before and after giving I.V. palonosetron.
- Use either the single-dose vial or the pre-filled syringe to administer a 0.25-mg dose. Do not use the pre-filled syringe to administer a dose other than 0.25 mg.

Mechanism of Action

Chemotherapy may induce nausea and vomiting by irritating the small intestine's mucosa, causing mucosal enterochromaffin cells to release serotonin (5-HT_3). The 5-HT_3 stimulates sympathetic receptors on afferent vagal nerve endings, and the vagus nerve causes the vomiting reflex.

Palonosetron selectively blocks these 5-HT_3 receptors. By keeping the vagus nerve from inducing the vomiting reflex, drug reduces or prevents nausea and vomiting. It also may block 5-HT_3 receptors centrally, in the brain's chemoreceptor trigger zone.

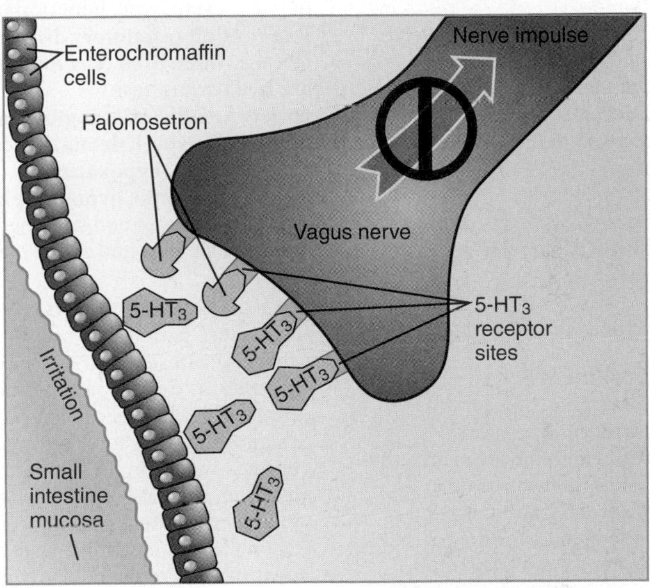

- Closely monitor any patient hypersensitive to other selective serotonin receptor antagonists for a similar reaction. If a reaction occurs, notify prescriber immediately.

WARNING Monitor patient closely for serotonin syndrome, which is characterized by agitation, coma, diarrhea, hallucinations, hyperreflexia, hyperthermia, incoordination, labile blood pressure, nausea, tachycardia, or vomiting. Notify prescriber immediately because serotonin syndrome may be life-threatening, and provide supportive care.

PATIENT TEACHING

- Advise patient to avoid hazardous activities until drug's CNS effects are known.
- Instruct patient to notify prescriber of any hypersensitivity reaction, such as allergic dermatitis or rash.

pamidronate disodium

Aredia

Class and Category

Pharmacologic class: Bisphosphonate
Therapeutic class: Antiosteoporotic
Pregnancy category: D

Indications and Dosages

➤ *To treat cancer-induced hypercalcemia that's inadequately managed by oral hydration alone*

I.V. INFUSION

Adults. 60 to 90 mg over 2 to 24 hr as a single dose when corrected serum calcium level is 12 to 13.5 mg/dl; 90 mg over 2 to 24 hr when corrected serum calcium level is greater than 13.5 mg/dl. May be repeated as prescribed after 7 days if hypercalcemia recurs.

DOSAGE ADJUSTMENT For patients with renal failure, dosage is limited to 30 mg over 4 to 24 hr, as prescribed. For patients with cardiac or renal failure, drug is given in a smaller volume of fluid or at a slower rate, as prescribed.

➤ *To treat moderate to severe Paget's disease of bone*

I.V. INFUSION

Adults. 30 mg daily over 4 hr on 3 consecutive days for a total dose of 90 mg. Repeated as needed and tolerated.

➤ *To treat osteolytic bone metastases of breast cancer*

I.V. INFUSION

Adults. 90 mg over 2 hr every 3 to 4 wk.

➤ *To treat osteolytic bone metastases of multiple myeloma*

I.V. INFUSION

Adults. 90 mg over 4 hr every mo.

Mechanism of Action

Inhibits bone resorption, possibly by impairing attachment of osteoclast precursors to mineralized bone matrix, thus reducing the rate of bone turnover in Paget's disease and osteolytic metastases. Pamidronate also reduces the flow of calcium from resorbing bone into bloodstream.

Incompatibilities

Don't mix pamidronate with calcium-containing infusion solutions, such as Ringer's solution.

Contraindications

Hypersensitivity to pamidronate, other bisphosphonates, or their components

Interactions

DRUGS

calcium-containing preparations; vitamin D preparations, such as calcifediol and calcitriol: Antagonized pamidronate effects when used to treat hypercalcemia

thalidomide: Increased risk of renal dysfunction in patients with multiple myeloma

Adverse Reactions

CNS: Confusion, fever, psychosis, visual hallucinations

CV: Hypotension

EENT: Conjunctivitis, ocular inflammation

GI: Abdominal cramps, anorexia, **GI bleeding**, indigestion, nausea, vomiting

GU: Azotemia, focal segmental glomerulosclerosis, glomerulonephropathies, hematuria, **nephritis, nephrotic syndrome, renal toxicity leading to failure**, renal tubular disorders

HEME: Leukopenia, lymphopenia

MS: Atypical fractures of femur; muscle spasms or stiffness; osteonecrosis (mainly of jaw); severe bone, joint or muscle pain

RESP: Adult respiratory distress syndrome, dyspnea, **interstitial lung disease**

SKIN: Pruritus, rash

Other: Anaphylaxis, angioedema, flu-like symptoms, **hyperkalemia, hypernatremia, hypocalcemia, hypokalemia, hypomagnesemia, hypophosphatemia**, injection-site pain and swelling, reactivation of herpes simplex and zoster infections

Nursing Considerations

- Make sure patient has had a dental checkup before invasive dental procedures during pamidronate therapy, especially if he has cancer; is receiving chemotherapy, a corticosteroid, or head or neck radiation; or has poor oral hygiene. Risk of osteonecrosis is increased in these patients.
- Obtain serum creatinine level before each treatment, as ordered. Notify prescriber of abnormal results because drug may have to be withheld or dosage adjusted until creatinine level returns to normal.

WARNING Be aware that no more than 90 mg should be given at any one time because of increased risk of serious adverse effect on kidneys.

- Monitor patient's CBC differential; hematocrit and hemoglobin; and serum electrolytes including calcium, magnesium, and phosphate levels, as ordered throughout therapy because abnormalities may occur.
- Monitor patient for hypocalcemia, especially if patient has had thyroid surgery.
- Stay alert for fever during first 3 days of therapy, especially in patients receiving high doses. If fever develops, obtain patient's CBC with differential, as ordered.
- Assess patient with anemia, leukopenia, or thrombocytopenia for worsening of the condition during first 2 weeks of therapy.

PATIENT TEACHING

- Emphasize need to comply with prescribed administration schedule for pamidronate.
- Advise patient to avoid calcium and vitamin D supplements during therapy.
- Instruct patient on proper oral hygiene and on need to notify prescriber about upcoming invasive dental procedures.
- Advise women of childbearing age to alert prescriber if she suspects or knows she is pregnant.
- Instruct patient to report to prescriber any new or unusual pain in hip or thigh in the absence of trauma.

pancreatin

Donnazyme: ***500 mg pancreatin, 1,000 units lipase, 12,500 units protease, 12,500 units amylase***
Hi-Vegi-Lip: ***2,400 mg pancreatin, 4,800 units lipase, 60,000 units protease, 60,000 units amylase***
4X Pancreatin: ***2,400 mg pancreatin, 12,000 units lipase, 60,000 units protease, 60,000 units amylase***
8X Pancreatin: ***7,200 mg pancreatin, 22,500 units lipase, 180,000 units protease, 180,000 units amylase***
Pancrezyme 4X: ***2,400 mg pancreatin, 12,000 units lipase, 60,000 units protease, 60,000 units amylase***

Class and Category

Pharmacologic class: Pancreatic enzyme
Therapeutic class: Digestive enzymes
Pregnancy category: C

Indications and Dosages

➤ *To treat pancreatic insufficiency, including steatorrhea*

CAPSULES, TABLETS

Adults. 8,000 to 24,000 units of lipase with meals or snacks, adjusted as prescribed, according to need for steatorrhea control. For severe insufficiency, up to 36,000 units of lipase with meals or snacks.

Mechanism of Action

Releases the enzymes amylase, lipase, pancreatin, and protease, mainly in the duodenum and upper jejunum. These enzymes facilitate the hydrolysis of fats into fatty acids and glycerol, starches into dextrins and sugars, and proteins into peptides. Pancreatin acts locally in the GI tract but is quickly inactivated by gastric acid.

Contraindications

Acute exacerbation of chronic pancreatic disease; acute pancreatitis; hypersensitivity to pancreatin, pancrelipase, or pork

Interactions

DRUGS

acarbose, miglitol: Decreased effectiveness of these drugs
aluminum hydroxide, H_2-receptor antagonists, omeprazole, sodium bicarbonate: Increased gastric pH, prolonged enzymatic action of pancreatin
calcium carbonate– and magnesium hydroxide–containing antacids: Decreased pancreatin effectiveness
iron supplements: Decreased iron absorption

Adverse Reactions

EENT: Stomatitis
GI: Abdominal cramps or pain, diarrhea, **intestinal obstruction**, nausea
SKIN: Rash, urticaria
Other: Hyperuricemia

Nursing Considerations

WARNING Don't administer pancreatin to patient who is allergic to pork.

- Assess patient for GI disturbances and hyperuricemia when giving high doses of pancreatin.
- Know that if patient opens capsules and sprinkles contents on food, patient should be watched for signs or symptoms of sensitization (chest tightness, dyspnea, nasal congestion, wheezing), which may result from repeated inadvertent inhalation of powder.
- Be aware that brands of pancreatin aren't interchangeable because the same doses don't contain equivalent amounts of drug.

PATIENT TEACHING

- Instruct patient to take pancreatin before or with meals or snacks to maximize effectiveness.
- Advise patient to take drug with a beverage while sitting upright, to swallow it quickly, and to follow with 1 or 2 mouthfuls of solid food.
- Caution patient not to chew tablets; doing so may irritate lips, mouth, and tongue.

- Tell patient if she has trouble swallowing capsules, she may open capsule and sprinkle its contents on food without inhaling them.
- Caution patient not to take antacids that contain calcium carbonate or magnesium hydroxide during therapy.

pancrelipase

Creon: ***3,000 units lipase, 9,500 units protease, 15,000 units amylase***
Creon: ***6,000 units lipase, 19,000 units protease, 30,000 units amylase***
Creon: ***12,000 units lipase, 38,000 units protease, 60,000 units amylase***
Creon: ***24,000 units lipase, 76,000 units protease, 120,000 units amylase***
Creon: ***36,000 units lipase, 114,000 units protease, 180,000 units amylase***
Pancreaze MT 4: ***4,200 units lipase, 10,000 units protease, 17,500 units amylase***
Pancreaze MT 10: ***10,500 units lipase, 25,000 units protease, 43,750 units amylase***
Pancreaze MT 16: ***16,800 units lipase, 40,000 units protease, 70,000 units amylase***
Pancreaze MT 20: ***21,000 units lipase, 37,000 units protease, 61,000 units amylase***
Pertzye: ***8,000 units lipase, 28,750 units protease, 30,250 units amylase***
Pertzye: ***16,000 units lipase, 57,500 units protease, 60,500 units amylase***
Pertzye: ***4,000 units lipase, 14,375 units protease, 15,125 units amylase***
Ultresa: ***13,800 units lipase, 27,600 units protease, 27,600 units amylase***
Ultresa: ***20,700 units lipase, 41,400 units protease, 41,400 units amylase***
Utresa: ***23,000 units lipase, 46,000 units protease, 46,000 units amylase***
Viokace: ***10,440 units lipase, 39,150 units protease, 39,150 units amylase***
Viokace: ***20,880 units lipase, 78,300 units protease, 78,300 units amylase***
Viokase Tablets: ***8,000 units lipase, 30,000 units protease, 30,000 units amylase***
Viokase Powder: ***16,800 units lipase, 70,000 units protease, 70,000 units amylase***
Zenpep: ***3,000 units lipase, 10,000 units protease, 16,000 units amylase***
Zenpep: ***5,000 units lipase, 17,000 units protease, 27,000 units amylase***
Zenpep: ***10,000 units lipase, 34,000 units protease, 55,000 units amylase***
Zenpep: ***15,000 units lipase, 51,000 units protease, 82,000 units amylase***
Zenpep: ***20,000 units lipase, 68,000 units protease, 109,000 units amylase***
Zenpep: ***25,000 units lipase, 85,000 units protease, 136,000 units amylase***
Zenpep: ***40,000 units lipase, 136,000 units protease, 218,000 units amylase***

Class and Category

Pharmacologic class: Pancreatic enzymes
Therapeutic class: Digestive enzymes
Pregnancy category: C

Indications and Dosages

➤ *To treat exocrine pancreatic insufficiency, including steatorrhea*

CAPSULES, POWDER, TABLETS

Adults and children age 4 and over. *Initial:* 500 lipase units/kg/meal, adjusted as needed and tolerated. *Maximum:* 2,500 lipase units/kg/meal (or less than or equal to 10,000 lipase units/kg/day), or less than 4,000 lipase units/g fat ingested/day.
Children ages 1 to 4. *Initial:* 1,000 lipase units/kg/meal, adjusted as needed and tolerated. *Maximum:* 2,500 lipase units/kg/meal (or less than or equal to 10,000 lipase units/kg/day), or less than 4,000 lipase units/g fat ingested/day.
Infants up to 12 months. 2,000 to 4,000 lipase units per breastfeeding or 120 ml of formula.

DELAYED-RELEASE CAPSULES

Adults and children age 4 and over. *Initial*: 500 lipase units/kg/meal, adjusted as needed and tolerated. *Maximum*: 2,500 lipase units/kg/meal (or less than or equal to 10,000 lipase units/kg/day), or less than 4,000 lipase units/g fat ingested/day.
Children ages 1 to 4. *Initial:* 1,000 lipase units/kg/meal, adjusted as needed and tolerated. *Maximum:* 2,500 lipase units/kg/meal (or less than or equal to 10,000 lipase units/kg/day), or less

than 4,000 lipase units/g fat ingested/day.
Infants up to 12 months. 3,000 lipase units per breastfeeding or 120 ml of formula.

➤ *To treat exocrine pancreatic insufficiency due to chronic pancreatitis or pancreatectomy*

DELAYED-RELEASE CAPSULES (CREON)
Adults. Highly individualized.

Mechanism of Action

Releases high levels of the enzymes amylase, lipase, and protease, mainly in duodenum and upper jejunum. These enzymes facilitate hydrolysis of fats into fatty acids and glycerol, proteins into peptides, and starches into dextrins and sugars.

Contraindications

Acute exacerbation of chronic pancreatic disease; acute pancreatitis; hypersensitivity to pancreatin, pancrelipase, or pork

Interactions

DRUGS
acarbose, miglitol: Decreased effectiveness of these drugs
aluminum hydroxide, H_2-receptor antagonists, omeprazole, sodium bicarbonate: Increased gastric pH, prolonged enzymatic action of pancrelipase
calcium carbonate– and magnesium hydroxide–containing antacids: Decreased pancrelipase effectiveness
iron supplements: Decreased iron absorption

Adverse Reactions

CNS: Dizziness, headache
EENT: Blurred vision, nasopharyngitis, stomatitis
ENDO: Hyperglycemia, **hypoglycemia**
GI: Abdominal cramps, distention, or pain; abnormal feces; constipation; diarrhea; elevated liver enzymes; fibrosing colonopathy; flatulence; **intestinal obstruction**; nausea; vomiting
HEME: Anemia
MS: Muscle spasm, myalgia
RESP: **Asthma**, cough
SKIN: Pruritus, rash, urticaria
Other: **Anaphylaxis**, hyperuricemia

Nursing Considerations

WARNING Don't administer pancrelipase to patient who is allergic to pork.

- Know that children older than 12 months and younger than 4 years who weigh less than 8 kg, and children 4 years and over weighing less than 16 kg, should not receive Pertzye brand of pancrelipase; nor should children older than 12 months and younger than 4 years who weigh under 14 kg, or children 4 years and over weighing less than 28 kg, receive Ultresa brand of pancrelipase because capsule dosage strength in these products cannot adequately provide correct dosing for these children.
- Use with caution in patients with gout, hyperuricemia, or renal impairment, because porcine-derived pancreatic enzyme products contain purines that may increase blood uric acid levels.
- Be aware that brands of pancrelipase aren't interchangeable because the same doses don't contain equivalent amounts of drug.
- Mix powder with fluid or soft, nondairy food.
- Know that if needed, capsules or delayed-release capsules may be opened and contents (enteric-coated spheres, microspheres, or microtablets) mixed with liquid or soft food that requires no chewing. Give immediately because enteric coating will dissolve after prolonged contact with foods at a pH > 6. Do not mix contents directly into formula or breast milk because effectiveness may be diminished. Instead, mix in a small amount of applesauce or other acidic food such as baby food, bananas, or pears, or place contents of capsule directly into infant's mouth, followed by breast milk or formula.
- Know that if patient opens capsules and sprinkles contents on food, patient should be assessed for signs of sensitization (chest tightness, dyspnea, nasal congestion, wheezing), which may result from repeated inadvertent inhalation of powder.
- Give drug before or with meals and snacks, and follow with a glass of water or juice.
- Expect drug to cause stomatitis if held in mouth.
- Monitor patient for allergic reactions when beginning therapy. Although rare, severe allergic reactions including anaphylaxis, asthma, hives, and pruritus may occur. Notify prescriber immediately and provide supportive care.

- Check stool for fecal fat content, as ordered.
- Monitor patient for iron deficiency anemia because serum iron level may decline during pancrelipase therapy.
- Monitor blood glucose levels more frequently in patients at risk for abnormal blood glucose levels because glycemic control may be affected by administration of pancreatic enzyme replacement therapy.

WARNING Monitor patient, especially children with cystic fibrosis, for abdominal pain because fibrosing colonopathy, although rare, may occur over a prolonged period of time, especially when doses of pancreatic enzyme products exceed 6,000 lipase units/kg/meal.

PATIENT TEACHING

- Instruct patient to take pancrelipase before or with meals and snacks and to follow with a glass of water or juice.
- Instruct patient not to chew capsules or capsule contents or to crush tablets; patient should swallow immediately because drug may cause irritation if held in mouth.
- Tell patient who is unable to swallow intact capsules to open capsules or delayed-release capsules and mix contents (enteric-coated spheres, microspheres, or microtablets) with liquid or soft food that requires no chewing. Tell patient to take immediately, because enteric coating will dissolve after prolonged contact with foods at a pH > 6. Tell parents not to mix contents directly into formula or breast milk, because effectiveness may be diminished. Instead, mix in a small amount of applesauce or other acidic food such as baby food, bananas, or pears, or place contents of capsule directly into infant's mouth, followed by breast milk or formula.
- Urge patient not to inhale powder from delayed-release capsules; doing so may cause chest tightness, shortness of breath, stuffy nose, trouble breathing, and wheezing.
- Inform patient that sneezing and tearing also may result from contact with powder.
- Caution patient not to use antacids; they may decrease drug effectiveness.
- Tell patient to seek immediate emergency care if she develops difficulty breathing, hives, or itching, as these may be signs of an allergic reaction.
- Inform patient that her stool may have foul smell.
- Instruct parents to notify prescriber if their child under the age of 12 complains of abdominal pain, bloating, constipation, or nausea, or exhibits diarrhea or vomiting, because stricture formation in the colon may occur in children under the age of 12 receiving high doses of pancreatic enzymes.

pantoprazole sodium

Pantoloc (CAN), Protonix, Protonix I.V.

Class and Category

Pharmacologic class: Proton pump inhibitor
Therapeutic class: Antiulcer
Pregnancy category: C

Indications and Dosages

➤ *To treat erosive esophagitis associated with gastroesophageal reflux disease (GERD) short-term*

DELAYED-RELEASE TABLETS

Adults. 40 mg daily for up to 8 wk. Repeated for another 4 to 8 wk if healing doesn't occur.

DELAYED-RELEASE ORAL SUSPENSION

Adults and children 5 years and over weighing 40 kg (88 lb) or more. 40 mg daily given 30 min before a meal for up to 8 wk. Repeated for another 4 to 8 wk if healing doesn't occur.

I.V. INFUSION

Adults. 40 mg daily infused over 2 or 15 min for 7 to 10 days, followed by oral doses.

➤ *To maintain healing of erosive esophagitis and reduce relapse of daytime and nighttime symptoms in patients with GERD*

DELAYED-RELEASE TABLETS

Adults. 40 mg daily for up to 12 mo.

DELAYED-RELEASE ORAL SUSPENSION

Adults. 40 mg daily given 30 min before a meal for up to 12 mo.

➤ *To treat pathological hypersecretion associated with Zollinger–Ellison syndrome or other neoplastic conditions*

DELAYED-RELEASE TABLETS

Adults. 40 mg twice daily. *Maximum:* 240 mg daily.

DELAYED-RELEASE ORAL SUSPENSION

Adults. 40 mg twice daily given 30 minutes before a meal. *Maximum:* 240 mg daily.

I.V. INFUSION

Adults. 80 mg every 12 hr infused over 2 or 15 min; adjusted based on patient's acid output measurements up to 80 mg every 8 hr.

Route	Onset	Peak	Duration
P.O.	1 day	1 wk	1 wk
I.V.	1 day	Unknown	1 wk

Mechanism of Action

Interferes with gastric acid secretion by inhibiting the hydrogen-potassium-adenosine triphosphatase (H^+-K^+-ATPase) enzyme system, or proton pump, in gastric parietal cells. Normally, the proton pump uses energy from hydrolysis of ATPase to drive H^+ and chloride (Cl^-) out of parietal cells and into the stomach lumen in exchange for potassium (K^+), which leaves the stomach lumen and enters parietal cells. After this exchange, H^+ and Cl^- combine in the stomach to form hydrochloric acid (HCl). Pantoprazole irreversibly inhibits the final step in gastric acid production by blocking the exchange of intracellular H^+ and extracellular K^+, thus preventing H^+ from entering the stomach and additional HCl from forming.

Incompatibilities

Midazolam and products containing zinc may cause precipitation or discoloration.

Contraindications

Concurrent therapy with rilpivirine-containing products, hypersensitivity to pantoprazole, substituted benzimidazoles (omeprazole, lansoprazole, rabeprazole sodium), or their components

Interactions

DRUGS

ampicillin, cyanocobalamin, digoxin, iron salts, ketoconazole: Possibly impaired absorption of these drugs
atazanavir, nelfinavir, rilpivirine: Significantly decreased plasma levels of these drugs reducing antiviral effect; possible increased risk of drug resistance
dasatinib, erlotinib, iron salts, itraconazole, ketoconazole, mycophenolate mofetil, nilotinib: Possible decreased absorption of these drugs and decreased effectiveness
digoxin, diuretics: Increased risk of hypomagnesemia
methotrexate: Increased risk of methotrexate toxicities
saquinavir: Possibly increased risk of antiretroviral toxicity
warfarin: Increased INR, PT, and bleeding risk

Adverse Reactions

CNS: Anxiety, asthenia, confusion, depression, dizziness, fatigue, fever, hallucinations, headache, hypertonia, hypokinesia, insomnia, malaise, migraine, somnolence, speech disorder, vertigo
CV: Chest pain, elevated triglycerides, hypercholesterolemia, hyperlipidemia
EENT: Anterior ischemic optic neuropathy, blurred vision, dry mouth, increased salivation, pharyngitis, rhinitis, sinusitis, taste disorder, tinnitus
ENDO: Hyperglycemia
GI: Abdominal pain, atrophic gastritis, ***Clostridium difficile*-associated diarrhea**, constipation, diarrhea, elevated liver enzymes, flatulence, fundic gland polyps (long-term use), gastroenteritis, **hepatic failure**, **hepatitis**, **hepatotoxicity**, indigestion, jaundice, nausea, **pancreatitis**, vomiting
GU: Elevated serum creatinine level, interstitial nephritis
HEME: Agranulocytosis, **leukopenia**, **pancytopenia**, **thrombocytopenia**
MS: Arthralgia, back or neck pain, bone fracture, myalgia, **rhabdomyolysis**
RESP: Bronchitis, dyspnea, increased cough, upper respiratory tract infection
SKIN: Cutaneous lupus erythematosus, **erythema multiforme**, photosensitivity, pruritus, rash, **Stevens–Johnson syndrome**, **toxic epidermal necrolysis**
Other: Anaphylaxis, **angioedema**, elevated creatine kinase and phosphokinase levels, flu-like symptoms, generalized pain, hyperuricemia, **hypomagnesemia**,

hyponatremia, infection, injection-site reaction, systemic lupus erythematosus, vitamin B_{12} deficiency weight changes

Nursing Considerations

- Ensure the continuity of gastric acid suppression during transition from oral to I.V. pantoprazole (or vice versa) because even a brief interruption of effective suppression can lead to serious complications.
- Don't give pantoprazole within 4 weeks of testing for *Helicobacter pylori* because antibiotics, bismuth preparations, and proton pump inhibitors suppress *H. pylori* and may lead to false-negative results. Drug also may cause false-positive results in urine screening tests for tetrahydrocannabinol. Consult guidelines for pantoprazole use before testing.
- Administer delayed-release oral suspension 30 minutes before a meal mixed in apple juice or applesauce or, if given through a nasogastric tube, mixed in apple juice only. Do not mix the oral suspension in liquids other than apple juice, or foods other than applesauce because proper pH is necessary for stability. When mixing with applesauce, administer within 10 minutes and encourage patient to take repeated sips of water to make sure granules are washed down into the stomach. When mixing with apple juice, use only 1 teaspoon of apple juice to mix granules in, stir for 5 seconds (granules will not dissolve) and give immediately to patient to drink. After administration, rinse the container once or twice with more apple juice and give to patient to drink to ensure full dose has been given.
- Flush I.V. line with D_5W, normal saline solution, or lactated Ringer's injection before and after giving drug.
- When giving I.V. over 2 minutes, reconstitute with 10 ml of normal saline injection. Solution may be stored up to 2 hours at room temperature.
- When giving I.V. over 15 minutes, reconstitute with 10 ml normal saline injection. Then, further reconstitute with 100 ml (for GERD) or 80 ml (for pathological hypersecretion in Zollinger–Ellison syndrome) of D_5W, normal saline injection, or lactated Ringer's injection. Solution may be stored up to 2 hours before further dilution and up to 22 hours before use.
- Expect to monitor PT or INR during therapy if patient takes an oral anticoagulant.
- Be aware that if therapy lasts more than 3 years, patient may not be able to absorb vitamin B_{12} because of achlorhydria or hypochlorhydria. Treatment for cyanocobalamin deficiency may be needed.
- Monitor patient's urine output because pantoprazole may cause acute interstitial nephritis. Notify prescriber if urine output decreases or there is blood in the patient's urine.
- Monitor patient for bone fracture, especially in patients receiving multiple daily doses for more than a year because proton pump inhibitors, such as pantoprazole, increase risk of osteoporosis-related fractures of the hip, spine, or wrist.
- Monitor patient for diarrhea from *C. difficile* which can occur with or without antibiotics in patients taking pantoprazole. If severe diarrhea occurs, notify prescriber and expect to withhold drug and treat with electrolytes, fluids, protein, and an antibiotic effective against *C. difficile*.
- Be aware that a symptomatic response to the drug does not rule out the presence of a gastric tumor.
- Monitor the patient, especially the patient on long-term therapy for hypomagnesemia. If patient is to remain on pantoprazole long-term, expect to monitor the patient's serum magnesium level, as ordered, and if level becomes low, anticipate magnesium replacement therapy to be given and pantoprazole to be discontinued.
- Know that both cutaneous and systemic lupus erythematosus have occurred within days to years after proton pump therapy such as pantoprazole was initiated. The most common symptoms presented were arthralgia, cytopenia, and rash. Report such findings to prescriber.

- Know that proton pump inhibitors such as pantoprazole should not be given longer than medically necessary.
- Expect drug to be withheld for at least 14 days before assessment of serum chromogranin A levels are performed, because levels increase when gastric acidity is decreased and thus interfere with diagnostic investigations for neuroendocrine tumors.
- Be aware that pantoprazole may result in false positive urine screening tests for tetrahydrocannabinol.

PATIENT TEACHING

- Instruct patient to swallow pantoprazole tablets whole and not to chew or crush them. Warn patient not to exceed dosage or take for longer than prescribed, as long-term use increases risk of serious adverse reactions.
- Tell patient to take delayed-release oral suspension 30 minutes before a meal mixed in apple juice or applesauce; no other liquid or food should be used. When mixing with applesauce, tell patient to take mixture within 10 minutes and then to take repeated sips of water to make sure granules are washed down into the stomach. When mixing with apple juice, tell patient to use only 1 teaspoon of apple juice to mix granules in, stir for 5 seconds (granules will not dissolve) and drink immediately. After drinking, tell patient to rinse the container once or twice with more apple juice and then drink to ensure full dose has been given.
- Advise patient to expect relief of symptoms within 2 weeks of starting therapy. Tell patient to notify prescriber if he has a suboptimal response to drug or an early symptomatic relapse.
- Advise patient who takes warfarin to follow bleeding precautions and to notify prescriber immediately if bleeding occurs.
- Instruct patient to notify prescriber if diarrhea occurs and becomes prolonged or severe.
- Advise patient to notify prescriber if patient notices he is experiencing a decrease in the amount of urine voided or there is blood in his urine. Also tell him to notify prescriber if he experiences new or worsening joint pain or a rash on his arms or cheeks that gets worse in the sun.
- Remind patient to notify all prescribers of pantoprazole use and not to take any over-the-counter medication, including herbal supplements, without discussing with prescriber.
- Advise patient taking pantoprazole for longer than 3 years to alert prescriber if he experiences signs and symptoms of vitamin B12 deficiency such as constipation or diarrhea, heart palpitations, mental problems such as depression or memory loss, pale skin, or feeling light-headed, tired, or weak. Also advise him to report any persistent, severe, or unusual signs or symptoms that may be suggestive of other adverse effects such as hypomagnesemia.
- Instruct women of childbearing age to notify prescriber if pregnancy is suspected or occurs, because drug may cause fetal harm.

paricalcitol

Zemplar

Class and Category

Pharmacologic class: Vitamin D analogue
Therapeutic class: Antihyperparathyroid
Pregnancy category: Not classified

Indications and Dosages

➤ *To prevent and treat secondary hyperparathyroidism in patients with chronic stage 3 or 4 renal failure*

CAPSULES

Adults and adolescents age 16 and over whose baseline iPTH level is 500 pg/ml or less. *Initial:* 1 mcg daily or 2 mcg three times weekly with doses separated by at least 1 day. *Maintenance:* Dosage adjusted at 2- to 4-wk intervals based on the intact parathyroid hormone (iPTH) level relative to baseline and serum calcium and phosphorus levels to maintain an iPTH level within target range.

Adults and adolescents age 16 and over whose baseline iPTH level exceeds 500 pg/ml. *Initial:* 2 mcg daily or 4 mcg three times weekly with doses separated by at least 1 day. *Maintenance:* Dosage adjusted at 2- to 4-wk intervals based on the iPTH level relative to baseline and serum calcium and

phosphorus levels to maintain an iPTH level within target range.
Children ages 10 to 16. *Initial:* 1 mcg three times weekly with doses separated by at least 1 day. *Maintenance:* Dosage adjusted every 4 wk based on the iPTH level relative to baseline and serum calcium and phosphorus levels to maintain an iPTH level within target range.

➤ *To prevent and treat secondary hyperparathyroidism associated with chronic stage 5 renal failure in patients on hemodialysis or peritoneal dialysis*

CAPSULES

Adults and adolescents age 16 and over. *Initial:* Baseline iPTH (pg/ml) divided by 80 three times weekly with doses separated by at least 1 day. *Maintenance:* Individualized based on most recent iPTH level (pg/ml) divided by 80 and current serum calcium and phosphorus levels to maintain iPTH level within target range.
Children ages 10 to 16. *Initial:* Baseline iPTH (pg/ml) divided by 120 rounding down to nearest whole number. *Maintenance:* Individualized and titrated based on most recent iPTH level and serum calcium and phosphorus levels to maintain an iPTH level within target range.

I.V. INJECTION

Adults. *Initial:* 0.04 to 0.1 mcg/kg (2.8–7 mcg) administered as a bolus no more frequently than every other day at any time during dialysis, with dosage increased by 2 to 4 mcg at 2- to 4-wk intervals, as needed. *Maintenance:* Individualized and titrated based on most recent iPTH level and serum calcium and phosphorus levels to maintain an iPTH level within target range.

Route	Onset	Peak	Duration
I.V.	Unknown	Unknown	15 hr

Mechanism of Action

Reduces serum PTH level by an unknown mechanism. In chronic renal failure, decreased renal synthesis of vitamin D leads to chronic hypocalcemia. In response, parathyroid glands secrete PTH to stimulate vitamin D synthesis, but serum calcium levels can't normalize because of renal failure.

Contraindications

Evidence of vitamin D toxicity, hypercalcemia, hypersensitivity to paricalcitol or components

Interactions

DRUGS

aluminum-containing preparations such as antacids or phosphate binders: Possibly increased blood levels of aluminum and aluminum bone toxicity
atazanavir, boceprevir, clarithromycin, conivaptan, indinavir, itraconazole, ketoconazole, lopinavir/ritonavir, mibefradil, nefazodone, nelfinavir, posaconazole, ritonavir, saquinavir, telaprevir, telithromycin, voriconazole: Increased effects of paricalcitol
cholestyramine, mineral oil: Possibly decreased absorption of oral paricalcitol
digoxin: Possibly increased risk of digitalis toxicity
drugs, such as cholestyramine, that impair absorption of fat-soluble vitamins: Possibly impaired absorption of oral paricalcitol
vitamin D or its derivatives (prescription-based doses): Increased risk of hypercalcemia

FOODS

grapefruit juice: Increased effects of paricalcitol

Adverse Reactions

CNS: Agitation, anxiety, asthenia, chills, confusion, **CVA**, delirium, depression, dizziness, fatigue, fever, gait disturbance, headache, insomnia, light-headedness, malaise, myoclonus, neuropathy, nervousness, paresthesia, restlessness, syncope, thirst, unresponsive to stimuli, vertigo
CV: Arrhythmia, **atrial flutter**, **cardiac arrest**, **cardiomyopathy**, chest pain, **congestive heart failure**, hypertension, **hypotension**, **MI**, orthostatic hypotension, palpitations, peripheral edema
EENT: Amblyopia, conjunctivitis, dry mouth, glaucoma, ear discomfort, epistaxis, **laryngeal edema**, ocular hyperemia, oropharyngeal pain, pharyngitis, retinal abnormality, rhinitis, sinusitis, taste perversion
ENDO: Breast tenderness, hyperpara-thyroidism, hypoparathyroidism, **hypoglycemia**

GI: Abdominal discomfort or pain, anorexia, constipation, diarrhea, dyspepsia, dysphagia, elevated liver enzymes, gastritis, gastroenteritis, gastroesophageal reflux disease, **GI bleeding**, **intestinal ischemia**, nausea, **rectal hemorrhage**, vomiting
GU: Abnormal kidney function, elevated blood creatinine level, erectile dysfunction, **renal failure**, uremia, urinary frequency, UTI
HEME: Anemia, lymphadenopathy, **prolonged bleeding time**
MS: Arthritis, back pain, joint stiffness, leg cramps, muscle spasms or twitching, myalgia
RESP: Increased cough, dyspnea, **exacerbation of asthma**, orthopnea, pneumonia, **pulmonary edema**, wheezing
SKIN: Acne, alopecia, burning sensation, ecchymosis, hirsutism, hypertrophy, night sweats, pruritus, rash (including vesiculobullous), ulceration, urticaria
Other: Acidosis, **angioedema**, dehydration, flu-like symptoms, fungal or viral infection, generalized edema or pain, gout, **hypercalcemia**, **hyperkalemia**, **hyperphosphatemia**, **hypersensitivity reactions**, **hypocalcemia**, **hypokalemia**, infections, injection-site pain or swelling, **sepsis**, weight loss

Nursing Considerations

- Assess parenteral form of paricalcitol for particles and discoloration before administering; if present, discard drug. Give as I.V. bolus; discard unused portion.

WARNING Know that paricalcitol may lead to vitamin D toxicity and hypercalcemia requiring emergency intervention. Early evidence includes arthralgia, constipation, dry mouth, headache, metallic taste, myalgia, nausea, somnolence, vomiting, and weakness. Late evidence includes albuminuria, anorexia, arrhythmias, azotemia, conjunctivitis (calcific), decreased libido, elevated BUN and serum ALT and AST levels, hypercholesterolemia, hypertension, hyperthermia, irritability, mild acidosis, nephrocalcinosis, nocturia, pancreatitis, photophobia, polydipsia, polyuria, pruritus, rhinorrhea, vascular calcification, and weight loss.

- If toxicity occurs, notify prescriber immediately and expect to decrease or stop drug. Place patient on bed rest and give fluids, low-calcium diet, and a laxative, as prescribed. If patient has a hypercalcemic crisis and dehydration, expect to infuse normal saline solution and a loop diuretic to prompt renal calcium excretion.
- Expect to check patient's serum PTH level, serum calcium, and serum phosphorus levels at least every 2 weeks for 3 months during the initial dosing of paricalcitol or following any dose adjustment, then monthly for 3 months, and then every 3 months thereafter.
- Know that increased serum creatinine levels may occur with paricalcitol therapy and will decrease the patient's estimated glomerular filtration rate, which is especially significant for predialysis patients.
- Be aware that if patient also takes digoxin, she should be monitored for evidence of digitalis glycoside toxicity, which is potentiated by hypercalcemia.

PATIENT TEACHING

- Advise patient to follow a diet high in calcium and low in phosphorus.
- Explain that phosphate binders may be needed to control serum phosphorus level.
- Review early evidence of hypercalcemia and vitamin D toxicity, such constipation, experiencing difficulty thinking clearly, feeling tired or unusually thirsty, increased urination, loss of appetite, nausea, vomiting, and weight loss. Tell patient to contact prescriber immediately if it develops.
- Urge patient to avoid hazardous activities until drug's CNS effects are known.
- Explain evidence of toxicity if patient takes digoxin and the need to contact prescriber immediately if it develops.
- Instruct patient on importance of routine monitoring of condition and not to skip laboratory tests or prescriber visits.
- Remind patient to notify all prescribers of all medications taken, including herbal preparations, prescription and nonprescription drugs, and supplements. Alert all prescribers of paricalcitol therapy.
- Inform women of childbearing age that breastfeeding is not recommended during paricalcitol therapy.

paroxetine hydrochloride

Paxil, Paxil CR

paroxetine mesylate

Brisdelle, Pexeva

Class and Category

Pharmacologic class: Selective serotonin reuptake inhibitor (SSRI)
Therapeutic class: Antianxiety, antidepressant, antiobsessional, antipanic, premenstrual analgesic
Pregnancy category: D

Indications and Dosages

➤ *To treat major depression*

C.R. TABLETS (PAXIL CR)

Adults. *Initial:* 25 mg daily, increased as prescribed and tolerated by 12.5 mg daily every wk. *Maximum:* 62.5 mg daily.

ORAL SUSPENSION, TABLETS

Adults. *Initial:* 20 mg daily, increased as prescribed and tolerated by 10 mg daily every wk. *Maximum:* 50 mg daily.

➤ *To treat obsessive-compulsive disorder*

ORAL SUSPENSION, TABLETS (PAXIL, PEXEVA)

Adults. *Initial:* 20 mg daily, increased as prescribed and tolerated by 10 mg daily every wk. *Usual:* 20 to 60 mg daily. *Maximum:* 60 mg daily.

➤ *To treat panic disorder*

C.R. TABLETS (PAXIL CR)

Adults. *Initial:* 12.5 mg daily, increased by 12.5 mg daily every wk as needed. *Maximum:* 75 mg daily.

ORAL SUSPENSION, TABLETS (PAXIL, PEXEVA)

Adults. *Initial:* 10 mg daily, increased as prescribed and tolerated by 10 mg daily every wk. *Usual:* 10 to 60 mg daily. *Maximum:* 60 mg daily.

➤ *To treat social anxiety disorder*

C.R. TABLETS (PAXIL CR)

Adults. *Initial:* 12.5 mg daily, increased by 12.5 mg daily every wk as needed. *Maximum:* 37.5 mg daily.

ORAL SUSPENSION, TABLETS (PAXIL)

Adults. *Initial:* 20 mg daily, increased as prescribed and tolerated by 10 mg daily every wk. *Usual:* 20 to 60 mg daily. *Maximum:* 60 mg daily.

➤ *To treat generalized anxiety disorder*

ORAL SUSPENSION, TABLETS (PAXIL, PEXEVA)

Adults. *Initial:* 20 mg daily, increased as prescribed and tolerated by 10 mg daily every wk. *Usual:* 20 to 50 mg daily. *Maximum:* 60 mg daily.

➤ *To treat posttraumatic stress disorder*

ORAL SUSPENSION, TABLETS (PAXIL)

Adults. *Initial:* 20 mg daily, increased as prescribed and tolerated by 10 mg daily every wk. *Usual:* 20 to 50 mg daily. *Maximum:* 50 mg daily.

➤ *To treat premenstrual dysphoric disorder*

C.R. TABLETS (PAXIL CR)

Adults. *Initial:* 12.5 mg daily in the morning, increased as needed after 1 wk to 25 mg daily. Or, 12.5 mg daily in the morning only during luteal phase of menstrual cycle (2-wk period before onset of monthly cycle), increased as needed after 1 wk to 25 mg daily in the morning during luteal phase of menstrual cycle.

DOSAGE ADJUSTMENT For patients who are debilitated, elderly, or have severe hepatic or renal dysfunction, initially 10 mg daily; maximum, 40 mg daily. Avoid C.R. form in these individuals. For patients taking severe hepatic or renal dysfunction who are taking C.R. tablets, initially 12.5 mg daily; maximum, 50 mg daily.

➤ *To treat moderate to severe vasomotor symptoms associated with menopause*

CAPSULES (BRISDELLE)

Adults. 7.5 mg once daily at bedtime.

Route	Onset	Peak	Duration
P.O.	1–4 wk	Unknown	Unknown

Mechanism of Action

Exerts antianxiety, antidepressant, antiobsessional, and antipanic effects as well as relieving symptoms associated with premenstrual dysphoric disorder and hot flashes associated with menopause by potentiating serotonin activity in CNS and inhibiting serotonin reuptake at presynaptic neuronal membrane. Blocked serotonin reuptake increases levels and prolongs activity of serotonin at synaptic receptor sites.

Contraindications

Hypersensitivity to paroxetine or its components, pimozide or thioridazine therapy, use within 14 days of an MAO inhibitor including linezolid or methylene blue I.V.

Interactions

DRUGS

amphetamines, buspirone, cisapride, fentanyl, isoniazid, linezolid, lithium, methylene blue (I.V.), MAO inhibitors, procarbazine, St. John's wort, tramadol, tricyclic antidepressants, triptans, tryptophan: Possibly increased risk of serotonin syndrome
antacids: Hastened release of C.R. paroxetine
aspirin, NSAIDs, warfarin: Increased anticoagulant activity and risk of bleeding
astemizole: Increased risk of arrhythmias
atomoxetine; risperidone; other drugs metabolized by CYP2D6, such as amitriptyline, desipramine, fluoxetine, imipramine, phenothiazines, tamoxifen, type IC antiarrhythmics: Increased plasma levels of these drugs
barbiturates, fosamprenavir, primidone, ritonavir: Decreased plasma paroxetine level
cimetidine: Possibly increased blood paroxetine level
codeine, haloperidol, metoprolol, perphenazine, propranolol, risperidone, thioridazine: Decreased metabolism and increased effects of these drugs
cyproheptadine: Decreased paroxetine effects
dextromethorphan: Decreased dextromethorphan metabolism and increased risk of toxicity
digoxin: Possibly decreased digoxin effects
encainide, flecainide, propafenone, quinidine: Potentiated toxicity of these drugs
lithium: Possibly increased blood paroxetine level, increased risk of serotonin syndrome
methadone: Decreased methadone metabolism, increased risk of adverse effects
phenytoin: Possibly phenytoin toxicity
pimozide: Increased risk of prolonged QT interval
procyclidine: Increased blood procyclidine level and anticholinergic effects
tamoxifen: Decreased tamoxifen effectiveness
theophylline: Possibly increased blood theophylline level and risk of toxicity
thioridazine: Increased thioridazine level, possibly leading to prolonged QT interval and life-threatening ventricular arrhythmias
tramadol: Increased risk of serotonin syndrome and seizures
tricyclic antidepressants: Increased metabolism and blood antidepressant levels; increased risk of toxicity, including seizures

Adverse Reactions

CNS: Agitation, akathisia, asthenia, confusion, decreased concentration, dizziness, drowsiness, emotional lability, hallucinations, headache, hypomania, insomnia, mania, **neuroleptic malignant syndrome**, psychomotor agitation, restlessness, **seizures**, **serotonin syndrome**, somnolence, **suicidal ideation**, tremor
CV: Palpitations, tachycardia, **torsades de pointes**, **ventricular fibrillation or ventricular tachycardia**
EENT: Angle-closure glaucoma, blurred vision, dry mouth, rhinitis, taste perversion
GI: Abdominal cramps or pain, anorexia, constipation, diarrhea, flatulence, nausea, vomiting
GU: Decreased libido, difficult ejaculation, impotence, sexual dysfunction, urine retention
HEME: Bleeding events
MS: Back pain, bone fracture, myalgia, myasthenia, myopathy
SKIN: Diaphoresis, rash, **Stevens–Johnson syndrome**
Other: Hyponatremia, weight gain or loss

Nursing Considerations

- Be aware that Brisdelle is not used to treat any psychiatric condition because it contains a lower dose of paroxetine.
- Shake oral suspension well. Measure with a calibrated device or an oral syringe.
- Don't give enteric-coated form with antacids.
- Watch for akathisia (inner sense of restlessness) and psychomotor agitation, especially during the first few weeks of therapy.
- Watch patient closely (especially young adults), for suicidal tendencies, particularly when therapy starts and dosage changes, because depression may worsen temporarily during these times, possibly leading to suicidal ideation.

- Watch for mania, which may result from any antidepressant in a susceptible patient.
- Monitor patient closely for evidence of GI bleeding, especially if patient also takes a drug known to cause GI bleeding, such as aspirin, an NSAID, or warfarin.

WARNING Monitor patient closely for serotonin syndrome exhibited by agitation, hallucinations, coma, diarrhea, hallucinations, hyperreflexia, hyperthermia, incoordination, labile blood pressure, nausea, tachycardia, or vomiting. Notify prescriber immediately because serotonin syndrome may be life-threatening, and provide supportive care.

WARNING Be aware that serotonin syndrome in its most severe form may resemble neuroleptic malignant syndrome, which includes autonomic instability with possibly rapid changes in mental status and vital signs, hyperthermia, and muscle rigidity. Stop drug immediately, and provide supportive care.

- To minimize adverse reactions, expect to taper drug rather than stop it abruptly.
- Be aware that pathological fractures have been associated with antidepressant therapy. Monitor patient for unexplained bone pain, bruising, joint tenderness, or swelling.

PATIENT TEACHING

- Advise patient to take paroxetine in the morning to minimize insomnia and to take it with food if adverse GI reactions develop.
- Instruct patient to avoid taking C.R. paroxetine within 2 hours of an antacid.
- Tell patient to swallow C.R. tablets whole and not to chew, crush, or cut them.
- Advise patient that drug may cause mild pupillary dilation, which may lead to an episode of acute closure glaucoma. Encourage patient to have eye exam before starting therapy to see if he is at risk.
- Suggest that patient avoid hazardous activities until drug's CNS effects are known.
- Tell family or caregiver to observe patient closely for suicidal tendencies, especially when therapy starts or dosage changes and especially if patient is a young adult.
- Explain that full effect may take 4 weeks.
- Urge patient to avoid alcohol during therapy; effects with paroxetine are unknown.
- Tell patient not to take aspirin or NSAIDs during therapy because they increase the risk of bleeding. If patient takes warfarin, tell her to use bleeding precautions and to notify prescriber at once if bleeding occurs.
- Inform patient that episodes of acute depression may persist for months or longer and that they require continued follow-up.
- Instruct patient not to stop drug abruptly but to taper dosage as instructed.
- Alert female patients of childbearing age that paroxetine may cause birth defects and persistent pulmonary hypertension in the newborn if taken during the first trimester of pregnancy. Emphasize the need to use effective contraception and to notify prescriber if pregnancy occurs or is suspected.
- Caution patient to alert all prescribers about paroxetine therapy because of potentially serious drug interactions.
- Tell patient to notify prescriber if she develops unexplained bone pain, bruising, joint tenderness, or swelling. Also advise patient to report any persistent, severe, or unusual signs and symptoms to prescriber.

patiromer sorbitex calcium

Veltassa

Class and Category

Pharmacologic class: Cation exchange polymer
Therapeutic class: Potassium binder
Pregnancy category: Not classified

Indications and Dosages

➤ *To treat hyperkalemia*

ORAL SUSPENSION

Adults. *Initial:* 8.4 g once daily, increased once a week or longer or decreased, as needed, in increments of 8.4 g to reach desired serum potassium concentration. *Maximum:* 25.2 g once daily.

Mechanism of Action

Binds potassium in the lumen of the gastrointestinal tract, which is then excreted in feces. This reduces the concentration of free potassium in the gastrointestinal lumen, reducing the serum potassium level.

Contraindications

Hypersensitivity to patiromer or its components

Interactions

DRUGS

orally administered medications: Possibly decreased oral drug absorption leading to reduced effectiveness

Adverse Reactions

GI: Abdominal discomfort, constipation, diarrhea, flatulence, nausea, vomiting
Other: Hypomagnesemia

Nursing Considerations

- Know that patiromer should not be given to patients with abnormal postoperative bowel motility disorders, bowel impaction or obstruction, or severe constipation because drug will worsen these conditions.
- Prepare each dose of the oral suspension immediately prior to administration by adding 30 ml (1 oz) of water to an empty glass or cup. Then empty entire contents of packet(s) into the cup or glass and stir thoroughly. Add an additional 60 ml (2 oz) of water to cup or glass and stir thoroughly again. Be aware that the powder will not dissolve and the mixture will look cloudy. Have patient drink the mixture immediately. If some powder remains in the cup or glass after drinking, add more water, stir, and have patient drink again. Repeat until the entire dose is administered.
- Give patiromer with food. However, do not heat the drug (i.e., microwave) or add to heated foods or liquids. Never administer drug in its dry form.
- Administer patiromer at least 3 hours before or 3 hours after other oral medications to prevent decreased absorption of these drugs.
- Monitor patient's serum magnesium level, as ordered, because drug binds to magnesium in the colon. Be aware patient may require a magnesium supplement if hypomagnesemia develops.

PATIENT TEACHING

- Instruct patient on how to mix patiromer immediately before taking. Remind him the powder will not dissolve and the mixture will appear cloudy. Make sure he understands the importance of adding additional water to container if any powder remains to ensure an accurate dose.
- Tell patient to take patiromer with food but not to add it to heated food or beverages. Also, tell patient not to heat the drug in any way and never ingest the dry powder.
- Instruct patient to take patiromer 3 hours before or 3 hours after other oral medication.
- Inform patient that drug should be stored in the refrigerator. Tell him that the drug must be used within 3 months of being taken out of the refrigerator.
- Alert patient that blood work to monitor his potassium level along with his magnesium level will be required periodically.

pegfilgrastim

Neulasta

pegfilgrastim-cbqv

Udenyca

pegfilgrastim-jmdb

Fulphila

Class and Category

Pharmacologic class: Colony stimulating factor
Therapeutic class: Hematopoietic
Pregnancy category: C

Indications and Dosages

➤ *To increase survival in patients acutely exposed to myelosuppressive doses of radiation.*

SUBCUTANEOUS INJECTION (NEULASTA)

Adults and children weighing 45 kg (99 lb) or more. 6 mg as soon as possible after exposure, followed by 6 mg 1 wk later.
Children weighing between 31 and 44 kg (68.2–96.8 lb): 4 mg as soon as possible after exposure, followed by 4 mg 1 wk later.
Children weighing between 21 and 30 kg (46.2–66 lb): 2.5 mg as soon as possible after exposure, followed by 2.5 mg 1 wk later.
Children weighing between 10 and 20 kg (22–44 lb): 1.5 mg as soon as possible after exposure, followed by 2.5 mg 1 wk later.

P

Children weighing less than 10 kg (22 lb): 0.1 mg/kg as soon as possible after exposure, followed by 0.1 mg/kg 1 wk later.

➤ *To reduce the risk of infection, as manifested by febrile neutropenia, in patients with nonmyeloid malignancies receiving myelosuppressive chemotherapy*

SUBCUTANEOUS INJECTION (FULPHILA, NEULASTA, UDENYCA)

Adults and children weighing more than 45 kg (99 lb). 6 mg with each chemotherapy cycle.

Children weighing between 31 and 44 kg (68.2–96.8 lb): 4 mg with each chemotherapy cycle.

Children weighing between 21 and 30 kg (46.2–66 lb): 2.5 mg with each chemotherapy cycle.

Children weighing between 10 and 20 kg (22–44 lb): 1.5 mg with each chemotherapy cycle.

Children weighing less than 10 kg (22 lb): 0.1 mg/kg with each chemotherapy cycle.

For both adults and children, dose given no sooner than 24 hr after chemotherapy administration and no later than 14 days before next chemotherapy administration.

Mechanism of Action

Induces formation of neutrophil progenitor cells by binding to receptors on granulocytes, which then divide. Pegfilgrastim also potentiates the effects of mature neutrophils, thus reducing fever and the risk of infection from severe neutropenia. It is pharmacologically identical to human granulocyte colony-stimulating factor.

Contraindications

Hypersensitivity to filgrastim, pegfilgrastim, or their components or to proteins derived from *Escherichia coli*

Interactions

DRUGS

lithium: Increased neutrophil production

Adverse Reactions

CNS: Fever

CV: Aortitis, edema, **hypotension**

GI: Elevated liver enzymes, **splenic rupture**, splenomegaly

GU: Elevated uric acid level glomerulonephritis

HEME: Capillary leak syndrome, hemoconcentration, leukocytosis, **sickle cell crisis**

MS: Bone or extremity pain

RESP: Acute respiratory distress syndrome, dyspnea, **hypoxia**, **pulmonary infiltrates**

SKIN: Acute febrile neutrophilic dermatosis (Sweet's syndrome), contact dermatitis (on-body injector), cutaneous vasculitis, erythema, flushing, pruritus, rash, urticaria

Other: Anaphylaxis, **angioedema**, antibody formation to pegfilgrastim, application-site reactions with on-body injector (bruising, discomfort, erythema, hemorrhage, pain), hypoalbuminemia, injection-site reactions (erythema, induration, pain)

Nursing Considerations

- Avoid giving pegfilgrastim for 14 days before and 24 hours after cytotoxic chemotherapy.
- Check CBC, hematocrit, and platelet count before and periodically during therapy.
- Let drug warm to room temperature for 30 minutes before injection. Administer subcutaneously via a single-dose prefilled syringe for manual use. Be aware, though, now that there is an on-body injector for Neulasta, which is co-packaged with a single-dose prefilled syringe, that the on-body injector form of Neulasta is not recommended for patients with hematopoietic subsyndrome or acute radiation syndrome.
- Don't shake the solution.
- Discard drug that contains particles, is discolored, or was stored more than 48 hours at room temperature. Be aware that the needle cap on the prefilled syringes contains dry natural rubber, which is a derivative of latex and should not be used by persons allergic to latex.

WARNING Monitor patient for signs of hypersensitivity. If signs of allergy occur, notify prescriber at once. If anaphylaxis occurs, give antihistamine, bronchodilator, corticosteroid, and epinephrine, as ordered. Be aware that the on-body injector of Neulasta may cause application-site and local skin reactions, including contact dermatitis.

WARNING Be aware that patients receiving filgrastim (parent drug) have had splenic rupture and acute respiratory distress syndrome, which may be life-threatening. Assess patient for fever, respiratory distress, and upper abdominal or shoulder tip pain and notify prescriber immediately, if present.

- Monitor patient's renal function, as ordered, because drug may cause glomerulonephritis. If renal dysfunction is suspected, notify prescriber and, if confirmed, expect drug to be withheld or dosage reduced.
- Monitor patient for signs and symptoms of aortitis such as abdominal pain, back pain, fever, increased inflammatory markers (C-reactive protein, white blood cell count), or malaise, as drug will have to be discontinued. Know that aortitis may occur as early as the first week after therapy is begun.
- Be aware that transient positive bone imaging changes may occur because of increased hematopoietic activity of the bone marrow in response to pegfilgrastim therapy.
- Assess patients with sickle cell disease for signs of sickle cell crisis; urge hydration. Know that drug should be discontinued if sickle cell crisis occurs.
- Give nonopioid and opioid analgesics, as ordered, if patient experiences bone pain.

WARNING Monitor patient for edema and hypotension that may indicate development of capillary leak syndrome. If present, notify prescriber and be prepared to provide supportive care, as ordered. Be aware that the on-body injector of Neulasta may cause application-site and local skin reactions, including contact dermatitis.

- Store drug at 2° to 8°C (36° to 46°F), and protect from freezing and light.
- Be aware that needle cover contains dry natural rubber and should not be handled by persons with a latex allergy.

PATIENT TEACHING

- Urge patient to report promptly any potentially serious reactions (breathing difficulty, chest tightness, left upper abdominal pain, rash, shoulder tip pain) and evidence of infection (chills, fever).
- Teach patient who will self-administer drug, how to prepare, give, and store drug. However, alert patient that the On-body Injector for drug uses acrylic adhesive, which can cause a significant reaction to those allergic to acrylic adhesive.
- Alert her that needle cover contains dry natural rubber and should not be handled if she has a latex allergy.
- Tell patient to rotate injection sites among abdomen (except for 2 inches around navel), buttocks, outer, upper arms and thighs. Caution her to avoid bruised, hard, red, or tender areas.
- Urge patient to discard used needles and syringes in a puncture-resistant container and not to reuse them.
- Alert patient that missed or partial doses have been reported with the on-body injector Neulasta due to potential device failure. Also tell patient not to reapply the on-body injector Neulasta if it comes off before the full dose is delivered. Instruct patient to notify prescriber immediately if the on-body injector Neulasta has come off or she suspects that the device may not have performed as intended, to get instructions on a possible replacement dose. Warn patient to avoid bumping the on-body injector Neulasta or knocking it off her body. Tell her she should not use additional materials to hold the on-body injector Neulasta in place, as this could dislodge the cannula and lead to a missed or incomplete dose.
- Tell patient to call prescriber immediately if the status light on the on-body injector Neulasta is flashing red. Also tell her not to remove the on-body injector Neulasta until the green light shines continuously. Tell patient to inform all healthcare workers of the presence of the on-body injector Neulasta, as it should not be exposed to medical imaging studies (CT scan, MRI, ultrasound, or X-ray), oxygen-rich environments, or radiation treatment.
- Remind patient not to use on-body injector Neulasta in the bathtub, hot tubs, saunas, or whirlpools and not to expose it to direct sunlight, as these may affect drug. Tell patient to avoid sleeping on the on-body injector Neulasta or getting cleaning agents, creams, lotions, or oils near the injector, as these products may loosen the adhesive.
- Advise patient to have a caregiver nearby when he administers the first dose and to avoid driving or operating heavy machinery during hours 26 to 29 following application of the on-body injector Neulasta.

- Warn patient to keep the on-body injector Neulasta at least 4 inches away from electrical equipment such as cell phones, cordless telephones, microwaves, and other common appliances, because of possible interference with its function.
- Emphasize the importance of follow-up tests.
- Advise patient to store pegfilgrastim in refrigerator and not to freeze it. Tell her to discard drug if left unrefrigerated for more than 48 hours.

peginesatide

Omontys

Class and Category

Pharmacologic class: Erythropoiesis stimulating agent
Therapeutic class: Hematopoietic
Pregnancy category: C

Indications and Dosages

➤ *To treat anemia due to chronic kidney disease in patients on dialysis*

I.V. OR SUBCUTANEOUS INJECTION

Adults not currently treated with another erythropoiesis-stimulating agent (ESA). 0.04 mg/kg once monthly.

Adults converting from epoetin alfa. Based on the weekly dose of epoetin alfa at the time of substitution, first dose given 1 wk after the last epoetin alfa dose was administered and then continued monthly.

Adults converting from darbepoetin alfa. Based on the weekly dose of darbepoetin alfa at the time of substitution, first dose given at the next scheduled dose of darbepoetin alfa in place of it.

DOSAGE ADJUSTMENT For patient experiencing a rapid rise in hemoglobin (more than 1 g/dl in the 2 wk prior to the next dose or more than 2 g/dl in 4 wk), dosage reduced by 25% or more. For the patient whose hemoglobin level is approaching or exceeding 11 g/dl, dosage reduced or drug withheld until hemoglobin levels begin to decrease. If drug was withheld, dosage restarted at a dosage that is 25% less than the previously administered dose. For patient who does not exhibit at least an increase in hemoglobin of more than 1 g/dl after 4 wk of therapy, dosage increased by 25%.

Mechanism of Action

Binds to and activates the human erythropoietin receptor and stimulates erythropoiesis in human red cell precursors to raise the reticulocyte count, which in turn increases hemoglobin.

Incompatibilities

Do not mix peginesatide with other drug solutions.

Contraindications

Hypersensitivity to peginesatide or any of its components, uncontrolled hypertension

Adverse Reactions

CNS: CVA, fever, headache, **seizures**
CV: Arteriovenous fistula-site complication, hypertension, **hypotension, MI, thromboembolism**
GI: Diarrhea, nausea, vomiting
MS: Arthralgia, back or extremity pain, muscle spasms
RESP: Bronchospasms, cough, dyspnea, upper respiratory tract infection
SKIN: Generalized pruritus
Other: Anaphylaxis, angioedema, hyperkalemia, infusion reactions, peginesatide-specific binding antibodies

Nursing Considerations

- Be aware that peginesatide therapy should not be used in patients with cancer whose anemia is not due to chronic renal failure, because peginesatide may increase risk of tumor progression or recurrence.
- Know that the iron status of the patient must be assessed before and during treatment with peginesatide. If patient has a bleeding condition, a chronic inflammatory or metabolic disorder, or a vitamin deficiency, expect these conditions to be treated and corrected before peginesatide treatment is begun.
- Obtain baseline blood pressure measurements prior to peginesatide therapy being started and regularly thereafter because drug may increase blood pressure. If blood pressure becomes difficult to control during drug therapy,

notify prescriber and expect drug to be withheld or dosage reduced.
- Know that peginesatide is initiated only in patients receiving dialysis and when the patient's hemoglobin level is less than 10 g/dl. Know that dosage increase should not be done more frequently than once every 4 weeks.
- Expect patient being converted from darbepoetin or epoetin alfa to maintain the same route of administration.
- Use peginesatide cautiously in patients with a history of cardiovascular disease or stroke, in patients with an insufficient hemoglobin response to other erythropoiesis-stimulating agents, and in patients who have a rate of hemoglobin rise of greater than 1 g/dl over 2 weeks with peginesatide therapy, because risk of developing life-threatening cardiovascular adverse effects or stroke is increased in these situations and death may occur.
- Use cautiously in patients receiving peginesatide who undergo coronary artery bypass graft surgery, because the risk of death is increased, and in patients who are undergoing orthopedic procedures because of increased risk for deep venous thrombosis.
- Do not dilute peginesatide or administer concurrently with other drugs.
- Monitor patient closely for allergic reactions to drug because serious and life-threatening hypersensitivity reactions may occur including anaphylaxis, angioedema, bronchospasm, generalized pruritis, and/or hypotension. At the first sign of hypersensitivity, notify prescriber and expect to provide supportive care.
- Expect patients to have adjustments made in their dialysis medications after peginesatide therapy is begun. Patients on hemodialysis may need increased anti-coagulation with heparin to prevent clotting of the extracorporeal circuit during hemodialysis.
- Monitor patient's hemoglobin response at least every 2 weeks, as ordered, until stable and then at least monthly thereafter because death, serious adverse cardiovascular effects, and stroke have occurred when the hemoglobin level became higher than 11 g/dl. Be aware that a patient who does not respond adequately over a 12-week escalation period should not have dosage increased further because effectiveness will not improve and risk of adverse reactions increases. Expect dose in this case to be the lowest possible to maintain a hemoglobin level low enough to reduce the need for red blood cell transfusions. If responsiveness does not improve, expect peginesatide therapy to be discontinued.
- Monitor patient's transferrin saturation and serum ferritin during therapy. Expect to give supplemental iron therapy when serum ferritin is less than 100 mcg/L or when serum transferrin saturation is less than 20%.
- Store unused drug contained in a multiple dose vial at 2° to 8°C (36° to 46°F) and discard after 28 days from date of opening vial or expiration date, whichever comes first. Remember to protect drug from light and store in original carton.

PATIENT TEACHING

- Instruct patient how to administer peginesatide subcutaneously, if prescribed, including how to withdraw drug solution into the syringe, how to administer a subcutaneous injection, sites to use and need for site rotation, storage of drug (in original carton), and proper disposal of equipment.
- Advise patient that if a dose is missed he should take it as soon as possible, and then restart peginesatide at the prescribed once-a-month schedule.
- Alert patient with a history of high blood pressure to comply with his antihypertensive therapy and dietary restrictions and to monitor his blood pressure regularly.
- Tell patient with a seizure disorder to alert prescriber of any new-onset neurologic symptoms or change in seizure frequency.
- Inform patient that he will need regular laboratory tests, and emphasize the importance of complying with testing schedule.

penicillamine

Cuprimine, Depen

Class and Category

Pharmacologic class: Heavy metal antagonist

Therapeutic class: Antirheumatic, antiurolithic, chelating agent
Pregnancy category: D

Indications and Dosages

➤ *To treat cystinuria*

CAPSULES, TABLETS

Adults and adolescents. *Initial:* 250 mg daily and increased slowly to 500 mg four times a day
Children. 7.5 mg/kg four times a day

➤ *To treat rheumatoid arthritis*

CAPSULES, TABLETS

Adults and adolescents. *Initial:* 125 or 250 mg daily. Dosage increased by 125 or 250 mg daily every 2 to 3 mo. *Maximum:* 1,500 mg daily.

➤ *To treat Wilson's disease*

CAPSULES, TABLETS

Adults and adolescents. Dosage individualized up to 2 g daily in divided doses four times a day by measuring urinary copper excretion.

DOSAGE ADJUSTMENT For elderly patients, 125 mg daily initially, then increased by 125 mg daily every 2 to 3 mo, up to maximum of 750 mg daily. For pregnant women with Wilson's disease, dosage reduced to 750 mg daily. For women having planned cesarean section, dosage limited to 250 mg daily during last 6 wk of pregnancy and until wound healing completed. For pregnant patients with cystinuria or rheumatoid arthritis, drug should be discontinued during pregnancy because of potential for fetal harm.

Route	Onset	Peak	Duration
P.O.*	2–3 mo	Unknown	Unknown

* For rheumatoid arthritis; 1 to 3 mo for Wilson's disease.

Mechanism of Action

Combines with copper to form a ring-shaped complex that's excreted in urine, thereby reducing copper levels in the body. Penicillamine also lowers urine cystine levels by binding with cystine to form penicillamine-cysteine disulfide, which is more soluble than cystine and more easily excreted in urine. The decrease in urine cystine level also helps prevent formation of cystine calculi and may help existing cystine calculi dissolve over time. In addition, penicillamine improves lymphocyte function by reducing IgM rheumatoid factor and immune complexes in serum and synovial fluid, which may play a role in treatment of rheumatoid arthritis.

Contraindications

Hypersensitivity to penicillin, penicillamine, or their components; penicillamine-related agranulocytosis or aplastic anemia; renal insufficiency (for patients with rheumatoid arthritis)

Interactions

DRUGS

4-aminoquinolines, bone marrow depressants, gold compounds, immunosuppressants (excluding glucocorticoids), phenylbutazone: Possibly increased risk of serious hematologic or renal adverse reactions
iron supplements: Possibly decreased effectiveness of penicillamine
pyridoxine: Decreased effectiveness of pyridoxine, possibly increased risk of anemia or peripheral neuritis reaction

Adverse Reactions

CNS: Agitation, anxiety, fever, mental changes, myasthenic syndrome, neuropathy
EENT: Altered or loss of taste, optic neuritis, stomatitis, tinnitus
GI: Anorexia, diarrhea, hepatic dysfunction, intrahepatic cholestasis, mild epigastric pain, **pancreatitis**, nausea, **toxic hepatitis**, vomiting
GU: Glomerulonephropathy, hematuria, proteinuria, **renal failure**
HEME: Agranulocytosis, **aplastic anemia**, **hemolytic anemia**, **leukopenia**, **thrombocytopenia**
MS: Arthralgia, dystonia, muscle weakness
SKIN: Pemphigus, pruritus, rash, urticaria
Other: Lupus-like symptoms, lymphadenopathy

Nursing Considerations

- Use penicillamine cautiously in elderly patients because they're at greater risk for altered taste, rash, and renal impairment.
- Give penicillamine 1 hour before or 2 hours after meals and at least 1 hour before or after any other drug, food, or

milk. Give last dose of day at least 3 hours after evening meal to maximize absorption.

- Be aware that for patient who has difficulty swallowing capsules or tablets, capsule may be opened and contents mixed in 15 to 30 ml of fruit juice or pureed fruit to mask drug's sulfur odor. Alternatively, ask pharmacist to prepare elixir for oral administration.
- Expect to give 25 mg pyridoxine, as prescribed, to patients receiving penicillamine because penicillamine increases intake requirements for this vitamin.
- Watch for febrile reactions in patients who developed a fever during previous penicillamine therapy. Expect to stop drug if patient develops drug-induced fever.
- Assess mucous membranes and skin for possible sensitivity reactions, such as mouth ulcers and skin lesions. Be prepared to discontinue drug as prescribed.
- Expect to monitor urine laboratory test results twice weekly during first month of therapy, then every 2 weeks for next 5 months, and monthly thereafter. Watch for hematuria or proteinuria, which may precipitate nephrotic syndrome, especially in patients with renal disease or history of renal insufficiency. Also, weigh patient daily, watch for edema, and monitor intake and output because penicillamine may worsen underlying renal disease.

WARNING **Monitor patient's hemoglobin, platelet count, and WBC and differential cell count, as ordered, and assess body temperature, lymph nodes, and skin for abnormalities twice weekly during first month of therapy, then every 2 weeks for next 5 months, and monthly thereafter because drug may cause potentially serious hematologic reactions.**

- Because of the potential for cross-sensitivity between penicillamine and penicillin, monitor for allergic reaction in patients with a history of penicillin allergy.
- Notify prescriber if patient reports decreased sense of taste, especially for salty and sweet foods. Expect normal taste sensation to be restored (except in patients with Wilson's disease) by giving 5 to 10 mg of copper a day, as prescribed.
- Monitor patients with diabetes mellitus for reduced insulin requirements to prevent risk of nighttime hypoglycemia because penicillamine may promote formation of anti-insulin antibodies.
- Check liver enzymes, as ordered, every 6 months (every 3 months for first year if patient has Wilson's disease) during penicillamine therapy because drug may cause serious hepatic dysfunction.

PATIENT TEACHING

- Advise patient to take penicillamine on an empty stomach.
- Instruct men and nonpregnant women with cystinuria to increase fluid intake and follow prescribed low-methionine diet to minimize cystine production and enhance drug's effectiveness. Urge patient to drink about 1 pint of fluid at bedtime and again during the night because this is when urine is more concentrated.
- Tell patient to notify prescriber immediately if he develops a bleeding, bruising, chills, fever, or sore throat because drug may have to be stopped.
- Instruct patient being treated for Wilson's disease to follow a diet low in copper, avoiding such foods as broccoli, chocolate, copper-enriched cereals, liver, molasses, mushrooms, nuts, and shellfish. Inform her that it may take 1 to 3 months of therapy for her condition to improve.
- Advise patient to consult prescriber before having dental work done during penicillamine therapy because drug can promote mouth ulcers.
- Instruct patient to avoid consuming iron during penicillamine therapy because iron can decrease drug's effectiveness.
- Explain that sense of taste may decrease during penicillamine therapy. Advise patient to notify prescriber if it becomes intolerable.
- Inform patient with rheumatoid arthritis that improvement may take 2 to 3 months of therapy.
- Caution female patient to notify prescriber immediately if she becomes or may be pregnant because dosage may have to be reduced or drug discontinued during pregnancy to prevent serious birth defects.

penicillin G benzathine

Bicillin C-R, Bicillin C-R 900/300, Bicillin L-A, Permapen

penicillin G potassium

Pfizerpen

penicillin G procaine

penicillin G sodium

penicillin V potassium

Apo-Pen-VK (CAN), Novo-Pen-VK (CAN), Penicillin-VK

Class and Category

Pharmacologic class: Penicillin
Therapeutic class: Antibiotic
Pregnancy category: B

Indications and Dosages

➤ *To treat systemic infections caused by gram-positive organisms (including* Bacillus anthracis, Corynebacterium diphtheriae, *enterococci,* Listeria monocytogenes, Staphylococcus aureus, *and* S. epidermidis), *gram-negative organisms (including* Neisseria gonorrhoeae, N. meningitidis, Pasteurella multocida, *and* Streptobacillus moniliformis [*rat-bite fever*]*), and gram-positive anaerobes (including* Actinomyces israelii [*actinomycosis*], Clostridium perfringens, C. tetani, Peptococcus *species,* Peptostreptococcus *species, and spirochetes, especially* Treponema carateum [*pinta*], T. pallidum, *and* T. pertenue [*yaws*]*)*

I.V. INFUSION, I.M. INJECTION (PENICILLIN G POTASSIUM, PENICILLIN G SODIUM)
Adults and children. Highly individualized based on type and severity of infection. Dosage ranges from 1 to 24 million units daily in divided doses usually every 4 to 6 hr, although some infections may require divided dosing every 2 hr. I.V. infusion given over 1 to 2 hr in adults and over 15 to 30 min in children.

I.M. INJECTION (PENICILLIN G PROCAINE)
Adults and adolescents. 600,000 to 1,200,000 units daily in divided doses every 12 to 24 hr.

➤ *To treat Group A streptococcal respiratory infections*

I.M. INJECTION (PENICILLIN G BENZATHINE)
Adults and children weighing more than 45 kg (100 lb). 1.2 million units as a single injection.
Children weighing 27 to 45 kg (59 to 100 lb). 900,000 units as a single injection.
Children weighing less than 27 kg (59 lb). 300,000 to 600,000 units as single injection.

➤ *To treat congenital syphilis*

I.M. INJECTION (PENICILLIN G BENZATHINE)
Children 2 years and over. Dosage adjusted based on adult dosing schedule.
Children under age 2. 50,000 units/kg as a single injection. *Maximum:* 2.4 million units/dose.

➤ *To treat syphilis of less than 1 year's duration*

I.M. INJECTION (PENICILLIN G BENZATHINE)
Adults and adolescents. 2.4 million units as a single injection.
Children. 50,000 units/kg up to adult dosage as a single injection. *Maximum:* 2.4 million units/dose.

➤ *To treat syphilis of more than 1 year's duration*

I.M. INJECTION (PENICILLIN G BENZATHINE)
Adults and adolescents. 2.4 million units every wk for 3 wk.
Children. 50,000 units/kg every wk for 3 wk. *Maximum:* 2.4 million units/dose.

➤ *To treat mild to moderate severe upper respiratory tract streptococcal infections, including erysipelas and scarlet fever*

TABLETS (PENICILLIN V POTASSIUM)
Adults and adolescents. 125 to 250 mg (200,000 to 400,000 units) every 6 to 8 hr for 10 days.

➤ *To treat mild to moderate pneumococcal infections, mild skin and soft tissue staphylococcal infections, mild to moderate staphylococcal (Vincent's) infection of the oropharynx*

TABLETS (PENICILLIN V POTASSIUM)
Adults and adolescents. 250 to 500 mg (400,000 to 800,000 units) every 6 to 8 hr.

DOSAGE ADJUSTMENT For patient with creatinine clearance of 10 to 50 ml/min, dosage reduced by 25%. For patient with creatinine clearance of less than 10 ml/min, dosage reduced up to 70%. For patient receiving hemodialysis, dosage administered after dialysis.

Mechanism of Action

Inhibits final stage of bacterial cell wall synthesis by competitively binding to penicillin-binding proteins inside the cell wall. Penicillin-binding proteins are responsible for various steps in bacterial cell wall synthesis. By binding to these proteins, penicillin leads to cell wall lysis.

Incompatibilities

Don't mix any penicillin in the same syringe or container with aminoglycosides because aminoglycosides will be inactivated. Don't mix penicillin G with drugs that may result in a pH < 5.5 or pH > 8.

Contraindications

Hypersensitivity to penicillin or its components

Interactions

DRUGS

ACE inhibitors, potassium-containing drugs, potassium-sparing diuretics: Increased risk of hyperkalemia (penicillin G potassium)
chloramphenicol, erythromycin, sulfonamides, tetracycline, thrombolytics: Possibly interference with penicillin's bactericidal effect
methotrexate: Decreased methotrexate clearance, increased risk of toxicity
oral contraceptives: Decreased contraceptive effectiveness (with penicillin V)
probenecid: Increased blood penicillin level

FOODS

acidic beverages, such as fruit juices: Possibly altered effects of oral penicillin G

Adverse Reactions

CNS: Confusion, dizziness, dysphasia, hallucinations, headache, lethargy, sciatic nerve irritation, **seizures**
CV: Labile blood pressure, palpitations
EENT: Black "hairy" tongue, oral candidiasis, stomatitis, taste perversion
GI: Abdominal pain, diarrhea, elevated liver enzymes (transient), indigestion, nausea, **pseudomembranous colitis**
GU: Acute interstitial nephritis, vaginal candidiasis
MS: Muscle twitching
SKIN: Rash
Other: Electrolyte imbalances; injection-site necrosis, pain, or redness

Nursing Considerations

- Obtain body tissue and fluid samples for culture and sensitivity tests as ordered before giving first dose. Expect to begin drug therapy before test results are known.
- Reconstitute vials of penicillin for injection with D_5W, or sodium chloride for injection, or sterile water for injection.
- Administer penicillin at least 1 hour before other antibiotics.
- Inject I.M. form deep into large muscle mass. Apply ice to relieve pain.

WARNING Give penicillin G benzathine and penicillin G procaine only by deep I.M. injection; I.V. injection may be fatal, and intra-arterial injection may cause extensive organ and tissue necrosis.

- Be aware that I.M. drug is absorbed slowly, which may make allergic reactions difficult to treat.
- Assess patient for signs of secondary infection, such as profuse, watery diarrhea. If such diarrhea develops, contact prescriber and expect to obtain a stool specimen to rule out pseudomembranous colitis caused by *Clostridium difficile.* If diarrhea occurs, notify prescriber and expect to withhold penicillin and treat with electrolytes, fluids, protein, and an antibiotic effective against *C. difficile.*
- Monitor serum sodium level and assess for early signs of heart failure in patients receiving high doses of penicillin G sodium.
- When giving penicillin G potassium to patient at risk for fluid overload or hypertension, be aware that each gram of penicillin G potassium also contains 1.02 mEq of sodium.

PATIENT TEACHING

- Instruct patient to report previous allergies to penicillins and to notify prescriber immediately about adverse reactions, including fever.
- Advise patient who uses oral contraceptives to use an additional form of contraception during penicillin V therapy.
- Urge patient to tell prescriber if diarrhea develops, even 2 months or more after penicillin therapy ends.

pentazocine lactate

Talwin

Class, Category, and Schedule

Pharmacologic class: Opioid
Therapeutic class: Opioid analgesic
Pregnancy category: C
Controlled substance schedule: IV

Indications and Dosages

➤ *To relieve pain severe enough to require opioid treatment and for which alternative treatment options such as nonopioid analgesics or opioid combination products are inadequate or not tolerated*

I.M., I.V., OR SUBCUTANEOUS INJECTION

Adults. *Initial:* 30 mg every 3 to 4 hr, as needed. *Maximum:* 30 mg/single dose I.V., 60 mg/single dose I.M. or subcutaneously, or 360 mg/24 hr for all parenteral forms. I.V. injection given slowly.

➤ *To relieve obstetric pain*

I.V. INJECTION

Adults. 20 mg given slowly when contractions become regular; repeated two or three times every 2 to 3 hr, as needed.

I.M. INJECTION

Adults. 30 mg as a single dose.

Route	Onset	Peak	Duration
I.V.	2–3 min	15–30 min	2–3 hr
I.M., SubQ	15–20 min	30–60 min	2–3 hr

Mechanism of Action

Binds with opioid receptors, mainly kappa and sigma receptors, at many CNS sites to alter perception of and emotional response to pain.

Incompatibilities

Don't mix pentazocine in same syringe with a soluble barbiturate because precipitation will occur.

Contraindications

Hypersensitivity to pentazocine or its components

Interactions

DRUGS

anticholinergics: Increased risk of urine retention and severe constipation
antidiarrheals, antiperistaltics: Increased risk of severe constipation and CNS depression
antihypertensives, diuretics, other hypotension-producing drugs: Additive hypotensive effects
antimigraine agents; cyclobenzaprine; dextromethorphan; dolasetron; granisetron; linezolid; MAO inhibitors; methylene blue; ondansetron; palonosetron; selected psychiatric drugs such as amoxapine, buspirone, lithium, maprotiline, mirtazapine, nefazodone, trazodone, vilazodone; selective serotonin reuptake inhibitors; serotonin-norepinephrine reuptake inhibitors; St. John's wort; tricyclic antidepressants; tryptophan: Increased risk of serotonin syndrome
benzodiazepines, CNS depressants, other opioids, sedating antihistamines, tricyclic antidepressants: Increased risk of severe respiratory depression and significant sedation and somnolence
buprenorphine: Decreased pentazocine effectiveness, increased respiratory depression
CNS depressants: Increased CNS depression, increased risk of habituation
hydroxyzine, other opioid analgesics: Increased analgesia, CNS depression, and hypotensive effects
MAO inhibitors: Increased risk of unpredictable, severe, even fatal adverse reactions
metoclopramide: Antagonized metoclopramide effects on GI motility
naloxone: Antagonized analgesic, CNS, and respiratory depressant effects of pentazocine
naltrexone: Withdrawal symptoms in patients physically dependent on pentazocine
neuromuscular blockers: Increased respiratory depression

ACTIVITIES

alcohol use: Additive CNS and respiratory depression that could be severe and increased risk of habituation
smoking: Decreased effectiveness

Adverse Reactions

CNS: Chills, confusion, depression, dizziness, drowsiness, euphoria, fatigue, headache, **increased intracranial pressure**, hallucinations, insomnia, light-headedness, nervousness, nightmares, paresthesia, restlessness, **seizures**, syncope, weakness

CV: Hypertension, **hypotension**, tachycardia
EENT: Blurred vision, diplopia, dry mouth, **laryngeal edema**, **laryngospasm**, miosis
ENDO: Adrenal insufficiency
GI: Anorexia, biliary tract spasm, constipation, diarrhea, **hepatotoxicity**, nausea, vomiting
GU: Decreased libido, decreased urine output, dysuria, erectile dysfunction, impotence, infertility, lack of menstruation, urinary frequency, urine retention
HEME: Agranulocytosis, transient eosinophilia
MS: Muscle rigidity (with large doses)
RESP: Atelectasis, **bronchospasm**, **depressed respirations**, dyspnea, **hypoventilation**, wheezing
SKIN: Diaphoresis, **erythema multiforme**, facial flushing, pruritus, rash, **Stevens–Johnson syndrome**, **toxic epidermal necrolysis**, urticaria
Other: Anaphylaxis; **angioedema**; injection-site burning, pain, redness, or swelling; physical and psychological dependence

Nursing Considerations

- Be aware that excessive use of opioids like pentazocine may lead to abuse, addiction, misuse, overdose, and possibly death. Monitor patient's intake of drug closely and for evidence of physical dependence.
- Know that chronic maternal use of pentazocine during pregnancy can result in neonatal opioid withdrawal syndrome (NOWS), which may be life-threatening if not recognized and treated appropriately. NOWS occurs when a newborn has been exposed to opioid drugs like pentazocine for a prolonged period while in utero.
- Use pentazocine with extreme caution in patients with head injury, increased intracranial pressure, or intracranial lesion. Drug may mask neurologic evidence.
- Use pentazocine cautiously: in patients physically dependent on opioid agonists because drug may prompt withdrawal symptoms; in patients with acute MI because drug's cardiovascular effects can increase cardiac workload; in patients with hepatic or renal dysfunction because drug is metabolized in liver and excreted in urine; and in patients with respiratory conditions or who are debilitated or elderly because drug depresses respiratory system.
- Know that when giving repeated parenteral doses, I.M. or I.V. route should be used when possible and as prescribed because subcutaneous route may cause severe tissue damage at injection site. Rotate I.M. sites to avoid tissue damage.

WARNING Know that many drugs may interact with opioids like pentazocine to cause serotonin syndrome. Monitor patient closely for signs and symptoms such as agitation, diaphoresis, diarrhea, fever, hallucinations, labile blood pressure, muscle twitching or stiffness, nausea, shakiness, shivering, tachycardia, trouble with coordination, or vomiting. Notify prescriber at once because serotonin syndrome may be life-threatening. Be prepared to discontinue drug, if possible and ordered, and provide supportive care.

- Monitor patient for adrenal insufficiency. Although rare, it can be life-threatening. Monitor patient for anorexia, dizziness, fatigue, hypotension, nausea, vomiting, or weakness. Notify prescriber if suspected and expect diagnostic testing to be done. If confirmed, expect to administer corticosteroids and wean patient off pentazocine, if possible.
- After giving parenteral form, expect to taper dosage gradually, as prescribed, to reduce the risk of withdrawal symptoms.

WARNING Be aware that pentazocine should only be used concomitantly with benzodiazepine therapy in patients for whom other treatment options are inadequate. If prescribed together, expect dosing and duration of pentazocine to be limited. Monitor patient closely for signs and symptoms of a decrease in consciousness, including coma, profound sedation, and significant respiratory depression. Notify prescriber immediately and provide emergency supportive care, as death may occur.

PATIENT TEACHING

- Caution patient that prolonged use of pentazocine may result in abuse, misuse, overdose, physical or psychological dependence, overdose, and possibly death.
- Advise patient to avoid hazardous activities until drug's CNS effects are known.

- Caution patient not to use alcohol, or take benzodiazepines or OTC drugs without consulting prescriber as severe respiratory depression can occur and may lead to death.
- Caution pregnant patient not to increase dosage or take pentazocine for a prolonged period, as adverse effects can cause infant to experience withdrawal when born.
- Advise patient to report possible allergic reaction, such as itching or a rash.
- Inform patient that long-term use of opioids like pentazocine may decrease sex hormone levels causing decreased libido, erectile dysfunction, impotence, infertility, or lack of menstruation. Encourage patient to report any symptoms to prescriber.
- Instruct patient to notify all prescribers of opioid use.

pentosan polysulfate sodium

Elmiron

Class and Category

Pharmacologic class: Bladder protectant
Therapeutic class: Bladder analgesic
Pregnancy category: B

Indications and Dosages

➤ *To relieve bladder discomfort or pain caused by interstitial cystitis*

CAPSULES

Adults. 100 mg three times a day for up to 3 mo, possibly followed by another 3 mo if no improvement and no adverse reactions.

Mechanism of Action

Adheres to mucosal membrane of bladder wall and may block irritating solutes from reaching cells, thereby decreasing local discomfort and pain.

Contraindications

Hypersensitivity to pentosan, other structurally related compounds, or their components

Interactions

DRUGS

alteplase (recombinant), aspirin (high doses), heparin, oral anticoagulants, streptokinase: Increased risk of hemorrhage

Adverse Reactions

CNS: Depression, dizziness, emotional lability, headache
GI: Abdominal pain, diarrhea, elevated liver enzymes, hepatic dysfunction, indigestion, nausea, **rectal hemorrhage**
HEME: Unusual bleeding or bruising
SKIN: Alopecia, rash

Nursing Considerations

- Use pentosan with extreme caution in patients with conditions that increase bleeding risk, such as aneurysm, diverticula, GI ulceration, hemophilia, polyps, and thrombocytopenia (especially heparin-induced).
- Use drug cautiously in patients with hepatic dysfunction because drug is desulfated in liver and spleen.
- Monitor patient for abnormal bleeding, such as unexplained bruises and epistaxis, because drug is a weak anticoagulant.

PATIENT TEACHING

- Instruct patient to take pentosan with a full glass of water at least 1 hour before or 2 hours after meals.
- Explain the pattern of exacerbations and remissions with interstitial cystitis. Reassure patient that symptoms should improve within 3 months after starting pentosan therapy.
- Advise patient to take bleeding precautions during therapy, such as using an electric shaver and a soft-bristled toothbrush.
- Alert patient that if alopecia develops, it's usually confined to a single area.

pentoxifylline

Pentoxil, Trental

Class and Category

Pharmacologic class: Xanthine derivative
Therapeutic class: Hemorrheologic agent
Pregnancy category: C

Indications and Dosages

➤ *To treat intermittent claudication in patients with peripheral vascular disease*

E.R. TABLETS
Adults. 400 mg three times a day with meals.
DOSAGE ADJUSTMENT For patients who have severe renal impairment (creatinine clearance below 30 ml/min), dosage reduced to 400 mg once a day. For patients who experience adverse GI or CNS reactions, dosage may be reduced to 400 mg twice daily.

Route	Onset	Peak	Duration
P.O.	2–4 wk	Unknown	Unknown

Mechanism of Action
Relieves symptoms of peripheral vascular disease by:
- reducing blood viscosity by decreasing plasma fibrinogen level and inhibiting RBC and platelet aggregation
- improving erythrocyte flexibility by inhibiting phosphodiesterase and increasing the amount of cAMP in RBCs
- decreasing peripheral vascular resistance and improving microcirculatory blood flow and tissue oxygenation.

Contraindications
Hypersensitivity to pentoxifylline, methylxanthines (such as caffeine, theobromine, and theophylline), or their components; recent cerebral or retinal hemorrhage

Interactions
DRUGS
antihypertensives: Potentiated antihypertensive effects
CYP1A2 inhibitors (strong) such as ciprofloxacin, fluvoxamine: Possibly increased exposure to pentoxifylline leading to increased adverse reactions
heparin, NSAIDs, oral anticoagulants, other platelet aggregation inhibitors, plicamycin, thrombolytics, valproic acid: Increased risk of bleeding
cimetidine: Increased blood pentoxifylline level, increased risk of adverse effects
insulin, oral antidiabetic agents: Potentiated blood-glucose lowering effect of these drugs
sympathomimetics, xanthines: Enhanced CNS stimulation
theophylline: Elevated theophylline plasma levels possibly leading to theophylline toxicity
vitamin K antagonists: Increased anticoagulant activity

ACTIVITIES
smoking: Possibly decreased therapeutic effects of pentoxifylline

Adverse Reactions
CNS: Agitation, anxiety, **aseptic meningitis**, confusion, depression, dizziness, drowsiness, headache, insomnia, malaise, nervousness, **seizures**, tremor
CV: Angina, **arrhythmia**, chest pain, edema, **hypotension**, palpitation, tachycardia
EENT: Bad taste, blurred vision, conjunctivitis, dry mouth, earache, epistaxis, excessive salivation, laryngitis, nasal congestion, scotoma, sore throat, swollen neck glands
GI: Abdominal discomfort, anorexia, belching, bloating, cholecystitis, constipation, diarrhea, dyspepsia, elevated liver enzymes, flatus, **hepatitis**, indigestion, jaundice, nausea, vomiting
HEME: **Aplastic anemia**, decreased serum fibrinogen, **leukemia**, **leukopenia**, **pancytopenia**, purpura, **thrombocytopenia**
RESP: Dyspnea
SKIN: Brittle nails, flushing, pruritus, rash, urticaria
Other: **Anaphylaxis**, **angioedema**, flu-like symptoms, thirst, weight changes

Nursing Considerations
- Use pentoxifylline cautiously in elderly patients and those with hepatic or renal dysfunction.
- Give drug with meals and an antacid, if needed, to reduce adverse GI reactions.

WARNING Monitor patient closely for hypersensitivity reactions that could be life-threatening. At the first sign of anaphylactic or anaphylactoid reaction, stop pentoxifylline therapy, notify prescriber, and provide supportive care.

PATIENT TEACHING
- Instruct patient to swallow pentoxifylline E.R. tablets whole and not to break, chew, or crush them.
- Advise patient to take drug with meals to reduce GI irritation. If adverse GI reactions occur anyway, advise her to also take an antacid with meals.
- Inform patient that although symptoms may not improve for several weeks, urge him to continue taking drug as

P

prescribed to achieve maximum therapeutic effect.
- Instruct patient not to smoke during therapy because smoking constricts blood vessels and may reduce drug effectiveness.
- Urge patient to report adverse reactions; dosage may have to be reduced.

peramivir

Rapivab

Class and Category

Pharmacologic class: Neuraminidase inhibitor
Therapeutic class: Antiviral
Pregnancy category: Not classified

Indications and Dosages

➤ *To treat acute uncomplicated influenza in patients who have been symptomatic for no more than 2 days*

I.V. INFUSION

Adults and adolescents. 600 mg as a single dose given over 15 to 30 min.
Children ages 2 to 13 years. 12 mg/kg as a single dose given over 15 to 30 min. *Maximum:* 600 mg as a single dose.

DOSAGE ADJUSTMENT For adult patients with a creatinine clearance between 30 and 49 ml/min, dosage reduced to 200 mg. For adult patients with a creatinine clearance between 10 and 29 ml/min, dosage reduced to 100 mg. For children with a creatinine clearance between 30 and 49 mg/kg, dosage reduced to 4 mg/kg. For children with a creatinine clearance between 10 and 29 ml/min, dosage reduced to 2 mg/kg.

Mechanism of Action

Inhibits influenza virus neuraminidase, affecting release of viral particles from the infected cells.

Incompatibilities

Do not mix or co-infuse peramivir with other intravenous medications and only dilute with 0.9% or 0.45% sodium chloride, 5% dextrose, or lactated Ringer's solution.

Contraindications

Hypersensitivity to peramivir or its components

Interactions

DRUGS

live attenuated influenza vaccine: Possibly decreased effectiveness

Adverse Reactions

CNS: Abnormal behavior, delirium, fever, hallucinations, insomnia
CV: Hypertension
EENT: Tympanic membrane erythema
ENDO: Hyperglycemia
GI: Constipation, diarrhea, elevated liver enzymes, vomiting
GU: Proteinuria
HEME: Neutropenia
MS: Elevated CPK level
SKIN: Erythema multiforme, **exfoliative dermatitis**, rash, **Stevens–Johnson syndrome**
Other: Anaphylaxis

Nursing Considerations

- Dilute an appropriate dose of peramivir 10 mg/ml solution in 0.9% or 0.45% sodium chloride, 5% dextrose or lactated Ringer's solution to a maximum volume of 100 ml. Administer immediately or administer refrigerated diluted solution up to 24 hours as an intravenous infusion over 15 to 30 min. If administering refrigerated diluted solution, allow diluted solution to reach room temperature, then administer immediately. Discard any unused diluted solution after 24 hours.

WARNING Monitor patient for serious hypersensitivity and skin reactions when administering peramivir. Know that anaphylaxis and skin reactions such as erythema multiforme and Stevens–Johnson syndrome have occurred. If present during infusion, discontinue peramivir therapy immediately, notify prescriber, and be prepared to provide emergency supportive care as ordered.

- Be aware that although uncommon, abnormal behavior and delirium have occurred after administration of peramivir, especially in children. Although the onset is abrupt, rapid resolution usually occurs once peramivir is discontinued.

PATIENT TEACHING

WARNING Advise patient to inform staff administering peramivir if he experiences any symptoms of an allergic reaction, such as itching. If he experiences any unusual

or severe adverse effects after infusion has been completed, instruct him to seek immediate medical attention.
- Alert patient and parents that, although uncommon, abnormal behavior and delirium have occurred, especially in children. Prescriber should be notified and child kept safe until behavior returns to normal.
- Inform patient that peramivir is not a substitute for receiving an annual flu vaccination.

perampanel

Fycompa

Class, Category, and Schedule

Pharmacologic class: AMPA glutamate receptor antagonist
Therapeutic class: Anticonvulsant
Pregnancy category: C
Controlled substance schedule: III

Indications and Dosages

➤ *Adjunct therapy for treatment of primary generalized tonic–clonic seizures in patients with epilepsy*

ORAL SUSPENSION, TABLETS

Adults and children age 12 and over. *Initial*: 2 mg once daily at bedtime, then increased in 2 mg increments weekly, as needed. *Usual:* 8 to 12 mg once daily at at bedtime. *Maximum:* 12 mg daily at bedtime.

➤ *To treat partial-onset seizures as adjunctive or monotherapy*

ORAL SUSPENSION, TABLETS

Adults and children age 4 and over. *Initial:* 2 mg once daily at bedtime, then increased in increments of 2 mg weekly, as needed. *Usual:* 8 to 12 mg.

DOSAGE ADJUSTMENT For elderly patients, dosage titration done every 2 wk. For patients with mild to moderate hepatic impairment, dosage increased every 2 wk in 2-mg increments until target dose is achieved. For patients with mild hepatic impairment, maximum daily dosage is 6 mg daily at bedtime; for patients with moderate hepatic impairment, maximum daily dosage is 4 mg daily at bedtime. For patients with moderate renal impairment, a slower titration may be considered. For patients taking moderate or strong CYP3A4 enzyme inducers, including enzyme-inducing AEDs such as carbamazepine, oxcarbazepine, or phenytoin, initial dosage increased to 4 mg once daily.

Mechanism of Action

Acts as a noncompetitive antagonist on the AMPA glutamate receptor on postsynaptic neurons. Glutamate is the primary excitatory neurotransmitter in the central nervous system. By preventing glutamate action, the central nervous system experiences less stimulation, resulting in less seizure activity in the brain.

Contraindications

Hypersensitivity to perampanel or its components

Interactions

DRUGS

CNS depressants: Possibly increased CNS depression
cytochrome P450 (CYP) inducers such as carbamazepine, phenytoin, oxcarbazepine, rifampin, St. John's wort: Significant decreased plasma perampanel levels
implant or oral contraceptives containing levonorgestrel: Possibly less effectiveness of contraceptive

ACTIVITIES

alcohol: Possibly increased CNS depression

Adverse Reactions

CNS: Abnormal coordination, affect lability, aggression, agitation, anger, anxiety, asthenia, ataxia, belligerence possibly leading to physical assault and **homicidal ideation**, confusion, delusions, depression, disorientation, dizziness, euphoria, fatigue, gait disturbance, hallucinations, headache, hostility, hypersomnia, hypoaesthesia, increased fall risk, irritability, memory impairment, mood alteration, paranoia, paresthesia, psychosis (acute), somnolence, **suicidal ideation**, worsening of preexisting psychiatric conditions, vertigo
CV: Peripheral edema
EENT: Blurred vision, diplopia, oropharyngeal pain
GI: Constipation, nausea, vomiting
MS: Arthralgia; back, extremity or musculoskeletal pain; dysarthria; myalgia

RESP: Cough, upper respiratory infections
Other: Drug reaction with eosinophilia and systemic symptoms (DRESS), hyponatremia, physical and psychological dependence, weight gain

Nursing Considerations

- Monitor patient closely for adverse reactions, especially the patient receiving 12 mg/day because of increased risk of adverse reactions at that dosage.
- Monitor patient for behavioral and psychiatric reactions, as perampanel may induce serious reactions leading to hostility and even become life-threatening, with possibility of homicidal ideation or physical assault occurring. These adverse reactions have occurred in patients without prior psychiatric history, prior aggressive behavior, or concomitant use of medications associated with aggression and hostility. Patients with pre-existing psychiatric conditions sometimes become worse, and use of alcohol significantly worsens mood and increases anger. Most often these reactions appear within the first 6 weeks of therapy, although new events may occur at any time during therapy. Notify prescriber immediately if adverse behavioral or psychiatric reactions occur. Perampanel dosage may have to be reduced or drug therapy temporarily withheld or discontinued.
- Monitor patient closely for depression that may lead to suicidal ideation, especially when perampanel therapy is begun and when dosage is increased.
- Monitor patient, especially the elderly, for dizziness and gait disturbance. Encourage patient to ask for help when getting out of bed or chair or when ambulating, especially during the titration phase. Notify prescriber if such reactions occur, as dosage may have to be altered or drug discontinued.
- Monitor patient for signs and symptoms of DRESS. Be aware that fever or lymphadenopathy may be present even if a rash is not. Notify prescriber immediately if DRESS is suspected and expect drug to be discontinued. Provide supportive care, as needed and prescribed.
- Be aware that perampanel therapy increases risk of falls, especially in the elderly. Monitor patient's movements closely and put safety measures in place to help prevent falls.
- Monitor patient's weight because drug can cause weight gain.

WARNING Be aware that perampanel has a potential for abuse and is classified as a controlled substance category III drug.

- Expect to withdraw perampanel therapy gradually when discontinued, if possible, because abrupt withdrawal can increase risk of seizures.

PATIENT TEACHING

- Advise patient to take drug exactly as prescribed as drug may cause physical and psychological dependency.
- Instruct patient taking oral suspension form to shake the bottle well and to use the adaptor and oral dosing syringe provided. Remind patient that a household teaspoon or tablespoon is not an adequate measuring device. Tell patient to discard any unused oral suspension remaining 90 days after first opening the bottle.
- Caution patient to avoid performing activities that require alertness, such as driving, until effects of drug are known. Review fall precautions with patient.
- Instruct patient to avoid ingesting alcohol products while taking perampanel because the combination can significantly worsen mood and increase anger, which may lead to physical assault and even homicidal ideation.
- Instruct patient and family members or caregivers to be on the alert for new onset or worsening of depression, any unusual changes in behavior or mood (e.g., confusion, difficulty with memory, hearing or seeing things that are not there), or expressions of thoughts about self-harm, especially when dosage of drug is being increased or higher doses are prescribed. Report changes to prescriber immediately.
- Tell patient to alert prescriber of any persistent, severe, or unusual signs and symptoms, especially a rash.
- Tell patient to notify prescriber if pregnancy is suspected or occurs while taking perampanel. If confirmed,

encourage patient to register pregnancy with the North American Antiepileptic Drug Pregnancy Registry by calling 1-888-233-2334 or visiting their website at http://www.aedprenancyregistry.org.
- Inform women of childbearing age taking a levonorgestrel-containing contraceptive to use an additional nonhormonal form of contraception while taking perampanel and for a month after drug is discontinued.
- Instruct patient not to stop taking perampanel abruptly, as seizure activity may increase.

perindopril erbumine

Aceon

Class and Category

Pharmacologic class: Angiotensin-converting enzyme (ACE) inhibitor
Therapeutic class: Antihypertensive
Pregnancy category: D

Indications and Dosages

➤ *To manage hypertension*

TABLETS

Adults. *Initial:* 4 mg daily as a single dose or in divided doses twice daily, increased as prescribed until blood pressure is controlled or maximum dosage is reached.
Maintenance: 4 to 8 mg daily. *Maximum:* 8 mg daily.
DOSAGE ADJUSTMENT If patient takes a diuretic, initial dosage possibly reduced to 2 to 4 mg daily; if patient has renal failure, initial dosage possibly reduced to 2 mg daily.

➤ *To reduce risk of cardiovascular death or nonfatal MI in patients with stable coronary artery disease*

TABLETS

Adults. *Initial:* 4 mg daily for 2 wk; then increased to 8 mg daily. *Maintenance:* 8 mg daily.
DOSAGE ADJUSTMENT If patient is elderly, 2 mg daily for 1 wk, increased to 4 mg daily for 1 wk and then to 8 mg daily if tolerated.

Mechanism of Action

Is converted to the active metabolite perindoprilat, which competes with angiotensin I binding sites, blocking conversion of angiotensin I to angiotensin II, a potent vasoconstrictor. As a result, this ACE inhibitor reduces vasoconstriction and blood pressure. Decreased angiotensin II also reduces aldosterone secretion, increasing renal excretion of water and sodium.

Contraindications

Concomitant therapy with a neprilysin inhibitor such as sacubitril or within 36 hours of its use; concurrent aliskiren therapy in patients with diabetes or renal impairment (GRF less than 60 ml/min); history of angioedema with ACE inhibitor treatment; hypersensitivity to perindopril, other ACE inhibitors, or their components

Interactions

DRUGS

aliskiren (patients with diabetes or renal impairment), angiotensin-converting-enzyme (ACE) inhibitors, angiotensin receptor blockers (ARDs): Increased risks of hyperkalemia, hypotension, or changes in renal function such as acute renal failure
diuretics: Increased risk of hypotension
lithium: Increased blood lithium level and risk of toxicity
mTOR inhibitors such as everolimus, sirolimus, temsirolimus; neprilysin inhibitors such as sacubitril: Possibly increased risk of angioedema
NSAIDs: Increased risk of renal impairment in patients who are elderly, volume-depleted, or already have renal dysfunction
potassium-sparing diuretics, potassium supplements: Increased risk of hyperkalemia
sodium aurothiomalate: Increased risk of nitritoid reaction with facial flushing, nausea, vomiting, and hypotension

Adverse Reactions

CNS: Amnesia, anxiety, dizziness, fatigue, fever, headache, hypertonia, migraine, syncope, vertigo
CV: Chest pain, **ECG changes**, heart murmur, **hypotension**, orthostatic hypotension, palpitations, **PVCs**
EENT: Conjunctivitis, earache, epistaxis, hoarseness, pharyngitis, rhinitis, sinusitis, sneezing, tinnitus
GI: Abdominal pain, diarrhea, elevated liver enzymes, flatulence, increased appetite, indigestion

GU: Flank pain, renal calculi, urinary frequency and urgency, vaginitis
HEME: Hematoma, **leukopenia, neutropenia**
MS: Arthritis, back pain, gout, limb pain, myalgia, neck pain
RESP: Cough
SKIN: Canker sores, diaphoresis, dry skin, ecchymosis, erythema, pruritus, rash
Other: Angioedema

Nursing Considerations

- Use cautiously with heart failure, renal artery stenosis, or renal dysfunction.
- Also use cautiously in elderly patients, and watch closely for adverse effects such as dizziness or vertigo, because these patients have an increased risk of falling.
- Monitor patients with hepatic dysfunction for enhanced therapeutic drug effects because drug's bioavailability is increased.
- Monitor serum potassium level to detect hyperkalemia, especially in patients with renal insufficiency or diabetes mellitus, and those who use a potassium-containing salt substitute or take a potassium-sparing diuretic or potassium supplement.

PATIENT TEACHING

- Instruct patient to take perindopril exactly as prescribed, even if she feels well.

WARNING Urge patient to stop taking drug and notify prescriber immediately if she experiences signs of angioedema.

- Advise patient to notify prescriber at once about fever, sore throat, or other signs that may indicate neutropenia.
- Urge patient to avoid potassium supplements and potassium-containing salt substitutes unless prescriber approves.
- Instruct patient to avoid hazardous activities until drug's CNS effects are known.
- Advise woman to report promptly suspected, known, or intended pregnancy. Drug will have to be discontinued.

perphenazine

Class and Category

Pharmacologic class: Phenothiazine
Therapeutic class: Antiemetic, antipsychotic
Pregnancy category: Not classified

Indications and Dosages

➤ *To treat psychotic disorders, such as schizophrenia*

ORAL SOLUTION

Hospitalized adults and adolescents. 8 to 16 mg twice daily to four times a day, adjusted as needed and tolerated. *Maximum:* 64 mg daily.

TABLETS

Adults and adolescents. 4 to 16 mg twice daily to four times daily, adjusted as needed and tolerated. *Maximum:* 64 mg daily.

➤ *To treat severe nausea and vomiting*

TABLETS

Adults and adolescents. 8 to 16 mg daily in divided doses, decreased as appropriate. *Maximum:* 24 mg daily.

DOSAGE ADJUSTMENT Initial dose possibly reduced and gradually increased for debilitated, elderly, or emaciated patients. Adolescents may need low adult dosage.

Route	Onset	Peak	Duration
P.O.	Several wk	4–7 days	Unknown

Mechanism of Action

Depresses areas of the brain that control activity and aggression, including cerebral cortex, hypothalamus, and limbic system, by an unknown mechanism. Perphenazine also prevents nausea and vomiting by blocking or inhibiting dopamine receptors in medullary chemoreceptor trigger zone and peripherally by blocking vagus nerve in the GI tract.

Incompatibilities

Don't mix perphenazine oral solution with beverages that contain caffeine or tannins (such as coffee, colas, and teas) or pectinates (such as apple juice) because they're physically incompatible.

Contraindications

Blood dyscrasias; bone marrow depression; cerebral arteriosclerosis; coma; concurrent use of CNS depressants (large doses); coronary artery disease; hepatic impairment; hypersensitivity to perphenazine, other phenothiazines, or their components; myeloproliferative disorders; severe CNS depression; severe hypertension or hypotension; subcortical brain damage

Interactions

DRUGS

aluminum- and magnesium-containing antacids, antidiarrheals (adsorbent): Decreased absorption of oral perphenazine
amantadine, anticholinergics, antidyskinetics, antihistamines: Increased adverse anticholinergic effects
amphetamines: Decreased therapeutic effects of both drugs
anticonvulsants: Decreased seizure threshold, inhibited metabolism and toxicity of anticonvulsant
antithyroid drugs: Increased risk of agranulocytosis
apomorphine: Additive CNS depression, decreased emetic response to apomorphine if perphenazine is given first
appetite suppressants (except phenmetrazine): Antagonized anorectic effect of appetite suppressants
beta blockers: Increased blood levels of both drugs and risk of arrhythmias, hypotension, irreversible retinopathy, and tardive dyskinesia
bromocriptine: Possibly interference with bromocriptine's effects
CNS depressants: Increased CNS and respiratory depression and hypotensive effects
dopamine: Antagonized peripheral vasoconstriction with high doses of dopamine
ephedrine: Decreased vasopressor response to ephedrine
epinephrine: Blocked alpha-adrenergic effects of epinephrine, possibly causing severe hypotension and tachycardia
hepatotoxic drugs: Increased risk of hepatotoxicity
hypotension-causing drugs: Increased risk of severe orthostatic hypotension
levodopa: Inhibited antidyskinetic effects of levodopa
lithium: Possibly neurotoxicity (disorientation, extrapyramidal symptoms, unconsciousness)
maprotiline, selective serotonin reuptake inhibitors, tricyclic antidepressants: Prolonged and intensified anticholinergic and sedative effects of these drugs or perphenazine
metrizamide: Decreased seizure threshold
opioid analgesics: Increased CNS and respiratory depression, increased risk of orthostatic hypotension and severe constipation
ototoxic drugs, especially antibiotics: Possibly masking of some symptoms of ototoxicity, such as dizziness, tinnitus, and vertigo
probucol, other drugs that prolong QT interval: Prolonged QT interval, which may increase risk of ventricular tachycardia
thiazide diuretics: Possibly hyponatremia and water intoxication

ACTIVITIES

alcohol use: Increased CNS and respiratory depression, hypotensive effects, and risk of heatstroke

Adverse Reactions

CNS: Behavioral changes, **cerebral edema**, dizziness, drowsiness, extrapyramidal reactions (such as akathisia, dystonia, pseudoparkinsonism), fever, headache, **neuroleptic malignant syndrome**, **seizures**, **suicidal ideation**, syncope, tardive dyskinesia (persistent)
CV: Bradycardia, **cardiac arrest**, hypertension, **hypotension**, orthostatic hypotension, tachycardia
EENT: Blurred vision, dry mouth, glaucoma, **laryngeal edema**, miosis, mydriasis, nasal congestion, ocular changes (corneal opacification, retinopathy)
ENDO: Decreased libido, galactorrhea, gynecomastia, syndrome of inappropriate ADH secretion
GI: Anorexia, constipation, diarrhea, fecal impaction, jaundice, nausea, vomiting
GU: Bladder paralysis, ejaculation failure, menstrual irregularities, polyuria, urinary frequency, urinary incontinence, urine retention
HEME: Agranulocytosis, eosinophilia, **hemolytic anemia**, **leukopenia**, **pancytopenia**, **thrombocytopenic purpura**
RESP: Asthma
SKIN: Diaphoresis, eczema, erythema, **exfoliative dermatitis**, hyperpigmentation, pallor, photosensitivity, pruritus, urticaria
Other: Anaphylaxis, **angioedema**

Nursing Considerations

- Know that perphenazine shouldn't be used to treat dementia-related psychosis in the elderly because of an increased mortality risk.

- Use perphenazine cautiously in patients with depression or hepatic, pulmonary, or renal dysfunction and in elderly patients, who are at increased risk for increased plasma concentrations and tardive dyskinesia.
- Obtain blood samples for CBC and liver and renal function tests, as ordered, to detect adverse reactions.
- Monitor temperature frequently, and notify prescriber if it rises; a significant increase suggests drug intolerance.
- Monitor blood pressure of patient who takes large doses of perphenazine, especially if surgery is indicated, because of the increased risk of hypotension.
- Watch patient closely (especially adolescents and young adults) for suicidal tendencies, particularly when perphenazine therapy starts and dosage changes, because depression may worsen temporarily during these times, possibly leading to suicidal ideation.

PATIENT TEACHING

- Instruct patient to take drug exactly as prescribed to ensure optimal effectiveness and minimize adverse reactions.
- Remind patient who takes oral solution to use a calibrated measuring device.
- Instruct patient taking oral solution to dilute every 5 ml (teaspoon) of drug in 2 fluid oz of carbonated beverage, fruit juice (except apple), milk, soup, tomato juice, or water. Caution against using beverages that contain caffeine or tannins (coffee, cola, tea).
- Caution patient not to spill oral solution on skin or clothing because it can cause contact dermatitis and damage clothing.
- Urge patient to avoid alcohol and other CNS depressants during perphenazine therapy and to avoid hazardous activities until drug's CNS effects are known.
- Advise patient to avoid excessive sun exposure and to protect skin when outdoors.
- Instruct patient to notify prescriber about persistent or severe adverse reactions.
- Urge patient to comply with long-term follow-up to detect adverse reactions and determine possible need for perphenazine dosage adjustments.
- Urge family or caregiver to watch patient closely for suicidal tendencies, especially when therapy starts or dosage changes and particularly if patient is a teenager or young adult.

phenazopyridine hydrochloride

Azo-Standard, Baridium, Phenazo (CAN), Pyridiate, Pyridium

Class and Category

Pharmacologic class: Alpha$_1$ agonist
Therapeutic class: Urinary analgesic
Pregnancy category: B

Indications and Dosages

➤ *To relieve burning and pain on urination, and urinary frequency and urgency*

TABLETS

Adults and adolescents. 200 mg three times daily with or without food for no longer than 2 days.

Mechanism of Action

Exerts a local anesthetic effect on urinary tract mucosa as drug is excreted in urine. Phenazopyridine's exact mechanism is unknown.

Contraindications

Hypersensitivity to phenazopyridine or its components, renal insufficiency

Adverse Reactions

CNS: Headache
GI: Indigestion, nausea, vomiting
GU: Reddish orange urine
SKIN: Pruritus, rash
Other: Discoloration of body fluids

Nursing Considerations

- Notify prescriber if yellowish skin or sclerae develop in patient taking phenazopyridine because this may indicate drug accumulation from impaired renal excretion. Expect prescriber to discontinue drug.
- Be aware that phenazopyridine treatment should be limited to 2 days.

PATIENT TEACHING

- Instruct patient not to take drug for longer than 2 days and to notify prescriber if symptoms persist beyond that time.
- Advise patient to take drug with meals if GI distress develops.

- Inform patient that drug turns urine orange to red and may discolor other body fluids, such as tears.
- Advise patient not to wear contact lenses during therapy because they may become stained.

phenelzine sulfate

Nardil

Class and Category

Pharmacologic class: Monoamine oxidase inhibitor (MAOI)
Therapeutic class: Antidepressant
Pregnancy category: C

Indications and Dosages

➤ *To treat depression after other drug therapies have failed*

TABLETS

Adults. *Initial:* 15 mg three times daily, increased rapidly as prescribed and tolerated. *Maintenance:* As tolerated. *Maximum:* 90 mg daily.

Route	Onset	Peak	Duration
P.O.	7–10 days	4–8 wk	10 days

Contraindications

Cardiovascular disease; cerebrovascular disease; heart failure; hepatic disease; history of headaches; hypersensitivity to phenelzine or its components; hypertension; pheochromocytoma; severe renal impairment; use of anesthetics, antihypertensives, bupropion, buspirone, carbamazepine, CNS depressants, cyclobenzaprine, dextromethorphan, meperidine, selective serotonin-reuptake inhibitors, sympathomimetics, or tricyclic antidepressants; use within 14 days of other MAO inhibitor

Interactions

DRUGS

anticholinergics, antidyskinetics, antihistamines: Increased anticholinergic effect, prolonged CNS depression (antihistamines)
anticonvulsants: Increased CNS depression, possibly altered pattern of seizures
beta blockers: Increased risk of bradycardia
bromocriptine: Possibly interference with bromocriptine effects
bupropion: Increased risk of bupropion toxicity
buspirone: Increased risk of hypertension
caffeine-containing drugs: Increased risk of dangerous arrhythmias and severe hypertension
carbamazepine, cyclobenzaprine, maprotiline, other MAO inhibitors: Increased risk of hyperpyretic crisis, hypertensive crisis, severe seizures, and death; altered pattern of seizures (with carbamazepine)
CNS depressants: Increased CNS depression
dextromethorphan: Increased risk of excitation, hyperpyrexia, and hypertension
diuretics: Increased hypotensive effect
doxapram: Increased vasopressor effects of either drug
fluoxetine: Increased risk of agitation, confusion, GI symptoms, hyperpyretic episodes, hypertensive crisis, potentially fatal serotonin syndrome, restlessness, and severe seizures.
guanadrel, guanethidine: Increased risk of hypertension
haloperidol, loxapine, molindone, phenothiazines, pimozide, thioxanthenes: Prolonged and intensified anticholinergic, hypotensive, and sedative effects of these drugs or phenelzine
insulin, oral antidiabetic drugs: Increased hypoglycemic effects
levodopa: Increased risk of sudden, moderate to severe hypertension
local anesthetics (with epinephrine or levonordefrin): Possibly severe hypertension
meperidine, other opioid analgesics: Increased risk of coma, hyperpyrexia, hypotension, immediate excitation, rigidity, seizures, severe hypertension, severe respiratory depression, sweating, vascular collapse, and death
methyldopa: Increased risk of hallucinations, headache, hyperexcitability, and severe hypertension
methylphenidate: Increased CNS stimulant effect of methylphenidate
metrizamide: Decreased seizure threshold, increased risk of seizures

Mechanism of Action

Phenelzine relieves symptoms of unipolar depressive disorders by inhibiting the enzyme monoamine oxidase (MAO). Normally, MAO breaks down monoamine neurotransmitters, such as serotonin, as shown below left. By inhibiting this enzyme, phenelzine increases the concentration of serotonin in the vesicles of monoamine nerve endings, allowing more serotonin to be released and engage with receptors on postsynaptic cells, as shown below right. A serotonin deficiency may be responsible in part for endogenous depression.

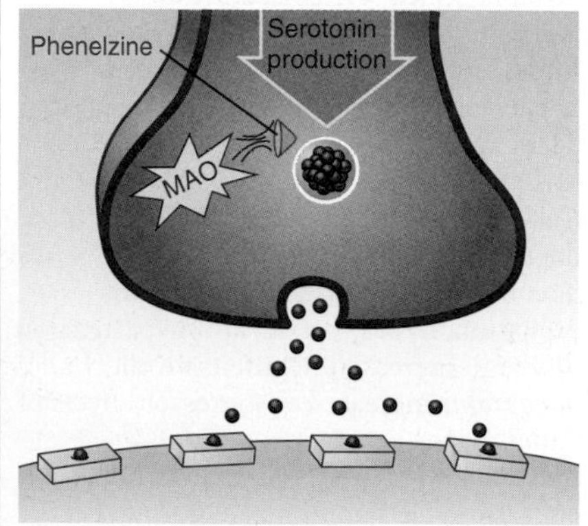

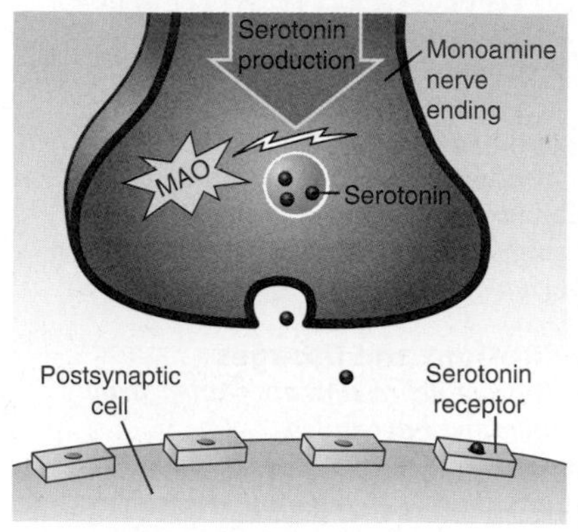

oral anticoagulants: Increased anticoagulant activity
paroxetine, sertraline, trazodone, tricyclic antidepressants: Increased risk of potentially fatal serotonin syndrome
phenylephrine (nasal or ophthalmic): Potentiated vasopressor effect of phenylephrine
rauwolfia alkaloids: Increased risk of moderate to severe hypertension, CNS depression (when phenelzine is added to rauwolfia alkaloid therapy), CNS excitation and hypertension (when rauwolfia alkaloid is added to phenelzine therapy)
spinal anesthetics: Increased risk of hypotension
succinylcholine: Possibly increased neuromuscular blockade of succinylcholine
sympathomimetics: Prolonged and intensified cardiac stimulant and vasopressor effects
tryptophan: Increased risk of confusion, disorientation, hyperreflexia, hyperthermia, hyperventilation, mania or hypomania, and shivering

FOODS
foods and beverages high in tyramine or other pressor amines, such as aged cheese; beer; broad beans such as fava beans; cured meat or sausage; liqueurs; overripe fruit; pickled or smoked fish, meat, and poultry; protein or yeast extracts; red and white wine; reduced-alcohol and alcohol-free beer and wine; sauerkraut; sherry: Increased risk of sudden, severe hypertension

ACTIVITIES
alcohol use: Increased CNS depressant effects and hypertensive crisis

Adverse Reactions

CNS: Agitation, dizziness, drowsiness, headache, overstimulation, restlessness, sedation, sleep disturbance, **suicidal ideation**, weakness
CV: Bradycardia, edema, **hypertensive crisis**, orthostatic hypotension, palpitations, tachycardia
EENT: Blurred vision, dry mouth, photophobia
ENDO: Hypoglycemia in diabetic patients

GI: Abdominal pain, constipation, diarrhea, elevated liver enzymes, increased appetite, nausea
GU: Impotence, priapism, sexual dysfunction, urinary frequency, urine retention
MS: Muscle twitching
SKIN: Diaphoresis, rash
Other: Hypernatremia, weight gain

Nursing Considerations

- Use phenelzine cautiously in patients with epilepsy because drug may alter seizure threshold.
- Use phenelzine cautiously in patients with diabetes mellitus because insulin sensitivity may increase, predisposing patient to hypoglycemia.
- Expect to observe some therapeutic effect within 7 to 10 days, but keep in mind that full effect may not occur for 4 to 8 weeks.
- Monitor cardiovascular status closely for changes in heart rate (especially if patient receives more than 30 mg daily) and signs of life-threatening hypertensive crisis. Question patient often about headaches and palpitations. If either occurs, notify prescriber and expect to discontinue drug.
- Keep phentolamine readily available to treat hypertensive crisis. Give 5 mg by slow I.V., as prescribed, to reduce blood pressure without causing excessive hypotension. Use external cooling measures, as prescribed, to manage fever.
- Be aware that to avoid hypertensive crisis, patient should expect to wait 10 to 14 days, as prescribed, when switching from one MAO inhibitor to another or when switching from a dibenzazepine-related drug, such as amitriptyline or perphenazine.
- Watch closely for suicidal tendencies, especially in young adults and especially when therapy starts or dosage changes.

PATIENT TEACHING

- Inform patient and family members that therapeutic effects of phenelzine may take several weeks to appear and that she should continue taking drug as prescribed.
- Caution patient to rise slowly from a lying or sitting position to minimize effects of orthostatic hypotension.

WARNING Instruct patient to avoid the following beverages, drugs, and foods during phenelzine therapy and for 2 weeks afterward: alcohol-free and reduced-alcohol beer and wine; appetite suppressants; beer; broad beans; cheese (except cottage and cream cheese); caffeine and chocolate in large quantities; dry sausage (including Genoa salami, hard salami, Lebanon bologna, and pepperoni); hay fever drugs; inhaled asthma drugs; liver; meat extract; OTC cold and cough preparations (including those containing dextromethorphan), nasal decongestants (drops, spray, or tablets); pickled herring; products that contain tryptophan; protein-rich foods that may have undergone protein changes by aging, fermenting, pickling, or smoking; sauerkraut; sinus drugs; weight-loss preparations; yeast extracts (including brewer's yeast in large quantities); yogurt; and wine.

- Advise patient to inform all healthcare providers (including dentists) that she takes an MAO inhibitor because certain drugs are contraindicated within 2 weeks of drug therapy.
- Urge patient to avoid hazardous activities until drug's CNS effects are known.
- Emphasize the importance of reporting headaches and other persistent, severe, or unusual symptoms.
- Tell family or caregiver to watch closely for suicidal tendencies, especially in young adults and especially when therapy starts or dosage changes.
- Urge patient with diabetes who's taking insulin or an oral antidiabetic to check blood glucose level often during therapy because phenelzine may affect glucose control.

P

phenobarbital sodium

Luminal

Class, Category, and Schedule

Pharmacologic class: Barbiturate
Therapeutic class: Anticonvulsant, sedative-hypnotic
Pregnancy category: D
Controlled substance schedule: IV

Indications and Dosages

➤ *To treat seizures*

ELIXIR, I.V. INFUSION, TABLETS

Adults. *Initial:* 1 to 3 mg/kg daily as a single dose or in divided doses. I.V. infused over 10 to 15 min (not to exceed 50 mg/min).

Children. Highly individualized. I.V. infused over 10 to 15 min.

➤ *To treat status epilepticus*

I.V. INFUSION OR INJECTION

Adults. *Initial:* 15 to 18 mg/kg given slowly over 10 to 15 min and repeated every 20 min as needed. *Maximum:* 30 mg/kg.

Children. 15 to 20 mg/kg at a rate not to exceed 2 mg/kg. *Maximum:* 1,000 mg/dose.

➤ *To provide short-term treatment of insomnia*

ELIXIR, TABLETS

Adults. 100 to 200 mg at bedtime. *Maximum:* 400 mg daily.

➤ *To provide daytime sedation*

ELIXIR, TABLETS

Adults. 30 to 120 mg daily in divided doses twice daily or three times a day. *Maximum:* 400 mg daily.

Children. 2 mg/kg three times a day.

➤ *To provide preoperative sedation*

ELIXIR, TABLETS

Children. 1 to 3 mg/kg before surgery.

I.M. INJECTION

Adults. 130 to 200 mg 60 to 90 min before surgery.

I.V. OR I.M. INJECTION

Children. 1 to 3 mg/kg 60 to 90 min before surgery.

DOSAGE ADJUSTMENT Dosage possibly reduced for debilitated or elderly patients to minimize confusion, depression, and excitement.

Route	Onset	Peak	Duration
P.O.	20–60 min	Unknown	Unknown
I.V.	5 min	30 min	4–6 hr
I.M.	5–20 min	Unknown	4–6 hr

Mechanism of Action

Inhibits ascending conduction of impulses in the reticular formation, which controls CNS arousal to produce drowsiness, hypnosis, and sedation. Phenobarbital also decreases the spread of seizure activity in cortex, limbic system, and thalamus. It promotes an increased threshold for electrical stimulation in the motor cortex, which may contribute to its anticonvulsant properties.

Contraindications

Hepatic disease; history of addiction to hypnotics or sedatives; hypersensitivity to phenobarbital, other barbiturates, or their components; nephritis; porphyria; severe respiratory disease with airway obstruction or dyspnea

Interactions

DRUGS

acetaminophen: Decreased acetaminophen effectiveness with long-term phenobarbital therapy

amphetamines: Delayed intestinal absorption of phenobarbital

anesthetics (halogenated hydrocarbon): Possibly hepatotoxicity

anticonvulsants (hydantoin): Unpredictable effects on metabolism of anticonvulsant

anticonvulsants (succinimide), including carbamazepine: Decreased blood levels and elimination half-lives of these drugs

calcium channel blockers: Possibly excessive hypotension

carbonic anhydrase inhibitors: Enhanced osteopenia induced by phenobarbital

chloramphenicol, corticosteroids, cyclosporine, dacarbazine, digoxin, metronidazole, quinidine: Decreased effectiveness of these drugs from enhanced metabolism

CNS depressants: Additive CNS depression

cyclophosphamide: Possibly reduced half-life and increased leukopenic activity of cyclophosphamide

disopyramide: Possibly ineffectiveness of disopyramide

doxycycline, fenoprofen: Shortened half-life of these drugs

griseofulvin: Possibly decreased absorption and effectiveness of griseofulvin

guanadrel, guanethidine: Possibly increased orthostatic hypotension

haloperidol: Decreased seizure threshold, decreased blood haloperidol level

ketamine (high doses): Increased risk of hypotension and respiratory depression

leucovorin: Interference with phenobarbital's anticonvulsant effect

levothyroxine, oral contraceptives, phenylbutazone, tricyclic antidepressants: Decreased effectiveness of these drugs

loxapine, phenothiazines, thioxanthenes: Decreased seizure threshold
MAO inhibitors: Prolonged phenobarbital effects, possibly altered pattern of seizure activity
maprotiline: Increased CNS depression, decreased seizure threshold at high doses, decreased phenobarbital effectiveness
methoxyflurane: Possibly hepatotoxicity and nephrotoxicity
methylphenidate: Increased risk of phenobarbital toxicity
mexiletine: Decreased blood mexiletine level
oral anticoagulants: Decreased anticoagulant activity, increased risk of bleeding when phenobarbital is discontinued
pituitary hormones (posterior): Increased risk of arrhythmias and coronary insufficiency
primidone: Altered pattern of seizures, increased CNS effects of both drugs
valproate, valproic acid: Decreased phenobarbital metabolism, increased risk of barbiturate toxicity
vitamin D: Decreased phenobarbital effectiveness
xanthines: Increased xanthine metabolism, antagonized hypnotic effect of phenobarbital

ACTIVITIES

alcohol use: Additive CNS depression

Adverse Reactions

CNS: Anxiety, depression, dizziness, drowsiness, headache, irritability, lethargy, mood changes, paradoxical stimulation, sedation, vertigo
CV: Bradycardia, hypotension
EENT: Miosis, ptosis
GI: Constipation, diarrhea, nausea, vomiting
GU: Decreased libido, impotence, sexual dysfunction
MS: Arthralgia, bone tenderness
RESP: Bronchospasm, respiratory depression
SKIN: Dermatitis, photosensitivity, rash, urticaria
Other: Injection-site phlebitis (I.V.), physical and psychological dependence

Nursing Considerations

- Be aware that phenobarbital shouldn't be given during third trimester of pregnancy because repeated use can cause dependence in neonate. It also shouldn't be given to breastfeeding women because it may cause CNS depression in infants.
- Use I.V. route cautiously in patients with CV disease, hypotension, pulmonary disease, or shock because drug may cause adverse hemodynamic or respiratory effects.
- Know that because drug can cause respiratory depression, respiratory rate and depth should be assessed before use, especially in patient with bronchopneumonia, pulmonary disease, respiratory tract infection, or status asthmaticus.
- Give elixir undiluted or mix with fruit juice, milk, or water. Use a calibrated device to measure doses.
- If necessary, crush tablets and mix with fluids or food.
- Reconstitute sterile powder with at least 10 ml sterile water for injection. Don't use reconstituted solution if it fails to clear within 5 minutes. Further dilute prescribed dose with normal saline solution or D_5W and infuse over 30 to 60 minutes.
- Don't give more rapidly than 60 mg/min by I.V. injection.
- For I.V. use, monitor blood pressure, heart rate and rhythm. Anticipate increased risk of hypotension, even at recommended rate. Keep resuscitation equipment readily available.
- For I.M. use, don't inject more than 5 ml into any one I.M. site to prevent sterile abscess formation.
- Be aware that drug may cause physical and psychological dependence.
- Expect that phenobarbital's CNS effects may exacerbate major depression, suicidal tendencies, or other mental disorders.
- Take safety precautions for elderly patients, as appropriate, because they're more likely to experience confusion, depression, and excitement as adverse CNS reactions.
- Anticipate that phenobarbital may cause paradoxical stimulation in children.
- Be aware that drug may trigger signs and symptoms in patients with acute intermittent porphyria.

PATIENT TEACHING

- Instruct patient to take phenobarbital elixir undiluted or to mix it with fruit

juice, milk, or water. Advise her to use a calibrated device to measure doses.
- If patient has trouble swallowing tablets, suggest crushing and adding to fluid or food.
- Caution patient about possible drowsiness and reduced alertness. Advise her to avoid potentially hazardous activities until drug's CNS effects are known.
- Urge patient to avoid alcohol during therapy.
- Inform parents that a child may react with paradoxical excitement. Tell them to notify prescriber if this occurs.
- Instruct woman to report suspected, known, or intended pregnancy. Advise against breastfeeding during therapy.

phentermine hydrochloride

Adipex-P, Lomaira

Class, Category, and Schedule

Chemical class: Sympathomimetic amine
Therapeutic class: Anorectic
Pregnancy category: X
Controlled substance schedule: IV

Indications and Dosages

➤ *Adjunct for short-term weight reduction in conjunction with behavioral modification, caloric restriction, and exercise in management of exogenous obesity in patients with an initial body mass index greater than or equal to 30 kg/m², or greater than or equal to 27 kg/m² in the presence of other risk factors such as controlled hypertension, diabetes, or hyperlipidemia*

TABLETS

Adults. Individualized. *Usual:* 8 mg three times daily half-hour before meals.

Mechanism of Action

Unknown, although thought to be related to its ability to suppress appetite.

Contraindications

Agitated states; breastfeeding; during or 14 days after MAO inhibitor therapy; glaucoma; history of cardiovascular disease such as arrhythmias, congestive heart failure, coronary artery disease, stroke, or uncontrolled hypertension; history of drug abuse; hypersensitivity to phentermine, other sympathomimetic amines, or their components; hyperthyroidism; pregnancy

Interactions

DRUGS

adrenergic neuron blocking drugs: Possibly decreased hypotensive effect of these drugs
dexfenfluramine, fenfluramine: Increased risk of primary pulmonary hypertension and regurgitant cardiac valvular disease
insulin, oral hypoglycemic drugs: Possibly increased risk of hypoglycemia
MAO inhibitors: Increased risk of hypertensive crisis

ACTIVITIES

alcohol use: Possibly increased incidence of serious adverse reactions

Adverse Reactions

CNS: Dizziness, dysphoria, euphoria, headache, insomnia, overstimulation, psychosis, restlessness, tremor
CV: Hypertension, ischemic events, palpitations, **regurgitant cardiac valvular disease**, tachycardia
EENT: Dry mouth, unpleasant taste
GI: Constipation, diarrhea, other gastrointestinal disturbances
GU: Changes in libido, impotence
RESP: Primary pulmonary hypertension
SKIN: Urticaria
Other: Physical and psychological dependence

Nursing Considerations

- Know that phentermine should not be given to women who are breastfeeding or pregnant because of serious adverse effects to fetus or baby.
- Use cautiously in patients with even mild hypertension, because drug can raise blood pressure; and in patients with diabetes who are taking insulin or oral hypoglycemic agents, as drug may enhance hypoglycemic effects.
- Use cautiously in patients with impaired renal function, especially the elderly, as phentermine is substantially excreted by the kidneys and can cause toxic effects in the presence of renal impairment.

WARNING Monitor patient for anginal pain, dyspnea (most common), lower extremity edema, or syncope because a life-threatening disorder, primary pulmonary hypertension, has occurred in patients taking phentermine alone or concomitantly with dexfenfluramine or fenfluramine. If signs or symptoms develop, notify prescriber, expect drug to be discontinued, and assist with diagnostic testing to confirm presence of disorder.

- Know that serious regurgitant cardiac valvular disease has occurred in otherwise healthy patients taking phentermine alone or in combination with dexfenfluramine or fenfluramine. Regularly evaluate patient's heart sounds for presence of murmurs, especially those associated with aortic, mitral, or tricuspid valvular disease.
- Monitor patient's blood pressure regularly, as phentermine therapy may cause hypertension.
- Assess patients with diabetes who are taking insulin or oral hypoglycemic agents for signs and symptoms of hypoglycemia. If persistent or serious hypoglycemia occurs, notify prescriber and expect to adjust the antidiabetic medication dosage, as ordered.

PATIENT TEACHING

- Caution patient to take phentermine exactly as prescribed and not to increase dosage or dosage interval if tolerance to drug develops. Instead, instruct patient to notify prescriber, as drug will have to be discontinued.
- Warn patient that drug is for short-term use only, as the drug may cause physical and/or psychological dependence and can be abused for these effects.
- Inform patient that phentermine therapy is not a substitute for behavioral changes, caloric restriction, and exercise.
- Warn patient not to combine phentermine therapy with other drug products for weight loss, including herbal products, over-the-counter drugs, and prescription drugs. Tell patient to inform all prescribers of phentermine use.
- Caution patient to avoid hazardous activities such as driving or operating machinery until the nervous system effects of the drug are known.
- Tell patient to keep drug out of reach of children and anyone who has a drug addiction and to take measures to prevent drug theft.
- Instruct patient to avoid drinking alcoholic beverages while taking phentermine, as serious adverse reactions may occur.
- Advise patients with diabetes who are taking medication to control their blood glucose levels to watch for low blood glucose reactions. If persistent or severe hypoglycemia occurs, instruct patient to notify prescriber, as dosage of the diabetic medication may have to be reduced. Also advise patient with high blood pressure to monitor blood pressure regularly.

WARNING Instruct patient to discontinue phentermine therapy and notify prescriber if chest pain, decrease in exercise tolerance, difficulty breathing, lower extremity swelling, or shortness of breath develop during phentermine therapy.

- Warn women of childbearing age to notify prescriber immediately if pregnancy occurs or is suspected, as drug will have to be discontinued immediately. Also inform women who are breastfeeding that breastfeeding must be avoided during phentermine therapy.

phentolamine mesylate

Regitine

Class and Category

Pharmacologic class: Alpha adrenergic blocker
Therapeutic class: Antihypertensive, diagnostic aid, vasodilator
Pregnancy category: Not classified

Indications and Dosages

➤ *To diagnose pheochromocytoma*

I.V. INJECTION

Adults. 5 mg as a single dose injected rapidly.
Children. 1 mg as a single dose injected rapidly.

➤ *To manage hypertension before or during pheochromocytomectomy*

I.V. OR I.M. INJECTION

Adults. 5 mg 1 to 2 hr before surgery, repeated as needed. During surgery, 5 mg I.V., as needed.

Children. 1 mg 1 to 2 hr before surgery, repeated as needed. During surgery, 1 mg I.V., as needed.

➤ *To prevent dermal necrosis or sloughing after extravasation of I.V. norepinephrine*

I.V. INJECTION

Adults. 10 mg/L of I.V. fluid that contains norepinephrine at rate determined by patient response.

➤ *To treat dermal necrosis or sloughing after extravasation of I.V. norepinephrine*

INTRADERMAL INJECTION

Adults. 5 to 10 mg in 10 ml of normal saline solution infiltrated in affected area within 12 hr of extravasation.

Mechanism of Action

Blocks the actions of circulating epinephrine and norepinephrine by antagonizing $alpha_1$ and $alpha_2$ receptors. Phentolamine causes peripheral vasodilation through direct relaxation of vascular smooth muscle and alpha blockade. Positive chronotropic and inotropic effects increase cardiac output. A positive inotropic effect primarily raises blood pressure, but in larger doses, phentolamine causes peripheral vasodilation and can reduce blood pressure.

In patients with pheochromocytoma, phentolamine causes systolic and diastolic blood pressures to fall dramatically. In those without pheochromocytoma, it causes blood pressure to fall or rise slightly or remain the same.

Contraindications

Angina, hypersensitivity to phentolamine or its components, MI

Interactions

DRUGS

antihypertensives: Additive hypotensive effect
dopamine: Antagonized vasopressor activity of dopamine
epinephrine, methoxamine, norepinephrine, phenylephrine: Inhibited alpha adrenergic effects of these drugs
metaraminol: Possibly decreased vasopressor effect of metaraminol

ACTIVITIES

alcohol use: Additive vasodilation, increased risk of hypotension and tachycardia

Adverse Reactions

CNS: Dizziness
CV: Angina, **arrhythmias**, **hypotension**, tachycardia
EENT: Nasal congestion
GI: Diarrhea, nausea, vomiting
GU: Ejaculation disorders, priapism
MS: Muscle weakness
SKIN: Flushing

Nursing Considerations

- Reconstitute each 5-mg vial phentolamine with 1 ml sterile water for injection.
- Use reconstituted solution immediately; don't store unused portion.
- Dilute 5 to 10 mg of reconstituted solution in 500 ml D_5W. Inspect drug for particles and discoloration before administering.
- When diagnosing pheochromocytoma, hold nonessential drugs, as ordered, for at least 24 hours (preferably 48 to 72) before test.
- Before giving I.V. test dose for pheochromocytoma, place patient in supine position and assess baseline blood pressure with readings every 10 minutes for at least 30 minutes.
- Know that in pheochromocytoma, expect excessive hypotension after patient receives drug.
- Take safety precautions according to facility policy if patient experiences dizziness.

PATIENT TEACHING

- Instruct patient to move slowly after phentolamine administration to minimize dizziness and avoid falls.

phenylephrine hydrochloride

Alconefrin Nasal Drops 12, Alconefrin Nasal Drops 25, Alconefrin Nasal Drops 50, Alconefrin Nasal Spray 25, Doktors, Duration, Neo-Synephrine, Neo-Synephrine Nasal Drops, Neo-Synephrine Nasal Jelly, Neo-Synephrine Nasal Spray, Neo-Synephrine Pediatric Nasal Drops, Nostril Spray Pump, Nostril Spray Pump Mild, Rhinall, Rhinall-10 Children's Flavored Nose Drops, Vicks Sinex

Class and Category

Pharmacologic class: Adrenergic
Therapeutic class: Antiarrhythmic, decongestant, vasoconstrictor, vasopressor
Pregnancy category: C (parenteral), Not classified (nasal)

Indications and Dosages

➤ *To manage mild to moderate hypotension*

I.V. INJECTION

Adults. *Initial:* 0.1 to 0.5 mg. *Usual:* 0.2 mg, repeated no more than every 10 to 15 min.

I.M. OR SUBCUTANEOUS INJECTION

Adults. *Initial:* 1 to 5 mg. *Usual:* 2 to 5 mg (range, 1 to 10 mg), repeated no more than every 10 to 15 min, as prescribed.

➤ *To treat severe hypotension or shock*

I.V. INFUSION

Adults. *Initial:* 100 to 180 mcg/min (0.1 to 0.18 mg/min) until blood pressure is stable. *Maintenance:* 40 to 60 mcg/min (0.04 to 0.06 mg/min). Infusion concentration and flow rate adjusted as needed, based on patient response.

➤ *To prevent hypotension during spinal anesthesia*

I.M. OR SUBCUTANEOUS INJECTION

Adults. 2 to 3 mg 3 or 4 min before injection of spinal anesthetic.
Children. 0.5 to 1 mg for each 11.3 kg (25 lb).

➤ *To treat hypotension during spinal anesthesia*

I.V. INJECTION

Adults. *Initial:* 0.2 mg, increased by no more than 0.2 mg, as needed. *Maximum:* 0.5 mg/dose.
Children. 0.5 to 1 mg for each 11.3 kg (25 lb).

➤ *To treat paroxysmal supraventricular tachycardia*

I.V. INJECTION

Adults. *Initial:* Up to 0.5 mg by rapid injection; later doses increased 0.1 to 0.2 mg higher than preceding dose, as needed. *Maximum:* 1 mg/dose.

➤ *To treat eustachian tube, nasal, and sinus congestion*

NASAL JELLY OR SOLUTION

Adults and children age 12 and over. 2 or 3 drops or sprays of 0.25% or 0.5% solution every 4 hr, as needed, or small quantity of 0.5% nasal jelly in each nostril every 3 to 4 hr, as needed. A 1% solution may be used for severe congestion.
Children ages 6 to 12. 2 or 3 drops or sprays of 0.25% solution in each nostril every 4 hr, as needed.
Children ages 2 to 6. 2 or 3 drops or sprays of 0.125% solution in each nostril every 4 hr, as needed.

Route	Onset	Peak	Duration
I.V.	Immediate	Unknown	15–20 min
I.M.	10–15 min	Unknown	30 min–2 hr
SubQ	10–15 min	Unknown	50 min–1 hr
Nasal	Unknown	Unknown	30 min–4 hr

Mechanism of Action

Directly stimulates alpha-adrenergic receptors and inhibits the intracellular enzyme adenyl cyclase, which then inhibits production of cAMP. Inhibition of cAMP causes arterial and venous constriction and increases peripheral vascular resistance and systolic blood pressure. With greater-than-therapeutic doses, phenylephrine directly stimulates beta-adrenergic receptors in the myocardium, which increases activity of adenyl cyclase and produces positive chronotropic and inotropic effect.
Intranasal use directly stimulates alpha-adrenergic receptors on the nasal mucosa, constricting local vessels and decreasing blood flow and mucosal edema.

Incompatibilities

Don't combine nasal form with alkalis, butacaine, ferrous salts, metals, or oxidizing agents.

Contraindications

Hypersensitivity to bisulfites, phenylephrine, or their components; severe coronary artery disease or hypertension; use within 14 days of MAO inhibitor; ventricular tachycardia

Interactions

DRUGS

alpha blockers, haloperidol, loxapine, phenothiazines, thioxanthenes: Possibly decreased vasoconstrictor effect of phenylephrine; decreased decongestant effect of nasal phenylephrine (with phenothiazines)

antihypertensives, diuretics: Possibly decreased antihypertensive effects
atropine: Possibly enhanced vasopressor effect of phenylephrine
beta blockers: Decreased therapeutic effects of both drugs
bretylium: Possibly potentiated vasopressor effect and arrhythmias
doxapram: Increased vasopressor effect of both drugs
ergot alkaloids: Possibly cerebral blood vessel rupture, increased vasopressor effect, peripheral vascular ischemia, and gangrene (with ergotamine)
guanadrel, guanethidine: Increased vasopressor effect of phenylephrine, increased risk of arrhythmias and severe hypertension
hydrocarbon inhalation anesthetics: Increased risk of serious arrhythmias
MAO inhibitors: Increased and prolonged cardiac stimulation, hyperpyrexia, increased risk of severe cardiovascular and cerebrovascular effects, increased vasopressor effect, vomiting
maprotiline, tricyclic antidepressants: Increased risk of severe cardiovascular effects (including arrhythmias, hyperpyrexia, severe hypertension); possibly decreased or increased sensitivity to I.V. phenylephrine
mecamylamine, methyldopa: Decreased hypotensive effects of these drugs, increased vasopressor effect of phenylephrine
nitrates: Possibly decreased vasopressor effect of phenylephrine and decreased antianginal effect of nitrates
oxytocin: Possibly severe, persistent hypertension
phenoxybenzamine: Decreased vasoconstrictor effect of phenylephrine, possibly hypotension and tachycardia
theophylline: Possibly enhanced toxicity (including cardiotoxicity); decreased theophylline level (with nasal phenylephrine)
thyroid hormones: Increased cardiovascular effects of both drugs
urinary acidifiers: Possibly decreased therapeutic effects and increased elimination (with nasal phenylephrine)
urinary alkalizers: Possibly decreased elimination and toxic effects (with nasal phenylephrine)

Adverse Reactions

CNS: Dizziness, headache, insomnia, nervousness, paresthesia, restlessness, sleep disturbance (nasal), tremor, weakness
CV: Angina, **bradycardia**, hypertension, **hypotension**, palpitations, peripheral vasoconstriction that may lead to necrosis or gangrene, tachycardia, **ventricular arrhythmias**
EENT: Burning, dry, or stinging nasal mucosa; rebound congestion; and rhinitis (nasal forms)
GI: Nausea, vomiting
RESP: Dyspnea
SKIN: Extravasation with tissue necrosis and sloughing, pallor
Other: **Hypersensitivity reactions**

Nursing Considerations

- Don't dilute phenylephrine for I.M. or subcutaneous use.
- Be aware that to reduce the risk of tissue extravasation, subcutaneous drug should not be injected intradermally.
- For I.V. use, dilute with D_5W or sodium chloride for injection and prepare as prescribed—usually 10 mg/500 ml.
- After nasal application, rinse spray bottle tip or nasal dropper with hot water and dry with clean tissue. Wipe tip of nasal jelly tube with clean tissue.
- Don't use nasal form on more than one patient to prevent transmission of infection.
- Assess for signs and symptoms of angina, arrhythmias, and hypertension because phenylephrine may increase myocardial oxygen demand and the risk of blood pressure changes and proarrhythmias.

WARNING If patient has thyroid disease, watch for increased sensitivity to catecholamines and possible cardiotoxicity or thyrotoxicity.

WARNING Be aware that extravasation may cause tissue necrosis, gangrene, and other reactions around injection site. Expect to use phentolamine if extravasation occurs.

PATIENT TEACHING

- Explain to patient using nasal form that excessive use may cause rebound congestion. Urge her not to exceed recommended dosage and to use for only 3 to 5 days.

- Teach patient who uses nasal form how to care for spray bottle, dropper, or tube.
- Advise patient to avoid hazardous activities until drug's CNS effects are known.

phenytoin

Dilantin-30 (CAN), Dilantin-125, Dilantin Infatabs

phenytoin sodium

Dilantin, Dilantin Kapseals, Phenytex

Class and Category

Pharmacologic class: Hydantoin derivative
Therapeutic class: Anticonvulsant
Pregnancy category: C

Indications and Dosages

➤ *To treat tonic–clonic or psychomotor (temporal) seizures in patients who have had no prior treatment*

CHEWABLE TABLETS, ORAL SUSPENSION (PHENYTOIN)

Adults and adolescents. *Initial:* 125 mg suspension or 100 to 125 mg tablet three times a day, adjusted every 7 to 10 days as needed and tolerated.
Children. *Initial:* 5 mg/kg daily in divided doses twice daily or three times a day, adjusted as needed and tolerated. *Maintenance:* 4 to 8 mg/kg daily in divided doses twice daily or three times daily. *Maximum for children over the age of 6:* 300 mg daily.

EXTENDED CAPSULES (PHENYTOIN SODIUM)

Adults and adolescents. *Initial:* 100 mg three times daily, adjusted every 7 to 10 days as needed and tolerated. *Maintenance:* Once seizures are controlled, adjusted dosage given daily if needed and tolerated.
DOSAGE ADJUSTMENT For hospitalized patients without hepatic or renal disease, oral loading dose of 400 mg followed in 2 hr by 300 mg, and then followed in 2 more hr by another 300 mg, for a total of 1 g.
Children. *Initial:* 5 mg/kg daily in divided doses twice daily or three times a day, adjusted as needed and tolerated. *Maintenance:* 4 to 8 mg/kg daily in divided doses twice daily or three times a day. *Maximum for children over the age of 6:* 300 mg daily.

PROMPT CAPSULES (PHENYTOIN SODIUM)

Adults and adolescents. 100 mg three times a day, adjusted every 7 to 10 days as needed and tolerated.
Children. *Initial:* 5 mg/kg daily in divided doses twice daily or three times a day, adjusted as needed and tolerated. *Maintenance:* 4 to 8 mg/kg daily in divided doses twice daily or three times a day. *Maximum:* 300 mg daily.

➤ *To treat status epilepticus*

I.V. INFUSION (PHENYTOIN SODIUM)

Adults and adolescents. *Initial:* 10 to 15 mg/kg in 50 ml sodium chloride injection at no more than 50 mg/min. *Maintenance:* 100 mg I.V. or P.O. every 6 to 8 hr.
Children. 15 to 20 mg/kg at no more than 1 to 3 mg/kg/min or 50 mg/min, whichever is slower.
DOSAGE ADJUSTMENT For elderly patients dosage reduced.

➤ *To prevent or treat seizures during neurosurgery*

I.V. INJECTION (PHENYTOIN SODIUM)

Adults. 100 to 200 mg every 4 hr at no more than 50 mg/min during or immediately after neurosurgery.

Mechanism of Action

Limits the spread of seizure activity and the start of new seizures by regulating voltage-dependent calcium and sodium channels in neurons, inhibiting calcium movement across neuronal membranes, and enhancing sodium-potassium ATP activity in neurons and glial cells. These actions all help stabilize the neurons.

Incompatibilities

Don't mix phenytoin in same syringe with any other drugs or with any I.V. solutions other than sodium chloride for injection because precipitate will form.

Contraindications

Adams–Stokes syndrome; concurrent use with delavirdine or non-nucleoside reverse transcriptase inhibitors; history of prior acute hepatotoxicity attributed to phenytoin; hypersensitivity to phenytoin, other hydantoins, or its components; SA block or second- or third-degree heart block; sinus bradycardia

Interactions

DRUGS

acetaminophen: Possibly hepatotoxicity, decreased acetaminophen effects
activated charcoal, antacids, calcium salts, enteral feedings, sucralfate: Decreased absorption of oral phenytoin
albendazole: Decreased plasma albendazole levels
allopurinol, benzodiazepines, chloramphenicol, cimetidine, disulfiram, fluconazole, isoniazid, itraconazole, methylphenidate, metronidazole, miconazole, omeprazole, phenacemide, ranitidine, sulfonamides, trazodone, trimethoprim: Decreased metabolism and increased effects of phenytoin
amiodarone; antiepileptic agents such as ethosuximide, felbamate, methsuximide, oxcarbazepine, or topiramate; capecitabine; chloramphenicol; chlordiazepoxide; disulfiram; estrogens; fluorouracil; fluoxetine; fluvastatin; fluvoxamine; H_2*-antagonists such as cimetidine; halothane; isoniazid; methsuximide, methylphenidate; omeprazole; phenothiazines; salicylates; sertraline; succinimides; sulfonamides; ticlopidine; tolbutamide; trazodone; warfarin:* Possibly increased blood phenytoin level
antiepileptics such as carbamazepine, felbamate, lamotrigine, topiramate, oxcarbazepine, quetiapine; antilipidemic drugs such as atorvastatin, fluvastatin, simvastatin; calcium channel blockers such as nifedipine, nimodipine, nisoldipine, verapamil: certain HIV antivirals such as amprenavir, efavirenz, indinavir, lopinavir/ritonavir, nelfinavir, ritonavir, saquinavir; chlorpropamide; clozapine; cyclosporine; digoxin; folic acid; methadone; mexiletine; praziquantel; quetiapine: Decreased plasma concentrations of these drugs
antifungals (azole): Increased blood phenytoin level, decreased blood antifungal level
antineoplastics, carbamazepine, diazepam, diazoxide, folic acid, fosamprenavir, nelfinavir, nitrofurantoin, pyridoxine, reserpine, rifampin, ritonavir, St. John's wort, sucralfate, theophylline, vigabatrin: Decreased phenytoin effects
barbiturates: Variable effects on blood phenytoin level
bupropion, clozapine, loxapine, MAO inhibitors, maprotiline, molindone, phenothiazines, pimozide, thioxanthenes, tricyclic antidepressants: Decreased seizure threshold, decreased anticonvulsant effects
calcium channel blockers: Increased metabolism and decreased effects of these drugs, possibly increased blood phenytoin level
carbamazepine: Decreased blood level and effects of carbamazepine, possibly phenytoin toxicity
carbonic anhydrase inhibitors: Increased risk of osteopenia from phenytoin
chlordiazepoxide, diazepam: Possibly increased blood phenytoin level, decreased effects of these drugs
clonazepam: Possibly decreased blood level and effects of clonazepam, possibly phenytoin toxicity
corticosteroids, cyclosporine, delavirdine, dicumarol, digoxin, disopyramide, doxycycline, estrogens, fluconazole, furosemide, irinotecan, itraconazole, ketoconazole, lamotrigine, levodopa, methadone, metyrapone, mexiletine, oral contraceptives, paclitaxel, paroxetine, posaconazole, quinidine, rifampin, sertraline, sirolimus, tacrolimus, teniposide, theophylline, vitamin D, voriconazole: Increased metabolism and decreased effects of these drugs
dopamine: Increased risk of severe hypotension and bradycardia (with I.V. phenytoin)
fluoxetine: Increased blood phenytoin level and risk of phenytoin toxicity
folic acid, leucovorin: Decreased blood phenytoin level, increased risk of seizures
fosamprenavir: Possibly decreased concentration of active metabolite, amprenavir
fosamprenavir/ritonavir: Possibly increased concentration of active metabolite, amprenavir
haloperidol: Decreased effects of haloperidol, decreased anticonvulsant effect of phenytoin
halothane anesthetics: Increased risk of hepatotoxicity and phenytoin toxicity
ifosfamide: Decreased phenytoin effects, possibly increased toxicity

influenza virus vaccine: Possibly decreased phenytoin effects
insulin, oral antidiabetic drugs: Possibly hyperglycemia, increased blood phenytoin level (with tolbutamide)
levonorgestrel, mebendazole, streptozocin, sulfonylureas: Decreased effects of these drugs
lidocaine, propranolol (possibly other beta blockers): Increased cardiac depressant effects (with I.V. phenytoin), possibly decreased blood level and increased adverse effects of phenytoin
lithium: Increased risk of lithium toxicity, increased risk of neurologic symptoms with normal blood lithium level
meperidine: Increased metabolism and decreased effects of meperidine, possibly meperidine toxicity
methadone: Possibly increased metabolism of methadone and withdrawal symptoms
neuromuscular blockers: Shorter duration of action and decreased effects of neuromuscular blockers
oral anticoagulants: Decreased metabolism and increased effects of phenytoin; early increase and then decrease in anticoagulation
paroxetine: Decreased bioavailability of both drugs
phenobarbital, sodium valproate, valproic acid: Decreased or increased serum phenytoin levels; unpredictable phenytoin effects on these drugs
phenylbutazone, salicylates: Increased phenytoin effects, possibly phenytoin toxicity
primidone: Increased primidone effects, possibly primidone toxicity
rifampin: Increased hepatic metabolism of phenytoin
vitamin D: Possibly decreased vitamin D effects, resulting in rickets or osteomalacia (with long-term use of phenytoin)
warfarin: Decreased or increased therapeutic response of warfarin

ACTIVITIES

alcohol use: Additive CNS depression, increased blood phenytoin levels with acute alcohol use; decreased blood phenytoin levels with chronic alcohol use

Adverse Reactions

CNS: Ataxia, cerebellar atrophy, confusion, depression, dizziness, drowsiness, excitement, fever, headache, involuntary motor activity, lethargy, nervousness, peripheral neuropathy, phenytoin-induced dyskinesias, restlessness, slurred speech, **suicidal ideation**, tremor, vertigo, weakness
CV: Bradycardia, cardiac arrest, hypotension, periarteritis nodosa, polyarteritis, vasculitis
EENT: Amblyopia, conjunctivitis, diplopia, earache, epistaxis, eye pain, gingival hyperplasia, hearing loss, loss of taste, nystagmus, pharyngitis, photophobia, rhinitis, sinusitis, taste perversion, tinnitus
ENDO: Gynecomastia, hyperglycemia
GI: Abdominal pain, **acute hepatic failure**, anorexia, constipation, diarrhea, epigastric pain, jaundice, hepatic dysfunction, **hepatic necrosis**, **hepatitis**, nausea, vomiting
GU: Glycosuria, Peyronie's disease, priapism, **renal failure**
HEME: Acute intermittent porphyria (exacerbation), **agranulocytosis**, anemia, eosinophilia, **granulocytopenia**, **leukopenia**, **pancytopenia**, **thrombocytopenia**
MS: Arthralgia, arthropathy, bone fractures, decreased bone mineral density, muscle twitching, osteomalacia, polymyositis
RESP: Apnea, **asthma**, bronchitis, cough, dyspnea, **hypoxia**, increased sputum production, pneumonia, **pneumothorax**, **pulmonary fibrosis**
SKIN: Bullous dermatitis, **exfoliative dermatitis**, maculopapular or morbilliform rash, purpuric dermatitis, **Stevens–Johnson syndrome**, **toxic epidermal necrolysis**, unusual hair growth, urticaria
Other: Facial feature coarsening or enlargement, immunoglobulin abnormalities, injection-site pain, lupus-like symptoms, lymphadenopathy, porphyria, weight gain or loss

Nursing Considerations

WARNING Know that patients of Asian ancestry who have the genetic allelic variant HLA-B 1502 develop serious and sometimes fatal dermatologic reactions 10 times more often than people without this variant when given carbamazepine, another antiepileptic drug. Because early data suggest a similar effect with phenytoin, this drug shouldn't be used as a substitute for carbamazepine in these patients.

- Be aware that preferred administration routes for phenytoin are oral and I.V. injection. With I.M. administration, phenytoin has a variable absorption rate.
- Know that if patient has difficulty swallowing, prompt (rapid-release) capsules may be opened and contents mixed with food or fluid.
- Shake oral suspension before measuring dose, and use a calibrated measuring device.
- Give phenytoin with or just after meals to minimize GI distress.
- Inspect I.V. form for particles and discoloration before administering.

WARNING **Avoid rapid I.V. injection because it may cause cardiac arrest, CNS depression, or severe hypotension.**

- To decrease vein irritation, follow I.V. injection with flush of sodium chloride for injection through same I.V. catheter.
- Continuously monitor blood pressure and ECG tracings when administering I.V. phenytoin. Be aware that bradycardia and cardiac arrest have occurred in patients receiving recommended dosages, in addition to patients experiencing phenytoin toxicity. Most cases of cardiac arrest occurred in patients with underlying cardiac disease.
- Frequently assess I.V. site for signs of extravasation because drug can cause tissue necrosis.
- Know that if patient has an NG tube in place, drug absorption by polyvinyl chloride tubing can be minimized by diluting suspension threefold with sodium chloride for injection, D_5W, or sterile water. After administration, flush tube with at least 20 ml diluent.
- Do not administer phenytoin concomitantly with an enteral feeding because feeding may lower phenytoin serum levels.
- Expect continuous enteral feedings to disrupt phenytoin absorption and, possibly, reduce blood phenytoin level. Discontinue tube feedings 1 to 2 hours before and after phenytoin administration, as prescribed. Anticipate giving increased phenytoin doses to compensate for reduced bioavailability during continuous tube feedings.
- Separate oral phenytoin administration by at least 2 hours from antacids and calcium salts.
- Monitor phenytoin level. Therapeutic level ranges from 10 to 20 mcg/L. Expect to monitor phenytoin serum levels based on the unbound fraction in patients with hepatic or renal disease or those with hypoalbuminemia because the fraction of unbound phenytoin is increased in these patients.
- Monitor patient closely for above therapeutic levels because high serum levels that are sustained may cause cerebellar atrophy (rare), delirium, encephalopathy, irreversible cerebellar dysfunction, or psychosis. Expect to obtain serum levels if early signs of dose-related CNS toxicity develops in any patient because some patients may be slow metabolizers of phenytoin. If above therapeutic range levels are found, expect phenytoin dosage to be reduced. If symptoms persist, expect drug to be discontinued.

WARNING **Monitor patient's hematologic status during therapy because phenytoin can cause blood dyscrasias. A patient with a history of agranulocytosis, leukopenia, or pancytopenia may have an increased risk of infection because phenytoin can cause myelosuppression.**

- Anticipate that drug may worsen intermittent porphyria.
- Frequently monitor blood glucose level of patient with diabetes mellitus because drug can stimulate glucagon secretion and impair insulin secretion, either of which can raise blood glucose level.
- Monitor thyroid hormone levels in patient receiving thyroid replacement therapy because phenytoin may decrease circulating thyroid hormone levels and increase thyroid-stimulating hormone level. Also know that drug may decrease dexamethasone or metyrapone test results or increase serum levels of alkaline phosphatase, gamma glutamyl transpeptidase (GGT), or glucose.
- Be aware that long-term phenytoin therapy may increase patient's requirements for folic acid or vitamin D

supplements. However, keep in mind that a diet high in folic acid may decrease seizure control.

- Know that phenytoin exposure may cause fetal harm and has been linked to congenital malformations and other adverse developmental outcomes. In addition, monitor pregnant patient close to term because a potentially life-threatening bleeding disorder related to decreased levels of vitamin K-dependent clotting factors may occur in newborns exposed to phenytoin in utero. Expect to administer vitamin K to the mother before delivery and to the neonate after birth.
- Monitor patient closely for evidence of suicidal thinking or behavior, especially when therapy starts or dosage changes.
- Know that phenytoin should not be stopped abruptly as status epilepticus may occur. Instead, expect drug to be discontinued gradually.

PATIENT TEACHING

- Instruct patient to crush or thoroughly chew phenytoin chewable tablets before swallowing or to shake oral solution well.
- Advise patient to take drug exactly as prescribed; she should not change brands, dosage, or stop taking drug unless instructed by prescriber.
- Instruct patients to use an accurately calibrated measuring device when using suspension form. Remind patient that a household teaspoon or tablespoon is not such a device.
- Instruct patient to avoid taking antacids or calcium products within 2 hours of phenytoin.
- Tell patient to report any signs of heart dysfunction such as dizziness, feeling heart skipping beats, slow pulse, or tiredness.
- Urge patient to avoid alcohol during therapy.
- Caution patient to avoid hazardous activities until drug's CNS effects are known.
- Inform patient with diabetes mellitus about the increased risk of hyperglycemia and the possible need for increased antidiabetic drug dosage during therapy. Advise her to check blood glucose level often.
- Emphasize the importance of good oral hygiene, and encourage patient to inform her dentist that she's taking phenytoin.
- Encourage patient to wear medical identification that indicates her diagnosis and drug therapy.
- Urge caregivers to watch patient closely for evidence of suicidal tendencies, especially when therapy starts or dosage changes, and to report concerns at once to prescriber.
- Instruct patient to notify prescriber at the first sign of a rash or if persistent, severe, or other unusual skin reactions occur.
- Inform women of childbearing age to notify prescriber immediately if pregnancy is suspected or occurs, as phenytoin may cause fetal harm. Encourage woman who becomes pregnant while taking phenytoin to enroll in the North American antiepileptic drug pregnancy registry by calling 1-888-233-2334. Explain that the registry is collecting information about the safety of antiepileptic drugs during pregnancy.

physostigmine salicylate

Antilirium

Class and Category

Pharmacologic class: Cholinesterase inhibitor
Therapeutic class: Anticholinergic antidote
Pregnancy category: Not classified

Indications and Dosages

➤ *To counteract toxic anticholinergic effects (anticholinergic syndrome)*

I.V. OR I.M. INJECTION

Adults and adolescents. 0.5 to 2 mg at no more than 1 mg/min and repeated every 20 min, as needed; then when effective 1 to 4 mg, repeated every 30 to 60 min if life-threatening signs recur.
Children. 0.02 mg/kg I.V., at no more than 0.5 mg/min, repeated every 5 to 10 min as needed. *Maximum:* 2 mg/dose.

Route	Onset	Peak	Duration
I.V.	3–8 min	5 min	30–60 min
I.M.	3–8 min	20–30 min	30–60 min

P

Mechanism of Action
Inhibits destruction of acetylcholine by acetylcholinesterase. This action increases acetylcholine concentration at cholinergic transmission sites and exaggerates and prolongs effects of acetylcholine that are blocked by toxic doses of anticholinergics.

Contraindications
Asthma; cardiovascular disease; diabetes mellitus; gangrene; GI or GU obstruction; hypersensitivity to physostigmine, sulfites, or their components

Interactions
DRUGS

choline esters: Enhanced effects of bethanechol and carbachol with concurrent use of physostigmine, enhanced effects of acetylcholine and methacholine with prior use of physostigmine
succinylcholine: Prolonged neuromuscular paralysis

Adverse Reactions
CNS: CNS stimulation, fatigue, hallucinations, restlessness, **seizures** (with too-rapid I.V. delivery), weakness
CV: Bradycardia (with too-rapid I.V. delivery), **irregular heartbeat**, palpitations
EENT: Increased salivation, lacrimation, miosis
GI: Abdominal pain, diarrhea, nausea, vomiting
GU: Urinary urgency
MS: Muscle twitching
RESP: Bronchospasm, chest tightness, dyspnea (with too-rapid I.V. administration), increased bronchial secretions, wheezing
SKIN: Diaphoresis

Nursing Considerations
- Use physostigmine cautiously in patients with bradycardia, epilepsy, or Parkinson's disease.
- Avoid rapid I.V. delivery, which may lead to bradycardia, respiratory distress, or seizures.
- Check blood pressure, neurologic status, and pulse and respiratory rates often.
- Monitor ECG tracing during I.V. use.
- Closely monitor patient with asthma for asthma attack because physostigmine may precipitate attack by causing bronchoconstriction.
- Watch for seizures in patient with a history of seizures because physostigmine can induce seizures by stimulating CNS.

WARNING Be alert for life-threatening cholinergic crisis, which may indicate physostigmine overdose and may include confusion, diaphoresis, hypotension, miosis, muscle weakness, nausea, paralysis (including respiratory paralysis), salivation, seizures, sinus bradycardia, and vomiting. If you detect such signs, prepare to give atropine (the antidote) and use resuscitation equipment. Keep in mind that atropine counteracts only muscarinic cholinergic effects; paralytic effects may continue.

PATIENT TEACHING
- Reassure patient that vital signs will be monitored often to help detect or prevent adverse reactions.
- Instruct patient to notify prescriber at once about evidence of cholinergic crisis.

pimavanserin
Nuplazid

Class and Category
Pharmacologic class: Serotonin 5-HT receptor inverse agonist and antagonist
Therapeutic class: Atypical antipsychotic
Pregnancy category: Not classified

Indications and Dosages
➤ *To treat delusions and hallucinations associated with Parkinson's disease psychosis*

TABLETS

Adults. 34 mg (two 17-mg tablets) once daily.

DOSAGE ADJUSTMENT For patients taking strong CYP3A4 inducers concurrently, dosage may have to be increased. For patients taking strong CYP3A4 inhibitors such as ketoconazole concurrently, dosage reduced to 10 mg once daily.

Mechanism of Action
Precise mechanism is unknown, but possibly mediates through a combination of inverse agonist and antagonist activity at

serotonin 5-HT2A receptors and to a lesser extent at serotonin 5-HT2C receptors to eradicate delusions and hallucinations associated with Parkinson's disease psychosis.

Contraindications

Hypersensitivity to pimavanserin or its components

Interactions

DRUGS

antibiotics such as gatifloxacin, moxifloxacin; antipsychotics such as chlorpromazine, thioridazine, ziprasidone; class 1A antiarrhythmics such as disopyramide, procainamide, quinidine; class 3 antiarrhythmics such as amiodarone, sotalol: Possible prolonged QT interval, increasing risk of cardiac arrhythmias

carbamazepine, phenytoin, rifampin, St. John's wort: Possibly reduced pimavanserin exposure, resulting in decreased effectiveness

clarithromycin, itraconazole, ketoconazole, indinavir: Increased pimavanserin exposure, leading to possible adverse reactions

Adverse Reactions

CNS: Confusion, fatigue, gait disturbance, hallucination, somnolence
CV: Peripheral edema, **QT prolongation interval**
EENT: Circumoral edema, **throat tightness**, tongue swelling
GI: Constipation, nausea
GU: UTI
RESP: Dyspnea
SKIN: Rash, urticaria
Other: Angioedema

Nursing Considerations

- Keep in mind that pimavanserin shouldn't be used to treat dementia-related psychosis in the elderly, because of an increased mortality risk.
- Know that pimavanserin therapy should be avoided in patients with a history of cardiac arrhythmias, known QT prolongation, or in combination with other drugs known to prolong the QT interval. Drug should also not be used in patients who are at risk for hypokalemia or hypomagnesemia or in the presence of congenital prolongation of the QT interval or symptomatic bradycardia. Monitor patient's EKG regularly for evidence of QT prolongation.
- Use cautiously in patients with renal impairment, including severe impairment and end-stage renal disease.

WARNING Monitor patient for evidence of a hypersensitivity reaction that could include angioedema, rash, or urticaria. If present, notify prescriber, expect drug to be discontinued, and provide supportive care, as needed and prescribed.

PATIENT TEACHING

- Tell patient or family to stop pimavanserin therapy and notify prescriber if an allergic reaction occurs. If reaction is severe, urge patient to seek immediate emergency medical care.
- Instruct patient or family to alert all prescribers to pimavanserin therapy and not to take any over-the-counter drugs (including herbal preparations) without prescriber knowledge.

pindolol

NovoPindol (CAN), SynPindol (CAN), Visken

Class and Category

Pharmacologic class: Beta blocker
Therapeutic class: Antihypertensive
Pregnancy category: B

Indications and Dosages

➤ *To manage hypertension*

TABLETS

Adults. *Initial:* 5 mg twice daily, increased by 10 mg daily every 3 to 4 wk, as prescribed. *Maintenance:* 10 to 30 mg daily. *Maximum:* 60 mg daily (U.S.), 45 mg daily (Canada).

Route	Onset	Peak	Duration
P.O.	Unknown	1–2 hr	Up to 24 hr

Mechanism of Action

Blocks sympathetic stimulation of $beta_1$ receptors in the heart and $beta_2$ receptors in vascular and bronchial smooth muscle by competing with adrenergic neurotransmitters, such as catecholamines. Pindolol's negative chronotropic effects

P

slow the resting heart rate and reduce exercise-induced tachycardia. Its negative inotropic effects reduce cardiac output, myocardial contractility, systolic and diastolic blood pressure, and myocardial oxygen consumption during stress or exercise. Among beta blockers, pindolol has the most intrinsic sympathomimetic activity and nonselective antagonism.

Contraindications

Advanced AV block; asthma; bronchospasm; cardiogenic shock; heart failure; hepatic disease; hypersensitivity to pindolol, other beta blockers, or their components; hypotension (with systolic pressure less than 100 mm Hg); sinus bradycardia

Interactions

DRUGS

allergy extracts or immunotherapy, iodinated contrast media: Increased risk of systemic reaction or anaphylaxis
aluminum salts, barbiturates, calcium salts, certain penicillins, cholestyramine, colestipol, NSAIDs, rifampin, salicylates, sulfinpyrazone: Decreased blood level and effects of pindolol
antihypertensives: Additive hypotensive effect
beta blockers, digoxin: Increased risk of bradycardia
calcium channel blockers, quinidine: Possibly increased effects of both drugs, symptomatic bradycardia (with diltiazem or verapamil), excessive hypertension or heart failure (with nifedipine)
cimetidine: Increased blood pindolol level
epinephrine: Possibly hypertension followed by bradycardia
ergotamine: Possibly severe peripheral vasoconstriction with pain and cyanosis
estrogens: Decreased antihypertensive effect
fentanyl, fentanyl derivatives: Risk of bradycardia after anesthesia induction
insulin, oral antidiabetic drugs: Masked symptoms of hypoglycemia, increased risk of hyperglycemia
lidocaine: Increased risk of lidocaine toxicity
MAO inhibitors: Possibly hypertension
neuromuscular blockers: Possibly increased or prolonged neuromuscular blockade
phenothiazines: Increased blood levels of both drugs
phenytoin: Possibly increased cardiac depressant effects
prazosin, reserpine: Increased risk of orthostatic hypotension, bradycardia (with reserpine)
quinolones: Possibly increased bioavailability of pindolol
xanthines: Possibly decreased effects of both drugs, decreased xanthine clearance

Adverse Reactions

CNS: Anxiety, confusion, **CVA**, depression, dizziness, fatigue, fever, hallucinations, **hypothermia**, insomnia, memory loss, paresthesia, peripheral neuropathy, syncope, weakness
CV: Arrhythmias (including AV block and bradycardia), chest pain, decreased peripheral circulation, **heart failure**, hyperlipidemia, **hypotension**, **MI**, orthostatic hypotension, peripheral edema and ischemia
EENT: Pharyngitis
ENDO: Hyperglycemia, **hypoglycemia**
GI: Colitis (ischemic), constipation, diarrhea, elevated liver enzymes, gastritis, **mesenteric artery thrombosis**, nausea, **pancreatitis**, vomiting
GU: Cystitis, decreased libido, renal colic, **renal artery thrombosis**, **renal failure**, urinary frequency, urine retention, UTI
HEME: Agranulocytosis, eosinophilia, **leukopenia**, nonthrombocytopenic purpura, **thrombocytopenia**, **thrombocytopenic purpura**, **unusual bleeding** or bruising
MS: Arthralgia, back pain
RESP: Bronchospasm, **pulmonary edema or pulmonary emboli**
SKIN: Acne; alopecia; crusted, red, or scaly skin; diaphoresis; eczema; **exfoliative dermatitis**; hyperpigmentation; pruritus; purpura; rash
Other: Angioedema, positive ANA titer

Nursing Considerations

- Check blood pressure and pulse rate often, especially at start of pindolol therapy. Also monitor fluid intake and output and daily weight, and assess for evidence of heart failure, such as dyspnea, edema, fatigue, and jugular vein distention.
- Be aware that drug shouldn't be stopped abruptly because MI, myocardial ischemia,

severe hypertension, or ventricular arrhythmias may result.
- Expect to discontinue drug up to 2 days before surgery, as prescribed, to reduce the risk of heart failure.
- Assess distal circulation and peripheral pulses in patient with Raynaud's phenomenon or other peripheral vascular disorder because drug can worsen these conditions.
- Be aware that pindolol can mask tachycardia from hyperthyroidism; abrupt withdrawal can cause thyroid storm. Drug also may potentiate diplopia and muscle weakness in patient with myasthenia gravis; decrease blood glucose level, prolong or mask symptoms of hypoglycemia, and promote hyperglycemia in patient with diabetes mellitus; and worsen psoriasis.

PATIENT TEACHING
- Instruct patient to weigh herself daily during pindolol therapy and to notify prescriber if she gains more than 2 lb (0.9 kg) in 1 day or 5 lb (2.3 kg) in 1 week.
- Caution patient not to stop drug abruptly.
- Advise patient to rise slowly from a seated or lying position to minimize effects of orthostatic hypotension.
- Advise patient to avoid hazardous activities until drug's CNS effects are known.
- Instruct patient to contact prescriber about bleeding or bruising, cough at night, depression, dizziness, edema, rash, shortness of breath, slow pulse rate, or sore throat.
- Advise diabetic patient to monitor her blood glucose level more often during pindolol therapy because drug may mask symptoms of hypoglycemia.
- Inform patient with psoriasis that drug may aggravate this condition.

pioglitazone hydrochloride

Actos

Class and Category
Pharmacologic class: Thiazolidinedione
Therapeutic class: Antidiabetic
Pregnancy category: C

Indications and Dosages
➤ *To achieve glucose control in type 2 diabetes mellitus as monotherapy or in combination with insulin, metformin, or a sulfonylurea*

TABLETS
Adults. *Initial:* 15 or 30 mg daily. *Maximum:* 45 mg daily.

DOSAGE ADJUSTMENT For patients with congestive heart failure, starting dose is 15 mg once daily. For patients receiving concomitant gemfibrozil or other strong CYP2C8 inhibitors, maximum dose should not exceed 15 mg once daily. For patients taking insulin, insulin dosage decreased by 10% to 25%, as prescribed, once glucose level reaches 100 mg/dl or less. If hypoglycemia occurs, dosage of any concurrent antidiabetic reduced, as prescribed.

Mechanism of Action
Decreases insulin resistance by enhancing the sensitivity of insulin-dependent tissues, such as adipose tissue, the liver, and skeletal muscle, and reduces glucose output from the liver. Drug activates peroxisome proliferator-activated receptor-gamma (PPARg) receptors, which modulate transcription of insulin-responsive genes involved in glucose control and lipid metabolism. In this way, pioglitazone reduces hyperglycemia, hyperinsulinemia, and hypertriglyceridemia in patients with type 2 diabetes mellitus and insulin resistance. However, to work effectively, pioglitazone needs endogenous insulin. Unlike sulfonylureas, it doesn't increase pancreatic insulin secretion.

Contraindications
Diabetic ketoacidosis, hypersensitivity to pioglitazone or its components, New York Heart Association (NYHA) Class III or IV heart failure, severe hepatic dysfunction, type 1 diabetes mellitus

Interactions
DRUGS
gemfibrozil and other strong CYP2C8 inhibitors: Increased pioglitazone effect
insulin, oral antidiabetic agents: Possibly increased risk of hypoglycemia
ketoconazole: Possibly decreased metabolism of pioglitazone
oral contraceptives: Possibly decreased effectiveness of oral contraceptives

rifampin: Possibly altered glucose control
topiramate: Decreased exposure of pioglitazone and its active metabolites

Adverse Reactions

CNS: Headache
CV: Congestive heart failure, edema
EENT: Blurred vision, decreased visual acuity, macular edema, pharyngitis, sinusitis, tooth disorders
GI: Elevated liver enzymes, jaundice
HEME: Decreased hemoglobin level and hematocrit
MS: Fractures, myalgia
RESP: Upper respiratory tract infection
Other: Weight gain

Nursing Considerations

- Be aware that pioglitazone isn't recommended for patients with symptomatic heart failure. It is also not recommended in patients with active bladder cancer because there is insufficient information regarding the drug's role in promoting bladder tumors and should only be used with extreme caution in patients with a history of bladder cancer.
- Be prepared to monitor liver enzymes before therapy begins, every 2 months during first year, and annually thereafter, as ordered, because drug is extensively metabolized in the liver. Expect to stop drug if jaundice develops or ALT values exceed 2.5 times normal.

WARNING Monitor patient for signs and symptoms of congestive heart failure—such as edema, rapid weight gain, or shortness of breath—because pioglitazone can cause fluid retention that may lead to or worsen heart failure. Notify prescriber immediately of any deterioration in the patient's cardiac status, and expect to discontinue the drug, as ordered.

- Assess for signs and symptoms of hypoglycemia, especially if patient is also taking another antidiabetic drug.
- Monitor fasting glucose level, as ordered, to evaluate effectiveness of therapy.
- Monitor glycosylated hemoglobin level to assess drug's long-term effectiveness.

PATIENT TEACHING

- Emphasize the need for patient to continue, diet control, exercise program, and weight management during pioglitazone therapy.
- Advise patient to notify prescriber immediately if she experiences fluid retention, shortness of breath, or sudden weight gain because drug may have to be discontinued.
- Urge patient to report vision changes promptly and expect to have an eye examination by an ophthalmologist, regardless of when the last examination occurred.
- Instruct patient to keep laboratory appointments for liver enzymes, as ordered, typically every 2 months during first year of therapy and annually thereafter.
- Inform female patient who uses oral contraceptives that drug decreases their effectiveness; suggest that she use another method of contraception while taking pioglitazone.
- Also inform female patient that she may be at risk for fractures during pioglitazone therapy, and urge her to take safety precautions to prevent falls and other injuries.

piroxicam

Apo-Piroxicam (CAN), Feldene, Novo-Pirocam (CAN)

Class and Category

Pharmacologic class: NSAID
Therapeutic class: Analgesic
Pregnancy category: C (first and second trimester), D (third trimester)

Indications and Dosages

➤ *To treat acute and chronic osteoarthritis and rheumatoid arthritis*

CAPSULES

Adults. *Initial:* 20 mg once daily or 10 mg twice daily.

Route	Onset	Peak	Duration
P.O.	Unknown	Several days to 1 wk*	Unknown

* With severe inflammation, 2 wk or more.

Mechanism of Action

Blocks the activity of cyclooxygenase, the enzyme needed for prostaglandin synthesis. Prostaglandins, important mediators of the inflammatory response, cause local vasodilation with pain and swelling. By blocking cyclooxygenase activity and inhibiting prostaglandins, this NSAID reduces inflammatory symptoms and pain.

Contraindications

Angioedema, asthma, bronchospasm, nasal polyps, rhinitis, or urticaria induced by aspirin, iodides, or other NSAIDs; hypersensitivity to piroxicam or its components; postoperatively after coronary artery bypass graft (CABG) surgery

Interactions

DRUGS

acetaminophen: Possibly increased adverse renal effects with long-term use of both drugs
ACE inhibitors: Decreased antihypertensive effects; increased risk of renal dysfunction, especially in the elderly and those with volume depletion or impaired renal function
antihypertensives: Possibly decreased or reversed effects of antihypertensives
aspirin, other NSAIDs: Increased risk of bleeding and adverse GI effects, possibly increased blood piroxicam level
cefamandole, cefoperazone, cefotetan: Increased risk of hypoprothrombinemia and bleeding
colchicine, platelet aggregation inhibitors: Increased risk of GI bleeding, hemorrhage, and ulcers
corticosteroids, potassium supplements: Increased risk of adverse GI effects
cyclosporine: Increased risk of nephrotoxicity from both drugs, increased blood cyclosporine level
diuretics: Decreased antihypertensive, diuretic, and natriuretic effects of diuretics
gold compounds, nephrotoxic drugs: Increased risk of adverse renal effects
heparin, oral anticoagulants, thrombolytics: Increased anticoagulant effects, increased risk of hemorrhage
insulin, oral antidiabetic drugs: Possibly increased hypoglycemic effect of these drugs
lithium: Possibly increased blood lithium level and toxicity
methotrexate: Decreased methotrexate clearance and increased risk of methotrexate toxicity
plicamycin, valproic acid: Increased risk of hypoprothrombinemia and GI bleeding, hemorrhage, and ulceration
probenecid: Possibly increased blood level, effectiveness, and risk of toxicity of piroxicam

ACTIVITIES

alcohol use: Increased risk of adverse GI effects

Adverse Reactions

CNS: Anxiety, **aseptic meningitis**, asthenia, confusion, **CVA**, depression, dizziness, dream disturbances, drowsiness, fever, headache, insomnia, malaise, nervousness, paresthesia, somnolence, syncope, transient ischemic attack, tremor, vertigo
CV: Deep vein thrombosis, edema, **heart failure**, hypertension, **MI**, peripheral edema, tachycardia
EENT: Blurred vision, dry mouth, epistaxis, glossitis, stomatitis, tinnitus
ENDO: Hypoglycemia
GI: Abdominal pain; anorexia; constipation; diarrhea; elevated liver enzymes; esophagitis; flatulence; gastritis; **GI bleeding**, **perforation**, or ulceration; **hematemesis**; **hepatitis**; indigestion; jaundice; **liver failure**; **melena**; nausea; vomiting
GU: Acute renal failure, cystitis, decreased female fertility, delayed reversible ovulation, dysuria, elevated serum creatinine level, hematuria, interstitial nephritis, **nephrotic syndrome**, oliguria, polyuria, proteinuria, **renal failure or insufficiency**
HEME: Agranulocytosis, anemia, **aplastic anemia**, **coagulation abnormalities**, eosinophilia, **leukopenia**, **pancytopenia**, **thrombocytopenia**
RESP: Asthma, dyspnea
SKIN: Alopecia, diaphoresis, ecchymosis, erythema, **erythema multiforme**, **exfoliative dermatitis**, photosensitivity, pruritus, purpura, rash, **Stevens–Johnson syndrome**, **toxic epidermal necrolysis**, urticaria
Other: Anaphylaxis, **angioedema**, flu-like symptoms, **hyperkalemia**, infection, **sepsis**, weight loss or gain

Nursing Considerations

- Be aware that NSAIDs like piroxicam should be avoided in patients with a recent MI because risk of reinfarction increases with NSAID therapy. If therapy is unavoidable, monitor patient closely for signs of cardiac ischemia.

- Know that the risk of heart failure increases with NSAID use. NSAIDs should not be used in patients with severe heart failure but, if unavoidable, monitor patient for worsening of heart failure.
- Administer piroxicam with food to decrease GI upset.
- Use piroxicam with extreme caution in patients with a history of GI bleeding or ulcer disease because NSAIDs such as piroxicam increase risk of GI bleeding and ulceration. Expect to use piroxicam for the shortest time possible in these patients.
- Be aware that serious GI tract, bleeding, perforation, and ulceration may occur without warning symptoms. Elderly patients are at greater risk. To minimize risk, give drug with food. If GI distress occurs, withhold drug and notify prescriber at once.
- Use piroxicam cautiously in patients with hypertension, and monitor blood pressure closely throughout therapy. Drug may cause hypertension or worsen it.

WARNING Monitor patient closely for thrombotic events, including MI and stroke, because NSAIDs increase the risk. These events have occurred even in patients who do not have a history or risk factors for cardiovascular disease. Monitor patient for warning signs such as chest pain, shortness of breath, slurring of speech, or weakness. If present, withhold piroxicam, alert prescriber immediately, and provide supportive care, as prescribed.

WARNING Keep in mind that if patient has bone marrow suppression or is receiving antineoplastic drug therapy, monitor laboratory results (including WBC count), and watch for evidence of infection because anti-inflammatory and antipyretic actions of piroxicam may mask signs and symptoms, such as fever and pain.

- Watch for less common but serious adverse GI reactions, including anorexia, constipation, diverticulitis, dysphagia, esophagitis, gastritis, gastroenteritis, gastroesophageal reflux disease, hemorrhoids, hiatal hernia, melena, stomatitis, and vomiting, especially if patient is elderly or taking drug long term.
- Monitor liver enzymes, as ordered, because, rarely, elevated levels may progress to severe hepatic reactions.
- Monitor BUN and serum creatinine levels in patients with heart failure, hepatic dysfunction, or impaired renal function; those taking ACE inhibitors or diuretics; and elderly patients because drug may cause renal failure.
- Monitor CBC for decreased hemoglobin level and hematocrit because drug may worsen anemia.
- Assess patient's skin routinely for rash or other signs of hypersensitivity reaction because piroxicam and other NSAIDs may cause serious skin reactions without warning, even in patients with no history of NSAID hypersensitivity. Stop drug at first sign of reaction, and notify prescriber.

WARNING Be aware that drug may cause premature closure of ductus arteriosus in growing fetus during third trimester of pregnancy. Be prepared to suggest referral for high-risk pregnancy.

PATIENT TEACHING

- Advise patient to take piroxicam with meals to minimize GI distress. Also direct her to take drug with a full glass of water and to remain upright for 30 minutes afterward to decrease risk of drug lodging in esophagus and causing irritation.
- Instruct patient to swallow capsules whole and not to break, chew, crush, or open them.
- Advise patient to avoid alcohol, aspirin, and other NSAIDs, unless prescribed, while taking piroxicam.
- Caution patient to avoid hazardous activities until drug's CNS effects are known.
- Keep in mind that if patient also takes an anticoagulant, advise her to watch for and immediately report bleeding problems, such as bloody or tarry stools and bloody vomitus.
- Advise patient who also takes insulin or an oral antidiabetic to closely monitor blood glucose level to prevent hypoglycemia. Urge her to carry candy or other simple sugars to treat mild hypoglycemia. Advise her to notify prescriber if

hypoglycemic episodes are frequent or severe.

- Explain that piroxicam may increase risk of serious adverse cardiovascular reactions; urge patient to seek immediate medical attention if signs or symptoms arise, such as chest pain, edema, shortness of breath, slurring of speech, unexplained weight gain, or weakness.
- Tell patient that piroxicam may increase risk of serious adverse GI reactions; stress the need to seek immediate medical attention for such signs and symptoms as abdominal or epigastric pain, black or tarry stools, indigestion or vomiting blood or material that looks like coffee grounds.
- Alert patient to possibility of rare but serious skin reactions. Urge her to seek immediate medical care for blisters, fever, itching, rash, or other signs of hypersensitivity.
- Alert female patient that drug may cause a reversible delay in ovulation. If she is planning a pregnancy, having difficulty conceiving, or experiencing infertility, she should notify prescriber.
- Instruct female patient to consult prescriber if she becomes pregnant because drug may cause premature closure of ductus arteriosus in growing fetus.

pitavastatin

Livalo, Nikita

Class and Category

Pharmacologic class: HMG-CoA reductase inhibitor (statin)
Therapeutic class: Antilipemic
Pregnancy category: X

Indications and Dosages

➤ *As adjunct to diet in patients with primary hyperlipidemia or mixed dyslipidemia*

TABLETS

Adults. *Initial:* 2 mg once daily, increased as needed. *Maximum:* 4 mg once daily

DOSAGE ADJUSTMENT For patients with moderate to severe renal impairment (glomerular filtration rate above 30 ml/min) or patients receiving dialysis, initial dosage reduced to 1 mg once daily, with maximum of 2 mg once daily. For patients taking erythromycin, dosage shouldn't exceed 1 mg daily; for patients taking rifampin, dosage shouldn't exceed 2 mg daily.

Route	Onset	Peak	Duration
P.O.	Unknown	1 hr	Unknown

Mechanism of Action

Reduces plasma cholesterol and lipoprotein levels by inhibiting cholesterol and HMG-CoA reductase synthesis in the liver. Consequently, number of LDL receptors on liver cells increases, and LDL uptake and breakdown are enhanced. With sustained inhibition of cholesterol synthesis in the liver, levels of very low-density lipoproteins are decreased.

Contraindications

Active liver disease (including unexplained persistent hepatic transaminase elevation), breastfeeding, concurrent cyclosporine therapy, hypersensitivity to pitavastatin or its components pregnancy.

Interactions

DRUGS

colchicine, fibrates such as gemfibrozil: Increased risk of myopathy, including rhabdomyolysis
cyclosporine, erythromycin, lopinavir and ritonavir, rifampin: Increased pitavastatin exposure
niacin: Increased risk of adverse skeletal muscle effects

Adverse Reactions

CNS: Asthenia, confusion, cognitive impairment, depression, dizziness, fatigue, headache, hypoesthenia, insomnia, malaise, memory loss, peripheral neuropathy
CV: Immune-mediated necrotizing myopathy (rare)
EENT: Nasopharyngitis
ENDO: Elevated glycosylated hemoglobin level, hyperglycemia
GI: Abdominal discomfort or pain, constipation, diarrhea, dyspepsia, elevated liver enzymes, **hepatic failure**, **hepatitis**, jaundice, nausea
GU: Acute renal failure, erectile dysfunction, **myoglobinuria**

P

MS: Arthralgia, back or extremity pain, muscle spasms, myopathy, myositis, **rhabdomyolysis**
RESP: **Interstitial lung disease**
SKIN: Pruritus, rash, urticaria
Other: Elevated creatine phosphokinase level, flu-like symptoms

Nursing Considerations

- Be aware that pitavastatin isn't recommended for patients receiving cyclosporine and lopinavir/ritonavir therapy because of increased risk of serious adverse effects.
- Note that pravastatin, another HMG-CoA reductase inhibitor, sounds similar to pitavastatin and could be confusing. Make sure of correct drug before giving.
- Monitor liver enzymes, as ordered, before pravastatin therapy starts and as indicated during therapy.
- Use pitavastatin cautiously in patients with risk factors for myopathy, such as concurrent use of niacin-containing products or fibrates, elderly (over age 65), presence of renal impairment, or in patients who are being inadequately treated for hypothyroidism. Monitor patient throughout therapy for muscular complaints and an elevated blood creatine kinase level. Drug should be discontinued if patient's creatine kinase level becomes markedly elevated, or if myopathy is suspected or confirmed.
- Expect to monitor patient's lipid levels after 4 weeks of therapy to determine drug effectiveness and periodically thereafter, as ordered. Expect dosage to be adjusted if lipid levels remain elevated.

PATIENT TEACHING

- Emphasize that pitavastatin is an adjunct to, not a substitute for, a low-cholesterol diet.
- Tell patient to take drug at the same time each day to maintain its effects.
- Instruct patient to report unexplained muscle pain, tenderness, or weakness, especially if accompanied by fever or malaise.
- Advise patient to limit alcohol ingestion while taking pitavastatin because alcohol-induced liver dysfunction may be difficult to differentiate from pitavastatin-induced liver dysfunction.
- Instruct patient to consult prescriber before taking OTC niacin products because of increased risk of adverse muscle effects.
- Caution women of childbearing age that drug is contraindicated in pregnancy because drug could be harmful to the baby. If pregnancy is suspected, patient should notify prescriber immediately.
- Advise women not to breastfeed during pitavastatin therapy.

plazomicin

Zemdri

Class and Category

Pharmacologic class: Aminoglycoside
Therapeutic class: Antibiotic
Pregnancy category: Not classified

Indications and Dosages

➤ *To treat complicated urinary tract infections, including pyelonephritis, caused by* Enterobacter cloacae, Escherichia coli, Klebsiella pneumoniae, *or* Proteus mirabilis

I.V. INFUSION

Adults and adolescents age 18 and over who have a creatinine clearance greater than or equal to 90 ml/min. 15 mg/kg infused over 30 min every 24 hr for 4 to 7 days.

DOSAGE ADJUSTMENT For patient with a creatinine clearance less than 90 ml/min but equal to or greater than 60 ml/min, dosage remains at 15 mg/kg every 24 hr. For patient with a creatinine clearance less than 60 ml/min but greater than or equal to 30 ml/min, dosage reduced to 10 mg/kg every 24 hr. For patient with a creatinine clearance less than 30 ml/min but greater than or equal to 15 ml/min, dosage reduced to 10 mg/kg and dosage interval increased to every 48 hr.

Mechanism of Action

Binds to bacterial 30S ribosomal subunit to inhibit protein synthesis, which exerts a bactericidal effect.

Incompatibilities

Do not mix plazomicin with other drugs or physically add to solutions containing other drugs, and do not infuse other drugs simultaneously with plazomicin, because incompatibilities are unknown.

Contraindications

Hypersensitivity to plazomicin, other aminoglycosides, or their components

Interactions

DRUGS

None reported

Adverse Reactions

CNS: Dizziness, headache, vertigo
CV: Hypertension, **hypotension**
EENT: Hearing loss, ototoxicity, tinnitus
GI: *Clostridium difficile*-associated diarrhea, constipation, diarrhea, elevated liver enzymes, gastritis, nausea, vomiting
GU: Elevated serum creatinine, hematuria, impaired renal function, **nephrotoxicity**
RESP: Dyspnea
Other: Hypersensitivity reactions, hypokalemia

Nursing Considerations

- Expect to assess creatinine clearance in all patients prior to first dose of plazomicin and daily during therapy. For patients with renal impairment with a creatinine clearance of 15 ml/min or greater but less than 90 ml/min, expect plasma trough concentrations to be below 3 mcg/ml. Plasma trough level should be measured about 30 min before administration of second dose. If level is greater than or equal to 3 mcg/ml, expect a dosage adjustment to be made by extending the dosing interval by 1.5-fold; for example, from every 24 hours to every 36 hours or from every 48 hours to every 72 hours. Know that patients at greater risk for nephrotoxicity are the elderly, patients with existing impaired renal function, and those who are receiving concomitant nephrotoxic drugs.
- Know that each drug vial contains 500 mg plazomicin freebase in 10 ml Water for Injection, giving a concentration of 50 mg/ml. Dilute drug vial solution in 0.9% sodium chloride injection, USP, or Lactated Ringer's Injection, USP, to achieve a final volume of 50 ml for intravenous infusion. After dilution, drug solution is stable for 24 hours at room temperature. Infuse each dose over 30 minutes.
- Monitor patient for hearing loss, tinnitus, and/or vertigo, because plazomicin may cause ototoxicity that may be irreversible and may not show up until after drug has been discontinued. Patients at higher risk include those with a family history of hearing loss, already have renal impairment, or are receiving higher doses and/or longer durations of therapy than recommended.

WARNING Monitor patient for adverse reactions associated with neuromuscular blockade, because aminoglycosides such as plazomicin have been associated with neuromuscular blockade. Patients at high risk include patients with underlying neuromuscular disorders (including myasthenia gravis) or patients who are receiving concomitantly neuromuscular blocking drugs.

WARNING Monitor patient for hypersensitivity reactions. Aminoglycosides have occasionally caused serious allergic reactions. Notify prescriber immediately and expect plazomicin to be discontinued. Provide supportive care, as ordered and needed.

- Assess patient for signs of secondary infection, such as profuse, watery diarrhea. If such diarrhea develops, contact prescriber and expect to obtain a stool specimen to rule out pseudomembranous colitis caused by *Clostridium difficile*. If diarrhea occurs, notify prescriber and expect to withhold plazomicin and treat with electrolytes, fluids, protein, and an antibiotic effective against *C. difficile*.

PATIENT TEACHING

- Tell patient that it is important to keep hydrated during plazomicin therapy, because dehydration increases the risk of kidney impairment.
- Alert patient that diarrhea is a common problem with antibacterial drugs. Tell patient that bloody or watery stools can occur even after plazomicin therapy has been discontinued. Stress importance of reporting diarrhea to prescriber.
- Instruct patient to report any adverse reactions that might indicate an allergic reaction (such as hives, itching, and rash), because an allergic reaction can become serious.

- Tell patient to report any changes in balance or hearing or if she experiences new onset or changes in preexisting buzzing or roaring in the ears, even after the course of plazomicin therapy has finished.
- Warn women of childbearing age to notify prescriber immediately if pregnancy is suspected or known, because aminoglycosides such as plazomicin can cause fetal harm.
- Inform patient with an underlying neuromuscular disease or patient who is receiving neuromuscular blocking agents that aggravation of muscle weakness has been reported with other aminoglycosides. Tell patient to report any muscle weakness that is abnormal for him to prescriber.

plecanatide

Trulance

Class and Category

Pharmacologic class: Guanylate cyclase-C agonist
Therapeutic class: Intestinal mobility agent
Pregnancy category: Not classified

Indications and Dosages

➤ *To treat chronic idiopathic constipation or irritable bowel syndrome with constipation*

TABLETS

Adults. 3 mg once daily.

Mechanism of Action

Acts locally on the luminal surface of the intestinal epithelium, resulting in an increase in both extracellular and intracellular concentrations of cyclic guanosine monophosphate (cGMP). Elevation of intracellular cGMP stimulates secretion of bicarbonate and chloride into the intestinal lumen. This increases intestinal fluid and accelerates transit time, which relieves constipation.

Contraindications

Children less than 6 years of age, hypersensitivity to plecanatide or its components, known or suspected mechanical gastrointestinal obstruction.

Interactions

DRUGS

None reported

Adverse Reactions

CNS: Dizziness
EENT: Nasopharyngitis, sinusitis
GI: Abdominal distention or tenderness, diarrhea, flatulence, elevated liver enzymes, nausea
GU: UTI
RESP: Upper respiratory tract infection
Other: Dehydration

Nursing Considerations

- Be aware that plecanatide therapy should be avoided in patients 6 years to less than 18 years of age and is contraindicated in patients who are less than 6 years of age because of the potential for serious dehydration from plecanatide use.
- Administer plecanatide in applesauce or water if patient has difficulty swallowing tablets whole. To administer in applesauce, crush tablet to a powder and mix with 1 teaspoon of room-temperature applesauce. Administer immediately. Do not store mixture for later use. To administer in water, place tablet in cup, add 30 ml of room-temperature water and gently swirl tablet and water mixture for at least 10 seconds. Have patient swallow entire contents of tablet/water mixture immediately. If any portion of the tablet is left in the cup, add another 30 ml of room-temperature water to the cup, swirl for at least 10 seconds, and have patient swallow the mixture immediately. Do not store the tablet/water mixture for later use.
- Know that plecanatide may be administered via a gastric or nasogastric feeding tube. Begin by placing plecanatide tablet in a cup; then add 30 ml of room-temperature water. Gently swirl the tablet and water mixture for at least 15 seconds. Flush the feeding tube with 30 ml of water. Draw up the drug mixture using the syringe and immediately administer via the feeding tube. Do not reserve for future use. If any portion of the tablet is left in the cup, add another 30 ml of room-temperature water, swirl for at least 15 seconds. Using the same syringe, administer via the feeding tube. Follow by flushing the feeding tube with at least 10 ml of water.

- Monitor patient for diarrhea, which can become severe. If severe diarrhea occurs, withhold drug. Notify prescriber and expect to follow measures to rehydrate patient, as ordered.

PATIENT TEACHING

- Caution patient not to exceed dosage, as severe dehydration may occur.
- Instruct patient to swallow tablet whole. If patient is unable to swallow tablet, tell patient how to mix in applesauce or room-temperature water. Warn patient to take mixture immediately and not to store for later use.
- Tell patient to store plecanatide in a dry place and protect from moisture. Also remind patient to keep drug in original bottle, with desiccant in the bottle, and not subdivide or repackage drug in any way. Instruct patient to keep bottle tightly closed when not in use.
- Tell patient to stop taking drug and notify prescriber if severe diarrhea occurs.
- Warn patient to keep plecanatide out of the reach of children, especially those who are less than 6 years of age.
- Tell patient if she misses a dose, she should skip the missed dose and take the next dose at the regular time. She should never double the dose.

posaconazole

Noxafil

Class and Category

Pharmacologic class: Triazole
Therapeutic class: Antifungal
Pregnancy category: C

Indications and Dosages

➤ *To prevent invasive* Aspergillus *and candida infections in patients at high risk because of severe immunocompromise from such conditions as graft-versus-host disease with hematopoietic stem-cell transplant or hematologic malignancies with prolonged neutropenia from chemotherapy*

ORAL SUSPENSION

Adults and adolescents. 200 mg (5 ml) three times a day until recovery from immunosuppression or neutropenia.

DELAYED RELEASE TABLETS

Adults and adolescents. *Initial:* 300 mg twice daily on first day, followed by 300 mg once daily starting on second day until recovery from immunosuppression or neutropenia.

I.V. INFUSION

Adults. *Initial:* 300 mg infused over 90 min via a central venous line or over 30 min for a peripheral venous line twice daily on first day, followed by 300 mg infused over 90 min via a central venous line or over 30 min for a peripheral venous line once daily starting on second day until recovery from neutropenia or immunosuppression.

➤ *To treat oropharyngeal candidiasis*

ORAL SUSPENSION

Adults. *Initial:* 100 mg (2.5 ml) twice daily on first day, followed by 100 mg (2.5 ml) once daily for 13 days.

➤ *To treat oropharyngeal candidiasis refractory to fluconazole and/or itraconazole*

ORAL SUSPENSION

Adults. 400 mg (10 ml) twice daily until underlying condition improves.

Route	Onset	Peak	Duration
P.O.	Unknown	3–5 hr	Unknown
I.V.	Unknown	Unknown	Unknown

Mechanism of Action

Blocks synthesis of ergosterol, an essential component of fungal cell membrane, by inhibiting 14 alpha-demethylase, an enzyme needed for conversion of lanosterol to ergosterol. Lack of ergosterol increases cellular permeability, and cell contents leak.

Incompatibilities

Do not dilute posaconazole in any solution other than 5% dextrose in water or 0.9% sodium chloride. The following drugs may be infused at the same time through the same cannula or intravenous line with posaconazole: amikacin, caspofungin, ciprofloxacin, daptomycin, dextrose in water 5%, dobutamine, famotidine, filgrastim, gentamicin, hydromorphone, levofloxacin, lorazepam, meropenem, micafungin, morphine sulfate, norepinephrine bitartrate, potassium chloride, sodium chloride 0.9%, and vancomycin. All other drugs and solutions may result in particulate formation and should not be coadministered through the same cannula or intravenous line.

Contraindications

Concurrent therapy with atorvastatin, lovastatin, simvastatin, sirolimus; hypersensitivity to posaconazole, its components, or other azole antifungals; use with ergot alkaloids or CYP3A4 substrates such as astemizole, cisapride, halofantrine, pimozide, quinidine, and terfenadine

Interactions

DRUGS

astemizole, cisapride, halofantrine, pimozide, quinidine, terfenadine: Increased risk of prolonged QT interval and torsades de pointes
atazanavir, atorvastatin, calcium channel blockers, cyclosporine, midazolam, phenytoin, rifabutin, ritonavir, simvastatin, sirolimus, tacrolimus: Increased plasma levels of these drugs, with increased risk of adverse reactions
cimetidine, efavirenz, fosamprenavir, phenytoin, rifabutin: Possibly decreased plasma level of posaconazole
digoxin: Increased risk of digitalis toxicity
ergot alkaloids: Increased plasma ergot alkaloid level and increased risk of ergotism
esomeprazole, metoclopramide: Possible breakthrough fungal infections
HMG-CoA reductase inhibitors: Increased plasma statin level and increased risk of rhabdomyolysis
vinca alkaloids: Increased plasma vinca alkaloid level and increased risk of neurotoxicity

Adverse Reactions

CNS: Anxiety, asthenia, dizziness, fatigue, fever, headache, insomnia, rigors, tremor, weakness
CV: Edema, hypertension, **hypotension**, **QT-interval prolongation**, tachycardia
EENT: Blurred vision, epistaxis, herpes simplex, mucositis, pharyngitis, taste perversion
ENDO: Hyperglycemia
GI: Abdominal pain, anorexia, bilirubinemia, constipation, diarrhea, dyspepsia, elevated liver enzymes, hepatomegaly, jaundice, nausea, **pancreatitis**, vomiting
GU: **Acute renal failure**, elevated blood creatinine level, vaginal hemorrhage
HEME: Anemia, **neutropenia**, **thrombocytopenia**
MS: Arthralgia, back or musculoskeletal pain
RESP: Coughing, dyspnea, pneumonia, upper respiratory tract infection
SKIN: Diaphoresis, petechiae, pruritus, rash
Other: **Bacteremia**, cytomegalovirus infection, dehydration, **hypocalcemia**, **hypokalemia**, **hypomagnesemia**, weight loss

Nursing Considerations

- Use cautiously in patients who have had a hypersensitivity reaction to other azoles because of risk for cross-sensitivity.
- Use cautiously in patients with hepatic or renal dysfunction. Know that posaconazole injection should be avoided, if possible, in patients with moderate or severe renal impairment (GFR less than 50 ml/min). If not possible, expect to monitor serum creatinine levels, as ordered, and if increases occur, anticipate patient being switched to oral posaconazole therapy.
- Use cautiously in patients with potentially proarrhythmic conditions because posaconazole may prolong QT interval.
- Obtain baseline assessment of liver function and check periodically during therapy, as ordered. If elevations occur or patient has evidence of elevated liver enzymes, notify prescriber.
- Shake oral suspension well before administering. Use only the spoon provided in the package to measure dosage. Each dose should be administered during or immediately following (within 20 minutes) a full meal to enhance absorption. If patient cannot eat a full meal, administer drug with an acidic carbonated beverage or a liquid nutritional supplement.
- Administer delayed-release tablets with food.
- Do not interchange delayed-release tablet and oral suspension because of differences in the dosing of each formulation.
- Prepare parenteral form of posaconazole by first removing vial from refrigerator and allowing it to warm to room temperature. Transfer 16.7 ml of the drug solution to an intravenous bag or bottle

containing about 150 ml of 5% dextrose in water or 0.9% sodium chloride. Once mixed, use immediately, or refrigerate for up to 24 hours. Discard any unused solution.

- Administer parenteral form of drug through a 0.22-micron polyethersulfone (PES) or polyvinylidene difluoride (PVD) filter using a central venous line by slow infusion over 90 minutes. Never administer drug by bolus injection. If a central venous line is not available, drug may be administered through a peripheral venous catheter only as a single dose in advance of a central venous line being placed or to bridge the period during which a central venous line is replaced or is in use for other treatment. When administering the drug through a peripheral venous catheter, infuse the drug over 30 minutes.
- Monitor patient experiencing severe diarrhea or vomiting for breakthrough fungal infections.

PATIENT TEACHING

- Advise patient prescribed oral suspension form to use the measuring spoon supplied by manufacturer and to rinse it with water after each use.
- Instruct patient to take posaconazole oral suspension with or within 20 minutes after a full meal or liquid nutritional supplement to increase drug absorption. Tell patient that he also may take posaconazole with an acidic carbonated beverage such as ginger ale.
- Advise patient prescribed delayed-release tablets to take with food; to swallow tablets whole; and to not chew, crush, or divide tablets.
- Tell patient to report severe diarrhea or vomiting because these conditions may interfere with drug effectiveness.
- Instruct patient to alert prescriber if he is already taking vinblastine, vincristine, or any other vinca alkaloids used to treat cancer.

potassium acetate

(contains 2 or 4 mEq of elemental potassium per 1 ml of injection)

potassium bicarbonate

(contains 6.5 mEq of elemental potassium per tablet, 20 or 25 mEq of elemental potassium per effervescent tablet for oral solution)
K+Care ET, K-Electrolyte, K-Ide, Klor-Con/EF, K-Lyte, K-Vescent

potassium bicarbonate and potassium chloride

(contains 20 mEq of elemental potassium per 2.8-g granule packet; 20, 25, or 50 mEq of elemental potassium per effervescent tablet for oral solution)
Klorvess Effervescent Granules, K-Lyte/Cl, K-Lyte/Cl 50, Neo-K (CAN), Potassium Sandoz (CAN)

potassium bicarbonate and potassium citrate

(contains 25 or 50 mEq of elemental potassium per effervescent tablet for oral solution)
Effer-K, K-Lyte DS

potassium chloride

(contains 8 or 10 mEq of elemental potassium per E.R. capsule; 6.7, 8, 10, 12, or 20 mEq of elemental potassium per E.R. tablet; 10, 20, 30, or 40 mEq of elemental potassium per 15 ml of oral solution; 10, 15, 20, or 25 mEq of elemental potassium per packet for oral solution; 20 mEq of elemental potassium per packet for oral suspension; 0.1, 0.2, 0.3, 0.4, 1.5, 2, 3, or 10 mEq of elemental potassium per 1 ml of injection)
Apo-K (CAN), Cena-K, Gen-K, K-8, K-10 (CAN), K+ 10, Kalium Durules (CAN), Kaochlor 10%, Kaochlor S-F 10%, Kaon-Cl, Kato, Kay Ciel, K+ Care, KCL 5% (CAN), K-Dur, K-Ide, K-Lease, K-Long (CAN), K-Lor, Klor-Con 10, Klor-Con Powder, Klor-

Con/25 Powder, Klorvess 10% Liquid, Klotrix, K-Lyte/Cl Powder, K-Med 900 (CAN), K-Norm, K-Sol, K-Tab, Micro-K, Micro-K 10, Potasalan, Roychlor 10% (CAN), Rum-K, Slow-K, Ten-K

potassium citrate

(contains 5 or 10 mEq of elemental potassium per tablet)
Urocit-K

potassium gluconate

(contains 20 mEq of elemental potassium per 15 ml of elixir; 2, 2.3, or 2.5 mEq of elemental potassium per tablet)
Glu-K, Kaon, Kaylixir, K-G Elixir, Potassium-Rougier (can)

potassium gluconate and potassium chloride

(contains 20 mEq of elemental potassium per 15 ml of oral solution; 20 mEq of elemental potassium per 5-g packet for oral solution)
Kolyum

potassium gluconate and potassium citrate

(contains 20 mEq of elemental potassium per 15 ml of oral solution)
Twin-K

trikates

(contains 15 mEq of elemental potassium per 5 ml of oral solution)
Tri-K

Class and Category

Pharmacologic class: Electrolyte cation
Therapeutic class: Electrolyte replacement
Pregnancy category: C

Indications and Dosages

➤ *To prevent or treat hypokalemia in patients who can't ingest sufficient dietary potassium or who are losing potassium because of a condition (such as hepatic cirrhosis or prolonged vomiting) or drug (such as potassium-wasting diuretics or certain antibiotics)*

EFFERVESCENT TABLETS (POTASSIUM BICARBONATE)
Adults and adolescents. 25 to 50 mEq/g once or twice daily, as needed and tolerated. *Maximum:* 100 mEq daily.

EFFERVESCENT TABLETS (POTASSIUM BICARBONATE AND POTASSIUM CHLORIDE)
Adults and adolescents. 20, 25, or 50 mEq once or twice daily, as needed and tolerated. *Maximum:* 100 mEq daily.

EFFERVESCENT TABLETS (POTASSIUM BICARBONATE AND POTASSIUM CITRATE)
Adults and adolescents. 25 or 50 mEq once or twice daily, as needed and tolerated. *Maximum:* 100 mEq daily.

ELIXIR (POTASSIUM GLUCONATE)
Adults and adolescents. 20 mEq twice daily to four times daily, as needed and tolerated. *Maximum:* 100 mEq daily.
Children. 2 to 3 mEq/kg daily in divided doses.

E.R. CAPSULES (POTASSIUM CHLORIDE)
Adults and adolescents. 40 to 100 mEq daily in divided doses twice daily or three times a day for treatment; 16 to 24 mEq daily in divided doses twice daily or three times a day for prevention. *Maximum:* 100 mEq daily.

E.R. TABLETS (POTASSIUM CHLORIDE)
Adults and adolescents. 6.7 to 20 mEq three times a day. *Maximum:* 100 mEq daily.

GRANULE PACKETS (POTASSIUM BICARBONATE AND POTASSIUM CHLORIDE)
Adults and adolescents. 20 mEq once or twice daily, as needed and tolerated. *Maximum:* 100 mEq daily.

GRANULES FOR ORAL SUSPENSION (POTASSIUM CHLORIDE)
Adults and adolescents. 20 mEq 1 to 5 times/day, as needed. *Maximum:* 100 mEq daily.

ORAL SOLUTION (POTASSIUM CHLORIDE)
Adults and adolescents. 20 mEq once daily to four times a day, as needed and tolerated. *Maximum:* 100 mEq daily.
Children. 1 to 3 mEq/kg daily in divided doses.

ORAL SOLUTION (POTASSIUM GLUCONATE AND POTASSIUM CHLORIDE, POTASSIUM GLUCONATE AND POTASSIUM CITRATE)
Adults and adolescents. 20 mEq twice daily to four times a day, as needed and tolerated. *Maximum:* 100 mEq daily.

Children. 2 to 3 mEq/kg daily in divided doses.

POWDER PACKET FOR ORAL SOLUTION (POTASSIUM CHLORIDE)

Adults. 15 to 25 mEq twice daily to four times a day, as needed and tolerated. *Maximum:* 100 mEq daily.

Children. 1 to 3 mEq/kg daily in divided doses, as needed and tolerated.

POWDER PACKET FOR ORAL SOLUTION (POTASSIUM GLUCONATE AND POTASSIUM CHLORIDE)

Adults and adolescents. 20 mEq twice daily to four times a day, as needed and tolerated. *Maximum:* 100 mEq daily.

Children. 2 to 3 mEq/kg daily in divided doses.

ORAL TRIKATES SOLUTION (POTASSIUM ACETATE, POTASSIUM BICARBONATE, AND POTASSIUM CITRATE)

Adults and adolescents. 15 mEq three times a day to four times a day, as needed and tolerated. *Maximum:* 100 mEq daily.

Children. 2 to 3 mEq/kg daily in divided doses.

TABLETS (POTASSIUM GLUCONATE)

Adults and adolescents. 5 to 10 mEq twice daily to four times a day, as needed and tolerated. *Maximum:* 100 mEq daily.

I.V. INFUSION (POTASSIUM ACETATE AND POTASSIUM CHLORIDE)

Adults and adolescents with serum potassium level above 2.5 mEq/L. Up to 10 mEq/ hr. *Maximum:* 200 mEq daily.

Adults and adolescents with serum potassium level below 2 mEq/L, ECG changes, or paralysis. Up to 20 mEq/hr. *Maximum:* 400 mEq daily.

Children. 3 mEq/kg daily infused at a rate no greater than 0.5 mEq/kg/hr.

DOSAGE ADJUSTMENT Dosage adjusted as prescribed based on patient's ECG patterns and serum potassium level.

➤ *To treat renal tubular acidosis with calcium stones, hypocitraturic calcium oxalate nephrolithiasis of any etiology, and uric acid lithiasis with or without calcium stones*

TABLETS (POTASSIUM CITRATE)

Adults. For patients with severe hypocitraturia, 15 mEq four times a day with meals or 20 mEq three times a day with meals. For patients with mild to moderate hypocitraturia, 10 mEq three times a day with meals.

DOSAGE ADJUSTMENT For patients with cirrhosis or renal impairment, dosage should be started at the lower end of the dosing range for all formulations of potassium.

Mechanism of Action

Acts as the major cation in intracellular fluid, activating many enzymatic reactions essential for physiologic processes, including nerve impulse transmission and cardiac and skeletal muscle contraction. Potassium also helps maintain electroneutrality in cells by controlling exchange of intracellular and extracellular ions. It also helps maintain normal renal function and acid–base balance.

Incompatibilities

Don't mix potassium chloride for injection in same syringe with amino acid solutions, lipid solutions, or mannitol because these drugs may precipitate from solution. Administration with blood or blood products can cause lysis of infused RBCs.

Contraindications

Acute dehydration, Addison's disease (untreated), concurrent use with amiloride or triamterene (potassium chloride), or potassium-sparing diuretics (all forms of potassium), crush syndrome, disorders that may delay drug passing through GI tract (potassium citrate), heat cramps, hyperkalemia, hypersensitivity to potassium salts or their components, peptic ulcer disease (potassium citrate), renal impairment with azotemia or oliguria, severe hemolytic anemia, UTI (potassium citrate)

P

Interactions

DRUGS

ACE inhibitors, aliskiren, amiloride, angiotensin II receptor antagonists, beta blockers, blood products, corticosteroids, cyclosporine, eplerenone, heparin, NSAIDs, potassium-containing drugs, potassium-sparing diuretics, tacrolimus, triamterene: Increased risk of hyperkalemia that can become severe

amphotericin B, corticosteroids (glucocorticoids, mineralocorticoids), gentamicin, penicillins, polymyxin B: Possibly hypokalemia

anticholinergics, drugs with anticholinergic activity: Increased risk of GI ulceration, stricture, and perforation

calcium salts (parenteral): Possibly arrhythmias
digoxin: Increased risk of digitalis toxicity
insulin, laxatives, sodium bicarbonate: Decreased serum potassium level
sodium polystyrene sulfonate: Possibly decreased serum potassium level and fluid retention
thiazide diuretics: Possibly hyperkalemia when diuretic is discontinued

FOODS

low-salt milk, salt substitutes: Increased risk of hyperkalemia

Adverse Reactions

CNS: Chills, confusion, fever, paralysis, paresthesia, weakness
CV: Arrhythmias, asystole, bradycardia, cardiac arrest, chest pain, **ECG changes, ventricular fibrillation**
EENT: Throat pain when swallowing
GI: Abdominal pain; **bloody stools**; diarrhea; flatulence; **GI bleeding, obstruction, perforation**, or ulceration; nausea; vomiting
RESP: Dyspnea
SKIN: Rash
Other: Anaphylaxis; angioedema; extravasation reactions such as necrosis, nerve or tendon injury, ulcers, or vascular injury; **hyperkalemia; hypokalemia**; infusion-site reactions such as burning sensation, erythema, irritation, pain, phlebitis, pruritus, rash, or **thrombosis**

Nursing Considerations

- Review patient's medical history before administering potassium chloride, because there are many conditions that may predispose patient to develop hyperkalemia and increased sensitivity to potassium.
- Administer oral potassium with or immediately after meals.
- Mix potassium chloride for oral solution or potassium gluconate elixir in cold water, orange juice, tomato juice (if patient isn't sodium restricted), or apple juice, and stir for 1 full minute before administering.
- Mix potassium bicarbonate, potassium bicarbonate and potassium chloride, and potassium bicarbonate and potassium citrate effervescent tablets with cold water and allow to dissolve completely.
- Be aware that liquid form of oral potassium is prescribed for patients with delayed gastric emptying, esophageal compression, or intestinal obstruction or stricture, as well as patients with dysphagia or swallowing disorders, to decrease the risk of tissue damage from solid forms of potassium that may remain in contact with the gastrointestinal mucosa for a prolonged period of time.
- Administer tablet forms of potassium with food to help prevent gastric irritation. Monitor patient receiving tablet forms of potassium for abdominal pain or distention, gastrointestinal bleeding, or severe vomiting, as this may indicate GI obstruction, perforation, or ulceration and should be reported immediately.
- Be aware that potassium chloride injection should be given with extreme caution, if at all, to patients with conditions that increase patient sensitivity to potassium or predispose patient to hyperkalemia, such as acute dehydration, congestive heart failure, extensive burns or tissue injury, or severe renal impairment. If use cannot be avoided, monitor patient closely.

WARNING Be aware that direct injection of a potassium concentrate may be immediately fatal. Dilute potassium concentrate for injection with adequate volume of solution before I.V. use. Maximum suggested concentration is 40 mEq/L, although stronger concentrations (up to 80 mEq/L) may be used for severe hypokalemia. Inappropriate solutions or improper technique may cause extravasation, fever, hyperkalemia, hypervolemia, I.V. site infection, phlebitis, venospasm, and venous thrombosis.

- Don't connect flexible plastic containers in series because of increased risk of residual air contained in the primary container that could cause an air embolism.
- Infuse potassium slowly at a controlled rate using a calibrated infusion device to avoid phlebitis and decrease risk of adverse cardiac reactions. Keep in mind that different forms of potassium salts contain different amounts of elemental potassium per gram and that not all forms are dosage equivalent. If possible, administer via a central intravenous route. Know that high concentrations of

potassium chloride only should be given through a central line.

- Monitor serum potassium level before and during administration of I.V. potassium. Be aware that mild or moderate hyperkalemia is asymptomatic and may be manifested only by increased serum potassium concentrations, and possibly by characteristic ECG changes. Arrhythmias can develop at any time during hyperkalemia.

WARNING Be aware that some forms of potassium contain tartrazine, which may cause an allergic reaction, such as asthma. Some forms may also contain aluminum, which may become toxic in a patient with impaired renal function.

- Regularly assess patient for signs of hypokalemia, such as arrhythmias, fatigue, and weakness, and for signs of hyperkalemia, such as arrhythmias, confusion, dyspnea, and paresthesia.
- Monitor serum creatinine level and urine output during administration, because adequate renal function is needed for potassium supplementation. Notify prescriber about signs of decreased renal function, because renal impairment may predispose patient to fluid overload and/or hyperkalemia.

PATIENT TEACHING

- Inform patient that potassium is part of a normal diet and that most meats, seafoods, fruits, and vegetables contain sufficient potassium to meet recommended daily intake. Also advise her not to exceed recommended daily amount of potassium.
- Teach patient the correct way to take prescribed potassium. This can vary from swallowing a tablet with a full glass of water to mixing certain preparations with half to full glass of cold water or juice.
- Caution patient not to crush or chew E.R. forms unless instructed otherwise.
- Instruct patient to take drug with or right after food.
- Teach patient how to take her radial pulse, and advise her to notify prescriber about significant changes in heart rate or rhythm.
- Advise patient to watch stools for changes in color and consistency and to notify prescriber if they become black, tarry, or red.
- Inform patient that although she may see waxy form of E.R. tablet in stools, she has received all of the potassium.
- Urge patient to keep follow-up laboratory appointments as directed by prescriber to determine serum potassium level.

potassium iodide
(KI, SSKI)

Pima, Thyro-Block

Class and Category

Pharmacologic class: Iodine
Therapeutic class: Antithyroid
Pregnancy category: D

Indications and Dosages

➤ *To prepare for thyroidectomy*

ORAL SOLUTION

Adults and children. 50 to 250 mg three times a day for 10 to 14 days before surgery.

➤ *To manage thyrotoxic crisis*

ORAL SOLUTION

Adults. 50 to 250 mg three times a day or 500 mg every 4 hr.

➤ *To protect thyroid gland during radiation exposure*

ORAL SOLUTION, SYRUP, TABLETS

Adults and adolescents. 100 to 150 mg 24 hr before administration of or exposure to radioactive isotopes of iodine and daily for 3 to 10 days afterward. *Maximum:* 12 g daily.
Children age 1 and over. 130 mg daily for 10 days after administration of or exposure to radioactive isotopes of iodine.
Children under age 1. 65 mg daily for 10 days after administration of or exposure to radioactive isotopes of iodine.

Route	Onset	Peak	Duration
P.O.*	24 hr	10–15 days	Up to 6 wk

* For antithyroid effects.

Mechanism of Action

Inhibits release of thyroid hormone into circulation, thus alleviating symptoms caused by excessive thyroid hormone stimulation. Potassium iodide also blocks thyroid uptake of radioactive iodine isotopes released as a result of radiation exposure.

P

Contraindications
Acute bronchitis, Addison's disease, dehydration, heat cramps, hyperkalemia, hypersensitivity to iodides or their components, hyperthyroidism, iodism, renal impairment, tuberculosis

Interactions
DRUGS
antithyroid drugs, lithium: Increased risk of hypothyroidism and goiter
captopril, enalapril, lisinopril, potassium-sparing diuretics: Increased risk of hyperkalemia

Adverse Reactions
CNS: Confusion, fatigue, headache, heaviness or weakness in legs, paresthesia
CV: Irregular heartbeat
EENT: Burning in mouth or throat, increased salivation, metallic taste, sore teeth or gums
GI: Diarrhea, epigastric pain, indigestion, nausea, vomiting
HEME: Eosinophilia
MS: Arthralgia
SKIN: Acneiform lesions, urticaria
Other: Angioedema, lymphadenopathy

Nursing Considerations
- Be aware that potassium iodide shouldn't be given to patients with tuberculosis because drug may cause pulmonary irritation and increased secretions.

WARNING Monitor serum potassium level regularly in patients with renal impairment because of the risk of hyperkalemia.
- Monitor thyroid function test results periodically to assess drug's effectiveness.

PATIENT TEACHING
- Advise patient taking potassium iodide oral solution or syrup to use a calibrated measuring device to ensure accurate doses.
- Urge patient to mix solution or syrup in a full glass (8 oz) of water, fruit juice, milk, or broth to improve taste and lessen GI reactions. Advise patient taking tablet form to dissolve each tablet in half a glass (4 oz) of water or milk before ingestion.
- If crystals form in solution, advise patient to place the closed container in warm water and gently shake to dissolve.
- Instruct patient to discard bottle and obtain a new one if solution turns brownish yellow.

potassium phosphates
K-Phos Original, Neutra-Phos-K

potassium and sodium phosphates
K-Phos M.F., K-Phos-Neutral, K-Phos No. 2, Neutra-Phos

sodium phosphates

Class and Category
Pharmacologic class: Soluble salts
Therapeutic class: Antiurolithic, electrolyte replenisher
Pregnancy category: C

Indications and Dosages
➤ *As adjunct to treat UTI, to prevent renal calculus formation*

MONOBASIC TABLETS (POTASSIUM PHOSPHATES)
Adults and adolescents. 1 g in 180 to 240 ml water four times a day, after meals and at bedtime.

MONOBASIC TABLETS (POTASSIUM AND SODIUM PHOSPHATES)
Adults and adolescents. 250 mg in 240 ml water four times a day, after meals and at bedtime. Dosage interval may be increased to every 2 hr if urine is difficult to acidify.
Maximum: 2 g/24 hr.

➤ *To prevent or treat hypophosphatemia*

CAPSULES (POTASSIUM PHOSPHATES)
Adults and children age 4 and over. 1.45 g in 75 ml water or juice four times a day, after meals and at bedtime.
Children up to age 4. 200 mg in 60 ml water or juice four times a day, after meals and at bedtime.

CAPSULES (POTASSIUM AND SODIUM PHOSPHATES)
Adults and children age 4 and over. 1.25 g in 75 ml water or juice four times a day, after meals and at bedtime.
Children up to age 4. 200 mg in 60 ml water or fruit juice four times a day, after meals and at bedtime.

MONOBASIC TABLETS (POTASSIUM PHOSPHATES)
Adults and children age 4 and over. 1 g in 180 to 240 ml water four times a day, after meals and at bedtime.

Children up to age 4. 200 mg in 60 ml water four times a day, after meals and at bedtime.

MONOBASIC TABLETS (POTASSIUM AND SODIUM PHOSPHATES)

Adults and children age 4 and over. 250 mg in 240 ml water four times a day, after meals and at bedtime.

Children up to age 4. 200 mg in 60 ml water four times a day, after meals and at bedtime.

ORAL SOLUTION (POTASSIUM PHOSPHATES, POTASSIUM AND SODIUM PHOSPHATES)

Adults and children age 4 and over. 250 mg four times a day, after meals and at bedtime.

Children up to age 4. 200 mg four times a day, after meals and at bedtime.

TABLETS (POTASSIUM AND SODIUM PHOSPHATES)

Adults and children age 4 and over. 250 mg in a full glass of water four times a day, after meals and at bedtime.

Children up to age 4. 200 mg in 60 ml water four times a day, after meals and at bedtime.

I.V. INFUSION (SODIUM PHOSPHATES)

Adults and adolescents. 10 to 15 mmol (310 to 465 mg) daily, infused over 4 to 6 hr.

Children. 1.5 to 2 mmol (46.5 to 62 mg)/kg daily, infused over 4 to 6 hr.

Mechanism of Action

Reverses symptoms of hypophosphatemia by replenishing the body's supply of phosphate; acidifies urine by causing hydrogen to be exchanged for sodium in renal distal tubule; and inhibits formation of calcium renal calculi by preventing solidification of calcium oxalate.

Incompatibilities

Don't add phosphates to calcium- or magnesium-containing solutions because precipitate may form.

Contraindications

Hyperkalemia (potassium formulations), hypernatremia (sodium formulations), hyperphosphatemia, magnesium ammonium phosphate urolithiasis accompanied by infection, severe renal insufficiency, UTI caused by urea-splitting organisms

Interactions

DRUGS

ACE inhibitors, cyclosporine, heparin (long-term use), NSAIDs, potassium-containing drugs, potassium-sparing diuretics: Increased risk of hyperkalemia (potassium forms only)

aluminum- or magnesium-containing antacids: Possibly impaired phosphate absorption

anabolic steroids, androgens, corticosteroids, estrogens: Increased risk of edema (sodium formulations only)

calcium-containing drugs: Increased risk of calcium deposition in soft tissues

iron supplements: Decreased absorption of oral iron

phosphate-containing drugs, vitamin D: Increased risk of hyperphosphatemia

salicylates: Increased blood salicylate level

zinc supplements: Reduced zinc absorption

FOODS

low-salt milk, salt substitutes: Increased risk of hyperkalemia

oxalates (in spinach and rhubarb), phytates (in bran and whole grains): Decreased absorption of phosphate

Adverse Reactions

CNS: Anxiety, confusion, dizziness, fatigue, headache, paresthesia, **seizures**, tremor, weakness

CV: **Arrhythmias**, edema of legs, tachycardia

GI: Diarrhea, epigastric pain, nausea, thirst, vomiting

GU: Decreased urine output

MS: Muscle cramps or weakness

RESP: Dyspnea

Other: **Hyperkalemia**, **hypernatremia**, **hyperphosphatemia**, **hypocalcemia**, weight gain

Nursing Considerations

- Monitor serum phosphorus level, as appropriate, in patient who receives phosphates and has a condition that may be associated with elevated phosphorus level, such as chronic renal disease, hypoparathyroidism, and rhabdomyolysis; phosphates may further increase serum phosphorus level.

P

- Monitor serum calcium level, as appropriate, in patient who receives phosphates and has a condition that may be associated with a low-calcium level, such as acute pancreatitis, chronic renal disease, hypoparathyroidism, osteomalacia, rhabdomyolysis, and rickets; phosphates may further decrease serum calcium level.
- Monitor serum potassium level, as appropriate, if patient who receives potassium phosphate has a condition linked to elevated potassium level, such as acute dehydration, adrenal insufficiency, extensive tissue breakdown (as in severe burns), myotonia congenita, pancreatitis, rhabdomyolysis, and severe renal insufficiency; she may have increased risk of hyperkalemia.
- Monitor serum sodium level in patient who receives sodium phosphates and has a condition that may be worsened by sodium excess, such as heart failure, hypernatremia, hypertension, peripheral or pulmonary edema, pre-eclampsia, renal impairment, and severe hepatic disease.
- Monitor urine pH, as ordered, to assess effectiveness of drug used to acidify urine.
- When administering sodium phosphates, monitor ECG tracing frequently during I.V. infusion to detect arrhythmias.

PATIENT TEACHING

- Instruct patient to take phosphates after meals to avoid GI upset and decrease laxative effect.
- Emphasize importance of not swallowing capsules or tablets whole; instead, advise patient to soak tablets in water or fruit juice for 2 to 3 minutes to dissolve them.
- Suggest chilling diluted drug to improve flavor, but caution against freezing.
- Encourage increased intake of fluids (8 oz/hr, if not contraindicated) to prevent renal calculi.
- Urge patient to notify prescriber immediately about muscle weakness or cramps, unexplained weight gain, or shortness of breath.
- Instruct patient who needs an iron supplement to take it 1 to 2 hours after taking phosphates.

pralidoxime chloride

(2-PAM chloride, 2-pyridine aldoxime methochloride)

Protopam Chloride

Class and Category

Pharmacologic class: Anticholinesterase
Therapeutic class: Anticholinesterase antidote
Pregnancy category: C

Indications and Dosages

➤ *As adjunct to reverse organophosphate pesticide toxicity*

I.V. INFUSION

Adults. *Initial:* 1 to 2 g in 100-ml normal saline solution infused over 15 to 30 min until muscarinic signs and symptoms disappear; may be repeated in 1 hr and then every 10 to 12 hr if muscle weakness persists
Children. *Initial:* 20 to 50 mg/kg (not to exceed 2,000 mg/dose) in 100-ml normal saline solution infused over 15 to 30 min followed by a continuous infusion of 10 to 20 mg/kg/hr. Alternatively, an initial intermittent infusion of 20 to 50 mg/kg (not to exceed 2,000 mg/dose) given over 15 to 30 min. Dosage may be repeated in 1 hr and then every 10 to 12 hr if muscle weakness persists.

DOSAGE ADJUSTMENT For patient with pulmonary edema, dosage given slowly (over not less than 5 min) as a 50 mg/ml solution in water.

I.M. INJECTION

Adults and children weighing 40 kg or more. For mild symptoms, 600 mg (2 ml). May repeat dose after 15 min and again after an additional 15 min, as needed. If at any time after the first dose patient develops severe symptoms, two additional 600-mg doses may be given in rapid succession for a total cumulative dose of 1,800 mg. For severe symptoms, 600 mg (2 ml) administered three times in rapid succession for a total dose of 1,800 mg. For persistent symptoms after three injections of 600 mg each have been given, series may be repeated beginning about 1 hr after administration of the last injection. **Children weighing less than 40 kg.** For mild symptoms, 15 mg/kg. May repeat dose after 15 min and again after an additional 15 min, as needed. If at any time after the first dose patient develops severe symptoms, two additional 15-mg/kg doses may be given in rapid succession for a total cumulative dose of 45 mg/kg. For severe symptoms, 15 mg/kg administered three times in rapid succession for a total dose of 45 mg/kg. For persistent symptoms after three injections of 15 mg/kg each have been given, series may be repeated beginning about 1 hr after administration of the last injection.

➤ *To treat anticholinesterase overdose secondary to myasthenic drugs (including ambenonium, neostigmine, and pyridostigmine)*

I.V. INJECTION

Adults. *Initial:* 1 to 2 g, followed by 250 mg every 5 min.

➤ *To treat exposure to nerve agents*

I.V. INJECTION

Adults. *Initial:* 1 atropine-containing autoinjector followed by 1 pralidoxime-containing autoinjector as soon as atropine's effects are evident; both injections repeated every 15 min for two additional doses if nerve agent symptoms persist.

DOSAGE ADJUSTMENT Dosage reduced for patients with renal insufficiency.

Mechanism of Action

Reverses muscle paralysis by removing phosphoryl group from inhibited cholinesterase molecules at neuromuscular junction of skeletal and respiratory muscles. Reactivation of cholinesterase restores body's ability to metabolize acetylcholine, which is inhibited by organophosphate pesticides, anticholinesterase overdose, or nerve agent poisoning.

Contraindications

Hypersensitivity to pralidoxime chloride or its components

Interactions

DRUGS

aminophylline, morphine, phenothiazines, reserpine, succinylcholine, theophylline: Increased symptoms of organophosphate poisoning

barbiturates: Potentiated barbiturate effects

Adverse Reactions

CNS: Dizziness, drowsiness, headache
CV: Increased systolic and diastolic blood pressure, tachycardia
EENT: Accommodation disturbances, blurred vision, diplopia
GI: Nausea, vomiting
MS: Muscle weakness
RESP: Hyperventilation
Other: Injection-site pain

Nursing Considerations

- Be aware that pralidoxime must be given within 36 hours of toxicity to be effective and atropine must be given as soon as possible after hypoxemia is improved.
- Use drug with extreme caution in patients with myasthenia gravis being treated for organophosphate poisoning because pralidoxime may precipitate myasthenic crisis.
- Reconstitute drug according to manufacturer's guidelines and administration route.
- For intermittent intravenous infusion, further dilute with normal saline solution to 100 ml and infuse over 15 to 30 minutes. Rate should not exceed 200 mg/min.
- Avoid too-rapid intravenous delivery, which may cause hypertension, laryngospasm, muscle spasms, neuromuscular blockade, and tachycardia. Also be sure to avoid intradermal injection.
- If intravenous route is not feasible, expect to administer the drug intramuscularly or subcutaneously.
- Closely monitor neuromuscular status during therapy.
- Monitor BUN and serum creatinine levels, as appropriate, in patients with renal insufficiency because drug is excreted in urine.
- When pralidoxime is administered with atropine, expect signs of atropination, such as dry mouth and nose, flushing, mydriasis, and tachycardia, to occur earlier than might be expected when atropine is given alone.

PATIENT TEACHING

- Inform patient receiving I.M. pralidoxime that she'll experience pain at the injection site for 40 to 60 minutes afterward.
- Reassure patient that she'll be closely monitored throughout therapy.

pramipexole dihydrochloride

Mirapex, Mirapex ER

Class and Category

Pharmacologic class: Nonergoline dopamine agonist
Therapeutic class: Antiparkinsonian
Pregnancy category: C

Indications and Dosages

➤ *To treat Parkinson's disease*

TABLETS

Adults. *Initial:* 0.125 mg three times a day for 1 wk, increased weekly thereafter as follows: for wk 2, 0.25 mg three times a day; for wk 3, 0.5 mg three times a day; for wk 4, 0.75 mg three times a day; for wk 5, 1 mg three times day; for wk 6, 1.25 mg three times a day; and for wk 7, 1.5 mg three times a day. *Maintenance:* 1.5 to 4.5 mg daily in divided doses three times a day. *Maximum:* 4.5 mg daily.

DOSAGE ADJUSTMENT For patients with renal impairment, dosage reduced as follows: for creatinine clearance greater than 50 ml/min, initial dosage of 0.125 mg three times a day with maximum dose limited to 1.5 mg three times a day; for creatinine clearance of 30 to 50 ml/min, initial dosage reduced to 0.125 mg twice a day and maximum dose limited to 0.75 mg three times a day; for creatinine clearance of 15 to less than 30 ml/min, initial dosage reduced to 0.125 mg once a day and maximum dose limited to 1.5 mg once a day. Drug shouldn't be given to patients with creatinine clearance of less than 15 ml/min.

E.R. TABLETS

Adults. *Initial:* 0.375 mg once daily, increased every 5 to 7 days, first to 0.75 mg and then by 0.75-mg increments, as needed. *Maximum:* 4.5 mg daily.

DOSAGE ADJUSTMENT For patients with moderate renal impairment (creatinine clearance between 30 and 50 ml/min), initial dosage taken every other day with dosage adjustment done after 1 wk in increments of 0.375 mg only, as needed, to maximum dosage of 2.25 mg daily.

➤ *To treat restless legs syndrome*

TABLETS

Adults. *Initial:* 0.125 mg once daily, 2 to 3 hr before bedtime. Increased in 4 to 7 days to 0.25 mg once daily 2 to 3 hr before bedtime, as needed. Further increased in 4 to 7 days to 0.5 mg once daily 2 to 3 hr before bedtime, as needed.

DOSAGE ADJUSTMENT For patients with moderate to severe renal impairment (creatinine clearance 20 to 60 ml/min) dosage interval for titration, if needed, increased to 14 days.

Mechanism of Action

May stimulate dopamine receptors in the brain, thereby easing symptoms of Parkinson's disease, which is thought to be caused by a dopamine deficiency.

Contraindications

Hypersensitivity to pramipexole or its components

Interactions

DRUGS

carbidopa, levodopa: Possibly increased peak blood levodopa level and potentiation of levodopa's dopaminergic adverse effects
diltiazem, quinidine, quinine, ranitidine, triamterene, verapamil: Decreased pramipexole clearance
haloperidol, metoclopramide, phenothiazines, thioxanthenes: Decreased pramipexole effectiveness

Adverse Reactions

CNS: Abnormal behavior, amnesia, anxiety, asthenia, compulsive behaviors such as pathological gambling or uncontrollable shopping or sexual activity, confusion, dream disturbances, drowsiness, dyskinesia, dystonia, fatigue, fever, hallucinations, headache, insomnia, malaise, paranoia, restlessness, syncope
CV: Cardiac failure, edema, orthostatic hypotension
EENT: Diplopia, dry mouth, rhinitis, vision changes
ENDO: Inappropriate antidiuretic hormone secretion (SIADH)

GI: Anorexia, constipation, dysphagia, eating disorders, nausea, vomiting
GU: Altered libido, hypersexuality, impotence, urinary frequency, urinary incontinence
MS: Arthralgia, myalgia, myasthenia, postural deformity, **rhabdomyolysis**
RESP: Pneumonia
SKIN: Diaphoresis, erythema, pruritis, rash, urticaria
Other: Weight gain or loss

Nursing Considerations

- Use pramipexole cautiously in patients with hallucinations, hypotension, or retinal problems (such as macular degeneration). Drug may worsen these conditions.
- Also use cautiously in patients with renal impairment because pramipexole elimination may be decreased.
- Monitor patient for postural deformity (antecollis, bent spine syndrome, Pisa syndrome) that may occur several months after pramipexole therapy has been initiated or after increasing dose. If present, notify prescriber and expect dosage to be decreased or drug discontinued, which may improve condition.
- Take safety precautions per facility policy until drug's CNS effects are known.
- Avoid stopping pramipexole abruptly because doing so may cause a symptom complex resembling neuroleptic malignant syndrome and consisting of altered level of consciousness, autonomic instability, hyperpyrexia, and muscle rigidity.
- Be aware that patient may be switched overnight from immediate-release pramipexole tablets to the extended-release tablets at the same daily dose. However, monitor effectiveness to determine if dosage adjustment may be necessary.
- Assess patient for skin changes regularly because melanomas may occur at a higher rate in patients with Parkinson's disease. It isn't clear if this is a result of the disease or drugs used to treat it.
- Know that some patients have reported worsening of their Parkinson's disease symptoms when tablet residue was visible in their stool. If this occurs, notify prescriber, as pramipexole therapy may have to be reevaluated.

PATIENT TEACHING

- Advise patient to take pramipexole with meals if nausea occurs.
- Caution patient about possible dizziness, drowsiness, or light-headedness, which may result from orthostatic hypotension. Advise her not to rise quickly from a lying or sitting position to minimize these effects.
- Instruct patient to notify prescriber immediately about vision problems or urinary frequency or incontinence.
- Inform patient that improvement in motor performance and activities of daily living may take 2 to 3 weeks.
- Urge patient to have regular skin examinations by a dermatologist or other qualified health professional.
- Advise patient and his family to notify prescriber about onset of compulsive and intense urges, such as eating binges, compulsive shopping, hypersexuality, or pathological gambling. Dosage may have to be reduced or drug discontinued.
- Caution patient not to stop taking pramipexole abruptly.
- Tell patient to alert prescriber if posture changes that cannot be controlled occur, such as neck bending forward; bending forward at the waist; or tilting sideways when sitting, standing, or walking.
- Remind patient that drug should be stored at room temperature.
- Advise patient to contact prescriber if he observes residue in his stool, which may resemble a swollen original E.R. tablet or swollen pieces of the original tablet.
- Advise patient to report unexplained muscle pain, tenderness, or weakness to prescriber.

pramlintide acetate

Symlin

Class and Category

Pharmacologic class: Human amylin analogue
Therapeutic class: Antidiabetic
Pregnancy category: C

Indications and Dosages

➤ *To achieve euglycemia in patients with type 1 diabetes who use mealtime insulin therapy but have not achieved desired glucose control*

SUBCUTANEOUS INJECTION

Adults. *Initial:* 15 mcg just before major meals with 50% reduced dosage of preprandial rapid-acting or short-acting insulin, including fixed-mix insulins such as 70/30. When nausea has abated at least 3 days, dosage increased in increments of 15 mcg. *Maintenance:* 30 to 60 mcg before major meals.

DOSAGE ADJUSTMENT Dosage decreased to 30 mcg if nausea occurs and persists at higher dosages.

➤ *To achieve euglycemia in patients with type 2 diabetes who use mealtime insulin, with or without a sulfonylurea and/or metformin, and have not achieved desire glucose control*

SUBCUTANEOUS INJECTION

Adults. *Initial:* 60 mcg immediately before major meals combined with dosage reduction of preprandial rapid-acting or short-acting insulin, including fixed-mix insulins such as 70/30, by 50%. When nausea has been absent for 3 to 7 days, dosage increased to 120 mcg before major meals.

DOSAGE ADJUSTMENT Dosage decreased to 60 mcg before major meals if nausea occurs and persists with 120-mcg dosage.

Route	Onset	Peak	Duration
SubQ	Unknown	19–21 min	3 hr

Mechanism of Action

Slows the rate at which food is released from stomach to small intestine, thus reducing initial postprandial rise in serum glucose level. Pramlintide also suppresses glucagon secretion and promotes satiety, thus furthering weight loss, which also lowers serum glucose level.

Pramlintide is a synthetic analogue of amylin, a naturally occurring neuroendocrine hormone secreted with insulin by pancreatic beta cells. In diabetes, secretion of insulin and amylin is reduced or absent.

Contraindications

Gastroparesis, hypersensitivity to pramlintide, cresol or its components; hypoglycemia unawareness

Incompatibilities

Don't mix in same syringe as insulin because pharmacokinetic parameters of pramlintide become altered.

Interactions

DRUGS

drugs that alter GI motility (such as anticholinergics) or slow intestinal absorption of nutrients (such as alpha-glucosidase inhibitors): Altered effects of these drugs

oral drugs: Delayed absorption

Adverse Reactions

CNS: Dizziness, fatigue, headache

EENT: Blurred vision, pharyngitis

GI: Abdominal pain, anorexia, nausea, **pancreatitis**, vomiting

MS: Arthralgia

RESP: Coughing

SKIN: Diaphoresis

Other: Hypersensitivity reactions; local injection-site reaction, such as redness, swelling, or pruritus

Nursing Considerations

- Because of the risks involved with pramlintide therapy, insulin-using patients with type 1 or 2 diabetes must have failed to achieve adequate glycemic control despite individualized insulin management and must be receiving ongoing care with guidance of insulin prescriber and a diabetes educator before pramlintide is prescribed.
- Expect that certain patients won't be prescribed pramlintide because its risks may outweigh its benefits. These include patients with poor compliance with current insulin regimen, poor compliance with monitoring blood glucose level, a glycosylated hemoglobin greater than 9%, recurrent severe hypoglycemia that required assistance during past 6 months, hypoglycemia unawareness, gastroparesis, concurrent therapy with drugs that stimulate GI motility, and pediatric patients.
- Before pramlintide therapy starts, make sure patient's premeal insulin dosage has been reduced by 50%.

- Give drug immediately before main meals.
- Monitor patient's premeal and postmeal blood glucose levels regularly to determine effectiveness of pramlintide and insulin therapy and to detect hypoglycemia.
- For 3 hours after each dose of pramlintide, monitor patient closely for hypoglycemia, which may be severe, especially in patients with type 1 diabetes. Effects may include hunger, headache, sweating, tremor, irritability, and trouble concentrating. They may occur with a rapid decrease in blood glucose level regardless of glucose values.
- Although pramlintide doesn't cause hypoglycemia, its use with insulin increases the risk of insulin-induced severe hypoglycemia, which can result in loss of consciousness, coma, or seizures. If hypoglycemia occurs, provide supportive care, including glucagon if prescribed, and notify prescriber. Expect insulin dosage accompanying pramlintide to be reduced.
- Keep in mind that early warning symptoms of hypoglycemia may be different or less severe if patient has had diabetes for a long time; has diabetic nerve disease; takes a beta blocker, clonidine, guanethidine, or reserpine; or is under intensified diabetes control.
- Closely monitor patients taking oral antidiabetics, ACE inhibitors, disopyramide, fibrates, fluoxetine, MAO inhibitors, pentoxifylline, propoxyphene, salicylates, or sulfonamide antibiotics because of an increased risk of hypoglycemia.
- Expect pramlintide to be stopped if patient develops recurrent hypoglycemia that requires medical assistance, develops persistent nausea, or becomes noncompliant with therapy or follow-up visits.

PATIENT TEACHING

- Alert patient that insulin-induced hypoglycemia may occur within 3 hours of injecting pramlintide. Review signs and symptoms and appropriate treatment. Tell patient to notify prescriber if hypoglycemia occurs because insulin dosage will have to be reduced.
- Emphasize need to monitor blood glucose level often, especially before and after eating.
- Tell patient to inject drug subcutaneously immediately before major meals using an insulin syringe to draw up dose and using the same technique as with insulin administration, including rotating sites. Or, if patient has been prescribed the Symlin Pen injector, show her how to use it. Advise patient to inject drug into her abdomen or thigh and not to use her arm as an injection site because absorption may be too variable.
- Warn patient not to mix pramlintide and insulin together in the same syringe.
- Warn patient that nausea is common with pramlintide; urge her to notify prescriber because dosage may have to be decreased.
- Caution patient that if she misses a dose, she should skip the missed dose and continue with the next scheduled dose.
- Instruct patient to keep unopened pramlintide vials in the refrigerator; vials that have been opened may be kept in the refrigerator or at room temperature. Vials should be discarded 28 days after opening.
- Caution patient to avoid hazardous activities that require mental alertness until effects of pramlintide are known.
- Reassure patient that pramlintide won't alter her awareness of or her body's response to insulin-induced hypoglycemia.
- Alert patient that she'll need close follow-up care, at least weekly until a target dose of pramlintide has been reached, she's tolerating the drug well, and her blood glucose level is stable.
- Instruct women of childbearing age to notify prescriber about planned, suspected, or known pregnancy because drug therapy will have to be adjusted.
- Explain that local injection-site reactions, such as redness, swelling or itching, may occur but usually resolve in a few weeks.
- Instruct patient using the SymlinPen to never share it with anyone else, even if the needle has been changed, because of a risk for transmission of bloodborne pathogens.

prasterone

Intrarosa

Class and Category

Pharmacologic class: Steroid

Therapeutic class: Intravaginal steroid
Pregnancy category: Not classified

Indications and Dosages

➤ *To treat moderate to severe dyspareunia, a symptom of vaginal and vulvar atrophy, due to menopause*

VAGINAL INSERTS

Adult postmenopausal women. 6.5 mg (1 insert) daily at bedtime.

Mechanism of Action

Converts into active androgens and/or estrogens to help relieve vaginal and vulvar atrophy responsible for painful sexual intercourse.

Contraindications

Current or history of breast cancer, hypersensitivity to prasterone or its components, undiagnosed abnormal genital bleeding

Interactions

DRUGS

None reported

Adverse Reactions

GU: Abnormal Pap smear, vaginal discharge

Nursing Considerations

- Know that prasterone should not be given to women with a current or past history of breast cancer because the drug has not been studied in women with a history of breast cancer.
- Know that drug should only be given to postmenopausal women.

PATIENT TEACHING

- Instruct patient how to insert a vaginal insert. Tell her to use one vaginal insert daily at bedtime, using the provided applicator.
- Alert patient that a vaginal discharge commonly occurs with use of the drug and to be prepared.
- Inform patient that an abnormal Pap smear may occur while using prasterone and, if present, will have to be investigated to rule out any potential underlying problems.

prasugrel

Effient

Class and Category

Pharmacologic class: $P2Y_{12}$ platelet inhibitor (thienopyridine)
Therapeutic class: Antiplatelet
Pregnancy category: B

Indications and Dosages

➤ *To reduce rate of thrombotic cardiovascular events (including stent thrombosis) in patients with acute coronary syndrome who will be managed with percutaneous coronary intervention because of non-ST-elevation MI, ST-elevation MI, or unstable angina*

TABLETS

Adults. *Initial:* 60 mg as a loading dose and then 10 mg once daily. *Maintenance:* 10 mg once daily.

DOSAGE ADJUSTMENT For patients weighing less than 60 kg (132 lb), daily maintenance dosage may be reduced to 5 mg once daily.

Route	Onset	Peak	Duration
P.O.	2 hr	30 min	7–10 days

Mechanism of Action

After forming active metabolite, irreversibly binds to ADP receptors on platelets to inhibit platelet activation and aggregation for the lifetime of the platelet, which is 7 to 10 days. Without platelet activation and aggregation, thrombus cannot form.

Contraindications

Active bleeding, history of transient ischemic attack or stroke, hypersensitivity to prasugrel or its components

Interactions

DRUGS

fibrinolytic agents, heparin, NSAIDs (chronic use), warfarin: Increased risk of bleeding
opioids: Decreased or delayed prasugrel absorption

Adverse Reactions

CNS: Dizziness, fatigue, fever, headache, **intracranial hemorrhage**
CV: Atrial fibrillation, bradycardia, hypercholesterolemia, hyperlipidemia, hypertension, **hypotension**, peripheral edema
EENT: Epistaxis, retinal hemorrhage
GI: Diarrhea, **GI or retroperitoneal hemorrhage**, hepatic dysfunction, nausea

HEME: Anemia, **leukopenia, bleeding, severe thrombocytopenia, thrombotic thrombocytopenia purpura**
MS: Back or limb pain
RESP: Cough, dyspnea, **hemoptysis**
SKIN: Subcutaneous hematoma, rash
Other: Anaphylaxis, angioedema, hypersensitivity reactions, malignancies, noncardiac chest pain

Nursing Considerations

- Be aware that patient should be receiving daily aspirin therapy (75 or 325 mg) throughout prasugrel therapy.
- Be aware that drug isn't recommended for patients age 75 or older (except in high-risk situations such as history of previous MI or presence of diabetes) or in patients who have active bleeding or a history of a transient ischemic attack or stroke. Monitor patients closely who have other risk factors for bleeding, which include a body weight less than 60 kg or a history of bleeding. Also monitor patients who are also taking drugs that increase risk of bleeding, such as chronic use of NSAIDs, fibrinolytic therapy, heparin, or warfarin.
- Know that prasugrel shouldn't be given to patients likely to undergo emergency coronary artery bypass graft (CABG) surgery because of increased bleeding risk. Drug should be discontinued at least 7 days before any surgery.

WARNING Monitor patient closely for bleeding because prasugrel can cause life-threatening hemorrhage. Report hypotension in patients who have recently undergone CABG surgery or other surgical procedures, coronary angiography, or percutaneous coronary intervention while taking drug. In this setting, expect therapy to continue because stopping prasugrel, especially in first few weeks after acute coronary syndrome, increases the risk of adverse cardiovascular effects.

- Be aware that because prasugrel inhibits platelet aggregation for the lifetime of the platelet, which is 7 to 10 days, withholding a dose is unlikely help in managing a bleeding event or the risk of bleeding associated with an invasive procedure. Expect to administer exogenous platelets but only 6 hours after prasugrel loading dose or 4 hours after maintenance dose was given.
- Monitor patient's CBC regularly, as ordered, watching for evidence of thrombotic thrombocytopenic purpura, such as abnormal blood counts, fever, neurologic abnormalities, or renal dysfunction. Notify prescriber immediately because condition can be fatal. Expect to implement emergency treatment, such as plasmapheresis.

PATIENT TEACHING

- Emphasize importance of taking prasugrel exactly as prescribed, without lapses in therapy, for drug to be effective and adverse reactions to be reduced.
- Instruct patient to take daily dose of aspirin as prescribed.
- Discourage use of NSAIDs, including OTC products, during prasugrel therapy because of risk of bleeding.
- Caution patient that bleeding may last longer than usual. Instruct him to report unusual bleeding or bruising.
- Instruct patient to inform healthcare providers that he takes prasugrel.
- Urge patient to take precautions against bleeding, such as using an electric shaver and a soft-bristled toothbrush.
- Advise patient to avoid activities that could cause traumatic injury and bleeding.
- Advise patient to seek immediate medical care if swelling of his face or throat occurs or if any signs of an allergic reaction develops that is persistent or becomes worse.

P

pravastatin sodium

Pravachol

Class and Category

Pharmacologic class: HMG-CoA reductase inhibitor (statin)
Therapeutic class: Antilipemic
Pregnancy category: X

Indications and Dosages

➤ *To prevent cardiovascular and coronary events in patients at risk, to treat hyperlipidemia*

TABLETS
Adults. *Initial:* 40 mg daily at bedtime, increased in 4 wk to 80 mg daily at bedtime, if needed.
DOSAGE ADJUSTMENT For patients with significant hepatic or renal impairment, those taking immunosuppressants, and elderly patients, initial dosage reduced to 10 mg daily at bedtime. For elderly patients and those taking immunosuppressants, maintenance dosage usually limited to 20 mg daily. For patients taking clarithromycin, dosage limited to 40 mg once daily.

➤ *To treat pediatric heterozygous familial hypercholesterolemia*

TABLETS
Adolescents ages 14 to 18. 40 mg daily at bedtime.
Children ages 8 to 14. 20 mg daily at bedtime.

Mechanism of Action

Inhibits cholesterol synthesis in liver by blocking the enzyme needed to convert hydroxymethylglutaryl-CoA (HMG-CoA) to mevalonate, a cholesterol precursor. When cholesterol synthesis is blocked, the liver also increases breakdown of LDL cholesterol.

Contraindications

Active hepatic disease or unexplained, persistent elevated liver enzymes; breastfeeding; hypersensitivity to pravastatin or its components; pregnancy

Interactions

DRUGS
cholestyramine, colestipol: Decreased pravastatin bioavailability
clarithromycin and other macrolide antibiotics, colchicine, cyclosporine, erythromycin, gemfibrozil, immunosuppressants, niacin, other fibrates: Increased risk of rhabdomyolysis and acute renal failure
oral anticoagulants: Increased bleeding or prolonged PT

Adverse Reactions

CNS: Anxiety, asthenia, chills, confusion, cognitive impairment, cranial nerve dysfunction, depression, dizziness, fatigue, headache, malaise, memory loss, nervousness, nightmare, peripheral nerve palsy, sleep disturbance
CV: Angina pectoris, chest pain, vasculitis
EENT: Blurred vision, diplopia, rhinitis
ENDO: Abnormal thyroid function, elevated glycosylated hemoglobin levels, gynecomastia, hyperglycemia
GI: Abdominal pain, cholestatic jaundice, cirrhosis, constipation, diarrhea, elevated liver enzymes, flatulence, **fulminant hepatic necrosis**, heartburn, hepatoma, **hepatic failure**, **hepatitis**, indigestion, nausea, **pancreatitis**, vomiting
GU: Dysuria, nocturia, urinary frequency
HEME: Hemolytic anemia, positive ANA, ESR elevation, purpura
MS: Arthralgia, musculoskeletal cramps or pain, myalgia, myopathy, polymyalgia rheumatica, **rhabdomyolysis**, tendon disorder
RESP: Cough, dyspnea, **interstitial lung disease**, upper respiratory tract infection
SKIN: Dermatomyositis, **erythema multiforme**, photosensitivity, rash, **Stevens–Johnson syndrome**, **toxic epidermal necrolysis**
Other: Anaphylaxis, **angioedema**, lupus-like syndrome

Nursing Considerations

- Use pravastatin cautiously in patients with hepatic or renal impairment and in elderly patients.
- Monitor liver enzymes before pravastatin therapy starts and as indicated during therapy.
- Give drug 1 hour before or 4 hours after giving cholestyramine or colestipol.
- Report unexplained muscle aches or weakness and significant increases in creatine kinase level to prescriber because in rare instances drug causes rhabdomyolysis with acute renal failure caused by myoglobinuria. Expect to stop drug and provide supportive care.
- Monitor patient's BUN and serum creatinine levels periodically for abnormal elevations.
- Monitor blood lipoprotein level, as indicated, to evaluate response to therapy.

PATIENT TEACHING
- Instruct patient to take drug at bedtime, without regard to meals.
- Caution patient not to perform hazardous activities such as driving until effects of drug is known.
- Advise patient to notify prescriber at once about muscle pain, tenderness, weakness, and other evidence of myopathy.

- Urge woman of childbearing age to use a reliable method of contraception during pravastatin therapy and to notify prescriber at once if she becomes pregnant or thinks she may be pregnant.
- Advise women not to breastfeed while on pravastatin therapy.
- Instruct patient not to stop taking pravastatin without consulting prescriber, even when cholesterol level returns to normal.

prazosin hydrochloride

Minipress

Class and Category

Pharmacologic class: Alpha blocker
Therapeutic class: Antihypertensive
Pregnancy category: C

Indications and Dosages

➤ *To manage hypertension*

CAPSULES

Adults. *Initial:* 1 mg twice daily or three times a day. *Maintenance:* 6 to 15 mg daily in divided doses twice daily or three times a day. *Maximum:* 40 mg daily.

DOSAGE ADJUSTMENT For elderly patients and those with renal impairment, initial dosage possibly reduced to 1 mg once to twice daily.

Route	Onset	Peak	Duration
P.O.	0.5–1.5 hr	2–4 hr*	7–10 hr

* For a single dose; 3 to 4 wk for multiple doses.

Mechanism of Action

Selectively and competitively inhibits $alpha_1$-adrenergic receptors. This action promotes peripheral arterial and venous dilation and reduces peripheral vascular resistance, thereby lowering blood pressure.

Contraindications

Hypersensitivity to prazosin, other quinazolines, or their components

Interactions

DRUGS

antihypertensives, beta blockers, diuretics, phosphodiesterase-5 inhibitors: Increased risk of hypotension and syncope
dopamine: Antagonized peripheral vasoconstrictive effect of dopamine (high doses)
ephedrine: Decreased vasopressor response to ephedrine
epinephrine: Possibly severe hypotension and tachycardia
metaraminol: Decreased vasopressor effect of metaraminol
methoxamine, phenylephrine: Possibly decreased vasopressor effect and shortened duration of action of these drugs
NSAIDs, sympathomimetics: Decreased effectiveness of prazosin

ACTIVITIES

alcohol use: Increased hypotensive effects

Adverse Reactions

CNS: Asthenia, dizziness, drowsiness, fatigue, headache, insomnia, malaise, nervousness, syncope
CV: Angina, **bradycardia**, edema, orthostatic hypotension, palpitations, vasculitis
EENT: Dry mouth, eye pain
ENDO: Gynecomastia
GI: Nausea
GU: Priapism, urinary frequency or incontinence
SKIN: Urticaria
Other: Hypersensitivity reactions

Nursing Considerations

- Use prazosin cautiously in patients with renal impairment because of increased sensitivity to prazosin's effects; in those with angina pectoris because drug may induce or aggravate angina; in those with narcolepsy because prazosin may worsen cataplexy; and in elderly patients because they're at increased risk for drug-induced hypotension.
- Monitor blood pressure regularly to evaluate effectiveness of therapy.

PATIENT TEACHING

- Instruct patient who is starting prazosin to take drug at bedtime to minimize effects of first-dose hypotension.
- Emphasize need to take drug even if feeling well.
- Advise patient to avoid drinking alcohol, exercising in hot weather, or standing for long periods because these activities increase risk of orthostatic hypotension.

- Suggest rising slowly from lying or sitting position to minimize orthostatic hypotension.
- Urge patient to avoid hazardous activities until drug's CNS effects are known.
- Advise patient to notify prescriber immediately about adverse reactions, especially dizziness and fainting.
- Instruct patient not to take any drugs, including OTC forms, without consulting prescriber, to avoid serious interactions.
- Instruct male patient that a prolonged erection may occur with prazosin therapy. If it lasts longer than 4 hours, stress importance of seeking immediate medical assistance.

prednisolone

Cotolone, Delta-Cortef, Prelone

prednisolone acetate

Articulose-50, Flo-Pred, Key-Pred, Predacort 50, Predalone 50, Predate 50, Predcor-25, Predcor-50, Pred-Ject 50

prednisolone sodium phosphate

Orapred ODT, Pediapred

prednisolone tebutate

Nor-Pred T.B.A., Predalone T.B.A., Predate TBA, Predcor-TBA

Class and Category

Pharmacologic class: Glucocorticoid
Therapeutic class: Immunosuppressant
Pregnancy category: C

Indications and Dosages

➤ *To treat adrenal insufficiency and acute and chronic inflammatory and immunosuppressive disorders*

SYRUP, TABLETS (PREDNISOLONE); DISINTEGRATING TABLETS, ORAL SOLUTION (PREDNISOLONE SODIUM PHOSPHATE); ORAL SUSPENSION (PREDNISOLONE ACETATE)
Adults and adolescents. 5 to 60 mg daily or in divided doses. *Maximum:* 250 mg daily.

I.M. INJECTION (PREDNISOLONE ACETATE)
Adults and adolescents. 4 to 60 mg daily.

INTRA-ARTICULAR, INTRALESIONAL, OR SOFT-TISSUE INJECTION (PREDNISOLONE ACETATE, PREDNISOLONE TEBUTATE)
Adults and adolescents. 4 to 100 mg of prednisolone acetate, repeated as needed, or 4 to 40 mg of prednisolone tebutate, repeated every 1 to 3 wk, as needed.

➤ *To treat adrenocortical insufficiency in children*

SYRUP, TABLETS (PREDNISOLONE); DISINTEGRATING TABLETS, ORAL SOLUTION (PREDNISOLONE SODIUM PHOSPHATE); ORAL SUSPENSION (PREDNISOLONE ACETATE)
Children. 0.14 mg/kg daily in divided doses three times a day.

I.M. INJECTION (PREDNISOLONE ACETATE)
Children. 0.14 mg/kg over a 24-hr period in divided doses three times a day every third day.

➤ *To treat acute exacerbations of multiple sclerosis*

SYRUP, TABLETS (PREDNISOLONE); DISINTEGRATING TABLETS, ORAL SOLUTION (PREDNISOLONE SODIUM PHOSPHATE); ORAL SUSPENSION (PREDNISOLONE ACETATE)
Adults. 200 mg daily for 1 wk, followed by 80 mg every other day for 1 mo.

Route	Onset	Peak	Duration
P.O.*	Unknown	1–2 hr	1.25–1.5 days
I.M.†	Slow	Unknown	Unknown
Intra-articular, intra-lesional, soft-tissue injection‡	1–2 days	Unknown	1–3 wk

* Prednisolone.
† Prednisolone acetate.
‡ Prednisolone tebutate.

Mechanism of Action

Binds to intracellular glucocorticoid receptors and suppresses inflammatory and immune responses by:

- inhibiting neutrophil and monocyte accumulation at inflammation site and suppressing their phagocytic and bactericidal activity

- stabilizing lysosomal membranes
- suppressing antigen response of macrophages and helper T cells
- inhibiting synthesis of inflammatory response mediators, such as cytokines, interleukins, and prostaglandins.

Contraindications

Hypersensitivity to prednisolone or its components, idiopathic thrombocytopenic purpura (I.M. form), systemic fungal infection

Interactions

DRUGS

acetaminophen: Possibly hepatotoxicity (long-term use or high acetaminophen doses)
acetazolamide: Possibly hypernatremia or edema
amphotericin B (parenteral): Possibly severe hypokalemia
anabolic steroids, androgens: Possibly edema and severe acne
anticholinergics: Increased intraocular pressure
asparaginase: Increased hyperglycemic effect of asparaginase, possibly neuropathy and disturbances in erythropoiesis
carbonic anhydrase inhibitors: Possibly hypocalcemia, hypokalemia, and osteoporosis
digoxin: Possibly arrhythmias and digitalis toxicity from hypokalemia
diuretics: Possibly decreased natriuretic and diuretic effects of diuretics, severe hypokalemia (with potassium-depleting diuretics)
ephedrine: Increased metabolic clearance of prednisolone
estrogens, oral contraceptives: Decreased clearance, increased elimination half-life, and increased therapeutic and toxic effects of prednisolone
folic acid: Increased folic acid requirements (with long-term prednisolone use)
heparin, oral anticoagulants, streptokinase, urokinase: Possibly decreased anticoagulant effect and increased risk of GI ulceration and bleeding
immunosuppressants: Increased risk of infection, lymphomas, and other lymphoproliferative disorders
isoniazid: Decreased blood isoniazid level
mexiletine: Possibly accelerated metabolism and decreased blood level of mexiletine
neuromuscular blockers: Increased neuromuscular blockade
NSAIDs: Increased risk of GI ulceration and bleeding, possibly added therapeutic effect when NSAIDs are used to treat arthritis
potassium supplements: Decreased effectiveness of both drugs
rifampin, other hepatic enzyme inducers: Decreased prednisolone effect
ritodrine: Increased risk of pulmonary edema in pregnant women
salicylates: Possibly decreased blood salicylate level, increased risk of GI ulceration and bleeding
sodium-containing drugs: Possibly edema and hypertension
somatrem, somatropin: Inhibited growth response to somatrem or somatropin
streptozocin: Increased risk of hyperglycemia
toxoids, vaccines: Possibly loss of antibody response, increased risk of neurologic complications
tricyclic antidepressants: Possibly worsened adverse psychiatric effects of prednisolone
troleandomycin: Increased therapeutic and toxic effects of prednisolone

FOODS

sodium-containing foods: Increased risk of edema and hypertension

ACTIVITIES

alcohol use: Increased risk of GI ulceration and bleeding

Adverse Reactions

CNS: Euphoria, headache, insomnia, nervousness, psychosis, restlessness, **seizures**, vertigo
CV: Edema, **heart failure**, hypertension
EENT: Cataracts, exophthalmos, glaucoma, increased ocular pressure
ENDO: Adrenal insufficiency, Cushing's syndrome, growth suppression in children, hyperglycemia
GI: Anorexia, **GI bleeding** and ulceration, increased appetite, indigestion, **intestinal perforation**, nausea, **pancreatitis**, vomiting
GU: Menstrual irregularities
MS: Avascular necrosis of joints, bone fractures, muscle atrophy or weakness, myalgia, osteoporosis, tendon rupture (local injection only)

SKIN: Acne; cutaneous or subcutaneous atrophy (with frequent repository injections); diaphoresis; ecchymosis; flushing; petechiae; striae; thin, fragile skin
Other: Delayed wound healing, **hypernatremia, hypokalemia**, injection-site scarring, negative nitrogen balance

Nursing Considerations

WARNING Avoid using prednisolone in patients with a history of active tuberculosis because drug can reactivate the disease.

- Give once-daily doses in the morning to mirror body's normal cortisol secretion.
- Inspect injectable form for particulates and discoloration before administering.
- For I.M. injection, shake suspension well before withdrawing. Keep in mind that I.M. injections are contraindicated in patients with idiopathic thrombocytopenic purpura.
- For intra-articular injection, attach a 20G to 24G needle to empty syringe, using aseptic technique, so prescriber can remove a few drops of synovial fluid to confirm that needle is in the joint. The aspirating syringe is then exchanged with a prednisolone-filled syringe to inject drug into joint.
- Because prednisolone can produce many adverse reactions, assess patient regularly for evidence of such reactions, including heart failure and hypertension. Also monitor patient's intake, output, and daily weight.
- Monitor growth pattern in children; prednisolone may retard bone growth.
- Prolonged use may cause hypothalamic-pituitary-adrenal suppression.

WARNING Withdraw drug gradually, as ordered, if therapy lasts longer than 2 weeks. Stopping abruptly may cause acute adrenal insufficiency or, possibly, death.

- Be aware that patient may be at risk for emotional instability or psychic disturbance while taking prednisolone, especially if predisposed to them or taking high doses.

PATIENT TEACHING

- Instruct patient to take oral prednisolone with food to decrease stomach upset and to take once-daily dose in the morning.
- Emphasize need to take drug exactly as prescribed; taking too much increases risk of serious adverse reactions.
- Instruct patient taking orally disintegrating tablets to remove tablet from blister pack only when ready to take drug and to place tablet on tongue. Warn her not to break, cut, or split tablets.
- Caution patient not to discontinue drug abruptly.
- Urge patient to avoid alcohol during therapy because of increased risk of GI ulcers and bleeding.
- Urge patient to avoid hazardous activities until drug's CNS effects are known.
- Advise patient to avoid people with contagious infections because drug has an immunosuppressant effect. Urge her to notify prescriber immediately about exposure to measles or chickenpox.
- Caution against receiving vaccinations or other immunizations and coming in contact with people who have recently received oral poliovirus vaccine.
- Teach patient about potential side effects of prednisolone therapy, including restlessness, mood swings, nervousness, and delayed wound healing.
- Instruct patient to notify prescriber immediately about joint pain, swelling, tarry stools, and visual disturbances. Also instruct her to report signs of infection or injury for up to 12 months after therapy.
- Advise patient to restrict joint use after intra-articular injection and to obtain activity guidelines from prescriber.
- Instruct diabetic patient to check her blood glucose level often because prednisolone may cause hyperglycemia.
- Advise patient to comply with follow-up visits to assess drug's effectiveness and detect adverse reactions.
- Urge patient to carry medical identification revealing prednisolone therapy.

prednisone

Apo-Prednisone (CAN), Deltasone Liquid Pred, Meticorten, Orasone 1, Orasone 5, Orasone 10, Prednicen-M, Prednicot, Prednisone Intensol, Rayos, Sterapred, Sterapred DS, Winpred (CAN)

Class and Category

Pharmacologic class: Glucocorticoid
Therapeutic class: Immunosuppressant
Pregnancy category: Not classified for oral solution, syrup, tablets; D for delayed-release tablets

Indications and Dosages

➤ *To treat adrenal insufficiency and acute and chronic inflammatory and immunosuppressive disorders*

DELAYED-RELEASE TABLETS, ORAL SOLUTION, SYRUP, TABLETS

Adults and adolescents. 5 to 60 mg daily as a single dose or in divided doses. *Maximum:* 250 mg daily.

➤ *To treat adrenogenital syndrome*

DELAYED-RELEASE TABLETS, ORAL SOLUTION, SYRUP, TABLETS

Adults and adolescents. 5 to 10 mg daily.
Children. 5 mg/m^2 daily in divided doses twice daily.

➤ *To treat acute exacerbations of multiple sclerosis*

DELAYED-RELEASE TABLETS, ORAL SOLUTION, SYRUP, TABLETS

Adults. 200 mg daily for 1 wk, then 80 mg every other day for 1 mo. *Maximum:* 250 mg daily.

➤ *To treat nephrosis in children*

DELAYED-RELEASE TABLETS, ORAL SOLUTION, SYRUP, TABLETS

Children age 10 and over. 20 mg four times a day.
Children ages 4 to 10. 15 mg four times a day.
Children ages 18 months to 4 years. 7.5 to 10 mg four times a day.

➤ *To treat rheumatic carditis, leukemia, and tumors in children*

DELAYED-RELEASE TABLETS, ORAL SOLUTION, SYRUP, TABLETS

Children. 0.5 mg/kg four times a day for 2 to 3 wk; then 0.375 mg/kg four times a day for 4 to 6 wk.

➤ *As adjunct to treat tuberculosis in children (with concurrent antitubercular therapy)*

DELAYED-RELEASE TABLETS, ORAL SOLUTION, SYRUP, TABLETS

Children. 0.5 mg/kg four times a day for 2 mo.

Route	Onset	Peak	Duration
P.O.	Rapid	1–2 hr	1.25–1.5 days

Mechanism of Action

Binds to intracellular glucocorticoid receptors and suppresses inflammatory and immune responses by:

- inhibiting neutrophil and monocyte accumulation at inflammation site and suppressing their phagocytic and bactericidal activity
- stabilizing lysosomal membranes
- suppressing antigen response of macrophages and helper T cells
- inhibiting synthesis of inflammatory response mediators, such as cytokines, interleukins, and prostaglandins.

Contraindications

Hypersensitivity to prednisone or its components, systemic fungal infection

Interactions

DRUGS

acetaminophen: Possibly hepatotoxicity (long-term use or high acetaminophen doses)
acetazolamide sodium: Possibly hypernatremia or edema
amphotericin B (parenteral): Possibly severe hypokalemia
anabolic steroids, androgens: Possibly edema and severe acne
antacids: Decreased absorption of prednisone (with long-term use)
anticholinergics: Increased intraocular pressure
asparaginase: Increased hyperglycemic effect of asparaginase, possibly neuropathy and disturbances in erythropoiesis
carbonic anhydrase inhibitors: Possibly hypocalcemia, hypokalemia, and osteoporosis
digoxin: Possibly arrhythmias and digitalis toxicity from hypokalemia
diuretics: Possibly decreased natriuretic and diuretic effects of diuretics, severe hypokalemia (with potassium-depleting diuretics)
ephedrine: Increased metabolic clearance of prednisone
estrogens, oral contraceptives: Decreased clearance, increased elimination half-life, and increased therapeutic and toxic effects of prednisone
folic acid: Increased folic acid requirements (with long-term prednisone use)
heparin, oral anticoagulants, streptokinase, urokinase: Possibly decreased anticoagulant

effect and increased risk of GI ulceration and bleeding
immunosuppressants: Increased risk of infection, lymphomas, and other lymphoproliferative disorders
isoniazid: Decreased blood isoniazid level
mexiletine: Possibly accelerated metabolism and decreased blood level of mexiletine
neuromuscular blockers: Increased neuromuscular blockade
NSAIDs: Increased risk of GI ulceration and bleeding, possibly added therapeutic effect when NSAIDs are used to treat arthritis
potassium supplements: Decreased effectiveness of both drugs
ritodrine: Increased risk of pulmonary edema in pregnant women
salicylates: Possibly decreased blood salicylate level, increased risk of GI ulceration and bleeding
sodium-containing drugs: Possibly edema and hypertension
somatrem, somatropin: Inhibited growth response to somatrem or somatropin
streptozocin: Increased risk of hyper-glycemia
toxoids, vaccines: Possibly loss of antibody response, increased risk of neurologic complications
tricyclic antidepressants: Possibly exacerbated adverse psychiatric effects of prednisone
troleandomycin: Increased therapeutic and toxic effects of prednisone

FOODS

sodium-containing foods: Increased risk of edema and hypertension

ACTIVITIES

alcohol use: Increased risk of GI ulceration and bleeding

Adverse Reactions

CNS: Euphoria, headache, insomnia, nervousness, psychosis, restlessness, **seizures**, vertigo
CV: Edema, **heart failure**, hypertension
EENT: Cataracts, exophthalmos, glaucoma, increased ocular pressure
ENDO: **Adrenal insufficiency**, Cushing's syndrome, growth suppression in children, hyperglycemia
GI: Anorexia, **GI bleeding** and ulceration, increased appetite, indigestion, **intestinal perforation**, nausea, **pancreatitis**, vomiting
GU: Menstrual irregularities
MS: Avascular necrosis of joints, bone fractures, muscle atrophy or weakness, myalgia, osteoporosis
SKIN: Acne; diaphoresis; ecchymosis; flushing; petechiae; striae; thin, fragile skin
Other: Delayed wound healing, **hypernatremia**, **hypokalemia**, negative nitrogen balance

Nursing Considerations

- Administer once-daily doses of prednisone in the morning to match body's normal cortisol secretion schedule.
- Because prednisone can produce many adverse reactions, assess regularly for signs and symptoms of such reactions as heart failure and hypertension. Also monitor fluid intake and output and daily weight.
- Monitor growth pattern in children. Prednisone may retard bone growth.
- Be aware that prolonged use of prednisone may cause hypothalamic-pituitary-adrenal suppression.

WARNING Withdraw prednisone gradually, as ordered, if therapy lasts longer than 2 weeks. Stopping abruptly may cause acute adrenal insufficiency and, possibly, death.

PATIENT TEACHING

- Instruct patient to take prednisone with food to decrease GI distress and to take once-daily dose in the morning.
- Emphasize importance of taking drug exactly as prescribed; taking more than prescribed increases risk of serious adverse reactions.
- Tell patient prescribed delayed-release tablet form not to break, divide, or chew tablet because the delayed-release action is dependent on an intact coating.
- Caution patient not to stop drug abruptly.
- Urge patient to avoid alcohol during therapy because of increased risk of GI ulcers and bleeding.
- Urge patient to avoid hazardous activities until drug's CNS effects are known.
- Advise patient to avoid people with contagious infections because drug has an immunosuppressant effect. Urge her to notify prescriber immediately about possible exposure to measles or chickenpox.
- Caution against receiving vaccinations or other immunizations and coming in contact with people who have recently received oral poliovirus vaccine.

- Instruct patient to notify prescriber immediately about joint pain, swelling, tarry stools, and visual disturbances. Also instruct her to report signs of infection or injury for up to 12 months after therapy.
- Instruct diabetic patient to check blood glucose level often because prednisone may cause hyperglycemia.
- Advise patient to comply with follow-up visits to assess drug effectiveness and detect adverse reactions.
- Urge patient to carry medical identification revealing prednisone therapy.

pregabalin

Lyrica, Lyrica CR

Class, Category, and Schedule

Pharmacologic class: Gamma-aminobutyric acid (GABA) analogue
Therapeutic class: Analgesic, anticonvulsant
Pregnancy category: C
Controlled substance schedule: V

Indications and Dosages

➤ *To relieve neuropathic pain associated with diabetic peripheral neuropathy*

CAPSULES, ORAL SOLUTION

Adults. *Initial:* 50 mg three times a day, increased to 100 mg three times a day, within 1 wk as needed.

E.R. TABLETS

Adults. *Initial:* 165 mg once daily after evening meal, then increased to 330 mg once daily after evening meal within 1 wk, as needed and tolerated. *Maximum:* 330 mg once daily.

➤ *To relieve postherpetic neuralgia; as adjunct therapy to manage partial-onset seizures*

CAPSULES, ORAL SOLUTION

Adults. *Initial:* 75 mg twice daily or 50 mg three times a day, increased to 150 mg twice daily or 100 mg three times a day within 1 wk as needed. Then increased to 300 mg twice daily or 200 mg three times a day in 2 to 4 wk as needed.

➤ *As adjunct therapy to manage partial-onset seizures*

CAPSULES, ORAL SOLUTION

Adults. *Initial:* 150 mg daily in two or three divided doses, then increased as needed. *Maximum:* 600 mg daily in two or three divided doses.
Children age 4 and over weighing 30 kg (66 lb) or more. *Initial:* 2.5 mg/kg/day in two or three divided doses, then increased as needed. *Maximum:* 10 mg/kg/day in two or three divided doses, not to exceed 600 mg/day.
Children age 4 and over weighing 11 kg (24.2 lb) to less than 30 kg (66 lb). *Initial:* 3.5 mg/kg/day in two or three divided doses. *Maximum:* 14 mg/kg/day in two or three divided doses.

➤ *To relieve postherpetic neuralgia*

E.R. TABLETS

Adults. *Initial:* 165 mg once daily after evening meal, then increased to 330 mg once daily after evening meal, if needed and tolerated. Dosage further increased to 660 mg once daily after evening meal after 2 to 4 wk, if needed and tolerated. *Maximum:* 660 mg once daily.

➤ *To manage fibromyalgia*

CAPSULES, ORAL SOLUTION

Adults. *Initial:* 75 mg twice daily, increased to 150 mg twice daily in 1 wk, as needed, and then to 225 mg twice daily in 1 wk as needed. *Maximum:* 450 mg daily.

➤ *To manage neuropathic pain associated with spinal cord injury*

CAPSULES, ORAL SOLUTION

Adults. *Initial:* 75 mg twice daily, increased to 150 mg twice daily in 1 wk, as needed, and then to 300 mg twice daily after 2 to 3 wk, as needed.

DOSAGE ADJUSTMENT For adult patient with renal impairment with a creatinine clearance of 30 to 60 ml/min, daily dosage reduced by 50%. Extended-release pregabalin should not be given to patients with creatinine clearance less than 30 ml/min. If clearance is 15 to 30 ml/min, daily dosage of immediate-release form reduced by 75% and frequency reduced to once or twice daily. If clearance is less than 15 ml/min, daily dosage of immediate-release form reduced to as low as 25 mg daily. If patient is having hemodialysis, daily dosage of immediate-release form is reduced and supplemental dose given immediately after every 4-hour hemodialysis session as follows: If reduced daily dosage is 25 mg daily, give supplemental dose of 25 or 50 mg. If reduced daily dosage is 25 to 50 mg daily, give supplemental dose of 50 or 75 mg. If reduced daily dosage is 50 to 75 mg daily, give supplemental dose of 75 or 100 mg. If reduced daily dosage is 75 mg, give supplemental dose of 100 or 150 mg.

Route	Onset	Peak	Duration
P.O.	Unknown	1.5 hr	Unknown

Mechanism of Action

Binds to alpha$_2$-delta site, an auxiliary subunit of voltage calcium channels, in CNS tissue where it may reduce calcium-dependent release of several neurotransmitters, possibly by modulating calcium channel function. With fewer neurotransmitters, pain sensation and seizure activity decline.

Contraindications

Hypersensitivity to pregabalin or its components

Interactions

DRUGS

ACE inhibitors: Increased risk of pregabalin-induced angioedema
CNS depressants: Additive CNS effects such as somnolence
lorazepam, oxycodone: Additive effects on cognitive and gross motor function
thiazolidinedione antidiabetics: Possibly increased risk of peripheral edema and weight gain

ACTIVITIES

alcohol use: Additive effects on cognitive and gross motor function

Adverse Reactions

CNS: Abnormal gait, amnesia, anxiety, asthenia, ataxia, balance disorder, confusion, depression, difficulty concentrating, dizziness, euphoria, extrapyramidal syndrome, fatigue, fever, headache, hypertonia, hypesthesia, incoordination, **intracranial hypertension**, myoclonus, nervousness, neuropathy, paresthesia, psychotic depression, schizophrenic reaction, somnolence, stupor, **suicidal ideation**, tremor, twitching, vertigo
CV: Chest pain, **heart failure**, peripheral edema, **ventricular fibrillation**
EENT: Amblyopia, blurred vision, conjunctivitis, decreased visual acuity, diplopia, dry mouth, nystagmus, otitis media, sinusitis, tinnitus, visual field defect
ENDO: Gynecomastia, **hypoglycemia**
GI: Abdominal distention or pain, constipation, diarrhea, flatulence, gastroenteritis, **GI hemorrhage**, increased appetite, nausea, vomiting
GU: **Acute renal failure**, anorgasmia, decreased libido, glomerulitis, impotence, **nephritis**, urinary frequency, urinary incontinence, urine retention
HEME: **Leukopenia**, **thrombocytopenia**
MS: Arthralgia, back pain, elevated creatine kinase level, leg or muscle cramps, myalgia, myasthenia
RESP: **Apnea**, dyspnea
SKIN: Ecchymosis, **exfoliative dermatitis**, pruritus, **Stevens–Johnson syndrome**
Other: **Anaphylaxis**, **angioedema**, **hypersensitivity reactions**, weight gain

Nursing Considerations

- Know that pregabalin therapy should be stopped gradually over at least 1 week to decrease risk of seizure activity and avoid unpleasant symptoms such as diarrhea, headache, insomnia, and nausea.
- Be aware that if patient has evidence of hypersensitivity (dyspnea, facial swelling, rash, red skin, urticaria, wheezing) drug should be stopped at once; notify prescriber, and give supportive care.
- Monitor patient closely for adverse reactions. Notify prescriber if significant adverse reactions persist.
- Monitor patient closely for evidence of suicidal behavior or thinking, especially when therapy starts or dosage changes.

PATIENT TEACHING

- Instruct patient prescribed extended-release tablets not to chew, crush, or split tablets but to swallow tablets whole. Tell patient to take tablets after evening meal.
- Tell patient converting from immediate-release formulation to extended release to take morning dose of immediate-release pregabalin and take first dose of

extended-release form in the evening on the day of the switch.
- Warn against stopping pregabalin abruptly. Tell patient that when pregabalin is no longer needed, the dosage should be tapered gradually over a minimum of one week before it is discontinued.
- Urge patient to avoid hazardous activities until she knows how drug affects her.
- Instruct patient to notify prescriber if she has changes in vision or unexplained muscle pain, tenderness, or weakness, especially if these muscle symptoms are accompanied by fever or malaise.
- Alert patient that drug may cause edema and weight gain.
- Tell patient who also takes a thiazolidinedione antidiabetic that these effects may be intensified. If significant, tell patient to notify prescriber.
- Inform male patient who plans to father a child that drug could impair his fertility.
- Instruct diabetic patients to inspect their skin while taking pregabalin.
- Urge caregivers to watch patient closely for evidence of suicidal tendencies, especially when therapy starts or dosage changes and to report concerns at once to prescriber.
- Urge woman who becomes pregnant while taking pregabalin for seizures to enroll in the North American antiepileptic drug pregnancy registry by calling 1-888-233-2334. Explain that the registry is collecting information about the safety of anti-epileptic drugs during pregnancy

primidone

Myidone, Mysoline, Sertan (CAN)

Class and Category

Pharmacologic class: Barbiturate
Therapeutic class: Anticonvulsant
Pregnancy category: Not classified

Indications and Dosages

➤ *To manage generalized tonic–clonic seizures, nocturnal myoclonic seizures, complex partial seizures, and simple partial seizures caused by epilepsy*

CHEWABLE TABLETS, ORAL SUSPENSION, TABLETS
Adults and children age 8 and over. *Initial:* 100 or 125 mg at bedtime for first 3 days; then increased to 100 or 125 mg twice daily for next 3 days, followed by 100 or 125 mg three times a day for next 3 days. On 10th day, begin maintenance dosage as prescribed. *Maintenance:* 250 mg three times a day or four times a day, adjusted as needed. *Maximum:* 2 g daily.
Children up to age 8. *Initial:* 50 mg at bedtime for first 3 days; then increased to 50 mg twice daily for next 3 days, followed by increase to 100 mg twice daily for next 3 days. On 10th day, begin maintenance dosage. *Maintenance:* 125 to 250 mg three times a day, adjusted as needed.

Mechanism of Action

Prevents seizures by decreasing excitability of neurons and increasing motor cortex's threshold of electrical stimulation.

Contraindications

Hypersensitivity to primidone, phenobarbital, or their components; porphyria

Interactions

DRUGS
acetaminophen: Decreased acetaminophen effectiveness, increased risk of hepatotoxicity
adrenocorticoids, chloramphenicol, cyclosporine, dacarbazine, disopyramide, doxycycline, levothyroxine, metronidazole, mexiletine, oral anticoagulants, oral contraceptives (estrogen-containing), quinidine, tricyclic antidepressants: Decreased effectiveness of these drugs
amphetamines: Possibly delayed absorption of primidone
anticonvulsants: Possibly altered pattern of seizures
carbamazepine: Decreased effectiveness of primidone
carbonic anhydrase inhibitors: Increased risk of osteopenia
CNS depressants: Possibly enhanced CNS and respiratory depressant effects of both drugs
cyclophosphamide: Reduced half-life and increased leukopenic activity of cyclophosphamide

enflurane, halothane, methoxyflurane: Increased risk of hepatotoxicity; increased risk of nephrotoxicity (with methoxyflurane)
fenoprofen: Decreased elimination half-life of fenoprofen
folic acid: Increased folic acid requirements
griseofulvin: Decreased antifungal effects of griseofulvin
guanadrel, guanethidine: Possibly aggravated orthostatic hypotension
haloperidol, loxapine, maprotiline, molindone, phenothiazines, thioxanthenes: Possibly lowered seizure threshold and increased CNS depression
leucovorin: Possibly decreased anticonvulsant effects of primidone (with large doses)
MAO inhibitors: Possibly prolonged primidone effects and altered seizure pattern
methylphenidate: Possibly increased blood primidone level, resulting in toxicity
phenobarbital: Increased sedative effects of either drug, possibly altered seizure pattern
phenylbutazone: Decreased primidone effectiveness, increased metabolism and decreased half-life of phenylbutazone
rifampin: Decreased blood primidone level
valproic acid: Increased blood primidone level, leading to increased CNS depression and neurotoxicity; decreased valproic acid half-life and increased hepatotoxicity risk
vitamin D: Decreased effects of vitamin D
xanthines: Increased metabolism and clearance of xanthines (except dyphylline)

ACTIVITIES

alcohol use: Possibly increased CNS and respiratory depressant effects of primidone

Adverse Reactions

CNS: Ataxia, confusion, dizziness, drowsiness, excitement, mental changes, mood changes, restlessness
EENT: Diplopia, nystagmus
GI: Anorexia, nausea, vomiting
GU: Impotence
RESP: Dyspnea
Other: Folic acid deficiency

Nursing Considerations

- Monitor blood levels of primidone and phenobarbital (its active metabolite), as ordered, to determine therapeutic level or detect toxic levels.
- Anticipate that drug may cause confusion, excitement, or mood changes in elderly patients and children.
- Assess for signs of folic acid deficiency: mental dysfunction, neuropathy, tiredness, and weakness.

PATIENT TEACHING

- Instruct patient to crush primidone tablets and mix with food or fluids, as needed.
- Advise patient taking oral suspension to shake bottle well and measure doses with a calibrated device.
- Suggest that patient take drug with meals to minimize adverse GI reactions.
- Urge patient not to stop taking primidone abruptly because doing so can precipitate seizures.
- Caution patient about possible decreased alertness.
- Advise her to avoid hazardous activities until drug's CNS effects are known.
- Urge patient to avoid consuming alcohol and other CNS depressants during primidone therapy.

probenecid

Benemid, Benuryl (CAN), Probalan

Class and Category

Pharmacologic class: Sulfonamide derivative
Therapeutic class: Uricosuric
Pregnancy category: Not classified

Indications and Dosages

➤ *To treat chronic gouty arthritis and hyperuricemia due to chronic gout*

TABLETS

Adults and adolescents. *Initial:* 250 mg twice daily for 1 wk; then increased to maintenance dosage. *Maintenance:* 500 mg twice daily; if not effective or 24-hr uric acid excretion isn't greater than 700 mg, dosage increased by 500 mg/day every 4 wk, as needed, up to a maximum of 3 g daily. If no acute attacks of gout occur over next 6 mo and serum uric acid level is within normal limits, dosage decreased by 500 mg every 6 mo until lowest effective maintenance dose is reached. *Maximum:* 3 g daily.

DOSAGE ADJUSTMENT Dosage possibly increased for patients with mild renal dysfunction, except for elderly patients, who require a dosage reduction.

➤ *As adjunct to antibiotic therapy with penicillins and some cephalosporins*

TABLETS

Adults, adolescents age 14 and over, and children weighing more than 50 kg (110 lb). 500 mg four times a day; if given with I.V. or I.M. antibiotic, administer at least 30 min before antibiotic.

Children ages 2 to 14 weighing up to 50 kg. 25 mg/kg as single dose, then 10 mg/kg four times a day; if given with I.V. or I.M. antibiotic, give at least 30 min before antibiotic.

➤ *As adjunct to treat sexually transmitted diseases*

TABLETS

Adults and adolescents. 1 g as single dose, given with appropriate antibiotic.

➤ *As adjunct to treat pediatric gonorrhea*

TABLETS

Postpubertal children and children weighing more than 45 kg (99 lb). 1 g as single dose, given with appropriate antibiotic.

➤ *As adjunct to treat neurosyphilis*

TABLETS

Adults and adolescents. 500 mg four times a day with 1 daily dose (2.4 million units) of penicillin G procaine for 10 to 14 days.

Route	Onset	Peak	Duration
P.O.	Unknown	30 min*	8 hr†

* For renal clearance of uric acid; 2 hr for effect on blood antibiotic level.

† For effect on blood antibiotic level; unknown for renal clearance of uric acid.

Mechanism of Action

Increases urinary excretion of uric acid and lowers serum uric acid level, which may prevent or resolve urate deposits, tophus formation, and joint changes. Eventually, incidence of acute gout attacks decreases. Probenecid also inhibits renal excretion of penicillins and some cephalosporins, thereby increasing their serum concentration and prolonging their duration of action.

Contraindications

Age less than 2 years, blood dyscrasias, hypersensitivity to probenecid or its components, renal calculi (urate)

Interactions

DRUGS

acyclovir: Decreased renal tubular secretion of acyclovir

allopurinol: Additive antihyperuricemic effects

aminosalicylate sodium, cephalosporins, ciprofloxacin, clofibrate, dapsone, ganciclovir, imipenem, methotrexate, nitrofurantoin, norfloxacin, penicillins: Increased and possibly prolonged blood levels of these drugs, increased risk of toxicity

antineoplastics (rapidly cytolytic): Possibly uric acid nephropathy

diazoxide, mecamylamine, pyrazinamide: Increased risk of hyperuricemia, decreased probenecid effectiveness

dyphylline: Increased half-life of dyphylline

furosemide: Increased blood furosemide level

heparin: Increased and prolonged anticoagulant effect

indomethacin, ketoprofen, other NSAIDs: Possibly increased adverse effects

lorazepam, oxazepam, temazepam: Increased effects of these drugs, possibly excessive sedation

riboflavin: Decreased GI absorption of riboflavin

rifampin, sulfonamides: Increased blood levels of these drugs and, possibly, toxicity

salicylates: Decreased uricosuric effects of probenecid

sodium benzoate and sodium phenylacetate: Decreased renal elimination of these drugs

sulfonylureas: Increased sulfonylurea half-life

thiopental: Prolonged thiopental effect

zidovudine: Increased risk of zidovudine toxicity

ACTIVITIES

alcohol use: Increased risk of hyperuricemia, decreased probenecid effectiveness

Adverse Reactions

CNS: Dizziness, headache

EENT: Sore gums

GI: Anorexia, nausea, vomiting

P

GU: Hematuria, renal calculi (urate), renal colic, urinary frequency
MS: Costovertebral pain; joint pain, redness, and swelling
SKIN: Facial flushing, pruritus, rash, urticaria

Nursing Considerations

- Be aware that probenecid therapy shouldn't start until acute gout attack has subsided. If acute attack starts during therapy, continue therapy as prescribed.
- Use drug cautiously in patients with peptic ulcer disease.
- Expect to give sodium bicarbonate (3 to 7.5 g daily) or potassium citrate (7.5 g daily), as prescribed, to keep urine alkaline and prevent renal calculus formation.
- Monitor CBC, serum uric acid level, and liver and renal function test results during therapy.
- Closely monitor patients receiving intermittent therapy because they're more likely to develop allergic reactions.
- Check blood glucose level often in diabetic patient who takes a sulfonylurea because of the risk of drug interactions.

PATIENT TEACHING

- Advise patient to take probenecid with meals to minimize GI distress.
- Encourage patient to increase fluid intake (up to 3 L daily, if not contraindicated) to help prevent renal calculus formation.
- Instruct patient to notify prescriber immediately if she has signs of an acute gout attack (joint pain, swelling, and redness) or of renal calculi (flank pain and blood in urine).
- Caution patient against taking salicylates while taking probenecid. Instead, advise acetaminophen to treat mild pain or fever.

procainamide hydrochloride

Procan SR, Promine, Pronestyl, Pronestyl-SR

Class and Category

Pharmacologic class: Sodium channel blocker of cardiomyocytes
Therapeutic class: Antiarrhythmic (Class 1a)
Pregnancy category: C

Indications and Dosages

➤ *To treat life-threatening ventricular arrhythmias*

CAPSULES, TABLETS

Adults. 50 mg/kg daily in 8 divided doses (every 3 hr), adjusted as needed and tolerated. *Maximum:* 6 g daily (maintenance).
Children. 12.5 mg/kg four times a day.

E.R. TABLETS

Adults. *Maintenance:* 50 mg/kg daily in divided doses four times a day (every 6 hr), adjusted as needed and tolerated. *Maximum:* 6 g daily (maintenance).

I.V. INFUSION OR INJECTION

Adults. *Initial:* 100 mg diluted in D_5W and given at no more than 50 mg/min. Repeated every 5 min until arrhythmia is controlled or maximum total dose of 1 g is reached. Or, 10 to 15 mg/kg I.V. bolus given at 25 to 50 mg/min. *Maintenance:* 1 to 4 mg/min by continuous infusion.

I.M. INJECTION

Adults. 50 mg/kg daily in divided doses every 3 to 6 hr.

➤ *To treat ventricular extrasystoles and arrhythmias associated with anesthesia and surgery*

I.V. INFUSION OR INJECTION

Adults. *Initial:* 100 mg diluted in D_5W and given at no more than 50 mg/min. Dosage repeated every 5 min until arrhythmia is controlled or maximum total dose of 1 g is reached. Or, 10 to 15 mg/kg I.V. bolus given at 25 to 50 mg/min. *Maintenance:* 1 to 4 mg/min by continuous infusion.

I.M. INJECTION

Adults. 100 to 500 mg every 3 to 6 hr.

DOSAGE ADJUSTMENT For elderly patients or those with cardiac or hepatic insufficiency, dosage possibly reduced or dosing intervals increased. For patients with creatinine clearance less than 50 ml/min/1.73 m^2, initial dosage reduced to 1 to 2 mg/min.

Route	Onset	Peak	Duration
P.O.	Unknown	Unknown	60–90 min
P.O. (E.R.)	Unknown	60–90 min	Unknown
I.V.	Unknown	Immediate	Unknown
I.M.	10–30 min	15–60 min	Unknown

Mechanism of Action

Prolongs recovery period after myocardial repolarization by inhibiting sodium influx through myocardial cell membranes. This action prolongs refractory period, causing myocardial automaticity, excitability, and conduction velocity to decline.

Contraindications

Complete heart block, concurrent therapy with a CYP2D6 inhibitor and hypersensitivity to procainamide or its components, systemic lupus erythematosus, torsades de pointes

Interactions

DRUGS

antiarrhythmics: Additive cardiac effects
anticholinergics, antidyskinetics, antihistamines: Possibly intensified atropine-like adverse effects, increased risk of ileus
antihypertensives: Additive hypotensive effects
antimyasthenics: Possibly antagonized effect of antimyasthenic on skeletal muscle
bethanechol: Possibly antagonized cholinergic effect of bethanechol
bone marrow depressants: Possibly increased leukopenic or thrombocytopenic effects
bretylium: Possibly decreased inotropic effect of bretylium and enhanced hypotension
neuromuscular blockers: Possibly increased or prolonged neuromuscular blockade
pimozide: Possibly prolonged QT interval, leading to life-threatening arrhythmias

Adverse Reactions

CNS: Chills, disorientation, dizziness, light-headedness
CV: Heart block (second-degree), hypotension, pericarditis, prolonged QT interval, tachycardia
EENT: Bitter taste
GI: Abdominal distress, anorexia, diarrhea, nausea, vomiting
HEME: Agranulocytosis, neutropenia, thrombocytopenia
MS: Arthralgia, myalgia
RESP: Pleural effusion
SKIN: Pruritus, rash
Other: Drug-induced fever

Nursing Considerations

- Place patient in a supine position before giving procainamide I.M. or I.V. to minimize hypotensive effects. Monitor blood pressure often and ECG tracings continuously during administration and for 30 minutes afterward.
- Inspect parenteral solution for particles and discoloration before giving drug; discard if particles are present or solution is darker than light amber.
- When possible, give drug by I.V. infusion or injection, as prescribed, rather than by I.M. injection.
- If drug is to be given I.M. and patient's platelet count is below $50,000/mm^3$, notify prescriber at once because patient may develop bleeding, bruising, or hematomas from procainamide-induced bone marrow suppression and thrombocytopenia. Expect to give procainamide I.V.
- For I.V. injection, dilute procainamide with D_5W according to manufacturer's instructions before administration.
- For I.V. infusion, dilute 200 to 1,000 mg of procainamide to a concentration of 2 or 4 mg/ml using 50 to 500 ml of D_5W.
- Administer I.V. infusion with an infusion pump or other controlled-delivery device.
- Don't exceed 500 mg in 30 minutes by I.V. infusion or 50 mg/min by I.V. injection because heart block or cardiac arrest may occur.
- Anticipate that patient has reached maximum clinical response when ventricular tachycardia resolves, hypotension develops, or QRS complex is 50% wider than original width.
- Expect to give first oral dose 3 to 4 hours after last I.V. dose.

PATIENT TEACHING

- Instruct patient to swallow E.R. procainamide tablets whole, without breaking, crushing, or chewing them.
- If patient has trouble swallowing, tell her to crush regular-release tablets or open capsules and mix contents with food or fluid.
- Instruct patient to take drug 1 hour before or 2 hours after meals with a full glass of water. Inform her that she may take drug with food if GI irritation develops.

- Urge patient to obtain needed dental work before therapy starts or after blood count returns to normal because drug can cause myelosuppression and increased risk of bleeding and infection. Encourage good oral hygiene during therapy, and urge patient to consult prescriber before having dental procedures.
- Advise patient to notify prescriber immediately about bruising, chills, diarrhea, fever, or rash.

prochlorperazine

Compazine, Stemetil (CAN)

prochlorperazine edisylate

Compazine

prochlorperazine maleate

Compazine Spansule, Nu-Prochlor (CAN), Stemetil (CAN)

Class and Category

Pharmacologic class: Piperaze phenothiazine
Therapeutic class: Antiemetic
Pregnancy category: Not classified

Indications and Dosages

➤ *To control nausea and vomiting related to surgery*

I.V. INFUSION OR INJECTION (PROCHLORPERAZINE EDISYLATE)

Adults and adolescents. 5 to 10 mg at a rate not to exceed 5 mg/ml 15 to 30 min before anesthesia or during or after surgery, as needed. Dosage repeated once, if necessary. *Maximum:* 10 mg/dose, 40 mg daily.

I.M. INJECTION (PROCHLORPERAZINE EDISYLATE)

Adults and adolescents. 5 to 10 mg 1 to 2 hr before anesthesia or during or after surgery, as needed. Repeated once in 30 min, if needed. *Maximum:* 10 mg/dose, 40 mg daily.

➤ *To control severe nausea and vomiting*

E.R. CAPSULES (PROCHLORPERAZINE MALEATE)

Adults and adolescents. 15 to 30 mg daily in the morning, or 10 mg every 12 hr. *Maximum:* 40 mg daily.

ORAL SOLUTION (PROCHLORPERAZINE EDISYLATE)

Adults and adolescents. 5 to 10 mg three times a day or four times a day. *Maximum:* 40 mg daily.
Children weighing 18 to 39 kg (40 to 86 lb). 2.5 mg three times a day or 5 mg twice daily. *Maximum:* 15 mg daily.
Children weighing 14 to 18 kg (31 to 40 lb). 2.5 mg twice daily or three times a day. *Maximum:* 10 mg daily.
Children weighing 9 to 14 kg (20 to 31 lb). 2.5 mg once or twice daily. *Maximum:* 7.5 mg daily.

TABLETS (PROCHLORPERAZINE MALEATE)

Adults and adolescents. 5 to 10 mg three times a day or four times a day. *Maximum:* 40 mg daily.

I.V. INFUSION OR INJECTION (PROCHLORPERAZINE EDISYLATE)

Adults and adolescents. 2.5 to 10 mg at a rate not to exceed 5 mg/min. *Maximum:* 40 mg daily.

I.M. INJECTION (PROCHLORPERAZINE EDISYLATE)

Adults and adolescents. 5 to 10 mg every 3 to 4 hr, as needed. *Maximum:* 40 mg daily.
Children ages 2 to 12. 132 mcg/kg/dose to maximum of 10 mg on day 1; then increased as needed. *Maximum:* On day 1, 10 mg; thereafter, 25 mg daily for children ages 6 to 12, 20 mg daily for children ages 2 to 6.

SUPPOSITORIES (PROCHLORPERAZINE)

Adults and adolescents. 25 mg twice daily.
Children weighing 18 to 39 kg. 2.5 mg three times a day or 5 mg twice daily. *Maximum:* 15 mg daily.
Children weighing 14 to 18 kg. 2.5 mg twice daily or three times a day. *Maximum:* 10 mg daily.
Children weighing 9 to 14 kg. 2.5 mg once or twice daily. *Maximum:* 7.5 mg daily.

➤ *To manage psychotic disorders, such as schizophrenia*

ORAL SOLUTION (PROCHLORPERAZINE EDISYLATE)

Adults and adolescents. 5 to 10 mg three times a day or four times a day, increased gradually every 2 to 3 days, as needed and tolerated. *Maximum:* 150 mg daily.

Children ages 2 to 12. 2.5 mg twice daily or three times a day. *Maximum:* On day 1, 10 mg for all children; thereafter, 25 mg daily for children ages 6 to 12, 20 mg daily for children ages 2 to 6.

TABLETS (PROCHLORPERAZINE MALEATE)

Adults and adolescents. 5 to 10 mg three times a day or four times a day, increased gradually every 2 to 3 days, as needed and tolerated. *Maximum:* 150 mg daily.

I.M. INJECTION (PROCHLORPERAZINE EDISYLATE)

Adults and adolescents.
Initial: 10 to 20 mg, repeated every 2 to 4 hr, as needed, to bring symptoms under control (usually 3 to 4 doses). *Maintenance:* 10 to 20 mg every 4 to 6 hr. *Maximum:* 200 mg daily.

Children ages 2 to 12. 132 mcg/kg/dose on day 1; then increased as needed. *Maximum:* On day 1, 10 mg for all children; thereafter, 25 mg daily for children ages 6 to 12, 20 mg/day for children ages 2 to 6.

➤ *To treat anxiety short-term*

E.R. CAPSULES (PROCHLORPERAZINE MALEATE)

Adults and adolescents. 15 mg daily in the morning, or 10 mg every 12 hr. *Maximum:* 20 mg/day for no longer than 12 wk.

ORAL SOLUTION, TABLETS (PROCHLORPERAZINE EDISYLATE)

Adults and adolescents. 5 mg three times a day or four times a day. *Maximum:* 20 mg daily for no longer than 12 wk.

I.V. INFUSION OR INJECTION (PROCHLORPERAZINE EDISYLATE)

Adults and adolescents. 2.5 to 10 mg at no more than 5 mg/min. *Maximum:* 40 mg daily.

I.M. INJECTION (PROCHLORPERAZINE EDISYLATE)

Adults and adolescents. 5 to 10 mg every 3 to 4 hr, as needed.

DOSAGE ADJUSTMENT Initial dose usually reduced and subsequent dosage increased more gradually for elderly, emaciated, and debilitated patients.

Route	Onset	Peak	Duration
P.O., I.V., I.M., P.R.	Up to several wk*	Up to 6 mo	Unknown

* For antipsychotic effects; unknown for other indications.

Mechanism of Action

Alleviates psychotic symptoms by blocking dopamine receptors, depressing release of selected hormones, and producing alpha-adrenergic blocking effect in the brain.

Prochlorperazine also alleviates nausea and vomiting by centrally blocking dopamine receptors in the medullary chemoreceptor trigger zone and by peripherally blocking the vagus nerve in the GI tract.

Anticholinergic effects and alpha-adrenergic blockade reduce anxiety by decreasing arousal and filtering internal stimuli to the brain stem reticular activating system.

Incompatibilities

Don't mix prochlorperazine in same syringe with other drugs. Precipitate may form when prochlorperazine edisylate is mixed in same syringe with morphine sulfate.

Contraindications

Age less than 2 years, blood dyscrasias, bone marrow depression, cerebral arteriosclerosis, coma, coronary artery disease, hepatic dysfunction, hypersensitivity to phenothiazines, myeloproliferative disorders, pediatric surgery, severe CNS depression, severe hypertension or hypotension, subcortical brain damage, use of large quantities of CNS depressants, weight less than 9 kg (20 lb)

Interactions

DRUGS

aluminum- or magnesium-containing antacids, antidiarrheals (adsorbent): Possibly inhibited absorption of oral prochlorperazine
amantadine, anticholinergics, antidyskinetics, antihistamines: Possibly intensified anticholinergic adverse effects, increased risk of prochlorperazine-induced hyperpyretic effect
amphetamines: Decreased stimulant effect of amphetamines, decreased antipsychotic effect of prochlorperazine
anticonvulsants: Lowered seizure threshold
antithyroid drugs: Increased risk of agranulocytosis
apomorphine: Possibly decreased emetic response to apomorphine, additive CNS depression

P

appetite suppressants: Possibly antagonized anorectic effect of appetite suppressants (except for phenmetrazine)
astemizole, cisapride, disopyramide, erythromycin, pimozide, probucol, procainamide: Additive QT-interval prolongation, increased risk of ventricular tachycardia
beta blockers: Increased risk of additive hypotensive effects, irreversible retinopathy, arrhythmias, and tardive dyskinesia
bromocriptine: Decreased effectiveness of bromocriptine
CNS depressants: Additive CNS depression
dopamine: Possibly antagonized peripheral vasoconstriction (high doses of dopamine)
ephedrine, epinephrine: Decreased vasopressor effects of these drugs
hepatotoxic drugs: Increased risk of hepatotoxicity
hypotension-producing drugs: Possibly severe hypotension with syncope
levodopa: Inhibited antidyskinetic effect of levodopa
lithium: Reduced absorption of oral prochlorperazine, increased lithium excretion, increased extrapyramidal effects, possibly masking of early symptoms of lithium toxicity
MAO inhibitors, maprotiline, tricyclic antidepressants: Possibly prolonged and intensified anticholinergic and sedative effects, increased antidepressant level, inhibited prochlorperazine metabolism, increased risk of neuroleptic malignant syndrome
mephentermine: Possibly antagonized antipsychotic effect of prochlorperazine and vasopressor effect of mephentermine
metrizamide: Increased risk of seizures
opioid analgesics: Increased risk of CNS and respiratory depression, orthostatic hypotension, severe constipation, urine retention
ototoxic drugs: Possibly masking of some symptoms of ototoxicity, such as dizziness, tinnitus, and vertigo
phenytoin: Possibly inhibited phenytoin metabolism, increased risk of phenytoin toxicity
thiazide diuretics: Possibly potentiated hyponatremia and water intoxication

ACTIVITIES

alcohol use: Additive CNS depression

Adverse Reactions

CNS: Akathisia, altered temperature regulation, dizziness, drowsiness, extrapyramidal reactions (such as dystonia, pseudoparkinsonism, tardive dyskinesia)
CV: **Hypotension**, orthostatic hypotension, tachycardia
EENT: Blurred vision, dry mouth, nasal congestion, ocular changes, pigmentary retinopathy
ENDO: Galactorrhea, gynecomastia
GI: Constipation, epigastric pain, nausea, vomiting
GU: Dysuria, ejaculation disorders, menstrual irregularities, urine retention
SKIN: Decreased sweating, photosensitivity, pruritus, rash
Other: Weight gain

Nursing Considerations

- Prochlorperazine shouldn't be used to treat dementia-related psychosis in the elderly because of increased mortality risk.
- Avoid contact between skin and solution forms of prochlorperazine because contact dermatitis could result.
- Inject I.M. form slowly, deep into upper outer quadrant of buttocks. Keep patient supine for 30 minutes after injection to minimize hypotensive effects.
- Rotate I.M. injection sites to prevent irritation and sterile abscesses.
- Be aware that I.V. form may be given undiluted as injection or diluted in isotonic solution as infusion (mesylate form requires dilution in at least 1 L). Both forms should be given at no more than 5 mg/min.
- Protect prochlorperazine from light.
- Parenteral solution may develop slight yellowing that won't affect potency. Don't use if discoloration is pronounced or precipitate is present.
- Expect antipsychotic effects to occur in 2 to 3 weeks, although range is days to months.

WARNING Monitor closely for numerous adverse reactions that may be serious.

- Adverse effects may occur up to 12 weeks after discontinuation of E.R. capsules.

PATIENT TEACHING

- Instruct patient to take prochlorperazine with food or a full glass of milk or water to minimize GI distress.

- Advise patient to swallow E.R. capsules whole, not to crush or chew them.
- Instruct patient using suppository to refrigerate it for 30 minutes or hold it under running cold water before removing the wrapper if it softens during storage.
- Teach patient correct administration technique for suppository.
- Caution patient on long-term therapy not to stop prochlorperazine abruptly; doing so may lead to such adverse reactions as nausea, vomiting, and trembling.
- Urge patient to avoid alcohol and OTC drugs that may contain CNS depressants.
- Advise patient to rise slowly from lying and sitting positions to minimize effects of orthostatic hypotension.
- Urge patient to avoid hazardous activities because of the risk of drowsiness and impaired judgment and coordination.
- Instruct patient to avoid excessive sun exposure and to wear sunscreen outdoors.
- Urge patient to notify prescriber about involuntary movements and restlessness.
- Explain that adverse effects may occur up to 12 weeks after stopping E.R. capsules.

progestins levonorgestrel

medroxy progesterone acetate

Alti-MPA (CAN), Gen-Medroxy (CAN), Novo-Medrone (CAN), Provera

megestrol acetate

Apo-Megestrol (CAN), Megace, Megace OS (CAN)

norethindrone acetate

Aygestin, Norlutate (CAN)

progesterone

Crinone, Gesterol 50, PMS-Progesterone (CAN), Prometrium

Class and Category

Pharmacologic class: Progesterone hormone
Therapeutic class: Ovarian hormone replacement
Pregnancy category: D (megestrol [tablets], progesterone); X (levonorgestrel, medroxyprogesterone [parenteral], megestrol [parenteral and suspension], norethindrone); NR (medroxyprogesterone [tablets])

Indications and Dosages

➤ *To treat renal cancer*

I.M. INJECTION (MEDROXYPROGESTERONE)
Adults and adolescents. *Initial:* 400 mg to 1 g every wk until improvement and stabilization. *Maintenance:* 400 mg or more every mo.

➤ *To treat breast cancer*

TABLETS (MEGESTROL)
Adults and adolescents. 40 mg four times daily.

➤ *To treat endometrial cancer*

TABLETS (MEGESTROL)
Adult and adolescent women. 40 to 320 mg daily in divided doses.

I.M. INJECTION (MEDROXYPROGESTERONE)
Adults and adolescents. *Initial:* 400 mg to 1 g every wk until improvement and stabilization. *Maintenance:* 400 mg or more every mo.

➤ *To treat anorexia, cachexia, or significant weight loss in patients who have AIDS*

SUSPENSION (MEGESTROL)
Adults and adolescents. 800 mg daily for the first mo, and then 400 or 800 mg daily for the next 3 mo.

➤ *To treat endometriosis*

TABLETS (NORETHINDRONE ACETATE)
Adult and adolescent women. *Initial:* 5 mg daily for 2 wk, increased by 2.5 mg daily at 2-wk intervals to total dose of 15 mg daily. *Maintenance:* 15 mg daily for 6 to 9 mo unless temporarily discontinued because of breakthrough menstrual bleeding.

P

➤ *To treat secondary amenorrhea*
TABLETS (MEDROXYPROGESTERONE)
Adult and adolescent women. 5 to 10 mg daily for 5 to 10 days, starting anytime during menstrual cycle.
TABLETS (NORETHINDRONE ACETATE)
Adult and adolescent women. 2.5 to 10 mg daily for 5 to 10 days during last half of menstrual cycle.
CAPSULES (PROGESTERONE)
Adult and adolescent women. 400 mg daily at bedtime for 10 days.
I.M. INJECTION (PROGESTERONE)
Adult and adolescent women. 5 to 10 mg daily for 6 to 10 days.
VAGINAL GEL (PROGESTERONE)
Adult and adolescent women. 45 mg (1 applicatorful of 4% vaginal gel) every other day for up to 6 doses. Dosage increased, as needed, to 90 mg (1 applicatorful of 8% vaginal gel) every other day for up to 6 doses.
➤ *To treat dysfunctional uterine bleeding*
TABLETS (MEDROXYPROGESTERONE)
Adult and adolescent women. 5 to 10 mg daily for 5 to 10 days, starting on day 16 or 21 of menstrual cycle.
TABLETS (NORETHINDRONE ACETATE)
Adult and adolescent women. 2.5 to 10 mg daily for 5 to 10 days during last half of menstrual cycle.
I.M. INJECTION (PROGESTERONE)
Adult and adolescent women. 5 to 10 mg daily for 6 consecutive days.
➤ *To induce menses*
TABLETS (MEDROXYPROGESTERONE)
Adult and adolescent women. 10 mg daily for 10 days, starting on day 16 of menstrual cycle. Repeated for 2 or more cycles if bleeding is satisfactorily controlled.
➤ *To prevent pregnancy (postcoital)*
TABLETS (LEVONORGESTREL)
Adult and adolescent women. 0.75 mg as soon as possible within 72 hr of intercourse. Second dose given 12 hr later.

Mechanism of Action

Progestins may diminish response to endogenous hormones in tumor cells by decreasing the number of steroid hormone receptors, causing a direct antiproliferative or cytotoxic effect on cell cycle growth and increased terminal cell differentiation. At higher doses, some progestins decrease adrenal production of androstenedione and estradiol, which may decrease estrogen- or testosterone-sensitive tumors. Megestrol stimulates appetite and metabolic effects, which promotes weight gain. Progestins also bind to cytosolic receptors that are loosely bound in cell nucleus, increasing protein synthesis and improving cachexia.

Progestins affect other hormones, especially estrogen, by reducing availability or stability of hormone receptor complex, shutting off estrogen-responsive genes, or causing negative feedback mechanism that decreases number of functioning estrogen receptors. These actions allow menstrual cycle to function normally, alleviating amenorrhea and dysfunctional uterine bleeding and inducing menses. Progestins also act to transform proliferative uterine endometrium into a more differentiated, secretory one, which is the basis for using medroxyprogesterone to treat some types of amenorrhea. In a normal ovulatory cycle not resulting in pregnancy, decline in progesterone secretion caused by degeneration of corpus luteum in late luteal phase results in endometrial sloughing. A similar sloughing occurs after 5 to 10 days of medroxyprogesterone, provided that adequate estrogen-stimulated proliferation has occurred during follicular phase.

The progestin, levonorgestrel, also inhibits secretion of gonadotropins from pituitary gland, which creates an atrophic endometrium, resulting in contraceptive effect.

Contraindications

Active thromboembolic disorder; thrombophlebitis; significant hepatic disease; hypersensitivity to peanuts or sesame oil/seeds (progesterone), progestins, or their components; known or suspected breast cancer; pregnancy; undiagnosed genital, uterine, or urinary tract bleeding

Interactions

DRUGS
aminoglutethimide: Possibly decreased blood level of medroxyprogesterone
atazanavir, clarithromycin, indinavir, itraconazole, ketoconazole, nefazodone, nelfinavir, ritonavir, saquinavir, telithromycin, voriconazole: Possibly

increased progestin level leading to potential for increased adverse reactions
carbamazepine, phenobarbital, phenytoin, rifabutin, rifampin, rifapentine, St. John's wort: Possibly decreased effectiveness of progestin
thyroid hormone: Decreased thyroid hormone effectiveness

Adverse Reactions

CNS: Altered or reduced coordination or speech, depression, dizziness, drowsiness, fatigue, headache, irritability, migraine, mood changes, nervousness, postmenopausal dementia, syncope, unusual tiredness or weakness
CV: Fluid retention; **hypotension**; numbness or pain in arm, chest, or leg; **thromboembolism**
ENDO: Adrenal insufficiency or suppression, breast pain or tenderness, Cushing's syndrome, decreased T_3 resin uptake, delayed return of fertility in women, elevated thyroid-binding globulin, galactorrhea, hyperglycemia
EENT: Gingival bleeding, swelling, or tenderness; vision changes or loss
GI: Abdominal cramps or pain, cholestatic jaundice, diarrhea, nausea, vomiting
GU: Amenorrhea, breakthrough bleeding or metromenorrhagia, changes in cervical erosion and secretions, decreased libido, hypermenorrhea, ovarian enlargement or cysts
HEME: Clotting and bleeding abnormalities
MS: Back pain, decreased bone density, osteoporosis, osteoporotic fractures
RESP: Acute eosinophilic pneumonia (progesterone in sesame oil), dyspnea
SKIN: Acne, alopecia, dermal edema, hirsutism, melasma, pruritus, rash, urticaria
Other: Anaphylaxis; **angioedema**; hot flashes; injection-site irritation, pain, or redness; weight gain or loss

Nursing Considerations

- Be aware that progestin/estrogen therapy shouldn't be used to prevent cardiovascular disease or dementia.
- Use progestins cautiously in patients with risk factors for arterial vascular disease, such as diabetes mellitus, hypercholesterolemia, hypertension, obesity, systemic lupus erythematosus, tobacco use, or a family or personal history of venous thromboembolism. Drug worsen these conditions.
- Use progestins cautiously in patients who have CNS disorders, such as depression or seizures, because progestins may worsen these conditions.
- Shake container vigorously for at least 1 minute before giving medroxyprogesterone acetate injection suspension or megestrol acetate oral suspension.
- Inject parenteral medroxyprogesterone slowly, over 5 to 7 seconds, into deltoid muscle. Don't inject into gluteal muscle to lessen absorption problems that may occur when patient sits on injection site. Pat site lightly after injection; don't rub it.

WARNING Notify prescriber immediately if patient develops signs of thrombotic events. Expect to discontinue progestin if such signs occur and provide emergency care, as ordered.

- Monitor patient for adrenal suppression, especially with megestrol therapy. If suspected, notify prescriber.
- Expect to stop progestin therapy in any woman who develops evidence of cancer; cardiovascular disease such as CVA, MI, pulmonary embolism, or venous thrombosis; or dementia.
- Be aware that acute eosinophilic pneumonia may occur in patients receiving progesterone in sesame oil. Monitor patient for dyspnea with hypoxic respiratory insufficiency and fever that may occur 2 to 4 weeks after patient starts progesterone in sesame oil therapy. If this reaction is suspected, notify prescriber and expect drug to be discontinued immediately.

PATIENT TEACHING

- Explain risks of progestin therapy, including breast, endometrial, or ovarian cancer; cardiovascular disease; dementia; and gallbladder disease, especially in postmenopausal women.
- Instruct woman to notify prescriber if uterine bleeding continues longer than 3 months or if menstruation is delayed by 45 days.

- Warn patient taking progestin for noncontraceptive purposes to use a contraceptive method to prevent pregnancy because drug may harm fetus.
- Advise female patient to contact prescriber immediately if she suspects pregnancy or misses a menstrual period.
- Advise patient that some products may contain peanut oil or sesame oil. If she is allergic to these, tell her to contact pharmacist to find out if prescribed progestin product contains peanut or sesame oil. Also tell patient to report difficulty breathing and fever to prescriber.
- Caution female patient who vomits within 1 hour of taking progestin for emergency contraception to contact prescriber about whether to repeat dose.
- Teach woman how to use vaginal gel, if prescribed. Tell her to avoid using other vaginal products for 6 hours before and after to ensure gel's complete absorption.
- Direct patient to alert all prescribers about progestin therapy because certain blood tests may be affected.
- Emphasize importance of good dental hygiene and regular dental checkups because elevated progestin level increases growth of normal oral flora, which may lead to gum tenderness, bleeding, or swelling.
- Caution postmenopausal women about increased risk of dementia associated with progestin therapy.

promethazine hydrochloride

Anergan 25, Anergan 50, Antinaus 50, Histantil (CAN), Pentazine, Phenazine 25, Phenazine 50, Phencen-50, Phenerzine, Phenoject-50, Pro-50, Promacot, Pro-Med 50, Promet, Prorex-25, Prorex-50, Prothazine, Shogan, V-Gan-25, V-Gan-50

Class and Category

Pharmacologic class: Phenothiazine
Therapeutic class: Antiemetic, antihistamine, antivertigo, sedative-hypnotic
Pregnancy category: C

Indications and Dosages

➤ *To prevent or treat motion sickness*

SYRUP, TABLETS

Adults and adolescents. 25 mg 30 to 60 min before travel and repeated 8 to 12 hr later, if needed. *Maximum:* 150 mg daily.

➤ *To treat vertigo*

SYRUP, TABLETS

Adults and adolescents. 25 mg twice daily, as needed. *Maximum:* 150 mg daily.
Children age 2 and over. 0.5 mg/kg or 10 to 25 mg every 12 hr, as needed.

SUPPOSITORIES

Adults and adolescents. 25 mg twice daily, as needed. *Maximum:* 150 mg daily.
Children age 2 and over. 0.5 mg/kg or 12.5 to 25 mg every 12 hr.

➤ *To prevent or treat nausea and vomiting in certain types of anesthesia and surgery*

SYRUP, TABLETS

Adults and adolescents. *Initial:* 25 mg; then 10 to 25 mg every 4 to 6 hr, as needed. *Maximum:* 150 mg daily.
Children age 2 and over. 0.25 to 0.5 mg/kg or 10 to 25 mg every 4 to 6 hr, as needed.

I.V. OR I.M. INJECTION

Adults and adolescents. 12.5 to 25 mg every 4 hr, as needed. *Maximum:* 150 mg daily. I.V. injection given slowly over 10 to 15 min.

I.M. INJECTION

Children age 2 and over. 0.25 to 0.5 mg/kg or 12.5 to 25 mg every 4 to 6 hr, as needed.

SUPPOSITORIES

Adults and adolescents. *Initial:* 25 mg; then 12.5 to 25 mg every 4 to 6 hr, as needed. *Maximum:* 150 mg daily.
Children age 2 and over. 0.25 to 0.5 mg/kg or 12.5 to 25 mg every 4 to 6 hr.

➤ *To treat signs and symptoms of allergic response*

SYRUP, TABLETS

Adults and adolescents. 10 to 12.5 mg four times a day before meals and at bedtime, as needed. Or, 25 mg at bedtime, as needed. *Maximum:* 150 mg daily.
Children age 2 and over. 0.125 mg/kg every 4 to 6 hr or 5 to 12.5 mg three times a

day, as needed. Or, 0.5 mg/kg or 25 mg at bedtime, as needed.

I.V. INJECTION

Adults and adolescents. 25 mg given slowly over 10 to 15 min, repeated within 2 hr, as needed.

I.M. INJECTION, SUPPOSITORIES

Adults and adolescents. 25 mg, repeated in 2 hr, as needed. *Maximum:* 150 mg daily.
Children age 2 and over. 0.125 mg/kg every 4 to 6 hr or 6.25 to 12.5 mg three times a day, as needed. Or, 0.5 mg/kg or 25 mg at bedtime, as needed.

➤ *To provide nighttime, preoperative, or postoperative sedation*

SYRUP, TABLETS

Adults and adolescents. 25 to 50 mg as a single dose. *Maximum:* 150 mg daily.
Children age 2 and over. 0.5 to 1 mg/kg or 10 to 25 mg as a single dose. Or, for preoperative sedation, 1.1 mg/kg along with 1.1 mg/kg of meperidine and appropriate dose of an atropine-like drug.

I.V. INJECTION

Adults and adolescents. 25 to 50 mg given slowly over 10 to 15 min as a single dose. Or, for preoperative and postoperative sedation, 25 to 50 mg combined with appropriately reduced dosages of analgesics and anticholinergics.

I.M. INJECTION, SUPPOSITORIES

Adults and adolescents. 25 to 50 mg as a single dose. Or, for preoperative and postoperative sedation, 25 to 50 mg combined with appropriately reduced dosages of analgesics and anticholinergics.
Children age 2 and over. 0.5 to 1 mg/kg or 12.5 to 25 mg as a single dose. Or, for preoperative sedation, 1.1 mg/kg along with 1.1 mg/kg of meperidine and an appropriate dose of an atropine-like drug.

➤ *To relieve apprehension and promote sleep the night before surgery*

SYRUP, TABLETS, SUPPOSITORIES

Adults and adolescents. 50 mg along with 50 mg of meperidine and an appropriate dose of an atropine-like drug at bedtime on the night before surgery.

DOSAGE ADJUSTMENT Dosage usually decreased for elderly patients.

➤ *To provide obstetric sedation*

I.V. OR I.M. INJECTION

Adults and adolescents. 50 mg for early stages of labor, followed by 1 or 2 doses of 25 to 75 mg after labor is established, repeated every 4 hr during normal labor. I.V. injection given slowly over 10 to 15 min.

Route	Onset	Peak	Duration
P.O.	15–60 min	Unknown	4–6 hr
I.V.	3–5 min	Unknown	4–6 hr
I.M., P.R.	20 min	Unknown	4–6 hr

Mechanism of Action

Competes with histamine for H_1-receptor sites, thereby antagonizing many histamine effects and reducing allergy signs and symptoms. Promethazine also prevents motion sickness, nausea, and vertigo by acting centrally on medullary chemoreceptive trigger zone and by decreasing vestibular stimulation and labyrinthine function in the inner ear. It also promotes sedation and relieves anxiety by blocking receptor sites in CNS, directly reducing stimuli to the brain.

Contraindications

Angle-closure glaucoma; benign prostatic hyperplasia; bladder neck obstruction; bone marrow depression; breastfeeding; children under age 2; coma; hypersensitivity or history of idiosyncratic reaction to promethazine, other phenothiazines, or their components; hypertensive crisis; lower respiratory tract disorders (including asthma) when used as an antihistamine; pyloroduodenal obstruction; stenosing peptic ulcer; use of large quantities of CNS depressants

Interactions

DRUGS

amphetamines: Decreased stimulant effect of amphetamines
anticholinergics: Possibly intensified anticholinergic adverse effects
anticonvulsants: Lowered seizure threshold
appetite suppressants: Possibly antagonized anorectic effect of appetite suppressants
beta blockers: Increased risk of additive hypotensive effects, irreversible retinopathy, arrhythmias, and tardive dyskinesia
bromocriptine: Decreased effectiveness of bromocriptine
CNS depressants: Additive CNS depression
dopamine: Possibly antagonized peripheral vasoconstriction (high doses of dopamine)

ephedrine, metaraminol, methoxamine: Decreased vasopressor response to these drugs
epinephrine: Blocked alpha-adrenergic effects of epinephrine, increased risk of hypotension
guanadrel, guanethidine: Decreased antihypertensive effects of these drugs
hepatotoxic drugs: Increased risk of hepatotoxicity
hypotension-producing drugs: Possibly severe hypotension with syncope
levodopa: Inhibited antidyskinetic effects of levodopa
MAO inhibitors: Possibly prolonged and intensified anticholinergic and CNS depressant effects of promethazine
metrizamide: Increased risk of seizures
ototoxic drugs: Possibly masking of some symptoms of ototoxicity, such as dizziness, tinnitus, and vertigo
quinidine: Additive cardiac effects
riboflavin: Increased riboflavin requirement

ACTIVITIES

alcohol use: Additive CNS depression

Adverse Reactions

CNS: Akathisia, CNS stimulation, confusion, dizziness, drowsiness, dystonia, euphoria, excitation, fatigue, hallucinations, hysteria, incoordination, insomnia, irritability, nervousness, **neuroleptic malignant syndrome**, paradoxical stimulation, pseudoparkinsonism, restlessness, sedation, **seizures**, syncope, tardive dyskinesia, tremor
CV: Bradycardia, hypertension, **hypotension**, tachycardia
EENT: Blurred vision; diplopia; dry mouth, nose, and throat; nasal congestion; tinnitus; vision changes
ENDO: Hyperglycemia
GI: Anorexia, cholestatic jaundice, ileus, nausea, rectal burning or stinging (suppository form), vomiting
GU: Dysuria
HEME: Agranulocytosis, **leukopenia**, **thrombocytopenia**, **thrombocytopenic purpura**
RESP: Apnea, **respiratory depression**, tenacious bronchial secretions
SKIN: Dermatitis, diaphoresis, jaundice, photosensitivity, rash, urticaria
Other: Angioedema, paradoxical reactions

Nursing Considerations

- Use promethazine cautiously in children and elderly patients because they may be more sensitive to its effects, patients with cardiovascular disease or hepatic dysfunction because of potential adverse effects, patients with asthma because of anticholinergic effects, and patients with seizure disorders or those who take drugs that may affect seizure threshold because drug may lower seizure threshold.
- Inject I.M. form deep into large muscle mass, and rotate sites.

WARNING Avoid inadvertent intra-arterial injection of promethazine because it can cause arteriospasm. Also avoid injecting drug under skin; severe tissue damage and gangrene may develop from impaired circulation.

- Give I.V. injection at no more than 25 mg/min; rapid I.V. administration may produce a transient drop in blood pressure.

WARNING Monitor respiratory function because drug may suppress cough reflex and cause thickening of bronchial secretions, aggravating such conditions as asthma and COPD. Rarely, it may depress respirations and induce apnea.

- Monitor patient's hematologic status as ordered because promethazine may cause bone marrow depression, especially when used with other known marrow-toxic agents. Assess patient for signs and symptoms of infection or bleeding.

WARNING Monitor patient for evidence of neuroleptic malignant syndrome, such as fever, hypertension or hypotension, involuntary motor activity, mental changes, muscle rigidity, tachycardia, and tachypnea. Be prepared to provide supportive treatment and drug therapy, as prescribed.

- Be aware that patient shouldn't have intradermal allergen tests within 72 hours of receiving promethazine because drug may significantly alter flare response.

PATIENT TEACHING

- Tell patient to use a calibrated device to ensure accurate doses of promethazine syrup.
- Teach patient correct administration technique for suppository, if needed.
- Advise patient to avoid OTC drugs unless approved by prescriber.

- Instruct patient to notify prescriber immediately if she has involuntary movements and restlessness.
- Urge patient to avoid alcohol and other CNS depressants during therapy.
- Instruct patient to avoid hazardous activities until drug's CNS effects are known.
- Suggest rinsing and use of sugarless gum or hard candy to relieve dry mouth.
- Urge patient to avoid excessive sun exposure and to use sunscreen when outdoors.

propafenone hydrochloride

Rythmol, Rythmol SR

Class and Category

Pharmacologic class: Sodium channel antagonist
Therapeutic class: Class IC antiarrhythmic
Pregnancy category: C

Indications and Dosages

➤ *To treat life-threatening ventricular arrhythmias*

TABLETS

Adults. *Initial:* 150 mg every 8 hr; after 3 or 4 days, increased to 225 mg every 8 hr (U.S.) or 300 mg every 12 hr (Canada), as needed; after an additional 3 or 4 days, further increased to 300 mg every 8 hr, as needed. *Maximum:* 900 mg daily.

➤ *To prolong time of recurrence of symptomatic atrial fibrillation in patients with episodic atrial fibrillation who do not have structural heart disease*

E.R. CAPSULES

Adults. *Initial:* 225 mg every 12 hr, increased after 5 or more days to 325 mg every 12 hr, as needed, and further increased to 425 mg every 12 hr, as needed.

DOSAGE ADJUSTMENT For patient with hepatic impairment, dosage may have to be reduced.

Mechanism of Action

Prolongs recovery period after myocardial repolarization by inhibiting sodium influx through myocardial cell membranes. This action prolongs the refractory period, causing myocardial automaticity, excitability, and conduction velocity to decline.

Contraindications

Bronchospastic disorders, such as asthma; Brugada syndrome; cardiogenic shock; concurrent use of both a CYP2D6 inhibitor and a CYP3A4 inhibitor (Rythmol SR); electrolyte imbalances; heart failure (uncontrolled); hypersensitivity to propafenone or its components; severe hypotension or obstructive pulmonary disease; sinus bradycardia or AV conduction disturbances (without artificial pacemaker)

Interactions

DRUGS

amiodarone: Possibly altered cardiac conduction and repolarization; possibly increased blood propafenone level
anesthetics (local): Increased risk of adverse CNS effects
antiarrhythmics, fluoxetine: Increased propafenone level and adverse CV effects
cimetidine, erythromycin, ketoconazole, paroxetine, ritonavir, saquinavir, sertraline: Possibly increased blood propafenone level
class IA and class III antiarrhythmics, oral macrolides, phenothiazines, tricyclic antidepressants: Possibly increased risk of prolonged QT interval
CYP2D6 inhibitors and CYP3A4 inhibitors combined: Significantly increased concentration of propafenone, increasing risk of proarrhythmias and other adverse reactions
desipramine: Possibly increased blood level of desipramine or propafenone
digoxin: Increased risk of digitalis toxicity
haloperidol, imipramine, venlafaxine: Possibly increased levels of these drugs
metoprolol, propranolol: Increased blood level and half-life of these drugs
orlistat: Possibly decreased absorption of propafenone
quinidine: Decreased propafenone metabolism
rifampin: Possibly decreased propafenone level
warfarin: Increased blood warfarin level and risk of bleeding

FOODS

grapefruit juice: Possibly increased blood propafenone level

Adverse Reactions

CNS: Anxiety, depression, dizziness, fatigue, headache, somnolence, tremor, weakness
CV: Angina, **atrial flutter**, **AV block**, **bradycardia**, chest pain, edema, **heart failure**, **hypotension**, **irregular heartbeat**, palpitations, **prolonged QT interval**, tachycardia, **ventricular arrhythmias**, **worsened supraventricular arrhythmias**
EENT: Altered taste, blurred vision, dry mouth
GI: Constipation, diarrhea, flatulence, nausea, vomiting
GU: Decreased sperm count, hematuria
HEME: **Agranulocytosis**
MS: Muscle weakness
RESP: Dyspnea, rales, upper respiratory tract infection, wheezes
SKIN: Ecchymosis, rash
Other: Elevated blood alkaline phosphatase, exacerbation of myasthenia gravis, flu-like symptoms, positive ANA titers

Nursing Considerations

- Assess patient for electrolyte imbalances, such as hyperkalemia, before starting propafenone or any antiarrhythmic to reduce risk of adverse cardiac reactions.
- Use propafenone cautiously in patients with heart failure or myocardial dysfunction because beta-blocking activity may further depress myocardial contractility.
- Use cautiously in patients with renal impairment because about 50% of the drug's metabolites are excreted in the urine, increasing risk of propafenone overdose.
- Monitor ECG tracings, blood pressure, and pulse rate, particularly at start of therapy and with dosage increases. Expect propafenone to be discontinued if Brugada syndrome is confirmed with ECG changes.
- Monitor patient for signs of infection such as fever, sore throat, or chills because propafenone may cause agranulocytosis, particularly during the initial 3 months of therapy. If present, notify prescriber.

PATIENT TEACHING

- Instruct patient to take a missed dose if she remembers within 4 hours; otherwise, tell her to skip missed dose and to resume the regular dosing schedule.
- Advise patient not to stop propafenone or change dosage without asking prescriber.
- Urge patient to carry medical identification showing she that takes propafenone.
- Advise patient to avoid hazardous activities until drug's CNS effects are known.
- Urge patient to increase fluid intake and dietary fiber if she becomes constipated.
- Explain that drug may cause an unusual taste. Advise patient to notify prescriber if taste interferes with compliance.
- Tell patient to notify prescriber promptly of any signs of infection such as fever, sore throat, or chills.

propantheline bromide

Pro-Banthine, Propanthel (CAN)

Class and Category

Pharmacologic class: Anticholinergic
Therapeutic class: Antiulcer
Pregnancy category: C

Indications and Dosages

➤ *As adjunct to treat peptic ulcer disease*

TABLETS

Adults. 15 mg three times a day before meals and 30 mg at bedtime, adjusted as needed and tolerated. *Maximum:* 120 mg daily.
Children. 0.375 mg/kg four times a day, adjusted as needed and tolerated.
DOSAGE ADJUSTMENT For elderly patients with mild symptoms or patients of below-average weight, dosage possibly reduced to 7.5 mg three times a day or four times a day.

Route	Onset	Peak	Duration
P.O.	Unknown	Unknown	6 hr

Mechanism of Action

Prevents the neurotransmitter acetylcholine from combining with receptors on postganglionic parasympathetic nerve terminal, thereby reducing smooth-muscle spasms in the GI system, slowing GI motility, and inhibiting gastric acid secretion. All these effects help to heal peptic ulcers.

Contraindications

Adhesions between iris and lens, angle-closure glaucoma, hemorrhage accompanied by hemodynamic instability, hepatic dysfunction, hypersensitivity to propantheline or its components, ileus, myasthenia gravis, myocardial ischemia, obstructive GI or urinary disease, renal dysfunction, severe ulcerative colitis, tachycardia

Interactions

DRUGS

amantadine, other anticholinergics, tricyclic antidepressants: Additive anticholinergic effects
antacids, antidiarrheals (adsorbent): Possibly reduced absorption of propantheline
antimyasthenics: Possibly further reduction in intestinal motility
atenolol: Increased effects of atenolol
cyclopropane: Possibly ventricular arrhythmias
digoxin: Possibly digitalis toxicity
haloperidol: Decreased antipsychotic effect of haloperidol in schizophrenic patients
ketoconazole: Decreased ketoconazole absorption
metoclopramide: Possibly decreased metoclopramide effect on GI motility
opioid analgesics: Increased risk of severe constipation and urine retention
phenothiazines: Possibly decreased antipsychotic effects
potassium chloride: Possibly increased severity of potassium chloride–induced GI ulceration, stricture, or perforation
urinary alkalizers: Delayed urinary excretion of propantheline

Adverse Reactions

CNS: Dizziness, excitement, insomnia, nervousness, paradoxical CNS stimulation
CV: Palpitations, tachycardia
EENT: Blurred vision; dry mouth, nose, and throat
GI: Constipation, dysphagia, heartburn, ileus, nausea, vomiting
GU: Impotence, urinary hesitancy, urine retention
SKIN: Decreased sweating, dry skin, flushing

Nursing Considerations

- Don't administer propantheline within 1 hour of antacids or antidiarrheals.
- Monitor elderly patients closely; they may respond to usual dose with agitation, confusion, drowsiness, or excitement.

WARNING Drug can interfere with sweating reflex, increasing the risk of heatstroke.

PATIENT TEACHING

- Instruct patient to take propantheline 30 to 60 minutes before meals and at bedtime, as prescribed.
- Inform patient that drug may cause dizziness. Urge her to avoid hazardous activities until drug's CNS effects are known.
- Encourage patient to increase fluid and fiber intake to decrease constipation. Instruct her to report persistent constipation and urine retention.
- Advise patient to avoid excessive exposure to heat to reduce risk of heat prostration and heatstroke.
- Suggest that patient relieve dry mouth with frequent rinsing and sugar-free hard candy or gum.

propofol
(disoprofol)

Diprivan

Class and Category

Pharmacologic class: Phenol derivative
Therapeutic class: Sedative-hypnotic
Pregnancy category: B

Indications and Dosages

➤ *To provide sedation for critically ill patients in intensive care*

I.V. INFUSION

Adults. 2.8 to 130 mcg/kg/min. *Usual:* 27 mcg/kg/min.

DOSAGE ADJUSTMENT For elderly, debilitated, or American Society of Anesthesiologists Physical Status (ASA-PS) III or IV patients, induction dose decreased and maintenance rate slower.

Route	Onset	Peak	Duration
I.V.	Within 40 sec	Unknown	3–5 min

Mechanism of Action

Decreases cerebral blood flow, cerebral metabolic oxygen consumption, and intracranial pressure and increases cerebrovascular resistance, which may play a role in propofol's hypnotic effects.

P

Incompatibilities

Don't mix propofol with other drugs before giving. Don't give propofol through same I.V. line as blood or plasma products because globular component of emulsion will aggregate.

Contraindications

Hypersensitivity to propofol or its components, to eggs or egg products, or to soybeans or soy products

Interactions

DRUGS

CNS depressants such as barbiturates, benzodiazepines, chloral hydrate, droperidol, fentanyl, meperidine, morphine: Additive CNS depressant, respiratory depressant, and hypotensive effects; possibly decreased emetic effects of opioids
droperidol: Possibly decreased control of nausea and vomiting
nitrous oxide, opioids, potent inhalational agents (enflurane, halothane, isoflurane): Increased anesthetic, cardiorespiratory, or sedative effects of propofol
valproate: Increased blood levels of propofol increasing risk of cardiorespiratory depression and sedation

ACTIVITIES

alcohol use: Additive CNS depressant, respiratory depressant, and hypotensive effects

Adverse Reactions

CV: Bradycardia, hypotension
GI: Nausea, vomiting
MS: Involuntary muscle movement (transient)
RESP: Apnea
Other: Anaphylaxis, injection-site burning, pain, or stinging

Nursing Considerations

- Know that repeated or lengthy (greater than 3 hours) use of sedation drugs such as propofol and general anesthetics during procedures or surgeries should be avoided, if possible, in children younger than 3 years of age or in pregnant women during their third trimester, because the combined use may affect the development of children's brains.
- Use propofol cautiously in patients with cardiac disease, peripheral vascular disease, impaired cerebral circulation, or increased intracranial pressure because drug may aggravate these disorders.
- To dilute before administration, use only D_5W for final solution of 2 mg/ml or more.
- Consult prescriber about pretreating injection site with 1 ml of 1% lidocaine to minimize pain, burning, or stinging that may occur. If ordered, lidocaine shouldn't be added to propofol solution in quantities greater than 20 mg/200 mg propofol because emulsion may become unstable. Giving drug through a larger vein in forearm or antecubital fossa also may minimize injection-site discomfort.
- Shake container well before using, administer drug promptly after opening, and use vial for a single patient. Use prefilled syringes within 6 hours of opening.
- Use a drop counter, syringe pump, or volumetric pump to safely control infusion rate. Don't infuse drug through filter with a pore size of less than 5 microns; doing so could cause emulsion to break down.
- Discard unused portion of propofol solution plus reservoirs, I.V. tubing, and solutions immediately after or within 12 hours of administration (6 hours if propofol was transferred from original container) to prevent bacterial growth in stagnant solution. Also, protect solution from light.
- Dosage must be tapered before stopping therapy. Stopping abruptly will cause rapid awakening, anxiety, agitation and resistance to mechanical ventilation.
- Expect patient to recover from sedation within 8 minutes.

WARNING Monitor patient for propofol infusion syndrome, especially with prolonged high-dose infusions. It may cause severe metabolic acidosis, hyperkalemia, lipemia, rhabdomyolysis, hepatomegaly and cardiac and renal failure. Alert prescriber at once and be prepared to provide emergency supportive care as ordered.

PATIENT TEACHING

- Urge patient and family to voice concerns and ask questions before administration.
- Reassure patient that she'll be monitored closely during administration and that vital functions will be supported as needed.
- Inform patient and family that caution is required when performing activities requiring mental alertness, such as driving, because mental alertness may be impaired for some time after general anesthesia or sedation such as propofol has been given.

propranolol hydrochloride

Detensol (CAN), Inderal, Inderal LA, InnoPran XL, Novopranol (CAN), pms Propranolol (CAN)

Class and Category

Pharmacologic class: Beta-adrenergic blocker
Therapeutic class: Antianginal, antiarrhythmic, antihypertensive, anti-MI, antimigraine, antitremor, hypertrophic cardiomyopathy, and pheochromocytoma therapy adjunct
Pregnancy category: C

Indications and Dosages

➤ *To manage hypertension*

E.R. TABLETS

Adults. *Initial:* 80 mg daily, increased gradually up to 160 mg daily. *Maximum:* 640 mg daily.

XL TABLETS (INNOPRAN XL)

Adults. *Initial:* 80 mg once daily at bedtime, increased, as needed, to 120 mg once daily at bedtime.

ORAL SOLUTION, TABLETS

Adults. *Initial:* 40 mg twice daily, increased gradually to 120 to 240 mg daily, as needed. *Maximum:* 640 mg daily.
Children. *Initial:* 0.5 to 1 mg/kg daily in divided doses twice daily to four times a day, adjusted as needed. *Maintenance:* 2 to 4 mg/kg daily in divided doses twice daily.

➤ *To treat chronic angina*

E.R. TABLETS

Adults. *Initial:* 80 mg daily, increased every 3 to 7 days, as prescribed. *Maximum:* 320 mg/day.

ORAL SOLUTION, TABLETS

Adults. 80 to 320 mg daily in divided doses twice daily, three times a day, or four times a day.

➤ *To treat supraventricular arrhythmias and ventricular tachycardia*

ORAL SOLUTION, TABLETS

Adults. 10 to 30 mg three times a day. or four times a day, adjusted as needed.

I.V. INJECTION

Adults. 1 to 3 mg at a rate not to exceed 1 mg/min; repeated after 2 min and again after 4 hr, as needed.
Children. 0.01 to 0.1 mg/kg at a rate not to exceed 1 mg/min; repeated every 6 to 8 hr, as needed. *Maximum:* 1 mg/dose.

➤ *To control tremor*

ORAL SOLUTION, TABLETS

Adults. *Initial:* 40 mg twice daily, adjusted as needed and prescribed. *Maximum:* 320 mg daily.

➤ *To prevent vascular migraine headaches*

E.R. TABLETS

Adults. *Initial:* 80 mg daily, increased gradually, as needed. *Maximum:* 240 mg daily.

ORAL SOLUTION, TABLETS

Adults. *Initial:* 20 mg four times a day, increased gradually, as needed. *Maximum:* 240 mg daily.

➤ *As adjunct to treat hypertrophic cardiomyopathy*

ORAL SOLUTION, TABLETS

Adults. 20 to 40 mg three times a day or four times a day adjusted, as needed.

➤ *As adjunct to manage pheochromocytoma*

ORAL SOLUTION, TABLETS

Adults. For operable tumors, 20 mg three times a day to 40 mg three times a day or four times a day for 3 days before surgery, concurrently with an alpha blocker. For inoperable tumors, 30 to 160 mg daily in divided doses.

➤ *To prevent MI*

ORAL SOLUTION, TABLETS

Adults. 180 to 240 mg daily in divided doses.

DOSAGE ADJUSTMENT Dosage increased or decreased for elderly patients, depending on sensitivity to propranolol.

Route	Onset	Peak	Duration
P.O.	Unknown	1–1.5 hr*	Unknown

* For regular-release form; unknown for E.R. form.

Mechanism of Action

Through beta-blocking action, propranolol:
- prevents arterial dilation and inhibits renin secretion, resulting in decreased blood pressure (in hypertension and pheochromocytoma) and relief of migraine headaches
- decreases heart rate, which helps resolve tachyarrhythmias

- improves myocardial contractility, which helps ease symptoms of hypertrophic cardiomyopathy
- decreases myocardial oxygen demand, which helps prevent anginal pain and death of myocardial tissue.

In addition, peripheral beta-adrenergic blockade may play a role in propranolol's ability to alleviate tremor.

Contraindications

Asthma, cardiogenic shock, greater than first-degree AV block, sick sinus syndrome, or sinus bradycardia (unless pacemaker in place); heart failure (unless secondary to tachyarrhythmia responsive to propranolol), hypersensitivity to propranolol or its components

Interactions

DRUGS

ACE inhibitors: Increased risk of hypotension, especially in presence of acute MI
allergen immunotherapy, allergenic extracts for skin testing: Increased risk of serious systemic adverse reactions or anaphylaxis
amiodarone: Additive depressant effects on conduction, negative inotropic effects
anesthetics (hydrocarbon inhalation): Increased risk of myocardial depression and hypotension
beta blockers: Additive beta blockade effects
bupivacaine, lidocaine, mepivacaine: Decreased clearance of these drugs, possibly increased risk of toxicity
calcium channel blockers, clonidine, diazoxide, guanabenz, reserpine, other hypotension-producing drugs: Additive hypotensive effect and, possibly, other beta blockade effects
catecholamine-depleting drugs, such as reserpine: Increased risk of hypotension, bradycardia, vertigo, syncope, and orthostatic hypotension
cimetidine: Possibly interference with propranolol clearance
digitalis glycosides: Increased risk of bradycardia
diltiazem: Increased risk of bradycardia, hypotension, high-degree heart block, and heart failure
dobutamine, isoproterenol: Reversed effects of propranolol
doxazosin, terazosin: Increased risk of orthostatic hypotension
epinephrine: Increased risk of uncontrolled hypertension
estrogens: Decreased antihypertensive effect of propranolol
fentanyl, fentanyl derivatives: Possibly increased risk of initial bradycardia after induction doses of fentanyl or a derivative (with long-term propranolol use)
glucagon: Possibly blunted hyperglycemic response
insulin, oral antidiabetic drugs: Possibly impaired glucose control, masking of tachycardia in response to hypoglycemia
MAO inhibitors, tricyclic antidepressants: Increased risk of significant hypertension
neuroleptic drugs: Increased risk of hypotension and cardiac arrest
neuromuscular blockers: Possibly potentiated and prolonged action of these drugs
NSAIDs: Possibly decreased hypotensive effects
phenothiazines: Increased blood levels of both drugs
phenytoin: Additive cardiac depressant effects (with parenteral phenytoin)
prazosin: Increased risk of first-dose hypotension
propafenone: Increased blood level and half-life of propranolol
quinidine: Increased propranolol level, resulting in higher degrees of beta blockade and orthostatic hypotension
sympathomimetics, xanthines: Possibly mutual inhibition of therapeutic effects
thyroxine: Possibly decreased T_3 level
verapamil: Increased risk of bradycardia, heart failure, and cardiovascular collapse
warfarin: Increased risk of bleeding

ACTIVITIES

alcohol: Possibly increased plasma propranolol level
nicotine chewing gum, smoking cessation, smoking deterrents: Increased therapeutic effects of propranolol

Adverse Reactions

CNS: Anxiety, depression, dizziness, drowsiness, fatigue, fever, insomnia, lethargy, nervousness, weakness
CV: AV conduction disorders, bradycardia, cold limbs, **heart failure, hypotension**

EENT: Dry eyes, **laryngospasm**, nasal congestion, pharyngitis
GI: Abdominal pain, constipation, diarrhea, nausea, vomiting
GU: Impotence, Peyronie's disease, sexual dysfunction
HEME: Agranulocytosis, nonthrombocytopenic purpura, **thrombocytopenic purpura**
MS: Muscle weakness, myopathy, myotonia
RESP: Bronchospasm, dyspnea, **respiratory distress**, wheezing
SKIN: Alopecia, **erythema multiforme**, erythematous rash, **exfoliative dermatitis**, psoriasiform rash, **Stevens–Johnson syndrome, toxic epidermal necrolysis**, urticaria
Other: Anaphylaxis, flu-like symptoms, systemic lupus-like reaction

Nursing Considerations

- Use propranolol cautiously in patients with bronchospastic lung disease because it may induce asthmatic attack, and in patients with underlying skeletal muscle disease; isolated reports of myopathy and myotonia have occurred with propranolol use.
- Monitor blood pressure, apical and radial pulses, fluid intake and output, daily weight, respiration, and circulation in extremities before and during therapy.
- Give I.V. injection at no more than 1 mg/min.

WARNING Monitor ECG continuously, as ordered, when giving I.V. injection. Have emergency drugs and equipment available in case of hypotension or cardiac arrest.

- Protect injection solution from light.
- Because drug's negative inotropic effect can depress cardiac output, monitor cardiac output in patients with heart failure, particularly those with severely compromised left ventricular dysfunction.
- Be aware that propranolol can mask tachycardia in hyperthyroidism and that abrupt withdrawal in patients with hyperthyroidism or thyrotoxicosis can cause thyroid storm.
- Monitor diabetic patient taking an antidiabetic because propranolol can prolong hypoglycemia or promote hyperglycemia. It also can mask signs of hypoglycemia, especially tachycardia, palpitations, and tremor, but it doesn't suppress diaphoresis or hypertensive response to hypoglycemia.

WARNING Be aware that stopping drug abruptly, even for surgery, may cause myocardial ischemia, MI, ventricular arrhythmias, or severe hypertension, especially in patients with cardiac disease. However, be aware that the heart may not be able to respond to reflex adrenergic stimuli normally during surgery, which increases the risks of general anesthesia and surgical procedures. It also may cause increased intraocular pressure to return. Dosage should be reduced gradually.

PATIENT TEACHING

- Instruct patient to take propranolol at the same time every day.
- Caution patient not to change dosage without consulting prescriber and not to stop taking drug abruptly.
- Advise patient to notify prescriber immediately if she has shortness of breath.
- Instruct diabetic patient to check blood glucose level and urine for ketones regularly.
- Advise patient to consult prescriber before taking OTC drugs, especially cold products.
- Urge patient to avoid hazardous activities until CNS effects of drug are known.
- Advise smoker to notify prescriber immediately if she stops smoking because cessation may decrease drug metabolism, calling for dosage adjustments.
- Tell patient to notify prescriber if she is or could be pregnant because drug may have to be discontinued.

propylthiouracil (PTU)

Propyl-Thyracil (CAN)

Class and Category

Pharmacologic class: Thyroid hormone antagonist
Therapeutic class: Antithyroid
Pregnancy category: D

Indications and Dosages

➤ *To treat Graves' disease with hyperthyroidism or toxic multinodular goiter in patients who are intolerant of methimazole and for whom radioactive iodine therapy or surgery is not an appropriate treatment option; to improve symptoms of hyperthyroidism in preparation for radioactive iodine therapy or thyroidectomy in patients who are intolerant of methimazole*

TABLETS

Adults. *Initial:* 300 to 900 mg daily in 3 divided doses until patient becomes euthyroid. *Maintenance:* 100 to 150 mg daily in 3 divided doses.

Route	Onset	Peak	Duration
P.O.	Unknown	17 wk	Unknown

Mechanism of Action

Inhibits conversion of peripheral thyroxine to triiodothyronine by interfering with incorporation of iodide into thyroglobulin; drug remains iodinated and degraded in thyroid gland. Diversion of oxidized iodine away from thyroglobulin diminishes thyroid hormone synthesis and levels of circulating thyroid hormone.

Contraindications

Hypersensitivity to propylthiouracil or its components

Interactions

DRUGS

amiodarone, iodinated glycerol, iodine, potassium iodide: Decreased efficacy of propylthiouracil
digoxin: Risk of digitalis toxicity
oral anticoagulants: Possibly enhanced anticoagulant effect
sodium iodide 131 (radioactive iodine, ^{131}I): Decreased thyroid uptake of ^{131}I

Adverse Reactions

CNS: Dizziness, drowsiness, headache, neuritis, paresthesia, peripheral neuropathy, vertigo
CV: Edema, periarteritis, vasculitis
EENT: Taste loss or perversion
ENDO: Hypothyroidism
GI: Abdominal pain, **acute liver failure**, epigastric distress, **hepatitis**, **hepatotoxicity**, nausea, vomiting
GU: Acute renal failure, glomerulonephritis, **nephritis**
HEME: Agranulocytosis, **aplastic anemia**, **bleeding**, **granulopenia**, **hypoprothrombinemia**, **leukopenia**, **thrombocytopenia**
MS: Arthralgia, joint redness or swelling, myalgia
RESP: Alveolar hemorrhage, **interstitial pneumonitis**, **pulmonary infiltrates**
SKIN: Alopecia, erythema nodosum, **exfoliative dermatitis**, leukocytoclastic vasculitis, pruritus, rash, **Stevens–Johnson syndrome**, **toxic epidermal necrolysis**, ulceration, urticaria
Other: Drug fever, lupus-like symptoms

Nursing Considerations

- Ensure that patient, parents, or caregivers have been informed about the risk of liver failure, before administering propylthiouracil.
- Monitor complete blood count (CBC), prothrombin time (PT), and thyroid function in patients taking propylthiouracil. Elevated serum triiodothyronine (T_3) level may be the sole indicator of inadequate treatment.
- Expect to stop drug 3 to 4 days before ^{131}I treatment to prevent decreased thyroid uptake of ^{131}I. Therapy may be resumed 3 to 5 days after radiation, if needed.
- Know that serum T_3 and thyroxine levels should decrease after about 3 weeks of therapy.
- Expect to decrease beta blocker or theophylline dosage once patient is euthyroid, as ordered.
- Monitor liver enzymes, especially during first 6 months of therapy, because drug may cause liver failure, need for liver transplant, or death. Expect to stop drug at first sign of liver dysfunction (easy bruising, fatigue, itching, jaundice, loss of appetite, vague abdominal pain, and weakness) and obtain liver enzymes, as ordered.
- Be aware that propylthiouracil may be the treatment of choice when an antithyroid drug is indicated during or just prior to the first trimester of pregnancy. However, after the first trimester of pregnancy, expect an alternative antithyroid medication to be prescribed because drug crosses the placenta and can cause fetal cretinism and goiter.

WARNING Be aware that cases of vasculitis resulting in severe complications and death have occurred in patients receiving propylthiouracil. If suspected, notify prescriber immediately and expect drug to be discontinued. For more severe cases, also expect patient to receive corticosteroids, immunosuppressant therapy, and plasmapheresis, as needed.

PATIENT TEACHING

- Instruct patient to take drug with meals to decrease risk of adverse GI reactions.
- Urge patient to avoid dietary sources of iodine, such as iodized salt and shellfish.
- Tell patient to check pulse rate and weight daily and to report increased heart rate and excessive weight loss to prescriber.
- Urge patient to report signs and symptoms of infection, such as fever and sore throat.
- Instruct patient to notify prescriber immediately if she becomes pregnant.
- Advise patient to report signs and symptoms of hypothyroidism, such as cold intolerance, depression, and increased fatigue.
- Tell patient to ask prescriber before using OTC cold drugs (some contain iodides).
- Advise patient to notify prescriber immediately if he has easy bruising, fatigue, itching, loss of appetite, vague right upper quadrant abdominal pain, weakness, or yellowing of eyes or skin.

protamine sulfate

Class and Category

Pharmacologic class: Heparin antagonist
Therapeutic class: Heparin antidote
Pregnancy category: C

Indications and Dosages

➤ *To treat heparin toxicity or hemorrhage associated with heparin therapy*

I.V. INJECTION

Adults and children. 1 mg for each 100 units of heparin to be neutralized, or as indicated by coagulation test results and given very slowly, not to exceed 50 mg in any 10-min period. *Maximum:* 100 mg (within 2-hr period).

Route	Onset	Peak	Duration
I.V.	5 min	Unknown	2 hr

Mechanism of Action

Neutralizes anticoagulant activity. A strong basic polypeptide, protamine combines with strongly acidic heparin complex to form an inactive stable salt, thereby neutralizing anticoagulant activity of both drugs.

Incompatibilities

Don't mix protamine sulfate in same syringe with other drugs unless they're known to be compatible. Several cephalosporins, penicillins, and other antibiotics are incompatible.

Contraindications

Allergy to fish, hypersensitivity to protamine or its components

Interactions

DRUGS

heparin: Neutralized anticoagulant effect of both drugs

Adverse Reactions

CNS: Weakness
CV: **Bradycardia**, hypertension, **hypotension**, **shock**
GI: Nausea, vomiting
HEME: **Unusual bleeding** or bruising
RESP: Dyspnea, **pulmonary edema (noncardiogenic)**, **pulmonary hypertension**
SKIN: Flushing, sensation of warmth
Other: **Anaphylaxis**

Nursing Considerations

- Expect to administer I.V. protamine undiluted. However, dilute drug if needed (for patients other than neonates) with 5 ml of bacteriostatic water for injection containing 0.9% benzyl alcohol. For neonates, reconstitute with preservative-free sterile water for injection.
- Inject drug slowly at 5 mg/min; administer no more than 50 mg in 10 minutes or 100 mg in 2 hours.

WARNING Be aware that rapid delivery may cause severe hypotension and anaphylaxis.

- Be prepared to obtain coagulation studies (APTT, activated clotting time) 5 to 15 minutes after giving drug and to repeat them in 2 to 8 hours to detect heparin-rebound hypotension, shock, and bleeding.
- Monitor vital signs, hemodynamic parameters, and fluid intake and output, and assess for flushing sensation.
- Have fluids—epinephrine 1:1,000, dobutamine, or dopamine—available for allergic or hypotensive reactions.

- Be aware that men with vasectomy have an increased risk of hypersensitivity reaction because of possible accumulation of antiprotamine antibodies.

PATIENT TEACHING

- Instruct patient to report adverse reactions immediately.

protriptyline hydrochloride

Triptil (CAN), Vivactil

Class and Category

Pharmacologic class: Tricyclic antidepressant
Therapeutic class: Antidepressant
Pregnancy category: Not classified

Indications and Dosages

➤ *To treat depression*

TABLETS

Adults. *Initial:* 5 to 10 mg three times a day or four times a day, increased every wk by 10 mg daily, as needed. *Maximum:* 60 mg daily.

Children age 12 and over. *Initial:* 5 mg three times a day, increased as needed.

DOSAGE ADJUSTMENT For elderly patients, initial dosage limited to 5 mg three times a day, then adjusted, as needed.

Route	Onset	Peak	Duration
P.O.	2–3 wk	Unknown	Unknown

Mechanism of Action

May block reuptake of norepinephrine and serotonin (and possibly other neurotransmitters) at neuronal membranes, thus enhancing their effects at postsynaptic receptors. These neurotransmitters may play a role in relieving depression symptoms.

Contraindications

Acute recovery phase after MI, hypersensitivity to protriptyline or its components, use within 14 days of MAO inhibitor therapy

Interactions

DRUGS

amantadine, anticholinergics, antidyskinetics, antihistamines: Additive anticholinergic effects, potentiated effects of antihistamines or protriptyline, possibly impaired detoxification of atropine and related drugs
anticonvulsants: Possibly lowered seizure threshold and decreased anticonvulsant effectiveness; enhanced CNS depression
antithyroid drugs: Possibly agranulocytosis
barbiturates, carbamazepine: Decreased therapeutic effects of protriptyline
bupropion, clozapine, cyclobenzaprine, haloperidol, loxapine, maprotiline, molindone, phenothiazines, thioxanthenes: Prolonged and intensified anticholinergic and sedative effects, lowered seizure threshold, increased risk of neuroleptic malignant syndrome; increased blood protriptyline level and inhibited phenothiazine metabolism (with phenothiazine use)
cimetidine: Increased risk of protriptyline toxicity
clonidine, guanadrel, guanethidine: Decreased hypotensive effects; increased CNS depression (with clonidine use)
CNS depressants: Possibly serious potentiation of CNS and respiratory depression and hypotensive effect
disulfiram, ethchlorvynol: Possibly transient delirium; increased CNS depression (with ethchlorvynol use)
fluoxetine: Increased protriptyline level
MAO inhibitors: Increased risk of hyperpyretic crisis, severe seizures, and death
methylphenidate: Possibly antagonized effects of methylphenidate and increased blood protriptyline level
metrizamide: Increased risk of seizures
naphazoline, oxymetazoline, phenylephrine, xylometazoline: Possibly increased vasopressor effects of these drugs
oral anticoagulants: Possibly increased anticoagulant activity
pimozide, probucol: Possibly prolonged QT interval and ventricular tachycardia
sympathomimetics: Possibly potentiated cardiovascular effects, decreased vasopressor effects of ephedrine and mephentermine
thyroid hormones: Increased therapeutic and toxic effects of both drugs

ACTIVITIES

alcohol use: Possibly increased response to alcohol

Adverse Reactions

CNS: Agitation, ataxia, confusion, **CVA**, dizziness, drowsiness, exacerbation of psychosis, extrapyramidal reactions, fatigue, lack of coordination, paresthesia, peripheral neuropathy, **suicidal ideation**, tremor, weakness
CV: Arrhythmias, including heart block; hypertension; **hypotension**; **MI**; orthostatic hypotension; palpitations; tachycardia
EENT: Angle closure glaucoma, black tongue, blurred vision, dry mouth, increased intraocular pressure, lacrimation, stomatitis, tongue swelling
ENDO: Hyperglycemia, **hypoglycemia**
GI: Abdominal cramps, anorexia, constipation, diarrhea, epigastric discomfort, hepatic dysfunction, nausea, vomiting
GU: Impotence, libido changes, nocturia, urinary frequency and hesitancy, urine retention
SKIN: Diaphoresis, petechiae, photosensitivity, rash, urticaria
Other: Angioedema, weight gain or loss

Nursing Considerations

- Use protriptyline cautiously in patients with a history of seizures because drug can lower seizure threshold.
- Use cautiously in patients with a history of urine retention or increased intraocular pressure because of drug's autonomic activity.

WARNING Avoid giving protriptyline with an MAO inhibitor. If patient is being switched from an MAO inhibitor to protriptyline, make sure MAO inhibitor has been discontinued for 14 days before starting protriptyline.

- Watch patients closely (especially children, adolescents, and young adults) for suicidal tendencies, particularly when therapy starts or dosage changes, because depression may worsen temporarily during these times, possibly leading to suicidal ideation.

PATIENT TEACHING

- Inform patient that protriptyline therapy may take several weeks to reach full effect.
- Advise patient that drug may cause mild pupillary dilation, which may lead to an episode of acute closure glaucoma. Encourage patient to have an eye exam before starting therapy to see if he is at risk.
- Instruct patient to avoid hazardous activities until drug's CNS effects are known.
- Advise patient to change position slowly to minimize orthostatic hypotension.
- Urge patient to avoid alcohol while taking drug.
- Suggest drinking water and using sugarless gum or hard candy to relieve dry mouth.
- Advise patient to avoid sunlight and tanning booths and to wear protective clothing, a hat, and sunscreen when outdoors.
- Instruct diabetic patient to check blood glucose level frequently during first few weeks of protriptyline therapy.
- Urge family or caregiver to watch patient for suicidal tendencies, especially when therapy starts or dosage changes and particularly if patient is a child, teenager, or young adult.

pyrazinamide

Tebrazid (CAN)

Class and Category

Pharmacologic class: Nicotinamide analogue
Therapeutic class: Antitubercular
Pregnancy category: C

Indications and Dosages

➤ *As adjunct to treat tuberculosis, along with other antitubercular drugs*

TABLETS

Adults and children. 15 to 30 mg/kg daily; or, 50 to 70 mg/kg 2 or 3 times/wk.
Maximum: For daily regimen, 2 g daily; for twice/wk regimen, 4 g daily; for 3-times/wk regimen, 3 g daily.

DOSAGE ADJUSTMENT For patients with HIV infection, 20 to 30 mg/kg daily for first 2 mo of therapy.

Mechanism of Action

Inhibits growth of *Mycobacterium tuberculosis* by decreasing pH level; exhibits bactericidal or bacteriostatic action, depending on blood pyrazinamide level.

Contraindications

Acute gout, hypersensitivity to pyrazinamide or its components, severe hepatic damage

Interactions

DRUGS

allopurinol, colchicine, probenecid, sulfinpyrazone: Possibly increased blood uric acid level and decreased antigout efficacy
cyclosporine: Possibly decreased blood level and therapeutic effects of cyclosporine

Adverse Reactions

CNS: Fever
GI: Anorexia, **hepatotoxicity**, nausea, vomiting
GU: Dysuria
HEME: Porphyria
MS: Arthralgia, gout, myalgia
SKIN: Acne, photosensitivity, pruritus, rash, urticaria

Nursing Considerations

- Review liver function test results before and every 2 to 4 weeks during therapy.
- Be aware that drug can affect the accuracy of certain urine ketone strip test results.
- Because drug is metabolized by liver, monitor patient for evidence of hepatotoxicity, such as darkened urine, fever, jaundice, malaise, nausea, severe pain in feet or toes, and vomiting.

PATIENT TEACHING

- Explain importance of complying with long-term pyrazinamide therapy.
- Tell diabetic patient about possible changes in ketone measurement during therapy.
- Instruct patient to report dark urine, fever, malaise, nausea, severe pain in feet or toes, vomiting, and yellowing of skin or eyes.
- Inform patient of need for regular blood tests and follow-up visits with prescriber.
- Urge patient to minimize exposure to sun and to wear protective clothing, hat, sunglasses, and sunscreen when outdoors.

pyridostigmine bromide

Mestinon, Mestinon-SR (CAN), Mestinon Timespans, Regonol (CAN)

Class and Category

Pharmacologic class: Cholinesterase inhibitor
Therapeutic class: Muscle stimulant
Pregnancy category: Not classified

Indications and Dosages

➤ *To treat symptoms of myasthenia gravis*

E.R. TABLETS

Adults and adolescents. 180 to 540 mg once or twice daily (at least 6 hr between doses).

SYRUP, TABLETS

Adults and adolescents. *Initial:* 30 to 60 mg every 3 to 4 hr, adjusted as needed. *Maintenance:* 60 mg to 1.5 g daily.
Children. 7 mg/kg daily in 5 or 6 divided doses.

I.V. OR I.M. INJECTION

Adults and adolescents. 2 mg every 2 to 3 hr. I.V. injection given no faster than 1 mg/min.

I.M. INJECTION

Neonates of myasthenic mothers. 0.05 to 0.15 mg/kg every 4 to 6 hr.

➤ *To reverse the effects of neuromuscular blockers*

I.V. INJECTION

Adults and adolescents. 10 to 20 mg given no faster than 1 mg/min after 0.6 to 1.2 mg of I.V. atropine has been given.
DOSAGE ADJUSTMENT Dosage possibly reduced for patients with renal impairment.

Route	Onset	Peak	Duration
P.O.	30–45 min	1–2 hr	3–6 hr
P.O. (E.R.)	30–60 min	1–2 hr	6–12 hr
I.V.	2–5 min	Unknown	2–4 hr
I.M.	15 min	Unknown	2–4 hr

Mechanism of Action

Improves muscle strength compromised by myasthenia gravis or neuromuscular blockade by competing with acetylcholine for its binding site on acetylcholinesterase. This action potentiates the effects of acetylcholine on skeletal muscle and the GI tract. Inhibited destruction of acetylcholine allows freer transmission of nerve impulses across the neuromuscular junction.

Contraindications

Hypersensitivity to pyridostigmine or its components, mechanical obstruction of GI or urinary tract

Interactions

DRUGS

aminoglycosides (systemic), anesthetics (hydrocarbon inhalation), capreomycin, lidocaine (I.V.), lincomycins, polymyxins, quinine: Possibly antagonized effect of pyridostigmine on skeletal muscle; possibly decreased neuromuscular blocking activity of these drugs (with large doses of pyridostigmine)
anesthetics (local): Inhibited neuronal transmission, increased anesthesia effects
anticholinergics: Possibly masked pyridostigmine overdose; reduced intestinal motility
cholinesterase inhibitors: Increased risk of additive toxicity
edrophonium: Possibly worsening of status
guanadrel, guanethidine, mecamylamine, neuromuscular blockers, procainamide: Possibly prolonged phase I blocking effect or reversal of nondepolarization blockade
quinidine, trimethaphan: Possibly antagonized effects of pyridostigmine

Adverse Reactions

EENT: Increased salivation, lacrimation, miosis
GI: Abdominal cramps, diarrhea, increased peristalsis, nausea, vomiting
GU: Urinary frequency, incontinence, or urgency
MS: Fasciculations, muscle spasms or weakness
RESP: Increased tracheobronchial secretions
SKIN: Diaphoresis

Nursing Considerations

- Use pyridostigmine cautiously in patients with renal disease because drug is mainly excreted unchanged by kidneys. Monitor BUN and serum creatinine levels.

WARNING Maintain a rigid dosing schedule because a missed or late dose can precipitate myasthenic crisis.

- Observe for cholinergic reactions when administering drug I.V. or I.M.

WARNING Pyridostigmine overdose may obscure diagnosis of myasthenic crisis because main symptom in both is muscle weakness. Treat cholinergic crisis by stopping anticholinesterase, giving atropine as prescribed, and helping with endotracheal intubation and mechanical ventilation, if needed.

- Be aware that reversal of neuromuscular blockade usually occurs in 15 to 30 minutes. Be prepared to maintain patent airway and ventilation until normal voluntary respiration returns completely. Assess respiratory measurements and muscle tone with peripheral nerve stimulator device, as indicated.

PATIENT TEACHING

- Instruct patient to take pyridostigmine as directed and on schedule. Explain that a late or missed dose can precipitate a crisis. Suggest the use of a battery-operated alarm clock as a reminder.
- Tell patient to take drug with a full glass of water or with food or milk if GI distress occurs.
- Warn patient not to crush or chew E.R. tablets.
- Ask patient to record pyridostigmine dosage, times taken, and drug effects to help determine optimal dosage and schedule.
- Urge patient to carry medical identification describing her condition and drug regimen.

QRS

quazepam

Doral

Class, Category, and Schedule

Pharmacologic class: Benzodiazepine
Therapeutic class: Sedative-hypnotic
Pregnancy category: C
Controlled substance schedule: IV

Indications and Dosages

➤ *To treat insomnia*

TABLETS

Adults. *Initial:* 7.5 mg at bedtime, increased, as needed to 15 mg at bedtime.
DOSAGE ADJUSTMENT Debilitated and elderly patients may be more sensitive to drug requiring a decreased dosage.

Mechanism of Action

May antagonize mu receptors at hypothalamic, limbic, and thalamic regions of the brain, blocking release of such inhibitory neurotransmitters as acetylcholine and gamma-aminobutyric acid (GABA). Central receptors interact with GABA receptors, allowing for greater influx of chloride into the neuron, thereby suppressing neuronal excitability. GABA effects may inhibit spinal afferent pathways and block the cortical and limbic arousal that normally occurs when reticular pathways are stimulated. These effects result in various levels of CNS depression, including sleep.

Contraindications

Hypersensitivity to quazepam or its components, pregnancy, sleep apnea (known or suspected)

Interactions

DRUGS

addictive drugs: Possibly habituation
carbamazepine: Decreased blood quazepam level, possibly increased blood carbamazepine level
cimetidine, diltiazem, disulfiram, erythromycin, fluoxetine, fluvoxamine, isoniazid, itraconazole, ketoconazole, nefazodone, oral contraceptives, propoxyphene, ranitidine, verapamil: Possibly potentiated effects of quazepam
clozapine: Possibly syncope, with respiratory depression or arrest
CNS depressants, opioids, other benzodiazepines, sedating antihistamines, tricyclic antidepressants: Increased CNS and respiratory depression that could become severe
CYP2B6 substrates such as bupropion and efavirenz: Possibly increased plasma levels of these agents leading to increased risk of adverse effects
digoxin: Possibly increased blood digoxin level and risk of digitalis toxicity
levodopa: Possibly decreased therapeutic effects of levodopa
phenytoin: Increased risk of phenytoin toxicity
theophyllines: Possibly antagonized effects of quazepam
zidovudine: Increased risk of zidovudine toxicity

FOODS

grapefruit juice: Increased quazepam level

ACTIVITIES

alcohol use: Additive CNS and respiratory depression that could become severe
smoking: Possibly decreased effectiveness of quazepam

Adverse Reactions

CNS: Abnormal complex behaviors, such as eating, having sex, sleep driving or talking on the phone without any recall; amnesia (anterograde); anxiety; ataxia; confusion; depression; dizziness; drowsiness; euphoria; fatigue; headache; light-headedness; paresthesia; slurred speech; **suicidal ideation**; tremor; weakness
CV: Chest pain, palpitations, tachycardia
EENT: Blurred vision, dry mouth, hyperacusis, photophobia, **throat tightness**, worsening of glaucoma
GI: Abdominal cramps, constipation, diarrhea, heartburn, nausea, thirst, vomiting
GU: Renal dysfunction, urinary incontinence, urine retention
MS: Muscle spasms
RESP: Dyspnea, increased tracheobronchial secretions
Other: Anaphylaxis, angioedema

Nursing Considerations

- Use quazepam cautiously in elderly patients because of age-related decreases in cardiac, hepatic, and renal function; in patients with angle-closure glaucoma because of drug's anticholinergic effects; in patients with hepatic dysfunction because this condition may prolong quazepam's half-life; in patients with myasthenia gravis because drug may worsen condition; in patients with renal dysfunction because accumulation of metabolites may result in toxicity; and in patients with severe COPD because adverse effects of quazepam may compromise respiratory function.

WARNING Monitor patient closely for signs and symptoms of hypersensitivity reactions, such as dyspnea, nausea, swelling, throat tightness, and vomiting. If present, discontinue quazepam immediately, notify prescriber, and provide supportive care.

WARNING Notify prescriber if eye pain develops in patient with angle-closure glaucoma.

WARNING Be aware that quazepam may intensify signs and symptoms of depression. Monitor patient closely for evidence of suicidal ideation, and institute suicide precautions, as needed.

WARNING Be aware that opioids should only be used concomitantly with benzodiazepine therapy in patients for whom other treatment options are inadequate. If prescribed together, expect dosing and duration of the opioid to be limited. Monitor patient closely for signs and symptoms of a decrease in consciousness including coma, profound sedation, and significant respiratory depression. Notify prescriber immediately and provide emergency supportive care, as death may occur.

PATIENT TEACHING

- Instruct patient to stop taking quazepam and seek emergency care if she has abnormal swelling, nausea, throat tightness, trouble breathing, or vomiting.
- Advise patient that drug may cause abnormal behaviors during sleep, such as driving a car, eating, having sex, or talking on the phone without recall of the event. If family members notice such behavior, or if patient sees evidence of it upon awakening, prescriber should be notified.
- Urge patient to avoid consuming alcohol during quazepam therapy because risk of abnormal behaviors, such as sleep driving and sedation, may increase.

WARNING Warn patient that taking quazepam with an opioid may lead to severe respiratory depression and possibly death. Tell him to inform all prescribers of quazepam use, especially when pain medication may be prescribed.

- Instruct patient not to stop drug abruptly after prolonged use (6 weeks or more).
- Instruct female patient of childbearing age to use effective contraception during therapy and to notify prescriber immediately of known or suspected pregnancy.
- Urge family or caregiver to watch patient closely for suicidal tendencies, especially when therapy starts or dosage changes.

quetiapine fumarate

Seroquel, Seroquel XR

Class and Category

Pharmacologic class: Dibenzothiazepine derivative
Therapeutic class: Antipsychotic
Pregnancy category: C

Indications and Dosages

➤ *To treat schizophrenia*

TABLETS

Adults. *Initial:* 25 mg twice daily on day 1. Increased by 25 to 50 twice daily or three times a day on days 2 and 3. *Usual:* 300 to 400 mg daily by day 4, in divided doses twice daily or three times a day. Increased every 2 days in increments of 25 to 50 mg twice daily, as needed. *Maximum:* 750 mg daily.

Adolescents. *Initial:* 25 mg twice daily on day 1; 50 mg twice daily on day 2; 100 mg twice daily on day 3; 150 mg twice daily on day 4; 200 mg twice daily on day 5. Increased further in increments no greater than 100 mg/day and no higher than a total daily dose of 800 mg, as needed.

E.R. TABLETS

Adults. *Initial:* 300 mg once daily in evening. Dosage increased daily in increments up to 300 mg, as needed. *Maximum:* 800 mg daily.

Adolescents. *Initial:* 50 mg daily on day 1; 100 mg daily on day 2; 200 mg daily on day 3; 300 mg daily on day 4; 400 mg daily on day 5. Increased further in increments no greater than 100 mg/day and no higher than a total daily dose of 800 mg, as needed.

➤ *To treat depressive episodes in bipolar disorder*

E.R. TABLETS

TABLETS

Adults. *Initial:* On day 1, 50 mg once at bedtime; day 2, 100 mg once at bedtime; day 3, 200 mg once at bedtime; day 4, 300 mg once at bedtime. *Maintenance:* 300 mg once daily at bedtime.

➤ *As adjunct therapy with antidepressants to treat major depressive disorder*

E.R. TABLETS

Adults. *Initial:* 50 mg once daily in evening, increased to 150 mg once daily in evening on day 3. *Maximum:* 300 mg daily in evening.

➤ *To treat acute manic episodes in bipolar I disorder as monotherapy*

TABLETS

Adults. *Initial:* 50 mg twice daily on day 1; 100 mg twice daily on day 2; 150 mg twice daily on day 3; 200 mg twice daily on day 4. Increased further in increments of no greater than 200 up to 800 mg/day by day 6, if needed.

Children age 10 and over. *Initial:* 25 mg twice daily on day 1; 50 mg twice daily on day 2; 100 mg twice daily on day 3; 150 mg twice daily on day 4; 200 mg twice daily on day 5. Further increased in increments no greater than 100 up to 600 mg/day, as needed.

E.R. TABLETS

Adults. *Initial:* 300 mg once daily in evening on day 1, followed by 600 mg once daily in evening on day 2 and 400 to 800 mg daily on day 3 and thereafter.

Children age 10 and over. *Initial:* 50 mg daily on day 1; 100 mg daily on day 2; 200 mg daily on day 3; 300 mg daily on day 4; 400 mg daily on day 5. Further increased in increments no greater than 100 up to 600 mg/day, as needed.

➤ *To treat acute manic episodes in bipolar I disorder as adjunct with lithium or divalproex*

E.R. TABLETS

Adults. *Initial:* 300 mg once daily in evening on day 1, followed by 600 mg once daily in evening on day 2 and 800 mg daily on day 3 and thereafter. *Maintenance:* 800 mg/day.

TABLETS

Adults. *Initial:* 50 mg twice daily on day 1; 100 mg twice daily on day 2; 150 mg twice daily on day 3; 200 mg twice daily on day 4. Increased further in increments of no greater than 200 up to 800 mg/day by day 6, if needed.

➤ *To maintain treatment in bipolar I disorder*

TABLETS

Adults. 400 to 800 mg daily given in 2 divided doses. *Maximum:* 800 mg daily.

DOSAGE ADJUSTMENT For elderly patients and patients with hepatic impairment, initial dosage no higher than 25 mg once daily for immediate-release (tablet) form and 50 mg once daily for extended-release tablet form and increased in increments of 25 to 50 mg/day depending on response and tolerance.

Mechanism of Action

May produce antipsychotic effects by interfering with dopamine binding to dopamine type 2 (D_2)-receptor sites in the brain and by antagonizing serotonin 5-HT_2, dopamine type 1 (D_1), histamine H_1, and adrenergic $alpha_1$ and $alpha_2$ receptors.

Contraindications

Hypersensitivity to quetiapine or its components

Interactions

DRUGS

antibiotics such as gatifloxacin or moxifloxacin; antipsychotic drugs such as chlorpromazine, thioridazine, ziprasidone; class 1A antiarrythmics such as procainamide or quinidine; class III antiarrythmics such as amiodarone or sotalol; levomethadyl acetate, methadone, pentamidine: Possibly increased risk of prolonged QT interval

antihypertensives: Possibly enhanced antihypertensive effects of these drugs
cimetidine, erythromycin, fluconazole, itraconazole, ketoconazole: Decreased clearance and possibly increased effects of quetiapine
CNS depressants: Possibly increased CNS depression
lorazepam: Possibly increased effects of lorazepam
phenytoin, thioridazine: Increased clearance and possibly decreased effectiveness of quetiapine

ACTIVITIES

alcohol use: Possibly enhanced CNS depression

Adverse Reactions

CNS: Depression, dizziness, drowsiness, dystonia, extrapyramidal reactions, hypertonia, **hypothermia**, lethargy, restless leg syndrome, retrograde amnesia, somnolence, **suicidal ideation**, tardive dyskinesia
CV: Cardiomyopathy, hypercholesterolemia, **myocarditis**, orthostatic hypotension, palpitations, **prolongation of QT interval**
EENT: Dry mouth, nasal congestion, pharyngitis, rhinitis
ENDO: Galactorrhea, hyperglycemia, syndrome of inappropriate ADH secretion
GI: Anorexia, constipation, indigestion, **pancreatitis**
GU: Nocturnal enuresis
HEME: Agranulocytosis, leukopenia, neutropenia, thrombocytopenia
MS: Dysarthria, muscle weakness, **rhabdomyolysis**
RESP: Cough, dyspnea
SKIN: Diaphoresis, **Stevens–Johnson syndrome, toxic epidermal necrolysis**
Other: Anaphylaxis, drug reaction with eosinophilia and systemic symptoms (DRESS), flu-like symptoms, **hyponatremia**, weight gain

Nursing Considerations

WARNING Know that quetiapine shouldn't be used for elderly patients with dementia-related psychosis because drug increases the risk of death in these patients.

- Know that quetiapine should not be given to patients who have a history of cardiac arrhythmias, such as bradycardia, or who experience hypokalemia or hypomagnesemia. The drug also should not be used with other drugs that prolong the QT interval or in a patient who has a congenital prolongation of the QT interval because quetiapine may increase the QT interval, which may increase the risk of torsades de pointes and/or sudden death.
- Use quetiapine cautiously in patients who have a history of cardiovascular disease, a family history of QT prolongation, or in patients who are elderly or take medications that may cause an electrolyte imbalance, such as diuretics, or who have congestive heart failure or heart hypertrophy, because these factors may increase the risk of a prolonged QT interval. Also use cautiously in cardiac patients because quetiapine may cause orthostatic hypotension.
- Monitor patients (particularly children and young adults) closely for suicidal tendencies, especially when therapy starts or dosage changes, because depression may worsen temporarily during these times.

WARNING Monitor patient taking quetiapine for predisposing factors for neuroleptic malignant syndrome, such as dehydration, heat stress, organic brain disease, and physical exhaustion. Neuroleptic malignant syndrome includes altered mental status, autonomic instability (which may include arrhythmias, blood pressure abnormalities, diaphoresis, irregular pulse, or tachycardia), hyperpyrexia, and muscle rigidity.

- Monitor patient for signs of tardive dyskinesia, a potentially irreversible complication characterized by involuntary, dyskinetic movements of eyelids, face, jaw, mouth, or tongue. Notify prescriber if such signs develop, because quetiapine therapy may need to be stopped.
- Monitor patient for orthostatic hypotension, especially during initial dosage titration period. Be prepared to correct underlying conditions, such as dehydration and hypovolemia, before starting quetiapine therapy, as prescribed.
- Monitor patient for prolonged abnormal muscle contractions, especially during the first few days of quetiapine therapy, in male patients and in younger patients.

- Assess patient for hypothyroidism because drug can cause dose-dependent decreases in total and free thyroxine (T_4) levels.
- Monitor laboratory results during first 3 weeks of therapy for transient elevations in hepatic enzyme levels. Notify prescriber if they persist or worsen.
- Monitor patient's blood glucose and lipid levels routinely, as ordered, because drug increases the risk of hyperglycemia and hypercholesterolemia.
- Check CBC often during the first few months of therapy, as ordered, in patients with a low white blood cell count or a history of drug-induced hematologic problems. If counts drop or patient develops a fever or other signs of infection, notify prescriber and expect to discontinue drug and provide supportive care.
- Institute fall precautions, because patients receiving quetiapine have a greater risk of falling.
- Expect to gradually taper off quetiapine therapy when discontinued, as ordered, to avoid acute withdrawal symptoms such as insomnia, nausea, and vomiting.

PATIENT TEACHING

- Instruct patient to take quetiapine with food to reduce stomach upset.
- Advise patient not to stop taking quetiapine suddenly because doing so may exacerbate his symptoms or produce withdrawal symptoms.
- Inform patient that quetiapine therapy may cause dizziness or drowsiness. Advise him not to drive or perform other activities that require alertness until drug's full CNS effects are known. Also, review fall precautions with patient.
- Instruct patient to rise slowly from a lying or seated position to reduce the risk of dizziness or fainting.
- Caution patient to avoid consuming alcoholic beverages because they can increase dizziness and drowsiness.
- Urge family or caregiver to watch patient closely for suicidal tendencies, especially when therapy starts or dosage changes and particularly if patient is a child or young adult.
- Encourage patient on long-term therapy to have regular eye examinations so that cataracts can be detected.
- Advise patient to contact prescriber if his pulse rate becomes abnormally slow or irregular.
- Alert patient that a false positive drug test for methadone or tricyclic antidepressants may occur with quetiapine use.

quinapril hydrochloride

Accupril

Class and Category

Pharmacologic class: Angiotensin converting enzyme (ACE) inhibitor
Therapeutic class: Antihypertensive
Pregnancy category: D

Indications and Dosages

➤ *To treat hypertension*

TABLETS

Adults not on diuretics. *Initial:* 10 or 20 mg daily, adjusted every 2 wk based on clinical response. *Maintenance:* 20 to 80 mg daily or in divided doses twice daily.

➤ *As adjunct to manage heart failure*

TABLETS

Adults. *Initial:* 5 mg twice daily, increased, weekly as needed and tolerated. *Maintenance:* 20 to 40 mg twice daily.

DOSAGE ADJUSTMENT For patients who are dehydrated from previous diuretic therapy, those who are still receiving diuretic therapy, and those with creatinine clearance of 30 to 60 ml/min, initial dosage reduced to 5 mg daily. For patients with creatinine clearance of 10 to 30 ml/min, initial dosage reduced to 2.5 mg daily. For elderly patients, initial dosage reduced to 10 mg once daily, then titrated slowly to optimal response.

Route	Onset	Peak	Duration
P.O.	In 1 hr	2–4 hr	Up to 24 hr

Mechanism of Action

Blocks conversion of angiotensin I to angiotensin II, leading to vasodilation, and reduces aldosterone secretion, which prevents water retention. Quinapril also reduces peripheral arterial resistance. These combined actions lead to a reduction in blood pressure. The reduction of aldosterone secretion also helps to relieve fluid buildup in heart failure.

Contraindications

Aliskiren therapy in patients with diabetes or patients with renal impairment (GRF less than 60 ml/min), history of angioedema related to previous treatment with ACE inhibitor, hypersensitivity to quinapril or its components, use of a neprilysin inhibitor such as sacubitril within 36 hours

Interactions

DRUGS

aliskiren (patients with diabetes and/or renal impairment), angiotensin receptor blockers, other ACE inhibitors: Increased risk of hyperkalemia, hypotension, and renal dysfunction
allopurinol, bone marrow depressants, corticosteroids (systemic), procainamide: Increased risk of fatal agranulocytosis or neutropenia
CNS depressants, other hypotension-producing drugs: Additive hypotensive effects
cyclosporine, potassium preparations, potassium-sparing diuretics: Possibly hyperkalemia
lithium: Possibly increased blood lithium level and risk of toxicity
mTOR inhibitors such as temsirolimus, neprilysin inhibitors such as sacubitril: Increased risk of angioedema
NSAIDs: Decreased antihypertensive effect of quinapril; increased risk of renal dysfunction in the elderly or patients who have preexisting renal dysfunction or are volume depleted
sodium aurothiomalate: Possibly nitritoid reactions such as facial flushing, hypotension, nausea, vomiting
sympathomimetics: Decreased antihypertensive effect of quinapril
tetracyclines: Reduced tetracycline absorption

FOODS

foods high in potassium such as milk or potatoes, potassium-containing, salt substitutes: Increased risk of hyperkalemia

ACTIVITIES

alcohol use: Additive hypotensive effects

Adverse Reactions

CNS: CVA, depression, dizziness, drowsiness, fatigue, fever, headache, insomnia, light-headedness, malaise, nervousness, paresthesia, sleep disturbance, somnolence, syncope, vertigo
CV: Angina pectoris, **arrhythmias**, **cardiogenic shock**, chest pain, edema, **heart failure**, **hypertensive crisis**, **hypotension**, orthostatic hypotension, **MI**, palpitations, tachycardia, vasodilation
EENT: Amblyopia, dry mouth or throat, loss of taste, pharyngitis
GI: Abdominal pain, constipation, diarrhea, dyspepsia, elevated liver enzymes, flatulence, **GI hemorrhage**, **hepatitis**, indigestion, nausea, **pancreatitis**, vomiting
GU: Acute renal failure, elevated blood urea nitrogen and creatinine, impotence, UTI, **worsening renal failure**
HEME: Agranulocytosis, **hemolytic anemia**, **thrombocytopenia**
MS: Arthralgia, back pain, myalgia
RESP: Cough, dyspnea, **eosinophilic pneumonitis**
SKIN: Alopecia, dermatopolymyositis, diaphoresis, **exfoliative dermatitis**, flushing, pemphigus, photosensitivity, pruritus, rash, urticaria
Other: Anaphylaxis, **angioedema**, **hyperkalemia**, **hyponatremia**

Nursing Considerations

- Use quinapril cautiously in patients with diabetes mellitus, renal impairment, or patients taking concomitant therapy with drugs that raise potassium levels. Monitor serum potassium levels, as ordered, in these patients and assess patient often for signs and symptoms of hyperkalemia.

WARNING Keep in mind patients with heart failure, hyponatremia, or severe salt or volume depletion; those who've recently received intensive diuresis or an increase in diuretic dosage; and those undergoing dialysis may be at risk for excessive hypotension. Monitor blood pressure often for first 2 weeks of therapy and whenever quinapril or diuretic dosage increases. If excessive hypotension occurs, notify prescriber immediately, place patient in a supine position, and, if prescribed, infuse normal saline solution.

WARNING Know that because of the risk of angioedema, be prepared to discontinue drug and administer emergency

measures, including subcutaneous epinephrine 1:1,000 (0.3 to 0.5 ml), if swelling of glottis, larynx, or tongue causes airway obstruction. Know that patients with a history of angioedema unrelated to ACE inhibitor therapy may be at increased risk of angioedema while receiving quinapril.
- Monitor patient's vital signs and cardiopulmonary status often to assess drug's effectiveness.

PATIENT TEACHING
- Instruct patient to notify prescriber immediately and stop taking quinapril if he has difficulty breathing or swallowing or he experiences swelling of the eyes, face, lips, or tongue.
- Explain that drug may cause dizziness and light-headedness, especially for first few days of therapy. Advise patient to avoid hazardous activities until drug's CNS effects are known and to notify prescriber if he faints.
- Inform women of childbearing age of risks of taking quinapril during pregnancy. Caution her to use effective contraception and to notify prescriber immediately of known or suspected pregnancy.
- Advise patient having surgery or receiving anesthesia to tell specialist that he takes quinapril.
- Instruct patient to consult prescriber before using potassium supplements or salt substitutes that contain potassium.

quinidine gluconate
quinidine sulfate

Class and Category
Pharmacologic class: Cinchona alkaloid
Therapeutic class: Class IA antiarrhythmic
Pregnancy category: C

Indications and Dosages
➤ *To restore normal sinus rhythm in patients with symptomatic atrial fibrillation or atrial flutter; to reduce frequency of relapse into atrial fibrillation or atrial flutter*

E.R. TABLETS (QUINIDINE GLUCONATE)
Adults. 324 to 648 mg every 8 to 12 hr. *Maximum:* 1,944 mg daily.

E.R. TABLETS (QUINIDINE SULFATE)
Adults. 300 every 8 to 12 hr with dosage cautiously increased if conversion not attained.

TABLETS (QUINIDINE SULFATE)
Adults. *Initial:* 400 mg every 6 hr with dosage cautiously increased if conversion not attained after 4 or 5 doses.

I.V. INFUSION (QUINIDINE GLUCONATE)
Adults. No faster than 0.25 mg/kg/min.

➤ *To treat life-threatening* Plasmodium falciparum *malaria*

I.V. INFUSION (QUINIDINE GLUCONATE)
Adults. *Loading dose:* 24 mg/kg in 250 ml of normal saline infused over 4 hr. *Maintenance:* 12 mg/kg infused over 4 hr every 8 hr, starting 8 hrs after the beginning of the loading dose for 7 days unless patient able to swallow, then dosage switched to oral form. Alternatively, *Loading dose:* 10/mg/kg in 250 ml of normal saline infused over 1 to 2 hr. *Maintenance:* 0.02 mg/kg/min for 72 hr or until parasitemia had decreased to 1% or less, whichever comes first.

Route	Onset	Peak	Duration
P.O.	Unknown	Unknown	6–8 hr
P.O. (E.R.)	Unknown	Unknown	12 hr
I.V.	Unknown	Unknown	Unknown

Mechanism of Action
Depresses conduction velocity, contractility, and excitability of the myocardium and increases the effective refractory period, thus suppressing arrhythmic activity in the atria, ventricles, and His-Purkinje system. In malaria, quinidine acts primarily as an intraerythrocytic schizonticide.

Contraindications
Digitalis toxicity; history of quinidine-induced thrombocytopenic purpura or torsades de pointes; hypersensitivity to quinidine, other cinchona derivatives, or their components; long-QT syndrome; myasthenia gravis; pacemaker-dependent conduction disturbances

Interactions

DRUGS

antiarrhythmics, phenothiazines, rauwolfia alkaloids: Additive cardiac effects
anticholinergics: Possibly intensified atropine-like adverse effects
antimyasthenics: Antagonized anti-myasthenic effects on skeletal muscle
barbiturates, rifampin: Possibly accelerated elimination and decreased effectiveness of quinidine
cimetidine: Increased elimination half-life, possibly leading to quinidine toxicity
digoxin: Possibly digitalis toxicity
hepatic enzyme inducers: Possibly decreased blood quinidine level
neuromuscular blockers: Possibly potentiated neuromuscular blockade
oral anticoagulants: Additive hypoprothrombinemia, increased risk of bleeding
pimozide: Risk of arrhythmias
quinine: Increased risk of quinidine toxicity
urinary alkalizers (such as antacids, carbonic anhydrase inhibitors, citrates, sodium bicarbonate, thiazide diuretics): Increased renal tubular reabsorption of quinidine, possibly leading to quinidine toxicity
verapamil: Possibly AV block, bradycardia, pulmonary edema, significant hypotension, and ventricular tachycardia

Adverse Reactions

CNS: Anxiety, asthenia, ataxia, confusion, delirium, difficulty speaking, dizziness, drowsiness, extrapyramidal reactions, fever, headache, hypertonia, syncope, vertigo
CV: **Complete heart block**, orthostatic hypotension, palpitations, peripheral edema, **prolonged QT interval**, **torsades de pointes**, vasculitis, **ventricular arrhythmias**, **widening QRS complex**
EENT: Blurred vision, change in color perception, diplopia, dry mouth, hearing loss (high-frequency), pharyngitis, photophobia, rhinitis, tinnitus
GI: Abdominal pain, anorexia, constipation, diarrhea, indigestion, nausea, vomiting
HEME: **Agranulocytosis**, **hemolytic anemia**, **leukopenia**, **neutropenia**, **thrombocytopenia**, **thrombocytopenic purpura**
MS: Arthralgia, myalgia
RESP: Dyspnea
SKIN: Diaphoresis, eczema, **exfoliative dermatitis**, flushing, hyperpigmentation, photosensitivity, pruritus, psoriasis, purpura, rash, urticaria
Other: **Angioedema**, flu-like symptoms, weight gain

Nursing Considerations

- For intermittent I.V. infusion, administer using an infusion pump at a rate of 0.25 mg/kg/min or less. Rapid administration may cause hypotension. Monitor blood pressure and ECG tracings throughout administration.
- Monitor therapeutic blood level of quinidine, as ordered.
- Monitor heart rate and rhythm closely because quinidine may cause serious adverse reactions and can be cardiotoxic, especially at dosages exceeding 2.4 g daily. Implement continuous cardiac monitoring, as ordered.
- Assess for early signs and symptoms of cinchonism, including blurred vision, change in color perception, confusion, diplopia, headache, and tinnitus, which may indicate quinidine toxicity.

PATIENT TEACHING

- Advise patient to take quinidine at the same times every day and at evenly spaced intervals.
- Instruct patient to swallow E.R. tablets whole, with a full glass of water, preferably while sitting upright.
- Advise patient to take drug with food if GI upset occurs.
- Urge patient to inform prescriber immediately of blurred or double vision, change in color perception, confusion, diarrhea, fever, headache, loss of hearing, or tinnitus.

rabeprazole sodium

AcipHex, AcipHex Sprinkle

Class and Category

Pharmacologic class: Proton pump inhibitor
Therapeutic class: Antiulcer
Pregnancy category: C

Indications and Dosages

➤ *To provide short-term treatment of erosive esophagitis or ulcerative gastroesophageal reflux disease (GERD)*

DELAYED-RELEASE TABLETS

Adults and adolescents age 12 and over. 20 mg daily for 4 to 8 wk; course may be repeated if healing has not occurred at the end of 8 wk.

➤ *To treat symptomatic GERD*

DELAYED-RELEASE TABLETS

Adults and adolescents age 12 and over. 20 mg daily for 4 wk. Course may be repeated if symptoms aren't completely resolved.

DELAYED-RELEASE CAPSULES (ACIPHEX SPRINKLE)

Children ages 1 to 11 weighing 15 kg (33 lb) or more. 10 mg once daily 30 min before a meal for up to 12 wk.

Children ages 1 to 11 weighing less than 15 kg (33 lb). 5 mg once daily 30 min before a meal up to 12 wk. Increased to 10 mg once daily, as needed.

➤ *To provide maintenance treatment of erosive esophagitis or GERD*

DELAYED-RELEASE TABLETS

Adults and adolescents age 12 and over. 20 mg daily for no longer than 12 months.

➤ *To promote healing of duodenal ulcer*

DELAYED-RELEASE TABLETS

Adults and adolescents age 12 and over. 20 mg daily after breakfast for up to 4 wk.

➤ *As adjunct to reduce the risk of duodenal ulcer recurrence by eradicating* Helicobacter pylori

DELAYED-RELEASE TABLETS

Adults and adolescents age 12 and over. 20 mg twice daily with morning and evening meals in conjunction with amoxicillin 1,000 mg and clarithromycin 500 mg twice daily for 7 days.

➤ *To treat hypersecretory conditions, such as Zollinger–Ellison syndrome*

DELAYED-RELEASE TABLETS

Adults and adolescents age 12 and over. *Initial:* 60 mg daily; may be increased, if needed, to 100 mg daily or 60 mg twice daily.

Mechanism of Action

Decreases gastric acid secretion by suppressing its release at the secretory surface of gastric parietal cells. Rabeprazole also increases gastric pH and decreases basal acid output, which helps to heal ulcerated areas. In gastric parietal cells, it's transformed to an active sulfonamide, which increases the clearance rate of *H. pylori.*

Contraindications

Concurrent therapy with rilpivirine-containing products; hypersensitivity to rabeprazole, other substituted benzimidazoles (lansoprazole, omeprazole), or their components

Interactions

DRUGS

atazanavir, nelfinavir, rilpivirine: Decreased exposure of these antiretrovirals with possible decreased antiviral effect and increased development of drug resistance
clarithromycin: Increased risk of serious adverse reactions, including possibly fatal arrhythmias
cyclosporine: Possibly inhibited cyclosporine metabolism
dasatinib, erlotinib, iron salts, itraconazole, ketoconazole, mycophenolate mofetil, nilotinib: Reduced absorption of these drugs decreasing effectiveness
digoxin: Increased risk of digitalis toxicity
methotrexate: Increased risk of methotrexate toxicities
saquinavir: Increased exposure resulting in possible increased toxicity
tacrolimus: Possibly increased exposure of tacrolimus, especially in transplant patients who are intermediate or poor metabolizers of CYP2C19
warfarin: Possibly increased prothrombin time (PT), international normalized ratio (INR)

Adverse Reactions

CNS: Coma, delirium, disorientation, dizziness, headache, malaise, vertigo
EENT: Blurred vision
ENDO: Elevated TSH levels
GI: Abdominal pain, ***Clostridium difficile*-associated diarrhea**, diarrhea, fundic gland polyps, jaundice, nausea, vomiting
GU: Interstitial nephritis
HEME: Agranulocytosis, hemolytic anemia, leukopenia, pancytopenia, thrombocytopenia
MS: Bone fracture, **rhabdomyolysis**
RESP: Bronchospasm, interstitial pneumonia

SKIN: Cutaneous lupus erythematosus, bullous and other drug skin eruptions, **erythema multiforme**, rash, **Stevens–Johnson syndrome, toxic epidermal necrolysis,** urticaria
Other: Anaphylaxis, angioedema, hyperammonemia, hypomagnesemia, systemic lupus erythematosus, vitamin B_{12} deficiency (long-term use)

Nursing Considerations

- Use rabeprazole cautiously in patients with hepatic dysfunction.
- Obtain a serum magnesium level, as ordered, prior to starting rabeprazole therapy for those patients expected to be on prolonged therapy or who also take digoxin or drugs that may cause hypomagnesemia such as diuretics when taken with rabeprazole.
- Expect to monitor serum gastrin level in long-term therapy to detect elevation.
- Closely monitor Japanese men receiving rabeprazole for adverse reactions because they're more likely than other patients to have increased blood drug levels.
- Be aware that symptomatic response to rabeprazole therapy does not preclude the presence of a gastric tumor. Expect patients who have a suboptimal response or an early symptomatic relapse after completing rabeprazole therapy to have further diagnostic testing done.
- Monitor patient for bone fracture, especially in patient receiving multiple daily doses for more than a year because proton pump inhibitors like rabeprazole increase risk of osteoporosis-related fractures of the hip, wrist, and spine.
- Monitor patient for diarrhea because diarrhea including *C. difficile*-associated diarrhea may occur with rabeprazole therapy. Notify prescriber if persistent or severe diarrhea develops.
- Monitor patient's magnesium level, as ordered during therapy, because hypomagnesemia may occur with rabeprazole therapy that has lasted longer than 3 months, although most cases have occurred after therapy had been given for more than a year. Notify prescriber if magnesium level drops below normal, as hypomagnesemia may cause tetany, arrhythmias, and seizures. Expect patient to receive magnesium replacement and drug to be discontinued.
- Monitor patient for arthralgia and rash, as rabeprazole may cause either cutaneous or systemic lupus erythematosus in patients as a new onset or an exacerbation of the existing autoimmune disease. Know that proton pump inhibitors like rabeprazole should not be given longer than necessary. If patient becomes symptomatic, notify prescriber. If confirmed, expect drug to be discontinued. Know that most patients improve within 12 weeks after drug is discontinued.
- Be aware that rabeprazole may produce false readings on the following tests: secretin stimulation test assessing for gastrinoma and serum chromogranin levels assessing for neuroendocrine tumors; these require rabeprazole to be withheld for at least 14 days before tests are performed. Urine tests for tetrahydrocannabinol may result in a false-positive result.

PATIENT TEACHING

- Tell patient to take rabeprazole 30 minutes before a meal.
- Instruct patient to swallow delayed-release rabeprazole tablets whole and not to chew, crush, or split tablets.
- Instruct parents whose child is prescribed delayed-release capsules to make sure that child swallows capsule whole and does not chew or crush granules. If patient is unable to swallow capsule, tell parents that delayed-release capsules may be opened and contents may be sprinkled on a small amount of soft food such, as applesauce or yogurt. Contents may also be emptied into a small amount of liquid, such as apple juice, infant formula, or pediatric electrolyte solution. The dose should be taken within 15 minutes of preparation. Remind parents that food or liquid used to mix granules in should be at or below room temperature. Unused mixture should be discarded.
- Instruct patient to notify prescriber immediately if he develops new or worsening joint pain or a rash on his arms or cheeks that gets worse in the sun.
- Inform patients with hypersecretory conditions, such as Zollinger–Ellison syndrome, that treatment can last for a year or longer.

- Tell patient to notify prescriber immediately if he experiences a decrease in the amount of urine voided or if urine has blood in it.
- Advise patient to contact prescriber if he develops persistent or severe diarrhea that is accompanied by abdominal pain and fever.
- Instruct patient to notify prescriber of any persistent, severe, or unusual adverse reactions.
- Tell patient to inform all prescribers of rabeprazole therapy.
- Inform patient that vitamin B_{12} deficiency may occur if drug is taken longer than 3 years.

raloxifene hydrochloride
(keoxifene hydrochloride)

Evista

Class and Category
Pharmacologic class: Selective estrogen receptor modulator (ISERM)
Therapeutic class: Antiosteoporotic
Pregnancy category: X

Indications and Dosages
➤ *To prevent osteoporosis in postmenopausal women; to reduce risk of invasive breast cancer in postmenopausal women with osteoporosis; to reduce risk of invasive breast cancer in postmenopausal women at high risk*

TABLETS

Adults. 60 mg daily.

Mechanism of Action
Prevents osteoporosis by binding to estrogen receptors, which decreases bone resorption and increases bone mineral density in postmenopausal women. May reduce risk of invasive breast cancer because of its binding effects on estrogen receptors.

Contraindications
History of thromboembolic disease, hypersensitivity to raloxifene or its components, pregnancy

Interactions
DRUGS

ampicillin, cholestyramine: Decreased raloxifene absorption
warfarin: Possibly decreased PT

Adverse Reactions
CNS: CVA, depression, fever, insomnia, migraine
CV: Chest pain, hot flashes, peripheral edema, **thromboembolism**, thrombophlebitis
EENT: Laryngitis, pharyngitis, sinusitis
ENDO: Hot flashes
GI: Abdominal pain, cholelithiasis, flatulence, indigestion, nausea, vomiting
GU: Cystitis, infertility, leukorrhea, UTI, vaginitis
MS: Arthralgia, arthritis, leg cramps or spasms, myalgia
RESP: Cough, pneumonia, **pulmonary embolism**
SKIN: Diaphoresis, rash
Other: Flu-like symptoms, weight gain

Nursing Considerations
- Be aware that raloxifene should not be used in premenopausal women.
- Use cautiously in patients who smoke or have a history of atrial fibrillation, hypertension stroke, or TIA because raloxifene may increase the risk of stroke.
- Use cautiously in patients with renal impairment because effects of raloxifene on renal system are unknown.

WARNING Monitor patient's limbs for impaired circulation and pain (possible thromboembolism).

- Expect prescriber to stop drug at least 72 hours before and during periods of prolonged immobilization. Resume raloxifene therapy as prescribed after patient is fully ambulatory.

PATIENT TEACHING

- Advise patient to avoid lengthy immobility during travel while taking raloxifene because of the increased risk of thromboembolism.
- Instruct patient to report adverse reactions to prescriber immediately, especially coughing up blood, leg pain or swelling, shortness of breath, a sudden change in vision, or sudden chest pain.
- Emphasize the importance of compliance with long-term raloxifene therapy.

- Advise patient that postmenopausal women require an average of 1,500 mg of elemental calcium and 400 to 800 international units of vitamin D daily. Vitamin D requirement is increased in women who are chronically ill or nursing-home bound, women with GI malabsorption syndromes, and women over age 70. Review dietary sources of calcium and vitamin D, and have patient discuss supplements with prescriber, as needed.

raltegravir

Isentress, Isentress HD

Class and Category

Pharmacologic class: HIV integrase strand transfer inhibitor
Therapeutic class: Antiretroviral
Pregnancy category: Not classified

Indications and Dosages

➤ *As adjunct to treat human immunodeficiency virus (HIV-1) infection*

CHEWABLE TABLETS, TABLETS

Adults who are treatment-naïve or who are virologically suppressed on an initial regimen of raltegravir of 400 mg twice daily. 1,200 mg once daily if using 600-mg film-coated tablets or 400 mg twice daily if using 400-mg film-coated tablets.
Adults who are treatment-experienced. 400 mg twice daily using 400-mg film-coated tablets.
Adults who are treatment-experienced or treatment-naïve and taking rifampin concomitantly. 800 mg twice daily using 400-mg film-coated tablets.
Children weighing at least 40 kg (88 lb), who are 4 weeks of age and over, and are treatment-naïve or virologically suppressed on an initial regimen of raltegravir 400 mg twice daily. 1,200 mg once daily using 600-mg film-coated tablets, 400 mg twice daily using 400-mg film-coated tablets, or 300 mg twice daily using chewable tablets.

CHEWABLE TABLETS, TABLETS

Children who weigh at least 28 kg (61.6 lb) but less than 40 kg (88 lb) and are 4 weeks of age and over. 400 mg twice daily using 400-mg film-coated tablets or 200 mg twice daily using chewable tablets.
Children who weigh at least 25 kg (55 lb) but less than 28 kg (61.6 lb)and are 4 weeks of age and over. 400 mg twice daily using 400-mg film-coated tablets or 150 mg twice daily using chewable tablets.

CHEWABLE TABLETS

Children who weigh 20 kg (44 lb) to less than 25 kg (55 lb) and are 4 weeks of age and over. 150 mg twice daily.

CHEWABLE TABLETS, ORAL SUSPENSION

Children who weigh 14 kg (30.8 lb) to less than 20 kg (44 lb) and are 4 weeks of age and over. 100 mg twice daily.
Children who weigh 11 kg (24.2 lb) to less than 20 kg (44 lb) and are 4 weeks of age and over. 75 mg twice daily using chewable tablets or 80 mg twice daily using oral suspension.

ORAL SUSPENSION

Children who weigh 8 kg (17.6 lb) to less than 11 (24.2 lb) and are 4 weeks of age and over. 60 mg twice daily.
Children who weigh 6 kg (13.2 lb) to less than 8 kg (17.6 lb) and are 4 weeks of age and over. 40 mg twice daily.
Children who weigh 4 kg (8.8 lb) to less than 6 kg (13.2 lb) and are 4 weeks of age and over. 30 mg twice daily.
Children who weigh 3 kg (6.6 lb) to less than 4 kg (8.8 kg) and are 4 weeks of age and over. 20 mg twice daily.
Neonates age 1 to 4 weeks weighing 4 kg (8.8 lb) to less than 5 kg (11 lb). 15 mg twice daily.
Neonates age 1 to 4 weeks weighing 3 kg (6.6 lb) to less than 4 kg (8.8 kg). 10 mg twice daily.
Neonates age 1 to 4 weeks weighing 2 kg (4.4 lb) to less than 3 kg (6.6 lb). 8 mg twice daily.
Neonates age birth to 1 week weighing 4 kg (8.8 lb) to less than 5 kg (11 lb). 7 mg once daily.
Neonates age birth to 1 week weighing 3 kg (6.6 lb) to less than 4 kg (8.8 lb). 5 mg once daily.
Neonates age birth to 1 week weighing 2 kg (4.4 lb) to less than 3 kg (6.6 lb). 4 mg once daily.
Note: If the mother has taken raltegravir 2 to 24 hours before delivery, then the

neonate, age birth to 4 weeks, should be given the first dose, regardless of weight, between 24 and 48 hr after birth.

Mechanism of Action

Inhibits HIV integrase by binding to the integrase active site and blocking the strand transfer step of retroviral DNA integration, which is needed for the HIV replication cycle.

Contraindications

Hypersensitivity to raltegravir or its components

Interactions

DRUGS

aluminum- and/or magnesium-containing antacids, calcium carbonate antacid, carbamazepine, etravirine, phenobarbital, phenytoin, rifampin: Decrease in plasma concentration of raltegravir and its effectiveness

Adverse Reactions

CNS: Abnormal dreams, asthenia, cerebellar ataxia, depression, dizziness, fatigue, fever, headaches, insomnia, malaise, nightmares, paranoia, **suicidal ideation**
CV: Elevated cholesterol and triglycerides
EENT: Conjunctivitis
ENDO: Hyperglycemia
GI: Abdominal pain, anorexia, bilirubin increase, diarrhea, dyspepsia, elevated liver and pancreatic enzymes, flatulence, gastritis, **hepatic failure**, **hepatitis**, nausea, vomiting
GU: Genital herpes, nephrolithiasis, **renal failure**
HEME: Decreased hemoglobin count, **neutropenia**, **thrombocytopenia**
MS: Elevated creatine kinase, myopathy, **rhabdomyolysis**
SKIN: Blisters, rash, **Stevens–Johnson syndrome**, **toxic epidermal necrolysis**
Other: **Angioedema**, herpes zoster, **hypersensitivity reactions**, immune reconstitution syndrome

Nursing Considerations

- Ask patient before starting raltegravir therapy if he has ever experienced an elevated creatine kinase level, myopathy, or rhabdomyolysis or is taking any drugs known to cause these conditions (such as fenofibrate, gemfibrozil, statins, or zidovudine), because drug may increase risk of developing these conditions.
- Know that chewable tablets and oral suspension cannot be substituted for the 400-mg or 800-mg film-coated tablets, because the formulations have different pharmacokinetic profiles.
- Be aware that raltegravir should not be given before dialysis, because the extent to which the drug is dialyzable is unknown.
- Mix oral suspension form by pouring packet contents into 5 ml of water and mixing. Once mixed, measure the recommended dose with a syringe and administer within 30 minutes of mixing. Discard any remaining suspension.

WARNING Monitor patient closely for severe skin reactions. Notify prescriber and expect raltegravir to be discontinued immediately if patient develops a rash that is accompanied by angioedema, blisters, conjunctivitis, eosinophilia, facial edema, fatigue, fever, joint or muscle aches, lip swelling, malaise, or oral lesions. Be aware that a delay in discontinuing drug may result in a life-threatening situation.

- Be aware that immune reconstitution syndrome has occurred in patients treated with combination antiretroviral therapy, including raltegravir. The inflammatory response predisposes susceptible patients to opportunistic infections such as cytomegalovirus, *Mycobacterium avium* infection, *Pneumocystis jiroveci* pneumonia, or tuberculosis. Autoimmune disorders such as Graves' disease, Guillain–Barré syndrome, or polymyositis have also occurred. Report sudden or unusual adverse reactions to prescriber.

PATIENT TEACHING

- Advise patient to avoid missing doses of raltegravir, as it can result in the development of resistance to the drug. If he misses a dose, he should take it as soon as he remembers, but should not double the next dose or take more than prescribed.
- Instruct patient to swallow film-coated tablets whole; chewable tablets may be swallowed whole or chewed.
- Tell patient or parents, if patient is prescribed oral suspension form, to pour

packet into 5 ml of water and mix. Dosage of drug should be measured with a syringe and administered within 30 minutes of mixing. Any leftover suspension should be discarded.

- Alert patient or parents that chewable tablet form contains phenylalanine and can be harmful to patients with phenylketonuria.

WARNING Inform patient to seek immediate medical attention if a rash develops or other signs and symptoms that are new, persistent, or severe appear, including evidence of an infection.

- Advise female patient to alert prescriber if pregnancy is suspected or has occurred and encourage her to register with the Antiretroviral Pregnancy Registry by calling 1-800-258-4263.
- Inform mothers that breastfeeding is not recommended during raltegravir therapy.
- Instruct patient to immediately report any unexplained muscle pain, tenderness, or weakness.

ramelteon

Rozerem

Class and Category

Pharmacologic class: Melatonin receptor agonist
Therapeutic class: Hypnotic
Pregnancy category: C

Indications and Dosages

➤ *To treat insomnia in patients having difficulty falling asleep*

TABLETS

Adults. 8 mg 30 min before at bedtime.

Route	Onset	Peak	Duration
P.O.	Unknown	0.5–1.5 hr	Unknown

Mechanism of Action

Binds to melatonin receptors MT1 and MT2 in the suprachiasmatic nucleus (SCN) of the hypothalamus. The SCN regulates the sleep–wake cycle, and endogenous melatonin probably is involved in maintaining the circadian rhythm underlying that cycle.

Contraindications

Concurrent therapy with fluvoxamine, history of angioedema with previous ramelteon treatment, hypersensitivity to ramelteon or its components, severe hepatic dysfunction

Interactions

DRUGS

benzodiazepines, melatonin, other sedative-hypnotics: Possible additive sedative effects
donepezil, doxepin, fluconazole, fluvoxamine, ketoconazole: Increased plasma ramelteon levels
rifampin: Decreased ramelteon effectiveness

ACTIVITIES

alcohol use: Possibly additive CNS effect

Adverse Reactions

CNS: Agitation, amnesia, anxiety, bizarre behavior, complex behaviors such as sleep driving, depression, dizziness, fatigue, hallucinations, headache, insomnia exacerbation, mania, somnolence, **suicidal ideation**
EENT: Throat tightness
ENDO: Decreased testosterone level, increased prolactin level
GI: Diarrhea, dysgeusia, nausea, vomiting
MS: Arthralgia, myalgia
RESP: Dyspnea, upper respiratory tract infection
Other: Anaphylaxis, angioedema

Nursing Considerations

- Be aware that ramelteon therapy is not recommended for patients with COPD or severe sleep apnea because its effects have not been studied in these patient populations.
- Use cautiously in patients with mild-to-moderate hepatic dysfunction. Drug is contraindicated in severe hepatic dysfunction.
- Ramelteon is the first approved hypnotic not classified as a controlled substance.

WARNING Monitor patient closely for hypersensitivity reactions such as dyspnea, nausea, swelling, throat tightness, and vomiting. If present, discontinue ramelteon immediately, notify prescriber, and provide supportive care.

- Watch patient closely for suicidal tendencies, particularly when therapy starts and dosage changes, because depression may worsen temporarily during these times, possibly leading to suicidal ideation.

PATIENT TEACHING

- Instruct patient not to take ramelteon with or immediately after eating a high-fat meal.
- Caution patient to avoid potentially hazardous activities after taking ramelteon; drug's intended effect is to decrease alertness.
- Advise patient that drug may cause abnormal behaviors during sleep, such as driving a car, eating, having sex, or talking on the phone without any recall of the event. If family members notice any such behavior or patient sees evidence of such behavior upon awakening, prescriber should be notified.
- Advise limiting alcohol during therapy.
- Tell patient to notify prescriber if insomnia worsens or new signs or symptoms occur.
- Inform patient that drug may affect reproductive hormones; urge patient to report cessation of menses or galactorrhea (females) or decreased libido or problems with infertility.
- Advise mothers who are breastfeeding while taking ramelteon to monitor infant for signs of feeding problems and sedation. Tell her to consider pumping and discarding breast milk during treatment and for 25 hours after ramelteon administration, to minimize drug exposure of her infant.
- Urge family or caregiver to watch patient closely for suicidal tendencies, especially when therapy starts or dosage changes.

ramipril

Altace

Class and Category

Pharmacologic class: Angiotensin converting enzyme (ACE) inhibitor
Therapeutic class: Antihypertensive
Pregnancy category: D

Indications and Dosages

➤ *To treat heart failure after MI*

CAPSULES

Adults. *Initial:* 2.5 mg twice daily with dose decreased to 1.25 mg twice daily if hypotension occurs. Dosage increased, as needed, about every 3 wk to maintenance dose. *Maintenance:* 5 mg twice daily.

➤ *To reduce risk of MI or stroke and death from cardiovascular causes*

CAPSULES

Adults age 55 and over. *Initial:* 2.5 mg once daily for 1 wk, followed by 5 mg once daily for 3 wk, and then increased, as tolerated to 10 mg once daily.

➤ *To treat hypertension*

CAPSULES

Adults not taking a diuretic. *Initial:* 2.5 mg daily. *Maintenance:* 2.5 to 20 mg once daily or in divided doses twice daily.

DOSAGE ADJUSTMENT For patients dehydrated from diuretics, those receiving diuretics, and those with creatinine clearance less than 40 ml/min; initial dosage reduced to 1.25 mg daily and then slowly increased until blood pressure is under control or maximum daily dose of 5 mg is reached. For patients with heart failure post myocardial infarction, who cannot tolerate the initial dosage of 2.5 mg, once daily dosage reduced to 1.25 mg daily. For patients who are hypertensive or had recent post myocardial infarction, daily dose may be given in divided doses to reduce risk of MI, stroke, or death from cardiovascular causes.

Route	Onset	Peak	Duration
P.O.	1–2 hr	4–6.5 hr	24 hr

Mechanism of Action

Blocks conversion of angiotensin I to angiotensin II, causing vasodilation, and reduces aldosterone secretion, which prevents water retention. Ramipril also reduces peripheral arterial resistance. Combined, these actions reduce blood pressure.

Contraindications

Aliskiren therapy in patients with diabetes or patients with renal impairment (GRF less than 60 ml/min); history of angioedema; hypersensitivity to ramipril, its components, or any other ACE inhibitors; use of neprilysin inhibitor such as sacubitril within 36 hours

Interactions

DRUGS

aliskiren (patients with diabetes and/or renal impairment), angiotensin receptor blockers, other ACE inhibitors: Increased risk of hyperkalemia, hypotension, and renal dysfunction
allopurinol, bone marrow depressants, corticosteroids (systemic), procainamide: Increased risk of fatal agranulocytosis or neutropenia
CNS depressants, other hypotension-producing drugs: Additive hypotensive effect
potassium preparations, potassium-sparing diuretics: Possibly hyperkalemia
insulin, oral antidiabetics: Increased risk of hypoglycemia
lithium: Increased risk of lithium toxicity
mTOR inhibitors such as temsirolimus, neprilysin inhibitor such as sacubitril: Increased risk of angioedema
NSAIDs: Decreased antihypertensive effect of ramipril; increased risk of renal dysfunction in the elderly and patients with preexisting renal dysfunction or volume depletion
sodium aurothiomalate: Increased risk of nitritoid reaction (facial flushing, hypotension, nausea, vomiting)
sympathomimetics: Decreased anti-hypertensive effect of ramipril
telmisartan: Possibly increased risk of adverse effects, especially renal dysfunction
tetracyclines: Reduced tetracycline absorption

FOODS

potassium-rich foods such as milk and potatoes, potassium-containing salt substitutes: Increased risk of hyperkalemia

ACTIVITIES

alcohol use: Additive hypotensive effects

Adverse Reactions

CNS: Depression, dizziness, drowsiness, fatigue, fever, headache, insomnia, light-headedness, malaise, paresthesia, sleep disturbance, syncope, vertigo
CV: Chest pain, **hypotension**, orthostatic hypotension, palpitations, tachycardia
EENT: Amblyopia, dry mouth, loss of taste, pharyngitis
GI: Abdominal pain, constipation, diarrhea, elevated liver enzymes, jaundice, **hepatic failure**, **hepatitis**, nausea, vomiting
GU: Acute renal failure, elevated BUN and serum creatinine levels, impotence, oliguria, **progressive azotemia**
HEME: Agranulocytosis, anemia, **bone marrow depression**, **pancytopenia**
MS: Arthralgia, back pain, myalgia
RESP: Cough, dyspnea
SKIN: Alopecia, diaphoresis, flushing, onycholysis, pemphigoid, photosensitivity, pruritus, rash, **Stevens–Johnson syndrome**, **toxic epidermal necrolysis**, urticaria
Other: Anaphylaxis, **angioedema**, **hyperkalemia**

Nursing Considerations

- Use ramipril cautiously in patients with renal or hepatic impairment.
- Monitor patient's serum potassium level, as ordered, and assess often for signs and symptoms of hyperkalemia, especially in patients with diabetes mellitus or renal insufficiency and those taking concomitantly other drugs that raise serum potassium levels.

WARNING Keep in mind patients with dehydration, heart failure, or hyponatremia; those who've recently received intensive diuresis or an increase in diuretic dosage; and those having dialysis may risk excessive hypotension. Monitor such patients closely the first 2 weeks of therapy and whenever ramipril or diuretic dosage increases. If excessive hypotension occurs, notify prescriber immediately, place patient in a supine position, and, if prescribed, infuse normal saline solution.

WARNING Know that because of the risk of angioedema, be prepared to stop drug and provide emergency measures, including subcutaneous epinephrine 1:1,000 (0.3 to 0.5 ml), if swelling of glottis, larynx, or tongue causes airway obstruction.

- Monitor blood pressure frequently during therapy to assess drug's effectiveness.
- Monitor patient's hepatic and renal function closely during therapy. If patient develops jaundice or marked elevations

of hepatic enzymes, notify prescriber and expect ramipril to be discontinued.

PATIENT TEACHING

- Advise patient to stop taking ramipril and inform prescriber immediately if she experiences difficulty breathing or swallowing or develops swelling of the eyes, face, lips, or tongue.
- Explain that drug may cause dizziness and light-headedness, especially during first few days of therapy. Instruct patient to notify prescriber immediately if she has fainting episode.
- Inform female patient of childbearing age of the risks of taking ramipril during pregnancy. Caution patient to use effective contraception and to report known or suspected pregnancy immediately.
- Urge patient to tell providers that she takes ramipril before having surgery or receiving anesthesia.
- Tell patient to ask prescriber before using supplements or salt substitutes that contain potassium.

ranitidine hydrochloride

Nu-Ranit (CAN), Zantac, Zantac EFFERdose

Class and Category

Pharmacologic class: H_2-receptor antagonist
Therapeutic class: Antiulcer agent, gastric acid secretion inhibitor
Pregnancy category: B

Indications and Dosages

➤ *To provide short-term treatment of active duodenal and benign gastric ulcers*

CAPSULES, EFFERVESCENT GRANULES, EFFERVESCENT TABLETS, SYRUP, TABLETS

Adults. 150 mg twice daily for gastric ulcers for 6 wks; 150 mg twice daily or 300 mg at bedtime for duodenal ulcers for 8 wks.
Children ages 1 month to 16 years. 2 to 4 mg/kg twice daily up to 300 mg daily. *Maintenance:* 2 to 4 mg/kg daily up to 150 mg daily.

CONTINUOUS I.V. INFUSION

Adults. 6.25 mg/hr over 24 hr. *Maximum:* 400 mg daily.
Children ages 1 month to 16 years. 2 to 4 mg/kg daily.

INTERMITTENT I.V. INFUSION

Adults and adolescents. 50 mg diluted to total volume of 100 ml and infused over 15 to 20 min every 6 to 8 hr. *Maximum:* 400 mg daily.
Children. 2 to 4 mg/kg daily diluted to a suitable volume and infused over 15 to 20 min given in divided doses every 6 to 8 hr. *Maximum:* 50 mg/dose.

I.V. INJECTION

Adults. 50 mg diluted up to 2.5 mg/ml and injected slowly at a rate of up to 4 ml/min every 6 to 8 hr. *Maximum:* 400 mg daily.

I.M. INJECTION

Adults. 50 mg every 6 to 8 hr. *Maximum:* 400 mg daily.

➤ *To treat acute gastroesophageal reflux disease*

CAPSULES, EFFERVESCENT GRANULES, EFFERVESCENT TABLETS, SYRUP, TABLETS

Adults. 150 mg twice daily.
Children ages 1 month to 16 years. 2.5 to 5 mg/kg twice daily.

➤ *To treat erosive esophagitis*

CAPSULES, EFFERVESCENT GRANULES, EFFERVESCENT TABLETS, SYRUP, TABLETS

Adults. 150 mg four times a day.
Children ages 1 month to 16 years. 2.5 to 5 mg/kg twice daily.

➤ *To treat hypersecretory GI conditions, such as Zollinger–Ellison syndrome, systemic mastocytosis, and multiple endocrine adenoma syndrome*

CAPSULES, EFFERVESCENT GRANULES, EFFERVESCENT TABLETS, SYRUP, TABLETS

Adults. *Initial:* 150 mg twice daily, adjusted as needed. *Maximum:* 6 g daily in divided doses.

CONTINUOUS I.V. INFUSION

Adults and adolescents. *Initial:* 1 mg/kg/hr, increased by 0.5 mg/kg/hr up to 2.5 mg/kg/hr, as needed.

➤ *To prevent acid indigestion, heartburn, and sour stomach caused by eating certain foods or drinking certain beverages*

TABLETS

Adults and adolescents. 75 to 150 mg 30 to 60 min before food or beverages expected to cause symptoms. *Maximum:* 150 mg daily over no more than 2 continuous wk.

➤ *To treat acid indigestion, heartburn, and sour stomach*

TABLETS

Adults and adolescents. 75 to 150 mg when symptoms start; repeated once within 24 hr, if needed.

DOSAGE ADJUSTMENT For patients whose creatinine clearance is less than 50 ml/min 150 mg P.O. every 24 hr with dosage interval increased thereafter to every 12 hr, as needed. Or 50 mg I.V. every 18 to 24 hr with dosage interval increased to every 12 hr, as needed.

Route	Onset	Peak	Duration
P.O., I.V., I.M.	Unknown	1–3 hr	13 hr

Mechanism of Action

Inhibits basal and nocturnal secretion of gastric acid and pepsin by competitively inhibiting the action of histamine at H_2 receptors on gastric parietal cells. This action reduces total volume of gastric juices and, thus, irritation of GI mucosa.

Contraindications

Acute porphyria, hypersensitivity to ranitidine or its components

Interactions

DRUGS

antacids: Decreased ranitidine absorption
atazanavir, delavirdine, diazepam, gefitinib, itraconazole, ketoconazole, sucralfate: Decreased absorption of these drugs
bone marrow depressants: Increased risk of neutropenia or other blood dyscrasias
glipizide, glyburide, metoprolol, midazolam, nifedipine, phenytoin, theophylline, triazolam: Increased effects of these drugs, possibly leading to toxic reactions
procainamide: Possibly increased risk of procainamide toxicity
warfarin: Possibly altered PT

ACTIVITIES

alcohol use: Increased blood alcohol level (with oral ranitidine)

Adverse Reactions

CNS: Dizziness, drowsiness, fever, headache, insomnia
CV: Vasculitis
GI: Abdominal distress, constipation, diarrhea, nausea, vomiting
GU: Acute interstitial nephritis, impotence
MS: Arthralgia, myalgia
RESP: Bronchospasm
SKIN: Alopecia, **erythema multiforme,** rash
Other: Anaphylaxis, angioedema

Nursing Considerations

- Be aware that ranitidine must be diluted for I.V. use if not using premixed solution. For I.V. injection, dilute to total of 20 ml with normal saline solution, D_5W, $D_{10}W$, lactated Ringer's solution, or 5% sodium bicarbonate. For I.V. infusion, dilute to total volume of 100 ml of same solutions.
- Give I.V. injection at no more than 4 ml/min, intermittent I.V. infusion at 5 to 7 ml/min, and continuous I.V. infusion at 6.25 mg/hr (except with hypersecretory conditions, when initial infusion rate is 1 mg/kg/hr, gradually increased after 4 hours, as needed, in increments of 0.5 mg/kg/hr).
- Don't add additives to premixed solution.
- Stop primary I.V. solution infusion during piggyback administration.

PATIENT TEACHING

- Tell patient to dissolve 150-mg effervescent tablets or granules in 6 to 8 oz water or 25-mg effervescent tablets in at least 5 ml water.
- Advise patient (or parent) to wait until effervescent tablet is completely dissolved before taking (or giving to child or infant).
- Caution patient not to chew effervescent tablets, let them dissolve on the tongue, or swallow them whole.
- Alert patients with phenylketonuria that effervescent granules and tablets contain phenylalanine.
- Tell patient that she may take drug with food.
- Tell patient to stop taking ranitidine and contact prescriber if she passes black or bloody stools, has trouble swallowing, or vomits blood.
- Advise patient to take antacids, 2 hours before or after ranitidine; advise against taking other acid reducers with drug.
- Instruct patient taking drug to prevent heartburn, to contact prescriber about frequent chest pain or wheezing with heartburn; stomach pain; unexplained weight loss; nausea; vomiting; heartburn lasting more than 3 months; heartburn with light-headedness, dizziness, or sweating;

chest or shoulder pain with shortness of breath, sweating, light-headedness, or pain spreading to arms, neck, or shoulders. These problems may be serious.
- Inform patient that healing of an ulcer may require 4 to 8 weeks of therapy.

ranolazine

Ranexa

Class and Category

Pharmacologic class: Cardiac agent
Therapeutic class: Antianginal
Pregnancy category: C

Indications and Dosages

➤ *To treat chronic angina*

E.R. TABLETS

Adults. *Initial:* 500 mg twice daily, increased to 1,000 mg twice daily, as needed. *Maximum:* 1,000 mg twice daily.
DOSAGE ADJUSTMENT For patients taking a moderate CYP3A inhibitor, such as diltiazem, erythromycin, or verapamil, maximum dosage reduced to 500 mg twice daily. For patients taking P-gp inhibitors, such as cyclosporine, dosage may need to be reduced.

Route	Onset	Peak	Duration
P.O.	Unknown	2–5 hr	Unknown

Mechanism of Action

Exerts antianginal and anti-ischemic effects by an unknown mechanism not dependent on reductions in blood pressure or heart rate. Ranolazine inhibits cardiac late sodium current, but how this action inhibits angina symptoms is also unknown.

Contraindications

Hypersensitivity to ranolazine or its components, liver cirrhosis, use of CYP3A inducers or strong inhibitors

Interactions

DRUGS

CYP2D6 such as antipsychotics, metoprolol, tricyclic antidepressants: Increased plasma levels of these drugs
CYP3A inducers, such as carbamazepine, phenobarbital, phenytoin, rifabutin, rifampin, rifapentine, St. John's wort: Decreased blood ranolazine level and decreased effectiveness
CYP3A substrates, such as cyclosporine, lovastatin, simvastatin, sirolimus, tacrolimus: Possibly increased blood levels of these drugs
CYP3A inhibitors, such as clarithromycin, diltiazem, erythromycin, fluconazole, indinavir, itraconazole, ketoconazole, nefazodone, nelfinavir, ritonavir, saquinavir, verapamil: Increased blood ranolazine level and increased risk of adverse reactions
digoxin: Increased blood digoxin level

ACTIVITIES

grapefruit juice, grapefruit containing products: Increased blood ranolazine level and increased risk of adverse reactions

Adverse Reactions

CNS: Abnormal coordination, asthenia, confusion, dizziness, hallucination, headache, hypoesthesia, paresthesia, syncope, tremor, vertigo
CV: **Bradycardia, hypotension**, orthostatic hypotension, palpitations, peripheral edema, **QT-interval prolongation**
EENT: Blurred vision, dry mouth, tinnitus
ENDO: Hypoglycemia
GI: Abdominal pain, anorexia, constipation, dyspepsia, nausea, vomiting
GU: Dysuria, elevated blood urea and creatinine levels, hematuria, **renal failure**, urinary retention
HEME: Eosinophilia, **leukopenia, pancytopenia, thrombocytopenia**
RESP: Dyspnea, **pulmonary fibrosis**
SKIN: Diaphoresis, pruritus, rash
Other: Angioedema

Nursing Considerations

- Monitor patient's QT interval, as ordered, because ranolazine prolongs it in a dose-related manner.
- Assess effectiveness of ranolazine at preventing anginal pain.
- Know that acute renal failure may occur in some patients with severe renal impairment (creatinine clearance less than 30 ml/min) while taking drug. Monitor patient's serum creatinine levels and blood urea nitrogen after drug therapy begins and then periodically, as ordered. If elevations occur, notify prescriber and expect drug to be discontinued.
- Monitor patient's serum magnesium, potassium, and liver enzyme levels.

PATIENT TEACHING

- Instruct patient to take ranolazine exactly as prescribed.
- Inform patient that drug may be taken with or without food.
- Caution patient to swallow tablets whole and not to break, chew, or crush them.
- Advise patient to limit the amount of grapefruit and grapefruit juice consumed while taking this drug.
- Advise patient to notify prescriber if persistent or severe adverse reactions occur.
- Instruct patient to notify all prescribers of ranolazine use.

rasagiline

Azilect

Class and Category

Pharmacologic class: Irreversible monoamine oxidase inhibitor (MAOI)
Therapeutic class: Antiparkinsonian
Pregnancy category: C

Indications and Dosages

➤ *To treat idiopathic Parkinson's disease as initial monotherapy in early-stage disease; adjunct in patients not taking levodopa*

TABLETS

Adults. 1 mg once daily.

➤ *As adjunct with levodopa or levodopa and carbidopa in treatment of later-stage idiopathic Parkinson's disease*

TABLETS

Adults. 0.5 mg once daily increased to 1 mg once daily, as needed.

DOSAGE ADJUSTMENT For patients with mild hepatic failure or taking ciprofloxacin or other CYP1A2 inhibitors, dosage shouldn't exceed 0.5 mg daily.

Route	Onset	Peak	Duration
P.O.	Unknown	1 hr	Unknown

Mechanism of Action

Inhibits metabolic degradation of catecholamines and serotonin in the CNS and peripheral tissues, increasing extracellular dopamine level in the striatum. The increased dopamine level helps control alterations in voluntary muscle movement (such as rigidity and tremors) in Parkinson's disease because dopamine, a neurotransmitter, is essential for normal motor function. By stimulating central and peripheral dopaminergic 2 (D_2) receptors on postsynaptic cells, dopamine inhibits firing of striatal neurons (such as cholinergic neurons), improving motor function.

Contraindications

Acute MI; angina; cardiac arrhythmias; cerebrovascular disease; coronary artery disease; elective surgery that requires general anesthesia; hypersensitivity to rasagiline or its components; moderate to severe hepatic impairment; pheochromocytoma; stroke; use within 14 days of cyclobenzaprine, dextromethorphan, MAO inhibitors, meperidine, methadone, mirtazapine, propoxyphene, St. John's wort, sympathomimetic amines, or tramadol

Interactions

DRUGS

ciprofloxacin and other CYP1A2 inhibitors: Increased rasagiline plasma level
dextromethorphan: Increased risk of bizarre or psychosis behavior
levodopa, levodopa, and carbidopa: Increased risk of dyskinesias
MAO inhibitors, sympathomimetics: Increased risk of hypertensive crisis
meperidine, methadone, propoxyphene, tramadol: Increased risk of life-threatening adverse reactions characterized by coma, excitation, hyperpyrexia, malignant hyperpyrexia, peripheral vascular collapse, seizures, severe hypertension or hypotension, and severe respiratory depression.
selective serotonin reuptake inhibitors, tetracyclic antidepressants, tricyclic antidepressants: Increased risk of severe CNS toxicity with behavioral and mental status changes, diaphoresis, hyperpyrexia, hypertension, muscle rigidity, syncope, and possible death

Adverse Reactions

CNS: Abnormal dreams, amnesia, anxiety, asthenia, ataxia, **cerebral ischemia, coma,** compulsive behaviors (binge eating,

increased sexual urges, intense urges to spend money), confusion, **CVA**, daytime sleepiness, depression, difficulty thinking, dizziness, dyskinesia, dystonia, fever, hallucinations, headache, malaise, manic depressive reaction, nightmares, paresthesia, psychotic-like behavior, **seizures**, **serotonin syndrome**, somnolence, stupor, syncope, vertigo
CV: Angina, bundle branch heart block, chest pain, **heart failure**, **MI**, **hypertensive crisis**, postural hypotension, thrombophlebitis, **ventricular fibrillation or tachycardia**
EENT: Blurred vision, conjunctivitis, dry mouth, epistaxis, gingivitis, **hemorrhage**, **laryngeal edema**, retinal detachment or hemorrhage, rhinitis
GI: Abdominal pain, anorexia, constipation, diarrhea, dyspepsia, dysphagia, elevated liver enzymes, gastroenteritis, **GI hemorrhage**, **intestinal obstruction or perforation**, nausea, vomiting
GU: **Acute renal failure**, albuminuria, decreased libido, hematuria, impotence, incontinence, priapism
HEME: Anemia, **leukopenia**, **thrombocytopenia**
MS: Arthralgia, arthritis, bone necrosis, bursitis, leg cramps, myasthenia, neck pain or stiffness, tenosynovitis
RESP: **Apnea**, **asthma**, cough, dyspnea, pleural effusion, **pneumothorax**, **interstitial pneumonia**
SKIN: Alopecia, **carcinoma**, diaphoresis, ecchymosis, **exfoliative dermatitis**, pruritus, ulcer, vesiculobullous rash
Other: **Angioedema**, flu-like symptoms, **hypersensitivity reactions**, **hypocalcemia**, weight loss

Nursing Considerations

WARNING Monitor patient's blood pressure closely throughout therapy. Notify prescriber immediately if patient has evidence of hypertensive crisis or signs and symptoms suggesting a stroke. Expect to stop drug immediately if these occur.

- Keep phentolamine readily available to treat hypertensive crisis. Give 5 mg by slow I.V. infusion, as prescribed, to reduce blood pressure without causing excessive hypotension. Use external cooling measures, as prescribed, to manage fever.
- Monitor patient receiving rasagiline with levodopa for worsening of preexisting dyskinesia. If it occurs, notify prescriber and expect levodopa dosage to be decreased.
- Be aware that patient may experience orthostatic hypotension, especially in the first 2 months of rasagiline therapy and that it may also occur while patient is supine.

PATIENT TEACHING

WARNING Inform patient taking recommended dosage of rasagiline that dietary tyramine restriction is no longer needed except for avoidance of very tyramine-rich foods such as aged cheese (e.g., Stilton), which may increase blood pressure greatly. If patient doesn't feel well soon after eating a suspected high-tyramine meal, he should contact prescriber immediately.

- Remind patient not to exceed the recommended dose because of risk of hypertension.
- Advise patient to stop taking rasagiline and to notify prescriber immediately if he develops blurred vision, chest pain, coma, nausea, palpitations, seizures, severe headache, stiff neck, stupor, trouble thinking, vomiting, or evidence of stroke.

WARNING Monitor patient closely for serotonin syndrome, a rare but serious adverse effect of rasagiline. Signs and symptoms include agitation, confusion, diaphoresis, diarrhea, fever, hyperactive reflexes, poor coordination, restlessness, shaking, talking or acting with uncontrolled excitement, tremor, and twitching. If symptoms occur, notify prescriber immediately, expect to discontinue drug, and provide supportive care.

- Suggest that patient change position slowly to minimize orthostatic hypotension.
- Alert patient that drug may cause changes in behavior that may be severe or hallucinations, especially at the initiation of drug therapy or when an increase in dosage occurs. If they occur, tell patient to notify prescriber promptly.
- Alert patient and caregivers that drug may cause compulsive or impulsive behaviors such as binge eating, gambling, increased sexual activities, or spending money inappropriately. If any questionable behavior occurs, instruct patient or caregiver to

notify prescriber, as dosage may need to be adjusted or drug discontinued.

- Instruct patient to notify all prescribers of rasagiline therapy, especially if antidepressants or antibiotics such as ciprofloxacin or a similar drug are being considered, and to avoid taking any over-the-counter cold medications.
- Caution patient not to perform hazardous activities until CNS effects of drug are known. Some patients have fallen asleep without warning while engaged in activities of daily living, including driving.
- Instruct patient to notify prescriber if pregnancy occurs.

repaglinide

Prandin

Class and Category

Pharmacologic class: Meglitinide
Therapeutic class: Antidiabetic
Pregnancy category: C

Indications and Dosages

➤ *To achieve glucose control in type 2 diabetes mellitus as monotherapy in patients whose glycosylated hemoglobin (HbA_{1c}) level is less than 8%*

TABLETS

Adults. *Initial:* 0.5 mg within 30 min before each meal. Dosage doubled, as needed, every wk until adequate glucose response obtained. *Maintenance:* 0.5 to 4 mg/dose up to four times a day. *Maximum:* 16 mg daily in divided doses of not more than 4 mg/dose.

➤ *To achieve glucose control in type 2 diabetes mellitus as monotherapy in patients whose HbA_{1c} is 8% or greater*

TABLETS

Adults. *Initial:* 1 or 2 mg within 30 min before each meal. Dosage doubled, as needed, every wk until adequate glucose response obtained. *Maintenance:* 1 to 4 mg/dose up to four times a day. *Maximum:* 16 mg daily in divided doses of not more than 4 mg/dose.

DOSAGE ADJUSTMENT For patients with severe renal impairment, dosage initiated at 0.5 mg before each meal and then titrated gradually, as needed. Concomitant use with clopidogrel should be avoided but if not possible, dosage initiated at 0.5 mg before each meal and total daily dose not to exceed 4 mg. Individualized dosing adjustments needed for patients taking concomitant strong CYP2C8 or CYP3A4 inducers or CYP2C8 or CYP3A4 inhibitors. Total daily dose of 6 mg should not be exceeded in patients receiving cyclosporine.

Mechanism of Action

Stimulates release of insulin from functioning pancreatic beta cells. In patients with type 2 diabetes mellitus, a shortage of these cells decreases blood insulin levels and causes glucose intolerance. By interacting with the adenosine triphosphatase (ATP)–potassium channel on the beta cell membrane, repaglinide prevents potassium from leaving the cell. This causes the beta cell to depolarize and the cell membrane's calcium channel to open. As a result, calcium moves into the cell and insulin moves out. The extent of insulin release is glucose dependent; the lower the glucose level, the less insulin is secreted from the cell.

Contraindications

Concurrent therapy with gemfibrozil, diabetic ketoacidosis, hypersensitivity to repaglinide or its components, severe hepatic impairment, type 1 diabetes mellitus

Interactions

DRUGS

antidiabetic agents, ACE inhibitors, angiotensin II receptor blocking agents, disopyramide, fibrates, fluoxetine, monoamine oxidase inhibitors, nonsteroidal anti-inflammatory agents (NSAIDs), pentoxifylline, pramlintide, propoxyphene, salicylates, somatostatin analogues (e.g., octreotide), and sulfonamide antibiotics: Increased risk of hypoglycemia

atypical antipsychotics, calcium channel blockers, corticosteroids, danazol, diuretics, estrogens, glucagon, isoniazid, niacin, oral contraceptives, phenothiazines, protease inhibitors, somatropin, sympathomimetics, thyroid hormones: Possibly loss of glucose control

barbiturates, carbamazepine, rifampin: Possibly increased repaglinide metabolism, decreasing effectiveness

beta blockers, clonidine, guanethidine, reserpine: Possibly blunt signs and symptoms of hypoglycemia
clarithromycin, clopidogrel, deferasirox, erythromycin, gemfibrozil, itraconazole, ketoconazole, montelukast, trimethoprim: Increased blood repaglinide level, resulting in enhanced and prolonged blood glucose–lowering effects
NPH insulin: Possibly increased risk of angina
OATP1B1 inhibitors such as cyclosporine, trimethoprim: Increased plasma repaglinide level

Adverse Reactions

CNS: Headache
CV: Angina
EENT: Rhinitis, sinusitis
ENDO: Hypoglycemia
GI: Diarrhea, elevated liver enzymes, **hepatitis**, nausea, **pancreatitis**
HEME: Hemolytic anemia, **leukopenia, thrombocytopenia**
MS: Arthralgia, back pain
RESP: Bronchitis, upper respiratory tract infection
SKIN: Alopecia, **Stevens–Johnson syndrome**
Other: Anaphylaxis

Nursing Considerations

- Be aware that repaglinide shouldn't be used with NPH insulin because the combination may increase the risk of angina.
- Expect to check HbA_{1c} level every 3 months, as ordered, to assess patient's long-term control of blood glucose level.
- During times of increased stress, such as from infection, surgery, or trauma, monitor blood glucose level often and assess need for additional insulin.

PATIENT TEACHING

- Instruct patient to take repaglinide within 30 minutes before meals and to skip dose whenever she skips a meal.
- Explain that repaglinide is an adjunct to diet in managing type 2 diabetes mellitus.
- Inform patient that changes in blood glucose level may cause blurred vision or visual disturbances, especially when repaglinide therapy starts. Reassure him that these changes are usually transient.
- Teach patient how to monitor her blood glucose level and when to notify prescriber about changes.
- Review signs and symptoms of hyperglycemia and hypoglycemia with patient and family. Instruct patient to notify prescriber immediately if she experiences anxiety, confusion, dizziness, excessive sweating, headache, increased thirst, increased urination, or nausea.
- Advise patient to wear or carry identification indicating that she has diabetes. Encourage her to carry candy or other simple carbohydrates with her to treat mild episodes of hypoglycemia.
- Inform patient that her HbA_{1c} level will be tested every 3 to 6 months until her blood glucose level is controlled.

reslizumab

Cinqair

Class and Category

Pharmacologic class: Interleukin-5 antagonist monoclonal antibody
Therapeutic class: Immunomodulator
Pregnancy category: Not classified

Indications and Dosages

➤ *Adjunct for add-on maintenance treatment in patients with severe asthma who have an eosinophilic phenotype*

I.V. INFUSION

Adults. 3 mg/kg over 20 to 50 min once every 4 wk.

Mechanism of Action

Inhibits IL-5 activity (the major cytokine responsible for activation and survival, differentiation, growth, and recruitment of eosinophils) by blocking its binding to the IL-5 receptor complex found on the eosinophil cell surface. Eosinophils are among many cell types involved in inflammation. By inhibiting IL-5 signaling, the production and survival of eosinophils are reduced, which then reduces inflammation present in asthma.

Incompatibilities

Don't mix reslizumab with any other drugs.

Contraindications

Hypersensitivity to reslizumab or its components

Interactions

DRUGS

None

Adverse Reactions

EENT: Oropharyngeal pain
GI: Vomiting
MS: Elevated CPK levels; chest, extremity, or neck musculoskeletal pain; muscle fatigue or spasms; myalgia
RESP: **Decreased oxygen saturation**, dyspnea, wheezing
SKIN: Urticaria
Other: Anaphylaxis, antibodies to reslizumab, **malignancy**

Nursing Considerations

- Know that reslizumab should not be used to treat acute asthma symptoms or acute exacerbations, including acute bronchospasm or status asthmaticus.
- Check to see that patient with an existing parasitic (helminth) infection has received treatment prior to starting reslizumab therapy because drug may interfere with resolving the infection. If patient becomes infected while receiving reslizumab and does not respond to antihelminth treatment, notify prescriber, as reslizumab will need to be discontinued until infection is resolved.
- Be aware that concurrent inhaled or systemic corticosteroid therapy should not be abruptly discontinued when reslizumab therapy is initiated, as systemic withdrawal symptoms may occur. Expect reductions to be done gradually, as ordered.
- Remove drug from refrigerator when ready to administer. To minimize foaming, do not shake vial. Inspect for particulate matter and discoloration. Know that because reslizumab is a protein, particles may be present that appear translucent to white and amorphous. Do not use if discolored or other foreign particulate matter is present. Withdraw proper volume and discard any unused portion. Inject drug slowly into an infusion bag containing 50 ml of 0.9% sodium chloride injection, USP, to minimize foaming. Know that drug is compatible with polyvinylchloride (PVC) or polyolefin infusion bags. Gently invert the bag to mix the solution. Do not shake. Do not mix or dilute with other drugs. Administer immediately after preparing. If not used immediately, drug may be stored in diluted solution in refrigerator or at room temperature, protected from light, for up to 16 hours, which must include the time for administration.
- Make sure diluted drug, if stored in refrigerator, is brought to room temperature before administering. Use an infusion set with an in-line, low-protein-binding filter (pore size of 0.2 micron). Know that drug is compatible with polyethersulfone (PES), polyvinylidence fluoride (PVDF), nylon, and cellulose acetate in-line infusion filters. Infuse drug over 20 to 50 min according to total volume to be infused and patient's weight. Do not infuse in the same intravenous line with other agents. After infusion is complete, flush the intravenous line with 0.9% sodium chloride injection, USP. Never administer drug by intravenous push.

WARNING **Monitor patient closely for allergic reactions to reslizumab, including anaphylaxis exhibited by decreased oxygen saturation, dyspnea, urticaria, vomiting, or wheezing. These reactions most often occurs during or within 20 minutes after completion of the infusion, although reactions have occurred before the second dose 4 weeks later. If severe symptoms, such as anaphylaxis, occur, stop infusion at once, notify prescriber, and provide supportive care, as ordered. Know that if anaphylaxis occurs, the drug should be permanently discontinued.**

- Be aware that, infrequently, malignancies of many different types have occurred within six months after patient's exposure to reslizumab. Report any persistent, severe, or unusual symptoms immediately to the prescriber.

PATIENT TEACHING

- Remind patient that reslizumab is not used to treat acute asthma symptoms or acute exacerbations. If asthma symptoms worsen or become acute, instruct patient to seek immediate emergency care.
- Inform patient that drug may cause an allergic reaction that could become life-threatening. Review signs and symptoms with patient and instruct her to seek immediate emergency care, if any occurs.

- Instruct patient to have any persistent, severe, or unusual symptoms checked out by prescriber.
- Tell patient not to change any concurrent inhaled or systemic corticosteroid dosage when starting reslizumab until instructed to do so by prescriber. Inform patient that if a dosage reduction is done, it will be done gradually to avoid withdrawal symptoms. Remind her that corticosteroids should never be abruptly stopped.

reteplase

Retavase

Class and Category

Pharmacologic class: Tissue plasminogen activator (tPA)
Therapeutic class: Thrombolytic
Pregnancy category: C

Indications and Dosages

➤ *To improve ventricular function, prevent heart failure, and reduce mortality after acute MI*

I.V. INJECTION

Adults. 10 units over 2 min; repeated after 30 min.

Mechanism of Action

Converts plasminogen to plasmin, which works to break up fibrin clots that have formed in the coronary arteries. Elimination of the clots improves cardiac blood and oxygen flow to the area, thus improving ventricular function.

Incompatibilities

Don't add other drugs to reteplase injection solution or administer them through same I.V. line as reteplase.

Contraindications

Active internal bleeding, aneurysm, arteriovenous malformation, bleeding diathesis, brain tumor, history of stroke or other cerebrovascular disease, hypersensitivity to reteplase or its components, intracranial or intraspinal surgery or trauma during previous 2 months, severe uncontrolled hypertension (systolic 200 mm Hg or higher, diastolic 110 mm Hg or higher)

Interactions

DRUGS

antifibrinolytics (including aminocaproic acid, aprotinin, and tranexamic acid): Decreased effectiveness of reteplase
antineoplastics, antithymocyte globulin, certain cephalosporins (such as cefamandole, cefoperazone, and cefotetan), heparin, oral anticoagulants, platelet aggregation inhibitors (such as abciximab, aspirin, and dipyridamole), strontium-89 chloride, sulfinpyrazone, valproic acid: Increased risk of bleeding

Adverse Reactions

CNS: Intracranial hemorrhage
GI: GI bleeding, nausea, vomiting
HEME: Thrombocytopenia
RESP: Hemoptysis
SKIN: Bleeding from wounds, ecchymosis, hematoma, purpura
Other: Hypersensitivity reactions, injection-site bleeding

Nursing Considerations

- Expect to start reteplase, as prescribed, as soon as possible after MI symptoms begin.
- Closely monitor patient with atrial fibrillation, severe hypertension, or other cardiac disease for signs and symptoms of cerebral embolism.
- To reconstitute, use diluent, syringe, needle, and dispensing pin provided. Withdraw 10 ml of preservative-free sterile water for injection. Remove and discard needle from syringe, and connect dispensing pin to syringe. Remove protective cap from spike end of dispensing pin, and insert spike into reteplase vial. Inject 10 ml of sterile water into the vial. With the spike still in the vial, swirl gently to dissolve the powder. Don't shake. Expect to see slight foaming. Let the vial stand for several minutes. When the bubbles dissipate, withdraw 10 ml of reconstituted solution into the syringe (about 0.7 ml may remain in the vial). Now detach the syringe from the dispensing pin and attach the 20G needle.
- Use the solution within 4 hours. Discard if it's discolored or contains particulates.
- Don't give heparin and reteplase in the same solution. Instead, flush the heparin line or D_5W or normal saline solution before and after reteplase injection.

- Closely monitor all possible bleeding sites (arterial and venous punctures, catheter insertions, cutdowns, and needle punctures) because fibrin is lysed during therapy.
- Avoid I.M. injections, venipunctures, and nonessential handling of patient during therapy.
- Know that if arterial puncture is needed, use an arm vessel that can be compressed, if possible. After sample is obtained, apply pressure for at least 30 minutes; then apply a pressure dressing. Check site often for bleeding.
- Know if bleeding occurs and can't be controlled by local pressure, notify prescriber immediately. Be prepared to stop anticoagulant therapy immediately and to discontinue second reteplase bolus, as prescribed.
- Anticipate that reperfusion arrhythmias, such as premature ventricular contractions or ventricular tachycardia, may follow coronary thrombolysis.

PATIENT TEACHING

- Advise patient to report adverse reactions immediately.

revefenacin

Yupelri

Class and Category

Pharmacologic class: Anticholinergic
Therapeutic class: Bronchodilator
Pregnancy category: Not classified

Indications and Dosages

➤ *To provide maintenance therapy for patients with chronic obstructive pulmonary disease (COPD)*

INHALATION SOLUTION

Adults. 175-mcg unit-dose vial once daily by nebulizer using a mouthpiece.

Mechanism of Action

Inhibits muscarinic receptor M3 in smooth muscles of the airways to produce bronchodilation

Contraindications

Hypersensitivity to revefenacin or its components

Interactions

DRUGS

OATP1B1 and OATP1B3 inhibitors such as cyclosporine, rifampicin: Possibly increased systemic exposure of revefenacin leading to increased adverse reactions
other anticholinergics: Possible additive anticholinergic effects leading to increased adverse reactions

Adverse Reactions

CNS: Dizziness, headache
CV: Hypertension
EENT: Nasopharyngitis, oropharyngeal pain
MS: Back pain
RESP: Bronchitis, cough, **paradoxical bronchospasms**, upper respiratory infection
Other: Immediate hypersensitivity reactions

Nursing Considerations

- Be aware that revefenacin should not be initiated in patients during acutely deteriorating or potentially life-threatening episodes of COPD. It should also not be used to relieve acute bronchospasms; know that acute symptoms should be treated with an inhaled, short-acting beta$_2$-agonist.
- Use cautiously in patients with narrow-angle glaucoma, because revefenacin may worsen the condition. Question patient frequently about presence of blurred vision, colored images, eye discomfort or pain, or visual halos in association with red eyes from conjunctival congestion and corneal edema. Notify prescriber immediately, if present.
- Use cautiously in patients with urinary retention, because revefenacin may worsen condition. Monitor patient for signs and symptoms of urinary retention such as difficulty passing urine or painful urination, especially in patients with bladder-neck obstruction or prostatic hyperplasia.
- Remove unit-dose vial from foil pouch and open immediately before use. Administer by the orally inhaled route via a standard jet nebulizer connected to an air compressor. Do not mix any other drugs in the nebulizer with revefenacin, as drug compatibility is unknown.

- Notify prescriber if revefenacin no longer controls symptoms of bronchoconstriction, because this may indicate that patient's condition is deteriorating and other forms of therapy may be required. The dosage or frequency of revefenacin should not be increased in this situation.

WARNING Monitor patient for paradoxical bronchospasm that may become life-threatening. If this should occur following a nebulizer treatment with revefenacin, notify prescriber immediately; expect to administer an inhaled, short-acting bronchodilator, as prescribed; and know that revefenacin should be discontinued immediately and alternative therapy substituted.

PATIENT TEACHING

- Inform patient that revefenacin therapy is not meant to relieve acute symptoms of COPD and extra doses should never be used for that purpose. Instead, acute symptoms should be treated with an inhaled short-acting $beta_2$ agonist such as albuterol.
- Teach patient how to administer drug using a standard jet nebulizer. Tell patient drug should only be administered via this device. Warn him not to inject or swallow the solution and not to mix it with other medications.
- Warn patient not to inhale more than one dose at any given time. Remind him the daily dosage should not exceed one unit-dose vial. Tell him to inhale the dosage via nebulization daily at the same time every day. He should throw the plastic dispensing vials away immediately after use.
- Stress importance of keeping plastic vials out of the reach of children, because the vials' small size poses a choking danger if swallowed.
- Instruct patient to notify prescriber immediately if he experiences decreased effectiveness or needs more of his inhaled short-acting $beta_2$ agonist or experiences a decrease in lung function. Warn him not to stop taking revefenacin without consulting prescriber, as symptoms may reoccur or become worse.
- Tell patient drug may cause allergic reactions that may occur after revefenacin has been administered. Instruct patient to notify prescriber, as drug will have to be discontinued, and to seek emergency care if reaction is severe.
- Instruct patient to report the presence of blurred vision, colored images, eye discomfort or pain, or visual halos in association with red eyes from conjunctival congestion and corneal edema.
- Tell patient, especially if he has bladder-neck obstruction or prostatic hyperplasia, to report difficulty passing urine or painful urination.

WARNING Inform patient that drug may cause paradoxical bronchospasm. If present, patient should use an inhaled, short-acting bronchodilator immediately, stop taking revefenacin, and notify prescriber.

ribavirin

Copegus, Moderiba, Rebetol, Ribasphere, Virazole

Class and Category

Pharmacologic class: Nucleoside analogue
Therapeutic class: Antiviral
Pregnancy category: X

Indications and Dosages

➤ *As adjunct to treat chronic hepatitis C (CHC) infection in combination with interferon alfa-2 b (pegylated and nonpegylated) in patients with compensated liver disease*

CAPSULES, ORAL SOLUTION (REBETOL)

Adults weighing more than 105 kg (231 lb). 600 mg in morning and 800 mg in evening for 24 to 48 wks depending on genotype.

Adults weighing between 81 and 105 kg (178 to 231 lb) and children ages 3 to 18 weighing more than 73 kg (162 lb). 600 mg in morning and 600 mg in evening for 24 to 48 wks depending on genotype.

Adults weighing between 66 and 80 kg (145 to 177 lb) and children ages 3 to 18 weighing 60 to 73 kg (132 to 162 lb). 400 mg in morning and 600 mg in evening for 24 to 48 wks depending on genotype.

Adults weighing less than 66 kg (144 lb) and children ages 3 to 18 weighing

between 47 and 59 kg (103 to 131 lb). 400 mg in morning and 400 mg in evening for 24 to 48 wks depending on genotype.

ORAL SOLUTION (REBETOL)

Children ages 3 to 18 weighing less than 47 kg (103 lb). 15 mg/kg/day divided and given in 2 doses for 24 to 48 wks depending on genotype.

➤ *As adjunct to treat chronic hepatitis C (CHC) infection in combination with peginterferon alfa-2a in patients with compensated liver disease who have not been previously treated with interferon alpha*

TABLETS (COPEGUS, MODERIBA, RIBASPHERE)

Adults with genotypes 1 or 4 weighing 75 kg (165 lb) or more. 600 mg in morning and 600 mg in evening for 48 wks.

Adults with genotypes 1 or 4 weighing less than 75 kg (165 lb). 400 mg in morning and 600 mg in evening for 48 wks.

Adults with genotypes 2 or 3. 400 mg in morning and 400 mg in evening for 24 wks.

Children ages 5 to 18 weighing 75 kg (165 lb) or more. 600 mg in morning and 600 mg in evening for 24 to 48 wks depending on genotype.

Children ages 5 to 18 weighing 60 to 74 kg (132 to 162.8 lb). 400 mg in morning and 600 mg in evening for 24 to 48 wks depending on genotype.

Children ages 5 to 18 weighing 47 to 59 kg (103.4 to 129.8. lb). 400 mg in morning and 400 mg in evening for 24 to 48 wks depending on genotype.

Children ages 5 to 18 weighing 34 to 46 kg (74.8 to 101.2 lb). 200 mg in morning and 400 mg in evening for 24 to 48 wks depending on genotype.

Children ages 5 to 18 weighing 23 to 33 kg (50.6 to 72.6 lb). 200 mg in morning and 200 mg in evening for 24 to 48 wks depending on genotype.

➤ *As adjunct to treat chronic hepatitis C with HIV co-infection in combination with peginterferon alfa-2a*

TABLETS (RIBASPHERE)

Adults. 400 mg in morning and 400 mg in evening for 48 wks.

➤ *To treat hospitalized infants and young children with severe lower respiratory tract infections due to respiratory syncytial virus (RSV)*

INHALATION SOLUTION (VIRAZOLE)

Hospitalized infants and young children. 20 mg/ml administered by SPAG-2 unit with continuous aerosol for 12 to 18 hr daily for 3 to 7 days.

DOSAGE ADJUSTMENT Dosage adjustment individualized for patients with renal dysfunction and severe adverse reactions.

Mechanism of Action

Precise action unknown, but may inhibit HCV polymerase or respiratory syncytial virus in a selective biochemical reaction.

Contraindications

Autoimmune hepatitis, coadministration with didanosine, creatinine clearance less than 50 ml/min, hemoglobinopathies (i.e., sickle-cell anemia, thalassemia major), hypersensitivity to ribavirin or its components, men whose female partners are pregnant, pregnancy

Interactions

DRUGS

azathioprine: Increased risk of azathioprine-related myelotoxicity and severe pancytopenia
didanosine: Increased risk of didanosine-induced toxicities such as hepatic failure, pancreatitis, peripheral neuropathy, and symptomatic hyperlactatemia/lactic acidosis
digoxin: Possibly digitalis toxicity with ribavirin inhalation solution
lamivudine, stavudine, zidovudine: Possibly decreased effectiveness of these drugs
nucleoside reverse transcriptase inhibitors: Increased risk of treatment-related toxicities, especially anemia and hepatic decompensation
zidovudine: Possibly increased risk of severe anemia and neutropenia

Adverse Reactions

CNS: Aggression, agitation, anger, anxiety, asthenia, chills, **CVA**, depression, dizziness, emotional swings in mood, fatigue, fever, hallucinations, headache, impaired concentration, insomnia, irritability, lethargy, malaise, memory impairment, nervousness, peripheral neuropathy, psychosis, rigors, **suicidal ideation**, vertigo
CV: Angina, **bigeminy**, **bradycardia** (inhalation solution), **cardiac arrest**, chest pain, **hypotension** (inhalation solution)

EENT: Blurred vision, conjunctivitis, dry mouth, hearing impairment or loss, pharyngitis, retinal detachment or exudates, rhinitis, significant ophthalmologic disorders, sinusitis, taste perversion, transient blindness
ENDO: Hyperglycemia, hypothyroidism, growth retardation (children)
GI: Abdominal pain, anorexia, cholangitis, colitis, constipation, diarrhea, dyspepsia, elevated liver enzymes, fatty liver, **GI bleeding, hepatic decompensation,** hepatomegaly, hyperbilirubinemia, nausea, **pancreatitis,** peptic ulcer, vomiting
GU: Menstrual disorder
HEME: Anemia, **hemolytic anemia, leukopenia, neutropenia, pure red cell aplasia,** reticulocytosis (inhalation solution), **thrombocytopenia, thrombotic thrombocytopenic purpura**
MS: Arthralgia, back pain, extremity pain, musculoskeletal pain, myalgia, myositis
RESP: Cough, dyspnea, **pulmonary embolism or hypertension** (inhalation solution in children); **apnea, atelectasis,** bacterial pneumonia, **bronchospasm, cyanosis,** dyspnea, **hypoventilation, pneumothorax, pulmonary edema, ventilator dependence, worsening of respiratory status** (inhalation solution)
SKIN: Alopecia, dermatitis, diaphoresis, dry skin, eczema, erythroderma, flushing, pruritus, rash, **Stevens-Johnson syndrome, toxic epidermal necrolysis,** urticaria
Other: Anaphylaxis; angioedema; autoimmune disorders; bacterial, fungal, or viral infections; dehydration; flu-like symptoms; graft rejection (liver or renal); hyperuricemia; weight loss

Nursing Considerations

- Know that patient requires the following tests to be performed before ribavirin therapy is started and then periodically thereafter, as ordered, to establish a baseline before treatment starts and allow early detection of adverse effects during treatment: ECG, standard hematologic tests including hemoglobin, liver function tests, monthly pregnancy tests for women of childbearing potential or partners of male patients, and TSH levels. Expect dosage to be temporarily withheld or discontinued, as ordered, if patient experiences severe adverse reactions or test abnormalities and drug to be discontinued immediately with confirmation of pregnancy.
- Be aware that ribavirin therapy should not be given to patients with a creatinine clearance less than 50 ml/min, because of risk of severe renal dysfunction. Ribavirin should not be given until a negative pregnancy test is obtained from women of childbearing age or the female partner of childbearing age of male patient. Also know that ribavirin should not be given to patient with a history of significant or unstable cardiac disease, because drug may cause a deterioration of cardiovascular status.
- Use caution when administering ribavirin to patient with preexisting but stable cardiac disease. Monitor these patients closely and expect that if there is any deterioration in cardiovascular status, ribavirin therapy will be discontinued.
- Be aware that the aerosol solution of ribavirin is for use in children only. It should not be mixed with or simultaneously given with other aerosolized medications. To prepare the powder for administration as a solution, reconstitute drug with a minimum of 75 ml of sterile water for injection, USP or inhalation in the original 100-ml glass vial. Shake well. Transfer solution to the clean, sterilized 500-ml SPAG-2 reservoir and further dilute to a final volume of 300 ml with sterile water for injection, USP or inhalation. The final concentration should be 20 mg/ml. Discard solutions in the SPAG-2 unit at least every 24 hours and when the liquid level is low before adding newly reconstituted solution.
- Monitor patients with impaired renal function and those over the age of 50 during therapy for anemia. Because anemia usually occurs early in treatment, expect to obtain a baseline of patient's hemoglobin and then assess at 2 and 4 weeks after therapy begins. Know that any patient who develops a decreased hemoglobin level below 10 g/dl should have dosage modified or drug discontinued, as ordered, because potentially fatal myocardial infarctions have occurred from anemia induced by ribavirin therapy. For patients with a history of stable cardiovascular disease, expect a permanent dosage reduction to occur if the

hemoglobin decreases by more than or equal to 2 g/dl during any 4-week period. If the hemoglobin remains less than 12 g/dl after 4 weeks of therapy on a reduced dose, expect drug to be discontinued. Also monitor patient taking azathioprine concomitantly for pancytopenia and bone marrow suppression, which usually occurs within 3 to 7 weeks after concomitant administration of pegylated interferon/ribavirin and azathioprine. Expect drug to be discontinued if pancytopenia develops.

- Monitor patient for signs and symptoms of pancreatitis (abdominal pain and tenderness, anorexia, fever, nausea, vomiting). If present, notify prescriber and expect drug to be discontinued.
- Expect patient's lungs to be assessed regularly for evidence of pulmonary function impairment or pulmonary infiltrates. If either develops, expect ribavirin therapy to be discontinued.
- Know that because ribavirin is used in conjunction with alpha interferons, serious and severe visual changes may occur. Know that patient should have a baseline ophthalmologic exam before therapy begins. Patients with preexisting ophthalmologic disorders such as diabetic or hypertensive retinopathy should receive periodic eye examinations throughout therapy or at any time ocular symptoms appear. Expect drug to be discontinued in patients who develop new or worsening ophthalmologic disorders.

PATIENT TEACHING

- Instruct patient to take ribavirin exactly as prescribed. If a dose is missed, tell patient to take the missed dose as soon as possible during the same day but not to double the next dose.
- Warn patient not to break open or crush Rebetol capsules.
- Tell patient to take oral ribavirin with food.

WARNING Instruct patients to use two reliable forms of contraception throughout treatment, because drug can cause fetal harm even in partner of male patient. Inform them that a pregnancy test must be performed monthly during ribavirin therapy and for 6 months after therapy is finished. Stress importance of notifying prescriber immediately if pregnancy occurs or is suspected.

- Tell mothers not to breastfeed during ribavirin therapy.
- Instruct patient to comply with dental checkups and to brush teeth thoroughly twice daily. If vomiting should occur, stress importance of rinsing out mouth thoroughly afterward.
- Inform patients that growth retardation often occurs with combination therapy that includes ribavirin. Reassure parents that following treatment, rebound growth and weight gain occur in most children.
- Stress importance of complying with scheduled laboratory tests.
- Tell patient to maintain adequate hydration throughout ribavirin therapy.
- Caution patient not to perform hazardous activities such as driving until effects of ribavirin on his nervous system are known and resolved.
- Caution patient or parents to watch for changes in behavior or mood as ribavirin may cause suicidal ideation. If changes are noted, stress importance of contacting prescriber.

rifampin
(rifampicin)

Rifadin, Rifadin IV, Rimactane, Rofact (CAN)

Class and Category

Pharmacologic class: Semisynthetic rifamycin
Therapeutic class: Antimycobacterial antitubercular
Pregnancy category: C

Indications and Dosages

➤ *As adjunct to treat tuberculosis caused by all strains of* Mycobacterium tuberculosis

CAPSULES, ORAL SUSPENSION, I.V. INFUSION

Adults. 10 mg/kg daily with other antitubercular drugs for 2 mo. with oral dosage given 1 hr before or 2 hr after a meal and IV dosage given over 3 hr if diluted in 500 ml of D_5W or 30 min if diluted in 100 ml of D_5W *Maximum:* 600 mg daily.
Children. 10 to 20 mg/kg daily in combination with other antitubercular drugs for 2 mo, with oral dosage given 1 hr

before or 2 hr after a meal and IV dosage given over 3 hr if diluted in 500 ml of D_5W or 30 min if diluted in 100 ml of D_5W. *Maximum:* 600 mg daily.

➤ *To eliminate meningococci from nasopharynx of asymptomatic carriers of* Neisseria meningitidis

CAPSULES, ORAL SUSPENSION, I.V. INFUSION

Adults. 600 mg every 12 hr for 2 days (total of 4 doses) with oral dosage given 1 hr before or 2 hr after a meal and IV dosage given over 3 hr if diluted in 500 ml of D_5W or 30 min if diluted in 100 ml of D_5W.

Infants age 1 month and over and children. 10 mg/kg every 12 hr for 2 days (total of 4 doses). *Maximum:* 600 mg daily.

Infants under age 1 month. 5 mg/kg every 12 hr for 2 days (total of 4 doses). *Maximum:* 600 mg daily.

Mechanism of Action

Inhibits bacterial and mycobacterial RNA synthesis by binding to DNA-dependent RNA polymerase, thereby blocking RNA transcription. Exhibits dose-dependent bactericidal or bacteriostatic action. Rifampin is highly effective against rapidly dividing bacilli in extracellular cavitary lesions, such as those found in the nasopharynx.

Incompatibilities

Don't administer rifampin in the same I.V. line as diltiazem.

Contraindications

Concurrent use of nonnucleoside reverse transcriptase inhibitors or protease inhibitors by patients with HIV; concurrent use with praziquantel or saquinavir/ritonavir; hypersensitivity to rifampin, other rifamycins or their components

Interactions

DRUGS

adrenal hormones, thyroid hormones: Possibly increased metabolism of these hormones, resulting in decreased effectiveness

aminophylline, oxtriphylline, theophylline: Increased metabolism and clearance of these theophylline preparations

anesthetics (hydrocarbon inhalation, except isoflurane), hepatotoxic drugs, isoniazid: Increased risk of hepatotoxicity

antacids: Possibly reduced oral absorption of rifampin

antiviral drugs such as atazanavir, darunavir, fosamprenavir, saquinavir, tipranavir: Decreased plasma concentration of antiviral drugs

atovaquone: Decreased plasma atovaquone levels and increased plasma rifampin levels

beta blockers, chloramphenicol, clofibrate, corticosteroids, cyclosporine, dapsone, digitalis glycosides, disopyramide, hexobarbital, itraconazole, ketoconazole, mexiletine, oral anticoagulants, oral antidiabetic drugs, phenytoin, propafenone, quinidine, tocainide, verapamil (oral): Increased metabolism, resulting in lower blood levels of these drugs

bone marrow depressants: Increased leukopenic or thrombocytopenic effects

clofazimine: Reduced absorption of rifampin, delaying its peak concentration and increasing its half-life

diazepam: Enhanced diazepam elimination, resulting in decreased drug effectiveness

estramustine, estrogens, oral contraceptives: Decreased estrogenic effects

methadone: Possibly impaired absorption of methadone, leading to withdrawal symptoms

nonnucleoside reverse transcriptase inhibitors, protease inhibitors (indinavir, nelfinavir, ritonavir, saquinavir): Accelerated metabolism of these drugs (by patients with HIV), resulting in subtherapeutic levels; delayed metabolism of rifampin, increasing risk of toxicity

other hepatotoxic drugs (saquinavir/ritonavir): Increased risk of hepatotoxicity that may become severe

praziquantel: Decreased blood levels of praziquantel, decreasing its effectiveness

probenecid: Increased blood level or prolonged duration of rifampin, increasing risk of toxicity

trimethoprim: Increased elimination and shortened elimination half-life of trimethoprim

vitamin D: Increased metabolism and decreased efficacy of vitamin D, leading to decreased serum calcium and phosphate levels and increased parathyroid hormone levels

ACTIVITIES

alcohol use: Increased risk of hepatotoxicity

Adverse Reactions

CNS: Ataxia, behavioral changes, chills, confusion, difficulty concentrating, dizzi-

ness, drowsiness, fatigue, fever, generalized numbness, headache, paresthesia, psychoses
CV: Hypotension, myopathy, vasculitis
EENT: Conjunctivitis; discolored saliva, sputum, tears, and teeth; mouth or tongue soreness; periorbital edema; visual disturbances
ENDO: Adrenal insufficiency (rare), hyperglycemia or **hypoglycemia** (in patients with diabetes)
GI: Abdominal cramps, anorexia, diarrhea, discolored feces, elevated liver enzymes, epigastric discomfort, flatulence, heartburn, **hepatitis**, jaundice, nausea, **pseudomembranous colitis**, vomiting
GU: Acute renal failure or tubular necrosis, discolored urine, elevated BUN and serum uric acid, hematuria, interstitial nephritis, menstrual disturbances, **renal insufficiency**
HEME: Agranulocytosis (rare), decreased hemoglobin, **disseminated intravascular coagulation (DIC)**, eosinophilia, **hemolytic anemia, leukopenia, neutropenia**, purpura, **thrombocytopenia** (rare)
MS: Arthralgia, extremity pain, muscle weakness, myalgia (rare)
RESP: Acute bronchospasm, shortness of breath, wheezing
SKIN: Acute generalized exanthematous pustulosis, discolored skin and sweat, **erythema multiforme**, flushing, pemphigoid reaction, pruritus, rash, **Stevens–Johnson syndrome, toxic epidermal necrolysis**, urticaria
Other: Anaphylaxis, angioedema, drug reaction with eosinophilia and systemic symptoms (DRESS), flu-like symptoms, lymphadenopathy

Nursing Considerations

- Obtain blood samples or other specimens for culture and sensitivity testing, as ordered, before giving rifampin and throughout therapy to monitor response to drug.
- Be aware that rifampin should not be used to treat meningococcal infection, because of the possibility of rapid emergence of resistant organisms.
- Expect to monitor liver enzymes and every 2 to 4 weeks during therapy. Immediately report abnormalities.
- Use rifampin cautiously in patients with diabetes mellitus because rifampin therapy may make diabetes management more difficult because of its effect on blood glucose levels.
- For I.V. infusion, reconstitute by adding 10 ml sterile water for injection to 600-mg vial of rifampin. Swirl gently to dissolve. Withdraw appropriate dose and add to 500 ml D_5W (preferred solution) or normal saline solution and infuse over 3 hours. Or, withdraw appropriate dose and add to 100 ml D_5W (preferred solution) or normal saline solution and infuse over 30 minutes. Use reconstituted drug promptly because rifampin may precipitate out of D_5W solution after 4 hours. In normal saline solution, drug is stable up to 24 hours at room temperature.
- Expect drug to discolor body fluids, skin, and teeth reddish orange to reddish brown.
- Be aware that rifampin can cause myelosuppression and increase risk of infection. Notify prescriber immediately if signs of infection, such as fever, develop.
- Monitor patient for signs and symptoms of hypersensitivity reactions. Notify prescriber if present, expect drug to be discontinued, and provide supportive care, as ordered.
- Monitor patient for rash or other skin abnormalities, as rifampin may cause severe skin reactions that could be life-threatening.

PATIENT TEACHING

- Instruct patient to take rifampin 1 hour before or 2 hours after a meal with a full glass of water.
- Emphasize the need to take drug exactly as prescribed. Explain that not completing the full course of therapy or skipping doses may decrease the effectiveness of the treatment and increase the chance that resistance to drug may develop, making it ineffective to treat an infection patient might develop in the future. Emphasize importance of compliance with the full course of therapy.
- Explain that drug may discolor feces, saliva, skin, sputum, sweat, tears, teeth, and urine reddish brown to reddish orange or yellow. Discoloration of teeth may be permanent.

- Caution patient against wearing soft contact lenses during therapy because drug may permanently stain them.
- Advise patient who takes an oral contraceptive to use an additional form of birth control during rifampin therapy.
- Urge patient to notify prescriber about anorexia, cough, darkened urine, fever, flu-like symptoms, joint pain or swelling, malaise, nausea, rash, shortness of breath, swollen lymph nodes, vomiting, wheezing, and yellowish eyes or skin.
- Advise patient to avoid alcohol during rifampin therapy.
- Instruct patient to notify prescriber if no improvement occurs within 2 to 3 weeks.
- Inform patient with diabetes mellitus that rifampin therapy may affect his blood glucose levels and to monitor his blood glucose levels closely.
- Tell patient to inform all prescribers of rifampin therapy.
- Instruct patient to notify prescriber immediately if rash or other skin abnormalities occur, as reaction may become severe.

rifamycin

Aemcolo

Class and Category

Pharmacologic class: Rifamycin antibacterial
Therapeutic class: Antibiotic
Pregnancy category: Not classified

Indications and Dosages

➤ *To treat travelers' diarrhea caused by noninvasive strains of* Escherichia coli

D.R. TABLETS

Adults. 388 mg twice daily (in morning and evening) for 3 days.

Mechanism of Action

As a semisynthetic derivative of rifampin, drug inhibits bacterial RNA synthesis by binding to DNA-dependent RNA polymerase, thereby blocking RNA transcription. This results in bacterial cell impairment or death.

Contraindications

Hypersensitivity to rifamycin, other rifamycin-class antimicrobial agents such as rifaximin, or their components

Interactions

DRUGS

None reported

ACTIVITIES

alcohol use: Possibly interference with effectiveness of rifamycin

Adverse Reactions

CNS: Fever, headache
GI: Abdominal pain, ***Clostridium difficile*-associated diarrhea**, constipation, dyspepsia

Nursing Considerations

- Be aware that rifamycin is not to be used in patients with diarrhea complicated by bloody stool or fever or due to pathogens other than noninvasive strains of *E. coli*.
- Administer rifamycin with 6 to 8 ounces of liquid.
- Know that drug should be discontinued if diarrhea gets worse or persists more than 48 hours.
- Assess patient for signs of secondary infection, such as profuse, watery diarrhea. If such diarrhea develops, contact prescriber and expect to obtain a stool specimen to rule out pseudomembranous colitis caused by *Clostridium difficile*. If diarrhea occurs, notify prescriber and expect to withhold rifamycin and treat with electrolytes, fluids, protein, and an antibiotic effective against *C. difficile*.

PATIENT TEACHING

- Tell patient to take rifamycin twice daily (once in morning and once in evening) with 6 to 8 ounces of liquid but not with alcohol.
- Caution patient not to break, chew, or crush tablets. Instead, tablets must be swallowed whole.
- Instruct patient to notify prescriber if diarrhea gets worse or persists for more than 48 hours, because drug will have to be discontinued and a different antibiotic prescribed.

rifaximin

Xifaxan

Class and Category

Pharmacologic class: Rifamycin

Therapeutic class: Antibiotic
Pregnancy category: Not classified

Indications and Dosages

➤ *To treat irritable bowel syndrome with diarrhea (IBS-D)*

TABLETS

Adults. 550 mg three times daily for 14 days. May be repeated up to two times for reoccurrence.

➤ *To treat travelers' diarrhea caused by noninvasive strains of* Escherichia coli

TABLETS

Adults and children age 12 and over. 200 mg three times daily for 3 days.

➤ *To reduce risk of overt hepatic encephalopathy*

TABLETS

Adults. 550 mg twice daily.

Mechanism of Action

As a semisynthetic derivative of rifampin, it inhibits bacterial RNA synthesis by binding to DNA-dependent RNA polymerase, thereby blocking RNA transcription. This results in bacterial cell impairment or death.

Contraindications

Hypersensitivity to rifaximin, any of the rifamycin antimicrobial agents, or their components

Interactions

DRUGS

P-glycoprotein inhibitors such as cyclosporine: Increased exposure to rifaximin leading to possible risk of increased adverse reactions
warfarin: Altered INR levels possibly requiring warfarin dosage adjustment

ACTIVITIES

alcohol use: Possibly increased risk of hepatotoxicity

Adverse Reactions

CNS: Depression, dizziness, fatigue, fever, headache
CV: Peripheral edema
EENT: Nasal passage irritation, nasopharyngitis, taste loss
GI: Abdominal pain, anorexia, ascites, ***Clostridium difficile*-associated colitis, dysentery**, elevated ALT liver enzyme, nausea
HEME: Anemia
MS: Arthralgia, muscle spasms, myalgia
RESP: Dyspnea
SKIN: Exfoliative dermatitis, flushing, pruritus, rash, urticaria
Other: Anaphylaxis, angioedema, elevated blood creatine phosphokinase, weight loss

Nursing Considerations

- Be aware that rifaximin should not be used in patients with travelers' diarrhea complicated by blood in the stool, diarrhea due to pathogens other than *E. coli*, or in the presence of fever.
- Use extreme caution in patients with severe hepatic impairment because of increased rifaximin exposure leading to possible increased risk of adverse reactions.
- Notify prescriber if diarrhea gets worse or persist for more than 48 hours in patients being treated for diarrhea or for a new onset of diarrhea in patients being treated for hepatic encephalopathy. The patient may be experiencing *C. difficile* colitis associated with antibiotic use requiring rifaximin to be discontinued and an antibiotic effective against *C. difficile* along with electrolytes, fluids, and protein replacement therapy, to be administered, as ordered.

PATIENT TEACHING

- Instruct patient to take drug for length of time prescribed, even when feeling better.
- Tell patient to report diarrhea that gets worse or persists for more than 48 hours or new onset or reoccurrence of diarrhea as *C. difficile*-associated diarrhea may occur even after rifaximin has been discontinued requiring additional treatment.

rilpivirine

Edurant

Class and Category

Pharmacologic class: Nonnucleoside reverse transcriptase inhibitor (NNRTI)
Therapeutic class: Antiretroviral
Pregnancy category: B

Indications and Dosages

➤ *As adjunct to treat human immunodeficiency virus type 1 (HIV-1) infection in antiretroviral treatment-*

naïve patients with NIV-1 RNA equal to or less than 100,000 copies/ml at the start of therapy

TABLETS

Adults and children age 12 years and over weighing at least 35 kg (77 lb). 25 mg once daily with food.

DOSAGE ADJUSTMENT For patient taking rifabutin concomitantly, dosage increased to 50 mg once daily with a meal.

Mechanism of Action

Inhibits HIV-1 replication by noncompetitive inhibition of HIV-1 reverse transcriptase.

Contraindications

Concomitant therapy with carbamazepine, dexamethasone (more than a single dose), esomeprazole, lansoprazole, omeprazole, oxcarbazepine, pantoprazole, phenobarbital, phenytoin, rabeprazole, rifampin, rifapentine, or St. John's wort; hypersensitivity to rilpivirine or its components

Interactions

DRUGS

aluminum- or magnesium-containing antacids, calcium carbonate, cimetidine, famotidine, nizatidine, ranitidine: Decreased rilpivirine concentration and significantly decreased effectiveness

atazanavir, atazanavir/ritonavir, clarithromycin, darunavir/ritonavir, delavirdine, erythromycin, fluconazole, fosamprenavir, fosamprenavir/ritonavir, indinavir, itraconazole, lopinavir/ritonavir, nelfinavir, posaconazole, saquinavir/ritonavir, telithromycin, tipranavir, voriconazole: Increased concentration of rilpivirine with possible prolonged action and risk of adverse reactions

carbamazepine, dexamethasone (more than a single-dose), phenobarbital, phenytoin, proton pump inhibitors, rifampin, rifapentine, St. John's wort: Possibly significant decrease in rilpivirine plasma concentrations, resulting in loss of virologic response

drugs that prolong QT interval: Increased risk of torsades de pointes

ketoconazole: Decreased ketoconazole concentration and effectiveness and increased rilpivirine concentration with possible prolonged action and risk of adverse reactions

methadone: Possible decreased methadone concentration with increased risk of opiate withdrawal

other NNRTIs (efavirenz, etravirine, nevirapine), rifabutin: Decreased concentration of rilpivirine with possible decreased effectiveness

Adverse Reactions

CNS: Abnormal dreams, anxiety, depression, dizziness, dysphoria, fatigue, fever, headache, insomnia, mood changes, sleep disorders, somnolence, **suicidal ideation**

CV: Elevated cholesterol and triglycerides

EENT: Conjunctivitis, oral ulceration

ENDO: Cushingoid appearance, fat redistribution

GI: Abdominal discomfort or pain, anorexia, bilirubin increase, cholecystitis, cholelithiasis, diarrhea, elevated liver enzymes, **hepatitis, hepatotoxicity**, nausea, vomiting

GU: Elevated creatinine, glomerulonephritis, nephrolithiasis, **nephrotic syndrome**

HEME: Eosinophilia

SKIN: Blisters, rash

Other: Angioedema, drug reaction with eosinophilia and systemic symptoms (DRESS), immune reconstitution syndrome

Nursing Considerations

- Administer rilpivirine with a meal. Know that a protein drink does not replace a meal.
- Know that drug should not be used in patients taking other medications with a known risk of torsades de pointes or in patients at higher risk of torsades de pointes, because rilpivirine may cause QT prolongation.

WARNING Obtain liver enzymes before therapy begins, as ordered, in patients with marked transaminase elevations, patients treated with other medications associated with liver toxicity, and patients with underlying hepatic disease, including hepatitis B or C viral infections. Also monitor liver enzymes throughout therapy, as ordered, on all patients, because rilpivirine may cause hepatotoxicity. Know that persistent elevations of serum transaminase levels may require rilpivirine therapy to be discontinued.

• Obtain cholesterol and triglyceride levels before rilpivirine is begun and periodically throughout therapy, because drug may cause an increase in total cholesterol and triglycerides.

WARNING Assess patient's skin regularly for rash or other abnormalities. Notify prescriber and expect rilpivirine to be discontinued immediately if a severe rash occurs and is accompanied by blisters, conjunctivitis, eosinophilia, facial edema, fever, joint or muscle aches, lip swelling, malaise, or oral lesions. Be aware that a delay in discontinuing the drug may result in a life-threatening situation.

• Monitor patient's mood and emotional status, as rilpivirine may cause significant depression, mood changes, and suicidal ideation. Report any changes to prescriber.

• Be aware that immune reconstitution syndrome has occurred in patients treated with combination antiretroviral therapy, including rilpivirine. The inflammatory response predisposes susceptible patients to opportunistic infections such as cytomegalovirus, *Mycobacterium avium* infection, *Pneumocystis jiroveci* pneumonia, or tuberculosis. Autoimmune disorders such as Graves' disease, Guillain–Barré syndrome, or polymyositis have also occurred. Report sudden or unusual adverse reactions to prescriber.

PATIENT TEACHING

• Advise patient to avoid missing doses of rilpivirine. If she misses a dose, she should take it as soon as she remembers, but should not double the next dose or take more than prescribed.

• Inform patient that rilpivirine must be taken with a meal. Remind patient that a protein drink does not replace a meal.

WARNING Inform patient about severe liver disease that may occur with rilpivirine. Tell her to report signs and symptoms of liver disease such as acholic stools, anorexia, fatigue, malaise, nausea, tenderness over liver area, or yellowing of skin or whites of the eyes and to seek immediate medical attention.

• Stress importance of being compliant with tests ordered to screen for adverse effects of rilpivirine therapy.

WARNING Advise patient that rilpivirine therapy may cause severe hypersensitivity or skin reactions. Tell her to report a rash, especially if it is accompanied by blisters, conjunctivitis, facial edema, fatigue, fever, joint or muscle aches, liver problems, or oral lesions and to seek immediate medical attention.

• Inform patient that rilpivirine therapy may cause changes in her body appearance because of fat redistribution. Prepare her for the possibility of developing breast enlargement, central obesity, dorsocervical fat enlargement (buffalo hump), facial wasting, and peripheral wasting.

• Instruct patient to report any persistent, severe, or unusual signs and symptoms.

• Encourage women of childbearing age to report known or suspected pregnancy. If pregnancy occurs, encourage patient to enroll in the Antiretroviral Pregnancy Registry by calling 1-800-258-4263.

• Alert mothers that breastfeeding is not recommended during rilpivirine therapy.

• Tell patient to report all drugs being taken, including over-the-counter medications and herbals, as serious drug interactions may occur. Advise patient not to begin any new drug therapy without first checking with prescriber.

• Tell patient or caregiver to report any signs of depression, mood changes, sleep disorders, or suicidal thoughts to prescriber.

riluzole

Rilutek, Tiglutik

Class and Category

Pharmacologic class: Benzothiazole
Therapeutic class: Amyotrophic lateral sclerosis treatment agent
Pregnancy category: C

Indications and Dosages

➤ *To treat amyotrophic lateral sclerosis*

ORAL SUSPENSION, TABLETS

Adults. 50 mg every 12 hr taken 1 hr before or 2 hr after a meal.

Mechanism of Action
Inhibits release of glutamic acid, an excitatory amino acid neurotransmitter, in the CNS, thus reducing its effects on target cells. Glutamic acid affects degeneration of neurons; reducing its level may help slow amyotrophic lateral sclerosis.

Contraindications
Hypersensitivity to riluzole or its components

Interactions
DRUGS
allopurinol, hepatotoxic drugs, methyldopa, sulfasalazine: Increased risk of hepatotoxicity
amitriptyline, phenacetin, quinolones, tacrine, theophylline: Delayed elimination of riluzole
omeprazole, rifampin: Increased riluzole clearance
FOODS
charbroiled foods: Increased riluzole elimination
ACTIVITIES
alcohol use: Increased risk of hepatotoxicity
smoking: Increased riluzole elimination

Adverse Reactions
CNS: Asthenia, dizziness, headache, insomnia, paresthesia (circumoral), somnolence, spasticity, vertigo
CV: Peripheral edema
EENT: Dry mouth, rhinitis, stomatitis
GI: Abdominal pain, anorexia, constipation, diarrhea, elevated liver enzymes, flatulence, **hepatitis**, indigestion, nausea, vomiting
HEME: Neutropenia
MS: Back or muscle pain or stiffness
RESP: Dyspnea, **hypersensitivity pneumonitis**, increased cough, **interstitial lung disorder**, pneumonia
SKIN: Alopecia, eczema, pruritus
Other: Anaphylaxis

Nursing Considerations
- Use riluzole cautiously in patients with impaired hepatic or renal function.
- Also use cautiously in elderly patients, Japanese patients and women because of increased risk of toxicity from decreased drug clearance.
- Monitor liver enzymes before and during riluzole therapy.
- Monitor patient for respiratory symptoms, such as dry cough or dyspnea. Notify prescriber if present, and expect patient to have a chest x-ray, as ordered. If evidence of hypersensitivity pneumonitis or interstitial lung disease is present, expect riluzole to be discontinued immediately.

PATIENT TEACHING
- Instruct patient to take riluzole regularly, every 12 hours, either 1 hour before or 2 hours after a meal, and at the same time each day.
- Instruct patient to store riluzole at room temperature, protected from bright light.
- Urge patient to minimize alcohol, charred foods, and smoking because they speed drug excretion.
- Tell patient to report cough, difficulty breathing, or fever.

risedronate sodium
Actonel, Atelvia

Class and Category
Pharmacologic class: Bisphosphonate
Therapeutic class: Antiosteoporotic
Pregnancy category: C

Indications and Dosages
➤ *To treat Paget's disease of bone*
TABLETS (ACTONEL)
Adults. 30 mg daily for 2 mo. Repeated after 2 mo if relapse occurs or if serum alkaline phosphatase level fails to normalize.
➤ *To prevent or treat glucocorticoid-induced osteoporosis*
TABLETS (ACTONEL)
Adults. 5 mg daily.
➤ *To prevent or treat postmenopausal osteoporosis*
TABLETS (ACTONEL)
Adults. 5 mg daily. Or, 35 mg once weekly, 75 mg taken on 2 consecutive days once a month, or 150 mg once a month
➤ *To treat osteoporosis in women*
E.R. TABLETS (ATELVIA)
Adults. 35 mg (1 tablet) once weekly.
➤ *To treat osteoporosis in men*
TABLETS (ACTONEL)
Adults. 35 mg once weekly.

Route	Onset	Peak	Duration
P.O.	Unknown	3 mo	16 mo

Mechanism of Action
Hinders excessive bone remodeling characteristic of Paget's disease by binding to bone and reducing the rate at which osteoclasts are resorbed by bone. Also, decreases elevated rate of bone turnover that is typically seen in osteoporosis.

Contraindications
Esophageal abnormalities that delay esophageal emptying, such as achalasia or stricture; hypersensitivity to risedronate or its components; hypocalcemia; inability to sit or stand upright for at least 30 minutes

Interactions
DRUGS
angiogenesis inhibitors, chemotherapy, corticosteroids: Possibly increased risk of osteonecrosis of the jaw
aspirin, NSAIDs: Increased risk of GI irritation
calcium-containing preparations, including antacids: Impaired absorption of risedronate
FOODS
all foods: Decreased risedronate bioavailability

Adverse Reactions
CNS: Anxiety, asthenia, depression, dizziness, fatigue, headache, insomnia, sciatica, syncope, vertigo, weakness
CV: Chest pain, hypercholesterolemia, hypertension, peripheral edema, vasodilation
EENT: Amblyopia, cataract, dry eyes, eye inflammation, nasopharyngitis, painful swallowing, pharyngitis, rhinitis, sinusitis, tinnitus
GI: Abdominal pain, colitis, constipation, diarrhea, dyspepsia, dysphagia, eructation, esophagitis, esophageal or gastric ulcers, flatulence, gastritis, nausea, vomiting
GU: UTI
MS: Arthralgia; atypical femur fractures; back, limb, neck, or shoulder pain; jaw osteonecrosis; leg cramps or spasms; myasthenia; myalgia; osteoarthritis; retrosternal pain; severe incapacitating bone, joint, or muscle pain
RESP: **Asthma exacerbation**; bronchitis, cough, pneumonia, upper respiratory tract infection
SKIN: Bullous reaction, pruritus, rash, **Stevens–Johnson syndrome, toxic epidermal necrolysis**
Other: **Anaphylaxis, angioedema**, flu-like symptoms, **hypersensitivity reactions, hypocalcemia**

Nursing Considerations
- Be aware that risedronate isn't recommended for patients with severe renal impairment.
- Make sure patient has had a dental checkup before having invasive dental procedures during risedronate therapy, especially if patient has cancer; is receiving angiogenesis inhibitors, chemotherapy, corticosteroids, or head or neck radiation; or has poor oral hygiene because risk of jaw osteonecrosis is increased in these patients.
- Give supplemental calcium and vitamin D, as prescribed, during risedronate therapy if patient's dietary intake is inadequate.
- Give calcium supplements and antacids at different time of day than risedronate administration to avoid impaired drug absorption and altered effectiveness.
- Watch for rare, but possibly severe hypersensitivity reactions such as angioedema, bullous skin reactions, or rash.

PATIENT TEACHING
- Instruct patient to take risedronate at least 1 hour before first food or drink of day (except water) while in an upright position and with 6 to 8 oz of water. Caution against lying down for at least 30 minutes after taking drug to keep it from lodging in esophagus and causing irritation. Also instruct patient not to chew or suck on tablet because doing so may irritate mouth or throat.
- Advise patient to stop taking risedronate and to notify prescriber if she develops dysphagia, new or worsening heartburn, or pain while swallowing, retrosternal pain. Also alert patient that drug may cause severe bone, joint, or muscle pain and to notify prescriber if present occurs.
- Alert patient that drugs in the same class as risedronate have caused severe bone,

joint, or muscle pain. If such symptoms appear while taking risedronate, advise patient to contact prescriber.
- Advise patient that if she takes 35 mg once weekly and misses a dose, tell her to take it the morning after she remembers and then to take the next dose on its usual day. If patient takes 75 mg on 2 consecutive days once monthly and she misses both doses with more than 7 days until the next scheduled dose, tell her to take the first missed dose on the morning after she remembers and the second dose the following day. If she misses only 1 of the 2 doses, tell her to take it the morning after she remembers and then resume her normal schedule. If patient takes 150 mg once monthly and misses a dose, urge her to contact prescriber for instructions. Caution patient not to take more than 150 mg within a 7-day period and not to take 2 tablets of any strength on the same day.
- Tell patient to take antacids or calcium supplements at different times than risedronate.
- Urge women of childbearing age to tell prescriber about planned, suspected, or known pregnancy because of risk to fetal skeleton.
- Tell patient to stop risedronate and contact prescriber if allergic reaction occurs. Stress importance of seeking immediate emergency care if she notices swelling or skin abnormalities.
- Instruct patient about proper oral hygiene and about the need to notify prescriber about invasive dental procedures.
- Instruct patient to notify prescriber immediately of any new groin or thigh pain that might be reflective of an atypical femur fracture.

risperidone

Perseris, Risperdal, Risperdal Consta

Class and Category

Pharmacologic class: Benzisoxazole derivative
Therapeutic class: Antipsychotic
Pregnancy category: C

Indications and Dosages

➤ *To treat schizophrenia*

ORAL SOLUTION, ORALLY DISINTEGRATING TABLETS, TABLETS

Adults. 1 mg twice daily on day 1; 2 mg twice daily on day 2; 3 mg twice daily on day 3. Or, 2 mg daily on day 1; 4 mg daily on day 2; 6 mg daily on day 3. Then increased by 1 to 2 mg daily at 1- to 2-wk intervals, as needed.
Maximum: 16 mg daily.
Adolescents ages 13 to 17. *Initial:* 0.5 mg once daily, increased as needed every 24 hr in 0.5- to 1-mg increments. *Maximum:* 3 mg once daily.

I.M. INJECTION (RISPERDAL CONSTA)

Adults. *Initial:* 25 mg every 2 wk, increased as needed every 4 wk to 37.5 or 50 mg.
Maximum: 50 mg every 2 wk.

SUBCUTANEOUS INJECTION (PERSERIS)

Adults. 90 mg or 120 mg once monthly injected into abdomen only.

➤ *To treat bipolar mania*

ORAL SOLUTION, ORALLY DISINTEGRATING TABLETS, TABLETS

Adults. *Initial:* 2 or 3 mg daily, increased as needed by 1 mg daily up to 6 mg. *Maximum:* 6 mg daily for no more than 3 wk.
Children and adolescents ages 10 to 17. *Initial:* 0.5 mg once daily, increased as needed every 24 hr in 0.5- to 1-mg increments. *Maximum:* 2.5 mg once daily.

➤ *To treat bipolar mania as monotherapy or as adjunct to lithium or valproate therapy*

I.M. INJECTION (RISPERDAL CONSTA)

Adults. 25 mg every 2 wk, increased, as needed to 37.5 or 50 mg. *Maximum:* 50 mg every 2 wk.

➤ *To treat irritability associated with autistic disorder*

ORAL SOLUTION, ORALLY DISINTEGRATING TABLETS, TABLETS

Children age 5 and over and adolescents weighing less than 20 kg (44 lb). *Initial:* 0.25 mg daily, increased after 4 days to 0.5 mg daily. Dosage further increased, as needed in 2-wk intervals in 0.25 mg increments.
Children age 5 and over and adolescents weighing 20 kg or more. *Initial:* 0.5 mg daily, increased after 4 days to 1 mg daily. Dosage further increased, as needed in 2 wk intervals in 0.5 mg increments.

DOSAGE ADJUSTMENT For elderly patients and patients with severe hepatic or renal impairment or who are taking CYP2D6 inhibitors, starting doses reduced as much as 50%. For patients taking CYP3A4 inducers such as carbamazepine, phenobarbital, phenytoin, or rifampin, dosage may have to be increased.

Mechanism of Action

Selectively blocks serotonin and dopamine receptors in the mesocortical tract of the CNS to suppress psychotic symptoms.

Incompatibilities

Don't mix oral solution with cola or tea.

Contraindications

Hypersensitivity to risperidone, paliperidone, or its components

Interactions

DRUGS

antihypertensives: Increased antihypertensive effects
bromocriptine, levodopa, pergolide: Possibly antagonized effects of these drugs
carbamazepine: Increased risperidone clearance with long-term concurrent use
clozapine: Decreased risperidone clearance with long-term concurrent use
CNS depressants: Additive CNS depression
fluoxetine, paroxetine: Increased plasma risperidone level

ACTIVITIES

alcohol use: Additive CNS depression

Adverse Reactions

CNS: Abnormal coordination, aggressiveness, agitation, akathisia, anxiety, asthenia, confusion, decreased concentration, depression, dizziness, dream disturbances, drooling, drowsiness, dyskinesia, dystonia, fatigue, fever, headache, **hypothermia**, insomnia, lassitude, malaise, mania, memory loss, nervousness, **neuroleptic malignant syndrome**, paresthesia, Parkinsonism, restlessness, **seizures**, shaking of head repeatedly, sleepwalking, somnolence, tardive dyskinesia, tremor, vertigo
CV: Atrial fibrillation, bradycardia, bundle branch block, **cardiopulmonary arrest**, chest pain, elevated triglyceride levels, first-degree AV block, hypercholesterolemia, orthostatic hypotension, palpitations, **QT-interval prolongation**, tachycardia
EENT: Conjunctivitis, decreased or increased salivation, dry mouth, ear pain, epistaxis, nasal congestion, pharyngitis, retinal artery occlusion, rhinitis, sinusitis, taste alteration, vision changes
ENDO: Diabetic ketoacidosis (patients with diabetes), elevated prolactin level, galactorrhea, hyperglycemia, hyperprolactinemia, **hypoglycemia**, inappropriate antidiuretic hormone secretion (SIADH), pituitary adenoma, precocious puberty
GI: Abdominal pain, anorexia, constipation, diarrhea, gastritis, ileus, indigestion, **intestinal obstruction**, jaundice, nausea, **pancreatitis**, vomiting
GU: Amenorrhea, decreased libido, delayed ejaculation, dysmenorrhea, dysuria, glucosuria, hypermenorrhea, incontinence, increased appetite, polyuria, priapism, sexual dysfunction, urinary incontinence or retention, UTI
HEME: Agranulocytosis, anemia, **leukopenia, neutropenia, thrombocytopenia**
MS: Arthralgia; back, buttock, or neck pain; dysarthria; muscle weakness; myalgia
RESP: Cough, dyspnea, **pulmonary embolism, sleep apnea**, upper respiratory tract infection
SKIN: Alopecia, diaphoresis, dry skin, eczema, hyperpigmentation, photosensitivity, pruritus, rash, seborrhea
Other: Anaphylaxis; angioedema; flu-like symptoms; infections; injection-site induration, pain, redness, or swelling; weight gain or loss

Nursing Considerations

- Use risperidone cautiously in debilitated patients, elderly patients, and patients with hepatic or renal dysfunction or hypotension because of their increased sensitivity to the drug. Also use risperidone cautiously in patients with a history of seizures; although rare, seizures may occur in those with schizophrenia.

WARNING Be aware that risperidone should not be used to treat elderly patients with dementia-related psychosis because it increases risk of death in these patients.

- Be aware that oral risperidone or another antipsychotic should be continued for 3 weeks after long-acting I.M. form of risperidone is first administered to provide an adequate therapeutic plasma level until risperidone release from injection site has begun. If the patient has never received oral risperidone, an oral trial should be prescribed before use of I.M. or subcutaneous forms to determine patient's tolerance of the drug.
- Know that patients with hepatic or renal impairment prescribed the long-acting subcutaneous form of risperidone will need to be carefully titrated up to at least 3 mg daily of oral risperidone. If patient can tolerate the oral dose and is psychiatrically stable, the long-acting subcutaneous form may be initiated at the lower dose of 90 mg once a month.
- Remove I.M. form (Risperdal Consta) from refrigerator and allow it to come to room temperature for at least 30 min before reconstitution. Follow manufacturer's guidelines for reconstitution, following the illustrations closely and, using only the diluent supplied in the dose pack.
- Give I.M. form using only the needle supplied in the dose pack. Inject entire contents of syringe into the upper outer quadrant of gluteal area using the 2-inch needle or into the deltoid muscle using the 1-inch needle within 2 minutes of reconstitution. Never combine the two different dose strengths for I.M. injection into a single administration. If drug can't be given right after reconstitution, shake the upright vial vigorously back and forth until particles are resuspended. Discard reconstituted drug if not used within 6 hours. Never administer I.M. form intravenously.
- Remove subcutaneous package (Perseris) from refrigerator and allow it to come to room temperature for at least 15 minutes before preparing drug for administration. Only prepare drug when ready to administer the dose, not before.
- To prepare a subcutaneous dose (Perseris), first hold the powder syringe in upright position and tap the barrel of the syringe to dislodge the packed powder. Then remove the cap first from the liquid syringe and then from the powder syringe. Place the liquid syringe on top of the powder syringe and connect the two syringes by twisting approximately 3/4 turn. Do not overtighten. Keep fingers off the plungers to avoid spillage of drug. Failure to fully mix drug can result in incorrect dosage. Transfer the contents of the liquid syringe into the powder syringe. Gently push the powder syringe plunger until resistance is felt. Repeat this gentle back-and-forth process for 5 cycles. Continue mixing the syringes for an additional 55 cycles. When fully mixed, drug should be a cloudy suspension that is uniform in color. It can vary from white to yellow-green. If any clear areas occur in the mixture, continue to mix it until the distribution of the color is uniform. Then transfer all the contents into the liquid syringe. After this, while maintaining slight pressure on the powder syringe plunger, pull back gently on the liquid syringe plunger while twisting the syringes apart. Finally, attach the safety needle by twisting until finger-tight.
- Administer subcutaneous form (Perseris) into the abdomen only after removing excess air from syringe; inject drug slowly and steadily. Do not rub the injection site after the injection. If there is bleeding, apply a bandage but use minimal pressure.
- Monitor for orthostatic hypotension, especially in patients with cardiac or cerebrovascular disease.

WARNING Immediately notify prescriber and expect to stop giving risperidone if patient shows evidence of neuroleptic malignant syndrome (altered mental status, autonomic instability, hyperpyrexia, muscle rigidity), which can be fatal.

- Monitor patient's blood glucose and lipid levels as ordered because drug increases the risk of hyperglycemia and hypercholesterolemia.
- Monitor patient's CBC, as ordered, because serious adverse hematologic reactions may occur, such as agranulocytosis, leukopenia, or neutropenia. More frequent monitoring during the first few months of risperidone therapy is recommended for patients with a history of drug-induced leukopenia or neutropenia, or those who have had a significantly low WBC count in the past.

If abnormalities occur during therapy, monitor patient for fever or other signs of infection, notify prescriber, and expect drug to be discontinued if severe.
- Institute fall precautions.

PATIENT TEACHING

- Instruct patient to dilute risperidone oral solution with water, coffee, orange juice, or low-fat milk, but not with cola or tea.
- Tell patient prescribed orally disintegrating tablets to break open the blister unit with dry hands by peeling the foil back to expose the tablet. Emphasize the importance of not pushing tablet through the foil because this could damage the tablet. Once patient has removed tablet, she should place immediately on her tongue, where it will dissolve within seconds. Tell patient not to chew orally disintegrating tablet or attempt to spit it out of her mouth.
- Urge patient to avoid alcohol because of its additive CNS effects.
- Caution diabetic patient to monitor blood glucose level closely, because risperidone may increase it.
- Caution patient that risperidone may cause sleepwalking
- Caution patient to avoid performing hazardous activities such as driving until CNS effects are known and subside. Review fall precautions with patient.
- Instruct mothers who are breastfeeding while taking risperidone to monitor the infant for abnormal muscle movements, excess sedation, failure to thrive, jitteriness, or tremors.
- Inform women of childbearing age that risperidone may reduce fertility, but that this is reversible after drug is discontinued.

ritonavir

Norvir

Class and Category

Pharmacologic class: Protease inhibitor
Therapeutic class: Antiretroviral
Pregnancy category: Not classified

Indications and Dosages

➤ *As adjunct to treat human immunodeficiency viral type 1 (HIV-1) infection*

CAPSULES, TABLETS

Adults. *Initial:* 300 mg twice daily with meals, increased by 100 mg twice daily every 2 to 3 days until maximum dose reached. *Maximum:* 600 mg twice daily.

Children able to swallow capsules or tablets. *Initial:* 250 mg/m^2 twice daily with meals, increased by 50 mg/m^2 twice daily every 2 to 3 days until a maintenance dosage is reached. *Maintenance:* 350 to 400 mg/m^2 twice daily with meals. *Maximum:* 600 mg twice daily.

ORAL SOLUTION

Adults. *Initial:* 300 mg twice daily with meals, increased by 100 mg twice daily every 2 to 3 days until maximum dose is reached. *Maximum:* 600 mg twice daily.

Infants at least 44 weeks old (calculated from first day of mother's last menstrual period to birth plus the time elapsed after birth) and children. *Initial:* 250 mg/m^2 twice daily with meals, increased by 50 mg/m^2 twice daily every 2 to 3 days until a maintenance dosage is reached. *Maintenance:* 350 to 400 mg/m^2 twice daily with meals. Maximum: 600 mg twice daily.

ORAL POWDER

Adults prescribed dosing in increments of 100 mg. *Initial:* 300 mg twice daily with meals, increased by 100 mg twice daily every 2 to 3 days until maximum dose reached. *Maximum:* 600 mg twice daily.

DOSAGE ADJUSTMENT For patient taking other protease inhibitors such as atazanavir, darunavir, fosamprenavir, saquinavir, and tipranavir, dosage reduced.

Mechanism of Action

Inhibits HIV protease to render the enzyme incapable of processing the Gag-Pol polyprotein precursor, which leads to the production of noninfectious immature HIV particles.

Contraindications

Concomitant therapy with other protease inhibitors, potent CYP3A inducers, or therapy that is highly dependent on CYP3A for drug clearance and for which elevated plasma concentrations have resulted in serious and/or life-threatening reactions (alfuzosin, amiodarone, cisapride, colchicine, dihydroergotamine, dronedarone, ergotamine, flecainide, lovastatin, lurasidone, methylergonovine, midazolam [oral], pimozide, propafenone, quinidine, ranolazine, St. John's wort, sildenafil [when used for treatment of pulmonary arterial hypertension], simvastatin, triazolam, voriconazole); hypersensitivity to ritonavir or its components

Interactions

DRUGS

amprenavir, atazanavir, atorvastatin, bedaquiline, bosentan, buspirone, carbamazepine, clarithromycin, clonazepam, clorazepate, colchicine, corticosteroids, cyclosporine, darunavir, dasatinib, desipramine, diazepam, diltiazem, disopyramide, dronabinol, estazolam, ethinyl estradiol, ethosuximide, fentanyl, fluoxetine, flurazepam, ibrutinib, indinavir, itraconazole, ketoconazole, lidocaine, maraviroc, methamphetamine, metoprolol, mexiletine, midazolam (parenteral), nefazodone, nifedipine, nilotinib, paroxetine, perphenazine, propoxyphene, quetiapine, quinine, rifabutin, risperidone, rosuvastatin, salmeterol, saquinavir, simeprevir, sirolimus, tacrolimus, thioridazine, timolol, tipranavir, trazodone, tricyclic antidepressants, venetoclax, verapamil, zolpidem: Increased concentration of these drugs with possible risk of prolonged action and adverse reactions
atovaquone, bupropion, divalproex, lamotrigine, phenytoin, raltegravir, rifampin, theophylline, voriconazole: Decreased concentration of these drugs with possible decreased efficacy
avanafil, sildenafil, tadalafil, vardenafil: Increased concentration of PDE5 inhibitors with possible increased risk of adverse reactions, including hypotension, prolonged erection, syncope, visual changes
delavirdine: Increased concentration of ritonavir with possible risk of prolonged action and adverse reactions
digoxin: Increased concentration of digoxin with possible increased risk of digitalis toxicity
disulfiram, metronidazole: Increased risk of adverse reactions, especially "hangover" symptoms, because ritonavir contains ethanol
methadone: Decreased concentration of methadone with increased risk of opiate withdrawal symptoms
meperidine: Increased concentrations of the metabolite of meperidine with possible risk of prolonged action and adverse reactions
rivaroxaban: Increased concentration of rivaroxaban with possible increased risk of bleeding
vinblastine, vincristine: Increased concentration of these drugs with increased risk of significant gastrointestinal or hematologic adverse reactions
warfarin: Altered INR in either direction requiring possible dosage adjustments

Adverse Reactions

CNS: Asthenia, attention disturbance, confusion, dizziness, fatigue, paresthesia, peripheral neuropathy, **seizures**, syncope
CV: AV block, elevated cholesterol and triglycerides, hypertension, **hypotension**, orthostatic hypotension, peripheral edema, right bundle branch block
EENT: Blurred vision, oral paresthesia, oropharyngeal pain
ENDO: Cushingoid appearance, fat redistribution, hot flashes
GI: Abdominal pain, bilirubin increase, diarrhea, dysgeusia, dyspepsia, elevated liver and pancreatic enzymes, flatulence, gastroesophageal reflux disease, **GI hemorrhage**, **hepatitis**, **hepatotoxicity**, jaundice, nausea, **pancreatitis**, vomiting
GU: Increased urination, **renal insufficiency**
HEME: Anemia, decreased red blood cells, **leukopenia**, **neutropenia**, **thrombocytopenia**
MS: Arthralgia, back pain, elevated creatine phosphokinase, myalgia, myopathy, peripheral coldness
RESP: Bronchospasm, coughing
SKIN: Acne, facial edema, flushing, pruritus, rash, skin eruptions, **Stevens-Johnson syndrome**, **toxic epidermal necrolysis**, urticaria
Other: Anaphylaxis, **angioedema**, dehydration, **electrolyte imbalances**, gout, immune reconstitution syndrome, lipodystrophy (acquired)

Nursing Considerations

- Use cautiously in patients with cardiomyopathies, ischemic heart disease, preexisting conduction system abnormalities, or structural heart disease, because ritonavir may prolong patient's PR interval.

- Use cautiously in patients with hepatitis (especially B and C), liver enzyme abnormalities, or preexisting liver disease, because of the increased risk of hepatotoxicity during ritonavir therapy. Expect to monitor liver enzymes, as ordered, in these patients more frequently during the first 3 months of ritonavir therapy.
- Expect to check patient's cholesterol and triglyceride levels prior to starting ritonavir therapy and then periodically throughout therapy. Notify prescriber if elevated, and expect patient to be treated for the lipid disorder.
- Be aware that oral powder form of ritonavir should only be used for dosing increments of 100 mg. If the dose is less than 100 mg or the dose falls between 100-mg intervals, other forms should be used instead of the powder.
- Administer ritonavir with meals. Mix oral solution with Advera, chocolate milk, or Ensure within 1 hour of administration to help improve the taste.
- Mix oral powder form with soft food such as applesauce or vanilla pudding or mix with liquids such as chocolate milk, infant formula, or water and use a calibrated dosing syringe to measure dosage, especially for infants and children. Once mixed, use within 2 hours or discard.
- Know that the oral powder form may be given via a feeding tube after being mixed with water.
- Do not use oral solution for use with polyurethane feeding tubes, because the presence of ethanol in the solution may be incompatible. Also know that oral solution should not be given to pregnant women because of the ethanol content. Be aware that the total amounts of ethanol and propylene glycol from all drugs given to infants 1 to 6 months of age should be taken into account to avoid toxicity.
- Be aware that a patient who takes 600-mg twice daily soft-gel capsule dose may experience more gastrointestinal adverse reactions (such as abdominal pain, diarrhea, nausea, and vomiting) when switching from the soft gel capsule to the tablet form, because of greater maximum plasma concentration in the tablet compared to the soft gel capsule. Know that these adverse events may diminish as ritonavir therapy continues.
- Know that dihydroergotamine or ergotamine should not be coadministered with ritonavir because acute ergot toxicity may occur, exhibited by ischemia of the extremities and other tissues including the central nervous system and vasospasm.
- Be aware that adrenal suppression and Cushing's syndrome may occur when ritonavir is coadministered with budesonide or fluticasone propionate.

WARNING Assess patient's skin regularly for signs of a hypersensitivity reaction. Know that angioedema, mild skin eruptions, and urticaria have occurred with ritonavir therapy. Cases of anaphylaxis, Stevens–Johnson syndrome, and toxic epidermal necrolysis have also occurred with ritonavir therapy. Report any abnormal findings and expect ritonavir to be discontinued if reaction is severe.

- Monitor patient's liver enzymes, as ordered, and patient for signs and symptoms of liver dysfunction.
- Monitor patient for pancreatitis such as the presence of abdominal pain, abnormal serum amylase or lipase values, nausea, or vomiting. If suspected, notify prescriber and expect ritonavir to be discontinued if confirmed.
- Monitor patient's blood glucose levels throughout ritonavir therapy, because some patients have experienced an exacerbation of diabetes mellitus or have developed hyperglycemia or new-onset diabetes mellitus with protease inhibitor therapy.
- Be aware that immune reconstitution syndrome has occurred in patients treated with combination antiretroviral therapy, including ritonavir. The inflammatory response predisposes susceptible patients to opportunistic infections such as cytomegalovirus, *Mycobacterium avium* infection, *Pneumocystis jiroveci* pneumonia, or tuberculosis. Autoimmune disorders such as Graves' disease, Guillain–Barré syndrome, or polymyositis have also occurred. Report sudden or unusual adverse reactions to prescriber.

- Observe patient for redistribution of body fat, including breast enlargement, central obesity, development of buffalo hump, facial wasting, and peripheral wasting, which may produce a cushingoid-type appearance.
- Monitor patients with hemophilia for increased bleeding, because spontaneous skin hemarthrosis and hematomas have occurred in these patients while taking ritonavir. Provide supportive care, as prescribed.

PATIENT TEACHING

- Instruct patient to swallow tablets whole and not to break, chew, or crush them.
- Tell patient prescribed the oral solution that the taste may be improved by mixing with Advera, chocolate milk, or Ensure within 1 hour of dosing.
- Instruct parents to mix oral powder with soft food such as applesauce or vanilla pudding or mix with liquid such as chocolate milk or water. The bitter aftertaste may be lessened if given with food.
- Warn patient switching from soft gel capsule form to tablets that he may experience an increase in gastrointestinal side effects such as abdominal pain, diarrhea, nausea, and vomiting, but that these adverse events may decrease over time.
- Instruct mothers not to breastfeed while receiving ritonavir therapy.
- Warn patient that fat distribution may occur with ritonavir therapy, altering appearance.
- Alert female patients using oral contraceptives or patch contraceptives containing ethinyl estradiol that alternative methods of contraception should be used.
- Tell women of childbearing age to report a known or suspected pregnancy.
- Inform patients with hemophilia of increased risk of bleeding and the need to seek immediate medical attention if bleeding occurs.

WARNING Instruct patient to report any signs of skin abnormalities, especially a skin rash, immediately to the prescriber.

- Warn patient to alert all prescribers of ritonavir therapy, because serious drug interactions can occur.

rivaroxaban

Xarelto

Class and Category

Pharmacologic class: Factor Xa inhibitor
Therapeutic class: Anticoagulant
Pregnancy category: C

Indications and Dosages

➤ *To reduce the risk of stroke and systemic embolism in patients with nonvalvular atrial fibrillation*

TABLETS

Adults with creatinine clearance greater than 50 ml/min. 20 mg once daily with evening meal.
Adults with creatinine clearance between 15 and 50 ml/min. 15 mg once daily with evening meal.

➤ *To prevent deep vein thrombosis, which may lead to pulmonary embolism following knee or hip replacement surgery*

TABLETS

Adults. 10 mg once daily begun 6 to 10 hr after surgery once hemostasis has been established and given for 12 days after knee replacement surgery and given 35 days after hip replacement surgery.

➤ *To treat deep vein thrombosis or pulmonary embolism*

TABLETS

Adults. 15 mg twice daily with food for 21 days, followed by 20 mg once daily with food.

➤ *To reduce risk of recurrence of deep vein thrombosis or pulmonary embolism*

TABLETS

Adults. 10 mg once daily with food for at least 6 months.

➤ *To reduce risk of major cardiovascular events in patients with chronic coronary artery disease or peripheral artery disease*

TABLETS

Adults. 2.5 mg twice daily with 75 or 100 mg aspirin once daily.

Mechanism of Action

Selectively blocks the active site of factor Xa, which plays a central role in the cascade of blood coagulation. Without the action of factor Xa, blood clotting is impaired.

Contraindications

Active pathological bleeding, hypersensitivity to rivaroxaban or its components

Interactions

DRUGS

anticoagulants, aspirin, clopidogrel, dual antiplatelet therapy, fibrinolytic therapy, heparin, NSAIDs, other antithrombotic agents or platelet aggregation inhibitors, selective serotonin reuptake inhibitors, serotonin-norepinephrine reuptake inhibitors, warfarin: Possibly increased bleeding risk

carbamazepine, phenytoin, rifampin, St. John's wort: Decreased effectiveness of rivaroxaban

conivaptan, diltiazem, dronedarone, erythromycin, fluconazole, indinavir/ritonavir, itraconazole, ketoconazole, lopinavir/ritonavir, ritonavir, verapamil: Increased rivaroxaban exposure resulting in increased bleeding risk

Adverse Reactions

CNS: Anxiety, **cerebral hemorrhage**, depression, dizziness, epidural hematoma, fatigue, hemiparesis, insomnia, **subdural hematoma**, syncope

GI: Abdominal pain, cholestasis, **cytolytic hepatitis**, **GI bleeding**, jaundice, **retroperitoneal hemorrhage**

HEME: **Agranulocytosis**, **excessive bleeding**, **hemorrhage**, **thrombocytopenia**

MS: Back or extremity pain, muscle spasm

RESP: **Pulmonary hemorrhage** with or without bronchiectasis

SKIN: Pruritus, **Stevens–Johnson syndrome**

Other: **Anaphylaxis**, **angioedema**, **drug reaction with eosinophilia and systemic symptoms (DRESS)**

Nursing Considerations

- Know that rivaroxaban used to reduce the risk of stroke and systemic embolism in nonvalvular atrial fibrillation should not be given to patients with moderate or severe hepatic impairment, to patients with any hepatic disease associated with coagulopathy, and to patients with a creatinine clearance that is less than 15 ml/min. Monitor patient's hepatic and renal function, as ordered, throughout rivaroxaban therapy.
- Know that rivaroxaban used to prevent or treat deep vein thrombosis, to treat pulmonary embolism, and to reduce risk of recurrence of deep vein thrombosis or pulmonary embolism should not be given to patients with a creatinine clearance less than 30 ml/min.
- Be aware that rivaroxaban should not be given to patients with prosthetic heart valves or as an alternative to unfractionated heparin in patients with pulmonary embolism who are hemodynamically unstable or who may receive pulmonary embolectomy or thrombolysis.
- Be aware that rivaroxaban should be used cautiously during pregnancy because drug has the potential to cross the placenta, causing bleeding at any site in the fetus and/or neonate.
- Monitor patient closely for signs and symptoms of a hypersensitivity reaction because severe hypersensitivity reactions have occurred following rivaroxaban therapy.
- Be aware that manufacturer guidelines should be followed when patient is switching from or to other anticoagulants. For example, when patient is switching from warfarin to rivaroxaban therapy, expect warfarin to be discontinued and rivaroxaban started when the International Normalized Ratio (INR) is below 3. For patients currently receiving an anticoagulant other than warfarin, such as low-molecular-weight heparin or nonwarfarin oral anticoagulant, expect to start rivaroxaban therapy within 2 hours of the next scheduled evening administration of the drug, and plan to omit administration of the other anticoagulant, as ordered. For unfractionated heparin being administered by continuous infusion, expect to stop the infusion and start rivaroxaban therapy at the same time. For patients currently taking rivaroxaban and transitioning to an anticoagulant with rapid onset, expect rivaroxaban to be discontinued and the first dose of the other anticoagulant given at the time the next rivaroxaban would have been given.
- Administering rivaroxaban via a nasogastric tube or gastric feeding tube

requires tablets to be crushed and suspended in 50 ml of water. Following administration, enteral feeding should be given immediately.

- Expect rivaroxaban to be discontinued if acute renal failure occurs.

WARNING Monitor patient closely for bleeding as rivaroxaban therapy may cause life-threatening bleeding. Expect to administer the antidote available to reverse the anti-factor Xa activity of rivaroxaban if bleeding is significant.

- Expect rivaroxaban to be discontinued 24 hours before an invasive procedure or surgery, if possible and restarted after adequate hemostasis has been established after the invasive surgery or procedure.
- Know that if patient has an epidural catheter inserted, it should not be removed any earlier than 18 hours for younger patients (less than 45 years) and 26 hours for older patients (60 years and over) after the last rivaroxaban dose was administered. Obtain specific guidelines for catheter removal from prescriber for patients between 45 and 60 years of age. The next rivaroxaban dose should not be administered any earlier than 6 hours after the removal of the catheter because an epidural or spinal hematoma can occur and can result in long-term or permanent paralysis. If traumatic puncture occurs, know that rivaroxaban should be withheld for 24 hours.
- Be aware that if rivaroxaban is discontinued and adequate alternative anticoagulation is not present, the risk for thrombosis increases. Monitor patient closely.

PATIENT TEACHING

- Emphasize the importance of taking rivaroxaban exactly as prescribed.
- Instruct patient taking 15- or 20-mg tablets to take with food; 10-mg tablets do not need to be taken with food. For patient unable to swallow tablets, tell patient to crush tablets and mix with applesauce immediately prior to taking and then follow with food.
- Tell patient not to stop taking rivaroxaban without first consulting prescriber.
- Instruct patient with atrial fibrillation to take the drug with the evening meal.
- Advise patient to report any unusual bleeding or bruising to the prescriber. Inform patient that it may take longer for him to stop bleeding and to take bleeding precautions, such as avoiding the use of a razor and using a soft-bristle toothbrush.
- Tell patient to alert all prescribers to use of rivaroxaban therapy before any invasive procedure, including dental work, is scheduled.
- Instruct patient who has had spinal anesthesia or puncture to watch for back pain, muscle weakness, numbness (especially in the lower limbs), stool or urine incontinence, or tingling. If present, stress importance of notifying prescriber immediately.
- Caution patient not to take any prescription or nonprescription medication, including over-the-counter and herbal medicines, without first consulting with prescriber.
- Advise female patient to notify prescriber immediately if pregnancy is suspected or known.
- Alert mothers wishing to breastfeed that drug has been found in breast milk. Advise patient to discuss breastfeeding with prescriber before doing so.

rivastigmine

Exelon Patch

rivastigmine tartrate

Exelon

Class and Category

Pharmacologic class: Cholinesterase inhibitor
Therapeutic class: Antidementia
Pregnancy category: B

Indications and Dosages

➤ *To treat mild-to-moderate Alzheimer's-type dementia*

CAPSULES, ORAL SOLUTION

Adults. *Initial:* 1.5 mg twice daily with morning and evening meals. Dosage increased by 3 mg daily every 2 wk, as needed. *Maximum:* 6 mg twice daily with morning and evening meals.

➤ *To treat mild, moderate, and severe Alzheimer's disease*

TRANSDERMAL

Adults. *Initial:* 4.6 mg/24 hr. After 4 wk, increased to 9.5 mg/24 hr. When therapeutic effect begins to decrease in and with at least 4 wk from last dosage increase, dosage increased to 13.3 mg/24 hr. *Maximum:* 13.3 mg/24 hr.

➤ *To treat mild-to-moderate dementia in Parkinson's disease*

CAPSULES, ORAL SOLUTION

Adults. *Initial:* 1.5 mg twice daily with morning and evening meals. Dosage increased by 3 mg daily every 4 wk, as needed. *Maximum:* 6 mg twice daily with morning and evening meals.

TRANSDERMAL

Adults. *Initial:* 4.6 mg/24 hr. After 4 wk, increased to 9.5 mg/24 hr. When therapeutic effect begins to decrease, dosage increased to 13.3 mg/24 hr. *Maximum:* 13.3 mg/24 hr.

➤ *To convert patient from oral to transdermal rivastigmine therapy*

TRANSDERMAL

Adults. If total oral dosage was less than 6 mg daily, use 4.6 mg/24 hr, with first transdermal patch applied the day after the last oral dose. If total oral dosage was 6 to 12 mg daily, use 9.5 mg/24 hr, with first transdermal patch applied the day after the last oral dose.

DOSAGE ADJUSTMENT If patient develops adverse effects (such as nausea or vomiting), treatment should be stopped for several doses, as prescribed and restarted at the same or next lower dose level. For patient with mild-to-moderate hepatic impairment, 4.6 mg/24 hr patch used for both initial and maximum dose. For patients with low body weight of less than 50 kg (110 lb) and experiencing excessive nausea and vomiting, maintenance dose kept at 4.6 mg/24 hr

Mechanism of Action

May slow the decline of cognitive function by increasing acetylcholine concentration at cholinergic transmission sites. This action prolongs and exaggerates the effects of acetylcholine that are otherwise blocked by toxic levels of anticholinergics. Cognitive decline is partially related to cholinergic deficits along neuronal pathways projecting from the basal forebrain to the cerebral cortex and hippocampus that are involved in attention, cognition, learning, and memory.

Contraindications

History of application-site reactions suggestive of allergic contact dermatitis (for patch form); hypersensitivity to carbamate derivatives, rivastigmine, or their components

Interactions

DRUGS

anticholinergics: Possibly decreased effectiveness of anticholinergics
beta blockers: Possible additive bradycardic effects resulting in syncope
bethanechol, succinylcholine: Possibly synergistic effects
metoclopramide: Increased risk of additive extrapyramidal adverse reactions.
other cholinomimetic drugs: Possibly increased cholinergic effects

Adverse Reactions

CNS: Aggression, anxiety, asthenia, confusion, depression, dizziness, extrapyramidal movements, fatigue, fever, hallucinations, headache, insomnia, malaise, nightmares, **seizures**, somnolence, tremor worsening of Parkinsonism
CV: Hypertension, tachycardia
EENT: Rhinitis
GI: Abdominal pain, anorexia, constipation, diarrhea, duodenal ulcers, elevated liver enzymes, flatulence, **hepatitis**, indigestion, nausea, vomiting
GU: UTI
SKIN: Allergic or disseminated dermatitis, increased sweating, reaction at patch application site (papule or vesicle formation, pruritus, redness, swelling), **Stevens–Johnson syndrome**, urticaria
Other: Dehydration, flu-like symptoms, weight loss

Nursing Considerations

WARNING Be aware that rivastigmine should be started at lowest recommended dosage and adjusted to effective maintenance dosage because initial therapy at high dosage can cause serious adverse GI reactions, including anorexia, nausea, and weight loss. Also, a higher than recommended starting dosage may cause severe vomiting and possibly esophageal rupture. If treatment is interrupted for longer than several days, expect to restart at lowest recommended dosage.

- Be aware that drug shouldn't be stopped abruptly because doing so may increase behavioral disturbances and precipitate a further decline in cognitive function.
- Monitor respiratory status of patients with pulmonary disease, including asthma, chronic bronchitis, and emphysema, because rivastigmine has a weak affinity for peripheral cholinesterase, which may increase bronchoconstriction and bronchial secretions.
- Monitor patient for adequate urine output because cholinomimetics, such as rivastigmine, may induce or exacerbate bladder or urinary tract obstruction.
- Monitor patients with Parkinson's disease for exaggerated parkinsonian symptoms, which may result from drug's increased cholinergic effects on CNS.

WARNING Monitor patient closely for hypersensitivity skin reactions regardless of route of administration. If suspected, notify prescriber, and expect drug to be discontinued.

PATIENT TEACHING

- Explain to patient and family that rivastigmine can't cure Alzheimer's or Parkinson's disease but may slow the progressive deterioration of memory and improve patient's ability to perform activities of daily living.
- Teach patient and family how to administer oral solution, if prescribed, emphasizing need to use the oral dosing syringe provided. Explain that dose may be swallowed directly from the syringe or mixed into a small glass of cold fruit juice, soda or water; stirred; and then drunk.
- Explain that oral drug should be taken with food to reduce adverse GI effects.
- Instruct patient or caregiver to apply transdermal patch to clean, dry, hairless, intact skin in a location, such as the back, that won't be rubbed by tight clothing and won't be affected by cream, lotion, or powder. Tell patient to remove the old patch before applying a new one and to use a new application site daily. Caution against using the same site within 14 days.
- Tell patient applying transdermal patch to press patch firmly against skin until the edges stick well. Reassure patient that patch may be worn while bathing or swimming.
- Instruct a family member to supervise patient's use of rivastigmine.
- Urge caregiver to contact prescriber and to withhold drug if patient stops taking it for more than several days.
- Emphasize importance of inspecting skin for signs of an allergic reaction, such as presence of hives, itching, rash, or redness. If present, instruct patient or family to notify prescriber, as drug will have to be discontinued.
- Advise women of childbearing age to notify prescriber if pregnancy occurs.

rizatriptan benzoate

Maxalt, Maxalt-MLT

Class and Category

Pharmacologic class: Selective serotonin receptor agonist
Therapeutic class: Antimigraine
Pregnancy category: C

Indications and Dosages

➤ *To relieve acute migraine headache*

DISINTEGRATING TABLETS, TABLETS

Adults. 5 to 10 mg when migraine headache starts; repeated every 2 hr, as needed. *Maximum:* 30 mg daily.
Children age 6 to 17 years weighing 40 kg (88 lb) or more. 10 mg when migraine headache starts.
Children age 6 to 17 years weighing less than 40 kg (88 lb). 5 mg when migraine headache starts.

DOSAGE ADJUSTMENT For adults taking propranolol, initial dosage reduced to 5 mg, then repeated every 2 hr, as needed, up to maximum of 15 mg daily.

Mechanism of Action

Binds to selective 5-hydroxytryptamine receptor sites on cerebral blood vessels, causing vessels to constrict. This may decrease the characteristic pulsing sensation and thus relieve the pain of migraine headaches. Rizatriptan may also relieve pain by inhibiting the release of proinflammatory neuropeptides and reducing transmission of trigeminal nerve impulses from sensory nerve endings during a migraine attack.

Contraindications

Basilar or hemiplegic migraine, hypersensitivity to rizatriptan or its components, ischemic coronary artery disease, uncontrolled hypertension, use within 14 days of MAO inhibitor therapy, use within 24 hours of ergotamine-containing or ergot-type drugs or other serotonin-receptor agonists

Interactions

DRUGS

ergot-containing drugs: Prolonged vasospastic reactions
MAO inhibitors, propranolol: Increased blood rizatriptan level
selective serotonin reuptake inhibitors, serotonin norepinephrine reuptake inhibitors, other triptans: Increased risk of serotonin syndrome
serotonin-receptor agonists: Additive vasospastic effects

Adverse Reactions

CNS: Altered temperature sensation, anxiety, asthenia, ataxia, chills, confusion, depression, disorientation, dizziness, dream disturbances, drowsiness, euphoria, fatigue, hangover, headache, hypoesthesia, insomnia, mental impairment, nervousness, paresthesia, somnolence, tremor, vertigo
CV: Bradycardia, chest pain, hot flashes, hypertension, palpitations, tachycardia
EENT: Blurred vision; burning eyes; dry eyes, mouth, and throat; earache; eye irritation; lacrimation; nasal congestion and irritation or pain; **pharyngeal edema**; pharyngitis; tinnitus; tongue swelling
GI: Abdominal distention, constipation, diarrhea, dysphagia, flatulence, heartburn, indigestion, nausea, thirst, vomiting
GU: Menstrual irregularities, polyuria, urinary frequency
MS: Arthralgia; dysarthria; muscle spasms, stiffness, or weakness; myalgia
RESP: Dyspnea, upper respiratory tract infection, wheezing
SKIN: Diaphoresis, flushing, pruritus, rash, urticaria
Other: Angioedema, dehydration

Nursing Considerations

- Use rizatriptan cautiously in patients with hepatic or renal dysfunction because of impaired drug excretion or metabolism. Monitor patient's BUN and serum creatinine levels and liver enzymes, as appropriate.
- Also use cautiously in patients with peripheral vascular disease because drug may cause vasospastic reactions, leading to colonic and vascular ischemia with abdominal pain and bloody diarrhea. Assess bowel sounds and peripheral circulation frequently during therapy.
- Assess patient's cardiovascular status and institute continuous ECG monitoring, as ordered, immediately after giving rizatriptan in patients with cardiovascular risk factors, because of possible asymptomatic cardiac ischemia.
- Monitor blood pressure regularly in patients with hypertension because rizatriptan may increase blood pressure.

WARNING Monitor patient closely for serotonin syndrome if she is taking rizatriptan along with a selective serotonin reuptake inhibitor or serotonin norepinephrine reuptake inhibitor. Notify prescriber immediately if the patient exhibits agitation, coma, diarrhea, hallucinations, hyperreflexia, hyperthermia, incoordination, labile blood pressure, nausea, tachycardia, or vomiting, as serotonin syndrome can be life-threatening. Provide supportive care.

PATIENT TEACHING

- Instruct patient taking rizatriptan-disintegrating tablets to remove tablet from blister pack with dry hands just before taking, to place tablet on tongue, and to allow it to dissolve and be swallowed with saliva.
- Advise phenylketonuric patient not to use disintegrating tablet form because it contains phenylalanine.
- Instruct patient to seek emergency care immediately if cardiac symptoms, such as chest pain, occur after administration.
- Caution patient about possible adverse CNS reactions, and advise her to avoid potentially hazardous activities until drug's CNS effects are known.
- Urge patient to inform all prescribers of rizatriptan therapy because serious drug interactions may occur.

roflumilast

Daliresp

Class and Category

Pharmacologic class: Selective phosphodiesterase 4 inhibitor
Therapeutic class: Antipulmonic obstructive agent
Pregnancy category: C

Indications and Dosages

➤ *To reduce the risk of COPD exacerbations in patients with severe COPD associated with chronic bronchitis and a history of exacerbations*

TABLETS

Adults. 500 mcg daily.

Mechanism of Action

Increases intracellular cyclic AMP in lung cells by inhibiting a major cyclic AMP-metabolizing enzyme in lung tissue to improve pulmonary function

Contraindications

Hypersensitivity to roflumilast or its components, moderate to severe liver impairment

Interactions

DRUGS

CYP450 inhibitors or dual inhibitors (both CYP1A2 and CYP3A4), such as cimetidine, enoxacin, erythromycin, fluvoxamine, ketoconazole; oral contraceptives containing gestodene and ethinyl estradiol: Increased roflumilast exposure with increased risk of adverse effects
cytochrome P450 enzyme inducers, such as carbamazepine, phenobarbital, phenytoin, rifampicin: Decreased effectiveness of roflumilast

Adverse Reactions

CNS: Anxiety, depression, dizziness, headache, insomnia, **suicidal ideation**, tremor
CV: Atrial fibrillation
EENT: Rhinitis, sinusitis
ENDO: Gynecomastia
GI: Abdominal pain, **acute pancreatitis**, anorexia, diarrhea, dyspepsia, gastritis, nausea, vomiting
GU: Acute renal failure, UTI
MS: Back pain, muscle spasms
SKIN: Rash, urticaria
Other: Angioedema, flu-like symptoms, weight loss

Nursing Considerations

- Monitor effectiveness of roflumilast to reduce COPD exacerbations.
- Watch patient closely for suicidal tendencies because roflumilast has been associated with an increase in psychiatric adverse reactions, such as depression and insomnia, as well as suicidal ideation.
- Monitor patient's weight and notify prescriber if significant weight loss occurs.

PATIENT TEACHING

- Tell family or caregiver to monitor patient for suicidal tendencies because drug may worsen depression during roflumilast and increase suicidal thinking.
- Warn patient that roflumilast is not a bronchodilator and should not be used to relieve acute bronchospasm.
- Inform women wishing to breastfeed their infants that drug is excreted in breast milk and breastfeeding should not be done.

rolapitant

Varubi, Varubi IV

Class and Category

Pharmacologic class: Substance P and neurokinin-1 receptor antagonist
Therapeutic class: Antiemetic
Pregnancy category: Not classified

Indications and Dosages

➤ *Adjunct to prevent delayed nausea and vomiting associated with emetogenic cancer chemotherapy*

TABLETS

Adults receiving cisplatin-based highly emetogenic cancer chemotherapy; adults receiving moderately emetogenic cancer chemotherapy and combinations of anthracycline and cyclophosphamide. 180 mg within 2 hr prior to chemotherapy in combination with dexamethasone and a 5-HT3 receptor antagonist.

I.V. INFUSION

Adults receiving cisplatin-based highly emetogenic cancer chemotherapy; adults receiving moderately emetogenic cancer chemotherapy and combinations of anthracycline and cyclophosphamide. 166.5 mg infused over 30 min within 2 hr prior to chemotherapy in combination with dexamethasone and a 5-HT3 receptor antagonist.

Mechanism of Action
Crosses the blood–brain barrier to occupy brain P/NK1 receptors, which prevents nerve transmission of signals that cause nausea and vomiting.

Contraindications
Concurrent therapy with CYP2D6 substrates with a narrow therapeutic index such as pimozide and thioridazine, hypersensitivity to rolapitant or its components

Interactions
DRUGS
digoxin and other P-gp substrates with a narrow therapeutic index; irinotecan, methotrexate, topotecan, and other BCRP substrates with a narrow therapeutic index: Increased plasma concentrations of these drugs, which increases risk of adverse reactions
pimozide, thioridazine, and other CYP2D6 substrates with a narrow therapeutic index: Increased plasma concentrations of these drugs, which can result in QT prolongation and torsades de pointes
rifampin and other strong CYP3A4 inducers: Decreased plasma concentrations and effectiveness of rolapitant

Adverse Reactions
CNS: Dizziness
CV: Chest pain, **hypotension**
EENT: Stomatitis
GI: Abdominal pain, anorexia, dyspepsia, hiccups
GU: UTI
HEME: Anemia, **neutropenia**
RESP: Dyspnea, wheezing
SKIN: Flushing, pruritus, urticaria
Other: Anaphylaxis including shock, **angioedema**

Nursing Considerations
- Know that rolapitant should not be given to patients with severe hepatic impairment but in the event its use cannot be avoided, monitor patient closely for rolapitant-related adverse reactions.

WARNING Use extreme caution when rolapitant is given concurrently with a CYP2D6 substrate with a narrow therapeutic index such as pimozide if use cannot be avoided. This is because an increase in plasma concentration of the substrate may result in QT prolongation. Monitor patient closely for this and other adverse reactions.

- Administer rolapitant within 2 hours of chemotherapy. Make sure dexamethasone and a 5-HT3 receptor antagonist has also been prescribed and is on hand ready to be given, as directed.
- Be aware that intravenous form of rolapitant does not require reconstitution or refrigeration. Once stopper is punctured in drug vial, use immediately. Do not add any diluents or medications directly into vial. Infuse over 30 minutes.

WARNING Monitor patient receiving rolapitant for hypersensitivity reactions that may occur within minutes during or after infusion of rolapitant injectable emulsion and can be life-threatening. If present, stop infusion immediately, notify prescriber, and be prepared to administer supportive emergency treatment, as ordered, that may include antihistamines and/or epinephrine.

PATIENT TEACHING
- Review with patient when rolapitant is to be administered in conjunction with the patient's chemotherapy. Also, instruct patient when to take dexamethasone if it is prescribed after his chemotherapy.
- Tell patient to inform all prescribers of rolapitant therapy.
- Advise women of childbearing age that rolapitant may impair fertility.

ropinirole hydrochloride
Requip, Requip XL

Class and Category
Pharmacologic class: Nonergot alkaloid dopamine agonist
Therapeutic class: Antiparkinsonian
Pregnancy category: C

Indications and Dosages
➤ *To treat signs and symptoms of Parkinson's disease*

TABLETS

Adults. *Initial:* 0.25 mg three times a day. Dosage titrated upward every wk according to the following schedule: 0.25 mg three times a day in wk 1; 0.5 mg three times a day in wk 2; 0.75 mg three times a day in wk 3; 1 mg three times a day in wk 4. After wk 4, if needed, dosage increased by 1.5 mg daily every wk up to 9 mg daily, then by 3 mg/day up to 24 mg daily. *Maximum:* 24 mg/day.

E.R. TABLETS

Adults. *Initial:* 2 mg once daily for 1 to 2 wk, increased, as needed, in increments of 2 mg/day at 1 wk or longer intervals. *Maximum:* 24 mg/day.

DOSAGE ADJUSTMENT For patient with end-stage renal disease on hemodialysis, dosage titration is based on tolerability and need for efficacy; maximum total daily dose reduced to 18 mg daily.

➤ *To treat moderate to severe primary restless legs syndrome*

TABLETS

Adults. *Initial:* 0.25 mg 1 to 3 hr before bedtime. Dosage increased, as needed, on day 3 to 0.5 mg and then to 1 mg at beginning of week 2 (day 8). If needed, dosage further increased in 0.5-mg increments every wk for 4 wk, followed by a 1 mg increase between wk 6 and 7, if needed. *Maximum:* 4 mg daily.

DOSAGE ADJUSTMENT For patients with end-stage renal disease on hemodialysis, dosage titration is based on tolerability and need for efficacy, with recommended maximum total daily dose reduced to 3 mg daily.

Mechanism of Action

Directly stimulates postsynaptic dopamine type 2 (D_2) receptors within the brain and acts as an agonist at peripheral D_2 receptors. These actions inhibit the firing of striatal cholinergic neurons, thus helping to control alterations in voluntary muscle movement (such as rigidity and tremors) associated with Parkinson's disease.

Contraindications

Hypersensitivity to ropinirole or its components

Interactions

DRUGS

carbamazepine, cimetidine, ciprofloxacin, clarithromycin, diltiazem, enoxacin, erythromycin, fluvoxamine, mexiletine, norfloxacin, omeprazole, phenobarbital, phenytoin, rifampin, ritonavir, troleandomycin: Altered drug clearance and increased blood level of ropinirole

chlorprothixene, domperidone, droperidol, haloperidol, metoclopramide, phenothiazines, thiothixene: Possibly decreased effectiveness of ropinirole

CNS depressants: Additive effects

ethinyl estradiol: Possibly reduced clearance of ropinirole

ACTIVITIES

alcohol use: Additive effects

Adverse Reactions

CNS: Abnormal dreaming, amnesia, anxiety, asthenia, compulsive behaviors, confusion, dizziness, dyskinesia, falling asleep during activities of daily living, fatigue, hallucinations, headache, hypoesthesia, hypokinesia, insomnia, malaise, nervousness, neuralgia, paresis, paresthesia, psychotic-like behaviors, rigors, somnolence, syncope, transient ischemic attack, tremor, vertigo

CV: Acute coronary syndrome, angina, **bradycardia**, **cardiac failure**, chest pain, hypertension, **MI**, orthostatic hypotension, palpitations, peripheral edema, **sick sinus syndrome**, tachycardia

EENT: Abnormal vision, diplopia, dry mouth, increased salivation, nasal congestion, nasopharyngitis, rhinitis, toothache

GI: Abdominal pain, constipation, diarrhea, dyspepsia, dysphagia, flatulence, **gastric hemorrhage**, gastroenteritis, indigestion, **intestinal obstruction**, **ischemic hepatitis**, nausea, **pancreatitis**, vomiting

GU: Elevated BUN level, erectile dysfunction, pyuria, urinary incontinence, UTI

HEME: Anemia

MS: Arthralgia; arthritis; back pain; exacerbation of restless leg syndrome limb pain; muscle cramps, spasms, or stiffness; myalgia; neck pain; osteoarthritis; tendinitis

RESP: Asthma, bronchitis, cough, dyspnea, upper respiratory tract infection

SKIN: Diaphoresis, flushing, hot flashes, **melanoma**, night sweats, pruritus, rash, urticaria

Other: Angioedema, elevation of serum creatine phosphokinase (CPK), flu-like symptoms, viral infection, weight loss

Nursing Considerations

WARNING Expect to reassess patient for excessive sedation periodically during therapy. Excessive, acute drowsiness may arise as late as 1 year after starting therapy.

- When ropinirole is given as adjunct to levodopa, expect concurrent dosage of levodopa to be gradually decreased as tolerated.
- Expect to stop ropinirole gradually over 7 days, as follows: over first 4 days, reduce from three times a day to twice daily; during last 3 days, reduce to once daily, followed by complete withdrawal of drug.

WARNING Watch for altered mental status during drug withdrawal. Rapid dose reduction may lead to a symptom complex resembling neuroleptic malignant syndrome that includes altered level of consciousness, autonomic instability, fever, and muscle rigidity.

- Watch for orthostatic hypotension, especially in patient with early Parkinson's disease. Orthostatic hypotension can occur more than 4 weeks after start of therapy or after a dosage reduction because ropinirole may impair systemic regulation of blood pressure.
- Monitor patient for hallucinations, especially if patient has Parkinson's disease, is elderly, or takes levodopa.
- Monitor patient for worsening of preexisting dyskinesia; ropinirole may potentiate dopaminergic adverse effects of levodopa.
- Avoid giving CNS depressants, other CNS-interacting drugs, and sleep aids during ropinirole therapy because they increase the risk of somnolence.
- Assess patient for skin changes regularly because risk of melanoma is higher in patients with Parkinson's disease. It isn't clear whether this results from disease or from the drugs used to treat it.

PATIENT TEACHING

- Inform patient with Parkinson's disease that ropinirole helps to improve muscle control and movement but doesn't cure Parkinson's disease.
- Encourage patient to take ropinirole with food to decrease risk of adverse GI effects. Tell her not to chew, crush, or divide extended-release tablets but to swallow them whole.
- Caution patient not to stop taking ropinirole abruptly. If concerns arise over ropinirole therapy, encourage her to speak with prescriber.
- Instruct patient to notify prescriber if allergic reactions occur, such as hives, itching, or rash. If facial swelling or difficulty breathing occurs, tell patient to seek immediate emergency treatment.
- Caution patient to avoid hazardous activities until CNS effects of drug—including sedation—are known.
- Tell the patient that if she falls asleep during normal activities, she should notify prescriber.
- Urge patient to avoid consuming alcohol and other sedating drugs (such as sleep aids) during therapy because they may increase drug's CNS depressant effects.
- Urge patient to stand up slowly from a lying or sitting position to avoid feeling dizzy, faint, nauseated, or sweaty.
- Explain to patient with restless legs syndrome that symptoms might appear in early morning or have an earlier onset in the evening or even the afternoon during ropinirole therapy and could be worse or spread to other limbs. Urge patient to notify prescriber if this occurs.
- Instruct patient to change positions slowly to minimize effect on blood pressure.
- Urge patient to have regular skin examinations by a dermatologist or other qualified health professional.
- Advise patient to notify prescriber about intense urges (as for gambling or sex) because dosage may have to be reduced or drug discontinued.
- Tell patient to inform all prescribers of ropinirole therapy.
- Inform patient that smoking may decrease effectiveness of ropinirole. If smoking is started or stopped during therapy, patient should notify prescriber.
- Tell female patients to notify prescriber if pregnancy occurs or is suspected.
- Instruct female patients wishing to breastfeed to discuss this with prescriber, as drug could inhibit lactation.

rosiglitazone maleate

Avandia

Class and Category

Pharmacologic class: Thiazolidinedione
Therapeutic class: Antidiabetic
Pregnancy category: C

Indications and Dosages

➤ *To achieve glucose control in type 2 diabetes mellitus*

TABLETS

Adults. *Initial:* 4 mg once daily or 2 mg twice daily, increased to 8 mg once daily or 4 mg twice daily. if glucose control is inadequate after 12 wk. *Maximum:* 8 mg daily.

Mechanism of Action

Increases tissue sensitivity to insulin. This peroxisome proliferator-activated receptor agonist regulates the transcription of insulin-responsive genes found in key target tissues, such as adipose tissue, the liver, and skeletal muscle. Enhanced tissue sensitivity to insulin lowers the blood glucose level.

Contraindications

Hypersensitivity to rosiglitazone or its components, New York Heart Association (NYHA) class III or IV heart failure

Interactions

DRUGS

CYP2C8 inducers, such as rifampin: Possibly decreased effects of rosiglitazone
CYP2C8 inhibitors, such as gemfibrozil: Possibly increased effects of rosiglitazone

Adverse Reactions

CNS: CVA, fatigue, headache
CV: Angina, **congestive heart failure**, edema, hypertension, **myocardial ischemia or infarction**
EENT: Blurred vision, decreased visual acuity, macular edema, nasopharyngitis, sinusitis
ENDO: Hyperglycemia, **hypoglycemia**
GI: Diarrhea, elevated liver enzymes, **hepatotoxicity**
HEME: Anemia
MS: Arthralgia, back pain, bone fracture (especially upper arm, foot, hand)
RESP: Dyspnea, upper respiratory tract infection
SKIN: Pruritus, rash, **Stevens–Johnson syndrome**, urticaria
Other: Anaphylaxis, **angioedema**, weight gain

Nursing Considerations

- Give rosiglitazone cautiously in patients with edema, heart failure, or hepatic impairment because of potential adverse reactions.
- Be aware that drug isn't recommended for patients with symptomatic heart failure.
- Evaluate patient's liver function before starting drug and periodically throughout therapy, as ordered. Notify prescriber about abnormalities, such as abdominal pain, anorexia, dark urine fatigue, nausea, and vomiting. Drug may have to be stopped.

WARNING Monitor patient for evidence of congestive heart failure—such as edema rapid weight gain, or shortness of breath—because rosiglitazone can cause fluid retention that may lead to or worsen heart failure. Notify prescriber immediately if the patient's cardiac status deteriorates, and expect to stop the drug, as ordered.

- Monitor fasting glucose and glycosylated hemoglobin A_{1c} levels periodically, as ordered, to evaluate rosiglitazone effectiveness.
- Be aware that drug is effective only in the presence of endogenous insulin.

PATIENT TEACHING

- Emphasize the need to follow an exercise program and a diet control program during rosiglitazone therapy.
- Advise patient to notify prescriber immediately if she has fluid retention, shortness of breath, or sudden weight gain, because drug may need to be discontinued.
- Instruct patient to have liver enzymes checked, as ordered, about every 2 months for first year and then annually.
- Inform anovulatory premenopausal patient that drug may induce ovulation, increasing risk of pregnancy.
- Urge patient, especially women, to take precautions against falling or experiencing trauma; drug increases

risk of fractures, particularly of the foot, hand, and upper arm.
- Instruct patient to notify all prescribers of rosiglitazone therapy and not to take any medication such as over-the-counter medicines, including herbal supplements and vitamins, without consulting prescriber first.

rosuvastatin calcium

Crestor

Class and Category

Pharmacologic class: HMG-CoA reductase inhibitor
Therapeutic class: Antilipemic
Pregnancy category: X

Indications and Dosages

➤ *To treat hyperlipidemia, mixed dyslipidemia, hypertriglyceridemia, and primary dysbetalipoproteinemia (type III hyperlipoproteinemia); to slow the progression of atherosclerosis; to prevent primary cardiovascular disease (reduce the risk of myocardial infarction, stroke, or need for arterial revascularization procedures) in patients without clinically evident CAD but with increased risk factors of cardiovascular disease such as age (men 50 years and over; women 60 years and over), hsCRP of 2 mg/l or greater, and the presence of at least one additional cardiovascular disease risk factor such as hypertension, low HDL-C, smoking, or a family history of premature CAD*

TABLETS

Adults with LDL-C level of 190 mg/dl or below. *Initial:* 10 mg daily, increased every 2 to 4 wk, as needed. *Maximum:* 40 mg daily.

Adults with LDL-C level greater than 190 mg/dl. *Initial:* 20 mg daily, increased every 2 to 4 wk, as needed. *Maximum:* 40 mg daily.

➤ *To treat homozygous familial hypercholesterolemia*

TABLETS

Adults. *Initial:* 20 mg daily, increased every 2 to 4 wk, as needed. *Maximum:* 40 mg daily.

Children ages 7 to 17. 20 mg daily.

➤ *To treat pediatric heterozygous familial hypercholesterolemia*

TABLETS

Children ages 10 to 17. 5 to 20 mg daily, increased every 4 wk, as needed. *Maximum:* 20 mg daily.

Children ages 8 to less than 10. 5 to 10 mg daily, increased every 4 wk, as needed. *Maximum:* 10 mg daily.

DOSAGE ADJUSTMENT For patients taking cyclosporine, dosage shouldn't exceed 5 mg daily. For Asian patients, initial dosage limited to 5 mg daily. For patients taking combined atazanavir and ritonavir lopinavir and ritonavir gemfibrozil, or simeprevir or for patients with severe renal impairment (creatinine clearance less than 30 ml/min) not on hemodialysis, initial dosage reduced to 5 mg daily with maintenance dose not to exceed 10 mg daily.

Route	Onset	Peak	Duration
P.O.	Unknown	3–5 hr	Unknown

Mechanism of Action

Cholesterol and triglycerides circulate in the blood as part of lipoprotein complexes. Rosuvastatin inhibits the enzyme 3-hydroxy-3-methylglutaryl-coenzyme A (HMG-CoA) reductase. This inhibition reduces lipid levels by increasing the number of hepatic low-density lipoprotein (LDL) receptors on the cell surface to increase uptake and catabolism of LDL. It also inhibits hepatic synthesis of very-low-density lipoprotein (VLDL), which decreases the total number of VLDL and LDL particles.

Contraindications

Active liver disease, breastfeeding, hypersensitivity to rosuvastatin or its components, pregnancy, unexplained persistent elevations of serum transaminase levels

Interactions

DRUGS

antacids: Decreased blood rosuvastatin level if given within 2 hours of rosuvastatin
atazanavir/ritonavir, cyclosporine, gemfibrozil, lopinavir/ritonavir, niacin (equal to or greater than 1 g/day), other lipid-

lowering drugs simeprevir: Increased rosuvastatin level and risk of myopathy
azole antifungals, clarithromycin, darunavir/ritonavir, erythromycin, fenofibrates, fosamprenavir, fosamprenavir/ritonavir, saquinavir/ritonavir, telaprevir, tipranavir/ritonavir: Possibly increased risk of myopathy
oral contraceptives: Increased blood ethinyl estradiol and norgestrel levels
warfarin: Increased INR

Adverse Reactions

CNS: Asthenia, cognitive impairment, confusion, depression, dizziness, headache, hypertonia, insomnia, memory loss, nightmares, paresthesia, peripheral neuropathy
CV: Chest pain, hypertension, peripheral edema
EENT: Pharyngitis, rhinitis, sinusitis
ENDO: Elevated glycosylated hemoglobin levels, gynecomastia, hyperglycemia, thyroid function abnormalities
GI: Abdominal pain, constipation, diarrhea, elevated liver enzymes, gastroenteritis, **hepatic failure**, **hepatitis**, jaundice, nausea, **pancreatitis**
GU: Acute renal failure, proteinuria, UTI
HEME: Thrombocytopenia
MS: Arthralgia, arthritis, back pain, immune-mediated necrotizing myopathy, myalgia, myopathy, **rhabdomyolysis**
RESP: Bronchitis, increased cough, **interstitial lung disease**
SKIN: Rash, urticaria
Other: Angioedema, flu-like symptoms, generalized pain, infection

Nursing Considerations

- Use rosuvastatin cautiously in patients who consume large quantities of alcohol or who have a history of liver disease, because drug is contraindicated in patients with active liver disease or unexplained persistent elevations of transaminase levels.
- Also use cautiously in patients with risk factors for myopathy, such as advanced age, hypothyroidism, or renal impairment.
- If ALT or AST levels increase to more than three times the normal range, expect dosage to be reduced or drug discontinued.
- Monitor serum lipoprotein level, as ordered, to evaluate response to therapy.
- Expect rosuvastatin to be discontinued if patient develops markedly elevated creatinine kinase levels, or if myopathy is diagnosed or suspected. Drug may be temporarily withheld if patient develops any condition that may be related to myopathy or that predisposes her to renal failure, such as hypotension; major surgery; sepsis; severe electrolyte, endocrine, or metabolic disorders; trauma, or uncontrolled seizures.
- Obtain baseline liver enzymes and expect to monitor them thereafter, as indicated. Notify prescriber if proteinuria or hematuria appears in patient's routine urinalysis, because rosuvastatin dosage may need to be reduced.

PATIENT TEACHING

- Encourage patient to follow a low-fat, low-cholesterol diet.
- Tell patient who takes antacids to wait at least 2 hours after taking rosuvastatin.
- Instruct patient to notify prescriber immediately about muscle pain, tenderness, or weakness, especially if accompanied by fever or malaise. He should also tell the prescriber if these symptoms occur even after drug is discontinued.
- Encourage patient or family to notify prescriber if patient begins to notice new onset or worsening of confusion, forgetfulness, or memory loss.
- Tell woman of childbearing age about the need to use reliable contraceptive method while taking drug. Instruct her to notify prescriber at once if she suspects she may be pregnant.
- Instruct patient with diabetes to test his blood glucose regularly and have a HbA_{1c} level checked routinely.

rotigotine

Neupro

Class and Category

Pharmacologic class: Nonergoline dopamine agonist
Therapeutic class: Antiparkinsonian
Pregnancy category: C

Indications and Dosages

➤ *To treat signs and symptoms of idiopathic Parkinson's disease*

TRANSDERMAL
Adults in early stage. *Initial:* Apply 2 mg every 24 hr once daily, increased weekly in increments of 2 mg every 24 hr, as needed. *Maximum:* 6 mg every 24 hr.
Adults in advanced stage. *Initial:* Apply 4 mg every 24 hr once daily, increased weekly in increments of 2 mg every 24 hr, as needed. *Maximum:* 8 mg every 24 hr.

➤ *To treat moderate-to-severe primary restless leg syndrome*

TRANSDERMAL
Adults. *Initial:* Apply 1 mg every 24 hr once daily, increased weekly in increments of 1 mg every 24 hr, as needed. *Maximum:* 3 mg every 24 hr.

Mechanism of Action

Thought to stimulate dopamine receptors within the caudate-putamen in the brain. Increased dopamine levels help relieve the signs and symptoms associated with Parkinson's disease and restless leg syndrome.

Contraindications

Hypersensitivity to rotigotine or the components of the transdermal system.

Interactions

DRUGS
dopamine antagonists (antipsychotics or metoclopramide): Possibly diminish effectiveness of rotigotine

Adverse Reactions

CNS: Abnormal dreams, aggressive behavior, agitation, asthenia, balance disorder, compulsive behaviors, confusion, delusions, depression, disorientation, dizziness, dysesthesias, dyskinesia, excessive sleepiness, fatigue, hallucinations, headache, insomnia, lethargy, paraesthesia, paranoid ideation, psychotic-like behavior, sleep disorders, somnolence, syncope, tremor, vertigo
CV: Cardiac valvulopathy, **ECG T-wave abnormality**, hypertension, orthostatic hypotension, **pericarditis**, peripheral edema, tachycardia
EENT: Dry mouth, nasal or sinus congestion, nasopharyngitis, pharyngolaryngeal pain, sinusitis, tinnitus
ENDO: Hot flashes, **hypoglycemia**
GI: Anorexia, constipation, diarrhea, dyspepsia, hiccups, nausea, retroperitoneal fibrosis, vomiting
GU: Elevated blood urea nitrogen, erectile dysfunction
HEME: Decreased hemoglobin and hematocrit or serum ferritin level
MS: Arthralgia, elevated serum creatine phosphokinase, exacerbation or worsening of restless leg syndrome, musculoskeletal pain, muscle spasms
RESP: Cough, pleural effusion or thickening, **pulmonary infiltrates**, upper respiratory infection
SKIN: Erythema, hyperhidrosis, **melanoma**, pruritis
Other: Application-site reactions (edema, erythema, pruritus, rash), weight gain or loss

Nursing Considerations

- Be aware that patients should be screened for a history of sleep disorders and usage of concomitant sedating medications because the risk of falling asleep with or without warning signs of sleepiness increases when these risk factors are present.
- Use caution when administering rotigotine to a patient with severe cardiovascular disease because syncope can occur. Also monitor patient for fluid retention, especially in a patient with a history of congestive heart failure.
- Monitor patient closely after rotigotine treatment is started for signs and symptoms of an allergic reaction to rotigotine or sulfite because the drug does contain a sulfite. Know that sulfite sensitivity is more frequent in asthmatic patients than in nonasthmatic patients.
- Take blood pressure and pulse frequently because drug can cause a significant increase in blood pressure, and pulse may become higher than 100 beats/minute. Also watch for orthostatic hypotension, especially in patients with early Parkinson's disease and in all patients during dosage titration.
- Monitor patient for dyskinesia, which may occur with rotigotine use. Notify prescriber if present because dosage adjustment may be needed or drug discontinued.

- Monitor patient for hallucinations, especially if patient has Parkinson's disease, is elderly, or takes levodopa.
- Monitor patient's blood glucose level, as ordered, even in patients who are not diabetic as drug may cause an abnormally low blood glucose level. This adverse effect can be especially pronounced in patients with advanced-stage Parkinson's disease. If hypoglycemia occurs, treat according to standard protocol and notify prescriber.
- Expect to gradually stop rotigotine therapy, as ordered. For patient with Parkinson's disease, daily dose reduced by a maximum of 2 mg in 24 hours every other day until complete withdrawal of rotigotine is achieved. For patient with restless leg syndrome, daily dose reduced by 1 mg every 24 hours every other day, until complete withdrawal of rotigotine is achieved.

PATIENT TEACHING

- Alert patient to the possibility of application-site reactions such as itchiness, puffiness, rash or redness. Using a different site when applying the patch can reduce these adverse effects. If application-site reactions become severe, tell patient to notify the prescriber.
- Advise patient to rise from a lying or sitting position slowly.
- Caution patient to avoid performing hazardous activities, such as driving until effects of drug are known.
- Inform him that some patients taking rotigotine have fallen asleep during activities of daily living, sometimes without warning.
- Instruct patient to weigh daily and report unexpected weight gain.
- Warn patient and family that drug may cause compulsive behaviors such as intense urges to binge eat, gamble, have sex, or shop. Prescriber should be notified if compulsive behaviors are exhibited.

rufinamide

Banzel

Class and Category

Pharmacologic class: Triazole derivative
Therapeutic class: Anticonvulsant
Pregnancy category: C

Indications and Dosages

➤ *As adjunct treatment of seizures associated with Lennox–Gastaut Syndrome*

TABLETS

Adults and adolescents age 17 and over. *Initial:* 200 to 400 mg twice daily, increased in daily increments of 200 to 400 mg twice daily, every 2 days until reaching 1,600 mg twice daily. *Maximum:* 1,600 mg twice daily.
Children age 1 to less than 17. *Initial:* 5 mg/kg twice daily, increased in daily increments of 5 mg/kg twice daily, every 2 days until reaching 22.5 mg/kg twice daily or 1,600 mg twice daily, whichever is less.

DOSAGE ADJUSTMENT For patients undergoing dialysis, dosage may need to be increased. For patients also receiving valproate, initial dosage reduced to less than 400 mg daily in adults and less than 10 mg/kg daily in children.

Route	Onset	Peak	Duration
P.O.	Unknown	4–6 hr	Unknown

Mechanism of Action

Unknown, although rufinamide is known to slow sodium channel recovery from inactivation after a prolonged prepulse and to limit repetitive firing of sodium-dependent action potentials in neurons in the brain. These actions may help limit seizure activity.

Contraindications

Familial short-QT syndrome, hypersensitivity to rufinamide or its components

Interactions

DRUGS

contraceptives containing ethinyl estradiol and norethindrone: Decreased effectiveness of the oral contraceptive
phenytoin: Increased plasma phenytoin level and risk of adverse reactions
valproate: Increased plasma rufinamide level and risk of adverse reactions

ACTIVITIES

alcohol use: Increased CNS effects

Adverse Reactions

CNS: Aggression, anxiety, ataxia, attention disturbance, dizziness, fatigue, headache, hyperactivity, **seizures**, somnolence, **status epilepticus**, **suicidal ideation**, tremor, vertigo
CV: First-degree AV block, right bundle branch block
EENT: Sinusitis
ENDO: Blurred vision, diplopia, nasopharyngitis, nystagmus
GI: Abdominal pain, anorexia, constipation, dyspepsia, nausea, vomiting
GU: Dysuria, enuresis, hematuria, incontinence, nephrolithiasis, pollakiuria, polyuria
HEME: Anemia, **leukopenia, neutropenia, thrombocytopenia**
MS: Back pain
RESP: Bronchitis
SKIN: Pruritus, rash including mucosal involvement, **Stevens–Johnson syndrome**
Other: Drug reaction with eosinophilia and systemic symptoms (DRESS), lymphadenopathy

Nursing Considerations

- Administer rufinamide with food because absorption is increased.
- Monitor patient's QT interval regularly, as ordered, because rufinamide may shorten the QT interval and possibly predispose patient to ventricular fibrillation if the interval falls below 300 msec.

WARNING Watch closely for multiorgan hypersensitivity, especially if patient develops a rash. Although uncommon, it may cause serious adverse effects, such as elevated eosinophils or liver enzymes, facial edema, fever, hematuria, lymphadenopathy, severe hepatitis, stupor, and urticaria, in addition to rash. Notify prescriber at once if such changes appear, and expect to stop drug and provide supportive care.

- Watch closely for suicidal tendencies, especially when therapy starts and dosage changes and particularly in children and adolescents.
- Expect to taper dosage off when no longer needed to minimize adverse effects rather than stopping abruptly.

PATIENT TEACHING

- Make sure patient receives medication guide describing drug use and possible suicidal tendencies.
- Instruct patient to take drug exactly as prescribed and to take each dose with food. If patient has trouble swallowing tablets, tell him they may be crushed.
- Inform woman that rufinamide decreases effectiveness of contraceptives containing ethinyl estradiol and norethindrone. Tell her to use a different contraceptive during therapy and to contact prescriber immediately if she thinks she's pregnant.
- Tell patient to report a rash accompanied by fever or other symptoms immediately.
- Warn family or caregiver to watch patient for suicidal tendencies, especially when therapy starts or dosage changes, and particularly if patient is a child or adolescent.
- Advise patient to avoid hazardous activities until drug's CNS effects are known.
- Caution patient not to stop taking drug abruptly. Explain that gradual tapering helps to avoid withdrawal symptoms.
- Explain that alcohol consumption may intensify drug effects.

safinamide

Xadago

Class and Category

Pharmacologic class: Monoamine oxidase type B (MAO-B) inhibitor
Therapeutic class: Antiparkinsonian
Pregnancy category: C

Indications and Dosages

➤ *As adjunct to levodopa/carbidopa in patients with Parkinson's disease experiencing "off" episodes*

TABLETS

Adults. *Initial:* 50 mg once daily at the same time of day, increased after 2 wk to 100 mg once daily, if needed and tolerated.

DOSAGE ADJUSTMENT For patient with moderate hepatic impairment, maximum dosage kept at 50 mg once daily.

Mechanism of Action

Precise mechanism unknown, but by inhibiting monoamine oxidase B activity through blocking the catabolism of dopamine, it is thought this action increases dopamine levels, which in turn increase dopaminergic activity in the brain to improve Parkinson symptoms.

Contraindications

Concurrent use with amphetamine, antidepressants (tetracyclic, triazolopyridine, or tricyclic), cyclobenzaprine, dextromethorphan, linezolid, methylphenidate, opioid drugs, other MAO inhibitors or other drugs that are potent inhibitors of MAOs; serotonin-norepinephrine reuptake inhibitors; St. John's wort; hypersensitivity to safinamide or its components; severe hepatic impairment

Interactions

DRUGS

amphetamine, antidepressants (tetracyclic, triazolopyridine, tricyclic), cyclobenzaprine, methylphenidate, opioid drugs, serotonin-norepinephrine reuptake inhibitors, St. John's wort: Increased risk of life-threatening serotonin syndrome
antipsychotics, metoclopramide: Possibly decreased effectiveness of safinamide; exacerbation of Parkinson's disease symptoms
dextromethorphan: Increased risk of abnormal behavior or psychosis
imatinib, irinotecan, lapatinib, methotrexate, mitoxantrone, rosuvastatin, sulfasalazine, topotecan: Possibly increased pharmacologic or adverse effect of substrates of breast cancer resistance protein (BCRP)
isoniazid, other MAO inhibitors, other drugs that are potent inhibitors of MAO, sympathomimetics, tyramine: Increased risk of hypertensive crisis

Adverse Reactions

CNS: Anxiety, compulsive behaviors, confusion, dyskinesia, falling asleep during activities of daily living, fever, hallucinations, insomnia, lack of impulse control, **serotonin syndrome**
CV: Hypertension, orthostatic hypotension
EENT: Gingival swelling, retinal pathology, tongue swelling
GI: Dyspepsia, elevated liver enzymes, nausea
RESP: Cough, dyspnea
SKIN: Rash

Nursing Considerations

- Be aware that safinamide therapy should not be used in patients with a major psychotic disorder because drug may exacerbate the psychosis.
- Monitor patient's blood pressure closely because safinamide may cause hypertension or exacerbate existing hypertension. Be aware that although dietary restriction is not necessary during treatment with recommended doses, certain foods that are very high in tyramine (more than 150 mg) could cause severe hypertension.

WARNING Monitor patient closely for serotonin syndrome, a rare but serious adverse effect of MAO inhibitors such as safinamide. Signs and symptoms include agitation, confusion, diaphoresis, diarrhea, fever, hyperactive reflexes, poor coordination, restlessness, shaking, talking or acting with uncontrolled excitement, tremor, and twitching. If symptoms occur, notify prescriber immediately, expect to discontinue drug, and provide supportive care.

- Monitor patient for dyskinesia because safinamide may cause dyskinesia or exacerbate preexisting dyskinesia. Notify prescriber, because reducing the patient's daily levodopa dosage or the dosage of another dopaminergic drug may lessen the dyskinesia.
- Monitor patient for hallucinations or psychotic behavior. If present, expect dosage to be reduced or drug discontinued.
- Monitor patient for visual changes, especially in patients with a history of certain eye disorders such as active retinopathy, albinism, family history of hereditary retinal disease, inherited retinal conditions, macular or retinal degeneration, retinitis pigmentosa, or uveitis. This is because retinal degeneration and loss of photoreceptor cells may occur with safinamide therapy.

WARNING Be aware that 100-mg dose should be tapered to 50 mg for 1 week before safinamide is discontinued. This is because a symptom complex resembling neuroleptic malignant syndrome, exhibited by altered consciousness, autonomic instability, elevated temperature, and muscular rigidity, has occurred with rapid dose reduction, withdrawal of, or changes in drugs that increase central dopaminergic tone.

PATIENT TEACHING

- Tell patient that if a dose is missed, he should take the next dose at the same time the next day.
- Instruct patient to avoid foods very high in tyramine, because consuming such may cause very high blood pressure.
- Advise patient to avoid performing hazardous activities, as drug may cause daytime sleepiness or episodes of falling asleep during activities that require full attention, such as driving. Tell patient to notify prescriber of any such occurrence.
- Tell patient drug may cause him to experience intense urges to perform compulsive behaviors such as binge eating, gambling excessively, having sex very frequently, or spending money uncontrollably. If present, tell him to notify prescriber, as dosage may have to be reduced or drug discontinued.
- Advise patient to inform all prescribers of safinamide therapy.
- Instruct patient and family to notify prescriber if persistent, severe, or unusual adverse effects occur, including dyskinesia, hallucinations, or psychotic behavior.
- Stress importance of not stopping drug abruptly. If patient has concerns about safinamide therapy, advise him to speak with prescriber.

salmeterol xinafoate

Serevent Diskus

Class and Category

Pharmacologic class: Long-acting $beta_2$ agonist (LABA)
Therapeutic class: Bronchodilator
Pregnancy category: C

Indications and Dosages

➤ *To treat asthma and prevent asthma-induced bronchospasm in patients with reversible obstructive airway disease who are currently using an inhaled corticosteroid but are inadequately controlled*

ORAL INHALATION POWDER

Adults and children age 4 and over. 1 inhalation (50 mcg) every 12 hr.

➤ *To provide maintenance treatment of bronchospasm associated with chronic obstructive pulmonary disease (COPD)*

ORAL INHALATION POWDER

Adults. 1 inhalation (50 mcg) every 12 hr.

➤ *To prevent exercise-induced bronchospasm in patients who do not have persistent asthma or, if persistent asthma present, used in conjunction with an inhaled corticosteroid*

ORAL INHALATION POWDER

Adults and children age 4 and over. 1 inhalation (50 mcg) at least 30 min before exercise. *Maximum:* No more than 1 inhalation (50 mcg) every 12 hr.

Route	Onset	Peak	Duration
Inhalation	10–20 min	3–4 hr	12 hr

Mechanism of Action

Attaches to $beta_2$ receptors on bronchial cell membranes, stimulating the intracellular enzyme adenylate cyclase to convert adenosine triphosphate to cAMP. The resulting increase in intracellular cAMP level inhibits histamine release, relaxes bronchial smooth-muscle cells, and stabilizes mast cells.

Contraindications

Hypersensitivity to salmeterol, its components, or to milk proteins (severe); primary treatment of status asthmaticus or other acute episodes of asthma or COPD where intensive measures are required; treatment of asthma without use of an inhaled corticosteroid

Interactions

DRUGS

atazanavir, clarithromycin, indinavir, itraconazole, ketoconazole, nefazodone, nelfinavir, ritonavir, saquinavir, telithromycin: Possibly increased risk of adverse cardiovascular effects
beta blockers: Mutual inhibition of therapeutic effects
loop or thiazide diuretics: Increased risk of hypokalemia and potentially life-threatening arrhythmias
MAO inhibitors, tricyclic antidepressants: Potentiated adverse vascular effects, such as hypertensive crisis

Adverse Reactions

CNS: Dizziness, fever, headache, nervousness, paresthesia, tremor
CV: Palpitations, tachycardia
EENT: Dry mouth, nose, and throat; sinus problems
GI: Nausea
MS: Arthralgia
RESP: Cough, **paradoxical bronchospasm**
SKIN: Contact dermatitis, eczema, rash, urticaria
Other: Angioedema, generalized aches and pains

Nursing Considerations

- Be aware that salmeterol shouldn't be used to relieve bronchospasm quickly because of its prolonged onset of action and that patients already taking drug twice daily shouldn't take additional doses for exercise-induced bronchospasm.

WARNING Be aware that a recent study suggests that asthma-related deaths may increase in asthmatics receiving salmeterol. Know that salmeterol should not be used in patients whose asthma is adequately controlled on low- or medium-dose inhaled corticosteroids and it should only be used as additional therapy for patients with asthma who are currently taking but are not adequately controlled on an inhaled corticosteroid. Salmeterol should never be used as monotherapy in the treatment of asthma. Monitor this patient population closely throughout salmeterol therapy, and notify prescriber immediately of any changes in patient's respiratory status. Expect to discontinue use as soon as possible.

- Watch for arrhythmias and changes in blood pressure after use in patients with cardiovascular disorders, including arrhythmias, hypertension, and ischemic cardiac disease, because of drug's beta-adrenergic effects.
- Monitor patient's compliance. Expect adults with poor compliance and children and adolescents who require the addition of a long-acting beta agonist such as salmeterol to be prescribed a combination product containing both an inhaled corticosteroid and a long-acting beta agonist to increase compliance.
- Be aware that Serevent Diskus delivers full dose of salmeterol in only 1 inhalation.

WARNING Stop salmeterol immediately and notify prescriber if patient develops paradoxical bronchospasm. Risk is greatest with first use of a new canister or vial used as an inhalant.

PATIENT TEACHING

- Instruct patient to use salmeterol exactly as prescribed and not to increase dosage or frequency of use.
- Advise patient with asthma or COPD to take doses 12 hours apart for optimum effect. Caution against using drug more than every 12 hours. Also, inform patients with asthma that salmeterol must be taken with an inhaled corticosteroid because a life-threatening reaction may occur if drug is taken alone. Tell patient using salmeterol to prevent exercise-induced bronchospasm to take drug at least 30 min before exercise.
- Teach patient how to use the diskus by instructing him to slide the lever only once when preparing dose to avoid wasting doses. Advise him to exhale immediately before using the diskus and then to place mouthpiece to his lips and inhale through his mouth, not his nose. Then he should remove mouthpiece from his mouth, hold his breath for at least 10 seconds, and exhale slowly.
- Advise patient to rinse mouth with water after each dose to minimize dry mouth.
- Advise patient to store drug in a dry place away from heat and sunlight in the unopened foil pouch until ready for use. Also tell patient to discard diskus 6 weeks after removing it from overwrap or when dose indicator reads zero.

WARNING Instruct patient to seek immediate medical attention if after taking salmeterol he develops breathing problems, a fast or irregular heartbeat, high blood glucose level, or any persistent, severe, or unusual side effects. Tell him that if he develops a low potassium level, that should also be reported to the prescriber.

- Instruct patient to notify prescriber if he needs four or more oral inhalations of rapid-acting inhaled bronchodilator a day for 2 or more consecutive days, or if he uses more than one canister of rapid-acting bronchodilator in an 8-week period.

- Caution patient not to use other drugs to treat his underlying respiratory condition without consulting prescriber and to let all prescribers know that he takes salmeterol.
- Caution patient to keep salmeterol diskus out of the reach of children. Also tell patient not to give the diskus to other people, even if they have the same symptoms, because it may harm them.

salsalate
(salicylic acid)

Class and Category

Pharmacologic class: Salicylate
Therapeutic class: Analgesic
Pregnancy category: C

Indications and Dosages

➤ *To relieve symptoms of osteoarthritis and rheumatoid arthritis and related rheumatic disorders*

CAPSULES

Adults and adolescents. *Initial:* 1,000 mg three times a day or 1,500 mg twice daily; dosage then titrated, as needed.

TABLETS

Adults and adolescents. *Initial:* 750 mg to 1,500 mg twice daily or 1,000 mg three times daily; dosage then titrated, as needed.

Route	Onset	Peak	Duration
P.O.	Unknown	2–3 wk	Unknown

Mechanism of Action

Exerts peripherally induced analgesic and anti-inflammatory effects by inhibiting prostaglandin synthesis and blocking pain impulses.

Contraindications

Bleeding disorders; hypersensitivity to NSAIDs, salicylates, or their components

Interactions

DRUGS

acetaminophen: Increased risk of renal dysfunction with prolonged use of both drugs
anticoagulants, thrombolytics: Increased risk and severity of GI bleeding
antiemetics: Masked symptoms of salicylate-induced ototoxicity
bismuth subsalicylate: Increased risk of salicylate toxicity with large doses of salsalate
cefamandole, cefoperazone, cefotetan, platelet aggregation inhibitors, plicamycin, valproic acid: Possibly hypoprothrombinemia
corticosteroids: Possibly decreased blood salsalate level; additive therapeutic effects when both drugs are used to treat arthritis
furosemide: Increased risk of ototoxicity and salicylate toxicity
hydantoins: Possibly decreased hydantoin metabolism, leading to toxicity
insulin, oral antidiabetic drugs: Potentiated hypoglycemic effect
laxatives (cellulose-containing): Possibly reduced salsalate effectiveness due to impaired absorption
methotrexate: Increased risk of methotrexate toxicity
NSAIDs: Increased risk of adverse GI effects
ototoxic drugs, vancomycin: Increased risk of ototoxicity
probenecid, sulfinpyrazone: Decreased uricosuric effects
topical salicylic acid, other salicylates: Increased risk of salicylate toxicity if significant quantities are absorbed
urinary acidifiers (ammonium chloride, ascorbic acid, potassium or sodium phosphates): Decreased salicylate excretion, possibly leading to salicylate toxicity
urinary alkalizers (antacids [long-term high-dose use], carbonic anhydrase inhibitors, citrates, sodium bicarbonate): Increased salicylate excretion, leading to reduced effectiveness and shortened half-life; increased risk of salicylate toxicity with carbonic anhydrase inhibitor–induced metabolic acidosis
vitamin K: Increased vitamin K requirements

ACTIVITIES

alcohol use: Increased risk of GI bleeding

Adverse Reactions

CNS: CNS depression, confusion, dizziness, drowsiness, fever, headache, lassitude
EENT: Hearing loss, tinnitus, vision changes

GI: Anorexia, diarrhea, epigastric discomfort, **GI bleeding**, **hepatotoxicity**, nausea, thirst, vomiting
HEME: Hemolytic anemia, **leukopenia**, **prolonged bleeding time**, **thrombocytopenia**
SKIN: Diaphoresis, purpura, rash, urticaria
Other: Angioedema, Reye's syndrome

Nursing Considerations

- Avoid using salsalate in patients with hypoprothrombinemia or vitamin K deficiency because drug's hypoprothrombinemic effect may precipitate bleeding.
- Monitor hepatic and renal function, as appropriate, during long-term therapy.
- Assess for signs and symptoms of GI bleeding, such as abdominal pain or black, tarry stools, especially in patient with peptic ulcer disease.
- Assess for symptoms of ototoxicity, such as ringing or roaring in ears.

PATIENT TEACHING

- Instruct patient to take salsalate with food or a full glass of water and to remain upright for 1 hour after administration to prevent drug from lodging in esophagus and causing irritation.
- Inform patient that therapeutic response may not occur for 2 to 3 weeks.
- Urge patient to notify prescriber immediately of abdominal pain or black, tarry stools; these symptoms may indicate GI bleeding or drug toxicity.

saquinavir mesylate

Invirase

Class and Category

Pharmacologic class: Protease inhibitor
Therapeutic class: Antiretroviral
Pregnancy category: B

Indications and Dosages

➤ *As adjunct to treat human immunodeficiency viral (HIV) infection in combination with ritonavir and other antiretroviral agents*

CAPSULES, TABLETS

Adults and adolescents over the age of 16 who are treatment-naïve or are switching from a regimen containing delavirdine. *Initial:* 500 mg within 2 hr after a meal twice daily in combination with ritonavir 100 mg twice daily for 7 days, then increased to 1,000 mg twice daily within 2 hr after a meal in combination with ritonavir 100 mg twice daily.
Adults and adolescents over the age of 16 who are not treatment-naïve or are not switching from a regimen containing delavirdine. 1,000 mg within 2 hr after a meal twice daily in combination with ritonavir 100 mg twice daily.

Mechanism of Action

Inhibits HIV protease to render the enzyme incapable of processing the Gag-Pol polyprotein precursor, which leads to the production of noninfectious immature HIV particles.

Contraindications

Combination with drugs that both increase saquinavir plasma concentrations and prolong the QT interval or CYP3A substrates that increase saquinavir levels resulting in serious or life-threatening adverse reactions; complete atrioventricular (AV) block without implanted pacemaker; concomitant therapy with alfuzosin, amiodarone, atazanavir, bepridil, clarithromycin, clozapine, dasatinib, dofetilide, disopyramide, ergot derivatives, erythromycin, flecainide, halofantrine, haloperidol, lidocaine, lovastatin, lurasidone, midazolam (oral), pentamidine, phenothiazines, pimozide, propafenone, quinidine, quinine, rifampin, rilpivirine (without a washout period of at least 2 weeks), sertindole, sildenafil (for treatment of pulmonary arterial hypertension), simvastatin, sunatinib, tacrolimus, trazodone, triazolam, ziprasidone; congenital long QT syndrome; high risk for complete AV block; hypersensitivity to saquinavir or its components; hypokalemia; hypomagnesemia; severe hepatic impairment

Interactions

DRUGS

alfentanil, alfuzosin, amiodarone, amitriptyline, atorvastatin, benzodiazepines, bepridil, bosentan, calcium channel blockers,

chlorpromazine, clarithromycin, clomipramine, clozapine, colchicine, dapsone, dasatinib, digoxin, disopyramide, dofetilide, ergot derivatives, erythromycin, fentanyl, flecainide, halofantrine, haloperidol, imipramine, immunosuppressants, ketoconazole, lidocaine (systemic), lovastatin, lurasidone, maprotiline, maraviroc, mesoridazine, midazolam, omeprazole, pimozide, propafenone, quetiapine, quinidine, quinine, rifabutin, rifampin, rilpivirine, salmeterol, sertindole, sildenafil, simvastatin, sunitinib, tacrolimus, tadalafil, thioridazine, trazodone, triazolam, vardenafil, vincamine, warfarin, ziprasidone: Increased concentration of these drugs
antiarrhythmics class 1A and class III, antidepressants, antihistaminics, antimicrobials, neuroleptics, PDE5 inhibitors (used for pulmonary arterial hypertension): Increased risk of prolonged PR and/or QT interval resulting in increased risk of ventricular arrhythmias, especially torsades de pointes
atazanavir: Increased concentration of atazanavir, ritonavir, and saquinavir
carbamazepine, efavirenz, garlic capsules, nevirapine, phenobarbital, phenytoin, St. John's wort, tipranavir/ritonavir: Decreased saquinavir concentration
corticosteroids: Decreased concentration of saquinavir and increased concentrations of corticosteroids
dalfopristin, quinupristin: Possibly increased saquinavir concentration
delavirdine, nefazodone, nelfinavir: Increased saquinavir concentration
ethinyl estradiol, methadone: Decreased concentration of these drugs
fusidic acid: Increased concentrations of fusidic acid, ritonavir, saquinavir
indinavir, itraconazole: Increased concentration of both drugs

Adverse Reactions

CNS: Abnormal coordination, anxiety, asthenia, confusion, depression, dizziness, fatigue, fever, headache, hypoesthesia, insomnia, **intracranial hemorrhage**, lethargy, loss of consciousness, paresthesia, peripheral neuropathy, psychotic disorder, **seizures**, somnolence, **suicidal ideation**, syncope, tremor
CV: Chest pain, edema, elevated LDH levels, hypertension, hypertriglyceridemia, heart murmur, **hypotension**, peripheral vasoconstriction, PR or **QT-interval prolongation**, **thrombophlebitis**
EENT: Sinusitis, taste distortion, tinnitus, visual impairment
ENDO: Diabetes mellitus (new-onset or worsening of existing condition), hyperglycemia
GI: Abdominal discomfort or pain, anorexia, ascites, constipation, diarrhea, dyspepsia, dysphagia, elevated liver and pancreatic enzymes, eructation, flatulence, gastritis, **gastrointestinal hemorrhage or obstruction**, **hepatitis**, hepatomegaly, hyperbilirubinemia, increased appetite, jaundice, nausea, **pancreatitis**, **portal hypertension**, vomiting
GU: Libido disorder, nephrolithiasis
HEME: Anemia including **hemolytic**, **leukopenia**, lymphadenopathy, **neutropenia**, **pancytopenia**, **thrombocytopenia**
MS: Arthralgia, back pain, muscle spasms, myalgia, polyarthritis
RESP: Bronchitis, cough, dyspnea, pneumonia
SKIN: Acne, alopecia, bullous dermatitis, diaphoresis, drug eruption, dry lips or skin, eczema, erythema, papillomatosis, pruritus, rash, **severe cutaneous reaction**, **Stevens–Johnson syndrome**, urticaria
Other: Acute myeloid leukemia, dehydration, elevated alkaline phosphatase, creatine phosphokinase, flu-like symptoms, **hypersensitivity reactions**, lipodystrophy, wasting syndrome, weight gain

Nursing Considerations

- Be aware that saquinavir must be used in combination with ritonavir because ritonavir significantly inhibits metabolism of saquinavir to provide increased plasma saquinavir levels. However, saquinavir is not recommended for use in combination with cobicistat because dosing recommendations for this combination have not been established.
- Be aware that if patient is unable to swallow capsules, capsules may be opened and emptied into a container. Add 15 ml of either sorbitol syrup or sugar syrup or 3 teaspoons of jam to the container. Stir with a spoon for 30 to 60 seconds. Administer the full amount prepared for

each dose. Know that the suspensions should be at room temperature before administering. Do not crush the tablet form.
- Administer ritonavir at the same time as saquinavir.
- Monitor patient closely because saquinavir interacts with many drugs. These interactions may cause serious adverse reactions that could be life-threatening or increase adverse reactions from greater exposure to saquinavir. In addition, some drug interactions can lower the therapeutic effect of saquinavir and possibly cause resistance to develop. Alert prescriber if a serious or severe toxicity occurs during treatment, as saquinavir will have to be discontinued.
- Obtain an ECG reading on all patients before starting saquinavir therapy, because of risk of PR or QT prolongation.
- Monitor patient's ECG for PR interval prolongation during therapy. Prolonged PR intervals can lead to conduction abnormalities including second- or third-degree atrioventricular block. Use caution with administering atazanavir, beta-adrenergic blockers, calcium channel blockers, or digoxin with saquinavir, because of the combined effect on the PR interval.
- Know that patients should also have ECG monitoring for QT-interval prolongation during therapy. Patients with long QT syndrome should not receive saquinavir, because of its effect on the QT interval. Risk factors for QT prolongation include presence of bradyarrhythmias, congestive heart failure, electrolyte abnormalities, or hepatic impairment. Know that hypokalemia or hypomagnesemia must be corrected before saquinavir therapy is begun. Expect to monitor patient's electrolyte levels throughout therapy. Know that saquinavir should be discontinued in any patient who develops a QT-interval prolongation greater than 20 msec over pretreatment measurement.
- Monitor patient's blood glucose levels, as new onset of diabetes mellitus, exacerbation of preexisting diabetes mellitus, and hyperglycemia have occurred with protease-inhibitor therapy such as saquinavir.
- Monitor patient with underlying chronic alcoholism, cirrhosis, hepatitis B or C, or other liver abnormalities, because portal hypertension has occurred after saquinavir therapy has been initiated. If severe hepatic dysfunction occurs, expect drug to be discontinued.
- Know that spontaneous bleeding in patients with hemophilia A and B has occurred during treatment with protease inhibitors such as saquinavir. Additional factor VIII may be required.
- Monitor patient's lipid profile, as ordered, because elevated cholesterol and/or triglyceride levels have occurred with the combination therapy of saquinavir and ritonavir.
- Be aware that immune reconstitution syndrome has occurred in patients treated with combination antiretroviral therapy, including saquinavir. The inflammatory response predisposes susceptible patients to opportunistic infections such as cytomegalovirus, *Mycobacterium avium* infection, *Pneumocystis jiroveci* pneumonia, or tuberculosis. Autoimmune disorders such as Graves' disease, Guillain–Barré syndrome, or polymyositis have also occurred. Report sudden or unusual adverse reactions to prescriber.

PATIENT TEACHING

- Instruct patient who is unable to swallow capsules to open capsules and place contents into an empty container. Tell patient to add 15 ml of room-temperature sorbitol syrup or sugar syrup or 3 teaspoons of jam to the container. Stir with spoon for 30 to 60 seconds before taking the entire amount.
- Instruct patient taking tablet form of saquinavir to swallow whole and never crush the tablets.
- Tell patient to take ritonavir at the same time as saquinavir and within 2 hours after a meal.
- Tell patient with diabetes to monitor his blood glucose levels closely, as saquinavir may cause blood glucose levels to rise.
- Inform patient that saquinavir therapy may cause changes in her body appearance because of fat redistribution. Prepare her for the possibility of developing breast enlargement, central obesity, dorsocervical fat enlargement

(buffalo hump), facial wasting, and peripheral wasting.
- Instruct patient to report any persistent, severe, or unusual signs and symptoms, such as dizziness, lightheadedness, or palpitations.
- Encourage women of childbearing age to report known or suspected pregnancy. Encourage patient to register with the antiretroviral pregnancy registry if pregnancy occurs.
- Alert mothers that breastfeeding is not recommended during saquinavir therapy, because drug is present in human breast milk.
- Inform patients with hemophilia that saquinavir may cause spontaneous bleeding and instruct them to seek immediate medical attention if bleeding occurs.
- Stress importance of compliance with ordered laboratory studies such as lipid profile to monitor for adverse reactions.
- Advise patient to notify all prescribers of saquinavir therapy, because of potential drug interactions, and advise patient not to take over-the-counter preparations (including herbal drugs and preparations) without consulting prescriber first.

sarecycline

Seysara

Class and Category

Pharmacologic class: Tetracycline
Therapeutic class: Antibacterial
Pregnancy category: Not classified

Indications and Dosages

➤ *To treat inflammatory lesions of non-nodular moderate to severe acne vulgaris*

TABLETS

Adults and children age 9 and over weighing 85 kg (187 lb) to 136 kg (299.2 lb). 150 mg once daily.
Adults and children age 9 and over weighing 55 kg (121 lb) to 84 kg (184.8 lb). 100 mg once daily.
Adults and children age 9 and over weighing 33 kg (72.6 lb) to 54 kg (118.8 lb). 60 mg once daily.

Mechanism of Action

Although the exact mechanism of action is unknown for the treatment of acne vulgaris, the tetracycline class of antibiotics exerts a bacteriostatic effect by passing through the bacterial lipid bilayer, where it binds reversibly to 30S ribosomal subunits. This blocks the binding of aminoacyl transfer RNA to messenger RNA, thus inhibiting bacterial protein synthesis, which may relieve the inflammation of acne vulgaris.

Contraindications

Hypersensitivity to sarecycline, other tetracyclines, or their components

Interactions

DRUGS

aluminum-, calcium-, or magnesium-containing antacids, bismuth subsalicylate, iron-containing preparations: Possibly altered absorption of sarecycline
anticoagulants: Possibly depressed plasma prothrombin activity, which may increase risk of bleeding
oral retinoids: Possibly additive increased risk of intracranial pressure
penicillin: Possible interference with bactericidal action of penicillin
P-glycoprotein substrates such as digoxin: Possibly increased concentrations of P-gp substrates

Adverse Reactions

GI: ***Clostridium difficile*-associated diarrhea**, nausea
GU: Vulvovaginal candidiasis, vulvovaginal mycotic infection

Nursing Considerations

- Assess patient for signs of secondary infection, such as profuse, watery diarrhea that has occurred with nearly all antibacterial agents. If such diarrhea develops, contact prescriber and expect to obtain a stool specimen to rule out pseudomembranous colitis caused by *C. difficile*. If diarrhea occurs, notify prescriber and expect to withhold penicillin and treat with electrolytes, fluids, protein, and an antibiotic effective against *C. difficile*.

• Monitor patient for central nervous system adverse reaction such as dizziness, lightheadedness, and vertigo, because although sarecycline has not been known to cause such reactions, other tetracyclines have.

WARNING Be aware that intracranial hypertension has occurred with the use of other tetracyclines. Monitor patient for blurred vision, headache, and papilledema. If present, notify prescriber immediately, because even though intracranial hypertension usually resolves with discontinuation of the tetracycline, vision loss may become severe or even permanent. Women of childbearing age who are overweight are at higher risk for developing intracranial hypertension.

• Monitor patient for superinfection such as mycotic or vulvovaginal candidiasis infections. If present, notify prescriber and expect sarecycline therapy to be discontinued.

PATIENT TEACHING

• Tell patient to take sarecycline therapy exactly as directed. Also stress importance of completing the full course of therapy and not skipping doses, because not doing so may decrease the effectiveness of current therapy and increase the likelihood that bacteria may develop resistance to other antibacterial drugs in the future.
• Instruct patient to take tablets with liberal amounts of fluid, to reduce risk of esophageal irritation and ulceration.
• Advise women of childbearing age that sarecycline may cause fetal harm. It may also cause permanent discoloration of teeth later on, and retardation of skeletal development in the developing fetus if exposed to the drug during the second or third trimesters of pregnancy. Suspected or known pregnancy should be reported immediately to prescriber.
• Urge patient to tell prescriber if diarrhea develops, even 2 months or more after sarecycline therapy ends.
• Caution patient not to perform hazardous activities such as driving until possible adverse reactions are known.
• Warn patient to avoid exposure to artificial or natural sunlight because photosensitivity, manifested as an exaggerated sunburn reaction, has occurred in patients taking other tetracycline products. Instruct patient to wear protective clothing and use sunscreen if natural sunlight cannot be avoided. If skin redness occurs, tell patient to report this to prescriber, as drug should be discontinued at the first sign of skin redness.
• Inform mothers wishing to breastfeed their infant that breastfeeding is not recommended during sarecycline therapy.

WARNING Instruct patient to report blurred vision or headaches immediately to prescriber.

sarilumab

Kevzara

Class and Category

Pharmacologic class: Monoclonal antibody
Therapeutic class: Antiarthritic
Pregnancy category: Not classified

Indications and Dosages

➤ *To treat moderate to severe active rheumatoid arthritis in patients who have had an inadequate response or intolerance to one or more disease-modifying antirheumatic drugs (DMARDs)*

SUBCUTANEOUS INJECTION

Adults. 200 mg once every 2 wk.

DOSAGE ADJUSTMENT For patients who experience an absolute neutrophil count (ANC) between 500 to 1,000 cells/mm^3, sarilumab withheld until ANC becomes greater than 1,000 cells/mm^3. Dosage restarted at 150 mg every 2 wk and then dosage increased to 200 mg and given every 2 wk, when clinically appropriate. For patients experiencing an ANC less than 500 cells/mm^3, drug discontinued. For patients who experience a low platelet count between 50,000 to 100,000 cells/mm^3, drug withheld until platelets become greater than 100,000 cells/mm^3. Dosage restarted at 150 mg every 2 wk and then dosage increased to 200 mg every 2 wk, when clinically appropriate. For patients experiencing a platelet count less than 50,000 cells/mm^3 and confirmed with repeat testing, drug discontinued. For patients experiencing an elevated (ALT) greater than upper level normal (ULN) to three times ULN or less, dosage may have to be modified on an individual basis. For patients who experience an ALT greater than three times ULN to five times ULN or less, drug withheld until ALT is less than three times ULN. Dosage restarted at 150 mg every 2 wk and then dosage increased to 200 mg every 2 wk, as clinically appropriate. For patient experiencing an ALT greater than five times ULN, drug discontinued.

Mechanism of Action

Binds to IL-6 receptors to inhibit IL-6 mediated signaling of inflammatory processes which occurs in rheumatoid arthritis. Without IL-6 mediated signaling, IL-6 as a pro-inflammatory cytokine cannot be produced by endothelial and synovial cells in joints. This helps relieve inflammation present in rheumatoid arthritis.

Contraindications

Hypersensitivity to sarilumab or its components

Interactions

DRUGS

atorvastatin, lovastatin, oral contraceptives: Possibly decreased effectiveness of these drugs
CYP450 substrates with narrow therapeutic index, such as theophylline, warfarin: Possibly altered dosage requirements
live vaccines: Increased risk of vaccine-related infection

Adverse Reactions

CV: Elevated cholesterol and triglyceride levels
EENT: Nasopharyngitis
GI: Elevated liver enzymes, **GI perforation**
GU: UTI
HEME: Neutropenia, **thrombocytopenia**
RESP: Upper respiratory infections
SKIN: Rash, urticaria
Other: Anaphylaxis; anti-sarilumab antibody formation; herpes zoster reactivation; **immunosuppression**; infections such as bacterial, invasive fungal, mycobacterial, tuberculosis, viral, or other opportunistic pathogens; injection-site erythema; pruritis, rash; **malignancies**

Nursing Considerations

- Be aware that sarilumab therapy should not be started in patients who have an elevated ALT or AST above 1.5 times the upper limit of normal, an absolute neutrophil count (ANC) less than 2,000/mm^3, or platelet count less than 150,000/mm^3.
- Expect patient to be tested for latent tuberculosis before sarilumab therapy is started. If result is positive, patient will need to be treated before sarilumab is initiated. In patient who has a history of active or latent tuberculosis and for whom an adequate course of treatment cannot be confirmed or results are negative, but patient has risk factors for tuberculosis infection, patient may need to be treated before beginning sarilumab therapy.
- Know that sarilumab should not be used with biological DMARDs because of increased immunosuppression and increased risk of infection.
- Be aware that sarilumab should be avoided in patients with active infections.
- Know that patients with active hepatic disease or hepatic impairment are not candidates for sarilumab therapy, because drug can have adverse effects on liver, as evidenced by elevation in liver enzymes.
- Allow prefilled syringe to sit at room temperature for 30 minutes prior to injecting drug subcutaneously. Syringe should not be warmed any other way. Inspect solution before administering. It should be clear and colorless to pale yellow. Discard if solution appears discolored, cloudy, or has particulate matter in it.

WARNING Monitor patient for signs and symptoms of infection because of sarilumab's immunosuppressant action. Serious and sometimes fatal infections due to bacterial, invasive fungal, mycobacterial, viral, or other opportunistic pathogens have occurred with sarilumab therapy. If infection occurs, notify prescriber, expect drug to be withheld for serious infections until infection is eradicated, and administer prescribed treatment for the infection.

- Expect to monitor patient's ALT, ANC, and platelet counts regularly. Expect dosage modifications or drug withholding until target levels are met.

- Monitor patient for hypersensitivity reactions, If present, notify prescriber, expect drug to be withheld or discontinued based upon severity of the reaction, and provide supportive care.

PATIENT TEACHING

- Teach patient or caregiver how to administer a subcutaneous injection. Tell patient to rotate injection sites with each injection and not to inject into skin that is bruised, damaged, scarred, or tender.
- Instruct patient to allow prefilled syringe to sit at room temperature for 30 minutes and the prefilled pen for 60 minutes prior to administering the injection. Warn patient not to warm syringe any other way. Have patient inspect the solution in the syringe before administering the injection. Solution should be clear and colorless to pale yellow. If solution is cloudy, discolored, or contains particles, instruct patient to discard it and use a new prefilled syringe. Also tell patient to discard the prefilled syringe or pen if not used within 14 days after being taken out of the refrigerator.
- Tell patient to inject the full amount in syringe to receive the prescribed dose.
- Instruct patient on infection precautions. Warn patient to avoid people with an active infection. Review signs and symptoms of an infection with patient and tell him to report any such evidence to prescriber immediately.
- Warn patient that allergic reactions can occur with sarilumab therapy. Tell patient to alert prescriber if present, as drug may have to be discontinued if reaction is serious.
- Inform patient that frequent blood tests will have to be performed to monitor for adverse effects. Stress importance of patient compliance with these appointments.
- Warn patient not to receive any live vaccines while taking sarilumab.
- Instruct patient to notify prescriber and seek immediate emergency medical attention if abdominal signs and symptoms such as pain occur.
- Tell women of childbearing age to notify prescriber if pregnancy occurs. Encourage female patient to enroll in the pregnancy registry.

saxagliptin monohydrate

Onglyza

Class and Category

Pharmacologic class: Dipeptidyl peptidase-4 (DPP-4) inhibitor
Therapeutic class: Antidiabetic
Pregnancy category: B

Indications and Dosages

➤ *To improve blood glucose control in type 2 diabetes mellitus as adjunct to diet and exercise*

TABLETS

Adults. 2.5 or 5 mg once daily

DOSAGE ADJUSTMENT For patients with moderate or severe renal impairment (creatinine clearance 50 ml/min or less), patients with end-stage renal disease, patients having hemodialysis, and patients receiving strong CYP3A4/5 inhibitors (i.e., atazanavir, clarithromycin, indinavir, itraconazole, ketoconazole, nefazodone, nelfinavir, ritonavir, saquinavir, telithromycin), dosage shouldn't exceed 2.5 mg once daily.

Route	Onset	Peak	Duration
P.O.	Unknown	2 hr	24 hr

Mechanism of Action

Incretin hormones, such as glucose-dependent insulintropic polypeptide (GIP) and glucagons-like peptide-1 (GLP-1), are released into bloodstream from small intestine in response to meals. Upon arrival at the pancreas, they stimulate pancreatic beta cells to release insulin. GLP-1 also reduces glucagon secretion from pancreatic alpha cells, which reduces hepatic glucose production. Incretin hormones become inactivated within minutes of release by the enzyme, dipeptidyl peptidase-4. Saxagliptin inhibits this enzyme, thereby slowing inactivation of incretin hormones, which provides more time for them to increase insulin levels and blunt glucagon secretion. More insulin and less hepatic glucose production work together to lower blood glucose levels.

Contraindications

Hypersensitivity to saxagliptin or its components

Interactions

DRUGS

aprepitant, diltiazem, erythromycin, fluconazole, fosamprenavir, verapamil: Possibly increased plasma saxagliptin level
atazanavir, clarithromycin, indinavir, itraconazole, ketoconazole, nefazodone, nelfinavir, ritonavir, saquinavir, telithromycin: Increased plasma saxagliptin level
insulin, sulfonylureas: Increased risk of hypoglycemia

FOODS

grapefruit juice: Possibly increased plasma saxagliptin levels

Adverse Reactions

CNS: Headache
CV: Heart failure, peripheral edema
EENT: Sinusitis, nasopharyngitis
ENDO: Hypoglycemia
GI: Acute pancreatitis, abdominal pain, gastroenteritis, vomiting
GU: Elevated plasma creatinine level, UTI
HEME: Lymphopenia
MS: Arthralgia (disabling, severe)
RESP: Upper respiratory tract infection
SKIN: Bullous pemphigoid, exfoliative skin conditions; rash; urticaria
Other: Anaphylaxis, angioedema

Nursing Considerations

- Know that saxagliptin shouldn't be used to treat type 1 diabetes mellitus or diabetic ketoacidosis.
- Use cautiously in patients who have experienced angioedema with another dipeptidyl peptidase-4 inhibitor because it is not known if a cross-sensitivity reaction may occur with saxagliptin.
- Obtain a serum creatinine level, as ordered, before starting saxagliptin therapy and then periodically thereafter to monitor patient's renal function.
- Monitor patient closely for hypersensitivity to saxagliptin, especially within the first 3 months of therapy beginning with first dose. These reactions can be serious and life-threatening and may include anaphylaxis, angioedema, and exfoliative skin conditions. Discontinue saxagliptin immediately if hypersensitivity occurs, and notify prescriber.
- Monitor patient's blood glucose level and hemoglobin A_{1c} to assess effectiveness of saxagliptin therapy.
- Monitor patient for signs and symptoms of heart failure during saxagliptin therapy because drug may increase risk. If present, notify prescriber, expect drug to be discontinued, and provide supportive care, as ordered.
- Watch for hypoglycemia in patients taking insulin or other antidiabetics, such as sulfonylureas. Expect dosage of insulin or other antidiabetics, such as sulfonylureas, to be decreased to reduce risk of hypoglycemia.
- Monitor patient for signs and symptoms of acute pancreatitis such as severe, sharp pain in the upper abdominal accompanied by fever, nausea, and vomiting. If present, notify prescriber, expect to stop saxagliptin, as ordered, and provide supportive care, as indicated and ordered.

PATIENT TEACHING

- Emphasize that saxagliptin isn't a replacement for diet and exercise therapy.
- Explain importance of self-monitoring glucose levels during saxagliptin therapy.
- Teach patient to recognize hypoglycemia and how to treat it if it should occur. Urge him to carry glucose with him at all times in case hypoglycemia occurs.
- Review signs and symptoms of heart failure with patient, such as difficulty breathing; swelling of feet, hands, or legs; or unexplained weight gain. Tell patient to notify prescriber immediately, if present.
- Instruct patient to notify prescriber if fever, illness, infection, surgery, trauma, or other stress occurs because blood glucose control may be altered, requiring temporary insulin therapy.
- Tell patient to watch for the development of blisters or breakdown of the outer layer of his skin. If present, he should notify prescriber, as drug may need to be discontinued.
- Instruct patient to seek immediate medical attention if he experiences persistent, acute abdominal pain, fever, nausea, and vomiting, as well as any sign of hypersensitivity, such as difficulty breathing or swallowing, hives, rash, skin flaking or

peeling, or swelling of any area on face or skin.
- Advise patient to seek medical attention if severe joint pain occurs. Tell patient that joint pain may develop within a day of taking saxagliptin or may develop years later.

scopolamine transdermal system

Transderm-Scop, Transderm-V (CAN)

Class and Category

Pharmacologic class: Belladonna alkaloid
Therapeutic class: Antiemetic
Pregnancy category: C

Indications and Dosages

➤ *To prevent nausea and vomiting associated with motion sickness or recovery from anesthesia and/or opiate analgesia and surgery*

TRANSDERMAL SYSTEM

Adults and adolescents. 1 U.S. transdermal system (1 mg) applied behind ear before antiemetic effect is required as follows: 4 hr before event known to cause motion sickness, evening before surgery, or 1 hr before caesarian section. Patch removed 24 hr postsurgical procedure. Patch may remain in place up to 3 days for prevention of motion sickness and may be replaced, as needed. Or, 1 Canadian transdermal system (1 mg) applied behind ear for 3-day period, beginning at least 12 hr before antiemetic effect is required.

DOSAGE ADJUSTMENT Dosage reduction possible for elderly patients because of their increased sensitivity to scopolamine.

Contraindications

Angle-closure glaucoma; hemorrhage with hemodynamic instability; hepatic dysfunction; hypersensitivity to barbiturates, scopolamine, other belladonna alkaloids, or their components; ileus; intestinal atony; myasthenia gravis; myocardial ischemia; obstructive GI disease, such as pyloric stenosis; obstructive uropathy, as in prostatic hyperplasia; renal impairment; tachycardia; toxic megacolon; ulcerative colitis

Route	Onset	Peak	Duration
Transdermal	4 hr	Unknown	72 hr

Mechanism of Action

Blocks neural pathways in the inner ear to relieve motion sickness.

Interactions

DRUGS

adsorbent antidiarrheals, antacids: Decreased absorption and therapeutic effects of scopolamine
anticholinergics (other): Possibly intensified anticholinergic effects
antimyasthenics: Possibly reduced intestinal motility
CNS depressants: Possibly potentiated effects of either drug, resulting in additive sedation
haloperidol: Decreased antipsychotic effect of haloperidol
ketoconazole: Decreased ketoconazole absorption
lorazepam (parenteral): Possibly hallucinations, irrational behavior, and sedation
metoclopramide: Possibly antagonized effect of metoclopramide on GI motility
opioid analgesics: Increased risk of severe constipation and ileus
potassium chloride: Possibly increased severity of potassium chloride–induced GI lesions
urinary alkalizers (antacids, carbonic anhydrase inhibitors, citrates, sodium bicarbonate): Delayed excretion of scopolamine, possibly leading to increased therapeutic and adverse effects

ACTIVITIES

alcohol use: Additive CNS effects

Adverse Reactions

CNS: Dizziness, drowsiness, euphoria, insomnia, memory loss, paradoxical stimulation
CV: Palpitations, tachycardia
EENT: Blurred vision; dry eyes, mouth, nose, and throat; mydriasis
GI: Constipation, dysphagia
GU: Urinary hesitancy, urine retention
SKIN: Decreased sweating, dry skin, flushing

Nursing Considerations

- Assess for bladder distention and monitor urine output because drug's antimuscarinic effects can cause urine retention.
- Monitor for pain. In presence of pain, drug may act as a stimulant and produce delirium if used without meperidine or morphine.
- Monitor heart rate for transient tachycardia, which may occur with high doses of drug. Rate should return to normal within 30 minutes.

PATIENT TEACHING

- Instruct patient to apply scopolamine transdermal patch on hairless area behind ear and to wash hands thoroughly with soap and water before and after applying.
- Advise patient to avoid hazardous activities until drug's CNS effects are known.
- Instruct patient to avoid alcohol while wearing the scopolamine patch.
- If patient complains of dry eyes, suggest lubricating drops.

secnidazole

Solosec

Class and Category

Pharmacologic class: 5-Nitroimidazole
Therapeutic class: Antibiotic
Pregnancy category: Not classified

Indications and Dosages

➤ *To treat bacterial vaginosis*

ORAL GRANULES

Adult women. 2 g taken once.

Route	Onset	Peak	Duration
P.O.	Unknown	4 hr	Unknown

Mechanism of Action

Enters the bacterial cell to reduce the nitro group to radical anions by bacterial enzymes. The radical anions then interfere with bacterial DNA synthesis to eradicate the infection.

Contraindications

Hypersensitivity to secnidazole, other nitroimidazole derivatives, or their components

Adverse Reactions

CNS: Headache
EENT: Distorted sense of taste
GI: Abdominal pain, diarrhea, nausea, vomiting
GU: Vulvovaginal candidiasis or pruritus

Nursing Considerations

- Open packet by folding over the corner and tearing across the top. Sprinkle entire contents onto applesauce, pudding, or yogurt. Be aware that the granules will not dissolve. Have patient consume all of the mixture within 30 minutes without chewing or crunching the granules. Provide a glass of water to aid in swallowing. Know that the granules are not intended to be dissolved in any liquid.
- Monitor patient for adverse reactions. Know that symptomatic vulvo-vaginal candidiasis may require treatment with an antifungal agent.

PATIENT TEACHING

- Tell patient that drug is taken only one time.
- Instruct patient to open packet by folding over the corner and tearing across the top. She should then sprinkle entire contents onto applesauce, pudding, or yogurt. Be aware that the granules will not dissolve. She should consume all of the mixture within 30 minutes without chewing or crunching the granules. Tell her to drink a glass of water afterward to aid in swallowing. Remind her that the granules are not intended to be dissolved in any liquid.
- Inform patient that vulvo-vaginal candidiasis may occur with secnidazole use. Tell her to notify prescriber if present because it may require treatment.
- Instruct a mother who is breastfeeding to pump and discard her milk for 96 hours after administration of secnidazole.

secobarbital sodium

Novosecobarb (CAN), Seconal

Class, Category, and Schedule

Pharmacologic class: Barbiturate

Therapeutic class: Sedative-hypnotic
Pregnancy category: D
Controlled substance schedule: II

Indications and Dosages

➤ *To induce sedation before surgery*

CAPSULES

Adults. 200 to 300 mg 1 to 2 hr before surgery.
Children. 2 to 6 mg/kg 1 to 2 hr before surgery. *Maximum:* 100 mg.

➤ *To provide short-term treatment of insomnia*

CAPSULES

Adults. 100 mg at bedtime.

DOSAGE ADJUSTMENT Reduced dosage required for debilitated or elderly patients and those with hepatic or renal dysfunction.

Route	Onset	Peak	Duration
P.O.	10–15 min	15–30 min	1–4 hr

Mechanism of Action

Inhibits upward conduction of nerve impulses to the reticular formation of the brain, thereby disrupting impulse transmission to the cortex. This action depresses the CNS, producing drowsiness, hypnosis, and sedation.

Contraindications

History of barbiturate addiction; hypersensitivity to secobarbital, other barbiturates, or their components; nephritis; porphyria; severe hepatic or respiratory impairment

Interactions

DRUGS

acetaminophen, adrenocorticoids, beta blockers, chloramphenicol, cyclosporine, dacarbazine, digoxin, disopyramide, estrogens, metronidazole, oral anticoagulants, oral contraceptives, quinidine, thyroid hormones, tricyclic antidepressants: Decreased effectiveness of these drugs
addictive drugs: Increased risk of addiction
calcium channel blockers: Possibly excessive hypotension
carbamazepine, succinimide anticonvulsants: Decreased blood levels and increased elimination of these drugs
carbonic anhydrase inhibitors: Increased risk of osteopenia
CNS depressants: Increased CNS depressant effects
cyclophosphamide: Increased risk of leukopenic activity and reduced half-life of cyclophosphamide
divalproex sodium, valproic acid: Increased CNS depression and neurologic toxicity
doxycycline, fenoprofen: Increased elimination of these drugs
general anesthetics (enflurane, halothane, methoxyflurane): Increased risk of hepatotoxicity; increased risk of nephrotoxicity (with methoxyflurane)
griseofulvin: Decreased griseofulvin absorption
guanadrel, guanethidine: Possibly increased orthostatic hypotension
haloperidol: Possibly altered frequency or pattern of seizures, decreased blood haloperidol level
ketamine: Increased risk of hypotension or respiratory depression (when secobarbital is used as preanesthetic)
leucovorin (large doses): Decreased anticonvulsant effect of secobarbital
loxapine, phenothiazines, thioxanthenes: Possibly lowered seizure threshold
MAO inhibitors: Possibly prolonged CNS depressant effects of secobarbital
maprotiline: Increased CNS depressant effect; possibly lowered seizure threshold and decreased anticonvulsant effect with high doses of maprotiline
methylphenidate: Increased risk of barbiturate toxicity
mexiletine: Decreased blood mexiletine level
phenylbutazone: Decreased effectiveness of secobarbital
posterior pituitary hormones: Increased risk of arrhythmias and coronary insufficiency
primidone: Increased sedative effect of either drug, change in seizure pattern
vitamin D: Decreased vitamin D effects
xanthines (aminophylline, oxtriphylline, theophylline): Increased metabolism of xanthines (except dyphylline), decreased hypnotic effect of secobarbital

FOODS

caffeine: Increased caffeine metabolism, decreased hypnotic effect of secobarbital

ACTIVITIES
alcohol use: Increased CNS depression

Adverse Reactions

CNS: Anxiety, clumsiness, confusion, depression, dizziness, drowsiness, hangover, headache, insomnia, irritability, lethargy, nervousness, nightmares, paradoxical stimulation, syncope
CV: Hypotension
EENT: Laryngospasm
GI: Anorexia, constipation, nausea, vomiting
MS: Arthralgia, muscle weakness
RESP: Apnea, **bronchospasm**, **respiratory depression**
SKIN: Jaundice
Other: Drug dependence, weight loss

Nursing Considerations

- Be aware that prolonged use of secobarbital may lead to tolerance and physical and psychological dependence.

WARNING To avoid withdrawal symptoms, expect to taper drug after long-term therapy. Withdrawal symptoms usually appear 8 to 12 hours after stopping drug and may include anxiety, insomnia, muscle twitching, nausea, orthostatic hypotension, vomiting, weakness, and weight loss. Severe symptoms may include delirium, hallucinations, and seizures. Generalized tonic–clonic seizures may occur within 16 hours or up to 5 days after last dose.

- Assess patient for signs and symptoms of barbiturate toxicity, including dyspnea, severe confusion, and severe drowsiness. Notify prescriber immediately if they appear because barbiturate toxicity may be life-threatening.
- Expect prescriber to provide patient with the least possible quantity of secobarbital to minimize the risk of acute or chronic overdosage. For patients who are depressed, drug-dependent, or suicidal or who have a history of drug abuse, institute precautions to prevent drug hoarding and overdosage.

PATIENT TEACHING

- Instruct patient to take secobarbital exactly as prescribed because of the risk of addiction.
- Inform patient that taking drug with food may reduce adverse GI effects.
- Advise patient to avoid alcohol and caffeine and potentially hazardous activities during therapy.
- Inform patient about possible hangover effect.
- Recommend to patient taking an oral contraceptive to use an additional form of birth control during therapy.
- Caution patient not to stop taking drug abruptly.
- Instruct patient to notify prescriber of bone pain, muscle weakness, or unexplained weight loss during therapy.

secukinumab

Cosentyx

Class and Category

Pharmacologic class: Monoclonal antibody
Therapeutic class: Immunosuppressant
Pregnancy category: B

Indications and Dosages

➤ *To treat moderate to severe plaque psoriasis in patients who are candidates for phototherapy or systemic therapy; to treat psoriatic arthritis in patients with coexistent moderate to severe plaque psoriasis*

SUBCUTANEOUS INJECTION
Adults. 150 or 300 mg once a wk for 5 doses, then 150 or 300 mg every 4 wk.

➤ *To treat active ankylosing spondylitis; to treat active psoriatic arthritis*

SUBCUTANEOUS INJECTION
Adults. *Initial:* 150 mg weekly for 5 doses, followed by 150 mg every 4 wk. Alternatively, 150 mg every 4 wk. *Maximum:* 150 mg every 4 wk (ankylosing spondylitis); 300 mg every 4 wk (psoriatic arthritis).

Mechanism of Action

Binds to interleukin-17A (IL-17A) cytokine and inhibits its interaction with the IL-17A receptor. Since IL-17A is a cytokine involved in normal immune and inflammatory responses, binding it inhibits the release of proinflammatory chemokines and cytokines. This action reduces immune and inflammatory responses in the body.

Contraindications

Hypersensitivity to secukinumab or its components

Interactions

DRUGS

CYP450 substrates with a narrow therapeutic index such as warfarin or drug concentration such as cyclosporine: Possibly change in therapeutic effect of these drugs
live vaccines: Increased risk of adverse vaccine effects
nonlive vaccines: Possibly an ineffective immune response

Adverse Reactions

CNS: Headache
CV: Hypercholesterolemia
EENT: Nasopharyngitis, oral herpes, pharyngitis, rhinitis, rhinorrhea
GI: Diarrhea, inflammatory bowel disease, nausea
HEME: Neutropenia
RESP: Upper respiratory tract infection
SKIN: Urticaria
Other: Anaphylaxis; antibody formation to secukinumab; increased incidence of infections such as candida infections, herpes viral infections, or staphylococcal skin infections

Nursing Considerations

- Ensure that patient has been tested for tuberculosis (TB) before secukinumab therapy is begun. Know that the drug should not be given to patients with active TB infection. Expect to initiate treatment of active or latent TB prior to giving secukinumab, as ordered.
- Use caution when administering secukinumab in patients with inflammatory bowel disease because exacerbations may occur. Monitor patient throughout drug therapy as a new onset of inflammatory bowel disease may also occur in patients who have never experienced the disease prior to secukinumab therapy.
- Know that patients receiving secukinumab should not receive live vaccines as adverse vaccine effects may occur. Also know that nonlive vaccinations may not produce an immune response sufficient to prevent disease during secukinumab therapy.
- Remove secukinumab Sensoready pen or prefilled syringe, if prescribed, from the refrigerator and allow it to warm to room temperature for 15 to 30 minutes without removing the needle cap. Be aware that the needle cap should not be handled by latex-sensitive individuals. Inspect the solution and do not use if the liquid is cloudy or discolored or contains visible particles. Administer the drug using the Sensoready pen or prefilled syringe within 1 hour after removing from refrigerator because it does not contain any preservatives.
- Reconstitute the lyophilized powder form taking no more than 90 minutes to do so. First, remove the secukinumab vial from refrigerator and allow it to warm to room temperature for 15 to 30 minutes. Make sure the sterile water for injection used to reconstitute the drug is also at room temperature. Then slowly inject 1 ml of sterile water for injection into the drug vial directing the stream of water onto the lyophilized powder. Tilt the vial at about 45 degrees and gently rotate between fingertips for about 1 minute. Do not shake or invert the vial. Allow the vial to stand for about 10 minutes at room temperature. Some foaming may occur. Repeat tilting the vial and gently rotating it between fingertips for about 1 minute without shaking or inverting the vial. Allow the vial to stand undisturbed at room temperature for about 5 minutes. Do not use if the powder has not fully dissolved or if the liquid is cloudy or discolored or contains visible particles. Prepare the number of vials needed (1 vial for the 150 mg dose or 2 vials for the 300 mg dose). The reconstituted solution contains 150 mg of secukinumab in 1 ml of solution.
- Administer immediately or store in the refrigerator for up to 24 hours. Do not freeze. If stored in the refrigerator, allow the reconstituted solution to reach room temperature for 15 to 30 minutes before administration. Administer within 1 hour after removal from refrigerator.
- Know that when administering a 300 mg dose, 2 separate injections consisting of 150 mg is required.
- Administer the subcutaneous injection into the patient's abdomen, thigh(s), or upper arm(s). Rotate the injection sites and do not administer into an area that is

affected by psoriasis or is bruised, indurated, redden, or tender.

WARNING Monitor patient closely for a hypersensitivity reaction as secukinumab has caused anaphylaxis and urticaria. If a serious allergic reaction occurs, stop drug therapy immediately, notify prescriber, and provide emergency supportive care.

- Monitor patient closely for signs and symptoms of infection. Know that some types of infections appear to be dose related. Notify prescriber as drug may need to be withheld until the infection resolves.
- Monitor patient closely for signs and symptoms of active TB during and after treatment.

PATIENT TEACHING

- Instruct patient how to administer a subcutaneous injection.
- Instruct patient on how to use the secukinumab Sensoready pen or prefilled syringe. Tell him to remove secukinumab Sensoready pen or prefilled syringe from the refrigerator and allow it to warm to room temperature for 15 to 30 minutes without removing the needle cap. Tell him to inspect the solution and not to use it if the liquid is cloudy or discolored or contains visible particles.
- Stress importance of administering drug within 1 hour after removing from refrigerator because it does not contain any preservatives.
- Tell patient that drug can be injected in the abdomen, upper arms, or thighs. Advise him to rotate the injection sites and not to administer into an area that is affected by psoriasis or is bruised, indurated, redden, or tender.

WARNING Advise patient to seek immediate medical attention if he experiences any symptoms of a serious allergic reaction.

- Warn patient that drug may lower his ability to fight infections. Review infection measures with the patient and advise him to avoid people with an infection. If he develops an infection, tell him to notify prescriber.
- Caution patient not to receive any live vaccines while he is taking secukinumab.

selegiline hydrochloride

Eldepryl, Zelapar

selegiline transdermal system

Emsam

Class and Category

Pharmacologic class: Monoamine oxidase inhibitor (MAOI)
Therapeutic class: Antidepressant (Emsam), antidyskinetic
Pregnancy category: C

Indications and Dosages

➤ *As adjunct to carbidopa–levodopa therapy to treat Parkinson's disease*

CAPSULES, TABLETS

Adults. 5 mg twice daily with breakfast and lunch.

➤ *As adjunct to carbidopa-levodopa therapy to treat Parkinson's disease in patients whose response to therapy has deteriorated*

ORALLY DISINTEGRATING TABLETS (ZELAPAR)

Adults. *Initial:* 1.25 mg once daily before breakfast for at least 6 wk; then increased to 2.5 mg once daily, as needed.

DOSAGE ADJUSTMENT For patients with mild-to-moderate hepatic dysfunction, dosage kept at 1.25 mg once daily.

➤ *To treat depression*

TRANSDERMAL SYSTEM (EMSAM)

Adults. *Initial:* 6 mg/24 hr with patch applied daily to upper torso, upper thigh, or outer surface of upper arm. Increased every 2 wk in increments of 3 mg/24 hr, as needed.
Maximum: 12 mg/24 hr.

Mechanism of Action

Reduces dopamine metabolism by noncompetitively inhibiting the brain enzyme monoamine oxidase type B. This increases the amount of dopamine available to relieve symptoms of Parkinsonism. Selegiline's metabolites may also enhance dopamine transmission by inhibiting its reuptake at synapses.

Contraindications

Hypersensitivity to selegiline or its components; pheochromocytoma; use within 14 days of meperidine; use within 10 days of general anesthesia; use with carbamazepine, oxcarbazepine, selective serotonin reuptake inhibitors (fluoxetine, paroxetine, sertraline), dual serotonin and norepinephrine reuptake inhibitors (duloxetine, venlafaxine), tricyclic antidepressants (amitriptyline, bupropion, imipramine), analgesics (tramadol, propoxyphene), dextromethorphan; use with cyclobenzaprine, mirtazapine, oral selegiline, other MAO inhibitors, St. John's wort, or sympathomimetic amines (Emsam only)

Interactions

DRUGS

carbamazepine, oxcarbazepine: Increased blood selegiline level
fluoxetine, fluvoxamine, nefazodone, paroxetine, sertraline, venlafaxine: Increased risk of adverse reactions similar to those of serotonin syndrome
levodopa: Increased risk of confusion, dyskinesia, hallucinations, nausea, and orthostatic hypotension
meperidine, possibly other opioid agonists: Increased risk of diaphoresis, excitation, muscle rigidity, and severe hypertension
serotonergic drugs: Increased risk of serotonin syndrome
sympathomimetics: Increased risk of severe hypertension
tricyclic antidepressants: Possibly serious CNS reactions

FOODS

caffeine: Increased risk of hypertension
foods that contain tyramine or other high-pressor amines: Increased risk of sudden and severe hypertension

ACTIVITIES

alcohol use: Increased risk of hypertension

Adverse Reactions

CNS: Anxiety, chills, compulsive behaviors such as intense urges to perform certain activities (such as gambling or sex), confusion, dizziness, drowsiness, dyskinesia, euphoria, extrapyramidal reactions, falling asleep during activities of daily living, fatigue, hallucinations, headache, insomnia, irritability, lethargy, memory loss, mood changes, nervousness, paresthesia, precipitation of manic/mixed episodes, restlessness, **suicidal ideation**, syncope, tremor, weakness
CV: **Arrhythmias**, chest pain, hypertension, orthostatic hypotension, palpitations, peripheral edema
EENT: Altered taste, blepharospasm, blurred vision, burning lips or mouth, diplopia, dry mouth, pharyngitis, sinusitis, tinnitus
GI: Abdominal pain, anorexia, constipation, diarrhea, **GI bleeding**, heartburn, nausea, vomiting
GU: Dysuria, urinary hesitancy, urinary urgency, urine retention
MS: Arthralgia, back and leg pain, muscle fatigue and spasms, neck stiffness
RESP: **Asthma**
SKIN: Diaphoresis, photosensitivity, rash
Other: Application site reactions (Emsam)

Nursing Considerations

- Expect to screen patient for a family or personal history of bipolar disorder, hypomania, or mania before selegiline therapy is begun, because drug may precipitate manic/mixed episodes.
- Assess patient for mental status and mood changes because selegiline can worsen such conditions as dementia, severe psychosis, tardive dyskinesia, and tremor. Be especially alert for suicidal tendencies, particularly when therapy starts or dosage changes.
- Monitor patient who is also taking levodopa for levodopa-induced adverse reactions, including confusion, dyskinesia, hallucinations, nausea, and orthostatic hypotension.
- Monitor for decreased symptoms of Parkinson's disease to evaluate drug's effectiveness.
- Be aware that drug can reactivate gastric ulcers because it prevents breakdown of gastric histamine. Assess for related signs and symptoms, such as abdominal pain.
- Assess patient for skin changes regularly because risk of melanoma is increased in patients with Parkinson's disease. It isn't clear whether increase results from disease or drugs used to treat it.

PATIENT TEACHING

- Caution patient to take only prescribed amount because increased dosage may cause severe adverse reactions.
- Advise patient to avoid taking selegiline in the late afternoon or evening because it may interfere with sleep.
- For orally disintegrating tablets, tell patient to take it before breakfast without any liquid. Caution him not to push tablet through the foil on the blister pack but instead to peel back the foil with dry hands and gently remove the tablet. He should then immediately place the tablet on top of his tongue and let it disintegrate. Advise him not to drink or ingest any food for 5 minutes before and after taking the drug.
- For transdermal form, explain how and where (outer surface of upper arm, upper torso below the neck and above the waist, or upper thigh) to apply patch, stressing need to rotate sites. Remind patient to apply patch at about the same time of day. Tell patient not to apply patch to broken, calloused, hairy, irritated, oily, or scarred skin. Also, patch should not be placed where clothing is tight. Have patient wash the area gently and thoroughly with soap and warm water, then rinse until all soap is removed. After drying area, patch is ready to be applied. Tell patient to wash hands well after application and to dispose of removed patch immediately.
- Emphasize that only one patch may be worn at a time. If a patch falls off, tell patient to apply a new patch to a new site and to resume previous schedule.
- Caution patient to avoid exposing transdermal patch to sources of direct heat, such as electric blankets, heat lamps, heating pads, hot tubs, prolonged sunlight exposure or saunas.
- Tell patient not to cut transdermal patch into smaller pieces.
- Urge caregiver to monitor patient closely for suicidal tendencies, especially when therapy starts or dosage changes.
- Urge patient to avoid tyramine-rich foods and beverages during and for 2 weeks after stopping selegiline therapy unless patient is prescribed the lowest dosage of transdermal system (6 mg/24 hours), which doesn't require diet modification. Review which foods are considered tyramine-rich. Stress importance of seeking immediate medical attention if the following acute symptoms occur: heart racing or palpitations, neck stiffness, severe headache, or other sudden or unusual symptoms.
- Urge patient to avoid hazardous activities until drug's CNS effects are known.
- Instruct patient to immediately report neck stiffness, palpitations, racing heart, severe headache, or other sudden or unusual symptoms.
- Advise patient to change positions slowly to minimize the effects of orthostatic hypotension.
- Suggest that patient elevate his legs when sitting to reduce ankle swelling.
- Urge patient to avoid excessive sun exposure.
- Instruct patient to notify prescriber if symptoms develop that could indicate overdose, including muscle twitching and eye spasms.
- Urge patient to notify prescriber if dry mouth lasts longer than 2 weeks. Advise him to have routine dental checkups.
- Urge patient to have regular skin examinations done by a dermatologist or other qualified health professional.
- Tell patient to inform prescriber of any new medications, including prescription drugs, over-the-counter drugs, and including herbal preparations.
- Advise patient to notify prescriber about intense urges (as for gambling or sex) because dosage may have to be reduced or drug discontinued.
- Inform mothers wishing to breastfeed their infants that breastfeeding is not recommended during treatment with selegiline and for 5 days after final dose.

semaglutide

Ozempic

Class and Category

Pharmacologic class: Glucagon-like peptide-1 (GLP-1) receptor agonist
Therapeutic class: Antidiabetic
Pregnancy category: Not classified

Indications and Dosages

➤ *As adjunct to diet and exercise to improve glycemic control in type 2 diabetes mellitus*

SUBCUTANEOUS INJECTION

Adults. *Initial:* 0.25 mg once a wk for 4 wk, then increased to 0.5 mg once a wk. Dosage further increased to 1 mg once a wk, if needed, after another 4 wk. *Maximum:* 1 mg once a wk.

Mechanism of Action

Selectively binds to and activates the GLP-1 receptor to reduce blood glucose through a mechanism that stimulates insulin secretion and lowers glucagon secretion, both in a glucose-dependent manner. Thus, when blood glucose is high, insulin secretion is stimulated and glucagon secretion is inhibited, to lower blood glucose levels. A minor delay in gastric emptying in the early postprandial phase may also cause a minor glucose lowering action.

Contraindications

Family or personal history of medullary thyroid carcinoma, hypersensitivity to semaglutide or its components, multiple endocrine neoplasia syndrome type 2 (MEN 2)

Interactions

DRUGS

insulin, insulin secretagogues such as sulfonylureas: Increased risk of hypoglycemia

oral drugs: Delayed absorption of these drugs

Adverse Reactions

CNS: Dizziness, fatigue

EENT: Distortion of taste

ENDO: Hypoglycemia

GI: Abdominal pain, cholelithiasis, constipation, diarrhea, dyspepsia, elevated pancreatic enzymes, flatulence, gastroesophageal reflux disease, gastritis, nausea, **pancreatitis**, vomiting

GU: Acute kidney injury, **worsening of chronic renal failure**

Other: Anti-semaglutide antibodies, injection-site reactions (discomfort, erythema)

Nursing Considerations

- Be aware that semaglutide is not recommended as a first-line therapy for patients who have inadequate glycemic control using diet and exercise, because of the uncertain relevance of possible tumor findings in animals.
- Know that semaglutide should not be given to patients with a history of pancreatitis, because effects are unknown. Monitor all patients for signs and symptoms of pancreatitis such as persistent severe abdominal pain which sometimes may radiate to the back and which may or may not be accompanied by vomiting. If pancreatitis is suspected, expect drug to be discontinued.
- Monitor patient with a history of diabetic retinopathy for progression of the disorder.
- Monitor patient for hypoglycemia, especially if patient is also taking insulin or an insulin secretagogue such as a sulfonylurea.
- Monitor patient closely for renal dysfunction, especially when initiating or escalating the dose of semaglutide or if patient develops severe adverse gastrointestinal reactions.

WARNING Know that other drugs in the same class as semaglutide have caused serious hypersensitivity reactions such as anaphylaxis and angioedema. Montior patient for such reactions. If present, stop drug therapy immediately and provide supportive care, as needed and prescribed.

PATIENT TEACHING

- Teach patient or caregiver how to administer a subcutaneous injection. Tell her to administer drug into the abdomen, thigh, or upper arm using a different injection site each time.
- Instruct patient to administer the once-weekly dosage at the same day each week at any time of the day and without regard to meals. However, let patient know that the day of weekly administration can be changed, if needed, as long as the time between two doses is more than 48 hours.
- Inform patient that if a dose is missed, she should take the drug as soon as possible if within 5 days after the missed dose. If more than 5 days have passed, she should skip the missed dose and administer the next dose on the regularly scheduled day.
- Tell patient who is also administering insulin to administer the two drugs as

separate injections and never to mix them. The two injections can be administered in the same body region, but injections should not be adjacent to each other.
- Remind patient never to share the semaglutide pen with anyone else, even if the needle has been changed, because of an increased risk of transmitting bloodborne pathogens.
- Review signs and symptoms of hypoglycemia with patient and how to treat if it should occur. This is especially important in patients at increased risk, such as patients taking concurrent insulin or a sulfonylurea.
- Tell patient to report acute gastrointestinal adverse reactions, severe abdominal pain that may or may not radiate to the back and possibly be accompanied by vomiting. Tell patient to report any visual changes to prescriber.
- Advise women of childbearing age to alert prescriber if pregnancy occurs.

WARNING Warn patient to seek immediate emergency care if severe or persistent signs and symptoms of an allergic reaction occur.

sertraline hydrochloride

Zoloft

Class and Category

Pharmacologic class: Selective serotonin reuptake inhibitor (SSRI)
Therapeutic class: Antianxiety, antidepressant, antiobsessant, antipanic, antiposttraumatic stress, antipremenstrual dysphoric
Pregnancy category: C

Indications and Dosages

➤ *To treat major depression*

ORAL CONCENTRATE, TABLETS

Adults. *Initial:* 50 mg daily, increased in increments of 25 to 50 mg daily every wk, as needed. *Maximum:* 200 mg daily.

➤ *To treat obsessive–compulsive disorder*

ORAL CONCENTRATE, TABLETS

Adults and adolescents. *Initial:* 50 mg daily, increased in increments of 25 to 50 mg daily every wk, as needed. *Maximum:* 200 mg daily.

Children ages 6 to 12. *Initial:* 25 mg daily, increased in increments of 25 mg every wk, as needed. *Maximum:* 200 mg daily.

➤ *To treat panic disorder, with or without agoraphobia; to treat posttraumatic stress disorder; to treat social anxiety disorder*

ORAL CONCENTRATE, TABLETS

Adults. *Initial:* 25 mg daily, increased by 25 to 50 mg daily every wk, as needed. *Maximum:* 200 mg daily.

➤ *To treat premenstrual dysphoric disorder (PMDD)*

ORAL CONCENTRATE, TABLETS

Adult women. *Initial:* 50 mg daily in morning or evening throughout menstrual cycle; or, 50 mg daily in morning or evening during luteal phase of menstrual cycle only. (starting 14 days prior to menses and continuing through onset of menses). Dosage increased each menstrual cycle in 50-mg increments up to 150 mg daily, or each luteal phase up to 100 mg daily, as needed. Once 100-mg daily dosage established for luteal phase, each successive cycle requires a dosage regimen of 50 mg daily for first 3 days followed by 100 mg daily during remaining dosage cycle. *Maximum:* 150 mg daily for dosing throughout menstrual cycle, or 100 mg daily for dosing during luteal phase only.

DOSAGE ADJUSTMENT For patients with mild hepatic dysfunction, all dosages reduced by 50%.

Route	Onset	Peak	Duration
P.O.	2–4 wk*	Unknown	Unknown

* For antidepressant and antipanic effects.

Mechanism of Action

Inhibits reuptake of the neurotransmitter serotonin by CNS neurons, thereby increasing the amount of serotonin available in nerve synapses. An elevated serotonin level may result in elevated mood and reduced depression. This action may also relieve symptoms of other psychiatric conditions attributed to serotonin deficiency and premenstrual dysphoric disorder.

Contraindications

Concurrent use of disulfiram (oral concentrate) or pimozide; hypersensitivity to sertraline or its components; use within

14 days of an MAO inhibitor, including intravenous methylene blue and linezolid for antiobsessant effect, longer than 4 wk.

Interactions

DRUGS

antibiotics (erythromycin, gatifloxacin, moxifloxacin, sparfloxacin), antipsychotics (chlorpromazine, droperidol, iloperidone, mesoridazine, ziprasidone), Class 1A antiarrhythmics (procainamide, quinidine), Class III antiarrhythmics (amiodarone, sotalol), dolasetron, halofantrine, levomethadyl, mefloquine, methadone, pentamidine, probucol, tacrolimus: Increased risk of QT-interval prolongation and/or ventricular arrhythmias

antidopaminergics, antipsychotics, moclobemide, serotonergics such as 5-HT agonists, buspirone, fenfluramine, fentanyl, lithium, St. John's wort, triptans, tryptophan: Increased risk of potentially fatal serotonin syndrome

antiplatelets, aspirin, NSAIDs, warfarin: Increased anticoagulant activity and risk of bleeding

astemizole, terfenadine: Possibly increased blood levels of these drugs, leading to increased risk of arrhythmias

cimetidine: Increased sertraline half-life

highly bound drugs to plasma protein: Increased free concentrations of sertraline, increasing risk of adverse reactions

MAO inhibitors: Possibly hyperpyretic episodes, hypertensive crisis, serotonin syndrome, and severe seizures

tolbutamide: Possibly hypoglycemia

tricyclic antidepressants: Possibly impaired metabolism of tricyclic antidepressants, resulting in increased risk of toxicity

Adverse Reactions

CNS: Abnormal dreams, aggressiveness, agitation, amnesia, anxiety, apathy, ataxia, **cerebrovascular spasm**, **coma**, confusion, delusions, depression, dizziness, drowsiness, emotional lability, euphoria, extrapyramidal symptoms, fatigue, fever, hallucination, headache, hyperkinesia, hypoesthesia, insomnia, lethargy, malaise, nervousness, **neuroleptic malignant syndrome-like reaction**, paranoid reaction, paresthesia, psychomotor hyperactivity, psychosis, **seizures**, **serotonin syndrome**, somnolence, **suicidal ideation**, syncope, tremor, weakness, yawning

CV: **Atrial arrhythmias**, **AV block**, **bradycardia**, hypertension, palpitations, **prolonged QT interval**, **torsades de pointes**, vasculitis, vasodilation, **ventricular tachycardia**

EENT: Abnormal accommodation, acute closure glaucoma, blindness, cataract, conjunctivitis, dry mouth, earache, epistaxis, eye pain, optic neuritis, rhinitis, sinusitis, teeth grinding, tinnitus, vision changes

ENDO: Galactorrhea, hyperglycemia, hyperprolactinemia, hypothyroidism, syndrome of inappropriate ADH secretion

GI: Abdominal cramps or pain, anorexia, constipation, diarrhea, elevated liver enzymes, flatulence, hepatic dysfunction, **hepatic failure**, **hepatitis**, increased appetite, indigestion, jaundice, nausea, **pancreatitis**, vomiting

GU: **Acute renal failure**; anorgasmia; decreased libido; ejaculation disorders; enuresis; hematuria; impotence; leucorrhea; menstrual disorders; priapism; polyuria; urinary frequency, incontinence, or retention; vaginal hemorrhage

HEME: **Agranulocytosis**, **altered platelet function**, **aplastic anemia**, **hemorrhage**, **leukopenia**, **pancytopenia**, **thrombocytopenia**

MS: Arthralgia, dystonia, lockjaw, muscle cramps or weakness, myalgia, **rhabdomyolysis**

RESP: **Bronchospasm**, coughing, dyspnea, **pulmonary hypertension**

SKIN: Alopecia, dermatitis including bullous, diaphoresis, flushing, photosensitivity, pruritus, purpura, rash, severe cutaneous disorders, **Stevens–Johnson syndrome**, **toxic epidermal necrolysis**, urticaria

Other: **Anaphylaxis**, **angioedema**, **hyponatremia**, lupus-like syndrome, serum sickness, weight loss

Nursing Considerations

- Be aware that sertraline should not be given to patients with bradycardia, congenital long QT syndrome, hypokalemia or hypomagnesemia, recent acute myocardial infarction, or uncompensated heart failure because of increased risk of prolonged QT interval and torsades de pointes. It should also not be given to patients who are taking other drugs that prolong the QT interval. Expect hypokalemia and hypomagnesemia to be corrected before sertraline therapy is begun.

- Monitor liver enzymes and BUN and serum creatinine levels, as appropriate, in patients with hepatic or renal dysfunction.

WARNING Monitor patient closely for evidence of serotonin syndrome, such as agitation, coma, diarrhea, hallucinations, hyperthermia, hyperreflexia, incoordination, labile blood pressure, nausea, tachycardia, and vomiting. Serotonin syndrome in its most severe form can resemble neuroleptic malignant syndrome, which includes autonomic instability, hyperthermia, mental status changes, muscle rigidity, and possibly rapid changes in vital signs. Notify prescriber immediately because serotonin syndrome reactions that resemble neuroleptic malignant syndrome may be life-threatening. Be prepared to provide supportive care.

- Monitor patient for hypo-osmolarity of serum and urine and for hyponatremia, which may indicate sertraline-induced syndrome of inappropriate ADH secretion.
- Be aware that effective antidepressant therapy can promote development of mania in predisposed people. If mania develops, notify prescriber immediately and expect to withhold sertraline.
- Watch closely for suicidal tendencies, especially when therapy starts and dosage changes and especially in children and adolescents.
- Monitor patient closely for evidence of GI bleeding, especially if patient takes a drug known to cause it, such as aspirin, an NSAID, or warfarin.
- When therapy stops, expect to taper dosage to minimize adverse effects rather than stopping drug abruptly.

PATIENT TEACHING

- Advise patient that drug may cause mild pupillary dilation, which may lead to an episode of acute closure glaucoma. Encourage patient to have an eye exam before starting therapy to see if he is at risk.
- Inform patient that oral solution contains alcohol and should not be taken with disulfiram.
- Teach patient to dilute oral concentrate before taking it. Tell him to use supplied dropper to remove prescribed amount and mix it with 4 oz (one-half cup) of ginger ale, lemon or lime soda, lemonade, orange juice, or water. Warn him not to mix oral concentrate with anything else. Explain that it's normal for mixture to be slightly hazy.
- Tell patient to take dose immediately after mixing it.
- Advise patient with a latex sensitivity to use an alternate dispenser because the supplied dropper dispenser contains dry natural rubber.
- Advise patient to avoid hazardous activities until drug's CNS effects are known.
- Inform patient that use of certain drugs, such as aspirin, NSAIDs, other antiplatelet drugs, warfarin, or other anticoagulants, with sertraline may increase his risk for bleeding.

WARNING Tell patient that sertraline increases the risk of serotonin syndrome and reactions that resemble neuroleptic malignant syndrome, rare but serious complications, when taken with some other drugs. Teach patient how to recognize signs and symptoms of these disorders and advise him to notify prescriber immediately if they occur.

- Warn family or caregiver to watch patient closely for evidence of suicidal thinking or behavior, especially when therapy starts or dosage changes, and especially if patient is a child or adolescent.
- Caution patient not to stop taking drug abruptly. Explain that gradual tapering helps to avoid withdrawal symptoms.
- Instruct female patients to notify prescriber if they are or could be pregnant and to discuss benefits and risks of continuing sertraline therapy throughout the pregnancy, as drug may cause withdrawal symptoms or persistent pulmonary hypertension in the newborn.
- Advise patient to consult prescriber before taking any OTC product, especially aspirin products or NSAIDs.
- Alert patient that false-positive urine testing for benzodiazepines may occur while taking sertraline, requiring a more sensitive test to be performed.

sevelamer hydrochloride

Renagel

sevelamer carbonate

Renvela

Class and Category

Pharmacologic class: Polymeric phosphate binder
Therapeutic class: Phosphate binder
Pregnancy category: C

Indications and Dosages

➤ *To control serum phosphate level in patients with chronic kidney disease on dialysis*

TABLETS (RENAGEL)

Adults. 800 mg three times a day if serum phosphorus level is 6 to 7.4 mg/dl; 1,200 mg three times a day if serum phosphorus level is 7.5 to 8.9 mg/dl; or 1,600 mg three times a day if serum phosphorus level is 9 mg/dl or more. Dosage increased or decreased every 2 weeks by 400 mg/meal as needed. *Maximum:* 13 g daily.

POWDER FOR SUSPENSION (RENVELA), TABLETS (RENVELA)

Adults not taking a phosphate binder. 800 mg three times a day with meals if serum phosphorus level is 5.5 to 7.5 mg/dl; 1,600 mg three times a day with meals if serum phosphorus level is 7.5 mg/dl or greater. Dosage increased or decreased by 800 mg/meal at 2-wk intervals, as needed.
Children age 6 years and over not taking a phosphate binder. 800 mg three times a day with meals if serum phosphorus level is 0.75 mg/dl to less than 1.2 mg/dl, with dosage titrated every 2 weeks by 400 mg/meal, as needed; 1,600 mg three times a day if serum phosphorus level is 1.2 mg/dl or greater, with dosage titrated every 2 weeks by 800 mg/meal, as needed.

DOSAGE ADJUSTMENT For adult patients being switched from calcium acetate to sevelamer carbonate, 800 mg of sevelamer can be substituted for every 667 mg of calcium being taken.

Mechanism of Action

Inhibits phosphate absorption in the intestine by binding dietary phosphate, thereby lowering serum phosphorus level.

Contraindications

Fecal impaction, GI obstruction, hypersensitivity to sevelamer or its components, hypophosphatemia, ileus

Interactions

DRUGS

antiarrhythmics, anticonvulsants, digoxin, levothyroxine, liothyronine, quinolones, tetracyclines, theophylline, warfarin: Possibly altered absorption of these drugs
phosphate salts, phosphorus salts: Neutralized therapeutic effects of sevelamer
ciprofloxacin: Decreased ciprofloxacin effectiveness

Adverse Reactions

CNS: Headache, fever
CV: Hypertension, **hypotension, thrombosis**
EENT: Nasopharyngitis
GI: Abdominal pain, constipation (severe), diarrhea, dysphagia, fecal impaction, flatulence, ileus, indigestion, **intestinal obstruction or perforation**, nausea, vomiting
RESP: Bronchitis, dyspnea, increased cough, upper respiratory tract infection
MS: Arthralgia, back or limb pain
SKIN: Pruritus, rash
Other: Hypersensitivity reactions, infection

Nursing Considerations

- Give other drugs at least 1 hour before or 3 hours after sevelamer to prevent interaction.
- Suggest suspension form be used in patients with swallowing disorders because tablet may get stuck in the esophagus in these individuals, and they may require hospitalization and emergency intervention to remove it.
- Be aware that severe hypophosphatemia may occur in patient with dysphagia, major GI tract surgery, or severe GI motility disorder (including severe constipation) because drug prevents phosphate absorption.
- Monitor blood pressure frequently.
- Monitor serum phosphorus level to determine drug's effectiveness; monitor

other serum electrolyte levels, especially bicarbonate and chloride, to detect imbalances.

PATIENT TEACHING

- Tell patient to take drug with meals and to swallow tablets whole with water and not to break, chew, crush, or open them.
- Instruct patient taking suspension form to mix entire contents of each packet of powder thoroughly with the amount of water indicated on packet. More than one packet can be mixed together. He should stir the mixture vigorously, even though it does not dissolve, and drink entire preparation immediately or up to 30 minutes later (but he will need to stir the mixture again vigorously right before drinking if it was not consumed immediately).
- Caution patient to take other drugs 1 hour before or 3 hours after sevelamer.
- Review symptoms of thrombosis, and advise patient to report them immediately.
- Instruct patient to report prolonged or severe constipation to prescriber because additional treatment may be needed to prevent serious complications.
- Inform patient of potential need for fat-soluble vitamins and folic acid supplements, especially if patient is pregnant.

sildenafil citrate

Revatio, Viagra

Class and Category

Pharmacologic class: Phosphodiesterase 5 (PDE5) inhibitor
Therapeutic class: Antihypertensive (pulmonary arterial), erectile dysfunction agent
Pregnancy category: B

Indications and Dosages

➤ *To treat erectile dysfunction*

TABLETS (VIAGRA)

Adults. *Initial:* 50 mg taken 30 min to 4 hr before sexual activity although best if taken 1 hr before sexual activity; decreased or increased as needed based upon response. *Usual range:* 25 to 100 mg daily. *Maximum:* Once per day with dosage not exceeding 100 mg, as needed based upon response.

DOSAGE ADJUSTMENT Initially, 25 mg for patients over 65 years of age, those with hepatic dysfunction or severe renal insufficiency (creatinine clearance less than 30 ml/min) and those taking an alpha blocker or potent cytochrome P-450 3A4 inhibitors, or ritonavir. Maximum dosage for patient taking ritonavir is 25 mg within a 48 hr period.

➤ *To treat pulmonary arterial hypertension in order to improve exercise ability and delay clinical worsening of condition in patients classified as group 1 by the World Health Organization*

ORAL SUSPENSION, TABLETS (REVATIO)

Adults. 5 or 20 mg three times a day 4 to 6 hr apart.

I.V. INJECTION (REVATIO)

Adults. 2.5 or 10 mg administered as bolus three times a day.

Route	Onset	Peak	Duration
P.O.	In 30 min	Unknown	4 hr

Mechanism of Action

Enhances the effect of nitric oxide released in the penis by stimulation. Nitric oxide increases cGMP level, relaxes smooth muscle, and increases blood flow to the corpus cavernosum, thus producing an erection.

By preventing breakdown of cyclic guanosine monophosphate by phosphodiesterase, levels increase leading to smooth muscle relaxation of the pulmonary vasculature and subsequently, vasodilation. Vasodilation causes the pressure within the pulmonary vasculature to decrease, which improves tolerance to exercise and delays worsening of pulmonary arterial hypertension.

Contraindications

Concomitant guanylate cyclase stimulator therapy, continuous or intermittent nitrate therapy, hypersensitivity to sildenafil or its components

Interactions

DRUGS

barbiturates, bosentan, carbamazepine, efavirenz, nevirapine, phenytoin, rifabutin, rifampin: Altered plasma level of either drug

cimetidine, erythromycin, itraconazole, ketoconazole, mibefradil: Prolonged sildenafil effect
doxazosin and other alpha-blockers, guanylate cyclase stimulators: Increased risk of symptomatic hypotension
nitrates: Profound hypotension
protease inhibitors: Increased sildenafil effect
rifampin: Decreased sildenafil effect
FOODS
high-fat meals: Oral drug absorption delayed by up to 60 minutes

Adverse Reactions

CNS: CVA, dizziness, headache, migraine, **seizures**, syncope, transient global amnesia, transient ischemic attack
CV: Heart failure, hypertension, **hypotension, myocardial infarction or ischemia**, orthostatic hypotension, palpitations, **sudden cardiac death**, tachycardia, vaso-occlusive crisis (presence of sickle cell disease), **ventricular arrhythmias**
EENT: Blurred vision; change in color perception; diplopia; epistaxis; hearing loss; increased intraocular pressure; nasal congestion; nonarteritic anterior ischemic optic neuropathy (NAION); ocular burning, pressure, redness or swelling; paramacular edema; photophobia; retinal vascular bleeding or disease; tinnitus, visual decrease or temporary vision loss; vitreous detachment
ENDO: Uncontrolled diabetes mellitus
GI: Diarrhea, indigestion
GU: Cystitis, dysuria, painful erection, priapism, UTI
MS: Arthralgia, back pain
RESP: Pulmonary hemorrhage, upper respiratory tract infection
SKIN: Flushing, photosensitivity rash, urticaria

Nursing Considerations

- Use sildenafil cautiously in the elderly and patients with hepatic or renal dysfunction, and men with penile abnormalities that may predispose them to priapism. In addition, use cautiously in patients who have suffered a life-threatening arrhythmia, myocardial infarction, or stroke within the last 6 months or in patients with cardiac failure, coronary artery disease causing unstable angina, hypertension (blood pressure greater than 170/110), related anemias, resting hypotension (blood pressure less than 90/50), retinitis pigmentosa, or sickle cell, as sildenafil therapy has not been studied in these patient groups.
- Also use cautiously in patients with left ventricular outflow obstruction, such as aortic stenosis and idiopathic hypertrophic subaortic stenosis, and those with severely impaired autonomic control of blood pressure because these conditions increase patient's sensitivity to vasodilators such as sildenafil.
- Reconstitute powder for oral suspension by tapping the bottle to release the powder, then remove the cap. Accurately measure out 60 ml of water and pour the water into the bottle, replace the cap, and shake the bottle vigorously for a minimum of 30 seconds. Solution should be clear and colorless and contain 10 mg sildenafil per 12.5 ml of solution. Store drug at room temperature. Discard any remaining oral suspension 60 days after constitution.
- Monitor patient's blood pressure and heart rate and rhythm before and often during therapy.
- Monitor vision, especially in patients over age 50; who have coronary artery disease, diabetes, hypertension, or hyperlipidemia; or who smoke, because, although rare, sildenafil may cause nonarteritic anterior ischemic optic neuropathy (NAION) that may lead to decreased vision or permanent vision loss. Patients at higher risk for NAION include those who have already experienced it in the past and those who have a low cup to optic disc ratio or retinitis pigmentosa.

WARNING Monitor patient being treated for pulmonary hypertension secondary to sickle cell disease for vaso-occlusive crisis (severe pain and change in color and temperature if extremity is involved). Notify prescriber immediately and prepare to provide supportive care.

PATIENT TEACHING

- Explain that sildenafil used to treat erectile dysfunction may be taken up to 4 hours before sexual activity, but that taking it 1 hour beforehand provides the most effective results.

WARNING Warn patient not to take sildenafil if he also takes any form of organic nitrate, either continuously or intermittently, or other PDE5 inhibitors, including REVATIO (a sildenafil product used to treat another condition), because profound hypotension and death could result. Also caution patient to inform prescriber of all medications taken as dosage may have to be decreased if a drug such as an alpha blocker has also been prescribed.

- Instruct patient prescribed oral suspension form how to mix it, store it, and discard any remaining suspension after 60 days. Stress importance of using the oral dosing syringe that accompanies the drug to measure dosage.
- Tell patient to stop taking drug and contact prescriber if vision decreases suddenly in one or both eyes or if he has a loss of hearing, possibly with dizziness or tinnitus.
- Advise patient taking sildenafil for erectile dysfunction to seek sexual counseling to enhance the drug's effects.
- Urge patient to notify prescriber immediately if erection is painful or lasts longer than 4 hours to avoid possible penile damage and permanent loss of erectile function.
- Instruct diabetic patient to monitor his blood glucose level frequently because drug may affect glucose control.

silodosin

Rapaflo

Class and Category

Pharmacologic class: Alpha adrenergic blocker
Therapeutic class: Benign prostatic antihyperplasia agent
Pregnancy category: B

Indications and Dosages

➤ *To treat symptomatic benign prostatic hyperplasia*

CAPSULES

Adult men. 8 mg daily. *Maximum:* 8 mg daily.

DOSAGE ADJUSTMENT For patients with moderate renal impairment (creatinine clearance between 30 and 50 ml/min), dosage reduced to 4 mg daily.

Mechanism of Action

Binds to postsynaptic $alpha_1$ adrenoreceptors located in the bladder base and neck, prostate gland, and prostatic capsule and urethra. Blocking action at these adrenoreceptor sites causes relaxation of smooth muscle in the local area, which improves urine flow and reduces other benign prostatic hyperplasia symptoms.

Contraindications

Hypersensitivity to silodosin and its components, severe hepatic insufficiency (Child-Pugh score 10 or above), severe renal insufficiency (creatinine clearance less than 30 ml/min), use with strong CYP3A4 inhibitors such as clarithromycin, ketoconazole, itraconazole, and ritonavir

Interactions

DRUGS

alpha blockers: Possibly increased effects and risk of adverse reactions
antihypertensives: Increased risk of dizziness and orthostatic hypotension
cyclosporine, CYP3A4 inhibitors such as clarithromycin, diltiazem, erythromycin, itraconazole, ketoconazole, ritonavir: Possibly increased serum silodosin levels and risk of adverse reactions
PDE5 inhibitors: Possibly increased risk of orthostatic hypotension

Adverse Reactions

CNS: Asthenia, dizziness, headache, insomnia, syncope
CV: Orthostatic hypotension
EENT: Nasal congestion, nasopharyngitis, rhinorrhea, sinusitis
GI: Abdominal pain, diarrhea, elevated liver enzymes, impaired hepatic function, jaundice
GU: Elevated prostate specific antigen level, retrograde ejaculation
SKIN: Pruritus, purpura, rash, **toxic skin eruption**, urticaria
Other: **Angioedema**

Nursing Considerations

- Use cautiously in patients with mild renal impairment and mild or moderate hepatic impairment. Patients with moderate renal impairment need dosage adjustment.

- Monitor patient's blood pressure for reduction, especially if he takes an antihypertensive with silodosin.

PATIENT TEACHING

- Instruct patient to take drug with a meal.
- Tell patient who has difficulty swallowing capsules that he may carefully open the capsule and sprinkle the powder on a tablespoonful of applesauce and take within 5 minutes without chewing. He should then drink an 8-oz glass of cool water immediately afterward. Inform him that the applesauce should not be hot and it should be soft enough to be swallowed without chewing.
- Advise patient to avoid hazardous activities until drug's CNS effects are known.
- Advise patient planning cataract surgery or other ocular procedure to tell ophthalmologist that he takes silodosin or has taken it in the past because of potential adverse reactions.

simeprevir

Olysio

Class and Category

Pharmacologic class: Protease inhibitor
Therapeutic class: Antiviral
Pregnancy category: Not classified

Indications and Dosages

➤ *As adjunct to treat chronic hepatitis C virus (HCV) infection in patients with genotype 1 or 4 who are without cirrhosis or who have compensated cirrhosis*

CAPSULES

Adults. 150 mg once daily with food for 12 wk; 24 wk in patients with genotype 1 infection taking sofosbuvir concomitantly and who also have compensated cirrhosis.

Mechanism of Action

Inhibits the HCV NS3/4A protease, which is essential for viral replication.

Contraindications

Hypersensitivity to simeprevir or its components

Interactions

DRUGS

amiodarone: Increased risk of serious symptomatic bradycardia when given in combination with sofosbuvir; increased plasma amiodarone level when used in a combination that does not contain sofosbuvir, increasing risk of adverse reactions
atazanavir, fosamprenavir, indinavir, lopinavir, nelfinavir, saquinavir, sirolimus, tipranavir: Change in plasma simeprevir levels, either decreasing it and possibly decreasing its effectiveness, or increasing it and increasing risk of adverse reactions
atorvastatin, fluvastatin, lovastatin, pitavastatin, pravastatin, rosuvastatin, simvastatin: Increased risk of myopathy, including rhabdomyolysis
calcium channel blockers, cisapride, cobicistat-containing products, disopyramide, flecainide, mexiletine, midazolam, milk thistle, propafenone, quinidine, triazolam: Increased plasma concentrations of these drugs with increased risk of adverse reactions
carbamazepine, dexamethasone, efavirenz, etravirine, nevirapine, oxcarbazepine, phenobarbital, phenytoin, rifabutin, rifampin, rifapentine, St. John's wort: Decreased plasma concentration of simeprevir, possibly reducing its effectiveness
clarithromycin, delavirdine, fluconazole, itraconazole, ketoconazole, posaconazole, ritonavir, telithromycin, voriconazole: Increased plasma concentration of simeprevir, increasing risk of adverse reactions
cyclosporine: Increased plasma concentration of both drugs, increasing risk of adverse reactions
darunavir/ritonavir: Increased plasma levels of both darunavir and simeprevir, increasing risk of adverse reactions
digoxin: Increased risk of digitalis toxicity
erythromycin: Increased plasma levels of both erythromycin and simeprevir, increasing risk of adverse reactions
ledipasvir: Increased plasma levels of both ledipasvir and simeprevir, increasing risk of adverse reactions
sildenafil, tadalafil: Increased plasma levels of these drugs when used chronically at doses used for the treatment of pulmonary arterial hypertension, increasing risk of adverse reactions

Adverse Reactions

CNS: Dizziness, fatigue, headache

CV: **Bradycardia (may become severe)**
GI: Diarrhea, elevated liver and pancreatic enzymes, **hepatic failure**, hyperbilirubinemia, nausea
MS: Myalgia
RESP: Dyspnea
SKIN: Photosensitivity, pruritus, rash
Other: Elevated alkaline phosphatase

Nursing Considerations

- Be aware that simeprevir should not be given to patients with moderate to severe hepatic impairment, because drug may cause hepatic decompensation and hepatic failure that may be fatal.
- Ensure that liver enzymes have been checked to provide a baseline of liver function prior to simeprevir use and then periodically as needed during simeprevir therapy. Closely monitor any patient who develops an increase in total bilirubin to greater than 2.5 times the upper limit of normal. Expect drug to be discontinued if any elevation in bilirubin is accompanied by elevated liver enzymes or signs and symptoms of hepatic decompensation.
- Know that patients with HCV genotype 1a infection containing the Q80K polymorphism should not be given simeprevir.
- Know that reducing the dosage of simeprevir or interrupting treatment should be avoided to prevent treatment failure. If treatment is discontinued because of adverse reactions or inadequate virologic response, know that simeprevir must not be restarted.

WARNING Ensure that all patients have been tested for current or prior HBV infection before simeprevir therapy is begun, because in patients coinfected with HBV and HCV, there is risk of hepatitis B virus reactivation that may result in fluminant hepatitis, hepatic failure, or even death. If patient tests positive for HBV, monitor patient closely for clinical and laboratory signs, as ordered, of hepatitis flare or HBV reactivation during treatment with simeprevir and during posttreatment follow-up. Expect treatment for HBV infection to be given, if needed.

- Monitor patient also receiving amiodarone and sofosbuvir for symptomatic bradycardia that may be severe enough to require pacemaker intervention. Be aware that bradycardia may occur up to 2 weeks after simeprevir therapy has begun. Patients at risk include those taking beta blockers or those with underlying advanced liver disease or cardiac disorders. Expect patient to be hospitalized for cardiac monitoring for the first 48 hours of simeprevir therapy. Notify prescriber if bradycardia occurs and expect drug to be discontinued. Known that bradycardia generally disappears after drug is discontinued.
- Assess patient's skin for a photosensitivity reaction that may appear as a severe sunburn or rash. These adverse reactions most often occur in the first 4 weeks of simeprevir therapy. If the photosensitivity reaction or rash is severe, expect drug to be discontinued. Know that patients at increased risk for these adverse reactions are patients with a sulfa allergy, because simeprevir contains a sulfonamide moiety.
- Monitor patient's HCV RNA levels, as ordered. Know that a sensitive assay with a lower limit of quantification of at least 25 IU/ml should be used. If patient experiences an inadequate virologic response at week 4, expect drug to be discontinued.

PATIENT TEACHING

- Instruct patient to take simeprevir exactly as ordered and not to discontinue it without prescriber knowledge.
- Tell patient to take simeprevir every day at a regularly scheduled time with food.
- Teach patient how to take his pulse and to report immediately a sudden decrease in pulse rate or signs and symptoms of serious bradycardia, such as chest pain, confusion, dizziness, excessive tiredness, fainting or near-fainting, malaise, memory problems, shortness of breath, or weakness.
- Instruct patient to notify prescriber if she experiences signs and symptoms of liver dysfunction such as discolored stools, fatigue, lack of appetite, nausea, vomiting, weakness, or yellowing of skin or whites of the eyes.
- Warn patient to take sun-protective measures and limit sun exposure during simeprevir therapy. If a sunburn reaction occurs, tell patient to notify prescriber, as further monitoring of condition may be

needed or simeprevir may have to be discontinued.
- Inform patient that a rash may occur within the first 4 weeks of therapy. Encourage him to notify prescriber so that the rash may be monitored for progression. If rash becomes severe, inform patient that the simeprevir will have to be discontinued.
- Tell patient to inform all prescribers of simeprevir therapy, because the drug reacts with many different drugs, which may cause reduced effectiveness or increased risk of adverse reactions.
- Advise female patients to notify prescriber if pregnancy occurs or is suspected. If patient is also taking ribavirin with simeprevir, tell patient to use two reliable contraceptives during treatment and for at least 6 months after stopping ribavirin.
- Tell mothers wishing to breastfeed to discuss the benefits versus risks with their prescriber.

simvastatin

Zocor

Class and Category

Pharmacologic class: HMG-CoA reductase inhibitor (statin)
Therapeutic class: Antilipemic
Pregnancy category: X

Indications and Dosages

➤ *To treat hyperlipidemia*

TABLETS

Adults. *Initial:* 10 to 40 mg daily in the evening. Dosage adjusted at 4-wk intervals, as needed, to achieve target LDL-cholesterol level. *Maintenance:* 5 to 40 mg daily.

➤ *To treat homozygous familial hypercholesterolemia; to reduce risk of cardiovascular events and coronary heart disease mortality in patients at high risk*

TABLETS

Adults. 40 mg daily in the evening. Dosage adjusted every 4 wk, as needed, to achieve target LDL-cholesterol level. *Maintenance:* 5 to 40 mg/day.

➤ *To treat adolescent heterozygous familial hypercholesterolemia*

TABLETS

Children ages 10 to 17 at least 1 year post-menarche. *Initial:* 10 mg daily in the evening. Adjusted every 4 wk, as needed, to achieve target LDL-cholesterol level. *Maintenance:* 10 to 40 mg daily. *Maximum:* 40 mg daily.

DOSAGE ADJUSTMENT For patients with severe renal impairment, initial dosage reduced to 5 mg daily. For patients who are taking diltiazem, dronedarone, or verapamil, daily dosage should not exceed 10 mg; for patients who take amiodarone, amlodipine, or ranolazine, daily dosage should not exceed 20 mg. For patient taking lomitapide, daily dosage reduced by 50% and maximum dosage should not exceed 20 mg. For Chinese patients taking lipid-modifying doses of niacin-containing products (1 g or more daily), dosage should not exceed 20 mg daily.

Route	Onset	Peak	Duration
P.O.	2 wk	4–6 wk	Unknown

Mechanism of Action

Interferes with the hepatic enzyme hydroxymethylglutaryl-coenzyme A reductase. This action reduces the formation of mevalonic acid, a cholesterol precursor, thus interrupting the pathway necessary for cholesterol synthesis. When the cholesterol level declines in hepatic cells, LDLs are consumed, which in turn reduces the levels of circulating total cholesterol and serum triglycerides.

Contraindications

Active hepatic disease; breastfeeding; concurrent use with cobicistat-containing products, cyclosporine, danazol, or gemfibrozil; concurrent use with strong CYP3A4 inhibitors such as boceprevir, clarithromycin, erythromycin, HIV protease inhibitors, itraconazole, ketoconazole, nefazodone, posaconazole, telaprevir, or telithromycin; hypersensitivity to simvastatin or its components; pregnancy

Interactions

DRUGS

amiodarone, amlodipine, antiretroviral protease inhibitors including combinations (amprenavir, boceprevir, indinavir, nelfinavir, ritonavir, saquinavir, telaprevir), azole antifungals, boceprevir, cobicistat-containing products, clarithromycin, colchicine, cyclosporine, danazol, dronedarone, erythromycin, gemfibrozil and other fibrates, itraconazole, ketoconazole, nefazodone, niacin (1 g daily or more), posaconazole, ranolazine, telithromycin, verapamil, voriconazole: Increased risk of myopathy or rhabdomyolysis
azole antifungals, cyclosporine, gemfibrozil, immunosuppressants, macrolide antibiotics (including erythromycin), niacin, verapamil: Increased risk of acute renal failure
bile acid sequestrants, cholestyramine, colestipol: Decreased simvastatin bioavailability
digoxin: Possibly slight elevation in blood digoxin level
diltiazem, lomitapide, verapamil: Possibly increased blood simvastatin level, increased risk of myopathy
oral anticoagulants: Increased bleeding or prolonged PT

FOODS

grapefruit juice (1 or more quarts daily): Increased risk of myopathy or rhabdomyolysis

Adverse Reactions

CNS: Asthenia, cognitive impairment, dizziness, fatigue, headache, insomnia, vertigo
CV: **Atrial fibrillation**, chest pain, edema
EENT: Cataracts, rhinitis, sinusitis
ENDO: Elevated hemoglobin A_{1c} levels, hyperglycemia
GI: Abdominal pain, constipation, diarrhea, elevated liver enzymes, flatulence, gastritis, heartburn, **hepatic failure**, indigestion, nausea, **pancreatitis**, vomiting
GU: Erectile dysfunction, UTI
MS: Immune-mediated necrotizing myopathy, myalgia, myopathy, **rhabdomyolysis**
RESP: Bronchitis, **interstitial lung disease**, upper respiratory tract infection
SKIN: Eczema, pruritus, rash

Nursing Considerations

- Use simvastatin cautiously in elderly patients and those with hepatic or renal impairment.
- Know that 80 mg of simvastatin should be used rarely, since it is associated with a high risk of myopathy. If 40 mg of simvastatin is not sufficiently efficacious, then an alternative agent should be used.
- Also, use cautiously in Chinese patients who are receiving more than 20 mg daily of simvastatin and are also receiving lipid-modifying doses of niacin-containing products because of increased risk for myopathy. Know that these patients should not receive 80 mg of simvastatin daily if they are taking concurrently 1 g or more of a niacin-containing product.
- Give drug 1 hour before or 4 hours after giving bile acid sequestrant, cholestyramine, or colestipol.
- Monitor serum lipoprotein level, as ordered, to evaluate response to therapy.
- Expect to obtain liver enzymes prior to initiation of simvastatin therapy and then thereafter, as needed.
- Monitor patient for elevated CPK level (as ordered) or for muscle pain, tenderness, or weakness and other symptoms of myopathy; if left unchecked, the more serious form—rhabdomyolysis—may occur, which may lead to renal failure. Risk factors for myopathy include being 65 years or older, of female gender, and having renal impairment or uncontrolled hypothyroidism. If CPK level is significantly elevated or patient has symptoms of myopathy, notify prescriber and expect to withhold drug, as ordered.

PATIENT TEACHING

- Urge patient to take drug in the evening.
- Urge patient to follow low-fat, cholesterol-lowering diet.
- Urge patient to notify prescriber immediately about muscle pain, tenderness, or weakness and other symptoms of myopathy and symptoms of abnormal liver function such as anorexia, dark urine, fatigue, right upper abdominal discomfort, or yellowing of skin.
- Inform female patient of childbearing age of need to use reliable contraceptive method while taking drug. Instruct her to

notify prescriber at once if she suspects pregnancy.
- Advise patient to avoid grapefruit juice to decrease risk of drug toxicity.
- Inform patient with diabetes of need to test his blood sugar regularly and to obtain an HbA_{1c} periodically.
- Encourage patient or family to notify prescriber if patient develops or exhibits confusion, forgetfulness, and worsening memory loss.
- Alert patient of increased risk for myopathy if he takes 80 mg of simvastatin daily.

sirolimus
(rapamycin)
Rapamune

Class and Category
Pharmacologic class: Macrocyclic lactone
Therapeutic class: Immunosuppressant
Pregnancy category: C

Indications and Dosages
➤ *To prevent rejection of kidney transplantation*

ORAL SOLUTION, TABLETS

Adults weighing 40 kg (88 lb) or more at high-immunologic risk. *Initial:* up to 15 mg loading dose on day 1 post-transplantation. *Maintenance:* 5 mg daily beginning on day 2 with dosage adjusted based on trough level taken 3 to 4 days after loading dose, as needed, with further adjustments made, as needed, every 7 to 14 days. *Maximum:* 40 mg daily.

Adults and adolescents weighing 40 kg (88 lb) or more at low- to moderate-immunologic risk. *Initial:* 6-mg loading dose. *Maintenance:* 2 mg daily, with dosage adjusted according to trough levels, every 7 to 14 days, as needed. *Maximum:* 40 mg daily.

Adolescents weighing less than 40 kg (88 lb) at low- to moderate-immunologic risk. *Initial:* 3-mg/m^2 loading dose. *Maintenance:* 1 mg/m^2 daily.

DOSAGE ADJUSTMENT Maintenance dosage reduced by one-third for patients with mild-to-moderate impaired hepatic function and one-half for patients with severe impaired hepatic function. Maintenance dosage increased for patients discontinuing concomitant cyclosporine therapy.

➤ *To treat lymphangioleiomyomatosis*

ORAL SOLUTION, TABLETS

Adults. 2 mg daily, dosage adjusted according to trough level 10 to 20 days later, then every 7 to 14 days, as needed, until a stable maintenance dose achieved.

Route	Onset	Peak	Duration
P.O.	Unknown	Unknown	Up to 6 mo after discontinuation

Mechanism of Action
Inhibits activation and proliferation of T lymphocytes and antibody production. Sirolimus also inhibits cell cycle progression from the G_1 to the S phase, possibly by inhibiting a key regulatory kinase believed to suppress cytokine-driven T-cell proliferation.

Contraindications
Hypersensitivity to sirolimus or its components, malignancy

Interactions
DRUGS

aminoglycosides, amphotericin B, cyclosporine: Possibly impaired renal function
boceprevir, bromocriptine, cimetidine, cisapride, clarithromycin, clotrimazole, cyclosporine, danazol, diltiazem, erythromycin, fluconazole, indinavir, itraconazole, ketoconazole, metoclopramide, nicardipine, ritonavir, telaprevir, troleandomycin, verapamil: Possibly increased blood sirolimus level and toxicity
calcineurin inhibitors: Increased risk of deteriorating renal function; development of hemolytic uremic syndrome (HUS), thrombotic microangiopathy (TMA), thrombotic thrombocytopenic purpura (TTP), or UTI; or serum lipid abnormalities
carbamazepine, phenobarbital, phenytoin, rifabutin, rifapentine, St. John's wort: Possibly decreased blood sirolimus level
corticosteroids: Increased risk of deteriorating renal function, serum lipid abnormalities, and UTI

Q R S

HMG-CoA reductase inhibitors: Increased risk of rhabdomyolysis when administered concurrently with sirolimus and cyclosporine
rifampin: Significantly increased sirolimus clearance
vaccines (killed virus): Possibly decreased immune response to vaccines
vaccines (live virus): Increased risk of contracting disease from live virus
verapamil: Possible increased verapamil concentration
FOODS
grapefruit juice: Possibly decreased metabolism of sirolimus
high-fat diet: Reduced rate of sirolimus absorption

Adverse Reactions
CNS: Asthenia, dizziness, fever, headache, insomnia, **posterior reversible encephalopathy syndrome**, **progressive multifocal leukoencephalopathy (PML)**, tremor
CV: Atrial fibrillation, chest pain, **deep vein thrombosis**, hyperlipidemia, hypersensitivity vasculitis, hypertension, hypertriglyceridemia, **pericardial effusion**, peripheral edema, tachycardia
EENT: Epistaxis, nasopharyngitis, stomatitis
ENDO: Hyperglycemia
GI: Abdominal pain, ascites, constipation, diarrhea, elevated liver enzymes, **hepatic artery thrombosis** (liver transplant), **hepatotoxicity**, nausea, **pancreatitis**, vomiting
GU: Azoospermia, BK viral nephritis, elevated serum creatinine level, focal segmental glomerulosclerosis, **hemolytic uremic syndrome**, menstrual disorders, **nephrotic syndrome**, ovarian cysts, proteinuria, pyelonephritis, UTI
HEME: Anemia, **leukopenia**, **neutropenia**, **pancytopenia**, **thrombocytopenia**, **thrombocytopenic purpura**
MS: Arthralgia, bone necrosis, low back or flank pain, joint abnormality, myalgia
RESP: Alveolar proteinosis, **bronchial anastomotic dehiscence** (lung transplant), dyspnea on exertion, **interstitial lung disease**, pleural effusion, pneumonia, **pulmonary embolism or hemorrhage**, upper respiratory tract infection
SKIN: Acne, **cancer including melanoma and Merkel cell carcinoma**, **exfoliative dermatitis**, rash
Other: Anaphylaxis; **angioedema**; cytomegalovirus; delayed wound healing; Epstein–Barr virus; herpes simplex or zoster; **hypokalemia**; **hypophosphatemia**; increased susceptibility to infection, including opportunistic infections such as tuberculosis and activation of latent viral infections; lymphedema; lymphocele; **lymphoma**; **sepsis**; weight gain or loss

Nursing Considerations
- Be aware that sirolimus isn't recommended in liver or lung transplant patients.
- Use sirolimus cautiously in patients who are receiving other drugs known to adversely affect renal function, such as aminoglycosides and amphotericin B; together, they may further decrease renal function.
- Monitor patients with existing or recent (including recent exposure to) chickenpox and patients with herpes zoster for worsening symptoms because they have an increased risk of developing severe generalized disease while taking sirolimus.
- Mix oral sirolimus with at least 2 oz (60 ml) of orange juice or water in a glass or plastic container. Don't dilute drug in grapefruit juice or any other liquid.
- Stir well and have patient drink solution immediately. Then rinse glass with at least 4 oz (120 ml) of additional liquid, stir well, and have patient drink that liquid to make sure that all of drug is taken.
- Give initial dose as soon after transplantation as possible and daily dose 4 hours after cyclosporine, as prescribed.
- Monitor whole blood sirolimus concentrations, as ordered, in patients receiving concentrated form of drug, patients with hepatic impairment or weighing less than 40 kg (88 lb), and those receiving potent CYP3A4 inducers or inhibitors concurrently.
- Know that when using trough level to determine drug's effectiveness, dosage adjustment should be made only after other factors are taken into account, such as signs, symptoms, and tissue biopsy findings. Keep in mind that interpretation

methods vary among laboratories and values aren't interchangeable.

- Monitor serum creatinine level, as ordered, because BK virus-associated nephropathy has occurred with sirolimus therapy. In addition, patients receiving sirolimus and cyclosporine may develop impaired renal function. Notify prescriber of any increases in serum creatinine level because sirolimus or cyclosporine dosage may have to be adjusted or drug discontinued.
- Monitor patient for urinary protein excretion, as ordered. If protein appears in urine, sirolimus may have to be discontinued.
- Monitor patient for signs and symptoms of infection and check CBC results, as ordered, to detect sirolimus-induced blood dyscrasias or changes in neutrophil count, which may indicate infection.
- Keep in mind for patients with hyperlipidemia, of the potential need to institute dietary changes, an exercise program, or a lipid-lowering drug regimen if blood cholesterol or triglyceride levels increase because drug may aggravate hyperlipidemia.
- Monitor patients with wounds who are taking sirolimus because drug may impair or delay wound healing, especially in patients with a body mass index greater than 30 kg/m^2.

PATIENT TEACHING

- Advise patient to take sirolimus consistently either with or without food (but not food high in fat) to prevent changes in absorption rate.
- Advise patient prescribed tablet form not to chew, crush, or split the tablets but to take whole.
- Instruct patient to take daily dose with at least 2 oz (60 ml) of orange juice or water. Caution him not to dilute drug in grapefruit juice or any other liquid. Advise him to stir mixture well and drink immediately, then to add at least another 4 oz (120 ml) of liquid to empty container, stir mixture again, and drink that liquid to ensure that he has swallowed all of drug.
- Urge patient to avoid people with cold, flu, or other infections because immunosuppression makes him more vulnerable.
- Instruct patient not to take live vaccines, during sirolimus therapy.
- Inform patient that sirolimus therapy may increase his risk of skin cancer. Tell him to avoid prolonged sun exposure, sun lamps, and tanning booths. He should use a sunscreen with a high protection factor and wear protective clothing when outdoors.
- Advise patient to keep follow-up appointments for blood tests, as ordered.
- Advise women of childbearing age that sirolimus may be harmful to unborn child. Stress importance of using an effective contraceptive before therapy starts, throughout therapy, and for 12 weeks after therapy is ended. If pregnancy does occur, instruct patient to notify prescriber immediately.

sitagliptin phosphate

Januvia

Class and Category

Pharmacologic class: Dipeptidyl peptidase-4 (DPP-4) inhibitor
Pregnancy category: C

Indications and Dosages

➤ *To achieve control of glucose level in type 2 diabetes mellitus as monotherapy or with metformin or other thiazolidinediones*

TABLETS

Adults. 100 mg once daily.
DOSAGE ADJUSTMENT For patients with moderate renal insufficiency (estimated glomerular filtration rate of 30 ml/min to less than 45 ml/min), dosage reduced to 50 mg once daily; for patients with severe renal insufficiency (estimated glomerular filtration rate less than 30 ml/min) or end-stage renal disease requiring hemodialysis or peritoneal dialysis, dosage reduced to 25 mg once daily.

Route	Onset	Peak	Duration
P.O.	Unknown	1–4 hr	Unknown

Mechanism of Action

Inhibits the dipeptidyl peptidase-4 enzyme to slow inactivation of incretin hormones.

These hormones are released by the intestine throughout the day but increase in response to a meal. When blood glucose level is normal or increased, incretin hormones increase insulin synthesis and release from pancreatic beta cells. One type of incretin hormone, glucagon-like peptide (GLP-1) also lowers glucagon secretion from pancreatic alpha cells, which reduces hepatic glucose production. These combined actions decrease blood glucose level in type 2 diabetes.

Contraindications

Hypersensitivity to sitagliptin or its components

Interactions

DRUGS

ACE inhibitors, disopyramide, fibric acid derivatives, fluoxetine, insulin or insulin secretagogue such as sulfonylureas: Possibly increased hypoglycemic effects
beta blockers: Possibly prolonged hypoglycemia or promotion of hyperglycemia
digoxin: Slightly increased plasma digoxin level
estrogens, oral contraceptives, phenytoin, progestins, thiazide diuretics, triamterene: Possibly decreased hypoglycemic effects

Adverse Reactions

CNS: Headache
EENT: Mouth ulceration, nasopharyngitis, stomatitis
GI: Abdominal pain, **acute pancreatitis**, constipation, diarrhea, elevated liver enzymes, nausea, vomiting
GU: Acute renal failure, worsening renal function
RESP: Upper respiratory tract infection
MS: Arthralgia (disabling, severe), back or extremity pain, myalgia
SKIN: Bullous pemphigoid, cutaneous vasculitis, rash, **Stevens–Johnson syndrome**, urticaria
Other: Anaphylaxis, **angioedema**

Nursing Considerations

- Assess patient's renal function before starting sitagliptin therapy, as ordered, and periodically thereafter. In moderate to severe renal dysfunction, dosage will be reduced and frequency of assessing renal function increased. Also know that renal function should be assessed more frequently in elderly patients because aging can be associated with reduced renal function.
- Monitor patient for hypersensitivity reactions that, although uncommon, may be severe. If present, notify prescriber and expect sitagliptin to be discontinued.
- Monitor patient's blood glucose level, as ordered, to determine effectiveness of sitagliptin therapy.
- Be aware that heart failure has occurred with two other drugs in the same class as sitagliptin. Monitor patient for signs and symptoms of heart failure and if present report immediately to prescriber; provide care according to standard protocols, as ordered; and know that sitagliptin may have to be discontinued.

PATIENT TEACHING

- Emphasize the need to follow a diet control program and an exercise program during sitagliptin therapy.
- Warn patient not to chew, crush, or split the tablet before swallowing.
- Advise patient to notify prescriber immediately if she has trouble breathing, or has hives, rash, or swelling.
- Inform patient that periodic blood tests will be done to determine effectiveness of drug and to assess kidney function.
- Teach patient how to monitor blood glucose level and when to report changes.
- Caution patient that taking other drugs in addition to sitagliptin to control his diabetes or taking certain drugs to treat other conditions may lead to hypoglycemia. Review signs, symptoms, and appropriate prescribed treatment for hypoglycemia with him.
- Instruct patient to contact prescriber if he develops other illnesses, such as infection, or experiences surgery or trauma because his diabetes medication may require adjustment.
- Advise patient to carry identification indicating that she has diabetes.
- Instruct patient to stop taking sitagliptin and report persistent severe abdominal pain, possibly radiating to the back and accompanied by vomiting.
- Review signs and symptoms of heart failure, such as rapid weight increase,

shortness of breath, or swelling in feet. Instruct patient to immediately report such to prescriber.
- Tell patient to report development of blisters or erosions while receiving sitagliptin therapy.
- Encourage women of childbearing age to enroll in the pregnancy exposure registry if pregnancy occurs while taking sitagliptin.

sodium bicarbonate

Baking Soda, Sellymin (CAN)

Class and Category

Pharmacologic class: Electrolyte
Therapeutic class: Antacid, electrolyte replenisher, systemic and urinary alkalizer
Pregnancy category: C

Indications and Dosages

➤ *To treat hyperacidity*

ORAL POWDER

Adults and adolescents. One-half teaspoon mixed in at least 120 ml of water every 2 hr, as needed. *Maximum:* 4 teaspoons daily.

TABLETS

Adults and adolescents. 325 mg to 2 g daily to four times a day, as needed. *Maximum:* 16 g daily.
Children ages 6 to 12. 520 mg, repeated once after 30 min, as needed.

➤ *To provide urinary alkalization*

ORAL POWDER

Adults and adolescents. 1 teaspoon mixed in at least 120 ml of water every 4 hr. *Maximum:* 4 teaspoons daily.

TABLETS

Adults and adolescents. *Initial:* 4 g, then 1 to 2 g every 4 hr. *Maximum:* 16 g daily.
Children. 23 to 230 mg/kg daily, adjusted as needed.

➤ *To treat metabolic acidosis during cardiac arrest in certain situations such as presence of hyperkalemia, pre-existing metabolic acidosis, or tricyclic antidepressant overdose*

I.V. INJECTION

Adults and children age 2 and over. *Initial:* 1 mEq/kg, followed by 0.5 mEq/kg every 10 min as needed and determined by blood gas analysis or laboratory measurement while arrest continues.
Neonates and children under age 2. 1 mEq/kg using a 4.2% solution given slowly over several min. *Maximum:* 8 mEq/kg in 24 hr.

➤ *To treat less urgent forms of metabolic acidosis*

I.V. INFUSION

Adults and children. 2 to 5 mEq/kg infused over 4 to 8 hr.

DOSAGE ADJUSTMENT Dosage reduction possible for elderly patients because of age-related renal impairment.

Mechanism of Action

Buffers excess hydrogen ions, increases plasma bicarbonate level, and raises blood pH, thereby reversing metabolic acidosis. Sodium bicarbonate also increases the excretion of free bicarbonate ions in urine, raising urine pH; increased alkalinity of urine may help to dissolve uric acid calculi. In addition, it relieves symptoms of hyperacidity by neutralizing or buffering existing stomach acid, thereby increasing the pH of stomach contents.

Incompatibilities

Don't admix I.V. form of sodium bicarbonate in same solution or administer through same I.V. line as other drugs because precipitate may form.

Contraindications

Hypocalcemia in which alkalosis may lead to tetany; hypochloremic alkalosis secondary to diuretics, nasogastric suction or vomiting; preexisting metabolic or respiratory alkalosis

Interactions

DRUGS

amphetamines, quinidine: Decreased urinary excretion of these drugs, possibly resulting in toxicity
anticholinergics: Decreased anticholinergic absorption and effectiveness
calcium-containing products: Increased risk of milk-alkali syndrome
chlorpropamide, lithium, salicylates, tetracyclines: Increased renal excretion and decreased absorption of these drugs

ciprofloxacin, norfloxacin, ofloxacin: Decreased solubility of these drugs, leading to crystalluria and nephrotoxicity
citrates: Increased risk of systemic alkalosis; increased risk of calcium calculus formation and hypernatremia in patients with history of uric acid calculi
digoxin: Possibly elevated digoxin level
enteric-coated drugs: Increased risk of duodenal or gastric irritation from rapid removal of enteric coating
ephedrine: Increased ephedrine half-life and duration of action
H_2-receptor antagonists, iron preparations or supplements, ketoconazole: Decreased absorption of these drugs
mecamylamine: Decreased excretion and prolonged effect of mecamylamine
methenamine: Decreased methenamine effectiveness
mexiletine: Possibly mexiletine toxicity
potassium supplements: Decreased serum potassium level
sucralfate: Interference with binding of sucralfate to gastric mucosa
urinary acidifiers (ammonium chloride, ascorbic acid, potassium and sodium phosphates): Counteracted effects of urinary acidifiers

FOODS

dairy products: Increased risk of milk-alkali syndrome with prolonged use of sodium bicarbonate

Adverse Reactions

CNS: Mental or mood changes
CV: Irregular heartbeat, peripheral edema (with large doses), weak pulse
EENT: Dry mouth
GI: Abdominal cramps, thirst
MS: Muscle spasms, myalgia
SKIN: Extravasation with necrosis, tissue sloughing, or ulceration

Nursing Considerations

- Monitor sodium intake of patient taking sodium bicarbonate oral powder contains 952 mg of sodium/tsp; and tablets contain 325 mg/3.9-mEq tablet, 520 mg/6.2-mEq tablet, and 650 mg/7.7-mEq tablet.
- For I.V. infusion, dilute drug with D_5W, normal saline solution, or other standard electrolyte solution before administration.
- Avoid rapid I.V. infusion, which can cause severe alkalosis. Be aware that during cardiac arrest, risk of death from acidosis may outweigh risks of rapid infusion.
- Monitor urine pH, as ordered, to determine drug's effectiveness as urine alkalizer.
- Know that if patient on long-term sodium bicarbonate therapy is consuming calcium or milk, watch for milk-alkali syndrome, characterized by anorexia, confusion, headache, hypercalcemia, metabolic acidosis, nausea, renal insufficiency, and vomiting.
- Be aware that parenteral forms are hypertonic and that increased sodium intake can produce edema and weight gain.
- Assess I.V. site often for evidence of extravasation. If it occurs, notify prescriber at once and remove I.V. catheter. Elevate the limb, apply warm compresses, and expect prescriber to administer a local injection of hyaluronidase or lidocaine.

PATIENT TEACHING

- Advise patient not to take sodium bicarbonate with large amounts of dairy products or for longer than 2 weeks, unless directed by prescriber.
- Caution patient not to take more drug than prescribed to avoid adverse reactions.
- Direct patient not to take drug within 2 hours of other oral drugs.
- Advise patient to avoid taking other prescribed or OTC drugs without prescriber's approval because many drugs interact with sodium bicarbonate.

sodium ferric gluconate

(contains 62.5 mg elemental iron per 5 ml)
Ferrlecit

Class and Category

Pharmacologic class: Iron salt, mineral
Therapeutic class: Hematinic
Pregnancy category: B

Indications and Dosages

➤ *To treat iron deficiency anemia in patients receiving long-term hemodialysis and supplemental epoetin therapy*

I.V. INFUSION OR INJECTION

Adults. 10 ml (125 mg of elemental iron.) diluted in 100 ml of 0.9% sodium chloride and infused over 1 hr per dialysis session or injected undiluted slowly at a rate of up to 12.5 mg/min per dialysis session. *Maximum:* 125 mg per dose. *Usual:* Minimum cumulative dose of 1 g elemental iron given over eight sequential dialysis treatments. Dosage repeated at lowest dosage needed to maintain target levels of hemoglobin and hematocrit and acceptable limits of blood iron level.

Children age 6 and over. 0.12 ml/kg (1.5 mg/kg of elemental iron) diluted in 25 ml of 0.9% sodium chloride infused over 1 hr per dialysis session. *Maximum:* 125 mg per dose.

Mechanism of Action

Acts to replenish iron stores lost during hemodialysis as a result of increased blood loss or increased iron utilization from epoetin therapy. Iron is an essential component of hemoglobin, myoglobin, and several enzymes, including catalase, cytochromes, and peroxidase, and is needed for catecholamine metabolism and normal neutrophil function. Sodium ferric gluconate also normalizes RBC production by binding with hemoglobin or being stored as ferritin in reticuloendothelial cells of the bone marrow, liver, and spleen.

Incompatibilities

Don't mix sodium ferric gluconate with other drugs or parenteral nutrition solutions for I.V. infusion.

Contraindications

Anemia other than iron deficiency; hypersensitivity to sodium ferric gluconate, other iron salts or their components; iron overload

Interactions

DRUGS

oral iron preparations: Possibly reduced absorption of oral iron supplements

Adverse Reactions

CNS: Asthenia, dizziness, fatigue, fever, headache, hypertonia, nervousness, paresthesia, syncope

CV: Chest pain, generalized edema, hypertension, **hypotension**, tachycardia

EENT: Dry mouth

GI: Abdominal pain, diarrhea, nausea, vomiting

HEME: Hemorrhage

MS: Back pain, leg cramps

RESP: Cough, dyspnea, upper respiratory tract infection, wheezing

SKIN: Diaphoresis, pruritus

Other: Anaphylaxis, generalized pain, **hyperkalemia**, **hypersensitivity reactions**, infusion or injection-site reaction

Nursing Considerations

- Reconstitute sodium ferric gluconate for I.V. infusion by diluting prescribed dosage in 100 ml of normal saline solution immediately before infusion. Infuse over 1 hour. Discard any unused diluted solution.
- Inspect drug for discoloration and particles before administration and discard if present.
- Give undiluted drug by slow I.V. injection at up to 12.5 mg/min, not to exceed 125 mg/injection.
- Be aware that most patients need a minimum cumulative dose of 1 g of elemental iron administered over eight sequential dialysis treatments.

WARNING Assess patient for evidence of allergic reaction, including chills, facial flushing, pruritus, and rash, and of a hypersensitivity reaction, including diaphoresis, dyspnea, nausea, severe lower back pain, vomiting, and wheezing. Discontinue drug and notify prescriber immediately if patient develops an allergic or hypersensitivity reaction, and be prepared to provide emergency interventions.

WARNING Assess blood pressure often after drug administration because hypotension may occur and may be related to infusion rate or total cumulative dose. Avoid rapid infusion, and be prepared to provide I.V. fluids for volume expansion.

- Expect to monitor blood hemoglobin level, hematocrit, serum ferritin level, and transferrin saturation, as ordered, before, during, and after sodium ferric gluconate therapy. Make sure serum iron level is tested 48 hours after last dose. To prevent

iron toxicity, notify prescriber and expect to end therapy if blood iron level is normal or elevated.
- Assess patient for possible iron overload, characterized by bleeding in GI tract and lungs, decreased activity, pale conjunctivae, and sedation.

PATIENT TEACHING
- Warn patient not to take any oral iron preparations during sodium ferric gluconate therapy without first consulting prescriber.
- Inform patient that symptoms of iron deficiency may include decreased stamina, fatigue, learning problems, and shortness of breath.

sodium polystyrene sulfonate

Kalexate, Kayexalate, K-Exit (CAN), Kionex, PMS-Sodium Polystyrene Sulfonate (CAN), SPS Suspension

Class and Category
Pharmacologic class: Sulfonated cation-exchange resin
Therapeutic class: Antihyperkalemic
Pregnancy category: C

Indications and Dosages
➤ *To treat hyperkalemia*

ORAL POWDER, SUSPENSION
Adults. 15 g (4 level tsp) once daily to four times a day.
Maximum: 40 g four times a day.
Children. 1 g/kg/dose, every 6 hr, as needed.

RECTAL POWDER, SUSPENSION
Adults. 30 to 50 g every 6 hr as retention enema, as needed.
Children. 1 g/kg/dose every 2 to 6 hr as retention enema, as needed.

Route	Onset	Peak	Duration
P.O.	2–12 hr	Unknown	Unknown

Mechanism of Action
Releases sodium ions in exchange for other cations in intestines. Resin enters large intestine and releases sodium ions in exchange for hydrogen ions. As the resin moves through the intestines, hydrogen ions are then exchanged for potassium ions, which are in greater concentration. Bound resin leaves the body in feces, carrying potassium and other ions with it, thereby reducing serum potassium level.

Contraindications
Hypersensitivity to sodium polystyrene sulfonate or its components, hypokalemia, obstructive bowel disease, reduced intestinal motility in neonates, oral administration in neonates

Interactions
DRUGS
aluminum hydroxide: Increased risk of intestinal obstruction
antacids, laxatives: Increased risk of metabolic alkalosis
potassium-sparing diuretics, potassium supplements: Increased risk of fluid retention
other orally administered medications: Decreased absorption and reduced effectiveness of these drugs

Adverse Reactions
CV: Peripheral edema
GI: Abdominal cramps, anorexia, **colonic necrosis**, constipation, diarrhea, epigastric pain, fecal impaction, gastric irritation, **GI bleeding**, indigestion, **intestinal necrosis or obstruction**, **ischemic colitis**, nausea, ulcerations, vomiting
GU: Decreased urine output
RESP: Aspiration
Other: Hypernatremia, **hypocalcemia**, **hypokalemia**, **hypomagnesemia**, **metabolic alkalosis**, weight gain

Nursing Considerations
- Know that sodium polystyrene sulfonate should not be given to a patient who has not had a bowel movement postsurgery, or in patients who are at risk for developing constipation or impaction (including patients with a history of chronic constipation, inflammatory bowel disease, impaction, ischemic colitis, previous bowel obstruction or resection, or vascular intestinal atherosclerosis) because these factors increase the risk for intestinal necrosis, which may be life-threatening.
- Use sodium polystyrene sulfonate cautiously in patients with heart failure, hypertension, or marked edema.

- Be aware that drug is available as powdered resin or as solution that contains sorbitol to facilitate movement of resin through intestines. As a result, patient may experience abdominal cramps, diarrhea, nausea, and vomiting.
- Be aware that because the drug doesn't take effect for several hours it's inappropriate for treating acute, life-threatening hyperkalemia.
- Assess patient for hypokalemia or hypocalcemia. If present, notify prescriber immediately and expect to withhold drug because it reduces calcium and potassium levels. Evidence of hypokalemia includes abdominal cramps, acidic urine, anorexia, drowsiness, ECG changes, hypotension, hypoventilation, muscle weakness, and tachycardia. Evidence of hypocalcemia includes abdominal pain, agitation, anxiety, ECG changes, hypotension, muscle twitching, psychosis, seizures, and tetany.
- Mix powdered resin to be given as oral suspension in food, syrup, or water and give promptly, being sure to follow full aspiration precautions (such as keeping patient in an upright position while giving drug), because patients may be at risk of aspiration caused by inhalation of sodium polystyrene sulfonate particles, especially patients with altered level of consciousness, impaired gag reflex, or who are prone to regurgitation. If needed, administer through gastric feeding tube.
- Administer other oral medication at least 3 hours before or 3 hours after sodium polystyrene sulfonate administration, because drug may interfere with the absorption of other orally administered medications. However, patients with gastroparesis may require a 6-hour separation.
- Precede rectal administration with a cleansing enema, as ordered.
- Know that when giving rectally, powdered resin in 100 ml of aqueous solution should be warmed to body temperature, in bag connected to soft, large (French 28) catheter. Have patient lie on his left side with his lower leg straight and upper leg flexed or with his knees to his chest. Gently insert the tube into the rectum and well into the sigmoid colon. The solution should flow into the colon by way of gravity and be retained for 30 to 60 minutes or longer, if possible. After patient is unable to retain the solution any longer, administer a non-sodium-containing cleansing enema, as prescribed.
- Use of sorbitol with sodium polystyrene sulfonate isn't recommended because of increased risk of colonic necrosis and other serious GI effects, such as bleeding, ischemic colitis, and perforation.
- Assess for constipation and fecal impaction after administration. If either occurs, notify prescriber, expect drug to be discontinued, and provide care, as ordered, to relieve constipation or fecal impaction.

PATIENT TEACHING

- Instruct patient not to mix oral form of sodium polystyrene sulfonate with foods and liquids high in potassium content, such as bananas and orange juice.
- Teach patient who will self-administer rectal solution, the correct technique and body position. Remind him to let the solution flow into the colon by gravity and to retain it for at least 30 to 60 minutes, longer if possible.
- Advise patient to notify prescriber immediately about abdominal cramps, nausea, and vomiting.

sodium zirconium cyclosilicate

Lokelma

Class and Category

Pharmacologic class: Potassium binder
Therapeutic class: Potassium reducer
Pregnancy category: Not classified

Indications and Dosages

➤ *To treat hyperkalemia in nonlife-threatening situations*

ORAL SUSPENSION

Adults. *Initial:* 10 mg three times daily for up to 48 hr. *Maintenance:* 10 mg once daily. Dosage increased during maintenance in increments of 5 mg at weekly or longer intervals, as needed, based on serum potassium.

Mechanism of Action

Increases fecal potassium excretion through binding of potassium in the lumen of the gastrointestinal tract. This reduces the concentration of free potassium in the gastrointestinal lumen, thereby lowering serum potassium levels.

Contraindications

Hypersensitivity to sodium zirconium cyclosilicate or its components

Interactions

DRUGS

oral drugs that have pH-dependent solubility: Altered absorption of these drugs, possibly causing altered efficacy or safety

Adverse Reactions

CV: Edema
Other: Hypokalemia

Nursing Considerations

- Know that sodium zirconium cyclosilicate should not be given to patients with abnormal postoperative bowel motility disorders, bowel obstruction, bowel impaction, or severe constipation, because drug may be ineffective or even worsen these gastrointestinal conditions.
- Empty entire contents of packet into a drinking glass containing about 3 tablespoons of water or more, if patient desires. Stir well and administer immediately. If powder remains in the drinking glass, add water, stir, and have patient drink immediately. Repeat until no powder remains, to ensure that entire dose has been given.
- Administer other oral drugs at least 2 hours before or after sodium zirconium cyclosilicate administration to prevent other drugs from not being absorbed properly.
- Monitor patient for edema, especially patients who should restrict their sodium intake or are prone to fluid retention, such as those with heart failure or renal disease.

PATIENT TEACHING

- Tell patient to empty entire contents of packet into a drinking glass containing about 3 tablespoons of water or more, if patient desires. Tell patient to stir well and drink immediately. If powder remains in the drinking glass, patient should add water, stir, and drink contents immediately. Repeat until no powder remains, to ensure that entire dose has been given.
- Instruct patient to take other oral drugs at least 2 hours before or after sodium zirconium cyclosilicate administration, to prevent other drugs from not being absorbed properly.
- Advise patient to limit dietary sodium intake, if needed, and to notify prescriber if fluid retention occurs.

sofosbuvir

Sovaldi

Class and Category

Pharmacologic class: NS5B polymerase inhibitor
Therapeutic class: Antiviral
Pregnancy category: Not classified

Indications and Dosages

➤ *As adjunct to treat chronic hepatitis C virus (HCV) infection in patients with genotype 1 or 4 who are without cirrhosis or who have compensated cirrhosis and used in combination with pegylated interferon and ribavirin*

TABLETS

Adults who are treatment-naïve. 400 mg once daily for 12 wk.

➤ *As adjunct to treat chronic hepatitis C virus (HCV) infection in patients with genotype 2 or 3 who are without cirrhosis or who have compensated cirrhosis and used in combination with ribavirin*

TABLETS

Adults and children age 12 years and over weighing at least 35 kg (77 lb). 400 mg once daily for 12 wk for genotype 2 and 24 wk for genotype 3.

➤ *As adjunct to treat chronic hepatitis C virus (HCV) infection in patients with hepatocellular carcinoma waiting for a liver transplant in combination with ribavirin*

TABLETS

Adults. 400 mg once daily for 48 wk or until liver transplant.

Mechanism of Action

Undergoes intracellular metabolism to form an active uridine analogue triphosphate, which is then incorporated into HCV RNA by the NS5B polymerase and acts as a chain terminator.

Contraindications

Hypersensitivity to sofosbuvir or its components

Interactions

DRUGS

amiodarone: Possibly development of serious symptomatic bradycardia
carbamazepine, oxcarbazepine, phenobarbital, phenytoin, rifabutin, rifampin, rifapentine, St. John's wort, tipranavir/ritonavir: Possibly decreased sofosbuvir plasma concentration, leading to reduced effectiveness

Adverse Reactions

CNS: Asthenia, chills, depression (severe), fatigue, fever, headache, insomnia, irritability, **suicidal ideation**
GI: Anorexia, diarrhea, elevated pancreatic enzymes, hyperbilirubinemia, nausea
HEME: Anemia, **neutropenia, pancytopenia, thrombocytopenia**
MS: Elevated creatine kinase, myalgia
SKIN: Pruritus, rash (sometimes with blisters or angioedema-like swelling)
Other: Angioedema, flu-like symptoms

Nursing Considerations

- Know that reducing the dosage of sofosbuvir or interrupting treatment should be avoided to prevent treatment failure. Also be aware that if other drugs used in combination with sofosbuvir are discontinued, sofosbuvir should also be discontinued.

WARNING Ensure that all patients have been tested for current or prior HBV infection before sofosbuvir therapy is begun, because in patients coinfected with HBV and HCV, there is risk of hepatitis B virus reactivation that may result in fluminant hepatitis, hepatic failure, or even death. If patient tests positive for HBV, monitor patient closely for clinical and laboratory signs, as ordered, of hepatitis flare or HBV reactivation during treatment with sofosbuvir and during posttreatment follow-up. Expect treatment for HBV infection to be given, if needed.

- Monitor patient also receiving amiodarone with sofosbuvir for symptomatic bradycardia that may be severe enough to require pacemaker intervention. Be aware that bradycardia may occur up to 2 weeks after sofosbuvir therapy has begun. Patients at risk include those taking beta blockers or those with underlying advanced liver disease or cardiac disorders. Expect patient to be hospitalized for cardiac monitoring for the first 48 hours of sofosbuvir therapy. Notify prescriber if bradycardia occurs and expect drug to be discontinued. Known that bradycardia generally disappears after the drug is discontinued.

PATIENT TEACHING

- Instruct patient to take sofosbuvir exactly as ordered and not to discontinue it without prescriber knowledge.
- Tell patient to take sofosbuvir every day at a regularly scheduled time.
- Teach patient how to take his pulse and to report immediately a sudden decrease in pulse rate or signs and symptoms of serious bradycardia, such as chest pain, confusion, dizziness, excessive tiredness, fainting or near-fainting, malaise, memory problems, shortness of breath, or weakness.
- Tell patient to inform all prescribers of sofosbuvir therapy, because the drug reacts with many different drugs, which may cause reduced effectiveness or increased risk of adverse reactions.
- Advise female patients to notify prescriber if pregnancy occurs or is suspected. If patient is also taking ribavirin with sofosbuvir, tell patient to use two reliable contraceptives during treatment and for at least 6 months after stopping ribavirin.
- Tell mothers wishing to breastfeed to discuss the benefits versus risks with their prescriber.

solifenacin succinate

VESIcare

Class and Category

Pharmacologic class: Antimuscarinic
Therapeutic class: Bladder antispasmodic
Pregnancy category: C

Indications and Dosages

➤ *To treat overactive urinary bladder with symptoms of frequency, urge incontinence, and urgency*

TABLETS

Adults. 5 mg daily; if tolerated well, increased to 10 mg daily.

DOSAGE ADJUSTMENT For patients with severe renal impairment or moderate hepatic impairment or patients taking ketoconazole or other potent CYP3A4 inhibitors, dosage limited to 5 mg daily.

Route	Onset	Peak	Duration
P.O.	Unknown	3–8 hr	Unknown

Mechanism of Action

Antagonizes the effect of acetylcholine on muscarinic receptors in detrusor muscle, decreasing the muscle spasms that cause inappropriate bladder emptying. This action increases bladder capacity and volume, which relieves the sensation of frequency and urgency and enhances bladder control.

Contraindications

Gastric retention, hypersensitivity to solifenacin or its components, uncontrolled angle-closure glaucoma, urine retention

Interactions

DRUGS

ketoconazole, other potent CYP3A4 inhibitors: Possibly decreased metabolism of solifenacin and increased risk of adverse effects

Adverse Reactions

CNS: Confusion, delirium, depression, dizziness, fatigue, hallucinations, headache, somnolence
CV: **Atrial fibrillation**, hypertension, palpitations, peripheral edema, **prolonged QT interval**, tachycardia, **torsades de pointes**
EENT: Blurred vision, dry eyes or mouth, glaucoma, pharyngitis
GI: Abdominal pain, anorexia, constipation, elevated liver enzymes gastroesophageal reflux disease, ileus, indigestion, nausea, vomiting
GU: Renal impairment, UTI, urinary retention
MS: Muscle weakness
RESP: **Airway obstruction from angioedema**, cough, dysphonia
SKIN: **Erythema multiforme, exfoliative dermatitis**, pruritus, rash, urticaria
Other: **Anaphylaxis, angioedema**, flu-like symptoms, **hyperkalemia**

Nursing Considerations

- Use cautiously in patients with intestinal atony, myasthenia gravis, or ulcerative colitis because solifenacin may decrease GI motility; in patients with significant bladder outflow obstruction because solifenacin may cause urine retention; in patients with hepatic impairment because solifenacin is metabolized in the liver; and in patients with renal impairment because solifenacin excretion may be impaired.
- Monitor patient closely, even after first dose, for hypersensitivity reactions. Although uncommon, anaphylactic reactions and angioedema have occurred with solifenacin therapy. Be prepared to manage these life-threatening reactions and expect drug to be discontinued if they occur.
- Monitor patient for signs of anticholinergic CNS adverse reactions, especially after treatment is begun or dosage increased.
- Monitor elderly patients, especially those age 75 and over, for adverse reactions because they're at increased risk for solifenacin-induced adverse reactions.

PATIENT TEACHING

- Instruct patient to take solifenacin with a full glass of water and to swallow the tablet whole.
- Caution patient to avoid exertion in a warm or hot environment because sweating may be delayed, which could increase body temperature and increase risk of heatstroke.
- Advise patient to avoid potentially hazardous activities until drug's CNS effects are known.
- Inform patient that alcohol may cause drowsiness, and urge patient to limit or avoid alcoholic beverages while taking solifenacin.

sotalol hydrochloride

Betapace, Betapace AF, Sorine, Sotacor (CAN), Sotalol I.V.

Class and Category

Pharmacologic class: Nonselective beta blocker

Therapeutic class: Class III antiarrhythmic
Pregnancy category: B

Indications and Dosages

➤ *To treat life-threatening ventricular arrhythmias*

TABLETS

Adults. *Initial:* 80 mg twice daily, increased, as needed, in increments of 80 mg every 3 days provided patient's QT interval is less than 500 msec. *Maintenance:* 160 to 320 mg daily in divided doses twice daily or three times a day. *Maximum:* 640 mg daily.

I.V. INFUSION (SOTALOL I.V.)

Adults. *Initial:* 75 mg over 5 hr every 12 hr, increased as needed, every 3 days. *Maximum:* 150mg daily.

➤ *To maintain normal sinus rhythm in patients with highly symptomatic atrial fibrillation who are currently in sinus rhythm*

TABLETS (BETAPACE AF)

Adults. *Initial:* 80 mg twice daily, increased after 3 days to 120 mg twice daily provided QTc interval is less than 500 msec. *Maximum:* 160 mg twice a day.

Children 2 years old and over: *Initial:* 30 mg/m^2 every 8 hr; may be titrated up to 60 mg/m^2/day allowing 36 hr between dosage adjustments. *Maximum:* 60 mg/m^2/day.

I.V. INFUSION (SOTALOL I.V.)

Adults. 75 mg over 5 hr every 12 hrs, increased as needed no sooner than every 3 days. *Maximum:* 150 mg twice daily.

DOSAGE ADJUSTMENT For adult patients treated for ventricular arrhythmias and with a creatinine clearance between 30 and 59 ml/min, oral dosage interval reduced to every 24 hours; if creatinine clearance is between 10 and 29 ml/min, oral dosage interval increased to 36 or 48 hours. For adult patients treated for atrial fibrillation or flutter, with a creatinine clearance between 40 to 59 ml/min, dosing interval increased to every 24 hours.

Route	Onset	Peak	Duration
P.O.	Unknown	2–3 hr	Unknown

Mechanism of Action

Combines class II and class III antiarrhythmic activity to increase sinus cycle length. This beta blocker decreases AV nodal conduction and increases AV nodal refractoriness. Suppression of SA node automaticity and AV node conductivity decreases atrial and ventricular ectopy.

Contraindications

Acquired or congenital QT syndromes, asthma, atrial arrhythmias (if baseline QT interval exceeds 450 msec or creatinine clearance is less than 40 ml/min), cardiogenic shock, COPD, heart failure (unless it results from tachyarrhythmia that's treatable by sotalol), hypersensitivity to sotalol or its components, second- or third-degree AV block without functioning pacemaker, sinus bradycardia

Interactions

DRUGS

allergen immunotherapy, allergenic extracts for skin testing: Increased risk of anaphylaxis or serious systemic adverse reaction
amiodarone: Additive depressant effect on conduction, negative inotropic effect
anesthetics (hydrocarbon inhalation): Increased risk of hypotension and myocardial depression
antacids: Altered sotalol effectiveness
astemizole, class I antiarrhythmics, phenothiazines, terfenadine, tricyclic antidepressants: Prolonged QT interval, life-threatening torsades de pointes
beta blockers (other): Additive beta blockade
$beta_2$-receptor stimulants: Decreased effectiveness of these drugs
calcium channel blockers, clonidine, diazoxide, guanabenz, reserpine, and other antihypertensives: Additive antihypertensive effect and, possibly, other beta-blocking effects
cimetidine: Possibly impaired sotalol clearance
digoxin: Increased risk of bradycardia
glucagon: Possibly blunted hyperglycemic response
insulin, oral antidiabetic drugs: Impaired glucose control, increased risk of hyperglycemia
lidocaine: Decreased lidocaine clearance, increased risk of lidocaine toxicity
MAO inhibitors: Increased risk of significant hypertension

neuromuscular blockers: Possibly potentiated and prolonged neuromuscular blockade
phenothiazines: Increased blood levels of both drugs
propafenone: Increased blood level and half-life of sotalol
sympathomimetics, xanthines: Possibly mutual inhibition of therapeutic effects

Adverse Reactions

CNS: Anxiety, depression, dizziness, drowsiness, fatigue, insomnia, lethargy, nervousness, weakness
CV: AV conduction disorders, bradycardia, **heart failure**, **hypotension**, peripheral vascular insufficiency
EENT: Nasal congestion
ENDO: Hyperglycemia, **hypoglycemia**
GI: Abdominal pain, constipation, diarrhea, nausea, vomiting
GU: Sexual dysfunction
MS: Muscle weakness
RESP: Bronchospasm, dyspnea, wheezing

Nursing Considerations

- Expect to obtain baseline creatinine clearance and QT interval before starting sotalol and periodically throughout therapy, as ordered.
- Monitor apical and radial pulses, blood pressure, circulation in limbs, daily weight, fluid intake and output, and respiratory rate, before and during sotalol therapy.
- Know that if prescriber is stopping amiodarone, sotalol shouldn't be started until QT interval has returned to baseline because of possible adverse cardiac effects.
- Be aware that stopping sotalol abruptly may cause life-threatening reactions. For this reason, chronic beta blocker therapy such as sotalol is not routinely withheld prior to major surgery. However, be aware that the impaired ability of the heart to respond to reflex adrenergic stimuli may increase the risks of general anesthesia and surgical procedures.
- Monitor serum electrolyte levels because drug can increase risk of torsades de pointes in patients with electrolyte imbalances, especially hypokalemia or hypomagnesemia.
- Assess carefully if patient has diabetes mellitus or thyrotoxicosis because they may mask hypoglycemia and hyperthyroidism.

PATIENT TEACHING

- Advise patient to notify prescriber immediately if he has difficulty breathing.
- Urge patient to consult prescriber before taking OTC drugs, especially cold remedies, which may decrease sotalol's effectiveness.
- Urge patient to avoid hazardous activities until drug's CNS effects are known.

spectinomycin hydrochloride

Trobicin

Class and Category

Pharmacologic class: Aminoglycoside
Therapeutic class: Antibiotic
Pregnancy category: Not classified

Indications and Dosages

➤ *To treat acute endocervical, rectal, and urethral gonorrhea caused by susceptible strains of* Neisseria gonorrhoeae

I.M. INJECTION

Adults. 2 g as a single dose.
DOSAGE ADJUSTMENT For patients living in geographic area where antibiotic resistance is known to be prevalent, dosage increased to 4 g as a single dose.

Mechanism of Action

Binds to negatively charged sites on bacterial outer cell membrane, disrupting cell integrity, and binds to bacterial ribosomal subunits, inhibiting protein synthesis. Both actions lead to bacterial cell death.

Contraindications

Hypersensitivity to spectinomycin or its components

Adverse Reactions

CNS: Dizziness, insomnia
GI: Abdominal cramps, nausea, vomiting
Other: Injection-site pain

Nursing Considerations

- To reconstitute spectinomycin, add 3.2 ml bacteriostatic water for injection (with benzyl alcohol) to each 2-g vial. Shake vial vigorously before withdrawing dose.

- Administer I.M. injection using a 20-gauge needle deep into large muscle mass, preferably upper outer quadrant of gluteal muscle. 4 g dose may be divided between two gluteal injection sites.

PATIENT TEACHING
- Tell patient he'll be tested for syphilis at the start of treatment and 3 months later because spectinomycin treatment may delay or mask syphilis symptoms.
- Explain risk factors for sexually transmitted diseases, and teach correct condom use.
- Advise patient to encourage sexual partner to be tested for gonorrhea.
- Instruct patient to notify prescriber if signs and symptoms persist after a few days.

spironolactone

Aldactone, Carospir

Class and Category

Pharmacologic class: Potassium-sparing diuretic
Therapeutic class: Diuretic
Pregnancy category: Not classified

Indications and Dosages

➤ *To increase survival and to reduce need for hospitalization for heart failure when used in addition to standard therapy in patients with severe heart failure (NYHA class III-IV)*

TABLETS
Adults. *Initial:* 25 mg once daily if patient's serum creatinine is equal to or less than 2.5 mg/dl and serum potassium is equal to or less than 5.0 mEq/L. Dosage increased to 50 mg once daily, as needed.
DOSAGE ADJUSTMENT If patient does not tolerate 25 mg once daily, dosage reduced to 25 mg every other day.

➤ *To treat edema caused by nephrotic syndrome*

TABLETS
Adults. *Initial:* 100 mg daily as a single dose or in divided doses, for at least 5 days if given as the only agent for diuresis. *Usual:* 25 to 200 mg daily as a single dose or in divided doses.

➤ *To treat heart failure*

TABLETS (ALDACTONE)
Adults. *Initial:* 100 mg daily as a single dose or in divided doses, for at least 5 days if given as the only agent for diuresis.
Usual: 25 to 200 mg daily as a single dose or in divided doses.

ORAL SUSPENSION (CAROSPIR)
Adults with a serum potassium of 5.0 mEq/l or greater and eGFR greater than 50 ml/min. *Initial:* 20 mg (4 ml) once daily, increased to 37.5 mg (7.5 ml) once daily, if needed.
Adults with an eGFR between 30 to 50 ml/min. 10 mg (2 ml) once daily.
DOSAGE ADJUSTMENT For heart failure patients who develop hyperkalemia while receiving a dose of 20 mg (4 ml) daily, dosage reduced to 20 mg (4 ml) every other day.

➤ *To treat hypertension*

TABLETS (ALDACTONE)
Adults. *Initial:* 50 to 100 mg daily as a single dose or in divided doses for at least 2 wk; gradually adjusted every 2 wk, as needed, to control blood pressure.

ORAL SUSPENSION (CAROSPIR)
Adults. *Initial:* 20 mg (4 ml) daily as a single dose or in divided doses for at least 2 wk; gradually adjusted every 2 wk as needed. *Maximum:* 75 mg (15 ml) daily.

➤ *To treat edema associated with hepatic cirrhosis*

TABLETS (ALDACTONE)
Adults. *Initial:* 100 mg daily as a single dose or in divided doses, for at least 5 days if given as the only agent for diuresis. *Usual:* 25 to 200 mg daily as a single dose or in divided doses.

ORAL SUSPENSION (CAROSPIR)
Adults. *Initial:* 75 mg (15 ml) daily as a single dose or in divided doses, for at least 5 days if given as the only agent for diuresis. Increased slowly to maximum dose, as needed. *Maximum:* 100 mg (20 ml) daily.

➤ *To aid in the diagnosis of primary hyperaldosteronism*

TABLETS
Adults. For long test, 400 mg daily for 3 to 4 wk; for short test, 400 mg daily for 4 days.

➤ *To treat primary hyperaldosteronism*

TABLETS
Adults. 100 to 400 mg daily.
DOSAGE ADJUSTMENT Long-term maintenance dosage decreased for

patients at risk for complications during surgery.

➤ *To substitute as therapy for diuretic-induced hypokalemia*

TABLETS

Adults. 25 to 100 mg daily.

Route	Onset	Peak	Duration
P.O.*	Unknown	2–3 days	2–3 days

* For diuretic effect; others unknown.

Contraindications

Acute renal insufficiency, Addison's disease or other conditions associated with hyperkalemia, anuria, concomitant use of eplerenone, hyperkalemia, hypersensitivity to spironolactone or its components

Interactions

DRUGS

ACE inhibitors, aldosterone blockers, angiotensin II antagonists, cyclosporine, heparin and low molecular weight heparin, NSAIDs, indomethacin, other potassium-sparing diuretics, potassium-containing drugs, potassium supplements, trimethoprim: Increased risk of severe hyperkalemia

aminoglycosides, cisplatin, NSAIDs: Increased risk of renal impairment

cholestyramine: Increased risk of hyperkalemic metabolic acidosis

digoxin: Possibly increased half-life of digoxin

exchange resins (sodium cycle), such as sodium polystyrene sulfonate: Increased risk of fluid retention and hypokalemia

heparin, oral anticoagulants: Decreased anticoagulant effect of these drugs

hypotension-producing drugs: Possibly potentiated antihypertensive or diuretic effect of spironolactone

lithium: Possibly lithium toxicity

NSAIDs, sympathomimetics: Decreased antihypertensive effect of spironolactone

FOODS

high potassium diet, low-salt milk, salt substitutes: Increased risk of severe hyperkalemia

Adverse Reactions

CNS: Ataxia, confusion, dizziness, drowsiness, **encephalopathy**, fatigue, fever, headache, lethargy, somnolence

CV: Hypotension, vasculitis

EENT: Increased intraocular pressure, nasal congestion, tinnitus, vision changes

Mechanism of Action

Normally, aldosterone attaches to receptors on the walls of distal convoluted tubule cells, causing sodium (Na^+) and water (H_2O) reabsorption in the blood, as shown at left. Spironolactone competes with aldosterone for these receptors, thereby preventing sodium and water reabsorption and causing their excretion through the distal convoluted tubules, as shown below right. Increased urinary excretion of sodium and water reduces blood volume and blood pressure.

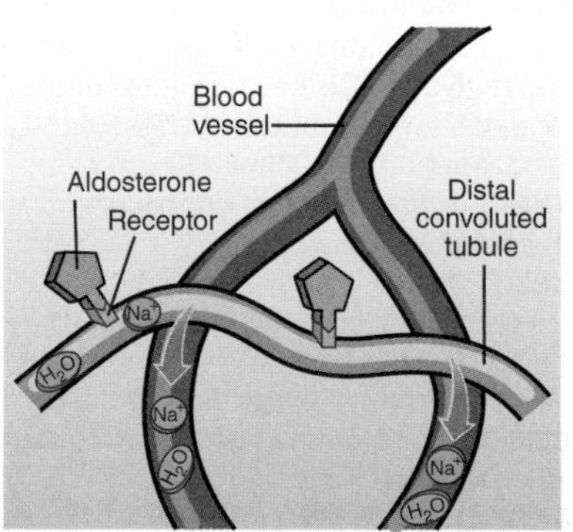

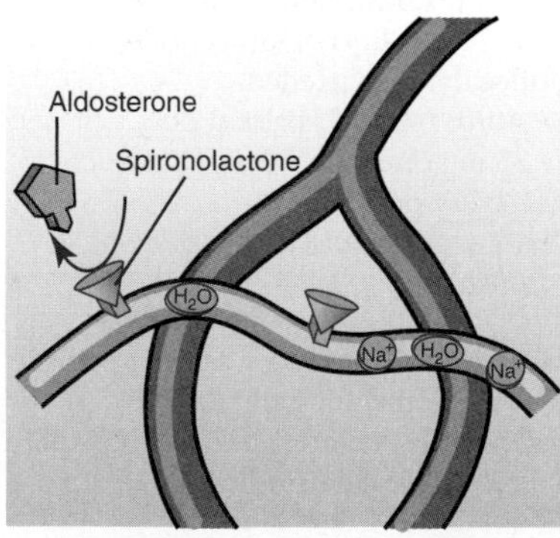

ENDO: Breast or nipple pain, gynecomastia, hyperglycemia
GI: Abdominal cramping or pain, anorexia, constipation, diarrhea, flatulence, **gastric bleeding** or ulceration, gastritis, **mixed cholestatic/hepatocellular toxicity**, nausea, vomiting
GU: Amenorrhea, decreased libido, impotence, irregular menses, postmenopausal bleeding, **renal failure**, worsening renal function
HEME: Agranulocytosis, **aplastic anemia**, **leukopenia**, **neutropenia**, **thrombocytopenia**
RESP: Cough, dyspnea
MS: Arthralgia, back and leg pain, leg cramps, muscle weakness, myalgia
SKIN: Alopecia, erythematous or maculopapular cutaneous eruptions, pruritus, **Stevens–Johnson syndrome**, **toxic epidermal necrolysis**, urticaria
Other: Anaphylaxis, dehydration, **drug reaction with eosinophilia and systemic symptoms (DRESS)**, **hyperkalemia**, hyperuricemia, **hypocalcemia**, **hypochloremic metabolic alkalosis**, **hypomagnesemia**, **hyponatremia**

Nursing Considerations

- Be aware that for patients who have trouble swallowing, pharmacist may crush spironolactone tablets, mix with flavored syrup, and dispense as a suspension. It's stable for 1 month when refrigerated.
- Know that in diagnosing primary aldosteronism, test is considered positive if patient's serum potassium level rises when spironolactone is given and falls when it's discontinued.
- Expect to evaluate patient's serum potassium level 1 week after spironolactone therapy begins, after each dosage adjustment, monthly for the first 3 months, quarterly for 1 year, and then every 6 months thereafter or as ordered. Notify prescriber if level exceeds 5 mEq/L or patient's renal function deteriorates (serum creatinine level exceeding 4 mg/dl). If patient has severe heart failure, know that potassium supplementation should be discontinued and patient followed closely, because hyperkalemia may be fatal in such patients.
- Evaluate spironolactone's effectiveness by assessing blood pressure and presence and degree of edema.
- Stop drug for several days, as prescribed, before patient undergoes adrenal vein catheterization to measure serum aldosterone level and plasma renin activity.
- Monitor patients with renal impairment closely because risk of adverse reactions is greater in these patients, as well as the elderly, because spironolactone is substantially excreted by the kidneys. Also be aware that patients with impaired renal function are at higher risk for hyperkalemia.

WARNING Monitor patient with hepatic impairment, especially if patient has ascites and cirrhosis, because spironolactone can cause sudden alterations in fluid and electrolyte balance which may cause coma, impaired neurological function, or worsening hepatic encephalopathy. Be aware that patients with hepatic impairment accompanied by ascites and cirrhosis should be given spironolactone initially in a hospital setting.

PATIENT TEACHING

- Instruct patient to take spironolactone with meals or milk.
- Tell patient who can't swallow tablets that drug is available as a suspension.
- Teach patient who takes spironolactone for hypertension how to measure his blood pressure. Urge him to monitor it regularly and report pressure greater than 140 mm Hg systolic or 90 mm Hg diastolic to prescriber.
- Caution patient that he may experience dizziness during spironolactone therapy if fluid balance is altered.
- Warn patient to avoid performing hazardous activities, such as driving, until adverse effects of drug are known.
- Instruct patient to inform prescriber of any new condition or new drug therapy, including over-the-counter medications so that prescriber can evaluate if the patient is at increased risk for hyperkalemia.
- Advise women to report suspected or known pregnancy to prescriber.

- Alert patient that there is a potential risk to the fetus if it is male because of the drug's anti-androgenic properties. Encourage her to use effective contraceptive measures throughout spironolactone therapy.

stavudine

Zerit

Class and Category

Pharmacologic class: Nucleoside analogue
Therapeutic class: Antiretroviral
Pregnancy category: C

Indications and Dosages

➤ *As adjunct to treat human immunodeficiency virus type 1 (HIV-1) infection*

CAPSULES, ORAL SOLUTION

Adults and children weighing at least 60 kg (132 lb). 40 mg every 12 hr.
Adults weighing less than 60 kg (132 lb) and children weighing at least 30 kg (66 lb) to less than 60 kg (132 lb). 30 mg every 12 hr.
Neonates at least 14 days old and children weighing less than 30 kg (66 lb). 1 mg/kg every 12 hr.
Neonates from birth to 13 days old. 0.5 mg/kg every 12 hr.

DOSAGE ADJUSTMENT For adults with a creatinine clearance between 26 and 50 ml/min and weighing at least 60 kg (132 lb), dosage reduced to 20 mg every 12 hr and if weighing less than 60 kg (132 lb), dosage reduced to 15 mg every 12 hr. For adults with a creatinine clearance between 10 and 25 ml/min and weighing at least 60 kg (132 lb), dosage reduced and interval increased to 20 mg every 24 hr and for adults weighing less than 60 kg (132 lb), dosage reduced and interval increased to 15 mg every 24 hr. For patients on hemodialysis, dosage and interval are the same as for patients with a creatinine clearance of 10 to 25 ml/min, but dosage is administered after the completion of hemodialysis on dialysis days and at the same time of day on nondialysis days. There are no specific recommendations for children with renal insufficiency.

Mechanism of Action

Inhibits the activity of HIV-1 reverse transcriptase by competing with the natural substrate thymidine triphosphate to cause DNA chain termination following its incorporation into viral DNA. It also inhibits selective cellular DNA polymerases to markedly reduce the synthesis of mitochondrial DNA.

Contraindications

Concomitant therapy with zidovudine, hypersensitivity to stavudine or its components

Interactions

DRUGS

doxorubicin, ribavirin: Possibly interfere with action of stavudine and its effectiveness
zidovudine: Interferes with action of stavudine, potentially rendering it ineffective

ACTIVITIES

alcohol use: Increased risk of liver damage or pancreatitis

Adverse Reactions

CNS: Chills, fever, headache, insomnia, motor weakness (severe), peripheral neurologic symptoms including neuropathy
ENDO: Cushingoid appearance, diabetes mellitus, fat redistribution, hyperglycemia
GI: Abdominal pain, anorexia, diarrhea, elevated liver and pancreatic enzymes, **hepatic failure or toxicity**, **hepatomegaly with steatosis** that may become severe, hyperlactatemia (symptomatic), nausea, **pancreatitis**, vomiting
HEME: Anemia, **leukopenia**, macrocytosis, **neutropenia**, **thrombocytopenia**
MS: Myalgia
SKIN: Rash
Other: Immune reconstitution syndrome, **hypersensitivity reactions**, **lactic acidosis**, lipoatrophy, lipodystrophy

Nursing Considerations

- Know that when stavudine is used with other agents with similar toxicities, the incidence of these toxicities may be higher than when stavudine is used alone. For example, use with didanosine may increase risk of hepatotoxicity, pancreatitis, and severe peripheral neuropathy. Know that the combination of didanosine and stavudine should be used with caution during pregnancy and is recommended only if the potential benefit clearly outweighs the potential risk.

- Know that extreme caution is needed when administering stavudine with patients with known risk factors for liver disease, because of increased risk of liver abnormalities that may become severe or even fatal. Be aware that the combination of stavudine along with didanosine and hydroxyurea should be avoided, because of increased risk of hepatotoxicity and hepatic failure that may result in death. Monitor liver enzymes and patient for evidence of worsening liver dysfunction. If present, notify prescriber and expect drug therapy to be interrupted or discontinued.

WARNING Monitor patient closely for signs and symptoms of symptomatic hyperlactatemia or lactic acidosis syndrome which may be severe, such as gastrointestinal (abdominal pain, nausea, vomiting, or unexplained weight loss), generalized fatigue, neurologic symptoms such as motor weakness, and respiratory symptoms (dyspnea, tachypnea). Although being of female gender, having prolonged nucleoside exposure, or obesity increases risk, patients without these risk factors have also developed lactic acidosis and severe hepatomegaly with steatosis. Notify prescriber immediately if patient becomes symptomatic or has laboratory values suggestive of lactic acidosis, pronounced hepatotoxicity, or symptomatic hyperlactatemia. Know that hepatomegaly and steatosis may occur without marked transaminase elevations. If confirmed, expect drug to be discontinued.

- Monitor patient for peripheral neuropathy. Know that motor weakness may mimic Guillain–Barré syndrome, including respiratory failure requiring drug to be discontinued immediately even though symptoms may continue or worsen after drug therapy has been stopped. Be aware that peripheral sensory neuropathy (numbness, pain, or tingling in feet or hands) most often occurs in patients with advanced HIV-1 disease or history of peripheral neuropathy, or in patients receiving other drugs that have been associated with neuropathy, including didanosine.
- Monitor patient for changes in appearance related to fat redistribution, such as the development of breast enlargement, central obesity, cushingoid appearance, dorsocervical fat enlargement (buffalo hump), and facial and peripheral wasting caused by antiretroviral therapy such as stavudine.
- Be aware that immune reconstitution syndrome has occurred in patients treated with combination antiretroviral therapy, including stavudine. The inflammatory response predisposes susceptible patients to opportunistic infections such as cytomegalovirus, *Mycobacterium avium* infection, *Pneumocystis jiroveci* pneumonia, or tuberculosis. Autoimmune disorders such as Graves' disease, Guillain–Barré syndrome, or polymyositis have also occurred. Report sudden or unusual adverse reactions to prescriber.

PATIENT TEACHING

- Advise patient to avoid missing doses of stavudine. If she misses a dose, she should take it as soon as she remembers, but should not double the next dose or take more than prescribed.

WARNING Inform patient about severe liver disease that may occur with stavudine. Tell her to report signs and symptoms of liver disease, such as acholic stools, anorexia, fatigue, malaise, nausea, tenderness over liver area, or yellowing of skin or whites of the eyes, and to seek immediate medical attention.

WARNING Instruct patient on early symptoms of lactic acidosis or symptomatic hyperlactatemia, such as abdominal discomfort, dyspnea, fatigue, nausea, motor weakness, unexplained weight loss, or vomiting. If present, tell patient to seek immediate medical attention, as drug may have to be discontinued.

- Warn patient to be alert for signs and symptoms of peripheral neuropathy such as numbness, pain, or tingling in feet or hands. If present, she should notify prescriber.
- Inform patient that stavudine therapy may cause changes in her body appearance because of fat redistribution. Prepare her

for the possibility of developing breast enlargement, central obesity, dorsocervical fat enlargement (buffalo hump), facial wasting, and peripheral wasting.
- Instruct patient to report any persistent, severe, or unusual signs and symptoms. Inform patient taking other drugs in combination with stavudine with similar adverse effects that the incidence of adverse reactions may be higher than when stavudine is used alone.
- Encourage women of childbearing age to report known or suspected pregnancy.
- Alert mothers that breastfeeding is not recommended during stavudine therapy.
- Tell patients with diabetes to monitor their blood glucose closely, as stavudine may increase blood glucose levels. Also tell patient taking oral solution that it contains 50 mg of sucrose (sugar) per ml.
- Warn patient to avoid alcohol intake while taking drug, because the combination may increase the risk of liver damage or pancreatitis.

streptomycin sulfate

Class and Category

Pharmacologic class: Aminoglycoside
Therapeutic class: Antibiotic
Pregnancy category: D

Indications and Dosages

➤ *To treat gram-negative bacillary bacteremia, meningeal infections, pneumonia, systemic infections, and UTI caused by susceptible strains of* Aerobacter aerogenes, Brucella, Calymmatobacterium granulomatis, Enterococcus faecalis, Escherichia coli, Haemophilus ducreyi, H. influenzae, Klebsiella pneumoniae, *and* Proteus

I.M. INJECTION

Adults. 1 to 2 g daily in divided doses every 6 to 12 hr. *Maximum:* 2 g daily.
Children. 20 to 40 mg/kg daily in divided doses every 6 to 12 hr.

➤ *As adjunct to treat endocarditis caused by* Streptococcus viridans *or* E. faecalis

I.M. INJECTION

Adults. 1 g twice daily for 1 wk (*S. viridans*) or 2 wk (*E. faecalis*) with penicillin. Then, 500 mg twice daily for 1 wk (*S. viridans*) or 4 wk (*E. faecalis*).

DOSAGE ADJUSTMENT For patients over 60 years of age being treated for streptococcal endocarditis, dosage reduced to 500 mg twice daily for entire 2 week period.

➤ *As adjunct to treat tuberculosis caused by* Mycobacterium tuberculosis

I.M. INJECTION

Adults. 15 mg/kg daily. *Maximum:* 1 g daily. Alternatively, 25 to 30 mg/kg twice weekly. *Maximum:* 1.5 g daily.
Children. 20 to 40 mg/kg daily. *Maximum:* 1 g daily. Alternatively, 25 to 30 mg/kg twice weekly. *Maximum:* 1.5 g daily.

➤ *To treat plague caused by* Yersinia pestis

I.M. INJECTION

Adults. 2 g daily in 2 equally divided doses for at least 10 days.
Children. 30 mg/kg daily in divided doses twice daily or three times a day for 10 days.

➤ *To treat tularemia caused by* Francisella tularensis

I.M. INJECTION

Adults. 1 to 2 g daily in divided doses for 7 to 14 days.

DOSAGE ADJUSTMENT If creatinine clearance is 50 to 80 ml/min dosage reduced to 7.5 mg/kg I.M. every 24 hr; if 10 to 49 ml/min 7.5 mg/kg I.M. every 24 to 72 hr; if less than 10 ml/min, 7.5 mg/kg I.M. every 72 to 96 hr.

Mechanism of Action

Binds to negatively charged sites on the bacteria's outer cell membrane, disrupting cell integrity. Streptomycin also binds to bacterial ribosomal subunits and inhibits protein synthesis. Both actions lead to bacterial cell death.

Incompatibilities

Don't mix streptomycin in same solution or administer through same I.V. line as other antibiotics.

Contraindications

Hypersensitivity to streptomycin, other aminoglycosides, or their components

Interactions

DRUGS

antimyasthenics: Possibly decreased effect of antimyasthenics on skeletal muscle
beta-lactam antibiotics: Inactivation of streptomycin

capreomycin, other aminoglycosides: Increased potential for nephrotoxicity, neuromuscular blockade, and ototoxicity
methoxyflurane, polymyxins (parenteral): Increased risk of nephrotoxicity and neuromuscular blockade
nephrotoxic and ototoxic drugs: Increased risk of nephrotoxicity and ototoxicity
neuromuscular blockers: Increased neuromuscular blockade

Adverse Reactions
CNS: Clumsiness, dizziness, **neurotoxicity**, paresthesia, peripheral neuropathy, **seizures**, unsteadiness, vertigo
EENT: Hearing loss, sensation of fullness in ears, tinnitus, vision loss
GI: Anorexia, nausea, thirst, vomiting
GU: Decreased or increased urine output, **nephrotoxicity**
MS: Muscle twitching
SKIN: Erythema, pruritus, rash, urticaria

Nursing Considerations
- Use streptomycin cautiously in patients with renal impairment. In severely uremic patients, single dose can produce high blood level of drug for several days; cumulative effects may produce ototoxicity.
- Expect prescriber to order baseline renal function studies and to assess cranial nerve VIII function (responsible for hearing) at start of streptomycin therapy to allow for later comparisons.
- Monitor serum peak and trough levels, as ordered, to ensure adequate, but not toxic, drug level.
- Be aware that streptomycin should be given only by I.M. injection.
- To reconstitute streptomycin, add between 4.2 and 4.5 ml of sodium chloride for injection or sterile water for injection to each 1-g vial to provide a concentration of 200 mg/ml, or add between 3.2 and 3.5 ml of diluent to each 5-g vial to provide a concentration of 250 mg/ml. Alternatively, add 6.5 ml of diluent to each 5-g vial to provide a concentration of 500 mg/ml.
- Don't give more than 500 mg/ml.
- Rotate injection sites to prevent sterile abscess formation.

PATIENT TEACHING
- Advise patient to refrigerate streptomycin solution at 2° to 8°C (36° to 46°F).
- Inform patient that treatment for tuberculosis lasts at least 1 year.
- Urge patient to notify prescriber if he has fullness or ringing in ears, hearing loss, or vertigo.

sucralfate
Carafate, Sulcrate (CAN)

Class and Category
Pharmacologic class: GI protectant
Therapeutic class: Antiulcer
Pregnancy category: B

Indications and Dosages
➤ *To prevent reoccurrence of duodenal ulcer*

ORAL SUSPENSION, TABLETS
Adults and adolescents. 1 g twice daily.

➤ *To treat active duodenal ulcer*

ORAL SUSPENSION, TABLETS
Adults. 1 g four times a day 1 hr before meals and at bedtime for 4 to 8 wk, possibly less.

Mechanism of Action
May react with hydrochloric acid in the stomach to form a complex that buffers acid. The complex adheres electrostatically to proteins on the ulcer's surface and creates a protective barrier at the ulcer site. Sucralfate also inhibits back-diffusion of hydrogen ions and adsorbs bile acids and pepsin, actions that promote healing of an existing duodenal ulcer and prevent reoccurring ulcer formation.

Interactions
DRUGS
aluminum-containing drugs (such as antacids, antidiarrheals, buffered aspirin with aluminum): Possibly aluminum toxicity in patients with renal failure
antacids: Possibly interference with binding of sucralfate to GI mucosa
cimetidine, ciprofloxacin, digoxin, norfloxacin, ofloxacin, phenytoin, ranitidine, tetracycline, theophylline: Decreased bioavailability of these drugs

Adverse Reactions
CNS: Dizziness, drowsiness, headache, insomnia, light-headedness, vertigo

EENT: Dry mouth
ENDO: Hyperglycemia
GI: Constipation, diarrhea, indigestion, nausea, vomiting
MS: Back pain
RESP: **Bronchospasm**, dyspnea
SKIN: Pruritus, rash, urticaria
OTHER: **Anaphylaxis, angioedema**

Nursing Considerations

- Use sucralfate cautiously in patients with chronic renal failure because of increased risk of aluminum toxicity.
- Administer drug to patient when he has an empty stomach.
- Monitor diabetic patient's blood glucose level closely because sucralfate may cause hyperglycemia significant enough to require an adjustment of antidiabetic drug therapy prescribed.

PATIENT TEACHING

- Instruct patient to take sucralfate on an empty stomach at least 1 hour before meals and at bedtime.
- Advise patient not to take antacids within 30 minutes of sucralfate.
- Caution patient to check with prescriber before taking another drug within 2 hours of sucralfate.

sucroferric oxyhydroxide

Velphoro

Class and Category

Pharmacologic class: Polynuclear iron(III) oxyhydroxide
Therapeutic class: Phosphate binder
Pregnancy category: B

Indications and Dosages

➤ *To control serum phosphorus levels in patients with chronic kidney disease on dialysis*

CHEWABLE TABLETS

Adults. *Initial:* 500 mg three times daily with meals, increasing or decreasing dosage in 500-mg increments weekly, as needed. *Maintenance:* 1,500 to 2,000 mg daily. *Maximum:* 3,000 mg daily.

Mechanism of Action

Phosphate binding takes place by ligand exchange between hydroxyl groups and/or water in sucroferric oxyhydroxide and phosphate in the diet. The bound phosphate is eliminated in feces. Both calcium phosphorus product levels and serum phosphorus levels are reduced as a consequence of the reduced dietary phosphate absorption.

Contraindications

Hypersensitivity to sucroferric oxyhydroxide or its components

Interactions

DRUGS

calcitriol, ciprofloxacin, digoxin, doxycycline, enalapril, furosemide, HMG-CoA reductase inhibitors, hydrochlorothiazide, levothyroxine, losartan, metoprolol, nifedipine, omeprazole, quinidine, warfarin: Absorption of these drugs may be affected

Adverse Reactions

EENT: Abnormal drug distaste, tooth discoloration
GI: Dark-colored feces, diarrhea, nausea
SKIN: Rash

Nursing Considerations

- Give sucroferric oxyhydroxide with meals and administer all other oral drugs prescribed for the patient at a different time because absorption of the other drugs may be affected.
- Monitor patient's serum phosphorus levels regularly, as ordered, to determine drug effectiveness and need for dosage adjustments.
- Monitor patients who have a history of hemochromatosis or other diseases characterized by iron accumulation, patients who develop peritonitis during peritoneal dialysis, and patients with significant gastric or hepatic disorders or following major gastrointestinal surgery, because sucroferric oxyhydroxide effects on these conditions are not known.

Patient Teaching

- Instruct patient to take sucroferric oxyhydroxide with meals.
- Tell patient tablets must be chewed and not swallowed whole. Tell him the tablets

may be crushed to aid chewing and swallowing them.
- Inform patient that drug may cause discolored (black) stool but this effect is harmless. Inform patient that drug may also stain teeth.
- Instruct patient to take any concomitant drug therapy at least 2 hours before sucroferric oxyhydroxide.
- Tell patient to report any rash to prescriber.

sufentanil

Dsuvia

Class, Category, and Schedule

Pharmacologic class: Opioid agonist
Therapeutic class: Opioid analgesic
Pregnancy category: Not classified
Controlled substance schedule: II

Indications and Dosages

➤ *To relieve acute pain severe enough to require an opioid analgesic and for which alternative treatments are inadequate in a medically supervised healthcare setting, such as emergency departments, hospitals, and surgical centers*

SUBLINGUAL TABLETS
Adults. 30 mcg, as needed, with a minimum of 1 hr between doses. *Maximum:* 360 mcg or 12 tablets in 24 hr, and not for use for more than 72 hr.

Mechanism of Action

Binds to and activates selective mu-opioid receptors found throughout the central nervous system to produce pain relief.

Contraindications

Acute or severe bronchial asthma in an unmonitored setting or in the absence of resuscitative equipment, gastrointestinal obstruction including paralytic ileus, hypersensitivity to sufentanil or its components, significant respiratory depression

Interactions

DRUGS
5-HT3 inhibitors (used to treat psychiatric disorders), linezolid, methylene blue (intravenous), MAO inhibitors, selective serotonin reuptake inhibitors, serotonin and norepinephrine reuptake inhibitors, tricyclic antidepressants, triptans: Increased risk of serotonin syndrome
anticholinergic drugs: Possibly increased risk of urinary retention and/or severe constipation, which may lead to paralytic ileus
benzodiazepines and other CNS depressants: Increased risk of serious adverse reactions such as coma, hypotension, profound sedation, and severe respiratory depression
CYP3A4 inducers such as carbamazepine, phenytoin, rifampin: Decreased plasma concentration of sufentanil, resulting in decreased efficacy or possible withdrawal symptoms in patients who have developed physical dependence to sufentanil
CYP3A4 inhibitors such as azole-antifungal agents, macrolide antibiotics, and protease inhibitors (ritonavir): Increased plasma concentration of sufentanil, resulting in increased or prolonged effects
diuretics: Reduced efficacy of diuretics
mixed agonist/antagonist or partial agonist opioid analgesics such as buprenorphine, butorphanol, nalbuphine, pentazocine: Possibly reduced analgesic effect of sufentanil and possible precipitation of withdrawal symptoms
muscle relaxants: Possibly enhanced neuromuscular blocking action of skeletal muscle relaxants; increased degree of respiratory depression

ACTIVITIES
alcohol use: Increased risk of serious adverse reactions such as coma, hypotension, profound sedation, and severe respiratory depression

Adverse Reactions

CNS: Agitation, anxiety, confusion, disorientation, dizziness, euphoric mood, hallucination, headache, hemiparesis, insomnia, lethargy, memory impairment, mental status changes, **seizures**, **serotonin syndrome**, somnolence, syncope
CV: Bradycardia, **electrocardiogram abnormalities,** hypertension, **hypotension (severe)**, orthostatic hypotension, tachycardia
EENT: Oral hypoesthesia
ENDO: Adrenal insufficiency

GI: Abdominal distention or pain, belching, constipation, diarrhea, dyspepsia, elevated liver enzymes, flatulence, gastritis, nausea, postoperative ileus, vomiting
GU: Decreased urine output, oliguria, **renal failure**, urinary hesitation or retention
MS: Muscle spasms
RESP: Apnea, atelectasis, bradypnea, decreased oxygen saturation and respiratory rate, hypoventilation, hypoxia, life-threatening respiratory depression, respiratory distress or failure
SKIN: Diaphoresis, flushing, pruritus, rash
Other: Anaphylaxis, physiological and physical dependence

Nursing Considerations

- Be aware that excessive use of sufentanil may lead to abuse, addiction, misuse, overdose, and possibly death. Know that sufentanil is available only through a restricted Risk Evaluation and Mitigation Strategy (REMS) program. Monitor patient's intake of drug closely. Alert prescriber if patient has a history of dependence on other opioids.
- Know that drug is only administered in a healthcare setting and never self-administered by patient.
- Use extreme caution when administering sufentanil to patients with significant chronic obstructive pulmonary disease or cor pulmonale, and to patients having a substantially decreased respiratory reserve, hypercapnia, hypoxia, or preexisting respiratory depression, especially when initiating or titrating therapy. These patients may develop respiratory depression, even with usual therapeutic doses, because sufentanil may decrease patient's respiratory drive to the point of apnea.
- Use sufentanil cautiously in cachectic, debilitated, or elderly patients, especially when initiating and titrating therapy, as these patients are at increased risk for adverse effects, especially respiratory depression.
- Put on gloves and tear open the notched pouch only when ready to administer sufentanil. Be aware that the pouch contains one clear plastic single-dose applicator (SDA) that houses a single blue-colored tablet in the tip. Remove the white lock from the green pusher by squeezing the sides together and detaching from pusher. To avoid accidentally ejecting the tablet, avoid touching the green pusher before placing the SDA in patient's mouth for administration. To administer, tell patient to open mouth and touch the tongue to the roof of the mouth, if possible. Rest the SDA lightly on patient's lips or lower teeth. Place the SDA tip under the tongue and aim at the floor of patient's mouth or sublingual space. Avoid direct mucosal contact with the SDA tip. Gently depress the green pusher to deliver the tablet to patient's sublingual space. Visually confirm tablet placement. Be aware that if tablet is not in patient's mouth, it must be retrieved and disposed of according to institutional CII waste procedures. Discard the used SDA in biohazard waste container after administration.

WARNING **Monitor patient for respiratory depression that could become life-threatening quickly, especially when drug is initiated or if patient is accidently exposed to drug. However, know that respiratory depression may occur at any time during sufentanil use and may occur even when used as recommended. If patient develops respiratory depression, expect to give naloxone. Watch for seizures, because naloxone may increase this risk. Take seizure precautions.**

- Be aware that sufentanil may increase the frequency of seizures in patients with seizure disorders and may increase risk of seizures in the presence of other conditions associated with seizures. Monitor patient closely.
- Be aware that opioids like sufentanil should not be given to women during pregnancy, while in labor, or when breastfeeding, as newborn or infant may experience neonatal opioid withdrawal syndrome (NOWS). This syndrome may exhibit as excessive or high-pitched crying, poor feeding, rapid breathing, or trembling. If not recognized and treated appropriately, it can become life-threatening.
- Monitor patients closely who may be susceptible to the intracranial effects of carbon dioxide retention from respiratory

depression caused by sufentanil therapy, such as patients with head injuries or those who have a preexisting elevation in intracranial pressure.

WARNING Know that many drugs may interact with opioids like sufentanil to cause serotonin syndrome. Monitor patient closely for signs and symptoms such as agitation, diaphoresis, diarrhea, fever, hallucinations, labile blood pressure, muscle twitching or stiffness, nausea, shakiness, shivering, tachycardia, trouble with coordination, or vomiting. Notify prescriber at once, because serotonin syndrome may be life-threatening. Be prepared to discontinue drug, if possible and ordered, and provide supportive care.

- Monitor effectiveness of sufentanil in relieving pain; consult prescriber as needed.
- Assess patient for constipation and provide a high-fiber diet and adequate fluid intake, if not contraindicated, because constipation can become severe.
- Monitor patient for evidence of physical dependence or abuse. Know that addiction can occur not only in those who obtain drug illicitly but also in patients who are appropriately prescribed drug at recommended doses. Be aware that excessive use of sufentanil may lead to abuse, addiction, misuse, overdose, and possibly death.
- Notify prescriber if serious adverse reactions occur with sufentanil therapy and expect dosage to be reduced.
- Monitor patient's vital signs closely. Know that in addition to respiratory depression, sufentanil may cause severe hypotension, especially in patients whose blood pressure is already compromised by a depleted blood volume or after concurrent administration of drugs that decrease blood pressure. Also be aware that the drug may cause bradycardia in some patients.
- Be aware that concomitant use with CYP3A4 inhibitors or discontinuation of CYP3A inducers can result in a fatal overdose of sufentanil.
- Monitor patient for adrenal insufficiency. Although rare, it can be life-threatening. Monitor patient for anorexia, dizziness, fatigue, hypotension, nausea, vomiting, or weakness. Notify prescriber if adrenal insufficiency is suspected and expect diagnostic testing to be done. If diagnosis is confirmed, expect to administer corticosteroids and discontinue sufentanil.
- Monitor patient for decreased bowel motility in postoperative patients receiving sufentanil, as drug may obscure the development of acute abdominal conditions.

WARNING Be aware that sufentanil should only be used concomitantly with benzodiazepine therapy in patients for whom other treatment options are inadequate. If prescribed together, expect dosing and duration of sufentanil to be limited. Monitor patient closely for signs and symptoms of a decrease in consciousness, including coma, profound sedation, and significant respiratory depression. Notify prescriber immediately and provide emergency supportive care, as death may occur.

PATIENT TEACHING

- Instruct patient to allow sufentanil tablet to dissolve under the tongue and not to chew or swallow the tablet. Also advise patient not to drink or eat and to minimize talking for 10 minutes after each dose of the drug.
- Warn patient of possibility of addiction even when taken as prescribed.
- Alert patient that respiratory depression may occur with sufentanil use, especially when drug is first given, and to report any breathing difficulties immediately.
- Warn patient to keep sufentanil away from the reach of children, as accidental consumption of even one tablet can cause significant respiratory depression and death.
- Caution patient to avoid having alcohol or other drugs brought to him in the healthcare setting because ingesting alcohol, including medications containing alcohol, increases the risk of overdose, respiratory depression, and death, as does taking other types of depressants, including benzodiazepines, together with sufentanil therapy.
- Advise women of childbearing age to notify prescriber if pregnancy is known or suspected, because a fetus exposed to sufentanil while in utero may require

treatment for neonatal opioid withdrawal syndrome (NOWS) when born. Also advise women not to breastfeed while taking sufentanil.

- Instruct patient to rise slowly from a lying or sitting position and to lie or sit down if he experiences light-headedness. If effect is frequent or severe, tell him to notify prescriber.
- Urge patient to consume plenty of fluids and high-fiber foods, if not contraindicated, to prevent constipation.

sulfadiazine

Class and Category

Pharmacologic class: Sulfonamide
Therapeutic class: Antibiotic
Pregnancy category: C

Indications and Dosages

➤ *As adjunct to treat chloroquine-resistant malaria,* Haemophilus influenzae *acute otitis media (with penicillin) or meningitis (with streptomycin), or toxoplasmosis encephalitis (with pyrimethamine); to prevent or treat meningococcal meningitis; to treat chancroid, inclusive conjunctivitis, nocardiosis, or trachoma; to treat urinary tract infections caused by* Enterobacter *species,* Escherichia coli, Klebsiella *species,* Proteus mirabilis, P. vulgaris, and Staphylococcus aureus *after failure with other sulfonamides*

TABLETS

Adults. *Initial:* 2 to 4 g. *Maintenance:* 2 to 4 g daily, divided into 3 to 6 doses.
Infants age 2 months and over and children. *Initial:* 75 mg/kg. *Maintenance:* 150 mg/kg daily divided into 4 to 6 doses. *Maximum:* 6 g daily.

➤ *To prevent rheumatic fever*

TABLETS

Children weighing more than 30 kg (66 lb). 1 g daily.
Children weighing less than 30 kg (66 lb). 500 mg daily.

Mechanism of Action

Inhibits para-aminobenzoic acid, a bacterial enzyme responsible for synthesizing folic acid, which susceptible bacteria require for growth. By inactivating bacteria, sulfadiazine prevents or alleviates infection.

Contraindications

Breastfeeding; hypersensitivity to sulfadiazine, its components, or other chemically related drugs, such as sulfonamides; infants under the age of two months except as adjunctive treatment for congenital toxoplasmosis; pregnancy at term

Interactions

DRUGS

bone marrow depressants such as methotrexate: Increased risk of leukopenic or thrombocytopenic effects
cyclosporine: Decreased blood cyclosporine level, increased risk of nephrotoxicity
estrogen-containing oral contraceptives: Increased risk of breakthrough bleeding and pregnancy
hemolytics: Increased risk of adverse effects
hepatotoxic drugs: Increased risk of hepatotoxicity
hydantoins, oral anticoagulants, oral antidiabetic drugs: Increased or prolonged effects of these drugs, possibly toxicity
indomethacin, probenecid, salicylates: Increased blood level of free sulfadiazine
phenylbutazone, sulfinpyrazone: Increased blood sulfadiazine level
uricosuric drugs: Potentiated uricosuric action

Adverse Reactions

CNS: Dizziness, fatigue, fever, headache, lethargy, weakness
EENT: Pharyngitis
GI: Anorexia, diarrhea, dysphagia, jaundice, nausea, vomiting
GU: Crystalluria
HEME: Agranulocytosis, aplastic anemia, hemolytic anemia, leukopenia, thrombocytopenia, unusual bleeding or bruising
MS: Arthralgia, myalgia
SKIN: Blisters, erythema, pallor, photosensitivity, pruritus, rash
Other: Drug-induced fever

Nursing Considerations

- Use sulfadiazine cautiously in patients with blood dyscrasias or megaloblastic anemia from folate deficiency because drug may cause blood dyscrasias; in those with G6PD deficiency because hemolysis may occur; in those with hepatic or renal impairment because of increased risk of toxicity; and in those with porphyria because drug may precipitate an acute attack.

- Obtain blood sample for CBC and body tissue or fluid specimen for culture and sensitivity tests, as ordered, before giving drug. Expect first dose to be given before results are available.

WARNING Monitor patient for drug-induced fever, which may develop 7 to 10 days after starting sulfadiazine therapy. Signs and symptoms may include abdominal pain, anorexia, ataxia, depression, diarrhea, headache, insomnia, nausea, peripheral neuropathy, tinnitus, and vomiting.

- Monitor fluid intake and output during therapy. Altered fluid balance may increase risk of crystalluria.
- Monitor patient's blood glucose level, and assess for signs and symptoms of hypoglycemia in patients who take an oral antidiabetic drug. Be prepared to respond if hypoglycemia develops.

PATIENT TEACHING

- Instruct patient to take sulfadiazine exactly as prescribed and to complete the full course, even if he feels better.
- Advise patient to take drug with a full glass of water and to drink plenty of fluids during therapy.
- Urge patient to notify prescriber if urine turns reddish brown; this may indicate crystalluria.
- Inform patient about possible dizziness, and urge him to avoid potentially hazardous activities until drug's CNS effects are known.
- Advise patient to avoid prolonged exposure to sunlight and to wear sunscreen and protective clothing when outdoors.
- Urge patient who takes oral contraceptives to use an additional method of birth control during therapy.
- Advise patient who takes an oral antidiabetic drug to check his blood glucose level frequently because of the increased risk of hypoglycemia during therapy.

sulfasalazine

Azulfidine, Azulfidine EN-Tabs, Salazopyrin, Salazopyrin EN-Tabs (CAN)

Class and Category

Pharmacologic class: Salicylate-sulfonamide
Therapeutic class: Anti-inflammatory
Pregnancy category: B

Indications and Dosages

➤ *To treat mild-to-moderate ulcerative colitis; as adjunct to treat severe ulcerative colitis; to prolong remission period between acute attacks of ulcerative colitis*

DELAYED-RELEASE TABLETS, TABLETS

Adults and adolescents. *Initial:* 500 to 1,000 mg every 6 to 8 hr. *Maintenance:* 500 mg every 6 hr.

Children age 6 and over. *Initial:* 40 to 60 mg/kg daily divided into 3 to 6 doses. *Maintenance:* 30 mg/kg daily divided into 4 doses.

➤ *To treat rheumatoid arthritis in patients who have not responded to salicylates or other NSAIDs*

DELAYED-RELEASE TABLETS

Adults. *Initial:* 500 to 1,000 mg daily during wk 1, increased by 500 mg daily every wk, as needed, up to 2,000 mg daily in divided doses. If no response after 12 wk, increased to 3,000 mg daily. *Maintenance:* 1,000 mg every 12 hr. *Maximum:* 3,000 mg daily.

➤ *To treat juvenile rheumatoid arthritis in patients who have not responded to salicylates or other NSAIDs*

DELAYED-RELEASE TABLETS

Children ages 6 and over. 30 to 50 mg/kg daily in divided doses twice daily. *Maximum:* 2 g daily.

DOSAGE ADJUSTMENT For patients with ulcerative colitis, initial dosage may be reduced if GI intolerance occurs. For adult patients with rheumatoid arthritis as a means to reduce possible GI intolerance, initial dosage may be reduced to 0.5 to 1 g daily and then increased weekly as needed. For children with juvenile rheumatoid arthritis as a means to reduce possible GI intolerance, initial dosage may be reduced to one-quarter to one-third of expected maintenance dose and then gradually increased weekly to reach maintenance dose.

Mechanism of Action

As a prodrug of sulfapyridine and 5-aminosalicylic acid (mesalamine), delivers more sulfapyridine and mesalamine to the colon than either metabolite could provide alone. Sulfapyridine provides antibacterial action along the intestinal wall; mesalamine inhibits cyclooxygenase, thereby decreasing the production of arachidonic acid metabolites and reducing colonic inflammation. It also reduces joint inflammation locally caused by rheumatoid arthritis.

Contraindications

Hypersensitivity to salicylates, sulfasalazine, sulfonamides, chemically related drugs, or their components; intestinal or urinary obstruction; porphyria

Interactions

DRUGS

bone marrow depressants: Increased leukopenic and thrombocytopenic effects of both drugs
digoxin: Possibly inhibited absorption and decreased blood level of digoxin
folic acid (vitamin B_9): Decreased folic acid absorption
hepatotoxic drugs: Increased risk of hepatotoxicity
hydantoins, oral anticoagulants, oral antidiabetic drugs: Increased, prolonged, or toxic effects of these drugs
methotrexate, phenylbutazone, sulfinpyrazone: Possibly potentiated effects of these drugs

Adverse Reactions

CNS: Ataxia, chills, depression, fatigue, fever, **Guillain–Barré syndrome**, headache, insomnia, **meningitis**, peripheral neuropathy, **seizures**, vertigo, weakness
CV: Myocarditis, **pericarditis**, vasculitis
EENT: Hearing loss, orange-yellow tears, oropharyngeal pain, pharyngitis, tinnitus
GI: Abdominal pain, anorexia, **cirrhosis**, diarrhea, elevated liver enzymes, **hepatitis**, **hepatotoxicity**, indigestion, jaundice, nausea, **pancreatitis**, ulcerative colitis exacerbation, vomiting
GU: Crystalluria, decreased ejaculatory volume, male infertility, **nephritis**, nephrolithiasis, **nephrotic syndrome**, orange-yellow urine, **toxic nephrosis**
HEME: Agranulocytosis, **aplastic anemia**, **hemolytic anemia**, **hematophagic histiocytosis**, **leukopenia**, **neutropenia**, **thrombocytopenia**, **unusual bleeding** or bruising
MS: Arthralgia, **rhabdomyolysis**
RESP: Cyanosis, **eosinophilic infiltration**, **idiopathic pulmonary fibrosis**, **lymphocytic interstitial pneumonitis**, pleuritis pneumonia
SKIN: Alopecia, **erythema multiforme**, **exfoliative dermatitis**, photosensitivity, pruritus, purpura, rash, **Stevens–Johnson syndrome**, **toxic epidermal necrolysis**, urticaria
Other: Anaphylaxis, **angioedema**, **drug rash with eosinophilia and systemic symptoms (DRESS)**, folate deficiency, infections (serious), lupus erythematosus-like syndrome, mononucleosis-like syndrome, **sepsis**, serum sickness syndrome

Nursing Considerations

- Use sulfasalazine cautiously in patients with a history of recurring or chronic infections because drug may predispose patient to infections. Monitor patients for new infections throughout therapy. If present, notify prescriber.
- Monitor BUN and serum creatinine levels, CBC, and liver enzymes, before and periodically during prolonged sulfasalazine therapy.
- Be aware that sulfasalazine doses over 4 g or a blood level over 50 mcg/ml increases the risk of adverse and toxic reactions.
- Monitor fluid intake and output and urine color, consistency, and pH. Acidic urine may require alkalization to prevent crystalluria.
- Be aware that measurements, by liquid chromatography, of urinary normetanephrine may cause a false-positive test result.

WARNING Monitor patient, especially during the first month of sulfasalazine therapy, for hypersensitivity reactions that may become life-threatening. At first sign of mucosal lesions, rash, or any other sign of hypersensitivity, stop sulfasalazine therapy and notify prescriber.

PATIENT TEACHING

- Instruct patient to take sulfasalazine with an antacid, meals, or milk to decrease GI distress, and to swallow tablets whole.
- Advise patient to prevent crystalluria by taking drug with a full glass of water and drinking at least 64 oz of fluid per day.
- Instruct patient and family to administer drug around the clock.
- Inform patient that symptom relief may take 2 to 5 days for ulcerative colitis and 4 to 12 weeks for rheumatoid arthritis.
- Alert patient that drug may turn skin and urine orange-yellow.
- Advise contact lens wearer to consider wearing glasses during therapy because drug can permanently stain contact lenses yellow.
- Instruct patient to avoid prolonged sun exposure and to wear protective clothing and sunscreen when outdoors.
- Advise patient to brush with a soft-bristled toothbrush and to use dental floss and toothpicks gently because leukopenic and thrombocytopenic drug effects increase risk of gingival bleeding and infection.
- Urge patient to return for laboratory tests and follow-up visits to monitor drug's effect.
- Instruct patient to report fever; jaundice; paleness; skin abnormalities such as skin blistering, discoloration, rash or hives; or sore throat. These may be signs of serious adverse effects. Explain that prescriber may order tests to determine their cause and that drug may be discontinued until test results are known.
- Instruct mothers who are breastfeeding to stop taking sulfasalazine or stop breastfeeding immediately if their infant develops bloody stools or diarrhea, and to notify prescriber.

sulindac

Clinoril

Class and Category

Pharmacologic class: NSAID
Therapeutic class: Analgesic, anti-inflammatory
Pregnancy category: C

Indications and Dosages

➤ *To decrease pain and inflammation in ankylosing spondylitis, acute attacks of gout or pseudogout, bursitis, moderately painful arthralgia, osteoarthritis, rheumatoid arthritis, and tendinitis*

TABLETS

Adults. *Initial:* 150 to 200 mg twice daily, adjusted based on patient's response. *Maximum:* 200 mg twice daily.

➤ *To relieve symptoms of acute gouty arthritis, acute subacromial bursitis, and supraspinatus tendinitis*

TABLETS

Adults. 200 mg twice daily for 7 to 14 days; decreased to lowest effective dosage after satisfactory response occurs.

DOSAGE ADJUSTMENT For elderly patients, dosage reduced to 50% of usual adult dosage, if needed.

Route	Onset	Peak	Duration
P.O.	In 1 wk*	2–3 wk*	Unknown

* For antirheumatic effects; unknown for antigout or anti-inflammatory effects.

Mechanism of Action

May block the activity of cyclooxygenase, an enzyme needed to synthesize prostaglandins, which mediate the inflammatory response that cause local vasodilation, pain, and swelling. By blocking cyclooxygenase and inhibiting prostaglandins, this NSAID reduces inflammatory symptoms and pain.

Contraindications

Angioedema, asthma, bronchospasm, nasal polyps, rhinitis, or urticaria induced by aspirin, iodides, or other NSAIDs; hypersensitivity to sulindac, other NSAIDs, and their components

Interactions

DRUGS

acetaminophen, cyclosporine, gold compounds, nephrotoxic drugs: Increased risk of adverse renal effects

angiotensin-converting enzyme (ACE) inhibitors, angiotensin II antagonists: Decreased antihypertensive effect of these drugs; increased risk of renal impairment in patients with already compromised renal function

antacids: Decreased blood level and effects of sulindac
antihypertensives: Risk of decreased antihypertensive effect
aspirin, salicylates: Decreased sulindac effects, increased risk of GI hemorrhage
bone marrow depressants: Increased risk of leukopenia and thrombocytopenia
cefamandole, cefoperazone, cefotetan, colchicine, oral anticoagulants, plicamycin, thrombolytics, valproic acid: Increased risk of bleeding
cimetidine, ranitidine: Increased bioavailability of both drugs
digoxin: Increased blood digoxin level and risk of digitalis toxicity
dimethyl sulfoxide (DMSO): Decreased sulindac effectiveness, possibly peripheral neuropathy with topical application of DMSO
diuretics: Possibly decreased loop diuretic effects and increased thiazide diuretic effects
glucocorticoids, other NSAIDs, potassium supplements: Increased risk of adverse GI effects
hydantoins: Increased blood hydantoin level and risk of phenytoin toxicity
insulin, oral antidiabetic drugs: Increased risk of hypoglycemia
lithium: Possibly increased blood level and toxic effects of lithium
methotrexate: Decreased methotrexate excretion, possibly leading to toxicity
platelet aggregation inhibitors: Increased risk of bleeding, additive effects of these drugs
probenecid: Increased blood level and adverse and toxic effects of sulindac

ACTIVITIES

alcohol use: Increased risk of adverse GI effects, including GI bleeding

Adverse Reactions

CNS: **Aseptic meningitis**, chills, **CVA**, drowsiness, fever, headache, malaise, nervousness, transient ischemic attack
CV: **Deep vein thrombosis**, edema, **heart failure**, hypertension, **MI**, palpitations, peripheral edema, vasculitis
EENT: Tinnitus
ENDO: **Hypoglycemia**
GI: Abdominal cramps or pain, anorexia, constipation, diarrhea, esophageal irritation, flatulence, gastritis, **GI bleeding** or ulceration, **hepatic failure**, **hepatitis**, **hepatotoxicity**, indigestion, jaundice, nausea, **perforation of intestines or stomach**, vomiting
GU: **Acute renal failure**, decreased urine output, interstitial nephritis, **nephrotic syndrome**, polyuria, proteinuria
HEME: **Agranulocytosis**, **aplastic anemia**, **leukopenia**, **pancytopenia**
RESP: **Bronchospasm**, dyspnea, **pulmonary edema**, wheezing
SKIN: Diaphoresis, **erythema multiforme**, **exfoliative dermatitis**, maculopapular rash, pruritus, purpura, **Stevens–Johnson syndrome**, **toxic epidermal necrolysis**, urticaria
Other: **Anaphylaxis**, **angioedema**, **hypersensitivity reactions**

Nursing Considerations

- Use sulindac with extreme caution in patients with a history of GI bleeding or ulcer disease because NSAIDs such as sulindac increase risk of GI bleeding and ulceration. Expect to use sulindac for the shortest time possible in these patients.
- Be aware that serious GI tract bleeding, perforation, and ulceration may occur without warning symptoms. Elderly patients are at greater risk. To minimize risk, give drug with food. If GI distress occurs, withhold drug and notify prescriber at once.
- Use sulindac cautiously in patients with hypertension, and monitor blood pressure closely throughout therapy. Drug may cause hypertension or worsen it.

WARNING Monitor patient closely for thrombotic events, including MI and stroke, because NSAIDs increase the risk.

- Be aware that if patient has systemic lupus erythematosus and mixed connective tissue disease, monitor him closely because sulindac increases the risk of aseptic meningitis.

WARNING Know that if patient has bone marrow suppression or is receiving antineoplastic drug therapy, monitor laboratory results (including WBC count), and watch for evidence of infection because anti-inflammatory and antipyretic actions of sulindac may mask signs and symptoms, such as fever and pain.

- Monitor patient closely, especially if patient is elderly or taking sulindac long

term, watch for less common but serious adverse GI reactions, including anorexia, constipation, diverticulitis, dysphagia, esophagitis, gastritis, gastroenteritis, gastroesophageal reflux disease, hemorrhoids, hiatal hernia, melena, stomatitis, and vomiting.
- Monitor liver enzymes because, in rare cases, elevated levels may progress to severe hepatic reactions, including fatal hepatitis, hepatic failure, and liver necrosis.
- Watch BUN and serum creatinine levels in elderly patients; those with heart failure, hepatic dysfunction, or impaired renal function; and those taking ACE inhibitors or diuretics; because drug may cause renal failure.
- Monitor CBC for decreased hemoglobin and hematocrit because drug may worsen anemia.
- Assess patient's skin routinely for rash or other signs of hypersensitivity reaction because sulindac and other NSAIDs may cause serious skin reactions without warning, even in patients with no history of NSAID hypersensitivity. Stop drug at first sign of reaction, and notify prescriber.

WARNING Monitor patient for adventitious breath sounds and dyspnea; sulindac may cause fluid retention, which may precipitate heart failure in susceptible patients.

- Expect patient to undergo audiometric examinations before and periodically during prolonged therapy, as ordered.

WARNING Monitor patient for evidence of hypersensitivity syndrome, which could become life-threatening. Report multiple occurring and multiorgan adverse reactions to prescriber and expect drug to be discontinued. Be prepared to provide emergency supportive care, as ordered.

PATIENT TEACHING

- Instruct patient to take sulindac exactly as prescribed. Explain that higher doses don't increase effectiveness and may increase risk of adverse reactions.
- Advise patient to crush tablet and mix with food, if needed, to aid in swallowing.
- Instruct patient to take drug with or immediately after meals to decrease GI distress, to take with a full glass of water, and to remain upright for 20 to 30 minutes after administration to prevent drug from lodging in esophagus and causing esophageal irritation.
- Urge patient to notify prescriber immediately of chills, fever, rash, or sweating, which may indicate hypersensitivity.
- Advise patient to consult prescriber before using acetaminophen, alcohol, aspirin, other NSAIDs, or any OTC drugs during sulindac therapy.
- Caution patient to avoid hazardous activities until drug's CNS effects are known.
- Explain the need for periodic laboratory tests and physical examinations during prolonged therapy to monitor drug effectiveness.
- Inform patient that sulindac may increase the risk of serious adverse cardiovascular reactions; urge patient to seek immediate medical attention if signs or symptoms arise, such as chest pain, shortness of breath, slurring of speech, or weakness.
- Tell patient that sulindac also may increase the risk of serious adverse GI reactions; stress the need to seek immediate medical attention for such signs and symptoms as abdominal or epigastric pain, black or tarry stools, indigestion, or vomiting blood or material that looks like coffee grounds.
- Alert patient to the possibility of rare but serious hypersensitivity reactions. Urge him to seek immediate medical attention for blisters, fever, itching, rash, or other indications of hypersensitivity.

sumatriptan succinate

Alsuma, Imitrex, Onzetra Xsail, Sumatriptan, Sumavel Dose Pro, Zembrace SymTouch

Class and Category

Pharmacologic class: Serotonin 5-HT_1-receptor agonist

Therapeutic class: Antimigraine
Pregnancy category: C

Indications and Dosages

➤ *To relieve acute migraine attacks, with or without aura*

TABLETS (SUMATRIPTAN)

Adults. 25 to 100 mg as a single dose as soon as possible after onset of symptoms, repeated every 2 hr, as needed. *Maximum:* 200 mg daily.

DOSAGE ADJUSTMENT For patients with mild-to-moderate hepatic dysfunction, 50 mg is maximum single dose.

SUBCUTANEOUS INJECTION (ZEMBRACE SYMTOUCH)

Adults. *Initial:* 3 mg, repeated after 1 hr, as needed. *Maximum:* 4 (3-mg) injections/24 hr with dosages separated by at least 1 hr.

SUBCUTANEOUS INJECTION (ALSUMA)

Adults. *Initial:* 6 mg, repeated after 1 or 2 hr, as needed. *Maximum:* 2 (6-mg) injections/24 hr with dosages separated by at least 1 hr. If migraine symptoms return after initial subcutaneous injection, 50 mg P.O. every 2 hr up to 200 mg daily.

SUBCUTANEOUS INJECTION (IMITREX, SUMAVEL DOSE PRO)

Adults. *Initial:* 1 to 6 mg (Imitrex) or 4 or 6 mg (Sumavel Dose Pro) depending on severity of headache, repeated after 1 hr, as needed, and only if response occurred to first dose. *Maximum:* 2 (6-mg) injections/24 hr with dosages separated by at least 1 hr.

NASAL SPRAY (SUMATRIPTAN)

Adults. 1 or 2 sprays (5 or 10 mg) into 1 nostril as a single dose or 1 spray (20 mg) into 1 nostril as a single dose. One additional dose may be taken if another attack occurs after at least 2 hr. *Maximum:* 40 mg daily.

NASAL POWDER (ONZETRA XSAIL)

Adults. 22 mg (1 11-mg nosepiece in each nostril) followed by 22 mg (1 11-mg nosepiece in each nostril) no sooner than 2 hr later if migraine not resolved or has returned. *Maximum:* 44 mg (4 nosepieces) daily with the 2 doses separated by at least 2 hr.

➤ *To relieve cluster headaches*

SUBCUTANEOUS INJECTION (IMITREX, SUMAVEL DOSE PRO)

Adults. *Initial:* 6 mg, repeated after 1 or 2 hr, as needed. *Maximum:* 2 (6-mg) injections/24 hr with dosages separated by at least 1 hr.

Route	Onset	Peak	Duration
P.O.	In 30 min	2–4 hr	Up to 24 hr
SubQ	In 10 min	1–2 hr	Up to 24 hr
Nasal	In 15 min	Unknown	Up to 24 hr

Mechanism of Action

May stimulate 5-HT_1 receptors, causing selective vasoconstriction of dilated and inflamed cranial blood vessels in carotid circulation, thus decreasing carotid arterial blood flow and relieving acute migraines and cluster headaches.

Contraindications

Basilar or hemiplegic migraine, cardiovascular disease, hypersensitivity to sumatriptan or its components, ischemic bowel disease, ischemic heart disease, peripheral vascular disease, Prinzmetal's angina, severe hepatic dysfunction, uncontrolled hypertension, use within 24 hours of ergotamine-containing or ergot-type drugs or another serotonin 5-HT_1 receptor agonist such as triptans, use within 14 days of MAO inhibitor therapy, Wolff–Parkinson–White syndrome or arrhythmias associated with other cardiac accessory conduction pathway disorders

Interactions

DRUGS

antidepressants, lithium: Increased risk of serious adverse effects
ergotamine-containing drugs: Possibly additive or prolonged vasoconstrictive effects
fluoxetine, fluvoxamine, paroxetine, sertraline: Possibly hyper-reflexia, incoordination, and weakness
MAO inhibitors: Risk of decreased sumatriptan clearance, increased risk of serious adverse effects
selective serotonin reuptake inhibitors, serotonin norepinephrine reuptake inhibitors, other triptans: Increased risk of serotonin syndrome

Adverse Reactions

CNS: Anxiety, atypical sensations, dizziness, drowsiness, fatigue, fever, headache, malaise, sedation, **serotonin syndrome**, **seizures**, vertigo, weakness
CV: **Arrhythmias**; chest heaviness, pain, pressure, or tightness; **coronary artery vasospasm**; **ECG changes**; hypertension; **hypotension**; palpitations; peripheral vascular ischemia
EENT: Abnormal vision, blindness or partial vision loss, jaw or mouth discomfort, nasal burning (P.O., subcutaneous), nasal irritation (nasal), nose or throat discomfort, photophobia (P.O., subcutaneous), taste perversion (nasal), tongue numbness or soreness
GI: Abdominal discomfort, **bloody diarrhea**, **colonic ischemia**, dysphagia
MS: Jaw discomfort, muscle cramps, myalgia, neck pain or stiffness
SKIN: Diaphoresis, erythema, flushing, pallor, photosensitivity (P.O., subcutaneous), pruritus, rash, urticaria
Other: **Anaphylaxis**, **angioedema**, injection-site burning, pain, and redness

Nursing Considerations

- Be aware that sumatriptan shouldn't be given to elderly patients because they're more likely to have coronary artery disease (CAD) and more pronounced blood pressure increases.
- Assess patient for arrhythmias, chest pain, or other signs of heart disease and monitor blood pressure in patients with CAD before and for at least 1 hour after sumatriptan administration.
- Don't give sumatriptan within 24 hours of another 5-HT_1-receptor agonist, such as naratriptan, rizatriptan, or zolmitriptan with the exception of a single dose of another sumatriptan product, provided the doses are separated by at least 1 to 2 hours depending on brand used. Don't give an ergotamine-containing or ergot-type drug within 24 hours of sumatriptan therapy. Doing so increases risk of serious adverse interactions and effects.
- After nasal spray administration, rinse tip of bottle with hot water (don't suction water into bottle) and dry with a clean tissue. Replace cap after cleaning.
- Inspect injection solution for discoloration and particles before administering. Discard solution if you detect these changes. Be aware that the needle shield of the prefilled syringe contains dry natural rubber, a latex derivative, that may cause allergic reactions in latex-sensitive persons.
- Be aware that parenteral form of drug shouldn't be administered I.V. because this may precipitate coronary artery vasospasm. Administer only as a subcutaneous injection.
- To use nasal powder, remove the clear device cap from the reusable delivery device, then remove a disposable nosepiece from its foil pouch and click the nosepiece into the device body. Then fully press and promptly release the white piercing button on the device body to pierce the capsule inside the nosepiece. The white piercing button should only be pressed once and released prior to administration to each nostril. Insert the nosepiece into the nostril so that it makes a tight seal. Keeping the nosepiece in the nose, rotate the device to place the mouthpiece into the mouth. Have patient blow forcefully through the mouthpiece to deliver the powder into the nasal cavity. A rattling noise may occur; this indicates that patient has blown forcefully. Once administered, have patient remove and discard the nosepiece. Repeat the procedure using a second 11-mg nosepiece into the other nostril.

WARNING Monitor patient closely for hypersensitivity reactions, including anaphylaxis and angioedema which may be life-threatening. If present, notify prescriber immediately and expect to provide emergency supportive care according to institution emergency protocols.

- Know that for patients with seizure disorder, seizure precautions should be instituted according to facility policy because sumatriptan may lower seizure threshold.

WARNING Monitor patient closely for serotonin syndrome exhibited by agitation, coma, diarrhea, hyperreflexia, hyperthermia, incoordination, labile blood pressure, nausea, tachycardia, or vomiting. Notify prescriber immediately because serotonin syndrome may be life-threatening and provide supportive care.

PATIENT TEACHING

- Advise patient to use sumatriptan as soon as possible after the onset of migraine symptoms.
- Urge patient to contact prescriber and avoid taking sumatriptan if headache symptoms aren't typical.
- Remind patient not to exceed prescribed daily dosage. Inform him that overuse of the drug for 10 or more days per month may lead to exacerbation of headache and may require detoxification. If his use of the drug increases, advise him to notify his prescriber.
- Advise patient to swallow tablets whole and drink fluids to disguise unpleasant taste.
- Show patient suitable sites for subcutaneous injection, and teach him how to load, administer, and discard autoinjector or how to use subcutaneous needle. Tell patient to alert prescriber if he is allergic to latex, as the needle cap of the prefilled syringe is made of a latex derivative. Or, explain how to administer drug using needle-free drug delivery system, Sumavel DosePro. (Snap off plastic tip, flip back lever into active position, and press end of device to the skin of abdomen or thigh.)
- Instruct patient not to exceed maximum doses and not to take a second dose if first dose doesn't provide significant relief.
- Inform patient that he may experience burning, pain, and redness for 10 to 30 minutes after subcutaneous injection. Suggest that he apply ice to relieve pain and redness.
- Teach patient prescribed the nasal powder or nasal spray forms how to use correctly.
- Advise patient never to share the medication with another person even if they have the same symptoms, as cross-contamination and severe adverse reactions could occur.
- Encourage patient to lie down in a dark, quiet room after taking drug to help relieve migraine.
- Instruct patient to seek emergency care for chest, jaw, or neck tightness after drug use because drug may cause coronary artery vasospasm; subsequent doses may require ECG monitoring.
- Urge patient to report palpitations or rash to prescriber.
- Advise patient to avoid potentially hazardous activities until drug's CNS effects are known.
- Alert patient with seizure disorder that drug may lower seizure threshold.
- Encourage yearly ophthalmologic examinations for patients who require prolonged drug therapy.
- Advise women of childbearing age to notify prescriber if pregnancy occurs.
- Inform woman who is breastfeeding that she should avoid breastfeeding for 12 hours after treatment with sumatriptan to minimize infant exposure to the drug.
- Urge patient to inform all prescribers of sumatriptan therapy because of potentially dangerous drug interactions.

suvorexant

Belsomra

Class, Category, and Schedule

Pharmacologic class: Orexin receptor antagonist
Therapeutic class: Hypnotic
Pregnancy category: C
Controlled substance schedule: IV

Indications and Dosages

➤ *To treat insomnia characterized by difficulties with sleep onset and/or sleep maintenance*

TABLETS

Adults. 10 mg once per night within 30 minutes of bedtime and with at least 7 hours remaining for sleep; increased, as needed, to 20 mg once daily. *Maximum:* 20 mg once daily at night.

DOSAGE ADJUSTMENT For patients taking moderate CYP3A inhibitors, dosage reduced to 5 mg once per night, with maximum dosage not exceeding 10 mg once per night. For patients taking CNS depressants concurrently, dosage may have to be decreased.

Mechanism of Action

Antagonism of orexin receptors blocks the binding of wake-promoting neuropeptides orexin A and orexin B to produce sleep.

Contraindications

Hypersensitivity to suvorexant and its components, narcolepsy

Interactions

DRUGS

benzodiazepines, opioids, other CNS depressants, tricyclic antidepressants: Additive CNS and respiratory depression; increased risk of abnormal behavior and thinking
CYP3A inducers: Decreased effectiveness of suvorexant
CYP3A inhibitors: Increased effect of suvorexant and incidence of adverse reactions
digoxin: Increased serum digoxin levels

ACTIVITIES

alcohol use: Additive CNS depression; increased risk of abnormal behavior and thinking

Adverse Reactions

CNS: Abnormal dreams, amnesia, anxiety, cataplexy-like behaviors (mild), dizziness, hallucinations, headache, impaired daytime wakefulness, leg weakness (temporarily), psychomotor hyperactivity, sleep paralysis (temporarily), somnolence, **suicidal ideation**, worsening of depression
CV: Palpitations, tachycardia
EENT: Dry mouth
GI: Diarrhea
RESP: Cough, upper respiratory tract infection
Other: Physical and psychological dependence

Nursing Considerations

- Use suvorexant with extreme caution in patients with a history of alcohol or drug abuse because of risk of addiction.
- Use suvorexant cautiously in debilitated or elderly patients and those with depression or impaired respiratory function.
- Monitor obese patients and women closely for adverse effects because these patients are at increased risk. Be aware that there is a dosage relationship to development of adverse reactions in general.
- Monitor respiratory status, especially in patients with respiratory compromise, who are at increased risk for respiratory depression.
- Watch patient closely for suicidal tendencies, particularly when therapy starts and dosage changes, because depression may worsen temporarily during these times, possibly leading to suicidal ideation.

PATIENT TEACHING

- Tell patient to take drug 30 minutes before bedtime on an empty stomach with at least 7 hours remaining for sleep time.
- Caution patient to avoid potentially hazardous activities after taking suvorexant; drug's intended effect is to decrease alertness. Tell patient that CNS depressant effects may persist in some patients for up to several days after the drug is discontinued.
- Advise patient that drug may cause abnormal behaviors during sleep that extend into daytime, causing wakefulness impairment. Such behaviors may include driving a car, eating, talking on the phone, or having sex without any recall of the event. If family members notice any such behavior or patient sees evidence of such behavior upon awakening, drug should be withheld and prescriber notified.
- Advise patient to avoid alcohol while taking suvorexant.
- Tell patient to notify prescriber if insomnia worsens or new signs or symptoms occur.
- Urge family or caregiver to watch patient closely for suicidal tendencies, especially when therapy starts or dosage changes.

T

tacrine hydrochloride (tetrahydroamino-acridine, THA)

Cognex

Class and Category

Pharmacologic class: Cholinesterase inhibitor
Therapeutic class: Antidementia agent
Pregnancy category: C

Indications and Dosages

➤ *To treat mild to moderate Alzheimer's-type dementia*

CAPSULES

Adults. *Initial:* 10 mg four times a day for 4 wk, increased to 20 mg four times a day, provided patient is tolerating drug and there are no significant transaminase elevations, and adjusted every 4 wk as prescribed. *Maximum:* 160 mg daily in four divided doses.

DOSAGE ADJUSTMENT For patients with transaminase levels elevated more than 3 to 5 times ULN, daily dosage reduced by 40 mg/day.

Contraindications

Hypersensitivity to tacrine, other acridine derivatives, or their components; jaundice from previous tacrine use; serum bilirubin level that exceeds 3 mg/dl

Interactions

DRUGS

anticholinergics: Decreased effects of both drugs

Mechanism of Action

Tacrine may relieve dementia in patients with Alzheimer's disease by increasing the acetylcholine level in the CNS. In Alzheimer's disease, some cholinergic neurons lose their ability to function, which decreases the acetylcholine level. The remaining functioning cholinergic neurons release acetylcholine, but it's enzymatically broken down by cholinesterases into acetic acid and choline, as shown below left. Without acetylcholine to activate muscarinic (M) and nicotinic (N) receptors on postsynaptic cell membranes, nerve transmission, and excitability decrease.

Tacrine binds with and inhibits cholinesterases, making more intact acetylcholine available in cholinergic synapses, as shown below right. This prolongs and enhances acetylcholine's effects, which increases nerve transmission and reduces symptoms of dementia.

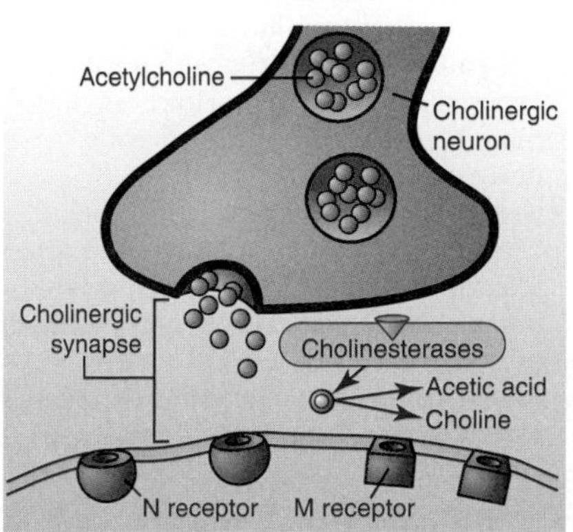

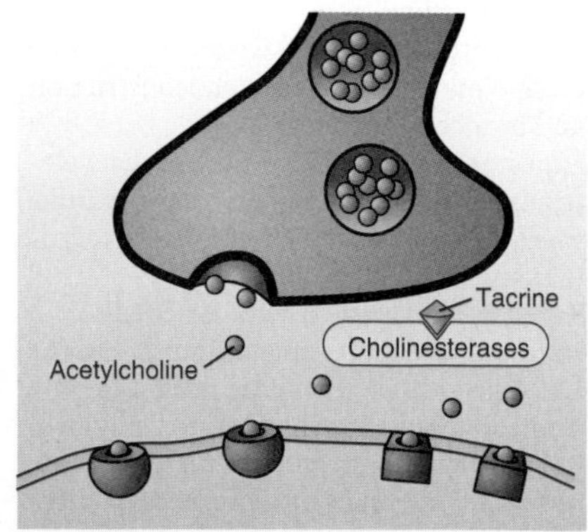

cholinergics, other cholinesterase inhibitors: Increased effects of these drugs and tacrine, possibly leading to toxicity
cimetidine: Increased blood tacrine level, possibly leading to toxicity
neuromuscular blockers: Exaggerated or prolonged muscle relaxation
NSAIDs: Increased gastric acid secretion, possibly GI bleeding and irritation
theophylline: Increased blood theophylline level, possibly leading to toxicity

FOODS

all foods: Reduced tacrine bioavailability

ACTIVITIES

smoking: Possibly decreased tacrine effectiveness

Adverse Reactions

CNS: Agitation, anxiety, asthenia, ataxia, confusion, depression, dizziness, fatigue, hallucinations, headache, hostility, insomnia, **seizures**, somnolence, syncope, tremor
CV: Arrhythmias, chest pain, **conduction disturbances**, hypertension, **hypotension**, palpitations, peripheral edema, **sick sinus syndrome**
EENT: Rhinitis
GI: Abdominal pain, anorexia, constipation, diarrhea, elevated liver enzymes, flatulence, indigestion, jaundice, nausea, vomiting
GU: Bladder obstruction, urinary frequency and incontinence, UTI
MS: Back pain, muscle stiffness, myalgia
RESP: Asthma, cough, upper respiratory tract infection, wheezing
SKIN: Flushing, purpura, rash
Other: Weight loss

Nursing Considerations

- Monitor asthmatic patients for increased mucus production and wheezing, because tacrine may increase bronchoconstriction and bronchial secretions.
- Expect to monitor hepatic enzyme levels (specifically ALT), as ordered, every other week from at least weeks 4 to 16 of tacrine therapy.
- Know that for patient with elevated transaminase levels greater than 5 times ULN, prescriber should be notified immediately, as tacrine therapy will have to be stopped until levels return to normal. Once transaminase levels return to normal, expect to begin tacrine therapy again (starting at 10 mg q.i.d.) as prescribed, and check patient's hepatic enzyme levels weekly for 16 weeks, monthly for 2 months, and then every 3 months thereafter, as ordered.
- Know that for patient experiencing jaundice confirmed by a bilirubin greater than 3 mg/dl and/or patient exhibiting signs of hypersensitivity such as fever or rash in association with elevated transaminase levels, drug may be expected to be discontinued immediately and not resumed.
- Monitor patient for bradyarrhythmias, conduction disturbances, and sick sinus syndrome because tacrine may have a vagotonic effect on the heart rate.

WARNING Be aware that tacrine's cholinergic effects may exacerbate parkinsonian symptoms or seizures.

- Monitor patient's urine output and assess for abdominal distention and abnormal bowel sounds, because drug's cholinergic effects may exacerbate conditions involving GI tract, such as ileus or obstruction, or urinary tract.
- Be aware that patients with peptic ulcer disease and those receiving NSAIDs are at increased risk for developing diarrhea, nausea, and vomiting because tacrine increases gastric acid secretion.
- Assess patient for increased signs and symptoms because drug becomes less effective as Alzheimer's disease progresses and the number of intact cholinergic neurons declines.

PATIENT TEACHING

- Instruct patient to take tacrine on an empty stomach, and advise caregiver to make sure that the patient swallows the drug.
- Tell patient to take drug with meals if he experiences GI distress. However, mention that drug's effects may be delayed.
- Urge patient to seek assistance when changing position or walking until drug's effects are known. Instruct her to avoid potentially hazardous activities during this period.
- Advise patient not to smoke because it may decrease drug's effectiveness.
- Caution patient not to stop taking drug abruptly. Doing so may impair cognitive ability.

- Inform caregiver that tacrine will become less effective as Alzheimer's disease progresses.
- Urge caregiver to make sure patient returns regularly for follow-up visits and laboratory tests to monitor drug effectiveness.

tacrolimus

Astagraf XL, Envarsus XR, Hecoria, Prograf

Class and Category

Pharmacologic class: Calcineurin inhibitor
Therapeutic class: Immunosuppressant
Pregnancy category: C

Indications and Dosages

➤ *To prevent organ rejection in patients undergoing allogeneic heart, kidney, or liver transplantation*

CAPSULES (HECORIA, PROGRAF), ORAL SUSPENSION

Adults having kidney transplantation in combination with azathioprine. 0.2 mg/kg/day given in two equally divided doses every 12 hr beginning with first dose begun between 6 and 24 hr post-transplant but only after renal function has recovered (serum creatinine level of 4 mg/dl or less).
Adults having kidney transplantation in combination with MMF/IL-2 receptor antagonist therapy. 0.1 mg/kg/day given in two equally divided doses every 12 hr beginning with first dose begun between 6 and 24 hr post-transplant but only after renal function has recovered (serum creatinine level of 4 mg/dl or less).
Children having kidney transplantation. 0.3 mg/kg/day given in two equally divided doses every 12 hr.
Adults having liver transplantation. 0.10 to 0.15 mg/kg/day given in two equally divided doses every 12 hr. Administer first dose 6 hr after transplantation.
Children having liver transplantation. 0.15 to 0.20 mg/kg/day (capsules) or 0.2 mg/kg/day (oral suspension) given in two equally divided doses every 12 hr. Administer first dose 6 hr after transplantation.
Adults having heart transplantation. 0.075 mg/kg/day given in two equally divided doses every 12 hr. Administer first dose 6 hr after transplantation.
Children having heart transplantation. 0.3 mg/kg/day (0.1 mg/kg/day if cell-depleting induction treatment is administered) given in two equally divided doses every 12 hr.

I.V. INFUSION (PROGRAF)

Adults having kidney or liver transplantation. 0.03 to 0.05 mg/kg/day as a continuous infusion beginning no sooner than 6 hr after transplantation.
Adults having heart transplantation. 0.01 mg/kg/day as a continuous infusion beginning no sooner than 6 hr after transplantation.
Children having liver transplantation. 0.03 to 0.05 mg/kg/day as a continuous infusion beginning no sooner than 6 hr after transplantation.
DOSAGE ADJUSTMENT For patients with hepatic or renal impairment, dosage kept at lower end of range with possible need for further reduction. Black patients may need higher doses after kidney transplantation to attain comparable trough concentrations compared to Caucasian patients.

➤ *To prevent organ rejection in patients undergoing allogeneic kidney transplantation*

EXTENDED-RELEASE CAPSULES (ASTAGRAF XL)

Adults with basiliximab induction. *Initial*: 0.15 to 0.2 mg/kg 1 hr before a meal or 2 hr after a meal and started prior to reperfusion or within 48 hr of completion of transplant procedure, but may be delayed until renal function has recovered. Dosage then adjusted to achieve target trough concentration range.
Adults without basiliximab induction. *Preoperatively*: 0.1 mg/kg as a single dose 1 hr before a meal or 2 hr after a meal within 12 hr prior to reperfusion. *Postoperatively*: 0.2 mg/kg as the second dose given 1 hr before a meal or 2 hr after a meal at least 4 hr after the preoperative dose and within 12 hr after reperfusion, then adjusted to achieve target trough concentration ranges.
DOSAGE ADJUSTMENT FOR ASTAGRAF XL Black patients may need higher doses to attain comparable trough concentrations compared to Caucasian patients. For patients who have developed

nephrotoxicity, dosage reduced. For patients with severe hepatic impairment, lower dosage may be required.

➤ *To prevent organ rejection in patients undergoing allogenic kidney transplantation and are converting from a tacrolimus immediate-release product*

XR TABLETS (ENVARSUS XR)

Adults. *Initial*: 80% of total daily dose of immediate-release product given once daily on an empty stomach, then adjusted to achieve target whole blood trough concentration ranges of 4 to 11 ng/ml.

Mechanism of Action

Inhibits T-lymphocyte activation, possibly by binding to an intracellular protein, FKBP-12. This binding results in formation of a complex of tacrolimus-FKBP-12, calcineurin, calcium, and calmodulin which inhibits phosphatase activity of calcineurin. This inhibition may prevent dephosphorylation and translocation of nuclear factor of activated T-cells, a nuclear component thought to initiate gene transcription for the formation of lymphokines. The result is inhibition of T-lymphocyte activation, which produces immunosuppression.

Incompatibilities

Don't store diluted drug in PVC containers because of increased instability of tacrolimus and possible extraction of phthalates. Don't mix or coinfuse tacrolimus with solutions of pH 9 or greater, such as with acyclovir or ganciclovir, because of chemical instability of tacrolimus in alkaline media.

Contraindications

Hypersensitivity to tacrolimus or its components, hypersensitivity to polyoxyl 60 hydrogenated castor oil (parenteral form)

Interactions

DRUGS

aminoglycosides, amphotericin B, cisplatin, cyclosporine, CYP3A4 inhibitors, ganciclovir, nucleotide reverse transcriptase inhibitors, other nephrotoxic drugs, protease inhibitors: Increased risk of renal impairment

amiodarone, boceprevir, bromocriptine, chloramphenicol, cimetidine, cisapride, clarithromycin, clotrimazole, cyclosporine, danazol, diltiazem, erythromycin, ethinyl estradiol, fluconazole, ganciclovir, itraconazole, ketoconazole, lansoprazole, magnesium-aluminum-hydroxide, methylprednisolone, metoclopramide, nefazodone, nelfinavir, nicardipine, nifedipine, omeprazole, protease inhibitors, ritonavir, Schisandra sphenanthera *extracts, telaprevir, troleandomycin, verapamil, voriconazole:* Possibly increased blood tacrolimus level

amiodarone, CYP3A4 inducers or inhibitors that have potential to prolong QT interval: Possibly prolonged QT interval

carbamazepine, methylprednisolone, phenobarbital, phenytoin, prednisone, rifabutin, rifampin, St. John's wort: Possibly decreased blood tacrolimus level

mycophenolic acid: Possibly increased plasma mycophenolic acid level

sirolimus: Increased risk of insulin-dependent post-transplant diabetes mellitus, renal dysfunction, and wound healing complications

vaccines (live or killed): Possibly suppressed immune response and increased adverse effects of vaccine

FOODS

grapefruit, grapefruit juice: Possibly increased blood tacrolimus trough levels in liver transplant patients

high-fat foods: Decreased absorption of oral tacrolimus

ACTIVITIES

alcohol use (Astagraf XL, Envarsus XR): Increased rate of release of tacrolimus

Adverse Reactions

CNS: Asthenia, **coma**, **CVA**, delirium, dizziness, fever, headache, hemiparesis, insomnia, jittery feeling, **leukoencephalopathy**, mental changes, motor and sensory dysfunction, mutism, **neurotoxicity**, paresthesia, **posterior reversible encephalopathy syndrome**, **progressive multifocal leukoencephalopathy**, **seizures**, speech disorder, syncope, tremor

CV: **Atrial and ventricular arrhythmias**, **cardiac arrest**, chest pain, hypercholesterolemia, hyperlipemia, hypertension, hypertriglyceridemia, myocardial hypertrophy, **MI**, **myocardial ischemia**, **pericardial effusion**, peripheral edema,

QT-interval prolongation, torsades de pointes, venous thrombosis
EENT: Blindness, cortical blindness, deafness, hearing loss, photophobia
ENDO: Cushingoid features, diabetes mellitus, hot flashes, hyperglycemia
GI: Abdominal pain, anorexia, ascites, bile duct stenosis, colitis, constipation, diarrhea, dyspepsia, enterocolitis, gastric ulcer, gastroenteritis, gastroesophageal reflux disease, **GI perforation, hepatic impairment or toxicity**, impaired gastric emptying, nausea, **pancreatitis, veno-occlusive liver disease**, vomiting
GU: BK virus nephropathy, elevated creatinine and BUN levels, hemorrhagic cystitis, **hemolytic-uremic syndrome**, micturition abnormality, **nephrotoxicity**, oliguria, **renal failure**, renal impairment, UTI
HEME: Agranulocytosis, anemia, **disseminated intravascular coagulation (DIC), hemolytic anemia**, leukocytosis, **leukopenia, neutropenia, pancytopenia, pure red cell aplasia, thrombocytopenia**
MS: Arthralgia, back pain, extremity pain including calcineurin-inhibitor induced pain syndrome
RESP: Acute respiratory distress syndrome, atelectasis, bronchitis, cough increase, dyspnea, **interstitial lung disease, lung infiltration**, pleural effusion, **pulmonary embolism or hypertension, respiratory distress or failure**
SKIN: Flushing, hyperpigmentation, **malignancy**, photosensitivity, pruritus, rash, **Stevens–Johnson syndrome, toxic epidermal necrolysis**
Other: Anaphylaxis, cytomegalovirus infection, **hyperkalemia, hypokalemia, hypomagnesemia, hypophosphatemia**, impaired wound healing, **lymphoproliferative or malignant disorders, multiorgan failure**, opportunistic infections (including activation of latent viral infections), primary graft dysfunction, weight loss

Nursing Considerations

- Know that tacrolimus should not be given to patients with congenital long QT syndrome because of increased risk of life-threatening ventricular arrhythmias.
- Know that tacrolimus therapy should not be started within 24 hours of cyclosporine, and vice versa. If tacrolimus or cyclosporine blood levels are elevated beyond 24 hours of either drug being discontinued, know that the other drug should not be started until elevation is resolved.
- Be aware that I.V. tacrolimus therapy should only be given if patient can't tolerate oral tacrolimus. Patient should be switched to oral therapy as soon as possible.
- Do not interchange oral immediate-release capsules with oral extended-release capsules or tablets. Also, do not interchange oral extended-release capsules with oral extended-release tablets, nor interchange capsules with granules.
- Know that drug should not be used simultaneously with cyclosporine, but when used to prevent kidney transplant rejection, it is recommended to be used concomitantly with mycophenolate mofetil. When Hecoria or Prograf formula is used to prevent either kidney or heart transplant rejection, azathioprine may be substituted for mycophenolate mofetil.
- Expect to give drug with adrenal corticosteroid therapy.
- Know that sirolimus should not be administered with tacrolimus because of the potential for severe adverse reactions.
- Be aware that tacrolimus can cause fetal harm. Take special precautions when handling drug.
- To prepare oral suspension, empty the entire contents of each Prograf granules packet into a glass cup. Add 15 to 30 milliters of room-temperature drinking water to the cup. Mix and administer entire contents of the cup. Know that the granules will not completely dissolve. The suspension should be given immediately after preparation. For younger patients, the suspension can be drawn up via a non-PVC oral syringe that is dispensed with drug. Rinse the cup or syringe with 15 to 30 ml of water and give to patient to ensure that all of the medication is taken. Do not sprinkle Prograf granules on food.
- Dilute intravenous drug with normal saline solution or 5% dextrose to 0.004 to 0.02 mg/ml following manufacturer

guidelines. Once diluted, drug should be stored in glass or polyethylene containers (not PVC, because of decreased stability and possible extraction of phthalates). Discard after 24 hours if not used.

- Keep in mind when converting patient from parenteral to oral therapy after heart transplantation, expect to give oral form 8 to 12 hours after infusion is discontinued.
- Be aware that children usually need higher doses of tacrolimus than adults.

WARNING Closely monitor patient for anaphylaxis at least during first 30 minutes of I.V. administration. Make sure emergency equipment and drugs, such as aqueous solution of epinephrine and oxygen, are immediately available.

- Monitor patient's blood tacrolimus trough levels regularly, as ordered. Higher trough levels increase risk of toxicity, especially nephrotoxicity and neurotoxicity.
- Monitor blood pressure, especially in patients with history of hypertension, because drug can worsen this condition.
- Monitor results of liver and renal function tests, as ordered, to detect signs of decreased function.
- Know that tacrolimus may increase serum cholesterol, lipid, and triglyceride levels.
- Monitor patient's blood glucose level closely because tacrolimus may cause post-transplant diabetes mellitus with the need for insulin therapy, especially in black and Hispanic patients.
- Monitor patient's serum potassium level, as ordered, because drug can alter it.
- Watch for evidence of neurotoxicity, especially in patients receiving high doses of drug. Evidence of encephalopathy includes headache, impaired consciousness, loss of motor function, psychiatric disturbance, seizures, and tremors.

WARNING Monitor patient's ECG and electrolytes, as ordered, periodically throughout tacrolimus therapy because drug may prolong the QT interval, especially in patients with bradyarrhythmias congestive heart failure, electrolyte disturbances, and concomitant use of certain antiarrhythmic drugs.

- Be aware that tacrolimus therapy increases the risk of patient developing serious infections and malignancies. Monitor patient closely, as patient may need to be hospitalized because of life-threatening severity.

PATIENT TEACHING

- Tell patient to inspect her tacrolimus medication when she receives a new prescription and before taking it. If it looks different or dosage instructions have changed, tell patient to alert prescriber, because tacrolimus products are not interchangeable.
- Advise patient to take oral doses of Prograf, 12 hours apart, at same time each day on an empty stomach. Advise patient to take oral doses of extended release form once daily in the morning either 1 hour before a meal or 2 hours after a meal on an empty stomach. Tell patient to swallow capsule or tablet whole and not to chew, divide, or crush capsule or tablet. Instruct patient or caregiver how to mix and administer Prograf oral granules used to make an oral suspension. Warn not to sprinkle granules on food and to take or administer the suspension immediately after preparation.
- Tell patient to avoid consuming alcohol or grapefruit juice or eating grapefruit while taking tacrolimus.
- Advise patient not to stop taking drug without consulting prescriber.
- Instruct patient not to receive virus vaccines during therapy. Urge him to avoid people who have received such vaccines or to wear a protective mask when he's around them.
- Caution patient to avoid having contact with people who have infections during therapy because tacrolimus causes immunosuppression. Stress importance of notifying prescriber if an infection occurs, as it can become severe. Tell patient to report chills; cough; fever; flu-like symptoms; muscle aches; or painful, red, or warm areas on the skin.
- Warn patient that tacrolimus may cause cancer because of its immunosuppressant action. Tell patient to report any unexplained or unusual signs and symptoms to prescriber.
- Emphasize the importance of having repeated laboratory tests while taking tacrolimus, and urge compliance.

- Inform patient that tacrolimus therapy may result in insulin-dependent diabetes. Tell him to report frequent urination or an increase in fatigue, hunger, or thirst.
- Tell patient to report shortness of breath, swelling anywhere on the body, or tiredness to prescriber.
- Instruct patient to alert all prescribers to tacrolimus therapy and not to take any over-the-counter drugs, including herbal products, without consulting prescriber first.
- Teach patient how to take his blood pressure and provide guidelines for when blood pressure readings should be reported to prescriber.
- Instruct patient to limit exposure to direct sunlight and to wear protective clothing and use sunscreen when exposure can't be avoided.
- Warn women of childbearing age and men who can father a child that tacrolimus can cause fetal harm and to use effective contraceptive measures before starting drug and continuing throughout therapy. If pregnancy occurs, tell both male and female patients to alert prescriber immediately and encourage pregnant women to enroll in the pregnancy exposure registry by calling 1-877-955-6877.
- Tell mothers who wish to breastfeed that tacrolimus has been reported in breast milk and to discuss breastfeeding with prescriber before doing so.

tadalafil

Adcirca, Cialis

Class and Category

Pharmacologic class: Phosphodiesterase-5 (PDE5) inhibitor
Therapeutic class: Erectile dysfunction agent
Pregnancy category: B

Indications and Dosages

➤ *To treat erectile dysfunction*

TABLETS (CIALIS)

Men. *Initial:* 10 mg taken 1 hr before sexual activity; dosage decreased to 5 mg or increased to 20 mg, based on clinical response. Alternatively, 2.5 mg once daily, increased to 5 mg once daily, as needed. *Maximum:* 20 mg daily.

DOSAGE ADJUSTMENT For patients who take drug on an as-needed basis and are taking potent CYP3A4 inhibitors such as itraconazole, ketoconazole, or ritonavir, dosage shouldn't exceed 10 mg every 72 hr. For patients taking potent CYP3A4 inhibitors and drug once daily, the maximum recommended dose is 2.5 mg daily. For patients with a creatinine clearance of 30 to 50 ml/min, who take drug on an as-needed basis, initial dosage decreased to 5 mg daily and maximum dosage not to exceed 10 mg every 48 hr. For patients with a creatinine clearance of less than 30 ml/min or who are on hemodialysis, who take drug on an as-needed basis, maximum dose should not exceed 5 mg every 72 hr. Once daily dosing is not recommended for patients with a creatinine clearance less than 30 ml/min. For patients with mild to moderate hepatic dysfunction who take drug on an as-needed basis, dosage should not exceed 10 mg once every day.

➤ *To treat benign prostatic hyperplasia*

TABLETS (CIALIS)

Men. 5 mg once daily at approximately the same time every day.

DOSAGE ADJUSTMENT For patients taking potent CYP3A4 inhibitors such as itraconazole, ketoconazole, or ritonavir, dosage reduced to 2.5 mg daily. For patients with a creatinine clearance of 30 to 50 mg/ml, initial dosage reduced to 2.5 mg once daily with possible increase to 5 mg, based upon individual response. Drug is not recommended for patients with a creatinine clearance less than 30 ml/min for this indication.

➤ *To treat benign prostatic hyperplasia and erectile dysfunction*

TABLETS (CIALIS)

Men. 5 mg once daily, at approximately the same time every day without regard to timing of sexual activity.

DOSAGE ADJUSTMENT For patients taking potent CYP3A4 inhibitors such as itraconazole, ketoconazole, or ritonavir, dosage reduced to 2.5 mg daily. For patients with a creatinine clearance of 30 to 50 mg/ml, initial dosage reduced to 2.5 mg once daily with possible increase to 5 mg, based upon individual response. Drug is not recommended for patients with a creatinine clearance less than 30 ml/min for this indication.

➤ *To treat pulmonary arterial hypertension in order to improve exercise ability in patients classified as group 1 by the World Health Organization*

TABLETS (ADCIRCA)

Adults. 40 mg once daily.

DOSAGE ADJUSTMENT For patients with mild to moderate hepatic or renal impairment or who have already taken ritonavir for at least 1 wk, initial dosage of 20 mg once daily and then increased as tolerated. For patient already taking tadalafil and being prescribed ritonavir, tadalafil temporarily discontinued for at least 24 hours before ritonavir starts. Then, after at least 1 week of ritonavir, tadalafil restarted at 20 mg once daily and then increased to 40 mg once daily, as tolerated.

Route	Onset	Peak	Duration
P.O.	Unknown	30 min–6 hr	Unknown

Mechanism of Action

Enhances the effect of nitric oxide released in the penis during sexual stimulation. Nitric oxide activates the enzyme guanylate cyclase, which causes increased levels of cGMP in the corpus cavernosum. This leads to increased blood flow to the penis, thus producing an erection.

By preventing breakdown of cyclic guanosine monophosphate by phosphodiesterase, levels increase leading to smooth muscle relaxation of the pulmonary vasculature and subsequently, vasodilation. Vasodilation causes the pressure within the pulmonary vasculature to decrease, which improves tolerance to exercise and delays worsening of pulmonary arterial hypertension.

Contraindications

Concomitant guanylate cyclase stimulator therapy, continuous or intermittent nitrate therapy, hypersensitivity to tadalafil or its components, retinitis pigmentosa

Interactions

DRUGS

carbamazepine, phenytoin, phenobarbital: Possibly decreased tadalafil effects

doxazosin, guanylate cyclase stimulators such as riociguat, tamsulosin and other alpha blockers: Increased risk of symptomatic hypotension

erythromycin, itraconazole, ketoconazole, ritonavir: Prolonged tadalafil effects

nitrates: Profound hypotension

protease inhibitors (other than ritonavir): Possibly prolonged tadalafil effects

rifampin: Decreased tadalafil effects

FOODS

grapefruit juice: Possibly prolonged tadalafil effects

ACTIVITIES

alcohol use: Potentiated blood pressure–lowering effects

Adverse Reactions

CNS: Asthenia, **CVA**, dizziness, fatigue, headache, hypesthesia, insomnia, migraine, paresthesia, **seizures**, somnolence, syncope, transient global amnesia, vertigo

CV: Angina pectoris, chest pain, hypertension, **hypotension**, **MI**, postural hypotension, palpitations, peripheral edema, **sudden cardiac death**, tachycardia

EENT: Blurred vision, changes in color vision, conjunctivitis, dry mouth, epistaxis, eyelid swelling, eye pain, hearing or visual loss, increased lacrimation, nasal congestion, nasopharyngitis, nonarteritic anterior ischemic optic neuropathy (NAION), pharyngitis, retinal artery or vein occlusion, tinnitus, visual field defects

GI: Diarrhea, dysphagia, dyspepsia, elevated liver enzymes, esophagitis, gastroesophageal reflux, gastritis, increased gamma-glutamyl transpeptidase levels, nausea, upper abdominal pain, vomiting

GU: Priapism, spontaneous penile erection, UTI

MS: Arthralgia, back or neck pain, extremity pain, myalgia

RESP: Bronchitis, cough, dyspnea, upper respiratory tract infection

SKIN: Diaphoresis, **exfoliative dermatitis**, flushing, pruritus, rash, **Stevens–Johnson syndrome**, urticaria

Other: Angioedema, flu-like symptoms, **hypersensitivity reactions**

Nursing Considerations

- Know that patients with hereditary degenerative retinal disorders, including retinitis pigmentosa, should not receive tadalafil because of the risk of serious ophthalmic adverse reactions.

- Be aware that patients with severe hepatic or renal impairment should not receive tadalafil because its effects in these patients are unknown.
- Use tadalafil cautiously in patients with left ventricular outflow obstruction, such as aortic stenosis and idiopathic hypertrophic subaortic stenosis, and those with severely impaired autonomic control of blood pressure because these conditions increase sensitivity to vasodilators, such as tadalafil.
- Use tadalafil cautiously in patients with conditions that may predispose them to priapism, such as leukemia, multiple myeloma, penile deformities (such as angulation, cavernosal fibrosis, or Peyronie's disease), or sickle cell anemia.
- Monitor blood pressure and heart rate and rhythm before and during therapy.

PATIENT TEACHING

- Explain that, when used as needed to treat erectile dysfunction, tadalafil should be taken 1 hour before sexual activity to provide the most effective results. Alternatively, if the patient chooses to take a smaller dose of tadalafil daily, encourage him to take it at about the same time every day, regardless of the timing of sexual activity.

WARNING Tell patient not to take tadalafil if he takes any form of organic nitrate, either continuously or intermittently, because profound hypotension and death could result.

- Advise patient taking tadalafil to treat erectile dysfunction to obtain sexual counseling to help enhance the drug's effects.
- Urge patient to notify prescriber immediately if erection is painful or lasts longer than 4 hours to avoid possible penile damage and permanent loss of erectile function.
- Advise patient to avoid alcohol or grapefruit juice consumption while taking tadalafil.
- Tell male patients taking tadalafil for pulmonary arterial hypertension not to take another form of tadalafil under the brand name of Cialis or any other PDE5 inhibitors to treat erectile dysfunction.

WARNING Tell patient to seek immediate medical attention if he experiences hearing loss that may be accompanied by dizziness or tinnitus or a sudden loss of vision in one or both eyes.

tamoxifen citrate

Apo-Tamox (CAN), Nolvadex, Soltamox

Class and Category

Pharmacologic class: Selective estrogen receptor modulator (SERM)
Therapeutic class: Anti-estrogen agent
Pregnancy category: D

Indications and Dosages

➤ *To treat estrogen receptor-positive metastatic breast cancer in men and women*

ORAL SOLUTION, TABLETS

Adults. 20 to 40 mg daily. Dosages greater than 20 mg administered twice daily.

➤ *As adjuvant treatment for early-stage estrogen receptor-positive breast cancer; to reduce occurrence of contralateral breast cancer when used as adjuvant therapy for the treatment of breast cancer*

ORAL SOLUTION, TABLETS

Adults. 20 mg daily for 5 to 10 years.

➤ *To reduce the risk of invasive breast cancer in women with ductal carcinoma in situ (DCIS) after radiation and surgery; to reduce the risk of breast cancer in women at high risk*

ORAL SOLUTION, TABLETS

Adults. 20 mg daily for 5 yr.

Mechanism of Action

May block the effects of estrogen on breast tissue by competing with estrogen for estrogen-receptor binding sites. Estrogen may stimulate the growth of cancer cells.

Contraindications

Hypersensitivity to tamoxifen or its components; women at high risk for breast cancer and women with DCIS and a history of deep vein thrombosis or pulmonary embolus or who need coumarin-type anticoagulant therapy

Interactions

DRUGS

bromocriptine: Possibly increased blood tamoxifen level
estrogens: Possibly altered therapeutic effect of tamoxifen
warfarin and other coumarin-type anticoagulants: Increased anticoagulant effect of these drugs

Adverse Reactions

CNS: Confusion, **CVA**, depression, dizziness, fatigue, headache, lightheadedness, somnolence, weakness
CV: Edema, hyperlipidemia, **thrombosis**
EENT: Keratopathy, ocular toxicity (including cataracts), optic neuritis, retinopathy
GI: Elevated liver enzymes, **hepatotoxicity**, nausea, vomiting
GU: Endometrial cancer, endometrial hyperplasia, endometrial polyps, genital itching, menstrual irregularities, ovarian cysts, vaginal discharge (females); impotence, decreased libido (males)
HEME: Anemia, **leukopenia, thrombocytopenia**
MS: Transient bone or tumor pain
RESP: Pulmonary embolism
SKIN: Bullous pemphigoid, dry skin, **erythema multiforme**, rash, **Stevens–Johnson syndrome**, thinning hair
Other: Angioedema, hot flashes, **hypercalcemia**, weight gain

Nursing Considerations

WARNING Make sure that patient has been informed about serious or potentially life-threatening adverse effects associated with tamoxifen before therapy begins. Be aware that women with ductal carcinoma in situ and those at high risk for breast cancer are more likely to develop pulmonary emboli, stroke, or uterine cancer than others receiving tamoxifen.

- Know that if patient is premenopausal, drug therapy should begin in the middle of menstruation; if patient's menstrual cycles are irregular, verify that she has had a negative pregnancy test before therapy starts.
- Expect patient to undergo an ophthalmic examination before and periodically during tamoxifen therapy. Also expect to monitor patient for adverse ocular reactions, such as cataracts.
- Assess patient for signs and symptoms of thromboembolic events, such as change in mental status, leg pain, or shortness of breath.
- Periodically monitor patient's cholesterol and triglyceride levels, liver enzymes, and platelet and WBC counts, as ordered.
- Monitor blood calcium level and assess patient for signs and symptoms of hypercalcemia, such as nausea, thirst, and vomiting; tamoxifen may cause hypercalcemia in breast cancer patients with bone metastasis within a few weeks of starting treatment.
- Store tamoxifen in a closed, light-resistant container at room temperature.

PATIENT TEACHING

- Advise patient to swallow tamoxifen tablet whole with water.
- Instruct premenopausal patient to use a nonhormonal form of contraception, such as a condom or diaphragm, during tamoxifen therapy. Emphasize that she shouldn't become pregnant while taking drug and for 2 months afterward. Advise her to notify prescriber at once if she becomes pregnant during therapy.
- Inform patient of the most common side effects—hot flashes, irregular menses, and vaginal discharge.
- Urge patient to immediately notify prescriber if she notices difficulty breathing, facial swelling, itching, or a rash, because they may signify a hypersensitivity reaction.
- Advise patient to notify prescriber if she experiences calf swelling or leg pain during tamoxifen therapy, because they may indicate a blood clot.
- Instruct patient to report signs of hepatotoxicity, such as flu-like symptoms, nausea, tiredness, or yellow skin.
- Advise patient to have regular gynecologic examinations and to notify prescriber about abnormal symptoms, including abdominal or pelvic pain, new breast lumps, and unusual vaginal bleeding or discharge.
- Urge patients who take tamoxifen for prophylaxis to have regular

mammograms, because tamoxifen doesn't prevent all breast cancers.
- Emphasize the importance of taking tamoxifen regularly. Urge patient to consult prescriber if adverse reactions, such as nausea and vomiting, are interfering with dosage schedule. These symptoms may be a sign of hypercalcemia.
- Inform women who wish to breastfeed that tamoxifen may appear in breast milk and cause serious adverse effects in the infant.

tamsulosin hydrochloride

Flomax

Class and Category

Pharmacologic class: Alpha adrenergic antagonist
Therapeutic class: Benign prostatic hyperplasia (BPH) agent
Pregnancy category: B

Indications and Dosages

➤ *To treat BPH*

CAPSULES

Adults. *Initial:* 0.4 mg daily 30 min after same daily meal for 2 to 4 wk, increased to 0.8 mg daily if no response to initial dosage. *Maximum:* 0.8 mg daily.

Mechanism of Action

Blocks alpha$_1$-adrenergic receptors in the prostate. This action inhibits smooth-muscle contraction in the bladder neck and prostate, prostatic capsule, and prostatic urethra, which improves the rate of urine flow and reduces symptoms of BPH.

Contraindications

Hypersensitivity to tamsulosin, quinazolines, or their components

Interactions

DRUGS

alpha blockers: Additive effects of both drugs
cimetidine: Risk of decreased tamsulosin clearance
CYP2D6 inhibitors (such as fluoxetine, paroxetine, terbinafine), CYP3A4 inhibitors (such as erythromycin, ketoconazole): Possibly increased plasma tamsulosin level
phosphodiesterase-5 inhibitors: Increased risk of hypotension

Adverse Reactions

CNS: Asthenia, dizziness, drowsiness, headache, insomnia, syncope, vertigo
CV: Arrhythmia, atrial fibrillation, chest pain, orthostatic hypotension, palpitations, tachycardia
EENT: Amblyopia, diplopia, dry mouth, epistaxis, intraoperative floppy iris syndrome (during cataract and glaucoma surgery), pharyngitis, rhinitis, visual impairment
GI: Constipation, diarrhea, nausea, vomiting
GU: Decreased libido, ejaculation disorders, priapism
MS: Back pain
RESP: Dyspnea, **respiratory impairment**
SKIN: Desquamation, **erythema multiforme, exfoliative dermatitis**, pruritus, rash, **Stevens-Johnson syndrome**, urticaria
Other: Angioedema

Nursing Considerations

- Be aware that prostate cancer should be ruled out before tamsulosin therapy begins.
- Give drug about 30 minutes after the same meal each day.
- Know that if patient takes drug on an empty stomach, his blood pressure should be monitored because of the increased risk of orthostatic hypotension.
- Be aware that if patient doesn't take drug for several days, therapy should be resumed at 0.4 mg/dose, as prescribed.

PATIENT TEACHING

- Instruct patient not to chew, crush, or open tamsulosin capsules and to take drug about 30 minutes after the same meal each day.
- Instruct patient to notify prescriber if he misses several days of therapy, and caution him against restarting drug at previous dosage.
- Advise patient to avoid potentially hazardous activities until drug's CNS effects are known. Mention the need for caution if dosage is increased.
- Advise patient to change position slowly, especially after initial dose and each

dosage increase, to minimize effects of orthostatic hypotension.
- Tell patient to inform ophthalmologist of tamsulosin therapy because drug may increase risk for complications with cataract surgery.

tapentadol
Nucynta, Nucynta ER

tapentadol hydrochloride
Nucynta Oral Solution

Class, Category, and Schedule
Pharmacologic class: Opioid
Therapeutic class: Opioid analgesic
Pregnancy category: C
Controlled substance schedule: II

Indications and Dosages
➤ *To relieve pain severe enough to require opioid treatment and for which alternative treatment options such as nonopioid analgesics or opioid combination products are inadequate or not tolerated*

ORAL SOLUTION, TABLETS

Adults. 50 to 100 mg repeated every 4 to 6 hr, as needed. *Maximum:* 700 mg on first day; 600 mg daily thereafter

DOSAGE ADJUSTMENT On first day of therapy, second dose may be given as soon as 1 hr after first dose, if needed. For patients with moderate hepatic impairment (Child–Pugh Class B), dosage should not exceed 50 mg for each episode, intervals between doses should be at least 8 hours, and no more than 3 doses should be given in a 24-hour period.

E.R. TABLETS

Adults. *Initial:* 50 mg every 12 hours, increased by 50 mg no more than twice daily every 3 days, as needed. *Maximum:* 250 mg twice daily.

DOSAGE ADJUSTMENT For patients with moderate hepatic impairment taking ER tablets, initial dosage reduced to 50 mg once daily and increased as needed to maximum dosage of 100 mg once daily.

➤ *To relieve neuropathic pain associated with diabetic peripheral neuropathy when a continuous, around-the-clock opioid analgesic is needed for an extended period of time*

E.R. TABLETS

Adults. *Initial:* 50 mg twice daily, increased as needed no sooner than every 3 days. *Maximum:* 250 mg twice daily.

DOSAGE ADJUSTMENT For patients with moderate hepatic impairment, initial dosage reduced to 50 mg once daily and increased as needed to maximum dosage of 100 mg once daily.

Route	Onset	Peak	Duration
P.O.	Unknown	1 hr	4 hr

Mechanism of Action
Binds with and activates opioid receptors (mainly mu receptors) in brain and spinal cord and inhibits norepinephrine reuptake to produce analgesia.

Contraindications
Acute or severe bronchial asthma, hypercapnia or significant respiratory depression not monitored or without available resuscitation equipment; gastrointestinal obstruction including paralytic ileus; hypersensitivity to tapentadol or its components; within 14 days of MAO inhibitor therapy

Interactions
DRUGS

antimigraine agents, cyclobenzaprine; dextromethorphan; dolasetron; granisetron; linezolid; MAO inhibitors; methylene blue; ondansetron; palonosetron; selected psychiatric drugs such as amoxapine, buspirone, lithium, maprotiline, mirtazapine, nefazodone, trazodone, vilazodone; selective serotonin reuptake inhibitors; serotonin-norepinephrine reuptake inhibitors; St. John's wort; tricyclic antidepressants; tryptophan: Increased risk of serotonin syndrome

benzodiazepines, CNS depressants, other opioids, sedating antihistamines, tricyclic antidepressants: Increased risk of severe respiratory depression and significant sedation and somnolence

CNS depressants: Increased risk of life-threatening effects from CNS or respiratory depression

MAO inhibitors: Possibly hyperpyretic episodes, hypertensive crisis, serotonin syndrome, and severe seizures
serotonergics: Increased risk of potentially fatal serotonin syndrome

ACTIVITIES

alcohol use: Increased serum tapentadol level possibly resulting in a fatal overdose from CNS and respiratory depression, risk of CNS depression

Adverse Reactions

CNS: Abnormal dreams, anxiety, confusion, dizziness, fatigue, hallucinations, headache, insomnia, lethargy, panic attack, **seizures**, **serotonin syndrome**, somnolence, **suicidal ideation**, syncope, tremor
CV: Hypotension, palpitations
EENT: Dry mouth, nasopharyngitis
ENDO: Adrenal insufficiency (rare), hot flashes
GI: Anorexia, constipation, diarrhea, dyspepsia, nausea, vomiting
GU: Decreased libido, erectile dysfunction, impotence, infertility, lack of menstruation, UTI
MS: Arthralgia
RESP: Respiratory depression, upper respiratory infection
SKIN: Diaphoresis, pruritus, rash, urticaria
Other: Anaphylaxis including anaphylactic shock, **angioedema**, physical or psychological dependence, withdrawal

Nursing Considerations

- Be aware that tapentadol isn't recommended for patients with severe renal impairment (creatinine clearance less than 30 ml/min) or severe hepatic dysfunction (Child–Pugh Class C).
- Use tapentadol with extreme caution in patients with decreased respiratory reserve, hypercapnia, or hypoxia such as may occur in asthma, CNS depression, coma, COPD, cor pulmonale, kyphoscoliosis, myxedema, severe obesity, or sleep apnea syndrome. Also use cautiously in patients with head injury or conditions in which increased intracranial pressure may occur because drug may obscure the signs and symptoms. Also use cautiously in patients with mild to moderate hepatic or renal dysfunction and in patients with biliary tract disease, including acute pancreatitis, because drug may cause spasm of the sphincter of Oddi.
- Be aware that excessive use of opioids like tapentadol may lead to abuse, addiction, misuse, overdose, and possibly death. For these reasons, a Risk Evaluation and Mitigation Strategy (REMS) is now required when tapentadol is prescribed. Monitor patient's intake of drug closely and for evidence of physical dependence.
- Know that chronic maternal use of tapentadol during pregnancy can result in neonatal opioid withdrawal syndrome (NOWS), which may be life-threatening if not recognized and treated appropriately. NOWS occurs when a newborn has been exposed to opioid drugs like tapentadol for a prolonged period while in utero.
- Expect to begin tapentadol therapy at lower doses in elderly patients because of age-related decreased hepatic and renal function.

WARNING Monitor patient's respiratory depth, effort, and rate during tapentadol therapy because drug may cause respiratory depression that may become severe, especially in debilitated or elderly patients and in those who have conditions accompanied by hypercapnia, hypoxia, or upper airway obstruction. If respiratory rate drops below 10 breaths/minute, notify prescriber, expect drug to be discontinued, and provide needed supportive care, which may include an opioid antagonist such as naloxone, as ordered.

- Monitor patient's blood pressure closely, especially when initiating tapentadol therapy and when titrating the dose because the drug may cause severe hypotension and syncope in ambulatory patients due to its vasodilatory effects. Risk of hypotension is greatest in patients who already have been compromised by a reduced blood volume or concurrent administration of certain CNS depressant drugs such as general anesthetics and phenothiazines.
- Monitor patients with seizure disorders closely because tapentadol may aggravate or induce seizures.
- Monitor patient for adrenal insufficiency. Although rare, it can be life-threatening. Monitor patient for anorexia, dizziness, fatigue, hypotension, nausea, vomiting, or weakness. Notify prescriber if adrenal insufficiency is suspected and expect diagnostic testing to be done. If confirmed,

expect to administer corticosteroids and wean patient off tapentadol, if possible.

WARNING Watch patient closely for evidence of serotonin syndrome, which can be life-threatening. Report autonomic instability (hyperthermia, labile blood pressure, tachycardia), GI disturbances (diarrhea, nausea, vomiting), mental status changes (agitation, coma, hallucinations), or neuromuscular abnormalities (hyperreflexia, incoordination).

- Don't stop tapentadol abruptly if used on a regular basis because withdrawal symptoms may occur.
- Be aware that tapentadol shouldn't be used just before or during labor and delivery.
- Watch patient closely for suicidal tendencies, particularly when therapy starts and after dosage changes.

WARNING Be aware that tapentadol should only be used concomitantly with benzodiazepine therapy in patients for whom other treatment options are inadequate. If prescribed together, expect dosing and duration of tapentadol to be limited. Monitor patient closely for signs and symptoms of a decrease in consciousness, including coma, profound sedation, and significant respiratory depression. Notify prescriber immediately and provide emergency supportive care, as death may occur.

PATIENT TEACHING

- Instruct patient to take tapentadol exactly as prescribed and not to adjust dose or frequency without consulting prescriber. Explain that excessive or prolonged use of drug may lead to abuse, addiction, misuse, overdose, and possibly death.
- Tell patient prescribed E.R. tablet form, to take tablet whole and not to chew, crush, cut, or dissolve the tablet because doing so could be fatal.
- Advise patient to avoid hazardous activities until drug's CNS effects are known.

WARNING Caution patient to avoid alcohol, benzodiazepines, or other CNS depressants while taking tapentadol because severe respiratory depression can occur and may lead to death.

- Advise patient who has been taking tapentadol regularly not to stop taking it abruptly; instead, patient should taper drug use gradually, based on prescriber instructions, to reduce the risk of withdrawal symptoms.
- Urge caregiver or family to watch patient closely for suicidal tendencies, especially when therapy starts or after dosage changes.
- Tell female patient to notify prescriber if pregnancy occurs, as prolonged use of tapentadol during pregnancy can result in neonatal opioid withdrawal syndrome, which may be life-threatening.
- Caution patient to keep drug out of the hands of children because accidental ingestion could be fatal.
- Inform patient that long-term use of opioids like tapentadol may decrease sex hormone levels, causing decreased libido, erectile dysfunction, impotence, infertility, or lack of menstruation. Encourage patient to report any symptoms to prescriber.
- Instruct patient to notify all prescribers of opioid use.

tedizolid

Sivextro

Class and Category

Pharmacologic class: Oxazolidinone
Therapeutic class: Antibiotic
Pregnancy category: C

Indications and Dosages

➤ *To treat acute bacterial skin and skin structure infections caused by the following gram-positive microorganisms:* Enterococcus faecalis, Staphylococcus aureus *(including methicillin-resistant and methicillin-susceptible isolates),* Streptococcus agalactiae, S. anginosus group *(including* S. anginosus, S. constellatus, *and* S. intermedius), *and* S. pyogenes

TABLETS

Adults. 200 mg once daily for 6 days.

I.V. INFUSION

Adults. 200 mg infused over 1 hr once daily for 6 days.

Mechanism of Action

Causes cell wall lysis and subsequent death of bacteria cell

Incompatibilities

Do not dilute tedizolid with any solution containing divalent cations (i.e., Ca^{2+}, Mg^{2+}), including lactated Ringer's injection and Hartmann's solution because of incompatibilities. Do not mix tedizolid with other drugs or reconstitute drug with any solution other than sterile water for injection because incompatibilities are unknown.

Contraindications

Hypersensitivity to tedizolid and its components

Interactions

DRUGS

breast cancer resistance protein (BCRP) substrates such as methotrexate, topotecan: Increased plasma concentrations of BCRP substrates with potential for adverse reactions

Adverse Reactions

CNS: Dizziness, headache, hypoesthesia, insomnia, paresthesia, peripheral neuropathy, VII nerve paralysis
CV: Hypertension, palpitations, tachycardia
EENT: Blurred vision, optic neuropathy, oral candidiasis, visual impairment, vitreous floaters
GI: ***Clostridium difficile*–associated diarrhea**, diarrhea, elevated liver enzymes, nausea, vomiting
GU: Vulvovaginal mycotic infection
HEME: Anemia, decreased hemoglobin, leukopenia, neutropenia, thrombocytopenia
SKIN: Dermatitis, flushing, pruritus, urticaria
Other: Hypersensitivity reactions, infusion-related reactions

Nursing Considerations

- Be aware that tedizolid may not be effective in the treatment of bacterial skin and skin structure infections in patients with neutropenia and should not be used.
- Reconstitute each vial with 4 ml of sterile water for injection. Gently swirl the contents (do not shake to minimize foaming) and let the vial stand until the cake has completely dissolved and any foam disperses. May be stored at room temperature or in the refrigerator for up to 24 hours.
- Withdraw 4 ml of reconstituted solution from vial (do not invert the vial during extraction). Slowly inject the 4 ml of reconstituted solution into an intravenous bag containing 250 ml of 0.9% sodium chloride. Invert bag gently to mix (do not shake).
- Administer parenteral form as an intravenous infusion over 1 hour. Never administer as an intravenous push or bolus. If the intravenous line is used for subsequent infusions of any other drugs, flush the line before and after tedizolid infusion with 0.9% sodium chloride injection, USP.
- Assess patient for signs of secondary infection, such as profuse, watery diarrhea. If such diarrhea develops, contact prescriber and expect to obtain a stool specimen to rule out pseudomembranous colitis caused by *C. difficile*. If diarrhea occurs, notify prescriber and expect to withhold drug and treat with electrolytes, fluids, protein, and an antibiotic effective against *C. difficile*.

PATIENT TEACHING

- Tell patient receiving oral tedizolid that it may be taken without regard to food.
- Instruct patient that if he misses a dose, to take it as soon as possible anytime up to 8 hours prior to his next scheduled dose. If less than 8 hours remain before the next dose, he should skip the missed dose and take the next dose on schedule.
- Stress the importance of completing the prescribed 6 days of therapy.
- Urge patient to tell prescriber if diarrhea develops, which may occur even as late as 2 or more months after tedizolid therapy has ended.

telavancin

Vibativ

T

Class and Category

Pharmacologic class: Lipoglycopeptide
Therapeutic class: Antibiotic
Pregnancy category: C

Indications and Dosages

➤ *To treat complicated skin and skin structure infections caused by gram-positive organisms*: Enterococcus faecalis *(vancomycin-susceptible isolates only)*, Staphylococcus aureus, Streptococcus agalactiae, S. anginosus *group (includes* S. anginosus, S. constellatus, *and* S. intermedius), *and* S. pyogenes *(*S. aureus, S. pyogenes, S. agalactiae, S. anginosus *group [includes* S. anginosus, S. intermedius, *and* S. constellatus*]), or* E. faecalis *(vancomycin-susceptible isolates only)*

I.V. INFUSION

Adults. 10 mg/kg administered over 60 min every 24 hr for 7 to 14 days

➤ *To treat hospital-acquired and ventilator-associated bacterial pneumonia caused by* S. aureus *when alternative treatments are not suitable*

I.V. INFUSION

Adults. 10 mg/kg administered over 60 min every 24 hr for 7 to 21 days.

DOSAGE ADJUSTMENT For patients with creatinine clearance of 30 to 50 ml/min/1.73m, dosage reduced to 7.5 mg/kg every 24 hours. For patient with creatinine clearance of at least 10 but less than 30 ml/min, 10 mg/kg every 48 hours.

Route	Onset	Peak	Duration
I.V.	Unknown	1–2 hr	24 hr

Mechanism of Action

Inhibits cell wall synthesis and alters the permeability of bacterial membranes, causing cell wall lysis and cell death.

Incompatibilities

Don't mix telavancin with other drugs or I.V. solutions containing additives. If administration must be through the same I.V. line, flush the line with 5% dextrose injection, 0.9% sodium chloride injection, or lactated Ringer's injection before and after infusing telavancin.

Contraindications

Hypersensitivity to telavancin or its components, intravenous unfractionated heparin sodium

Interactions

DRUGS

ACE inhibitors, loop diuretics, NSAIDs: Increased risk of nephrotoxicity

drugs known to prolong the QT interval, such as clarithromycin, disopyramide, erythromycin, quinidine: Increased risk of prolonged QT interval

Adverse Reactions

CNS: Dizziness, rigors
CV: Prolonged QT interval
EENT: Taste disturbance
GI: Abdominal pain, anorexia, diarrhea, ***Clostridium difficile*–associated diarrhea**, nausea, vomiting
GU: Elevated creatinine level, foamy urine, **nephrotoxicity**
HEME: Abnormal coagulation
SKIN: Pruritus, rash
Other: Anaphylaxis, infusion-related reactions such as erythema or pain

Nursing Considerations

- Know that telavancin isn't recommended for patients with congenital long-QT syndrome, severe left ventricular hypertrophy, uncompensated heart failure or who currently have a prolonged QT interval because it may prolong the QT interval, causing life-threatening complications.
- Know that use of intravenous unfractionated heparin sodium is contraindicated with telavancin because the activated partial thromboplastin time (aPTT) test results may be falsely prolonged for up to 18 hours after telavancin administration.
- Use cautiously in patients taking drugs known to prolong the QT interval because of increased risk of a prolonged QT interval.
- Make sure woman of childbearing age has a negative pregnancy test result before starting telavancin because of risk of fetal harm.
- Obtain baseline serum creatinine level before telavancin therapy starts because preexisting moderate to severe renal impairment may increase mortality in the presence of telavancin therapy and is not recommended in such patients unless the benefit outweighs the potential risk. Expect to, monitor patient's serum creatinine level throughout therapy, as ordered, because drug may cause nephrotoxicity, especially in patients with congestive heart failure, diabetes mellitus, hypertension, or preexisting renal disease and in patients taking such nephrotoxic drugs as ACE inhibitors, loop diuretics, and NSAIDs. If

renal function declines, notify prescriber and expect to discontinue telavancin.

- Dilute a 250-mg vial with 15 ml or a 750-mg vial with 45 ml of a diluent such as 5% dextrose injection, sterile water for injection, or 0.9% sodium chloride injection to obtain a solution of 15 mg/ml. When ready to administer drug, further dilute doses of 150 to 800 mg in 100 to 250 ml of 5% dextrose injection, 0.9% sodium chloride injection, or lactated Ringer's injection before infusion. Doses less than 150 mg or greater than 800 mg should be further diluted in a volume that yields a final concentration of 0.6 to 0.8 mg/ml.
- Use telavancin within 4 hours of the time it is reconstituted in the vial (including its transfer to an infusion bag for further dilution) if kept at room temperature and 72 hours if refrigerated. Discard if time limit exceeds these parameters.
- Infuse telavancin over 60 minutes because more rapid infusion may cause a reaction like red-man syndrome, which causes flushing of upper body, pruritus, rash or urticaria. If present, stop or slow infusion to resolve.
- Monitor patient for hypersensitivity reactions during and after infusion of drug. Stop infusion at first sign of skin rash or any other hypersensitivity sign and notify prescriber.
- Monitor patient for diarrhea, which may range from mild to severe and may occur more than 2 months after antibiotic is discontinued. Report diarrhea and, if *C. difficile* is suspected, expect telavancin to be discontinued. Provide supportive care, such as antibiotic therapy to treat *C. difficile*, electrolyte and fluid replacement, protein supplementation, and possibly surgical intervention, as needed.
- Be aware that while telavancin doesn't interfere with coagulation, it does interfere with certain tests used to monitor coagulation, such as activated clotting time, APTT, coagulation-based factor Xa tests, INR, and PT. Collect blood samples for coagulation tests as close as possible to administration of next dose of telavancin to minimize interference.

PATIENT TEACHING

- Instruct women of childbearing age to use effective contraception during telavancin therapy.
- Caution patient that diarrhea may occur more than 2 months after antibiotic has been discontinued and to report any persistent or severe episodes to prescriber.
- Warn patient that drug may cause urine to be foamy and taste to be altered.
- Advise patient to alert all prescribers that he takes telavancin because some drugs may interact with it, causing serious adverse effects.

telbivudine

Tyzeka

Class and Category

Pharmacologic class: Nucleoside analogue
Therapeutic class: Antiviral
Pregnancy category: B

Indications and Dosages

➤ *To treat chronic hepatitis B in patients with evidence of viral replication and either evidence of persistent elevations in serum aminotransferases (ALT or AST) or histologically active disease*

ORAL SOLUTION, TABLETS

Adults and adolescents age 16 and over. 600 mg tablet or 30 ml of oral solution once daily.

DOSAGE ADJUSTMENT For patient with renal impairment and a creatinine clearance between 30 and 40 ml/min, oral solution dosage decreased to 20 ml once daily or 600-mg tablet taken every 48 hours. For patient with renal impairment and a creatinine clearance less than 30 ml/min but not requiring dialysis, oral solution dosage decreased to 10 ml once daily or 600-mg tablet taken every 72 hours. For patient with end-stage renal disease, oral solution decreased to 6 ml once daily or 600-mg tablet taken every 96 hours.

Mechanism of Action

After being phosphorylated by cellular kinases to the active triphosphate form, telbivudine is incorporated into hepatitis B viral DNA, causing DNA chain termination.

Contraindications

Coadministration with pegylated interferon alfa-2a, hypersensitivity to telbivudine or its components

Interactions

DRUGS

drugs that alter renal function, such as aminoglycosides and NSAIDs: Possibly increased risk of nephrotoxicity
pegylated interferon alfa-2a: Increased risk of peripheral neuropathy occurrence and severity

Adverse Reactions

CNS: Dizziness, fatigue, fever, headache, hypoesthesia, insomnia, paresthesia, peripheral neuropathy
EENT: Pharyngolaryngeal pain
GI: Abdominal distention or pain, diarrhea, dyspepsia, elevated liver and pancreatic enzymes, **hepatitis B exacerbation**, hyperbilirubinemia, nausea, **severe hepatomegaly with steatosis**
HEME: Neutropenia, **thrombocytopenia**
MS: Arthralgia, back pain, elevated creatine kinase (CK) level, myalgia, myopathy, myositis, muscle weakness, **rhabdomyolysis**
RESP: Cough
SKIN: Pruritus, rash
Other: Lactic acidosis

Nursing Considerations

- Expect to monitor HBV DNA every 6 months to check effectiveness of telbivudine. If patient tests positive for HBV DNA at any time during treatment, expect telbivudine to be discontinued and alternative therapy prescribed. In addition, if patient demonstrates incomplete viral suppression (HBV DNA greater than or equal to 300 copies per ml) after 24 weeks of treatment, expect drug to be discontinued and an alternate therapy prescribed.

WARNING Know that lactic acidosis and severe hepatomegaly with steatosis have occurred with telbivudine therapy and that death has occurred in some patients. Risk factors include presence of obesity, prolonged nucleoside exposure, and being a woman. However, know that lactic acidosis and severe hepatomegaly with steatosis have also occurred in patients with no known risk factors. Expect drug to be discontinued in any patient who develops clinical or laboratory findings suggestive of lactic acidosis or pronounced hepatotoxicity, even in the absence of marked transaminase elevations.

- Expect to monitor patient's liver enzymes, as ordered, throughout therapy and for several months after telbivudine has been discontinued, because severe acute exacerbations of hepatitis B have occurred in patients who have discontinued anti-hepatitis B therapy, including telbivudine.
- Monitor patient for unexplained persistent muscle aches and/or muscle weakness in conjunction with increases in CK values, because telbivudine therapy has been associated with myopathy and rhabdomyolysis. If present, notify prescriber and expect drug to be withheld during testing and discontinued if myopathy is confirmed.
- Be aware that if patient develops signs and symptoms of peripheral neuropathy (burning, numbness, or tingling sensations in the arms and/or legs with or without gait disturbance), telbivudine can be expected to be withheld during testing and discontinued if peripheral neuropathy is confirmed.

PATIENT TEACHING

- Stress importance of not missing a dose, as resistance to drug can develop. Also tell patient to take drug exactly as prescribed.
- Tell patient to keep tablets and oral solution in their original container and store at room temperature. Remind patients taking oral solution to use the oral solution within 2 months after opening the bottle.
- Advise patient to dispose of drug when it is outdated or no longer needed by taking it to a community take-back disposal program, if available, or by placing it in a closed container such as a sealed bag in the household trash after removing all identifying information from the original container before throwing it out.
- Instruct patient not to discontinue telbivudine therapy without consulting prescriber, because deterioration of liver disease may occur.

- Remind patient that telbivudine therapy is not a cure for hepatitis B.
- Stress importance of promptly reporting unexplained muscle aches, pain, tenderness, or weakness, as well as any persistent, severe, or unusual signs and symptoms.
- Tell patient to report any burning sensations, numbness, or tingling in his arms and/or legs with or without gait disturbance.
- Emphasize importance of keeping telbivudine out of the reach of children.
- Alert patient on a low-sodium diet that telbivudine oral solution contains about 47 mg of sodium per 30 ml.
- Encourage women who become pregnant while taking telbivudine to enroll in the pregnancy exposure registry by calling 1-800-258-4263.

telmisartan

Micardis

Class and Category

Pharmacologic class: Angiotensin II receptor blocker (ARB)
Therapeutic class: Antihypertensive
Pregnancy category: D

Indications and Dosages

➤ *To manage hypertension, alone or with other antihypertensives*

TABLETS

Adults. *Initial:* 40 mg daily. *Maintenance:* 20 to 80 mg daily. *Maximum:* 80 mg daily.

➤ *To reduce risk of MI, stroke, or death from cardiovascular causes in patients at high risk who are unable to take ACE inhibitors*

TABLETS

Adults age 55 and over. 80 mg once daily.

Route	Onset	Peak	Duration
P.O.	Unknown	In 4 wk	Unknown

Mechanism of Action

Blocks angiotensin II from binding to receptor sites in many tissues, including adrenal glands and vascular smooth muscle. This action inhibits the aldosterone-secreting and vasoconstrictive effects of angiotensin II, which reduces blood pressure.

Contraindications

Concurrent aliskiren therapy in patients with diabetes or renal impairment (GFR less than 60 ml/min), hypersensitivity to telmisartan or its components

Interactions

DRUGS

ACE inhibitors, aliskiren, other angiotensin receptor blockers: Increased risk of hyperkalemia, hypotension, and renal dysfunction
digoxin: Increased peak blood digoxin level and risk of digitalis toxicity
diuretics, other antihypertensives: Enhanced hypotensive effect
lithium: Increased serum lithium levels and toxicity
NSAIDs: Increased risk of renal dysfunction in elderly patients and those with volume depletion and existing renal dysfunction
potassium-sparing diuretics, potassium supplements: Increased risk of hyperkalemia
ramipril: Increased serum ramipril level; decreased telmisartan level

FOOD

salt substitutes containing potassium: Increased risk of hyperkalemia

Adverse Reactions

CNS: Asthenia, dizziness, fatigue, headache, syncope, weakness
CV: **Atrial fibrillation**, **bradycardia**, chest pain, **congestive heart failure**, hypertension, **hypotension**, **MI**, orthostatic hypotension, peripheral edema
EENT: Pharyngitis, sinusitis
ENDO: **Hypoglycemia** (in diabetics)
GI: Abdominal pain, diarrhea, elevated liver enzymes, indigestion, nausea, vomiting
GU: **Acute renal failure**, erectile dysfunction, renal dysfunction, UTI
HEME: Anemia, eosinophilia, **thrombocytopenia**
MS: Back pain, leg or muscle cramps, myalgia, tendinitis, tendon pain, tenosynovitis
RESP: ACE cough, upper respiratory tract infection
SKIN: Diaphoresis, erythema, rash, urticaria

Other: **Anaphylaxis**, **angioedema**, elevated uric acid level, flu-like symptoms, **hyperkalemia**, hypovolemia

Nursing Considerations

- Give telmisartan cautiously to patients with dehydration or hyponatremia.
- Expect prescriber to add a diuretic to regimen if patient's blood pressure isn't well controlled by telmisartan.
- Check patient's blood pressure regularly. Be prepared to treat symptomatic hypotension by placing patient in supine position and giving normal saline solution, as ordered.
- Monitor BUN and serum creatinine levels and urine output in patients with impaired renal function because they're at increased risk for oliguria, progressive azotemia, and possibly acute renal failure.
- Monitor liver enzymes, as appropriate, and assess for evidence of drug toxicity in patients with severe hepatic disease because they're at increased risk for toxicity from increased drug accumulation.
- Avoid using telmisartan in pregnant women during second and third trimesters because drug can increase the risk of fetal harm.

PATIENT TEACHING

- Advise patient to avoid hazardous activities until telmisartan's CNS effects are known.
- Instruct patient to change position slowly to minimize effects of orthostatic hypotension.
- Urge patient to immediately notify prescriber about diarrhea, dizziness, severe nausea, or vomiting.
- Instruct patient to consult prescriber before taking any new drug.
- Advise patient not to use potassium supplements or salt substitutes that contain potassium without checking with prescriber first.
- Advise patient to drink adequate amounts of fluid during hot weather and when exercising.
- Advise female patients of childbearing age to notify prescriber immediately about known or suspected pregnancy.
- Inform mothers not to breastfeed their infant because serious adverse reactions may occur in the breastfed infant.

temazepam

Restoril

Class, Category, and Schedule

Pharmacologic class: Benzodiazepine
Therapeutic class: Sedative-hypnotic
Pregnancy category: X
Controlled substance schedule: IV

Indications and Dosages

➤ *To provide short-term management of insomnia*

CAPSULES

Adults. 7.5 to 30 mg 30 min before bedtime. *Maximum:* 30 mg daily.

DOSAGE ADJUSTMENT For elderly or debilitated patients, 7.5 mg 30 min before bedtime. *Maximum:* 15 mg daily.

Mechanism of Action

May potentiate the effects of gamma-aminobutyric acid (GABA) and other inhibitory neurotransmitters by binding to specific benzodiazepine receptor sites in cortical and limbic areas of the CNS. By binding to these receptor sites, temazepam increases GABA's inhibitory effects and blocks cortical and limbic arousal.

Contraindications

Hypersensitivity to temazepam, other benzodiazepines, or their components; pregnancy

Interactions

DRUGS

antihistamines (such as brompheniramine, carbinoxamine, chlorpheniramine, clemastine, cyproheptadine, diphenhydramine, trimeprazine), anxiolytics, barbiturates, general anesthetics, opioid analgesics, other benzodiazepines, phenothiazines, promethazine, sedating antihistamines, sedative-hypnotics, tramadol, tricyclic antidepressants: Increased respiratory depression or sedation, which could become severe

clozapine: Risk of respiratory depression or arrest

digoxin: Increased risk of elevated blood digoxin level and digitalis toxicity
flumazenil: Increased risk of withdrawal symptoms
levodopa: Possibly decreased levodopa effects
oral contraceptives: Decreased response to temazepam
phenytoin: Possibly phenytoin toxicity
probenecid: Increased response to temazepam
zidovudine: Possibly zidovudine toxicity

ACTIVITIES

alcohol use: Increased CNS and respiratory depression including apnea
smoking: Increased temazepam clearance

Adverse Reactions

CNS: Aggressiveness, anxiety (in daytime), ataxia, complex behaviors (such as sleep driving), confusion, decreased concentration, depression, dizziness, drowsiness, euphoria, fatigue, headache, insomnia, nightmares, slurred speech, **suicidal ideation**, syncope, talkativeness, tremor, vertigo, wakefulness during last third of night
CV: Palpitations, tachycardia
EENT: Abnormal or blurred vision, increased salivation, **throat tightness**
GI: Abdominal pain, constipation, diarrhea, hepatic dysfunction, jaundice, nausea, thirst, vomiting
GU: Decreased libido
HEME: Agranulocytosis, anemia, **leukopenia, neutropenia, thrombocytopenia**
MS: Muscle spasm or weakness
RESP: Dyspnea, increased bronchial secretions
SKIN: Diaphoresis, flushing, pruritus, rash
Other: Anaphylaxis, angioedema, physical and psychological dependence

Nursing Considerations

- Use temazepam cautiously in patients with a history of depression or suicidal thoughts.

WARNING Monitor patient closely for evidence of hypersensitivity reaction, such as dyspnea, nausea, swelling, throat tightness, and vomiting. If present, discontinue temazepam immediately, notify prescriber, and provide supportive care.

- Watch patient closely for suicidal tendencies, particularly when therapy starts and dosage changes, because depression may worsen temporarily during these times and could lead to suicidal ideation.

WARNING Monitor patient for evidence of physical and psychological dependence during therapy.

- Implement safety precautions, according to facility policy, especially in elderly patients, because they're more sensitive to drug's CNS effects.
- Assess patients with respiratory depression, severe COPD, or sleep apnea for signs of ventilatory failure.
- Be aware that temazepam can aggravate acute intermittent porphyria, myasthenia gravis, and severe renal impairment.
- Be aware that temazepam may cause deterioration of cognition or coordination in patients with late-stage Parkinson's disease or worsening psychosis.
- Be aware that drug shouldn't be discontinued abruptly, even after only 1 to 2 weeks of therapy, because doing so may cause seizures or withdrawal symptoms, such as insomnia, irritability, and nervousness.

WARNING Know that opioids should only be used concomitantly with benzodiazepine therapy in patients for whom other treatment options are inadequate. If prescribed together, expect dosing and duration of the opioid to be limited. Monitor patient closely for signs and symptoms of a decrease in consciousness, including coma, profound sedation, and significant respiratory depression. Notify prescriber immediately and provide emergency supportive care, as death may occur.

PATIENT TEACHING

- Instruct patient to take temazepam exactly as prescribed and not to stop or change dosage without consulting prescriber.
- Explain the risks associated with abrupt cessation, including abdominal cramps, acute sense of hearing, confusion, depression, nausea, numbness, perceptual disturbances, photophobia, sweating, tachycardia, tingling, trembling, and vomiting.
- Advise patient to avoid consuming alcohol because it increases drug's sedative effects and the risk of such abnormal behaviors as sleep driving. Also, tell patient that combining alcohol or a benzodiazepine such as temazepam with an opioid could

result in severe respiratory depression and even death.

- Caution patient about possible drowsiness. Advise her to avoid potentially hazardous activities until drug's CNS effects are known.
- Urge patient to notify prescriber immediately about excessive drowsiness, nausea, and known or suspected pregnancy.
- Instruct patient to stop taking temazepam and seek emergency care if she experiences abnormal swelling, difficulty breathing, nausea, throat tightness, or vomiting.
- Advise patient that drug may cause abnormal behaviors during sleep, such as driving a car, eating, talking on the phone, or having sex without any recall of the event. If family notices any such behavior or patient sees evidence of such behavior upon awakening, the prescriber should be notified.
- Urge family or caregiver to watch patient closely for suicidal tendencies, especially when therapy starts or dosage changes.
- Instruct patient to inform all prescribers of temazepam use, especially when pain medication may be prescribed.

tenecteplase

TNKase

Class and Category

Pharmacologic class: Tissue plasminogen activator (tPA)
Therapeutic class: Thrombolytic
Pregnancy category: C

Indications and Dosages

➤ *To reduce mortality associated with acute MI*

I.V. INJECTION

Adults. Single bolus administered over 5 sec in individualized dosage based on patient's weight, as follows: 50 mg (10 ml) for patients weighing 90 kg (198 lb) or more; 45 mg (9 ml) for patients weighing 80 to 89 kg (176 to 196 lb); 40 mg (8 ml) for patients weighing 70 to 79 kg (154 to 174 lb); 35 mg (7 ml) for patients weighing 60 to 69 kg (132 to 152 lb); 30 mg (6 ml) for patients weighing less than 60 kg (132 lb). *Maximum:* 50 mg total dose.

Mechanism of Action

Binds to fibrin and converts plasminogen to plasmin. Plasmin breaks down fibrin, fibrinogen, and other clotting factors, resulting in dissolution of a coronary artery thrombus.

Incompatibilities

Don't administer tenecteplase through an I.V. line containing dextrose because precipitation may occur.

Contraindications

Active internal bleeding, aneurysm, arteriovenous malformation, bleeding disorders, brain tumor, history of cerebrovascular accident, hypersensitivity to tenecteplase or its components, intracranial or intraspinal surgery or trauma within past 2 months, severe uncontrolled hypertension

Interactions

DRUGS

abciximab, aspirin, clopidogrel, dipyridamole, heparin, oral anticoagulants, ticlopidine: Possibly increased risk of bleeding

Adverse Reactions

CNS: **Intracranial hemorrhage**
EENT: Epistaxis, gingival bleeding, **laryngeal edema**, pharyngeal bleeding
GI: **GI and retroperitoneal bleeding**
GU: **Genitourinary bleeding**, prolonged or heavy menstrual bleeding
HEME: Hematoma
RESP: **Hemoptysis**
SKIN: Bleeding at puncture sites, surgical incision sites, or venous cutdown sites; rash; urticaria
OTHER: **Anaphylaxis, angioedema**

Nursing Considerations

WARNING Reconstitute tenecteplase for injection immediately before use because drug contains no antibacterial preservatives. If reconstituted drug isn't used immediately, refrigerate vial at 2° to 8° C (36° to 46° F). Discard solution if not used within 8 hours.

- Use the supplied 10-ml syringe with dual cannula device to reconstitute and administer drug. Withdraw 10 ml of supplied (preservative-free) sterile water for injection into syringe, and inject entire contents into vial containing tenecteplase dry powder, directing stream of diluent into powder. Gently swirl—don't shake—vial until contents are completely dissolved. If slight foaming occurs during reconstitution, allow drug to stand undisturbed for a few minutes to allow large bubbles to dissipate. Then withdraw prescribed dose of tenecteplase from reconstituted drug in vial, using supplied syringe. Make sure that reconstituted preparation is a colorless to pale yellow transparent solution. Discard any unused solution.

- Give drug as a single I.V. bolus over 5 seconds. Although supplied syringe is intended for use with needleless I.V. systems, be aware that it is also compatible with a conventional needle. Follow manufacturer's directions for use with each system. Flush any dextrose-containing I.V. lines with saline solution before and after administering tenecteplase.
- Monitor patient during and for several hours after tenecteplase has been administered for hypersensitivity reactions which may include anaphylaxis, angioedema, laryngeal edema, rash, and urticaria. If symptoms occur, notify prescriber, expect drug therapy to be discontinued, and provide supportive care, as prescribed.

WARNING Monitor patient for evidence of GI bleeding, including bloody or black, tarry stools; bloody or coffee-ground vomitus; and severe stomach pain. Notify prescriber immediately if any of these signs or symptoms develops.

- Assess tenecteplase injection site for signs and symptoms of hematoma, including dark, deep purple bruises under skin and itching, pain, redness, or swelling. Also monitor patient for delayed bleeding at puncture sites, bleeding from surgical incisions, and superficial bleeding.
- Assess for signs and symptoms of genitourinary bleeding (such as hematuria), intracranial bleeding (such as decreased level of consciousness), respiratory tract bleeding (such as hemoptysis), or retroperitoneal bleeding (such as abdominal pain or swelling or back pain). Notify prescriber immediately if patient develops any of these signs or symptoms.
- If serious bleeding (not controllable by local pressure) occurs, expect to discontinue concomitant heparin or oral antiplatelet therapy immediately.
- Avoid I.M. injections and nonessential handling of patient, if possible, for first few hours after drug administration.
- Know that if arterial puncture becomes necessary during first few hours after tenecteplase administration, you should expect to use an upper extremity that's accessible to manual compression. Apply pressure for at least 30 minutes after procedure, use a pressure dressing, and frequently monitor puncture site for signs of bleeding.
- Monitor patients at higher risk for thromboembolism, such as patients with atrial fibrillation or mitral stenosis, while receiving a thrombolytic such as tenecteplase.

PATIENT TEACHING

- Advise patient to immediately report any bleeding, including from gums or nose.
- Instruct patient to limit physical activity during tenecteplase administration to reduce the risk of bleeding or injury.

tenofovir disoproxil fumarate

Viread

Class and Category

Pharmacologic class: Nucleoside reverse transcriptase inhibitor (NRTI)
Therapeutic class: Antiretroviral
Pregnancy category: B

Indications and Dosages

➤ *As adjunct to treat human immunodeficiency virus type 1 (HIV-1) infection; to treat chronic hepatitis B virus (HBV)*

ORAL POWDER, TABLETS

Adults and children weighing at least 35 kg (77 lb). 300 mg once daily.
Adults and children age 2 and over weighing less than 35 kg (77 lb) but at

least 10 kg (22 lb). 8 mg/kg once daily. *Maximum:* 300 mg once daily.
DOSAGE ADJUSTMENT For adult patient with a creatinine clearance between 30 and 49 ml/min, dosage interval increased to every 48 hr. For adult patient with a creatinine clearance between 10 and 29 ml/min, dosage interval increased to every 72 to 96 hr. For hemodialysis patient, dosage interval increased to every 7 days or after a total of approximately 12 hours of dialysis. There are no specific recommendations for children with renal dysfunction.

Mechanism of Action

Inhibits the activity of HIV-1 reverse transcriptase and HBV reverse transcriptase by competing with the natural substrate deoxyadenosine 5′ triphosphate and, after incorporation into DNA, by DNA chain termination.

Contraindications

Hypersensitivity to tenofovir disoproxil fumarate or its components

Interactions

DRUGS

adefovir dipivoxil: Increased blood tenofovir level increasing risk of adverse reactions
atazanavir: Decreased atazanavir concentration decreasing drug effectiveness
atazanavir/ritonavir, darunavir/ritonavir, ledipasvir/sofosbuvir, lopinavir/ritonavir, sofosbuvir/velpatasvir, sofosbuvir/velpatasvir/voxilaprevir: Increased tenofovir concentration with increased risk of adverse reactions
didanosine: Increased concentration of didanosine with increased risk of adverse reactions
drugs affecting renal function, such as aminoglycosides, acyclovir, cidofovir, ganciclovir, high-dose or multiple NSAIDs use, valacyclovir, valganciclovir: Possibly increased concentration of tenofovir and/or increased concentration of other renally eliminated drugs

Adverse Reactions

CNS: Anxiety, asthenia, depression, dizziness, fatigue, fever, headache, insomnia, peripheral neuropathy
CV: Chest pain, elevated cholesterol and triglycerides
EENT: Nasopharyngitis, sinusitis
ENDO: Hyperglycemia
GI: Abdominal pain, **acute hepatitis (severe)**, anorexia, diarrhea, dyspepsia, elevated liver and pancreatic enzymes, flatulence, **hepatomegaly with steatosis (severe)**, nausea, **pancreatitis**, vomiting
GU: Acute renal failure, acute tubular necrosis, elevated creatinine, **Fanconi syndrome**, hematuria, interstitial nephritis, **renal impairment**
HEME: Anemia, **neutropenia**
MS: Arthralgia, back pain, decreased bone density, elevated bone specific alkaline phosphatase and creatine kinase, muscular weakness, myalgia, myopathy, osteomalacia, **rhabdomyolysis**
RESP: Dyspnea, pneumonia, upper respiratory infections
SKIN: Diaphoresis, maculopapular rash, pruritus, pustular rash, rash, urticaria, vesiculobullous rash
Other: Angioedema, hypokalemia, hypophosphatemia, immune reconstitution syndrome, **lactic acidosis**, lipodystrophy, pain, weight loss

Nursing Considerations

- Know that HIV-1 antibody testing should be done on all HBV-infected patients before initiating therapy with tenofovir, to avoid the development of HIV-1 resistance.
- Obtain an estimated creatinine clearance, serum creatinine, urine glucose, and urine protein in all patients prior to initiating tenofovir therapy and periodically throughout, as ordered, because drug is principally eliminated by the kidneys. Renal impairment may occur, which may become severe in patients with chronic kidney disease. Also know that patient's serum phosphorus level should be assessed before and during therapy. Report at any time throughout therapy patient complaints of bone, extremity, or muscle pain or weakness or if patient sustains a fracture, as these may be manifestations of proximal renal tubulopathy and require a prompt evaluation of renal function.

- Be aware that tenofovir should not be used in combination with any other drug containing tenofovir or adefovir dipivoxil. Also know that tenofovir should not be administered with nephrotoxic agents such as high-dose or multiple NSAIDs, because of increased risk of renal dysfunction.
- Measure oral powder using only the supplied dosing scoop. Mix with 2 to 4 ounces of soft food not requiring chewing, such as applesauce, baby food, or yogurt. Administer mixture immediately to avoid a bitter taste. Do not mix powder in a liquid because the powder may float on top of the liquid even after stirring.

WARNING Monitor patient being treated for hepatitis B upon discontinuation of tenofovir for several months, because severe acute exacerbations of hepatitis have occurred when drug has been stopped. Monitoring should include not only an assessment for signs and symptoms of hepatitis, but also laboratory studies such as liver enzymes, as ordered.

- Notify prescriber if patient develops a fracture and/or muscular pain or weakness, persistent or worsening bone pain, or pain in extremities, as these may be signs and symptoms of proximal renal tubulopathy and require further evaluation.

WARNING Monitor patient for signs and symptoms, as well as laboratory findings, of lactic acidosis or pronounced hepatotoxicity that may develop with tenofovir therapy. Know that hepatomegaly and steatosis may occur even in the absence of marked transaminase elevations.

- Be aware that patients who have a history of pathologic bone fracture or other risk factors for bone loss or osteoporosis should be assessed regularly for bone density loss. Patient may benefit from calcium and vitamin D supplementation.
- Be aware that immune reconstitution syndrome has occurred in patients treated with combination antiretroviral therapy, including tenofovir. The inflammatory response predisposes susceptible patients to opportunistic infections such as cytomegalovirus, *Mycobacterium avium* infection, *Pneumocystis jiroveci* pneumonia, or tuberculosis. Autoimmune disorders such as Graves' disease, Guillain–Barré syndrome, or polymyositis have also occurred. Report sudden or unusual adverse reactions to prescriber.

PATIENT TEACHING

- Instruct patient to take tenofovir exactly as prescribed and to avoid missing doses. If a dose is missed, tell patient to take the dose as soon as she remembers it, but not to double the dose. Warn patient not to discontinue the drug without consulting prescriber.
- Remind patient or caregiver measuring oral powder to use only the supplied dosing scoop, to ensure an accurate dose. Tell him to mix with 2 to 4 ounces of soft food not requiring chewing, such as applesauce, baby food, or yogurt, and to take mixture immediately to avoid a bitter taste. Tell patient not to mix powder in a liquid.
- Inform patient that bone density scanning may be ordered during tenofovir therapy.
- Tell patient to avoid high-dose or multiple NSAIDs while taking tenofovir, because of the risk of renal dysfunction.
- Caution patient to report any persistent, severe, or unusual signs and symptoms, including infection, to prescriber.
- Tell patient to inform all prescribers of tenofovir therapy, as other drugs containing tenofovir should not be prescribed during therapy.
- Tell woman of childbearing age to notify prescriber if pregnancy occurs. Encourage her to enroll in the Antiretroviral Pregnancy Registry by calling 1-800-258-4263.
- Inform mothers not to breastfeed during tenofovir therapy.

WARNING Inform patients who are discontinuing tenofovir after being treated for hepatitis B virus to seek medical attention if signs and symptoms of hepatitis reappear. This is because severe acute exacerbations of hepatitis may occur for many months after drug has been discontinued.

terazosin hydrochloride

Class and Category

Pharmacologic class: Alpha adrenergic blocker
Therapeutic class: Antihypertensive, benign prostatic hyperplasia (BPH) agent
Pregnancy category: C

Indications and Dosages

➤ *To manage hypertension*

CAPSULES

Adults. *Initial:* 1 mg at bedtime. *Maintenance:* 1 to 5 mg daily as a single dose or in divided doses every 12 hr. *Maximum:* 20 mg daily.

➤ *To treat symptomatic BPH*

CAPSULES

Adults. *Initial:* 1 mg at bedtime, increased in increments to 2, 5, and then 10 mg, as needed, based on symptom improvement and urine flow rate. *Maintenance:* 10 mg daily as a single dose or in divided doses every 12 hr. *Maximum:* 20 mg daily.

Route	Onset	Peak	Duration
P.O.	15 min	2–3 hr	24 hr

Mechanism of Action

Blocks postsynaptic $alpha_1$-adrenergic receptors in many tissues, including the bladder neck, the prostate and vascular smooth muscle. This action promotes vasodilation, which reduces blood pressure and improves urine flow.

Contraindications

Hypersensitivity to terazosin, other quinazolines, or their components

Interactions

DRUGS

clonidine: Possibly decreased clonidine effects
diuretics, other antihypertensives: Additive hypotensive effect
dopamine: Risk of decreased terazosin effects and antagonized vasoconstrictive effect of dopamine (in high doses)
epinephrine: Risk of decreased terazosin effects, possibly severe hypotension and tachycardia
indomethacin, other NSAIDs: Altered terazosin effects related to sodium and fluid retention
methoxamine, phenylephrine: Decreased vasopressor effects, and shortened duration of action of these drugs
phosphodiesterase-5 inhibitors, verapamil: Additive blood pressure–lowering effects and symptomatic hypotension
sympathomimetics: Decreased terazosin effects

Adverse Reactions

CNS: Asthenia, dizziness, headache, lethargy, nervousness, paresthesia, somnolence, syncope, vertigo
CV: Chest pain, **hypotension**, orthostatic hypotension, palpitations, peripheral edema, sinus tachycardia
EENT: Blurred vision, dry mouth, intraoperative floppy iris syndrome, nasal congestion, sinusitis
GI: Constipation, diarrhea, nausea, vomiting
MS: Arthralgia, back pain
Other: Flu-like symptoms, weight gain

Nursing Considerations

- Be aware that prostate cancer should be ruled out before giving terazosin for BPH.
- Expect prescriber to reduce terazosin dosage if a diuretic or another antihypertensive is added to patient's regimen.
- Monitor blood pressure 2 to 3 hours after initial dose because of possible first-dose hypotension and again after 24 hours to evaluate patient's response.
- If patient requires administration by feeding tube, place capsule in 60 ml of warm tap water. Stir until capsule shell dissolves and liquid contents are released into water (5 to 10 minutes).
- Be aware that elderly patients may have exaggerated hypotension and other adverse reactions.

PATIENT TEACHING

- Instruct patient to take terazosin at the same time each night.
- Explain possible first-dose hypotension. Advise patient to change position and rise slowly to prevent syncope early in therapy. Suggest lying down or sitting if dizziness or light-headedness occurs.

- Advise patient to avoid hazardous activities until drug's CNS effects are known.
- Instruct patient to notify prescriber if she misses several doses in a row; caution her against resuming therapy at previous dose.
- Inform patient that drug may take 2 to 6 weeks to improve urinary hesitancy.
- Advise patient to avoid alcohol use, excessive exercise, exposure to hot weather, or prolonged standing, because these activities can worsen orthostatic hypotension.
- Emphasize the importance of regular follow-up visits with prescriber to evaluate patient's response to drug.

terbinafine hydrochloride

Lamisil

Class and Category

Pharmacologic class: Allylamine derivative
Therapeutic class: Antifungal
Pregnancy category: B

Indications and Dosages

➤ *To treat onychomycosis of fingernails and toenails due to dermatophytes*

TABLETS

Adults and adolescents. 250 mg once daily for 6 wk for fingernail onychomycosis and 12 wk for toenail onychomycosis.

➤ *To treat tinea capitis*

ORAL GRANULES

Adults and children age 4 and over weighing more than 35 kg (77 lb). 250 mg once daily for 6 wk.
Children age 4 and over weighing 25 kg (55 lb) to 35 kg (77 lb). 187.5 mg once daily for 6 wk.
Children age 4 and over weighing less than 25 kg (55 lb). 125 mg once daily for 6 wk.

Mechanism of Action

Inhibits the conversion of squalene monooxygenase to squalene epoxidase, a key enzyme in fungal biosynthesis. The resulting squalene accumulation weakens cell membranes and creates a deficiency of ergosterol, the fungal membrane component necessary for normal fungal growth.

Contraindications

Active or chronic liver disease, hypersensitivity to terbinafine or its components

Interactions

DRUGS

beta blockers, class 1C antiarrhythmics such as flecainide and propafenone, MAO inhibitors (type B), selective serotonin reuptake inhibitors, tricyclic antidepressants: Possibly increased blood levels of these drugs
cimetidine, other hepatic enzyme inhibitors: Significantly decreased terbinafine clearance, possibly increased adverse reactions
cyclosporine: Increased clearance of cyclosporine and decreased effectiveness of cyclosporine
CYP2C and CYP3A4 inhibitors such as amiodarone and ketoconazole: Possibly increased systemic exposure of terbinafine
hepatotoxic drugs: Increased risk of hepatotoxicity
rifampin: Increased clearance and decreased effectiveness of terbinafine
warfarin: Altered prothrombin time

FOODS

caffeine: Decreased caffeine clearance

ACTIVITIES

alcohol use: Increased risk of severe hepatitis

Adverse Reactions

CNS: Anxiety, depression, fatigue, fever, headache, hypoesthesia, malaise, paresthesia, vertigo
CV: **Myocarditis**, **pericarditis**, **thrombotic microangiopathy**, vasculitis
EENT: Hearing impairment, loss of smell, reduced visual acuity, taste loss or perversion (possibly severe), tinnitus, visual field defect
GI: Abdominal pain, anorexia, cholestasis, diarrhea, elevated liver enzymes, flatulence, **hepatic failure**, **hepatitis**, **hepatotoxicity**, indigestion, jaundice, nausea, **pancreatitis**, vomiting
GU: **Hemolytic uremic syndrome**, **nephritis**
HEME: **Agranulocytosis**, anemia, **neutropenia (severe)**, **pancytopenia**, **thrombocytopenia**, **thrombotic thrombocytopenic purpura**
MS: Arthralgia, myalgia, **rhabdomyolysis**

RESP: Pneumonitis
SKIN: Acute generalized exanthematous pustulosis, alopecia, bullous dermatitis, cutaneous lupus erythematosus, **erythema multiforme**, exacerbation of psoriasis, **exfoliative dermatitis**, photosensitivity, psoriasiform eruptions, pruritus, rash, **Stevens–Johnson syndrome**, **toxic epidermal necrolysis**, urticaria
Other: Anaphylaxis, **angioedema**, **drug reaction with eosinophilia and systemic symptoms (DRESS)**, elevated blood creatine phosphokinase, influenza-like illness, serum sickness-like reaction, systemic lupus erythematosus

Nursing Considerations

- Know that because terbinafine has been linked to serious adverse hepatic effects, expect to send nail specimens for laboratory testing to confirm onychomycosis before starting therapy. Also expect to check liver enzymes, as ordered, prior to starting therapy.
- Ensure that patient's liver enzymes have been checked before terbinafine therapy is begun, to rule out preexisting liver disease. Expect to monitor liver enzymes regularly throughout therapy if baseline enzymes are normal.
- Sprinkle entire contents of each packet of oral granules on a spoonful of nonacidic food such as mashed potatoes or pudding and have patient swallow contents in its entirety.
- Administer oral granules by sprinkling the contents of each packet on a spoonful of pudding or other soft, nonacidic food such as mashed potatoes and have patient swallow the entire spoonful without chewing. Do not use applesauce or fruit-based foods. If patient is taking 2 packets of oral granules, both packets may be sprinkled on one spoonful of food or each packet may be sprinkled on a separate spoonful. Give drug with food.
- Monitor patient for hepatic failure (anorexia, dark urine, fatigue, jaundice, nausea, pale stools, right upper abdominal pain, and vomiting). Know that periodic monitoring of liver enzymes should be done throughout therapy because hepatotoxicity may also occur in patients without preexisting liver disease. Expect to stop drug and obtain liver enzyme tests if these problems develop.

WARNING Monitor patient for serious hypersensitivity or skin reactions such as Stevens–Johnson syndrome or drug reaction with eosinophilia and systemic symptoms (DRESS) syndrome. Know that in addition to skin abnormalities such as rash and urticaria, DRESS may also involve one or more organs. If hypersensitivity reactions persist or progress, notify prescriber and expect drug to be discontinued.

- Monitor patient's complete blood count, as ordered. Know that thrombotic microangiopathy has occurred with terbinafine use and can be life-threatening. Notify prescriber promptly of any abnormalities, especially unexplained anemia and thrombocytopenia. If thrombotic microangiopathy is confirmed, expect drug to be discontinued.

PATIENT TEACHING

- Tell patient or parents to sprinkle each packet of oral granules onto a spoonful of nonacidic food such as mashed potatoes or pudding and have patient swallow it in its entirety.
- Emphasize the need to complete the full course of terbinafine therapy to prevent relapse of infection.
- Instruct patient prescribed oral granules to sprinkle the contents of each packet on a spoonful of pudding or other soft, nonacidic food such as mashed potatoes and swallow the entire spoonful without chewing. Caution patient not to use applesauce or fruit-based foods. If patient is taking 2 packets of oral granules, tell him that both packets may be sprinkled on one spoonful or each packet may be sprinkled on a separate spoonful. Stress importance of taking drug with food.
- Discourage consumption of alcohol during therapy.
- Tell patient to contact prescriber if onychomycosis doesn't improve in a few weeks.
- Instruct patient to notify prescriber if he develops persistent anorexia, dark urine, fatigue, jaundice, nausea, pale stools, or right upper abdominal pain. Stress importance of stopping terbinafine

therapy immediately if any of these symptoms occur.
• Instruct patient to avoid direct sunlight or UV light and to wear sunscreen when outdoors.
• Tell patient to watch for skin reactions, such as hives, itching, or rash suggestive of a hypersensitivity reaction. If present, tell patient to notify prescriber.
• Instruct patient to inform prescriber of any unexplained bleeding or bruising that may occur.
• Advise patient to alert prescriber if loss or perversion of taste occurs and becomes severe enough to cause anxiety, depression, or weight loss.

terbutaline sulfate

Brethaire, Brethine, Bricanyl, Bricanyl Turbuhaler (CAN)

Class and Category

Pharmacologic class: Beta adrenergic receptor agonist
Therapeutic class: Bronchodilator
Pregnancy category: B

Indications and Dosages

➤ *To prevent or reverse bronchospasm from asthma, bronchitis, or emphysema*

TABLETS (BRETHINE, BRICANYL)
Adults and adolescents age 15 and over. 2.5 to 5 mg three times a day at 6-hr intervals while awake. *Maximum:* 15 mg daily.
Children ages 12 to 15. 2.5 mg three times a day at 6-hr intervals while awake. *Maximum:* 7.5 mg daily.
Children ages 6 to 11. 50 to 75 mcg/kg three times a day at 6-hr intervals while awake. *Maximum:* 150 mcg/kg/dose or 5 mg daily.

SUBCUTANEOUS INJECTION (BRICANYL)
Adults and children age 12 and over. *Initial:* 0.25 mg, repeated in 15 to 30 min as needed. *Maximum:* 0.5 mg/4-hr period.
Children ages 6 to 12. 5 to 10 mcg (0.005 to 0.01 mg)/kg every 15 to 20 min, up to three doses. *Maximum:* 400 mcg (0.4 mg)/dose.

INHALATION AEROSOL (BRETHAIRE)
Adults and children. 2 inhalations (400 mcg) every 4 to 6 hr, as needed.

INHALATION AEROSOL (BRICANYL TURBUHALER)
Adults and children. 1 inhalation (500 mcg), repeated after 5 min, as needed. *Maximum:* 6 inhalations daily.

Route	Onset	Peak	Duration
P.O.	30–90 min	2–3 hr	4–8 hr
SubQ	15–30 min	30–60 min	1.5–4 hr
Inhalation	In 5 min	30–90 min	3–6 hr

Mechanism of Action

Stimulates $beta_2$-adrenergic receptors in the lungs, which is believed to increase production of cAMP. The increased cAMP level relaxes bronchial smooth muscles, thereby increasing bronchial airflow and relieving bronchospasm.

Contraindications

Hypersensitivity to terbutaline, other sympathomimetic amines, or their components

Interactions

DRUGS
antihypertensives, diuretics: Decreased antihypertensive effect
beta blockers: Mutual inhibition of therapeutic effects, increased risk of bronchospasm
CNS stimulants: Additive CNS stimulation, possibly resulting in adverse effects
digoxin: Increased risk of arrhythmias, possibly digitalis toxicity
halogenated anesthetics: Possibly ventricular arrhythmias
MAO inhibitors: Possibly potentiated action of terbutaline; headache, hyperpyrexia, hypertension, possible hypertensive crisis
maprotiline, tricyclic antidepressants: Possibly potentiated action of terbutaline
nitrates: Decreased effectiveness of nitrates
ritodrine: Increased effects of either drug and potential for adverse effects
sympathomimetics: Increased CNS stimulation and risk of adverse cardiovascular effects, including prolonged QT interval
thyroid hormones: Increased effects of either drug, risk of coronary insufficiency in patients with coronary artery disease

xanthines (theophylline): Increased CNS stimulation and other additive toxic effects

FOODS

caffeine: Increased CNS stimulation and other additive toxic effects

Adverse Reactions

CNS: Anxiety, dizziness, drowsiness, headache, insomnia, light-headedness, nervousness, restlessness, tremor, weakness
CV: Chest pain, **irregular heartbeat**, palpitations, tachycardia
EENT: Dry mouth, taste perversion
ENDO: Hyperglycemia
GI: Heartburn, nausea, vomiting
MS: Muscle spasms
RESP: Dyspnea
SKIN: Diaphoresis, flushing, rash

Nursing Considerations

- Use terbutaline cautiously in patients with cardiovascular disease because drug can adversely affect cardiovascular function. Monitor patient's heart rate and rhythm and blood pressure, and assess for chest pain.
- For subcutaneous use, inject into lateral deltoid area.
- Assess patient's respiratory rate, depth, and quality; oxygen saturation; and activity tolerance at regular intervals because continuous use of beta$_2$-agonists for 12 months or longer accelerates the decline in pulmonary function.

PATIENT TEACHING

- Teach patient how to use terbutaline aerosol inhaler or give subcutaneous injection, as needed.
- Instruct patient not to increase dose or frequency without consulting prescriber.
- Urge patient to seek immediate medical attention if symptoms worsen.
- Inform patient that she may experience transient nervousness or tremors during terbutaline therapy.

teriflunomide

Aubagio

Class and Category

Pharmacologic class: Pyrimidine synthesis inhibitor
Therapeutic class: Immunomodulator
Pregnancy category: X

Indications and Dosages

➤ *To treat relapsing forms of multiple sclerosis*

TABLETS

Adults. 7 or 14 mg once daily.

Mechanism of Action

Inhibits dihydroorotate dehydrogenase, a mitochondrial enzyme involved in de novo pyrimidine synthesis to possibly reduce the number of activated lymphocytes in the central nervous system responsible for the signs and symptoms of multiple sclerosis.

Contraindications

Concurrent therapy with leflunomide; hypersensitivity to teriflunomide, leflunomide, or their components; pregnancy; severe hepatic impairment; women of childbearing age not using reliable contraception

Interactions

DRUGS

alosetron, caffeine, duloxetine, theophylline, tizanidine: Reduced effectiveness of these drugs
ethinylestradiol, levonorgestrel: Increased risk of adverse reactions related to these drugs
paclitaxel, pioglitazone, repaglinide, rosiglitazone: Possibly increased exposure of these drugs with potential for leading to adverse effects
warfarin: Decreased peak international normalized ratio

Adverse Reactions

CNS: Anxiety, burning sensation, headache, paresthesia, peripheral neuropathy, sciatica
CV: Hypertension, palpitations
EENT: Blurred vision, conjunctivitis, oral herpes, sinusitis, toothache
GI: Abdominal distention, diarrhea, elevated liver enzymes, gastroenteritis, **hepatic dysfunction or failure**, nausea, **pancreatitis**, upper abdominal pain
GU: Acute renal failure, acute uric acid nephropathy, cystitis, elevated serum creatinine levels
HEME: Leukopenia, **neutropenia**, **thrombocytopenia**
MS: Manifestation of carpal tunnel syndrome, musculoskeletal pain, myalgia

RESP: Acute interstitial pneumonitis, bronchitis, dyspnea, **interstitial lung disease**, upper respiratory infection
SKIN: Acne, alopecia, pruritus, **Stevens–Johnson syndrome**, **toxic epidermal necrolysis**, urticaria
Other: Anaphylaxis, **angioedema**, flu-like symptoms, **hyperkalemia**, onset of seasonal allergies, weight loss

Nursing Considerations

- Know that teriflunomide isn't recommended for patients with bone marrow dysplasia, severe immunodeficiency, or severe, uncontrolled infections because of its immunosuppressant effect. It is also not recommended for patients with liver disease or those with a serum alanine aminotransferase level greater than two times the upper level normal prior to initiation of therapy because drug may worsen liver dysfunction.
- Obtain a pregnancy test on all women of childbearing age, as ordered, prior to starting teriflunomide therapy. Know that drug should not be started if pregnancy is suspected or confirmed and in women who refuse to use a reliable contraceptive.
- Use cautiously in patients who are over 60 years of age, patients with diabetes, or in patients taking concomitant neurotoxic drugs because of an increased risk of developing peripheral neuropathy. If peripheral neuropathy occurs during teriflunomide therapy, notify prescriber and expect drug to be discontinued and possibly cholestyramine washout ordered.
- Test patient for latent tuberculosis before starting leflunomide, as ordered. If positive, expect standard medical treatment to be given before teriflunomide therapy starts.
- Obtain baseline blood pressure before starting teriflunomide, and monitor periodically thereafter because drug may cause hypertension.
- Assess liver enzyme (ALT and AST) levels at start of therapy, monthly during first 6 months, and if stable, every 6 to 8 weeks thereafter, as ordered. If levels become elevated greater than threefold upper level normal, notify prescriber and expect teriflunomide therapy to be withheld until underlying cause is determined. If the elevation is thought to be teriflunomide induced, expect to start cholestyramine washout, as ordered, and monitor liver test weekly until normalized. If another cause is found for the elevation, expect to resume teriflunomide therapy.
- Ensure that a complete CBC has been done within the past 6 months prior to starting teriflunomide therapy to use as a baseline. Repeat CBC, as ordered, thereafter if signs and symptoms of bone marrow suppression occur.
- Notify prescriber if patient develops a serious infection or skin condition because drug may need to be interrupted and charcoal or cholestyramine given to eliminate drug rapidly.

WARNING Monitor patient's respiratory function closely because drug may cause interstitial lung disease that could become life-threatening. If patient develops a cough and dyspnea, notify prescriber; drug may need to be stopped, and patient may need charcoal or cholestyramine to eliminate drug rapidly.

- Check patient's serum potassium level, as ordered, if symptoms of acute renal failure or hyperkalemia occur.

PATIENT TEACHING

- Tell patient to report signs of respiratory dysfunction, such as cough and dyspnea.

WARNING Caution woman of childbearing potential not to become pregnant while taking drug because of the high risk of birth defects. Emphasize importance of using reliable forms of birth control and to notify prescriber immediately if pregnancy is suspected. Also advise men not wishing to father a child and their female partners to use effective contraception to minimize any possible risk to the fetus.

- Inform women to discuss breastfeeding with their prescriber, because they cannot breastfeed while taking teriflunomide.
- Advise patient to avoid live vaccines during teriflunomide therapy.
- Instruct patient to notify prescriber if she develops an infection or skin condition.
- Instruct patient to stop taking teriflunomide if he develops an allergic reaction, including difficulty breathing; itching or swelling of eyes, face, lips, throat, or tongue; fever, rash, or swollen glands; or signs of liver dysfunction such

as darkened urine, fatigue, and yellow eyes or skin. In addition, patient should seek immediate medical attention.

teriparatide

Forteo

Class and Category

Pharmacologic class: Recombinant human parathyroid hormone (PTH)
Therapeutic class: Antiosteoporotic
Pregnancy category: C

Indications and Dosages

➤ *To treat osteoporosis in postmenopausal women and primary or hypogonadal osteoporosis in men at high risk for fracture; to treat men and women with glucocorticoid-induced osteoporosis at high risk for fracture*

SUBCUTANEOUS INJECTION
Adults. 20 mcg daily for up to 2 yr.

Route	Onset	Peak	Duration
SubQ	2 hr	4–6 hr	16–24 hr

Contraindications

Hypersensitivity to teriparatide or its components

Interactions

DRUGS
digitalis glycosides: Possibly increased risk of digitalis toxicity

Adverse Reactions

CNS: Asthenia, depression, dizziness, headache, insomnia, paresthesia, syncope, vertigo
CV: Angina pectoris, chest pain, hypertension, transient orthostatic hypotension

Mechanism of Action

Teriparatide, which contains recombinant PTH, stimulates new bone growth and increases bone density. In a patient with osteoporosis, bone density and mass are diminished by an imbalance between bone destruction and formation. Normally, osteoclasts break down and resorb bone, leaving behind a cavity in a section of bone. Then bone-building cells, called osteoblasts, line the walls of the cavity and stimulate new bone formation. PTH stimulates these actions by attaching to receptors on osteoclasts and osteoblasts, as shown below. Teriparatide binds to cell-surface receptors on osteoblasts and preferentially stimulates osteoblastic over osteoclastic activity. Also, the drug increases the amount of circulating calcium available for bone formation by increasing the intestinal absorption of calcium and phosphate, thus enhancing the rate of calcium resorption from bone, increasing the reabsorption of calcium, and inhibiting the reabsorption of phosphate in the kidneys. These actions stimulate new bone formation and increase bone density to reduce osteoporotic bone changes.

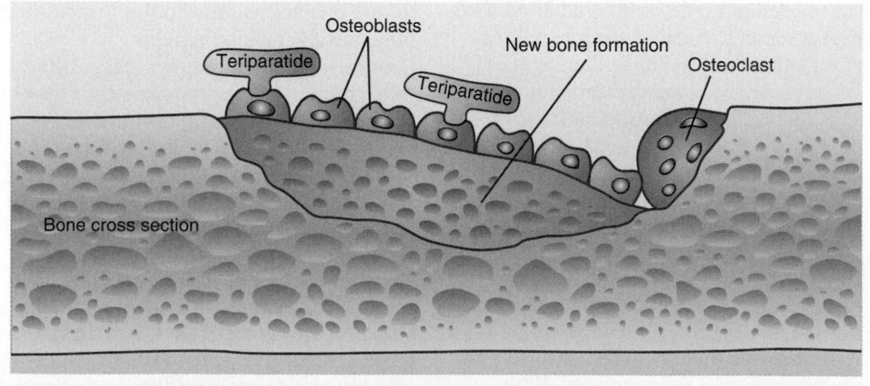

EENT: Pharyngitis, rhinitis, taste perversion, tooth disorder
ENDO: Hypoparathyroidism
GI: Constipation, diarrhea, indigestion, vomiting
MS: Arthralgia, muscle cramps or spasms in back or leg, neck pain
RESP: Cough, dyspnea, pneumonia
SKIN: Diaphoresis, pruritus, rash, urticaria
Other: **Angioedema,** generalized pain, **hypercalcemia, hypocalcemia** injection-site reactions (erythema, localized bruising, minor bleeding, pain, pruritus, swelling)

Nursing Considerations

WARNING Be aware that teriparatide shouldn't be used to treat patients at risk for osteosarcoma (such as those with Paget's disease or a metabolic bone disease other than osteoporosis), unexplained elevations of alkaline phosphatase, open epiphyses, or prior skeletal radiation or malignancy.

WARNING Be aware that patients with hypercalcemia shouldn't receive teriparatide because drug may worsen hypercalcemia.

- Use drug cautiously in patients with active or recent urolithiasis because drug could worsen this condition.
- Monitor patient closely for allergic reactions because teriparatide is a peptide agent.
- Monitor patient's blood calcium level, and notify prescriber of any elevation; in persistent hypercalcemia, the drug may have to be stopped.
- Monitor patient's blood pressure during the first several doses of drug therapy because of a risk of transient orthostatic hypotension. If this occurs, place patient in a reclining position and alert prescriber.

PATIENT TEACHING

- Teach patient how to administer teriparatide by subcutaneous injection and how to properly use the delivery pen device and dispose of needles. Advise her not to share pen device with others.
- Inform patient that each delivery pen can be used for up to 28 days after the first injection but then should be discarded even if it still contains solution.
- Instruct patient to store the delivery pen in the refrigerator and to recap it when not in use to protect it from damage and light.
- Tell patient that delivery pen may be used immediately after removal from refrigerator and should be put back in refrigerator as soon as the injection is given.
- Instruct patient to inject drug into thigh or abdominal wall and to rotate injection sites.
- Caution patient to administer drug in a room where she can immediately sit or lie down if light-headedness or palpitations occur. Advise her to notify prescriber if these symptoms persist or worsen.
- Instruct patient to notify prescriber of persistent symptoms of hypercalcemia, such as nausea, vomiting, constipation, lethargy, and muscle weakness.
- Caution patient about potential developing osteosarcoma.

tesamorelin

Egrifta

Class and Category

Pharmacologic class: Growth hormone releasing factor analogue
Therapeutic class: Endocrine metabolic agent
Pregnancy category: X

Indications and Dosages

➤ *To reduce excess abdominal fat in HIV-infected patients with lipodystrophy*

SUBCUTANEOUS INJECTION

Adults. 2 mg once daily.

Mechanism of Action

Stimulates growth hormone secretion, which is both anabolic and lipolytic. By interacting with specific receptors on adipocytes, fat breakdown occurs.

Contraindications

Active malignancy; disruption of the hypothalamic-pituitary axis due to head irradiation, head trauma, hypophysectomy, hypopituitarism, or pituitary tumor or surgery; hypersensitivity to tesamorelin or its components; pregnancy

T

Interactions

DRUGS

anticonvulsants, corticosteroids, cyclosporine, sex steroids: Possibly altered metabolization of these drugs
glucocorticoids: Possibly decreased effectiveness requiring larger dosages

Adverse Reactions

CNS: Depression, hypoesthesia, insomnia, paresthesia, peripheral neuropathy
CV: Chest pain, hypertension, palpitations, peripheral edema
ENDO: Hot flashes, hyperglycemia
GI: Abdominal pain (upper), dyspepsia, nausea, vomiting
MS: Arthralgia, carpel tunnel syndrome, elevated blood creatine phosphokinase, extremity pain, joint stiffness or swelling, muscle spasms or strain, musculoskeletal pain or stiffness, myalgia
SKIN: Erythema, flushing, night sweats, pruritus, rash, urticaria
Other: Antitesamorelin IgG antibodies, injection-site reactions (erythema, hemorrhage, irritation, pain, pruritis, rash, swelling, urticaria)

Nursing Considerations

- Do not administer tesamorelin to any patient with an active malignancy, and expect drug to be discontinued if patient becomes critically ill for any reason during tesamorelin therapy.
- Use cautiously in patients with a history of nonmalignant neoplasms or patients with a history of treated and stable malignancies because tesamorelin therapy could reactivate the underlying malignancy.
- Evaluate patient's glucose status prior to initiating tesamorelin therapy to obtain a baseline because the drug may cause glucose intolerance. Continue to monitor glucose levels throughout therapy and treat accordingly, as prescribed.
- Follow instructions provided with the medication for reconstituting tesamorelin. Once reconstituted, drug must be administered immediately. If a delay occurs, the reconstituted solution must be discarded.
- Administer as a subcutaneous injection into the abdomen. Rotate sites to different areas of the abdomen. Do not inject drug into bruises, the navel, or scar tissue.
- Monitor serum IGF-1 levels, as ordered, because tesamorelin stimulates growth hormone production and increases serum IGF-1 levels. If persistent elevations occur (greater than 3 SDS), notify prescriber because drug may have to be discontinued.
- Ensure patient with diabetes undergoes ophthalmologic examinations regularly because drug may cause retinopathy to develop or worsen because of the increased drug-induced IGF-1 levels.
- Monitor patient closely for hypersensitivity reactions such as the development of erythema, flushing, pruritus, rash, or urticaria. If present, notify prescriber and expect tesamorelin to be discontinued.

PATIENT TEACHING

- Teach patient how to reconstitute drug and administer a subcutaneous injection. Emphasize importance of rotating sites within the abdomen to reduce incidence of injection reactions.
- Instruct patient to notify prescriber immediately and to stop taking tesamorelin if he develops a hypersensitivity reaction such as hives or a rash.
- Inform patient with diabetes that drug may alter his glucose control and that he should test his blood glucose regularly. Medical attention should be sought if glucose control becomes affected.

tetracycline hydrochloride

Class and Category

Pharmacologic class: Tetracycline
Therapeutic class: Antibiotic
Pregnancy category: D

Indications and Dosages

➤ *To treat infections caused by gram-negative and gram-positive organisms*

CAPSULES

Adults. 250 mg four times daily or 500 mg twice daily increased to 500 mg four times daily, as needed for severe infections or those not responding to lower doses.
Children age 9 and over. 25 to 50 mg/kg daily divided into four equal doses.

➤ *To treat moderate to severe acne vulgaris in patients requiring long-term treatment*

CAPSULES

Adults. *Initial:* 1,000 mg daily in divided doses until improvement occurs (usually in 3 wk); then dosage reduced gradually. *Maintenance:* 125 to 500 mg daily, every other day, or intermittently.

➤ *To treat brucellosis caused by susceptible organisms*

CAPSULES

Adults. 500 mg every 6 hr for 3 wk, given with 1 g of streptomycin I.M. every 12 hr in wk 1 and daily in wk 2.

➤ *To treat gonorrhea caused by* Neisseria gonorrhoeae

CAPSULES

Adults. 500 mg every 6 hr for 5 days.

➤ *To treat syphilis in patients allergic to penicillin*

CAPSULES

Adults. 500 mg every 6 hr for 15 days (for early syphilis of less than 1 yr duration) or 30 days (for late syphilis with more than 1 yr duration except for neurosyphilis).

➤ *To treat uncomplicated endocervical, rectal, or urethral infections caused by* Chlamydia trachomatis

CAPSULES

Adults. 500 mg four times a day for at least 7 days.

DOSAGE ADJUSTMENT For patients with renal impairment, dosage reduced or time intervals extended between doses because of extended half-life.

Mechanism of Action

Exerts a bacteriostatic effect against a wide variety of gram-negative and gram-positive organisms by passing through the bacterial lipid bilayer, where it binds reversibly to 30S ribosomal subunits. Bound tetracycline blocks the binding of aminoacyl transfer RNA to messenger RNA, thus inhibiting bacterial protein synthesis.

Contraindications

Hypersensitivity to tetracycline or its components

Interactions

DRUGS

aluminum-, calcium-, or magnesium-containing antacids; iron supplements (oral); magnesium-containing laxatives; magnesium salicylate; multivitamins (containing manganese or zinc salts); sodium bicarbonate: Possibly impaired absorption of oral tetracycline and formation of nonabsorbable complexes
cholestyramine, colestipol: Possibly impaired absorption of oral tetracycline
digoxin: Possibly increased digoxin level
methoxyflurane: Possibly nephrotoxicity
oral contraceptives (containing estrogen): Possibly reduced contraceptive reliability and increased risk of breakthrough bleeding (with long-term tetracycline use)
penicillins: Possibly decreased bactericidal effect of penicillins
vitamin A: Possibly benign intracranial hypertension

FOODS

dairy products and other foods: Possibly impaired absorption of oral tetracycline

Adverse Reactions

CNS: Dizziness, light-headedness, unsteadiness
EENT: Darkened or discolored tongue, enamel hypoplasia, oral candidiasis, tooth discoloration (in children)
GI: Abdominal pain, diarrhea, **hepatotoxicity**, nausea, rectal candidiasis, vomiting
GU: Vaginal candidiasis
SKIN: Photosensitivity

Nursing Considerations

- Avoid giving tetracycline to children age 8 and under because drug may cause permanent brown or yellow tooth discoloration and enamel hypoplasia.
- Be aware that enamel hypoplasia and tooth discoloration may occur in breastfed infants, along with inhibition of linear skeletal growth, oral and vaginal candidiasis, and photosensitivity.
- Know that to reduce the risk of esophageal irritation or ulceration, bedtime dosing of tetracycline should be avoided for patient with esophageal obstruction or compression.
- Assess for photosensitivity, which can develop within a few minutes or up to several hours after exposure to sunlight or other ultraviolet (UV) light. Effects may last for 1 to 2 days after discontinuation of drug.

- Be aware that citric acid in tetracycline preparations may accelerate drug deterioration and that using outdated drug may cause Fanconi's syndrome, characterized by multiple defects in renal tubular function. Symptoms include acidosis, bicarbonate wasting, glycosuria, hypokalemia, osteomalacia, and phosphaturia.

PATIENT TEACHING

- Instruct patient to take oral tetracycline at least 1 hour before meals or 2 hours after meals because dairy products and some foods may interfere with absorption.
- Advise patient to take each dose with a full glass of water while in an upright position to avoid esophageal or GI irritation.
- Advise patient to avoid taking other drugs, including OTC antacids and other preparations, within 3 hours of oral tetracycline.
- Urge patient to complete entire course of tetracycline therapy even if she feels better.
- Caution her to avoid direct sunlight or UV light and to wear sunscreen when outdoors.
- Advise women who use oral contraceptives containing estrogen to use another method of contraception while taking tetracycline because contraceptives may be less effective. Tell patient to notify prescriber immediately if pregnancy is known or suspected.
- Emphasize the need to discard outdated tetracycline because of the risk of toxic effects.
- Encourage patient to take safety precautions if she experiences dizziness or other adverse CNS reactions.

theophylline

Elixophyllin, Theo-24, Theochron, Theolair, Uniphyl

Class and Category

Pharmacologic class: Xanthine derivative
Therapeutic class: Bronchodilator
[Preg]nancy category: C

Indications and Dosages

➤ *As adjunct to inhaled beta-2 selective agonists and systemically administered corticosteroids to treat acute exacerbations of symptoms and reversible airflow obstruction associated with asthma and other chronic lung diseases such as chronic bronchitis and emphysema*

ELIXIR, I.V. INFUSION, TABLETS

Adults, children, and infants. Loading and maintenance doses highly individualized based upon the following factors: age and weight of patient; currently using or not using a theophylline drug; nonsmoker or smoker; presence or absence of sepsis with multi-organ failure, or shock; and presence of underlying heart, liver, or lung conditions.

➤ *To treat symptoms and reversible airflow obstruction associated with chronic asthma and other chronic lung diseases such as chronic bronchitis and emphysema*

ELIXIR, ER CAPSULES, ER TABLETS, TABLETS

Adults, children, and infants. Highly individualized based upon age and weight of patient, serum theophylline concentrations, and underlying heart, liver, or lung conditions.

Mechanism of Action

Inhibits phosphodiesterase enzymes, causing bronchodilation. Normally, these enzymes inactivate cAMP and cGMP, which are responsible for bronchial smooth-muscle relaxation. Theophylline also may antagonize adenosine and prostaglandins receptors, cause calcium translocation, inhibit cGMP metabolism, and stimulate catecholamines.

Incompatibilities

Don't mix parenteral theophylline solution with any additives. Don't infuse theophylline through same I.V. line as Hetastarch (Hespan), a colloidal plasma volume expander, which is incompatible with theophylline.

Contraindications

Hypersensitivity to theophylline or its components, peptic ulcer disease, uncontrolled seizure disorder

Interactions

DRUGS

adenosine: Decreased adenosine effectiveness
allopurinol, cimetidine, ciprofloxacin, clarithromycin, disulfiram, enoxacin, erythromycin, fluvoxamine, interferon alpha (human recombinant), methotrexate, mexiletine, pentoxifylline, propafenone, propranolol, tacrine, thiabendazole, ticlopidine, troleandomycin, verapamil: Increased blood theophylline level and risk of toxicity
aminoglutethimide, carbamazepine, isoproterenol (I.V.), moricizine, oral contraceptives (containing estrogen), phenobarbital, phenytoin, rifampin: Decreased blood theophylline level and possibly drug effectiveness
benzodiazepines: Possibly reversal of benzodiazepine sedation
beta blockers: Possibly decreased bronchodilator effect of theophylline
ephedrine: Increased adverse effects, including insomnia, nausea, and nervousness
halothane anesthetics: Increased risk of ventricular arrhythmias
ketamine: Lowered seizure threshold
lithium: Decreased lithium effectiveness
neuromuscular blockers: Possibly antagonized neuromuscular blockade
sucralfate: Decreased absorption of oral theophylline

FOODS

high-carbohydrate, low-protein diet: Possibly decreased theophylline elimination
low-carbohydrate, high-protein diet; daily intake of charbroiled beef: Possibly increased theophylline elimination

ACTIVITIES

alcohol use: Increased blood theophylline level and risk of toxicity
smoking: Increased drug clearance, decreased drug effectiveness

Adverse Reactions

CNS: Agitation, anxiety (I.V. form), behavioral changes, confusion, disorientation, headache, insomnia, nervousness, **nonconvulsive status epilepticus**, **seizures**, tremor
CV: Hypotension, tachycardia, **ventricular arrhythmias**
ENDO: Hyperglycemia
GI: Abdominal pain, diarrhea, heartburn, nausea, vomiting
GU: Increased urine output
Other: Hypercalcemia

Nursing Considerations

- Be aware that ideal body weight is used to calculate theophylline dosages because drug doesn't bind well in body fat.
- Be aware that E.R. capsules and tablets shouldn't be used for oral loading doses.
- Administer continuous theophylline infusion with rate-controlled infusion device. Administer loading dose given intravenously over 30 minutes. Be aware that a continuous infusion rate is highly individualized and based on serum theophylline concentrations.
- Monitor blood theophylline level, as ordered, to gauge therapeutic level and detect toxicity. Know that patients with uncorrected acidemia have an increased risk of toxicity.
- Frequently assess heart rate and rhythm because theophylline can exacerbate existing arrhythmias.
- Be especially alert for signs of toxicity in patient with acute pulmonary edema, hypothyroidism, influenza vaccination, prolonged fever, sepsis with multiple organ failure, shock, or viral pulmonary infection because of decreased drug clearance.
- Expect patient with cystic fibrosis or hyperthyroidism to have increased theophylline clearance and decreased drug effectiveness. Monitor blood theophylline level in these patients, as ordered.
- Suspect toxicity if patient experiences vomiting, and be prepared to obtain blood theophylline level.

PATIENT TEACHING

- Instruct patient to swallow theophylline tablets whole and not to chew or crush them, unless scored for breaking.
- Instruct patient to take drug with a full glass of water on an empty stomach (30 to 60 minutes before meals or 2 hours after meals). However, suggest that she take drug with antacids or food if GI distress occurs.
- Encourage patient to take drug at the same time every day.

- Advise patient to notify prescriber if she develops a fever, makes a significant dietary change, or starts or stops smoking or taking other drugs because these factors may alter blood theophylline level.
- Tell female patient to notify prescriber if she is or could be pregnant.

tiagabine hydrochloride

Gabitril

Class and Category

Pharmacologic class: Gamma aminobutyric acid (GABA) reuptake inhibitor
Therapeutic class: Anticonvulsant
Pregnancy category: C

Indications and Dosages

➤ *As adjunct to treat partial seizures*

TABLETS

Adults already taking enzyme-inducing antiepileptic drugs. *Initial:* 4 mg daily; increased by 4 to 8 mg/wk until desired response occurs given in two to four divided doses daily. *Usual:* 32 to 56 mg daily. *Maximum:* 56 mg daily in two to four divided doses.

Children ages 12 to 18 already taking enzyme-inducing antiepileptic drugs. *Initial:* 4 mg daily for 1 wk, then increased to 8 mg, followed a wk later by increases of 8 mg/wk until desired response occurs and given in two to four divided doses daily. *Maximum:* 32 mg daily in two to four divided doses.

DOSAGE ADJUSTMENT For patients taking only non-enzyme-inducing antiepileptic drugs, dosage reduced and possibly a slower titration schedule required. For patients with impaired hepatic function, dosage individualized and reduced, or interval extended if needed.

Mechanism of Action

Appears to inhibit neuronal and glial uptake of gamma-aminobutyric acid (GABA), the major inhibitory neurotransmitter in the CNS. Tiagabine makes more GABA available in the CNS to open chloride channels in postsynaptic membranes, thereby leading to membrane hyperpolarization and preventing transmission of nerve impulses.

Contraindications

Hypersensitivity to tiagabine or its components

Interactions

DRUGS

benzodiazepines, CNS depressants: Possibly additive CNS depression
carbamazepine, phenobarbital, phenytoin: Possibly decreased tiagabine effectiveness
St. John's wort: Possibly enhanced metabolism of tiagabine

ACTIVITIES

alcohol use: Possibly additive CNS depression

Adverse Reactions

CNS: Amnesia, anxiety, asthenia, ataxia, confusion, depression, dizziness, drowsiness, EEG abnormalities, hostility, impaired cognition, insomnia, lightheadedness, paresthesia, **seizures**, **status epilepticus**, **suicidal ideation**, tremor, weakness
EENT: Blurred vision, pharyngitis, stomatitis
GI: Abdominal pain, diarrhea, increased appetite, nausea, vomiting
GU: UTI
MS: Dysarthria
SKIN: Bullous dermatitis, ecchymosis, rash

Nursing Considerations

- Give tiagabine with food.

WARNING Expect to taper dosage gradually, as prescribed, because stopping drug abruptly may increase seizure frequency.

- Take seizure precautions because tiagabine has caused seizures and status epilepticus in patients with no history of seizures.
- Watch patient closely for evidence of suicidal tendencies, especially when therapy starts or dosage changes, and report concerns at once.

PATIENT TEACHING

- Instruct patient to take drug with food.
- Advise patient to avoid hazardous activities until drug's CNS effects are known. Also urge her to avoid alcohol use.

- Inform patient who takes a CNS depressant, that drug may increase depressant effect.
- Instruct patient not to stop taking tiagabine abruptly. Explain that prescriber usually tapers dosage over 4 weeks to reduce the risk of withdrawal seizures.
- Urge caregivers to watch patient closely for evidence of suicidal tendencies, especially when therapy starts or dosage changes, and to report concerns immediately.
- Encourage woman who becomes pregnant while taking tiagabine to enroll in the North American antiepileptic drug pregnancy registry by calling 1-888-233-2334. Explain that the registry is collecting information about the safety of antiepileptic drugs during pregnancy.

ticagrelor

Brilinta

Class and Category

Pharmacologic class: $P2Y_{12}$ platelet inhibitor
Therapeutic class: Antiplatelet
Pregnancy category: C

Indications and Dosages

➤ *To reduce the rate of thrombotic cardiovascular events such as cardiovascular death, myocardial infarction, and stroke in patients with acute coronary syndrome (ACS) or history of myocardial infarction; reduce rate of stent thrombosis in patients who have been stented for treatment of ACS*

TABLETS

Adults. *Initial:* 180 mg as a loading dose followed by 90 mg twice daily for 1 yr, then 60 mg twice daily.

Mechanism of Action

Reversibly interacts with the platelet $P2Y_{12}$ ADP-receptor to prevent platelet activation.

Contraindications

Active bleeding, history of intracranial hemorrhage, hypersensitivity to ticagrelor or its components, severe hepatic impairment

Interactions

DRUGS

aspirin (daily doses above 100 mg): Reduced effectiveness of ticagrelor
CYP3A inducers such as carbamazepine, dexamethasone, phenobarbital, phenytoin, rifampin: Elevated ticagrelor levels and risk of adverse effects
CYP3A inhibitors such as atazanavir, clarithromycin, indinavir, itraconazole, ketoconazole, nefazodone, nelfinavir, ritonavir, saquinavir, voriconazole: Substantially reduced blood ticagrelor levels and effectiveness
digoxin: Altered blood digoxin levels
lovastatin, simvastatin: Increased serum levels of these drugs
opioids: Delayed or reduced absorption of ticagrelor

Adverse Reactions

CNS: Dizziness, fatigue, headache, **intracranial bleeding**
CV: Atrial fibrillation, bradycardia including AV block, chest pain, hypertension, **hypotension (may be severe), intracardiac bleed with cardiac tamponade**
EENT: Epistaxis, intraocular bleeding with permanent vision loss
ENDO: Gynecomastia
GI: Diarrhea, nausea
GU: Elevated serum creatinine level
HEME: Minor or **major bleeding**
MS: Back or noncardiac chest pain
RESP: Cough, dyspnea
SKIN: Bruising, rash
Other: Angioedema, elevated uric acid, **hypovolemic shock**

Nursing Considerations

- Be aware that ticagrelor shouldn't be given to patients with active pathological bleeding or who have a history of intracranial hemorrhage. It should also not be started in patients who are undergoing urgent coronary artery bypass graft (CABG) surgery or who have severe hepatic impairment.
- Know that patients with a history of bradycardia-related syncope not protected by a pacemaker, second or third AV block, or sick sinus syndrome may be at a higher risk of developing bradyarrhythmias with ticagrelor.

• Be aware that aspirin is used with ticagrelor therapy. Expect to administer 325 mg of aspirin initially followed by a maintenance dose of aspirin of 75 to 100 mg daily. Know that a patient who has already received a loading dose of clopidogrel may be started on ticagrelor therapy immediately.
• Be prepared to crush tablets and mix with water for patients who are unable to swallow tablets whole. Know that the mixture can also be administered via a nasogastric tube.
• Monitor patient closely for bleeding tendencies. Know that risk of bleeding increases with ticagrelor use in older patients as well as patients with a history of bleeding disorders or performance of percutaneous invasive procedures. Risk of bleeding also increases with concomitant use of drugs such as anticoagulant and fibrinolytic therapy, chronic use of nonsteroidal anti-inflammatory drugs, and higher doses of aspirin.
• Be prepared to discontinue ticagrelor therapy, as ordered, 5 days before surgery, if possible.
• Be suspicious of bleeding in a patient who becomes hypotensive and has recently undergone coronary angiography, CABG, PCI, or other surgical procedures, even if the patient does not have any signs of bleeding. Notify prescriber immediately if patient becomes hypotensive, and expect to provide supportive care. Be aware that attempts to manage bleeding should be made without discontinuing drug, if possible, because stopping ticagrelor increases risk of subsequent cardiovascular events.
• Monitor patient for dyspnea that may occur with ticagrelor therapy. If dyspnea is determined to be caused by the drug, expect to continue therapy as no specific treatment is needed and often resolves on its own.
• Avoid abrupt interruption of ticagrelor therapy because doing so increases the risk of myocardial infarction, stent thrombosis, and death.

PATIENT TEACHING

• Warn patient not to discontinue ticagrelor therapy abruptly because of increased risk of life-threatening adverse effects.
• Advise patient unable to swallow the tablet whole to crush it and mix with water immediately before taking the drug.
• Advise patient to seek immediate emergency care if bleeding occurs and is serious.
• Instruct patient to take bleeding precautions such as avoiding the use of a razor and brushing teeth with a soft-bristled toothbrush.
• Tell patient to alert all prescribers of ticagrelor therapy.

tigecycline

Tygacil

Class and Category

Pharmacologic class: Glycylcycline
Therapeutic class: Antibiotic
Pregnancy category: D

Indications and Dosages

➤ *To treat community-acquired bacterial pneumonia caused by* Haemophilus influenzae *(beta-lactamase negative isolates),* Legionella pneumophila, *and* Streptococcus pneumoniae *(penicillin-susceptible isolates), including cases with concurrent bacteremia; to treat complicated intra-abdominal infections caused by* Bacteroides fragilis, B. thetaiotaomicron, B. uniformis, B. vulgatus, Citrobacter freundii, Clostridium perfringens, Enterobacter cloacae, Enterococcus faecalis *(vancomycin-susceptible isolates only),* Escherichia coli, Klebsiella oxytoca, K. pneumoniae, Peptostreptococcus micros, Staphylococcus aureus *(methicillin-susceptible isolates only), and* Streptococcus anginosus *group only); to treat complicated skin and skin structure infections caused by* B. fragilis, E. coli, E. faecalis *(vancomycin-susceptible isolates only),* S. aureus *(methicillin-susceptible and resistant isolates),* S. agalactiae, S. anginosus *group (includes* S. anginosus, S. constellatus, *and* S. intermedius), *and* S. pyogenes

I.V. INFUSION

Adults. *Initial:* 100 mg infused over 30 to 60 min followed by 50 mg infused over 30 to 60 min every 12 hr for 5 to 14 days for complicated skin and skin structure infections and intra-abdominal infections (7 to 14 days for community-acquired bacterial pneumonia).

DOSAGE ADJUSTMENT For patients with severe hepatic impairment, initial dosage of 100 mg should be followed by a reduced maintenance dosage of 25 mg every 12 hr.

Mechanism of Action

Inhibits protein translation in bacteria by binding to the 30S ribosomal subunit, which prevents binding of aminoacyl tRNA molecules to the ribosome complex, thus interfering with protein synthesis. Through this bacteriostatic action, bacteria are weakened.

Incompatibilities

Don't give amphotericin B, chlorpromazine, methylprednisolone, or voriconazole simultaneously through the same Y-site.

Contraindications

Hypersensitivity to tigecycline or its components

Adverse Reactions

CNS: Asthenia, chills, dizziness, fever, headache, insomnia, somnolence
CV: **Bradycardia**, hypertension, **hypotension**, peripheral edema, phlebitis, tachycardia, thrombophlebitis, vasodilation
EENT: Dry mouth, taste perversion
ENDO: Hyperglycemia, **hypoglycemia**
GI: Abdominal pain, **acute pancreatitis**, anorexia, cholestasis (hepatic), constipation, diarrhea, dyspepsia, elevated liver enzymes, hepatic dysfunction, **hepatic failure**, jaundice, nausea, **pseudomembranous colitis**, stool abnormality, vomiting
GU: Elevated BUN and creatinine levels, leukorrhea, vaginal candidiasis, vaginitis
HEME: Anemia, eosinophilia, **increased international normalized ratio (INR)**, leukocytosis, **prolonged activated partial thromboplastin time (aPTT)**, **prolonged prothrombin time (PT)**, **thrombocytopenia**
MS: Back pain
RESP: Increased cough, dyspnea
SKIN: Diaphoresis, photosensitivity, pruritus, rash, **Stevens–Johnson syndrome**
Other: **Anaphylaxis**; **hypersensitivity reactions**; **hypocalcemia**; **hypokalemia**; **hyponatremia**; hypoproteinemia; injection-site reaction, such as edema, inflammation, pain, and phlebitis; **septic shock**

Nursing Considerations

- Know that tigecycline should only be prescribed when alternative treatments are not suitable because an increase in all-cause mortality has been observed in clinical trials.
- Obtain body tissue and fluid samples for culture and sensitivity tests as ordered before giving first dose of tigecycline. Expect to begin drug therapy before test results are known.
- Use tigecycline cautiously in patients hypersensitive to tetracycline antibiotics because glycylcycline antibiotics are structurally similar to tetracyclines.
- Also use cautiously in patients with complicated intra-abdominal infections secondary to intestinal perforation because of the risk of septic shock.
- Determine whether female patients could be pregnant before starting tigecycline therapy because the drug may cause harm to fetus.
- Reconstitute each vial of tigecycline with 5.3 ml of 0.9% sodium chloride injection or 5% dextrose injection to achieve a concentration of 10 mg/ml. Note that the color will be yellow to orange. If it's not, the solution should be discarded. Immediately withdraw reconstituted solution from the vial and add to a 100-ml I.V. bag for infusion. Drug may be stored in the I.V. bag at room temperature for up to 6 hours or refrigerated up to 24 hours before use.
- Know that if patient's I.V. line is used to infuse other drugs, the line should be flushed with either 0.9% sodium chloride injection or 5% dextrose injection before and after tigecycline infusion.
- Infuse tigecycline over 30 to 60 minutes.
- Monitor patient closely for diarrhea, which may indicate pseudomembranous colitis, which is known to occur with many antibiotics. If diarrhea occurs during tigecycline therapy, notify prescriber and

expect to withhold drug. Expect to treat pseudomembranous colitis, if confirmed, with an antibiotic effective against *Clostridium difficile*, as well as administration of electrolytes, fluids, and protein.

- Monitor patient for adverse reactions, keeping in mind the similarity between tigecycline and tetracycline.
- Assess patient for superinfection, such as vaginal candidiasis, that may result from overgrowth of nonsusceptible organisms, including fungi. If signs of infection are present, notify prescriber and provide supportive care, as prescribed.
- Monitor patient's liver function closely. If enzyme levels become elevated, notify prescriber because dosage may need to be decreased or drug discontinued.
- Be aware that adverse reactions may continue after therapy stops.

PATIENT TEACHING

- Instruct patient to report adverse reactions, especially hypersensitivity reactions, such as a itching or a rash, as well as diarrhea.
- Tell patient to report discomfort at the infusion site because the site may need to be changed.
- Urge patient to report diarrhea that's severe or prolonged. Remind patient that watery or bloody stools can occur 2 or more months after antibiotic therapy and can be serious, requiring prompt treatment.

tildrakizumab-asmn

Ilumya

Class and Category

Pharmacologic class: Monoclonal antibody
Therapeutic class: Immunomodulator
Pregnancy category: Not classified

Indications and Dosages

➤ *To treat moderate to severe plaque psoriasis in patients who are candidates for systemic therapy or phototherapy*

SUBCUTANEOUS INJECTION

Adults. 100 mg followed by 100 mg in 4 wk and then 100 mg every 12 wk thereafter.

Mechanism of Action

Selectively binds to the p19 subunit of IL-23 and inhibits its interaction with the IL-23 receptor to inhibit the release of proinflammatory chemokines and cytokines, which reduces inflammation.

Contraindications

Hypersensitivity to tidrakizumab-asmn or its components

Interactions

DRUGS

live vaccines: Increased risk of infection from live vaccine

Adverse Reactions

GI: Diarrhea
RESP: Upper respiratory infections
SKIN: Urticaria
Other: Angioedema, antibody formation to tildrakizumab-asmn, injection-site reactions (bruising, edema, erythema, hematoma, hemorrhage, inflammation, pain, pruritus, swelling)

Nursing Considerations

- Ensure that patient has been evaluated for tuberculosis prior to start of tidrakizumab-asmn therapy. Know that drug should not be given to patients with active tuberculosis. Know that patients with a past history of active or latent tuberculosis in whom an adequate course of treatment cannot be confirmed may need antituberculosis treatment before tidrakizumab-asmn is given.
- Know that tidrakizumab-asmn should not be given to patient with a serious infection until the infection resolves or is adequately treated.
- Check patient's immunization history to ensure that patient is current on immunizations before tidrakizumab-asmn therapy is begun. Do not administer a live vaccine while patient is taking tidrakizumab-asmn because of risk of infection.
- Remove tildrakizumab-asmn from refrigerator and let prefilled syringe sit, in the carton with lid closed, at room temperature for 30 minutes. Follow instructions on carton to remove syringe correctly, and remove only when ready to inject. Do not pull off needle cover until

ready to inject. Inspect syringe contents. Solution should appear clear to slightly opalescent, colorless to slightly yellow. Air bubbles may be present, but there is no need to remove them.

- Pull needle cover straight off (do not twist) and discard. Inject drug subcutaneously into abdomen, thighs, or upper arm by pushing down the blue plunger until it can go no further. Remove needle from the skin entirely before letting go of the blue plunger. After the blue plunger is released, the safety lock will draw the needle inside the needle guard. If a dose is missed, administer the dose as soon as possible and then resume dosing at the regularly scheduled interval.

WARNING Monitor patient for angioedema and urticaria. If present, notify prescriber, expect drug to be discontinued, and provide supportive care, as ordered.

- Monitor patient for infections, especially respiratory infections. If patient develops a serious infection or is not responding to standard treatment for an infection, alert prescriber, as drug may have to be discontinued.

PATIENT TEACHING

- Inform patient that tidrakizumab-asmn will be given by a health professional. Stress importance of keeping appointments for drug administration.
- Instruct patient to seek immediate medical attention if she experiences any serious allergic reactions after drug has been administered.
- Review signs and symptoms of infection with patient and tell patient to notify prescriber if present.

tiludronate disodium

Skelid

Class and Category

Pharmacologic class: Aminobiphosphonate
Therapeutic class: Bone resorption inhibitor
Pregnancy category: C

Indications and Dosages

➤ *To treat Paget's disease in patients with serum alkaline phosphatase levels at least twice the upper limit of normal, who are symptomatic or at risk for future complications of the disease*

TABLETS

Adults. *Initial:* 400 mg daily 2 hr before or after meals for 3 mo. *Maximum:* 400 mg of tiludronic acid daily.

Mechanism of Action

Reduces the activity of cells that cause bone loss; increases bone mass. Tiludronate may act by inhibiting osteoclast activity on newly formed bone resorption surfaces. This activity reduces the number of sites at which bone is remodeled. When bone formation exceeds bone resorption at these remodeling sites, bone mass increases. Tiludronate may also inhibit bone destruction by binding to hydroxyapatite crystals, which give bone its rigidity.

Contraindications

Creatinine clearance less than 30 ml/min, esophageal abnormalities that delay esophageal emptying, hypersensitivity to tiludronate or its components, inability to sit upright or stand for at least 30 minutes

Interactions

DRUGS

aluminum- or magnesium-containing antacids, mineral supplements (such as calcium, iron), salicylates, salicylate-containing compounds: Decreased absorption of tiludronate
indomethacin: Possibly increased bioavailability of tiludronate

FOODS

all foods and beverages (except plain water): Decreased absorption of tiludronate

Adverse Reactions

CNS: Dizziness, headache
CV: Chest pain, edema
EENT: Cataracts, conjunctivitis, difficulty swallowing, glaucoma, pharyngitis, rhinitis
GI: Diarrhea, esophageal irritation and ulceration, flatulence, indigestion, nausea, vomiting

MS: Arthralgia, atypical femoral fractures, back pain, myalgia, osteonecrosis of jaw, retrosternal pain
RESP: Cough, upper respiratory tract infection
SKIN: Rash
Other: Flu-like symptoms

Nursing Considerations

- Be prepared to monitor serum calcium levels before, during, and after tiludronate therapy because drug may exacerbate such conditions as hyperparathyroidism, hypocalcemia, and vitamin D deficiency. Ensure adequate dietary intake of calcium and vitamin D during and after treatment. If hypocalcemia occurs, expect to administer a calcium supplement, as prescribed.
- Use cautiously in patients with active upper gastrointestinal conditions such as Barrett's esophagus, dysphagia, other esophageal disease, duodenitis, gastritis, or ulcers because tiludronate therapy may worsen these conditions because of its irritating effect on upper GI mucosa.

WARNING Know that to help minimize tiludronate's irritation on the patient's upper GI mucosa, patient should drug with full glass of plain water and remain upright for at least 30 minutes.

PATIENT TEACHING

- Instruct patient to take drug with 6 to 8 oz of plain water on an empty stomach (at least 2 hours before or after beverages, food, other drugs, or mineral supplements, including mineral water) because beverages and food may severely reduce drug's effect. Also, advise her to remain upright for at least 30 minutes after taking drug.
- Advise patient not to chew or suck on tablet to reduce the risk of esophageal irritation.
- Instruct patient to notify prescriber immediately if she develops signs or symptoms of esophageal irritation, such as painful swallowing, retrosternal pain, trouble swallowing, or worsening heartburn; these may indicate a serious esophageal disorder.
- Caution patient not to take salicylate-containing drugs, such as aspirin, during tiludronate therapy.
- Encourage patient to maintain adequate calcium and vitamin D intake during tiludronate therapy. Calcium supplements should not be taken within 2 hours before or 2 hours after taking tiludronate. Aluminum- or magnesium-containing antacids should also be taken at least 2 hours after taking tiludronate.
- Instruct patient to notify prescriber of new or worsening groin or thigh pain.

timolol maleate

Apo-Timol (CAN), Novo-Timol (CAN)

Class and Category

Pharmacologic class: Beta blocker
Therapeutic class: Antihypertensive, MI prophylactic, vascular headache prophylactic
Pregnancy category: C

Indications and Dosages

➤ *To manage hypertension*

TABLETS

Adults. *Initial:* 10 mg twice daily, increased every wk as prescribed. *Maintenance:* 20 to 40 mg daily in divided doses. *Maximum:* 60 mg daily.

➤ *To provide long-term prophylaxis after MI*

TABLETS

Adults. 10 mg twice daily, beginning 1 to 4 wk after MI and continuing for at least 2 yr.

➤ *To prevent migraine headache*

TABLETS

Adults. *Initial:* 10 mg twice daily. *Maintenance:* 20 mg daily as a single dose or in divided doses. *Maximum:* 30 mg daily; discontinued after 8 wk, as prescribed, if maximum dose is ineffective.

Route	Onset	Peak	Duration
P.O.	30 min	1–2 hr	4–8 hr

Mechanism of Action

Selectively blocks $alpha_1$ and $beta_2$ receptors in vascular smooth muscle and $beta_1$ receptors in the heart. This reduces peripheral vascular resistance and in turn blood pressure and relieves migraine headaches. Timolol's potent beta blockade prevents the reflex tachycardia that typically occurs with most alpha blockers, and decreases cardiac excitability, cardiac output, and myocardial oxygen demand, thus preventing MI.

Contraindications

Acute bronchospasm; asthma; cardiogenic shock; children; COPD (severe); heart failure; hypersensitivity to timolol, other beta blockers, or their components; second- or third-degree AV block; severe sinus bradycardia

Interactions

DRUGS

allergen immunotherapy, allergenic extracts for skin testing: Increased risk of serious systemic adverse reactions or anaphylaxis
amiodarone: Additive depressant effect on cardiac conduction, negative inotropic effect
anesthetics (hydrocarbon inhalation): Increased risk of hypotension and myocardial depression
beta blockers: Additive beta blockade effects
calcium channel blockers, clonidine, diazoxide, guanabenz, reserpine, other hypotension-producing drugs: Additive hypotensive effect and, possibly, other beta blockade effects
cimetidine: Possibly interference with timolol clearance
estrogens: Decreased antihypertensive effect of timolol
fentanyl, fentanyl derivatives: Possibly increased risk of initial bradycardia after induction doses of fentanyl or derivative (with long-term timolol use)
glucagon: Possibly blunted hyperglycemic response
insulin, oral antidiabetic drugs: Possibly masking of tachycardia in response to hypoglycemia, impaired glucose control
lidocaine: Decreased lidocaine clearance, increased risk of lidocaine toxicity
MAO inhibitors: Increased risk of significant hypertension
neuromuscular blockers: Possibly potentiated and prolonged action of these drugs
NSAIDs: Possibly decreased hypotensive effect
phenothiazines: Increased blood levels of both drugs
phenytoin (parenteral): Additive cardiac depressant effect
sympathomimetics, xanthines: Possibly mutual inhibition of therapeutic effects

Adverse Reactions

CNS: Asthenia, **CVA**, decreased concentration, depression, dizziness, fatigue, fever, hallucinations, headache, insomnia, nervousness, nightmares, paresthesia, syncope, vertigo
CV: Angina, **arrhythmias**, **bradycardia**, **cardiac arrest**, chest pain, edema, palpitations, Raynaud's phenomenon, vasodilation
EENT: Diplopia, dry eyes, eye irritation, ptosis, tinnitus, vision changes
ENDO: Hyperglycemia, **hypoglycemia**
GI: Abdominal pain, diarrhea, hepatomegaly, indigestion, nausea, vomiting
GU: Decreased libido, impotence
MS: Arthralgia, decreased tolerance to exercise, extremity pain, muscle weakness
RESP: Bronchospasm, cough, crackles, dyspnea
SKIN: Alopecia, diaphoresis, hyperpigmentation, pruritus, purpura, rash
Other: Anaphylaxis, weight loss

Nursing Considerations

WARNING Be aware that timolol may mask evidence of acute hypoglycemia in diabetic patient. It also may mask certain signs of hyperthyroidism, such as tachycardia.

- Be aware that timolol may prolong hypoglycemia by interfering with glycogenolysis or may promote hyperglycemia by decreasing tissue sensitivity to insulin.
- Monitor blood pressure and cardiac output, as appropriate, for patient with a history of left ventricular dysfunction or systolic heart failure, because timolol's negative inotropic effect can depress cardiac output.

WARNING Be aware that timolol shouldn't be discontinued abruptly because this may produce MI, myocardial ischemia, severe hypertension, or ventricular arrhythmias, particularly in patient with known cardiovascular disease.

- Expect varied drug effectiveness in elderly patients; they may be less sensitive to drug's antihypertensive effect or more sensitive because of reduced drug clearance.
- Monitor for impaired circulation in elderly patients with age-related peripheral vascular disease or patients with Raynaud's phenomenon. Such patients

may experience exacerbated symptoms from increased alpha stimulation. Elderly patients also are at increased risk for beta blocker–induced hypothermia.
- Know that if timolol worsens skin condition, such as psoriasis, prescriber should be notified.

PATIENT TEACHING
- Instruct patient taking timolol to inform prescriber of chest pain, fainting, light-headedness, or shortness of breath, which may indicate the need for dosage change.
- Caution patient not to stop taking drug abruptly. Timolol dosage must be tapered gradually under prescriber's supervision.
- Instruct patient with diabetes to monitor blood glucose level often during therapy.
- Warn patient with psoriasis about possible flare-ups of skin condition.

tinidazole

Tindamax

Class and Category

Pharmacologic class: **Nitroimidazole**
Therapeutic class: Antiprotozoal
Pregnancy category: C

Indications and Dosages

➤ *To treat trichomoniasis caused by* Trichomonas vaginalis

TABLETS
Adults. 2 g one time with food.

➤ *To treat giardiasis caused by* Giardia duodenalis (G. lamblia)

TABLETS
Adults. 2 g one time with food.
Children age 4 and over. 50 mg/kg (up to 2 g) one time with food.

➤ *To treat intestinal amebiasis caused by* Entamoeba histolytica

TABLETS
Adults. 2 g daily for 3 days with food.
Children age 4 and over. 50 mg/kg (up to 2 g) daily for 3 days with food.

➤ *To treat amebic liver abscess caused by* E. histolytica

TABLETS
Adults. 2 g daily for 3 to 5 days with food.
Children age 4 and over. 50 mg/kg (up to 2 g) daily for 3 to 5 days with food.

➤ *To treat bacterial vaginosis in non-pregnant women*

TABLETS
Non-pregnant women. 2 g once daily for 2 days with food. Alternatively, 1 g once daily for 5 days with food.

DOSAGE ADJUSTMENT For patients receiving hemodialysis, an additional dose equivalent to one-half the dose prescribed should be given after the dialysis treatment on the days dialysis is performed.

Mechanism of Action

Undergoes intracellular chemical reduction during anaerobic metabolism. After tinidazole is reduced, it damages DNA's helical structure and breaks its strands, which inhibits bacterial nucleic acid synthesis and causes cell death.

Contraindications

Breastfeeding, hypersensitivity to tinidazole or its components, treatment of trichomoniasis during first trimester of pregnancy

Interactions

DRUGS
cholestyramine: Possibly decreased bio-availability of tinidazole
cimetidine, ketoconazole: Possibly delayed elimination and increased blood level of tinidazole
cyclosporine, tacrolimus: Possibly increased serum cyclosporine and tacrolimus levels
disulfiram: Possibly combined toxicity, resulting in confusion and psychosis
fluorouracil: Possibly decreased fluorouracil clearance
lithium: Possibly increased serum lithium levels
oral anticoagulants: Possibly increased anticoagulant effect
oxytetracycline: Possibly diminished effect of tinidazole
phenobarbital, phenytoin, rifampin: Possibly increased metabolism and decreased blood level of tinidazole

ACTIVITIES
alcohol use: Possibly disulfiram-like effects

Adverse Reactions

CNS: Ataxia, **coma**, confusion, depression, dizziness, drowsiness, fatigue, fever, headache, insomnia, malaise, peripheral neuropathy, **seizures**, vertigo, weakness
CV: Palpitations
EENT: Bitter or metallic taste, dry mouth, excessive salivation, furry tongue, oral candidiasis, pharyngitis, stomatitis, tongue discoloration
GI: Abdominal cramps, anorexia, constipation, diarrhea, epigastric discomfort, flatulence, hepatic abnormalities, indigestion, nausea, thirst, vomiting
GU: Darkened urine, dysuria, increased vaginal discharge, menorrhagia, UTI, vaginal candidiasis or odor, vulvo-vaginal discomfort
HEME: Leukopenia, neutropenia, thrombocytopenia
MS: Arthralgia, arthritis, myalgia, pelvic pain
RESP: Bronchospasm, dyspnea, upper respiratory tract infection
SKIN: Diaphoresis, **erythema multiforme**, flushing, pruritus, rash, **Stevens–Johnson syndrome**, urticaria
Other: Angioedema

Nursing Considerations

- Use tinidazole cautiously in patients with blood dyscrasias or CNS disease because tinidazole's adverse effects may worsen these disorders. Also use cautiously in patients with hepatic impairment because a chemically related drug has reduced elimination.
- Take seizure precautions. If a seizure or other abnormal neurologic symptoms occur, notify prescriber and expect to stop drug.
- Treat a patient diagnosed with trichomoniasis and her sexual partner with the same dose of tinidazole and at the same time, as ordered, because trichomoniasis is a sexually transmitted disease.
- Monitor patient's total WBC count and differential if retreatment with tinidazole is needed because adverse hematologic reactions may occur with repeated use.

PATIENT TEACHING

- Tell patient to take tinidazole with food to minimize gastric discomfort.
- Instruct patient unable to swallow tablets to crush tinidazole and mix in artificial cherry syrup and then take with food.
- Advise patient to avoid alcohol while taking tinidazole and for 3 days afterward because alcohol can cause intense flushing.
- Tell patient to alert prescriber before taking tinidazole if she thinks or knows she is pregnant because tinidazole crosses the placental barrier during the first trimester and its effects on the fetus are unknown.
- Instruct breastfeeding patient not to breastfeed during therapy and for 3 days after taking last dose.

tiotropium bromide

Spiriva HandiHaler, Spiriva Respimat

Class and Category

Pharmacologic class: Anticholinergic
Therapeutic class: Bronchodilator
Pregnancy category: C

Indications and Dosages

➤ *To provide long-term maintenance treatment of asthma*

ORAL INHALATION (RESPIMAT)

Adults and children age 6 and over. 2.5 mcg (2 inhalations) once daily. *Maximum:* 2.5 mcg every 24 hr.

➤ *To provide long-term maintenance treatment of bronchospasm associated with COPD, including chronic bronchitis and emphysema; to reduce COPD exacerbations*

ORAL INHALATION (HANDIHALER)

Adults. 18 mcg (2 inhalations) once daily. *Maximum*: 18 mcg every 24 hr.

ORAL INHALATION (RESPIMAT)

Adults.
5 mcg (2 inhalations) once daily. *Maximum:* 5 mcg every 24 hr.

➤ *To provide maintenance treatment of asthma*

ORAL INHALATION (RESPIMAT)

Adults and children age 6 and over. 2.5 mcg (2 inhalations) once daily. *Maximum:* 2.5 mcg every 24 hr.

Mechanism of Action

Prevents acetylcholine from attaching to muscarinic receptors on membranes of smooth-muscle cells. By blocking acetylcholine's effects in the bronchi and bronchioles, tiotropium relaxes smooth muscles and causes bronchodilation.

Contraindications

Hypersensitivity to atropine or its derivatives, including ipratropium, tiotropium, or their components

Interactions

DRUGS

anticholinergics: Possibly increased anticholinergic effects

Adverse Reactions

CNS: CVA, depression, difficulty speaking, dizziness, insomnia, paresthesia
CV: Angina, **atrial fibrillation**, chest pain, hypercholesterolemia, hypertension, palpitations, peripheral edema, **supraventricular tachycardia**, tachycardia
EENT: Application site irritation (glossitis, mouth ulceration, pharyngolaryngeal pain), blurred vision, cataract, dry mouth, dysphonia, epistaxis, eye pain, glaucoma, glossitis, hoarseness, increased intraocular pressure, laryngitis, oral candidiasis, pharyngitis, rhinitis, sinusitis, stomatitis, throat irritation, visual halos
ENDO: Hyperglycemia
GI: Abdominal pain, constipation, diarrhea, dysphagia, gastroesophageal reflux, indigestion, **intestinal obstruction**, ileus, vomiting
GU: Difficulty urinating, urine retention, UTI
MS: Arthritis, leg or skeletal pain, myalgia
RESP: Cough, **paradoxical bronchospasm**, upper respiratory tract infection
SKIN: Pruritus, rash, urticaria
Other: Anaphylaxis, **angioedema**, candidiasis, dehydration, flu-like symptoms, **hypersensitivity reaction (immediate)**, infection

Nursing Considerations

- Use tiotropium cautiously in patients with angle-closure glaucoma, benign prostatic hyperplasia, or bladder neck obstruction.

WARNING Monitor patient closely after giving first dose of tiotropium for immediate hypersensitivity reactions, including anaphylaxis, angioedema , bronchospasm, and skin reactions. If reaction occurs, notify prescriber and expect to stop tiotropium and provide supportive care. Know that patients with a hypersensitivity to atropine should not receive tiotropium, because tiotropium is a derivative of atropine. Also use tiotropium cautiously in patients who have severe hypersensitivity to milk proteins.

- Know that when tiotropium is used for maintenance therapy in patients with asthma, it may take up to 8 weeks to realize maximum benefits.
- Be aware that tiotropium should never be used to relieve acute bronchospasm.
- Monitor patient's renal function, as ordered, especially in patients with moderate to severe renal impairment, because tiotropium is excreted mainly by the kidneys. Monitor patient with renal dysfunction closely for anticholinergic effects.
- Monitor patient's pulmonary function, as ordered, to evaluate the effectiveness of tiotropium.

PATIENT TEACHING

- Caution patient not to use tiotropium to treat acute bronchospasm and that drug should not be used more often than every 24 hours.
- Instruct patient on the proper use of the HandiHaler inhalation device, if prescribed. Tell patient to place the capsule into the center chamber of the inhalation device and then to press and release the button on the side of the inhalation device to pierce the capsule. Then have the patient exhale completely, close her lips around the mouthpiece, inhale slowly and deeply, and hold her breath for as long as is comfortable.
- Alert patient that the HandiHaler device should not be used to take any other drug and that the tiotropium capsule must be taken only using the device and never swallowed.
- Tell patient not to expose capsules used in the HandiHaler device to air until ready for use. To remove a capsule from the blister pack, tell patient to open the foil only as far as the stop line to avoid exposing the rest of the capsules in the blister pack to air. Instruct patient to discard capsules used in the HandiHaler device if they are inadvertently exposed to air and won't be used immediately.

- Advise patient to keep powder found in the capsule used with the HandiHaler device out of her eyes because it may irritate them or blur her vision.
- Tell patient prescribed the Respimat inhaler to insert the cartridge into the inhaler prior to first use and prime the device by actuating the inhaler (pointed toward the ground) until an aerosol cloud is visible and then repeat the process three more times. Remind patient that if the inhaler is not used for more than 3 days, the inhaler should be actuated once prior to use; if not used for more than 21 days, the inhaler should be activated three times prior to use.
- Inform patient that the Respimat inhaler should not be used to take any other drug.
- Instruct patient to rinse her mouth after each treatment to help minimize throat dryness and irritation.

WARNING Instruct patient to stop using drug and seek immediate emergency care if an acute allergic reaction occurs.

- Advise patient to tell prescriber about decreased response to tiotropium as well as difficulty urinating, eye pain, palpitations, and vision changes.

tipranavir

Aptivus

Class and Category

Pharmacologic class: Protease inhibitor
Therapeutic class: Antiretroviral
Pregnancy category: C

Indications and Dosages

➤ *As adjunct to treat human immunodeficiency virus type 1 (HIV-1) infection in patients who are treatment-experienced and infected with HIV-1 strains resistant to more than one protease inhibitor*

CAPSULES, ORAL SOLUTION

Adults. 500 mg (2 capsules or 5 ml oral solution) coadministered with 200 mg of ritonavir twice daily, taken with or without meals.

Children ages 2 to 18. 14 mg/kg with 6 mg/kg of ritonavir (or 375 mg/m^2 coadministered with ritonavir 150 mg/m^2) twice daily, taken with or without meals. *Maximum:* 500 mg coadministered with ritonavir 200 mg twice daily.

DOSAGE ADJUSTMENT For children who develop intolerance or toxicity, dosage reduced to 12 mg/kg with 5 mg/kg ritonavir (or 290 mg/m^2 coadministered with 115 mg/m^2 ritonavir) twice daily, provided their virus is not resistant to multiple protease inhibitors.

Mechanism of Action

Selectively inhibits the virus-specific processing of specific polyproteins in HIV-1 infected cells to prevent formation of mature virions.

Contraindications

Coadministration with alfuzosin, amiodarone, bepridil, cisapride, dihydroergotamine, ergonovine, ergotamine, flecainide, lurasidone, lovastatin, methylergonovine, midazolam (oral), pimozide, propafenone, quinidine, rifampin, St. John's wort, sildenafil (for treatment of pulmonary arterial hypertension), simvastatin, triazolam; hypersensitivity to tipranavir or its components; moderate to severe hepatic impairment

Interactions

DRUGS

abacavir, amprenavir, didanosine, etravirine, fosamprenavir, lopinavir, meperidine, methadone, omeprazole, raltegravir, saquinavir, valproic acid, zidovudine: Decreased concentration of these drugs with possible loss of therapeutic effect

atazanavir: Decreased concentration of atazanavir with possible decreased effectiveness and increased tipranavir concentration with possible increased effect and incidence of adverse reactions

atorvastatin, bosentan, colchicine, desipramine, fluticasone, fluoxetine, itraconazole, ketoconazole, midazolam (parenteral), paroxetine, quetiapine, rifabutin, rilpivirine, rosuvastatin, salmeterol, sertraline, sildenafil, tadalafil, trazodone, vardenafil: Increased concentration of these drugs, with possible increased effect and incidence of adverse reactions

T

buprenorphine/naloxone, carbamazepine, phenobarbital, phenytoin: Decreased concentration of tipranavir with possible decreased effectiveness
calcium channel blockers, cyclosporine, pioglitazone, repaglinide, sirolimus, tacrolimus: Possibly decreased concentration of these drugs with possible decreased effectiveness, or increased concentrations of these drugs with possible increased effect and incidence of adverse reactions
clarithromycin: Increased concentration of both drugs, with possible increased effects and incidences of adverse reactions
disulfiram, metronidazole: Possible increased disulfiram effect with tipranavir capsules because of alcohol content
enfuvirtide, fluconazole: Increased tipranavir concentration with possible increased effect and incidence of adverse reactions
ethinyl estradiol-containing drugs: Ethinyl estradiol concentrations decreased by as much as 50%, making oral contraceptive use ineffective; increased risk of estrogen deficiency in women taking drug as hormone replacement; increased risk of nonserious rash
warfarin: Possibly change in international normalized ratio (INR), with possible need for dosage change

Adverse Reactions

CNS: Dizziness, fatigue, fever, headache, insomnia, **intracranial hemorrhage**, malaise, peripheral neuropathy, sleep disorder, somnolence
CV: Elevated cholesterol and triglyceride levels
ENDO: Diabetes mellitus, hyperglycemia
GI: Abdominal distention or pain, anorexia, diarrhea, dyspepsia, elevated liver and pancreatic enzymes, flatulence, gastroesophageal reflux disease, **hepatic failure**, **hepatic steatosis**, **hepatitis**, hyperbilirubinemia, nausea, **pancreatitis**, vomiting
GU: Renal insufficiency
HEME: Anemia, **leukopenia**, **neutropenia**, **thrombocytopenia**
MS: Myalgia, muscle cramp
RESP: Cough, dyspnea
SKIN: Exanthema, photosensitivity, pruritus, rash
Other: Dehydration, facial wasting, flu-like illness, **hypersensitivity reactions**, lipoatrophy, lipodystrophy (acquired), lipohypertrophy, **mitochondrial toxicity**, weight loss

Nursing Considerations

- Know that use of tipranavir and ritonavir in treatment-naïve patients is not recommended.
- Be aware that genotypic or phenotypic testing and/or treatment history should guide tipranavir use.
- Use cautiously in patients with a co-infection with hepatitis B or C or who have elevated transaminase levels or mild hepatic impairment, because these patients are at greater risk of experiencing tipranavir's adverse effect on the liver. Expect to have liver function tests done at initiation of therapy and then monitored frequently throughout course of treatment. Know that with asymptomatic elevations in ALT or AST greater than 10 times the upper normal limit or elevations between 5 and 10 times the upper normal limit, and patient's total bilirubin greater than 2.5 times the upper normal limit, expect drug to be discontinued. Also monitor patient for clinical signs and symptoms of hepatic dysfunction, such as acholic stools, anorexia, fatigue, jaundice, liver tenderness or enlargement, or nausea. Report findings to prescriber.
- Use cautiously in patients who are at risk for increased bleeding or who are receiving drugs known to increase risk of bleeding, because tipranavir may cause intracranial bleeding.
- Use cautiously in patients with a sulfa allergy, because tipranavir contains a sulfonamide moiety and cross-sensitivity between the two types of drugs is unknown.
- Expect patient's cholesterol and triglyceride levels to be checked before tipranavir therapy is begun and periodically throughout therapy, because drug may cause elevated lipid levels that may require treatment.

- Know that pediatric dosage of tipranavir is based on body weight or body surface area and should not exceed the recommended adult dose.
- Monitor patient for rash, which may become severe, though this is uncommon. If severe, notify prescriber, expect drug to be discontinued, and provide supportive care, as prescribed.
- Monitor patient's blood glucose level. Exacerbation of preexisting diabetes or new-onset diabetes mellitus has occurred in patients receiving protease inhibitor therapy such as tipranavir.
- Be aware that immune reconstitution syndrome has occurred in patients treated with combination antiretroviral therapy, including tipranavir. The inflammatory response predisposes susceptible patients to opportunistic infections such as cytomegalovirus, *Mycobacterium avium* infection, *Pneumocystis jiroveci* pneumonia, or tuberculosis. Autoimmune disorders such as Graves' disease, Guillain–Barré syndrome, or polymyositis have also occurred. Report sudden or unusual adverse reactions to prescriber.
- Monitor patients with hemophilia, especially type A and B, because hemarthrosis and spontaneous skin hematomas have occurred with protease inhibitors.

PATIENT TEACHING

- Tell patient to take tipranavir exactly as prescribed and not to alter dosage without prescriber knowledge. Also instruct patient to swallow capsule whole and not to chew or open capsules.
- Instruct patient to report a skin rash, sensitivity to the sun, or other symptoms such as blister formation, fever, generalized itching, joint pain or stiffness, peeling of skin, redness, or throat tightness and seek immediate medical attention. Also, advise patient to seek medical attention immediately if any unexplained or unusual bleeding or other reaction occurs.
- Tell patient prescribed oral solution form not to take supplemental vitamin E greater than a standard multivitamin, as oral solution of tipranavir contains higher amounts of vitamin E.
- Instruct patient to report any signs and symptoms of liver dysfunction, such as fatigue, loss of appetite, malaise, or yellowing of skin or white areas of her eyes.
- Tell patient to inform all prescribers of tipranavir therapy, because of multiple drug interactions associated with this drug. Stress importance of not taking any over-the-counter preparations, including herbals, without consulting prescriber.
- Inform women receiving estrogen-based hormonal contraceptives to use additional or alternative nonhormonal contraceptives during tipranavir therapy. Also, alert these women that they are at increased risk of developing a rash with tipranavir therapy.
- Inform mothers that breastfeeding should not be done during tipranavir therapy.

tirofiban hydrochloride

Aggrastat

Class and Category

Pharmacologic class: Glycoprotein IIb/IIIa receptor antagonist
Therapeutic class: Antiplatelet
Pregnancy category: B

Indications and Dosages

➤ *To reduce the rate of thrombotic cardiovascular events (combined endpoint of death, myocardial infarction, or refractory ischemia/repeat cardiac procedure) in patients with non-ST elevation acute coronary syndrome (NSTE-ACS)*

I.V. INFUSION

Adults. *Initial*: 25 mcg/kg within 5 minutes and then 0.15 mcg/kg/min for up to 18 hr.
DOSAGE ADJUSTMENT For patients with creatinine clearance of 60 ml/min or less, infusion rate reduced to 0.075 mcg/kg/min, for up to 18 hr.

Route	Onset	Peak	Duration
I.V.	Immediate	30 min	4–8 hr

T

Mechanism of Action

Binds to glycoprotein IIb/IIIa receptor sites on the surface of activated platelets. Circulating fibrinogen can bind to these receptor sites and link platelets together, forming a clot that eventually blocks a coronary artery. By binding to receptor sites, tirofiban prevents the normal binding of fibrinogen and other factors and inhibits platelet aggregation.

Incompatibilities

Don't infuse tirofiban in same I.V. line with any drug other than atropine sulfate, dobutamine, dopamine, epinephrine hydrochloride, furosemide, heparin, lidocaine, midazolam hydrochloride, morphine sulfate, nitroglycerin, potassium chloride, propranolol hydrochloride, or famotidine (Pepcid injection).

Contraindications

Acute pericarditis; arteriovenous malformation; coagulopathy; stroke that occurred within previous 30 days or a history of hemorrhagic stroke; GI or GU bleeding; hemophilia; history of thrombocytopenia after tirofiban use; hypersensitivity to tirofiban or its components; intracranial aneurysm or mass, intracranial bleeding, retinal bleeding, aortic dissection, or any evidence of active abnormal bleeding within previous 30 days; major surgery or trauma within previous 6 weeks; severe uncontrolled hypertension (systolic blood pressure above 180 mm Hg, diastolic blood pressure above 110 mm Hg)

Interactions

DRUGS

antineoplastics, antithymocyte globulin, NSAIDs, oral anticoagulants, platelet aggregation inhibitors, strontium-89 chloride, thrombolytics: Increased risk of bleeding

levothyroxine, omeprazole: Increased rate of tirofiban clearance

porfimer: Decreased effectiveness of porfimer photodynamic therapy

salicylates: Increased risk of bleeding, possibly hypoprothrombinemia

Adverse Reactions

CNS: Chills, dizziness, fever, headache, **intracranial hemorrhage**

CV: Edema, **hemopericardium**, peripheral edema, sinus bradycardia

GI: Hematemesis, nausea, **retroperitoneal bleeding**, vomiting

GU: Hematuria, pelvic pain

HEME: Severe bleeding, thrombocytopenia

RESP: Pulmonary hemorrhage

SKIN: Diaphoresis, rash, urticaria

Other: Anaphylaxis, hypersensitivity reactions, infusion-site bleeding

Nursing Considerations

WARNING Dilute 50-ml vial of tirofiban before use; don't dilute 500-ml container because it holds premixed solution ready for I.V. infusion. Don't use solution unless it's clear and the seal is intact.

WARNING Keep in mind that if patient is also receiving a heparin infusion, expect to monitor APTT before treatment, 6 hours after heparin infusion starts, and regularly thereafter. Expect to adjust heparin dosage to maintain APTT at about two times the control, as ordered. Notify prescriber immediately if patient develops an abnormally high APTT. Also, assess patient for signs and symptoms of abnormal bleeding and report them to prescriber immediately because potentially life-threatening bleeding may occur.

- Know that after cardiac catheterization or percutaneous transluminal coronary angioplasty, keep patient on bed rest with head of bed elevated. Ensure hemostasis of percutaneous site for at least 4 hours before discharge. Minimize invasive procedures, including epidural procedures, to reduce the risk of bleeding.
- Monitor patient's hemoglobin level, hematocrit, and platelet count, as ordered. Expect to discontinue tirofiban if patient's platelet count is less than $90,000/mm^3$. Expect to give a platelet transfusion, as prescribed, if platelet count falls below $50,000/mm^3$.

PATIENT TEACHING

- Advise patient to immediately report any bleeding, bruising, headache, pain, or swelling during I.V. infusion of tirofiban.

tizanidine hydrochloride

Zanaflex

Class and Category

Pharmacologic class: Alpha$_2$ adrenergic agonist
Therapeutic class: Antispasmodic
Pregnancy category: C

Indications and Dosages

➤ *To manage acute and intermittent increases of muscle tone with spasticity*

CAPSULES, TABLETS

Adults. *Initial:* 2 to 4 mg every 6 to 8 hr, as needed, for maximum of 3 doses in 24 hr and then increased gradually by 2 to 4 mg/dose after 1 to 4 days, as needed and as prescribed. *Maximum:* 16 mg as a single dose or 36 mg total daily.

DOSAGE ADJUSTMENT For patients with hepatic dysfunction or renal insufficiency, dosage reduced when drug is being titrated upward.

Route	Onset	Peak	Duration
P.O.	Unknown	1–2 hr	3–6 hr

Mechanism of Action

Reduces spasticity by decreasing the release of excitatory amino acids. This alpha$_2$-adrenergic agonist's action increases presynaptic inhibition of spinal motor neurons, with the greatest effects on polysynaptic pathways.

Contraindications

Hypersensitivity to tizanidine or its components, use with ciprofloxacin or fluvoxamine

Interactions

DRUGS

acetaminophen: Delayed peak effects of acetaminophen
alpha$_2$-adrenergic agonists: Possibly significant hypotension
antihypertensives: Additive hypotensive effects
CYP1A2 inhibitors (such as acyclovir, amiodarone, cimetidine, famotidine, mexiletine, propafenone, ticlopidine, verapamil, zileuton), fluoroquinolones (including ciprofloxacin, fluvoxamine): Possibly increased plasma tizanidine level; increased risk of hypotension and sedation
oral contraceptives: Decreased tizanidine clearance
rofecoxib: Possibly increased adverse reactions

ACTIVITIES

alcohol use: Increased adverse effects of tizanidine, additive CNS depression

Adverse Reactions

CNS: Anxiety, delusions, drowsiness, dyskinesia, fatigue, fever, hallucinations, slurred speech
CV: Orthostatic hypotension
EENT: Dry mouth, pharyngitis, rhinitis
GI: Abdominal pain, anorexia, constipation, diarrhea, dyspepsia, elevated liver enzymes, **hepatic failure**, **hepatomegaly**, jaundice, nausea, vomiting
GU: Urinary frequency, UTI
MS: Back pain, muscle weakness, myasthenia
SKIN: Diaphoresis, rash, ulceration

Nursing Considerations

- Be aware that extreme caution is required if tizanidine is prescribed for a patient with hepatic impairment because the drug is extensively metabolized in the liver.
- Monitor hepatic and renal function for first 6 months and periodically thereafter.
- Expect prolonged drug use to inhibit saliva.
- Be aware that tizanidine should be stopped slowly to prevent rebound hypertension, tachycardia, and hypertonia as well as withdrawal.

PATIENT TEACHING

- Caution patient not to stop taking tizanidine suddenly to prevent adverse effects.
- Advise patient to change positions slowly to minimize effects of orthostatic hypotension.
- Urge patient to avoid alcohol during drug therapy because of its additive CNS effects.
- Tell patient to notify dentist or prescriber if dry mouth lasts longer than 2 weeks.
- Instruct patient to inform all pharmacists and prescribers about any drug he starts or stops taking.

tobramycin sulfate

Bethkis, Kitabis Pak, Tobi, Tobi Podhaler, Tobramycin

Class and Category

Pharmacologic class: Aminoglycoside
Therapeutic class: Antibiotic
Pregnancy category: D

Indications and Dosages

➤ *To treat bacteremia; bone and joint, gynecologic, intra-abdominal, lower respiratory tract, skin and soft-tissue, and urinary tract infections; endocarditis; meningitis; neonatal sepsis; pyelonephritis; and septicemia caused by susceptible strains of* Acinetobacter *species,* Aeromonas *species,* Citrobacter *species,* Enterobacter *species,* Escherichia coli, Haemophilus influenzae *(beta lactamase–negative and –positive),* Klebsiella *species,* Morganella morganii, Proteus mirabilis, Proteus vulgaris, Providencia rettgeri, Pseudomonas aeruginosa, Salmonella *species,* Serratia *species,* Shigella *species,* Staphylococcus aureus, *and* Staphylococcus epidermidis; *to treat febrile neutropenia*

I.V. INFUSION, I.M. INJECTION (TOBRAMYCIN)

Adults with serious infection. 1 mg/kg (over 20 to 60 minutes for I.V. infusion) every 8 hr.

Adults with life-threatening infections. 5 mg/kg (over 20 to 60 min for I.V. infusion) daily in three to four divided doses, reduced to 3 mg/kg (over 20 to 60 min for I.V. infusion) daily divided into 3 equal doses and given every 8 hr as soon as possible.

Children and neonates over age 7 days. 2 to 2.5 mg/kg (over 20 to 60 min for I.V. infusion) every 8 hr or 1.5 mg/kg every 6 hr.

Premature or full term neonates age 7 days or less. Up to 2 mg/kg (over 20 to 60 min for I.V. infusion) every 12 hr.

➤ *To treat pulmonary infection caused by* P. aeruginosa *in patients with cystic fibrosis*

I.M. INJECTION, I.V. INFUSION (TOBRAMYCIN)

Adults and children. 2.5 mg/kg every 6 hr; dosage adjusted to achieve peak blood drug level of 8 to 12 mcg/ml and trough blood drug level below 2 mcg/ml. I.V. infusion given over 20 to 60 min.

INHALATION (BETHKIS, KITABIS PAK, TOBI)

Adults and children over age 6. 1 ampule (300 mg) twice daily 12 hours apart in alternating periods of 28 days on and 28 days off.

INHALATION (TOBI PODHALER)

Adults and children 6 years and over. Four 28 mg capsules inhaled using Podhaler every 12 hr in alternating periods of 28 days on and 28 days off.

DOSAGE ADJUSTMENT For patients with renal impairment, dosage possibly reduced or dosage interval increased.

Mechanism of Action

Inhibits bacterial protein synthesis by binding irreversibly to one of two aminoglycoside-binding sites on the 30S ribosomal subunit, resulting in bacteriostatic effects. Bactericidal effects may stem from tobramycin's ability to accumulate within cells so that the intracellular drug level exceeds the extracellular level.

Incompatibilities

Don't mix tobramycin in same solution with parenteral aminoglycosides or beta-lactam antibiotics because mutual inactivation may result. Don't dilute or mix inhalation solution in nebulizer with dornase alfa.

Contraindications

Concurrent cidofovir, ethacrynic acid, furosemide, intravenous mannitol, or urea therapy; hypersensitivity to tobramycin, aminoglycosides, sodium bisulfite, or their components

Interactions

DRUGS

acyclovir, aminoglycosides, amphotericin B, carboplatin, cisplatin, NSAIDs, vancomycin: Additive nephrotoxicity
carbenicillin, ticarcillin: Possibly inactivation of tobramycin
dimenhydrinate: Possibly masking of symptoms of ototoxicity
ethacrynic acid, furosemide: Additive ototoxicity

ethacrynic acid, furosemide, mannitol, urea: Increased risk of aminoglycoside toxicity
general anesthetics, neuromuscular blockers: Possibly increased neuromuscular blockade
other drugs with nephrotoxic, neurotoxic, or ototoxic potential including systemic aminoglycosides: Increased risk of nephrotoxicity, neurotoxicity, and ototoxicity

Adverse Reactions

CNS: Confusion, dizziness, headache, inability to speak, lethargy, malaise **neurotoxicity**, vertigo
EENT: Hearing loss, laryngitis, oropharyngeal pain, ototoxicity, taste perversion, tinnitus, voice alteration
GI: Anorexia, ***Clostridium difficile*–associated diarrhea**, diarrhea, elevated liver enzymes, nausea, vomiting
GU: Elevated BUN and serum creatinine levels, **nephrotoxicity**, oliguria, proteinuria, **renal failure**
HEME: Anemia, leukocytosis, **leukopenia**, **neutropenia**, **thrombocytopenia**
MS: Myalgia
RESP: **Bronchospasm**, discolored sputum, wheezing
SKIN: **Exfoliative dermatitis**, pruritus, rash, urticaria
Other: **Hypersensitivity reactions**, **hypocalcemia**, **hypokalemia**, **hypomagnesemia**, **hyponatremia**, injection-site pain

Nursing Considerations

- Obtain fluid and tissue samples for culture and sensitivity testing before and during tobramycin therapy, as ordered. Review results, if available, before therapy starts.
- For I.V. administration, after reconstituting drug with 30 ml of sterile or bacteriostatic water for injection, dilute further with normal saline solution or D_5W in volumes of 50 to 100 ml for adults. Less volume will be needed when diluting drug to be administered to infant or child. Check manufacturer guidelines for specific volume to use.
- Give each I.V. dose over 20 to 60 minutes.

WARNING Don't infuse tobramycin over less than 20 minutes to avoid neuromuscular blockade and excessive peak drug level.

- Don't expose ampules for inhalation solution to intense light. Refrigerate them at 2° to 8° C (36° to 46° F).
- Know that capsules for inhalation should be stored in the blister and each capsule removed immediately before use. Always administer tobramycin by Podhaler last, if other inhaled medications are being administered.
- Expect the serum concentration of tobramycin to be monitored only through venipuncture, as a finger-stick sample may lead to falsely increased measurements of serum levels of the drug, which cannot be completely avoided with handwashing before testing is done.
- Keep in mind that because drug can cause bilateral and irreversible hearing loss, assess for early signs of cochlear and vestibular ototoxicity, including ataxia, dizziness, high-frequency hearing loss, tinnitus, and vertigo. If present, expect an audiogram to be ordered. Drug may have to be discontinued.
- Monitor patient for bronchospasms and wheezing. Notify prescriber immediately if present and be prepared to treat, as prescribed.
- Monitor serum calcium, magnesium, potassium, and sodium levels to detect electrolyte imbalances.

WARNING Be alert for allergic reactions, including anaphylaxis.

- Stop tobramycin therapy 7 days before starting cidofovir therapy, as prescribed. Know that diuretics can increase risk of aminoglycoside toxicity by altering antibiotic concentrations in serum and tissue and therefore should not be administered with tobramycin.
- Watch for signs of nephrotoxicity, such as elevated BUN and serum creatinine levels. Be aware that patients with renal dysfunction or who are taking nephrotoxic drugs should have measurements of serum concentrations of tobramycin and renal function done as ordered by prescriber. If nephrotoxicity occurs, drug may have to be discontinued.

- Expect dehydration to increase the risk of nephrotoxicity.

WARNING Monitor patient with myasthenia gravis or Parkinsonism for increased muscle weakness because of tobramycin's potential curare-like effect.

- Monitor patient closely for diarrhea, which may indicate pseudomembranous colitis caused by *C. difficile.* If diarrhea occurs, notify prescriber, expect to withhold tobramycin, and treat with electrolytes, fluids, protein, and an antibiotic effective against *C. difficile.*

PATIENT TEACHING

- Instruct patient on how to administer drug by inhalation. For inhaled tobramycin using ampules, instruct patient to inhale over 10 to 15 minutes, using a handheld nebulizer with a compressor. For inhaled tobramycin using capsules, instruct patient always to store capsules in the blister, not to remove capsules until immediately before use, and to use only with the Podhaler.
- Teach patient how to use nebulizer while sitting or standing upright and to breathe normally through its mouthpiece. Nose clips may help patient breathe through her mouth.
- Instruct patient to disinfect her nebulizer every other treatment day by boiling the nebulizer parts (except tubing) for a full 10 minutes and then drying the parts on a clean, lint-free cloth.
- Advise patient to notify prescriber if shortness of breath or wheezing occurs after administration of tobramycin inhalation solution.
- Urge patient to immediately report high-frequency hearing loss and vertigo.
- Instruct female patient to notify prescriber immediately about known or suspected pregnancy because drug poses danger to fetus.
- Advise mothers who are breastfeeding to monitor their infants for bloody or loose stools and for diaper rash or thrush, because tobramycin may cause intestinal flora alteration in the breastfed infant.
- Urge patient to tell prescriber about diarrhea that's severe or lasts longer than 3 days. Remind patient that watery or bloody stools may occur 2 or more months after antibiotic therapy and may be serious, requiring prompt treatment.
- Remind patient to alert all prescribers about tobramycin therapy, because drug interacts with many other drugs.

tocilizumab

Actemra

Class and Category

Pharmacologic class: Monoclonal antibody (interleukin-6 receptor inhibitor)
Therapeutic class: Antiarthritic (disease-modifying antirheumatic drug [DMARD])
Pregnancy category: C

Indications and Dosages

➤ *To treat moderate to severe active rheumatoid arthritis as monotherapy in patients who have had an inadequate response to one or more disease-modifying anti-rheumatic drugs (DMARDs) or as adjunct with methotrexate or other DMARDs*

I.V. INFUSION

Adults. 4 mg/kg over 60 min every 4 wk, increased, as needed, to 8 mg/kg over 60 min every 4 wk. *Maximum:* 800 mg per infusion.

SUBCUTANEOUS INJECTION

Adults weighing 100 kg (220 lb) or more. 162 mg every wk.
Adults weighing less than 100 kg (220 lb). 162 mg every other wk, followed by increased dosage frequency to every wk, as needed.

➤ *To treat active systemic juvenile idiopathic arthritis as monotherapy or as adjunct with methotrexate*

I.V. INFUSION

Children age 2 and over weighing 30 kg (66 lb) or more. 8 mg/kg over 60 min every 2 wk.
Children age 2 and over weighing less than 30 kg (66 lb). 12 mg/kg over 60 min every 2 wk.

SUBCUTANEOUS INJECTION

Children age 2 and over weighing 30 kg (66 lb) or more. 162 mg once every wk.
Children age 2 and over weighing less than 30 kg (66 lb). 162 mg every 2 wk.

➤ *To treat active polyarticular juvenile idiopathic arthritis*

I.V. INFUSION

Children age 2 and over weighing 30 kg (66 lb) or more. 8 mg/kg over 60 min every 4 wk.

Children age 2 and over weighing less than 30 kg (66 lb). 10 mg/kg over 60 min every 4 wk.

SUBCUTANEOUS INJECTION

Children age 2 and over weighing 30 kg (66 lb) or more. 162 mg once every 2 wk.

Children age 2 and over weighing less than 30 kg (66 lb). 162 mg once every 3 wk.

DOSAGE ADJUSTMENT Dosage reduction or interruption of dosing for treatment of rheumatoid arthritis or interruption of dosing for polyarticular juvenile idiopathic arthritis and systemic juvenile idiopathic arthritis may be needed to manage dose-related laboratory abnormalities, including elevated liver enzymes, neutropenia, and thrombocytopenia.

➤ *To treat giant cell arteritis*

SUBCUTANEOUS INJECTION

Adults. 162 mg once wk in combination with a tapering course of glucocorticoids. Alternatively, 162 mg once every other wk in combination with a tapering course of glucocorticoids.

➤ *To treat chimeric antigen receptor T-cell-induced severe or life-threatening cytokine release syndrome*

I.V. INFUSION

Adults and children age 2 and over weighing 30 kg (66 lb) or more. 8 mg/kg infused over 1 hr with up to 3 more doses administered with at least 8 hours between doses, if needed. *Maximum:* 800 mg per infusion.

Adults and children age 2 and over weighing less than 30 kg (66 lb). 12 mg/kg infused over 1 hr with up to 3 more doses administered at least 8 hr between doses, if needed. *Maximum:* 800 mg per infusion.

Mechanism of Action

Binds to interleukin 6 (IL-6) receptors to interrupt signaling through them. IL-6 is a proinflammatory cytokine produced by various cells, such as B- and T-cells, fibroblasts, lymphocytes, and monocytes. It is also produced by endothelial and synovial cells, leading to local production of IL-6 in joints affected by inflammatory processes such as polyarticular juvenile idiopathic arthritis, rheumatoid arthritis, and systemic juvenile idiopathic arthritis. Binding of IL-6 receptors prevents inflammation-related signals from being relayed, which reduces inflammatory response and relieves signs and symptoms of inflammatory-related arthritis.

Incompatibilities

Don't mix tocilizumab with other drugs.

Contraindications

Absolute neutrophil count below 2,000/mm^3, hypersensitivity to tocilizumab or its components, liver enzymes (ALT or AST) above 1.5 times upper limit of normal, platelet count below 100,000/mm^3

Interactions

DRUGS

anti-CD20 monoclonal antibodies, IL-1R antagonists, selective co-stimulation modulators, TNF antagonists: Increased risk of immunosuppression and infection

atorvastatin; cytochrome P-450 substrates with a narrow therapeutic index such as cyclosporine, theophylline, warfarin; CYP3A4 substrates such as lovastatin, oral contraceptives, simvastatin; omeprazole: Possibly decreased plasma levels of these drugs with decreased effectiveness

live vaccines: Increased risk of adverse vaccine effects

Adverse Reactions

CNS: Demyelinating disorders, dizziness, headache

CV: Elevated lipid levels, hypertension

EENT: Nasopharyngitis, oral ulceration

GI: Diverticulitis, elevated liver enzymes, gastritis, gastroenteritis, hepatic impairment, **pancreatitis**, **perforation**, upper abdominal pain

GU: UTI

HEME: Neutropenia, **thrombocytopenia**

MS: Bacterial arthritis

RESP: Bronchitis, pneumonia, upper respiratory tract infection

SKIN: Cellulitis, generalized erythema, pruritus, rash, **Stevens–Johnson syndrome**, urticaria

Other: Anaphylaxis, anti-tocilizumab antibodies, herpes zoster,

immunosuppression, injection-site reactions (erythema, pain, pruritus, swelling), **malignancies**, infections including activation of latent infections, **sepsis**, tuberculosis with pulmonary or extrapulmonary disease

Nursing Considerations

- Know that tocilizumab isn't recommended for patients with active liver disease or impairment because drug may adversely affect liver function.
- Make sure patient has a tuberculin skin test before therapy starts. If skin test is positive, tuberculosis treatment will need to be started before tocilizumab therapy can begin. Even patients who have tested negative for tuberculosis may develop tuberculosis during therapy. Monitor patient for low-grade fever, persistent cough, and wasting or weight loss; report such findings to prescriber.

WARNING Know that if patient has evidence of an active infection when drug is prescribed, therapy shouldn't start until infection has been treated. Monitor all patients for infections, including invasive fungal infections such as aspergillosis, candidiasis, or pneumocystis; or bacterial, myobacterial, protozoal, or viral opportunistic infections during and after therapy, especially patients who are taking immunosuppressants. If a serious infection develops, expect prescriber to interrupt drug therapy until infection is controlled.

- Obtain a baseline of patient's absolute neutrophil count, liver enzymes, and platelet count before starting tocilizumab therapy, as ordered. Therapy shouldn't begin if patient's absolute neutrophil count is below 2,000/mm^3, ALT or AST level is above 1.5 times the upper limit of normal, or platelet count is below 100,000/mm^3. Monitor these values, as ordered, 4 to 8 weeks (2 to 4 weeks for systemic juvenile idiopathic arthritis) after drug is initiated and then every 3 months after that, and report abnormalities. Dosage adjustment may be required or drug may have to be discontinued if abnormalities occur. For example, drug should be discontinued if absolute neutrophil count drops below 500 per mm^3.
- Use tocilizumab cautiously in patients with recurrent infection or increased risk of infection, patients who live in regions where histoplasmosis and tuberculosis are endemic, and patients with a history of CNS demyelinating disorders because they may occur, although rarely, during tocilizumab therapy.
- Know that when to give tocilizumab intravenously, use either a 100-ml infusion bag or bottle (patients weighing 30 kg or more) or a 50-ml infusion bag or bottle (patients weighing less than 30 kg) containing 0.9% sodium chloride injection. Begin by withdrawing a volume equal to the volume of tocilizumab solution (patient's dose). Slowly add drug from each vial into infusion bag or bottle and gently invert bag to mix while avoiding foaming. Discard any unused drug left in vials. Once fully diluted, solution may be stored in the refrigerator or at room temperature for up to 24 hours.
- Give tocilizumab with an infusion set, and never as I.V. push or bolus. Don't infuse concurrently with other drugs in same I.V. line.
- Know that when transitioning from intravenous therapy to subcutaneous therapy, the first subcutaneous dose should be given instead of next scheduled intravenous dose.

WARNING Stop tocilizumab immediately and notify prescriber if patient has an allergic reaction. Provide supportive care, as needed.

PATIENT TEACHING

- Instruct patient or caregiver on how to administer drug subcutaneously, if prescribed. Remind patient or caregiver to rotate sites and never give injection into moles, scars, or areas where the skin is bruised, hard, not intact, red, or tender. Tell how to dispose of syringe properly and to keep syringes, including those discarded, out of reach of children and pets.
- Review the signs and symptoms of an allergic reaction (difficulty breathing, rash, swollen face), and tell patient to seek emergency care immediately if these occur.
- Stress importance of compliance with laboratory tests ordered to monitor for adverse reactions.

- Inform patient that infections, including activation of latent infections such as tuberculosis, may occur during tocilizumab therapy. Instruct him to report persistent, severe, or unusual signs and symptoms to prescriber.
- Instruct patient to contact a healthcare provider immediately about persistent, severe abdominal pain because it could reflect GI perforation.
- Advise patient to avoid people with infections and to have all prescribed laboratory tests performed.
- Inform patient that risk of developing a malignancy is higher in patients taking tocilizumab, but it is still rare. Emphasize importance of follow-up visits and reporting any sudden or unusual signs or symptoms.
- Caution against receiving live-virus vaccines while taking tocilizumab.
- Advise patient to inform all healthcare providers about tocilizumab use and to inform prescriber about any OTC medications being taken, including herbal remedies and mineral and vitamin supplements.
- Urge woman who becomes pregnant while receiving tocilizumab to contact prescriber and to join the pregnancy registry by calling 1-877-311-8972 so that exposure to tocilizumab can be monitored.
- Inform women to alert pediatrician of tocilizumab use during pregnancy before live or live-attenuated vaccines are given to the infant.

tofacitinib citrate

Xeljanz, Xeljanz XR

Class and Category

Pharmacologic class: Janus kinase inhibitor
Therapeutic class: Antirheumatic (disease-modifying antirheumatic drug [DMARD])
Pregnancy category: C

Indications and Dosages

➤ *To treat moderate to severe active rheumatoid arthritis as monotherapy in patients who have had an inadequate response or intolerance to methotrexate; or as adjunct to methotrexate or other nonbiologic disease-modifying antirheumatic drugs (DMARDs); to treat psoriatic arthritis in patients who have had an inadequate response or intolerance to methotrexate or other DMARDs.*

TABLETS

Adults. 5 mg twice daily.

E.R. TABLETS

Adults. 11 mg once daily.

DOSAGE ADJUSTMENT For patients with moderate hepatic impairment or moderate or severe renal insufficiency, or patients taking concomitant CYP3A4 inhibitors such as ketoconazole, or concomitant use with one or more drugs that result in both potent inhibition of CYP2C19 such as fluconazole and moderate inhibition of CYP3A4, dosage reduced to 5 mg once daily.

➤ *To treat moderate to severe active ulcerative colitis*

TABLETS

Adults. 10 mg twice daily for at least 8 wk followed by 5 or 10 mg twice daily, depending on therapeutic response.

DOSAGE ADJUSTMENT For patients taking a strong CYP3A4 inhibitor such as ketoconazole or a moderate CYP3A4 inhibitor with a strong CYP2C19 inhibitor such as fluconazole and for patients with moderate hepatic impairment or moderate to severe renal impairment, dosage reduced to 5 mg twice daily if patient was taking 10 mg twice daily, and dosage reduced to 5 mg once daily if patient was taking 5 mg twice daily. For patients with an absolute neutrophil count (ANC) between 500 and 1000 cells/mm^3, dosage reduced to 5 mg twice daily if patient was taking 10 mg twice daily and dosage increased back to 10 mg twice daily when ANC is greater than 1000. For patients with a hemoglobin less than 8 g/dl or for patient who experiences a decrease of more than 2 g/dl, drug therapy interrupted until hemoglobin values have normalized. For patients who experience an ANC or lympohocyte count less than 500 cells/mm^3, drug discontinued.

Mechanism of Action

Modulates the signaling pathway by inhibiting the enzyme, Janus kinase (JAK). JAK is an intracellular enzyme which transmits signals arising from cytokine or growth factor–receptor interactions on the cellular membrane to influence cellular processes of hematopoiesis and immune cell function. Inhibiting the phosphorylation and activation of Signal Transducers and Activator of Transcription (STATs) needed to influence cellular processes lessens some of the signs and symptoms of rheumatoid arthritis.

Contraindications

Hypersensitivity to tofacitinib or its components

Interactions

DRUGS

azathioprine, cyclosporine, tacrolimus: Potentiated immunosuppression
CYP3A4 potent inducers such as rifampin: Possibly loss or reduced effectiveness of tofacitinib
live vaccines: Increased risk of infection
potent CYP3A4 inhibitors such as ketoconazole, moderate CYP34A inhibitors/ potent CYP2C19 inhibitors such as fluconazole: Increased tofacitinib exposure and adverse drug reactions

Adverse Reactions

CNS: Fatigue, fever, headache, insomnia, paresthesia
CV: Elevated lipid levels, hypertension, peripheral edema
EENT: Esophageal candidiasis, nasopharyngitis, sinus congestion
GI: Abdominal pain, diarrhea, diverticulitis, dyspepsia, elevated liver enzymes, gastritis, hepatic steatosis, liver injury, nausea, vomiting
GU: Elevated serum creatinine levels, UTI
HEME: Anemia, **lymphopenia, neutropenia**
MS: Arthralgia, elevated creatine phosphokinase, joint swelling, musculoskeletal pain, tendonitis
RESP: Cough, dyspnea, **interstitial lung disease**, pneumonia, **pneumocystosis**, upper respiratory infection
SKIN: Cellulitis, erythema, **melanoma**, multidermatomal herpes zoster, **nonmelanoma skin cancers**, rash, pruritus
Other: Bacteria, myobacterial, invasive fungal, viral or other opportunistic infections such as tuberculosis and other BK viral, cytomegalovirus, cryptococcus, or mycobacterial infections; dehydration; herpes zoster; **lymphoproliferative disorder; malignancies such as breast, colorectal, gastric, lung, lymphoma, malignant melanoma, prostate, and renal cell**

Nursing Considerations

- Be aware tofacitinib therapy should not be given to a patient who has an active infection, including localized infections.
- Know that tofacitinib should not be given to patients with severe hepatic impairment; tofacitinib should not be initiated in patients with a lymphocyte count less than 500 cells/mm^3, an absolute neutrophil count (ANC) less than 1,000 cells/mm^3, or hemoglobin levels less than 9 g/dl.
- Check with patient to be sure past immunizations received are in line with current immunization guidelines before starting tofacitinib therapy. If the patient needs further immunizations, ensure that it is done before drug therapy begins.
- Screen patient for viral hepatitis, as ordered, prior to starting tofacitinib therapy.
- Check to be sure that the patient has been tested for latent or active tuberculosis before tofacitinib therapy begins. Antituberculosis therapy might be prescribed for patients with a past history of active or latent tuberculosis if completion of treatment cannot be verified. Also, patients who have a negative test for latent tuberculosis may also be prescribed antituberculosis therapy if they have risk factors for tuberculosis.
- Use extreme caution when administering drug to patients with a history of chronic or recurrent infections, exposure to tuberculosis, history of a serious infection or an opportunistic infection, have resided or traveled in areas of endemic mycoses or endemic tuberculosis, or have underlying conditions that may predispose them to infection.
- Use cautiously in patients with a known malignancy, other than successfully treated nonmelanoma skin cancer. The prescriber may choose to discontinue the

drug in patients who develop a malignancy during tofacitinib therapy.
- Use cautiously in patients who may be at increased risk for gastrointestinal perforation, such as a patient with a history of diverticulitis. Monitor patient closely throughout tofacitinib therapy. Notify prescriber if patient experiences new onset abdominal symptoms suggestive of perforation.
- Use caution when administering nondeformable extended-release form of drug to patients with preexisting severe gastrointestinal narrowing. Rare reports of obstructive symptoms in patients with known strictures have occurred with other drugs utilizing a nondeformable extended-release formula.
- Obtain a CBC to determine patient's baseline, as ordered. Once the baseline is established, expect prescriber to order a lymphocyte level every 3 months; an ANC level after 4 to 8 weeks of therapy and then every 3 months; and a hemoglobin level after 4 to 8 weeks and then every 3 months. These test results will guide the prescriber in making modifications in the patient's treatment plan.
- Be aware that patient taking higher doses for the treatment of rheumatoid arthritis is at increased risk for developing a pulmonary embolism.
- Monitor the patient's liver enzymes routinely, as ordered, because drug has been associated with liver damage. Alert prescriber of any abnormalities and expect drug to be withheld during the investigation as to the cause of the elevated liver enzymes. If no other cause can be found, expect prescriber to discontinue the drug.
- Know that viral reactivation, including herpes virus reactivation (herpes zoster), has occurred with tofacitinib therapy.
- Expect prescriber to order a lipid profile on the patient 4 to 8 weeks after tofacitinib therapy has begun, because the drug has caused increases in lipid parameters generally within the first 6 weeks of therapy. Expect to manage hyperlipidemia, if present, according to clinical guidelines, as prescribed.
- Monitor patient for signs and symptoms of infection during and after tofacitinib therapy. Know that patients with diabetes mellitus are at increased risk for infection. Notify prescriber if an infection develops and expect to obtain a complete blood count, if ordered. Be aware that drug should be discontinued if the patient has an ANC count or lymphocyte count less than 500. If the patient has an ANC level between 500 and 1,000 or a hemoglobin level greater than a 2 g/dl decrease or less than 8 g/dl, expect drug therapy to be interrupted until the ANC and hemoglobin levels have returned to target range.

PATIENT TEACHING
- Instruct patient to take tofacitinib exactly as prescribed.
- Alert patient that an inert tablet shell may be passed in her stool or via colostomy. If present, reassure her that the active medication has already been absorbed by the time patient sees the shell.
- Review infection control measures with patient as well as the signs and symptoms of an infection. If an infection occurs, tell patient to notify prescriber immediately.
- Make sure patient understands the serious adverse reactions associated with tofacitinib such as the development of malignancies and serious infections.
- Stress importance for women of childbearing age to use effective contraception during treatment and for at least 4 weeks after the last dose of tofacitinib. Tell female patient to notify prescriber if pregnancy is suspected or known because drug effect on the fetus is unknown. Encourage her to enroll in the pregnancy registry by calling 1-877-311-8972.
- Make women of childbearing age aware that breastfeeding should not be done while taking tofacitinib.
- Inform female patients that tofacitinib therapy may reduce fertility.
- Encourage patient to comply with laboratory blood tests needed to monitor patient's reaction to tofacitinib.
- Advise patient at increased risk for skin cancer to have a periodic skin examination.
- Warn patient to avoid live vaccines while taking tofacitinib.

tolcapone

Tasmar

Class and Category

Pharmacologic class: Catechol-O-Methyltransferase (COMPT) inhibitor
Therapeutic class: Antiparkinsonian
Pregnancy category: C

Indications and Dosages

➤ *As adjunct (with levodopa and carbidopa) to treat idiopathic Parkinson's disease in patients who are experiencing symptom fluctuations and are not responding satisfactorily to or are not appropriate candidates for other adjunctive treatment*

TABLETS

Adults. *Initial:* 100 mg three times a day. *Maximum:* 200 mg three times a day.

Mechanism of Action

Prolongs plasma half-life of levodopa by inhibiting catechol-*O*-methyltransferase (COMT), an enzyme responsible for metabolizing catecholamines—including dopa, dopamine, epinephrine, norepinephrine, and their hydroxylated metabolites. COMT inhibition decreases the metabolizing enzyme for levodopa, which yields a more sustained plasma levodopa level, making more available for diffusion into the CNS to be converted to dopamine.

Contraindications

Confusion, hyperpyrexia, or rhabdomyolysis with previous use of tolcapone; hepatic dysfunction; hypersensitivity to tolcapone or its components

Interactions

DRUGS

desipramine: Possibly increased frequency of adverse effects
levodopa: Increased levodopa bioavailability, with increased risk of orthostatic hypotension and syncope
MAO inhibitors: Possibly inhibited catecholamine metabolism

Adverse Reactions

CNS: Aggression, agitation, compulsive behaviors such as intense urges to perform certain activities excessively (binge eating, gambling, sex, or spending money), confusion, delirium, delusions, disorientation, dizziness, drowsiness, dyskinesia, fatigue, fever, hallucinations, headache, lethargy, loss of balance, paranoid ideation, psychotic-like behavior, somnolence
CV: Chest pain, orthostatic hypotension
EENT: Dry mouth
GI: Abdominal pain, **acute fulminant liver failure**, anorexia, cholestasis, constipation, diarrhea, elevated liver enzymes, jaundice, vomiting
GU: Bright yellow urine, hematuria
MS: Muscle cramps, **rhabdomyolysis**
RESP: Dyspnea, upper respiratory tract infection
SKIN: Diaphoresis

Nursing Considerations

- Ensure that patient has had the risks of tolcapone therapy explained fully to him and has signed the acknowledgment form before starting therapy.
- Know that tolcapone should not be given to patient with a major psychotic disorder because of the increased risk of exacerbating psychosis.
- Use cautiously in patient with severe dyskinesia or dystonia because drug is known to cause rhabdomyolysis.
- Monitor liver enzymes, as ordered, during tolcapone therapy to detect hepatic impairment. Expect to discontinue drug if patient's liver enzymes exceed twice the upper limit of normal or if patient has any signs or symptoms of liver dysfunction, such as persistent anorexia, dark urine, fatigue, jaundice, lethargy, nausea, pruritus, or right upper quadrant tenderness.
- Assess patient for behavioral changes, hallucinations, or new or worsening mental status during tolcapone therapy or after starting or increasing the dose, especially in patients over age 75. If present, notify prescriber as dosage may need to be reduced or drug discontinued.
- Anticipate that drug may precipitate or exaggerate preexisting dyskinesia.
- Expect tolcapone to be discontinued if no improvement occurs after 3 weeks of drug therapy.

- Assess patient for skin changes regularly because risk of melanoma is higher in patients with Parkinson's disease. It isn't clear whether risk results from disease or drugs used to treat it.

PATIENT TEACHING

- Inform patient that urine may turn bright yellow during tolcapone therapy.
- Advise patient to avoid hazardous activities until drug's CNS effects are known. Inform patient that tolcapone therapy may cause him to fall asleep suddenly during activities of daily living without warning and can occur for the first time even a year after therapy has begun. If this happens, tell patient to notify prescriber and continue to avoid hazardous activities until prescriber has deemed such activities safe. Also warn patient and family that behavioral changes, hallucinations, or new or worsening mental status have occurred with use of tolcapone, especially in patients over the age of 75.
- Urge patient to notify prescriber immediately about darkened urine, decreased appetite, fatigue, jaundice, lethargy, and right sided abdominal pain.
- Caution patient not to stop taking drug abruptly. Explain that prescriber will supervise tapering of drug dosage.
- Urge patient to have regular follow-up appointments and laboratory tests.
- Urge patient to have regular skin examinations by a dermatologist or other qualified health professional.
- Advise patient to notify prescriber about intense urges that result in performing certain behaviors excessively (such as binge eating, uncontrolled gambling, sex, or spending money) because dosage may need to be reduced or drug discontinued.

tolterodine tartrate

Detrol, Detrol LA

Class and Category

Pharmacologic class: Cholinergic receptor blocker
Therapeutic class: Antispasmodic
Pregnancy category: C

Indications and Dosages

➤ *To treat overactive bladder*

TABLETS

Adults. 2 mg twice daily. Reduced to 1 mg twice daily based on patient response and tolerance.

DOSAGE ADJUSTMENT Dosage reduced to 1 mg twice daily for patients with significant hepatic or renal dysfunction and for patients who are also receiving cytochrome P-450 3A4 inhibitors, such as antifungals (itraconazole, ketoconazole, and miconazole), clarithromycin, cyclosporine, erythromycin, and vinblastine.

E.R. CAPSULES

Adults. 4 mg daily. Reduced to 2 mg daily based on individual response and tolerance.

DOSAGE ADJUSTMENT For patients with mild to moderate hepatic dysfunction, severe renal dysfunction, and for patients receiving cytochrome P-450 3A4 inhibitors, such as clarithromycin, itraconazole, ketoconazole, or ritonavir, dosage reduced to 2 mg once daily.

Mechanism of Action

Exerts antimuscarinic (atropine-like) and potent direct antispasmodic (papaverine-like) actions on smooth muscle in the bladder, which decreases detrusor muscle contractions. This helps reduce urinary frequency and urgency as well as urge-related incontinence.

Contraindications

Gastric retention; hypersensitivity to tolterodine tartrate, its components, or to fesoterodine fumarate extended-release tablets; uncontrolled angle-closure glaucoma; urine retention

Interactions

DRUGS

class IA antiarrhythmics (such as procainamide, quinidine) or class III antiarrhythmics (such as amiodarone, sotalol): Possibly increased risk of prolonged QT interval
fluoxetine: Possibly decreased tolterodine metabolism
potent CYP3A4 inhibitors such as clarithromycin, cyclosporine, erythromycin, itraconazole, ketoconazole, miconazole ritonavir, vinblastine: Possibly increased blood tolterodine level

Adverse Reactions

CNS: Confusion, disorientation, dizziness, drowsiness, fatigue, hallucinations, headache, memory impairment, somnolence, worsening of dementia
CV: Chest pain, edema, hypertension, palpitations, **QT prolongation**, tachycardia
EENT: Abnormal vision, blurred vision, dry eyes, dry mouth
GI: Abdominal pain, constipation, diarrhea, flatulence, indigestion, nausea
GU: Dysuria, urine retention, UTI
Other: Anaphylaxis, angioedema, flu-like symptoms

Nursing Considerations

- Use cautiously in patients with decreased GI motility, myasthenia gravis, or narrow-angle glaucoma because tolterodine could make these conditions worse.

WARNING Monitor patients with a history of bladder outflow obstruction for bladder distention or decreased urine output because tolterodine poses a risk of urine retention.

- Monitor patients for abdominal bloating or distention or patients with a history of GI obstructive disorders, such as pyloric stenosis, because of increased risk of gastric retention.
- Be aware that drug's antimuscarinic effects may produce blurred vision, dizziness, and drowsiness. If these occur, institute fall precautions according to facility policy.

PATIENT TEACHING

- Instruct patient taking tolterodine to report immediately to prescriber any difficulty urinating or infrequent urination, as well as difficulty breathing or swelling that involves the face, lips, throat or tongue, and to seek emergency medical care.
- Advise patient not to drive or perform activities that require high alertness until drug's CNS and vision effects are known. Instruct her to notify prescriber if blurred vision, dizziness, or drowsiness persists.
- Encourage patient to use sugarless candy, gum, or ice to relieve dry mouth. Advise her to notify prescriber or dentist if dry mouth persists or worsens over 2 weeks.

tolvaptan

Samsca

Class and Category

Pharmacologic class: Vasopressin receptor antagonist
Therapeutic class: Vasopressin antagonist
Pregnancy category: C

Indications and Dosages

➤ *To treat significant hypervolemic and euvolemic hyponatremia (serum sodium level less than 125 mEq/L or symptomatic but less-marked hyponatremia that has resisted correction with fluid restriction), including patients with heart failure or syndrome of inappropriate antidiuretic hormone (SIADH)*

TABLETS

Adults. *Initial:* 15 mg once daily, increased after at least 24 hours to 30 mg once daily. *Maximum:* 60 mg once daily for 30 days or less.

Mechanism of Action

Raises serum sodium levels by decreasing urine osmolality and increasing urine output. Tolvaptan does this by preventing attachment of vasopressin to vasopressin V2 receptors on cell membranes in the nephron's collecting duct. Without vasopressin activity, urinary water excretion increases.

Contraindications

Acute need to raise serum sodium urgently; anuria; concomitant use of strong CYP3A inhibitors such as clarithromycin, ketoconazole, indinavir, itraconazole, nefazodone, nelfinavir, ritonavir, saquinavir, telithromycin; hypovolemic hyponatremia; hypersensitivity to tolvaptan or its components; inability of patient to sense or respond appropriately to thirst

Interactions

DRUGS

ACE inhibitors, angiotensin receptor blockers, potassium sparing diuretics, potassium supplements: Increased risk of hyperkalemia

CYP3A inducers such as barbiturates, carbamazepine, phenytoin, rifabutin, rifampin, rifapentine, St. John's wort: Decreased serum tolvaptan level and decreased effectiveness
CYP3A inhibitors such as aprepitant, clarithromycin, diltiazem, erythromycin, fluconazole, ketoconazole, indinavir, itraconazole, nefazodone, nelfinavir, ritonavir, saquinavir, telithromycin, verapamil; P-gp inhibitors such as cyclosporine: Increased serum tolvaptan level and risk of adverse reactions
desmopressin: Possibly altered desmopressin activity
digoxin: Increased digoxin level

FOODS

grapefruit juice: Increased serum tolvaptan level

Adverse Reactions

CNS: Asthenia, **CVA**, fever, **osmotic demyelination syndrome**, thirst
CV: Deep vein thrombosis, **intracardiac thrombus**, **ventricular fibrillation**
EENT: Dry mouth
ENDO: Diabetic ketoacidosis, hyperglycemia
GI: Anorexia, constipation, **GI bleeding**, hepatic dysfunction, **hepatic injury**, **ischemic colitis**, nausea
GU: Nocturia, polyuria, **urethral or vaginal hemorrhage**
HEME: Disseminated intravascular coagulation (DIC), prolonged prothrombin time
MS: Rhabdomyolysis
RESP: Pulmonary embolism, **respiratory failure**
SKIN: Rash
Other: Anaphylaxis, dehydration, **hyperkalemia**, **hypernatremia**, **hyponatremia**, hypovolemia

Nursing Considerations

- Be aware that tolvaptan should not be given to patients with a creatine clearance of less than 10 ml/min because no benefit can be expected in patients who are anuric. Also know that tolvaptan should not be used to treat autosomal dominant polycystic kidney disease, because of the risk of hepatoxicity.
- Use cautiously in patients with cirrhosis because of increased risk of GI bleeding.

WARNING Give tolvaptan, initially or if reintroduced, in a hospital setting because too-rapid correction of hyponatremia (more than 12 mEq/L in 24 hour) causes osmotic demyelination (affective changes, coma, dysarthria, dysphagia, lethargy, mutism, spastic quadriparesis, seizures, death). If present, notify prescriber immediately and expect to stop tolvaptan and give hypotonic fluids.

- Monitor fluid and electrolyte balance regularly, especially when starting tolvaptan and adjusting dosage, as ordered. If patient develops hypernatremia, notify prescriber and expect to decrease dose or withhold drug and modify the patient's free-water infusion or intake, as ordered.
- Don't restrict fluids during first 24 hours of therapy because doing so may increase the risk of overly rapid correction of dehydration, hypovolemia, and serum sodium.
- Use of hypertonic saline isn't recommended during tolvaptan therapy because effects are unknown.
- Monitor patient for signs and symptoms of hepatic dysfunction such as anorexia, dark urine, fatigue, jaundice, and right upper abdominal pain; if present, notify prescriber, and obtain liver enzymes immediately, as ordered. Be aware that to minimize risk of liver injury that could become life-threatening, drug should not be given longer than 30 days. If hepatic dysfunction is confirmed, expect drug to be discontinued. Know that if the cause of hepatic dysfunction is found to be due to something other than tolvaptan therapy, expect drug to be resumed.

PATIENT TEACHING

- Instruct patient to consume fluids according to thirst during first 24 hours of therapy and not to try to limit fluid intake.
- Tell patient that he'll need to resume fluid restriction and will need continued monitoring of sodium level and fluid status when drug is discontinued.
- Tell patient to notify prescriber if he experiences dark urine or yellowing of eyes and skin, fatigue, loss of appetite, or right upper abdominal pain.

topiramate

Qudexy XR, Topamax, Trokendi XR

Class and Category

Pharmacologic class: Sulfamate-substituted monosaccharide
Therapeutic class: Anticonvulsant
Pregnancy category: D

Indications and Dosages

➤ *To treat partial-onset or primary generalized tonic–clonic seizures*

CAPSULES, TABLETS (TOPAMAX)

Adults and children age 10 and over. *Initial:* 25 mg twice daily in morning and evening for wk 1; 50 mg twice daily in morning and evening for wk 2; 75 mg twice daily in morning and evening for wk 3; 100 mg twice daily in morning and evening for wk 4; 150 mg twice daily in morning and evening for wk 5; and 200 mg twice daily in morning and evening for wk 6. *Maintenance:* 200 mg twice daily in morning and evening.

Children age 2 to 10 years of age. *Initial:* 25 mg once daily in evening for wk 1. Increased to 25 mg twice daily in morning and evening for wk 2. Increased thereafter by 25 to 50 mg/day each subsequent wk, as tolerated, over the next 5 wk. *Maintenance:* For children weighing up to 11 kg (up to 24.2 lb), 75 to 125 mg twice daily; for children weighing 12 to 22 kg (26.4 to 48.4 lb), 100 to 150 mg twice daily; for children weighing 23 to 31 kg (50.6 to 68.2 lb), 100 to 175 mg twice daily; for children weighing 32 to 38 kg (70.4 to 83.6 lb), 125 to 175 mg twice daily; and for children weighing more than 38 kg (more than 83.6 lb), 125 to 200 mg twice daily. *Maximum:* Highest maintenance dosage for weight.

EXTENDED-RELEASE CAPSULES (QUDEXY XR, TROKENDI XR)

Adults and children age 10 and over. *Initial:* 50 mg once daily for wk 1; 100 mg once daily for wk 2; 150 mg once daily for wk 3; 200 mg once daily for wk 4; 300 mg once daily for wk 5; and 400 mg once daily for wk 6 and beyond. *Maintenance:* 400 mg once daily.

EXTENDED-RELEASE CAPSULES (QUDEXY XR, TROKENDI XR)

Children age 2 to less than 10 (Qudexy XR) and children age 6 to less than 10 (Trokendi XR). *Initial:* 25 mg once daily at night for wk 1; 50 mg once daily at night for wk 2; then increased weekly in increments of 25 to 50 mg until minimum maintenance dose reached, usually within 5 to 7 wk. Additional increases in increments of 25 to 50 mg made weekly to maximum maintenance dose, as needed. *Maintenance:* For children weighing up to 11 kg (24.2 lb), 150 to 250 mg once daily at night; for children weighing 12 to 22 kg (26.4 to 48.4 lb), 200 to 300 mg once daily at night; for children weighing 23 to 31 kg (50.6 to 68.2 lb), 200 to 350 mg once daily at night; for children weighing 32 to 38 kg (70.4 to 83.6 lb), 250 to 350 mg once daily at night; and for children weighing more than 38 kg (83.6 lb), 250 to 400 mg once daily at night. *Maximum:* Highest maximum maintenance dose for weight.

➤ *As adjunct to treat partial seizures and primary generalized tonic–clonic seizures*

CAPSULES, TABLETS (TOPAMAX)

Adults and adolescents age 17 and over. *Initial:* 25 to 50 mg daily in divided doses twice daily for 1 wk. Increased by 25 to 50 mg daily every wk thereafter until maintenance dose is reached. *Maintenance:* 200 to 400 mg daily in divided doses twice daily for partial onset seizures and 400 mg daily in divided doses twice daily for primary generalized tonic–clonic seizures.

Children ages 2 to 16. *Initial:* 1 mg/kg/day to 3 mg/kg daily at night for 1 wk. Increased every 1 to 2 wk by 1 to 3 mg/kg daily in divided doses twice daily until maintenance dose is reached. *Maintenance:* 5 to 9 mg/kg daily in divided doses twice daily.

EXTENDED-RELEASE CAPSULES (QUDEXY XR)

Adults and adolescents age 17 and over. *Initial:* 25 to 50 mg once daily, increased weekly in increments of 25 to 50 mg once daily, as needed. *Maximum:* 400 mg once daily.

Children age 2 to 16 years of age. *Initial:* 1 to 3 mg/kg/day once daily at night for 1 wk, increased every 1 to 2 wk in increments of 1 to 3 mg/kg/day, as needed. *Maximum:* 9 mg/kg/day.

EXTENDED-RELEASE CAPSULES (TROKENDI XR)

Children age 6 to 16 years of age. *Initial:* 1 to 3 mg/kg/day once daily at night for

1 wk, increased every 1 to 2 wk in increments of 1 to 3 mg/kg/day, as needed. *Maximum*: 9 mg/kg/day.

➤ *As adjunct to treat seizures associated with Lennox–Gastaut syndrome*

CAPSULES, TABLETS (TOPAMAX)

Adults and adolescents age 17 and over. 25 to 50 mg daily in divided doses twice daily for 1 wk. Increased by 25 to 50 mg daily every wk thereafter until maintenance dose is reached. *Maintenance*: 200 to 400 mg daily in divided doses twice daily.

Children ages 2 to 16. *Initial*: 1 to 3 mg/kg/day at night for 1 wk. Increased every 1 to 2 wk by 1 to 3 mg/kg daily in divided doses twice daily until maintenance dose is reached *Maintenance:* 5 to 9 mg/kg daily in divided doses twice daily.

EXTENDED-RELEASE CAPSULES (TROKENDI XR)

Adults and adolescents age 17 and over. *Initial:* 25 to 50 mg once daily, increased weekly in increments of 25 to 50 mg once daily, as needed. *Maximum:* 400 mg once daily.

Children age 6 to 16 years of age. *Initial:* 1 to 3 mg/kg/day once daily at night for 1 wk, increased every 1 to 2 wk in increments of 1 to 3 mg/kg/day, as needed. *Maximum*: 9 mg/kg/day.

EXTENDED-RELEASE CAPSULES (QUDEXY XR)

Adults and adolescents age 17 and over. *Initial*: 25 to 50 mg once daily, increased weekly in increments of 25 to 50 mg once daily, as needed. *Maximum:* 400 mg once daily.

Children age 2 to 16 years of age. *Initial*: 1 to 3 mg/kg/day once daily at night for 1 wk., increased every 1 to 2 wk in increments of 1 to 3 mg/kg/day, as needed. *Maximum*: 9 mg/kg/day.

➤ *To prevent migraine headache*

CAPSULES, TABLETS (QUDEXY XR, TOPAMAX)

Adults and children age 12 and over. *Initial:* 25 mg daily in evening for wk 1; then 25 mg twice daily morning and evening for wk 2; then 25 mg in morning and 50 mg in evening for wk 3, then 50 mg twice daily in morning and evening. *Maintenance:* 50 mg twice daily.

DOSAGE ADJUSTMENT For patients with moderate to severe renal impairment, dosage possibly reduced by 50%. For patients undergoing hemodialysis, a supplemental dose may be required during a prolonged period of dialysis. For patients taking carbamazepine and/or phenytoin, a dosage adjustment may be required.

Mechanism of Action

May block the spread of seizures by reducing the length and frequency of excitatory transmission. Topiramate increases the availability of the inhibitory neurotransmitter gamma-aminobutyric acid by blocking voltage-sensitive sodium channels. This action promotes the movement of chloride ions into neurons.

Contraindications

Hypersensitivity to topiramate or its components, metabolic acidosis with concurrent metformin use (Trokendi XR), recent alcohol use defined as within 6 hours prior to and 6 hours after taking topiramate (Trokendi XR)

Interactions

DRUGS

amitriptyline: Possibly high increase in amitriptyline blood concentration increasing risk of adverse reactions

antihistamines, barbiturates, benzodiazepines, CNS depressants, opioid analgesics, skeletal muscle relaxants, tricyclic antidepressants: Additive CNS depression

carbamazepine, phenytoin: Decreased blood topiramate level

digoxin: Possibly decreased blood digoxin level

ethinyl estradiol: Increased risk of break-through bleeding

hydrochlorothiazide: Possibly increased blood topiramate levels

lithium: Increased risk of lithium toxicity

oral contraceptives: Increased risk of breakthrough bleeding, decreased contraceptive efficacy

other carbonic anhydrase inhibitors such as acetazolamide, dichlorphenamide, zonisamide: Increased risk of kidney stone formation; increased severity of metabolic acidosis

phenobarbital: Altered blood phenobarbital level

pioglitazone: Possibly decreased exposure of pioglitazone with decreased effectiveness

probenecid: Possibly blocked renal tubular reabsorption of topiramate and decreased blood topiramate level
valproic acid: Decreased blood levels of both drugs, increased risk of hyperammonemia or hypothermia
warfarin: Decreased International Normalized Ratio (INR) or prothrombin time

ACTIVITIES

alcohol use: Additive CNS depression

Adverse Reactions

CNS: Abnormal coordination, aggression, agitation, anxiety, aphasia, apathy, asthenia, ataxia, confusion, decreased concentration, depersonalization, depression, dizziness, dysphasia, emotional lability, **encephalopathy**, fatigue, fever, gait abnormality, hallucinations, headache, hyperkinesia, hyperthermia, hypoesthesia, hyporeflexia, insomnia, irritability, language problems, memory alterations or loss, mood changes, nervousness, neurosis, paresthesia, personality disorder, psychomotor slowing, psychosis, rigors, **seizures**, slurred or other abnormalities of speech, somnolence, stupor, **suicidal ideation**, syncope, thirst, tremor, vertigo
CV: Bradycardia, **cardiac arrest**, chest pain, edema, hypertension, **hypotension**, palpitations, vasodilation
EENT: Blurred vision, conjunctivitis, diplopia, dry mouth, edema of the pharynx, gingivitis, glossitis, gum hyperplasia, hearing loss, increased saliva, laryngitis, maculopathy, myopia, nystagmus, otitis media, periorbital pain, pharyngitis, rhinitis, secondary angle-closure glaucoma with acute myopia, sinusitis, taste loss or perversion, tinnitus, tongue edema, vision changes including visual field defects
ENDO: Breast pain, hot flashes, hyperglycemia, **hypoglycemia**, hypothyroidism
GI: Abdominal pain, anorexia, constipation, diarrhea, dyspepsia, fecal incontinence, flatulence, gastroenteritis, gastroesophageal reflux, **hepatic failure**, **hepatitis**, increased appetite, indigestion, nausea, **pancreatitis**, vomiting
GU: Cystitis, decreased libido, dysmenorrhea, dysuria, frequent urination, hematuria, impotence, leukorrhea, menstrual irregularities, nocturia, premature ejaculation, prostatic disorder, renal calculi, renal tubular acidosis, urinary frequency or incontinence, UTI, vaginitis
HEME: Anemia, **bleeding events**, **increased prothrombin time**, **leukopenia**, purpura, **thrombocytopenia**
MS: Arthralgia, back pain, dysarthria, involuntary muscle contractions, leg cramps or pain, muscle weakness, myalgia, skeletal pain
RESP: Bronchitis, cough, dyspnea, pneumonia, **pulmonary embolism**, upper respiratory tract infection
SKIN: Abnormal hair growth, acne, alopecia, bullous skin reactions, decreased or increased sweating, dermatitis, **erythema multiforme**, eczema, flushing, pallor, pemphigus, pruritus, rash, seborrhea, skin discoloration, **Stevens–Johnson syndrome**, **toxic epidermal necrolysis**
Other: Body odor, **decreased serum bicarbonate levels**, dehydration, elevated serum alkaline phosphatase, flu-like symptoms, **hyperammonemia**, **hypersensitivity reactions**, **hyponatremia**, **hypophosphatemia**, increased susceptibility to infection, **metabolic acidosis**, moniliasis, weight gain or loss

Nursing Considerations

- Obtain baseline serum bicarbonate level before topiramate therapy and monitor periodically throughout therapy, as ordered.
- Use topiramate cautiously in patients with impaired hepatic function, or inborn errors of metabolism, or those who are taking valproic acid; these patients may be at higher risk for hyperammonemia, with or without encephalopathy, while taking topiramate. In addition, hypothermia may occur in patients taking valproic acid concomitantly. If present, notify prescriber and expect topiramate or valproic acid therapy to be discontinued.
- Give capsule with water and have patient swallow it whole. If needed, open capsules and empty contents onto a spoonful of soft food. Discard unused portion.
- Never store food sprinkled with drug for use at a later time.

WARNING Anticipate an increase in seizure activity if topiramate therapy for seizures stops abruptly. Take seizure precautions, as appropriate. Expect drug to be withdrawn gradually if time permits.

- Keep in mind that if patient reports ocular pain or decreased visual acuity, notify prescriber immediately; topiramate may cause increased intraocular pressure and secondary angle-closure glaucoma as well as visual field defects. Expect to stop drug immediately.
- Monitor patient for cognitive-related dysfunction, especially patients who are started on a higher initial dose or have a rapid titration rate.
- Assess for signs of recurrence of renal calculi if patient has a history of this condition.
- Monitor patient for bleeding events, especially patients who have conditions that increase risk of bleeding, who take drugs that cause thrombocytopenia such as other antiepileptic drugs, or who take drugs that affect platelet function or coagulation such as anticoagulants aspirin, nonsteroidal anti-inflammatory drugs, or selective serotonin reuptake inhibitors.

PATIENT TEACHING

- Instruct patient to swallow topiramate tablets whole.
- Urge patient to avoid potentially hazardous activities until drug's CNS effects are known.
- Advise patient to watch for decreased sweating and significantly increased body temperature, especially during hot weather, and to notify prescriber immediately if they occur.
- Tell patient to maintain adequate fluid intake to minimize the risk of developing kidney stones.
- Instruct patient to avoid alcohol use completely within 6 hours before and after taking topiramate.
- Advise female patient of possible break-through bleeding. If she takes an oral contraceptive, encourage her to use another form of contraception during therapy.
- Caution patient not to stop taking topiramate abruptly because seizures may occur. Instead, patient should expect drug to be withdrawn gradually if it must be discontinued.
- Instruct patient to seek immediate emergency care for blurred vision, other visual disturbances, or periorbital pain.
- Tell patient to notify prescriber if he develops changes in mental status, unexplained lethargy, or vomiting.
- Urge caregivers to watch patient closely for evidence of suicidal tendencies, especially when topiramate therapy starts or dosage changes, and to report concerns at once to prescriber.
- Counsel female patient of childbearing age to use effective birth control, as topiramate therapy may cause cleft lip or palate as well as low body weight if the fetus is exposed to drug in utero.
- Urge woman who becomes pregnant while taking topiramate to enroll in the North American antiepileptic drug pregnancy registry by calling 1-888-233-2334. Explain that the registry is collecting information about the safety of antiepileptic drugs during pregnancy.
- Alert mothers wishing to breastfeed that topiramate is excreted in breast milk, and to talk to prescriber before doing so while taking topiramate.

torsemide

Demadex

Class and Category

Pharmacologic class: Loop diuretic
Therapeutic class: Antihypertensive, diuretic
Pregnancy category: B

Indications and Dosages

➤ *To treat edema in heart failure*

TABLETS, I.V. INJECTION

Adults. *Initial:* 10 to 20 mg daily (I.V. injected slowly over 2 min), adjusted by doubling, as prescribed, to achieve desired effect. *Maximum:* 200 mg daily.

➤ *To treat edema in chronic renal failure*

TABLETS, I.V. INJECTION

Adults. *Initial:* 20 mg daily (I.V. injected slowly over 2 min), adjusted by doubling, as prescribed, to achieve desired effect. *Maximum:* 200 mg daily.

➤ *To treat ascites, alone or with amiloride or spironolactone*

TABLETS, I.V. INJECTION

Adults. *Initial:* 5 to 10 mg daily (I.V. injected slowly over 2 min), adjusted by doubling, as needed to achieve desired effect. *Maximum:* 40 mg daily.

➤ *To manage hypertension*

TABLETS

Adults. *Initial:* 5 mg daily, increased to 10 mg daily after 4 to 6 wk, if response is inadequate. *Maximum:* 10 mg daily.

Route	Onset	Peak	Duration
P.O.	1 hr	1–2 hr	6–8 hr
I.V.	10 min	1 hr	6–8 hr

Mechanism of Action

Blocks active chloride and sodium reabsorption in the ascending loop of Henle by promoting rapid excretion of chloride, sodium, and water. Torsemide also increases the production of renal prostaglandins, increasing the plasma renin level and renal vasodilation. As a result, blood pressure falls, reducing preload and afterload.

Contraindications

Anuric patients; hepatic coma; hypersensitivity to torsemide, povidone, sulfonamides, or their components

Interactions

DRUGS

ACE inhibitors, angiotensin receptor blockers, antihypertensives: Additive hypotension; increased risk of renal impairment
ACTH, corticosteroids: Possibly increased risk of hypokalemia
amiloride, spironolactone, triamterene: Possibly counteracted torsemide-induced hypokalemia
aminoglycoside antibiotics, ethacrynic acid: Increased risk of ototoxicity
amphotericin B: Increased risk of nephrotoxicity and severe, prolonged hypokalemia or hypomagnesemia
cholestyramine: Possibly decreased absorption of orally administered torsemide
cisplatin: Increased risk of significant hypokalemia or hypomagnesemia, possibly permanent ototoxicity
cortisone, fludrocortisone, hydrocortisone: Increased risk of hypokalemia and sodium retention
CYP2C9 inducers such as rifampin: Decreased plasma concentrations of torsemide possibly decreasing effectiveness
CYP2C9 inhibitors such as amiodarone, fluconazole, miconazole, oxandrolone: Increased plasma concentrations of torsemide and possibly increased risk of adverse reactions
CYP2C9 substrates such as celecoxib or substrates with a narrow therapeutic range, such as phenytoin, warfarin: Possibly decreased effectiveness and safety of these drugs
digoxin: Increased risk of arrhythmias and digitalis toxicity due to hypokalemia or hypomagnesemia
indomethacin: Possibly decreased antihypertensive and diuretic effects of torsemide and increased risk of renal failure
lithium: Possibly lithium toxicity
metolazone, thiazide diuretics: Increased risk of severe fluid and electrolyte loss
nephrotoxic drugs such as aminoglycosides, cisplatin, NSAIDs: Increased risk of worsening renal function
NSAIDS, salicylates: Increased risk of nephrotoxicity and salicylate toxicity
neuromuscular blockers: Possibly increased neuromuscular blockade due to hypokalemia
probenecid, other organic anion drugs: Possibly decreased diuretic effect of torsemide
quinidine and other ototoxic drugs: Increased risk of ototoxicity
radiocontrast agents: Increased risk of renal toxicity

ACTIVITIES

alcohol use: Additive diuresis and, possibly, dehydration

Adverse Reactions

CNS: Confusion, dizziness, drowsiness, fatigue, headache, insomnia, lethargy, nervousness, paresthesia, restlessness, thirst, weakness
CV: Chest pain, **ECG abnormalities**, edema, **hypotension**, tachycardia
EENT: Dry mouth, hearing loss, ototoxicity, pharyngitis, rhinitis, tinnitus, visual impairment

ENDO: Hyperglycemia
GI: Abdominal pain, anorexia, constipation, diarrhea, elevated liver enzymes, indigestion, nausea, **pancreatitis**, vomiting
GU: Azotemia, elevated blood urea creatinine and nitrogen levels, oliguria, urinary frequency or retention, worsening renal function
HEME: Anemia, **leukopenia, thrombocytopenia**
MS: Muscle spasms, myalgia
RESP: Cough
SKIN: Photosensitivity, pruritus, **Stevens–Johnson syndrome, toxic epidermal necrolysis**
Other: Elevated uric acid levels, **hypocalcemia**, hypochloremic alkalosis, **hypokalemia, hypomagnesemia, hyponatremia**, hypovolemia, thiamine (vitamin B1) deficiency

Nursing Considerations

- Inject I.V. torsemide slowly over 2 minutes. Flush I.V. line with normal saline solution before and afterward.
- Don't exceed 200 mg in a single I.V. dose of torsemide.
- Monitor patient's serum electrolyte levels and fluid intake and output to detect hypovolemia, because dehydration can worsen renal function, causing acute renal failure. Patients at higher risk include patients who are taking renin-angiotensin aldosterone inhibitors or other nephrotoxic drugs or who are salt-depleted. Expect to monitor renal function in patients who experience dehydration.
- Monitor patient with hepatic disease who has ascites or cirrhosis, because a sudden shift in fluid and electrolyte balance may precipitate hepatic coma. Diuretic therapy can also contribute to a variety of disorders such as azotemia, hypokalemia, hyponatremia, hypovolemia, or metabolic alkalosis in these patients, which can cause or worsen hepatic encephalopathy. Know that if this occurs, drug should be withheld or discontinued.

WARNING Expect torsemide-induced electrolyte imbalances, such as hypokalemia and hypomagnesemia, to increase the risk of toxicity and fatal arrhythmias in a patient who takes a digitalis glycoside. Hypokalemia also potentiates the neuromuscular blockade effects of nondepolarizing neuromuscular blockers.

PATIENT TEACHING

- Advise patient to change position slowly to minimize the effects of orthostatic hypotension. Instruct patient to notify prescriber if fainting occurs.
- Tell patient to maintain an adequate fluid intake and to be aware that diarrhea, excessive perspiration, or vomiting can lower blood pressure, possibly causing fainting to occur. Instruct patient to notify prescriber if excessive fluid loss occurs.
- Warn patient not to take any over-the-counter NSAID drug without consulting prescriber first.
- Instruct patient to notify prescriber at once about drowsiness, dry mouth, hearing changes, lethargy, muscle pain, nausea, restlessness, thirst, vomiting, or weakness.
- Advise diabetic patient to monitor her blood glucose level often because drug may raise it.

tramadol hydrochloride

ConZip, Ultram, Ultram ER

Class, Category, and Schedule

Pharmacologic class: Opioid agonist
Therapeutic class: Opioid analgesic
Pregnancy category: C
Controlled substance schedule: IV

Indications and Dosages

➤ *To relieve pain severe enough to require opioid-like treatment and for which alternative treatment options such as nonopioid analgesics or opioid combination products are inadequate or not tolerated*

TABLETS

Adults with chronic pain not requiring rapid onset of analgesic effect. *Initial:* 25 mg daily in morning, then titrated every 3 days in 25 mg increments in separate doses to reach 100 mg daily given as 25 mg four times daily. Then, if further analgesia is needed, total daily dose increased by 50 mg every 3 days to reach 200 mg daily given as 50 mg four times daily.

Adults requiring rapid pain relief. 50 to 100 mg every 4 to 6 hr, as needed. *Maximum:* 400 mg daily.

➤ *To manage moderate to moderately severe chronic pain in patients who require around-the-clock treatment for an extended period of time*

E.R. TABLETS

Adults not currently treated with immediate-release form of tramadol. 100 mg once daily, increased in 100-mg increments once daily every 5 days, as needed. *Maximum:* 300 mg once daily.

Adults maintained on tramadol immediate-release form. Dosage calculated using the 24-hr immediate-release dosage rounded down to the next lowest 100-mg increment. Dosage then adjusted as needed. *Maximum:* 300 mg once daily.

DOSAGE ADJUSTMENT For patients with creatinine clearance less than 30 ml/min, dosing interval increased to 12 hr with maximum daily dosage not to exceed 200 mg. For patients with cirrhosis, dosage reduced to 50 mg every 12 hr. For patients over 75 years of age, maximum dosage reduced to 300 mg daily.

Route	Onset	Peak	Duration
P.O. -immediate release	1 hr	2–3 hr	7–14 hr
P.O. -extended release	Unknown	12 hr	24 hr

Mechanism of Action

Binds with mu receptors and inhibits the reuptake of norepinephrine and serotonin, which may account for tramadol's analgesic effect.

Contraindications

Acute or severe bronchial asthma in the absence of resuscitative equipment or unmonitored setting, alcohol intoxication; children under the age of 12; excessive use of central-acting analgesics, hypnotics, opioids, or other psychotropic drugs; hypersensitivity to tramadol or its components; known or suspected gastrointestinal obstruction, including paralytic ileus; postoperative management in children ages 12 to 18 following adenoidectomy and/or tonsillectomy; significant respiratory depression; use within 14 days of MAO inhibitor therapy

Interactions

DRUGS

alpha blockers, CYP2D6 and CYP3A4 inhibitors, linezolid, lithium, MAO inhibitors, St. John's wort, selective serotonin and norepinephrine reuptake inhibitors, tricyclic antidepressants, triptans: Increased risk of serotonin syndrome

amiodarone, cimetidine, clomipramine, CYP2D6 inhibitors (bupropion, fluoxetine, paroxetine), desipramine, fluphenazine, haloperidol, propafenone, quinidine, ritonavir, thioridazine: Decreased analgesia, increased adverse effects of tramadol

amitriptyline, amphetamines, antipsychotics, bupropion, cyclobenzaprine, dextro-amphetamine, erythromycin, fluoxetine, ketoconazole, paroxetine, quinidine, MAO inhibitors, naloxone, tricyclic antidepressants: Increased risk of seizures

antimigraine agents, cyclobenzaprine; dextromethorphan; dolasetron; granisetron; linezolid; MAO inhibitors; methylene blue; ondansetron; palonosetron; selected psychiatric drugs such as amoxapine, buspirone, lithium, maprotiline, mirtazapine, nefazodone, trazodone, vilazodone; selective serotonin reuptake inhibitors; serotonin-norepinephrine reuptake inhibitors; St. John's wort; tricyclic antidepressants; tryptophan: Increased risk of serotonin syndrome

benzodiazepines, CNS depressants, opioids, sedating antihistamines, tricyclic antidepressants: Increased risk of severe respiratory depression and significant sedation and somnolence

carbamazepine: Increased tramadol metabolism

CNS depressants such as barbiturates, benzodiazepines, opioid analgesics, phenothiazines, sedative-hypnotics, tranquilizers: Additive CNS depression including coma, profound sedation, and respiratory depression

CYP3A4 inducers such as carbamazepine, phenytoin, rifampin: Decreased plasma concentration of tramadol and effectiveness
CYP3A4 inhibitors such as azole antifungal agents, macrolide antibiotics, protease inhibitors: Increased plasma concentration of tramadol and risk of adverse reactions
general anesthetics: Increased CNS and respiratory depression
phenothiazines, rifampin: Additive CNS depression, increased risk of seizures
warfarin: Possibly increased INR

ACTIVITIES

alcohol use: Additive CNS depression and respiratory depression that may become severe

Adverse Reactions

CNS: Agitation, anxiety, asthenia, depression, dizziness, emotional lability, euphoria, fatigue, fever, hallucinations, headache, hypertonia, hypoesthesia, insomnia, lethargy, nervousness, paresthesia, restlessness, rigors, **seizures**, **serotonin syndrome**, somnolence, **suicidal ideation**, tremor, vertigo, weakness
CV: Chest pain, orthostatic hypotension, **prolonged QT interval**, **torsades de pointes**, vasodilation
EENT: Blurred vision, dry mouth, nasal or sinus congestion, sore throat, vision changes
ENDO: Adrenal insufficiency, hot flashes
GI: Abdominal pain, anorexia, constipation, diarrhea, indigestion, nausea, vomiting
GU: Androgen deficiency, decreased libido, erectile dysfunction, impotence, infertility, lack of menstruation, urinary frequency, urine retention
MS: Arthralgia; back, limb, or neck pain
RESP: Cough, dyspnea, **respiratory depression (severe)**
SKIN: Diaphoresis, dermatitis, flushing, pruritus, rash
Other: Anaphylaxis, flu-like illness, physical and psychological dependence

Nursing Considerations

- Be aware that tramadol shouldn't be given to patients with a history of anaphylactoid reactions to codeine or other opioids.
- Avoid giving tramadol to patients with acute abdominal conditions because it may mask evidence and disrupt assessment of the abdomen.
- Be aware that tramadol should not be given to children under the age of 12, children ages 12 to 18 who have undergone an adenoidectomy and/or tonsillectomy, and children who have other risk factors that may increase their sensitivity to the respiratory depressant effects of drug. Risk factors to be alert for include concomitant use of other medications that cause respiratory depression or conditions associated with hypoventilation, such as neuromuscular disease, obesity, obstructive sleep apnea, postoperative status, or severe pulmonary disease.
- Be aware that excessive use of tramadol may lead to abuse, addiction, misuse, overdose, and possibly death. Monitor patient's intake of drug closely and for evidence of physical dependence. Alert prescriber if patient has a history of dependence on other opioids. Be aware that a Risk Evaluation and Mitigation Strategy (REMS) is required before tramadol can be prescribed.
- Know that chronic maternal use of tramadol during pregnancy can result in neonatal opioid withdrawal syndrome (NOWS), which may be life-threatening if not recognized and treated appropriately. NOWS occurs when a newborn has been exposed to tramadol for a prolonged period while in utero.
- Use tramadol cautiously in patients who are taking antidepressant drugs or tranquilizers and in patients who use alcohol in excess or who suffer from depression or emotional disturbance.
- Watch for allergic reactions after giving first dose of tramadol, including angioedema, bronchospasm, pruritus, Stevens–Johnson syndrome, toxic epidermal necrolysis, and urticaria. Also watch for signs and symptoms of anaphylaxis, such as dyspnea and hypotension.

WARNING Monitor patient for respiratory depression that could become life-threatening quickly, especially when drug is initiated or dosage is increased. If patient develops respiratory depression, expect to give naloxone. Watch for seizures because naloxone may increase this risk. Take seizure precautions.

- Assess respiratory status often if patient has head injury or increased intracranial pressure because of possible increased carbon dioxide retention and CSF pressure, either of which may cause respiratory depression. Also, be aware that tramadol may constrict pupils, obscuring evidence of intracranial complications.

WARNING Watch for seizures in patients with epilepsy, a history of seizures, or an increased risk of seizures, such as those with alcohol or drug withdrawal, CNS infection, head injury, or metabolic disorder.

- Expect to taper tramadol rather than stopping it abruptly to avoid acute withdrawal symptoms such as anxiety, diarrhea, insomnia, nausea, pain, panic attacks, paresthesias, piloerection, rigors, sweating, tremor, and upper respiratory symptoms.

WARNING Know that many drugs may interact with tramadol to cause serotonin syndrome. Monitor patient closely for signs and symptoms such as agitation, diaphoresis, diarrhea, fever, hallucinations, labile blood pressure, muscle twitching or stiffness, nausea, shakiness, shivering, tachycardia, trouble with coordination, or vomiting. Notify prescriber at once because serotonin syndrome may be life-threatening. Be prepared to discontinue drug, if possible and ordered, and provide supportive care.

- Monitor patient for adrenal insufficiency. Although rare, it can be life-threatening. Monitor patient for anorexia, dizziness, fatigue, hypotension, nausea, vomiting, or weakness. Notify prescriber if adrenal insufficiency is suspected and expect diagnostic testing to be done. If confirmed, expect to administer corticosteroids and wean patient off tramadol, if possible.
- Monitor patient closely for evidence of suicidal thinking or behavior, especially when therapy starts or dosage changes.

WARNING Be aware that tramadol should only be used concomitantly with benzodiazepine therapy in patients for whom other treatment options are inadequate. If prescribed together, expect dosing and duration of tramadol to be limited. Monitor patient closely for signs and symptoms of a decrease in consciousness, including coma, profound sedation, and significant respiratory depression. Notify prescriber immediately and provide emergency supportive care, as death may occur.

PATIENT TEACHING

- Urge patient to follow prescribed dose limits and dosing intervals to prevent respiratory depression and seizures. Warn patient that excessive or prolonged use can lead to abuse, addiction, misuse, overdose, and possibly death.
- Instruct patient prescribed extended-release form to swallow tablet whole and not to chew, crush, or split tablet.
- Instruct patient to seek immediate emergency medical care and to stop taking tramadol if a serious allergic reaction occurs.
- Caution patient not to stop tramadol abruptly.
- Instruct patient to avoid hazardous activities until drug's CNS effects are known.
- Warn patient not to consume alcohol or take a benzodiazepine without prescriber knowledge, as severe respiratory depression can occur and may lead to death.
- Inform patient that long-term use of tramadol may decrease sex hormone levels, causing decreased libido, erectile dysfunction, impotence, infertility, or lack of menstruation. Encourage patient to report any symptoms to prescriber.
- Urge patient to notify prescriber about known, suspected, or intended pregnancy.
- Tell mothers wishing to breastfeed to consult prescriber before doing so, because if mother is an ultra-rapid metabolizer, infant could experience life-threatening respiratory depression.
- Urge caregivers to watch patient closely for evidence of suicidal tendencies, especially when therapy starts or dosage changes and to report concerns at once to prescriber.
- Tell patient to notify prescriber immediately if he develops any persistent, severe, sudden, or unusual adverse reactions.
- Instruct patient to inform all prescribers of tramadol therapy because of potential drug interactions.

- Caution patient to keep tramadol out of the reach of children because even one dose could result in a fatal overdose in a child.
- Warn patient that tramadol may cause severe constipation. Advise patient to maintain adequate hydration, increase fiber in diet, and to seek treatment instructions from prescriber if constipation occurs and is not relieved soon after onset.
- Instruct patient how to dispose of unused tramadol in accordance with local state guidelines and/or regulations.

trandolapril

Mavik

Class and Category

Pharmacologic class: Angiotensin converting enzyme (ACE) inhibitor
Therapeutic class: Antihypertensive, vasodilator
Pregnancy category: D

Indications and Dosages

➤ *To manage hypertension*

TABLETS

Adults. *Initial:* 1 mg daily, increased every wk based on clinical response. Dosage may be given in two daily doses if antihypertensive effect diminishes before 24 hr. *Usual:* 2 to 4 mg daily. *Maximum:* 8 mg daily.

➤ *To treat heart failure or left-ventricular dysfunction after MI*

TABLETS

Adults. *Initial:* 1 mg daily, increased as needed toward target dose of 4 mg once daily.

DOSAGE ADJUSTMENT Initial dosage increased to 2 mg daily for blacks with hypertension. Initial dosage reduced to 0.5 mg for patients also receiving a diuretic, those with cirrhosis, or those with a creatinine clearance of less than or equal to 30 ml/min.

Route	Onset	Peak	Duration
P.O.	2 hr	8 hr	24 hr

Mechanism of Action

Reduces blood pressure by inhibiting the conversion of angiotensin I to angiotensin II. Angiotensin II is a potent vasoconstrictor that stimulates the renal cortex to secrete aldosterone. Decreased release of aldosterone reduces sodium and water retention and increases their excretion, thereby reducing blood pressure and edema associated with heart failure. Trandolapril may also inhibit renal and vascular production of angiotensin II.

Contraindications

Aliskiren therapy in patients with diabetes or renal impairment (GFR less than 60 ml/min), hereditary or idiopathic angioedema, history of angioedema related to previous treatment with ACE inhibitor, hypersensitivity to trandolapril or its components, use within 36 hours of an mTOR inhibitor (everolimus, sirolimus, temsirolimus) or a neprilysin inhibitor (sacubitril) therapy

Interactions

DRUGS

aliskiren (in patients with diabetes), angiotensin receptor blockers, other ACE inhibitors: Increased risk of hyperkalemia, hypotension, and renal dysfunction
allopurinol, bone marrow depressants (such as methotrexate), corticosteroids (systemic), cytostatic drugs, procainamide: Increased risk of potentially fatal neutropenia or agranulocytosis
antacids: Decreased blood trandolapril level
cyclosporine, potassium-containing drugs, potassium-sparing diuretics, potassium supplements: Increased risk of hyperkalemia
diuretics, other antihypertensives: Increased hypotensive effects
inhalation anesthetics (selected): Enhanced hypotensive effect of selected inhalation anesthetics
insulin, oral hypoglycemic agents: Possibly increased risk of hypoglycemia
lithium: Increased blood lithium level and risk of lithium toxicity
mTOR inhibitor such as everolimus, sirolimus, temsirolimus; neprilysin inhibitor such as sacubitril: Increased risk of angioedema
NSAIDs: Possibly reduced antihypertensive effects; increased risk of renal dysfunction especially in the elderly and patients with preexisting renal dysfunction or volume depletion

sodium aurothiomalate: Increased risk of nitroid reactions, such as facial flushing, hypotension, nausea, vomiting
sympathomimetics: Possibly reduced antihypertensive effects

FOODS

high-potassium diet, low-sodium milk, potassium-containing salt substitutes: Increased risk of hyperkalemia

ACTIVITIES

alcohol use: Possibly increased hypotensive effect

Adverse Reactions

CNS: Anxiety, **CVA**, depression, dizziness, drowsiness, fatigue, fever, hallucination, headache, insomnia, malaise, paresthesia, syncope, transient ischemic attack, vertigo
CV: Angina, **arrhythmia**, **bradycardia**, **cardiac failure**, chest pain, edema, first-degree AV block, **hypotension**, **MI**, **myocardial ischemia**, orthostatic hypotension, palpitations, tachycardia, **ventricular tachycardia**
EENT: Dry mouth, epistaxis, loss of taste, throat inflammation
GI: Abdominal cramps, distention, or pain; constipation; diarrhea; dyspepsia; elevated liver enzymes; **hepatitis**; jaundice; nausea; **pancreatitis**; vomiting
GU: Decreased libido, elevated blood urea nitrogen and creatinine, impotence, **renal failure**
HEME: Agranulocytosis, **leukopenia**, **neutropenia**, **pancytopenia**, **thrombocytopenia**
MS: Extremity pain, muscle cramps, myalgia
RESP: Bronchitis, cough, dyspnea, upper respiratory tract infection
SKIN: Alopecia, diaphoresis, flushing, pemphigus, pruritus, rash, **Stevens–Johnson syndrome**, **toxic epidermal necrolysis**
Other: Angioedema, elevated SGOT levels, gout, **hyperkalemia**, **hypocalcemia**, **hyponatremia**

Nursing Considerations

WARNING Closely monitor blood pressure during first 2 weeks of therapy and whenever dosage is adjusted, especially in patients with heart failure, hyponatremia, or severe sodium or volume loss. If excessive hypotension occurs, notify prescriber immediately, place patient in supine position, and infuse I.V. with a normal saline solution, as prescribed.

WARNING Be alert for signs and symptoms of angioedema. If swelling of glottis, larynx, or tongue causes airway obstruction, notify prescriber and be prepared to discontinue drug and administer emergency measures, including subcutaneous epinephrine 1:1,000 (0.3 to 0.5 ml).

- Continue to monitor patient's blood pressure to assess drug's long-term effectiveness.

PATIENT TEACHING

- Instruct patient to notify prescriber immediately and stop taking trandolapril if she experiences swelling of eyes, face, lips, or tongue or has difficulty breathing.
- Explain that drug may cause dizziness and light-headedness, especially during first few days of therapy. Advise patient to avoid driving and other potentially hazardous activities until drug's CNS effects are known and to notify prescriber immediately if she faints.
- Inform female patient of childbearing age about risks of taking trandolapril during pregnancy. Urge her to use effective contraceptive method and to notify prescriber immediately if she becomes or thinks she might be pregnant.
- Advise patient planning to undergo anesthesia or surgery to inform specialist that she's taking trandolapril.
- Instruct patient to consult prescriber before using potassium supplements or salt substitutes containing potassium.
- Inform patient about possible loss of taste, which may result in weight loss. Reassure her that loss of taste is usually reversed after 2 to 3 months.

tranexamic acid

Cyklokapron, Lysteda

Class and Category

Pharmacologic class: Plasminogen activation inhibitor
Therapeutic class: Antifibrinolytic
Pregnancy category: B

Indications and Dosages

➤ *To treat cyclic heavy menstrual bleeding*

TABLETS

Adults. 1,300 mg three times daily for a maximum of 5 days during monthly menstruation

DOSAGE ADJUSTMENT For patient with a serum creatinine level above 1.4 mg/dl but equal to or less than 2.8 mg/dl, 1,300 mg two times a day for a maximum of 5 days during menstruation; for patient with a serum creatinine level above 2.8 mg/dl but equal to or less than 5.7 mg/dl, 1,300 mg once daily for a maximum of 5 days during menstruation; for patient with a serum creatinine level above 5.7 mg/dl, 650 mg once daily for a maximum of 5 days during menstruation.

➤ *To treat patients with hemophilia to reduce or prevent hemorrhage and reduce need for replacement therapy during and following tooth extraction*

I.V. INFUSION

Adults. *Initial:* 10 mg/kg infused at 50 mg/min immediately before tooth extraction together with replacement therapy, followed by 10 mg/kg three times a day or four times a day, as needed, for up to 8 days.

DOSAGE ADJUSTMENT For patients with moderate to severe renal impairment with a serum creatinine of 1.36 to 2.83 mg/dl, dosage reduced to 10 mg/kg twice daily. For patients with a serum creatinine of 2.83 to 5.66 mg/dl, dosage reduced to 10 mg/kg daily. For patient with serum creatinine greater than 5.66 mg/dl, dosage reduced to 5 mg/kg every 24 hours or 10 mg/kg every 48 hours.

Route	Onset	Peak	Duration
P.O.	Unknown	3 hr	Unknown
I.V.	Unknown	Unknown	7–17 hr

Mechanism of Action

Displaces plasminogen from surface of fibrin by binding to high-affinity lysine site of plasminogen. This diminishes dissolution of hemostatic fibrin, which decreases bleeding.

Incompatibilities

Do not administer tranexamic acid intravenously with blood or solutions containing penicillin.

Contraindications

Acquired defective color vision; active thromboembolic disease; history or intrinsic risk of thromboembolism or thrombosis, including retinal artery or vein occlusion; hypersensitivity to tranexamic acid or its components; subarachnoid hemorrhage; use of combination hormonal contraception

Interactions

DRUGS

anti-inhibitor coagulant concentrates, factor IX complex concentrates, hormonal contraceptives: Increased thrombotic risk

tissue plasminogen activators: Possibly decreased effectiveness of both tranexamic acid and the tissue plasminogen activator

tretinoin (oral): Possibly exacerbation of the procoagulant effect of tretinoin

Adverse Reactions

CNS: Cerebral thrombosis, dizziness, fatigue, headache, migraine, **seizures**

CV: Deep vein thrombosis, **MI**

EENT: Central retinal artery and vein obstruction, impaired color vision, ligneous conjunctivitis, nasal and sinus congestion, sinusitis, **throat tightness**, visual abnormalities

GI: Abdominal pain, diarrhea, nausea, vomiting

GU: Acute renal cortical necrosis

HEME: Anemia

MS: Arthralgia, back pain, muscle cramps and spasms, myalgia

RESP: Dyspnea, **pulmonary embolism**, respiratory congestion

SKIN: Allergic skin reactions, facial flushing

Other: Anaphylaxis, **hypersensitivity reactions**

Nursing Considerations

- Know that tranexamic acid therapy isn't recommended for women who use hormonal contraceptives or who take factor IX complex concentrates or anti-inhibitor coagulant concentrates because of the increased risk of thromboembolism, especially if she is obese, a smoker, or over the age of 35.
- Use tranexamic acid cautiously in patients with acute promyelocytic leukemia who

are taking oral tretinoin for remission induction; they could be susceptible to possible exacerbation of the procoagulant effect of tretinoin.

- Be aware that intravenous form of drug may be diluted with most solutions such as amino acid, carbohydrate, Dextran, or electrolyte solutions. Diluted solution may be stored for up to 4 hours at room temperature prior to patient administration. Administer at a rate of 50 mg/min.
- Be aware that cerebral edema and cerebral infarction may occur in women taking tranexamic acid if a subarachnoid hemorrhage occurs.

WARNING Monitor patient closely for allergic reactions to tranexamic acid such as dyspnea, facial flushing, or a feeling of tightness in the throat. Be aware that severe allergic reactions such as anaphylaxis have occurred after intravenous administration of tranexamic acid. Monitor patient closely and be prepared to provide emergency supportive care according to standard protocol, as ordered.

PATIENT TEACHING

- Instruct patient to swallow tranexamic acid tablets whole, without breaking or chewing them. Therapy shouldn't exceed 5 days during menstruation.
- Tell patient to seek emergency care immediately if she has any signs of allergic reaction, especially dyspnea, facial flushing, or a feeling of tightness in the throat; if any of these occur, she should stop taking drug.
- Advise patient to report any changes in vision or ocular discomfort.

trazodone hydrochloride

Desyrel, Oleptro

Class and Category

Pharmacologic class: Triazolopyridine derivative
Therapeutic class: Antidepressant
Pregnancy category: C

Indications and Dosages

➤ *To treat major depression*

E.R. TABLETS

Adults. *Initial:* 150 mg once daily, increased by 75 mg daily every 3 days, as needed. *Maximum:* 375 mg daily.

TABLETS

Adults. *150 mg in divided doses daily following a meal or light snack, increased by 50 mg/day every 3 to 4 days. Maximum:* 400 mg daily in divided doses.

Route	Onset	Peak	Duration
P.O.	1–2 wk	Unknown	Unknown

Mechanism of Action

Blocks serotonin reuptake along the presynaptic neuronal membrane, causing an antidepressant effect. Trazodone exerts an alpha-adrenergic blocking action and produces modest histamine blockade, causing a sedative effect. It also inhibits the vasopressor response to norepinephrine, which reduces blood pressure.

Contraindications

Hypersensitivity to trazodone or its components, recovery from acute MI, use within 14 days of an MAO inhibitor including intravenous methylene blue and linezolid

Interactions

DRUGS

aspirin, NSAIDs: Possibly increased risk of bleeding
barbiturates and other CNS depressants: Enhanced effect of CNS depressants
carbamazepine: Decreased trazodone level
CYP3A4 inhibitors such as indinavir, ketoconazole, and ritonavir: Possibly increased plasma trazodone levels with increased risk of adverse reactions
digoxin, phenytoin: Possibly increased blood levels of these drugs and increased risk of toxicity
MAO inhibitors: Increased serotonin effects
serotonergic drugs: Increased risk of serotonin syndrome
warfarin: Altered anticoagulation response

ACTIVITIES

alcohol use: Increased CNS depression, risk of hypotension and respiratory depression

Adverse Reactions

CNS: Abnormal coordination or dreams, agitation, anxiety, aphasia, ataxia, balance disorder, chills, confusion, **CVA**, dizziness, drowsiness, extrapyramidal symptoms, fatigue, hallucinations, headache, insomnia, light-headedness, memory impairment, migraine, nervousness, paresthesia, paranoid reaction, psychosis, **seizures**, **serotonin syndrome**, somnolence, stupor, **suicidal ideation**, syncope, tardive dyskinesia, tremor, vertigo, weakness
CV: **Arrhythmias**, **congestive heart failure**, edema, **hypotension**, orthostatic hypotension, palpitations, **prolonged QT interval**, vasodilation
EENT: Angle-closure glaucoma, blurred vision, diplopia, dry mouth
ENDO: Inappropriate ADH syndrome
GI: Abdominal pain, cholestasis, constipation, diarrhea, elevated bilirubin or liver enzymes, indigestion, jaundice, nausea, vomiting
GU: Anorgasmia; ejaculation disorders; decreased libido; priapism; urinary incontinence, retention, or urgency
HEME: **Hemolytic anemia**, leukocytosis
MS: Back pain, myalgia
RESP: **Apnea**, dyspnea
SKIN: Alopecia, hirsutism, night sweats, pruritus, psoriasis, rash, urticaria
Other: **Hyponatremia**

Nursing Considerations

- Use trazodone cautiously in patients with cardiac disease because drug can cause arrhythmias.
- Give trazodone shortly after the patient has a meal or light snack to reduce nausea.
- Give larger portion of daily dose at bedtime if drowsiness occurs.
- Expect most patients who respond to trazodone to do so by the end of the second week of therapy.
- Closely monitor depressed patients for suicidal thoughts and tendencies. Notify prescriber if they occur, and take suicide precautions according to facility policy.

WARNING Monitor patient closely for serotonin syndrome exhibited by agitation, coma, diarrhea, hallucinations, hyperreflexia, hyperthermia, incoordination, labile blood pressure, nausea, tachycardia, and vomiting. Notify prescriber immediately because serotonin syndrome may be life-threatening and provide supportive care.

WARNING Be aware that serotonin syndrome in its most severe form may resemble neuroleptic malignant syndrome, which includes autonomic instability with possibly rapid changes in vital signs and mental status, or hyperthermia and muscle rigidity. Stop drug immediately and provide supportive care.

- Be aware that adverse CNS reactions usually improve after patient completes a few weeks of therapy.

WARNING Be aware that trazodone therapy may increase the risk of priapism.

PATIENT TEACHING

- Urge patient to avoid taking trazodone on an empty stomach because doing so may increase the risk of dizziness or light-headedness.
- Advise patient that drug may cause mild pupillary dilation, which may lead to an episode of acute closure glaucoma. Encourage patient to have an eye exam before starting therapy to see if he is at risk.
- Caution patient to avoid potentially hazardous activities during therapy until nervous system effects have abated.
- Advise patient not to fast during trazodone therapy because of possible adverse CNS reactions.
- Instruct male patient to notify prescriber immediately about priapism.
- Caution patient not to take aspirin or nonsteroidal anti-inflammatory agents without first discussing use with the prescriber.
- Instruct patient not to stop trazodone therapy abruptly.
- Urge family and caregivers to watch patient closely for abnormal thinking or behavior or increased aggression or hostility. Emphasize importance of notifying prescriber about unusual changes.
- Advise women of childbearing age to notify prescriber if pregnancy occurs or is suspected. If pregnancy is confirmed, encourage patient to enroll in the pregnancy exposure registry.

triamcinolone

triamcinolone acetonide

Azmacort, Kenalog-10, Kenalog-40, Nasacort Allergy 24 Hour, Zilretta

triamcinolone diacetate

triamcinolone hexacetonide

Aristospan

Class and Category

Pharmacologic class: Glucocorticoid
Therapeutic class: Corticosteroid
Pregnancy category: C (nasal and oral inhalation), Not classified

Indications and Dosages

➤ *To prevent bronchospasm or provide long-term corticosteroid treatment to control asthma*

ORAL INHALATION (AZMACORT)

Adults and children age 12 and over. *Initial:* 2 metered sprays (150 mcg) three times a day or four times a day. Alternatively, 4 metered sprays (300 mcg) twice daily. *Maximum:* 16 metered sprays (1,200 mcg) daily in divided doses.
Children ages 6 to 11. 1 to 2 metered sprays (75 to 150 mcg) three to four times daily. Alternatively, 2 to 4 metered sprays (150 to 300 mcg) twice daily. *Maximum:* 12 metered sprays (900 mcg) daily.

➤ *To treat a multitude of disorders exhibiting severe inflammation or need for immunosuppression*

I.M. INJECTION (KENALOG-40)

Adults. 2.5 to 100 mg daily depending on specific disease entity being treated. Dosage adjusted as needed.
Children. *Initial:* 0.11 to 1.6 mg/kg daily in 3 or 4 divided doses. Dosage adjusted as needed.

I.M. INJECTION (ARISTOCORT FORTE)

Adults. 3 to 48 mg daily depending on specific disease entity being treated. Dosage adjusted as needed.
Children. 0.11 to 1.6 mg/kg daily in three or four divided doses. Dosage adjusted as needed.

➤ *To relieve inflammation caused by acute gouty arthritis, acute nonspecific tenosynovitis, acute or subacute bursitis, epicondylitis, osteoarthritis, post-traumatic osteoarthritis, rheumatoid arthritis, and synovitis*

INTRA-ARTICULAR INJECTION (KENALOG-10)

Adults. 2.5 to 5 mg for smaller joints and 5 to 15 mg for larger joints, as needed.

INTRA-ARTICULAR INJECTION (ARISTOCORT FORTE)

Adults. 5 to 40 mg, and repeated, as needed 1 wk to 2 months.

INTRA-ARTICULAR INJECTION (ARISTOSPAN)

Adults. 2 to 20 mg, repeated as prescribed every 3 to 4 wk, as needed.

➤ *To relieve osteoarthritis pain of the knee*

E.R. INTRA-ARTICULAR INJECTION (ZILRETTA)

Adults. 32 mg injected once in the knee.

➤ *To relieve symptoms of perennial and seasonal allergic rhinitis*

NASAL INHALATION (NASACORT ALLERGY 24 HOUR)

Adults and children age 12 and over. *Initial:* 110 mcg daily in 2 sprays (55 mcg each)/nostril.
Children ages 6 to 11. 110 mcg daily in 1 spray (55 mcg each)/nostril. *Maximum:* 220 mcg or 4 sprays daily.
Children ages 2 to 5. 110 mcg daily in 1 spray (55 mcg)/nostril.

Route	Onset	Peak	Duration
I.M.	24–48 hr	Unknown	1–6 wk
Inhalation-	12 hr	3–4 hr	Unknown
Intra-articular	Unknown	Unknown	Several wk
Nasal	Unknown	1.5–4 hr	Unknown

Mechanism of Action

Inhibits the release of leukotrienes and prostaglandins, thus reducing immediate and late-phase allergic responses in chronic asthma. Triamcinolone also:

- decreases peribronchial edema and mucus secretion by inhibiting the binding of allergens to immunoglobulin E antibodies on

the surface of mast cells, thereby inactivating the release of chemotactic substances
- decreases inflammation by interfering with leukocyte adhesion to capillary walls
- inhibits the release of leukocytic acid hydrolases, preventing macrophage accumulation at the infection site
- inhibits histamine and kinin release, preventing the formation of scar tissue.

Incompatibilities

Don't mix triamcinolone hexacetonide with parenteral local anesthetics because precipitation can occur.

Contraindications

Acute status asthmaticus (inhalation form), administered as an intrathecal injection, hypersensitivity to triamcinolone or its components, live-virus vaccine therapy, systemic fungal infection (except Aristocort Forte when administered as an intra-articular injection for localized joint conditions), idiopathic thrombocytopenic purpura (given as I.M. injection)

Interactions

DRUGS

amphotericin B, ethacrynic acid, furosemide, thiazide diuretics: Increased potassium-wasting effect, severe hypokalemia
aspirin: Increased blood salicylate level, increased risk of salicylate toxicity
cholinesterase inhibitors: Increased risk of severe muscle weakness in patients with myasthenia gravis
CYP3A4 inhibitors such as atazanavir, clarithromycin, cobicistat-containing products, indinavir, itraconazole, ketoconazole, nefazodine, nelfinavir, ritonavir, saquinavir, telithromycin: Decreased triamcinolone clearance, increased risk of adverse effects
digitalis glycosides: Increased risk of arrhythmias and digitalis toxicity
estrogens: Increased triamcinolone effects
hepatic enzyme inducers such as barbiturates, carbamazepine, phenytoin, rifampin: Increased triamcinolone metabolism with decreased effectiveness
insulin, oral antidiabetic drugs: Increased blood glucose level
isoproterenol: Increased risk of cardiotoxicity
live-virus vaccines: Decreased antibody response, increased risk of neurologic complications
neuromuscular blockers: Increased risk of hypokalemia and enhanced neuromuscular blockade
NSAIDs: Increased risk of adverse GI effects
toxoids: Decreased resistance to toxoids

Adverse Reactions

CNS: Depression, dizziness, emotional lability, exacerbated psychosis, fatigue, headache, **increased intracranial pressure with papilledema (pseudotumor cerebri)**, insomnia, malaise, neuritis, neuropathy, paresthesia, personality changes, psychiatric disorders, restlessness, **seizures**, vertigo
CV: Edema, **heart failure**, hypertension
EENT: Altered sense of smell or taste, cataracts, dry mouth, epistaxis (nasal form), glaucoma, hoarseness, nasal congestion, nasal irritation (inhalation form), nasal septal perforation (nasal form), oropharyngeal candidiasis, pharyngitis, posterior subcapsular cataracts, rhinorrhea, secondary ocular infection, sinusitis, sneezing
ENDO: Cushing's syndrome, diabetes mellitus, growth retardation (children)
GI: Abdominal pain, constipation, diarrhea, dyspepsia, esophageal ulceration, gastritis, nausea, vomiting
GU: Altered motility and number of spermatozoa, cystitis, postmenopausal **vaginal hemorrhage**, renal disease, UTI, vaginitis
MS: Bone mineral density loss, bursitis, muscle wasting or weakness, myalgia, osteoporosis, tenosynovitis
RESP: Asthma, bronchitis, **bronchospasm** (inhalation form), chest congestion, dyspnea, increased cough
SKIN: Ecchymosis, petechiae (parenteral form), photosensitivity, pruritus, rash, striae, urticaria
Other: Anaphylaxis; **angioedema**; decreased resistance to infections; flu-like symptoms; herpes infection; hiccups; impaired wound healing; injection-site atrophy, induration, pain, soreness, and sterile abscess; moon face; weight gain

Nursing Considerations

- Be aware that high doses of corticosteroids such as triamcinolone aren't recommended for patients with cranial trauma who don't require a corticosteroid for another condition because they increase risk of death.
- Know that triamcinolone should be administered with extreme caution, if at all, in patients who have active or quiescent tuberculosis infection of the respiratory tract, ocular herpes simplex, systemic parasitic or viral infection, or untreated bacterial or fungal infection, because this drug can make these infections worse.
- Use cautiously in patients with active or latent peptic ulcer, diverticulitis, fresh intestinal anastomoses, and nonspecific ulcerative colitis; there is increased risk of a perforation for these patients. Be aware that signs of peritoneal irritation following gastrointestinal perforation in patients receiving steroid therapy may be minimal or absent.
- Monitor patient with cirrhosis carefully for an enhanced drug effect because increased metabolism of steroids may occur in the presence of cirrhosis.
- Know that triamcinolone acetonide parenteral formulation with trade name Kenalog-40 can be administered I.M. Other parenteral triamcinolone acetonide forms should never be injected I.M. Shake I.M. suspension thoroughly before drawing it into syringe.
- Be aware that specialized training may be needed to administer parenteral triamcinolone.
- Don't administer parenteral forms of triamcinolone intravenously.

WARNING Know that drug should not be administered via the epidural or intrathecal route because severe neurologic adverse reactions may occur

- Know that drug should not be administered intra-articularly into an infected site, and injection into a previously infected joint is usually not recommended.
- Be aware that triamcinolone may reactivate tuberculosis in patients who have a history of it.
- Monitor patient for hypersensitivity. Although rare, triamcinolone has caused anaphylaxis that ended in death. Notify prescriber immediately if hypersensitivity occurs; expect to discontinue triamcinolone therapy and provide emergency supportive care.
- Monitor patients for exposure to high doses, which may result in toxicity evidenced by life-threatening hypotension and metabolic acidosis.

WARNING Know that patients on corticosteroid therapy require an increased dosage of rapidly acting corticosteroids when unusual stress is anticipated, during the stressful event, and for a period after the stressful situation. Assess patient for signs and symptoms of adrenal insufficiency (fatigue, hypotension, lassitude, nausea, vomiting, and weakness) during times of stress, such as infection, surgery, or trauma. Notify prescriber immediately if you detect these signs and symptoms because adrenal insufficiency may be life-threatening. Drug-induced secondary adrenocortical insufficiency may be minimized by gradual reduction of dosage.

- Be aware that, although rare, bone mineral density loss and osteoporosis may occur, which may increase risk of fractures, especially in patients on prolonged triamcinolone therapy.
- Adjust triamcinolone dosage, as prescribed, in patients with changes in thyroid status because metabolic clearance of corticosteroids is decreased in hypothyroid patients and increased in hyperthyroid patients.
- Assess patient for signs and symptoms of infection (abnormal symptoms in particular body system, fever, or malaise), because steroid therapy such as triamcinolone increases risk of susceptibility to infections, especially with higher dosages.

PATIENT TEACHING

- Caution patient not to adjust dosage for prescription triamcinolone without consulting prescriber and to follow dosage recommendations when using an over-the-counter preparation.
- Teach patient how to administer nasal aerosols properly, using

manufacturer's instructions, to avoid nasal irritation.

- Teach patient how to use nasal spray, including how to prime spray pump bottle before use. Caution patient not to get nasal spray in eyes. If this occurs, patient should rinse his eyes well with water.
- Inform patient that maximum benefit of triamcinolone therapy may not occur for up to 2 weeks.
- Advise patient to notify prescriber immediately if asthma fails to respond to inhaled drug; additional systemic therapy may be needed.
- Caution patient to avoid exposure to people who have chickenpox or measles, as well as other contagious infections, throughout triamcinolone therapy and for 12 months afterward.
- Advise patient to have periodic eye examinations during long-term therapy because triamcinolone can cause glaucoma or ocular nerve damage.

triamterene

Dyrenium

Class and Category

Pharmacologic class: Potassium-sparing diuretic
Therapeutic class: Diuretic
Pregnancy category: B

Indications and Dosages

➤ *To treat edema in cirrhosis, heart failure, and nephrotic syndrome, as well as edema secondary to hyperaldosteronism, idiopathic edema, and steroid-induced edema*

CAPSULES

Adults. *Initial:* 100 mg twice daily after meals and adjusted as needed. *Maximum:* 300 mg daily.

Route	Onset	Peak	Duration
P.O.	2–4 hr	1 to several days	7–9 hr

Mechanism of Action

Inhibits sodium reabsorption in distal convoluted tubules and cortical collecting ducts, causing sodium and water loss and enhancing potassium retention.

Contraindications

Anuria, diabetic nephropathy or renal disease linked to renal insufficiency, hyperkalemia (potassium level of 5.5 mEq/L or more), hypersensitivity to triamterene or its components, severe hepatic dysfunction

Interactions

DRUGS

ACE inhibitors, amiloride, angiotensin-II receptor antagonists, cyclosporine, heparin, potassium-containing drugs, potassium salts, potassium-sparing diuretics, potassium supplements: Increased risk of hyperkalemia
amantadine: Decreased amantadine clearance, possibly amantadine toxicity
antihypertensives: Increased antihypertensive effect
diuretics: Increased diuretic effect
folic acid: Possibly antagonized action of folic acid
indomethacin: Increased risk of renal impairment
lithium: Increased risk of lithium toxicity
NSAIDs: Decreased diuretic effect of triamterene, increased risk of hyperkalemia
oral antidiabetic drugs: Altered blood glucose control

Adverse Reactions

CNS: Dizziness, fatigue, headache, weakness
EENT: Dry mouth
ENDO: Hyperglycemia, **hypoglycemia**
GI: Diarrhea, jaundice, nausea, vomiting
GU: **Azotemia**, elevated BUN and serum creatinine levels, renal calculi
SKIN: Photosensitivity, rash

Nursing Considerations

- Be aware that triamterene shouldn't be given to patient with creatinine clearance below 10 ml/min because this condition increases the risk of drug-induced hyperkalemia.
- Monitor serum potassium level during therapy, especially in patient with

diabetes mellitus or renal impairment. Also monitor patient's BUN and serum creatinine levels to assess renal function and prevent hyperkalemia.
- Monitor patient for irregular heartbeat, which is usually the first sign of hyperkalemia. If you suspect hyperkalemia, obtain an ECG tracing, as ordered. A widened QRS complex or an arrhythmia requires prompt additional therapy.
- Monitor laboratory test results and watch for signs of metabolic or respiratory acidosis, which may occur suddenly in patient with cardiac disease or uncontrolled diabetes mellitus.
- Monitor patient's serum sodium and uric acid levels, as ordered, because triamterene may worsen preexisting hyponatremia and reduce uric acid clearance, increasing the risk of gout and hyperuricemia.
- Monitor CBC with differential because drug may increase the risk of megaloblastic anemia in patient with folic acid deficiency.

PATIENT TEACHING
- Advise patient to take triamterene with food or milk.
- Instruct patient to avoid exposure to excessive heat or sunlight to prevent dehydration and, possibly, photosensitivity.
- Explain to patient with a history of gout that drug may increase the risk of attack.
- Advise patient to notify prescriber about ineffective diuresis and unexplained weight gain during therapy.

triazolam

Halcion

Class, Category, and Schedule

Pharmacologic class: Benzodiazepine
Therapeutic class: Sedative-hypnotic
Pregnancy category: X
Controlled substance schedule: IV

Indications and Dosages

➤ *To provide short-term management of insomnia*

TABLETS

Adults. 0.125 to 0.25 mg at bedtime. *Maximum:* 0.5 mg daily (for patients with inadequate response to usual dose).
DOSAGE ADJUSTMENT For elderly or debilitated patients, initial dosage not to exceed 0.125 mg at bedtime and maximum dosage limited to 0.25 mg daily.

Route	Onset	Peak	Duration
P.O.	15–30 min	Unknown	Unknown

Mechanism of Action

Potentiates effects of the inhibitory neurotransmitter gamma-aminobutyric acid, which increases inhibition of the ascending reticular activating system and produces varying levels of CNS depression, including anticonvulsant activity, coma, hypnosis, sedation, and skeletal muscle relaxation.

Contraindications

Concurrent therapy with azoles such as fluconazole, itraconazole, ketoconazole, or nefazodone, and selected HIV protease inhibitors such as indinavir, lopinavir, nelfinavir, ritonavir, or saquinavir; hypersensitivity to triazolam, other benzodiazepines, or their components; pregnancy

Interactions

DRUGS

anxiolytics, barbiturates, brompheniramine, carbinoxamine, cetirizine, chlorpheniramine, clemastine, cyproheptadine, dimenhydrinate, diphenhydramine, doxylamine, general anesthetics, methdilazine, opioid analgesics, other benzodiazepines and CNS depressants, phenothiazines, promethazine, sedating antihistamines, sedative-hypnotics, tramadol, tricyclic antidepressants, trimeprazine: Increased sedation, respiratory depression that could become severe
azoles such as itraconazole, ketoconazole, or nefazodone; selected HIV protease inhibitors such as indinavir, lopinavir, nelfinavir, ritonavir, or saquinavir: Possibly increased plasma triazolam levels and increased risk of adverse reactions
cimetidine, diltiazem, disulfiram, erythromycin, probenecid, verapamil: Increased sedation

flumazenil: Increased risk of withdrawal symptoms
oral contraceptives: Increased blood triazolam level

FOODS

grapefruit juice: Increased blood triazolam level and sedation

ACTIVITIES

alcohol use: Increased sedation, respiratory depression that could become severe

Adverse Reactions

CNS: Anxiety, ataxia, complex behaviors (such as sleep driving), confusion, depression, dizziness, drowsiness, fatigue, headache, insomnia, nightmares, syncope, talkativeness, tremor, vertigo
EENT: **Throat tightness**
GI: Nausea, vomiting
RESP: Dyspnea
Other: **Anaphylaxis, angioedema**, physical and psychological dependence

Nursing Considerations

- Be aware that triazolam shouldn't be discontinued abruptly, even after only 1 to 2 weeks of therapy. Doing so can cause withdrawal symptoms, including abdominal cramps, confusion, depression, diaphoresis, hyperacusis, insomnia, irritability, nausea, nervousness, paresthesia, perceptual disturbances, photophobia, tachycardia, tremor, and vomiting.

WARNING Assess patient for signs of physical and psychological dependence, and notify prescriber if they occur.

- Monitor patient's ABG results and respiratory depth and rate, as appropriate, because drug may worsen ventilatory failure in patient with pulmonary disease, such as respiratory depression, severe COPD, or sleep apnea. Use drug cautiously in patients with acute intermittent porphyria, myasthenia gravis, and severe renal impairment because it may aggravate these conditions.
- Take safety precautions for elderly patients because triazolam may impair cognitive and motor function and increase the risk for falls.
- Use drug cautiously in patients with advanced Parkinson's disease because it may worsen cognition, coordination, and psychosis.

WARNING Monitor patient closely for hypersensitivity reactions such as dyspnea, nausea, swelling, throat tightness, and vomiting. If present, stop triazolam immediately, notify prescriber, and provide supportive care.

WARNING Be aware that opioids should only be used concomitantly with benzodiazepine therapy like triazolam in patients for whom other treatment options are inadequate. If prescribed together, expect dosing and duration of the opioid to be limited. Monitor patient closely for signs and symptoms of a decrease in consciousness, including coma, profound sedation, and significant respiratory depression. Notify prescriber immediately and provide emergency supportive care, as death may occur.

PATIENT TEACHING

- Instruct patient to take triazolam exactly as prescribed and not to stop taking it abruptly because of the risk of having withdrawal symptoms.
- Instruct patient to stop taking triazolam and seek emergency care if she has abnormal swelling, nausea, throat tightness, trouble breathing, or vomiting.
- Advise patient that drug may cause abnormal behaviors during sleep, such as driving a car, eating, having sex, or talking on the phone without any recall of the event. If family notices any such behavior or patient sees evidence of such behavior upon awakening, the prescriber should be notified.
- Caution patient about possible drowsiness during therapy and to avoid performing hazardous activities, if present.
- Urge patient to avoid alcohol consumption and opioid use because these increase drug's sedative effects, including respiratory depression which can become severe, and risk of abnormal behaviors, such as sleep driving.
- Advise patient to notify prescriber about excessive drowsiness, known or suspected pregnancy, and nausea.
- Instruct patient to inform all prescribers of triazolam use, especially when pain medication may be prescribed.

trospium chloride

Sanctura, Sanctura XR

Class and Category

Pharmacologic class: Antimuscarinic
Therapeutic class: Bladder antispasmodic
Pregnancy category: C

Indications and Dosages

➤ *To treat overactive bladder with symptoms of urge urinary incontinence, urgency, and urinary frequency*

TABLETS

Adults. 20 mg twice daily 1 hr before meals or on empty stomach.

DOSAGE ADJUSTMENT For patients with severe renal insufficiency (creatinine clearance less than 30 ml/min/1.73 m^2) and patients age 75 or over, dosage reduced to 20 mg daily at bedtime.

E.R. CAPSULES

Adults. 60 mg daily in the morning, 1 hr before a meal or on empty stomach.

Route	Onset	Peak	Duration
P.O.	Unknown	5–6 hr	Unknown

Mechanism of Action

Antagonizes the effect of acetylcholine on muscarinic receptors in the bladder. Trospium's parasympatholytic action reduces the tonus of smooth muscle in the bladder. These actions increase maximum cystometric bladder capacity and volume with the first detrusor contraction, which relieves the sensation of frequency and urgency and enhances bladder control.

Contraindications

Gastric retention, hypersensitivity to trospium or its components, uncontrolled angle-closure glaucoma, urine retention

Interactions

DRUGS

anticholinergics: Increased frequency or severity of adverse effects; possibly reduced absorption of trospium
digoxin, metformin, morphine, pancuronium, procainamide: Possibly increased plasma concentration of all these drugs as well as trospium

ACTIVITIES

alcohol use: Possibly increased drowsiness

Adverse Reactions

CNS: Confusion, delirium, dizziness, drowsiness, fatigue, fever, hallucinations, headache, insomnia, light-headedness, syncope
CV: Chest pain, **hypertensive crisis**, palpitations, tachycardia
EENT: Blurred vision; dry eyes, mouth, or throat; visual abnormalities
GI: Abdominal distention or pain, constipation, flatulence, gastritis, indigestion, vomiting
GU: Urine retention
MS: Rhabdomyolysis
SKIN: Decreased sweating, dry skin, flushing, rash, **Stevens–Johnson syndrome**
Other: Anaphylaxis, angioedema

Nursing Considerations

- Use trospium cautiously in patients with intestinal atony, myasthenia gravis, or ulcerative colitis, because drug may decrease GI motility; patients with significant bladder outflow obstruction because drug may cause urine retention; patients with hepatic impairment because drug's effects on the liver are unknown; and patients with renal impairment because drug excretion may be impaired.
- Monitor elderly patients carefully, especially those age 75 or over, for adverse reactions because elderly patients have an increased risk of trospium-induced adverse reactions.
- Monitor patient for anticholinergic central nervous system adverse effects such as confusion, dizziness, hallucinations, and somnolence. If present, notify prescriber and expect a dose reduction or drug to be discontinued.

PATIENT TEACHING

- Instruct patient to take trospium on an empty stomach or at least 1 hour before eating because food delays its absorption.
- Caution patient to avoid performing activities in a warm or hot environment because sweating may be delayed, which could cause a sudden increase in body temperature and heatstroke.

- Advise patient to avoid hazardous activities until drug's CNS effects are known.
- Inform patient that alcohol may increase the risk of drowsiness; urge patient to limit or abstain from alcoholic beverages while taking trospium.
- Emphasize importance of reporting allergic reactions, including swelling of her face, lips, throat, or tongue; stopping trospium therapy; and seeking emergency medical care immediately.
- Advise patient to notify prescriber if he develops confusion, dizziness, hallucinations, or somnolence, as dosage may have to be altered or drug discontinued.

U V W

umeclidinium

Incruse Ellipta

Class and Category

Pharmacologic class: Anticholinergic
Therapeutic class: Bronchodilator
Pregnancy category: C

Indications and Dosages

➤ *To provide long-term maintenance treatment of airflow obstruction in chronic obstructive pulmonary disease (COPD), including chronic bronchitis and/or emphysema*

ORAL INHALATION

Adults. 62.5 mcg (1 inhalation) daily.
Maximum: 62.5 mcg in a 24-hr period.

Mechanism of Action

Inhibits the muscarinic M_3 receptor in smooth muscle to cause bronchodilation.

Contraindications

Hypersensitivity to umeclidinium or its components, severe hypersensitivity to milk proteins

Interactions

DRUGS

anticholinergics: Possibly additive effects

Adverse Reactions

CNS: Depression, dizziness, headache, vertigo
CV: Atrial fibrillation, idioventricular rhythm, supraventricular extrasystole, tachycardia
EENT: Blurred vision, eye pain, nasopharyngitis, pharyngitis, rhinitis, worsening of narrow-angle glaucoma
GI: Abdominal pain (upper), diarrhea, dyspepsia, nausea
GU: Dysuria, urinary retention, UTI, worsening of urinary retention
MS: Arthralgia; back, extremity, or neck pain; myalgia
RESP: Cough, **paradoxical bronchospasm**, respiratory tract infection
SKIN: Pruritus, rash, urticaria
Other: Anaphylaxis, angioedema

Nursing Considerations

- Know that umeclidinium should not be initiated in patients who are experiencing a rapidly deteriorating or potentially life-threatening episode of COPD.
- Do not administer umeclidinium for relief of acute symptoms. Drug is not a rescue inhaler. Instead, acute symptoms should be treated with an inhaled, short-acting $beta_2$-agonist, as ordered.
- Monitor patient for hypersensitivity reactions such as anaphylaxis, pruritus, rash, swelling in any area of the body, or urticaria. Expect drug to be discontinued if present. Be prepared to treat according to protocol standards. Know that patients with a severe milk protein allergy should not receive umeclidinium therapy because after inhaling other powder products containing lactose, some patients with a severe milk protein allergy have developed serious hypersensitivity reactions.
- Use with caution in patients with narrow-angle glaucoma or urinary retention because these conditions may worsen with umeclidinium therapy.

WARNING Monitor patient's respiratory status for paradoxical bronchospasm. Because of its life-threatening nature, notify prescriber immediately, withhold umeclidinium, and prepare to treat patient with an inhaled, short-acting bronchodilator, as ordered. If bronchospasm develops during umeclidinium therapy, expect drug to be permanently discontinued.

PATIENT TEACHING

- Tell patient to take umeclidinium at about the same time every day and not to use more than once in a 24-hour period.
- Remind patient that umeclidinium cannot be used to relieve acute symptoms of COPD. Instead, tell patient to treat acute symptoms with a prescribed inhaled, short-acting $beta_2$ agonist such as albuterol, as prescribed.
- Teach patient how to use the inhaler.
- Urge patient to notify prescriber if her symptoms worsen, if umeclidinium becomes less effective, or if she needs more inhalations of her prescribed short-acting $beta_2$-agonist than usual. This may

indicate that patient's condition is worsening.
- Inform patient that drug may cause paradoxical bronchospasms. If present, tell patient to discontinue drug and notify prescriber.
- Tell patient to notify prescriber immediately if she develops blurred vision; colored images in association with red eyes; eye discomfort, pain, or visual halos.
- Advise patient to notify prescriber immediately if she develops any difficulty passing urine or painful urination, especially if she has a bladder-neck obstruction or if, in a male patient, prostatic hyperplasia is present.
- Instruct patient not to stop taking umeclidinium without prescriber knowledge, because symptoms may recur.

ursodiol
(ursodeoxycholic acid)

Actigall, Urso Forte, URSO 250, Ursofalk (CAN)

Class and Category
Pharmacologic class: Bile acid
Therapeutic class: Bile salt replenisher, cholelitholytic
Pregnancy category: B

Indications and Dosages
➤ *To prevent gallstone formation in obese patients during rapid weight loss*

CAPSULES (ACTIGALL, URSO FORTE)

Adults and adolescents. 300 mg twice daily.

➤ *To dissolve gallstones*

CAPSULES (ACTIGALL, URSO FORTE)

Adults and adolescents. 8 to 10 mg/kg daily in divided doses twice daily or three times a day.

➤ *To treat primary biliary cirrhosis*

TABLETS (URSO 250)

Adults. 13 to 15 mg/kg daily in two to four divided doses.

Mechanism of Action
Suppresses biliary secretion, hepatic synthesis, and intestinal reabsorption of cholesterol. Prolonged use promotes dissolution of gallstones.

Contraindications
Acute cholangitis; gallstone complications (such as biliary GI fistula; biliary obstruction; calcified, radiopaque, or radiotranslucent bile-pigment gallstones; cholecystitis; pancreatitis); hypersensitivity to ursodiol, other bile acids, or their components

Interactions
DRUGS

aluminum-containing antacids, cholestyramine, colestipol: Decreased absorption and therapeutic effects of ursodiol
clofibrate, estrogens, neomycin, oral contraceptives, progestins: Interference with ursodiol's therapeutic effects; increased risk of gallstone formation

FOODS

any foods: Increased dissolution of drug

Adverse Reactions
CNS: Anxiety, asthenia, depression, dizziness, fatigue, fever, headache, malaise, sleep disturbance
CV: Chest pain, hypertension, peripheral edema
ENDO: Hyperglycemia
EENT: Laryngeal edema, metallic taste, rhinitis, stomatitis
GI: Abdominal discomfort or pain, cholecystitis, constipation, diarrhea, elevated liver enzymes, esophagitis, flatulence, indigestion, jaundice, nausea, peptic ulcer, vomiting
GU: Elevated creatinine level
HEME: Leukopenia, thrombocytopenia
MS: Arthralgia, back pain, myalgia
RESP: Cough
SKIN: Alopecia, diaphoresis, dry skin, pruritus, rash, urticaria
Other: Angioedema

Nursing Considerations
- Administer ursodiol with food to increase drug dissolution.
- Give aluminum-containing antacids, cholestyramine, and colestipol at least 1 hour before or 4 hours after ursodiol because they may decrease drug's effects.
- Monitor patient's liver enzymes every month for 3 months after ursodiol therapy

is begun and then every 6 months thereafter, as ordered. If elevation occurs, notify prescriber as drug may have to be discontinued.

- Expect drug to be discontinued if gallstones haven't partially dissolved after 12 months of therapy.
- If patient inadvertently takes too much ursodiol, diarrhea will most likely result and may warrant systemic treatment.

PATIENT TEACHING

- Tell patient to take ursodiol with meals.
- Urge patient to take aluminum-containing antacids at least 1 hour before or 4 hours after ursodiol to support absorption.
- Urge patient to notify prescriber immediately if evidence of acute cholecystitis develops, such as acute right-upper-quadrant abdominal pain.
- Inform patient that he may need to take ursodiol for a prolonged period before gallstones dissolve.
- Advise diabetic patient to monitor blood glucose levels during therapy because ursodiol may alter blood glucose control.

ustekinumab

Stelara

Class and Category

Pharmacologic class: Monoclonal antibody
Therapeutic class: Immunomodulator
Pregnancy category: B

Indications and Dosages

➤ *To treat moderate to severe plaque psoriasis in patients who are candidates for phototherapy or systemic therapy*

SUBCUTANEOUS INJECTION

Adults and children ages 12 to 18 weighing more than 100 kg (220 lb). *Initial:* 90 mg followed by 90 mg 4 wk later and then 90 mg every 12 wk.
Adults weighing 100 kg (220 lb) or less. *Initial:* 45 mg followed by 45 mg 4 wk later and then 45 mg every 12 wk.
Children ages 12 to 18 weighing 60 kg (132 lb) to 100 kg (220 lb). *Initial:* 45 mg, followed by 45 mg 4 wk later, and then 45 mg every 12 wk.
Children ages 12 to 18 weighing less than 60 kg (132 lb). 0.75 mg/kg, followed by 0.75 mg/kg 4 wk later and then 0.75 mg/kg every 12 wk.

➤ *To treat active psoriatic arthritis as monotherapy or in combination with methotrexate.*

SUBCUTANEOUS INJECTION

Adults. *Initial:* 45 mg, followed by 45 mg 4 wk later, and then 45 mg every 12 wk.
DOSAGE ADJUSTMENT For patients who weigh more than 100 kg (220 lb) and also have coexistent moderate to severe plaque psoriasis in addition to psoriatic arthritis, initial dosage increased to 90 mg followed by 90 mg 4 wk later, and then 90 mg every 12 wk.

➤ *To treat moderate to severe active Crohn's disease in patients who have either failed or were intolerant of treatment with corticosteroids or immunomodulators but never failed treatment with a tumor necrosis factor (TNF) blocker or failed or were intolerant of treatment with one or more TNF blockers*

I.V. INFUSION

Adults who weigh more than 85 kg (187 lb). *Initial:* 520 mg as a single infusion infused over at least 60 min.
Adults who weigh more than 55 kg (121 lb) but less than 86 kg (189 lb). *Initial:* 390 mg as a single infusion infused over at least 60 min.
Adults who weigh 55 kg (121 lb) or less. *Initial:* 260 mg as a single infusion infused over at least 60 min.

SUBCUTANEOUS INJECTION

Adults. *Maintenance:* 90 mg 8 wk after initial intravenous dose, then every 8 wk thereafter.

Route	Onset	Peak	Duration
SubQ	Unknown	7–13.5 days	Unknown
I.V.	Unknown	Unknown	Unknown

Mechanism of Action

Binds to p40 protein subunit used by interleukin (IL)-12 and IL-23 cytokines. These specific cytokines are involved in inflammatory and immune responses, such as natural killer cell activation and $CD4^+$ T-cell differentiation and activation.

By disrupting signaling mediated by IL-12 and IL-23, signs and symptoms caused by inflammatory and immune responses are diminished or relieved.

Contraindications

Hypersensitivity to ustekinumab or its components

Interactions

DRUGS

cytochrome P-450 substrates such as cyclosporine, theophylline, warfarin: Possibly altered effects or blood levels of these drugs when ustekinumab is started or stopped
live-virus vaccines: Increased risk of adverse vaccine effects

Adverse Reactions

CNS: Depression, dizziness, fatigue, headache, **reversible posterior leukoencephalopathy syndrome**
ENDO: Nasopharyngitis, pharyngolaryngeal pain
GI: Diarrhea, diverticulitis, gastroenteritis
GU: UTI
MS: Back pain, myalgia, osteomyelitis
RESP: Pneumonia, upper respiratory tract infection
SKIN: Cellulitis, erythrodermic psoriasis, pruritus, pustular psoriasis, rash, urticaria
Other: Anaphylaxis, **angioedema**, anti-ustekinumab antibodies, injection-site reactions (bruising, erythema, hemorrhage, induration, irritation, pain, pruritus, swelling), **malignancies (breast, colorectal, head and neck, kidney, melanoma and nonmelanoma disorders of skin, prostate, or thyroid)**, serious infection, including bacterial, fungal, and viral infections and reactivation of latent infections

Nursing Considerations

- Make sure patient has a tuberculin skin test before therapy starts. If skin test is positive, treatment of latent tuberculosis should start before ustekinumab therapy starts. Also expect antituberculosis therapy to start if patient has a history of latent or active tuberculosis but adequate therapy can't be confirmed or if patient has a negative test for latent tuberculosis but has risk factors for tuberculosis.
- Make sure patient is current with all immunizations before starting ustekinumab therapy because patient shouldn't receive live vaccines during treatment. BCG vaccines shouldn't be given for 1 year before or after ustekinumab therapy.
- Use caution when administering ustekinumab to a patient undergoing allergen immunotherapy because drug may decrease the protective effect of allergen immunotherapy which in turn may increase the risk of an allergic reaction to a dose of allergen immunotherapy.
- Use ustekinumab cautiously in patients with recurrent infection or increased risk of infection and in patients who live in regions where histoplasmosis and tuberculosis are endemic.

WARNING Know that if patient has evidence of an active infection when drug is prescribed, therapy shouldn't start until infection has been treated. Monitor all patients for infection during therapy, especially those receiving immunosuppressants. Be on the alert for cough, dyspnea, and interstitial infiltrates following one to three doses that may suggest pneumonia has developed. If a serious infection, an opportunistic infection, or sepsis develops, expect prescriber to stop ustekinumab and start appropriate antimicrobial therapy.

- Be aware that patients with a history of cancer or who have genetic deficiencies in IL-12 or IL-23 should be thoroughly evaluated before ustekinumab therapy starts because various cancers have occurred in patients being treated with ustekinumab. Monitor patients throughout therapy for persistent, severe, or unusual signs and symptoms.
- Give ustekinumab subcutaneously by using a 27G, half-inch needle into gluteal region, thighs, upper arms, or any quadrant of abdomen. Rotate sites, and avoid areas that are bruised, erythematous, indurated, or tender.
- Note that needle cover on prefilled syringe used for subcutaneous injections contains a latex derivative and shouldn't be handled by persons with a latex allergy.
- Prepare intravenous infusion by first determining the number of ustekinumab

vials needed based on patient's weight (each 26-ml vial contains 130 mg of ustekinumab). Withdraw, and then discard a volume of the 0.9% sodium chloride injection, USP, from the 250-ml infusion bag equal to the volume of drug to be added. Withdraw the dose from each vial needed and add it to the 250-ml infusion bag. The final volume in the infusion bag should be 250 ml. Gently mix. Diluted solution may be stored for up to 4 hours prior to infusion.

- Use only an infusion set for intravenous administration that has an in-line, sterile, nonpyrogenic, low protein-binding filter (pore size 0.2 micrometer). Do not infuse ustekinumab concomitantly in the same intravenous line with other agents. Infuse diluted solution to be given intravenously over at least 1 hour.
- Know that comparison of the incidence of antibodies to ustekinumab with the incidence of antibodies to other products may be misleading.
- Monitor patient for hypersensitivity reactions that could become life threatening. At first sign of hypersensitivity, notify prescriber, expect drug to be discontinued, and provide supportive care.
- Monitor patient for confusion, headache, seizures, and vision disturbances, which may signal reversible posterior leukoencephalopathy syndrome, a rare neurologic disorder that may occur with ustekinumab therapy. If present, notify prescriber, discontinue ustekinumab therapy, and provide appropriate treatment, as ordered.
- Inspect patient's skin regularly for evidence of abnormalities because rapid appearance of multiple cutaneous squamous cell carcinoma has occurred in patients who had preexisting risk factors for nonmelanoma skin cancer. Patients who are over 60 years of age, have a medical history of prolonged immunosuppressant therapy, and those with a history of psoralen plus ultraviolet radiation using UVA bands (PUVA) treatment should be closely monitored.

PATIENT TEACHING

- Inform patient that treatment must be supervised by a healthcare professional.
- Teach patient how to administer the drug subcutaneously, if self-administration is ordered by prescriber.
- Inform patient that tuberculosis may occur during ustekinumab therapy. Instruct him to report low-grade fever, persistent cough, or wasting or weight loss to prescriber.
- Teach patient to recognize and report evidence of infection; drug may need to be stopped. Advise patient to avoid people with infections and to have all prescribed laboratory tests performed.
- Inform patient that the risk of developing certain kinds of cancer is higher in patients taking ustekinumab. Emphasize importance of follow-up visits and reporting any persistent, sudden-onset, or unusual signs or symptoms.
- Caution against receiving live-virus vaccines while taking ustekinumab; doing so may adversely affect the immune system.
- Urge patient to inform all healthcare providers about ustekinumab use and to inform prescriber about all OTC medications being taken, including herbal remedies and mineral and vitamin supplements.
- Encourage any woman who becomes pregnant while receiving ustekinumab to enroll in the pregnancy registry.

valacyclovir hydrochloride

Valtrex

Class and Category

Pharmacologic class: Nucleoside nucleotide
Therapeutic class: Antiviral
Pregnancy category: B

Indications and Dosages

➤ *To treat herpes labialis*

CAPLETS, ORAL SUSPENSION

Adults and children age 12 and over. 2 g twice daily for 1 day given 12 hr apart with therapy begun at the earliest symptom (burning, itching, tingling).

➤ *To treat initial episode of genital herpes in immunocompetent patients*

CAPLETS, ORAL SUSPENSION

Adults. 1 g twice daily for 10 days.

➤ *To treat recurrent episodes of genital herpes in immunocompetent patients*

CAPLETS, ORAL SUSPENSION

Adults. 500 mg twice daily for 3 days, with therapy begun at the first sign of recurrence.

➤ *To suppress chronic recurrent episodes of genital herpes in immunocompetent patients*

CAPLETS, ORAL SUSPENSION

Adults. 1 g once daily. Alternatively, for patient with history of 9 or fewer episodes per year, 500 mg once daily.

➤ *To suppress chronic recurrent episodes of genital herpes in patients with HIV-1 viral infection who have a CD4+ cell count equal to or greater than 100 cells/mm^3*

CAPLETS, ORAL SUSPENSION

Adults. 500 mg twice daily.

➤ *To reduce transmission of genital herpes for immunocompetent source partner in patient with history of 9 or fewer episodes per year*

CAPLETS, ORAL SUSPENSION

Adults. 500 mg once daily.

➤ *To treat herpes zoster*

CAPLETS, ORAL SUSPENSION

Adults. 1 g three times daily for 7 days begun at the earliest sign or symptom of herpes zoster.

Children ages 2 to 18. 20 mg/kg three times daily for 5 days. *Maximum:* 1 g three times daily.

DOSAGE ADJUSTMENT For adult patients with renal impairment being treated for herpes labialis, dosage reduced to 1 g twice daily for 1 day if creatinine clearance is between 30 and 49 ml/min; dosage reduced to 500 mg twice daily for 1 day if creatinine clearance is between 10 and 29 ml/min; and dosage reduced to a 500-mg single dose if creatinine clearance is less than 10 ml/min. For patients with renal impairment being treated for initial episode of genital herpes, dosage reduced to 1 g every 24 hr if creatinine clearance is between 10 and 29 ml/min, and dosage reduced to 500 mg every 24 hr if creatinine clearance is less than 10 ml/min. For immunocompetent patients with renal impairment being treated for recurrent episode of genital herpes, or for suppressive therapy, dosage reduced to 500 mg every 24 hr if creatinine clearance is 29 ml/min or less, and for alternate therapy if renal-impaired patient has had 9 or fewer recurrences per year, dosage reduced to 500 mg every 48 hr. For HIV-1 infected patients with renal impairment using drug to suppress chronic recurrent episodes of genital herpes, dosage reduced to 500 mg every 24 hr if creatinine clearance is 29 ml/min or less. For adult patients with renal impairment being treated for herpes zoster, dosage reduced to 1 g every 12 hr if creatinine clearance is between 30 and 49 ml/min; dosage reduced to 1 g every 24 hr if creatinine clearance is between 10 and 29 ml/min, and reduced to 500 mg every 24 hr if creatinine clearance is less than 10 ml/min.

Mechanism of Action

After conversion to acyclovir, several actions (inhibition of DNA polymerase, premature termination of DNA synthesis, and the thymidine kinase specificity) combine to inhibit herpes virus replication

Contraindications

Hypersensitivity to valacyclovir or its hydrochloride salt, acyclovir, or their components

Interactions

DRUGS

cimetidine, probenecid: Possibly increased valacyclovir plasma concentrations
other nephrotoxic drugs: Increased risk of renal impairment

Adverse Reactions

CNS: Aggressive behavior, agitation, ataxia, auditory and visual hallucinations, **coma**, confusion, depression, dizziness, **encephalopathy**, fatigue, fever, headache, mania, psychosis, **seizures**, tremors
CV: Hypertension, tachycardia
EENT: Nasopharyngitis, rhinorrhea, visual abnormalities
GI: Abdominal pain, diarrhea, elevated liver enzymes, **hepatitis**, nausea, vomiting
GU: Anuria, dysmenorrhea, **hemolytic-uremic syndrome**, **renal failure**, renal pain

HEME: Anemia, **aplastic anemia**, leukocytoclastic vasculitis, **leukopenia**, **neutropenia**, **thrombocytopenia**, **thrombotic thrombocytopenic purpura**
MS: Arthralgia, dysarthria
RESP: Dyspnea, upper respiratory infection
SKIN: Alopecia, **erythema multiforme**, photosensitivity, pruritus, rash, urticaria
Other: Anaphylaxis, **angioedema**, dehydration, elevated alkaline phosphatase, herpes simplex

Nursing Considerations

- Use valacyclovir cautiously in patients who are elderly and those with impaired renal function. Also use caution when patients are receiving other nephrotoxic drugs or have inadequate hydration. Expect dosage to be decreased when renal dysfunction is present.

WARNING Know that thrombotic thrombocytopenic purpura/hemolytic uremic syndrome has occurred in patients with advanced HIV-1 infection, or who have received an allogeneic bone marrow transplant or renal transplant while taking valacyclovir. Notify prescriber immediately if signs and symptoms of this disorder occur. Expect laboratory tests to be done to confirm diagnosis and, if confirmed, know that valacyclovir therapy should be stopped immediately.

- Maintain adequate hydration for patient throughout valacyclovir therapy because precipitation of the prodrug, acyclovir, may occur in the renal tubules, causing renal impairment. Know that the patient may need hemodialysis in the event anuria and acute renal failure occur.
- Monitor patients closely throughout valacyclovir therapy for central nervous system adverse reactions, especially elderly patients.

PATIENT TEACHING

- Instruct patient to begin therapy at the earliest symptom of a cold sore or recurrent genital herpes, such as burning, itching, or tingling in the area.
- Stress importance of maintaining adequate hydration throughout valacyclovir therapy.
- Remind patient being treated for a cold sore that only two doses of valacyclovir are needed and the two doses should be taken 12 hours apart.
- Instruct patient with genital herpes to avoid contact with lesions or intercourse when lesions and/or symptoms are present, to avoid infecting partners. However, remind patient to use safer sex practices in combination with suppressive therapy, because genital herpes is frequently transmitted in the absence of symptoms. Instruct male patient or partner to use a latex or polyurethane condom whenever sexual contact occurs.
- Inform patient that valacyclovir is not a cure for herpes.
- Tell mothers not to breastfeed during valacyclovir therapy.

WARNING Warn patient to get emergency help immediately if an allergic reaction occurs, such as difficulty breathing, hives, or swelling of face, lips, tongue, or throat.

- Tell patient to stop taking valacyclovir and seek immediate medical attention if the following signs and symptoms appear: bleeding easily, bloody diarrhea, easy bruising, fainting, fever, pale or yellowed skin, red spots on the skin (not related to chickenpox or herpes), urinating less than usual or not at all, or weakness.

valbenazine

Ingrezza

Class and Category

Pharmacologic class: Vesicular monoamine transporter 2 (VMAT2) inhibitor
Therapeutic class: Antidyskinesic
Pregnancy category: Not classified

Indications and Dosages

➤ To treat tardive dyskinesia

CAPSULES

Adults. *Initial:* 40 mg once daily, increased after 1 wk to 80 mg once daily.

DOSAGE ADJUSTMENT For patients with moderate or severe hepatic impairment or for patients taking a strong CYP3A4 inhibitor concomitantly, dosage kept at 40 mg once daily. For patients who are known CYP2D6 poor metabolizers or who are taking strong CYP2D6 inhibitors concomitantly, dosage reduction maybe considered.

Route	Onset	Peak	Duration
P.O.	Unknown	0.51 hr	Unknown

Mechanism of Action
Unknown, but thought to regulate monoamine uptake from the cytoplasm to the synaptic vesicle for storage and release. This action may relieve symptoms of tardive dyskinesia.

Contraindications
Hypersensitivity to valbenazine or its components

Interactions
DRUGS
CYP2D6 strong inhibitors such as fluoxetine, paroxetine, quinidine; CYP3A4 strong inhibitors such as clarithromycin, itraconazole, ketoconazole: Increased exposure of valbenazine with possible increase in adverse reactions
CYP3A4 strong inducers such as carbamazepine, phenytoin, St. John's wort: Decreased exposure of valbenazine with possible reduced effectiveness
digoxin: Increased digoxin levels with potential for digitalis toxicity
MAO inhibitors: Possibly increased concentration of monoamine neurotransmitters in synapses, possibly leading to increased risk of adverse reactions such as serotonin syndrome or increased effect of valbenazine

Adverse Reactions
CNS: Akathisia, anxiety, attention and gait disturbances, balance disorder, dizziness, dyskinesia, extrapyramidal symptoms (nonakathisic), fatigue, headache, insomnia, restlessness, sedation, somnolence
CV: QT-interval prolongation
EENT: Blurred vision, drooling, dry mouth
ENDO: Elevated prolactin levels, hyperglycemia
GI: Constipation, elevated bilirubin levels, nausea, vomiting
GU: Urinary retention
MS: Arthralgia
RESP: Respiratory infections
SKIN: Allergic dermatitis, pruritus, rash, urticaria
Other: Angioedema, elevated alkaline phosphatase levels, weight gain

Nursing Considerations
- Know that valbenazine should not be given to patients with arrhythmias associated with a prolonged QT interval or who have congenital long QT syndrome, because drug may increase the QT interval.
- Be aware that patients who are taking a strong CYP2D6 or CYP3A4 inhibitors or who are CYP2D6 poor metabolizers are at risk for prolonged QT interval as a result of valbenazine therapy. Expect to assess the QT interval in these patients before the dosage is increased.
- Institute fall precautions, because valbenazine can cause somnolence.

PATIENT TEACHING
- Caution patient not to perform activities requiring mental alertness, such as driving, if somnolence or other adverse central nervous system effects are present.
- Review fall precautions with patient.
- Instruct patient to tell all prescribers about valbenazine therapy and not to take any over-the-counter medications, including herbal products, without prescriber consent.
- Advise mothers not to breastfeed during valbenazine therapy and for 5 days after drug is discontinued.
- Tell women of childbearing age to alert prescriber if pregnancy is suspected or known, because risk to fetus is unknown with exposure to valbenazine.

valganciclovir hydrochloride

Valcyte

Class and Category
Pharmacologic class: Nucleoside nucleotide
Therapeutic class: Antiviral
Pregnancy category: Not classified

Indications and Dosages
➤ *To treat cytomegalovirus (CMV) retinitis*
TABLETS
Adults. *Induction:* 900 mg twice daily for 21 days with food. *Maintenance:* 900 mg once daily.
➤ *To prevent CMA disease in heart, kidney, and kidney-pancreas transplant adults at high risk*
TABLETS
Adults who have received a heart or kidney-pancreas transplant. 900 mg once daily with food starting within 10 days of transplantation until 100 days post-transplantation.

Adults who have received a kidney transplant. 900 mg once daily with food starting within 10 days of transplantation until 200 days post-transplantation.

➤ *To prevent CMA disease in children with a heart or kidney transplant*

ORAL SOLUTION, TABLETS

Infants 1 month of age and over, children up to 16 years who have received a heart transplant. Dosage calculated individually (7 × body surface area (BSA) × creatinine clearance (CrCl)) given once daily with food and started within 10 days of transplantation until 100 days post-transplantation. *Maximum:* 900 mg daily.

Infants 4 months of age and over, children up to 16 years who have received a kidney transplant. Dosage calculated individually (7 × BSA × CrCl) given once daily with food and started within 10 days of transplantation until 200 days post-transplantation. *Maximum:* 900 mg daily.

DOSAGE ADJUSTMENT For pediatric patients, the maximum calculated creatinine clearance to be used in the formula is 150 mg/min. For adult patients with a creatinine clearance between 40 and 59 ml/min, induction dosage reduced to 450 mg twice daily and maintenance dosage reduced to 450 mg once daily. For adult patients with a creatinine clearance between 25 and 39 ml/min, induction dosage reduced to 450 mg once daily and maintenance dosage reduced to 450 mg every 2 days. For adult patients with a creatinine clearance between 10 and 24 ml/min, induction dosage reduced to 450 mg every 2 days and maintenance dosage reduced to 450 mg twice weekly.

Mechanism of Action

After being rapidly converted to ganciclovir, drug is phosphorylated to ganciclovir monophosphate primarily in virus-infected cells to inhibit viral DNA polymerase, which in turn inhibits replication of CMV.

Contraindications

Hypersensitivity to valganciclovir, ganciclovir, or any of their components

Interactions

DRUGS

amphotericin B, cyclosporine: Possibly increased serum creatinine level
didanosine: Increased risk of didanosine toxicity such as pancreatitis
imipenem-cilastatin: Possibly increased risk of generalized seizures
mycophenolate mofetil: Increased risk for hematological and renal toxicities
other myelosuppression or nephrotoxic drugs such as adriamycin, dapsone, doxorubicin, flucytosine, hydroxyurea, pentamidine, tacrolimus, trimethoprim/sulfamethoxazole, vinblastine, vincristine, zidovudine: Increased risk of higher toxicity
probenecid: Increased risk of toxicity

Adverse Reactions

CNS: Agitation, asthenia, chills, confusion, dizziness, fatigue, fever, hallucinations, headache, insomnia, malaise, paresthesia, peripheral neuropathy, psychotic disorder, **seizures**, tremor
CV: Arrhythmias, **hypotension**, peripheral edema
EENT: Deafness, eye pain, macular edema, mouth ulceration, nasopharyngitis, oral candidiasis, pharyngitis, retinal detachment, taste disturbance
GI: Abdominal distention or pain, anorexia, constipation, diarrhea, dyspepsia, elevated liver enzymes, hepatic dysfunction, nausea, **pancreatitis**, vomiting
GU: Acute renal failure, decreased creatinine clearance, elevated serum creatinine levels, hematuria, impaired fertility, UTI
HEME: Agranulocytosis, anemia, **aplastic anemia**, **bone marrow failure**, **granulocytopenia**, **leukopenia**, **life-threatening bleeding**, **neutropenia**, **pancytopenia**, **thrombocytopenia**
MS: Arthralgia, back or extremity pain, muscle spasms, myalgia
RESP: Cough, dyspnea, upper respiratory infection
SKIN: Cellulitis, dermatitis, night sweats, pruritus
Other: Anaphylaxis, **fetal toxicity**, flu-like symptoms, generalized pain, **hyperkalemia**, **hypersensitivity reactions**, **hypophosphatemia**, **increased risk of developing cancer**, postoperative wound infections, **sepsis**, weight loss

Nursing Considerations

- Use valganciclovir cautiously in patients with preexisting cytopenias and in patients receiving irradiation or myelosuppressive drugs, because of the potential for severe hematological toxicity to develop with valganciclovir use.
- Use caution in handling tablets and oral solution, because valganciclovir is considered a potential carcinogen and teratogen in humans. Tablets should not be broken or crushed. If contact occurs, wash area thoroughly with soap and water and rinse eyes thoroughly with plain water. Dispose of valganciclovir using the guidelines for antineoplastic drugs.
- Know that all calculated doses should be rounded to the nearest 10-mg increment. If calculated dosage exceeds 900 mg, expect to administer only 900 mg as the maximum dose.
- Be aware that adults should use the tablet form of valganciclovir and not the oral solution.
- Administer valganciclovir with food to enhance its absorption.

WARNING Monitor patient's hematologic status, especially patients with renal impairment and patients in whom ganciclovir or other nucleoside analogues have previously resulted in leukopenia, or in whom neutrophil counts are less than 1000 cells/μL at the beginning of treatment. Expect to monitor complete blood counts with differential and platelet counts frequently, as ordered, because valganciclovir may cause severe hematologic toxicity, such as severe anemia including aplastic anemia, bone marrow failure, leukopenia, neutropenia, and pancytopenia. Expect valganciclovir therapy to be stopped if patient's absolute neutrophil count drops below 500 cells/μL, hemoglobin is less than 8 g/dl, or platelet count becomes less than 25,000/μL. Be prepared to provide supportive care including administering hematopoietic growth factors, as ordered. Expect to see cell counts begin to recover within 3 to 7 days after valganciclovir has been discontinued.

- Monitor patient's serum creatinine levels regularly, as ordered, because drug may cause renal dysfunction. Be aware that acute renal failure may occur in elderly patients with or without reduced renal function. Use caution when using valganciclovir in these patients or in patients receiving potential nephrotoxic drugs. Ensure that patient is adequately hydrated at all times.

PATIENT TEACHING

- Inform patient being treated for CMV retinitis that valganciclovir is not a cure for CMV retinitis and that patient will continue to need ophthalmologic follow-up examinations at a minimum of every 4 to 6 weeks while being treated.
- Instruct patient to take valganciclovir with food.
- Tell patient that adequate hydration must be maintained throughout drug therapy, to help prevent kidney dysfunction.
- Inform patient that frequent laboratory tests will be needed throughout valganciclovir therapy, for early detection of adverse reactions. Compliance with these appointments is very important.
- Inform patient that valganciclovir is considered a carcinogenic drug and to report any persistent, severe, or unusual signs and symptoms to prescriber.

WARNING Stress importance of using appropriate and effective birth control measures throughout valganciclovir therapy, because valganciclovir may be toxic to the fetus and has the potential to cause birth defects. Tell female patients to use effective contraception during and for at least 30 days following treatment and for males to use condoms during and for at least 90 days following treatment. Notify prescriber immediately if pregnancy is known or suspected in patient or partner.

- Alert patient regarding valganciclovir's possible effects on fertility, such as temporary or permanent inhibition of spermatogenesis in males and suppression of fertility in females.
- Caution mothers not to breastfeed while taking valganciclovir.
- Tell patient to avoid performing tasks that require alertness, such as driving or operating machinery, as confusion, dizziness, sedation, or seizures can occur with drug use.

valproic acid

Alti-Valproic (CAN), Depakene, Stavzor

valproate sodium

Depacon

divalproex sodium

Depakote, Depakote ER, Depakote Sprinkle, Epival (CAN)

Class and Category

Pharmacologic class: Carboxylic acid derivative
Therapeutic class: Anticonvulsant
Pregnancy category: D (epilepsy, manic episodes associated with bipolar disorder), X (prevention of migraine headaches)

Indications and Dosages

➤ *To treat as monotherapy or as adjunct complex partial seizures that occur in isolation or associated with other types of seizures*

CAPSULES, DELAYED-RELEASE SPRINKLE CAPSULES, DELAYED-RELEASE TABLETS, SYRUP, I.V. INFUSION (VALPROIC ACID, VALPROATE SODIUM, DIVALPROEX SODIUM)

Adults and children age 10 and over. *Initial:* 10 to 15 mg/kg/day, increased by 5 to 10 mg/kg daily every wk, as needed. *Maximum:* 60 mg/kg daily.

➤ *To treat as monotherapy or as adjunct simple and complex absence seizures*

CAPSULES, DELAYED-RELEASE SPRINKLE CAPSULES, DELAYED-RELEASE TABLETS, SYRUP, I.V. INFUSION (VALPROIC ACID, VALPROATE SODIUM, DIVALPROEX SODIUM)

Adults. *Initial:* 15 mg/kg/day, increased by 5 to 10 mg/kg daily every wk, as needed. *Maximum*: 60 mg/kg/day.

DOSAGE ADJUSTMENT For adults being converted from immediate-release divalproex tablets to delayed-release tablets, dosage increased by 8% to 20% more than total daily dose of immediate-release tablets and given once daily.

➤ *To treat acute manic phase of bipolar disorder*

DELAYED-RELEASE TABLETS (DIVALPROEX SODIUM), DELAYED-RELEASE CAPSULES (STAVZOR)

Adults. *Initial:* 750 mg daily in divided doses. *Maximum:* 60 mg/kg daily.

EXTENDED-RELEASE TABLETS (DIVALPROEX SODIUM)

Adults. *Initial:* 25 mg/kg/day once daily, increased as rapidly as possible to achieve therapeutic dose. *Maximum*: 60 mg/kg/day.

➤ *To prevent migraine headache*

DELAYED-RELEASE TABLETS (DIVALPROEX SODIUM), DELAYED-RELEASE CAPSULES (STAVZOR)

Adults. *Initial:* 250 mg every 12 hr, increased as needed. *Maximum:* 1 g daily.

EXTENDED-RELEASE TABLETS (DIVALPROEX SODIUM)

Adults. *Initial:* 500 mg daily for 1 wk, increased, as needed, up to 1 g daily. *Maximum:* 1 g daily.

Mechanism of Action

May decrease seizure activity by blocking reuptake of gamma-aminobutyric acid (GABA), the most common inhibitory neurotransmitter in the brain. GABA suppresses the rapid firing of neurons by inhibiting voltage-sensitive sodium channels.

Contraindications

Hepatic impairment; hypersensitivity to valproic acid, valproate sodium, divalproex sodium, or their components; mitochondrial disease caused by POLG mutations; pregnancy or women of childbearing age who are not using effective contraception (for prevention of migraine headaches); urea cycle disorders

Interactions

DRUGS

aspirin: Increased valproic acid level with possible increased risk of adverse reactions
aspirin, heparin, NSAIDs, oral anticoagulants, thrombolytics: Increased inhibition of platelet aggregation and risk of bleeding
barbiturates, primidone: Increased blood levels of both drugs, additive CNS effects
carbamazepine, phenobarbital, phenytoin, primidone, rifampin, ritonavir: Possibly decreased valproic acid effectiveness
carbapenem antibiotics (ertapenem, imipenem, meropenem): Reduced serum valproic acid level, causing loss of seizure control
chlorpromazine: Increased trough plasma levels of valproate
cholestyramine: Decreased bioavailability of valproic acid
clonazepam: Increased risk of absence seizures
CNS depressants: Increased CNS depression
diazepam: Inhibited diazepam metabolism
estrogen-containing hormonal contraceptives: Possibly increased clearance of valproate,

which may decrease effectiveness and increase risk of seizures
ethosuximide: Unpredictable blood ethosuximide level
felbamate: Impaired valproic acid metabolism and increased valproate level
haloperidol, loxapine, MAO inhibitors, maprotiline, phenothiazines, thioxanthenes, tricyclic antidepressants: Increased CNS depression, lowered seizure threshold
lamotrigine: Decreased lamotrigine clearance
mefloquine: Decreased blood levels of divalproex, valproate sodium, and valproic acid; increased risk of seizures
phenytoin: Increased risk of phenytoin toxicity, loss of seizure control
propofol: Possibly increased blood levels of propofol
rufinamide: Increased rufinamide concentrations
topiramate: Increased risk of hyper-ammonemia with or without encephalopathy

ACTIVITIES

alcohol use: Additive CNS depression

Adverse Reactions

CNS: Abnormal dreams or thinking, aggression, agitation, amnesia, apathy, asthenia, ataxia, attention disturbance, behavioral deterioration, catatonic reaction, cerebral pseudoatrophy, chills, cognitive decline, confusion, depression, dizziness, drowsiness, emotional upset, **encephalopathy**, euphoria, fever, gait abnormality, hallucinations, headache, hostility, hyperactivity, hyperesthesia, hypertonia, hypokinesia, **hypothermia**, increased reflexes, insomnia, irritability, lack of coordination, learning disorder, lethargy, **loss of seizure control**, malaise, nervousness, **paradoxical seizures**, paresthesia, parkinsonism, psychomotor hyperactivity, psychosis, sedation, speech disorder, somnolence, **suicidal ideation**, tardive dyskinesia, tremor, twitching, vertigo, weakness
CV: Bradycardia, chest pain, edema, hypertension, **hypotension**, orthostatic hypotension, palpitations, peripheral edema, tachycardia, vasodilation
EENT: Amblyopia, conjunctivitis, diplopia, dry eyes, ear or eye pain, glossitis, hearing loss, nystagmus, parotid gland swelling, pharyngitis, rhinitis, sinusitis, spots before eyes, stomatitis, taste perversion, tinnitus
ENDO: Breast enlargement, elevated testosterone level, galactorrhea, hyperandrogenism, hyperglycemia, inappropriate ADH secretion, parotid gland swelling
GI: Abdominal pain, anorexia, constipation, diarrhea, dyspepsia, elevated liver enzymes, fecal incontinence, flatulence, gastroenteritis, **hepatotoxicity**, increased appetite, indigestion, jaundice, nausea, **pancreatitis**, vomiting
GU: Aspermia, azoospermia, cystitis, decreased sperm count or spermatozoa motility, dysuria, enuresis, male infertility, menstrual irregularities, polycystic ovary disease, urinary incontinence, UTI, **vaginal hemorrhage**
HEME: Agranulocytosis, anemia, **aplastic anemia, bone marrow suppression**, eosinophilia, hematoma, **hypofibrinogenemia, leukopenia**, lymphocytosis, macrocytosis, **pancytopenia**, porphyria (acute, intermittent), **prolonged bleeding time, thrombocytopenia**
MS: Arthralgia, arthrosis, back pain, bone pain, decreased bone mineral density, dysarthria, fractures, leg cramps, myalgia, neck pain or rigidity, osteopenia, osteoporosis
RESP: Dyspnea, increased cough
SKIN: Alopecia, changes in hair color or texture, cutaneous vasculitis, diaphoresis, discoid lupus erythematosus, dry skin, ecchymosis, **erythema multiforme**, furunculosis, hair color or texture changes, hirsutism, maculopapular rash, nail and nail bed disorders, petechiae, photosensitivity, pruritus, rash, seborrhea, **Stevens–Johnson syndrome, toxic epidermal necrolysis**
Other: Anaphylaxis, decreased carnitine concentration, developmental delay (children), **drug reaction with eosinophilia and systemic symptoms (DRESS), hyperammonemia, hyponatremia**, injection-site pain, weight gain or loss

Nursing Considerations

- Know that women of childbearing age should not be prescribed divalproex, valproate sodium, or valproic acid, unless other treatments have failed or are

unacceptable because drug exposure very early on in pregnancy may cause decreased IQ and major congenital malformations in the fetus.
- Use caution when administering drug to children or patient with history of hepatic disease, patient receiving multiple anticonvulsants, patient with congenital metabolic disorders, severe seizure disorder accompanied by mental retardation, and organic brain disease, because they may be at increased risk for developing hepatotoxicity.
- Give oral divalproex or valproic acid with food to minimize GI irritation, if needed.
- Administer drug at least 2 hours before or 6 hours after cholestyramine.
- Don't mix syrup with carbonated beverages; result may be an unpleasant-tasting mixture and irritate mouth and throat.
- Don't break or let patient chew delayed-release or extended-release tablets.
- Know that, if needed, sprinkle contents of delayed-release sprinkle capsules on small amount of semisolid food just before administration. Instruct patient not to chew contents of delayed-release sprinkle capsules.
- For I.V. administration, dilute prescribed dose with at least 50 ml compatible diluent and infuse over 60 minutes.
- Know that patient should be switched from I.V. to P.O. form of valproic acid as soon as possible.
- Be aware that patient with hypoalbuminemia or another protein-binding deficiency is at increased risk for valproic acid toxicity.
- Watch for evidence of decreased hepatic function, including anorexia, facial edema, jaundice, lethargy, loss of seizure control, malaise, vomiting, and weakness, especially during the first 6 months of treatment.
- Monitor liver enzymes, as ordered. Notify prescriber immediately if hepatotoxicity is suspected and, if confirmed, expect drug to be discontinued immediately.
- Monitor platelet count, as ordered, for signs of thrombocytopenia, and notify prescriber if they appear.

WARNING Keep in mind hyperammonemia may occur even if liver function test results are normal. Monitor ammonia levels, as ordered. If patient develops unexplained lethargy, vomiting, or changes in mental status with an increase in ammonia level; if asymptomatic ammonia elevations are detected and persist; or if patient develops hypothermia even without hyperammonemia, expect to discontinue valproic acid.

- Watch patient closely for suicidal tendencies, particularly when therapy starts and dosage changes, because depression may worsen temporarily during these times, possibly leading to suicidal ideation.
- Monitor patient's drug level, as ordered, especially early in therapy and if patient takes other drugs, because interactions can alter the blood level.
- Be aware drug may alter urine ketone test and thyroid function tests.

PATIENT TEACHING

- Instruct patient to swallow capsules whole to prevent irritation to mouth and throat. However, delayed-release sprinkle capsules may be opened and contents mixed with food for easier swallowing. Instruct patient not to chew contents of delayed-release sprinkle capsules.
- Tell patient to notify prescriber immediately and withhold further doses of drug, unless advised otherwise by prescriber, if symptoms such as anorexia, facial edema, lethargy, malaise, weakness, and vomiting occur.
- Advise patient to avoid hazardous activities during therapy because drug may affect mental and motor performance.
- Urge patient to avoid alcohol during therapy.
- Advise patient to notify prescriber if tremor develops during therapy; it may be dose-related.
- Urge family or caregiver to watch patient closely for suicidal tendencies, especially when therapy starts or dosage changes.
- Instruct women of childbearing age to use effective contraception while taking drug and to notify prescriber if pregnancy is suspected or occurs, as valproate exposure in utero can cause adverse effects on the cognitive development of the unborn child. Encourage woman who becomes pregnant while taking valproic acid to enroll in the North American antiepileptic drug pregnancy registry by calling 1-888-233-2334. Explain that the registry is collecting information about the safety of antiepileptic drugs during pregnancy.

valsartan

Diovan, Prexxartan

Class and Category

Pharmacologic class: Angiotensin II receptor blocker (ARB)
Therapeutic class: Antihypertensive
Pregnancy category: D

Indications and Dosages

➤ *To manage hypertension, alone or with other antihypertensives*

ORAL SUSPENSION, TABLETS (DIOVAN)

Adults. *Initial:* 80 or 160 mg daily, increased as needed and prescribed. *Maximum:* 320 mg/day.
Children ages 6 to 16. 1.3 mg/kg (up to 40 mg total) once daily, increased as needed and prescribed. *Maximum:* 2.7 mg/kg (up to 160 mg) daily.

ORAL SOLUTION (PREXXARTAN)

Adults. *Initial:* 40 mg or 80 mg twice daily, increased as needed and prescribed. *Maximum:* 320 mg/day.
Children ages 6 to 16. *Initial:* 0.65 mg/kg (up to maximum of 40 mg) twice daily, increased as needed and prescribed. *Maximum:* 1.35 mg/kg twice daily.

➤ *To treat New York Heart Association (NYHA) class II to IV heart failure*

ORAL SOLUTION (PREXXARTAN), ORAL SUSPENSION, TABLETS (DIOVAN)

Adults. *Initial:* 40 mg twice daily, increased to 80 mg twice daily and then 160 mg twice daily, as needed. *Maximum:* 320 mg daily.

➤ *To reduce cardiovascular mortality in stable patients with left ventricular failure or dysfunction following an MI*

ORAL SOLUTION (PREXXARTAN), ORAL SUSPENSION, TABLETS (DIOVAN)

Adults. *Initial:* 20 mg twice daily starting as early as 12 hr after MI, increased to 40 mg twice daily within 7 days, followed by subsequent adjustments to 160 mg twice daily as tolerated. *Maintenance:* 160 mg twice daily.

DOSAGE ADJUSTMENT If patient develops symptomatic hypotension or renal dysfunction, dosage decreased.

Route	Onset	Peak	Duration
P.O.	2 hr	6 hr	24 hr

Mechanism of Action

Blocks the hormone angiotensin II from binding to receptor sites in adrenal glands, vascular smooth muscle, and other tissues. This action inhibits aldosterone-secreting and vasoconstrictive effects of angiotensin II, thereby reducing blood pressure. It also reduces renal reabsorption of sodium, which helps to reduce fluid retention that occurs in heart failure.

Contraindications

Concurrent aliskiren therapy in diabetic patients, hypersensitivity to valsartan or its components

Interactions

DRUGS

ACE inhibitors, aliskiren, other angiotensin receptor blockers: Increased risk of hypotension, hyperkalemia, and renal dysfunction
antihypertensives, diuretics: Additive hypotensive effect
cyclosporine, rifampin, ritonavir: Possibly increased blood valsartan level
lithium: Possibly increased serum lithium concentration and toxicity
NSAIDs: Increased risk of renal dysfunction, especially in the elderly and patients with or existing renal dysfunction or volume depletion
potassium salts, potassium-sparing diuretics, potassium supplements: Possibly hyperkalemia

FOODS

high potassium foods such as bananas or potatoes, potassium-containing salt substitutes: Possibly hyperkalemia

Adverse Reactions

CNS: Dizziness, fatigue, headache, insomnia, syncope, vertigo
CV: Edema, **hypotension**, orthostatic hypotension, vasculitis
EENT: Blurred vision, pharyngitis, rhinitis, sinusitis
GI: Abdominal pain, diarrhea, elevated liver enzymes, **hepatitis**, indigestion, nausea, vomiting
GU: **Acute renal failure**, increased blood creatinine level
HEME: **Thrombocytopenia**
MS: Arthralgia, back pain, **rhabdomyolysis**
RESP: Cough, upper respiratory tract infection

SKIN: Alopecia, bullous dermatitis, rash
Other: **Angioedema**, **hyperkalemia**, increased incidence of viral infection

Nursing Considerations

- Know that valsartan shouldn't be given to patients who are taking a diuretic or have hypovolemia, because there is increased risk of severe hypotension from volume depletion. If severe hypotension occurs, place patient in a supine position, notify prescriber, and expect to give an intravenous infusion of normal saline.
- Be aware that Diovan tablets including the oral suspension form made from the tablets are not interchangeable with Prexxartan oral solution.
- Check patient's blood pressure often
- Be aware that maximal blood pressure reduction typically occurs after 4 weeks.
- during therapy.
- Monitor serum potassium level because drug may elevate potassium level by blocking aldosterone secretion.
- Obtain a serum creatinine level periodically, as ordered, because changes in renal function can occur during valsartan therapy. Know that patients who are at high risk for renal dysfunction are patients with chronic kidney disease, renal artery stenosis, severe congestive heart failure, or who are volume-depleted. Notify prescriber of an elevated serum creatinine level and changes in voiding patterns because renal dysfunction could lead to acute renal failure.

PATIENT TEACHING

- Instruct patient to take valsartan exactly as prescribed at the same time each day to maintain therapeutic effect.
- Advise patient to avoid hazardous activities until drug's CNS effects are known.
- Advise patient to avoid using potassium-containing salt substitutes without consulting prescriber.
- Instruct female patient of childbearing age to use reliable birth control during therapy and to notify prescriber at once about known or suspected pregnancy, because valsartan will have to be discontinued.
- Urge patient to keep follow-up appointments to monitor progress.
- Tell patients to inform all prescribers of valsartan therapy and any other drug therapy they are taking, including drugs such as ibuprofen and naproxen.

vancomycin hydrochloride

Firvanq, Vancocin

Class and Category

Pharmacologic class: Glycopeptide
Therapeutic class: Antibiotic
Pregnancy category: B (oral), C (parenteral)

Indications and Dosages

➤ *To treat pseudomembranous colitis caused by* Clostridium difficile

CAPSULES, ORAL SOLUTION

Adults. 125 mg every 6 hr for 7 to 10 days (capsules) or 10 days (oral solution). *Maximum:* 2 g daily.
Children. 40 mg/kg daily in three or four divided doses for 7 to 10 days. *Maximum:* 2 g daily.

➤ *To treat staphylococcal enterocolitis caused by* Staphylococcus aureus

CAPSULES, ORAL SOLUTION

Adults. 500 mg to 2 g daily in three or four divided doses for 7 to 10 days.
Children. 40 mg/kg daily in three or four divided doses for 7 to 10 days. *Maximum:* 2 g daily.

➤ *To treat bacterial endocarditis caused by methicillin-resistant* Staphylococcus aureus

I.V. INFUSION

Adults. 30 mg/kg daily infused at a rate of no more than 10 mg/min or over at least 1 hr, whichever is longer, in equally divided doses twice daily for 4 to 6 wk. *Maximum:* 2 g daily.

➤ *As adjunct to treat bacterial endocarditis caused by methicillin-resistant* S. aureus *in patients with prosthetic heart valve*

I.V. INFUSION

Adults. 30 mg/kg daily infused at a rate of no more than 10 mg/min or over at least 1 hr, whichever is longer, in equally divided doses twice daily to four times a day for 6 wk or longer in conjunction with rifampin and gentamicin. *Maximum:* 2 g daily.

➤ *To treat bacterial endocarditis caused by* Streptococcus bovis *or* Streptococcus viridans

I.V. INFUSION

Adults. 30 mg/kg daily infused at a rate of no more than 10 mg/min or over at least 1 hr, whichever is longer, in equally divided doses twice daily for 4 wk. *Maximum:* 2 g daily.

➤ *As adjunct to treat bacterial endocarditis caused by enterococci*

I.V. INFUSION

Adults. 30 mg/kg daily infused at a rate of no more than 10 mg/min or over at least 1 hr, whichever is longer, in equally divided doses twice daily for 4 to 6 wk in conjunction with gentamicin. *Maximum:* 2 g daily.

➤ *To treat bacterial septicemia, bone and joint infections, pneumonia, and skin and soft-tissue infections caused by staphylococcus, including methicillin-resistant strains, and life-threatening infections*

I.V. INFUSION

Adults and children age 12 and over. 500 mg every 6 hr or 1 g every 12 hr, infused at a rate of no more than 10 mg/min or over at least 1 hr, whichever is longer. *Maximum:* 4 g daily.

Children ages 1 month to 12 years. 10 mg/ kg every 6 hr, infused over at least 60 min.

Neonates ages 1 week to 1 month. *Initial:* 15 mg/kg followed by 10 mg/kg every 8 hr, infused over at least 60 min.

Neonates under age 1 week. *Initial:* 15 mg/kg followed by 10 mg/kg every 12 hr, infused over at least 60 min.

Mechanism of Action

Inhibits bacterial RNA and cell wall synthesis; alters permeability of bacterial membranes, causing cell wall lysis and cell death.

Incompatibilities

Don't give I.V. vancomycin through same I.V. line as other drugs. Don't add to albumin-containing solutions, alkaline solutions, aminophylline, amobarbital sodium, aztreonam, cefepime, ceftazidime, chloramphenicol sodium succinate, chlorothiazide sodium, dexamethasone sodium phosphate, foscarnet sodium, heparin sodium, methicillin sodium, penicillin G, pentobarbital sodium, phenobarbital sodium, piperacillin sodium and tazobactam sodium, secobarbital sodium, and sodium bicarbonate. Vancomycin may precipitate with heavy metals.

Contraindications

Hypersensitivity to corn or corn products when given with dextrose solutions, hypersensitivity to vancomycin or its components

Interactions

DRUGS

aminoglycosides (amikacin, gentamicin, tobramycin), amphotericin B, bacitracin (parenteral), bumetanide, capreomycin, carmustine, cidofovir, cisplatin, cyclosporine, ethacrynic acid, furosemide, paromomycin, pentamidine (parenteral), polymyxin B, salicylates (parenteral), streptozocin viomycin: Additive nephrotoxicity or ototoxicity

antihistamines, buclizine, cyclizine, meclizine, phenothiazines, thioxanthenes, trimethobenzamide: Masked symptoms of ototoxicity

cholestyramine, colestipol: Decreased antibacterial activity of oral vancomycin

dexamethasone: Decreased penetration of vancomycin into cerebrospinal fluid

nephrotoxic drugs: Increased risk of nephrotoxicity

Adverse Reactions

CNS: Chills, depression, dizziness, fatigue, fever, headache, insomnia, vertigo

CV: **Hypotension**, peripheral edema, vasculitis

EENT: Ototoxicity

GI: Abdominal pain, constipation, ***Clostridium difficile*- associated diarrhea**, diarrhea, flatulence, nausea, vomiting

GU: **Acute kidney injury**, interstitial nephritis, **nephrotoxicity**, UTI

HEME: Anemia, eosinophilia, **neutropenia, thrombocytopenia**

MS: Back pain

RESP: Dyspnea, wheezing

SKIN: **Exfoliative dermatitis**; extravasation with pain, tenderness, thrombophlebitis, and tissue necrosis; pruritus; rash; **Stevens–Johnson syndrome**; **toxic epidermal necrolysis**; urticaria

Other: **Anaphylaxis, drug reaction with eosinophilia and systemic symptoms**

(DRESS), drug-induced fever, **hypokalemia**, injection-site inflammation, superinfection

Nursing Considerations

- Be aware that vancomycin is not indicated for prophylaxis of endophthalmitis, nor should it be administered intracamerally or intravitreally, especially during or after cataract surgery, because it may cause hemorrhagic occlusive retinal vasculitis which may result in permanent vision loss.
- Reconstitute 500-mg vial of vancomycin for I.V. use by adding 10 ml of sterile water for injection; further dilute with at least 100 ml of compatible I.V. solution. For 1-g vial of dry, sterile powder, add 20 ml of sterile water for injection; further dilute with at least 200 ml of compatible I.V. solution.

WARNING Infuse over at least 1 hr/g of vancomycin. Rapid delivery may cause hypotension or transient "red man syndrome," characterized by chills; fainting; fever; flushing of face, neck, torso and upper arms; hypotension; nausea; tachycardia; and vomiting.

- Expect to monitor blood vancomycin concentrations frequently. Higher trough concentrations of 15 to 20 mg/L are commonly targeted now, though they are associated with more nephrotoxicity than the lower trough concentrations previously used.
- Monitor serum vancomycin concentration in patients with colitis or renal impairment because significant increases in blood drug level have occurred in such patients taking multiple oral doses of vancomycin.
- Know that if patient has an inflammatory intestinal disorder, he should be assessed often for adverse reactions because vancomycin absorption may be increased in these conditions.
- Check CBC results and BUN and serum creatinine levels during therapy, especially if patient has renal impairment or takes an aminoglycoside, because systemic vancomycin may cause acute kidney injury.
- Observe I.V. infusion site for evidence of extravasation, including necrosis, pain, tenderness, and thrombophlebitis. If extravasation occurs, discontinue infusion immediately and notify prescriber.
- Assess hearing during therapy. Transient or permanent ototoxicity may occur if patient receives an excessive amount of drug, has an underlying hearing loss, or receives concurrent aminoglycosides.
- Monitor patient closely for diarrhea when receiving intravenous form of vancomycin, because it may indicate pseudomembranous colitis caused by *C. difficile,* a risk with many antibiotics. If diarrhea occurs during therapy, notify prescriber and expect to withhold drug. If confirmed, treat with fluids, electrolytes, protein, and an antibiotic effective against *C. difficile.*
- Know that oral vancomycin is only used for gastrointestinal *C. difficile* and staphylococcal infections, as it is not absorbed. Patients cannot be converted from I.V. to oral vancomycin for other infections.

PATIENT TEACHING

- Instruct patient to use a calibrated measuring device to measure accurate doses of oral solution.
- Advise patient to notify prescriber if no improvement occurs after a few days.
- Instruct patient to complete full course of vancomycin, as prescribed.
- Instruct patient to notify prescriber if she develops persistent or severe diarrhea.
- Instruct patient to keep follow-up appointments during and after treatment.

vardenafil hydrochloride

Levitra, Staxyn

Class and Category

Pharmacologic class: Phosphodiesterase type 5 (PDE5) inhibitor
Therapeutic class: Anti-impotence agent
Pregnancy category: B

Indications and Dosages

➤ *To treat erectile dysfunction*

TABLETS (LEVITRA)

Adults. 10 mg taken 1 hr before sexual activity; increased to 20 mg or decreased to 5 mg, as needed. *Maximum:* 20 mg and once-daily limit regardless of dosage.

DOSAGE ADJUSTMENT If patient takes ritonavir, vardenafil dosage shouldn't exceed 2.5 mg in 72 hr. If patient takes atazanavir, clarithromycin, indinavir, itraconazole 400 mg daily, ketoconazole 400 mg daily, saquinavir, or another potent CYP3A4 inhibitor, vardenafil dosage shouldn't exceed 2.5 mg in 24 hr. If patient takes erythromycin, itraconazole 200 mg daily, or ketoconazole 200 mg daily, vardenafil dosage shouldn't exceed 5 mg in 24 hr.

ORALLY DISINTEGRATING TABLETS (STAXYN)

Adults. 10 mg taken 1 hr before sexual activity. *Maximum:* 10 mg within 24-hr period.

Route	Onset	Peak	Duration
P.O.	30 min	30 min–2 hr	4–5 hr

Mechanism of Action

Enhances effect of nitric oxide (released in the penis by sexual stimulation) and inhibits phosphodiesterase type 5, which increases cGMP level, relaxes smooth muscle, increasing blood flow into the corpus cavernosum to produce an erection.

Contraindications

Concurrent administration of alpha blockers or guanylate cyclase stimulators (riociguat), concurrent continuous or intermittent nitrate therapy, hypersensitivity to vardenafil or its components

Interactions

DRUGS

alpha blockers, guanylate cyclase stimulators, nitrates: Profound hypotension

atazanavir, clarithromycin, erythromycin, indinavir, itraconazole, ketoconazole, ritonavir, saquinavir: Increased vardenafil effects

class IA (procainamide, quinidine) and class III (amiodarone, sotalol) antiarrhythmics: Possibly increased QT-interval prolongation

indinavir, ritonavir: Reduced blood levels of indinavir and ritonavir

FOODS

grapefruit juice: Possibly increased vardenafil effect

Adverse Reactions

CNS: Dizziness, headache, **seizures**, transient global amnesia

CV: Hypotension, prolonged QT interval

EENT: Decreased vision, hearing loss, loss of vision in one or both eyes, nasal congestion, nonarteritic anterior ischemic optic neuropathy (NAION), rhinitis, sinusitis, tinnitus

GI: Indigestion, nausea

GU: Priapism

MS: Back pain

SKIN: Flushing

Other: Flu-like symptoms

Nursing Considerations

- Know that vardenafil shouldn't be used by men taking class IA (procainamide, quinidine) or class III (amiodarone, sotalol) antiarrhythmics or by men who have congenital prolonged QT interval. Drug may potentiate prolonged QT interval. It should also not be used in men who have hypotension (resting systolic blood pressure of less than 90 mm Hg), myocardial infarction (within last 6 months), presence of life-threatening arrhythmia, recent history of stroke, severe cardiac failure, uncontrolled hypertension (greater than 170/110 mm Hg), or unstable angina, because drug use could worsen these conditions.
- Use vardenafil cautiously in elderly men, men with penile abnormalities that may predispose them to priapism, or men with mild hepatic impairment (should not be used if patient has moderate to severe hepatic impairment), or renal dysfunction (although it should not be used if patient is on dialysis).
- Also use cautiously in patients with left ventricular outflow obstruction, such as aortic stenosis, and those with severely impaired autonomic control of blood pressure. These conditions increase sensitivity to vasodilators, such as vardenafil.
- Be aware that Levitra tablets are not interchangeable with Staxyn tablets.
- Monitor blood pressure and heart rate before and after giving drug, especially if patient takes an alpha blocker, because of increased risk of symptomatic hypotension.
- Monitor patient's vision, especially if he's over age 50; has coronary artery disease, diabetes, hyperlipidemia, or hypertension; or smokes, because vardenafil rarely leads to nonarteritic ischemic optic neuropathy and vision that is decreased, possibly permanently.
- Monitor patient's hearing. Sudden decrease or loss, possibly with dizziness

and tinnitus, may occur with vardenafil use. Report such changes immediately, and expect drug to be discontinued.

PATIENT TEACHING

- Alert patient that orally disintegrating tablets contain phenylalanine and should not be taken by patients with phenylketonuria. It also contains sorbitol and should not be taken if he has hereditary problems with fructose intolerance.
- Tell patient to take drug 1 hour before anticipated sexual activity for best results.
- Instruct patient to place a prescribed orally disintegrating tablet on his tongue immediately after removing it from the blister package and allow it to dissolve. He should not crush or split the tablet, and tablet should not be taken with any liquid.

WARNING Tell patient not to take vardenafil if he takes an organic nitrate, continuously or intermittently, or within 4 hours of taking an alpha blocker because profound hypotension and death could result.

- Caution patient not to take vardenafil more than once daily or to exceed 20 mg daily for oral tablet or 10 mg for orally disintegrating tablet. Tell him to call his prescriber or go to the emergency department immediately if he accidentally takes more vardenafil than prescribed.
- Tell patient to stop taking vardenafil and notify prescriber if he has a sudden hearing loss, sudden loss of vision in one or both eyes, or trouble remembering.
- Advise patient to seek sexual counseling to enhance drug's effects.
- Inform patient taking Staxyn that some form of sexual stimulation is needed for an erection to happen.
- Urge patient to notify prescriber at once if erection is painful or lasts longer than 4 hours, to avoid possible penile damage and permanent loss of erectile function.
- Instruct patient to alert all prescribers of vardenafil use.

varenicline

Chantix

Class and Category

Pharmacologic class: Nicotinic receptor partial agonist
Therapeutic class: Nicotinic blocker
Pregnancy classification: C

Indications and Dosages

➤ *As adjunct to smoking cessation treatment*

TABLETS

Adults. *Initial:* 0.5 mg daily for 3 days; then increased to 0.5 mg twice daily for 4 days, and then increased to 1 mg twice daily for a total of 12 wk of therapy. If effective, an additional 12 wk of therapy may be given.

DOSAGE ADJUSTMENT If patient has severe renal impairment, maximum dosage is 0.5 mg twice daily. If patient is having hemodialysis for end-stage renal disease, maximum dosage is 0.5 mg daily.

Mechanism of Action

Blocks nicotine from activating $alpha_4beta_2$ receptors by binding to them. This inhibits nicotine stimulation of the central nervous mesolimbic dopamine system, which probably is the area that produces pleasure in and reinforcement of smoking.

Contraindications

Hypersensitivity to varenicline or its components

Interactions

DRUGS

nicotine (transdermal): Increased adverse reactions

ACTIVITIES

alcohol use: Increased intoxicating effects of alcohol including aggressive behavior and sometimes amnesia of event

Adverse Reactions

CNS: Abnormal dreams, aggression, agitation, anxiety, asthenia, attention difficulties, behavior changes, **CVA**, delusions, depression, dizziness, dysgeusia, fatigue, hallucinations, headache, **homicidal ideation**, hostility, insomnia, irritability, lethargy, loss of consciousness, malaise, mania, mental impairment, panic, paranoia, psychosis, restlessness, **seizures**, sensory disturbances, sleep disorder, sleepwalking, somnambulism, somnolence, **suicidal ideation**, thirst
CV: Angina, chest pain, edema, hypertension, **MI**, peripheral ischemia, **thrombosis**, **ventricular extrasystole**

EENT: Dry mouth, epistaxis, gingivitis, rhinorrhea
ENDO: Hot flashes, hyperglycemia
GI: Abdominal pain, **acute pancreatitis**, anorexia, constipation, diarrhea, dyspepsia, flatulence, gastroesophageal reflux disease, **GI hemorrhage**, increased appetite, liver enzyme abnormalities, nausea, splenomegaly, vomiting
GU: **Acute renal failure**, polyuria, urine retention
HEME: Leukocytosis, **thrombocytopenia**
MS: Arthralgia, back pain, muscle cramp, musculoskeletal pain, myalgia
RESP: **Asthma**, dyspnea, **pulmonary embolism**
SKIN: Diaphoresis, **erythema multiforme**, pruritus, rash, **Stevens–Johnson syndrome**, urticaria
Other: **Angioedema**, flu-like syndrome, **hyperkalemia**, **hypersensitivity reactions**, **hypokalemia**, lymphadenopathy

Nursing Considerations

- Use cautiously in patients with renal disease because varenicline is substantially excreted by the kidneys.
- Review patient's medication history before starting varenicline because dosage adjustments may be needed for drugs such as insulin, theophylline, and warfarin.

WARNING Monitor patient for angioedema, difficult breathing, rash with mucosal lesions, or other signs of hypersensitivity. Report immediately, stop varenicline therapy, and provide supportive emergency care, as prescribed.

- If patient has nausea, the most common adverse reaction to varenicline, notify prescriber. Dosage reduction may help.

WARNING Know that serious neuropsychiatric adverse effects have occurred with varenicline use, even in patients with no prior psychiatric history. Aggressive or unusual behavior directed to self or others may be exhibited. Observe patient closely. If present, stop drug therapy immediately, notify prescriber, and provide safety measures to protect patient and others.

- Even with varenicline therapy, nicotine withdrawal symptoms and worsening of underlying psychiatric illness may occur with smoking cessation. If present, notify prescriber immediately, institute safety measures, and expect drug to be discontinued.
- Watch patient closely for suicidal tendencies, particularly when therapy starts and dosage changes, because depression may worsen temporarily during these times, possibly leading to suicidal ideation.
- Monitor patient for seizures, especially within the first month of therapy, and in patients with a history of seizures or other factors that could lower their seizure threshold.

PATIENT TEACHING

- Explain that using nicotine patches while taking varenicline won't increase its effectiveness and may increase adverse reactions such as dizziness, nausea, and vomiting.
- Instruct patient to set a date to quit smoking and then start taking varenicline 1 week before the quit date. Or, patient can begin therapy and then set a date to quit smoking between days 8 and 35 of treatment. Or, if patient is unable or unwilling to quit smoking right away, inform him that he can start taking varenicline and reduce smoking during the first 12 weeks of treatment as follows: during weeks 1–4, reduce number of cigarettes smoked daily by half; during weeks 5–8, reduce number of cigarettes smoked daily to reach one-quarter of the starting daily cigarettes smoked; and during weeks 9–12, keep reducing number of cigarettes smoked until zero is reached by week 12. Know that varenicline can be taken for an additional 12 weeks of therapy after smoking has stopped, if needed.
- Explain how to adjust dose when drug is used for smoking cessation. Tell patient to take drug after eating and with a full glass of water.
- Encourage patient to continue trying to stop smoking even if an early relapse occurs during varenicline therapy.

WARNING Tell patient to seek medical attention immediately if he develops difficulty breathing; mucosal lesions; rash or other skin reaction; swelling of his eyes, face, lips, mouth or neck; or any other signs of hypersensitivity during therapy.

- Inform patient that the most common adverse reactions to varenicline therapy are insomnia and nausea, usually transient. If they persist, patient should notify prescriber; dosage reduction may help.
- Caution patient to avoid hazardous activities until CNS effects of drug are known. Explain that near-miss traffic accidents and other accidental injuries have occurred in patients taking varenicline.
- Explain that strange, unusual, or vivid dreams may occur during therapy. Also inform patient that sleepwalking may occur that can lead to behavior that may be harmful to self, others, or property. If sleepwalking occurs, tell patient to stop taking drug and notify prescriber.

WARNING Tell patient and family or caregiver that nicotine withdrawal can occur even with varenicline use and that aggressive or unusual behavior can occur in patients with or without a history of mental illness. Tell them that if patient has an existing mental illness, varenicline therapy may worsen it. Inform them that sometimes these behaviors may become serious and can be directed to self or others and may be worsened by concomitant use of alcohol. Advise patient to avoid alcohol during varenicline therapy and urge family or caregiver to monitor patient closely for suicidal or homicidal tendencies, especially when therapy starts or dosage changes. Advise patient, family, or caregiver to notify prescriber about abnormal thinking or behavior and to stop taking drug immediately if this occurs.

- Instruct patient to seek emergency medical care if she experiences a seizure or new or worsening symptoms of cardiovascular disease such as calf pain when walking, chest pain, shortness of breath, or sudden onset of difficulty speaking, numbness, or weakness.
- Advise women who are breastfeeding while taking varenicline to monitor infant for excessive vomiting and seizures. If present, tell patient to stop taking varenicline and have infant seen by a pediatrician.

vasopressin (antidiuretic hormone [ADH])

Pressyn (CAN)

Class and Category

Pharmacologic class: Posterior pituitary hormone
Therapeutic class: Antidiuretic hormone
Pregnancy category: C

Indications and Dosages

➤ *To prevent or control symptoms of central diabetes insipidus caused by insufficient ADH*

SUBCUTANEOUS INJECTION

Adults. 5 to 10 units twice daily or three times a day, as needed.

I.M. INJECTION

Adults. 5 to 10 units twice daily or three times a day, as needed.
Children. 2.5 to 10 units three times a day or four times a day, as needed.

I.V. INFUSION

Adults and children. 0.0005 units/kg/hr. Dosage doubled every 30 min, as needed. *Maximum:* 0.01 units/kg/hr.

➤ *To prevent or treat abdominal distention postoperatively*

I.M. INJECTION

Adults. 5 units, increased to 10 units every 3 to 4 hr, as needed.

Route	Onset	Peak	Duration
I.M., SubQ	Unknown	Unknown	2–8 hr
I.V.	Unknown	Unknown	30–60 min

Contraindications

Chronic nephritis with nitrogen retention, hypersensitivity to vasopressin or its components

Interactions

DRUGS

carbamazepine, chlorpropamide, clofibrate, fludrocortisone, tricyclic antidepressants: Increased antidiuretic effect
demeclocycline, lithium, norepinephrine: Decreased antidiuretic effect

Mechanism of Action

Vasopressin, a synthetic form of antidiuretic hormone, treats diabetes insipidus by decreasing urine output and raising urine osmolality. When vasopressin attaches to vasopressin 2 (V_2) receptors on cell membranes in the nephron's collecting duct, it activates the enzyme adenyl cyclase to convert adenosine triphosphate (ATP) to cyclic adenosine monophosphate (cAMP). This action increases the collecting duct's permeability and enhances water reabsorption into the blood.

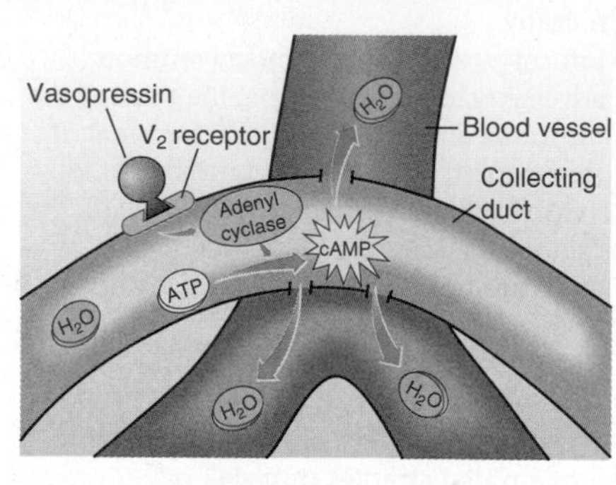

Adverse Reactions

CNS: Dizziness, headache, lightheadedness, tremor
CV: Angina, **MI**
EENT: Circumoral pallor
ENDO: Water intoxication
GI: Abdominal cramps, diarrhea, eructation, flatulence, intestinal hypermotility, nausea, vomiting
SKIN: Diaphoresis, pallor
Other: Hypersensitivity reaction

Nursing Considerations

- Use vasopressin with extreme caution in patients with asthma, epilepsy, heart failure, or migraine headache because extracellular fluid may increase rapidly; in those with coronary artery disease because it may cause angina or MI; and in those with hypertension because it may increase blood pressure.
- Monitor fluid and electrolyte balance during therapy. Check intake and output at least every 8 hours, and watch for evidence of water intoxication and hyponatremia, including anuria, confusion, drowsiness, headache, listlessness, and weight gain.

PATIENT TEACHING

- Teach patient how to administer vasopressin, if needed; stress the need to rotate injection sites.
- Urge patient to notify prescriber immediately if he has evidence of possible water intoxication, including anuria, confusion, drowsiness, headache, listlessness, and unexplained weight gain.
- Inform patient that abdominal cramps, nausea, and skin blanching will subside after a few minutes and can be minimized by drinking one or two glasses of water.

vedolizumab

Entyvio

Class and Category

Pharmacologic class: Monoclonal antibody
Therapeutic class: Anti-inflammatory
Pregnancy category: B

Indications and Dosages

➤ *To treat moderate to severe ulcerative colitis or Crohn's disease in patients who have had an inadequate response, lost response, were intolerant to a tumor necrosis factor blocker or immunomodulator, or were intolerant to or demonstrated dependence on corticosteroids; to improve endoscopic appearance of the mucosa in ulcerative colitis*

I.V. INFUSION

Adults. 300 mg infused over 30 min, followed by 300 mg 2 and 6 wk later, and then every 8 wk thereafter.

Mechanism of Action

Binds to a specific integrin and blocks its action with mucosal addressin cell adhesion molecule 1. It also inhibits the migration of memory T lymphocytes across the endothelium into the inflamed gastrointestinal parenchymal tissue. These actions are thought to help relieve the chronic inflammation that occurs with ulcerative colitis and Crohn's disease.

Incompatibilities

Do not mix any other drug with vedolizumab, and do not use any other solution for reconstitution of the drug except sterile water for injection and 0.9% sodium chloride for dilution because incompatibilities are unknown.

Contraindications

Hypersensitivity to vedolizumab or its components

Interactions

DRUGS

natalizumab: Increased risk of progressive multifocal leukoencephalopathy (PML) and other infections
tumor necrosis factor blockers: Increased risk of infections

Adverse Reactions

CNS: Dizziness, fatigue, fever, headache
CV: Hypertension, tachycardia
EENT: Nasopharyngitis, oropharyngeal pain, sinusitis
GI: Elevated bilirubin and liver enzymes, jaundice, **hepatic injury (severe)**, **hepatitis**, nausea, vomiting
MS: Arthralgia, back or extremity pain
RESP: Bronchitis, **bronchospasm**, cough, dyspnea, upper respiratory tract infection
SKIN: Flushing, pruritus, rash, urticaria
Other: Anaphylaxis, antivedolizumab antibodies, flu-like symptoms, infections, infusion-related reactions, **malignancies**, **sepsis**, **septic shock**

Nursing Considerations

- Ensure patient is up-to-date with all immunizations prior to initiating vedolizumab therapy.
- Know that vedolizumab is not recommended for use in patients with active, severe infections until the infections are controlled. Ensure that patient has been screened for tuberculosis.
- Use caution when administering vedolizumab to patient with a history of recurring severe infections.
- Reconstitute vedolizumab powder by injecting 4.8 ml of sterile water for injection, using a syringe with a 21G to 25G needle. Gently swirl the vial for at least 15 seconds to dissolve the powder. Do not vigorously shake or invert the vial. Allow solution to sit for up to 20 minutes at room temperature to allow for reconstitution and for any foam to settle; swirl vial, if needed, during this time. If not fully dissolved after 20 minutes, allow another 10 minutes for dissolution. Do not use if the powder is not dissolved after 30 minutes. Solution should be clear or opalescent, colorless to light brownish yellow, and free of visible particulates. Prior to withdrawing drug solution from the vial, gently invert vial three times. Withdraw 5 ml (300 mg) of reconstituted solution and add to 250 ml of sterile 0.9% sodium chloride; then gently mix in the infusion bag. Infusion solution may be stored up to 4 hours in the refrigerator prior to administration.
- Administer as an intravenous infusion over 30 minutes. Never administer as an intravenous push or bolus. Do not add any other drugs to the prepared solution. Flush the intravenous line with 30 ml of sterile 0.9% sodium chloride injection before and after the infusion.

WARNING Monitor patient closely for hypersensitivity reactions during infusion and up to several hours post infusion. Allergic reactions may include bronchospasm, dyspnea, flushing, rash, and urticaria. Blood pressure and heart rate may become elevated. If present, stop infusion, notify prescriber, expect to discontinue drug therapy, as ordered, and provide appropriate treatment according to standard of care.

- Monitor patient for infections because vedolizumab increases risk for infection. Notify prescriber if signs and symptoms occur, as drug may need to be withheld if infection is severe.

WARNING Monitor patient for any new onset or worsening of neurologic signs and symptoms, which may include changes in memory, orientation, or thinking; clumsiness of extremities; progressive weakness on one side of the body; or visual disturbances, because another drug in the same class has been associated with progressive multifocal leukoencephalopathy (PML), a rare and often fatal infection of the central nervous system. If PML is suspected, expect drug to be withheld and patient referred to a neurologist. If PML is confirmed, expect drug to be discontinued.

PATIENT TEACHING

- Stress importance of keeping appointments for vedolizumab administration.
- Instruct patient to notify prescriber immediately if allergic reaction occurs, such as difficulty breathing, hives, or rash.
- Review signs and symptoms of infection and tell patient to notify prescriber immediately if present, as drug may need to be withheld or discontinued.
- Encourage female patients who become pregnant during vedolizumab therapy to register with the pregnancy exposure registry by calling 1-877-825-3327.

venlafaxine hydrochloride

Effexor, Effexor XR, Venlafaxine E.R.

desvenlafaxine

Khedezla

desvenlafaxine fumarate

Desvenlafaxine ER

desvenlafaxine succinate

Pristiq

Class and Category

Pharmacologic class: Selective serotonin and norepinephrine reuptake inhibitor (SSNRI)
Therapeutic class: Antidepressant
Pregnancy category: C

Indications and Dosages

➤ *To treat and prevent relapse of major depression*

E.R. CAPSULES (EFFEXOR XR)

Adults. 75 mg daily with a meal at same time each day, morning or evening (for some patients, 37.5 mg daily for 4 to 7 days before increasing to 75 mg daily); then increased by 75 mg daily every 4 days, as prescribed. *Maximum:* 225 mg daily.
DOSAGE ADJUSTMENT Initial daily dose decreased by 25% to 50% for patients with mild to moderate renal impairment and by 50% for patients with hepatic impairment.

E.R. TABLETS (DESVENLAFAXINE ER, KHEDEZLA, PRISTIQ)

Adults. 50 mg daily, with a meal, at the same time each day morning or evening

E.R. TABLETS (VENLAFAXINE ER)

Adults. *Initial:* 75 mg daily as single dose (for some patients, 37.5 mg daily for 4 to 7 days before increasing to 75 mg daily); then increased by 75 mg daily every 4 days, as prescribed. *Maximum:* 225 mg daily.
DOSAGE ADJUSTMENT For patient with moderate to severe hepatic impairment or moderate renal impairment taking Pristiq, maximum dosage is 50 mg daily. For patient with severe renal impairment, 50 mg every other day or, with Pristiq brand, dosage reduced to 25 mg daily or 50 mg every other day.

TABLETS (EFFEXOR)

Adults. 75 mg daily in divided doses twice daily or three times a day, increased by 75 mg daily every 4 days, as needed. *Maximum:* 375 mg daily (225 mg/day for outpatients).
DOSAGE ADJUSTMENT For patients with mild to moderate hepatic impairment, dosage reduced by 50% or more. For patients with mild to moderate renal impairment, dosage reduced by 25% or, if patient is undergoing hemodialysis, dosage reduced by 50%.

➤ *To treat generalized anxiety disorder*

E.R. CAPSULES (EFFEXOR XR)

Adults. 75 mg daily with a meal at same time each day, morning or evening (for some patients, 37.5 mg daily for 4 to 7 days before increasing to 75 mg daily); then increased by 75 mg daily every 4 days, as needed. *Maximum:* 225 mg daily.

➤ *To treat social anxiety disorder*

E.R. CAPSULES (EFFEXOR XR)

Adults. 75 mg daily.

E.R. TABLETS (VENLAFAXINE ER)

Adults. 75 mg daily as a single dose.

➤ *To treat panic disorder*

E.R. CAPSULES (EFFEXOR XR)

Adults. *Initial:* 37.5 mg daily for 7 days, increased to 75 mg daily, as needed; then increased by 75 mg daily every 4 days, as needed. *Maximum:* 225 mg daily.

DOSAGE ADJUSTMENT Initial daily dose of E.R. capsules decreased by 25% to 50% for patients with mild to moderate renal impairment and by 50% for patients with hepatic impairment.

Route	Onset	Peak	Duration
P.O.	2 wk	Unknown	Unknown

Mechanism of Action

Inhibits neuronal reuptake of norepinephrine and serotonin, along with its active metabolite, *O*-desmethylvenlafaxine. These actions raise norepinephrine and serotonin levels at nerve synapses, elevating mood and reducing depression.

Contraindications

Hypersensitivity to desvenlafaxine, venlafaxine, or their components; use of an MAO inhibitor within 14 days, including intravenous methylene blue and linezolid

Interactions

DRUGS

aspirin, NSAIDs, other serotonin-norepinephrine reuptake inhibitors, selective serotonin reuptake inhibitors, warfarin and other anticoagulants: Increased risk of bleeding
cimetidine: Decreased clearance and increased levels of desvenlafaxine and venlafaxine
clozapine: Possibly increased blood clozapine level and serious adverse reactions, including seizures
CYP3A4 inhibitors, ketoconazole: Increased plasma venlafaxine level and risk of adverse reactions
MAO inhibitors: Increased risk of hypertension; hyperthermia; mental status changes, including coma and delirium; muscle rigidity; and severe myoclonus
metoprolol: Increased plasma metoprolol level, but decreased effectiveness in lowering blood pressure
serotonergic drugs such as amitriptyline, amphetamines, buspirone, clomipramine, desipramine, doxepin, fentanyl, haloperidol, imipramine, linezolid, lithium, nortriptyline, protriptyline, St. John's wort, tramadol, trazodone, triptans: Possibly serotonin syndrome
warfarin: Possibly increased PT, partial thromboplastin time, and INR

ACTIVITIES

alcohol use: Increased CNS effects

Adverse Reactions

CNS: Abnormal dreams, agitation, amnesia, anxiety, asthenia, attention disturbance, bruxism, **cerebral ischemia**, chills, confusion, delirium, delusions, depersonalization, depression, dizziness, dream disturbances, drowsiness, dyskinesia, extrapyramidal disorder, fatigue, fever, hallucinations, headache, hypesthesia, hypomania, impaired balance and coordination, insomnia, irritability, mania, migraine, mood changes, nervousness, **neuroleptic malignant syndrome**, paresthesia, **seizures**, **serotonin syndrome**, somnolence, **suicidal ideation**, syncope, tardive dyskinesia, tremor, vertigo
CV: Arrhythmias, **AV block**, chest pain, **congestive heart failure**, elevated cholesterol and triglyceride levels, edema, **extrasystoles**, hypertension, **hypotension**, **MI**, palpitations, **prolonged QT interval**, sinus tachycardia, **Takotsubo cardiomyopathy**, thrombophlebitis, **torsades de pointes**, vasodilation, **ventricular fibrillation or tachycardia**, worsening of peripheral vascular disease
EENT: Abnormal vision, accommodation abnormality, angle-closure glaucoma, blurred vision, dry mouth, mucous membrane bleeding, mydriasis, pharyngitis, rhinitis, taste alteration, tinnitus
ENDO: Elevated blood prolactin levels, hot flashes, hyperglycemia, syndrome of inappropriate ADH secretion
GI: Abdominal pain, anorexia, colitis, constipation, diarrhea, elevated liver enzymes, flatulence, **GI hemorrhage**, **hepatitis**, indigestion, nausea, **pancreatitis**, vomiting
GU: Anorgasmia (women), decreased libido, ejaculation disorder, impotence, urinary incontinence or urgency, urine hesitancy or retention
HEME: Abnormal bleeding, **agranulocytosis**, anemia, **aplastic anemia**, leukocytosis, **leukopenia**, **neutropenia**, **pancytopenia**, **prolonged bleeding time**, **thrombocytopenia**
MS: Neck pain, musculoskeletal stiffness, **rhabdomyolysis**

RESP: Cough, eosinophilic pneumonia, increased dyspnea, **interstitial lung disease**
SKIN: Diaphoresis, ecchymosis, **erythema multiforme**, pruritus, rash, **Stevens–Johnson syndrome**, **toxic epidermal necrolysis**
Other: **Angioedema**, **hypersensitivity reactions**, **hyponatremia**, lymphadenopathy, weight gain or loss

Nursing Considerations

- Be aware that desvenlafaxine and venlafaxine should not be given to patients with bradycardia, congenital long QT syndrome, hypokalemia or hypomagnesemia, recent acute myocardial infarction, or uncompensated heart failure because of increased risk of prolonged QT interval and torsades de pointes. It should also not be given to patients who are taking other drugs that prolong the QT interval. Expect hypokalemia and hypomagnesemia to be corrected before drug therapy is begun.
- Use cautiously in patients with a history of mania because desvenlafaxine and venlafaxine therapy may worsen condition. Also use cautiously in patients with a history of seizures, and expect to discontinue drug, as ordered, if seizures occur.
- Use cautiously in patients who have medical conditions that might be made worse by an increased heart rate, as in heart failure, hyperthyroidism, or recent MI.

WARNING **Be aware that serotonin syndrome in its most severe form may resemble neuroleptic malignant syndrome, which includes autonomic instability with possibly rapid changes in vital signs, hyperthermia, mental status changes, and muscle rigidity. Notify prescriber, withhold drug immediately, and provide supportive care. Expect drug to be discontinued.**

- Monitor blood pressure often during therapy because it may cause dose-related sustained increase in supine diastolic pressure. Expect to reduce or stop drug, as prescribed, if increase develops.
- Assess patient's electrolyte balance, as ordered, because drug can cause hyponatremia, especially in elderly patients and in patients who take diuretics or are volume-depleted. If patient has evidence of hyponatremia (confusion, headache, trouble concentrating, unsteadiness, weakness), notify prescriber. If imbalance is confirmed, expect to stop drug and give appropriate care.
- Watch patient for suicidal tendencies, especially when therapy starts and dosage changes.
- Be aware that false-positive urine immunoassay screening tests for amphetamine and phencyclidine (PCP) have been found in patients taking desvenlafaxine or venlafaxine. Expect different testing to be done to distinguish drug from PCP and amphetamine.

WARNING **Know that drug shouldn't be stopped abruptly, because doing so may cause multiple adverse effects, including asthenia, dizziness, flu-like symptoms, headache, insomnia, and nervousness.**

- Monitor patient closely for abnormal bleeding that may range from ecchymosis to life-threatening hemorrhage. Know that concomitant use of desvenlafaxine and venlafaxine and drugs known to affect bleeding or coagulation increases the risk of bleeding.

PATIENT TEACHING

- Instruct patient not to chew or crush E.R. capsules or tablets. If she has trouble swallowing capsules, tell her to open capsule, sprinkle contents on a spoonful of applesauce, and swallow immediately without chewing, followed by a glass of water.
- Advise patient that drug may cause mild pupillary dilation, which may lead to an episode of acute closure glaucoma. Encourage patient to have an eye exam before starting therapy to see if he is at risk.
- Advise patient to avoid alcohol during desvenlafaxine or venlafaxine therapy.
- Advise patient not to stop taking desvenlafaxine or venlafaxine abruptly.
- Caution patient to notify prescriber if she becomes pregnant during therapy because she'll need a different antidepressant. Taking desvenlafaxine or venlafaxine during third trimester of pregnancy increases risk of complications in the newborn.
- Advise patient to tell prescriber about all other prescribed drugs or OTC products she takes because of risk of interactions.

- Urge caregivers to monitor patient closely for suicidal tendencies, especially when therapy starts or dosage changes.
- Alert patient that fertility impairment may occur while taking desvenlafaxine or venlafaxine. If this is a concern for the patient, instruct her to discuss with prescriber.
- Caution patient to avoid aspirin and NSAIDs, if possible, while taking desvenlafaxine or venlafaxine.
- Inform patient that urine screening tests for amphetamine and phencyclidine (PCP) may produce a false positive for several days following discontinuation of desvenlafaxine or venlafaxine therapy, but that other tests may be done to distinguish drug from amphetamine and PCP.

WARNING Tell patient to report immediately sudden-onset, persistent, severe, or unusual symptoms.

- Tell patient to inform all prescribers of desvenlafaxine or venlafaxine therapy and not to take any over-the-counter medications, including herbal preparations, without prescriber knowledge.

verapamil

Apo-Verap (CAN), Calan, Novo-Veramil (CAN), Nu-Verap (CAN)

verapamil hydrochloride

Calan SR, Covera-HS, Verelan, Verelan PM

Class and Category

Pharmacologic class: Calcium channel blocker
Therapeutic class: Antianginal, antiarrhythmic, antihypertensive
Pregnancy category: C

Indications and Dosages

➤ *To treat chronic angina pectoris*

TABLETS (VERAPAMIL)
Adults and adolescents age 15 and over. *Initial:* 80 to 120 mg three times a day, increased every day or wk, as needed. *Maximum:* 480 mg daily in divided doses.

TABLETS (COVERA-HS)
Adults. *Initial:* 180 mg at bedtime. If response inadequate, dosage may be titrated to 180 mg at bedtime, then to 360 mg at bedtime, and 480 mg at bedtime, as needed. *Maximum:* 480 mg daily at bedtime.

➤ *To manage hypertension*

E.R. CAPSULES (VERAPAMIL HYDROCHLORIDE)
Adults and adolescents. *Initial:* 240 mg daily, increased every day or wk, as needed. *Maximum:* 480 mg daily.

E.R. TABLETS (VERAPAMIL HYDROCHLORIDE)
Adults and adolescents. *Initial:* 180 mg daily, increased every day or wk, as needed, according to following schedule: 240 mg daily in the morning; 180 mg every 12 hr or 240 mg in the morning and 120 mg in the evening; then 240 mg every 12 hr. *Maximum:* 480 mg daily in divided doses.

TABLETS (VERAPAMIL)
Adults and adolescents age 15 and over. *Initial:* 80 to 120 mg three times a day, increased every day or wk, as needed. *Maximum:* 480 mg daily in divided doses.

E.R. CAPSULES (VERELAN PM)
Adults. *Initial:* 200 mg at bedtime, increased to 300 mg at bedtime, then to 400 mg at bedtime, if needed.

E.R. TABLETS (COVERA-HS)
Adults. *Initial:* 180 mg at bedtime. If response inadequate, dosage may be titrated to 180 mg at bedtime, then to 360 mg at bedtime, and 480 mg at bedtime, as needed. *Maximum:* 480 mg daily at bedtime.

➤ *To prevent or treat supraventricular tachycardia*

TABLETS (VERAPAMIL)
Adults and adolescents age 15 and over. *Initial:* 80 to 120 mg three times a day, increased every day or wk, as needed. *Maximum:* 480 mg daily in divided doses.

DOSAGE ADJUSTMENT Initial P.O. dosage, possibly reduced for elderly and low-weight patients and those with impaired hepatic or left ventricular function. Dosage may need to be reduced in patients with decreased neuromuscular transmission.

I.V. INJECTION (VERAPAMIL HYDROCHLORIDE)
Adults and adolescents age 15 and over. *Initial:* 5 to 10 mg slowly over 2 min; then 10 mg, as needed, if response isn't adequate after 30 min.

Children ages 1 to 15. *Initial:* 100 to 300 mcg/kg slowly over 2 min, up to maximum of 5 mg; then dosage repeated as needed, if response isn't adequate after 30 min.
Infants up to age 1. *Initial:* 100 to 200 mcg/kg slowly over 2 min; then dosage repeated, as needed, if response isn't adequate after 30 min.
DOSAGE ADJUSTMENT I.V. drug administered over 3 minutes in elderly patients.

Route	Onset	Peak	Duration
P.O.	1–2 hr	30–90 min	6–8 hr
P.O. (E.R.)	1–2 hr	30–90 min	Unknown
I.V.	1–5 min	3–5 min	10 min–6 hr

Mechanism of Action

Inhibits calcium movement into coronary and vascular smooth-muscle cells by blocking slow calcium channels in cell membranes. The resulting decrease in intracellular calcium level has the following effects:

- inhibits smooth-muscle cell contractions
- decreases myocardial oxygen demand by relaxing coronary and vascular smooth muscle, reducing peripheral vascular resistance, and decreasing systolic and diastolic pressures
- slows AV conduction time and prolongs AV nodal refractoriness
- interrupts reentry circuit in AV nodal reentrant tachycardias.

Incompatibilities

Don't mix I.V. verapamil with albumin, amphotericin B injection, hydralazine hydrochloride injection, nafcillin, or sulfamethoxazole and trimethoprim injection. Solutions with pH above 6.0 cause precipitation.

Contraindications

Cardiogenic shock, concomitant use of beta blockers (with I.V. verapamil) or ivabradine, hypersensitivity to verapamil or its components, hypotension, severe heart failure unless secondary to supraventricular tachycardia that responds to verapamil, severe left ventricular dysfunction, sick sinus syndrome or second- or third-degree heart block unless artificial pacemaker is in place, ventricular tachycardia (with I.V. verapamil)

Interactions

DRUGS

alpha blockers, antihypertensives, general anesthetics (hydrocarbon), prazosin: Hypotensive effects
aspirin: Increased bleeding time
beta blockers: Increased risk of heart failure, hypotension, and severe bradycardia
calcium supplements: Decreased response to verapamil
carbamazepine, cyclosporine, theophylline, valproate: Increased risk of toxicity from these drugs
cimetidine: Decreased metabolism and increased blood level of verapamil
clonidine: Increased risk of severe sinus bradycardia
cyclophosphamide, oncovin, procarbazine, prednisone (COPP) regimen; vindesine, adriamycin, cisplatin (VAC) regimen: Decreased verapamil absorption
dantrolene: Increased risk of hyperkalemia and myocardial depression
digoxin: Increased blood digoxin level and risk of digitalis toxicity
disopyramide, flecainide: Additive negative inotropic effects
doxorubicin: Increased plasma doxorubicin level
erythromycin, ritonavir: Increased blood verapamil level
HMG-CoA reductase inhibitors such as atorvastatin, lovastatin, and simvastatin: Increased risk of myopathy and rhabdomyolysis
ivabradine: Increased exposure to ivabradine with possible exacerbation of bradycardia and conduction disturbances
lithium: Increased risk of neurotoxicity
neuromuscular blockers: Prolonged recovery from neuromuscular blockade
NSAIDs, sympathomimetics: Decreased antihypertensive effect of verapamil
paclitaxel: Decreased paclitaxel clearance
phenobarbital: Increased verapamil clearance
procainamide: Increased QT interval, additive negative inotropic effects
protein-bound drugs (hydantoins, salicylates, sulfonamides, sulfonylureas, and warfarin

and other oral anticoagulants): Altered blood levels of these drugs
quinidine: Increased risk of quinidine toxicity, increased QT interval, additive negative inotropic effects
rifampin: Decreased bioavailability of oral verapamil
telithromycin: Increased risk of brady-arrhythmias, hypotension, and lactic acidosis

FOODS

grapefruit juice: Increased verapamil level

ACTIVITIES

alcohol use: Increased blood alcohol level and prolonged CNS effects

Adverse Reactions

CNS: Asthenia, confusion, **CVA**, disequilibrium, dizziness, equilibrium disorders, extrapyramidal reactions, fatigue, headache, insomnia, paresthesia, psychosis, shakiness, somnolence, syncope
CV: Abnormal ECG, angina, **AV conduction disorders**, **bradycardia**, claudication, **heart failure**, hypertension, **hypotension**, **MI**, palpitations, peripheral edema, tachycardia, vasculitis
EENT: Blurred vision, dry mouth, tinnitus
ENDO: Gynecomastia, hyperprolactinemia
GI: Constipation, diarrhea, elevated liver enzymes, GI distress, nausea
GU: Galactorrhea, impotence, increased urination, menstrual irregularities
MS: Arthralgia, muscle spasms
RESP: Dyspnea, **pulmonary edema**
SKIN: Alopecia, diaphoresis, ecchymosis, **erythema multiforme**, exanthema, flushing, hyperkeratosis, rash, **Stevens–Johnson syndrome**, urticaria
Other: Allergy aggravated

Nursing Considerations

- Administer I.V. verapamil with compatible solutions, including D_5W, normal saline solution, or Ringer's injection.
- Maintain continuous ECG monitoring and keep emergency resuscitative equipment and drugs readily available during I.V. therapy.
- Assess patient with hypertrophic cardiomyopathy or idiopathic hypertrophic subaortic stenosis for early development of hypotension and pulmonary edema, because second-degree AV block and sinus arrest can result.
- Assess for bradycardia and hypotension, and notify prescriber if blood pressure or heart rate declines significantly.
- Know that disopyramide or flecainide shouldn't be given within 48 hours before or 24 hours after verapamil because additive negative inotropic effects can result.
- Institute measures to prevent constipation, including a high-fiber diet and a stool softener, as prescribed.

PATIENT TEACHING

- Instruct patient not to chew or crush verapamil E.R. capsules or tablets. Inform her that she may break E.R. tablets in half if necessary to aid swallowing.
- Direct patient to check her pulse before taking verapamil and to notify prescriber if it's below 50 beats/minute or as instructed by prescriber.
- Caution patient about possible dizziness and the need to avoid potentially hazardous activities until drug's CNS effects are known.
- Inform patient that adverse skin reactions may subside with continued verapamil use. Advise her to notify prescriber if rash persists.
- Encourage patient to increase dietary fiber intake to help prevent constipation. Advise her to notify prescriber if problem becomes persistent or severe.

vigabatrin

Sabril

Class and Category

Pharmacologic class: Gamma aminobutyric acid (GABA) transaminase inhibitor
Therapeutic class: Anticonvulsant
Pregnancy category: C

Indications and Dosages

➤ *As adjunct therapy for refractory complex partial seizures in patients with inadequate response to several alternative treatments and for whom potential benefits outweigh the risk of vision loss*

TABLETS

Adults, adolescents 17 years and over, and children age 10 to 16 weighing more than 60 kg (132 lb). *Initial:* 500 mg twice daily, increased weekly in 500 mg increments, as needed. *Maximum:* 1.5 g twice daily.

Children age 10 to 16 years of age weighing 60 kg (132 lb) or less. *Initial:* 250 mg twice daily, increased weekly in 500 mg/day increments, as needed. *Maximum:* 1 g twice daily.

DOSAGE ADJUSTMENT For patient with mild renal impairment (creatinine clearance 51 to 80 ml/min), reduce dose by 25%. For patients with moderate renal impairment (creatinine clearance 31 to 50 ml/min), reduce dose by 50%. For patients with severe renal impairment (creatinine clearance 11 to 30 ml/min), reduce dose by 75%.

➤ *As monotherapy for pediatric patients with infantile spasms for whom potential benefits outweigh risk of vision loss*

ORAL SOLUTION

Children age 1 month to 2 years. *Initial:* 50 mg/kg/day in two divided doses, increased every 3 days by 25 to 50 mg/kg/day, as needed. *Maximum:* 150 mg/kg/day in two divided doses.

Route	Onset	Peak	Duration
P.O.	Unknown	1 hr	Unknown

Mechanism of Action

Inhibits the action of gamma aminobutyric acid transaminase (GABA-T), the enzyme responsible for metabolism of the inhibitory neurotransmitter GABA. This increases GABA level in the CNS, which may play a role in suppression of seizure activity.

Contraindications

Hypersensitivity to vigabatrin and its components

Interactions

DRUGS

phenytoin: Decreased serum phenytoin level

Adverse Reactions

CNS: Abnormal behavior or dreams, abnormal magnetic resonance imaging (MRI), acute psychosis, anxiety, apathy, asthenia, attention disturbance, confusion, coordination abnormality, delirium, depression, dizziness, dystonia, **encephalopathy**, expressive language disorder, fatigue, fever, gait disturbance, headache, hyperreflexia, hypertonia, hypoesthesia, hyporeflexia, hypomania, hypotonia, insomnia, irritability, lethargy, malaise, **malignant hyperthermia**, memory loss, myoclonus, nervousness, paresthesia, peripheral neuropathy, postictal state, **seizures**, sensory disturbance, somnolence, **status epilepticus**, **suicidal ideation**, thirst, tremor, vertigo

CV: Chest pain, edema, peripheral edema

EENT: Asthenopia, blurred vision, deafness, diplopia, eye pain, **laryngeal edema**, nasopharyngitis, nystagmus, optic neuritis, pharyngolaryngeal pain, **stridor**, tinnitus, toothache, tunnel vision, vision loss (permanent and severe), visual field defect

ENDO: Delayed puberty

GI: Abdominal or stomach pain, cholestasis, constipation, decreased liver enzymes, diarrhea, distention, dyspepsia, esophagitis, **GI hemorrhage**, nausea, vomiting

GU: Dysmenorrhea, erectile dysfunction, UTI

HEME: Anemia

MS: Arthralgia; back or limb pain; dysarthria; muscle spasticity, spasms or twitching

RESP: Bronchitis, cough, **pulmonary edema**, **respiratory failure**, upper respiratory infection

SKIN: Alopecia, maculopapular rash, pruritus, **Stevens–Johnson syndrome**, **toxic epidermal necrolysis**

Other: **Angioedema**, birth defects, developmental delay, flu-like symptoms, **multiorgan failure**, weight gain

Nursing Considerations

- Be aware that vigabatrin therapy is only available under a restricted distribution program called the Sabril REMS program (1-888-457-4273).

WARNING Monitor patient's vision, and make sure patient has been examined by an ophthalmic professional in which visual fields and retinal examination has been performed no later than 4 weeks after vigabatrin therapy has begun and then every 3 months throughout therapy and 3 to 6 months after therapy has been discontinued, because drug can cause progressive and permanent bilateral concentric visual field constriction and severely reduce visual acuity. Be aware that while risk increases with total dose and duration of therapy, all patients are at risk for visual abnormalities even after drug has been stopped. Because of the risk of permanent and possibly severe vision loss, drug can be prescribed and obtained only through the REMS distribution program. Report any visual abnormalities immediately, and expect drug to be discontinued.

- Know that abnormal MRI results have been noted in some infants receiving vigabatrin.
- Monitor patient for suicidal ideation throughout therapy but especially when therapy starts or dosage changes.
- When discontinuing vigabatrin therapy, expect to do so gradually by decreasing daily dose by 1 g each week until drug is discontinued, as ordered.
- When discontinuing vigabatrin therapy in children, expect to do so gradually by decreasing dose by 25 to 50 mg/kg/day every 3 to 4 days.
- Monitor patient for evidence of peripheral neuropathy, such as numbness or tingling in feet or toes, progressive loss of reflexes, starting at the ankles, or reduced distal lower limb position sense or vibration. Alert prescriber if abnormalities are present.
- Assess patient routinely for edema, including peripheral edema.

PATIENT TEACHING

- Explain the risk of possibly permanent vision loss that may occur as blurred vision or tunnel vision before patient starts vigabatrin. Stress the importance of having vision checked every 3 months throughout therapy and 3 to 6 months after drug is discontinued even if patient is an infant. However, inform patient that vision testing may be insensitive and may not detect vision loss before it is severe and has become permanent.
- Warn patient not to stop taking vigabatrin abruptly; she will need to be weaned off drug gradually over several weeks.
- Instruct parents how to mix the oral solution by emptying the entire contents of each 500-mg packet needed into a clean cup and dissolved in 10 ml of cold or room-temperature water per packet. Show parents how to administer the resulting solution using the 10-ml oral syringe supplied with the medication. Remind them that the concentration of the final solution is 50 mg/ml. Stress importance of checking dosage before administering.
- Advise female patient of childbearing age to use effective contraception if sexually active and to report suspected or confirmed pregnancy immediately.
- Advise patient or caregiver to notify prescriber if patient has unusual behaviors or feelings, especially if related to suicidal ideation and particularly at the beginning of therapy and during dosage adjustments.
- Caution patient not to perform hazardous activities such as operating equipment until CNS effects of the drug are known.
- Alert patient to monitor his weight because drug may cause weight gain.

vilazodone hydrochloride

Viibryd

Class and Category

Pharmacologic class: Selective serotonin reuptake inhibitor (SSRI)
Therapeutic class: Antidepressant
Pregnancy category: C

Indications and Dosages

➤ *To treat major depressive disorder*

TABLETS

Adults. *Initial:* 10 mg once daily for 7 days, followed by 20 mg once daily for 7 days, then increased to 40 mg once daily as needed.

DOSAGE ADJUSTMENT For patients taking a strong inhibitor of CYP3A4 such as ketoconazole, dosage should not exceed 20 mg daily. For patients taking a strong CYP3A4 inducer such as carbamazepine for more than 14 days, dosage may be increased up to twofold but not exceeding 80 mg daily.

Mechanism of Action
Exerts antidepressant effects by potentiating serotonin activity in CNS and inhibiting serotonin reuptake at the presynaptic neuronal membrane. Blocked serotonin reuptake increases levels and prolongs activity of serotonin at synaptic receptor sites.

Contraindications
Hypersensitivity to vilazodone or its components, use within 14 days of MAO inhibitor therapy

Interactions
DRUGS

amphetamines, buspirone, fentanyl, lithium, MAO inhibitors, serotonin norepinephrine reuptake inhibitors, serotonin reuptake inhibitors, St. John's wort, tramadol, tricyclic antidepressants, triptans, tryptophan: Increased risk of life-threatening adverse effects such as serotonin syndrome

aspirin, NSAIDs, warfarin, and other anticoagulants: Increased risk of bleeding

CYP2C8 substrate, highly protein bound drugs: Possibly increased blood concentration of the CYP2C8 substrate or highly protein bound drug

CYP3A4 inhibitors such as erythromycin, ketoconazole: Increased blood vilazodone levels with increased risk of adverse effects

Adverse Reactions
CNS: Abnormal dreams, dizziness, fatigue, feeling jittery, hallucinations, insomnia, irritability, mania, migraine, **neuroleptic malignant syndrome-like reactions**, panic attack, paresthesia, restlessness, **seizures**, **serotonin syndrome**, sleep paralysis, **suicidal ideation**, tremor

CV: Palpitations, **prolonged QT interval**, **torsades de pointes**, **ventricular extrasystoles**

EENT: Angle-closure glaucoma, blurred vision, cataracts, dry eyes or mouth

GI: **Acute pancreatitis**, anorexia, diarrhea, dyspepsia, flatulence, gastroenteritis, **GI bleeding**, increased appetite, nausea, vomiting

GU: Decreased libido, delayed ejaculation, erectile dysfunction, pollakiuria

HEME: **Bleeding events**

MS: Arthralgia

SKIN: Diaphoresis, drug eruption, night sweats, rash, urticaria

Nursing Considerations
- Be aware that vilazodone should not be given to patients with bradycardia, congenital long QT syndrome, hypokalemia or hypomagnesemia, recent acute myocardial infarction, or uncompensated heart failure because of increased risk of prolonged QT interval and torsades de pointes. It should also not be given to patients who are taking other drugs that prolong the QT interval. Expect hypokalemia and hypomagnesemia to be corrected before vilazodone therapy is begun.
- Use vilazodone cautiously in a patient with a seizure disorder because drug effect has not been studied in patients with seizures.
- Expect to taper vilazodone therapy gradually when drug is no longer required; abrupt discontinuation can precipitate withdrawal symptoms.

WARNING Monitor patient closely for serotonin syndrome exhibited by agitation, coma, diarrhea, hallucinations, hyperreflexia, hyperthermia, incoordination, labile blood pressure, nausea, tachycardia, or vomiting. Notify prescriber immediately because serotonin syndrome may be life-threatening; provide supportive care.

WARNING Be aware that serotonin syndrome in its most severe form may resemble neuroleptic malignant syndrome, which includes autonomic instability with possibly rapid changes in mental status and vital signs, hyperthermia, and muscle rigidity. Stop drug immediately, and provide supportive care.

- Watch patient closely for suicidal tendencies, particularly when therapy starts and dosage changes, because depression may worsen temporarily during these times, possibly leading to suicidal ideation.
- Watch for mania, which may result from any antidepressant in a susceptible patient.
- Monitor patient closely for evidence of GI bleeding, especially if patient also takes a

drug known to cause GI bleeding, such as aspirin, an NSAID, or warfarin.
- Monitor patient's serum sodium level, as ordered, especially in the elderly and patients with volume depletion, because selective serotonin reuptake inhibitors, the class of drugs vilazodone belongs to, have caused hyponatremia. If patient develops a confusion, difficulty concentrating, headache, memory impairment, unsteadiness, and weakness, and sodium level has decreased, notify prescriber and expect drug to be discontinued. Be prepared to provide supportive care.

PATIENT TEACHING
- Instruct patient to take vilazodone with food because drug may not be as effective if taken on an empty stomach.
- Advise patient that drug may cause mild pupillary dilation, which may lead to an episode of acute closure glaucoma. Encourage patient to have an eye exam before starting therapy to see if he is at risk.
- Tell family or caregiver to observe patient closely for suicidal tendencies, especially when therapy starts or dosage changes.
- Tell patient not to take aspirin or NSAIDs during therapy because they increase the risk of bleeding. If patient takes warfarin, tell her to use bleeding precautions and to notify prescriber at once if bleeding occurs.
- Caution patient to alert all prescribers about vilazodone therapy because of potentially serious drug interactions.
- Advise patient to notify prescriber of any persistent, severe, or unusual adverse reactions.

vorapaxar

Zontivity

Class and Category

Pharmacologic class: Protease activated receptor-1 (PAR-1) inhibitor
Therapeutic class: Antiplatelet
Pregnancy category: B

Indications and Dosages

➤ *To reduce thrombotic cardiovascular events in patients with a history of myocardial infarction or peripheral arterial disease*

TABLETS
Adults. 2.08 mg once daily.

Mechanism of Action

Inhibits thrombin-induced and thrombin receptor agonist peptide-induced platelet aggregation.

Contraindications

Active pathologic bleeding; history of intracranial hemorrhage, stroke, or transient ischemic attack; hypersensitivity to vorapaxar or its components

Interactions

DRUGS
strong CYP3A inducers such as carbamazepine, phenytoin, rifampin, St. John's wort: Decreased vorapaxar effectiveness
strong CYP3A inhibitors such as boceprevir, clarithromycin, conivaptan, indinavir, itraconazole, ketoconazole, nelfinavir, posaconazole, ritonavir, saquinavir: Increased vorapaxar exposure and adverse reactions

Adverse Reactions

CNS: Depression, **intracranial hemorrhage**
EENT: Diplopia, oculomotor disturbance, retinal disorder including retinopathy
GI: GI bleeding
HEME: Anemia, **bleeding events that may become severe**, iron deficiency
SKIN: Eruptions, exanthema, rash

Nursing Considerations

- Be aware that vorapaxar is usually prescribed along with other antiplatelet agents such as aspirin and/or clopidogrel.
- Know that vorapaxar should not be given to patients with a history of intracranial hemorrhage, stroke, or transient ischemic attack because of an increased risk for intracranial hemorrhage. The drug should be discontinued in a patient who experiences a stroke while taking vorapaxar.
- Assess patient's bleeding risk before beginning vorapaxar therapy, because vorapaxar increases the risk of bleeding in proportion to the patient's underlying bleeding risk. Factors that may increase the patient's risk of bleeding include the

use of certain concomitant drugs such as anticoagulants, chronic nonsteroidal anti-inflammatory drugs, fibrinolytic therapy, selective serotonin reuptake inhibitors, or serotonin–norepinephrine reuptake inhibitors; history of bleeding disorders; low body weight; older age; or reduced hepatic or renal function.

- Know that vorapaxar should not be given to patients with severe hepatic impairment because of increased risk for bleeding.

WARNING Monitor patient for bleeding throughout vorapaxar therapy. Suspect bleeding in patient who is hypotensive and has recently undergone coronary angiography, coronary artery bypass graft surgery, percutaneous coronary intervention, or other surgical procedures. Stop vorapaxar therapy and notify prescriber immediately of suspected or known bleeding. Prepare to support patient according to standard of care, as there is no known treatment to reverse the antiplatelet effect of the drug because of its long half-life. Significant inhibition of platelet aggregation has been known to persist for at least 4 weeks after the drug has been discontinued.

PATIENT TEACHING

- Tell patient to take vorapaxar exactly as prescribed and not to discontinue the drug without discussing it with the prescriber.
- Inform patient that he may bleed or bruise more easily. Stress importance of promptly reporting any excessive, prolonged, or unanticipated bleeding, or blood in the stool or urine.
- Review safety precautions to avoid bleeding events, such as using an electric razor and soft toothbrush.
- Remind patient to inform all dentists and physicians of vorapaxar use prior to any dental procedure or surgery. Emphasize that the dentist or doctor performing the procedure should talk to the prescriber before stopping the drug.
- Tell patient to keep prescriber informed of all dietary supplements, over-the-counter drugs, or prescription drugs he takes.

voriconazole

Vfend

Class and Category

Pharmacologic class: Triazole
Therapeutic class: Antifungal
Pregnancy category: D

Indications and Dosages

➤ *To treat invasive aspergillosis; to treat serious fungal infections caused by* Scedosporium apiospermum *and* Fusarium *species, including* Fusarium solani, *in patients intolerant of or refractory to other therapy*

I.V. INFUSION

Adults. *Initial:* 6 mg/kg over 1 to 2 hr at no more than 3 mg/kg/hr every 12 hr for two doses followed by 4 mg/kg over 1 to 2 hr at no more than 3 mg/kg/hr every 12 hr for at least 7 days before being switched to an oral form.

ORAL SUSPENSION, TABLETS

Adults weighing 40 kg (88 lb) or more. *Maintenance:* 200 mg every 12 hr, increased to 300 mg every 12 hr, as needed, and taken at least 1 hr before or after a meal.

Adults weighing less than 40 kg (88 lb). *Maintenance:* 100 mg every 12 hr, increased to 150 mg every 12 hr, as needed, and taken at least 1 hr before or after a meal.

➤ *To treat candidemia in nonneutropenic patients and other deep-tissue disseminated* Candida *infections involving the abdomen, bladder wall, kidney, skin, or a wound*

I.V. INFUSION

Adults. *Initial:* 6 mg/kg over 1 to 2 hr at no more than 3 mg/kg/hr every 12 hr for two doses, followed by 3 to 4 mg/kg over 1 to 2 hr at no more than 3 mg/kg/hr every 12 hr and then switched to oral form when feasible. If it's not possible to switch to oral form, IV therapy given for at least 14 days after symptoms resolve or last positive culture, whichever takes longer.

ORAL SUSPENSION, TABLETS

Adults. *Maintenance:* 200 mg every 12 hr taken at least 1 hr before or after a meal for at least 14 days after symptoms resolve or last positive culture, whichever takes longer.

➤ *To treat esophageal candidiasis*

ORAL SUSPENSION, TABLETS

Adults. 200 mg every 12 hr taken at least 1 hr before or after a meal for at least 14 days and at least 7 days after signs and symptoms resolve.

DOSAGE ADJUSTMENT If patient can't tolerate drug, I.V. maintenance dose may be reduced to 3 mg/kg every 12 hr and oral maintenance dose by 50-mg decrements to at least 200 mg every 12 hr (100 mg every 12 hr for patients weighing less than 40 kg). For use with efavirenz or phenytoin, maintenance dose increased. For patients with mild to moderate hepatic cirrhosis, maintenance dosage reduced.

Mechanism of Action

Prevents fungal ergosterol biosynthesis by inhibiting fungal cytochrome P-450–mediated 14 alpha-lanosterol demethylation. The loss of ergosterol in the fungal cell wall renders the fungal cell inactive.

Incompatibilities

Don't infuse into the same cannula or line with other drugs, including parenteral nutrition, to prevent an increase in subvisible particulate matter. Avoid infusion with blood products and any electrolyte supplements. Don't dilute with 4.2% sodium bicarbonate infusion because the mildly alkaline nature of the diluent causes slight degradation of voriconazole after 24 hours of storage at room temperature.

Contraindications

Coadministration with long-acting barbiturates, carbamazepine, CYP3A4 substrates (astemizole, cisapride, pimozide, quinidine, or terfenadine), efavirenz, ergot alkaloids, rifabutin, rifampin, ritonavir, sirolimus, or St. John's wort; hypersensitivity to voriconazole or its components; galactose intolerance, glucose-galactose malabsorption, or Lapp lactase deficiency (oral form only contains lactose)

Interactions

DRUGS

alfentanil: Increased plasma alfentanil level and increased risk of adverse reactions

benzodiazepines: Possibly prolonged sedative effect of benzodiazepines

calcium channel blockers; HMG-CoA reductase inhibitors, such as lovastatin; omeprazole; sirolimus: Possibly increased plasma levels of these drugs, leading to increased risk of adverse reactions and toxicity

carbamazepine, long-acting barbiturates, rifampin, ritonavir, St. John's wort: Decreased plasma voriconazole concentration

cyclosporine, sirolimus, tacrolimus: Increased serum concentrations of these drugs and risk of toxicity, especially nephrotoxicity

CYP3A4 substrates (astemizole, cisapride, pimozide, quinidine, terfenadine): Increased plasma levels of these drugs, which may lead to prolonged QT interval and, rarely, torsades de pointes

efavirenz: Possibly decreased plasma voriconazole levels and increased plasma efavirenz levels

ergot alkaloids (dihydroergotamine, ergotamine): May increase plasma level of ergot alkaloids, leading to ergotism

fentanyl and other long-acting opiates metabolized by CYP3A4 such as oxycodone: Increased plasma level of fentanyl and other long-acting opiates with increased risk of adverse reactions

everolimus, fluconazole, oral contraceptives: Increased plasma voriconazole level and risk of toxicity

HIV protease inhibitors (amprenavir, nelfinavir, ritonavir, saquinavir), non-nucleoside reverse transcriptase inhibitors (delavirdine): Possibly inhibited metabolism of voriconazole possibly leading to increased plasma voriconazole levels

methadone: Increased plasma level of methadone, possibly leading to toxicity, including QT-interval prolongation

NSAIDs: Increased plasma NSAID levels leading to possible increased adverse reactions, including toxicity

oral contraceptives: Increased plasma voriconazole level and risk of toxicity ; toxicity; increased plasma levels of oral contraceptives and risk of adverse reactions

phenytoin: Decreased plasma level of voriconazole and increased plasma level of phenytoin

rifabutin: Increased rifabutin plasma level; decreased voriconazole plasma level
sulfonylureas: Possibly increased plasma level of sulfonylureas and increased risk of hypoglycemia
vinca alkaloids: Possibly increased risk of neurotoxicity
warfarin: Possibly increased PTT

Adverse Reactions

CNS: Chills, dizziness, fever, hallucinations, headache
CV: **Cardiac arrest**, chest pain, hypertension, **hypotension**, peripheral edema, **prolonged QT interval**, tachycardia, **torsades de pointes**, vasodilation, **ventricular tachycardia**
EENT: Abnormal or blurred vision, altered or enhanced visual perception, change in color perception, chromatopsia, dry mouth, eye hemorrhage, photophobia, visual disturbances
GI: Abdominal pain, cholestatic jaundice, diarrhea, elevated liver enzymes, **fulminant hepatic failure**, **hepatitis**, jaundice, nausea, **pancreatitis**, vomiting
GU: Abnormal kidney function, **acute renal failure**, elevated serum creatinine level
HEME: Anemia, **leukopenia**, **pancytopenia**, **thrombocytopenia**
MS: Fluorosis, periostitis, skeletal pain
RESP: Respiratory disorders
SKIN: **Erythema multiforme**, maculopapular rash, photosensitivity, pruritus, rash, **Stevens–Johnson syndrome**, **toxic epidermal necrolysis**
Other: **Anaphylaxis**, elevated alkaline phosphatase, **hypokalemia**, **hypomagnesemia**, **sepsis**

Nursing Considerations

- Use voriconazole cautiously in patients hypersensitive to other azoles and in patients at risk for proarrhythmic events (such as those receiving cardiotoxic chemotherapy or concomitant drug therapy known to prolong QT interval, or those who have acquired or congenital QT prolongation, cardiomyopathy, hypokalemia, sinus bradycardia, or symptomatic arrhythmias [existing]). because drug may prolong the QT interval. Know that calcium, magnesium, and potassium imbalances should be corrected before starting voriconazole therapy as well as any time an imbalance occurs during voriconazole therapy. Monitor patient's electrolyte balance closely.
- Determine if patient has any problems with galactose intolerance, glucose-galactose malabsorption, or Lapp lactase deficiency before starting therapy because voriconazole tablets contain lactose and shouldn't be given to patients with these conditions.
- Obtain specimens for fungal culture and other relevant laboratory studies (including histopathology), as ordered, before giving first dose. Expect to begin drug before test results are known.
- Assess patient's liver function, including bilirubin, as ordered, at the start of voriconazole therapy and at least weekly for the first month of treatment then monthly thereafter because, although uncommon, drug has caused serious hepatic reactions, including fatalities. Be aware that drug may be discontinued if liver abnormalities occur.
- For I.V. infusion, reconstitute powder with 19 ml water for injection to obtain 20 ml of concentrate containing 10 mg/ml voriconazole. To make sure exact amount of water is injected into vial, use a standard 10-ml nonautomated syringe. Shake vial until all powder is dissolved. Further dilute so final concentration is no less than 0.5 mg/ml and no more than 5 mg/ml. This requires withdrawing and discarding at least an equal volume of diluent from infusion bag or bottle before instillation of concentrate.
- Discard partially used vials after mixing. If infusion isn't administered immediately, store at 2° to 8°C (37° to 46°F) for no longer than 24 hours.
- Administer I.V. infusion over 1 to 2 hours at no more than 3 mg/kg/hr.
- Monitor renal function, especially serum creatinine level, when giving I.V. form of voriconazole because drug may accumulate in body when creatinine clearance is less than 50 ml/min, increasing the risk of adverse reactions.

WARNING Observe patient receiving I.V. voriconazole closely for anaphylactoid-type reactions, such as chest tightness,

dyspnea, faintness, fever, flushing, nausea, pruritus, rash, sweating, and tachycardia, which may occur immediately after starting infusion. Stop infusion if these reactions occur, and notify prescriber immediately.
- Monitor patient closely throughout therapy for rash, which may indicate a serious cutaneous reaction, such as Stevens–Johnson syndrome. If rash occurs, notify prescriber, and expect that voriconazole may be discontinued.
- Monitor cyclosporine, tacrolimus, and warfarin closely for elevated levels when voriconazole is given with any of these drugs.
- Monitor diabetic patients also taking sulfonylureas closely for hypoglycemia, and check blood glucose levels regularly.
- Keep in mind voriconazole dosage will need to be adjusted when given with efavirenz or phenytoin. Expect to monitor plasma phenytoin level and observe patient closely for adverse reactions.
- Assess patient's visual function, including color perception, visual acuity, and visual field, if voriconazole therapy continues longer than 28 days.
- Monitor patient closely for pancreatitis, especially if patient is a child or has risk factors for acute pancreatitis, such as recent chemotherapy or hematopoietic stem cell transplantation.
- Report skeletal pain to prescriber and expect skeletal x-rays to be done. If fluorosis or periostitis is found, anticipate voriconazole therapy to be discontinued.

PATIENT TEACHING
- Instruct patient taking oral voriconazole to take oral suspension or tablets at least 1 hour before or 1 hour after a meal.
- Inform female patient of possible fetal risk, and emphasize need to avoid pregnancy. Tell her to use effective contraception during therapy and to notify prescriber immediately if pregnancy is suspected.
- Caution patient not to drive at night and to avoid hazardous activities because drug may cause visual disturbances, including blurring or photophobia.
- Advise patient to avoid exposure to direct sunlight or UV light and to wear sunscreen when outdoors.

vortioxetine hydrobromide

Trintellix

Class and Category

Pharmacologic class: Serotonin modulator
Therapeutic class: Antidepressant
Pregnancy category: C

Indications and Dosages

➤ *To treat major depressive disorder (MDD)*

TABLETS

Adults. *Initial:* 10 mg once daily, then increased to 20 mg once daily, as tolerated. *Maximum:* 20 mg once daily.

DOSAGE ADJUSTMENT For patients who cannot tolerate higher doses, dosage may be decreased down to 5 mg once daily. For patients taking strong CYP inducers, such as carbamazepine, phenytoin, or rifampin concurrently for longer than 14 days, dosage increased up to three times the original dose and when inducer is discontinued, dosage decreased to original level within 14 days. For patients taking strong CYP2D6 inhibitors such as bupropion, fluoxetine, paroxetine, or quinidine concurrently, dosage reduced by one half, and when inhibitor is discontinued, dosage increased to original level within 14 days. For patients who are known CYP2D6 poor metabolizers, maximum dosage is 10 mg once daily.

Mechanism of Action

Enhances serotonergic activity in the central nervous system through inhibiting the reuptake of serotonin. Enhanced serotonergic activity is thought to relieve symptoms of depression.

Contraindications

Hypersensitivity to vortioxetine or its components; use within 14 days of a MAO inhibitor, including intravenous methylene blue and linezolid

Interactions

DRUGS

aspirin, NSAIDs, warfarin, and other anticoagulants: Increased risk of bleeding

buspirone, MAO inhibitors, SNRIs, SSRIs, tramadol, triptans, tryptophans: Increased risk of serotonin toxicity
CYP2D6 inducers (strong) such as carbamazepine, phenytoin, rifampin: Decreased plasma vortioxetine levels with possible decreased effectiveness
CYP2D6 inhibitors (strong) such as bupropion, fluoxetine, paroxetine, and quinidine: Increased plasma vortioxetine levels with increased risk of adverse reactions

Adverse Reactions

CNS: Abnormal dreams, activation of hypomania/mania, dizziness, **seizures**, **serotonin syndrome**, **suicidal ideation**, vertigo
EENT: Altered taste, angle-closure glaucoma, dry mouth
GI: **Acute pancreatitis**, constipation, diarrhea, dyspepsia, flatulence, nausea, vomiting
GU: Decreased libido, sexual performance, or sexual satisfaction
HEME: **Abnormal bleeding**
RESP: Difficulty breathing
SKIN: Flushing, pruritus, rash, urticaria
Other: **Hyponatremia**, weight gain

Nursing Considerations

- Be aware that at least 14 days should elapse between discontinuing a MAO inhibitor used to treat psychiatric disorders and initiation of vortioxetine therapy to avoid risk of patient developing serotonin syndrome. Also, know that at least 21 days should elapse after vortioxetine is discontinued and therapy with a MAO inhibitor used to treat a psychiatric disorder is begun.
- Expect dosage to be decreased to 10 mg once daily for 1 week before vortioxetine is discontinued to avoid patient experiencing dizziness, headaches, mood swings, including muscle tension, runny nose, or sudden outbursts of anger that may occur in the first week of abrupt discontinuation of the drug.
- Watch patient closely for suicidal tendencies, particularly when therapy starts and dosage changes, because depression may worsen temporarily during these times, possibly leading to suicidal ideation.
- Watch for mania, which may result from use of any antidepressant in a susceptible patient.
- Monitor patient closely for evidence of GI bleeding, especially if patient also takes a drug known to cause GI bleeding, such as aspirin, a NSAID, warfarin, or other anticoagulants.

WARNING Monitor patient closely for serotonin syndrome exhibited by agitation, coma, diarrhea, hallucinations, hyperreflexia, hyperthermia, incoordination, labile blood pressure, nausea, or vomiting. Notify prescriber immediately because serotonin syndrome may be life-threatening, and provide supportive care.

- Monitor patient's serum sodium level because hyponatremia has occurred with use of serotonergic drugs, including vortioxetine. Patients at greater risk include the elderly and patients taking diuretics or who are volume-depleted. Report signs and symptoms of hyponatremia, such as confusion, difficulty concentrating, headache, memory impairment, unsteadiness, or weakness. If left untreated, coma, death, hallucinations, respiratory arrest, seizures, or syncope may occur.

PATIENT TEACHING

- Instruct patient to take drug exactly as prescribed and to alert prescriber with concerns.
- Inform patient that nausea is the most common side effect of vortioxetine therapy, and it commonly occurs within the first week of treatment.
- Advise patient that drug may cause mild pupillary dilation, which may lead to an episode of acute closure glaucoma. Encourage patient to have an eye exam before starting therapy to see if he is at risk.
- Tell family or caregiver to observe patient closely for suicidal tendencies, especially when therapy starts or dosage changes.
- Warn patient not to discontinue drug abruptly.
- Advise patient to inform all prescribers of vortioxetine therapy.
- Emphasize importance of reporting any persistent, severe, or sudden symptoms to prescriber.

- Alert patients about risk of bleeding when taking drugs known to increase risk of bleeding, such as aspirin, blood thinners, or NSAIDs.
- Tell patient and caregivers to report any signs of abnormal behavior.
- Inform elderly patient or patient who is taking drugs, such as diuretics, that cause him to be dehydrated of the risk of a low sodium level; tell patient to alert prescriber if he experiences new or sudden onset of symptoms.
- Advise patient to seek emergency medical attention if an allergic reaction such as difficulty breathing, hives, rash, or swelling occurs.
- Instruct female patients of childbearing age to notify prescriber if pregnancy occurs or is suspected.
- Tell patient to inform all prescribers of vortioxetine therapy and not to take any over-the-counter medications, including herbal products, without prescriber knowledge.

warfarin sodium

Coumadin

Class and Category

Pharmacologic class: Coumarin derivative
Therapeutic class: Anticoagulant
Pregnancy category: X

Indications and Dosages

➤ *To prevent or treat pulmonary embolism; recurrent MI; thromboembolic complications from atrial fibrillation, heart valve replacement, or MI; and venous thrombosis (and its extension)*

TABLETS

Adults. *Initial:* 2 to 5 mg daily for 2 to 4 days. *Usual:* 2 to 10 mg daily based on target INR and PT results. *Maximum:* Determined by target INR and PT results, as prescribed.

I.V. INJECTION

Adults. *Initial:* 2 to 5 mg daily infused over 1 to 2 min. *Usual:* 2 to 10 mg daily infused over 1 to 2 min based on target INR and PT results. *Maximum:* Determined by target INR and PT results, as prescribed.

DOSAGE ADJUSTMENT For Asian, debilitated, or elderly patients, dosage reduced and then adjusted based on INR and PT results.

Route	Onset	Peak	Duration
P.O.	24 hr	3–4 days	2–5 days
I.V.	Unknown	3–4 days	2–5 days

Mechanism of Action

Interferes with the liver's ability to synthesize vitamin K–dependent clotting factors, depleting clotting factors II (prothrombin), VII, IX, and X. This action, in turn, interferes with the clotting cascade. By depleting vitamin K–dependent clotting factors and interfering with the clotting cascade, warfarin prevents coagulation.

Incompatibilities

Don't mix warfarin in solution with amikacin sulfate, epinephrine hydrochloride, metaraminol tartrate, oxytocin, promazine hydrochloride, tetracycline hydrochloride, or vancomycin hydrochloride.

Contraindications

Bleeding or bleeding tendencies; blood dyscrasias; cerebral or dissecting aneurysm; cerebrovascular hemorrhage; diverticulitis; eclampsia or preeclampsia; history of warfarin-induced necrosis; hypersensitivity to warfarin or its components; malignant or severe uncontrolled hypertension; malnutrition and emaciation; mental state or condition that leads to lack of patient cooperation, or unsupervised situation; pericardial effusion; pericarditis; polyarthritis; pregnancy except in women with mechanical heart valves, who are at high risk of thromboembolism; prostatectomy; recent or planned neurosurgery, ophthalmic surgery, or spinal puncture; severe hepatic or renal disease

Interactions

DRUGS

acetaminophen, agrimony, aminoglycosides, amiodarone, androgens, argatroban, beta blockers, bivalirudin, capecitabine, cephalosporins, chloral hydrate, chloramphenicol, chlorpropamide, cimetidine, clofibrate, corticosteroids, cyclophosphamide, dextrothyroxine, diflunisal, disulfiram, erythromycin, ezetimibe, fluconazole, gemfibrozil, glucagon, hydantoins, ifosfamide, influenza virus vaccine, isoniazid, ketoconazole, lepirudin, loop diuretics, lovastatin, metronidazole, miconazole, mineral oil, moricizine, nalidixic acid, NSAIDs, omeprazole, penicillins, phenylbutazones, propafenone, propoxyphene, quinidine, quinine, quinolones, salicylates, streptokinase, sulfamethoxazole-trimethoprim, sulfinpyrazone, sulfonamides, tamoxifen, tetracyclines, thyroid hormones, urokinase, valdecoxib, vitamin E: Increased anticoagulant effect of warfarin, increased risk of bleeding

aminoglutethimide, barbiturates, carbamazepine, cholestyramine, dicloxacillin, estrogens, ethchlorvynol, etretinate, glutethimide, griseofulvin, multivitamins (selected ones), nafcillin, oral contraceptives, rifampin, spironolactone, sucralfate, thiazide diuretics, trazodone, vitamin C, vitamin K: Decreased anticoagulant effect of warfarin

atorvastatin, pravastatin: Increased or decreased anticoagulant effect of warfarin

herbal remedies (including bromelains, danshen, dong quai, garlic, ginkgo biloba, and ginseng): Increased anticoagulant effect of warfarin, increased risk of bleeding

I.V. lipid emulsion, other medical products that contain soybean oil: Possibly decreased vitamin K absorption and increased anticoagulant effect of warfarin

nicotine patch: Altered response to warfarin

FOODS

certain enteral feedings, vitamin K–rich foods: Decreased warfarin effects

ACTIVITIES

alcohol use: Increased risk of hypoprothrombinemia

smoking, smoking cessation aids: Altered response to warfarin

Adverse Reactions

CNS: Coma, intracranial hemorrhage, loss of consciousness, syncope, weakness
CV: Angina, calcium uremic arteriolopathy (calciphylaxis), chest pain, **hypotension**
EENT: Epistaxis, intraocular hemorrhage
GI: Abdominal cramps and pain, diarrhea, **hepatitis**, jaundice, nausea, vomiting
GU: Hematuria, vaginal bleeding (abnormal)
HEME: Anemia, **potentially fatal hemorrhage**
SKIN: Alopecia, ecchymosis, petechiae, pruritus, purple-toe syndrome, tissue necrosis
Other: Anaphylaxis

Nursing Considerations

- Ensure that women of childbearing age has a negative pregnancy test result before warfarin therapy is initiated because drug may cause fetal harm even in the first trimester.
- Reconstitute parenteral warfarin just before administration with 2.7 ml sterile water for injection to yield 2 mg/ml. Then give slowly over 1 to 2 minutes through peripheral I.V.
- Expect to give another parenteral anticoagulant, such as enoxaparin or heparin, with oral warfarin for at least 3 days, or until desired response occurs, before giving warfarin only.
- Avoid I.M. injections during warfarin therapy, if possible, because they can result in bleeding, bruising, and hematoma.
- Monitor INR (daily in acute care setting) and assess for therapeutic effects, as prescribed. Therapeutic INR levels are 2.0 to 3.0 for bioprosthetic heart valve, nonvalvular atrial fibrillation, and venous thromboembolism, and 2.5 to 3.5 after MI and for mechanical heart valve.
- Monitor patient with hepatic impairment closely for bleeding, because hepatic impairment decreases metabolism of warfarin and impairs synthesis of clotting factors. Expect to monitor patient's INR more frequently.
- Expect treatment to last up to 12 weeks for bioprosthetic heart valve, 1 to 3 months for nonvalvular atrial fibrillation or venous thromboembolism, and for rest of life after MI and for mechanical heart valve replacement.

WARNING Be aware of the increased risk for intracranial hemorrhage if patient has cerebral ischemia (such as recent transient ischemic attack or minor ischemic stroke) and INR of 3 to 4.5. As prescribed, withhold next warfarin dose and give vitamin K, as ordered, if INR exceeds 4 because of the risk of bleeding.

- Assess for occult bleeding if patient receives I.V. lipid emulsion or other medical product that contains soybean oil. Such products can decrease vitamin K absorption and increase warfarin's anticoagulant effect.
- Monitor patient for persistent, severe, sudden, or unusual signs and symptoms, as warfarin therapy may cause many adverse reactions, including calciphylaxis, a syndrome of blood clots, calcification of blood vessels, and skin necrosis. If diagnosed, expect warfarin therapy to be discontinued and alternative anticoagulation therapy prescribed.

PATIENT TEACHING

- Explain that warfarin therapy aims to prevent thrombosis by decreasing clotting ability while avoiding the risk of spontaneous bleeding.
- Instruct patient to take drug exactly as prescribed at the same time each evening.
- Advise patient if a dose is missed to take it as soon as it is remembered on the same day, but not to take a double dose the next day to make up for it.
- Urge patient to keep weekly follow-up appointments for blood tests after discharge until PT and INR levels are stabilized.
- Advise patient to avoid alcohol during warfarin therapy.
- Urge patient to take precautions against bleeding, such as using an electric shaver and a soft-bristled toothbrush. Advise him to continue these precautions for 2 to 5 days after therapy stops, as directed, because anticoagulant effect may persist during this time.
- Caution patient to avoid activities that could cause traumatic injury and bleeding.
- Advise patient to avoid drastic changes in dietary habits, such as eating large amounts of leafy, green vegetables. Explain that dark green, leafy vegetables contain vitamin K that counteracts the effects of warfarin.
- Urge patient to notify prescriber immediately about unusual bleeding and any unexplained symptoms, such as abnormal vaginal bleeding; dizziness; easy bruising; gum bleeding; headache; nosebleeds; prolonged bleeding from cuts; red, black, or tarry stool; red or dark brown urine; swelling; and weakness.
- Advise patient to consult prescriber before taking other drugs—including OTC drugs and herbal remedies—during therapy. Also instruct him to not discontinue any drug, including over-the-counter drugs and herbal products he takes regularly, without consulting the prescriber.
- Instruct female patient of childbearing age to use an effective contraceptive during warfarin therapy and for at least 1 month after warfarin has been discontinued. Stress importance because drug may cause fetal harm. Also tell patient to notify prescriber immediately if pregnancy occurs or is suspected.
- Tell patient who is breastfeeding to monitor her infant for bleeding or bruising and to notify prescriber immediately if either occurs.

WARNING **Tell patient to contact prescriber immediately if he experiences pain and discoloration of the skin mostly on areas of the body with a high fat content, such as abdomen, breasts, buttocks, hips, and thighs or if he experiences any unusual symptoms. Explain that drug may cause reversible purple-toe syndrome but that this syndrome isn't harmful.**

- Urge patient to carry medical identification that reveals he's taking warfarin.
- Tell patient to inform all dentists and healthcare professionals that he is taking warfarin, especially before any procedure or surgery, including dental, is performed.

XYZ

zafirlukast

Accolate

Class and Category

Pharmacologic class: Leukotriene receptor antagonist
Therapeutic class: Antiasthmatic
Pregnancy category: B

Indications and Dosages

➤ *To prevent or treat chronic asthma*

TABLETS

Adults and children over age 11. 20 mg twice daily.
Children ages 5 to 11. 10 mg twice daily.

Route	Onset	Peak	Duration
P.O.	1 wk	Unknown	Unknown

Mechanism of Action

Inhibits the selective binding of cysteinyl leukotrienes (arachidonic acid derivatives that usually mediate inflammation in asthma and other inflammatory disorders) by competitively blocking receptor sites. This action causes bronchial relaxation and decreases bronchial hyperresponsiveness, eosinophil movement, mucus secretion, and vascular leakage.

Contraindications

Hepatic impairment including hepatic cirrhosis, hypersensitivity to zafirlukast or its components

Interactions

DRUGS

alprazolam, amitriptyline, calcium channel blockers, carbamazepine, citalopram, corticosteroids, cyclosporine, diazepam, diclofenac, ibuprofen, imipramine, irbesartan, lidocaine, lovastatin, midazolam, phenytoin, quinidine, simvastatin, tolbutamide, tolterodine, triazolam: Inhibited metabolism and, possibly, additive adverse effects of these drugs
aspirin: Increased blood zafirlukast level
erythromycin, terfenadine: Decreased response to zafirlukast
sildenafil: Increased adverse sildenafil effects
theophylline: Decreased zafirlukast level; possibly increased theophylline levels
warfarin: Prolonged PT

FOODS

any food: Possibly decreased bioavailability of zafirlukast

Adverse Reactions

CNS: Asthenia, depression, dizziness, fever, headache, insomnia, malaise
CV: Edema, vasculitis
GI: Abdominal pain, diarrhea, edema, elevated liver enzymes, **hepatic failure**, **hepatitis**, hyperbilirubinemia, indigestion, nausea, vomiting
HEME: Agranulocytosis, bleeding, eosinophilia
MS: Arthralgia, back pain, myalgia
RESP: Eosinophilic pneumonia
SKIN: Bruising, pruritus, rash, urticaria
Other: Angioedema, generalized pain, **hypersensitivity reactions**, infections

Nursing Considerations

- Know that zafirlukast shouldn't be used to treat bronchospasm during an acute asthma attack or status asthmaticus; it can't relieve symptoms quickly enough.
- Assess respiratory depth, quality, and rate, as well as breath sounds, before and during treatment to evaluate response to therapy.
- Be aware that if patient is being weaned from corticosteroids while taking zafirlukast, she should be monitored for Churg–Strauss syndrome—a rare allergic reaction characterized by eosinophilia, fever, myalgia, and weight loss—for cardiac complications, neuropathy, and worsening pulmonary symptoms.

PATIENT TEACHING

- Instruct patient to take drug exactly as prescribed, in evenly spaced doses, every day, even during acute exacerbations and symptom-free periods.
- Instruct patient to take drug on an empty stomach at least 1 hour before meals, or 2 hours after.
- Urge patient to continue using prescribed rescue inhalants for acute asthma attacks.

- Teach patient how to use peak-flow meter to monitor pulmonary function.
- Tell patient to report immediately any evidence of liver dysfunction, such as anorexia, fatigue, flu-like symptoms, jaundice, lethargy, nausea, right upper-quadrant abdominal pain, or pruritus.

zaleplon

Sonata

Class, Category, and Schedule

Pharmacologic class: Pyrazolopyrimidine
Therapeutic class: Hypnotic
Pregnancy category: C
Controlled substance schedule: IV

Indications and Dosages

➤ *Short-term treatment of insomnia*

CAPSULES

Adults up to age 65. 10 mg daily at bedtime, as needed, for up to 35 days. *Usual:* 10 mg daily at bedtime for 7 to 10 days. *Maximum:* 20 mg daily.

DOSAGE ADJUSTMENT For patients who are debilitated, elderly, have hepatic impairment or low weight, or take cimetidine, dosage reduced to 5 mg daily.

Route	Onset	Peak	Duration
P.O.	30 min	Unknown	4 hr

Mechanism of Action

Selectively binds with type 1 benzodiazepine (BZ1 or omega$_1$) receptors on the gamma-aminobutyric acid-A receptor complex. This binding produces muscle relaxation and sedation as well as antianxiety and anticonvulsant effects.

Contraindications

Hypersensitivity to zaleplon or its components

Interactions

DRUGS

amitriptyline; amoxapine; azatadine; benzodiazepines; brompheniramine; chlorpheniramine; clemastine; clomipramine; clozapine; cyproheptadine; dexchlorpheniramine; diphenhydramine; doxepin; entacapone; haloperidol; hydroxyzine; imipramine; maprotiline; mirtazapine; molindone; nefazodone; nortriptyline; olanzapine; opioid analgesics; other anxiolytics, hypnotics and sedatives; phenindamine; phenothiazines; pimozide; pramipexole; promethazine; quetiapine; risperidone; ropinirole; thioridazine; trazodone; trimipramine; tripelennamine: Possibly additive CNS depression
carbamazepine, phenobarbital, phenytoin, rifampin: Reduced zaleplon effects
cimetidine: Increased blood zaleplon level
flumazenil: Reversal of zaleplon's sedation

FOODS

high-fat foods: Prolonged absorption time and reduced effectiveness of zaleplon

ACTIVITIES

alcohol use: Increased CNS depression

Adverse Reactions

CNS: Amnesia, anxiety, complex behaviors (such as sleep driving), depression, dizziness, drowsiness, fever, hallucinations, hypertonia, insomnia, nightmares, paresthesia, **seizures**, **suicidal ideation**, tremor, vertigo
EENT: Dry mouth, gingivitis, glossitis, mouth ulcers, stomatitis, **throat tightness**
GI: Anorexia, colitis, constipation, eructation, esophagitis, flatulence, gastritis, gastroenteritis, increased appetite, indigestion, **melena**, nausea, **rectal bleeding**, vomiting
MS: Back pain
RESP: Dyspnea
SKIN: Photosensitivity, pruritus, rash
Other: Anaphylaxis, **angioedema**, physical and psychological dependence

Nursing Considerations

- Give zaleplon just before bedtime because its onset of action is rapid.
- Avoid giving drug with or after a heavy, high-fat meal because decreased absorption may reduce drug's effects.
- Watch patient closely for suicidal tendencies, particularly when therapy starts and dosage changes, because depression may worsen temporarily during these times, possibly leading to suicidal ideation.
- Monitor patient for signs of drug abuse because zaleplon has an abuse potential similar to that of benzodiazepines and benzodiazepine-like hypnotics.

WARNING Monitor patient closely for hypersensitivity reactions, such as dyspnea, nausea, throat tightness, vomiting, and swelling. If present, discontinue zaleplon immediately, notify prescriber, and provide supportive care.

PATIENT TEACHING

- Explain that zaleplon is intended for short-term use. Advise against using it for any condition other than insomnia.
- Caution patient against exceeding prescribed dosage.
- Instruct patient to take zaleplon immediately before bedtime or right after having trouble falling asleep because of drug's rapid onset of action.
- Teach patient alternative measures for relaxation and sleep induction.
- Advise patient to consult prescriber before taking other CNS depressants.
- Urge patient to avoid alcohol during zaleplon therapy because it increases risk of abnormal behaviors, such as sleep driving.
- Warn patient that zaleplon contains FD & C Yellow No. 5 (tartrazine), which can cause an allergic reaction, especially in those with an aspirin sensitivity. Instruct patient to immediately report allergic reactions, such as difficulty breathing or rash, to prescriber.
- Instruct patient to notify prescriber if inability to sleep continues. Dosage may need to be adjusted.
- Instruct patient to stop taking zaleplon and seek emergency care if she has abnormal swelling, nausea, throat tightness, trouble breathing, or vomiting.
- Explain that drug may cause abnormal behaviors during sleep, such as driving a car, eating, having sex, or talking on the phone without any recall of the event. If family notices any such behavior or patient sees evidence of such behavior upon awakening, prescriber should be notified.
- Urge family or caregiver to watch patient closely for suicidal tendencies, especially when therapy starts or dosage changes.

zanamivir

Relenza

Class and Category

Pharmacologic class: Neuraminidase inhibitor
Therapeutic class: Antiviral
Pregnancy category: Not classified

Indications and Dosages

➤ *To treat acute uncomplicated illness due to influenza A and B viral infection in patients who have been symptomatic for no more than 2 days*

ORAL INHALATION

Adults and children ages 7 years and over. 10 mg twice daily about 12 hr apart for 5 days. The first two doses should be taken on the first day with at least 2 hr separating the doses if 12-hr stretch is not feasible.

➤ *To prevent influenza*

ORAL INHALATION

Adults and children ages 5 years and over. 10 mg daily for 10 days.
Adults and adolescents in a community setting. 10 mg once daily for 28 days.

Mechanism of Action

Inhibits influenza virus neuraminidase, affecting release of viral particles of infected cells.

Contraindications

Hypersensitivity to zanamivir or its components or to milk proteins

Interactions

DRUGS

live attenuated influenza vaccine: Possibly decreased effectiveness

Adverse Reactions

CNS: Abnormal behavior, agitation, altered level of consciousness, anxiety, chills, confusion, delirium, dizziness, fatigue, fever, hallucinations, headache, malaise, nightmares, **seizures**, syncope, vasovagal episode
CV: Arrhythmias
EENT: Ear, nose, **throat hemorrhage** or infection; oropharyngeal edema; sinusitis
GI: Abdominal pain, anorexia, diarrhea, elevated liver enzymes, increased appetite, nausea, vomiting
HEME: Lymphopenia, neutropenia
MS: Arthralgia, elevated CPK level, muscle pain, myalgia
RESP: Asthma, bronchitis, **bronchospasm**, cough, dyspnea
SKIN: Erythema multiforme, rash, **Stevens–Johnson syndrome, toxic epidermal necrolysis**, urticaria

Other: Anaphylaxis, angioedema

Nursing Considerations

- Know that zanamivir is not recommended for prevention or treatment of influenza in patients with underlying airway disease such as asthma or chronic obstructive pulmonary disease, because of increased risk of bronchospasm. If used, it should be done with extreme caution.
- Be aware that zanamivir has not been shown to be effective for preventing influenza in a nursing home setting.
- Do not make zanamivir inhalation powder into an extemporaneous solution for administration by mechanical ventilation or nebulization. It must only be administered using the device provided.
- Be aware that the drug comes packaged in medicine disks and is inhaled by mouth using the delivery device contained in the package. Begin by locating the half-circle flap with the name "Relenza" on top. Lift this flap from the outer edge until it cannot go any farther. Flap must be straight up for the plastic needle to puncture both the top and bottom of the silver medicine disk inside. Keeping the Diskhaler level, click the flap down into place.
- Administer zanamivir by having patient breathe all the way out before putting the white mouthpiece into her mouth, while keeping the Diskhaler level so the medicine does not spill out. Have patient close lips firmly around the mouthpiece but not to cover the small holes on either side of it. A breath through the mouth should be taken as steadily and as deeply as possible; then patient should hold breath for a few seconds. To take another inhalation, move to the next blister and repeat the steps again.

WARNING Monitor patient closely following administration for bronchospasms. In the event patient develops bronchospasms, stop zanamivir therapy immediately, notify prescriber, and provide supportive emergency care, as ordered.

WARNING Observe patient closely for an allergic reaction when zanamivir is administered, such as the development of hives, oropharyngeal edema, or rash. Know that anaphylaxis and skin reactions such as erythema multiforme, Stevens–Johnson syndrome, and toxic epidermal necrolysis have occurred. If present, stop zanamivir therapy immediately, notify prescriber, and provide supportive emergency care, as ordered.

- Be aware that although uncommon, abnormal behavior and delirium have occurred after administration of zanamivir, especially in children. Although the onset is abrupt, rapid resolution usually occurs once drug is discontinued.

PATIENT TEACHING

- Instruct patient who is scheduled to use an inhaled bronchodilator at the same time as zanamivir to use the bronchodilator before taking zanamivir.
- Tell patient to administer zanamivir doses at the same times each day. Instruct patient that if a dose is missed, it should be taken as soon as remembered. However, if it is within 2 hours of the next dose, patient should wait and take the next dose at the scheduled time. The dose should not be doubled.
- Instruct patient, parents, or caregivers on how to administer zanamivir using the device provided. Tell patient that drug comes packaged in medicine disks and is inhaled by mouth using the delivery device contained in the package. She should begin by locating the half-circle flap with the name "Relenza" on top. She should then lift this flap from the outer edge until it cannot go any farther. Flap must be straight up for the plastic needle to puncture both the top and bottom of the silver medicine disk inside. Keeping the Diskhaler level, she should click the flap down into place.
- Instruct patient, when ready to administer drug, to breathe all the way out before putting the white mouthpiece into her mouth. She should keep the Diskhaler level so the medicine does not spill out. Then tell her to close her lips firmly around the mouthpiece but not to cover the small holes on either side of it and breathe in through her mouth steadily and as deeply as she can. She should then hold her breath for a few seconds. To take another inhalation, she should move to the next blister and repeat the steps again.
- Advise patient that if bronchospasms occur, she should stop taking zanamivir, notify prescriber, and seek immediate medical attention. Instruct patient with

underlying asthma or chronic obstructive pulmonary disease to have a fast-acting bronchodilator available.
- Alert patient and parents that, although uncommon, abnormal behavior, confusion, delirium, and seizures have occurred, especially in children. Notify prescriber if present and expect drug to be discontinued. Keep child safe until behavior returns to normal.
- Inform patient that zanamivir is not a substitute for receiving an annual flu vaccination. Also tell patient that drug does not reduce the risk of transmission of influenza to others.

ziconotide

Prialt

Class and Category

Pharmacologic class: Nonopioid N-type calcium channel blocker
Therapeutic class: Analgesic
Pregnancy category: C

Indications and Dosages

➤ *To manage severe chronic pain in patients intolerant of or refractory to other pain management measures*

INTRATHECAL

Adults. *Initial:* 2.4 mcg daily (0.1 mcg/hr), increased as needed by 2.4 mcg daily but no more than three times/wk. *Maximum:* 19.2 mcg/day (0.8 mcg/hr).

Contraindications

Conditions or treatments that make intrathecal use hazardous (infection at microinfusion site, spinal canal obstruction that impairs CSF circulation , uncontrolled bleeding diathesis), history of psychosis, hypersensitivity to ziconotide or its components.

Interactions

DRUGS

CNS depressants: Increased risk of adverse CNS reactions

Adverse Reactions

CNS: Abnormal gait, agitation, anxiety, aphasia, asthenia, ataxia, chills, confusion, CSF abnormality, **CVA**, decreased reflexes, depression, difficulty concentrating, dizziness, dysesthesia, emotional lability, fever, hallucinations, headache, hostility, hyperesthesia, hypertonia, incoordination, insomnia, malaise, memory loss, **meningitis**, nervousness, neuralgia, paranoia, paresthesia, psychosis, **seizures**, somnolence, speech disorder, stupor, **suicidal ideation**, syncope, tremor, twitching, unusual dreams, vertigo
CV: Atrial fibrillation, **bradycardia**, chest pain, edema, hypertension, **hypotension**, orthostatic hypotension, peripheral edema, tachycardia, T-wave changes on ECG, vasodilation
EENT: Abnormal vision, diplopia, dry mouth, nystagmus, pharyngitis, photophobia, rhinitis, sinusitis, taste perversion, tinnitus
GI: Abdominal pain, anorexia, constipation, diarrhea, indigestion, nausea, vomiting
GU: Acute renal failure, dysuria, urinary hesitancy or incontinence, urine retention, UTI
HEME: Anemia
MS: Arthralgia, arthritis, back pain, leg cramps, muscle spasms or weakness, myalgia, myasthenia, neck pain or rigidity, **rhabdomyolysis**
RESP: Aspiration pneumonia, bronchitis, cough, dyspnea, lung disorder, pneumonia, **respiratory distress**
SKIN: Cellulitis, diaphoresis, dry skin, ecchymosis, pruritus, rash
Other: Catheter site infection or pain, dehydration, elevated CK level, flu-like symptoms, generalized pain, **hypokalemia**, **sepsis**, viral infection, weight loss

Nursing Considerations

- Determine if patient will receive ziconotide therapy by external microinfusion device and catheter or implanted variable-rate microinfusion device. Then, follow manufacturer guidelines for programming the microinfusion devise and doing an initial pump fill, including priming using only undiluted 25-mcg/ml solution and rinsing the internal pump surfaces with 2 ml of drug three times.
- Use strict aseptic technique when preparing ziconotide solution and filling, refilling, or handling the microinfusion device.
- Be aware that initial ziconotide dosage shouldn't exceed 2.4 mcg daily.
- Know that refills can use diluted or undiluted ziconotide solutions. If diluting

Mechanism of Action

Pain sensations are transmitted by sensory neurons that travel through N-type calcium channels in the dorsal horn of the spinal cord and ascend to the brain, as shown below.

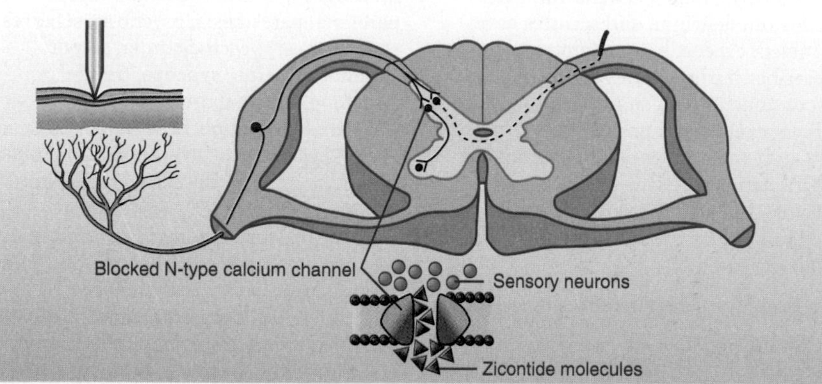

Ziconotide binds to N-type calcium channels on primary nociceptive afferent nerves in superficial layers of the dorsal horn, as shown below. By blocking these channels, the drug prevents excitatory neurotransmitter release in primary afferent nerve terminals and relieves pain.

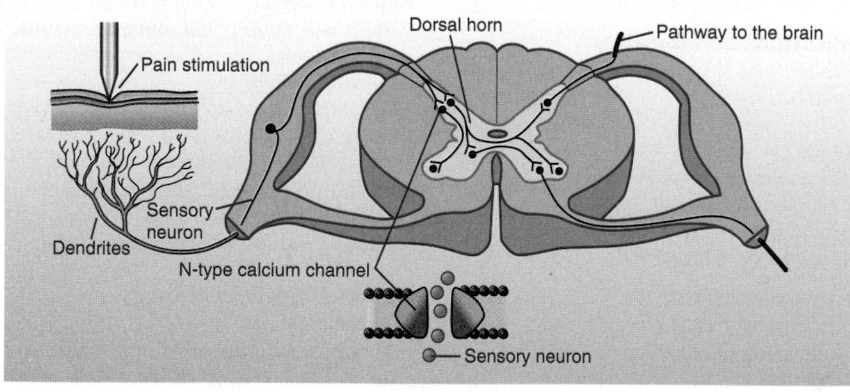

ziconotide, use only normal saline solution without preservatives, following manufacturer guidelines. Refrigerate solution up to 24 hours if it isn't used immediately. Expect device to need refilling about every 40 days if ziconotide is given diluted or about 60 days if given undiluted.

- Assess patient's response to ziconotide regularly. Notify prescriber if pain relief isn't adequate, and expect to increase dosage.
- Check infusion site regularly, and be aware that meningitis can occur within 24 hours after contamination of delivery system; a disconnected catheter is the most common problem with external devices.
- Monitor patient closely for evidence of meningitis, such as altered mental status,

headache, nausea, stiff neck, vomiting, and occasionally seizures caused by inadvertent contamination of microinfusion device or catheter tract used to deliver ziconotide. Notify prescriber immediately if you suspect meningitis.
- Monitor patient closely for changes in consciousness or mood, cognitive impairment, or hallucinations, because ziconotide may cause severe psychiatric symptoms. If present, notify prescriber and expect to decrease dosage or stop ziconotide. Provide supportive care, as prescribed, for adverse effects. Tell prescriber again if adverse effects are still present after 2 weeks.
- Expect to stop ziconotide temporarily if patient becomes stuporous or unresponsive during therapy; drug may be continued when patient reverts to previous mental status.
- Know that ziconotide can be stopped abruptly without causing withdrawal symptoms.
- Monitor patient's serum CK level every other week for first month of therapy and monthly thereafter, as ordered. If levels become elevated, notify prescriber and expect to decrease ziconotide dosage or stop drug until levels return to normal.

PATIENT TEACHING
- Teach caregiver how to care for external device, if present. Emphasize the need for strict aseptic technique with the microinfusion device and connections and the need to check the site often for problems, such as a disconnected catheter, which increase the risk of meningitis.
- Review evidence of meningitis with caregiver, and tell her to contact prescriber immediately if she suspects meningitis.
- Advise patient to notify prescriber if pain relief isn't adequate.
- Tell patient and caregiver to notify prescriber immediately about muscle pain, soreness, and weakness with or without a change in mental status including depression, mood changes, or suicidal ideation, or dark urine.
- Advise patient to avoid hazardous activities that require mental alertness or motor coordination while receiving ziconotide.
- Caution patient to avoid taking OTC preparations that contain CNS depressants because of the risk of adverse CNS effects.

zidovudine

Retrovir

Class and Category

Pharmacologic class: Nucleoside reverse transcriptase inhibitor
Therapeutic class: Antiretroviral
Pregnancy category: Not classified

Indications and Dosages

➤ *As adjunct to treat human immunodeficiency viral type (HIV-1) infection*

CAPSULES, SYRUP

Adults. 300 mg twice daily.
Children less than 18 years weighing 30 kg (66 lb) or more. 300 mg twice daily or 200 mg three times daily. Alternatively, 240 mg/m^2 body surface area (BSA) twice daily or 160 mg/m^2 BSA three times daily. *Maximum:* 600 mg daily.
Infants at least 4 weeks old and children less than 18 years weighing 9 kg (19.8 lb) to less than 30 kg (66 lb). 9 mg/kg twice daily or 6 mg/kg three times daily. Alternatively, 240 mg/m^2 body surface area (BSA) twice daily or 160 mg/m^2 BSA three times daily. *Maximum:* 300 mg twice daily.
Infants at least 4 weeks old and weighing at least 4 kg (8.8 lb) but less than 9 kg (19.8 lb). 12 mg/kg twice daily or 8 mg/kg three times daily. Alternatively, 240 mg/m^2 BSA twice daily or 160 mg/m^2 BSA three times daily. *Maximum:* 300 mg twice daily.

I.V. INFUSION

Adults. 1 mg/kg at a constant rate over 1 hr every 4 hr.

➤ *To prevent maternal-fetal HIV-1 transmission*

CAPSULES, SYRUP

Pregnant women at greater than 14 weeks of pregnancy. 100 mg five times daily until start of labor.

I.V. INFUSION

Pregnant women during labor and delivery. 2 mg/kg infused over 1 hr followed by a continuous I.V. infusion of 1 mg/kg/hr until umbilical cord is clamped.

SYRUP

Neonate 12 hr after birth. 2 mg/kg every 6 hr for 6 wk.

I.V. INFUSION

Neonate 12 hr after birth. 1.5 mg/kg infused over 30 min, every 6 hr for 6 wk.

DOSAGE ADJUSTMENT For adult patients on dialysis or who have a creatinine clearance of less than 15 ml/min, oral dosage reduced to 100 mg every 6 to 8 hr and the intravenous dosage interval increased to every 6 to 8 hr.

Mechanism of Action

After being phosphorylated to its active metabolite, the metabolite inhibits the DNA- and RNA-dependent polymerase activities of HIV-1 reverse transcriptases via DNA chain termination after incorporation of the nucleotide analogue into viral DNA. This destroys activity of the HIV-1 viruses.

Contraindications

Hypersensitivity to zidovudine or its components

Interactions

DRUGS

bone marrow suppressive or cytotoxic agents, ganciclovir, interferon alfa, ribavirin: Possibly increased hematologic toxicity of zidovudine

doxorubicin, nucleoside analogues affecting DNA replication such as ribavirin, stavudine: Antagonistic relationship between the two drugs

Adverse Reactions

CNS: Anxiety, asthenia, chills, confusion, decreased reflexes, depression, dizziness, fatigue, headache, insomnia, irritability, loss of mental acuity, malaise, mania, nervousness, neuropathy, paresthesia, **seizures**, somnolence, syncope, tremor, vertigo

CV: Cardiomyopathy, chest pain, **congestive heart failure**, **ECG abnormalities**, edema, left ventricular dilation, vasculitis

EENT: Amblyopia; ear discharge, erythema, pain, or swelling; hearing loss; macular edema; mouth ulcers; nasal congestion or discharge; oral mucosa pigmentation; photophobia; rhinitis; sinusitis; stomatitis; taste perversion

ENDO: Cushingoid appearance, fat redistribution, gynecomastia

GI: Abdominal cramps or pain, anorexia, constipation, diarrhea, dyspepsia, dysphagia, elevated liver or pancreatic enzymes, flatulence, **hepatic decompensation**, **hepatitis**, hyperbilirubinemia, jaundice, nausea, **pancreatitis**, **severe hepatomegaly with steatosis**, splenomegaly, vomiting

GU: Hematuria, urinary frequency or hesitancy

HEME: Anemia, **aplastic anemia**, **granulocytopenia**, **hemolytic anemia**, **leukopenia**, macrocytosis, **neutropenia**, **pancytopenia with marrow hypoplasia**, **pure red cell aplasia**, **thrombocytopenia**

MS: Arthralgia, back pain, elevated CPK and LDH levels, musculoskeletal pain, muscle spasm, myalgia, myopathy, myositis, **rhabdomyolysis**

RESP: Abnormal breath sounds, cough, dyspnea, wheezing

SKIN: Diaphoresis, pigmentation changes in nail and skin, pruritus, rash, **Stevens–Johnson syndrome**, **toxic epidermal necrolysis**, urticaria

Other: Anaphylaxis, **angioedema**, flu-like symptoms, generalized pain, intravenous site irritation or pain, **lactic acidosis**, lymphadenopathy, weight loss

Nursing Considerations

- Use zidovudine cautiously in patients with hepatic dysfunction, including liver cirrhosis, because of potential for hepatic dysfunction during zidovudine therapy.
- Be aware that dosing regimen for the prevention of maternal-fetal HIV-1 transmission includes three phases. First, oral zidovudine is given to the mother beginning after 14 weeks of pregnancy and continued throughout the remainder of pregnancy, stopping at the start of labor. Then drug is given intravenously to the mother during labor until the umbilical cord is cut. Lastly, drug is then given to the newborn beginning 12 hours after birth and continued for 6 weeks. Use an appropriate-sized syringe with 0.1-ml graduation to ensure dosing of the syrup formulation in neonates.
- Know that pediatric dosage is based upon body weight in kg or alternatively on BSA. In some cases, the dosage calculated by body weight will not be the same as that calculated by BSA.

- Dilute intravenous injection solution by adding drug to 5% dextrose injection solution to achieve a concentration no greater than 4 mg/ml. Use within 8 hours if left at room temperature and 24 hours if refrigerated.
- Be aware that zidovudine injection solution should never be given as a bolus injection or by rapid infusion, nor should it be administered intramuscularly.
- Be aware that the vial stoppers on zidovudine injection bottles contain natural rubber latex and could cause a hypersensitivity reaction if touched by someone with a latex allergy.

WARNING Know that lactic acidosis and severe hepatomegaly with steatosis have occurred with zidovudine therapy, and death has occurred in some patients. Risk factors include presence of obesity, prolonged nucleoside exposure, and being a woman. However, know that lactic acidosis and severe hepatomegaly with steatosis have also occurred in patients with no known risk factors. Expect drug to be discontinued in any patient who develops clinical or laboratory findings suggestive of lactic acidosis or pronounced hepatotoxicity, even in the absence of marked transaminase elevations.

- Monitor patient's hematologic status closely during zidovudine therapy, as ordered. Know that if patient's hemoglobin falls to less than 7.5 g/dl or the reduction is greater than 25% of baseline and/or granulocyte count falls to less than 750 cells/mm^3 or the reduction is greater than 50% of baseline, notify prescriber and expect zidovudine therapy to be withheld until marrow recovery occurs. Even with marrow recovery, adjunctive supportive measures such as epoetin alfa might be required when zidovudine therapy is restarted.
- Know that coadministration of ribavirin and zidovudine is not advised, because ribavirin exacerbates the development of zidovudine-induced anemia.
- Be aware that patients receiving interferon alfa and/or ribavirin in addition to zidovudine should be monitored closely for treatment-associated toxicities, especially anemia, hepatic decompensation, and neutropenia. Dosage reduction or discontinuation of interferon alfa, ribavirin, or both may be required if zidovudine toxicities become serious.
- Be aware that prolonged therapy increases the risk of myopathy and myositis.
- Be aware that immune reconstitution syndrome has occurred in patients treated with combination antiretroviral therapy, including zidovudine. The inflammatory response predisposes susceptible patients to opportunistic infections such as cytomegalovirus, *Mycobacterium avium* infection, *Pneumocystis jiroveci* pneumonia, or tuberculosis. Autoimmune disorders such as Graves' disease, Guillain–Barré syndrome, or polymyositis have also occurred. Report sudden or unusual adverse reactions to prescriber.
- Observe patient for redistribution of body fat, including breast enlargement, central obesity, development of buffalo hump, facial wasting, and peripheral wasting, which may produce a cushingoid-type appearance.

PATIENT TEACHING

- Instruct parents or caregivers to take extra care in measuring dosage when using syrup that will be given to babies and children, to avoid dosage errors. Caution them to use an appropriately sized syringe with 0.1-ml graduation to ensure accurate dosing of the syrup formulation. Do not use the common household teaspoon.
- Tell patient that if she misses a dose of zidovudine, she should take it as soon as she remembers, but should not double the next dose or take more than prescribed.

WARNING Instruct patient to seek immediate medical attention if she experiences a serious allergic reaction, such as having difficulty breathing, hives, or swelling of her face, lips, tongue, or throat.

- Inform patient that periodic laboratory studies will have to be performed and that compliance with these appointments is essential for early detection of adverse reactions. If toxicity develops, inform her that she may need transfusions or zidovudine to be discontinued.
- Alert patient that fat accumulation and redistribution may occur during zidovudine therapy.

WARNING Alert patient that severe conditions may develop while taking zidovudine. Encourage her to stop taking drug and seek medical attention immediately if she experiences any persistent, severe, or unusual symptoms.

- Advise patient to inform all prescribers of zidovudine therapy.

WARNING Inform patient that zidovudine may cause lactic acidosis, which if not treated, could be fatal. Tell patient to seek immediate medical attention if she develops breathing difficulty, cold or numb feeling in her arms and legs, dizziness, fast or uneven heart rate, muscle pain or weakness, nausea, vomiting, or any other unexpected or unusual signs or symptoms.

- Tell mothers that breastfeeding should not be done during zidovudine therapy.

zileuton

Zyflo CR

Class and Category

Pharmacologic class: Leukotriene inhibitor
Therapeutic class: Antiasthmatic
Pregnancy category: C

Indications and Dosages

➤ *To prevent or treat chronic asthma*

E.R. TABLETS

Adults and adolescents. 1,200 mg twice daily. *Maximum:* 2,400 mg daily.

Route	Onset	Peak	Duration
P.O.	2 hr	Unknown	Unknown

Mechanism of Action

Inhibits formation of leukotrienes found mainly in eosinophils, macrophages, mast cells, monocytes, and neutrophils. Normally, leukotrienes augment capillary permeability, eosinophil and neutrophil migration, leukocyte adhesion, monocyte and neutrophil aggregation, and smooth-muscle contraction. By inhibiting leukotriene formation, zileuton causes bronchial relaxation and decreases bronchial hyperresponsiveness, edema and vascular leakage, eosinophil movement, and mucus secretion.

Contraindications

Hepatic impairment, hypersensitivity to zileuton or its components

Interactions

DRUGS

propranolol, terfenadine: Increased effects of these drugs
theophylline: Doubled theophylline level
warfarin: Prolonged INR and PT

Adverse Reactions

CNS: Asthenia, dizziness, fever, headache, hypertonia, insomnia, malaise, nervousness, neuropsychiatric events, sleep disorders, somnolence
CV: Chest pain
EENT: Conjunctivitis
GI: Abdominal pain, constipation, flatulence, indigestion, nausea, vomiting
GU: UTI, vaginitis
MS: Arthralgia, myalgia, neck pain or rigidity
SKIN: Pruritus, rash, urticaria
Other: Lymphadenopathy

Nursing Considerations

- Be aware that zileuton should not be used in children under the age of 12 because of the risk of hepatotoxicity.
- Know that zileuton shouldn't be used to treat bronchospasm during an acute asthma attack or status asthmaticus; it can't relieve symptoms quickly enough.
- Monitor serum ALT level, as ordered, usually before treatment starts, once a month for 3 months, every 2 to 3 months for remainder of first year, and periodically thereafter during therapy.
- Monitor results of CBC and liver and pulmonary function tests during therapy.
- Monitor patient taking zileuton for neuropsychiatric symptoms including worsening of preexisting psychiatric illness. If present, notify prescriber immediately, institute safety measures and expect drug to be discontinued.

PATIENT TEACHING

- Advise patient to take drug exactly as prescribed, in evenly spaced doses, every day. Emphasize need to take drug even during acute exacerbations and symptom-free periods.
- Urge patient not to chew, crush, or cut capsule but to swallow it whole.

- Instruct patient to continue using rescue inhalants, as prescribed, for acute attacks.
- Teach patient how to use peak-flow meter to assess and monitor pulmonary function.
- Instruct patient to report any abnormal behavior or thoughts.
- Encourage women who become pregnant while taking zileuton to enroll in the pregnancy exposure registry by calling 1-877-311-8972. Also, advise mothers wishing to breastfeed their infant to discuss breastfeeding with prescriber before doing so.

zinc acetate

Galzin

zinc chloride

zinc gluconate

Orazinc

zinc sulfate

Orazinc, Verazinc, Zinc 15, Zinc-220, Zinca-Pak, Zincate

Class and Category

Pharmacologic class: Trace element, mineral
Therapeutic class: Nutritional supplement
Pregnancy category: A (oral), C (I.V.)

Indications and Dosages

➤ *To prevent zinc deficiency based on recommended daily allowances*

CAPSULES, E.R. TABLETS, LOZENGES, TABLETS

Men and boys age 14 and over. 11 mg daily.
Women. 8 mg daily.
Pregnant women. 11 mg daily.
Breastfeeding women. 12 mg daily.
Adolescent females ages 14 to 18. 9 mg daily.
Pregnant adolescents ages 14 to 18. 12 mg daily.
Breastfeeding adolescents ages 14 to 18. 13 mg daily.
Children ages 9 to 13. 8 mg daily.
Children ages 4 to 8. 5 mg daily.
Children ages 1 to 3. 3 mg daily.
Infants ages 7 to 13 months. 3 mg daily.
Newborns to 6 months. 2 mg daily.

I.V. INFUSION

Adults and children. 2.5 to 4 mg daily added to total parenteral nutrition (TPN) solution. *Maximum:* 12 mg daily.
Children from birth to age 5. 100 mcg/kg daily added to TPN solution.
Premature infants weighing up to 3 kg. 300 mcg/kg daily added to TPN solution.

➤ *To treat zinc deficiency*

CAPSULES, E.R. TABLETS, LOZENGES, TABLETS

Adults and children. Dosage individualized based on severity of deficiency.

I.V. INFUSION

Adults and adolescents. 2.5 to 4 mg daily added to TPN solution. *Maximum:* 12 mg daily.
Children from birth to age 5. 100 mcg/kg daily added to TPN solution.
Premature infants weighing up to 3 kg. 300 mcg/kg daily added to TPN solution.

➤ *As adjunct maintenance therapy for patients previously treated for Wilson's disease*

CAPSULES

Adults. 50 mg three times a day.
Pregnant women. 25 mg three times a day, increased to 50 mg three times a day if drug effectiveness decreases.
Children age 10 and over. 25 mg three times a day, increased to 50 mg three times a day if drug effectiveness decreases.

Mechanism of Action

Needed for proper function of more than 200 metalloenzymes (those with tightly bound zinc atoms as an integral part of their structure), including alcohol dehydrogenase, alkaline phosphatase, carbonic anhydrase, carboxypeptidase A, and RNA polymerase. Zinc also helps maintain cell membrane, nucleic acid, and protein structure and is essential for certain physiologic functions, including cell growth and division, dark adaptation and night vision, host immunity, sexual maturation and reproduction, taste acuity, and wound healing. This mineral also provides cellular antioxidant protection by scavenging free radicals.

In addition, zinc acetate interferes with intestinal absorption of copper and produces a protein that binds with copper, preventing its transfer to blood. Bound copper is then excreted in stools, thus decreasing copper toxicity in Wilson's disease.

Contraindications

Hypersensitivity to zinc or its components

Interactions

DRUGS

copper supplements: Impaired copper absorption (with large doses of zinc)
oral iron supplements, oral phosphate salts, penicillamine, phosphorus-containing drugs: Decreased zinc absorption
quinolones, tetracyclines: Decreased absorption and possibly decreased effectiveness of these antibiotics
thiazide diuretics: Increased urinary excretion of zinc
zinc-containing preparations: Increased blood zinc level

FOODS

fiber- or phylate-containing foods (such as bran, cereals, whole-grain breads), phosphorus-containing foods (including milk, poultry): Decreased zinc absorption

Adverse Reactions

CNS: Neurologic deterioration
GI: Elevated alkaline phosphate, amylase, and lipase; gastric irritation; nausea; vomiting

Nursing Considerations

WARNING Don't give I.V. zinc preparations that contain benzyl alcohol to neonates or premature infants because this preservative may cause a fatal toxic syndrome characterized by metabolic acidosis and CNS, circulatory, renal and respiratory function impairment.

- Give oral zinc supplements 1 hour before or 2 to 3 hours after meals; at least 2 hours after giving oral iron supplements (to prevent decreased zinc absorption) or copper supplements (to prevent decreased copper absorption); and at least 6 hours before or 2 hours after administering quinolone or tetracycline antibiotics (to prevent decreased absorption of these drugs).
- Monitor patient receiving long-term zinc therapy for sideroblastic anemia, which may result from zinc-induced copper deficiency and is characterized by anemia, bone marrow problems, granulocytopenia, leukopenia, and neutropenia. Be aware that these effects are reversible after zinc is discontinued.
- Monitor patient with preexisting copper deficiency for exacerbation of this condition; zinc can decrease serum copper level.
- Monitor blood alkaline phosphatase level monthly, as ordered; it may increase.
- Be aware that zinc chloride contains aluminum, which may accumulate to the point of toxicity if patient's kidney function is impaired. Assess kidney function regularly.

PATIENT TEACHING

- Explain the need for a zinc supplement.
- Instruct patient to take zinc on an empty stomach, at least 1 hour before or 2 hours after meals. Caution her not to take zinc within 2 hours of iron or copper supplements or phosphorus-containing drugs.
- Instruct patient to let zinc lozenge dissolve in mouth slowly and completely and not to swallow it whole or chew it. Advise her not to take zinc lozenges more often than directed.

ziprasidone hydrochloride

Geodon, Zeldox (CAN)

ziprasidone mesylate

Geodon for Injection

Class and Category

Pharmacologic class: Benzisoxazole
Therapeutic class: Antipsychotic
Pregnancy category: C

Indications and Dosages

➤ *To treat schizophrenia*

CAPSULES

Adults. *Initial:* 20 mg twice daily with food. Dosage increased as indicated every 2 or more days. *Usual:* 20 to 80 mg twice daily with food. *Maximum:* 80 mg twice daily.

➤ *To treat acute agitation in schizophrenic patients*

I.M. INJECTION

Adults. *Initial:* 10 to 20 mg. 10 mg dose may be given every 2 hr up to maximum dose; 20 mg dose may be given every 4 hr up to maximum dose. *Maximum:* 40 mg daily for no longer than 3 consecutive days.

➤ *To treat acute manic or mixed episodes of bipolar disorder*

CAPSULES

Adults. *Initial:* 40 mg twice daily. with food on day 1; then increased to 60 or 80 mg on day 2 with food with further adjustments as needed.

➤ *As adjunct to lithium or valproate for maintenance treatment of bipolar I disorder*

CAPSULES

Adults. Same dose patient was initially stabilized on that falls within 40 to 80 mg twice daily and taken with food.

Mechanism of Action

Selectively blocks dopamine and serotonin receptors in the mesocortical tract of the CNS, thereby suppressing psychotic symptoms.

Incompatibilities

Don't mix injection form with drugs or solvents other than sterile water for injection.

Contraindications

Concurrent use of other drugs that prolong QT interval, history of arrhythmia or prolonged QT interval, hypersensitivity to ziprasidone or its components, recent acute MI, uncompensated heart failure

Interactions

DRUGS

antihypertensives: Additive antihypertensive effects
carbamazepine: Possibly decreased blood ziprasidone level
CNS depressants: Increased CNS depression
dopamine agonists, levodopa: Decreased therapeutic effects of these drugs
drugs that prolong QT interval (including dofetilide, pimozide, quinidine, sotalol, sparfloxacin, and thioridazine): Increased risk of prolonged QT interval, torsades de pointes, and sudden death
ketoconazole: Possibly increased blood ziprasidone level

FOODS

all foods: Increased ziprasidone absorption

Adverse Reactions

CNS: Agitation, akathisia, amnesia, anxiety, asthenia, **CVA**, depression, dizziness, dystonia, extrapyramidal reactions, headache, hypertonia, hypomania, insomnia, mania, **neuroleptic malignant syndrome**, paresthesia, personality or speech disorder, **serotonin syndrome**, somnolence, syncope, **suicidal ideation**, tardive dyskinesia, tremor
CV: Bradycardia, chest pain, hypercholesterolemia, hypertension, orthostatic hypotension, **prolonged QT interval**, tachycardia, thrombophlebitis, vasodilation
EENT: Abnormal vision, dry mouth, increased salivation, rhinitis, tongue swelling
ENDO: Dysmenorrhea, hyperglycemia, hyperprolactinemia
GI: Abdominal pain, anorexia, constipation, diarrhea, dysphagia, indigestion, nausea, **rectal bleeding**, vomiting
GU: Priapism, urinary incontinence
HEME: Agranulocytosis, **leukopenia**, **neutropenia**
MS: Arthralgia, back pain, dysarthria, myalgia
RESP: Cough, **pulmonary embolism**, upper respiratory tract infection
SKIN: Allergic dermatitis, diaphoresis, **exfoliative dermatitis**, furunculosis, rash, **Stevens–Johnson syndrome**, urticaria
Other: Accidental injury, **angioedema**, **drug reaction with eosinophilia and systemic symptoms (DRESS)**, flu-like symptoms, injection-site pain, weight gain

Nursing Considerations

WARNING Know that ziprasidone shouldn't be used to treat elderly patients with dementia-related psychosis because drug increases the risk of death in these patients.

- Protect ziprasidone vials from light. Reconstitute by adding 1.2 ml sterile water for injection to vial and shaking vigorously until drug is dissolved. Each ml of reconstituted solution contains 20 mg ziprasidone. Discard any unused portion.
- Give parenteral form only by I.M. route and administer cautiously to patients with renal dysfunction.
- Reconstituted drug may be stored 24 hours protected from light or up to 7 days if refrigerated and protected from light.

WARNING Assess cardiac rhythm in patients with hypokalemia or hypomagnesemia. Dizziness, palpitations, and syncope may indicate life-threatening torsades de pointes. Be prepared to stop ziprasidone if QT interval is greater than 500 msec.

- Monitor patient, especially elderly women, for involuntary movements, which may become irreversible tardive dyskinesia. If symptoms develop, notify prescriber immediately and be prepared to stop drug.
- Immediately report evidence of neuroleptic malignant syndrome, a rare but potentially fatal adverse reaction including acute renal failure, altered mental status, arrhythmia, blood pressure changes, diaphoresis, hyperpyrexia, irregular pulse, muscle rigidity, myoglobinuria (rhabdomyolysis), and tachycardia.
- Monitor patient's blood glucose and lipid levels routinely, as ordered, because drug increases risk of hypercholesterolemia and hyperglycemia.
- Monitor patient's CBC, as ordered, because serious adverse hematologic reactions may occur, such as agranulocytosis, leukopenia, and neutropenia. Monitor more frequently during first few months of therapy if patient has a history of drug-induced leukopenia, neutropenia, or significantly low WBC count. If abnormalities occur during ziprasidone therapy, watch for fever and other evidence of infection, notify prescriber, and expect to discontinue drug if severe.
- Monitor patient closely for evidence of suicidal thinking or behavior, especially when therapy starts or dosage changes.
- Know that long-standing hyperprolactinemia caused by ziprasidone therapy may cause decreased bone density if associated with hypogonadism.
- Institute fall precautions.

PATIENT TEACHING

- Instruct patient to take ziprasidone with food to increase absorption.
- Advise patient to avoid hazardous activities until CNS effects are known. Review fall precautions with patient and family or caregiver.
- Tell family to monitor patient closely for suicidal tendencies; patients with bipolar disorder or psychotic illness are at greater risk.
- Urge patient to rise slowly from lying or seated position to minimize orthostatic hypotension.
- Urge patient to notify prescriber immediately if he develops persistent, severe, sudden-onset, or unusual adverse reactions, especially a fever, rash, or swollen lymph nodes. If present, tell him to stop taking ziprasidone and seek urgent medical care.

zoledronic acid

Reclast, Zometa

Class and Category

Pharmacologic class: Bisphosphonate
Therapeutic class: Antiosteoporotic
Pregnancy category: D

Indications and Dosages

➤ *To treat hypercalcemia caused by cancer*

I.V. INFUSION (ZOMETA)

Adults. 4 mg infused over at least 15 min. After 7 days, retreatment with 4 mg if serum calcium level doesn't remain at or return to normal. *Maximum:* 4 mg/dose.

➤ *As adjunct treatment for patients with multiple myeloma or bony metastasis who are receiving standard antineoplastic therapy and have a creatinine clearance above 60 ml/min*

I.V. INFUSION (ZOMETA)

Adults. 4 mg infused over at least 15 min every 3 to 4 wk.

DOSAGE ADJUSTMENT If patient's creatinine clearance is 50 to 60 ml/min dosage decreased to 3.5 mg; if it's 40 to 49 ml/min dosage decreased to 3.3 mg; and if it's 30 to 39 ml/min/dosage decreased to 3 mg.

➤ *To treat postmenopausal osteoporosis in women; to treat osteoporosis in men; to treat and prevent glucocorticoid-induced osteoporosis in patients receiving daily prednisone doses of 7.5 mg or greater for at least 12 months*

I.V. INFUSION (RECLAST)
Adults. 5 mg infused over at least 15 min once yearly.

➤ *To treat Paget's disease of the bone*

I.V. INFUSION (RECLAST)
Adults. 5 mg infused over at least 15 min followed by 1,500 mg elemental calcium daily in divided doses and 800 international units of vitamin D daily for 2 wk.

➤ *To prevent osteoporosis in postmenopausal women*

I.V. INFUSION (RECLAST)
Adults. 5 mg infused over at least 15 min every 2 yr.

Mechanism of Action

Inhibits resorption of mineralized bone and cartilage by osteoclasts and induces osteoclast breakdown. In cancer-related hypercalcemia, hyperactive osteoclasts cause bone resorption and release of calcium into blood, which causes polyuria, GI disruption, progressive dehydration, and decreasing GFR. This, in turn, increases renal calcium resorption and worsens hypercalcemia. Zoledronic acid interrupts this process.

Incompatibilities

Don't mix zoledronic acid with calcium-containing I.V. solutions, such as lactated Ringer's solution.

Contraindications

Acute renal impairment, creatinine clearance less than 35 ml/min; hypersensitivity to zoledronic acid, other bisphosphonates, or their components

Interactions

DRUGS

aminoglycosides, calcitonin: Possibly additive serum calcium–lowering effect *angiogenesis inhibitors, chemotherapy, corticosteroids:* Increased risk of osteonecrosis of the jaw
loop diuretics, such as furosemide: Possibly increased risk of hypocalcemia
nephrotoxic drugs, NSAIDs: Increased risk of nephrotoxicity

Adverse Reactions

CNS: Anxiety, asthenia, chills, confusion, depression, dizziness, fatigue, fever, headache, hyperesthesia, hypoesthesia, insomnia, malaise, paresthesia, tremor, vertigo, weakness
CV: Atrial fibrillation, bradycardia, chest pain, hypertension, **hypotension,** peripheral edema
EENT: Blurred vision, conjunctivitis, dry mouth, episcleritis, iritis, orbital edema or inflammation, osteonecrosis of external auditory canal, scleritis, sore throat, stomatitis, taste disturbance, uveitis
GI: Abdominal pain, anorexia, constipation, diarrhea, dyspepsia, nausea, vomiting
GU: Acquired Fanconi syndrome, elevated serum creatinine level, hematuria, proteinuria, **renal insufficiency or failure,** UTI
HEME: Anemia, **neutropenia, thrombocytopenia**
MS: Arthralgia; atypical subtrochanteric and diaphyseal femoral fractures; incapacitating bone, joint, or muscle pain; muscle cramps or spasms; myalgia; osteonecrosis of the jaw, femur, or hip
RESP: Bronchospasm, cough, dyspnea, **exacerbation of asthma, interstitial lung disease,** upper respiratory tract infection
SKIN: Alopecia, dermatitis, diaphoresis, flushing, **Stevens–Johnson syndrome, toxic epidermal necrolysis,** urticaria
Other: Aggravated malignant neoplasm, anaphylaxis, angioedema, flu-like illness, **hypersensitivity reactions, hyperkalemia, hypernatremia, hypocalcemia, hypomagnesemia, hypophosphatemia,** infusion-site redness and swelling, weight gain

Nursing Considerations

- Be aware that zoledronic acid isn't indicated for hypercalcemia from hyperparathyroidism or other nontumor conditions.
- Verify pregnancy status of women of childbearing age before zoledronic acid therapy is initiated, because drug can cause fetal harm.
- Use cautiously in patients with aspirin sensitivity because biphosphonates such as zoledronic acid have caused bronchoconstriction in these patients.
- Make sure patient has had a dental checkup before zoledronic acid starts, especially if patient has cancer; is receiving chemotherapy, head or neck radiation, or

a corticosteroid; or has poor oral hygiene because risk of jaw osteonecrosis is increased in these patients, and invasive dental procedures during zoledronic acid therapy may worsen osteonecrosis.

- Expect to aggressively hydrate hypercalcemic patient with I.V. normal saline solution before and during zoledronic acid therapy, as prescribed, to achieve and maintain urine output of about 2 L daily.

WARNING Monitor fluid intake and output often during hydration, and assess patient, especially one with heart failure, for evidence of life-threatening overhydration.

- Expect to give acetaminophen, if not contraindicated, before zoledronic acid to reduce adverse reactions, such as fever, flu-like symptoms, headache, and myalgia. Joint swelling may also occur. These reactions usually occur within first 3 days after zoledronic acid administration and resolve within 3 days (although resolution may take up to 14 days for some patients).
- Be aware that Reclast doesn't require reconstitution.
- Know that hypocalcemia and mineral metabolism disorders must be treated before zoledronic acid therapy begins.
- Reconstitute Zometa by adding 5 ml of sterile water for injection to drug vial to yield solution that contains 4 mg of zoledronic acid. Make sure drug is completely dissolved before withdrawing prescribed dose. Further dilute in 100 ml normal saline solution or 5% dextrose injection, and infuse over no less than 15 minutes.
- Inspect reconstituted and diluted solution before giving drug, and discard it if particles or discoloration are present.
- Refrigerate reconstituted drug at 2° to 8° C (36° to 46° F) and discard after 24 hours.
- Give drug as a single I.V. solution in a separate I.V. line.

WARNING Be aware that a single dose of Zometa shouldn't exceed 4 mg, and that neither Zometa nor Reclast should be infused over less than 15 minutes; exceeding these limits may lead to significant renal function deterioration, which may progress to renal failure.

WARNING Assess patient's renal function, as ordered, before and during zoledronic acid therapy to detect renal deterioration. For patient with a normal serum creatinine level who develops an increase of 0.5 mg/dl within 2 weeks of receiving zoledronic acid, expect to withhold next dose until serum creatinine level is within 10% of patient's baseline value. For patient with an abnormal serum creatinine level who develops an increase of 1.0 mg/dl within 2 weeks of receiving drug, expect to withhold next dose until serum creatinine level is within 10% of baseline value.

- Monitor patient's serum calcium, magnesium, and phosphate levels, as ordered, during zoledronic acid therapy. If hypocalcemia, hypomagnesemia, or hypophosphatemia occurs, expect to give short-term supplemental therapy.
- Assess aspirin-sensitive asthma patients for worsening of respiratory symptoms during zoledronic acid therapy because other bisphosphonates have caused bronchoconstriction in these patients.
- Monitor patient for dehydration. If present, notify prescriber and expect drug to be withheld until dehydration has been corrected.
- Monitor patient for acute phase reaction (APR) that may occur within 3 days following intravenous administration of zoledronic acid. If patient develops flu-like symptoms such as arthralgias, bone pain, chills, fever, flushing, and myalgias, notify prescriber.
- Store drug at 25° C (77° F).
- Monitor patient closely for severe and occasionally incapacitating bone, joint, and/or muscle pain. If present, notify prescriber and expect to provide supportive care, as ordered, for pain relief.

PATIENT TEACHING

- Teach patient the importance of eating a nutritious diet, including adequate amounts of calcium and vitamin D. Tell patients with multiple myeloma and bone metastasis of solid tumors to check with prescriber about the need for an oral calcium supplement containing 500 mg of calcium and a multivitamin containing 400 international units of vitamin D.
- Instruct patient to drink at least two glasses of fluid within a few hours before receiving zoledronic acid intravenously.

- Advise patient to alert prescriber about bone, joint, or muscle pain or new or worsening groin, hip, or thigh pain.
- Instruct patient on proper oral hygiene and on need to notify prescriber before undergoing invasive dental procedures.
- Tell patient to notify prescriber if he notices blood or other changes in his urine or a change in amount of urine voided or frequency of voiding pattern. Stress importance of compliance in having regular blood tests that have been ordered to check his kidney function.
- Advise women of childbearing age to use effective contraception during and after zoledronic acid therapy and to notify prescriber immediately if they are or could be pregnant, because drug will have to be stopped. Alert female patients that drug may also impair fertility. Also inform these patients that breastfeeding is also not recommended during zoledronic acid therapy.
- Inform patient not to take other bisphosphonates concurrently, including Reclast if they are prescribed Zometa or Zometa if they are prescribed Reclast.

zolmitriptan

Zomig, Zomig ZMT

Class and Category

Pharmacologic class: Selective 5-hydroxytryptamine agonist
Therapeutic class: Antimigraine
Pregnancy category: C

Indications and Dosages

➤ *To treat acute migraine headache with or without aura*

ORAL DISINTEGRATING TABLETS, TABLETS

Adults. *Initial:* 1.25 or 2.5 mg, repeated in 2 hr as needed. *Maximum:* 5 mg as a single dose, 10 mg in 24 hr, or 3 headaches/mo.

NASAL SPRAY

Adults and children age 12 and over. *Initial:* 2.5 mg repeated in 2 hr as needed. Dosage increased to 5 mg/episode, as needed. *Maximum:* 5 mg as single dose; 10 mg/24 hr; or 4 headaches/mo.

DOSAGE ADJUSTMENT For patient with moderate to severe hepatic impairment, initial oral dosage using tablet form should not be higher than 1.25 mg and maximum dose should not exceed 5 mg in 24 hr. Nasal spray or oral disintegrating tablets are not recommended for these patients. For patient receiving cimetidine concurrently, single dosage should not exceed 2.5 mg and the maximum dosage should not exceed 5 mg in a 24-hr period.

Mechanism of Action

Constricts dilated and inflamed cranial blood vessels in the carotid circulation and inhibits production of proinflammatory neuropeptides by binding to receptors on intracranial blood vessels and sensory nerves in the trigeminal-vascular system to stimulate negative feedback, which halts the release of serotonin.

Contraindications

Basilar or hemiplegic migraine, cardiovascular disease, concurrent use of ergotamine-containing drugs, hypersensitivity to zolmitriptan or its components, ischemic heart disease, peripheral vascular disease, Prinzmetal's angina, symptomatic Wolff–Parkinson–White syndrome or other accessory pathway conduction disorder, use of another 5-hydroxytryptamine agonist within past 24 hours, use of an MAO inhibitor within 14 days

Interactions

DRUGS

acetaminophen: Delayed peak effect of acetaminophen (by 1 hour)
cimetidine: Prolonged zolmitriptan half-life
ergot alkaloids: Prolonged vasoconstriction effects
fluoxetine, fluvoxamine, paroxetine, sertraline: Hyperreflexia, lack of coordination, and weakness
MAO inhibitors: Increased zolmitriptan effects
naratriptan, rizatriptan, sumatriptan: Prolonged zolmitriptan effects
norepinephrine and serotonin reuptake inhibitors: Increased risk of developing serotonin syndrome
oral contraceptives, propranolol: Increased blood zolmitriptan level

Adverse Reactions

CNS: Asthenia, dizziness, hyperesthesia, paresthesia, somnolence, vertigo
CV: Angina, **coronary artery vasospasm**, hypertension, **MI**, palpitations, transient myocardial ischemia, **ventricular fibrillation or tachycardia**
EENT: Dry mouth, vision disturbance
GI: Abdominal pain, **bloody diarrhea**, dysphagia, **GI or splenic infarction**, indigestion, **ischemic colitis**, nausea, vomiting
MS: Myalgia; myasthenia; pain, pressure, or tightness in jaw, neck, or throat
SKIN: Diaphoresis, flushing
Other: Anaphylaxis, **angioedema**

Nursing Considerations

WARNING Monitor patient for signs and symptoms of vasoconstriction, which may lead to colonic and vascular ischemia with abdominal pain and bloody diarrhea, especially if patient has ischemic bowel disease or peripheral vascular disease (including Raynaud's phenomenon).

- Monitor elderly patients and those with hepatic impairment for increased blood pressure, and notify prescriber immediately if it occurs.
- Monitor patient closely for signs and symptoms of angina. If patient develops chest pain, notify prescriber.

WARNING Monitor patient closely for signs and symptoms of serotonin syndrome, which may include agitation, coma, diarrhea, hallucinations, hyperreflexia, hyperthermia, incoordination, labile blood pressure, nausea, tachycardia, and vomiting. Notify prescriber immediately because serotonin syndrome may be life-threatening. Be prepared to provide supportive care and discontinue zolmitriptan.

PATIENT TEACHING

- Instruct patient to take zolmitriptan exactly as prescribed. Tell her also not to take more than 10 mg in any 24-hour period, nor should she take drug for more than recommended number of times per month because overuse of drug may lead to exacerbation of headache. Tell her to be alert for migraine-like daily headaches developing or marked increase in frequency of migraine headaches that signals overuse may be occurring. Tell her to notify prescriber, as drug may no longer be as effective and drug withdrawal may be needed.
- Advise patient not to remove disintegrating tablet from blister pack until just before taking the tablet. Instruct her to peel open pack, let tablet dissolve on her tongue, and then swallow. Remind her not to break orally disintegrating tablet. However, if she is prescribed the regular 2.5-mg tablet form, she may break it in half, if needed for a 1.25-mg dose.
- Urge patient to notify prescriber about severe or unusual adverse reactions.
- Caution patient using nasal spray to avoid spraying drug into her eyes.
- Instruct patient not to take zolmitriptan within 24 hours of other drugs in the same class.
- Tell patient to inform all prescribers of zolmitriptan therapy because serious drug interactions may occur.
- Advise women of childbearing age to notify prescriber if pregnancy occurs, because of increased risk of preeclampsia during pregnancy. Also tell mothers wishing to breastfeed to discuss this with prescriber before doing so.

zolpidem tartrate

Ambien, Ambien CR, Edluar, Intermezzo, Zolpimist

Class, Category, and Schedule

Pharmacologic class: Imidazopyridine
Therapeutic class: Hypnotic
Pregnancy category: C
Controlled substance schedule: IV

Indications and Dosages

➤ *To provide short-term treatment of insomnia*

ORAL SPRAY, S.L. TABLETS, TABLETS

Adult men. 5 to 10 mg at bedtime for 7 to 10 days. *Maximum:* 10 mg daily.
Adult women. 5 mg at bedtime for 7 to 10 days. *Maximum:* 5 mg daily.

DOSAGE ADJUSTMENT For elderly men or debilitated male patients and men with mild to moderate hepatic impairment, dosage possibly reduced to 5 mg at bedtime, with a maximum of 5 mg daily for nursing facility residents.

E.R. TABLETS

Adult men. 6.25 or 12.5 mg immediately before bedtime.

Adult women. 6.25 mg immediately before bedtime.

DOSAGE ADJUSTMENT For elderly or debilitated patients and those with mild to moderate hepatic impairment, dosage reduced to 6.25 mg immediately before bedtime.

➤ *To treat insomnia when a middle-of-the-night awakening occurs and patient cannot get back to sleep and has more than 4 hours of sleep remaining before planned time of waking.*

S.L. TABLETS (INTERMEZZO)

Adult women. 1.75 mg once nightly, as needed.

Adult men. 3.5 mg once nightly, as needed.

DOSAGE ADJUSTMENT For elderly men or male patients with hepatic impairment or who take concomitant CNS depressants, dosage reduced to 1.75 mg once nightly, as needed.

Mechanism of Action

May potentiate the effects of gamma-aminobutyric acid (GABA) and other inhibitory neurotransmitters. By binding to specific benzodiazepine receptors in the limbic and cortical areas of the CNS, zolpidem increases GABA's inhibitory effects, blocks cortical and limbic arousal, and preserves deep sleep (stages 3 and 4).

Contraindications

Hypersensitivity to zolpidem or its components, ritonavir therapy, severe hepatic impairment

Interactions

DRUGS

barbiturates, chlorpromazine, general anesthetics, opioid agonists, other CNS depressants, phenothiazines, tramadol, tricyclic antidepressants: Possibly increased CNS depression and reduced psychomotor function

bupropion: Increased blood zolpidem level, possibly visual hallucinations, loss of alertness

CYP3A4 inducers such as rifampin, St. John's wort: Decreased effectiveness of zolpidem

CYP3A4 inhibitors such as ketoconazole: Increased risk of zolpidem-induced adverse reactions

desipramine, imipramine: Increased risk of visual hallucinations and reduced alertness

flumazenil: Antagonized sedative effect

haloperidol: Increased CNS depression

nevirapine: Decreased blood zolpidem level

selective serotonin-reuptake inhibitors: Increased risk of delusions, disorientation, and hallucinations

FOOD

all foods: Increased time to peak blood zolpidem level, decreased effects of zolpidem

ACTIVITIES

alcohol use: Increased CNS depression

Adverse Reactions

CNS: Abnormal thinking, aggressiveness, amnesia, asthenia, ataxia, behavioral changes, complex behaviors (such as sleep driving), confusion, decreased level of consciousness or inhibition, dizziness, drowsiness, euphoria, hallucinations, headache, insomnia, lethargy, paradoxical CNS stimulation (including agitation, euphoria, hallucinations, hyperactivity, and nightmares), **suicidal ideation**, vertigo, worsening of depression
EENT: Application site reactions from sublingual dose form (blisters, mucosal inflammation, oral ulcers), blurred vision, diplopia, **throat tightness**, visual abnormality
GI: Constipation, diarrhea, elevated liver enzymes, **hepatic injury**, hiccups, indigestion, jaundice, nausea, vomiting
GU: UTI
MS: Arthralgia, myalgia
RESP: Dyspnea, **respiratory depression**, upper or lower respiratory infection
Other: **Anaphylaxis**, **angioedema**, withdrawal symptoms

Nursing Considerations

- Use zolpidem cautiously in patients with additional disorders because it isn't known if zolpidem therapy might aggravate these conditions, especially conditions with respiratory impairment.
- Administer zolpidem just before patient's bedtime because drug has a rapid onset of action.
- Expect patient to receive no more than a 1-month supply of zolpidem for outpatient therapy.

WARNING Keep in mind if zolpidem is withdrawn abruptly (especially after prolonged therapy), monitor patient for withdrawal symptoms, such as abdominal cramps or discomfort, fatigue, flushing, inconsolable crying, light-headedness, nausea, nervousness, panic attack, rebound insomnia, and vomiting.
- Expect that zolpidem will produce anticonvulsant and muscle relaxant effects at high doses.
- Know that if patient takes other CNS depressants, expect to reduce zolpidem dosage, as prescribed.
- Monitor patient closely for suicidal tendencies, particularly when therapy starts or dosage increases because depression may worsen temporarily during these times, possibly leading to suicide.

WARNING Monitor patient closely for hypersensitivity reactions such as dyspnea, nausea, swelling, throat tightness, or vomiting. If present, discontinue zolpidem immediately, notify prescriber, and provide supportive care.
- Monitor neonates born to mothers using zolpidem late in the third trimester of pregnancy for hypotonia, respiratory depression, and sedation.

PATIENT TEACHING
- Caution patient to take drug exactly as prescribed and not to increase dosage unless directed by prescriber.
- Advise patient taking extended-release form to swallow tablet whole and not to break, chew, or crush it.
- Instruct patient to take zolpidem (except for Intermezzo brand of sublingual tablets) immediately before going to bed, on an empty stomach.
- Tell patient prescribed Intermezzo brand of sublingual tablets to keep tablets at bedside and take only once if awaken during the night but has more than 4 hours of sleep time remaining. Instruct patient to place tablet under his tongue and allow it to dissolve completely before swallowing. Tell him never to swallow the sublingual tablet whole.
- Advise patient to notify prescriber immediately about abdominal cramps or discomfort, fatigue, flushing, inconsolable crying, light-headedness, nausea, nervousness, panic attack, and vomiting.
- Instruct patient to stop taking zolpidem and seek emergency care if she has abnormal swelling, nausea, throat tightness, trouble breathing, or vomiting.
- Advise patient that zolpidem may produce abnormal behaviors during sleep, such as driving a car, eating, talking on the phone, or having sex without any recall of the event. If patient's family notices any such behavior or if patient sees evidence of such behavior upon awakening, prescriber should be notified.
- Tell patient that drug may cause drowsiness or decreased level of consciousness and even next-morning impairment from zolpidem use despite feeling fully awake. Advise patient to get a good night's sleep of at least 7 or 8 hours to help minimize this adverse effect. Tell her to take precautions against falling and not to perform any hazardous activity such as driving, especially after taking the drug and during the morning hours.
- Tell family or caregiver to observe patient closely for suicidal tendencies, especially when therapy starts or dosage changes.
- Advise mothers breastfeeding during zolpidem therapy to monitor the infant for excess sedation, hypotonia, and slower-than-normal breathing, because drug passes through into breast milk. Encourage mother instead to interrupt breastfeeding, if possible, and pump and then discard breast milk during zolpidem therapy and for 23 hours after drug administration in order to minimize drug exposure of the breastfed infant.

zonisamide

Zonegran

Class and Category

Pharmacologic class: Sulfonamide
Therapeutic class: Anticonvulsant
Pregnancy category: C

Indications and Dosages

➤ *As adjunct to treat partial seizures*

CAPSULES

Adults. *Initial:* 100 mg daily. Dosage increased by 100 mg daily every 2 wk, as needed. *Usual:* 200 to 400 mg daily. *Maximum:* 400 mg daily.

Mechanism of Action

May stop seizures and suppress their foci by blocking sodium channels and reducing voltage-dependent, inward currents from calcium channels. This action stabilizes neuronal membranes and suppresses synchronized neuronal hyperactivity.

Contraindications

Hypersensitivity to zonisamide, other sulfonamides, or their components

Interactions

DRUGS

carbamazepine, phenobarbital, phenytoin, valproate: Possibly decreased blood zonisamide level

CNS depressants: Additive CNS depressant effects

FOODS

grapefruit juice: Possibly decreased metabolism of zonisamide

Adverse Reactions

CNS: Abnormal gait, agitation, anxiety, asthenia, ataxia, confusion, depression, difficulty concentrating, dizziness, fatigue, headache, incoordination, insomnia, irritability, memory loss, nervousness, paresthesia, schizophrenia, **seizures**, somnolence, speech abnormalities, **suicidal ideation**, tremor

CV: Chest pain

EENT: Amblyopia, diplopia, dry mouth, nystagmus, pharyngitis, rhinitis, taste alteration, tinnitus

GI: Abdominal pain, **acute pancreatitis**, anorexia, constipation, diarrhea, dyspepsia, nausea, vomiting

GU: Renal calculi

HEME: Anemia, **leukopenia**, **thrombocytopenia**

MS: Elevated creatine phosphokinase levels, **rhabdomyolysis**

RESP: Increased cough

SKIN: Ecchymosis, pruritus, rash

Other: Angioedema, **drug reaction with eosinophilia and systemic symptoms (DRESS)**, flu-like symptoms, **metabolic acidosis**, weight loss

Nursing Considerations

- Obtain a serum bicarbonate level before starting zonisamide and then periodically during therapy, as prescribed because drug may cause metabolic acidosis, especially in patients with predisposing conditions or therapies or who are younger in age.

WARNING Monitor results of patient's CBC and other laboratory tests for signs of blood dyscrasias because zonisamide is a sulfonamide and can be absorbed systemically. Systemic absorption may result in life-threatening reactions, including agranulocytosis, aplastic anemia, and other blood dyscrasias; fulminant hepatic necrosis; Stevens–Johnson syndrome; and toxic epidermal necrolysis.

- Be aware that patients receiving doses of 300 mg daily or more are at increased risk for adverse CNS reactions, including decreased concentration, drowsiness, fatigue, and impaired speech.
- Monitor BUN and serum creatinine levels for signs of abnormally decreased glomerular filtration rate (GFR). Expect some decrease in GFR during first 4 weeks of treatment and return to baseline within 2 to 3 weeks after drug is discontinued.
- Monitor patient for signs and symptoms of renal calculi.
- Be aware that zonisamide shouldn't be discontinued abruptly because doing so may increase frequency of seizures.
- Monitor patient closely for evidence of suicidal thinking or behavior, especially when therapy starts or dosage changes.

PATIENT TEACHING

- Inform patient that zonisamide is usually prescribed with other anticonvulsants and that she should continue to take all drugs as prescribed.
- Instruct patient to swallow zonisamide capsules whole and not to break them open or chew them.
- Inform patient that prescriber may have to adjust zonisamide dosage over several

weeks or months before stable dose is achieved.

- Advise patient to use caution when driving or performing other activities that are hazardous or require mental alertness because zonisamide commonly causes decreased concentration, dizziness, and somnolence, particularly during first month of therapy.
- Advise patient to wear a medical identification bracelet or necklace or carry medical identification with information about her seizure disorder.
- Encourage patient to drink six to eight glasses of water each day to prevent kidney stones, unless contraindicated.
- Advise patient to rise slowly from a lying or seated position to reduce the risk of dizziness.
- Urge caregivers to watch closely for evidence of suicidal tendencies, especially when therapy starts or dosage changes, and to report concerns immediately to prescriber.
- Encourage woman who becomes pregnant while taking zonisamide to enroll in the North American antiepileptic drug pregnancy registry by calling 1-888-233-2334. Explain that the registry is collecting information about the safety of antiepileptic drugs during pregnancy.
- Instruct patient to notify prescriber immediately if seizures worsen, signs of blood abnormalities (fever, sore throat, oral ulcers, easy bruising) are present, signs of kidney stones occur (abdominal pain, blood in urine, sudden back pain), or a skin rash develops. She should also report signs and symptoms such as fast breathing, fatigue, irregular heart beat, loss of appetite, or palpitations.

Appendices

Safety Guidelines for Opioid Use

Pain relief has been a long-standing goal in health care for patients with pain. Patients may experience short-term pain as a result of an illness, injury, or medical or surgical procedure. Others experience chronic or persistent pain, defined as pain that lasts longer than 3 months or beyond normal tissue healing, which can drastically alter quality of life.

Opioids are powerful pain-reducing drugs, and their efficacy has made them increasingly popular for both short- and long-term pain management. However, opioids are also addictive, especially when used inappropriately. This has led to their abuse and misuse in society, along with a sharp increase in recent years of opioid-related overdoses and deaths.

In an effort to address the opioid crisis in the United States, the Food and Drug Administration (FDA) has formulated and implemented a plan called the *FDA Opioids Action Plan*. This plan details seven measures the FDA is using to combat this problem and includes:

- Expanding the use of advisory committees to approve any new drug application for an opioid that does not have abuse-deterrent properties, as well as seeking expert advice on opioid labeling regarding use by children.
- Providing clearer information to prescribers of opioids by making certain changes to immediate-release opioid labeling similar to those issued in 2013 for extended-release or long-acting opioid analgesics.
- Requiring drug companies to address issues of abuse and misuse associated with long-term use of their opioid drug products, provide predictors of opioid addiction, and explore other important issues related to opioid addiction through adherence to postmarketing requirements.
- Increasing training for prescribers on pain management and safe prescription use of opioid drugs.
- Encouraging the development of abuse-deterrent formulations, especially generic opioid formulations.
- Making naloxone more accessible to treat opioid overdose while at the same time encouraging drug companies to develop new classes of analgesics that would be as effective as opioids but not carry the same risks.
- Increasing the patient's understanding of the risks associated with opioids, and the risks of misuse by other persons who obtain them.

As a result of the FDA Opioids Action Plan, drug companies are now required to address several safety issues in their opioid drug labels (package inserts). Changes to individual sections of the drug label reflective of these safety issues are summarized here:

- **Boxed Warning**—Now includes warnings about addiction, abuse, and misuse; life-threatening respiratory depression; accidental ingestion; neonatal opioid withdrawal syndrome (NOWS); and any significant drug product-specific interactions that could raise the risk of adverse reactions associated with opioid use.
- **Indications and Usage**—Modified to emphasize that opioids are to be reserved for the management of pain only if alternative treatment options such as nonopioid analgesics cannot be used or are ineffective and the pain is severe enough to require an opioid analgesic.
- **Contraindications**—Includes patients with significant respiratory depression and patients with acute or severe bronchial asthma in an unmonitored setting or in the absence of resuscitative equipment.
- **Warning and Precautions**—Addresses each of the components found in the boxed warning as well as risks associated with concurrently administered central nervous system depressants; life-threatening respiratory depression in patients with chronic pulmonary disease, in the elderly or patients who are cachectic or debilitated; and the potential development of adrenal insufficiency with opioid use.
- **Adverse Reactions**—Lists all the serious adverse reactions addressed in the "Warnings and Precautions" section of the drug label as well as adding adrenal insufficiency and serotonin syndrome to the postmarketing section.
- **Drug Interactions**—Includes any significant drug-specific interactions that would increase the opioid effect as well as interactions between opioids and central nervous system depressants, including alcohol and between opioids and serotonergic drugs.
- **Specific Populations**—Additional information included regarding NOWS and potential for neonatal respiratory depression during delivery or with breastfeeding; potential risk for infertility with chronic use; and increased risk for respiratory depression in the elderly.
- **Drug Abuse and Dependence**—Details information about opioid abuse and dependence.
- **Overdosage**—Adds or modifies information to address seriousness and current treatment of opioid overdose.

- **Patient Counseling**—Includes information to be given to the patient on addiction, abuse, and misuse of opioids; risk of life-threatening respiratory depression or accidental ingestion; interactions with alcohol and other CNS depressants; potential for adrenal insufficiency and serotonin syndrome and what to report; potential for development of NOWS and embryo-fetal toxicity during pregnancy, respiratory depression in infants during delivery and with breastfeeding; how to dispose of the unused opioid; and the addition of a medication guide.

In addition, the Centers for Disease Control (CDC) has also released recommendations for use of opioids in treating chronic pain. These recommendations exclude patients who are in active cancer treatment, palliative care, or end-of-life care.

The CDC recommends that opioids not be used as first-line therapy in the treatment of chronic pain. Instead, nonpharmacologic therapies such as cognitive behavioral therapy or exercise, or nonopioid pharmacologic therapies such as NSAIDs, should be tried first. If opioids are prescribed, the CDC recommends that they be combined with nonpharmacologic or nonopioid pharmacologic therapy to provide greater benefits and lower opioid dosage requirements.

When opioids are used, the lowest possible effective dosage should be prescribed and therapy should start with immediate-release opioids rather than extended-release or long-acting opioids. In addition, the quantity prescribed should not go beyond the expected need for pain relief.

Closer follow-up is also recommended, with regular monitoring of patients to determine effectiveness of the prescribed pain measures. It is especially important to ascertain that the opioid is not causing harm. If benefits do not outweigh harm, it is recommended that the opioid dosage be reduced and then discontinued, if needed.

It is very important that the patient's response to pain relief measures be accurately measured and assessed. Only then can the goal to provide effective pain relief without causing the patient harm be achieved. Although opioid therapy has its place in pain management, it is important to understand that opioids are not always necessary and, if used inappropriately, can cause much harm, not only to the patient but to society in general.

Data from Food and Drug Administration. (2016). Fact sheet—FDA opioids action plan. Retrieved from https://www.fda.gov/newsevents/newsroom/factsheets/ucm484714.htm

Parenteral Insulin Preparations

For each category of insulin, the following table lists the species; common trade names; onset, peak, and duration; and key nursing considerations.

CATEGORY, SPECIES, AND TRADE NAMES	KEY NURSING CONSIDERATIONS
Rapid-acting insulin	
Onset: 10–20 min* **Peak:** 30–90 min	**Duration:** 2–5 hr
Human • Apidra (insulin glulisine) • Humalog (insulin lispro) • NovoLog (insulin aspart) • NovoRapid (insulin aspart) (CAN) • Fiasp (insulin aspart) (CAN) **Concentrated** • Humalog U-200	• Only mix with NPH (intermediate-type) insulin, if needed, except for Humalog U-200, which should not be mixed with any other insulin. Administer immediately after mixing. • When mixing rapid-acting insulin with a longer-acting insulin, always draw the rapid-acting insulin into the syringe first to avoid dosage errors. • When giving SubQ, give Humalog up to 15 minutes before a meal or immediately after a meal; give NovoLog and NovoRapid 5 to 10 minutes before a meal; give Apidra up to 15 to 20 minutes before a meal, and give Fiasp up to 2 minutes before a meal or up to 20 minutes after starting a meal. When giving rapid-acting insulin (except for Fiasp) via an insulin pump, do not dilute or mix with any other insulin, change the insulin in the reservoir at least every 48 hours (Apidra), 6 days (NovoLog, NovoRapid), and 7 days (Humalog). Change the infusion sets and insertion site at least every 3 days. • Be aware that 1 unit of rapid-acting insulin has the same glucose-lowering ability as 1 unit of short-acting insulin. • Rapid-acting insulin is available as a cartridge. Make sure to use the correct device for the brand of insulin prescribed, and don't add any other insulin to the cartridge. • Assess patient taking insulin concurrently with a thiazolidinedione for signs and symptoms of heart failure. If heart failure develops, provide supportive care, as ordered, and expect the thiazolidinedione to be discontinued or dosage reduced. • Know that Fiasp's onset is 5 to 10 minutes.
Short-acting insulin	
Onset: 30–60 min **Peak:** 1.5–4 hr	**Duration:** 5–8 hr
Human • Humulin-R • Novolin ge Toronto (CAN) • Novolin R • ReliOn Novolin R **Concentrated** • Humulin R U-500	• Don't use short-acting insulin if it's cloudy, discolored, or unusually viscous. • Use the U-500 strength to treat insulin resistance, as prescribed. Be very careful to use conversion chart if U-500 strength is being administered using U-100 syringes. Also, make sure the right strength of the short-acting insulin is being administered, as severe hypoglycemia and death have occurred because of dispensing, prescribing, and administration errors. • Mix short-acting insulin with other insulin types, if needed.

CATEGORY, SPECIES, AND TRADE NAMES	KEY NURSING CONSIDERATIONS
Short-acting insulin *(continued)*	
Onset: 30–60 min **Peak:** 1.5–4 hr **Duration:** 5–8 hr	
	• Administer SubQ, I.M., or I.V., as prescribed. Use a continuous SubQ infusion pump, if ordered. The catheter tubing and reservoir insulin should be changed every 48 hours or as specified by the pump manufacturer. • When giving SubQ or I.M. injections, give the short-acting insulin 15 to 30 minutes before a meal or bedtime snack. • Assess patient taking insulin concurrently with a thiazolidinedione for signs and symptoms of heart failure. If heart failure develops, provide supportive care, as ordered, and expect the thiazolidinedione to be discontinued or dosage reduced.
Intermediate-acting insulin	
Onset: 1–3 hr **Peak:** 4–12 hr **Duration:** 12–24 hr	
Human • Humulin N • Novolin ge NPH (CAN) • Novolin N • ReliOn Novolin N	• Don't use intermediate-acting insulin if it contains precipitate that is clumped or granular or that clings to the sides of the vial. • Roll the vial gently between your palms to mix; don't shake it. Also gently turn the prefilled syringe up and down several times before using to achieve a uniform mixture. • Administer by SubQ injection only, 30 minutes before a meal or bedtime snack. • Be aware that intermediate-acting insulin rarely produces a blood glucose level that's as close to normal as possible. So expect to mix it with a rapid-acting or short-acting insulin, as prescribed, for optimum blood glucose control. • Assess patient taking insulin concurrently with a thiazolidinedione for signs and symptoms of heart failure. If heart failure develops, provide supportive care, as ordered, and expect the thiazolidinedione to be discontinued or dosage reduced.

(continues)

Parenteral Insulin Preparations *(continued)*

CATEGORY, SPECIES, AND TRADE NAMES	KEY NURSING CONSIDERATIONS
Long-acting insulin	
Onset: 1–1.5 hr **Peak:** None **Duration:** 24–28 hr	
Human • Basaglar (insulin glargine) • Detemir (insulin detemir) (CAN) • Glargine (insulin glargine) (CAN) • Lantus (insulin glargine) • Levemir (insulin detemir)	• Don't use long-acting insulin if it contains precipitate that is clumped or granular or that clings to the sides of the vial. • Do not mix insulin detemir or insulin glargine with another insulin or solution. • Know that insulin degludec is now approved for use in children age 1 year and over. • Roll the vial gently between your palms to obtain a uniform mixture; don't shake it. • Administer by the SubQ route only. Inject insulin glargine once daily at any time, keeping the daily injection time consistent. Inject insulin detemir prescribed once daily with the evening meal or at bedtime; inject insulin detemir prescribed twice daily with the morning meal and with the evening meal, at bedtime, or 12 hours after the morning dose. • Give insulin glargine at bedtime, if possible, so that additional insulin can be given while patient is awake if effects decline before 24 hours pass. If insulin glargine is given in the morning and its effects don't last 24 hours, hyperglycemia may occur while patient sleeps. • Assess patient taking insulin concurrently with a thiazolidinedione for signs and symptoms of heart failure. If heart failure develops, provide supportive care, as ordered, and expect the thiazolidinedione to be discontinued or dosage reduced.
Ultra long-acting insulins	
Onset: 1–6 hr **Peak:** None **Duration:** 36–42 hr	
• Toujeo (insulin glargine) • Tresiba (insulin degludec) **Concentrated** • Tresiba U-200	• Don't use ultra long-acting insulin if it contains precipitate that is clumped or granular or that clings to the sides of the vial. • Roll the vial gently between your palms to obtain a uniform mixture; don't shake it. • Be aware that Toujeo contains 3 times as much insulin (300 units/ml) in 1 ml as standard insulin (100 units/ml) and is not for use in children. Toujeo Max SoloStar holds 900 units of insulin glargine—more than any other long-acting insulin pen in the United States—and provides up to 160 units/ml in a single injection and allows for 2-unit increment adjustment. In comparison, Toujeo Solo Star pen contains 450 units of insulin glargine with a maximum dose of 80 units per injection, and dosage must be adjusted in 1-unit increments. • Administer by the SubQ route only. Inject once daily at any time of day but keep time consistent. • Assess patient taking insulin concurrently with a thiazolidinedione for signs and symptoms of heart failure. If heart failure develops, provide supportive care, as ordered, and expect the thiazolidinedione to be discontinued or dosage reduced.

CATEGORY, SPECIES, AND TRADE NAMES	KEY NURSING CONSIDERATIONS
Combination insulins	
Onset: 30 min **Peak:** 1–12 hr **Duration:** 18–24 hr	
Human **Intermediate-acting/short-acting** • Humalog Mix 25 (CAN) • Humalog Mix 50 (CAN) • Humalog Mix 75/25 • Humalog Mix 50/50 • Humulin 30/70 (CAN) • Humulin 70/30 • Novolin 70/30 • Novolin ge 30/70 (CAN) • Novolin ge 40/60 (CAN) • Novolin ge 50/50 (CAN) • NovoLog Mix 70/30 • NovoMix 30 (CAN) • ReliOn Novolin 70/30 **Ultra long-acting/rapid-acting** • Ryzodeg 70/30	• Don't use combination insulin if it contains precipitate that is clumped or granular. • Know that Ryzodeg 70/30 is now approved for use in children age 1 year and over. • Roll the vial gently between your palms to mix; don't shake it. Also gently turn the prefilled syringe up and down several times before using to achieve a uniform mixture. • Administer combination insulin by the SubQ route only, 30 minutes before a meal. • Be aware that Canadian and American products contain the same insulin ratio but express it differently. For example, the Canadian Humulin 30/70 and the American Humulin 70/30 both contain 30 units of a short-acting insulin and 70 units of an intermediate-acting insulin. Canadian products list the short-acting insulin first; American products list it second. • Know that Ryzodeg 70/30 is composed of 70% long-acting insulin and 30% rapid-acting insulin. • Assess patient taking insulin concurrently with a thiazolidinedione for signs and symptoms of heart failure. If heart failure develops, provide supportive care, as ordered, and expect the thiazolidinedione to be discontinued or dosage reduced.
Combination insulins and glucagon-like peptide-1 receptor agonists	
Onset: 4–6 hr **Peak:** 8–20 hr **Duration:** 24–28 hr	
Long-acting insulin/GLP-1 receptor agonist • Xultophy 100/3.6 (insulin degludec/liraglutide) • Soliqua 100/33 (insulin glargine/lixisenatide)	• Know that onset, peak, and duration are determined by the insulin contained in the combination. • Expect the same adverse reactions that occur with the individual drugs making up the combination product. • Monitor for hypoglycemia that may become life-threatening, especially with lifestyle or medication changes. • Monitor renal function in patients with renal impairment or severe GI adverse reactions, as acute kidney injury can occur. • Evaluate patient's serum potassium level as ordered, because severe hypokalemia has occurred. • Assess patient concurrently taking a thiazolidinedione for signs and symptoms of heart failure. If heart failure develops, provide supportive care, as ordered, and expect dosage to be reduced or drug discontinued. • Monitor patient for signs and symptoms of pancreatitis.

Oral Allergen Extracts

Prevention of allergy symptoms in patients diagnosed with an allergy has historically required an extended period of desensitization through the administration of injections given in a healthcare setting. Many patients do not have the time or resources required to undergo such a rigorous desensitization process. A new form of treatment using a sublingual route that the patient can self-administer (after the first dose) is now available for certain types of allergens as summarized in the following chart.

GENERIC AND TRADE NAMES	INDICATIONS	USUAL ADULT DOSAGES	NURSING CONSIDERATIONS FOR ALLERGEN EXTRACTS
grass pollen Grastek	To treat grass pollen–induced allergic rhinitis	2800 Bioequivalent Allergy Unit (1 tablet) sublingual once daily	• Know that allergen extracts are contraindicated in patients with severe, unstable asthma; in patients with a history of any severe systemic allergic reaction, severe local reaction after taking any sublingual allergen immunotherapy, or eosinophilic esophagitis; or in patients with a hypersensitivity to any of the inactive ingredients (gelatin, mannitol, or sodium hydroxide).
mixed pollens allergen extract Oralair	To treat grass pollen–induced allergic rhinitis	300 Index of Reactivity (1 tablet) sublingual once daily	• Monitor patient closely for allergic reactions that could become severe and life threatening, such as anaphylaxis and severe laryngopharyngeal constriction.
ragweed extract Ragwitek	To treat short-term ragweed pollen–induced allergic rhinitis	12 AMB a 1-Unit (1 tablet) sublingual once daily	• First dose must be administered in a healthcare setting and patient observed for at least 30 minutes after administration for signs and symptoms of an allergic reaction.

Selected Antihistamines

Antihistamines are usually used to relieve immediate hypersensitivity reactions. They're also used as antiemetics (especially in motion sickness), antidyskinetics, antitussives, sedatives, and adjuncts to preoperative or postoperative analgesia.

Antihistamines are contraindicated in patients taking drugs that prolong the QT interval (including itraconazole, ketoconazole, mibefradil, some macrolide antibiotics, quinidine, and zileuton). They're also contraindicated in patients hypersensitive to antihistamines or their components.

The table below includes trade names; usual dosages; and onset, peak, and duration for antihistamines that your patient is most likely to use daily or intermittently to control symptoms of allergic rhinitis. When caring for a patient who takes an antihistamine, individualize your plan of care but be sure to include these general interventions:

- Use antihistamines cautiously in patients with a history of glaucoma, peptic ulcer, or urine retention because anticholinergic effects may worsen these conditions.
- Assess patient for hypokalemia and correct the imbalance, as prescribed, before antihistamine therapy to reduce the risk of arrhythmias.
- Obtain a detailed medication history before antihistamine therapy to help prevent drug interactions.
- Give antihistamines with food if GI distress occurs.
- Urge patient to avoid alcohol and other CNS depressants during antihistamine use because the combination can cause additive CNS depression.
- Monitor blood pressure because these drugs' anticholinergic effects may cause hypertension.
- Be aware that short- and long-acting antihistamines may be combined and H_2 blockers added to increase antihistamine effects.
- Be aware that products containing pseudoephedrine should be used for less than 7 days.

GENERIC AND TRADE NAMES	USUAL ADULT DOSAGE	ONSET, PEAK, AND DURATION
acrivastine Semprex-D (also include pseudoephedrine)	8 mg/60 mg P.O. every 4 to 6 hr. *Maximum:* Four times a day	**Onset:** 30 min **Peak:** Unknown **Duration:** 6 to 8 hr
azatadine Optimine	1 to 2 mg P.O. every 8 to 12 hr. *Maximum:* 2 mg in 24 hr	**Onset:** 15 to 60 min **Peak:** 4 hr **Duration:** 12 hr
azelastine Astelin	1 to 2 sprays (137 mcg/spray) in each nostril twice daily	**Onset:** In 3 hr **Peak:** Unknown **Duration:** 12 hr
Astepro 0.1%	1 to 2 sprays (137 mcg/spray) in each nostril twice daily	
Astepro 0.15%	2 sprays (205.5 mcg/spray) in each nostril once daily	
carbinoxamine maleate Arbinoxa, Palgic	4 to 8 mg P.O. three times a day or four times a day. *Maximum:* 24 mg in 24 hr (Immediate Release)	**Onset:** 30 min **Peak:** Unknown **Duration:** 4 hr (Arbinoxa, Palgic), 17 hr (Karbinal ER)
Karbinal ER	6 to 16 mg P.O. every 12 hr (Extended Release)	

(continues)

Selected Antihistamines *(continued)*

GENERIC AND TRADE NAMES	USUAL ADULT DOSAGE	ONSET, PEAK, AND DURATION
cetirizine hydrochloride		**Onset:** 30 to 60 min
Zyrtec	5 to 10 mg P.O. daily	**Peak:** 1 hr
Zyrtec D (also includes pseudoephedrine)	5 mg/120 mg every 12 hr	**Duration:** Up to 24 hr
desloratadine		**Onset:** Unknown
Clarinex, Clarinex Reditabs	5 mg P.O. daily	**Peak:** 3 hr (Clarinex Reditabs); unknown for other types
Clarinex-D 12 hr (also contains pseudoephedrine)	2.5 mg/120 mg P.O. twice daily	**Duration:** Unknown
Clarinex-D 24 hr (also contains pseudoephedrine)	2.5 mg/240 mg P.O. once daily	
fexofenadine hydrochloride		**Onset:** 1 hr
Allegra	60 mg P.O. twice daily or 180 mg P.O. daily	**Peak:** 2 to 3 hr **Duration:** 12 hr
Allegra-D-12 hr (also includes pseudoephedrine)	60 mg/120 mg P.O. every 12 hr	
Allegra-D-24 hr (also includes pseudoephedrine)	180 mg/240 mg P.O. once daily	
levocetirizine dihydrochloride		**Onset:** Less than 1 hr
Xyzal	2.5 to 5 mg P.O. daily in evening	**Peak:** 0.9 hr **Duration:** 24 hr
loratadine		**Onset:** 1 to 3 hr
Claritin	10 mg P.O. daily	**Peak:** 8 to 12 hr
Claritin-D12 (also includes pseudoephedrine)	5 mg/120 mg P.O. every 12 hr	**Duration:** At least 24 hr
Claritin-D24 (also includes pseudoephedrine)	10 mg/240 mg P.O. every 24 hr	
olopatadine hydrochloride		**Onset:** Unknown
Patanase	2 sprays (665 mcg/spray) in each nostril twice daily	**Peak:** 15 to 120 min **Duration:** Unknown

Selected Ophthalmic Drugs

Although less commonly prescribed than oral drugs, drugs instilled into the eyes are frequently brought into the clinical setting by patients with chronic conditions. In most cases, the patient or a family member has administered these preparations at home. Your patient teaching should include a review of proper administration and storage of these drugs. Have the patient or a family member demonstrate proper use of the drug to make sure it will be administered correctly at home. Use this time to reassess the patient's ability to continue self-medication. Also, instruct him to report any changes in the condition being treated, either negative or positive. A properly educated patient not only ensures safe drug administration, but also is more likely to detect adverse reactions that require a dosage reduction or drug discontinuation, thus preventing the development of more serious health problems.

The following chart lists the generic and trade names, FDA-approved indications, and usual adult dosages for those ophthalmic preparations you're most likely to see in your practice setting. The drugs are divided according to therapeutic use.

GENERIC AND TRADE NAMES	INDICATIONS	USUAL ADULT DOSAGES
Ophthalmic antibiotics		
bacitracin AK-Tracin	To treat surface bacterial infections affecting the conjunctiva and cornea	1/4-in to 1/2-in strip of ointment applied to conjunctival sac, 1 to 3 times daily or as needed
besifoxacin 0.6% Besivance	To treat bacterial conjunctivitis due to susceptible organisms	1 gtt in affected eye(s) three times a day 4 to 14 hr apart for 7 days
chloramphenicol 1% Diochloram, Pentamycetin /HC, Sopamycetin (CAN)	To treat severe surface bacterial infections affecting the conjunctiva and cornea	Apply small amount of ointment to lower conjunctival sac every 3 to 6 hr and as needed for at least 48 hr after eye resumes normal appearance
ciprofloxacin hydrochloride 0.3% Ciloxan	To treat corneal ulcers due to *Pseudomonas aeruginosa, Staphylococcus aureus, S. epidermidis, Streptococcus pneumoniae,* and possibly *Serratia marcescens* and *S. viridans*	2 gtt in affected eye every 15 min for first 6 hr, then 2 gtt every 30 min for rest of first day; on day 2, 2 gtt in affected eye every hr; on days 3 to 14, 2 gtt in affected eye every 4 hr
	To treat bacterial conjunctivitis due to *Haemophilus influenzae, S. aureus, S. epidermidis, S. pneumoniae* and *S. viridans*	1 or 2 gtt in conjunctival sac of affected eye every 2 hr while awake for first 2 days and then 1 or 2 gtt every 4 hr while awake for next 5 days; or 1/2-in strip of ointment in affected eye three times a day for 2 days, then twice daily for next 5 days
erythromycin Ilotycin	To treat superficial eye infections involving conjunctiva and/or cornea	1 cm (0.39 in) of ointment applied in infected eye up to 6 times/day, depending on severity of infection
	As adjunct to prevent ophthalmia neonatorum due to *Neisseria gonorrhoeae* or *Chlamydia trachomatis*	1 cm (0.39 in) of ointment applied in each eye
ganciclovir gel 0.15% Zirgan	To treat acute herpes keratitis (dendritic ulcers)	1 gtt five times daily (about every 3 hr while awake) until corneal ulcer heals; then 1 gtt three times a day for 7 days

(continues)

Selected Ophthalmic Drugs *(continued)*

GENERIC AND TRADE NAMES	INDICATIONS	USUAL ADULT DOSAGES
Ophthalmic antibiotics *(continued)*		
gatifloxacin 0.5% Zymaxid	To treat bacterial conjunctivitis due to *Staphylococcus aureus, S. epidermidis, Streptococcus mitis, S. pneumoniae, and Haemophilus influenzae*	1 gtt in affected eye every 2 hr while awake, up to eight times daily on day 1; then 1 gtt twice daily to four times a day while awake on days 2 to 7
gentamicin sulfate Garamycin, Genoptic, Gentacidin, Gentak	To treat bacterial infections such as blepharitis, blepharoconjunctivitis, conjunctivitis, corneal ulcers, dacryocystitis, keratoconjunctivitis, or meibomianitis due to susceptible organisms	1 or 2 gtt every 4 hr or, for severe infection, up to 2 gtt/hr; alternatively, 1/2-in strip of ointment applied to lower conjunctival sac twice daily or three times daily
levofloxacin 0.5% Quixin	To treat bacterial conjunctivitis due to susceptible organisms	On days 1 and 2: 1 or 2 gtt every 2 hr while awake, up to 8 times/day; on days 3 to 7: 1 or 2 gtt every 4 hr while awake, up to 4 times/day
moxifloxacin 0.5% Vigamox	To treat bacterial conjunctivitis due to *Staphylococcus aureus, S. epidermidis, S. haemolyticus, S. hominis, Streptococcus pneumoniae, S. viridans* group, *Haemophilus influenzae, and Chlamydia trachomatis*	1 gtt three times a day for 7 days
ofloxacin 0.3% Ocuflox	To treat conjunctivitis due to *Staphylococcus aureus, S. epidermidis, Streptococcus pneumoniae, Enterobacter cloacae, Haemophilus influenzae, Proteus mirabilis,* and *Pseudomonas aeruginosa*	1 or 2 gtt in conjunctival sac every 2 to 4 hr for first 2 days; then 1 to 2 gtt four times a day for up to 5 more days
	To treat bacterial corneal ulcers due to *S. aureus, S. epidermidis, S. pneumoniae, E. cloacae, H. influenzae, Propionibacterium mirabilis, Propionibacterium aeruginosa, Serratia marcescens,* and *Propionibacterium acnes*	1 or 2 gtt every 30 min while awake and 1 or 2 gtt every 4 to 6 hr after retiring for 2 days; then 1 or 2 gtt/hr while awake for up to 7 more days; then 1 to 2 gtt four times a day until end of treatment
sulfacetamide sodium 10% Bleph-10, Ocu-Sol 10, Ocu-Sol 15, Ocu-Sol 30, Sodium Sulamyd, Sulf-10, Sulfac 10%	To treat conjunctivitis and other superficial eye infections due to susceptible organisms	1 or 2 gtt solution in lower conjunctival sac every 2 to 3 hr initially, with dosage tapered by increasing time interval between doses as condition improves for up to 10 days; or 1/4-in to 1/2-in strip of ointment in conjunctival sac four times a day and bedtime

GENERIC AND TRADE NAMES	INDICATIONS	USUAL ADULT DOSAGES
Ophthalmic antibiotics *(continued)*		
sulfacetamide sodium ointment 10%, solution 15% Isopto Cetamide	As adjunct to treat trachoma	2 gtt in lower conjunctival sac every 2 hr
tobramycin Tobrasol 0.3%, Tobrex, Tomycine (CAN)	To treat external superficial ocular infections and its adnexa due to susceptible organisms	1 to 2 gtt every 1 to 4 hr, depending on severity of infection; or 1/2-in strip of ointment applied to lower conjunctival sac every 8 to 12 hr for mild to moderate infections or every 3 to 4 hr for severe infections
tobramycin 0.3% (3 mg) and dexamethasone 0.1% (1 mg) TobraDex	To treat steroid-responsive inflammatory ocular conditions for which a corticosteroid is indicated and where superficial bacterial ocular infection or a risk of bacterial ocular infection exists	1 to 2 gtt every 4 to 6 hr; during first 24 to 48 hr, dosage may be increased to 1 to 2 gtt every 2 hr; or apply 1/2-in strip of ointment into the conjunctival sac up to four times a day
Ophthalmic anti-inflammatory drugs		
bromfenac 0.09% Xibrom (0.09%)	To treat postoperative inflammation and reduce ocular pain after cataract extraction	1 gtt in operative eye twice daily starting 24 hr after cataract surgery and continuing through first 2 wk of postoperative period
Bromday (0.09%) Prolensa (0.07%)	To treat postoperative inflammation and reduce ocular pain after cataract extraction	1 gtt in operative eye once daily, starting 24 hr before cataract surgery and continuing through first 2 wk of postoperative period
BromSite	To treat postoperative inflammation and prevent ocular pain associated with cataract extraction	1 gtt in operative eye twice daily (morning and evening) 1 day before surgery, day of surgery, and 14 days postoperatively
dexamethasone Maxidex **dexamethasone sodium phosphate 0.1%** AK-Dex	To treat allergic conjunctivitis; corneal injury from chemical or thermal burns or from penetration of foreign bodies; inflammatory conditions of the anterior segment of globe, conjunctiva, cornea, or eyelids; iridocyclitis; suppression of graft rejection after keratoplasty; and uveitis	1 or 2 gtt of suspension or solution every hr during day and every 2 hr at night initially. When response occurs, 1 gtt every 4 hr; or apply 1/2-in to 1-in strip of ointment up to four times daily, then tapered to once daily

(continues)

Selected Ophthalmic Drugs *(continued)*

GENERIC AND TRADE NAMES	INDICATIONS	USUAL ADULT DOSAGES
Ophthalmic anti-inflammatory drugs *(continued)*		
diclofenac sodium 0.1% Voltaren, Voltaren Ophtha (CAN)	To treat postoperative inflammation after removal of cataract	1 gtt in conjunctival sac four times a day, starting 24 hr after surgery through first 2 postoperative wk
	To provide temporary relief of pain and photophobia in corneal refractive surgery	1 or 2 gtt in operative eye 1 hr before surgery. Then 1 or 2 gtt 15 min after surgery. Then 1 gtt four times a day, starting 4 to 6 hr after surgery for up to 3 days, as needed
difluprednate 0.05% Durezol	To treat inflammation and pain associated with ocular surgery	1 gtt in conjunctival sac of affected eye(s) four times a day for 2 wk starting 24 hr after surgery. Then 1 gtt twice daily for 1 wk
	To treat endogenous anterior uveitis	1 gtt into conjunctival sac of affected eye four times a day for 14 days, then tapered as needed
fluorometholone 0.1% Fluor-Op, FML Forte, FML Liquifilm, FML S.O.P.	To treat corticosteroid-responsive inflammation of the anterior segment of the globe, bulbar and palpebral conjunctiva, and cornea	1 gtt in conjunctival sac twice daily to four times a day or, in severe conditions, up to every 4 hr during first 1 to 2 days, as needed; or 1.5-in strip of ointment in conjunctival sac once daily to three times a day
fluorometholone acetate Eflone, Flarex		1 or 2 gtt in conjunctival sac four times daily or, in severe conditions, up to every 2 hr during first 1 or 2 days, as needed
flurbiprofen sodium 0.03% Ocufen	To inhibit intraoperative miosis	1 gtt in affected eye every 30 min, beginning 2 hr before surgery, up to total of 4 gtt
ketorolac tromethamine Acular 0.5%	To relieve ocular itching due to seasonal allergic conjunctivitis	1 gtt in conjunctival sac of each eye four times a day
	To treat postoperative inflammation in patients who have undergone cataract extraction	1 gtt in operative eye four times a day, starting 24 hr after surgery through first 2 postoperative wk
Acuvail 0.45%	To relieve pain and treat postoperative inflammation in patients who have undergone cataract extraction	1 gtt in affected eye twice daily, starting 1 day before surgery, continuing through day of surgery and first 2 wk of postoperative period

GENERIC AND TRADE NAMES	INDICATIONS	USUAL ADULT DOSAGES
Ophthalmic anti-inflammatory drugs *(continued)*		
loteprednol etabonate Alrex 0.2%	To relieve seasonal allergic conjunctivitis	1 gtt of 0.2% suspension in affected eyes four times a day
Lotemax 0.5% Inveltys 1%	To treat postoperative inflammation following ocular surgery	1 or 2 gtt in conjunctival sac of operated eye four times a day, beginning 24 hr after surgery and continuing through first 2 wk of postoperative period
	To treat steroid-responsive inflammatory conditions of the anterior segment of the globe, bulbar and palpebral conjunctiva, and cornea	1 or 2 gtt in conjunctival sac of affected eye four times a day. Initially, dosage may be increased during first week to 1 gtt every hour, as needed
medrysone 1.0% HMS Liquifilm	To treat allergic conjunctivitis, episcleritis, epinephrine sensitivity, and vernal conjunctivitis	1 gtt into conjunctival sac up to every 4 hr
olopatadine hydrochloride 0.1% Patanol	To treat signs and symptoms of allergic conjunctivitis	1 gtt twice daily at 6- to 8-hr intervals
olopatadine hydrochloride 0.7% Pazeo	To treat ocular itching associated with allergic conjunctivitis	1 gtt into conjunctival sac in each affected eye once daily
prednisolone acetate suspension 1% Econopred Plus, Omnipred, Pred Forte, Pred Mild **prednisolone sodium phosphate solution 1%** AK-Pred, Prednisol	To treat steroid-responsive inflammation of the anterior segment of globe, cornea, and bulbar and palpebral conjunctiva; to treat corneal injury from chemical, radiation, or thermal burns, or penetration of foreign bodies	1 or 2 gtt in conjunctival sac twice daily to four times a day (suspension) or 1 gtt in conjunctival sac every 4 hr (solution) unless severe, then initially every hr during day and every 2 hr at night until response noted, then decreased to 1 gtt every 4 hr
rimexolone 1% Vexol	To treat anterior uveitis	1 or 2 gtt in conjunctival sac every hr while awake in first wk; 1 gtt every 2 hr while awake in second wk; then tapered until uveitis resolves
	To treat postoperative inflammation after ocular surgery	1 or 2 gtt in conjunctival sac of affected eye four times a day, starting 24 hr after surgery and continuing through first 2 postoperative wk

(continues)

Selected Ophthalmic Drugs *(continued)*

GENERIC AND TRADE NAMES	INDICATIONS	USUAL ADULT DOSAGES
Ophthalmic cycloplegic mydriatics		
atropine sulfate 1% Isopto Atropine, Minims Atropine (CAN)	To treat acute iritis or uveitis	Small strip of ointment applied to conjunctival sac up to twice daily
	To produce dilation for cycloplegic refraction	1 gtt 40 min before refraction. *Maximum:* 2 gtt
cyclopentolate hydrochloride 0.5%, 1%, 2% AK-Pentolate, Cyclogyl, Minims Cyclopentolate (CAN), Pentolair	To produce mydriasis and cycloplegia required in specific diagnostic procedures	1 or 2 gtt of 0.5%, 1%, or 2% solution in each eye; then 1 or 2 gtt in 5 to 10 min, as needed
homatropine hydrobromide 2%, 5% Isopto Homatropine, Minims Homatropine (CAN)	To dilate pupils for cycloplegic refraction	1 or 2 gtt in each eye, repeated in 5 to 10 min as needed
	To treat uveitis	1 or 2 gtt in affected eye(s) every 3 to 4 hr
tropicamide 0.5%, 1% Mydriacyl, Opticyl, Tropicacyl	To produce mydriasis	1 to 2 gtt of 1% solution, repeated in 5 min, as needed
	To dilate pupils for cycloplegic funduscopic exam	1 to 2 gtt of 0.5% solution in eyes 15 to 20 min before exam, repeated every 30 min as needed
Ophthalmic miotics		
acetylcholine chloride Miochol-E	To produce papillary miosis in cataract surgery, penetrating keratoplasty, iridectomy, and other anterior segment surgery	0.5 to 2 ml gently into anterior chamber before or after sutures secured or after lens placement in cataract surgery
carbachol 0.01% Carbastat, Miostat	To produce papillary miosis in ocular surgery; to reduce intensity of intraocular pressure elevation in first 24 hr after cataract surgery	0.5 ml (solution) into anterior chamber before or after sutures secured or after lens placement in cataract surgery
carbachol 0.75%, 1.5%, 2.25%, 3% Carboptic, Isopto Carbachol	To treat open-angle glaucoma	1 or 2 gtt up to three times a day

GENERIC AND TRADE NAMES	INDICATIONS	USUAL ADULT DOSAGES
Ophthalmic miotics *(continued)*		
naphazoline hydrochloride Ak-Con 0.1%, Albalon 0.1%, Clear Eyes 0.012%, Naphcon A 0.025%, Vasocon 0.05%	To treat ocular congestion, irritation, or itching	1 gtt of 0.1% solution every 3 to 4 hr; or 1 gtt of 0.012% to 0.03% solution up to four times a day for no more than 72 hr
oxymetazoline hydrochloride	To provide relief from eye redness due to minor eye irritations	1 or 2 gtt in conjunctival sac four times a day (at least 6 hr apart) for no more than 72 hr
phenylephrine hydrochloride 2.5%, 10% Ak-Dilate, 2.5% (CAN), Mydfrin 2.5%, Neofrin 2.5%, Ocu-Phrin 2.5%, Phenoptic 2.5%, Prefrin 2.5%	To produce mydriasis without cycloplegia	1 gtt of 2.5% or 10% solution before eye exam, then repeated in 1 hr, as needed
	To produce mydriasis and vasoconstriction	1 gtt of 2.5% or 10% solution as single dose
	To treat chronic mydriasis	1 gtt of 2.5% or 10% solution or three times a day
	To prevent posterior synechiae in anterior uveitis or post iridectomy	1 gtt of 10% solution three times daily or more (anterior uveitis) or 1 gtt of 10% solution once or twice daily (post iridectomy)
pilocarpine 1%, 2%, 4% Akarpine, Isopto Carpine, Miocarpine (CAN), Pilocar, Pilopine HS, Pilostat	To treat primary open-angle glaucoma	1 gtt up to four times a day; or 1-cm (0.39-in) ribbon of 4% gel at bedtime
pilocarpine hydrochloride Akarpine, Isopto Carpine, Minocarpine (CAN), Pilocar, Pilopine HS, Pilostat	To treat acute angle-closure glaucoma as emergency therapy	1 gtt of 2% solution every 15 to 60 min for up to four doses
pilocarpine nitrate 1% Minims Pilocarpine (CAN)	To treat mydriasis due to mydriatic or cycloplegic drug therapy	1 gtt of 1% solution
proparacaine hydrochloride 0.5% AK-Taine, Alcaine, Ophthetic, Parcaine	To provide deep anesthesia during cataract extraction	1 gtt every 5 to 10 min for 5 to 7 doses
	To provide anesthesia during removal of eye sutures	1 or 2 gtt 2 to 3 min before procedure
	To provide anesthesia during removal of foreign bodies	1 or 2 gtt in affected eye before surgery
	To provide anesthesia during tonometry	1 or 2 gtt immediately before measurement
tetracaine 0.5% Pontocaine	To provide eye anesthesia (short term)	1 or 2 gtt, as needed

(continues)

Selected Ophthalmic Drugs *(continued)*

GENERIC AND TRADE NAMES	INDICATIONS	USUAL ADULT DOSAGES
Miscellaneous ophthalmic drugs		
alcaftadine 0.25% Lastacaft	To prevent itching associated with allergic conjunctivitis	1 gtt in each eye once daily
apraclonidine hydrochloride 0.5% Iopidine	As adjunct in patients on maximally tolerated medical therapy who require additional intraocular pressure (IOP) reduction	1 or 2 gtt in affected eye(s) three times daily
azelastine hydrochloride 0.05% Optivar	To treat itching of the eye associated with allergic conjunctivitis	1 gtt in affected eye twice daily
bepotastine besilate 1.5% Bepreve	To treat itching of the eye associated with allergic conjunctivitis	1 gtt in affected eye twice daily
betaxolol hydrochloride Betoptic 0.5%, Betoptic S 0.25%	To treat chronic open-angle glaucoma or ocular hypertension	1 or 2 gtt of 0.5% solution twice daily or 1 gtt of 0.25% solution twice daily
bimatoprost 0.01%, 0.03% Lumigan	To reduce elevated IOP in patients with open-angle glaucoma or ocular hypertension	1 gtt in affected eye daily in evening
brimonidine tartrate Alphagan 0.2%, Alphagan P 0.1%, 0.15%	To reduce IOP in open-angle glaucoma or ocular hypertension	1 gtt in affected eye three times daily, about 8 hr apart
brinzolamide 1% Azopt	To reduce IOP in ocular hypertension or open-angle glaucoma	1 gtt three times a day
brinzolamide 1% and brimonidine tartrate 0.2% Simbrinza	To reduce IOP in open-angle glaucoma or ocular hypertension	1 gtt in affected eye three times a day
carteolol hydrochloride 1% Ocupress	To treat chronic open-angle glaucoma or intraocular hypertension	1 gtt in conjunctival sac of affected eye twice daily
cyclosporine 0.09% cyclosporine emulsion 0.05% Restasis	To increase tear production in keratoconjunctivitis sicca	1 gtt every 12 hr

GENERIC AND TRADE NAMES	INDICATIONS	USUAL ADULT DOSAGES
Miscellaneous ophthalmic drugs *(continued)*		
cysteamine 0.44% Cystaran	To treat corneal cystine crystal accumulation in patients with cystinosis	1 gtt in each eye, every waking hr
dipivefrin hydrochloride 0.1% Ophto-Dipivefrin (CAN), Propine	To reduce IOP in chronic open-angle glaucoma	1 gtt every 12 hr
dorzolamide hydrochloride Trusopt	To treat increased IOP in ocular hypertension or open-angle glaucoma	1 gtt in conjunctival sac of affected eye three times a day
emedastine difumarate Emadine	To treat allergic conjunctivitis	1 gtt in affected eye up to four times a day
ketotifen fumarate Zaditor	To treat allergic conjunctivitis	1 gtt in affected eye twice daily every 8 to 12 hr, but no more than twice daily
latanoprost 0.005% Xalatan, Xelpros	To reduce IOP in ocular hypertension or open-angle glaucoma	1 gtt in conjunctival sac of affected eye daily in evening
latanoprostene bunod 0.024% Vyzulta	To reduce IOP in ocular hypertension or open-angle glaucoma	1 gtt in affected eye(s) once daily in evening
levobunolol hydrochloride AKBeta, Betagan, Novo-Levobunolol (CAN)	To treat chronic open-angle glaucoma or ocular hypertension	1 or 2 gtt of 0.5% solution once daily or 0.25% solution twice daily
levocabastine hydrochloride 0.05% Livostin	To treat signs and symptoms of seasonal allergic conjunctivitis	1 gtt four times a day
lifitegrast 5% Xiidra	To treat dry eye disease	1 gtt twice daily (about 12 hr apart) in each eye
metipranolol 0.3% OptiPranolol	To reduce IOP in ocular hypertension or open-angle glaucoma	1 gtt in affected eye twice daily
nedocromil sodium 2% Alocril	To treat itching associated with both seasonal and perennial allergic conjunctivitis	1 or 2 gtt twice daily

(continues)

Selected Ophthalmic Drugs *(continued)*

GENERIC AND TRADE NAMES	INDICATIONS	USUAL ADULT DOSAGES
Miscellaneous ophthalmic drugs *(continued)*		
netarsudil 0.02% Rhopressa	To reduce IOP in ocular hypertension or open-angle glaucoma	1 gtt in affected eye(s) once daily in evening
sodium chloride, hypertonic Altachlore, Muro-128 2%, Muro-128 5%, Muroptic-5	To provide temporary relief from corneal edema	1 or 2 gtt every 3 to 4 hr; or 1/4-in of ointment applied every 3 to 4 hr
tafluprost 0.0015% Zioptan	To reduce IOP in ocular hypertension or open-angle glaucoma	1 gtt in conjunctival sac in affected eye(s) once daily in evening
tetrahydrozoline hydrochloride 0.05% Eye-Sine, Murine Plus, Optigene 3, Tetrasine, Visine	To treat allergic conditions, conjunctival congestion, and irritation	1 gtt up to four times a day or as directed
timolol hemihydrate 0.25%, 0.5% Betimol **timolol maleate 0.25%, 0.5%** Apo-Timop (CAN), Timoptic **timolol maleate extended- release gel solution 0.25%, 0.5%** Timoptic-XE	To reduce IOP in ocular hypertension or open-angle glaucoma	1 gtt of 0.25% solution in affected eye twice daily, increased to 1 gtt of 0.5% solution, as needed; then 1 gtt daily; or 1 gtt extended-release gel solution in affected eye daily
travoprost 0.004% Travatan	To reduce elevated IOP in patients with open-angle glaucoma or ocular hypertension	1 gtt in affected eye daily in evening
unoprostone isopropyl 0.15% Rescula	To reduce elevated IOP in patients with open-angle glaucoma or ocular hypertension	1 gtt in affected eye twice daily

Selected Topical Drugs

Topical drugs consist of an active drug prepared in a specified medium that promotes absorption through the skin. Media commonly are chosen based on drug solubility; rate of drug release; ability to hydrate the outer skin layer; ability to enhance penetration; drug stability; and interactions between the chosen medium, skin, and active ingredient.

Topical media include aerosols, creams, gels, lotions, ointments, powders, tinctures, and wet dressings. Aerosols, gels, lotions, and tinctures are convenient for application to the scalp and other hairy areas. Acutely inflamed areas are best treated with drying preparations, such as lotions, tinctures, and wet dressings. Chronic inflammation does well with applications of lubricating preparations, including creams and ointments.

Because of its physical properties, the skin can act as a holding area for many drugs, allowing slow penetration and prolonged duration of action. (This characteristic makes it important to understand the patient's allergies.) However, when administering topical or transdermal drugs that aren't prescribed for a specific location, keep in mind that penetration properties may vary in different areas of the body. For example, the axillae, face, scalp, and scrotum are more permeable than the limbs, and ventral surfaces typically are more permeable than dorsal surfaces.

Topical Drug Types

Topical drugs are classified as antibacterials, antifungals, antivirals, corticosteroids, retinoids, and other miscellaneous preparations.

- *Antibacterials* may be useful in the early treatment of minor skin infections and wounds. Minor skin infections may respond well to topical drugs applied at the infection site. Minor wounds should be treated at the site and in the immediately surrounding area to prevent other pathogens from colonizing the area.
- *Antifungals* usually are used to treat mucocutaneous infections, such as tineas, primarily ringworm and athlete's foot. Systemic use of antifungals is limited by their potentially toxic adverse effects, most commonly hepatic or renal damage. All fungi are completely resistant to conventional antibacterial drugs.
- *Antivirals* are used to inhibit viral replication. They work by targeting any one of the steps involved in viral replication: penetration into susceptible host cells; uncoating of the viral nucleic acid; synthesis of regulatory proteins, RNA and DNA, and structural proteins; assembly of viral particles; and release of the virus from the cell. Topical antivirals such as penciclovir can shorten the duration of herpetic lesions, lessen lesion pain, and minimize viral shedding.
- *Corticosteroids* reduce the signs and symptoms of inflammation. Topical corticosteroids cause vasoconstriction, probably by suppressing cell degranulation. They also cause decreased cell permeability by reducing histamine release from basal and mast cells.
- *Retinoids,* typically derivatives of vitamin A, are very effective in treating acne vulgaris, although the acne may appear to worsen before it improves. Retinoids are also useful for reducing wrinkles. When applied to the skin, retinoids remain primarily in the dermis; less than 10% of the drug is absorbed into the circulation. Prolonged use of retinoids promotes new dermal growth, new blood vessel formation, and thickening of the epidermis. Because these drugs are absorbed systemically and may have teratogenic effects, they shouldn't be used by pregnant women.
- *Miscellaneous topical drugs* are used to treat a variety of topical skin conditions, including dry skin, ichthyosis, parasitic infestations, psoriasis, and unwanted hair growth.

Administration Tips

Before you apply a topical drug, clean the site and let it dry. Use gloves or a finger cot during application to prevent the drug from being absorbed through your own skin. Inform your patient of any expected discomfort, such as temporary burning or stinging. After application, cover the site only if required; some topical drugs shouldn't be covered with an occlusive dressing.

Be sure to teach the patient and a family member correct administration technique. Also, review possible adverse reactions, highlighting those that should be reported to the prescriber. Stress the importance of complying with the drug regimen because some topical drugs require weeks or months of therapy to eradicate the underlying condition.

The following table includes the generic and trade names of many commonly prescribed topical drugs as well as their FDA-approved indications and usual adult dosages.

Selected Topical Drugs *(continued)*

GENERIC AND TRADE NAMES	INDICATIONS	USUAL ADULT DOSAGES
Antibacterials		
azelaic acid cream 20% Azelex	To treat mild to moderate inflammatory acne vulgaris	Gently massage thin film into affected area twice daily, morning and evening.
azelaic acid foam 15% Finacea Foam **azelaic acid gel 15%** Finacea Gel	To treat inflammatory papules and pustules of mild to moderate rosacea	Apply thin layer to entire facial area twice daily, morning and evening.
bacitracin zinc	To treat topical infections; to prevent infection in minor skin wounds such as abrasions, minor burns, and cuts	Apply light dusting of powder or thin film of ointment to affected area once daily to three times a day up to 1 wk.
benzoyl peroxide Benzac, Brevoxyl, Clearasil, Desquam, Fostex, Triaz, ZoDerm	To treat mild to moderate inflammatory acne vulgaris	Apply to affected area once daily, gradually increasing to twice daily or three times a day.
clindamycin and benzoyl peroxide Acanya 1.2%/2.5%, Benzaclin 1%/5%, Duac 1.2%/5%, Nevac 1.2%/5%	To treat acne vulgaris	Apply once or twice daily (morning and/or evening) to affected areas.
clindamycin 1.2% and tretinoin 0.025% Veltin Gel, Ziana Gel	To treat acne vulgaris	Apply pea-sized amount to affected areas once daily in evening.
clindamycin phosphate Cleocin 1%, Clinda-Derm 1%, Clindaget 1%, Clindesse 2%, Clindets 1%, Dalacin T Topical Solution 1% (CAN), Evoclin 1%	To treat inflammatory acne vulgaris To treat bacterial vaginosis	Apply to affected area once or twice daily (morning and evening). 1 applicatorful (100 mg) intravaginally at bedtime for 7 days.
dapsone gel 7.5% Aczone	To treat acne vulgaris	Apply pea-sized amount in thin layer to entire face or other affected areas once daily.
dapsone gel 5% Aczone	To treat acne vulgaris	Apply pea-sized amount in thin layer to entire face or other affected areas twice daily.
erythromycin 1.5%, 2% Akne-Mycin, A/T/S, EryDerm, Erygel, Erythrogel, ETS (CAN), Sans-Acne (CAN), Staticin	To treat inflammatory acne vulgaris	Apply to affected areas once or twice daily (morning and evening).
erythromycin 3% and benzoyl peroxide 5% Benzamycin	To treat moderate inflammatory acne vulgaris	Apply to affected areas twice daily, morning and evening.

GENERIC AND TRADE NAMES	INDICATIONS	USUAL ADULT DOSAGES
Antibacterials *(continued)*		
gentamicin sulfate Garamycin, G-myticin	To prevent or treat superficial skin infections due to susceptible bacteria; to treat superficial burns	Apply small amount to skin in affected area three or four times a day.
mafenide acetate Sulfamylon	As adjunct to treat second- and third-degree burns	Apply 1/16-in layer aseptically to affected areas once or twice daily.
metronidazole 0.75%, 1% MetroCream, MetroGel, MetroGel-Vaginal, MetroLotion, Noritate	To treat inflammatory papules and pustules of acne rosacea	Apply thin film to affected area once or twice daily (morning and evening).
	To treat bacterial vaginosis	1 applicatorful (37.5 mg) intravaginally at bedtime or twice daily for 5 days.
mupirocin 2% Bactroban, Bactroban Cream, Bactroban Nasal, Bactroban Ointment, Centany Nasal	To treat impetigo due to *Staphylococcus aureus* and *Streptococcus pyogenes*	Apply to affected areas three times a day up to 10 days.
	To treat secondary infections of traumatic skin lesions due to *S. aureus* and *S. pyogenes*	Apply thin film and cover with a gauze dressing three times a day for 10 days.
	To eradicate nasal colonization of methicillin-resistant *S. aureus*	Apply half of the contents of a unit-dose tube to each nostril twice daily for 5 days.
neomycin sulfate Myciguent	To prevent or treat superficial bacterial infections	Rub fingertip-size dose into affected area once daily to three times a day for no more than 1 week.
ozenoxacin Xepi	To treat impetigo due to *Staphylococcus aureus* or *Streptococcus pyogenes*	Apply thin layer to affected area (not exceeding 100 cm^2) twice daily for 5 days.
povidone-iodine 0.75%, 10% Betadine, Betadine Cream, Betadine Spray	To disinfect wounds and burns	Apply or spray to affected area, as needed.
	To prepare skin for surgical incision	Wet skin with water, then apply 1 cc/20–30 sq inches using 7.5% solution. Lather and scrub site for 5 minutes, then rinse. Follow with 10% solution painted on skin and allowed to dry.
silver sulfadiazine 1% Flamazine (CAN), Silvadene, Thermazine	To prevent and treat wound sepsis in second- and third-degree burns	Apply 1/16-in layer aseptically once to twice daily to clean debrided burns; reapply promptly if removed.
sulfacetamide sodium 10% Klaron	To treat acne vulgaris	Apply thin film twice daily.

(continues)

Selected Topical Drugs *(continued)*

GENERIC AND TRADE NAMES	INDICATIONS	USUAL ADULT DOSAGES
Antifungals		
butenafine hydrochloride 1% Lotrimin Ultra, Mentax	To treat tinea corporis, tinea cruris, or tinea versicolor	Apply to affected surrounding area once daily for 2 wk.
Lotrimin Ultra, Mentax	To treat interdigital tinea pedis due to *Epidermophyton floccosum, Trychophyton mentagrophytes,* or *T. rubrum*	Apply to affected and immediately surrounding area once daily for 4 wk or twice daily for 1 wk.
butoconazole nitrate 2% Femstat 3	To treat vulvovaginal mycotic infections caused by *Candida* species	1 applicatorful (100 mg) intravaginally at bedtime for 3 days.
Gynazole-1	To treat vulvovaginal infections caused by *Candida albicans*	1 applicatorful (100 mg) intravaginally once anytime day or night; may repeat course for total of 6 days in pregnant women (second and third trimester only).
ciclopirox olamine Loprox Cream 0.77%	To treat candidiasis, tinea corporis, tinea cruris, tinea pedis, and tinea versicolor	Massage gently into affected and surrounding area twice daily, morning and evening.
Loprox Shampoo 1%	To treat seborrheic dermatitis	Apply 5 ml to scalp (10 ml for long hair), lather and leave on scalp for 3 minutes, then rinse. Repeat twice weekly for 4 weeks with minimum of 3 days between applications.
ciclopirox olamine 8% Penlac	To treat onychomycosis of the fingernails and toenails	Apply evenly to entire nail surface and surrounding 5 mm of skin at bedtime for up to 48 wk.
clotrimazole Canesten (CAN), Desenex, Femcare, FungiCURE, Fungoid, Gyne-Lotrimin, Lotrimin, Mycelex, Trivagizole	To treat superficial fungal infections (tinea corporis, tinea cruris, tinea pedis, tinea versicolor, candidiasis)	Apply thin film and massage into affected and surrounding area twice daily, morning and evening, for 2 to 8 wk.
	To treat vulvovaginal candidiasis	Insert 100-mg vaginal tablet at bedtime for 7 days; or 500-mg vaginal tablet at bedtime for 1 day; or 1 applicatorful intravaginally at bedtime for 7 days (or 3 days if using Trivagizole).
	To treat oropharyngeal candidiasis	Dissolve oral troche over 15 to 30 min 5 times/day for 14 days.
	To prevent oropharyngeal candidiasis	Dissolve oral troche over 15 to 30 min three times a day for duration of chemotherapy or until corticosteroid dosage is reduced to maintenance levels.

GENERIC AND TRADE NAMES	INDICATIONS	USUAL ADULT DOSAGES
Antifungals *(continued)*		
econazole nitrate 1% Ecostatin (CAN)	To treat tinea corporis, tinea cruris, tinea pedis, tinea versicolor	Rub into affected area once or twice daily for at least 2 wk (4 wk for tinea pedis).
	To treat cutaneous candidiasis	Rub into affected area twice daily (morning and evening) for 2 wk.
Ecoza	To treat interdigital tinea pedis	Apply to affected areas once daily for 4 wk.
gentian violet 1%, 2%	To treat candidiasis	Apply 1% solution to affected area two or three times daily for 3 days.
	To help protect against skin infection in minor burns, cuts, or scrapes	Apply small amount of 2% solution to affected area once to three times daily.
ketoconazole 1%, 2% Ketozole, Nizoral	To treat tinea corporis, tinea cruris, tinea pedis, and tinea versicolor due to susceptible organisms; to treat cutaneous candidiasis	Apply thin film to affected and immediately surrounding area daily for at least 2 wk (6 wk for tinea pedis).
Ketozole Shampoo 2%, Nizoral AD Shampoo 1%	To treat tinea versicolor	Apply Nizoral AD Shampoo 1% to wet hair, lather, massage for 1 min, leave drug on scalp for 3 min, then rinse and repeat 2 times/wk for 4 up to 8 wk (with at least 3 days between shampoos), then intermittently, as needed. Alternatively, apply Ketozole Shampoo 2% one time only to wet hair, lather, massage for 1 min, leave drug on scalp for 5 min, then rinse.
Extina 2%, Xolegel 2%	To treat seborrheic dermatitis	Apply to affected and immediately surrounding area twice daily for 4 wk.
luliconazole 1% Luzu	To treat interdigital tinea pedis	Apply to affected area and about 1 in of the immediate surround area(s) once daily for 2 wk.
	To treat tinea cruris and tinea corporis	Apply to affected area and about 1 in of the immediate surrounding area(s) once daily for 1 wk.

(continues)

Selected Topical Drugs *(continued)*

GENERIC AND TRADE NAMES	INDICATIONS	USUAL ADULT DOSAGES
Antifungals *(continued)*		
miconazole nitrate 2% Fungoid, Micatin, Monistat 1, Monistat 3, Monistat 7, Zeasorb-AF	To treat tinea corporis, tinea cruris, tinea pedis; cutaneous candidiasis; and common dermatophyte infections	Apply cream sparingly (or powder or spray liberally) over affected area twice daily for 2 wk (4 wk for tinea corporis and tinea pedis).
	To treat tinea versicolor	Apply sparingly to affected area daily for 2 wk.
	To treat vulvovaginal candidiasis	Insert into vaginal canal at bedtime for 7 days (100 mg), repeated, as needed; insert 200-mg strength into vaginal canal at bedtime for 3 days; or insert 1,200-mg strength into vaginal canal as a single treatment.
	To treat onychomycosis	Brush tincture on affected areas of nail surface, beds, and edges and under nail surface once or twice daily for up to several months; or spray on clean, dry, affected nails, holding actuator down for 1 or 2 sec once or twice daily.
naftifine hydrochloride 2% Naftin	To treat tinea corporis, tinea cruris, and interdigital tinea pedis	Apply to affected area and 1/2-in margin surrounding area once daily for 2 wk.
nystatin Nadostine (CAN), Nilstat, Nystop	To treat cutaneous and mucocutaneous infections due to *Candida albicans*	Apply cream to affected area twice daily or as indicated; or apply powder twice daily or three times a day.
oxiconazole nitrate Oxistat, Oxizold (CAN)	To treat tinea corporis, tinea cruris, and tinea pedis	Apply to affected and surrounding area once or twice daily for 2 wk (4 wk for tinea pedis).
	To treat tinea versicolor	Apply cream to affected and surrounding area daily for 2 wk.
selenium sulfide 1%, 2.5% Selsun, Versel (CAN)	To treat tinea versicolor	Apply to scalp, lather with small amount of water, wait 10 min, then rinse, once daily for 7 days.
	To treat dandruff and seborrheic scalp dermatitis	Massage into wet scalp, wait 2 to 3 min, rinse, and repeat 2 times/wk for 2 wk, then once daily for 2, 3, or 4 wk.
sulconazole nitrate 1% Exelderm	To treat tinea corporis, tinea cruris, and tinea versicolor	Massage small amount gently into affected and surrounding areas once or twice daily (tinea pedis) for 3 wk.

GENERIC AND TRADE NAMES	INDICATIONS	USUAL ADULT DOSAGES
Antifungals *(continued)*		
tavaborole Kerydin	To treat onychomycosis of the toenails due to *Trichophyton mentagrophytes* or *Trichophyton rubrum*	Apply to affected toenails, including under the tip of each toenail, once daily for 48 wk.
terbinafine hydrochloride 1% Lamisil	To treat tinea versicolor	Apply to affected area twice daily for 1 or 2 wk.
	To treat tinea corporis and tinea cruris	Apply thin film to affected area once or twice daily for 1 wk.
	To treat interdigital tinea pedis	Apply between the toes twice daily for 1 wk (interdigital tinea pedis) or to affected area daily for 1 wk.
	To treat tinea pedis involving bottom or sides of feet	Apply to affected area twice daily (morning and evening) for 2 wk.
terconazole 0.4%, 0.8% Terazol 3, Terazol 7	To treat vulvovaginal candidiasis	1 applicatorful (20 mg) intravaginally at bedtime for 3 days (0.4%) or 1 applicatorful (40 mg) for 7 days (0.8%); or insert 80-mg vaginal suppository at bedtime for 3 consecutive days.
tioconazole GyneCure Ovules (CAN), Vagistat-1	To treat vulvovaginal candidiasis	Insert 1 applicatorful (300 mg) or 1 suppository (300 mg) intravaginally at bedtime as a single dose.
tolnaftate 1% Absorbine Footcare, Aftate for Athlete's Foot, Aftate for Jock Itch, Dr. Scholl's Athlete's Foot, Genaspore, NP-27, Pitrex, Quinsana Plus, Tinactin, Ting, Zeasorb-AF	To treat tinea corporis, tinea cruris, tinea manuum, tinea pedis, and tinea versicolor	Apply to affected and surrounding areas twice daily, morning and evening, for 4 wk (2 wk for tinea cruris); continue for 2 wk after symptoms subside or up to 6 wk.
Antivirals		
acyclovir 5% Zovirax	To treat initial genital herpes and selectively for non-life–threatening mucocutaneous herpes simplex in immunocompromised patients	Apply ointment every 3 hr (6 times/day) for 7 days. Use finger cot, rubber glove, or applicator stick for both forms to prevent herpetic whitlow.
	To treat herpes labialis in immunocompentent patients	Apply cream to affected area 5 times a day for 4 days.
docosanol 10% Abreva	To treat recurrent herpes labialis of lips and face	Apply cream gently and completely to affected area five times daily, starting with first visible sign of lesion and continuing until lesion is healed.
penciclovir 1% Denavir	To treat recurrent herpes labialis of lips and face	Apply every 2 hr while awake for 4 days.

(continues)

Selected Topical Drugs *(continued)*

GENERIC AND TRADE NAMES	INDICATIONS	USUAL ADULT DOSAGES
Corticosteroids		
alclometasone dipropionate 0.05% Aclovate	To relieve inflammatory and pruritic manifestations of corticosteroid-responsive dermatoses	Apply thin film to affected area and massage twice daily to three times a day.
amcinonide 0.01% Cyclocort	To relieve inflammatory and pruritic manifestations of corticosteroid-responsive dermatoses	Apply thin film to affected area and massage twice daily (lotion) or twice daily to three times a day (cream, ointment).
betamethasone benzoate 0.05% Beben (CAN), Uticort	To relieve inflammatory and pruritic manifestations of corticosteroid-responsive dermatoses	Apply thin film or a few drops to affected area once or twice daily up to 45 g/wk (ointment, cream), 50 g/wk (gel), or 50 ml (lotion).
betamethasone dipropionate 0.05% Diprolene, Diprolene AF, Diprosone, Topilene (CAN)	To relieve inflammatory and pruritic manifestations of corticosteroid-responsive dermatoses	Apply thin film or a few drops to affected area once or twice daily.
betamethasone valerate 0.1% Betatrex, Beta-Val, Luxiq, Valisone	To relieve inflammatory and pruritic manifestations of corticosteroid-responsive dermatoses	Apply foam to scalp, and massage until foam disappears, twice daily (morning and evening). Apply thin film of cream or ointment 1 to 3 times daily. Apply a few drops of lotion twice daily (morning and evening).
clobetasol propionate 0.025% Impoyz	To treat moderate to severe plaque psoriasis	Apply thin layer to affected skin and rub in gently twice daily, up to 50 g/wk for 2 wk.
clobetasol propionate 0.05% Dermovate (CAN), Embeline, Temovate	To relieve inflammatory and pruritic manifestations of corticosteroid-responsive dermatoses	Apply thin film to affected area and rub in gently twice daily (morning and evening), up to 50 g/wk, for 2 wk.
Olux	To relieve moderate to severe inflammatory and pruritic manifestations of corticosteroid-responsive dermatoses of scalp	Apply to affected area of scalp twice daily, once in morning and once at night, up to 50 g/wk, for 2 wk.
desonide 0.05% DesOwen, Tridesilon	To relieve inflammatory and pruritic manifestations of corticosteroid-responsive dermatoses	Apply thin film to affected area twice daily to four times a day.

GENERIC AND TRADE NAMES	INDICATIONS	USUAL ADULT DOSAGES
Corticosteroids *(continued)*		
desoximetasone 0.05% Topicort	To relieve inflammatory and pruritic manifestations of corticosteroid-responsive dermatoses	Apply thin film to affected skin areas twice daily.
diflorasone diacetate 0.05% Florone, Psorcon	To relieve inflammatory and pruritic manifestations of corticosteroid-responsive dermatoses	Apply thin film to affected area once daily to four times a day.
fluocinolone acetonide 0.01% Derma Smooth FS, Fluoderm (CAN), Fluolar (CAN), Fluonid (CAN), Synalar, Synamol (CAN)	To relieve inflammatory and pruritic manifestations of corticosteroid-responsive dermatoses	Apply thin film to affected area twice daily to four times a day.
	To treat seborrheic dermatoses	Use shampoo on scalp daily.
	To treat scalp psoriasis	Apply oil to affected areas on scalp and leave overnight.
fluocinonide 0.05% Lidemol (CAN), Lidex	To relieve inflammatory and pruritic manifestations of corticosteroid-responsive dermatoses	Apply thin film to affected area twice daily to four times a day.
flurandrenolide Cordran 0.05%, Cordran Tape, Drenison 0.05% (CAN)	To relieve inflammatory and pruritic manifestations of corticosteroid-responsive dermatoses	Apply thin film to affected area and massage twice daily to three times a day; or apply tape every 12 to 24 hr.
fluticasone propionate 0.05% Cutivate	To treat atopic dermatitis; to relieve inflammatory and pruritic manifestations of corticosteroid-responsive dermatoses	Apply thin film once or twice daily (atopic dermatitis) or twice daily (dermatoses).
halcinonide 0.1% Halog	To relieve inflammatory and pruritic manifestations of corticosteroid-responsive dermatoses	Apply sparingly and massage two to three times a day.
halobetasol propionate 0.05% Ultravate	To treat plaque psoriasis	Apply thin film to affected area and rub in gently twice daily, up to 50 g/wk, for 2 wk.
halobetasol propionate 0.01% Bryhali		Apply thin layer to affected area and rub in gently once daily, up to 50 g/wk and for no longer than 8 wk.

(continues)

Selected Topical Drugs *(continued)*

GENERIC AND TRADE NAMES	INDICATIONS	USUAL ADULT DOSAGES
Corticosteroids *(continued)*		
hydrocortisone 0.25% Cetacort **hydrocortisone 0.5%** Cetacort, Cortate (CAN), Delacort, Dermtex HC, Emo-Cort (CAN), Hydro-Tex **hydrocortisone 1%** Ala-Cort, Cort-Dome, Cortizone 10, Emo-Cort (CAN), Nutracort, Synacort **hydrocortisone 2%** Ala-Scalp HP, Dermasorb HC **hydrocortisone 2.5%** Anusol-HC, Emo-Cort (CAN), Hytone, Nutracort, Stie-Cort, Synacort, Texacort **hydrocortisone acetate 0.1%** Corticreme (CAN) **hydrocortisone acetate 0.5%** Corticaine, Cortacet (CAN), Cortoderm (CAN), Hyderm, Lanacort, Novohydrocort (CAN)	To relieve inflammatory and pruritic manifestations of corticosteroid-responsive dermatoses	Apply thin film (aerosol foam, cream, lotion, ointment, solution) to affected area once daily to four times a day.
hydrocortisone acetate 1%, 2%, 2.5% Cortaid, Corticreme (CAN), Cortoderm (CAN), Hyderm (CAN), Maximum Strength Cortaid, Micort HC-Lipocream, Novohydrocort (CAN) **hydrocortisone acetate 1% and pramoxine hydrochloride 1% topical aerosol foam** Epifoam	To relieve inflammatory and pruritic manifestations of corticosteroid-responsive dermatoses	Apply thin film (aerosol foam, cream, lotion, ointment, solution) to affected area once daily to four times a day.
hydrocortisone butyrate 0.1% Locoid **hydrocortisone probutate 0.1%**	To relieve inflammatory and pruritic manifestations of corticosteroid-responsive dermatoses	Apply to affected area twice daily to three times a day.
hydrocortisone probutate 0.1% Pandel		Apply to affected area once or twice daily.
hydrocortisone valerate 0.2% Westcort		Apply to affected area two to three times daily.

GENERIC AND TRADE NAMES	INDICATIONS	USUAL ADULT DOSAGES
Corticosteroids *(continued)*		
hydrocortisone acetate, polymyxin B sulfate, and neomycin sulfate Cortisporin	To treat corticosteroid-responsive dermatoses (short term) with mild bacterial infection	Apply sparingly and massage twice daily to four times a day.
mometasone furoate 0.1% Elocom (CAN), Elocon	To relieve inflammatory and pruritic manifestations of corticosteroid-responsive dermatoses	Apply thin film or a few drops to affected area daily.
prednicarbate 0.1% Dermatop	To relieve inflammatory and pruritic manifestations of corticosteroid-responsive dermatoses	Apply thin film to affected area twice daily.
triamcinolone acetonide 0.025%, 0.5% Aristocort, Aristocort A, Aristocort D (CAN), Kenalog, Triacet, Triaderm (CAN), Trianide Mild (CAN)	To relieve inflammatory and pruritic manifestations of corticosteroid-responsive dermatoses	Apply thin film of 0.025% to affected area twice daily to four times a day; apply 0.1% or 0.5% two to three times daily.
triamcinolone acetonide 0.1% Aristocort, Aristocort A, Aristocort R (CAN), Delta-Tritex, Flutex, Kenac, Kenalog, Kenalog-H, Triacet, Triaderm (CAN), Trianide Regular (CAN) **triamcinolone acetonide 0.5%** Aristocort, Aristocort A, Aristocort C (CAN), Flutex, Kenalog, Triacet	To relieve inflammatory and pruritic manifestations of corticosteroid-responsive dermatoses	Apply thin film (cream) to affected area twice daily to four times a day; 0.025% lotion or ointment once or twice daily; 0.1% lotion or ointment once daily; or 0.5% ointment once daily.
triamcinolone acetonide topical aerosol 0.2% Kenalog	To relieve inflammatory and pruritic manifestations of corticosteroid-responsive dermatoses	Spray affected area three times a day to four times a day.
Retinoids		
adapalene 0.1% Differin	To treat acne vulgaris	Apply thin film to affected area at bedtime.
tazarotene 0.1% Avage	As adjunct to treat mitigation of facial fine wrinkling, facial mottled hyper- and hypopigmentation, and benign facial lentigines	Apply pea-size amount to affected area at bedtime.

(continues)

Selected Topical Drugs *(continued)*

GENERIC AND TRADE NAMES	INDICATIONS	USUAL ADULT DOSAGES
Retinoids *(continued)*		
tazarotene 0.05%, 0.1% Avage, Tazorac	To treat acne; to treat mild to moderately severe facial acne vulgaris	Apply thin film to affected area at bedtime.
tazarotene 0.1% Fabior	To treat acne vulgaris	Apply thin layer to affected areas of the face and upper trunk once daily in the evening.
tretinoin 0.025% Avita, Renova, Retin-A, Retin-A Micro, Stieva-A (CAN), Tretin-X **tretinoin 0.05%** Altreno	To treat acne vulgaris	Apply pea-size amount to clean, dry affected area at bedtime.
Miscellaneous topical drugs		
adapalene 0.1% and benzoyl peroxide 2.5% gel Epiduo **adapalene 0.3% and benzoyl peroxide 2.5% gel** Epiduo Forte	To treat acne vulgaris	Apply pea-size amount to each clean, dry affected area once daily.
ammonium lactate 12% Lac-Hydrin	To treat dry, scaly skin and ichthyosis vulgaris	Apply to affected area, and rub in twice daily.
anthralin Anthranol 1 (CAN), Anthranol 2 (CAN), Anthranol 3 (CAN), Anthrascalp (CAN), Drithocreme, Dritho-Scalp, Psoriatec, Zithranol, Zithranol-RR	To treat chronic psoriasis To treat chronic scalp psoriasis	Apply sparingly and massage into affected lesions daily. Apply to lesions daily for 1 wk.
becaplermin Regranex	To treat lower-extremity diabetic neuropathic ulcers that extend into the subcutaneous tissue or beyond and that have an adequate blood supply	Amount applied to ulcers daily calculated based on size of ulcer.
brimonidine 0.33% Mirvaso	To treat rosacea	Apply pea-sized amount onto each of the five areas of the face once daily. Do not apply to eyes or lips.
calcipotriene 0.005% Dovonex, Sorilux	To treat plaque psoriasis	Apply cream or scalp lotion in a thin layer twice daily up to 8 wk. Apply thin layer of ointment once or twice daily up to 8 wk.

GENERIC AND TRADE NAMES	INDICATIONS	USUAL ADULT DOSAGES
Miscellaneous topical drugs *(continued)*		
calcipotriene hydrate 0.005% and betamethasone dipropionate 0.064% Taclonex	To treat plaque psoriasis	Apply suspension to affected areas and rub in gently once daily for up to 8 wk.
Taclonex Scalp	To treat moderate to severe plaque psoriasis of the scalp	Apply suspension to affected scalp areas and rub in gently once daily for 2 to 8 wk or until skin clears.
	To treat psoriasis vulgaris	Apply ointment to affected skin; rub in gently and completely once daily for up to 4 wk.
capsaicin 0.025%, 0.075%, 0.1% Capsin, Zostrix	To provide temporary pain relief from rheumatoid arthritis and osteoarthritis; to relieve neuralgias from pain following shingles (herpes zoster) infection	Apply to affected area no more than four times a day.
chlorhexidine gluconate 4% Betasept, Hibiclens	To clean skin wounds	Rinse area, apply minimal amount to cover, then wash and rinse thoroughly.
	To prepare skin for surgical incision	Apply liberally to surgical site and swab for at least 2 minutes. Dry with sterile towel and repeat once.
clotrimazole and betamethasone dipropionate 0.05%/1% Lotrisone	To treat symptomatic inflammatory tinea corporis, tinea cruris, and tinea pedis	Apply thin layer and massage cream gently into affected and surrounding skin areas twice daily for 2 wk (tinea corporis, tinea cruris) or for 4 wk (tinea pedis).
coal tar Denorex, Pentrax, Zetar, Zetar Shampoo	To treat psoriasis	Add 15 to 20 ml to lukewarm bath, immerse affected area for 15 to 20 min, and rinse thoroughly 3 to 7 times/wk.
	To treat dandruff or scalp seborrhea	Massage into wet scalp, rinse, repeat application and wait 5 min, then rinse again.
crotamiton 10% Eurax	To treat scabies	Massage into cleansed body from chin to soles of feet, and reapply after 24 hr; change bed linens next day, and bathe 48 hr after second dose; repeat in 7 to 10 days if new lesions appear.
	To treat symptomatic pruritic skin	Massage gently into affected areas until absorbed. Repeat as needed.

(continues)

Selected Topical Drugs *(continued)*

GENERIC AND TRADE NAMES	INDICATIONS	USUAL ADULT DOSAGES
Miscellaneous topical drugs *(continued)*		
desoximetasone 0.05% Topicort	To relieve inflammatory and pruritic manifestations of corticosteroid-responsive dermatoses	Apply thin film twice daily to affected areas.
diclofenac sodium 3% Solaraze	To treat actinic keratoses	Massage gel gently onto affected lesion areas twice daily for 60 to 90 days.
doxepin hydrochloride 5% Zonalon	To treat moderate pruritus associated with atopic dermatitis and chronic lichen simplex	Apply thin film to affected area four times a day (every 3 to 4 hr) for up to 8 days.
eflornithine hydrochloride 13.9% Vaniqa	To retard unwanted hair growth	Apply thin film to affected area of face and chin twice daily (at least 8 hr apart); don't wash treated area for at least 4 hr.
fluocinolone acetonide 0.01%, hydroquinone 4%, tretinoin 0.05% TRI-LUMA Cream	To treat severe facial melasma	Apply a thin film lightly and uniformly to hyperpigmented areas of melasma including about 1/2 in of skin surrounding each lesion daily at least 30 min before bedtime.
fluorouracil cream Carac 0.5%	To treat actinic and solar keratoses of face and anterior scalp	Apply to lesions twice daily for 4 wk.
Efudex 2%, 5%	To treat actinic or solar keratosis	Apply to lesions twice daily for 2 to 4 wk.
	To treat superficial basal cell carcinoma	Apply 5% preparation twice daily in sufficient amounts to cover lesions for up to 12 wks.
Fluoroplex 1%	To treat actinic or solar keratosis	Apply to lesions twice daily for 2 to 6 wk.
glycopyrronium 2.4% Qbrexza	To treat primary axillary hyperhidrosis	Apply once daily to both axillae using a single cloth.
hexachlorophene 3% Phisohex	To use as a surgical scrub	Wet hands and forearms with water, apply 5 ml of solution and rub into a copious lather for 3 min, then rinse; repeat once.
	To use for bacteriostatic cleansing	Wet hands with water, pour 5 ml into palm and work up a lather, then apply to area to be cleaned. Rinse thoroughly.

GENERIC AND TRADE NAMES	INDICATIONS	USUAL ADULT DOSAGES
Miscellaneous topical drugs *(continued)*		
hydrocortisone acetate 1%, polymyxin B sulfate, bacitracin zinc, and neomycin sulfate Cortisporin	To treat corticosteroid-responsive dermatoses associated with secondary bacterial infection	Apply small amount to affected areas twice daily to four times a day for up to 7 days.
hydroquinone Claripel 4%, Eldopaque 2%, Eldoquin 2% and 4%, Melanex 3%	To treat hyperpigmentation and melanin	Apply twice daily to the affected areas for no longer than 2 mo.
imiquimod 2.5%, 3.75% Zyclara	To treat facial or scalp actinic keratoses	Apply 2.5% or 3.75% to affected area daily for two 2-wk treatment cycles separated by a 2-wk no-treatment period.
	To treat external genital and perianal warts	Apply 3.75% cream to the external genital and perianal warts until total clearance or up to 8 wk.
imiquimod 5% Aldara	To treat external genital and perianal warts	Apply thin layer to affected area and rub in 3 times/wk at bedtime for up to 16 wk; remove with soap and water after 6 to 10 hr.
	To treat actinic keratosis on face and scalp	Apply to affected area on face or scalp (but not both concurrently) for 16 wk.
	To treat superficial basal cell carcinoma	Apply to affected area 5 times per wk for 6 wk prior to bedtime and leave on skin for about 8 hrs, then wash area with mild soap and water.
ingenol mebutate 0.015%, 0.05% Picato	To treat actinic keratosis	Apply 0.015% gel to face and scalp once daily for 3 consecutive days; apply 0.05% gel to trunk and extremities once daily for 2 consecutive days.
ivermectin 0.5% Sklice	To treat head lice	Apply to dry hair in amount sufficient to coat the hair and scalp thoroughly; leave on for 10 minutes, then rinse off with water.
ivermectin 1% Soolantra	To treat inflammatory lesions of rosacea	Apply pea-sized amount for each affected area of the face (chin, each cheek, forehead) once daily.
lidocaine 2.5% and prilocaine 2.5% EMLA	For local anesthesia	Apply 1 disk or thick layer of 2- to 2.5-g cream occlusively for at least 1 hr before the start of routine procedure or 2 hr before the start of painful procedure.

(continues)

Selected Topical Drugs *(continued)*

GENERIC AND TRADE NAMES	INDICATIONS	USUAL ADULT DOSAGES
Miscellaneous topical drugs *(continued)*		
malathion 0.5% Ovide	To treat pediculus humanus capitis (head lice and their ova) of scalp hair	Apply to dry hair in amount just sufficient to wet the hair and scalp thoroughly; then let hair dry naturally. After 8 to 12 hr, shampoo and rinse hair and use a fine-toothed comb to remove dead lice and eggs. If lice are still present after 7 to 9 days, repeat application.
mequinol 2%, tretinoin 0.01% Solage	To treat solar lentigines	Apply solution twice daily, morning and evening, at least 8 hr apart. Avoid application to surrounding skin, and do not bathe for 6 hr after application.
minoxidil 2%, 5% Rogaine	To treat alopecia and androgenetica of the scalp	For women: Apply 1/2 capful of 5% foam, aerosol once daily or 1 ml of 2% solution twice daily for up to 4 months. For men: Apply 1/2 capful of 5% foam, aerosol twice daily, or 1 ml of 2% or 5% solution twice daily for up to 4 months.
nitroglycerin 0.4% Rectiv	To treat moderate to severe pain associated with chronic anal fissure	Apply 1 in of ointment intra-anally every 12 hr for up to 3 wk.
oxybutynin chloride 10% Gelnique	To treat overactive bladder with symptoms of urge urinary incontinence, urgency, and frequency	Apply 1 sachet of gel or 1 activation of metered-dose pump once daily to clean, dry, intact skin on abdomen, upper arms/shoulders, or thighs.
permethrin 1% Nix	To prevent or treat head lice	Wash and dry hair, saturate scalp, leave on hair for 10 min, then rinse; remove nits with provided comb; repeat in 7 days if living mites are still present.
permethrin 5% Acticin, Elimite	To treat scabies	Massage into skin from head to soles of feet, and remove after 8 to 10 hr; repeat in 14 days if living mites are still present.
pimecrolimus 1% Elidel	To treat mild-to-moderate atopic dermatitis as a second-line therapy	Apply to affected areas twice daily for up to 6 wk.

GENERIC AND TRADE NAMES	INDICATIONS	USUAL ADULT DOSAGES
Miscellaneous topical drugs *(continued)*		
podofilox 0.5% Condylox	To treat anogenital warts (gel)	Apply gel to anogenital warts for 3 days, then withhold for 4 days; repeat cycle up to four times.
	To treat external genital warts (gel or solution)	Apply gel or solution to external genital warts every 12 hr in the morning and evening for 3 days, then withhold for 4 days; repeat cycle up to four times.
pyrethrin and piperonyl butoxide Licide, Pronto, RID	To treat body, head, and pubic lice	Apply to dry hair or affected body area. Massage through all hairy areas until hair is wet. Leave on hair for 10 min; then wash with warm water and rinse thoroughly. Repeat in 7 to 10 days.
spinosad 0.9% Natroba	To treat head lice	Apply to dry scalp and hair using only the amount needed to cover the scalp and hair. Rinse off with warm water after 10 min. Repeat in 7 days if live lice are still seen.
tacrolimus 0.03% and 0.1% Protopic	To treat moderate to severe atopic dermatitis in patients unresponsive to other therapies	Apply thin layer to affected areas twice daily, rubbing in gently and completely.
urea 41%, 45% Utopic	To treat hyperkeratotic conditions	Apply to affected area twice daily and rub in.

Selected Combination Antiviral Drugs

Combination antiviral drugs are used to treat viral infections, such as human immunodeficiency virus (HIV) and hepatitis C infections.

The following table lists the generic and trade names, indications, and usual adult dosages for some commonly used combination antivirals. Although you must individualize your care for a patient who receives an antiviral, be sure to include these general interventions in your plan of care:

- Avoid administering HIV drugs all at once.
- If patient takes an antacid, administer it 1 hour before or 2 hours after an antiviral because antacids may reduce antiviral absorption.
- Monitor hepatic enzyme levels to detect elevations and help prevent hepatotoxicity.
- Monitor BUN and serum creatinine levels to detect signs of impaired renal function.
- Monitor I.V. injection site for pain or phlebitis, which may result from the high pH of reconstituted solutions.
- Assess the immunosuppressed patient for opportunistic infections during antiviral therapy.
- Inform female patient that oral contraceptives may be ineffective when taken with HIV drugs. Suggest alternate contraceptive methods.

GENERIC AND TRADE NAMES	INDICATIONS	USUAL ADULT DOSAGES
Antivirals used for HIV infection		
abacavir sulfate, dolutegravir, and lamivudine Triumeq	To treat HIV-1 infection	600 mg abacavir, 50 mg dolutegravir, and 300 mg lamivudine (1 tablet) P.O. once daily
abacavir sulfate and lamivudine Epzicom	As adjunct to treat HIV-1 infection	600 mg abacavir and 300 mg lamivudine (1 tablet) P.O. daily
abacavir sulfate, lamivudine, and zidovudine Trizivir	As adjunct or as monotherapy to treat HIV-1 infection	300 mg abacavir, 150 mg lamivudine, and 300 mg zidovudine (1 tablet) P.O. twice daily
atazanavir sulfate and cobicistat Evotaz	As adjunct to treat HIV-1 infection	300 mg atazanavir and 150 mg cobicistat (1 tablet) P.O. once daily
bictegravir, emtricitabine, and tenofovir alafenamide Biktarvy	To treat HIV-1 infection	50 mg bictegravir, 200 mg emtricitabine, and 25 mg tenofovir alafenamide (1 tablet) P.O. once daily.
darunavir and cobicistat Prezcobix	As adjunct to treat HIV-1 infection	800 mg darunavir and 150 mg cobicistat (1 tablet) P.O. once daily
darunavir, cobicistat, emtricitabine, and tenofovir alafenamide Symtuza	To treat HIV-1 infection	800 mg darunavir, 150 mg cobicistat, 200 mg emtricitabine, and 10 mg tenofovir alafenamide (1 tablet) P.O. once daily.
doravirine, lamivudine, and tenofovir disoproxil fumarate Delstrigo	To treat HIV-1 infection	100 mg doravirine, 300 mg lamivudine, and 300 mg tenofovir disoproxil fumarate (1 tablet) P.O. once daily

GENERIC AND TRADE NAMES	INDICATIONS	USUAL ADULT DOSAGES
Antivirals used for HIV infection *(continued)*		
efavirenz, emtricitabine, and tenofovir disoproxil fumarate Atripla	As adjunct or monotherapy to treat HIV-1 infection in adults weighing at least 40 kg (88 lb) or more	600 mg efavirenz, 200 mg emtricitabine, and 300 mg tenofovir disoproxil fumarate (1 tablet) P.O. once daily, at bedtime
efavirenz, lamivudine, and tenofovir disoproxil fumarate Symfi	To treat HIV-1 infection in patients weighing at least 40 kg (88 lb) or more	600 mg efavirenz, 300 mg lamivudine, and 300 mg tenofovir disoproxil fumarate (1 tablet) P.O. once daily
Symfi Lo	To treat HIV-1 infection in adults and children weighing at least 35 kg (77 lb)	400 mg efavirenz, 300 mg lamivudine, and 300 mg tenofovir disoproxil fumarate (1 tablet) P.O. once daily
elvitegravir, cobicistat, emtricitabline, tenofovir alafenamide Genvoya	To treat HIV-1 infection	150 mg elvitegravir, 150 mg cobicistat, 200 mg emtricitabine, and 10 mg tenofovir alafenamide (1 tablet) once daily
elvitegravir, cobicistat, emtricitabine, tenofovir disoproxil fumarate Stribild	To treat HIV-1 infection	150 mg elvitegravir, 150 mg cobicistat, 200 mg emtricitabine, 300 mg tenofovir (1 tablet) P.O. once daily with food
emtricitabine, rilpivirine, tenofovir disoproxil fumarate Complera	To treat HIV-1 infection	200 mg emtricitabine, 25 mg rilpivirine, 300 mg tenofovir (1 tablet) P.O. daily with meal
emtricitabine, rilpivirine, tenofovir alafenamide Odefsey	To treat HIV-1 infection	200 mg emtricitabine, 25 mg rilpivirine, and 25 mg tenofovir alafenamide (1 tablet) P.O. once daily
emtricitabine and tenofovir alafenamide Descovy	To treat HIV-1 infection	200 mg emtricitabine and 25 mg tenofovir alafenamide (1 tablet) P.O. once daily in combination with other antiretrovirals
emtricitabine and tenofovir disoproxil fumarate Truvada	As adjunct to treat HIV-1 infection in patients weighing at least 17 kg (37.4 lb)	*Weighing at least 35 kg (77 lb):* 200 mg emtricitabine and 300 mg tenofovir disoproxil fumarate (1 tablet) P.O. once daily *Weighing 28 kg (61.6 lb) to less than 35 kg (77 lb):* 167 mg emtricitabine and 250 mg tenofovir disoproxil fumarate (1 tablet) P.O. once daily

(continues)

Selected Combination Antiviral Drugs *(continued)*

GENERIC AND TRADE NAMES	INDICATIONS	USUAL ADULT DOSAGES
Antivirals used for HIV infection *(continued)*		
		Weighing 22 kg (48.4 lb) to less than 28 kg (61.6 lb): 133 mg emtricitabine, 200 mg tenofovir disoproxil fumarate (1 tablet) P.O. once daily *Weighing 17 kg (37.4 lb) to less than 22 (48.4 lb):* 100 mg emtricitabine and 150 mg tenofovir disoproxil fumarate (1 tablet) P.O. once daily
lamivudine and raltegravir Dutrebis	As adjunct to treat HIV-1 infection	150 mg lamivudine and 300 mg raltegravir (1 tablet) P.O. twice daily
lamivudine and tenofovir disoproxil fumarate Cimduo	As adjunct to treat HIV-1 infection in patients weighing 35 kg (77 lb) or more	300 mg lamivudine and 300 mg tenofovir disproxil fumarate (1 tablet) P.O. once daily
lamivudine and zidovudine (3TC/AZT, 3TC/ZDV) Combivir	As adjunct to treat HIV-1 infection in patients who weigh 50 kg (110 lb) or more	150 mg of lamivudine and 300 mg of zidovudine P.O. twice daily
lopinavir and ritonavir Kaletra	As adjunct to treat HIV-1 infection	800 mg lopinavir and 200 mg ritonavir once daily or 400 mg lopinavir and 100 mg ritonavir P.O. twice daily
Antivirals used for hepatitis C infection		
elbasivir and grazoprevir Zepatier	To treat chronic hepatitis C with genotype 1 or 4	50 mg elbasivir and 100 mg grazoprevir (1 tablet) P.O. once daily
ledipasvir and sofosbuvir Harvoni	To treat chronic hepatitis C genotype 1, 4, 5, or 6 in patients without cirrhosis or with compensated cirrhosis; as adjunct to treat chronic hepatitis C genotype 1 in patients with decompensated cirrhosis or genotype 1 or 4 in liver transplant recipients without cirrhosis or compensated cirrhosis	90 mg ledipasvir and 400 mg sofosbuvir (1 tablet) P.O. once daily
ombitasvir, paritaprevir, and ritonavir Technivie	As adjunct to treat chronic hepatitis C genotype 4 in patients without cirrhosis	25 mg ombitasvir, 150 mg paritaprevir, and 100 mg ritonavir (2 tablets) P.O. once daily in morning
sofosbuvir and velpatasvir Epclusa	To treat chronic hepatitis C genotype 1, 2, 3, 4, 5, or 6 in patients with compensated cirrhosis or without cirrhosis, or with decompensated cirrhosis when used in combination with ribavirin	400 mg sofosbuvir and 100 mg velpatasvir (1 tablet) P.O once daily

GENERIC AND TRADE NAMES	INDICATIONS	USUAL ADULT DOSAGES
Antivirals used for hepatitis C infection *(continued)*		
sofosbuvir, velpatasvir, and voxilaprevir Vosevi	To treat chronic hepatitis C genotype 1, 2, 3, 4, 5, or 6 in patients with compensated cirrhosis or without cirrhosis in patients previously treated with an HCV regimen containing an NS5A inhibitor or genotype 1a or 3 infection previously treated with an HCV regimen containing sofosbuvir without an NS5A inhibitor	400 mg sofosbuvir, 100 mg velpatasvir, and 100 mg voxilaprevir (1 tablet) P.O. once daily

Common Cancers and Antineoplastic Drug Therapy

Antineoplastic drugs are commonly used in the treatment of many types of cancer today. Most of these drugs work by inhibiting cell proliferation, which leads to cell death. They're most effective at killing actively dividing cells.

Cell-specific antineoplastics exert their actions during one or more phases of the cell cycle. S-phase antineoplastics interfere with deoxyribonucleic acid (DNA) synthesis; M-phase drugs interfere with the formation of microtubules and disrupt mitosis.

Most antineoplastics impair DNA in one of the following four ways:

- preventing separation of DNA strands
- inhibiting DNA repair
- mimicking DNA bases
- disrupting the triplicate codons or producing oxygen-free radicals that damage the DNA.

Antineoplastic drugs are cytotoxic, which means that they affect both neoplastic cells and normal cells. As a result, they may cause serious and sometimes life-threatening adverse reactions.

Antineoplastics are most harmful to normal cells that exhibit rapid activity and growth, such as bone marrow tissue, the epithelium of the GI mucosa, and hair follicles. When these drugs suppress bone marrow activity, the patient may develop leukopenia, thrombocytopenia, or anemia. When they affect the GI mucosa, the patient may experience nausea, vomiting, anorexia, bowel dysfunction, and mucosal ulcerations. When antineoplastic drugs affect the hair follicles, the result is hair loss (alopecia), one of the most common adverse reactions. Although not life-threatening, hair loss can be emotionally traumatic for patients, especially women. However, the recent FDA approval of scalp-cooling caps to spare hair loss as a result of chemotherapy can help to prevent baldness in many patients.

The following chart lists the most common cancers (excluding nonmelanoma skin cancers) in the order of prevalence according to the American Cancer Society. The most common type of cancer for women is breast cancer and the most common type of cancer for men is prostate cancer.

The antineoplastic drugs that may be used initially to treat these common cancers are listed under each cancer type. Adult dosages for these cancers are usually based on body weight in kilograms and subsequent dosages are adjusted according to the type and severity of adverse reactions that have occurred during the last cycle. Antineoplastic therapy is given in cycles of a certain number of days or weeks based on protocol for that type of cancer and the patient's reaction to the drugs given during the previous cycle. For example, if the patient experiences bone marrow suppression from the previous cycle, the degree of suppression will determine if the antineoplastic drug regimen is withheld until the blood counts improve or the dosages of the drugs used are decreased.

It is imperative that the nurse monitor patients receiving antineoplastic therapy closely for adverse reactions, because reactions can occur suddenly and can often become serious or life-threatening quickly.

Common Cancers and Antineoplastic Drug Therapy

CANCER TYPE	COMMON ANTINEOPLASTIC DRUG THERAPY
Breast cancer	• Anthracyclines: Examples include doxorubicin (Adriamycin) and epirubicin (Ellence) • Taxanes: Examples include paclitaxel (Taxol) and docetaxel (Taxotere) • 5-fluorouracil (5-FU) • carboplatin (Paraplatin) • cyclophosphamide (Cytoxan) Combinations of 2 or 3 of these drugs are most often administered. Advanced breast cancer • Anthracyclines: Examples include doxorubicin (Adriamycin), epirubicin (Ellence), and pegylated liposomal doxorubicin (Doxil) • Platinum agents: Examples include carboplatin (Paraplatin) and cisplatin (Platinol, Platinol-AQ) • Taxanes: Examples include albumin-bound paclitaxel (Abraxane), docetaxel (Taxotere), and paclitaxel (Taxol) • capecitabine (Xeloda) • eribulin (Halaven) • gemcitabine (Gemzar) • ixabepilone (Ixempra) • nab-paclitaxel (Abraxane) • vinorelbine (Navelbine) Most often, advanced breast cancer is treated with a single antineoplastic agent, although a combination such as carboplatin plus paclitaxel may be administered depending on the clinical status of the patient.
Prostate cancer	• cabazitaxel (Jevtana) • docetaxel (Taxotere) • estramustine (Emcyt) • mitoxantrone (Novantrone)
Lung cancer	• carboplatin (Paraplatin) • cisplatin (Platinol, Platinol-AQ) • docetaxel (Taxotere) • doxorubicin (Adriamycin) • etoposide (VePesid, VP-16) • gemcitabine (Gemzar) • paclitaxel (Taxol) • pemetrexed (Alimta) • vinorelbine (Navelbine) Various combinations of these drugs are often administered.

(continues)

Common Cancers and Antineoplastic Drug Therapy *(continued)*

CANCER TYPE	COMMON ANTINEOPLASTIC DRUG THERAPY
Colorectal cancer	• 5-fluorouracil (5-FU) • capecitabine (Xeloda) • irinotecan (Camptosar) • oxaliplatin (Eloxatin) • trifluridine and tipiracil (Lonsurf) Combinations of 2 or more of these drugs are often administered.
Melanoma	• carboplatin (Paraplatin) • cisplatin (Platinol, Platinol-AQ) • dacarbazine (DTIC) • nab-paclitaxel (Abraxane) • paclitaxel (Taxol) • temozolomide (Temodar) • vinblastine (Alkaban-AQ, Velban)
Bladder cancer	Used with radiation: • 5-fluorouracil (5-FU) • cisplatin (Platinol, Platinol-AQ) • mitomycin (Mitomycin-C, MTC) Used without radiation: • carboplatin (Paraplatin) • cisplatin (Platinol, Platinol-AQ) • docetaxel (Taxotere) • doxorubicin (Adriamycin) • gemcitabine (Gemzar) • methotrexate (MTX, Otrexup, Trexall) • paclitaxel (Taxol) • vinblastine (Alkaban-AQ, Velban) Combinations such as carboplatin and either paclitaxel or docetaxel (for patients with poor kidney function); cisplatin and gemcitabine; methotrexate, vinblastine, doxorubicin, and cisplatin (called MVAC); or cisplatin, methotrexate, and vinblastine (called CMV) may be used. However, if adverse reactions are severe, single drugs as listed earlier may have to be administered instead.
Lymphoma (Non-Hodgkin)	• cyclophosphamide (Cytoxan, Neosar) • doxorubicin (Adriamycin) • vincristine (Oncovin, Vincasar)

CANCER TYPE	COMMON ANTINEOPLASTIC DRUG THERAPY
Kidney (renal cell) cancer	Antineoplastic drugs are usually not effective in treating kidney cancer and are not standard treatment. However, the following drugs may be used after targeted drugs and/or immunotherapy have already been tried. • 5-fluorouracil (5-FU) • capecitabine (Xeloda) • floxuridine (FUDR) • gemcitabine (Gemzar) • vinblastine (Alkaban-AQ, Velban)
Acute myeloid leukemia	• cytarabine (Cytosar-U) • daunorubicin (Cerubidine) • idarubicin (Idamycin) • mitoxantrone (Novantrone, OTN Mitoxantrone) Additional antineoplastic drugs that may be used include: • 6-mercaptopurine (6-MP, Purinethol) • 6-thioguanine (6-TG, Tabloid) • azacitidine (Vidaza) • cladribine (Leustatin, 2-CdA) • decitabine (Dacogen) • etoposide (VePeside, VP-16) • fludarabine (Fludara) • hydroxyurea (Hydrea) • methotrexate (MTX, Otrexup, Trexall) • topotecan (Hycamtin)
Endometrial cancer	• carboplatin (Paraplatin) • doxorubicin (Adriamycin) • liposomal doxorubicin (Doxil) • paclitaxel (Taxol)

Selected Antihypertensive Combinations

Antihypertensive drugs are used along with lifestyle changes to manage hypertension. Antihypertensive combinations, which commonly include one or two antihypertensives and a diuretic, are used to simplify patients' drug regimens and, in some cases, to enhance drug actions.

The table below lists the generic and trade names; functional classes; usual adult

ANTIHYPERTENSIVE COMBINATION TRADE NAMES	ANTIHYPERTENSIVE GENERIC NAMES	DIURETIC GENERIC NAMES
Aldoril-15	methyldopa 250 mg	hydrochlorothiazide (HCTZ) 15 mg
Aldoril-25	methyldopa 250 mg	HCTZ 25 mg
Aldoril D30	methyldopa 500 mg	HCTZ 30 mg
Aldoril D50	methyldopa 500 mg	HCTZ 50 mg
Amturnide 150/5/12.5	aliskiren 150 mg, amlodipine 5 mg	HCTZ 12.5 mg
Amturnide 300/5/12.5	aliskiren 300 mg, amlodipine 5 mg	HCTZ 12.5 mg
Amturnide 300/5/25	aliskiren 300 mg, amlodipine 5 mg	HCTZ 25 mg
Amturnide 300/10/12.5	aliskiren 300 mg, amlodipine 10 mg	HCTZ 12.5 mg
Amturnide 300/10/25	aliskiren 300 mg, amlodipine 10 mg	HCTZ 25 mg
Apresazide 25/25	hydralazine hydrochloride (HCL) 25 mg	HCTZ 25 mg
Apresazide 50/50	hydralazine HCl 50 mg	HCTZ 50 mg
Apresazide 100/50	hydralazine HCl 100 mg	HCTZ 50 mg
Atacand HCT 16/12.5	candesartan cilexetil 16 mg	HCTZ 12.5 mg
Atacand HCT 32/12.5	candesartan cilexetil 32 mg	HCTZ 12.5 mg
Atacand HCT 32/25	candesartan cilexetil 32 mg	HCTZ 25 mg
Avalide-150	irbesartan 150 mg	HCTZ 12.5 mg
Avalide-300	irbesartan 300 mg	HCTZ 12.5 mg
Azor 5/20	amlopidine 5 mg, olmesartan 20 mg	None
Azor 5/40	amlodipine 5 mg, olmesartan 40 mg	
Azor 10/20	amlodipine 10 mg, olmesartan 20 mg	
Azor 10/40	amlodipine 10 mg, olmesartan 40 mg	
Benicar HCT 20/12.5	olmesartan medoxomil 20 mg	HCTZ 12.5 mg
Benicar HCT 40/12.5	olmesartan medoxomil 40 mg	HCTZ 12.5 mg
Benicar HCT 40/25	olmesartan medoxomil 40 mg	HCTZ 25 mg
Capozide 25/15	captopril 25 mg	HCTZ 15 mg
Capozide 25/25	captopril 25 mg	HCTZ 25 mg
Capozide 50/15	captopril 50 mg	HCTZ 15 mg
Capozide 50/25	captopril 50 mg	HCTZ 25 mg

dosages; and onset, peak, and duration for commonly used antihypertensive combinations. For information about the mechanisms of action, interactions, adverse reactions, and nursing considerations related to antihypertensive combinations, review the entries for the specific antihypertensives and diuretics that they contain.

FUNCTIONAL CLASSES	USUAL ADULT DOSAGES	ONSET, PEAK, AND DURATION
Centrally acting antiadrenergic and thiazide diuretic	1 tab twice daily or three times daily 1 tab twice daily 1 tab daily 1 tab daily	**Onset:** Unknown **Peak:** 4 to 6 hr **Duration:** 12 to 24 hr
Direct renin inhibitor, calcium channel blocker, and thiazide diuretic	1 tab once daily 1 tab once daily 1 tab once daily 1 tab once daily 1 tab once daily	**Onset:** Unknown **Peak:** 3 to 8 hr **Duration:** Unknown
Peripherally acting arterial dilator and thiazide diuretic	1 cap once or twice daily 1 cap once or twice daily 1 cap once or twice daily	**Onset:** 20 to 30 min **Peak:** 1 to 2 hr **Duration:** 2 to 4 hr
Angiotensin II receptor antagonist and thiazide diuretic	1 tab once or twice daily 1 tab daily 1 tab daily	**Onset:** 1 to 2 wk **Peak:** Within 4 wk **Duration:** Unknown
ACE inhibitor and thiazide diuretic	1 tab daily 1 tab daily	**Onset:** Unknown **Peak:** Unknown **Duration:** Unknown
Calcium channel blocker and angiotensin II receptor antagonist	1 tab daily 1 tab daily 1 tab daily 1 tab daily	**Onset:** Unknown **Peak:** 1 to 6 hr **Duration:** 24 hr
Angiotensin II receptor antagonist and thiazide diuretic	1 tab daily 1 tab daily 1 tab daily	**Onset:** Unknown **Peak:** Unknown **Duration:** Unknown
ACE inhibitor and thiazide diuretic	1 tab daily to three times a day 1 tab once or twice daily 1 tab once daily to three times a day 1 tab once or twice daily	**Onset:** 15 to 60 min **Peak:** 60 to 90 min **Duration:** 6 to 12 hr

(continues)

Selected Antihypertensive Combinations *(continued)*

ANTIHYPERTENSIVE COMBINATION TRADE NAMES	ANTIHYPERTENSIVE GENERIC NAMES	DIURETIC GENERIC NAMES
Diovan HCT 80/12.5	valsartan 80 mg	HCTZ 12.5 mg
Diovan HCT 160/12.5	valsartan 160 mg	HCTZ 12.5 mg
Diovan HCT 160/25	valsartan 160 mg	HCTZ 25 mg
Diovan HCT 320/12.5	valsartan 320 mg	HCTZ 12.5 mg
Diovan HCT 320/25	valsartan 320 mg	HCTZ 25 mg
Dyazide 37.5/25	triamterene 37.5 mg	HCTZ 25 mg
Edarbyclor 40/12.5	azilsartan 40 mg	chlorthalidone 12.5 mg
Edarbyclor 40/25	azilsartan 40 mg	chlorthalidone 25 mg
Exforge 5/160	amlodipine 5 mg, valsartan 160 mg	None
Exforge 10/160	amlodipine 10 mg, valsartan 160 mg	
Exforge 5/320	amlodipine 5 mg, valsartan 320 mg	
Exforge 10/320	amlodipine 10 mg, valsartan 320 mg	
Exforge HCT 5/160/12.5	amlodipine 5 mg, valsartan 160 mg	HCTZ 12.5 mg
Exforge HCT 10/160/12.5	amlodipine 10 mg, valsartan 160 mg	HCTZ 12.5 mg
Exforge HCT 5/160/25	amlodipine 5 mg, valsartan 160 mg	HCTZ 25 mg
Exforge HCT 10/160/25	amlodipine 10 mg, valsartan 160 mg	HCTZ 25 mg
Exforge HCT 10/320/25	amlodipine 10 mg, valsartan 320 mg	HCTZ 25 mg
Hyzaar 50/12.5	losartan potassium 50 mg	HCTZ 12.5 mg
Hyzaar 100/12.5	losartan potassium 100 mg	HCTZ 12.5 mg
Hyzaar 100/25	losartan potassium 100 mg	HCTZ 25 mg
Inderide 40/25	propranolol HCL 40 mg	HCTZ 25 mg
Inderide 80/25	propranolol HCl 80 mg	HCTZ 25 mg
Inderide LA 80/50	propranolol HCl 80 mg	HCTZ 50 mg
Inderide LA 120/50	propranolol HCl 120 mg	HCTZ 50 mg
Inderide LA 160/50	propranolol HCl 160 mg	HCTZ 50 mg
Lopressor HCT 50/25	metoprolol tartrate 50 mg	HCTZ 25 mg
Lopressor HCT 100/25	metoprolol tartrate 100 mg	HCTZ 25 mg
Lopressor HCT 100/50	metoprolol tartrate 100 mg	HCTZ 50 mg
Lotensin HCT 5/6.25	benazepril HCl 5 mg	HCTZ 6.25 mg
Lotensin HCT 10/12.5	benazepril HCl 10 mg	HCTZ 12.5 mg
Lotensin HCT 20/12.5	benazepril HCl 20 mg	HCTZ 12.5 mg
Lotensin HCT 20/25	benazepril HCl 20 mg	HCTZ 25 mg

FUNCTIONAL CLASSES	USUAL ADULT DOSAGES	ONSET, PEAK, AND DURATION
Angiotensin II receptor blocker and thiazide diuretic	1 or 2 tabs daily 1 tab daily 1 tab daily 1 tab daily 1 tab daily	**Onset:** 2 hr **Peak:** 6 hr **Duration:** 24 hr
Potassium-sparing diuretic and thiazide diuretic	1 or 2 caps or tabs daily	**Onset:** 2 to 4 hr **Peak:** 1 day **Duration:** 7 to 9 hr
ACE inhibitor and thiazide-like diuretic	1 tab daily 1 tab daily	**Onset:** Unknown **Peak:** 6 hr **Duration:** 24 hr
Calcium channel blocker and angiotensin II receptor blocker	1 or 2 tabs daily 1 tab daily 1 tab daily 1 tab daily	**Onset:** Unknown **Peak:** 6 to 12 hr **Duration:** 24 hr
Calcium channel blocker, angiotensin II receptor blocker, and thiazide diuretic	1 tab daily 1 tab daily 1 tab daily 1 tab daily 1 tab daily	**Onset:** Unknown **Peak:** 2 to 6 hr **Duration:** Unknown
Angiotensin II receptor blocker and thiazide diuretic	1 or 2 tabs daily 1 tab daily 1 tab daily	**Onset:** Unknown **Peak:** 6 hr **Duration:** 24 hr or more
Beta blocker and thiazide diuretic	1 or 2 tabs twice daily 1 or 2 tabs twice daily 1 cap daily 1 cap daily 1 cap daily	**Onset:** Unknown **Peak:** 1 to 1.5 hr **Duration:** Unknown
Beta blocker and thiazide diuretic	2 tabs daily or 1 tab twice daily 1 or 2 tabs daily or 1 tab twice daily 2 tabs daily or 1 tab twice daily	**Onset:** 1 hr **Peak:** 1 to 2 hr **Duration:** Unknown
ACE inhibitor and thiazide diuretic	1 tab daily 1 tab daily 1 tab daily 1 tab daily	**Onset:** 1 hr **Peak:** 2 to 4 hr **Duration:** 24 hr

(continues)

Selected Antihypertensive Combinations *(continued)*

ANTIHYPERTENSIVE COMBINATION TRADE NAMES	ANTIHYPERTENSIVE GENERIC NAMES	DIURETIC GENERIC NAMES
Lotrel 2.5/10	amlodipine 2.5 mg, benazepril HCl 10 mg	None
Lotrel 5/10	amlodipine 5 mg, benazepril HCl 10 mg	None
Lotrel 5/20	amlodipine 5 mg, benazepril HCl 20 mg	None
Lotrel 5/40	amlodipine 5 mg, benazepril 40 mg	None
Lotrel 10/20	amlodipine 10 mg, benazepril HCl 20 mg	None
Lotrel 10/40	amlodipine 10 mg, benazepril 40 mg	None
Maxzide-25 37.5/25	triamterene 37.5 mg	HCTZ 25 mg
Maxzide 75/50	triamterene 75 mg	HCTZ 50 mg
Micardis HCT 40/12.5	telmisartan 40 mg	HCTZ 12.5 mg
Micardis HCT 80/12.5	telmisartan 80 mg	HCTZ 12.5 mg
Micardis HCT 80/25	telmisartan 80 mg	HCTZ 25 mg
Moduretic	amiloride 5 mg	HCTZ 50 mg
Prinzide 10/12.5	lisinopril 10 mg	HCTZ 12.5 mg
Prinzide 20/12.5	lisinopril 20 mg	HCTZ 12.5 mg
Tekamlo 150/5	aliskiren 150 mg, amlodipine 5 mg	None
Tekamlo 150/10	aliskiren 150 mg, amlodipine 10 mg	None
Tekamlo 300/5	aliskiren 300 mg, amlodipine 5 mg	None
Tekamlo 300/10	aliskiren 300 mg, amlodipine 10 mg	None
Tekturna HCT 150/12.5	aliskiren 150 mg	HCTZ 12.5 mg
Tekturna HCT 150/25	aliskiren 150 mg	HCTZ 25 mg
Tekturna HCT 300/12.5	aliskiren 300 mg	HCTZ 12.5 mg
Tekturna HCT 300/25	aliskiren 300 mg	HCTZ 25 mg

FUNCTIONAL CLASSES	USUAL ADULT DOSAGES	ONSET, PEAK, AND DURATION
Calcium channel blocker and ACE inhibitor	1 or 2 caps daily 1 cap daily 1 cap daily 1 cap daily 1 cap daily 1 cap daily	**Onset:** Unknown **Peak:** Unknown **Duration:** 24 hr
Potassium-sparing diuretic and thiazide diuretic	1 tab daily 1 tab daily	**Onset:** 2 to 4 hr **Peak:** 1 day **Duration:** 7 to 9 hr
Angiotensin II receptor antagonist and thiazide diuretic	1 tab once or twice daily 1 tab once or twice daily 1 tab once daily	**Onset:** Within 3 hr **Peak:** In 4 wk **Duration:** Several days to 1 wk
Potassium-sparing diuretic and thiazide diuretic	1 or 2 tabs daily	**Onset:** 2 hr **Peak:** 6 to 10 hr **Duration:** 24 hr
ACE inhibitor and thiazide diuretic	1 or 2 tabs daily 1 or 2 tabs daily	**Onset:** 1 hr **Peak:** 6 hr **Duration:** 24 hr
Direct renin inhibitor and calcium channel blocker	1 or 2 tabs daily 1 tab daily 1 tab daily 1 tab daily	**Onset:** Unknown **Peak:** 3 to 8 hr **Duration:** 24 hr
Direct renin inhibitor and thiazide diuretic	1 tab daily 1 tab daily 1 tab daily 1 tab daily	**Onset:** Unknown **Peak:** 1 to 2.5 hr **Duration:** Unknown

(continues)

Selected Antihypertensive Combinations *(continued)*

ANTIHYPERTENSIVE COMBINATION TRADE NAMES	ANTIHYPERTENSIVE GENERIC NAMES	DIURETIC GENERIC NAMES
Timolide 10/25	timolol maleate 10 mg	HCTZ 25 mg
Tribenzor 20/5/12.5	amlodipine 5 mg, olmesartan 20 mg	HCTZ 12.5 mg
Tribenzor 40/5/12.5	amlodipine 5 mg, olmesartan 40 mg	HCTZ 12.5 mg
Tribenzor 40/5/25	amlodipine 5 mg, olmesartan 40 mg	HCTZ 25 mg
Tribenzor 40/10/12.5	amlodipine 10 mg, olmesartan 40 mg	HCTZ 12.5 mg
Tribenzor 40/10/25	amlodipine 10 mg, olmesartan 40 mg	HCTZ 25 mg
Twynsta 40/5	telmisartan 40 mg, amlodipine 5 mg	None
Twynsta 40/10	telmisartan 40 mg, amlodipine 10 mg	None
Twynsta 80/5	telmisartan 80 mg, amlodipine 5 mg	None
Twynsta 80/10	telmisartan 80 mg, amlodipine 10 mg	None
Uniretic 7.5/12.5	moexipril HCL 7.5 mg	HCTZ 12.5 mg
Uniretic 15/12.5	moexipril 15 mg	HCTZ 12.5 mg
Uniretic 15/25	moexipril HCl 15 mg	HCTZ 25 mg
Valturna 150/160	aliskiren 150 mg, valsartan 160 mg	None
Valturna 300/320	aliskiren 300 mg, valsartan 320 mg	None
Vaseretic 10/25	enalapril maleate 10 mg	HCTZ 25 mg
Zestoretic 10/12.5	lisinopril 10 mg	HCTZ 12.5 mg
Zestoretic 20/12.5	lisinopril 20 mg	HCTZ 12.5 mg
Zestoretic 20/25	lisinopril 20 mg	HCTZ 25 mg
Ziac 2.5/6.25	bisoprolol fumarate 2.5 mg	HCTZ 6.25 mg
Ziac 5/6.25	bisoprolol fumarate 5 mg	HCTZ 6.25 mg
Ziac 10/6.25	bisoprolol fumarate 10 mg	HCTZ 6.25 mg

FUNCTIONAL CLASSES	USUAL ADULT DOSAGES	ONSET, PEAK, AND DURATION
Beta blocker and thiazide diuretic	2 tabs daily or 1 tab twice daily	**Onset:** Unknown **Peak:** 1 to 2 hr **Duration:** Unknown
Angiotensin II receptor antagonist, calcium channel blocker, and thiazide diuretic	1 tab daily 1 tab daily 1 tab daily 1 tab daily 1 tab daily	**Onset:** Unknown **Peak:** 1 to 6 hr **Duration:** 24 hr
Angiotensin II receptor antagonist and calcium channel blocker	1 tab daily 1 tab daily 1 tab daily 1 tab daily	**Onset:** Unknown **Peak:** 1 to 6 hr **Duration:** Unknown
Potassium-sparing diuretic and thiazide diuretic	1 tab daily 1 tab daily 1 tab daily	**Onset:** 1 hr **Peak:** 3 to 6 hr **Duration:** 24 hr
Direct renin inhibitor and angiotensin II antagonist	1 tab daily 1 tab daily	**Onset:** Unknown **Peak:** 1 to 3 hr **Duration:** Unknown
ACE inhibitor and thiazide diuretic	1 tab once or twice daily	**Onset:** 1 hr **Peak:** 4 to 6 hr **Duration:** 24 hr
ACE inhibitor and thiazide diuretic	1 or 2 tabs daily 1 or 2 tabs daily 1 or 2 tabs daily	**Onset:** 1 hr **Peak:** 6 hr **Duration:** 24 hr
Beta blocker and thiazide diuretic	1 or 2 tabs daily 1 or 2 tabs daily 1 or 2 tabs daily	**Onset:** Unknown **Peak:** Unknown **Duration:** Unknown

Selected Obstetrical Drugs

Obstetrical drugs are used during pregnancy for a variety of reasons, such as control of nausea and vomiting, pain relief, and assistance in the labor and delivery process. Drugs used to control nausea and vomiting throughout pregnancy and analgesics used to provide pain relief, especially during the labor and delivery process, are covered in the main section of the *Nurse's Drug Handbook*. While other drugs may be used during pregnancy, not all have FDA approval for such use. For example, misoprostol, a synthetic prostaglandin, is used to treat ulcers. However, it may also be used for indications not approved by the FDA, such as assisting in the termination of a pregnancy, evacuation of the uterine contents in a missed abortion, and dilating the cervix prior to labor. These uses are considered "off-label" uses because they have not been FDA approved. In adherence with the standard of only including FDA-approved indications in the *Nurse's Drug Handbook*, following are selected obstetrical drugs that are FDA approved for use with pregnancy issues.

GENERIC NAME AND TRADE NAME	INDICATIONS	ADULT DOSAGES
dinoprostone Cervidil, Prepidil, Prostin E_2	Initiation and/or continuation of cervical ripening in patients at or near term in whom there is a medical or obstetrical indication for the induction of labor	10 mg intravaginally designed to release 0.3 mg/hr of the drug over a 12-hr period; removed upon onset of active labor or 12 hr after insertion
hydroxyprogesterone caproate Makena	To reduce risk of preterm birth in women who are carrying only one fetus and who have a history of singleton spontaneous preterm birth	250 mg (1 ml) I.M. once weekly begun between16 wk, 0 days and 20 wk, 6 days of gestation and continued weekly until wk 37 or delivery, whichever comes first
oxytocin Pitocin	To initiate or improve uterine contractions in situations where there are fetal or maternal concerns, so as to achieve a vaginal delivery	*Initial:* 0.5 mU (milliunits)/min to 1 mU/min I.V., increased in increments of 1 to 2 mU/min every 30 to 60 min, as needed; once desired frequency of contractions has been reached and labor has progressed to 5 to 6 cm dilation, dosage may be decreased by 1 to 2 mU/min every 30 to 60 min

GENERIC NAME AND TRADE NAME	INDICATIONS	ADULT DOSAGES
	To produce uterine contractions during the third stage of labor and to control postpartum bleeding or hemorrhage	10 to 40 units added to existing intravenous solution being infused (maximum 40 units to 1,000 ml of solution) and infused at a rate to sustain uterine contraction and control atony *Alternatively,* 10 units (1 ml) I.M. after delivery of placenta
	To treat incomplete, inevitable, or elective abortion	*Initial:* I.V. infusion rate highly individualized (10 units mixed in 500 ml of saline or 5% dextrose-in-water solution) *Maximum:* 30 units in a 12-hr period
ulipristal acetate ELLA	To prevent pregnancy following unprotected intercourse or contraceptive failure	30 mg (1 tablet) as soon as possible within 120 hours (5 days) after unprotected intercourse or contraceptive failure

Vitamins

As you know, an adequate daily intake of vitamins is essential to vital bodily functions, such as embryonic development (vitamin A), regulation of serum calcium and phosphate (vitamin D), and blood clotting (vitamin K).

Vitamins are classified as one of two types: fat soluble (vitamins A, D, E, and K) and water soluble (vitamin C and all forms of vitamin B). Fat-soluble vitamins can accumulate in body tissue over time; when excessive amounts are ingested through diet or supplementation,

GENERIC AND TRADE NAMES	RECOMMENDED DAILY INTAKE
vitamin A (retinol) Aquasol A	***Adult men and boys over age 10.*** 1,000 mcg/day. ***Adult women and girls over age 10.*** 800 mcg/day. ***Pregnant women.*** 800 mcg/day. (900 mcg/day [CAN].) ***Breastfeeding women.*** 1,200 to 1,300 mcg/day. (1,200 mcg/day [CAN].) ***Children ages 7 to 10.*** 700 mcg/day. (700 to 800 mcg/day [CAN].) ***Children ages 4 to 7.*** 500 mcg/day. ***Neonates and children to age 4.*** 375 to 400 mcg/day. (400 mcg/day [CAN].)
vitamin B_1 (thiamine hydrochloride) Betaxin (CAN), Bewon (CAN), Biamine	***Adult men and boys over age 10.*** 1.2 to 1.5 mg/day. (0.8 to 1.3 mg/day [CAN].) ***Adult women and girls over age 10.*** 1 to 1.1 mg/day. (0.8 to 0.9 mg/day [CAN].) ***Pregnant women.*** 1.5 mg/day. (0.9 to 1 mg/day [CAN].) ***Breastfeeding women.*** 1.6 mg/day. (1 to 1.2 mg/day [CAN].)

severe and life-threatening toxicity can develop. Water-soluble vitamins don't accumulate in the body; they are excreted daily so that toxicity is not usually a concern with excessive intake.

The following chart lists the generic and trade names of fat-soluble and water-soluble vitamins, the recommended daily intake to prevent vitamin deficiency, dosages when deficiency occurs, other indications and dosages for vitamin therapy, and guidelines for parenteral administration of vitamins.

OTHER INDICATIONS AND DOSAGES	PARENTERAL ADMINISTRATION GUIDELINES
TO TREAT VITAMIN A DEFICIENCY CAPSULES, ORAL SOLUTION, TABLETS ***Adults and adolescents.*** Dosage individualized based on severity of deficiency, as prescribed. I.M. INJECTION ***Adults and children age 8 and over.*** 15,000 to 30,000 retinol equivalent (RE)/day (50,000 to 100,000 IU/day) for 3 days, followed by 15,000 RE/day (50,000 IU/day) for 2 wk. ***Children ages 1 to 8.*** 1,500 to 4,500 RE/day (5,000 to 15,000 IU/day) for 10 days; for severe deficiency, 5,250 to 10,500 RE/day (17,500 to 35,000 IU/day) for 10 days. ***Infants to age 1 year.*** 1,500 to 3,000 RE/day (5,000 to 10,000 IU/day) for 10 days; for severe deficiency, 2,250 to 4,500 RE/day (7,500 to 15,000 IU/day) for 10 days. I.V. INFUSION ***Adults and children.*** Dosage individualized as part of total parenteral nutrition solution, as prescribed. ***TO TREAT XEROPHTHALMIA*** CAPSULES, ORAL SOLUTION, TABLETS ***Children age 1 and over.*** 60,000 RE (200,000 IU) as a single dose. Dose repeated on day 2 and again in 4 wk. ***Children ages 6 months to 1 year.*** 30,000 RE (100,000 IU) as a single dose. Dose repeated on day 2 and again in 4 wk. ***AS AN ADJUNCT TO TREAT MEASLES*** CAPSULES, ORAL SOLUTION, TABLETS ***Children age 1 and over.*** 60,000 RE (200,000 IU) as a single dose when measles are diagnosed. ***Children ages 6 months to 1 year.*** 30,000 RE (100,000 IU) as a single dose when measles are diagnosed.	• Be aware that anaphylaxis and death have occurred after I.V. administration of vitamin A; I.V. administration is restricted to special solutions, such as in total parenteral nutrition solution. Typically, parenteral administration of vitamin A is by I.M. injection. • Take precautions to protect vitamin A solution from exposure to light because it's light sensitive.
TO TREAT VITAMIN B_1 DEFICIENCY (BERIBERI) ELIXIR, TABLETS ***Adults.*** 5 to 10 mg t.i.d. ***Children and infants.*** 10 mg/day. I.V. OR I.M. INJECTION ***Adults.*** *Initial:* 5 to 100 mg every 8 hr, switched to P.O. vitamin B_1 therapy as soon as possible and continued for total of 1 mo.	• Be aware that I.V. administration of vitamin B_1 has caused severe and life-threatening reactions, especially with repeat administration. Monitor patient closely for angioedema, GI bleeding, respiratory distress, throat tightness, urticaria, vascular collapse, and weakness during and after administration.

(continues)

Vitamins *(continued)*

GENERIC AND TRADE NAMES	RECOMMENDED DAILY INTAKE
vitamin B_1 *(continued)*	***Children ages 7 to 10.*** 1 mg/day. (0.8 to 1 mg/day [CAN].) ***Children ages 4 to 7.*** 0.9 mg/day. (0.7 mg/day [CAN].) ***Children ages 1 to 4.*** 0.3 to 0.7 mg/day. (0.3 to 0.6 mg/day [CAN].)
vitamin B_3 (niacin) Endur-Acin, Nia-Bid, Niac, Niacels, Niacor, Nico-400, Nicobid Tempules, Nicolar, Nicotinex Elixir, Novo-Niacin (CAN), Slo-Niacin	***Adult men and boys age 11 and over.*** 15 to 20 mg/day. (14 to 23 mg/day [CAN].) ***Adult women and girls age 11 and over.*** 13 to 15 mg/day. (14 to 16 mg/day [CAN].) ***Pregnant women.*** 17 mg/day. (14 to 16 mg/day [CAN].) ***Breastfeeding women.*** 20 mg/day. (14 to 16 mg/day [CAN].) ***Children ages 7 to 11.*** 13 mg/day. (14 to 18 mg/day [CAN].) ***Children ages 4 to 7.*** 12 mg/day. (13 mg/day [CAN].) ***Neonates and children to age 4.*** 5 to 9 mg/day. (4 to 9 mg/day [CAN].)
vitamin B_6 (pyridoxine hydrochloride) Beesix, Doxine, Nestrex, Pyri, Rodex, Vita-bee 6	***Adult men and boys age 11 and over.*** 1.7 to 2 mg/day. ***Adult women and girls age 11 and over.*** 1.4 to 1.6 mg/day. ***Pregnant women.*** 2.2 mg/day. ***Breastfeeding women.*** 2.1 mg/day. ***Children ages 7 to 10.*** 1.4 mg/day. ***Children ages 4 to 6.*** 1.1 mg/day. ***Neonates and children to age 3.*** 0.3 to 1 mg/day.

OTHER INDICATIONS AND DOSAGES	PARENTERAL ADMINISTRATION GUIDELINES
TO TREAT WERNICKE'S ENCEPHALOPATHY I.V. OR I.M. INJECTION **Adults.** *Initial:* 100 mg I.V. *Maintenance:* 50 to 100 mg I.V. or I.M. daily until normal recommended daily intake is achieved.	• Rotate sites for I.M. administration of vitamin B_1 to help prevent induration and tenderness that may occur following administration. • Be aware that I.M. administration may be painful; use the Z-track method of administration. • Know that because of incompatibilities, parenteral vitamin B_1 shouldn't be added to alkaline or neutral solutions; also, don't mix it with oxidizing and reducing agents, including barbiturates, carbonates, citrates, and copper. • Take precautions to protect vitamin B_1 solution from exposure to light because it's light sensitive.
TO TREAT VITAMIN B_3 DEFICIENCY E.R. CAPSULES, E.R. TABLETS, ORAL SOLUTION, TABLETS ***Adults and children age 11 and over.*** Dosage individualized based on severity of deficiency, as prescribed. *Maximum:* 6 g/day. I.V. INJECTION ***Adults and children age 11 and over.*** 25 to 100 mg at least twice daily. ***Children to age 11.*** Up to 300 mg daily I.M. INJECTION ***Adults and children age 11 and over.*** 50 to 100 mg at least 5 times/day. ***Children to age 11.*** Dosage individualized based on severity of deficiency. ***TO TREAT HYPERLIPIDEMIA (NIACIN ONLY)*** E.R. CAPSULES, E.R. TABLETS, ORAL SOLUTION, TABLETS **Adults.** *Initial:* 1,000 mg t.i.d. Dosage increased by 500 mg/day every 2 to 4 wk, as needed. *Maintenance:* 1 to 2 g t.i.d. *Maximum:* 6 g/day. ***DOSAGE ADJUSTMENT*** To reduce or prevent facial flushing, initial dosage reduced to 100 mg/day (tab) or 500 mg/day (E.R. tab), and then gradually increased to 3 to 4 g/day.	• Be aware that I.V. administration of vitamin B_3 may cause CNS or CV adverse reactions, such as arrhythmias, dizziness, headache, peripheral vasodilation, and syncope. Rate of I.V. administration shouldn't exceed 2 mg/min, regardless of method of I.V. administration. • Know that vitamin B_3 must be diluted for I.V. use. For direct injection, dilute to 2 mg/ml; for intermittent or continuous infusion, dilute dose in 500 ml of normal saline or other compatible solution. • Give I.M. injection following routine I.M. administration guidelines. Vitamin B_3 doesn't need to be diluted for I.M. injection. • Be aware that parenteral administration shouldn't be used to treat hyperlipidemia.
TO TREAT VITAMIN B_6 DEFICIENCY E.R. CAPSULES, TABLETS ***Adults and children.*** Dosage individualized based on severity of deficiency, as prescribed. E.R. TABLETS **Adults.** Dosage individualized based on severity of deficiency, as prescribed. I.V. INFUSION ***Adults and children.*** Dosage individualized as part of total parenteral nutrition.	• Be aware that I.M. or SubQ administration of vitamin B_6 may cause injection-site burning or stinging. Before giving injection, alert patient that this adverse effect may occur. • Know that I.V. administration is given as part of a multivitamin solution; follow the guidelines for administering an I.V. multivitamin solution as recommended for the product being used.

(continues)

Vitamins *(continued)*

GENERIC AND TRADE NAMES	RECOMMENDED DAILY INTAKE
vitamin B_6 *(continued)*	***Children ages 7 to 10.*** 1.4 mg/day. ***Children ages 4 to 6.*** 1.1 mg/day. ***Neonates and children to age 3.*** 0.3 to 1 mg/day. ***Adult men and boys age 11 and over.*** 1.7 to 2 mg/day. ***Adult women and girls age 11 and over.*** 1.4 to 1.6 mg/day. ***Pregnant women.*** 2.2 mg/day. ***Breastfeeding women.*** 2.1 mg/day.
vitamin B_9 (folic acid) Apo-Folic (CAN), Folvite, Novo-Folacid (CAN)	***Adult men and boys age 11 and over.*** 150 to 400 mcg/day. (150 to 220 mcg/day [CAN].) ***Adult women and girls age 11 and over.*** 150 to 400 mcg/day. (145 to 190 mcg/day [CAN].) ***Pregnant women.*** 400 to 800 mcg/day. (445 to 475 mcg/day [CAN].) ***Breastfeeding women.*** 260 to 800 mcg/day. (245 to 275 mcg/day [CAN].) ***Children ages 7 to 11.*** 100 to 400 mcg/day. (125 to 180 mcg/day [CAN].) ***Children ages 4 to 7.*** 75 to 400 mcg/day. (90 mcg/day [CAN].) ***Neonates and children to age 4.*** 25 mcg/day. (50 to 80 mcg/day [CAN].)
vitamin B_{12} (cyanocobalamin, hydroxycobalamin)	***Adults age 19 and over.*** 2.4 mcg/day. ***Pregnant women.*** 2.6 mcg/day. ***Breastfeeding women.*** 2.8 mcg/day. ***Adolescents ages 14 to 19.*** 2.4 mcg/day. ***Children ages 9 to 14.*** 1.8 mcg/day. ***Children ages 4 to 9.*** 1.2 mcg/day. ***Children ages 1 to 4.*** 0.9 mcg/day. ***Infants ages 6 to 12 months.*** 0.4 mcg/day. ***Neonates and infants to 6 months.*** 0.5 mcg/day.

OTHER INDICATIONS AND DOSAGES	PARENTERAL ADMINISTRATION GUIDELINES
TO TREAT PYRIDOXINE DEPENDENCY SYNDROME I.V. OR I.M. INJECTION ***Adults and children age 11 and over.*** 30 to 600 mg daily. ***Infants with seizures.*** *Initial:* 10 to 100 mg, then individualized based on severity of deficiency, as prescribed. ***TO TREAT DRUG-INDUCED PYRIDOXINE DEFICIENCY*** I.V. OR I.M. INJECTION ***Adults and children age 11 and over.*** 50 to 200 mg/day for 3 wk, then 25 to 100 mg/day, as needed.	• Know that vitamin B_6 may increase AST (SGOT) levels. Be aware that at least one manufacturer warns against I.V. administration of vitamin B_6 to patients with heart disease. • Take precautions to protect vitamin B_6 solution from exposure to light because it's light sensitive.
TO TREAT VITAMIN B_9 DEFICIENCY TABLETS ***Adults and children.*** Dosage individualized based on severity of deficiency, as prescribed. I.V. INFUSION, I.M. OR SUBCUTANEOUS INJECTION ***Adults and children.*** 0.25 to 1 mg daily until hematologic response occurs.	• Be aware that some vitamin B_9 solutions contain benzyl alcohol. Don't administer these solutions to neonates or immature infants because of a risk of fatal toxic syndrome, which may include circulatory, CNS, renal, and respiratory impairment and metabolic acidosis. • Know that unless ordered otherwise, you should dilute 5 mg/ml of vitamin B_9 with 49 ml of sterile water for injection to provide a solution containing 0.1 mg of vitamin/ml. • Know that parenteral administration may cause anaphylaxis. Parenteral administration should be used only in patients with severe vitamin deficiency or in those with severely impaired GI absorption. • Be aware that SubQ administration should be injected deep. • Take precautions to protect vitamin B_9 solution from exposure to light because it's light sensitive.
TO TREAT VITAMIN B_{12} DEFICIENCY *Caused by nutritional intake imbalance (not for use to treat pernicious anemia)* lozenges, tablets ***Adults and children.*** Dosage individualized based on severity of deficiency, as prescribed. *Caused by pernicious anemia; malabsorption disorders (tropical or nontropical sprue, partial or total gastrectomy, regional enteritis, gastroenterostomy, ileal resection); or malignancies, granulomas, strictures, or anastomoses involving the ileum.* SUBCUTANEOUS INJECTION (CYANOCOBALAMIN) ***Adults.*** *Initial:* 30 mcg daily for 5 to 10 days, then switched to I.M. administration for maintenance therapy.	• Be aware that parenteral vitamin B_{12} solution is incompatible with many drugs, including ascorbic acid, chlorpromazine hydrochloride, dextrose, heavy metals, phytonadione, prochlorperazine edisylate, and warfarin sodium. Also know that alkaline or strongly acidic solutions and oxidizing or reducing agents are also incompatible with vitamin B_{12} solution. Do not administer vitamin with other drugs. • Know that both cyanocobalamin and hydroxycobalamin may be administered by I.M. injection, but only cyanocobalamin may be administered as a SubQ injection. Be alert to which form is being administered to ensure correct route of administration.

(continues)

Vitamins *(continued)*

GENERIC AND TRADE NAMES	RECOMMENDED DAILY INTAKE
vitamin B_{12} *(continued)*	**Children ages 7 to 10**. 1 mg/day. (0.8 to 1 mg/day [CAN].) **Children ages 4 to 7**. 0.9 mg/day. (0.7 mg/day [CAN].) **Children ages 1 to 4**. 0.3 to 0.7 mg/day. (0.3 to 0.6 mg/day [CAN].)
vitamin C (ascorbic acid) Ascorbic Acid, Cecon Drops, Cenolate, Cevi-Bid, Vicks Vitamin C Drops	***Adult men.*** 90 mg/day. ***Adult women.*** 75 mg/day. ***Pregnant women age 19 and over.*** 85 mg/day. ***Breastfeeding women age 19 and over.*** 120 mg/day. ***Adolescent boys ages 14 to 19.*** 75 mg/day. ***Adolescent girls ages 14 to 19.*** 65 mg/day. ***Pregnant girls ages 14 to 19.*** 80 mg/day. ***Breastfeeding girls ages 14 to 19.*** 115 mg/day. ***Children ages 9 to 14.*** 45 mg/day. ***Children ages 4 to 9.*** 25 mg/day. ***Children ages 1 to 4.*** 15 mg/day. ***Infants ages 7 to 12 months.*** 50 mg/day. ***Neonates and infants to age 7 months.*** 40 mg/day. ***DOSAGE ADJUSTMENT*** Recommended daily intake for people who smoke is 100 mg/day because of an increased utilization of vitamin C. Recommended daily intake should be increased to promote wound healing and for those with a chronic illness, fever, hemovascular disorder, or infection; the amount of vitamin C increase depends on the severity of the underlying condition.

OTHER INDICATIONS AND DOSAGES	PARENTERAL ADMINISTRATION GUIDELINES
Children. *Initial:* 1,000 to 5,000 mcg given in single daily doses of 100 mcg over 2 or more wk. *Maintenance:* 60 or more mcg/mo. I.M. INJECTION (CYANOCOBALAMIN OR HYDROXYCOBALAMIN) ***Adults.*** *Initial:* 30 mcg daily for 5 to 10 days. *Maintenance:* 100 to 200 mcg every mo. ***Children.*** *Initial:* 1,000 to 5,000 mcg, given in single daily doses of 100 mcg over 2 or more wk. *Maintenance:* 60 or more mcg/mo. ***DOSAGE ADJUSTMENT*** Dosage adjusted, as needed, to maintain normal hematologic morphology and an erythrocyte count greater than 4.5 million/mm. ***Adults.*** *Initial.* 1 mg/wk for 3 wk. *Maintenance:* 250 mcg/mo. ***TO TREAT FAMILIAL SELECTIVE B_{12} MALABSORPTION*** I.M. INJECTION (CYANOCOBALAMIN) ***TO TREAT HEREDITARY DEFICIENCY OF TRANSCOBALAMIN II*** I.M. INJECTION (CYANOCOBALAMIN) ***Adults.*** 1 to 2 mg/wk.	• Be aware that SubQ administration of cyanocobalamin should be injected deeply. • Know that vitamin B_{12} is excreted more rapidly after I.V. injection; I.V. administration isn't recommended. • Take precautions to protect vitamin B_{12} solution from exposure to light because it's light sensitive.
TO TREAT VITAMIN C DEFICIENCY (SCURVY) E.R. CAPSULES; LOZENGES; ORAL SOLUTION; E.R. TABLETS; TABLETS; SUBCUTANEOUS, I.M., OR I.V. INJECTION ***Adults.*** 100 to 250 mg once or twice daily until skeletal changes and signs and symptoms of hemorrhagic disorder are reversed (usually within 2 to 21 days). ORAL SOLUTION; TABLETS; SUBCUTANEOUS, I.M.,OR I.V. INJECTION ***Infants and children.*** 100 to 300 mg/day in divided doses until skeletal changes and signs and symptoms of hemorrhagic disorder are reversed (usually within days).	• Be aware that I.M. injection is the preferred parenteral route for administering vitamin C, although it may be administered I.V. or SubQ when necessary. • Rotate sites for I.M. and SubQ administration to help prevent transient mild soreness that may occur following administration. Inform patient that this adverse effect may occur. • Avoid rapid administration, if giving I.V. vitamin C, to prevent dizziness or faintness. • Administer vitamin C solution by itself because it's incompatible with many drugs. • Be aware that vitamin C solution rapidly oxidizes in air and in alkaline solutions. Take precautions to protect vitamin solution from exposure to air and light. • Open vitamin C ampules carefully because increased pressure may develop after prolonged storage.

(continues)

Vitamins *(continued)*

GENERIC AND TRADE NAMES	RECOMMENDED DAILY INTAKE
vitamin D_2 (ergocalciferol) Calciferol, Calciferol Drops, Drisdol, Drisdol Drops, Ostoforte (CAN), Radiostol Forte (CAN)	***Adults and children ages 11 and over.*** 200 to 400 IU/day. (100 to 200 IU/day [CAN].) ***Pregnant and breastfeeding women.*** 400 IU/day. (200 to 300 IU/day [CAN].) ***Children ages 7 to 11.*** 400 IU/day. (100 to 200 IU/day [CAN].) ***Children ages 4 to 7.*** 400 IU/day. (200 IU/day [CAN].) ***Neonates and children to age 4.*** 300 to 400 IU/day. (200 to 400 IU/day [CAN].)
vitamin E (alpha tocopherol) Amino-Opti-E, Aquasol E, E-Complex 600, E-Vitamin succinate, Liqui-E, Pheryl E, Vita-Plus E, Webber Vitamin E (CAN)	***Adult men and adolescent boys.*** 16.7 IU/day. (10 to 16.7 IU/day [CAN].) ***Adult women and adolescent girls.*** 13 IU/day. (8.3 to 11.7 IU/day [CAN].) ***Pregnant women.*** 16.7 IU/day. (13 to 15 IU/day [CAN].) ***Breastfeeding women.*** 18 to 20 IU/day. (15 to 16.7 IU/day [CAN].) ***Children ages 7 to 10.*** 11.7 IU/day. (10 to 13 IU/day [CAN].) ***Children ages 4 to 7.*** 11.7 IU/day. (8.3 IU/day [CAN].) ***Infants and children to age 4.*** 5 to 10 IU/day. (5 to 6.7 IU/day [CAN].)

OTHER INDICATIONS AND DOSAGES	PARENTERAL ADMINISTRATION GUIDELINES
TO TREAT VITAMIN D_2 DEFICIENCY CAPSULES, ORAL SOLUTION, TABLETS ***Adults and children.*** Dosage individualized based on severity of deficiency, as prescribed. ***TO TREAT VITAMIN D-RESISTANT RICKETS*** CAPSULES, ORAL SOLUTION, TABLETS ***Adults.*** 12,000 to 150,000 IU units daily ***TO TREAT VITAMIN D-DEPENDENT RICKETS*** CAPSULES, ORAL SOLUTION, TABLETS ***Adults.*** 10,000 to 60,000 IU daily. *Maximum:* 150,000 IU daily. ***Children.*** 3,000 to 10,000 IU daily. *Maximum:* 50,000 IU daily. ***TO TREAT OSTEOMALACIA CAUSED BY LONG-TERM ANTICONVULSANT USE*** CAPSULES, ORAL SOLUTION, TABLETS ***Adults.*** 1,000 to 4,000 IU daily. ***Children.*** 1,000 IU daily. ***TO TREAT FAMILIAL HYPOPHOSPHATEMIA*** CAPSULES ***Adults.*** 50,000 to 100,000 IU daily. ***TO TREAT HYPOPARATHYROIDISM*** CAPSULES ***Adults.*** 50,000 to 150,000 IU daily. ***Children.*** 50,000 to 200,000 IU daily. ***TO TREAT INTESTINAL MALABSORPTION*** I.M. INJECTION ***Adults and children.*** 10,000 IU daily.	• Be aware that vitamin D_2 is usually given orally. However, I.M. injection may be required for patients with biliary, GI, or liver disease associated with malabsorption of vitamin D analogues. • Take precautions to protect parenteral vitamin D_2 solution from exposure to light because light causes it to decompose.
TO TREAT VITAMIN E DEFICIENCY CAPSULES (ADULTS ONLY), ORAL SOLUTION, TABLETS ***Adults and children.*** Dosage individualized based on severity of deficiency, as prescribed.	Know that vitamin E isn't administered parenterally.

(continues)

Vitamins *(continued)*

GENERIC AND TRADE NAMES	RECOMMENDED DAILY INTAKE
vitamin K_1 (phytonadione) AquaMEPHYTON, Mephyton	*Recommended daily intake hasn't been established for vitamin K_1. However, adequate intake is suggested as follows:* ***Adult men age 19 and over.*** 120 mcg/day. ***Adult women age 19 and over, pregnant and breast-feeding women.*** 90 mcg/day. ***Adolescents ages 14 to 19.*** 75 mcg/day. ***Children ages 9 to 14.*** 60 mcg/day. ***Children ages 4 to 9.*** 55 mcg/day. ***Children ages 1 to 4.*** 30 mcg/day. ***Infants ages 7 to 12 months.*** 2.5 mcg/day. ***Neonates and infants to age 7 months.*** 2 mcg/day.

OTHER INDICATIONS AND DOSAGES

TO PREVENT HYPOPROTHROMBINEMIA DURING PROLONGED USE OF TOTAL PARENTERAL NUTRITION

I.M. INJECTION

Adults. 5 to 10 mg/wk.
Children. 2 to 5 mg/wk.

TO PREVENT HYPOPROTHROMBINEMIA IN INFANTS WITH DIETS DEFICIENT IN VITAMIN K (LESS THAN 100 MCG/L)

I.M. INJECTION

Infants. 1 mg/mo.

TO TREAT ANTICOAGULANT-INDUCED HYPOPROTHROMBINEMIA

TABLETS, I.M. OR SUBCUTANEOUS INJECTION

Adults. 2.5 to 25 mg, repeated 12 to 48 hr after P.O. dose or 6 to 8 hr after SubQ or I.M. dose, as prescribed. *Maximum:* 50 mg/dose.
Children. 2.5 to 10 mg SubQ or I.M., repeated in 6 to 8 hr, as prescribed.
Infants. 1 to 2 mg SubQ or I.M., repeated in 4 to 8 hr, as prescribed.

TO TREAT HYPOPROTHROMBINEMIA FROM OTHER CAUSES

TABLETS, I.M. OR SUBCUTANEOUS INJECTION

Adults. 2 to 25 mg. *Usual:* 25 mg. *Maximum:* 50 mg/dose.
Children. 5 to 10 mg SubQ or I.M.
Infants. 2 mg SubQ or I.M.

TO PREVENT HEMORRHAGIC DISEASE IN NEONATES

I.M. OR SUBCUTANEOUS INJECTION

Neonates. 0.5 to 1 mg within 1 hr after birth, repeated in 6 to 8 hr, as prescribed.

TO TREAT HEMORRHAGIC DISEASE IN NEONATES

I.M. OR SUBCUTANEOUS INJECTION

Neonates. 1 mg (or higher dose if mother took an oral anticoagulant or anticonvulsant during pregnancy).

PARENTERAL ADMINISTRATION GUIDELINES

- Be aware that severe adverse reactions, including anaphylaxis, cardiac and respiratory arrest, hypersensitivity, and shock, may occur during or immediately after I.M. or I.V. administration of vitamin K_1, even if it's diluted to avoid rapid infusion. Administer vitamin by SubQ route whenever possible.
- Know that if vitamin K_1 must be administered I.V., you should not exceed rate of 1 mg/min, as prescribed.
- Be aware that some vitamin K_1 solutions contain benzyl alcohol. Don't administer these solutions to neonates or immature infants because of a risk of fatal toxic syndrome, which may include circulatory, CNS, renal, and respiratory impairment and metabolic acidosis.
- Take precautions to protect vitamin K_1 solution from exposure to light because it's light sensitive.

Interferons

Interferons are classified as biological response modifiers or antineoplastics. They fall into three major categories—alpha, beta, and gamma—which are described below.

The table on the following pages lists the trade names, indications, usual adult dosages, adverse reactions, and nursing considerations for these interferons.

Interferon alpha

Highly purified proteins produced by a recombinant DNA process, drugs in this category exhibit antiviral and antitumor activity. Antiviral activity depends on their inhibition of viral protein synthesis. Antitumor activity results from their ability to exert a cytostatic effect, reducing the rate of cell proliferation by delaying RNA and protein production. This delay induces cells to enter a resting stage. These drugs also increase the activity of human natural killer (NK) cells, which have the ability to lyse certain tumor cells and normal targets. They also selectively increase the number of cytotoxic T-cells, thereby affecting tumor growth. Phagocytic activity of macrophages also is increased.

Interferon alfacon

This specific form of interferon is produced by fermentation of genetically engineered *Escherichia coli.* It's structurally and functionally related to interferon beta and has greater biological activity than other interferon alfas.

Interferon beta

Produced by fibroblasts and epithelial cells, drugs in this category neutralize the activity

GENERIC AND TRADE NAMES	INDICATIONS AND USUAL ADULT DOSAGES
Interferon alpha drugs	
interferon alfa-n3 Alferon N	*To treat condyloma acuminatum:* 250,000 international units intralesionally at base of wart 2 times/wk for up to 8 wk.
peginterferon alfa-2a PEGASYS	*As monotherapy to treat patients with chronic heptatitis C who have compensated liver disease and contraindications or significant intolerance to other hepatitis C virus antiviral drugs; as adjunct to treat patients with chronic hepatitis C and compensated liver disease in combination with other antiviral drugs; to treat patients with chronic hepatitis B who have compensated liver disease and evidence of viral replication and liver inflammation:* 180 mcg/wk SubQ for individualized length of time for chronic hepatitis C and 48 wk for chronic hepatitis B.
peginterferon alfa-2b PEG-Intron Sylatron	*As adjunct to treat patients with chronic hepatitis C who have compensated liver disease and have never received an interferon alpha:* 180 mcg/wk SubQ for 48 wk. *To treat patients with chronic hepatitis C:* 1 mcg/kg/wk (PEG-Intron) SubQ every wk on the same day of the wk for 1 yr. *As adjunct to treat patients with chronic hepatitis C in combination with ribavirin:* 1.5 mcg/kg (PEG-Intron) SubQ every wk on the same day of the wk for 48 wk for genotype 1 and 24 wk for genotype 2 or 3. *As adjunct treatment of melanoma with microscopic or gross nodal involvement within 84 days of definitive surgical resection:* 6 mcg/kg/wk (Sylatron) SubQ for 8 doses followed by 3 mcg/kg/wk (Sylatron) SubQ for up to 5 yr.
recombinant interferon alfa-2b Intron A	*To treat hairy cell leukemia:* 2 million international units/m^2 I.M. or SubQ 3 times/wk for up to 6 mo. *To treat condyloma acuminatum:* 1 million international units (using only the 10-million units/ml strength) intralesionally at base of wart (up to 5 warts/course) 3 times/wk on alternate days for 3 wk. If response is inadequate 12 to 16 wk after initial treatment, repeat course, as prescribed.

of endogenous interferon gamma (IFNG), the substance believed to be responsible for triggering the autoimmune process that leads to multiple sclerosis. In multiple sclerosis, an initial viral infection may stimulate IFNG production by T cells. Then IFNG induces macrophages to produce proteinases that degrade the myelin sheath around the nerves and spinal cord. Cytotoxic T cells then move to the site of inflammation, recognizing antigens as receptor sites, where they attack the tissue affected by IFNG, resulting in progressive neurologic dysfunction. Interferon beta drugs interfere with IFNG production by lymphocytes and the mRNA transcription caused by IFNG. As a result, cytotoxic T cells can't locate receptor sites and cause further damage in the CNS.

Interferon gamma

Produced from genetically engineered *E. coli,* this type of interferon is chemically and therapeutically distinct from interferon alpha. Drugs in this category have potent phagocyte-activating properties. By enhancing oxidative metabolism, they produce toxic oxygen metabolites in phagocytes, which permits more efficient killing of certain fungi, bacteria, and protozoal microbes. Enhanced antibody-dependent cellular cytotoxicity and NK-cell activity reduce the risk of developing a serious infection in patients with chronic disease. These drugs also stimulate production of cytokines, such as interleukin-1-beta, and regulate the immune system by suppressing the IgE level and inhibiting collagen production.

ADVERSE REACTIONS	NURSING CONSIDERATIONS
CNS: Depression, dizziness, fatigue, headache, **homicidal or suicidal ideation**, psychosis, peripheral neuropathy, **seizures**, vertigo **CV:** Hypertriglyceridemia, hypertension, **hypotension**, palpitations **EENT:** Dry mouth, hearing loss **GI:** Anorexia, diarrhea, **hepatotoxicity**, nausea, vomiting **GU: Renal failure** **HEME:** Anemia, **leukopenia**, **pure red cell aplasia**, **thrombocytopenia**, **thrombotic thrombocytopenic purpura** **MS:** Myositis, **rhabdomyolysis** **RESP: Pulmonary fibrosis** **SKIN:** Alopecia, rash, **Stevens–Johnson syndrome**, **toxic epidermal necrolysis**, urticaria **Other: Anaphylaxis**, **angioedema**, bacterial infections, flu-like symptoms, liver or renal graft rejection, **sepsis**, systemic lupus erythematosus	• Use interferon alpha drugs cautiously in patients with renal impairment and in elderly patients. • Be aware that cross-sensitivity may occur among interferon alpha drugs. • Be aware that interferon alpha drugs aren't interchangeable. • Be aware that patients who are sensitive to mouse immunoglobulin also may be sensitive to recombinant interferon alfa-2a. • Ensure that patient is well hydrated, if not contraindicated, at the start of and throughout therapy to reduce the risk of hypotension. • Reconstitute by adding 3 ml of diluent provided by manufacturer and swirling gently to dissolve. • Be aware that reconstitution of peginterferon alfa-2a and interferon alfa-n3 is not necessary. • Don't shake vial. • Be aware that cross-sensitivity with interferon alfa-n3 to egg protein, mouse immunoglobulin, or neomycin may occur. ***WARNING*** Know that because interferon alpha drugs may cause or aggravate fatal or life-threatening autoimmune, ischemic, infectious, or neuropsychiatric disorders, patient should be monitored periodically with clinical and laboratory evaluations; expect drug to be discontinued if he develops severe or worsening signs and symptoms of these conditions.

(continues)

Interferons *(continued)*

GENERIC AND TRADE NAMES	INDICATIONS AND USUAL ADULT DOSAGES
Interferon alpha drugs *(continued)*	
	To treat AIDS-related Kaposi's sarcoma: 30 million international units/m^2 (using 50 million international units/ml) I.M. or SubQ 3 times/wk. *To treat chronic hepatitis B:* 5 million international units/day or 10 million international units 3 times/wk I.M. or SubQ for 16 wk. *To treat chronic hepatitis C:* 3 million international units I.M. or SubQ 3 times/wk. *To treat malignant melanoma:* 20 million international units/m^2 as I.V. infusion over 20 min for 5 consecutive days/wk for 4 wk, followed by 10 million international units/m^2 SubQ 3 times/wk for 48 wk. *As adjunct to treat follicular lymphoma:* 5 million international units/m^2 3 times/wk SubQ for up to 18 months.
Interferon alfacon-1 drugs	
interferon alfacon-1 Infergen	*To treat chronic hepatitis C in patients with compensated liver disease:* 9 mcg SubQ 3 times/wk, at intervals of at least 48 hr, for 24 wk. If inadequate response or relapse occurs, 15 mcg SubQ 3 times/wk, for up to 48 wk. *As adjunct with ribavirin to treat chronic hepatitis C:* 15 mcg daily for up to 48 wk.
Interferon beta drugs	
interferon beta-1a Avonex	*To treat relapsing forms of multiple sclerosis:* 30 mcg I.M. once/wk.
Rebif	*To treat relapsing forms of multiple sclerosis: Initial:* 20% of maintenance dose 3 times/wk SubQ, and increased over 4-wk period to the targeted maintenance dose. *Maintenance:* 22 mcg or 44 mcg SubQ 3 times/wk.
interferon beta-1b Betaseron, Extavia	*To treat relapsing forms of multiple sclerosis:* 0.0625 mg SubQ every other day for wk 1 and 2, increased to 0.125 mg SubQ every other day for wk 3 and 4, increased to 0.1875 mg SubQ every other day for wk 5 and 6, and increased to 0.25 mg SubQ every other day on wk 7 and thereafter.
peginterferon beta-1a Plegridy	*To treat relapsing forms of multiple sclerosis:* 63 mcg on day 1, 94 mcg on day 15, and 125 mcg on day 29 and every 14 days thereafter.

ADVERSE REACTIONS	NURSING CONSIDERATIONS
	• Obtain CBC before and regularly during treatment, as ordered, because interferon alpha drugs may cause bone marrow suppression. Expect drug to be discontinued if patient develops severe decreases in neutrophil or platelet count. • Implement bleeding and infection-control measures, according to facility policy. • Be aware that cross-sensitivity may occur with *Escherichia coli*–derived products. • Discard vial if left at room temperature for more than 12 hours. • Implement bleeding and infection-control measures, according to facility policy. • Administer acetaminophen, as prescribed, to prevent or treat fever or headache.
CNS: Anxiety, confusion, decreased concentration, depression, insomnia, nervousness **EENT:** Abnormal vision **HEME: Leukopenia**, **thrombocytopenia**	• Be aware that use of interferon alfacon-1 isn't recommended for patients with autoimmune hepatitis or psychiatric disorders. • Be aware that cross-sensitivity may occur with other interferon alfa drugs or *E. coli*–derived products. • Don't shake vial. • Implement bleeding and infection-control measures, according to facility policy. • Monitor patient for signs and symptoms of vision abnormalities.
CNS: Anxiety, confusion, depression, dizziness, emotional lability, fatigue, headache, **seizures**, **suicidal ideation**, weakness **CV: Cardiomyopathy**, palpitations, tachycardia, vasodilation **EENT:** Retinal vascular disorders **ENDO:** Thyroid dysfunction **GI: Autoimmune hepatitis**, diarrhea, elevated liver enzyme levels, nausea, **pancreatitis**, vomiting **GU: Hemolytic-uremic syndrome** **HEME:** Anemia, **leukopenia, pancytopenia**, **thrombocytopenia** **RESP: Bronchospasm** **SKIN:** Alopecia, pruritus, skin discoloration, urticaria **Other: Anaphylaxis**, flu-like symptoms, infection, injection-site reactions (including necrosis), systemic lupus erythematosus, weight changes	• Use beta interferons with extreme caution in patients with depression or seizure disorder. • Be aware that cross-sensitivity may occur with human albumin or natural or recombinant interferon beta. • Reconstitute following manufacturer's directions and refrigerate. Use interferon beta-1a within 6 hours of reconstitution. Use interferon beta-1b within 3 hours of reconstitution. • Implement bleeding and infection-control measures, according to facility policy.

(continues)

Interferons *(continued)*

GENERIC AND TRADE NAMES	INDICATIONS AND USUAL ADULT DOSAGES
Interferon gamma drugs	
interferon gamma-1b Actimmune	*To reduce frequency and severity of serious infections associated with chronic granulomatous disease or to delay progression of severe, malignant osteopetrosis in patients with body surface area greater than 0.5 m²:* 50 mcg/m² (1 million international units/m²) SubQ 3 times/wk. *To reduce frequency and severity of serious infections associated with chronic granulomatous disease or to delay progression of severe, malignant osteopetrosis in patients with body surface area of 0.5 m² or less:* 1.5 mcg/kg/dose SubQ 3 times/wk.

ADVERSE REACTIONS	NURSING CONSIDERATIONS
CNS: Fatigue, headache **GI:** Diarrhea, nausea, vomiting **HEME: Leukopenia** **SKIN:** Rash **Other:** Flu-like symptoms	• Use gamma interferon cautiously in patients previously exposed to cytotoxic drugs or radiation therapy. • Be aware that cross-sensitivity may occur with *Escherichia coli*–derived products. • Know that stopper on vial is a derivative of latex, which may cause allergic reactions to those sensitive to latex. • Discard vial if left at room temperature for more than 12 hours. • Implement bleeding and infection-control measures, according to facility policy. • Administer acetaminophen, as prescribed, to prevent or treat fever and headache.

Compatible Drugs in a Syringe

The table below lets you know at a glance whether particular drugs are compatible for at least 15 minutes when mixed together in a syringe for immediate administration. However, keep in mind that drugs listed as compatible when mixed in a syringe may not be compatible when prepared for other routes of administration. Drug combinations prepared for immediate administration usually require a more concentrated solution than those prepared for infusion.

Key: C = Compatible; I = Incompatible; n/a = Compatibility information not available, no recommendations can be given.

	atropine	chlorpromazine	dexamethasone	diazepam	diphenhydramine	droperidol	furosemide	glycopyrrolate	haloperidol
atropine		C	n/a	n/a	C	C	n/a	C	I
chlorpromazine	C		n/a	n/a	C	C	n/a	C	n/a
dexamethasone	n/a	n/a		n/a	I	n/a	n/a	n/a	n/a
diazepam	n/a	n/a	n/a		n/a	n/a	n/a	I	n/a
diphenhydramine	C	C	I	n/a		C	n/a	C	I
droperidol	C	C	n/a	n/a	C		I	C	n/a
furosemide	n/a	n/a	n/a	n/a	n/a	I		n/a	n/a
glycopyrrolate	C	C	I	C	C	C	n/a		C
haloperidol	n/a	n/a	n/a	n/a	C	n/a	n/a	n/a	
heparin	C	I	n/a	I	n/a	I	C	n/a	I
hydromorphone	C	C	n/a	n/a	C	n/a	n/a	C	C
hydroxyzine	C	C	n/a	n/a	C	C	n/a	C	I
ketorolac	n/a	n/a	n/a	I	n/a	n/a	n/a	n/a	I
lidocaine	n/a	n/a	n/a	n/a	n/a	n/a	n/a	C	n/a
lorazepam	n/a	n/a	n/a	n/a	n/a	n/a	n/a	n/a	n/a
meperidine	C	C	n/a	C	C	C	n/a	C	n/a
metoclopramide	C	C	n/a	n/a	C	C	I	n/a	n/a
midazolam	C	C	n/a	n/a	C	n/a	n/a	C	C
morphine	C	C	n/a	n/a	C	C	n/a	C	I
pentobarbital	C	I	n/a	n/a	I	I	n/a	I	n/a
prochlorperazine	C	n/a	n/a	n/a	C	C	n/a	C	n/a
ranitidine	C	I	C	n/a	C	n/a	n/a	C	n/a
scopolamine	C	C	n/a	n/a	C	C	n/a	C	n/a

	heparin	hydromorphone	hydroxyzine	ketorolac	lidocaine	lorazepam	meperidine	metoclopramide	midazolam	morphine	pentobarbital	prochlorperazine	ranitidine	scopolamine
	n/a	C	C	n/a	n/a	n/a	C	C	C	C	C	C	C	C
	I	C	C	n/a	n/a	n/a	C	C	C	I	I	C	C	C
	n/a	C	n/a	n/a	n/a	n/a	n/a	C	n/a	n/a	n/a	n/a	C	n/a
	I	n/a	n/a	I	n/a	n/a	n/a	n/a	n/a	n/a	n/a	n/a	I	n/a
	n/a	C	C	n/a	n/a	n/a	C	C	C	C	I	C	C	C
	I	n/a	C	n/a	n/a	n/a	C	C	C	C	I	C	n/a	C
	C	n/a	n/a	n/a	n/a	n/a	n/a	I	n/a	n/a	n/a	n/a	n/a	n/a
	n/a	C	C	n/a	C	n/a	C	n/a	C	C	I	C	C	C
	I	C	I	I	n/a	n/a	n/a	n/a	n/a	I	n/a	n/a	n/a	n/a
		n/a	n/a	n/a	C	n/a	I	C	n/a	C	n/a	n/a	n/a	n/a
	n/a		C	I	n/a	C	n/a	n/a	C	n/a	C	I	C	C
	n/a	C		I	C	n/a	C	C	C	C	I	C	C	C
	n/a	I	I		n/a	n/a	n/a	n/a	n/a	n/a	n/a	I	n/a	n/a
	C	n/a	C	n/a		n/a	n/a	C	n/a	n/a	n/a	n/a	n/a	n/a
	n/a	C	n/a	n/a	n/a		n/a	n/a	n/a	n/a	n/a	n/a	I	n/a
	I	n/a	C	n/a	n/a	n/a		C	I	I	C	C	C	C
	C	C	n/a	n/a	C	n/a	C		C	C	n/a	C	C	C
	n/a	C	C	n/a	n/a	n/a	C	C		C	I	I	I	C
	C*	n/a	C	n/a	n/a	n/a	n/a	C	C		I	C	C	C
	n/a	C	I	n/a	n/a	n/a	I	I	I	I		I	I	C
	n/a	I	C	I	n/a	n/a	C	C	I	C	I		C	C
	n/a	C	I	n/a	n/a	I	C	C	I	C	I	C		C
	n/a	C	C	n/a	n/a	n/a	C	C	C	C	C	C	C	

* Compatible only with morphine doses of 1, 2, and 5 mg.

Drug Formulas and Calculations

When giving drugs, you must be familiar with drug formulas and calculation methods to make sure your patient receives the prescribed drug in the correct dosage, strength, or flow rate. This appendix offers a quick review of ways to calculate the strength of a solution, drug dosages, and I.V. flow rates.

Calculating the Strength of a Solution

Most solutions are prepared in the required strength by the pharmacy or medical supply source.

But sometimes only a concentrated form is available, and you'll need to dilute the solution or solid to administer the prescribed strength.

When a solid form of a drug is used to prepare a solution, the drug must be completely dissolved. Solid drug forms, such as tablets, crystals, and powders, are considered 100% strength. (An exception to this is boric acid, which is only 5% at full strength.) The final diluted solution is stated in terms of liquid measurement. To prepare a solution, you'll need to add the prescribed solid or liquid form of the drug (the solute) to the prescribed amount of diluent (the solvent). Two of the most common clinical diluents are normal saline solution and sterile water.

You can use two formulas to calculate the strength of a solution, as shown in the examples below.

Method 1: Calculating percentage and volume

Use the following formula:

$$\frac{\text{Weaker solution}}{\text{Stronger solution}} = \frac{\text{Solute}}{\text{Solvent}}$$

Example: You need to dilute a stock solution of 100% strength to a 5% solution. How much solute will you need to add to obtain 500 ml of the 5% solution?

Calculate as follows:

$$\frac{5\ (\%)\ (\text{Weaker solution})}{100\ (\%)\ (\text{Stronger solution})} = \frac{X\ (\text{g})\ \ (\text{solute})}{500\ \text{ml}\ (\text{solvent})}$$

$$100\,X = (500)(5) \text{ or } 2{,}500$$

$$X = 25 \text{ g}$$

Answer: You'll need to add 25 g of solute to each 500 ml of solvent to prepare a 5% solution.

Method 2: Calculating percentage and volume

Use the following formula:

$$\frac{(\text{Desired strength})}{(\text{Available strength})} \times \begin{matrix}\text{Total amount of}\\ \text{desired solution}\end{matrix} = X \begin{matrix}\text{(amount of undiluted drug}\\ \text{needed to make solution)}\end{matrix}$$

Example: You need to make 100 ml of a 20% solution, using an 80% solution. How much of the 80% solution must you add to the sterile water to yield a final volume of 100 ml of a 20% solution?

Calculate as follows:

$$\frac{20\ (\%)(\text{Desired strength})}{80\ (\%)(\text{Available strength})} \times \begin{matrix}\text{100 ml (Total amount}\\ \text{of desired solution)}\end{matrix} = X$$

$$\frac{0.20}{0.80} = 0.25$$

$$0.25 \times 100\ (\text{ml}) = X$$

$$X = 25\ \text{ml of } 80\%\ \text{solution}$$

Answer: You'll need to add 25 ml of the 80% solution to the water to make a final volume of 100 ml of a 20% solution.

Calculating Drug Dosages

You may be required to calculate drug dosages when you need to administer a drug that's available only in one measure, but prescribed in another. You should also be prepared to convert various units of measure, such as milligrams (mg) to grains (gr), and dry measurements to liquid. You can use three common methods of ratio and proportion to calculate drug dosages, as shown in the examples below.

CALCULATING ORAL DRUG DOSAGES

Example: You need to give a patient 0.25 mg of digoxin, which comes only in 0.125-mg tablets. How many tablets will you need to give him to attain the proper dosage?

Method 1: Using labeled amount of drug

In this method, true proportions between the drug label and the prescribed dose are used to determine ratio and proportion. The drug label, which states the amount of drug in one unit of measurement—in this case, 0.125 mg in each tablet of digoxin—is the first ratio, expressed as follows:

$$\text{milligrams} : \text{tablets} = \text{milligrams} : \text{tablets}$$

$$0.125\ \text{mg (amount of drug)} : 1\ \text{tablet (unit of measure)}$$

The prescribed dose—in this case, 0.25 mg—is the second ratio; it must be stated in the same order and units of measure as the first, as follows:

$$0.125\ \text{mg} : 1\ \text{tablet} = 0.25\ \text{mg} : X\ (\text{tablets})$$

Calculate as follows:

$$0.125\,X = 0.25$$

$$X = \frac{0.25}{0.125}$$

$$X = 2$$

Answer: You'll need to give the patient 2 tablets of digoxin 0.125 mg.

Be sure to use critical thinking to assess whether your answer is correct. Because the amount of drug prescribed is greater than the amount of drug in one tablet, it's reasonable to expect the required number of tablets to be greater than one.

Method 2: Using an established formula

To determine the correct number of digoxin tablets to give using this method, use the following formula:

$$\frac{\text{Prescribed dose}}{\text{Dose available}} \times \text{Quantity (unit of measure)} = X\ (\text{unknown quantity to be given})$$

Calculate as follows:

$$\frac{0.25\ \text{mg}}{0.125\ \text{mg}} \times 1\ \text{tablet} = X\ \text{(number of 0.125-mg tablets)}$$

$$\frac{0.25}{0.125} = X$$

$$2 = X$$

Answer: You'll need to give the patient 2 tablets of digoxin 0.125 mg.

Method 3: Calculating according to proportion size

This method uses the same components as method #1, but the ratio is based on proportions according to size. To determine the correct number of digoxin tablets to give using this method, use the following formula:

$$\frac{\text{Smaller}}{\text{Larger}} = \frac{\text{Smaller}}{\text{Larger}}$$

Substitute 0.125 into the smaller part and 0.25 into the greater part of the first ratio. Critical thinking leads us to believe that you'll need more than 1 tablet of the weaker 0.125-mg strength to equal the stronger 0.25 mg. Set up the proportion as follows:

$$\frac{0.125\ \text{mg}}{0.25\ \text{mg}} = \frac{1\ \text{(tablet)}}{X\ \text{(tablets)}}$$

Calculate as follows:

$$0.125\ X = 0.25$$

$$X = \frac{0.25}{0.125}$$

$$X = 2\ \text{tablets}$$

Answer: You'll need to give the patient 2 tablets of digoxin 0.125 mg.

CALCULATING PARENTERAL DRUG DOSAGES

The same methods used for calculating oral drugs and solutions can be used for preparing parenteral injections.

Example: You need to administer a prescribed dose of 1 mg morphine sulfate from a unit-dose cartridge containing 4 mg/2 ml. How many milliliters will you need to give to equal the prescribed dose of 1 mg?

Method 1: Using labeled amount of drug

Using the same ratio as for oral drugs, the drug label—in this case, 4 mg—is the first ratio, and the prescribed dose—in this case, 1 mg—is the second ratio, expressed as follows:

4 mg (the amount of drug) : 2 ml (the unit of measure)

Calculate as follows:

$$4\ \text{mg} : 2\ \text{ml} = 1\ \text{mg} : X\ \text{ml}$$

$$4X = 2$$

$$X = \frac{2}{4}$$

$$X = 0.5\ \text{ml}$$

Answer: You'll need to give 0.5 ml of morphine sulfate to equal the prescribed dose of 1 mg.

Method 2: Using an established formula

Use this formula:

$$\frac{\text{Prescribed dose}}{\text{Dose available}} \times \text{Quantity (unit of measure)} = \text{X (unknown quantity to be given)}$$

Calculate as follows:

$$\frac{1 \text{ mg}}{4 \text{ mg}} \times 2 \text{ ml} = \text{X (number of ml)}$$

$$\frac{2}{4} = 0.5$$

Answer: You'll need to give 0.5 ml of morphine sulfate to equal the prescribed dose of 1 mg.

Method 3: Calculating according to proportion size

To determine the correct amount of morphine sulfate to give using this method, use the following formula:

smaller : greater = smaller : greater

milligrams : milligrams = milliliters : milliliters

Critical thinking leads us to believe that 1 mg is less than 4 mg and that you'll need less than 2 ml to give 1 mg of the drug; therefore, 1 mg goes into the smaller part of the first ratio, and X goes into the smaller part of the second ratio. Set up the proportion as follows:

$$1 \text{ mg} : 4 \text{ mg} = \text{X (ml)} : 2 \text{ ml}$$

$$4X = 2$$

$$X = \frac{2}{4}$$

$$X = 0.5$$

Answer: You'll need to give 0.5 ml of morphine sulfate to equal the prescribed dose of 1 mg.

Calculating I.V. Flow Rates

When an I.V. solution is delivered by gravity, you must calculate the number of drops needed per minute for proper infusion. To calculate I.V. flow rates, you need to know three things:

- The drip factor—or the number of drops contained in 1 ml for the type of I.V. set you'll be using. This information is provided on the individual package label.
- The amount and type of fluid that you'll infuse as prescribed on the physician's order sheet
- The infusion duration time in minutes.

Once you've gathered this information, you can calculate the I.V. flow rate using the following equation:

$$\frac{\text{Total number of ml}}{\text{Total number of minutes}} \times \text{drip factor (gtt/ml)} = \text{flow rate (gtt/min)}$$

Example 1: If the physician prescribes 1,000 ml of D_5W to infuse over 10 hours, and the drip rate for your administration set is 15 drops (gtt)/ml, calculate as follows:

$$\frac{1{,}000 \text{ ml}}{10 \text{ hours} \times 60 \text{ minutes}} \times 15 \text{ gtt/ml} = X \text{ gtt/minute}$$

$$\frac{1{,}000 \text{ ml}}{600 \text{ minutes}} \times 15 \text{ gtt/ml} = X \text{ gtt/minute}$$

$$1.67 \text{ ml/minute} \times 15 \text{ gtt/ml} = X \text{ gtt/minute}$$

$$25.05 \text{ gtt/minute} = X$$

Answer: To infuse, round off 25.05 to 25 gtt/minute or according to your institution's policy.

Example 2: If the physician prescribes 500 ml of half-normal (0.45%) saline solution to infuse over 2 hours, and the drip rate for your administration set delivers 10 gtt/ml, calculate as follows:

$$\frac{500 \text{ ml}}{2 \text{ hours} \times 60 \text{ minutes}} \times 10 \text{ gtt/ml} = X \text{ gtt/minute}$$

$$\frac{500 \text{ ml}}{120 \text{ minutes}} \times 10 \text{ gtt/ml} = X \text{ gtt/minute}$$

$$4.17 \text{ ml/minute} \times 10 \text{ gtt/ml} = X \text{ gtt/minute}$$

$$41.7 \text{ gtt/minute} = X$$

Answer: To infuse, round off 41.7 to 42 gtt/minute or according to your institution's policy.

Note: When preparing for I.V. administration using a controlled infusion device, the electronic flow-regulator will either count drops using an electronic eye or use a controlled pumping action to deliver the fluid in milliliters. Your final calculation will be based on the unit of measure used by the device: drops per minute or ml per hour.

Weights and Equivalents

The following three tables show approximate equivalents among systems of measurement.

Table 1 Liquid Equivalents Among Household, Apothecaries', and Metric Systems

HOUSEHOLD	APOTHECARIES'	METRIC
1 teaspoon (tsp)	1 fluid dram	5 milliliters (ml)
1 tablespoon (tbs)	0.5 fluid oz	15 ml
2 tbs (1 ounce [oz])	1 fluid oz	30 ml
1 cupful	8 fluid oz	240 ml
1 pint	16 fluid oz	473 ml
1 quart (qt)	32 fluid oz	946 ml (1 liter)

Table 2 Solid Equivalents Among Apothecaries' and Metric Systems

APOTHECARIES'	METRIC
15 grains (gr)	1 gram (g) (1,000 milligrams [mg])
10 gr	0.6 g (600 mg)
7.5 gr	0.5 g (500 mg)
5 gr	0.3 g (300 mg)
3 gr	0.2 g (200 mg)
1.5 gr	0.1 g (100 mg)
1 gr	0.06 g (60 mg) or 0.065 g (65 mg)
0.75 gr	0.05 g (50 mg)
0.5 gr	0.03 g (30 mg)
0.25 gr	0.015 g (15 mg)
1/60 gr	0.001 g (1 mg)
1/100 gr	0.6 mg
1/120 gr	0.5 mg
1/150 gr	0.4 mg

(continues)

Table 3 Solid Equivalents Among Avoirdupois, Apothecaries', and Metric Systems

AVOIRDUPOIS	APOTHECARIES'	METRIC
1 gr	1 gr	0.065 g
15.4 gr	15 gr	1 g
1 ounce (oz)	480 gr	28.35 g
437.5 gr	1 oz	31 g
1 pound (lb)	1.33 lb	454 g
0.75 lb	1 lb	373 g
2.2 lb	2.7 lb	1 kg

Equianalgesic Doses for Opioid Agonists

An equianalgesic dose of a synthetic opioid agonist is the dose that produces the same level of analgesia as 10 mg of I.M. or subQ morphine, the prinicipal opioid obtained from opium poppies. If your patient is switched from one opioid to another, expect to use the equianalgesic dose to decrease the risk of adverse reactions while increasing the likelihood of adequate pain relief. The chart below compares equianalgesic doses (oral and parenteral) for adults and children who weigh 50 kg (110 lb) or more.

OPIOID	ORAL DOSE	PARENTERAL DOSE
codeine	200 mg (not recommended)	120 to 130 mg
hydrocodone	30 mg	Not applicable
hydromorphone	7.5 mg	1.5 mg
levorphanol	4 mg	2 mg
meperidine	300 mg	75 to 100 mg
morphine (around-the-clock dosing)	30 mg	10 mg
morphine (single or intermittent dosing)	60 mg	10 mg
oxycodone	30 mg	Not applicable

Abbreviations

The following abbreviations, which are common to nursing practice, may be used throughout the text.

ABG	arterial blood gas
ACE	angiotensin-converting enzyme
ADH	antidiuretic hormone
AIDS	acquired immunodeficiency syndrome
ALT	alanine aminotransferase
ANA	antinuclear antibodies
APTT	activated partial thromboplastin time
AST	aspartate aminotransferase
ATP	adenosine triphosphate
AV	atrioventricular
BUN	blood urea nitrogen
°C	degrees Celsius
cAMP	cyclic adenosine monophosphate
(CAN)	Canadian drug trade name
cap	capsule
CBC	complete blood count
cGMP	cyclic guanosine monophosphate
CK	creatine kinase
Cl	chloride
cm	centimeter
CMV	cytomegalovirus
CNS	central nervous system
COPD	chronic obstructive pulmonary disease
CSF	cerebrospinal fluid
CV	cardiovascular
CVA	cerebrovascular accident
D_5LR	dextrose 5% in lactated Ringer's solution
D_5NS	dextrose 5% in normal saline solution
$D_5/0.2NS$	dextrose 5% in quarter-normal saline solution
$D_5/0.45NS$	dextrose 5% in half-normal saline solution
D_5W	dextrose 5% in water
$D_{10}W$	dextrose 10% in water
$D_{50}W$	dextrose 50% in water
dl	deciliter
DNA	deoxyribonucleic acid
DS	double-strength
EC	enteric-coated
ECG	electrocardiogram
EEG	electroencephalogram
EENT	eyes, ears, nose, and throat
ENDO	endocrine
E.R.	extended-release
°F	degrees Fahrenheit
FDA	Food and Drug Administration
g	gram
GABA	gamma aminobutyric acid
GFR	glomerular filtration rate
GI	gastrointestinal
gtt	drop
GU	genitourinary
H_1	histamine$_1$
H_2	histamine$_2$
HDL	high-density lipoprotein
HEME	hematologic
HIV	human immunodeficiency virus
HMG-CoA	hydroxymethylglutaryl-coenzyme A
HPV	human papilloma virus
hr	hour
HSV	herpes simplex virus
HZV	herpes zoster virus
ICP	intracranial pressure
I.D.	intradermal
IgA	immunoglobulin A
IgE	immunoglobulin E
I.M.	intramuscular
INR	international normalized ratio
I.V.	intravenous
IVPB	intravenous piggyback
kg	kilogram
KIU	kallikrein inactivator units
L	liter
LA	long-acting
lb	pound
LD	lactate dehydrogenase
LDL	low-density lipoprotein
LOC	level of consciousness
LR	lactated Ringer's solution
M	molar
m^2	square meter
MAO	monoamine oxidase
mcg	microgram
mEq	milliequivalent
mg	milligram
MI	myocardial infarction
min	minute
ml	milliliter
mm	millimeter
mm^3	cubic millimeter
mmol	millimole
mo	month
MS	musculoskeletal
msec	millisecond
Na	sodium
NaCl	sodium chloride
NG	nasogastric
ng	nanogram
NPH	human isophane insulin
NPO	nothing by mouth

NS	normal saline solution
0.225NS	quarter-normal saline (0.225%) solution
0.45NS	half-normal saline (0.45%) solution
NSAID	nonsteroidal anti-inflammatory drug
NYHA	New York Heart Association
OTC	over the counter
oz	ounce
PCA	patient-controlled analgesia
P.O.	by mouth
P.R.	by rectum
PSVT	paroxysmal supraventricular tachycardia
PT	prothrombin time
PTCA	percutaneous transluminal coronary angioplasty
PTT	partial thromboplastin time
PVC	premature ventricular contraction
RBC	red blood cell
REM	rapid eye movement
RESP	respiratory
RNA	ribonucleic acid
RSV	respiratory syncytial virus
SA	sinoatrial
sec	second
S.L.	sublingual
S.R.	sustained-release
stat	immediately
SubQ	subcutaneous
supp	suppository
tab	tablet
T_3	triiodothyronine
T_4	thyroxine
USP	United States Pharmacopeia
UTI	urinary tract infection
VLDL	very-low-density lipoprotein
WBC	white blood cell
WK	week

Index

• Generic and alternate names: lowercase initial letter
• Trade names: uppercase initial letter
• Illustrations: *i* after page number
• Tables: *t* after page number

A

B

C

D

E

F

G

H

I

J

K

L

M

N

P

Q

R

S

T

U

V

W

X

Y

Z

Body Mass Index Calculation

Body mass index (BMI) is a formula used to determine obesity; it's calculated by dividing a person's weight in kilograms by height in meters squared (kg/m^2). A BMI of 25 or higher increases your patient's risk of developing hypertension, cardiovascular disease, type 2 diabetes mellitus, and stroke. It also increases the risk that he won't respond effectively to the usual drug dosages. If your patient has an abnormal BMI, be prepared to make dosage adjustments that are individualized based on body weight, as prescribed.

The table below will help you find your patient's BMI easily. The table converts pounds to kilograms and inches to meters, and then it shows the BMI. To use it, simply find the patient's height on either side of the table, then move across the row to the weight that matches your patient's most closely. At the bottom of the column containing the weight, you'll find the BMI for that patient. For example, the BMI for a patient who is 70 inches tall and weighs 208 lb is 30.

WEIGHT (POUNDS)

HEIGHT (INCHES)																		
58	91	96	100	105	110	115	119	124	129	134	138	143	148	153	158	162	167	172
59	94	99	104	109	114	119	124	128	133	138	143	148	153	158	163	168	173	178
60	97	102	107	112	118	123	128	133	138	143	148	153	158	163	168	174	179	184
61	100	106	111	116	122	127	132	137	143	148	153	158	164	169	174	180	185	190
62	104	109	115	120	126	131	136	142	147	153	158	164	169	175	180	186	191	196
63	107	113	118	124	130	135	141	146	152	158	163	169	175	180	186	191	197	203
64	110	116	122	128	134	140	145	151	157	163	169	174	180	186	192	197	204	209
65	114	120	126	132	138	144	150	156	162	168	174	180	186	192	198	204	210	216
66	118	124	130	136	142	148	155	161	167	173	179	186	192	198	204	210	216	223
67	121	127	134	140	146	153	159	166	172	178	185	191	198	204	211	217	223	230
68	125	131	138	144	151	158	164	171	177	184	190	197	203	210	216	223	230	236
69	128	135	142	149	155	162	169	176	182	189	196	203	209	216	223	230	236	243
70	132	139	146	153	160	167	174	181	188	195	202	209	216	222	229	236	243	250
71	136	143	150	157	165	172	179	186	193	200	208	215	222	229	236	243	250	257
72	140	147	154	162	169	177	184	191	199	206	213	221	228	235	242	250	258	265
73	144	151	159	166	174	182	189	197	204	212	219	227	235	242	250	257	265	272
74	148	155	163	171	179	186	194	202	210	218	225	233	241	249	256	264	272	280
75	152	160	168	176	184	192	200	208	216	224	232	240	248	256	264	272	279	287
76	156	164	172	180	189	197	205	213	221	230	238	246	254	263	271	279	287	295
BODY MASS INDEX	**19**	**20**	**21**	**22**	**23**	**24**	**25**	**26**	**27**	**28**	**29**	**30**	**31**	**32**	**33**	**34**	**35**	**36**